Patrick C. Walsh, M.D.

Urologist-in-Chief, James Buchanan Brady
  Urological Institute
The Johns Hopkins Hospital
Professor and Director
  Department of Urology
The Johns Hopkins University
  School of Medicine
Baltimore, Maryland

Ruben F. Gittes, M.D.

Urologist-in-Chief
Brighman and Women's Hospital
Professor of Urological Surgery
Harvard Medical School
Boston, Massachusetts

Alan D. Perlmutter, M.D.

Chief, Department of Pediatric Urology
Children's Hospital of Michigan
Professor of Urology
Wayne State University School of Medicine
Detroit, Michigan

Thomas A. Stamey, M.D.

Professor of Surgery and
Chairman, Division of Urology
Stanford University School of Medicine
Stanford, California

Volume 1

Campbell's

UROLOGY

FIFTH EDITION

1986
W.B. SAUNDERS COMPANY

Philadelphia • London • Toronto • Mexico City • Rio de Janeiro • Sydney • Tokyo • Hong Kong

W. B. Saunders Company: West Washington Square
Philadelphia, PA   19105

Library of Congress Cataloging in Publication Data

Urology.

Campbell's Urology.

1. Urology.   I. Campbell, Meredith Fairfax, 1894-
1968.   II. Walsh, Patrick C.   III. Title. [DNLM:
1. Urologic diseases. WJ 100 C192]

RC871.U758 1986   616.6   83–20427

ISBN 0–7216–9088–2 (set)

Listed here is the latest translated edition of this book together with the language of the translation and the publisher.

Italian (3rd Edition)—   Casa Editrice Universo,
Rome, Italy

Portuguese (1st Edition)—Editora Guanabara Koogan,
Rio de Janeiro, Brazil

Editor: Carroll Cann
Cover Designer: Terri Siegel
Production Manager: Bob Butler
Manuscript Editor: Connie Burton
Illustration Coordinator: Walt Verbitski

Volume 1 ISBN   0–7216–9085–8
Volume 2 ISBN   0–7216–9086–6
Volume 3 ISBN   0–7216–9087–4
Set ISBN   0–7216–9088–2

Campbell's Urology

Last digit is the print number: 9   8   7   6   5   4   3   2   1

CONTRIBUTORS

HERBERT L. ABRAMS, M.D.

Philip H. Cook Professor of Radiology, Harvard Medical School; Senior Radiologist, Brigham and Women's Hospital, Boston, Massachusetts.

Computed Tomography of the Kidney; Renal and Adrenal Angiography; Renal Venography

DOUGLASS E. ADAMS, M.D.

Professor of Radiology, Harvard Medical School; Director, NMR Division, Department of Radiology, Brigham and Women's Hospital, Boston, Massachusetts.

Renal and Adrenal Angiography

S. JAMES ADELSTEIN, M.D., Ph.D.

Professor of Radiology, Harvard Medical School; Director, Joint Program in Nuclear Medicine, Brigham and Women's Hospital, Beth Israel Hospital, The Children's Hospital, Dana Farber Cancer Institute, Boston, Massachusetts.

Radionuclides in Genitourinary Disorders

ERNEST H. AGATSTEIN, M.D.

Senior Resident, Division of Urology, University of California, Los Angeles, School of Medicine; Staff, UCLA Medical Center, Los Angeles, California.

Imperforate Anus, Persistent Cloaca, and Urogenital Sinus Outlet Obstruction

RODNEY U. ANDERSON, M.D.

Associate Professor of Surgery (Urology), Stanford University School of Medicine; Chief of Urology, Santa Clara Valley Medical Center, San Jose, California.

Urinary Tract Infections in Spinal Cord Injury Patients

STUART B. BAUER, M.D.

Assistant Professor of Urology (Surgery), Harvard Medical School; Associate in Surgery (Urology), The Children's Hospital Medical Center, Boston, Massachusetts.

Anomalies of the Upper Urinary Tract

RICHARD E. BERGER, M.D.

Associate Professor, Department of Urology, University of Washington School of Medicine; Chief, Department of Urology, Harborview Medical Center, Seattle, Washington.

Sexually Transmitted Diseases

JAY BERNSTEIN, M.D.

Clinical Professor of Pathology, Wayne State University School of Medicine; Director, Department of Anatomic Pathology, William Beaumont Hospital, Royal Oak, Michigan.

Renal Cystic Disease and Renal Dysplasia

WILLIAM E. BRADLEY, M.D.

Professor, Department of Neurology, University of California, Irvine, School of Medicine; Neurology Service, Veterans Administration Medical Center, Long Beach, California.

Physiology of the Urinary Bladder

CHARLES B. BRENDLER, M.D.

Assistant Professor of Urology, The Johns Hopkins University School of Medicine, Baltimore, Maryland.

Perioperative Care

v

C. EUGENE CARLTON, Jr., M.D.

Russell and Mary Hugh Scott Professor and Chairman, Department of Urology, Baylor College of Medicine; Chief, Urology Service, Methodist Hospital; Active Staff, Ben Taub General Hospital, St. Luke's Episcopal Hospital, Texas Children's Hospital; Consulting Staff, Veterans Administration Hospital, Houston, Texas.

Initial Evaluation, Including History, Physical Examination, and Urinalysis.

WILLIAM J. CATALONA, M.D.

Professor and Chief, Division of Urologic Surgery, Washington University Medical Center; Attending Urologist, Barnes Hospital, Jewish Hospital, St. Louis Children's Hospital, St. Louis County Hospital, Veterans Administration Hospital, St. Louis, Missouri.

Carcinoma of the Prostate

THOMAS S. K. CHANG, Ph.D.

Assistant Professor, James Buchanan Brady Urological Institute, The Johns Hopkins University School of Medicine, Baltimore, Maryland.

The Testis, Epididymis, and Ductus Deferens

DONALD S. COFFEY, Ph.D.

Professor of Urology, Professor of Oncology, and Professor of Pharmacology and Experimental Therapeutics, The Johns Hopkins University School of Medicine; Director of the Research Laboratories of the Department of Urology, The Johns Hopkins Hospital, Baltimore, Maryland.

Biochemistry and Physiology of the Prostate and Seminal Vesicles.

GIULIO J. D'ANGIO, M.D.

Professor of Radiology, Radiation Therapy, and Pediatric Oncology, University of Pennsylvania School of Medicine; Director, Children's Cancer Research Center, Children's Hospital of Philadelphia, Philadelphia, Pennsylvania.

Pediatric Oncology

JEAN B. DE KERNION, M.D.

Professor of Surgery/Urology, and Head of Urologic Oncology, University of California, Los Angeles, School of Medicine; Director for Clinical Programs, Jonsson Cancer Center; Attending Physician, UCLA Hospital, Wadsworth Veterans Administration Hospital, Los Angeles, California.

Renal Tumors

FRANCESCO DEL GRECO, M.D.

Chief, Section of Nephrology-Hypertension, and Professor of Medicine, Northwestern University Medical School, Chicago, Illinois.

Other Renal Diseases of Urologic Significance

CHARLES J. DEVINE, Jr., M.D., F.A.C.S., F.A.A.P.

Professor and Chairman, Department of Urology, Eastern Virginia Medical School; Staff, Medical Center Hospitals, Norfolk General Hospital, De Paul Hospital, Leigh Memorial Hospital; Consultant in Urology, U.S. Naval Regional Medical Center, Portsmouth; Chief of Urology, Children's Hospital of the King's Daughters, Norfolk, Virginia.

Surgery of the Urethra

ROBERT G. DLUHY, M.D.

Associate Professor of Medicine, Harvard Medical School; Physician, Brigham and Women's Hospital, Boston, Massachusetts.

The Adrenals.

GEORGE W. DRACH, M.D.

Professor of Surgery and Chief of Urology, University of Arizona College of Medicine, Tucson, Arizona.

Urinary Lithiasis.

MICHAEL J. DROLLER, M.D.

Professor and Chairman, Department of Urology, Mount Sinai Medical School; Consultant, Bronx Veterans Administration Medical Center, Elmhurst General Hospital; Director of Urology, Mount Sinai Medical Center, New York, New York.

Transitional Cell Cancer: Upper Tracts and Bladder

JOHN W. DUCKETT, M.D.

Professor of Urology, University of Pennsylvania School of Medicine; Director, Division of Urology, Children's Hospital of Philadelphia, Philadelphia, Pennsylvania.

Hypospadias; Disorders of the Urethra and Penis

RICHARD M. EHRLICH, M.D., F.A.C.S., F.A.A.P.

Professor of Surgery/Urology, University of California, Los Angeles, School of Medicine; Staff, UCLA Medical Center, Los Angeles, California.

Imperforate Anus, Persistent Cloaca, and Urogenital Sinus Outlet Obstruction

AUDREY E. EVANS, M.D.

Professor of Pediatrics, University of Pennsylvania School of Medicine; Director, Division of Oncology, Children's Hospital of Philadelphia, Philadelphia, Pennsylvania.

Pediatric Oncology

LARRY L. EWING, Ph.D.

Professor, The Johns Hopkins University School of Hygiene and Public Health, Baltimore, Maryland.

The Testis, Epididymis, and Ductus Deferens

STEWART FELDMAN, M.D.

Formerly, Resident in Urology, Case Western Reserve University School of Medicine, Cleveland, Ohio.

Extrinsic Obstruction of the Ureter

JOHN F. GAETA, M.D.

Professor of Pathology and Associate Professor of Urology, State University of New York at Buffalo School of Medicine; Director, Tissue Pathology, Buffalo General Hospital, Buffalo, New York.

Tumors of Testicular Adnexal Structures and Seminal Vesicles

KENNETH D. GARDNER, Jr., M.D.

Professor of Medicine, University of New Mexico School of Medicine; Chief of Renal Diseases, Department of Medicine, University of New Mexico Hospital, Albuquerque, New Mexico.

Renal Cystic Disease and Renal Dysplasia

FREDRICK W. GEORGE, Ph.D.

Assistant Professor of Cell Biology, University of Texas Health Science Center at Dallas, Southwestern Medical School, Dallas, Texas.

Embryology of the Genital Tract

JAY Y. GILLENWATER, M.D.

Professor and Chairman, Department of Urology, University of Virginia School of Medicine; Chief of Urology, University of Virginia Hospital, Charlottesville, Virginia.

The Pathophysiology of Urinary Obstruction

RUBEN F. GITTES, M.D.

Elliot C. Cutler Professor of Urological Surgery, Harvard Medical School; Chief of Urology, Brigham and Women's Hospital, Boston, Massachusetts.

Partial Nephrectomy: In Situ or Extracorporeal; The Adrenals

JAMES G. GOW, M.D., Ch.M., F.R.C.S.

Formerly, Clinical Lecturer, University of Liverpool; Lourdes Private Hospital, Liverpool, England.

Genitourinary Tuberculosis

HARRY GRABSTALD, M.D., F.A.C.S.

Professor of Urology, Mount Sinai School of Medicine; Acting Director, Department of Urology, Beth Israel Medical Center, New York, New York.

Benign and Malignant Tumors of the Male and Female Urethra; Surgery of Penile and Urethral Carcinoma

JOHN T. GRAYHACK, M.D.

Professor and Chairman, Department of Urology, Northwestern University Medical School; Chief, Northwestern Memorial Hospital; Consultant, Veterans Administration Lakeside Hospital, Chicago, Illinois.

Surgical Management of Ureteropelvic Junction Obstruction.

LAWRENCE F. GREENE, M.D., Ph.D.*

Formerly, Clinical Professor of Surgery/Urology, University of California, San Diego, School of Medicine; Chief of Urology, Veterans Administration Hospital, San Diego, California.

Transurethral Surgery

JAMES E. GRIFFIN, M.D.

Associate Professor of Internal Medicine, University of Texas Health Science Center at Dallas, Southwestern Medical School; Attending Physician, Parkland Memorial Hospital, Dallas, Texas.

Disorders of Sexual Differentiation

H. ROGER HADLEY, M.D.

Assistant Professor, Loma Linda University School of Medicine; Consultant, Riverside General Hospital; Staff, Jerry Pettis Veterans Hospital, San Bernardino County Hospital, Loma Linda University Medical Center, Loma Linda, California.

The Treatment of Male Urinary Incontinence

W. HARDY HENDREN, M.D.

Professor of Surgery, Harvard Medical School; Chief of Surgery, The Children's Hospital; Visiting Surgeon, Massachusetts General Hospital, Boston, Massachusetts.

Urinary Undiversion: Refunctionalization of the Previously Diverted Urinary Tract

STANLEY C. HOPKINS, M.D., C.M., F.R.C.S.(C)

Assistant Professor of Surgery, Division of Urology, University of South Florida College of Medicine; Acting Chief, Urology Section, James A. Haley Veterans Administration Hospital, Tampa, Florida.

Benign and Malignant Tumors of the Male and Female Urethra

---

*Deceased.

STUART S. HOWARDS, M.D.

Professor of Urology and Physiology, University of Virginia School of Medicine; Urologist, University of Virginia Medical Center, Charlottesville, Virginia.

Male Infertility; Surgery of the Scrotum and Its Contents

DOMINIK J. HUBER, M.D.

Radiologist, Long Island Jewish Medical Center, New Hyde Park, New York.

Computed Tomography of the Kidney

PERRY B. HUDSON, M.D.

Professor of Surgery, University of South Florida College of Medicine; Chief, Urology Section, Veterans Administration Medical Center, Bay Pines, Florida

Perineal Prostatectomy

SARWAT HUSSAIN, M.B.B.S.

Department of Radiology, Aga Khan University Medical College, Islamabad, Pakistan.

Computed Tomography of the Adrenal Gland

ROBERT D. JEFFS, M.D., F.R.C.S.(C).

Professor of Pediatric Urology, The Johns Hopkins University School of Medicine; Director of Pediatric Urology, The Johns Hopkins Hospital; Consultant in Pediatric Urology, Francis Scott Key Medical Center, University of Maryland Hospital, John F. Kennedy Institute, Baltimore, Maryland.

Management of the Exstrophy-Epispadias Complex and Urachal Anomalies

JOSEPH J. KAUFMAN, M.D.

Professor of Surgery/Urology, and Chief, Division of Urology, University of California, Los Angeles, School of Medicine; Chief, UCLA Urology Hospital; Director, Clark UCLA Urological Center; Consultant, Wadsworth Veterans Administration Hospital, Sepulveda Veterans Administration Hospital, Cedars/Sinai Hospital, Los Angeles, California.

Surgical Treatment of Renovascular Hypertension

ROBERT W. KINDRACHUK, M.D.

Chief Resident in Urology, Stanford University Medical School; Staff, Stanford University Medical Center, Stanford, California.

Urinalysis

LOWELL R. KING, M.D.

Professor of Urology and Associate Professor of Pediatrics; Head, Section on Pediatric Urology, Duke University School of Medicine; Division of Urology, Duke University Medical Center, Durham, North Carolina.

Vesicoureteral Reflux, Megaureter, and Ureteral Reimplantation

FREDERICK A. KLEIN, M.D.

Assistant Professor of Urology, Virginia Commonwealth University Medical College of Virginia School of Medicine; Staff, Medical College of Virginia Hospitals, Richmond, Virginia.

Surgery of the Ureter

STEPHEN A. KOFF, M.D.

Associate Professor of Surgery; Head, Section of Pediatric Urology, Ohio State University Medical College, Columbus, Ohio.

Enuresis

WARREN W. KOONTZ, Jr., M.D.

Professor and Chairman, Division of Urology, Associate Dean for Clinical Affairs, Virginia Commonwealth University Medical College of Virginia School of Medicine; Staff, Medical College of Virginia Hospitals, Richmond, Virginia.

Surgery of the Ureter

ROBERT J. KRANE, M.D.

Professor and Chairman, Department of Urology, Boston University School of Medicine; Urologist-in-Chief, University Hospital, Boston, Massachusetts.

Sexual Function and Dysfunction.

R. LAWRENCE KROOVAND, M.D.

Associate Professor of Surgery (Pediatric Urology) and Pediatrics, and Director of Pediatric and Reconstructive Urology, Bowman Gray School of Medicine of Wake Forest University; Director of Pediatric and Reconstructive Urology, North Carolina Baptist Hospital, Winston-Salem, North Carolina.

Myelomeningocele

ELROY D. KURSH, M.D.

Associate Professor of Urology, Case Western Reserve University School of Medicine; Staff, University Hospitals of Cleveland, Cleveland, Ohio.

Extrinsic Obstruction of the Ureter

PAUL H. LANGE, M.D.

Professor of Urologic Surgery, University of Minnesota Medical School; Chief, Urology Section, Veterans Administration Medical Center, Minneapolis, Minnesota.

Diagnostic and Therapeutic Urologic Instrumentation

JAY STAUFFER LEHMAN, M.D.*

Formerly, Assistant Director, The Edna McConnell Clark Foundation, New York, New York.

Parasitic Diseases of the Genitourinary System

---

*Deceased.

HERBERT LEPOR, M.D.

Postdoctoral Fellow, Department of Urology, The Johns Hopkins University School of Medicine; Chief Resident, Department of Urology, The Johns Hopkins Hospital, Baltimore, Maryland.

Management of the Exstrophy-Epispadias Complex and Urachal Anomalies

BRUCE R. LESLIE, M.D.

Staff Physician, Division of Hypertensive Diseases, Ochsner Medical Institutions, New Orleans, Lousiana.

Normal Renal Physiology

SELWYN B. LEVITT, M.D.

Adjunct Clinical Professor of Urology, New York Medical College; Attending Pediatric Urologist, Albert Einstein College Hospital; Co-Director, Section of Pediatric Urology, Westchester County Medical Center; Attending Pediatric Urologist, Montefiore Hospital and Medical Center and Bronx Municipal Hospital Center, New York, New York.

Vesicoureteral Reflux, Megaureter, and Ureteral Reimplantation

MICHAEL M. LIEBER, M.D.

Associate Professor of Urology, Mayo Medical School, Consultant in Urology, Mayo Clinic; Staff, Methodist Hospital, St. Mary's Hospital, Rochester, Minnesota.

Open Bladder Surgery

GARY LIESKOVSKY, M.D.

Assistant Professor of Surgery/Urology, University of Southern California School of Medicine, Los Angeles, California.

Use of Intestinal Segments in the Urinary Tract

BERNARD LYTTON, M.B., F.R.C.S.

Professor of Surgery/Urology, Yale University School of Medicine; Chief of Urology, Yale–New Haven Medical Center, New Haven, Connecticut.

Surgery of the Kidney

MAX MAIZELS, M.D.

Assistant Professor of Urology, Northwestern University Medical School; Staff, Children's Memorial Hospital, Northwestern Memorial Hospital, Chicago, Illinois.

Normal Development of the Urinary Tract

TERRENCE R. MALLOY, M.D.

Professor of Urology, University of Pennsylvania School of Medicine; Chief, Section of Urology, Pennsylvania Hospital, Philadelphia, Pennsylvania.

Surgery of the Penis

FRAY F. MARSHALL, M.D.

Associate Professor of Urology, The Johns Hopkins University School of Medicine; Active Staff, The Johns Hopkins Hospital, Baltimore, Maryland.

Anatomy of the Retroperitoneum and Adrenal

VICTOR F. MARSHALL, M.D., D.Sc.

Emeritus Professor of Surgery (Urology), Cornell University Medical College; Professor of Urology, University of Virginia; Emeritus Attending Surgeon, Memorial Hospital for Cancer and Allied Diseases; Consultant in Urology, University of Virginia Hospital, Charlottesville, Virginia.

Suprapubic Vesicourethral Suspension (Marshall-Marchetti-Krantz) for Stress Incontinence.

EDWARD J. McGUIRE, M.D.

Professor of Surgery and Head, Section of Urology, University of Michigan Medical School, Ann Arbor, Michigan.

Neuromuscular Dysfunction of the Lower Urinary Tract

EDWIN M. MEARES, Jr., M.D.

Charles M. Whitney Professor of Urology, and Chairman, Division of Urology, Tufts University School of Medicine; Chairman, Department of Urology, and Urologist-in-Chief, New England Medical Center Hospitals, Boston, Massachusetts.

Prostatitis and Related Disorders

HARRY Z. MELLINS, M.D.

Professor of Radiology, Harvard Medical School; Director, Diagnostic Radiology, Brigham and Women's Hospital, Boston, Massachusetts.

Urography and Cystourethrography

EDWARD M. MESSING, M.D.

Assistant Professor of Surgery and Human Oncology, Division of Urology, University of Wisconsin School of Medicine; Attending Surgeon, University of Wisconsin Hospital and Clinics; Consulting Surgeon, Middleton Veterans Administration Hospital, Madison, Wisconsin.

Interstitial Cystitis and Related Syndromes

BRUCE A. MOLITORIS, M.D.

Assistant Professor of Medicine, Division of Renal Diseases, University of Colorado School of Medicine; Staff, University Hospital, Denver Veterans Administration Medical Center, Denver, Colorado.

Etiology, Pathogenesis, and Management of Renal Failure

MICHAEL J. MORSE, M.D.

Assistant Professor of Surgery (Urology), Cornell University Medical College; Clinical Assistant Attending, Urologic Service, Memorial Sloan-Kettering Cancer Center, New York, New York.

Neoplasms of the Testis; Surgery of Testicular Neoplasms

EDWARD C. MUECKE, M.D.

Clinical Professor of Surgery (Urology), Cornell University Medical College; Attending Surgeon (Urology), The New York Hospital; Associate Attending Surgeon (Urology), Lenox Hill Hospital, New York, New York.

Exstrophy, Epispadias, and Other Anomalies of the Bladder

GERALD P. MURPHY, M.D.

Professor of Surgery, State University of New York at Buffalo School of Medicine; Director, Roswell Park Memorial Institute, Buffalo, New York.

Tumors of Testicular Adnexal Structures and Seminal Vesicles

JOHN B. NANNINGA, M.D.

Associate Professor of Urology, Northwestern University Medical School; Attending Urologist, Northwestern Memorial Hospital; Consultant in Urology, Veterans Administration Lakeside Hospital; Chief, Division of Surgery, Rehabilitation Institute of Chicago, Chicago, Illinois.

Suprapubic and Retropubic Prostatectomy

WALTER R. NICKEL, M.D.

Clinical Professor of Dermatology and Pathology, University of California, San Diego, School of Medicine; Civilian Consultant, U.S. Naval Regional Medical Center, San Diego, California.

Visible Lesions of the Male Genitalia; Cutaneous Diseases of External Genitalia

VINCENT J. O'CONOR, Jr., M.D.

Professor of Urology, Northwestern University Medical School; Chief of Urology, Northwestern Memorial Hospital; Attending Urologist, Veterans Administration Lakeside Hospital, Chicago, Illinois.

Suprapubic and Retropubic Prostatectomy

CARL A. OLSSON, M.D.

Lattimer Professor and Chairman, Department of Urology, College of Physicians and Surgeons, Columbia University; Chief of Urology and Director, Squier Urologic Clinic, Presbyterian Hospital, New York, New York.

Anatomy of the Upper Urinary Tract

JOHN M. PALMER, M.D.

Professor of Urology, University of California, Davis, School of Medicine; Consultant, Veterans Administration Medical Center, Kaiser Permanente Medical Center, Sutter Community Hospitals Cancer Center, Sacramento, California.

Surgery of The Seminal Vesicles

JEROME P. PARNELL, II, M.D.

Clinical Assistant Professor of Surgery-Urology, University of North Carolina at Chapel Hill School of Medicine, Chapel Hill, North Carolina.

Suprapubic Vesicourethral Suspension (Marshall-Marchetti-Krantz) for Stress Incontinence

DAVID F. PAULSON, M.D.

Professor and Chief, Division of Urology, Department of Surgery, Duke University Medical Center, Durham, North Carolina.

Principles of Oncology

ALAN D. PERLMUTTER, M.D.

Professor of Urology, Wayne State University School of Medicine; Chief, Department of Pediatric Urology, Children's Hospital of Michigan, Detroit, Michigan.

Anomalies of the Upper Urinary Tract; Management of Intersexuality; Temporary Urinary Diversion in Infants and Young Children

LESTER PERSKY, M.D.

Clinical Professor of Urology, Case Western Reserve University School of Medicine; Staff, University Hospitals of Cleveland, St. Luke's Hospital, Cleveland, Ohio.

Extrinsic Obstruction of the Ureter

PAUL C. PETERS, M.D.

Professor and Chairman, Division of Urology, The University of Texas Health Science Center at Dallas, Southwestern Medical School; Chief of Urology, Parkland Memorial Hospital, Children's Medical Center; Attending Staff, Baylor University Medical Center, Presbyterian Hospital, Medical Arts Hospital, John Peter Smith Hospital (Ft. Worth), Dallas Veterans Administration Hospital, Dallas, Texas.

Genitourinary Trauma

ROBERT T. PLUMB, M.D.

Clinical Professor of Surgery (Urology), University of California, San Diego, School of Medicine; Senior Staff, Mercy Hospital, Donald N. Sharp Memorial Community Hospital, Coronado Hospital, San Diego, California.

Visible Lesions of the Male Genitalia; Cutaneous Diseases of External Genitalia

JACOB RAJFER, M.D.

Associate Professor of Surgery/Urology, University of California, Los Angeles; School of Medicine; Chief, Division of Urology, Harbor/UCLA Medical Center, Los Angeles, California.

Congenital Anomalies of the Testis

R. BEVERLY RANEY, Jr., M.D.

Associate Professor of Pediatrics, The University of Pennsylvania School of Medicine; Associate Director for Education and Training, and Senior Physician, Division of Oncology, Department of Pediatrics, Children's Hospital of Philadelphia, Philadelphia, Pennsylvania.

Pediatric Oncology

VASSILIOS RAPTOPOULOS, M.D.

University of Massachusetts Medical School; University of Massachusetts Medical Center, Worcester, Massachusetts.

Ultrasound

SHLOMO RAZ, M.D.

Associate Professor of Surgery/Urology, University of California, Los Angeles, School of Medicine; UCLA Center for the Health Sciences, Los Angeles, California.

The Treatment of Male Urinary Incontinence

MARTIN I. RESNICK, M.D.

Professor and Chairman, Division of Urology, Case Western Reserve University School of Medicine; Staff, University Hospitals of Cleveland, Cleveland, Ohio.

Extrinsic Obstruction of the Ureter

ALAN B. RETIK, M.D.

Professor of Surgery (Urology), Harvard Medical School; Chief, Division of Urology, The Children's Hospital, Boston, Massachusetts.

Anomalies of the Upper Urinary Tract; Ectopic Ureter and Ureterocele; Temporary Urinary Diversion in Infants and Young Children

JEROME P. RICHIE, M.D.

Associate Professor of Urological Surgery, Harvard Medical School; Chief, Urologic Oncology, Brigham and Women's Hospital, Boston, Massachusetts.

Ureterointestinal Diversion

ARTHUR I. SAGALOWSKY, M.D.

Associate Professor, Division of Urology, and Surgical Director, Renal Transplant, The University of Texas Health Science Center at Dallas, Southwestern Medical School; Attending Staff, Dallas Veterans Administration Hospital, Children's Medical Center, St. Paul Hospital, Baylor University Medical Center Hospital, Parkland Memorial Hospital, Dallas, Texas.

Genitourinary Trauma

OSCAR SALVATIERRA, Jr., M.D.

Professor of Surgery and Urology, and Chief, Transplant Service, University of California, San Francisco, School of Medicine, San Francisco, California.

Renal Transplantation

PETER T. SCARDINO, M.D.

Associate Professor of Urology, Baylor College of Medicine; Active Staff, The Methodist Hospital, Ben Taub General Hospital; Assistant Staff, St. Luke's Episcopal Hospital; Courtesy Staff, Veterans Administration Hospital, Texas Children's Hospital, Houston, Texas.

Initial Evaluation, Including History, Physical Examination, and Urinalysis

ANTHONY J. SCHAEFFER, M.D.

Associate Professor, Northwestern University Medical School; Attending, Northwestern Memorial Hospital; Associate Attending, Children's Memorial Hospital; Consultant in Urology, Veterans Administration Lakeside Hospital, Chicago, Illinois.

Other Renal Diseases of Urologic Significance; Surgical Management of Ureteropelvic Junction Obstruction

PAUL F. SCHELLHAMMER, M.D.

Professor of Urology, Eastern Virginia Medical School; Director, Urology Training Program, Eastern Virginia Graduate School of Medicine; Active Staff, General Hospital of Virginia Beach, Norfolk General Hospital, Leigh Memorial Hospital, Children's Hospital of the King's Daughters, DePaul Hospital, Norfolk, Virginia.

Tumors of the Penis

JAN SCHÖNEBECK, M.D.

Associate Professor of Urology, University of Linköping, Sweden; Head of Urology, Department of Surgery, Central Hospital, Norrköping, Sweden.

Fungal Infections of the Urinary Tract

ROBERT W. SCHRIER, M.D.

Professor and Chairman, Department of Medicine, University of Colorado School of Medicine; Head, Division of Renal Diseases; Staff, University Hospital, Denver Veterans Administration Medical Center, Denver General Hospital, Rose Medical Center, Denver, Colorado

Etiology, Pathogenesis, and Management of Renal Failure

WILLIAM W. SCOTT, Ph.D., M.D., D.Sc.

Professor of Urology, Emeritus, The Johns Hopkins University School of Medicine; The Johns Hopkins Hospital, Baltimore, Maryland.

Carcinoma of the Prostate

STEVEN E. SELTZER, M.D.

Associate Professor of Radiology, Harvard Medical School; Radiologist and Director, Computed Tomography, Brigham and Women's Hospital, Boston, Massachusetts.

Computed Tomography of the Kidney

RICHARD J. SHERINS, M.D.

Chief, Section on Reproductive Endocrinology, Developmental Endocrinology Branch, National Institute of Child Health and Human Development, Bethesda, Maryland.

Male Infertility

LINDA M. DAIRIKI SHORTLIFFE, M.D.

Assistant Professor of Surgery (Urology), Stanford University School of Medicine; Chief, Urology Section, Veterans Administration Medical Center, Palo Alto, California.

Infections of the Urinary Tract: Introduction and General Principles; Urinary Infections in Adult Women; Urinary Incontinence in the Female: Stress Urinary Incontinence

DONALD G. SKINNER, M.D.

Professor and Chairman, Division of Urology (Surgery), University of Southern California School of Medicine; Chief of Staff, Kenneth Norris, Jr., Cancer Hospital and Research Institute, Los Angeles, California.

Ureterointestinal Diversion; Use of Intestinal Segments in the Urinary Tract

EDWARD H. SMITH, M.D.

Professor and Chairman, Department of Radiology, University of Massachusetts Medical School, Worcester, Massachusetts.

Ultrasound

BRENT W. SNOW, M.D.

Assistant Professor, University of Utah School of Medicine, Salt Lake City, Utah.

Disorders of the Urethra and Penis

HOWARD McC. SNYDER, III, M.D.

Assistant Professor of Urology in Surgery, University of Pennsylvania School of Medicine; Assistant Surgeon, Division of Urology, Children's Hospital of Philadelphia, Philadelphia, Pennsylvania.

Pediatric Oncology

JOSEPH T. SPAULDING, M.D.

Assistant Clinical Professor of Urology, University of California, San Francisco, School of Medicine; Active Staff, St. Francis Memorial Hospital, St. Mary's Medical Center, Pacific Presbyterian Medical Center, San Francisco, California.

Surgery of Penile and Urethral Carcinoma

THOMAS A. STAMEY, M.D.

Professor of Surgery and Chairman, Division of Urology, Stanford University School of Medicine, Stanford, California.

Urinalysis; Infections of the Urinary Tract: Introduction and General Principles; Urinary Infections in Adult Women; Urinary Incontinence in the Female: Stress Urinary Incontinence

RALPH A. STRAFFON, M.D.

Chairman, Division of Surgery; Member, Department of Urology, Cleveland Clinic Foundation, Cleveland, Ohio.

Surgery for Calculus Disease of the Urinary Tract

RONALD S. SWERDLOFF, M.D.

Professor of Medicine, University of California, Los Angeles, School of Medicine; Chief, Division of Endocrinology, Harbor-UCLA Medical Center, Los Angeles, California.

Physiology of Male Reproduction: Hypothalamic-Pituitary Function

EMIL A. TANAGHO, M.D.

Professor and Chairman, Department of Urology, University of California, San Francisco, School of Medicine, San Francisco, California.

Anatomy of the Lower Urinary Tract

SALVATOR TREVES, M.D.

Associate Professor of Radiology, Harvard Medical School; Chief, Division of Nuclear Medicine, The Children's Hospital Medical Center, Boston, Massachusetts.

Radionuclides in Genitourinary Disorders

TIMOTHY S. TRULOCK, M.D.

Fellow in Pediatric Urology, Emory University School of Medicine, Atlanta, Georgia.

Prune-Belly Syndrome

SABAH S. TUMEH, M.D.

Assistant Professor of Radiology, Harvard Medical School; Radiologist, Brigham and Women's Hospital; Consultant in Oncodiagnostic Radiology and Nuclear Medicine; Dana Farber Cancer Institute, Boston, Massachusetts.

Radionuclides in Genitourinary Disorders

RICHARD TURNER-WARWICK,
B.Sc., D.M. (Oxon.), M.Ch.,
F.R.C.S., F.R.C.P., F.A.C.S.

Consultant Urological Surgeon, The London University Institute of Urology, Middlesex Hospital, St. Peter's Group Hospitals, Royal National Orthopaedic Hospital, London, England.

Urinary Fistulae in the Female

DAVID C. UTZ, M.D.

Anson L. Clark Professor of Urology, Mayo Clinic and Mayo Medical School; Staff, Methodist Hospital, Saint Mary's Hospital, Rochester, Minnesota.

Open Bladder Surgery

E. DARRACOTT VAUGHAN, Jr., M.D.

James J. Colt Professor of Urology in Surgery, Cornell University Medical College; Attending Surgeon, The New York Hospital, Memorial Sloan-Kettering Cancer Center; Visiting Physician, The Rockefeller University Hospital, New York, New York

Normal Renal Physiology; Renovascular Hypertension; Suprapubic Vesicourethral Suspension (Marshall-Marchetti-Krantz) for Stress Incontinence

M. J. VERNON SMITH, M.D., Ph.D.

Professor of Urology, Virginia Commonwealth University Medical College of Virginia School of Medicine; Staff, Medical College of Virginia Hospitals, Richmond, Virginia.

Surgery of the Ureter

FRANZ VON LICHTENBERG, M.D.

Professor of Pathology, Harvard Medical School; Pathologist, Brigham and Women's Hospital, Boston, Massachusetts.

Parasitic Diseases of the Genitourinary System

PATRICK C. WALSH, M.D.

David Hall McConnell Professor and Director, Department of Urology, The Johns Hopkins University School of Medicine; Urologist-In-Chief, The James Buchanan Brady Urological Institute, the Johns Hopkins Hospital, Baltimore, Maryland.

Benign Prostatic Hyperplasia; Radical Retropubic Prostatectomy

ALAN J. WEIN, M.D.

Professor of Urology and Chairman, Section of Urology, University of Pennsylvania School of Medicine, Philadelphia, Pennsylvania.

Surgery of the Penis

LESTER WEISS, M.D.

Clinical Professor of Pediatrics, University of Michigan, Medical School; Director, Medical Genetics and Birth Defects Center, Henry Ford Hospital, Detroit, Michigan.

Genetic Determinants of Urologic Disease

ROBERT M. WEISS, M.D.

Professor, Department of Surgery/Urology, Yale University School of Medicine; Adjunct Professor, Department of Pharmacology, Columbia University, College of Physicians and Surgeons, New York, New York; Medical Staff, Gaylord Hospital, Wallingford; Attending, Yale–New Haven Hospital; Consulting, West Haven Veterans Administration Hospital, Waterbury Hospital, Sharon Hospital, William Backus Hospital, Norwalk Hospital, St. Raphael's Hospital, New Haven, Connecticut.

Physiology and Pharmacology of the Renal Pelvis and Ureter

WILLET F. WHITMORE, Jr., M.D.

Professor of Surgery (Urology), Cornell University Medical College; Attending Surgeon, Urologic Service, Memorial Sloan-Kettering Cancer Center, New York, New York.

Neoplasms of the Testis; Surgery of Testicular Neoplasms

JEAN D. WILSON, M.D.

Professor of Internal Medicine, University of Texas Health Science Center at Dallas, Southwestern Medical School; Attending Physician, Parkland Memorial Hospital, Dallas, Texas.

Embryology of the Genital Tract; Disorders of Sexual Differentiation

JAN WINBERG, M.D.

Professor of Pediatrics, Karolinska Institute; Chairman, Department of Pediatrics, Karolinska Hospital, Stockholm, Sweden.

Urinary Tract Infections in Infants and Children

JOHN R. WOODARD, M.D.

Professor of Surgery (Urology) and Director of Pediatric Urology, Emory University School of Medicine; Chief, Urology Service, Henrietta Egleston Hospital for Children, Atlanta, Georgia.

Prune-Belly Syndrome; Neonatal and Perinatal Emergencies

PHILIPPE E. ZIMMERN, M.D.

Resident in Urology, University of California, Los Angeles, School of Medicine, Los Angeles, California.

The Treatment of Male Urinary Incontinence

PREFACE

Urology has undergone remarkable growth and change since the Fourth Edition of this textbook was published. In creating this edition we recognized the need for an authoritative textbook incorporating the new advances in basic science, clinical medicine, instrumentation, and surgical technique. At the outset we knew we had the opportunity to create the best textbook of urology ever written and, in doing so, to improve the quality of care provided by all urologists for their patients.

We began by re-evaluating every chapter in the Fourth Edition with the help of our residents. No one is more critical or frank than the resident in training, and these evaluations were helpful in focusing new goals. We recognized that it was possible to consolidate the pathophysiologic material contained in the early chapters into a smaller space while providing more information. This enabled us to expand the clinical and surgical sections.

In keeping with past tradition there has been a significant turnover of participants in the book in order to ensure fresh approaches to specific topics. In this edition, for example, there are 26 new authors and 9 new chapters. The anatomy chapter has been subdivided into three sections: the retroperitoneum and adrenal, the upper urinary tract, and the lower urinary tract and genitalia. All three sections are now under new authorship and have new illustrations, new depth, and new emphasis on surgical considerations. The sections on normal renal function; renovascular hypertension; the etiology, pathogenesis, and management of renal failure; and renal diseases of urologic significance have new authorship. They have been completely updated and modernized and contain succinct, factual, specific applications for the urologist. A new chapter on diagnostic and therapeutic urologic instrumentation has been provided. This excellent chapter on endourology incorporates all the new information in this rapidly developing field. The section on sexual function and dysfunction, which also has new authorship, contains the newer concepts of physiology of penile erection along with extensive recommendations regarding the evaluation and management of patients with sexual dysfunction. In the recognition that a major portion of the urologist's practice involves the management of patients with cancer, a new chapter, "Principles of Oncology," has been included. Urologists have been called upon to provide an ever increasing level of sophisticated care for cancer patients. This chapter will enable the urologist to have a more informed understanding of the principles of oncology and their applications to clinical care. A new chapter on pre- and postoperative care of the urologic patient is also included. This chapter amounts to a "mini-textbook" of medicine and is an excellent synopsis of the modern concepts of pre- and postoperative care that the urologic surgeon should know.

Over 50 per cent of the chapters on urologic surgery have new authors and new illustrations. Examples from this section of the book include new chapters on urinary undiversion and the surgery of calculus disease. In addition, new approaches are presented to the management of extracorporeal renal surgery and partial nephrectomy, the surgical management of ureteropelvic junction obstruction, the surgical management of the ureter, open bladder surgery, transurethral prostatectomy, surgery of the penis, and surgery of the scrotum and its contents. The chapter on the use of intestinal segments provides an excellent description of the Kock pouch, a technique that has received widespread attention from urologists because it provides a form of urinary diversion that does not require an external appliance. In addition, the chapter on radical retropubic prostatectomy emphasizes the new "nerve-sparing" modifications that preserve postoperative potency following radical prostatectomy and cystoprostatectomy.

We wish to thank the authors of prior editions, since this new edition has been built upon the solid foundation they laid. Our gratitude is greatest for the contingent of contributing authors who collectively represent the finest scientists and clinicians associated with the field of urology. We wish to pay tribute to the late J. Hartwell Harrison, who coedited the Third Edition with the late Meredith Campbell and who led all of us through the major transition incorporated in the Fourth Edition. His untimely death prevents his witnessing our present efforts.

A work of this scope and magnitude cannot be accomplished without the assistance of a great number of persons whose efforts may not be specifically attributed within this book. Finally, we wish to express our thanks to Carroll C. Cann, Robert Butler, Constance Burton, Carolyn Naylor, and the staff of the W. B. Saunders Company for their patience and help in bringing this ambitious undertaking to publication.

PATRICK C. WALSH, M.D.
For the Editors

CONTENTS

VOLUME 1

SECTION I. ANATOMY AND PHYSIOLOGY

1
ANATOMY AND SURGICAL APPROACH TO THE UROGENITAL TRACT

SECTION II. THE UROLOGIC EXAMINATION AND DIAGNOSTIC TECHNIQUES

6
INITIAL EVALUATION, INCLUDING HISTORY, PHYSICAL EXAMINATION, AND URINALYSIS

7
RADIOLOGY OF THE URINARY TRACT

SECTION III. THE PATHOPHYSIOLOGY OF URINARY OBSTRUCTION

9

Jay Y. Gillenwater, M.D.

10

*Lester Persky, M.D., Elroy D. Kursh, M.D., Stewart Feldman, M.D.,
and Martin I. Resnick, M.D.*

SECTION IV. NEUROGENIC BLADDER

SECTION V. INFERTILITY

SECTION VI. SEXUAL FUNCTION

SECTION VII. INFECTIONS AND INFLAMMATIONS OF THE GENITOURINARY TRACT

SECTION VIII. URINARY LITHIASIS

SECTION IX. GENITOURINARY TRAUMA

VOLUME 2

SECTION X. BENIGN PROSTATIC HYPERPLASIA

SECTION XI. TUMORS OF THE GENITOURINARY TRACT IN THE ADULT

SECTION XII. EMBRYOLOGY AND ANOMALIES OF THE GENITOURINARY TRACT

SECTION XIII. PEDIATRIC UROLOGIC SURGERY

56
NEONATAL AND PERINATAL EMERGENCIES 2217
John R. Woodard, M.D.

57
PEDIATRIC ONCOLOGY 2244
*Howard McC. Snyder, III, M.D., Giulio J. D'Angio, M.D.,
Audrey E. Evans, M.D., and R. Beverly Raney, M.D.*

VOLUME III

SECTION XIV. RENAL DISEASES OF UROLOGIC SIGNIFICANCE

58
RENOVASCULAR HYPERTENSION 2298
E. Darracott Vaughan, Jr., M.D.

59
ETIOLOGY, PATHOGENESIS, AND MANAGEMENT OF RENAL FAILURE 2326
Bruce A. Molitoris, M.D., and Robert W. Schrier, M.D.

SECTION XV. UROLOGIC SURGERY

ANATOMY AND PHYSIOLOGY

Anatomy and Surgical Approach to the Urogenital Tract

Anatomy of the Retroperitoneum and Adrenal

FRAY F. MARSHALL, M.D.

The retroperitoneal space remains the frequent domain of the genitourinary surgeon. Surgical management of diseases of the kidney, ureter, adrenal gland, and retroperitoneum requires detailed anatomic knowledge of this area. The retroperitoneum above the pelvis will be considered in this section, starting with a description of the musculoskeletal shell of the retroperitoneum. Within the retroperitoneum, the organs, vasculature, lymphatics, nerves, and their relationships will be demonstrated.

MUSCULOSKELETAL BOUNDARIES OF RETROPERITONEUM

The musculotendinous diaphragm (Fig. 1–1) divides the thorax and abdomen and provides the superior boundary of the retroperitoneum. The transversalis fascia resides on the inner aspect of the transversus abdominis muscle and extends onto the inferior aspect of the diaphragm. It also extends over the quadratus lumborum and psoas muscles. The muscular fibers of the diaphragm extend radially around a central tendon and attach to the inferior six ribs. The crura attach to the anterior aspect of the lumbar vertebra. The right and left crura of the diaphragm unite in front of the aortic hiatus and form the median arcuate ligament. The diaphragm is also perforated by the vena cava and esophagus as well as by nerves and lymphatics. The primary blood supply to the diaphragm arises from the inferior phrenic arteries, and the innervation is supplied by the phrenic nerve (C_3, C_4, C_5). The vasculature and innervation extend from medial to lateral, so that there is less surgical damage to the diaphragm if it is divided laterally. On the right side inferiorly, the diaphragm has primary contact with the liver, and peritoneum covers the majority of the inferior aspect of the diaphragm. On the left side, the stomach and spleen reside immediately under the diaphragm. The adrenal glands as well as the kidneys lie very close to the diaphragm, but connective tissue and fat separate these structures from the diaphragm.

Posteriorly, the retroperitoneum is bordered by the vertebral column, the psoas muscle, and the quadratus lumborum muscle, with their fascial coverings. Inferior and lateral is the iliacus muscle. The fascia over all of these muscles is continuous with the transversalis fas-

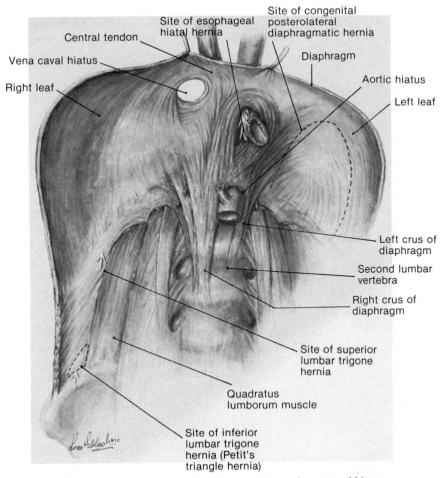

Figure 1–1. The diaphragm with its muscular attachments and hiatus.

cia. The iliopsoas muscles are primary hip flexors, and pain may result when an inflammatory process occurs on this muscle or on the genitofemoral nerve, which runs along its anterior surface. Laterally, the confines of the retroperitoneum include the transversus abdominis muscle external to the transversalis fascia. The internal oblique muscle overlies the transversus abdominis. In the area of the lumbar triangle, the latissimus dorsi muscle may not cover completely the external oblique muscle, and the lumbar triangle (Petit's triangle) is formed at the superior aspect of the ilium. It is through this potentially weak area of the lateral muscle wall that perinephric or retroperitoneal abscesses may present (Fig. 1–1).

URINARY ORGANS

Internal to the fascia covering the muscles surrounding the retroperitoneum there is the pararenal fat. Within this fat is Gerota's fascia

(renal fascia), which surrounds the kidney and adrenal gland (Fig. 1–2). The fascia is somewhat thicker posteriorly and then curves anteriorly where it is contiguous with the peritoneum. Then the anterior and posterior leaves of Gerota's fascia meet medially at the level of the great vessels and fuse, so that it is unusual for retroperitoneal infection on one side to spread to the contralateral side. In contrast, the inferior aspect of Gerota's fascia is open, as demonstrated by visualization of the adrenal glands from presacral retroperitoneal gas insufflation (Fig. 1–2). Within Gerota's fascia is the usually more abundant perirenal fat. Fibrous trabeculae that provide support for the kidney extend within this fat.

The kidneys are the largest retroperitoneal structures. They usually are 11 to 12 cm in length and are located from the level of the twelfth thoracic vertebra to the third lumbar vertebra (Fig. 1–3). In some patients there can be considerable mobility of the kidney. The kidney is in close relationship with adjacent

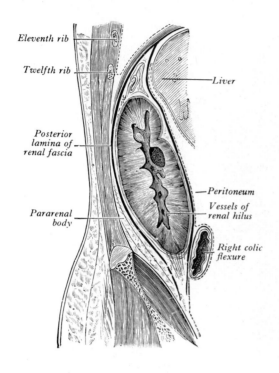

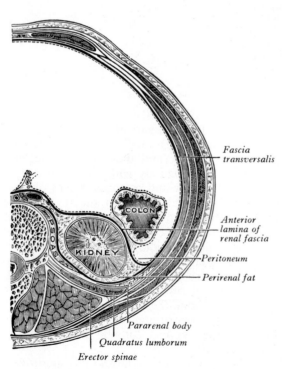

Figure 1–2. *A,* Transverse section at level of the second lumbar vertebra, demonstrating renal fascia and organ relationships. *B,* A sagittal section demonstrating relations of renal or Gerota's fascia to the right kidney.

organs (Fig. 1–4). On the right, the adrenal gland is superior, the liver covers a major portion of the anterior surface, the duodenum extends over the hilum and medial aspect of the kidney, and the lower aspect of the kidney may be covered by a portion of colon (Figs. 1–2 and 1–4). The kidney also lies in close proximity to the vena cava. On the left side, the adrenal gland is located on the superior but more medial aspect of the kidney. The spleen covers a major lateral area of the kidney. The tail of the pancreas extends over the area of the renal hilum. The stomach may be just above this area, and the jejunum and colon may be adjacent to the inferior aspect of the left kidney. Posteriorly, the diaphragm covers the kidney superiorly, and each kidney rests on the quadratus lumborum and psoas muscles.

The ureters are a continuation of the renal pelvis and generally are 28 to 34 cm in length. The ureters run inferiorly over the psoas muscle and cross the iliac vessels at the bifurcation of the internal and external iliac arteries. The right ureter is covered by the duodenum and the right colic and ileocolic vessels and lies within Gerota's fascia. The left ureter is covered by the left colic vessels. The gonadal vessels are initially medial to the ureter and then cross over them. They also provide accessory vasculature to the ureter, although the primary superior arterial supply comes from the renal artery.

MAJOR ARTERIAL AND VENOUS VASCULATURE OF THE RETROPERITONEUM

The aorta enters the abdomen through the aortic hiatus of the diaphragm and extends inferiorly in front of the vertebrae to bifurcate at the level of the fourth lumbar vertebra. Proceeding from a superior to an inferior direction, the first paired arterial branches of the aorta include the left and right inferior phrenic arteries. Often there are multiple adrenal branches extending off these arteries just as the aorta comes through the diaphragm. The arterial supply of the adrenal is extensive and diffuse. The celiac trunk (hepatic, splenic, left gastric branches) is the next major branch, and the single superior mesenteric artery arises just underneath it in the midline. Then the paired right and left adrenal arteries (middle adrenal arteries), which are often rather small, arise just above the renal arteries (Fig. 1–5). The gonadal

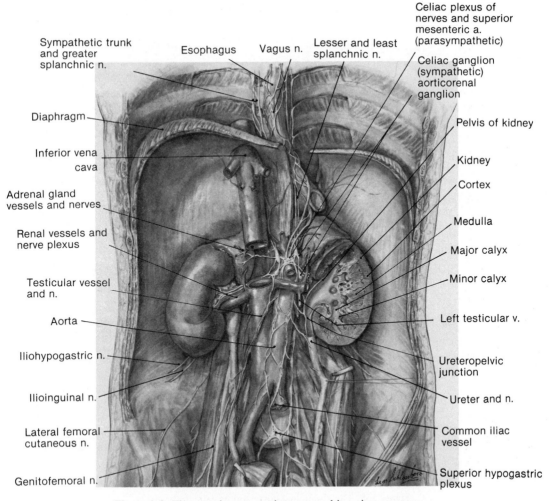

Figure 1–3. The superior retroperitoneum and its primary organs.

Sympathetic trunk and greater splanchnic n.

Esophagus

Vagus n.

Lesser and least splanchnic n.

Celiac plexus of nerves and superior mesenteric a. (parasympathetic)

Celiac ganglion (sympathetic) aorticorenal ganglion

Diaphragm

Inferior vena cava

Adrenal gland vessels and nerves

Renal vessels and nerve plexus

Testicular vessel and n.

Aorta

Iliohypogastric n.

Ilioinguinal n.

Lateral femoral cutaneous n.

Genitofemoral n.

Pelvis of kidney

Kidney

Cortex

Medulla

Major calyx

Minor calyx

Left testicular v.

Ureteropelvic junction

Ureter and n.

Common iliac vessel

Superior hypogastric plexus

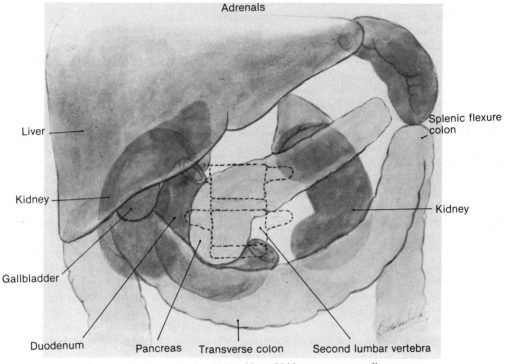

Figure 1–4. The anatomic relationships of kidneys to surrounding organs.

Adrenals

Liver

Kidney

Gallbladder

Duodenum

Pancreas

Transverse colon

Second lumbar vertebra

Splenic flexure colon

Kidney

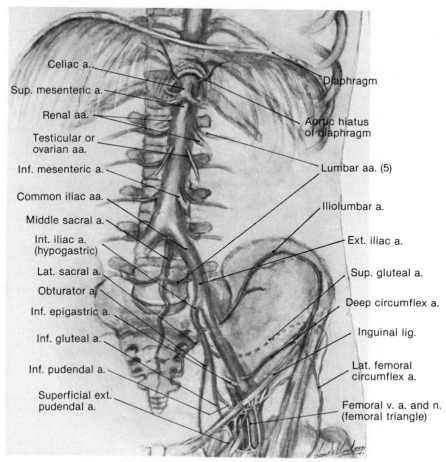

Figure 1–5. The abdominal aorta and its primary branches.

arteries (testicular or ovarian) usually arise from the aorta several centimeters below the renal arteries. These vessels are small and their origin is somewhat variable. They may even arise from a single trunk, a branch off the renal, or an accessory renal artery. The inferior mesenteric artery arises considerably more inferiorly. Last, there are usually at least four sets of lumbar arteries, which constitute the remainder of the primary abdominal aortic branches. The aorta terminates into the right and left common iliac artery and a much smaller middle sacral artery.

Anomalous development of the major arterial system is relatively frequent, but major arterial malformations are less well tolerated embryologically than venous abnormalities, so there is less variation than in the venous system. For example, the inferior phrenic arteries may arise from the abdominal aorta, the celiac trunk, or other abdominal aortic branches. The celiac axis also can have a wide variation; supernumerary renal arteries occur in one third of patients. Frequently there are double renal ar-

teries or an artery to the lower pole. More than 10 per cent of kidneys have two or more arteries originating at the aorta and entering close to the renal hilum, another 10 per cent have two arteries, one entering the hilus and the other entering one pole of the kidney (Pick and Anson, 1940). Kidneys that are ectopic almost always have anomalous and frequently multiple arteries. The gonadal arteries have been reported to be duplicated in 17 per cent of patients, and in 14 per cent they have arisen from the renal artery (Notkovitch, 1956).

The inferior vena cava and its branches generally parallel the arterial system (Fig. 1–6). The internal and external iliac veins join to form the common iliac veins, which then converge to form the vena cava. The right common iliac vein lies behind and slightly lateral to the right common iliac artery. The left common iliac vein lies medial to or slightly below the left common iliac artery. Additional venous tributaries include the right gonadal vein (ovarian or testicular), which enters below the level of the right

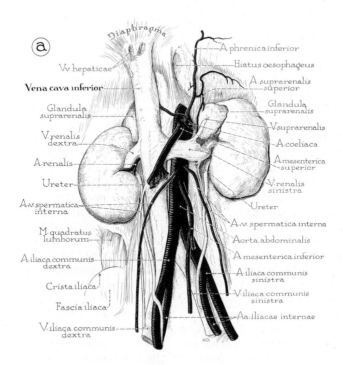

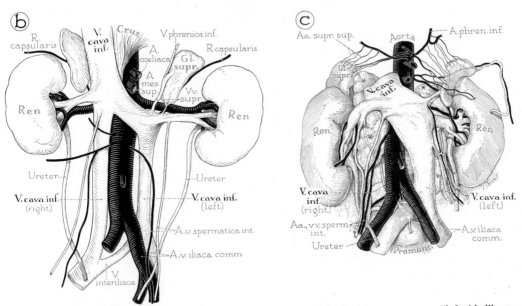

Figure 1–6. The inferior vena cava: typical and aberrant forms: a. normal, b. double vena cava, c. "left-sided" vena cava.

renal vein. The left gonadal vein generally enters the left renal vein. Above the gonadal vein the right and left renal veins enter the vena cava. Supernumerary renal veins are more common on the right side. The most common anomaly of the left renal vein is a circumaortic left renal vein. This anomaly has been found in as many as 6 per cent of patients (Reis and Esenther, 1959). Above the renal vein is the right adrenal vein, which can sometimes reside a surprising distance above the right renal vein. It is quite short and drains directly into the inferior vena cava. The left adrenal vein enters the left renal vein. Just above this level on the vena cava there may be multiple smaller hepatic venous branches, often to the caudate lobe. The two or three major hepatic veins insert superiorly just as the vena cava penetrates the diaphragm. In addition, there are phrenic veins that insert superiorly. Last, there are four or five paired lumbar veins on each side, which establish connections with the posterior vertebral venous plexus. The lumbar veins entering the vena cava have frequent variability in their anatomic patterns. Some may unite and enter the vena cava together, or they may unite with the ascending lumbar vein, which lies behind the psoas muscle. There may be communications with the common iliac vein or iliolumbar vein, which may lead into the azygos or hemiazygos veins.

Embryologic development of the inferior vena cava is complex. The area of the bifurcation of the vena cava is derived from the posterior cardinal veins. The vena cava to the level of the renal veins is derived from the supracardinal veins. The area of the renal veins is derived from the anastomotic segment of the subcardinal and supracardinal venous system. Subcardinal and hepatic segments are the origin for the remainder of the vena cava. Anomalies of the vena cava are common. Persistence of a subcardinal vein rather than a supracardinal vein below the level of the kidneys leads to a retrocaval ureter. Another relatively common occurrence is persistence of the cardinal system on the left side, which results in vena caval duplication or a left-sided vena cava. Double vena cava has been estimated to occur in 2 to 3 per cent of patients (Fig. 1–6).

Multiple collaterals develop when vena caval obstruction occurs, because of the diffuse nature of the venous system. This obstruction may be due to a tumor thrombus from renal cell carcinoma or surgical ligation for multiple pulmonary emboli. Multiple anastomoses with the vertebral, lumbar, azygous, and hemiazy-gous systems allow drainage to the superior vena cava. Anastomotic channels with the superior and inferior rectal veins allow drainage through the portal system as well.

LYMPHATICS

Lymphatics tend to follow blood vessels. This concept is especially important if there is anomalous vascular drainage, because the lymphatics will tend to follow these vessels, and any lymph node dissection should be altered accordingly. The lymphatics from the lower extremities, abdomen, and pelvis drain into the perivenacaval and periaortic lymphatic channels (Parker, 1935). These lymphatics start along common iliac vessels and enter the common iliac nodes. They ascend along the vena cava to the lumbar nodes. Multiple tributaries enter the cisterna chyli, which is formed by the union of the right and left lumbar trunks from the right and left lumbar nodal chain and an intestinal trunk derived from the celiac and superior mesenteric lymph node chain. In addition to these main trunks, a trunk from the upper retroaortic nodes may enter the cisterna chyli. The cisterna chyli is usually found on the anterior surface of the first and second lumbar vertebrae, with the thoracic duct starting at the level of the twelfth thoracic vertebra.

Two organs with major lymphatic drainage to the retroperitoneum include the testis and kidney. The right testis has lymphatic drainage to the perivenacaval lymph nodes below the right renal vein with crossover drainage to the interaortocaval and left renal hilar lymph nodes. Again, lymphatic drainage tends to parallel the venous drainage on the right side. The lymphatic drainage from the left testis is primarily to the area just inferior to the left renal vein. There is much less likely to be interaortocaval nodal drainage on the left unless there is a lymphatic obstruction from tumor or inflammation. There is more lymphatic crossover from right to left than from left to right.

The lymphatic drainage of the kidneys also varies on each side (Marshall and Powell, 1982). From the right kidney there are lymphatic channels that drain posterior to the vena cava (Fig. 1–7) and course superiorly to the interaortocaval area and lateral caval nodes. There is additional drainage anteriorly that may extend on the surface of the vena cava or to the interaortocaval area. The regional lymphatic drainage of the right kidney is basically circumvenacaval.

On the left side, however (Fig. 1–8), the

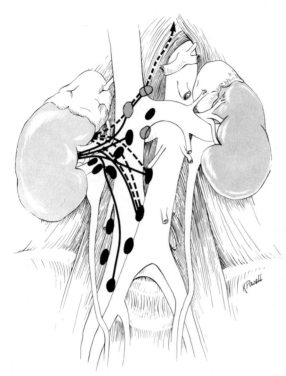

Figure 1–7. Right renal efferent lymphatics and regional lymph drainage. Dark nodes = anterior; shaded nodes = posterior; solid lines = anterior vessels; dotted lines = posterior vessels; directional arrows lead to cisterna chyli.

is the subcostal nerve, usually formed primarily from T_{12} extending inferiorly. The iliohypogastric nerve, which arises primarily from the first lumbar nerve, comes through the psoas muscle and crosses the quadratus lumborum (Fig. 1–4) to the crest of the ilium. There it divides into a lateral cutaneous branch, which is distributed to the skin of the gluteal region, and an anterior cutaneous branch, which supplies the skin in the hypogastric region. There are also muscle branches supplied to the internal oblique and transversus abdominis muscles. The ilioinguinal nerve arises inferiorly to the iliohypogastric and has muscle branches as well as cutaneous branches to the skin over the penis, scrotum, and medial portion of the thigh. The genitofemoral nerve arises from the first and second lumbar nerves and emerges on the ventral surface of the psoas muscle. It divides into a genital branch that supplies the cremaster muscle and the skin of the scrotum and the thigh; a femoral branch enters the femoral sheath and supplies the skin of the anterior surface of the thigh. The lateral femoral cutaneous nerve arises from the second and third lumbar nerves and passes

posterior lymphatic drainage tends to stay in the left lateral lumbar nodes, and there may be several additional nodes on the left crus of the diaphragm that extend around the aortic hiatus. Anteriorly, there is again drainage into the lateral lumbar nodes, but the regional drainage of the left kidney usually does not extend to the interaortocaval area. The regional nodal drainage extends basically from the diaphragm to just below the inferior mesenteric artery. If there are supernumerary renal vessels, the nodal drainage follows the vascular pattern. Consequently, there are obvious implications for altering a lymph node dissection for neoplasm (Marshall and Powell, 1982).

NERVES

Much of the innervation of the lower extremity arises in the retroperitoneal space. The lumbar plexus originates within the psoas muscle by the union of the ventral rami of the first three lumbar nerves (Fig. 1–9). There is often a contribution from the fourth lumbar and possibly the twelfth thoracic nerves. The first nerve

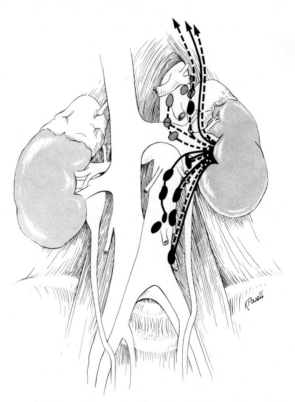

Figure 1–8. Left renal efferent lymphatics and regional lymph node drainage. Dark nodes = anterior; shaded nodes = posterior; solid lines = anterior vessels; dotted lines = posteror vessels; directional arrows lead to cisterna chyli.

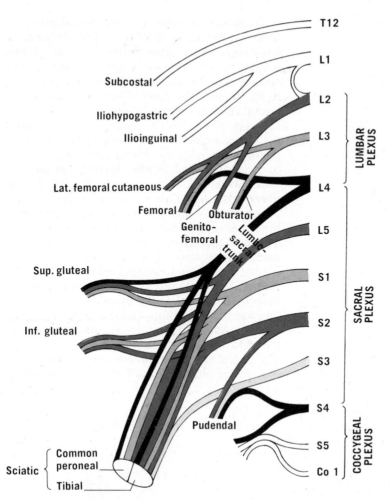

Figure 1–9. Lumbosacral plexus.

under the inguinal ligament and over the sartorius muscle into the thigh. Additional branches of the lumbar plexus include the femoral nerve and the accessory obturator nerve and lumbosacral trunk.

The abdominal portion of the sympathetic trunk lies ventral to the lumbar vertebrae along the medial aspect of the psoas muscle and adjacent to the aorta or vena cava. The lumbar ganglia vary in number from two to six and have no fixed pattern. The roots of the lumbar ganglia extend only as far as the second lumbar nerve, which is the caudal limit of the thoracolumbar outflow. The preganglionic fibers for the rest of the lumbar sacral ganglia run caudally and distally in the trunk. The ganglia of the lumbar trunk generally lie on the corresponding vertebrae, the second ganglion being the most consistent. The branches of the lumbar trunk include the gray rami communicantes, the lumbar splanchnic nerves, and the visceral branches of the celiac plexus. The celiac ganglion may be 2

cm in diameter and superficially resembles a lymph node. It usually resides at the level of the first lumbar vertebra. The aorticorenal and superior mesenteric ganglia may be attached to or detached from the celiac ganglion. The roots of these ganglia are splanchnic nerves. Postganglionic fibers arising in the celiac ganglion form an extensive plexus of nerves, which in general follow the branches of the abdominal aorta. some of these nerves converge and meet at the bifurcation of the aorta and continue with the right and left hypogastric nerves.

ADRENAL

The adrenal is composed of two primary elements; the adrenal cortex constitutes a much greater segment of the adrenal gland than does the medulla. The suprarenal or adrenal glands weigh 7 to 12 gm and are 2.5 to 3.0 cm in length (Fig. 1–10). They reside on the upper antero-

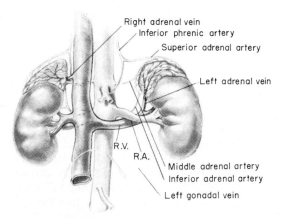

Right adrenal vein
Inferior phrenic artery
Superior adrenal artery
Left adrenal vein
R.V.
R.A.
Middle adrenal artery
Inferior adrenal artery
Left gonadal vein

Figure 1–10. Right and left adrenals with adrenal veins.

medial surface of the kidney within Gerota's fascia. The right adrenal gland tends to be shaped somewhat like a pyramid, while the left one is usually more flattened, with a crescent shape because of extensive contact with the left kidney. Embryologically, the adrenal glands develop behind the peritoneum, with the cortex being a derivative of the coelomic epithelium and the medulla arising from the same cells that give rise to the sympathetic ganglia—neural crest cells. Because of the separate embryologic derivation of the kidney, the adrenal gland is usually present in patients with renal agenesis. In addition, with ectopic kidneys, the adrenal gland may be slightly lower but generally stays in its approximate normal position.

Posteriorly, the right adrenal gland rests against the diaphragm (Fig. 1–3). Anteriorly, it is crossed by the posterior layer of the coronary ligament from the liver to the diaphragm. The lower part of the right adrenal gland is covered by inferior vena cava and peritoneum. The left adrenal gland is only partially covered by peritoneum. The upper half of the left adrenal gland is in contact with peritoneum, and the lower part is covered by the pancreas.

The arterial supply is diffuse and comes from three sources. The superior branches arise from the inferior phrenic artery. The middle adrenal branches come from the aorta, and the inferior branches arise from the renal artery. Adrenal veins are more consistent (Fig. 1–10); the right adrenal vein rises directly from the vena cava, and the left adrenal vein arises from the left renal vein. The lymphatic drainage includes the right or left lumbar nodes, which then drain into the cisterna chyli. There may be a few perforating branches into low thoracic nodes. The innervation of the adrenal comes from the lower end splanchnic nerves and from the celiac plexus, which enter posteriorly and connect with the medulla.

References

Marshall, F. F., and Powell, K. C.: Lymphadenectomy for renal cell carcinoma: anatomical and therapeutic considerations. J. Urol., *128*:677, 1982.
Notkovitch, H.: Variations of the testicular and ovarian arteries in relation to the renal pedicle. Surg. Gynecol. Obstet., *103*:487, 1956.
Parker, A. E.: Studies on the main posterior lymph channels of the abdomen and their connections with the lymphatics of the genitourinary system. Am. J. Anat., *56*:409, 1935.
Pick, J. W., and Anson, B. J.: The renal vascular pedicle. An anatomical study of 430 body halves. J. Urol., *44*:411, 1940.
Reis, R. H., and Esenther, G.: Variations in the pattern of renal vessels and their relation to the type of posterior vena cava in man. Am. J. Anat., *104*:295, 1959.

General References

Anson, B. J., and McVay, C. B.: Surgical Anatomy. Vol. I. 5th ed. Philadelphia, W. B. Saunders Co., 1971.
Hollinshead, W. H.: Anatomy for Surgeons. Vol. 2. 2nd ed. Chapters 10 and 11. The Thorax, Abdomen, and Pelvis. New York, Harper & Row, 1971.
Hollinshead, W. H.: Textbook of Anatomy. 3rd ed. New York, Harper & Row, 1974.
Warwick, R., and Williams, P. L.: Gray's Anatomy. 36th ed. Philadelphia, W. B. Saunders Co., 1980.

Anatomy of the Upper Urinary Tract

CARL A. OLSSON, M.D.

RENAL ANATOMY

The kidneys are paired solid organs situated on each side of the midline in the retroperitoneal space. Each kidney is oval, although thicker and rounder at its upper pole. The size and weight of the kidneys are generally proportional to body dimensions. In the newborn, the two kidneys constitute 1/80 of total body weight, whereas in the adult the proportion of both kidneys to total body weight is 1/240. Thus, in the adult male the weight of each kidney averages about 150 gm, and in the adult female the average weight of each kidney is 135 gm. The kidneys measure approximately 12 × 7 cm, with a thickness of approximately 3 cm. The left kidney is usually longer and narrower than the right.

The lateral border of each kidney is convex, while the medial border is S-shaped (convex at each pole and concave between the poles) (Fig. 1–11). This concave region of the medial border is termed the renal hilum and is, in effect, a vertical fissure in the medial renal border through which the renal vessels, the nerves, the lymphatics, and a portion of the renal pelvis traverse. The hilum of the kidney leads into a central cavity called the renal sinus. This cavity expands radially within the renal substance and, at its innermost aspect, is studded with conelike projections, termed the renal papillae. These projections cannot be seen during surgical dissections, since each papillary projection is encompassed by smooth muscular sleeves (calyces) leading to the renal pelvis. Within the renal sinus, the renal pelvis divides into two or three branches termed the major calyces, which, in turn, divide into several shorter minor calyces that expand distally to encompass one or two renal papillae. The necks of the renal calyces are often termed by the clinician the infundibula of the renal pelvis. Outside the hilum, the renal pelvis tapers abruptly to merge imperceptibly with the ureter.

Numerous variations of calyceal and pelvic anatomy are possible. In some instances the renal pelvis may lie entirely within the renal sinus, whereas in other circumstances the caly-ceal branches are sufficiently long that the entire pelvis is extrarenal (Fig. 1–12). These normal variations must be considered by the clinician when interpreting urographic studies. It should also be realized that there is a tendency for variations in renal pelvic and calyceal anatomy to be symmetric bilaterally, so that greater clinical suspicion is warranted in instances in which a unilateral variant is found (Fig. 1–13).

Despite the foregoing variations, the inter-relationship of hilar structures remains relatively constant, with the renal vein situated anteriorly and the renal pelvis posteriorly. The main renal artery occupies a position in between but gives off major anterior and posterior divisional branches that flank the upper portion of the renal pelvis.

With anomalies of incomplete ascent or

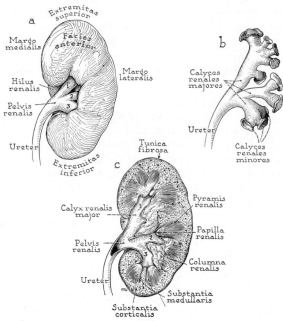

Figure 1–11. Kidney and ureter: external and internal structure. *a,* The kidney, renal pelvis, and proximal portion of the ureter; anterior surface. *b,* The renal pelvis and calices. *c,* The structure of the kidney, seen in section. The major calices are numbered to correspond with the enumeration in *a.* (From McVay; C.: Anson & McVay Surgical Anatomy. 6th ed. Philadelphia, W. B. Saunders Co, 1984.)

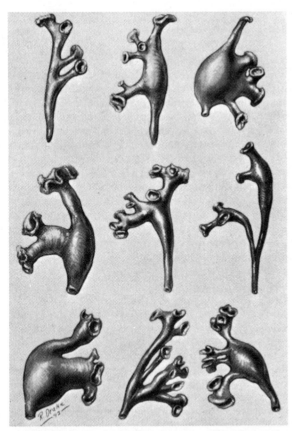

Figure 1–12. Three-dimensional drawing illustrating few of many variations in contour of normal renal pelvis (after Hauch). (From Kelly, H. A., and Burnam, C. F.: Diseases of the Kidneys, Ureters and Bladder, With Special Reference to the Diseases in Women. New York, D. Appleton and Company, 1914.)

rotation of the kidney, the entire anatomy of the renal sinus may be significantly altered such that these anatomic relations no longer pertain. In such instances the entire renal sinus may be effaced anteriorly, and the relationship between the resultant extrarenal calyces and the renal vasculature is highly variable.

The kidney is covered by a fibroelastic membranous capsule that extends within the renal sinus, merging with the expanded ends of the renal calyces as they encompass the papillae. This fibroelastic membrane is connected to the renal parenchyma by delicate strands of connective tissue and capillaries, such that it may be easily stripped from the renal surface except when scarring has resulted from renal disease. The strength of the renal capsule is of considerable significance. This resilient membrane acts as a barrier to separate intrarenal from extrarenal disease processes (abscess, hemorrhage); furthermore, it is the structure that allows the surgeon to suture the otherwise friable renal parenchyma.

The renal parenchyma may be divided into an internal medullary and an external cortical substance (Figs. 1–11 and 1–14). The medulla is composed of 8 to 18 striated cones, called the renal pyramids. These pyramids are arranged with their bases directed toward the periphery, while their apices, known as the renal papillae, are directed into the lumina of the minor calyces within the renal sinus. The striated appearance of the cut section of the renal pyramids results from the parallel linear arrangement of renal tubules in the medulla (ascending and descending loops of Henle and collecting ducts). The renal cortex is more granular than striated in appearance. It constitutes the portion of kidney between the bases of the pyramids and the renal capsule as well as occupying the spaces between adjacent pyramids. Tongues of cortical tissue extending between adjacent pyramids are known as the renal columns (of Bertin). When there is a large aggregation of such cortical tissue in this location (so-called hypertrophic renal column), an infundibular or calyceal distortion, similar to that caused by a space-occupying lesion, may be seen on urographic examination.

A detailed description of the microanatomy of the kidney is beyond the scope of this section.

Figure 1–13. Three-dimensional drawing illustrating tendency to symmetry of renal pelves in same individual (after Hauch). (From Kelly, H. A., and Burnam, C. F.: Diseases of the Kidneys, Ureters and Bladder, With Special Reference to the Diseases in Women. New York, D. Appleton and Company, 1914.)

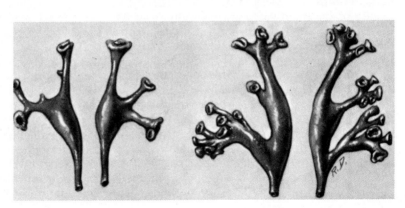

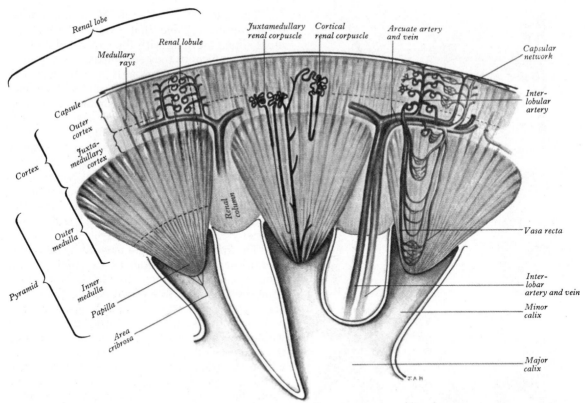

Figure 1–14. A diagram illustrating the major structures in the kidney cortex and medulla (left), the position of cortical and juxtamedullary nephrons (middle), and the major blood vessels (right). (From Williams, P. L., and Warwick, R. (Eds.): Gray's Anatomy. 36th ed. Philadelphia, W. B. Saunders Co., 1980.)

The reader is referred to any of a number of standard texts as well as to Figure 1–15, which reviews the renal microstructure in diagrammatic fashion.

Renal Arteries

Variations in the renal vasculature are very common and usually so complex that the standard concept of a simple renal pedicle is erroneous in most instances (Fig. 1–16). The complexity of the renal vasculature results from its development in a richly plexiform fashion from numerous sources in embryonic life, such that a variety of persistent postnatal transitional channels are frequently found. Most commonly (in about 70 per cent of individuals), there are single left and right renal arteries arising from the aorta. The origin of the right renal artery is somewhat higher than that of the left. Before reaching the kidney, each renal artery gives off one or more inferior adrenal arteries as well as smaller, unnamed branches supplying the perinephric tissue, renal capsule, renal pelvis, and proximal ureter (Fig. 1–16). Accessory renal arteries may be found in approximately 30 per cent of individuals. These arteries usually arise from the aorta above or below the main renal artery and run a course parallel with it to the renal hilum. Often, however, accessory arteries are found that directly enter the lower or, more commonly, the upper renal pole. On occasion, particularly in the case of errors in complete ascent (ectopic kidneys), accessory vessels may arise from the celiac axis or superior mesenteric or common iliac arteries. When there are accessory renal arteries to the lower pole of the kidney, they often cross the collecting system of the kidney at the level of the ureteropelvic junction. In this location, they have been implicated as a cause of congenital ureteropelvic junction obstruction. This etiologic relationship is far from clear in all cases, as accessory vessels in this location are often found in the absence of any hydronephrosis. Furthermore, microdissection of the ureteropelvic junction allegedly obstructed by these aberrant vessels often demonstrates intrinsic abnormalities of the smooth musculature in the region.

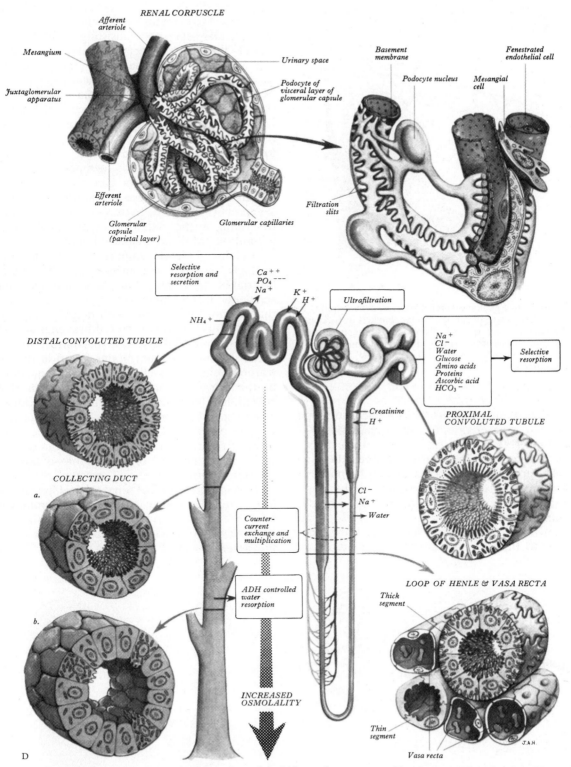

Figure 1–15. Diagrammatic representation of portions of the kidney microanatomy with reference to functional significance of each. (From Williams, P. L., and Warwick, R. (Eds.): Gray's Anatomy. 36th ed. Philadelphia, W. B. Saunders Co., 1980.)

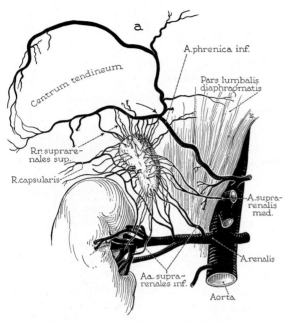

Figure 1–16. Renal and adrenal arteries, demonstrating the plexus-like arrangement of vascular channels distributed to the renal capsule, adrenal, diaphragm, perinephric tissues, and (not shown) ureter. (From McVay, C.: Anson & McVay Surgical Anatomy. 6th ed. Philadelphia, W. B. Saunders Co., 1984.)

The main renal arteries on each side separate into a larger anterior and a smaller posterior division (Fig. 1–17). As mentioned previously, the anterior division courses between the renal pelvis and the renal vein, whereas the posterior division courses posteriorly behind the upper portion of the renal pelvis or superior infundibulum. Primary branches of each division are known as segmental arteries, distributing blood flow to the various vascular segments of the kidney. Various classifications are used to describe the division of the kidney into vascular segments. Most authorities accept a division into five vascular segments, consisting of the following: (1) the apical segment, including the medial side and anterior portion of the upper pole; (2) the upper anterior division, occupying the remaining portion of the upper pole as well as the superior aspect of the anterior central region; (3) the middle anterior division, comprising the remainder of the anterior central region; (4) the lower division, consisting of the entire lower pole; and (5) the posterior segment, occupying the whole of the posterior aspect of the central region of kidney between the apical and lower segments (Fig. 1–18). Systems of nomenclature describing further subdivisions of vascular segmentation are of little clinical import.

There are many important issues for the urologic surgeon to consider regarding renal arterial blood supply. First, the various vascular segments of the kidney are supplied by arteries that do not interconnect with neighboring segments. Thus, the renal arterial branches should be considered end-arteries, in contrast to the extensive intercommunications found in the intrarenal veins. The lack of collateral connections in the intrarenal arterial supply is such that cessation of blood flow to a portion of the kidney results in infarction of that vascular segment. On the other hand, the rich capillary network distributed around the renal capsule can deliver a significant amount of arterial blood flow to the outer cortical glomeruli, particularly in situations in which gradual renal arterial narrowing has occurred, as when arteriosclerosis impinges upon the renal arterial lumen. Second, there is a relatively avascular line of cleavage between the anterior and the posterior portions of the

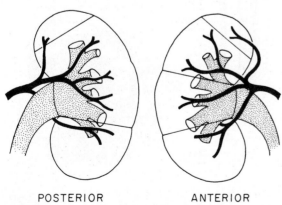

Figure 1–17. Segmental distribution of the renal arterial supply. Anterior and posterior branches are shown separately. (After Graves.)

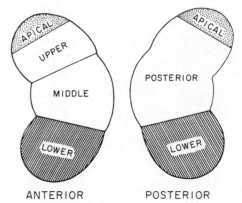

Figure 1–18. Segments of the left kidney as seen from anterior and posterior planes. (After Graves.)

kidney. This cleavage plane originates in the posterolateral border of the kidney, approximately one third of the distance between the posterior and anterior surfaces. A plane radiating centrally from this line toward the renal pelvis is unlikely to traverse major intrarenal arterial branches. It should be emphasized, however, that the intrarenal arterial supply to both renal poles may be damaged by extending an incision in this so-called avascular plane to either of the renal poles. Furthermore, the urologic surgeon should be aware of the safest method whereby he can incise the renal parenchyma so as to secure an extended pyelotomy approach (as advocated by Gil-Vernet). This incision is best conducted along the lower border of the renal pelvis posteriorly into the inferior infundibulum, as this is a region in which the surgeon is least likely to produce any significant damage to intrarenal blood supply (Fig. 1–19). A final point of clinical significance regarding the intrarenal vasculature is the relationship of renal arteries and veins as they cross the upper portion of the renal pelvis or the superior infundibulum. Such anatomic variations may be misinterpreted as renal pelvic filling defects during intravenous or retrograde urographic examinations. These are rarely of any clinical import, except that they must be differentiated from other radiolucent filling defects affecting the collecting system. Such differentiation can be easily made by digital subtraction or standard angiographic examination. Obstruction of the

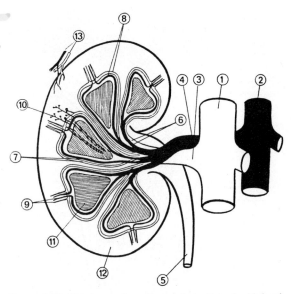

Figure 1–20. Diagram of renal vascularization. 1, Abdominal aorta; 2, inferior vena cava; 3, renal artery; 4, renal vein; 5, ureter; 6, main branches of the renal artery; 7, interlobar arteries and veins; 8, arcuate artery and vein; 9, interlobular artery and vein; 10, afferent arterioles; 11, malpighian pyramids; 12, renal cortex; 13, perforating capsular vessels. (From Hamburger, J., et al. (Eds.): Nephrology. New York, John Wiley & Sons, 1979.)

superior infundibulum has been ascribed to these crossing vessels in rare instances, but the existence of this condition and its described cause have been questioned by some.

The branching of segmental arteries within the kidney is relatively constant (Figs. 1–20 and 1–21). The initial branches of the segmental vessels constitute lobar arteries, usually distributed one to each pyramid. These again divide into two or three interlobar arteries that traverse between the renal pyramids toward the renal cortex. At the corticomedullary junction of the kidney, the interlobar arteries give rise to arcuate vessels, which, as their name implies, arch over the bases of the pyramids. Each of the arcuate arteries gives rise to a series of interlobular arteries. The termination of the arcuate artery constitutes an additional interlobular vessel that does not interconnect with other similar arcuate arteries. The interlobular arteries usually pursue a straight course toward the renal cortex, with some terminal twigs passing through the renal capsule to anastomose with the renal capsular plexus of vessels receiving blood supply from other nonrenal sources (adrenal, phrenic, and gonadal arteries). The major branches of the interlobular arteries are the afferent glomerular arterioles that usually are distributed to one or more glomeruli. After

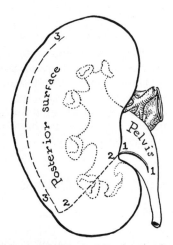

Figure 1–19. Most bloodless incision for opening the kidney pelvis and kidney substance.

1–1 indicates pyelotomy incision; this can be carried obliquely through renal parenchyma as shown in 2–2, thus opening the lower calices; continued incision along 3–3 opens the entire pelvis. (After Kelly, Burnam.) (From McVay, C.: Anson & McVay Surgical Anatomy. 6th ed. Philadelphia, W. B. Saunders Co., 1984.)

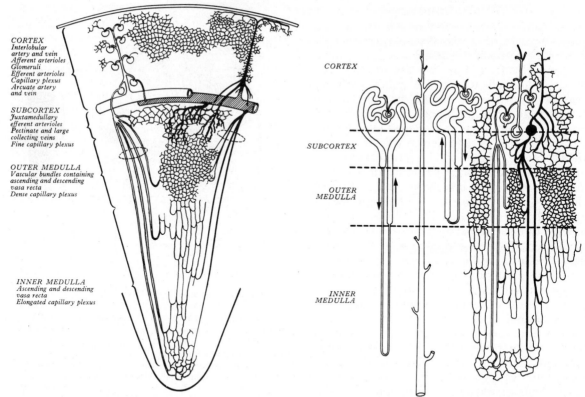

Figure 1–21. *A,* A diagram of the basic arrangements of the blood vessels in the mammalian kidney. Arteries—black outlines; capillaries—single black lines; veins—cross-hatched or full black. Note the variations in the pattern of the meshes in the capillary networks. *B,* A diagram to illustrate the arrangement of the tubules (left) and blood vessels (right) in various structural zones of the kidney. Note the variations in the pattern of the tubules with either long or short medullary loops; tubules of intermediate length also occur. Compare the different structural and functional segments of the tubules that occur together in the cortical, subcortical, and outer and inner medullary zones, with their related vascular patterns. Arteries—black outlines; capillaries—single black lines; veins—full black. (From Fourman, J., and Moffat, D. B.: The Blood Vessels of the Kidney. Oxford, Blackwell Scientific Publications, 1971.)

passing through the capillary network in the glomerulus, an efferent glomerular arteriole arises. In most regions of the renal cortex, these arterioles divide to form a peritubular capillary plexus running among the proximal and distal convoluted tubules of the kidney. This capillary plexus emerges at its venous end and drains into interlobular veins that accompany the course of the interlobular arteries.

The blood supply to the kidney medulla is derived from the vasa recta, a few of which arise from the arcuate or interlobar arteries, with the majority arising from the efferent arterioles of juxtamedullary glomeruli. These straight branches, as their name implies, descend in a straight course into the renal medulla, contributing side branches to a capillary plexus closely applied to the descending and ascending limbs of Henle's loop as well as to the collecting tubules. The venous end of this capillary plexus converges to form ascending vasa recta that drain into intralobular or intra-arcuate veins. The parallel relationship of the descending and ascending vasa recta with themselves and with the duct system results in the anatomic basis for a countercurrent exchange mechanism that is important in renal physiology.

Renal Venous Drainage

The interlobular veins drain into arcuate veins, which, unlike their arterial counterparts, freely interconnect with neighboring arcuate venous structures. Arcuate veins drain into interlobar veins, paralleling the course of the arteries of the same name, and converge into the major renal branches, finally forming the renal vein. Immediately beneath the renal capsule is a stellate plexus of venous capillaries that serve

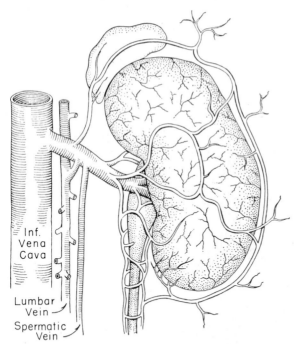

Inf.
Vena
Cava

Lumbar
Vein

Spermatic
Vein

Figure 1–22. The venous anastomosis of the perinephric area and renal surface with the ureteral plexus, showing the lumbar vein with its many branches—an important potential source of bleeding during renal surgery. (After Albarran.)

as the origin of some of the interlobular veins (Fig. 1–22). This capsular plexus serves as an additional means by which renal venous supply may be drained, particularly from the outer renal cortex, to vessels freely interconnecting with the inferior phrenic, adrenal, gonadal, and ureteral veins.

The renal veins, rather than representing single vascular channels, should be considered as parts of a richly interconnecting network of vascular tributaries from various structures, ultimately draining into the inferior vena cava (Fig. 1–23). The right renal vein is short and enters the cava directly, without receiving many tributaries. When a branch vessel does enter the right renal vein, it is usually on its inferior border and represents aberrant drainage from the right gonadal vein. The longer left renal vein, on the other hand, regularly receives branches from the inferior phrenic and adrenal veins on its superior border and from the gonadal vein and second or third lumbar vein on its inferior border. The right renal vein is usually single, although two (and, rarely, three) veins of equal diameter often course from the right renal hilum. On the left side, in contrast, there is frequently a more complicated arrangement known as the circumaortic venous plexus (Figs. 1–23 [g–l] to 1–25). Here again, there is usually

a single trunk that courses anterior to the aorta to drain into the vena cava; however, behind the aorta there may be a set of venous channels of varying size, freely communicating with lumbar veins (particularly the left ascending lumbar vein), the hemiazygous system, and smaller veins draining the prevertebral plexus before reaching the vena cava posteriorly. The lumbar connections of the left renal vein, constituting a retroaortic portion of the circumaortic venous ring, assume widely variable patterns. There is often a large single lumbar connection that may pierce the psoas muscle after connecting with the hemiazygous system in its course to the vena cava.

The clinical implications of the renal venous anatomy are obvious. Tumor extension into the vena cava is much more commonly seen on the right side, owing to the shorter length of the right renal vein. Although varicose dilatation of the left spermatic vein may represent a common anatomic variant, when this condition appears de novo on either side in adult life, one should be wary of renal venous or caval obstruction (such as by tumor). The size and length of the left renal vein make it the most common of the four major vascular tributaries of the kidneys to be afflicted by penetrating injuries of the renal pedicle. Because of extensive communicating vessels on the left side, renal vein thrombosis or ligation is more readily tolerated by the left kidney than by the right. If, in the course of surgical procedures, the left renal vein must be sacrificed, the extensive circumaortic venous channels existing on the left, in addition to the pericapsular drainage into diaphragmatic, adrenal, lumbar, and gonadal veins, will result in sufficient venous effluent to preserve the functional status of the kidney in 85 per cent of cases or more. Finally, urologists should be constantly aware of the circumaortic venous plexus when carrying out left nephrectomy, since the accidental avulsion of lumbar tributaries may be a prominent source of blood loss.

Lymphatic Drainage of the Kidney

There are three plexuses of lymphatic vessels draining the kidney and its surrounding structures. An extensive plexus originating in the substance of the kidney courses between the renal tubules to drain into four or five large trunks that emerge at the renal hilum, follow the course of the renal vein, and end by draining into the lateral aortic nodes. A subcapsular plexus drains the tissue immediately beneath

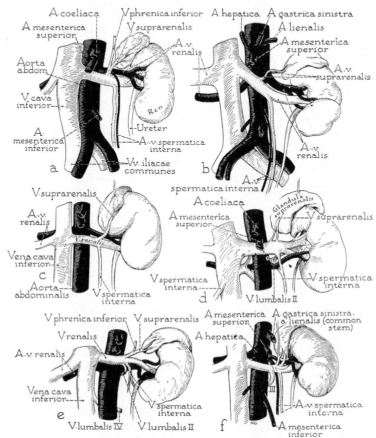

Figure 1–23. Common variations in the renal blood supply. Selected examples from a study of 33 consecutive laboratory specimens.

a, The most frequent arrangement of renal tributaries, in which the inferior phrenic and suprarenal veins (combined in a common vessel) and the internal spermatic vein enter the left renal; and in which the vessel that terminates on the caudal (inferior) border of the transversely coursing renal vein is situated lateral to the point at which the confluent stem enters on the cranial (superior) border. The internal spermatic artery is unusual in accompanying the renal vessel in the medial half of the pedicle. *b,* The suprarenal vein enters the renal independently, and the left internal spermatic artery arises at the usual level. In the presence of these common features a rare arterial variation occurs in which the three vessels regularly derived from a celiac axis take origin independently from the aorta. *c,* The regular tributaries enter the renal vein opposite each other. *d,* The suprarenal and internal spermatic veins are bifid; the latter sends its divergent channels into the renal vein on superficial level and into the second lumbar vein on deep level. The renal artery courses between the arms of the Y-shaped division. *e,* The second left lumbar vein ends independently in the renal, but the fourth lumbar crosses to the opposite side to become a caval tributary. *f,* The third left lumbar vein ends in the renal; the suprarenal vein is double, one of the pair being confluent with the inferior phrenic. On the arterial side the left gastric and splenic arteries arise from a common aortic stem, while the hepatic (in the absence of a celiac source) leaves the aorta independently. An accessory renal artery arises as a common stem with the internal spermatic, both becoming constituents of the renal pedicle. (Legend continues on opposite page.)

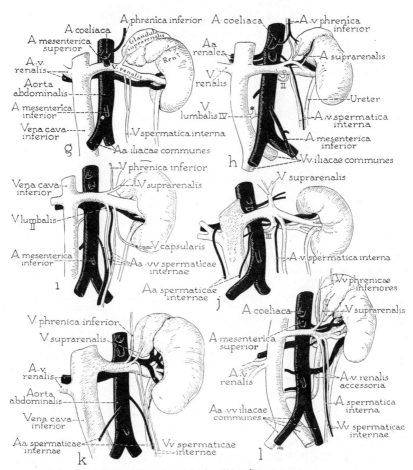

Figure 1–23. Common variations in the renal blood supply *(continued).*

g, Bifurcation of the internal spermatic vein, the separate channels entering the renal lateral to the point of termination of the suprarenal vein. *h,* The left renal vein divides. An internal spermatic artery of high origin passes through the hiatus thus formed, to become a constituent of the renal pedicle. The cranial element of the divided vein receives two suprarenal tributaries, one of which is confluent with the inferior phrenic vein, while the caudal division receives a large second lumbar and an internal spermatic vein. One of the lower lumbar veins receives lesser tributaries from prevertebral level (at*). *i,* On its caudal margin the left renal vein receives the divisions of a *bifid* internal spermatic (the lateral one of the pair being a common tributary with a capsular vessel) and the second lumbar vein. The spermatic artery is also double in the upper portion; the cranial one of the pair, being renal in origin, emerges from the pedicle. *j,* Doubling of the left renal vein through the lateral half of its course; the superficial limb receives the visceral tributaries (suprarenal and internal spermatic), the deep limb receives the parietal tributary (third lumbar vein). The left internal spermatic artery, after a short transverse course as a constituent of the renal pedicle, hooks around the Y-shaped confluens of the renal limbs to descend vertically with the corresponding vein. On the right side an internal spermatic artery of aortic origin gives rise to a lumbar vessel; the other arising from the renal, arches over the renal vein. *k,* One of a pair of internal spermatic veins enters the left renal vein independently; the other forms a common channel with the suprarenal. *l,* One of a pair of inferior phrenic veins joins the suprarenal in the customary way; the other courses through the gland before establishing connection with the suprarenal drainage. Caudally the tributaries are elements of, or vessels related to, an elongate type of so-called circumaortic venous ring. The postaortic limb of the "ring" (serving as an accessory renal vein and matching the course of a supernumerary artery) joins the preaortic limb just as the latter receives two internal spermatic veins and a single second lumbar vein. Additionally, an internal spermatic artery loops around the lumbar tributary. The pedicle is exceptionally long (10 cm) and consists of the following vessels: three renal arteries, two renal veins; three internal spermatic vessels (two veins, one artery); a lumbar vein; a combined vessel formed by meeting of the suprarenal and inferior phrenic veins. (From Anson and Kurth: Surg. Gynecol. Obstet. *100:*156, 1955. By permission of Surgery, Gynecology & Obstetrics.)

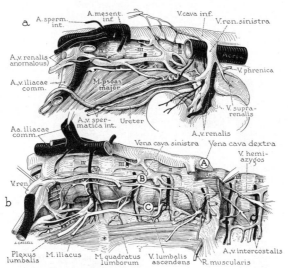

Figure 1–24. Renal venous communications, parietal (lumbar) and visceral.

In this specimen a pelvic kidney occurred on the right side, and a circumaortic venous ring and peristent caval channel on the left. From the aorta, in *a,* a segment has been excised to expose the postaortic limb of the ring. In *b* the left kidney and portions of both venous limbs have been removed; the psoas major muscle has been dissected away. In *a* the arrow points to an accessory loop of the left inferior vena cava, which passed ventral to the common iliac artery. In *b* the asterisk marks the crest of the ilium. *A,* Inferior vena cava; *B,* persistent left vena cava; *C,* ascending lumbar vein.

The ascending lumbar vein is connected with the left inferior vena cava by segmentally arranged lumbar veins. The latter are brought into connection with the azygos vein system through the intermediation of a trunk that passes behind the diaphragm. Here the three vertical venous channels occur: a large right inferior vena cava, a smaller left, and an intramuscular ascending vein. The ascending lumbar vein is in close proximity to the nerves of the lumbar plexus. The renal vein divides to form a circumaortic venous ring; the deep division receives the left inferior vena cava and communicates with the hemiazygos vein. (From Anson, Cauldwell, Pick, and Beaton: Surg. Gynecol. Obstet., *84*:313, 1947; J. Urol., *60*:714, 1948. By permission of Surgery, Gynecology & Obstetrics.)

the renal capsule. This plexus emerges within the renal hilum to join the same vessels emptying the substance of the kidney. A perinephric plexus of lymphatics communicates freely with the subcapsular plexus but drains independently to the lateral aortic nodes by multiple small channels. The lateral aortic nodes are distributed on each side of the great vessels and lie in front of the medial edge of the psoas major (Fig. 1–26). On the right side, these nodes are situated just lateral to the vena cava and anterior to this structure near the right renal vein. Efferent drainage from the lateral aortic lymph nodes is by means of a lumbar trunk on each side, both of which end in the cisterna chyli. However, smaller branches of efferent vessels can be found running behind and in front of the aorta, in a freely intercommunicating fashion, with crossover drainage fairly common, particularly from the right to the left sides.

The clinical significance of this pattern of lymphatic drainage is clear. The lateral aortic lymph nodes are those most likely to be involved by metastatic cancer from the renal parenchyma, its capsule, or its coverings. When such tumor spread is encountered by the surgeon, the free interconnections with the contralateral side and with superior efferent distributions are such that one is most likely dealing with systemic illness that is not amenable to local extirpative control. The renal lymphatics may play a role in harboring so-called passenger leukocytes that serve as a stimulus to rejection in renal homotransplantation. Finally, chyluria, or the leakage of lymphatic fluid into the urinary collecting system, is a documented entity both in filariasis and in situations in which a lymphatic varix has spontaneously discharged into the collecting system. In both circumstances, leakage from the major abdominal lymphatics may gain access to the urine, usually at the level of the renal calyx, and result in a moderately large amount of insensible protein loss.

Renal and Ureteral Nerve Supply

Subdivisions of the celiac plexus, called the renal plexuses, are collections of nerve cells usually situated behind the origin of each renal artery. Contributing to these nerve collections are branches from the aorticorenal ganglion, the celiac ganglia, the aortic plexus, and the lowest thoracic as well as first lumbar splanchnic nerve (Fig. 1–27). Efferent vessels from this plexus

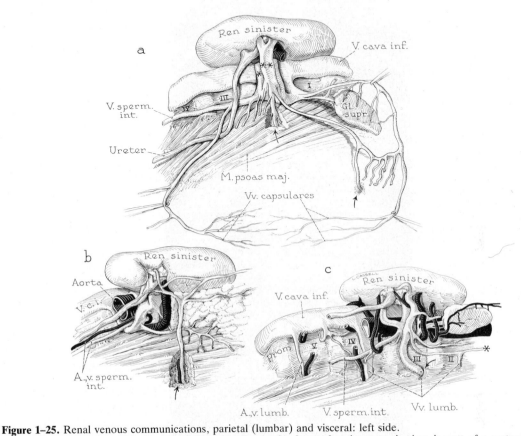

Figure 1–25. Renal venous communications, parietal (lumbar) and visceral: left side.

a, A specimen in which the bifid left renal vein, in the form of a circumaortic ring, is part of a system of venous return from parietal musculature, viscera, and retroperitoneal connective tissue. Here, and in *b* and *c,* the left kidney has been rolled medialward over the inferior vena cava. Division of the renal vein of the left side forms a preaortic segment (at*) and a retroaortic segment (at**) of a circumaortic ring (the aorta excised in this specimen). The capsular veins, in oval form, are peripheral to the "bed" of the kidney; they receive lumbar and intercostal tributaries (the latter indicated by arrow.) The lower capsular vein terminates in the internal spermatic. The upper one divides, one limb forming a common trunk with the internal spermatic vein; the other, after receiving the intercostal tributary, joins the second lumbar vein (at arrow, upper middle). *b,* A lumbar vein communicates with the left renal vein and receives capsular tributaries from the retroperitoneal connective tissue. The deep course of the second lumbar vein is demonstrated by dissecting away a portion of the psoas major muscle. *c,* Here the left renal vein is brought into communication with vessels from the thoracic, lumbar, and pelvic regions. The hemiazygos vein (at*), after receiving the second lumbar, joins the third lumbar (at the arrow); the combined trunk becomes continuous with the renal. The internal spermatic terminates in the left renal vein.(From Anson: Atlas of Human Anatomy. Philadelphia, W. B. Saunders Co., 1963.)

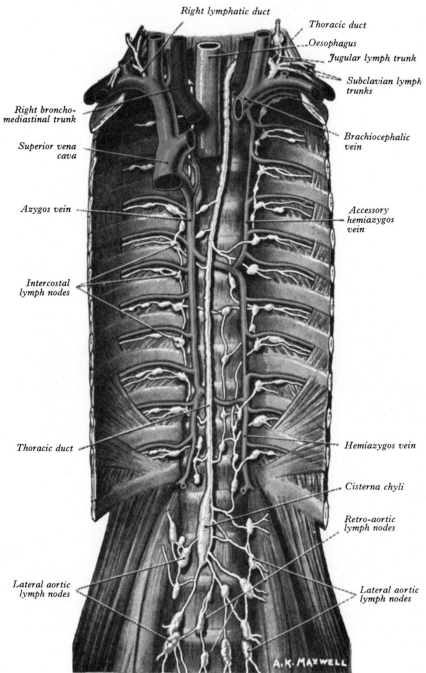

Figure 1–26. The lateral aortic lymph nodes demonstrating their intercommunications across the midline and drainage to the cisterna chyli. (From Williams, P. L., and Warwick, R. (Eds.): Gray's Anatomy. 36th ed. Philadelphia, W. B. Saunders Co., 1980.)

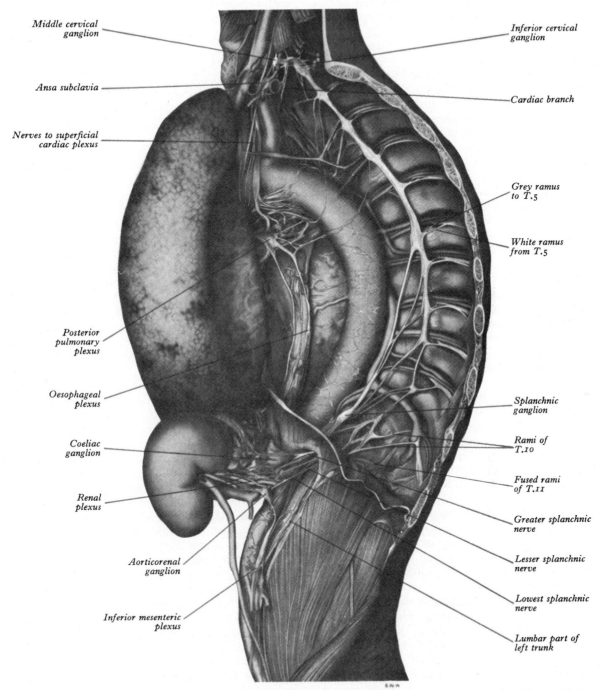

Figure 1–27. The thoracic and upper retroperitoneal sympathetic nerves. Note the position of the renal plexus and its association with celiac and aorticorenal ganglia. (From Williams, P. L., and Warwick, R. (Eds.): Gray's Anatomy. 36th ed. Philadelphia, W. B. Saunders Co., 1980.)

are continued into the kidney along the course of the renal arteries, supplying the vessels, glomerular structures, and tubules of the kidney, particularly in the region of the renal cortex. Autonomic afferent fibers course through the same pathway, some traveling with the sympathetic nerve distribution and some with the vagus nerve.

The full clinical import of renal innervation is poorly understood. Efferent fibers are thought to be predominantly vasomotor in nature. However, recent observations have demonstrated that acute unilateral renal denervation experiments result in diuresis and natriuresis without alterations in either glomerular filtration rate or renal plasma flow, suggesting that these nerves may affect nonvascular functions as well. The distribution of afferent sensory fibers with these autonomic nerves is such that renal pain is perceived in a vague fashion in the region of the costovertebral angle. In addition, however, somatic sensory nerve fibers from the groin and thigh, entering the spinal cord at the same level as the autonomic afferent fibers, result in the production of referred pain to these regions. Finally, the nausea, vomiting, and intestinal hypoperistalsis that are seen with renal pain are possibly due to some of the afferent sensory fibers traveling along the course of the vagus nerve.

The ureteric nerve plexus receives branches from the renal and aortic plexuses in its upper third, from the superior hypogastric plexus in its middle third, and from branches of the hypogastric nerve and inferior hypogastric plexus in its lower third. The function of these nerves is unknown except that they serve to conduct sensory afferent stimuli. Ureteral motility is thought to be triggered in the region of the renal calyx, although stimulation of the ureter at any point along its course will induce a peristaltic wave emanating from the point of stimulus, even if all the ureteral nerves are stripped away.

Since pain originating in the ureter is conducted along visceral afferent fibers in a fashion similar to that of the kidney, direct as well as referred pain is usually experienced when ureteral distention or inflammation occurs. The segments of spinal cord entered by these visceral afferent nerves are T11 to L2. Thus, pain referred from the ureter parallels the course of that from the kidney, to the regions of the groin, genitalia, and proximal thigh.

URETERAL ANATOMY

The renal pelvis tapers down into a muscular tube, the ureter, on each side. This tube extends through the retroperitoneum such that its peristaltic contractions can deliver urine from the kidney to the urinary bladder. The average ureter is about 30 cm in length and may be divided into approximately equal abdominal and pelvic portions. Each portion, in turn, may be further classified, somewhat artificially, into two divisions. The abdominal ureter consists of lumbar and iliac divisions, each approximating 8 cm in length, traversing the lumbar and iliac fossae, respectively. The pelvic ureter is divided into the longer parietal and shorter intravesical divisions.

The abdominal ureter assumes a vertical course downward and medially on the anterior surface of the psoas muscle, which separates it from the transverse processes (Fig. 1–28). As will be described later, the abdominal ureter is well encompassed within an extension of Gerota's fascial space. Unless the cleavage plane between the mesocolon or parietal peritoneum and the anterior leaf of Gerota's fascia has been well developed and dissected distally, the iliac abdominal and entire pelvic portions of ureter usually remain closely attached to the peritoneum when it is reflected anteriorly, rather than remaining adherent to the fascial structures overlying the posterior abdominal and pelvic musculature.

The above-mentioned anatomic relations should be borne in mind in a number of clinical circumstances. The medially directed course of the ureters inferiorly is such that so-called medial deviation of the ureters described in retroperitoneal fibrosis is often not substantially different from the normal ureteral course or, at least, variants thereof. It is only when the ureters become shifted medially well above the pelvic brim that a deviation from normal course becomes apparent. This normally assumed medial course brings the ureters into close proximity with the great vessels and their surrounding lymphatics such that lateral bowing of the ureters may be seen when the retroperitoneal lymph nodes are enlarged by neoplastic processes or when aortic aneurysmal dilatation exists. Because of the intimate relationship of the abdominal ureter to the psoas muscle, there may be alterations in the ureteral course due to hypertrophy of this structure in athletic individuals.

The pelvic ureter on each side is approximately 15 cm in length. The anatomy of the intramural division of the pelvic ureter will be described in the section on anatomy of the bladder. The longer parietal division of the pelvic ureter continues in its close relationship with the peritoneum, crossing the brim of the pelvis just lateral to the bifurcation of the com-

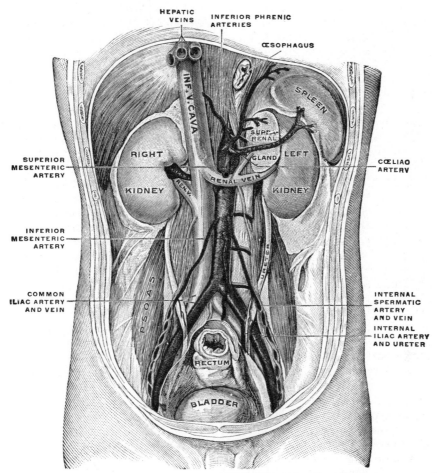

HEPATIC VEINS

INFERIOR PHRENIC ARTERIES

ŒSOPHAGUS

INF. V. CAVA

SPLEEN

SUPRA-RENAL

RIGHT

GLAND   LEFT

SUPERIOR MESENTERIC ARTERY

CŒLIAC ARTERY

KIDNEY   RENAL VEIN   KIDNEY

INFERIOR MESENTERIC ARTERY

COMMON ILIAC ARTERY AND VEIN

PSOAS

URETER

INTERNAL SPERMATIC ARTERY AND VEIN

INTERNAL ILIAC ARTERY AND URETER

RECTUM

BLADDER

Figure 1–28. Posterior abdominal wall after removal of the peritoneum, showing kidneys, ureters, and great vessels. (Corning.)

mon iliac arteries (Fig. 1–28). It descends posterolaterally between the hypogastric artery and the peritoneum and is separated by the hypogastric artery from the pelvic musculature and nerves. As it approaches the bladder base, the superior vesical artery crosses above the ureteral course, which then becomes medially directed once again (approximately at the level of the ischial spine) to reach the urinary bladder.

The ureter is composed of three layers easily detected on cross-sectional views: fibrous, muscular, and mucosal (Fig. 1–29). The fibrous layer is continuous with the renal capsule within the renal sinus and continues to merge imperceptibly with tissues surrounding the urinary bladder. The muscular layer is composed of circular and longitudinally arranged fibers varying in location and predominance depending upon the level of the collecting system. Circular fibers are predominant around the bases of the renal papillae; longitudinal fibers then become intermingled with the circular fibers along the

course of the renal pelvis and ureter; longitudinal fibers finally predominate in its intravesical portion. The inner mucosal layer is composed of transitional epithelium continuous with that of the urinary bladder and merges with a cuboidal lining covering the surface of the renal papillae. This mucosa is characterized by variously developed longitudinal folds that can become unfolded during ureteral dilatation. These longitudinal folds may be exaggerated in normal individuals as well as in patients with ureteritis, giving a striated appearance to the ureter on urographic examination.

The fact that the ureter and renal pelvis share the same mucosa with the urinary bladder is the anatomic basis explaining the relationship of urothelial cancers of the upper and lower urinary tract. Because of either distal seeding of tumor cells or the effect of similar carcinogenic stimuli on similar epithelia, approximately 50 per cent of patients with upper tract urothelial cancer develop bladder cancer; however, a

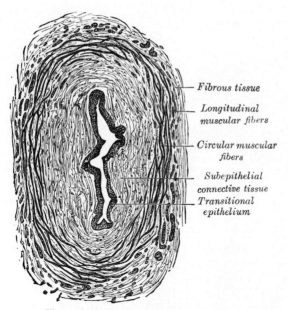

Fibrous tissue

Longitudinal muscular fibers

Circular muscular fibers

Subepithelial connective tissue
Transitional epithelium

Figure 1–29. Transverse section of ureter.

smaller number (3 per cent) of bladder cancer patients develop upper tract urothelial malignancy.

The ureter is not of uniform caliber, but rather displays three points of physiologic narrowing at: (1) the ureteropelvic junction, (2) the crossing of the iliac artery, and (3) the ureterovesical junction (Fig. 1–30). The internal diameter of the ureter tends to be smallest at the ureterovesical junction. These three narrow points correlate well with the areas prone to impaction of ureteral calculi. The fact that the intramural ureter is the narrowest region is important to the new field of ureteroscopic surgery. If this most narrow area can be dilated so as to admit the available instruments (No. 9 to 11 French), the rest of the ureteral path can usually be negotiated without difficulty. In the male with prostatic hypertrophy, there may be significant elevation of the bladder floor, such that the intramural ureter curves superiorly (hockey-stick sign in urographic examination), resulting in significant angulation between the parietal and intramural segments of the pelvic ureter. Such angulation constitutes another zone of ureteral narrowing in these individuals.

Ureteral Blood Supply

The arteries supplying the ureter arise from renal, abdominal aortic, gonadal, hypogastric, vesical, and uterine arterial branches (Fig.

1–31). Branches from the main renal artery or renosuprarenal plexus serve as a rich contribution to proximal ureteral and renal pelvic blood supply. Similarly, the numerous branches to the pelvic ureter from hypogastric, vesical, and uterine arterial sources result in a heavily vascularized region. The intermediate, or iliac abdominal, region of the ureter receives the fewest direct arterial contributions. However, there is a richly intercommunicating anastomotic network of smaller vessels surrounding the ureter throughout its length that ensures its nutrition and viability. Venous drainage of the ureter is multiform and tends to follow a pattern similar to that seen in arterial distribution.

Because of the richly intercommunicating plexus of arteries and veins surrounding the ureter, distention of these vessels can sometimes be detected on urographic examination (so-called ureteral notching). These convex indentations of ureteral caliber may result from ureteral vein dilatation (secondary to renal vein thrombosis) or from compensatory expansion of ureteral arteries (secondary to renal artery stenosis).

Final points of clinical concern regarding

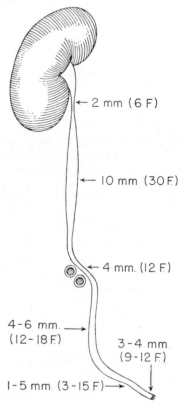

← 2 mm (6 F)

← 10 mm (30 F.)

← 4 mm. (12 F.)

4-6 mm. → (12-18 F.)

3-4 mm. (9-12 F.)

1-5 mm. (3-15 F.) →

Figure 1–30. The ureter, showing its variations of caliber. (After Eisendrath and Rolnick.)

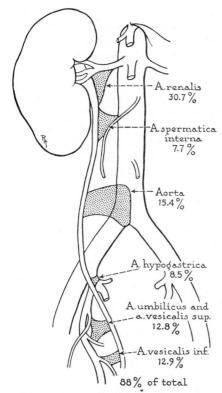

Figure 1–31. Ureteric arteries, schematic.
Sources of supply indicated, with percentage of vessels from each of the important contributory vessels, in 50 specimens.
The combined percentages cover 88 per cent of the vessels (remaining 12 per cent include vessels derived from the capsular, suprarenal, uterine and urethral arteries). (From McCormack and Anson: Quart. Bull., Northwestern Univ. M. School, 24:291–4, 1950)

ureteral blood supply consist of caveats to the surgeon. First, overzealous mobilization of the ureter and stripping of periureteral tissues should be avoided at all times, particularly in the iliac fossa, where the blood supply of the ureter is heavily dependent upon the longitudinal anastomotic network. Second, in harvesting kidneys for renal transplantation, one must take care not to skeletonize the main renal artery and never to sacrifice a lower polar vessel, because resultant ureteral complications related to devascularization will be significant.

Lymphatic Drainage of the Ureter

There is a freely interconnecting plexus of vessels draining the submucosa, muscularis, and adventitia of the ureter along its entire length. Various collecting vessels may be found from these plexuses. In the upper third of the ureter, the collecting vessels either intercommunicate with the four or five lymphatic trunks draining the kidney or drain directly to the lateral aortic lymph nodes. In the middle third of the ureter, the collecting vessels empty into the common iliac node chain. From the pelvic portion of the ureter, however, the lymphatic drainage merges with that of the urinary bladder to drain into the internal iliac lymph node group, outlying members of which include the presacral lymph nodes and the obturator nodes.

The clinical significance of ureteral lymphatic drainage consists entirely of an understanding of the lymphatic drainage of ureteral neoplasms. In the upper portion of the ureter, the drainage would be anticipated to affect the lateral aortic nodes; in the middle region of the ureter, the common iliac nodes may well be involved as a primary avenue for metastatic spread. In the pelvis, the hypogastric, obturator, and presacral lymph node groups might be anticipated to reflect tumor spread.

ANATOMIC RELATIONS OF THE KIDNEYS, THE URETERS, AND THEIR COVERINGS

The kidney and ureter are surrounded and protected by various fascial, muscular, and skeletal structures, an understanding of which is essential to the urologist's knowledge of the surgical approaches to these organs. They themselves are in juxtaposition to various other organs, relationships that are essential to the clinician's understanding of various disease processes affecting the kidney and ureter as well as the symptomatic presentations of these conditions.

Perirenal Fascia

Each kidney is surrounded by an envelope of retroperitoneal connective tissue (Fig. 1–32). This structure splits into a prerenal and postrenal leaf at the lateral border of the kidney to form the perirenal fascial space of Gerota, which encompasses the kidney and adrenal gland as well as an abundant amount of protective perirenal protective fatty tissue on both sides. There is usually a thin, indistinct layer of connective tissue subdividing Gerota's space into renal and adrenal compartments. Both the anterior and the posterior layers of Gerota's fascia probably continue across the midline. The posterior layer

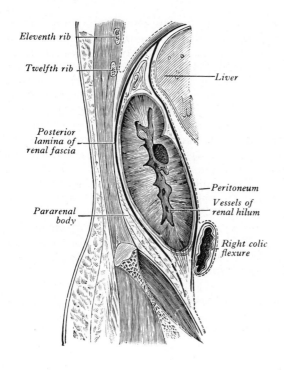

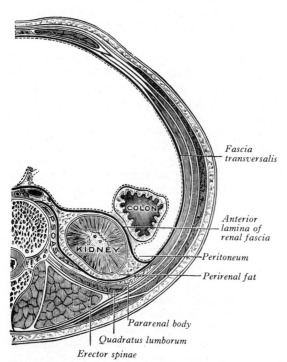

Figure 1–32. *A,* A sagittal section through the posterior abdominal wall showing the relations of the renal fascia of the right kidney. *B,* A transverse section, showing the relations of the renal fascia. (From Williams, P. L., and Warwick, R. (Eds.): Gray's Anatomy. 36th ed. Philadelphia, W. B. Saunders Co., 1980.)

extends across the midline behind the great vessels, whereas the anterior layer extends to the contralateral side anterior to these structures. Superiorly, the layers are reapproximated at the level of the diaphragm. Inferiorly, the leaflets of Gerota's fascia descend into the true pelvis, encompassing the ureter within its circumscribed compartment. On each side, the anterior layer of the perirenal fascia, toward its lateral extent, fuses with the parietal peritoneum in the region of Toldt's line.

The clinical significance of the fascial coverings of the kidney and ureter is obvious. Urinary extravasation, renal tumors, abscess, or hemorrhage that escapes beneath the kidney capsule or its collecting system are usually contained within Gerota's compartment. Neoplastic processes are usually confined to the region of the kidney, whereas fluid collections, such as blood, urine, or infectious fluid, may extend superiorly toward the diaphragm and inferiorly along the ureter. Such extensions do not usually cross the midline because there is often partial fusion between the fascial layers that encompass the great vessels and the vessels themselves. Abscesses in the perinephric tissues are similarly confined as blood and urine; however, destruction of Gerota's fascia may occur posteriorly, allowing extension of infection to the trunk musculature (Fig. 1–33).

In surgical approaches to the kidney, one can readily find a dissection plane between the mesocolon and the anterior leaf of Gerota's fascia by incising along the line of Toldt and reflecting the corresponding colon and its mesocolon (and adjacent posterior parietal peritoneum) anteriorly (Figs. 1–34 and 1–35). This maneuver may be utilized in either transabdominal or flank approaches so as to gain access to the major renal vasculature prior to carrying out dissection within Gerota's fascial compartment.

As mentioned previously, there is a substantial fat pad, known as the perirenal fat, contained within Gerota's fascia. This is more abundant at the borders of the kidney as well as posterior to this organ. The kidney and ureter move with respiration, protected by this fatty tissue, within the relatively stationary Gerota's fascial leaves. Outside Gerota's fascia is a layer of pararenal fat, again most abundant posteriorly, which is continuous with the extraperitoneal fatty plane of the anterolateral abdominal wall as well as with the extrapleural areoloadipose tissue above the edge of the diaphragm.

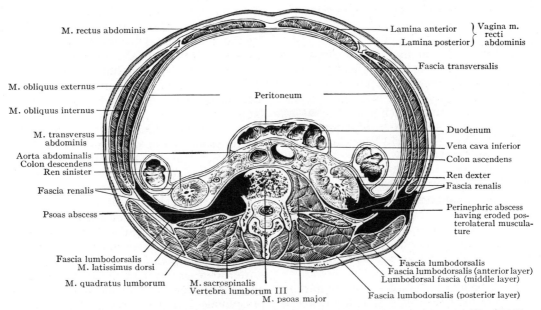

Figure 1–33. Cross section to show extension of iliolumbar abscesses: perinephric and psoas abscesses. (From McVay, C.: Anson & McVay Surgical Anatomy. 6th ed. Philadelphia, W. B. Saunders Co., 1984.)

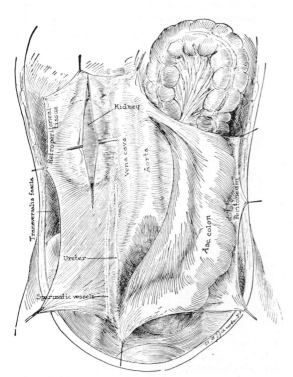

Figure 1–34. Peritoneum associated with ascending colon dissected free and displaced to expose the deeper stratum of subserous fascia associated with kidney and great vessels. (Tobin, courtesy of Anat. Record.)

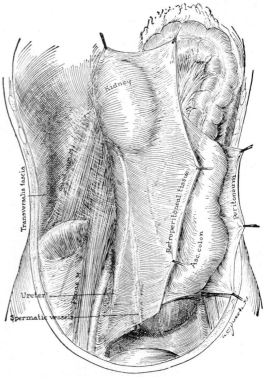

Figure 1–35. Deeper stratum of subserous fascia dissected free and displaced to expose the transversalis fascia. (Tobin, courtesy of Anat. Record.)

Muscular Coverings of the Kidney and Ureter

The kidneys lie in the lumbar fossae on each side (Figs. 1–36 to 1–38). This is a somewhat artificial space beginning just beneath the diaphragm and extending to the base of the sacrum and iliac crest on each side. The lateral margin of the lumbar fossa is the lateral edge of the quadratus lumborum muscle, which, along with the psoas major muscle, forms the floor of this cavity. The fascia overlying the quadratus lumborum muscle is the anterior sheath of the lumbodorsal fascia, and the fascia of the psoas muscle is continuous inferiorly with the fascia of the iliacus muscle. The roof of the fossa is constituted by the posterior parietal layer of the peritoneum as well as the mesocolon.

The lumbodorsal fascia is an important constituent of the posterolateral abdominal wall (Fig. 1–31). It consists of three divisions that fuse lateral to the sacrospinalis and quadratus lumborum muscles to form a broad aponeurosis, which serves as the origin of the transversus abdominal muscle. The anterior layer of lumbodorsal fascia is its least resistant component and arises from the anterior surface of the lumbar transverse processes and, as previously mentioned, courses anteriorly over the quadratus lumborum muscle. It is strengthened above by the lumbocostal ligament, which, in turn, gives rise to fibers of the diaphragm. The anterior layer meets the middle layer of fusion at the lateral margin of the quadratus lumborum. The middle layer attaches to the posterior surfaces and tips of the lumbar transverse processes, coursing behind the quadratus lumborum and in front of the sacrospinalis muscles. This layer fuses with the posterior layer of lumbodorsal fascia lateral to the sacrospinalis muscle. In its upper portion it is strengthened by the posterior lumbocostal ligament (which runs between the transverse processes of the first two lumbar vertebrae to the lowest rib). The lower margin of the lumbocostal ligament demarcates the posterior plane of pleural reflection. The posterior thick layer of the lumbodorsal fascia originates over the lumbar spines and the supraspinous ligaments and dorsally invests the sacrospinalis muscle. It is covered by the latissimus dorsi and the serratus posterior inferior muscles to which it gives origin.

The posterior abdominal musculature consists of superficial, middle, and deep groups. The deep muscles are constituted by the quadratus lumborum and psoas muscles. The quadratus lumborum is a quadrilateral muscular

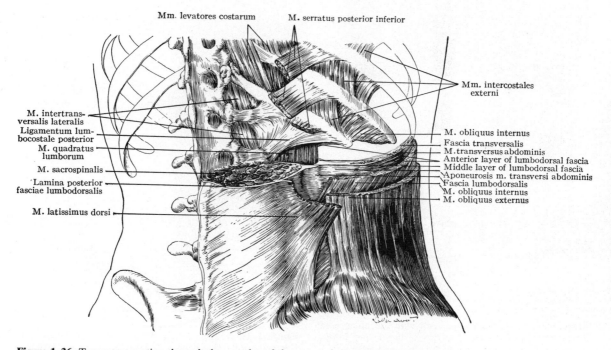

Figure 1–36. Transverse section through the muscles of the posterolateral abdominal wall.
Attention is called to the three layers of lumbodorsal fascia, which fuse at the lateral margin of the quadratus lumborum muscle to form the aponeurosis of the transversus abdominis muscle. (After Kelly, Burnam.) (From McVay, C.: Anson & McVay Surgical Anatomy. 6th ed. Philadelphia, W. B. Saunders Co., 1984.)

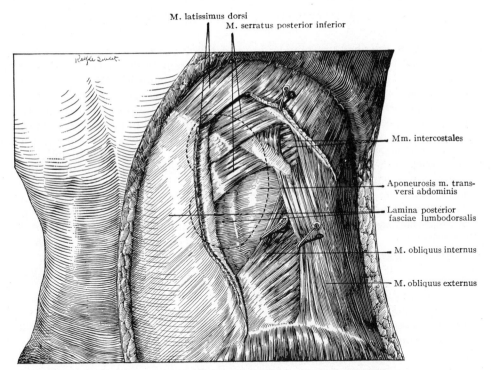

M. latissimus dorsi

M. serratus posterior inferior

Mm. intercostales

Aponeurosis m. transversi abdominis

Lamina posterior fasciae lumbodorsalis

M. obliquus internus

M. obliquus externus

Figure 1–37. Deeper structures of the posterolateral abdominal wall.
Part of the latissimus dorsi muscle has been removed to show the aponeurosis of the tranversus abdominis, which all posterolateral kidney incisions must traverse. (After Kelly, Burnam.) (From Anson, B. J., and McVay, C.: Surgical Anatomy. 5th ed. Philadelphia, W. B. Saunders Co., 1971.)

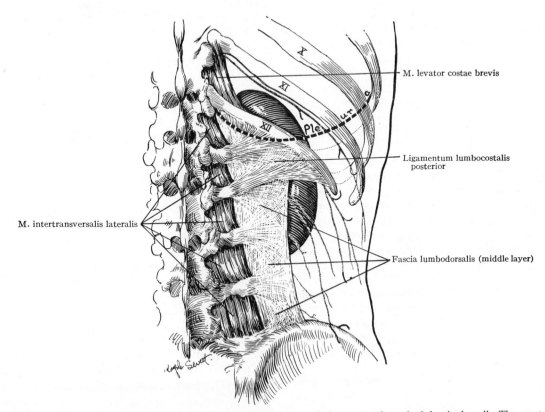

M. levator costae brevis

Ligamentum lumbocostalis posterior

M. intertransversalis lateralis

Fascia lumbodorsalis (middle layer)

Figure 1–38. Relations of the kidney with the deep structures of the posterolateral abdominal wall. The posterior lumbocostal ligament and its relations to the inferior pleural reflection are emphasized. (From McVay, C.: Anson & McVay Surgical Anatomy. 6th ed. Philadelphia, W. B. Saunders Co., 1984.)

structure arising from the iliac crest and ilio-lumbar ligament and, coursing superiorly, inserting on the twelfth rib. The kidney usually extends 1 to 3 cm beyond the lateral margin of this muscle. The psoas muscle receives fibers from the twelfth thoracic vertebra and all lumber vertebrae, gaining bulk as it descends to occupy the trough between the transverse processes and the bodies of the lumbar vertebrae. It tapers into a fusiform shape distally, courses over the pelvic brim, and terminates beneath the inguinal ligament as a tendinous structure entering the thigh and inserting into the lesser trochanter of the femur.

The middle muscular layer of the posterior abdominal wall consists of the sacrospinalis, internal oblique, and serratus posterior inferior muscles. The latter is a four-sided, thin, flat muscle arising from the lumbodorsal fascia and running laterally to insert on the lower four ribs. It forms the upper edge of the superior lumbar triangle and is covered externally by the latissimus dorsi muscle. The internal oblique muscle arises from the iliac crest and the lower portion of the lumbodorsal fascia. Its superior margin forms the lateral border of the superior lumbar triangle. The sacrospinalis muscle is an elongated structure occupying the compartment formed by the split dorsal and middle layers of lumbodorsal fascia. It lies in the groove along the spinous processes. The surgeon should be aware that the lateral and ventral branches of the last thoracic and first lumbar nerves traverse through the body of this muscle, so that, if it is cut at all, the incision should be situated in an oblique plane below and parallel to the twelfth rib.

The superficial layer of posterior abdominal musculature consists of the latissimus dorsi and the external oblique muscles. The latissimus muscle arises from the outer ridge of the posterior third of the iliac crest and from the lumbar and sacral spinous processes as well as the posterior leaf of the lumbodorsal fascia. The fibers of this muscle run upward and laterally to insert by a flat tendon into the bicipital groove of the humerus. This muscle can be cut with impunity, in the expectation that good healing will result. Its anterior border constitutes the posterior edge of Petit's triangle, which is based on the posterolateral portion of the iliac crest. The final muscle in the superficial portion of the posterior abdominal wall is the external oblique muscle, which arises from the ninth through eleventh ribs and courses downward and around the flank to insert in an aponeurosis that forms the anterior rectus sheath. The lateral margin of this muscle constitutes the anterior edge of Petit's triangle, the floor of which is the internal oblique aponeurosis.

The iliac fossa is much less complicated than the lumbar fossa. It delimits the region of the retroperitoneum between the lumbar fossa and the true pelvis. Its floor is formed by the iliacus and psoas muscles, and its roof is the posterior parietal peritoneum. The iliac fascia overlies the iliacus muscle and continues cephalad over the psoas muscle, medially attaches to the linea terminalis or pelvic brim, and anterolaterally fuses with the transversalis fascia. The iliac fossa is traversed by the iliac portion of the ureter, the iliac and gonadal vessels, and the ilioinguinal genitofemoral nerves (Fig. 1–39).

Renal Relations with Ribs, Pleura, and Spine

The kidneys are situated in oblique planes when viewed both anteroposteriorly and laterally. In the former circumstance, the rather bulky body of the psoas muscle causes the renal axis to tilt laterally at its caudal end, such that an imaginary line drawn through the midline of each kidney would intersect at approximately the level of the tenth thoracic vertebra (Fig. 1–40). In the latter circumstance, there is a slight anterior tilt of the caudal end of the kidney owing to its relationship with the spine and trunk musculature (Fig. 1–41).

The kidneys are located on a level from the twelfth thoracic to the third lumbar vertebrae. Some variations in this positioning are observed (Fig. 1–42). The right kidney is situated 1 to 2 cm lower than the left, probably because of interference with renal ascent by the bulk of the liver on the right. In general, the kidneys are situated lower in the female than in the male (by approximately one-half the height of a lumbar vertebra).

The reflection of the posterior costal pleura assumes a transverse plane at the level of the base of the twelfth thoracic vertebra below the origin of the twelfth rib (Fig. 1–43). Therefore, the twelfth rib, extending obliquely downward, crosses the pleural reflection at approximately three fingerbreadths lateral to the midline on each side. Stated in a different fashion, the proximal 4 cm of each twelfth rib is above the pleural reflection, whereas the remainder is usually below this plane. Because of the higher anatomic location of the left kidney, approximately one half of the left kidney and one third

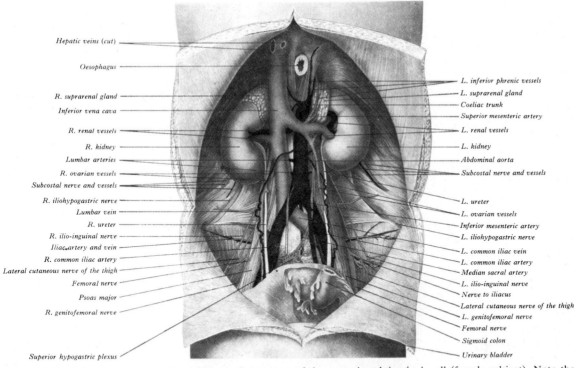

Hepatic veins (cut)
Oesophagus
R. suprarenal gland
Inferior vena cava
R. renal vessels
R. kidney
Lumbar arteries
R. ovarian vessels
Subcostal nerve and vessels
R. iliohypogastric nerve
Lumbar vein
R. ureter
R. ilio-inguinal nerve
Iliac artery and vein
R. common iliac artery
Lateral cutaneous nerve of the thigh
Femoral nerve
Psoas major
R. genitofemoral nerve
Superior hypogastric plexus

L. inferior phrenic vessels
L. suprarenal gland
Coeliac trunk
Superior mesenteric artery
L. renal vessels
L. kidney
Abdominal aorta
Subcostal nerve and vessels
L. ureter
L. ovarian vessels
Inferior mesenteric artery
L. iliohypogastric nerve
L. common iliac vein
L. common iliac artery
Median sacral artery
L. ilio-inguinal nerve
Nerve to iliacus
Lateral cutaneous nerve of the thigh
L. genitofemoral nerve
Femoral nerve
Sigmoid colon
Urinary bladder

Figure 1–39. A dissection to show the relations of structures of the posterior abdominal wall (female subject). Note the iliac fossa occupied by the iliacus and lower portion of psoas muscles. (From Williams, P. L., and Warwick, R. (Eds.): Gray's Anatomy. 36th ed. Philadelphia, W. B. Saunders Co., 1980.)

Figure 1–40. The anteroposterior surface projection of the kidneys and ureters, emphasizing the medial position of the kidneys, the renal axis, and the pleural reflection.

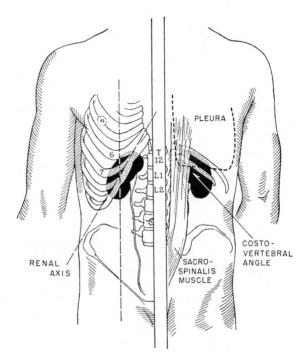

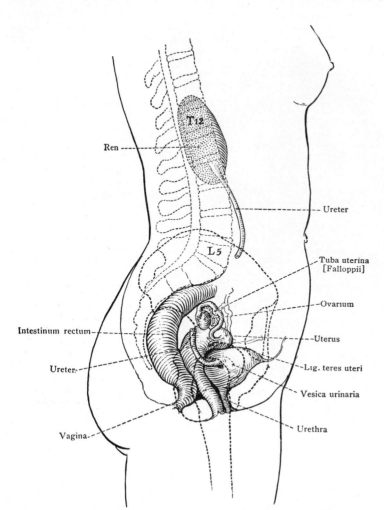

Ren

T12

Ureter

L5

Tuba uterina
[Falloppii]

Ovarium

Intestinum rectum

Uterus

Ureter

Lig. teres uteri

Vesica urinaria

Vagina

Urethra

Figure 1–41. Projection showing the oblique position of the kidney. Lateral view. (Eycleshymer and Jones.)

of the right kidney are above the pleural reflection and therefore separated from the diaphragm by only a single fascial plane. In fact, in some individuals, weakened portions of the diaphragm allow the perirenal fascia to come into direct contact with the pleural reflection. This is particularly true on the left side, in comparison with the right.

Because of the location of the kidneys, tenderness in these organs is usually reproduced by percussing the costovertebral angle. The obliquity of the renal axis is a relatively constant landmark, variations in which seen in urographic examinations may be caused by renal or pararenal masses. The closeness of the kidney and its coverings to the diaphragmatic pleura frequently produces a sympathetic pleural effusion in response to renal or perirenal inflammatory processes. At times, infection from the perinephric space may extend to within the pleural cavity, resulting in an empyema.

The relationship of the lower ribs to the kidneys is important to a consideration of traumatic injuries of the kidneys. The ribs generally protect the upper portion of the kidneys from blunt injury. In contrast, with fractures of the lower ribs, contusions or lacerations of the renal cortex may result. Furthermore, the location of the kidneys beneath the ribs, particularly on the left side, produces a region (the upper portion of the left kidney) that may be difficult to evaluate by ultrasonography because of interference with the transmission of sound waves by the overlying ribs.

Perinephric infections, since they are contained in Gerota's fascial space, may extend upward toward the diaphragm and down into the iliac fossa. Filling of Gerota's space with infection, blood, or urine may cause obliteration of the psoas margin seen on x-ray examination of the abdomen. The proximity of Gerota's fascia to the psoas muscle results in the possibility of a positive psoas sign when inflammatory processes are located in the perirenal region.

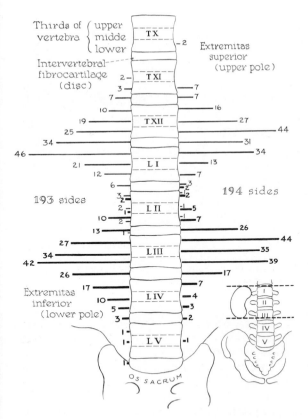

Thirds of { upper
vertebra { midde
{ lower

Intervertebral
fibrocartilage
(disc)

193 sides

Extremitas
inferior
(lower pole)

Extremitas
superior
(upper pole)

194 sides

Figure 1–42. Relation of the extremities of the kidneys to the vertebrae and the intervening fibrocartilages.

The vertebrae, for purposes of topography, are shown divided into thirds; the fibrocartilage would be the fourth part of a segment. The lighter cross-bars represent the upper pole; the heavy bars represent the lower pole. Considered together (right and left sides), the highest point of renal extent was the lower third of the tenth thoracic vertebra; the lowermost was the disc between the vertebral column and the sacrum. (Anson and Daseler: Surg. Gynecol. & Obstet., *112*:439, 1961. By permission of Surgery, Gynecology & Obstetrics.)

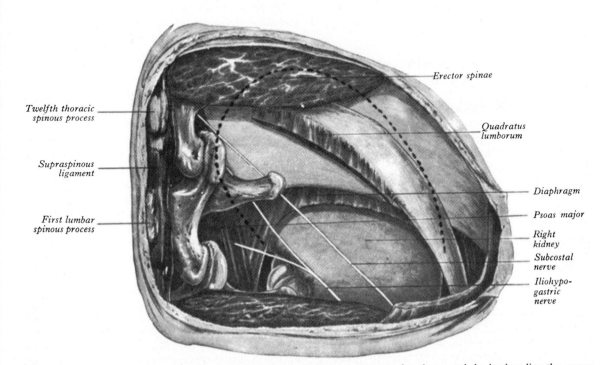

Figure 1–43. The right kidney, posterior exposure. The shaded area represents the pleura and the broken line the upper part of the kidney. The subcostal nerve has been displaced downwards. Parts of the diaphragm and the quadratus lumborum have been resected. (From Williams, P.L., and Warwick, R. (Eds.): Gray's Anatomy. 36th ed. Philadelphia, W.B. Saunders Co., 1980.)

Contiguity of the psoas compartment with the iliohypogastric and ilioinguinal nerves is one means by which referral of pain into the groin or thigh may result from retroperitoneal disease processes. The relationship of the kidneys and perinephric tissues to the spinal column is such that inflammatory processes or hemorrhage on one side may result in an involuntary curvature of the spine away from the involved side.

An understanding of the foregoing anatomic relationships helps the urologic surgeon to plan operative approaches to the kidney. Access to the kidney is usually obtained by subcostal or rib-resecting procedures. Subcostal incisions are unlikely to damage the pleura. These should be situated so as to run a course parallel to the twelfth intercostal nerve in order to avoid damaging this structure. This approach gives good operative access to the lower half of the left kidney and the lower two thirds of the right kidney as well as to both upper ureters. For improved operative access to the upper portions of the kidney, an eleventh or twelfth rib-resecting incision may be employed. In these incisions, the pleura may be damaged if not reflected upward prior to transection of diaphragmatic fibers. In contrast, one may use even higher approaches, purposefully traversing the pleural cavity so as to gain improved operative access to the adrenal glands or upper renal poles.

Renal Relations with Other Organs

The anterior surface of each kidney is juxtaposed to a number of retro- and intraperitoneal structures. These relationships are essential to an understanding of symptom complexes associated with renal disease as well as being the anatomic basis for explaining renal involvement by conditions affecting these organs. These renal surface relationships are represented diagrammatically in Figure 1–44 and shown more pictorially in Figure 1–45.

Along the upper medial border of each kidney lies the adrenal gland. Although it is separated from the kidney by an individual compartmentalization of Gerota's fascial space, malignant lesions of the adrenal may result in renal involvement by direct extension of neoplastic tissue across this attenuated connective tissue plane. Adrenal masses tend to produce alterations in renal position. Straightening of the oblique axis and depression of the entire kidney may be detected urographically in patients with large adrenal lesions of any sort.

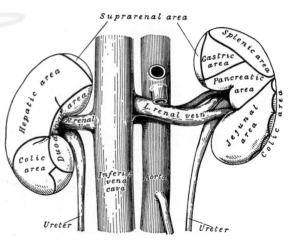

Figure 1–44. The anterior surfaces of the kidneys, showing the areas related to neighboring viscera. (From Williams, P.L., and Warwick, R. (Eds.): Gray's Anatomy. 36th ed. Philadelphia, W.B. Saunders Co., 1980.)

The descending duodenum is in direct contact with the medial portion of the right kidney and right renal pelvis. Laterally, the majority of the anterior renal surface on the right is overlaid by the right lobe of the liver. These relationships explain the confusion of symptoms of renal disease with those resulting from duodenal ulcer, cholecystitis, and hepatitis (or vice versa). They also explain the rather frequent association between traumatic injuries of kidney and liver. Finally, a knowledge of the relationships of the liver to the diaphragm and intrahepatic vena cava (as well as to the kidney) is essential to the urologist carrying out thorocoabdominal surgery on the right side, particularly when there is intracaval extension of a right renal cancer (Figs. 1–46 and 1–47). In these circumstances, the liver must be separated from the diaphragm by incision of the right triangular ligament. The bare area may then be exposed bluntly and reflected anteriorly to expose the intrahepatic cava with its communicating short hepatic veins.

On the left side the upper pole of the kidney rests against the spleen on its anterolateral aspect. This relationship is important to a proper interpretation of urographic shape of the left kidney, for there is often an indentation in this region that gives the appearance of a masslike hump of renal parenchyma just below, along the lateral border of the kidney (so-called splenic hump). The proximity of the kidney and spleen accounts for the frequent association between traumatic injuries of these organs. Furthermore, the surgeon must take care not to injure the spleen in the course of left renal surgery. Finally, the juxtaposition of splenic artery and renal artery is the anatomic basis for

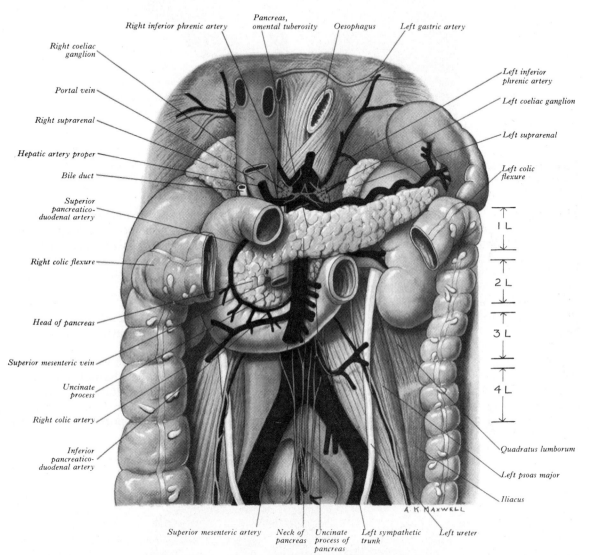

Right inferior phrenic artery

Pancreas, omental tuberosity

Oesophagus

Left gastric artery

Right coeliac ganglion

Portal vein

Right suprarenal

Hepatic artery proper

Bile duct

Superior pancreatico- duodenal artery

Right colic flexure

Head of pancreas

Superior mesenteric vein

Uncinate process

Right colic artery

Inferior pancreatico- duodenal artery

Left inferior phrenic artery

Left coeliac ganglion

Left suprarenal

Left colic flexure

Quadratus lumborum

Left psoas major

Iliacus

A K MAXWELL

Superior mesenteric artery

Neck of pancreas

Uncinate process of pancreas

Left sympathetic trunk

Left ureter

Figure 1–45. A dissection to show the relationships between the kidneys and adrenals, duodenum, pancreas, stem arterial rami of the gastrointestinal tract, and surrounding structures. The right and left hepatic veins have been cut away at their points of entry into the inferior vena cava. (In this specimen the left renal artery is situated anterior to the left renal vein at the hilum of the kidney.) (From Williams, P.L., and Warwick, R. (Eds.): Gray's Anatomy. 36th ed. Philadelphia, W.B. Saunders Co., 1980.)

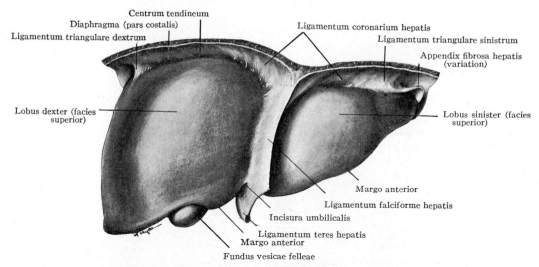

Figure 1–46. Anterosuperior surface of the liver and its connection with the diaphragm. (From McVay, C.: Anson & McVay Surgical Anatomy. 6th ed. Philadelphia, W.B. Saunders Co., 1984.)

the validity of splenorenal arterial shunts in cases of renal artery constriction.

The left kidney also contacts the stomach over a variable region of its anterior surface. The gastric fundus lies directly above the medial aspect of the kidney, and tomographic radiologic studies sometimes confuse the mass of gastric tissue in this region with a suprarenal mass lesion.

Finally, the left kidney is overlaid by a significant portion of the body or tail of the pancreas, a fact the surgeon must keep in mind in order to avoid trauma to this structure during dissections of the anterior leaf of Gerota's fascia on the left. Pancreatitis may result in symptoms

predominating posteriorly in rare circumstances, mimicking left renal disease. Pancreatic lesions, such as pseudocyst, may distort the position of the left kidney and be misinterpreted as renal masses, even with the most sophisticated radiologic studies.

Ureteral Relations

On the right side, the abdominal ureter lies deep to the peritoneum of the right mesocolon and the right infracolonic compartment (Figs. 1–39, 1–45, and 1–48). Above, it lies behind the descending and transverse portions of the duo-

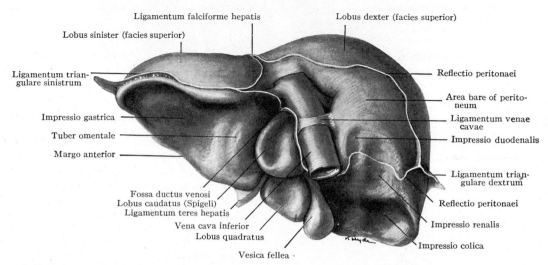

Figure 1–47. Demonstrating the bare area and the peritoneal reflections that suspend the liver from the diaphragm. (From McVay, C.: Anson & McVay Surgical Anatomy. 6th ed. Philadelphia, W.B. Saunders Co., 1984.)

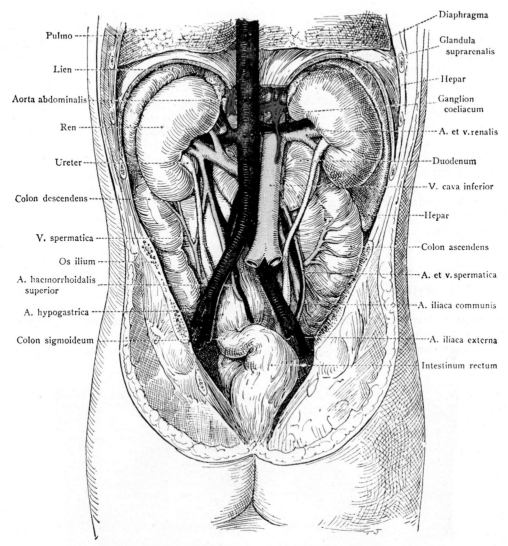

Pulmo

Lien

Aorta abdominalis

Ren

Ureter

Colon descendens

V. spermatica

Os ilium

A. haemorrhoidalis superior

A. hypogastrica

Colon sigmoideum

Diaphragma

Glandula suprarenalis

Hepar

Ganglion coeliacum

A. et v. renalis

Duodenum

V. cava inferior

Hepar

Colon ascendens

A. et v. spermatica

A. iliaca communis

A. iliaca externa

Intestinum rectum

Figure 1–48. Dissection of abdominal viscera, dorsal view, showing relations of the kidneys and ureters. (After Corning's Topographischen Anatomie in Eycleshymer and Jones.)

denum. More distally, it is crossed anteriorly by the gonadal artery and vein as well as by the right colic and ileocolic vessels. The abdominal portion of the right ureter is also crossed by the root of the mesentery and terminal ileum below. On the left side, the gonadal vessels initially parallel and then cross the ureteral course, and the left colic and sigmoid vasculature cross over the ureter anteriorly. Portions of the sigmoid colon approach juxtaposition with the abdominal ureter.

Flank extraperitoneal approaches to abdominal ureteral surgery are easier than transperitoneal approaches because anteriorly situated vessels and bowel do not require mobilization. The anatomic relationship between the duodenum and the right renal pelvis

and proximal right ureter explains the rare case of duodenal renal fistula. On the right side, the proximity of the ureter to the appendix is such that, particularly in the case of a retrocecal appendicitis, a misdiagnosis of ureteral calculus may be made. Perforated appendicitis or tuberculous or regional enteritis may result in right ureteral obstruction at the level of the crossing ileum. Also on the right side, the relationships of the gonadal vessels to the ureter account for those rare circumstances in which ovarian vein dilatation results in interference with ureteral drainage (so-called ovarian vein syndrome). Proximity of the sigmoid colon to the left ureter is such that various diseases affecting this region of bowel, such as diverticulitis or malignancy, can result in left ureteral obstruction.

Operative injuries of the abdominal ureter are predominantly associated with colon surgery. The adherence of the ureter and its surrounding fascia to the mesosigmoid may be exaggerated by inflammation or neoplasm in the surrounding tissues. The proximity of the inferior mesenteric artery and its branches to the left ureter results in another mechanism whereby the ureter may be traumatized inadvertently during operations on the colon. Other operative injuries of the abdominal ureter have been reported during aortic resection or grafting, vena caval plication or ligature, and sympathectomy, all resulting from the contiguity of the ureter to the aorta, vena cava, and sympathetic nerve chains.

Renal and Ureteral Relations with Somatic Nerves

The major nerves traversing the lumbar fossa are the twelfth thoracic (subcostal) and first and second lumbar nerves (Fig. 1–49). The ventral division of the former first appears in the retroperitoneum at the lateral border of the superior lumbar triangle, running behind the kidney in front of the quadratus lumborum. It then perforates the aponeurosis of the transversus abdominis muscle, running thence anteriorly between that muscle and the internal oblique, paralleling the course of the lower intercostal nerves. The subcostal nerve supplies the anterior abdominal muscles and gives rise to a lateral cutaneous branch, which, after piercing the internal and external oblique muscles, descends over the iliac crest, supplying the skin of the front of the gluteal region.

The ventral division of the first lumbar nerve, supplemented by a twig from the subcostal nerve, further divides into a larger iliohypogastric and smaller ilioinguinal branch, which emerge in the retroperitoneum at the lateral border of the psoas muscle and also course anterior to the quadratus lumborum muscle. The iliohypogastric perforates the transversus abdominis muscle just above the iliac crest. It sends fibers to the flat abdominal muscles and

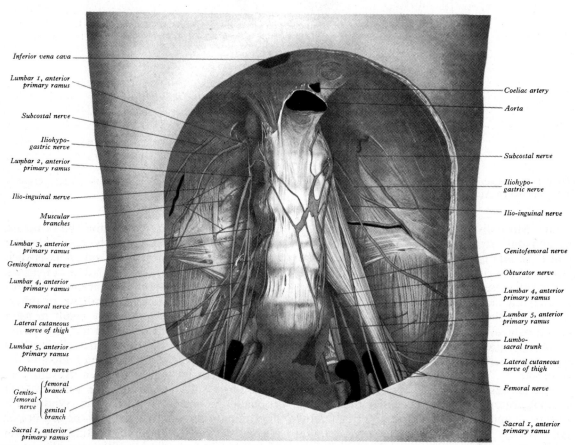

Figure 1–49. A dissection of the posterior abdominal wall to show the lumbar plexus and sympathetic trunks. The right psoas major has been removed. (From Williams, P.L., and Warwick, R. (Eds.): Gray's Anatomy. 36th ed. Philadelphia, W.B. Saunders Co., 1980.)

then divides into a lateral branch that supplies the skin of the posterior gluteal region and an anterior branch that supplies the skin of the abdomen above the pubis. The ilioinguinal nerve runs along the lower aspect of the quadratus lumborum and the iliacus muscles to perforate the transversus abdominis near the anterior portion of the iliac crest, giving rise to twigs supplying the abdominal muscles and subsequently traversing the internal oblique muscle and entering the inguinal canal. It is distributed to the skin of the proximal penis and scrotum (or labia in the female) as well as to the superomedial aspect of the thigh. The genitofemoral (lumboinguinal) nerve, arising from the ventral roots of the first and second lumbar nerves, emerges from the anterior surface of the psoas muscle at the level of the third or fourth lumbar vertebra. It courses downward, crossing behind the ureter, and divides into genital and femoral branches. The former supplies the cremaster muscle and the skin of the scrotum (or labia in the female); the latter accompanies the external iliac artery to supply the skin overlying the femoral triangle.

The importance of all these somatic nerve relationships is threefold: (1) their contribution to patterns of pain referral from the kidney and ureter; (2) their actual involvement in retroperitoneal processes that may give rise to pain or paresthesias in the regions innervated; and (3) their importance to the surgeon whose task it is to identify and preserve these structures in carrying out surgical procedures on the kidney and ureter.

Pelvic Ureteral Relations

The anatomic relations of the pelvic ureteral course depend on sex. In the male, the ureter is crossed in a lateral to medial direction anteriorly by the vas deferens. The vas at this point separates the ureter from the peritoneum (Fig. 1–50). The ureter then continues medially to reach the seromuscular layer of bladder in the lateral aspect of the angle formed by the vas and seminal vesicle (Figs. 1–51 and 1–52).

In the female, the parietal division of the pelvic ureter enters the pelvis in close association with the suspensory ligament of the ovary (containing the ovarian vessels) (Fig. 1–53). It then descends along the posterior peritoneal surface of the broad ligament. It enters the parametrium, through which it proceeds forward around the cervix and, coursing anteromedially, reaches the urinary bladder. Typically, it is separated laterally from the cervix by ap-

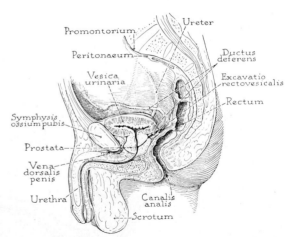

Figure 1–50. Median view of male pelvis showing relationship of vas deferens to ureteral course. (From McVay, C.: Anson & McVay Surgical Anatomy. 6th ed. Philadelphia, W.B. Saunders Co., 1984.)

proximately 2 cm and is about 1 cm above the vaginal fornix at this point. In this region it is enveloped by the veins of the vaginal and perivesical plexus of venous drainage. The anteromedial direction of the ureteral course from the cervix to the bladder results in the distalmost ureter lying anterior to the vaginal wall just prior to reaching the urinary bladder (Fig. 1–54).

These anatomic relations must be borne in mind when pelvic disease exists or when pelvic surgery is under consideration. The proximity of the ureter to the ovary, cervix, and uterus in the female, to the prostate and seminal vesicles in the male, and to the bladder and rectum in both sexes is such that conditions affecting these structures can either result in involvement of the ureter or produce symptoms reminiscent of ureteral obstruction.

The contiguity of the ureters to the cervix, uterus, and ovary means that disease in these structures may result in ureteral involvement, usually manifested by obstruction. Thus, pelvic endometriosis or inflammatory disease, cervical cancer, uterine cancer, and benign as well as malignant lesions of the ovary may result in ureteral blockage. Similarly, rectal lesions, bladder diverticula, or cancer as well as prostatic malignancy can affect ureteral drainage.

Surgery in the pelvis always produces potential danger points wherein inadvertent injury to the ureter may result. The gynecologic surgeon should use extreme care in transecting and ligating the ovarian vessels as well as the uterine artery because of the proximity of the ureter to these vascular structures. The rectal surgeon should be aware of the relationship of the ureter

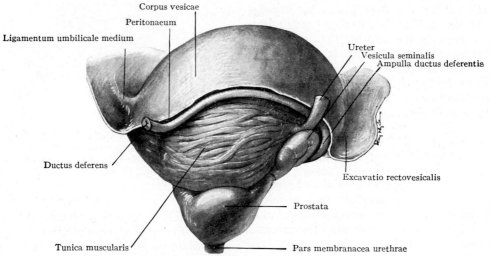

Figure 1–51. Lateral view of the ureter, bladder, and male pelvic genitals. (From McVay, C.: Anson & McVay Surgical Anatomy. Philadelphia, W.B. Saunders Co., 1984.)

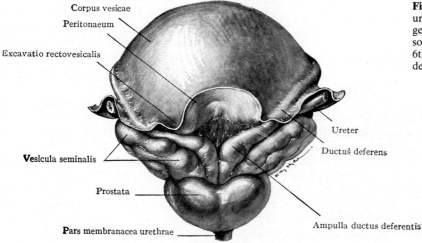

Figure 1–52. Posterior view of the ureter, bladder, and male pelvic genitals. (From McVay, C.: Anson & McVay Surgical Anatomy. 6th ed. Philadelphia, W.B. Saunders Co., 1984.)

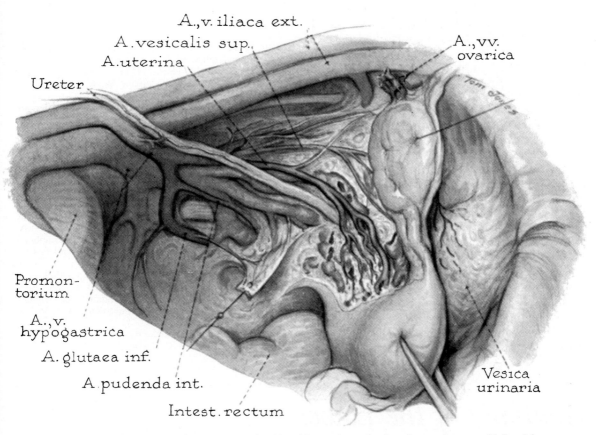

Figure 1–53. Female pelvis: ureteral relationship with arteries and veins of posterior part of left pelvis.

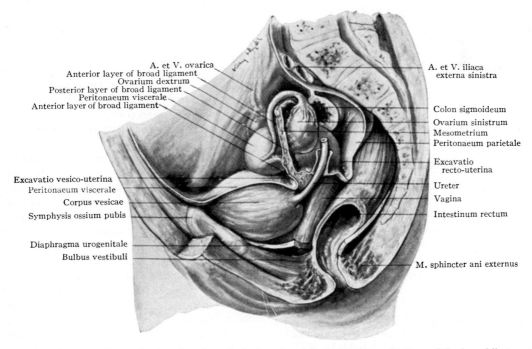

Figure 1–54. Left paramedian sagittal section through the female pelvis to show the reflections of the broad ligament and the pelvic peritoneum.

to the overlying branches of inferior mesenteric artery crossing the ureteral course and, in particular, be wary of the adherence of the ureter to the reflected peritoneum or mesosigmoid. The urologist should take heed of the intimate relationship that may pertain between a bladder diverticular wall and the ureter.

Surgery on the pelvic ureter in both sexes is best carried out through a retroperitoneal approach. An oblique incision in the groin region above the inguinal canal is the favored route. After incision of the transversus abdominis muscle and tranversalis fascia, the peritoneal envelope may be swept medially to reveal the proximal half of the pelvic ureter quite clearly. At about this level it is crossed by the superior vesical artery, which may be sacrificed to expose the rest of the ureteral course (in the male) and at least to the region of the parametrium in the female. This approach can be carried out without extensively encircling the ureter so as to avoid vascular injury to its blood supply.

References

Anson, B. J., and McVay, C. B.: Surgical Anatomy. 5th ed. Philadelphia, W. B. Saunders Co., 1971.
Anson, B. J., and Maddock, W. G.: Collander's Surgical Anatomy. 3rd ed. Philadelphia, W. B. Saunders Co., 1952.
Emmet, J. L., and Witten, D. M.: Clinical Urography. 3rd ed. Philadelphia, W. B. Saunders Co., 1971.
Goss, C. M.: Anatomy of the Human Body by Henry Gray. 27th ed. Philadelphia, Lea & Febiger, 1959.
Hamburger, J., Richet, G., Crosnier, J., Funk-Brentano, J. L., Antoine, B., Ducrot, H., Mery, J. P., and deMontera, H.: Nephrology. (Translated by A. Walsh.) Philadelphia, W. B. Saunders Co., 1968.
Lich, R., Jr., Howerton, L. W., and Amin, M.: Anatomy and surgical approach to the urogenital tract in the male. *In* Harrison, J. H., Gittes, R. F., Perlmutter, A. D., Stamey, T. A., and Walsh, P. C. (Eds.): Campbell's Urology. 4th ed. Philadelphia, W. B. Saunders Co., 1978, Vol. 1, pp. 3–33.
Notley, R. G.: The anatomy of the ureter and pathology of congenital obstructions. *In* Williams, D. I., and Chisholm, G. D. (Eds.): Scientific Foundations of Urology. Chicago, Year Book Medical Publishers, 1976, Vol. 2, pp. 1–17.
Williams, P. L., and Warwick, R.: Gray's Anatomy. 36th ed. Philadelphia, W. B. Saunders Co., 1980.

Anatomy of the Lower Urinary Tract

EMIL A. TANAGHO, M. D.

THE URINARY BLADDER

The Bladder Proper

EMBRYOLOGIC ORIGIN

Early in fetal life, when cloacal dilatation first appears and the hindgut ends in a blind sac, an ectodermal depression develops under the root of the tail and sinks in toward the gut until only a thin layer of tissue remains between the gut and the outside of the body. This ectodermal depression is known as proctodeum, and the thin layer of tissue is called the cloacal membrane. The division of the cloaca is effected by the development of the urorectal fold, which closes caudally toward the cloacal membrane. As the urorectal fold cuts progressively deeper into the cloaca, a wedge-shaped mass of mesenchyme accompanies it and forms a dense septum between the urogenital sinus anteriorly and the rectum posteriorly. This separation of the cloaca is completed before the cloacal membrane ruptures so that its two parts open independently (Fig. 1–55).

When it first opens to the outside, the urogenital sinus, which is the ventral division of the cloaca, is tubular and continuous with the allantois. At this stage it can be divided into a ventral or pelvic portion, which will become the bladder proper, and a urethral portion, which receives the mesonephric and the fused müllerian ducts, to later become the prostatic and membranous urethra in the male and the whole urethra in the female. The sequence of differentiation in both sexes at 8 and 12 weeks is demonstrated in Figures 1–56 and 1–57. Both portions have the same origin and are continuous.

After the 8-week stage, the ventral part of

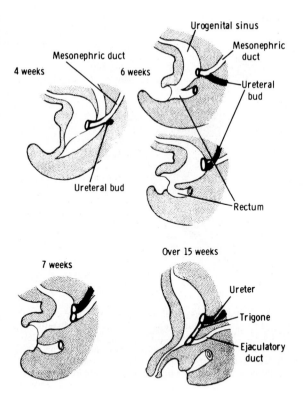

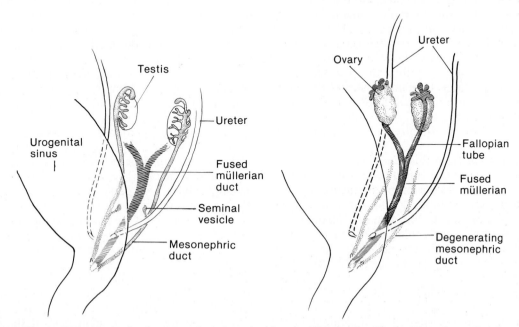

Figure 1–55. Embryologic sequence of development of the urogenital sinus as it separates from the cloaca. Ureteral bud (first appearance at 4 weeks of gestation) at the bend of the mesonephric duct; the common nephric duct becomes incorporated into the urogenital sinus when the latter separates from the rectum. When this separation is complete, the cloacal membrane will rupture to form two independent openings for the urogenital sinus and the rectum. (From Tanagho, E.A.: *In* Raz, S. (Ed.): Female Urology. Philadelphia, W.B. Saunders Co., 1983.)

Figure 1–56. *A,* Embryologic development of an 8-week-old male. The fused müllerian ducts have already met the urogenital sinus at Müller's tubercle. On either side is the opening of the mesonephric ducts. The ureteral buds have started their ascent on the urogenital sinus; the gonads have started to differentiate and now connect to the mesonephric duct. *B,* Development of the fused müllerian ducts in a 8-week-old female embryo: Their cranial ends attach to the ovary, while the mesonephric ducts are degenerating. Again, the fused müllerian ducts already join the urogenital sinus at the level of Müller's tubercle.

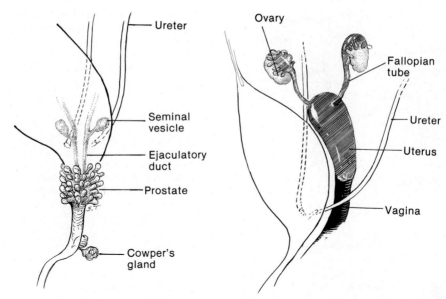

Figure 1–57. *A,* Development of the prostatic gland in a 12-week-old male embryo: Several buds originate out of the proximal part of the urethral segment of the urogenital sinus. Cowper's glands begin to appear slightly more distally. The seminal vesicles develop from the caudal end of the mesonephric ducts. These changes are happening under the influence of testicular differentiation. *B,* Further differentiation of the fused müllerian ducts into the upper two thirds of the vagina as well as the uterus and the fallopian tubes, which are now directly related to the differentiated ovaries (12-week-old female embryo). The müllerian tubercle has moved more caudally and now opens into the vaginal vestibule, which is formed by the most distal segment of the urogenital sinus.

the urogenital sinus starts to expand to form an epithelial sac, the apex of which tapers into an elongated narrowed urachus, and the splanchnic mesoderm surrounding both segments begins to differentiate into interlacing bands of smooth muscle fibers and an outer fibroconnective tissue coat. By the 12-week stage, the layers characteristic of the adult urethra and bladder can be recognized. Figure 1–58 demonstrates the entire urinary system in the lamb fetus at midterm (75 gestational days), showing the slight expansion of the bladder and its direct continuity with the urethra.

It is clear from this sequence of events that the detrusor muscle and the urethral musculature have the same origin, constituting one uninterrupted structure. This arrangement is easily visualized in the female, bladder and urethra being one tubular unit with expansion of the upper part. In the male, the structure is complicated by the simultaneous development of the prostatic gland. Yet the developmental sequence is the same in both sexes, and the structural arrangement in the male is not much different from the simpler arrangement in the female.

GROSS CONFIGURATION

The bladder is a hollow muscular organ, its main function being that of a reservoir.

POSITION

When empty, the adult bladder lies behind the pubic symphysis and is largely a pelvic organ. In infants and children it is situated higher. When full, the bladder rises well above the symphysis and can readily be palpated or percussed. When overdistended, as in acute or chronic urinary retention, it may cause the lower abdomen to bulge visibly and it is easily palpable in the suprapubic region.

The empty bladder is described as having an apex, a superior surface, two infralateral or anterolateral surfaces, a base or posterior surface, and a neck. The apex reaches a short distance above the pubic bone and ends as a fibrous cord derivative of the urachus, which originally connected the bladder to the allantois. This fibrous cord extends from the apex of the bladder to the umbilicus between the peritoneum and the transversalis fascia. It raises a ridge of peritoneum called the median umbilical ligament. The superior surface is the only surface of the bladder covered by peritoneum, although in the male a small part of the base also has a peritoneal covering.

ANATOMIC RELATIONSHIP

The superior surface of the bladder is in relation with the uterus and ileum in the female

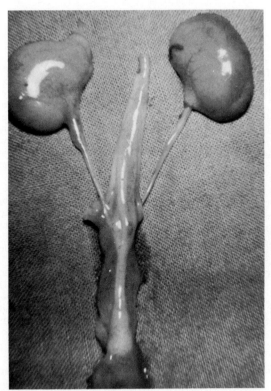

Figure 1–58. Entire urinary system of the lamb fetus at midterm (75 gestational days): The cylindrical urogenital sinus narrows at the bladder neck and continues uninterrupted as the urethral canal to the opening in the vaginal vestibule. The ureters are well formed, and the renal masses are well defined. The urogenital sinus tapers off to the allantois, where it joins the umbilicus. (From Tanagho, E.A.: *In* Raz, S. (Ed.): Female Urology. Philadelphia, W.B. Saunders Co., 1983.)

and with the ileum and any portion of the colon that is in the pelvic cavity in the male. The base of the bladder faces posteriorly and is separated from the rectum by the vasa deferentia, seminal vesicles, and ureters in the male, and by the uterus and vagina in the female. The anterolateral surfaces on each side of the bladder are in relation to the pubic bone and with the levator ani and obturator internus muscles, but the bladder is actually separated from the pubic bone by the retropubic space, which contains an abundance of fat and venous plexus (Fig. 1–59).

The neck of the bladder, its most inferior part, leads to the urethra. The bladder is a distensible cavity; when it is filled with urine, although the position of the neck remains stationary, the dome rises into the pelvic cavity and then into the lower abdomen. As the bladder rises into the lower abdomen, it comes in touch with the posterior aspect of the lower part of the anterior abdominal wall and its perito-

neally covered surface becomes in relation to the intra-abdominal contents, mainly the small and large bowel.

LINING OF THE BLADDER

The interior of the bladder is completely covered by transitional epithelium several layers deep. There is a loose underlying connective tissue that permits considerable stretching of the mucosa; for that reason the mucosal lining is wrinkled when the bladder is empty but quite smooth and flat when the bladder is distended. This arrangement exists throughout except over the trigonal area, where the mucous membrane is firmly adherent to the underlying musculature of the superficial trigone—this is why the trigone is always smooth, whether the bladder is full or empty.

MUSCULATURE

Muscular Wall. The bladder wall is frequently described as having three muscular coats. This is true only around the bladder outlet. In the remaining part there is no layering, and muscle fibers move freely from one coat to another (Fig. 1–60).

Muscular Lining. The bladder musculature itself is arranged in relatively coarse muscle bundles, widely separated, with no sheet formation. The bundles cross each other freely and have no definite orientation, being longitudinal

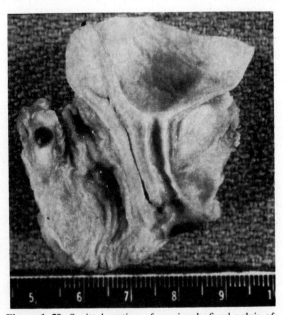

Figure 1–59. Sagittal section of previously fixed pelvis of a newborn female: It is split exactly in the midline, showing the anatomic relation of the pubic bone to the urethra and the bladder neck as well as the bladder cavity, rectum, and anal sphincter.

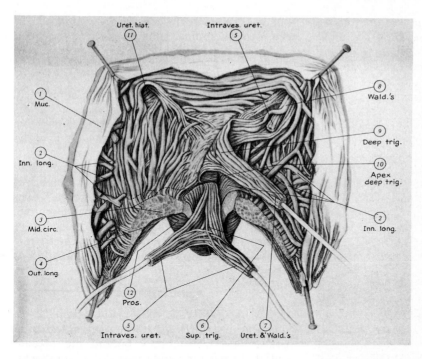

Figure 1–60. Muscle layers around the bladder neck as seen from the inside of a male bladder: (1) remaining edge of the bladder mucosa; (2) inner longitudinal layer with meshlike arrangement of fibers that continue in the urethra; (3) middle circular fibers condensed anteriorly and fanning out dorsocranially; (4) outer longitudinal coat; (5) intravesical ureter cut and reflected downward; (6) superficial trigone dissected and reflected; (7) intramural ureter with Waldeyer's sheath; (8) Waldeyer's sheath; (9) deep trigone (direct continuation of Waldeyer's sheath); (10) apex of deep trigone ending at the internal meatus; (11) the ureteral hiatus; (12) the prostate. (From Tanagho, E.A., and Smith, D.R.: Br. J. Urol., *38*:54, 1966.)

or circular except around the bladder neck, where three definite layers can be separated. However, if these three layers are traced cranially in any direction, it will be noted that the muscle bundles gradually mingle into their layering as they start to move from one plane to another. For a distance they might be on the inside of the bladder, then reach its middle part, to appear on the outer surface and return back to the inside, weaving their way in a true mesh fashion. These muscle bundles not only change levels in the bladder wall but also branch out and unite with adjoining bundles (Fig. 1–61). If one views the muscular structure of the bladder wall in this sense, one can consider its entire musculature as a single bundle weaving its way in and out, changing planes, changing direction, and changing levels, but still as a directly continuous filament.

This configuration, however, does not hold true near and at the bladder neck. As they approach this area, the muscle bundles on the inner side of the bladder are arranged in a radial fashion, all converging toward the internal meatus; they form a definite inner coat, which continues its course after sweeping over the

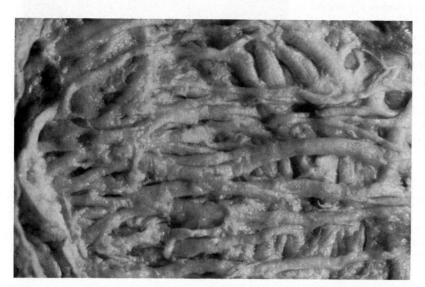

Figure 1–61. Detrusor musculature as seen from the inside after the bladder mucosa has been peeled off: The heavy muscle bundles of the hypertrophied bladder wall are widely separated and change their course as well as their level in the bladder wall. Note the fusion between the adjacent muscle bundles as they pursue their course.

internal ring into the urethra, to lie in its inner aspect as the urethral inner longitudinal muscle layer (Fig. 1–60). The other bundles in the middle portion of the bladder, again close to its neck, condense in a dense, circular orientation that is prominent in the midline anteriorly; these bundles fan out and spread apart as they proceed laterally and then dorsally. The most caudal muscle bundle reaches the extreme proximal end of the urethra but does not extend into it, while the most cranial bundle passes over the ureteral hiatus and forms a complete ring around the bladder base. The fibers in between, as they proceed laterally and dorsally, fuse with the lateral border and the dorsal aspect of the deep trigone; some of them progress a fair distance behind the deep trigone before they fuse with it.

The muscle fibers of the outer side of the bladder form the outer longitudinal coat and, close to the bladder neck, a complete sheet of radially disposed muscle bundles surrounding the vesical wall above the level of the internal meatus. In the male, a few of the dorsal and longitudinal fibers fuse with the deep surface of the apex of the trigone; others penetrate the base of the prostate gland and mix with its musculature; others again descend and loop around the proximal urethra and turn back again to its outer surface. This happens from every direction—360 degrees around the bladder neck. The muscle fibers descending to wrap themselves around the urethra constitute its outer coat but return to the bladder to constitute the outer longitudinal coat of the bladder musculature (Fig. 1–62).

LIGAMENTS AND FASCIAL ATTACHMENTS

The loose subserous fascia of the pelvic cavity is continuous superiorly over all pelvic organs, and this is true for the bladder. The condensation of this fascia forms attachments for the bladder with the anterior abdominal wall and lateral pelvic wall. Dorsolaterally, there is excessive condensation of this connective areolar tissue to form the dorsolateral ligament, where the main blood and nerve supplies enter the bladder base. The median umbilical ligament, which is representative of the urachal remnant, attaches the bladder to the umbilicus. Inferiorly, the condensations of the fascia running from the levator ani muscle and the pubic bones to the bladder are called pubovesical ligaments in the female and puboprostatic ligaments in the male.

RADIOGRAPHIC ANATOMY

The bladder is visualized radiographically by intravenous urography or retrograde cystography. When full, it assumes a rounded configuration filling a great portion of the pelvic cavity and then rising into the lower abdominal cavity. Its outline is usually smooth, central, and symmetric. In a lateral exposure, normally the bladder base is flat and lies behind the pubic bone. The urethrovesical junction is well supported by the pubocervical ligaments or puboprostatic ligaments; so are the pelvic floor and the genitourinary diaphragm. The urethrovesical segment usually lies opposite the lower third of the pubic bone; this feature is important in the diagnosis of pelvic floor weakness and bladder

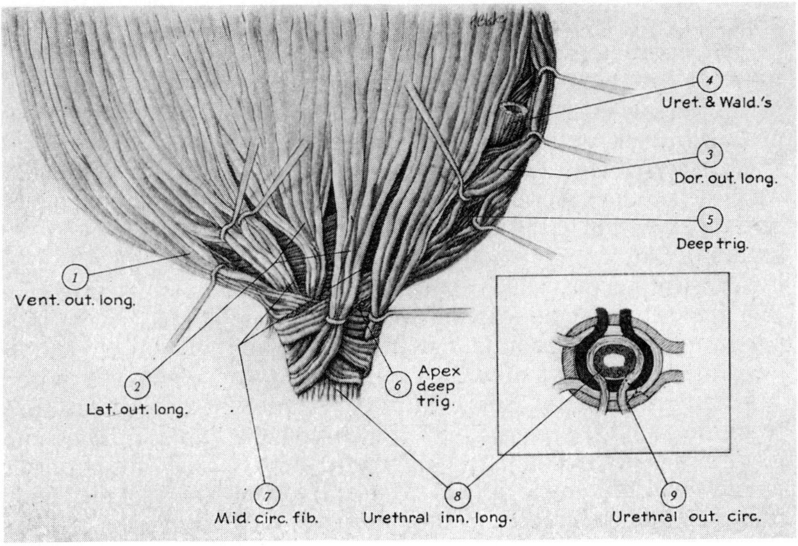

Figure 1–62. Arrangement of the muscle layers as seen from the lateral aspect of a female bladder: (1) ventral outer longitudinal fibers; (2) lateral outer longitudinal fibers; (3) dorsal outer longitudinal fibers; (4) juxtavesical ureter surrounded by Waldeyer's sheath; (5) deep trigone as seen through the outer longitudinal coat; (6) apex of the deep trigone at the internal meatus; (7) urethral inner longitudinal coat; (8) urethral outer circular or oblique fibers. *Insert*: Cross section of the proximal urethra with diagrammatic representation of the outer longitudinal fibers of the detrusor looping around the urethra. (From Tanagho, E.A., and Smith, D. R.: Br. J. Urol., *38*:55, 1966.)

support in patients with questionable stress urinary incontinence.

BLOOD SUPPLY

Arterial Supply. The arterial blood supply to the bladder comes from the superior, middle, and inferior vesical arteries, which are branches from the anterior division of the hypogastric artery. Smaller branches from the obturator and inferior gluteal arteries also reach the urinary bladder. In the female, the uterine and vaginal arteries send some branches to the bladder base. The bladder is a very vascular organ, well supplied by all these vessels, with rich anastomosis between all of them.

Venous Drainage. Surrounding the bladder there is a rich plexus of veins usually lying between the bladder wall proper and the adventitial layer covering it. These veins ultimately terminate in the hypogastric veins after gathering together in several main trunks; some of them accompany the arteries, others do not. The vesicovenous plexus also communicates with the retropubic venous plexus or plexus of Santorini, which drains the penis as well as other perineal organs.

LYMPHATIC DRAINAGE

The bladder lymphatics drain into the external iliac, hypogastric, and common iliac lymph nodes. There is a rich lymphatic anastomosis between all pelvic organs and between the lymphatics of the genital organs as well as the vesical lymphatics and the lower gastrointestinal lymphatics.

NEUROANATOMY

The bladder and urethra receive a rich nerve supply from both divisions of the autonomic nervous system.

Sympathetic Nerve Supply. It originates from the lower thoracic and upper lumbar segments, mainly T11–T12 and L1–L2. These sympathetic fibers descend into the sympathetic trunk, then to the lumbar splanchnic nerves, which reach the superior hypogastric plexus, an inferior extension of the aortic plexus. The latter separates into a right and a left plexus, the hypogastric nerves, which extend inferiorly to join the pelvic plexus coming from the pelvic parasympathetic, and adjoin it to proceed toward the bladder and urethra.

Parasympathetic Nerve Supply. It arises from the sacral segments S2–S4, which proceed to form the rich pelvic parasympathetic plexus, joined by the hypogastric plexus; vesical branches then emerge from this plexus toward the bladder base. The vesical plexus, essentially the main extension of the pelvic plexus, reaches the lateral side of the bladder, innervating both bladder and urethra. In the male, a separate segment will reach the prostate, forming the prostatic plexus. From the latter, the cavernous nerves emerge to supply the penile erectile tissue in the male or the clitoris in the female. These nerves carry both efferent and afferent pathways, and they are combined motor and sensory.

Branches of the vesical plexus ramify in the adventitia and penetrate the muscular coat as they travel throughout the entire bladder wall. Ganglia are present along the nerve trunks of the vesical plexus and also in its deeper branches. By repetitive branching, progressively smaller nerves are distributed throughout the muscular coat. The parasympathetic cholinergic nerve fibers are believed to be in the ratio of 1:1 to each muscle fiber. The sympathetic nerve fibers, more richly distributed in the bladder base and proximal urethra than in the bladder dome and lateral walls, show a much lower ratio. Within the bladder wall, the nerves pursue a tortuous course that will enable them to accommodate stretching during bladder filling. It is assumed that the motor nerve supply to the detrusor muscle is primarily the pelvic parasympathetic plexus (all are cholinergic fibers), while the motor nerve supply to the trigone and the lower end of the ureters is of sympathetic origin (mainly adrenergic).

The Sensory Pathways. It is believed that the sensation of stretch and fullness in the bladder is carried along the pelvic parasympathetic innervation, while the sensations of pain, touch, and temperature are carried along the sympathetic innervation. The sympathetic adrenergic nerve endings are both alpha- and beta-adrenergic, with alpha-adrenergic predominance in the bladder base and proximal urethra, and beta-adrenergic preponderance in the bladder dome and lateral wall. The functional value of this arrangement is discussed in the chapter on neurogenic bladder.

The Ureterovesical Junction

It is clear that the ureterovesical junction comprises more than the ureteral orifice or the submucosal ureter (Fig. 1–63). For proper anatomic discussion of the ureterovesical junction one must consider separately (1) the lower ureter, (2) the trigone, and (3) the adjacent bladder wall (Fig. 1–64).

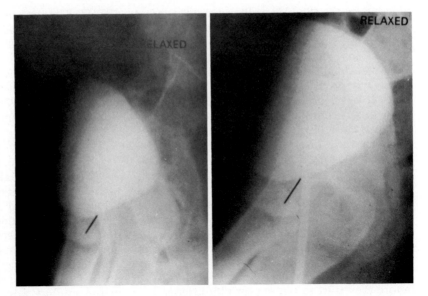

Figure 1–63. Lateral exposure of a full bladder in a normal female shows the relationship of the bladder base to the urethra and the pubic bone. A perpendicular drop from the ureterovesical junction on the long axis of the pubic bone will hit the latter opposite its lower third. (From Tanagho, E.A.: *In* Raz, S. (Ed.): Female Urology. Philadelphia, W.B. Saunders Co., 1983.)

THE LOWER URETER

The ureter proper has only one muscular coat; because of the irregular helical pattern of its muscle bundles, the fibers are oriented in almost every direction. As the ureter approaches the bladder and finally enters the bladder wall, its helical fibers elongate and become parallel to the lumen throughout the intravesical ureter. These fibers continue uninterrupted but in a pure longitudinal course. Because of this

pure longitudinal orientation, it has been believed that the circular and oblique fibers outside the bladder end before the ureter enters the bladder wall, so that the intravesical ureter is less muscularized than the juxtavesical ureter. This happens not to be true. All the muscle fibers of the juxtavesical ureter continue in the intravesical ureter after changing their orientation and becoming parallel to their lumen. The intravesical ureter is about 1.5 cm long and is divided into an intramural segment totally sur-

Figure 1–64. Normal ureterovesico-trigonal complex. *A,* Side view with Waldeyer's muscular sheath surrounding vestige of the intravesical ureter and continuing downward as the deep trigone, which extends to the bladder neck. The ureteral musculature becomes the superficial trigone, which extends to the verumontanum in the male and stops just short of the external meatus in the female. *B,* Waldeyer's sheath connected by a few fibers to the detrusor muscle in the ureteral hiatus. This muscular sheath inferior to the ureteral orifice becomes the deep trigone. The musculature of the ureters continues downward as the superficial trigone. (From Tanagho, E.A., and Pugh, R.C.B.: Br. J Urol., *35:*151, 1963.)

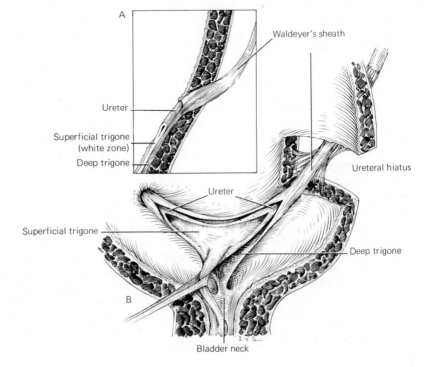

rounded by the bladder wall and a submucosal segment (about 0.8 cm long) directly under the bladder mucosa.

The longitudinal fibers of the lower end of the ureter do not end at the level of the ureteral orifice but proceed uninterrupted into the trigone. It was long believed that the floor fibers of the ureter continued into the trigone, to what is known as Bell's muscle, while the roof fibers ended or were inserted into the vesicoureteral mucosal reflection at the roof of the orifice. This assumption proved not to be true. The fact is that all ureteral muscles extend uninterrupted into the base of the bladder and continue as the trigone, where they approach the ureteral orifice, the roof fibers splitting and swinging to the side, thus forming the lips of the ureteral orifice. They then join the floor fibers, where they accumulate just distal to the ureteral orifice before they start to fan out into the trigone.

The juxtavesical ureter (distal 3 to 4 cm) as well as the intramural segment of the intravesical ureter is surrounded by a fibromuscular sheath, Waldeyer's sheath (Waldeyer, 1891; Wesson, 1920). As the sheath is traced upward, its muscular element gradually fuses with the ureteral musculature and becomes an integral part of the ureteral wall. Distally, the sheath surrounds the intramural ureter, but, when the ureter emerges into the bladder and the intramural ureter becomes a submucosal ureter, the fibers of Waldeyer's sheath diverge from each other, very much like those of the ureter itself at the level of the ureteral orifice, and they sweep around the sides of the ureter to meet and fuse with the fibers forming the floor of the sheath. The sheath then continues downward, deep to the superficial trigone formed by the continuation of the ureteral muscles. This deep trigone ends at the level of the internal meatus. In this manner, Waldeyer's sheath proximally fuses with the intrinsic musculature of the ureter and distally acts as an added fixation linking the ureter proper and the detrusor. Part of the deep trigone is derived from the detrusor, which joins Waldeyer's sheath at the level of the ureteral hiatus. Also, detrusor fibers from the ventral condensation of the middle circular layer just above the internal meatus merge with the sides and the dorsum of the deep trigone, securing its fixation and possibly establishing the morphologic link between the bladder and trigone so the latter can physiologically influence the former.

There is much controversy over Waldeyer's description. Is it a sheath or a space (Woodburn, 1964; Elbadawi, 1972; Elbadawi and Schenk 1974)? The debate is pointless, for even if Waldeyer described a space, there has to be a layer on either side of the space and this outside layer is the lower ureteral sheath, well known as Waldeyer's sheath. It is also wondered whether Waldeyer's sheath is of ureteral or detrusor origin. We think that it is primarily ureteral, with a contribution from the detrusor.

THE TRIGONE

The trigone is composed of two layers.

The Superficial Trigone. The longitudinal fibers of the intravesical ureter diverge at the ureteral orifice and continue uninterrupted into the base of the bladder as the superficial trigone. Some fibers run across the base of the trigone between one submucosal ureter and the other. The rest fan out and converge at the internal meatus to proceed downward into the urethra in the midline posteriorly. In the male, these fibers terminate at the level of the verumontanum and possibly join the musculature of the ejaculatory ducts, and they form the crista urethralis. In the female, the same fibers terminate at the level of the external meatus.

The Deep Trigone. All the fibers forming Waldeyer's sheath continue downward uninterrupted into the base of the bladder, forming the deep trigone. Again, the only change is that the tubular sheath has become flat and its muscle bundles have become more compact and more firmly bound together. This flattening-and-fanning begins shortly before the ureter loses its lumen at the ureteral orifice. The upper fibers proceed medially to meet those from the other side, forming the base of the trigonal structure, the interureteral ridge or Mercier's bar. The lower fibers proceed medially and downward at various degrees of obliquity to meet and fuse with the fibers from the other side. The deep trigone ends at the internal meatus as a dense muscular fibrocollagenous structure. There is no muscular communication between the superficial and deep trigones, and they can be dissected easily from one another. The deep trigone is also easily dissected from the detrusor muscle behind it in its upper half. However, in its lower half, it is progressively more adherent and firmly attached to the underlying detrusor and the middle circular layer of the bladder. The superficial trigone adheres firmly to the overlying mucosal layer. The two layers of the trigone are in direct continuation with the lower ureter, with no interruption or loss of any of the musculature. The ureter has merely changed from a tubular to a sheetlike form. One may say that the ureter does not end at the ureteral orifice but continues uninterrupted as a flat sheet instead of a tubular structure.

THE ADJACENT BLADDER WALL

The ureter wrapped with its sheath pierces the bladder wall to gain access to the inside. As a result, it is completely surrounded by detrusor muscle. The latter contributes a few fibers to the ureteral sheath. Thus, the first connection between ureter and bladder is established, and a certain degree of fixation is imparted to the sheath while the ureter is free to slide in and out within it. If it were not for its fixation to Waldeyer's sheath cranially and the internal meatus and proximal urethra distally, the ureter could easily pull out from within the bladder. The site of penetration of the detrusor by the ureter, known as the ureteral hiatus, is probably the weakest part of the bladder wall. As the ureter emerges into the bladder, it lies directly submucosally, with the detrusor musculature behind. It maintains its tubular shape for a distance (the submucosal ureter) before it loses its lumen and becomes a trigone, both superficial and deep. The detrusor lies behind the submucosal ureter as well as behind the trigone. The trigone seems to be superimposed over the detrusor, which at that level is composed of two layers. Immediately behind the deep trigone, some detrusor circular fibers are firmly adherent or actually fuse with it, while the rest are unattached to the trigone but form a definite layer of circular orientation deeper to the deep trigone. Still deeper, the detrusor outer longitudinal muscular coat is very well developed posteriorly and forms a complete sheet behind the deep trigone. Through the connection between the deep trigone and the detrusor circular fibers, the trigone gains its firm fixation. At the midline posteriorly, at the level of the trigone and from inside out, four layers are to be distinguished: (1) the superficial trigone; (2) the deep trigone; (3) the detrusor circular coat; and (4) the detrusor outer longitudinal coat. This segment of the bladder is its strongest, least resilient, and most fixed part.

FUNCTIONAL ANATOMY OF THE URETEROVESICAL JUNCTION

The main function of the ureterovesical (UV) junction is to allow free efflux of urine from the ureter to the bladder but prevent any reflux of urine from the bladder to the ureter. The morphologic arrangement of the ureterovesical junction, as outlined, permits this balance between free flow from above downward, and no backflow from below upward. Considering the anatomic arrangement discussed, it can readily be appreciated that the resting tone of the trigone and intravesical ureter can keep the latter closed, except when a ureteral peristaltic wave forces it open and pushes up urine against minimal resistance. As the bladder fills and is gradually distended, the trigone is progressively stretched; this is instantaneously reflected in increasing resistance at the intravesical ureter, with firmer closure guarding against reflux during bladder filling. No matter how great the degree of bladder distention, reflux will never occur because of the simultaneously increasing degree of closure of the ureterovesical junction. During the act of voiding, when active detrusor contraction and sharp rise in intravesical pressure occur, contraction of the trigone happens synchronously, completely sealing the intravesical ureter against both reflux and efflux. Fortunately, that is a very temporary phase, and at its completion the resistance will drop and the urine flow will resume its passage from the ureter to the bladder.

The Bladder Neck

The anatomy of the bladder neck will be discussed under three headings: (1) the trigonal musculature, (2) the detrusor muscle, and (3) the urethral musculature.

THE TRIGONAL MUSCULATURE

The trigone has just been discussed in relation to the vesicoureteral junction. In relation to the bladder neck, it must be emphasized that the trigone has two muscular layers: a superficial layer, a direct continuation of the ureteral muscle; and a deeper layer, a direct continuation of Waldeyer's sheath. As the superficial trigone continues downward toward the bladder neck, its muscle fibers accumulate closer to the midline posteriorly, pass over the posterior lip of the internal meatus, then continue through almost the entire length of the urethra in the female; in the male, most of these fibers end at the level of the verumontanum, where they fuse with the musculature of the ejaculatory duct. The deep trigone forms a dense compact layer in the base of the bladder, which gains a certain degree of fusion with the detrusor muscle fibers acting as an anchoring mechanism for the ureterotrigonal unit. The muscle fibers of the deep trigone accumulate and terminate at the level of the internal meatus in the midline posteriorly.

THE DETRUSOR MUSCLE

The bladder wall is frequently described as having three muscular coats. This is true only around the bladder outlet. In the rest of the bladder, there is no layering and muscle fibers move freely from one coat to another, as discussed earlier. Around the internal meatus, the muscle bundles of the bladder are distributed into three distinct muscular coats.

The inner coat consists of purely longitudinal fibers. After their wide separation and multiple directions, as they get closer to the bladder neck they are arranged in a radial fashion; they form a compact sheet of muscle fibers that converges over the internal meatus and then sweeps over its lips into the urethra, forming the latter's inner longitudinal layer.

The middle circular layer is prominent in the midline ventrally and least developed in the midline dorsally. This appreciable condensation of muscle fibers, in circularly oriented bundles (about 2 cm wide), is complete ventrally, then sweeps through the sides of the bladder neck and fans outward as it moves dorsocranially (See Fig. 1–60). The most caudal muscle bundles reach the extreme proximal end of the urethra but do not extend into it. These bundles partly fuse with the lateral border or dorsal aspect of the deep trigone. While some higher bundles of this condensation pass uninterrupted behind the deep trigone, the highest pass over the ureteral orifice, forming a complete circle around the bladder base, closer to the internal meatus anteriorly than posteriorly. The outer longitudinal layer forms almost a complete sheet of radially disposed muscle bundles all around the vesical wall above the level of the internal meatus segment, close to the bladder neck. In the male, a few of the dorsal longitudinal fibers fuse with the deep surface of the apex of the trigone. Other fibers penetrate the base of the prostate gland and mix with its musculature. Some descend and loop around the proximal urethra and then turn back again to the outer surface of the bladder. These bundles can be quite prominent as they proceed obliquely downward and ventrally on each side of the urethra, looping around its ventral surface. New fibers in the ventral segment of this loop run almost transversely and surround a good segment of proximal urethra.

In the female, the arrangement is essentially the same, except that instead of penetrating the substance of the prostate, the fibers end in the vesicovaginal septum. This arrangement is very close to Wesson's (1920) description of the outer loop, which is complete ventrally and open dorsally. However, it is not the only loop around the urethra, since the ventral outer longitudinal coat has almost the same disposi-tion as the dorsal one. Definite muscle bundles from the ventral outer longitudinal coats move downward and dorsally around the sides of the proximal urethra to loop around its dorsal surface. This is true from either side. Thus, there are not one or two loops around the urethra, but many, all of them in direct continuation with the outer longitudinal coat of the bladder. None of these loops is continuous with the middle circular layer. Some are quite closed, with narrow necks, while others are widely open.

The Urethra

MUSCULATURE

The urethra and bladder have the same origin and their musculatures are directly continuous. While the bladder is a muscular sac, the urethra is a muscular tube. This is true in the entire female urethra and in the proximal segment of the male urethra. In the female, the urethral musculature is easily demonstrated; it consists of two coats—an inner longitudinal coat and an outer semicircular coat. The adult female urethra is about 4 cm long and is muscular in its entire length, except for the terminal few millimeters, which are dense collagen and act as a point of fixation for the insertion into the urethral musculature. The inner longitudinal coat of the urethra is a direct continuation of the inner longitudinal muscle layer of the bladder. It is relatively thick, formed of very delicate muscle bundles, in contradistinction to the coarse arrangement on the bladder side. Its thick coat and the muscle bundles are firmly bound together by dense, compact collagen tissue and elastic fibers. The outer coat consists of semicircular fibers, which are part of the fibers looping around the urethra and returning back to the detrusor. This circular coat also is quite thick, mostly near the internal meatus, and progressively less so caudally until it ends at the distal end of the urethra and the external meatal segment.

In the male, the developing prostatic epithelial buds meet the developing muscle fibers around the urogenital sinus, incorporating most of them into the prostatic gland and thus forming its muscular stroma (See Fig. 1–57A). Histologically, the urethral musculature is very compact and contains abundant collagen tissue with widespread elastic fibers throughout its entire length.

It is clear from this muscular arrangement that the only fibers that could exert any sphincteric action are the semicircular fibers surrounding the entire female urethra and the proximal part of the male urethra. No separate anatomic entity located at the level of the internal meatus or at any other level can be delineated as the internal sphincter. The sphincteric mechanism is not localized in one place or at one level but involves practically the entire urethral length in the female and the entire prostatomembranous urethra in the male (Fig. 1–65).

The Voluntary External Sphincter. Striated skeletal muscle fibers encircle the membranous urethra in the male and the midurethral segment in the female. Although embryologically related to the musculature of the pelvic floor, these fibers are anatomically separate—a differentiated segment of the cloacal sphincter, which gives the urethral, vaginal, and anal orifices each its own specialized sphincteric func-

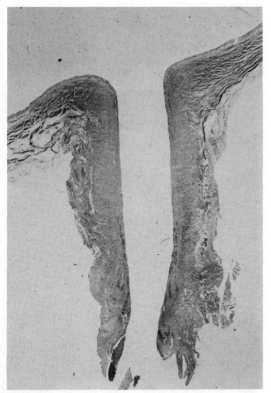

Figure 1–65. Sagittal sections of the entire female urethra from the internal to the external meatus. Note the muscular nature of the entire urethral tube except at its most distal end, which is fibrous and opens to the outside at the level of the vaginal vestibule. The inner longitudinal fibers are embedded in dense collagen, while the outer semicircular fibers constitute the bulk of the musculature of the urethral canal from the level of the internal meatus all the way down to the external meatus, as a direct continuation of the outer longitudinal fibers of the bladder wall. (From Tanagho, E.A., and Smith, D.R.: J. Urol., *100*: 640, 1968.)

tion. The striated external sphincter is a more or less complete ring in the female, with the median raphe in the midline posteriorly. It has an omega-shaped configuration in the male, again deficient in the midline posteriorly. It probably gains insertion in the perineal body (Fig. 1–66). Striated muscle fibers extend over the apex of the prostate in the male, and a few fibers may wander up to the level of the bladder neck. The bulk of the external sphincter is around the membranous urethra in the male and the midurethral third in the female.

Histologically, the striated muscle fibers can be classified into two main groups: slow-twitch fibers, which on contraction attain a low amplitude and can sustain it for a relatively long time; and fast-twitch fibers, which usually attain a higher amplitude but sustain it for a shorter period of time. The slow-twitch fibers constitute about 35 per cent of the overall striated muscle mass and the fast-twitch fibers the remaining 65 per cent. Detailed study of the histochemistry of these striated muscle fibers differentiated two subgroups in the fast-twitch fibers: (1) fast-twitch fatigable fibers, and (2) an intermediate type, which is fast-twitch fatigue-resistant. Of the 65 per cent fast-twitch fibers, 50 per cent are fatigable and 15 per cent are fatigue-resistant. This mixture of muscle fibers accounts for the varied contribution of the striated sphincter to the continence mechanism. A portion (slow-twitch) is needed for sustained tonus, and another (fast-twitch) for emergency (stress). The presence of fast-twitch fatigue-resistant fibers provides the combination of these two properties in an effective way—high amplitude, sustained for a longer time.

There is a tendency to underestimate the sphincteric contribution of the striated sphincter, especially in the female since it is less bulky and less developed than in the male. However, urodynamic evaluation shows its significance. There is also a tendency to underestimate the bulk and the extent of the external sphincter. Most illustrations show the male external sphincter as a short segment of about 1 cm, whereas in reality it is about 1 inch long. This is clearly seen in sagittal sections of the intact pelvis (Fig. 1–67) as well as in the recent NMR studies (Fig. 1–68), which delineate the anatomy very accurately. The segment is also a few millimeters deep; thus, to do a sphincterotomy in the male, the incision should be at least 1 inch long (from just below the level of the verumontanum toward the bulbous urethra) and at least 6 mm deep in order to get the entire thickness of the striated muscular sphincter

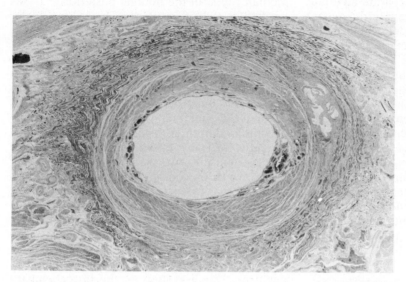

Figure 1–66. Histologic section of the membranous urethra of a normal adult male shows the distribution of the smooth intrinsic musculature in the urethral wall, with circular fiber orientation; it is surrounded by an equally thick intrinsic coat of striated muscle fibers, essentially omega-shaped, with a defect in the midline posteriorly where it inserts in the perineal body. Note that the external sphincter constitutes an integral part of the musculature of the urethral wall at the level of the membranous urethra.

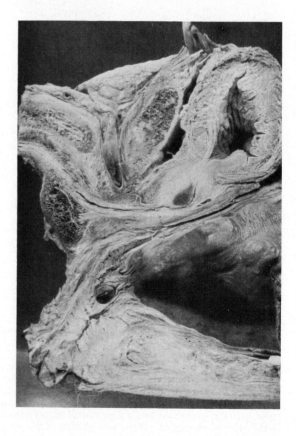

Figure 1–67. Sagittal section of a fixed adult male pelvis, cut exactly in the midline to show the anatomic relationship of the pubic bone to the bladder, bladder neck, and prostatic segment as well as the membranous urethra and the penile urethra when it enters the spongy tissue of the penis. Also note the prominent anal sphincter as well as the rectum. Most significant is the length of the urethral segment traversing the pelvic floor before entering the spongy tissue of the penis. The distance between the apex of the prostate and the bulbous part of the urethra constitutes the membranous urethra, which is roughly the same length as the prostatic urethra—a fact confirmed by NMR studies (see Figure 1–68).

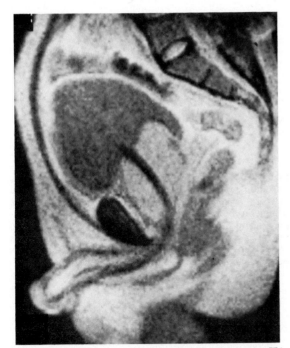

Figure 1–68. NMR demonstration of a sagittal cut in an adult male with BPH. Note the size of the prostate as well as the prostatomembranous urethra before it enters the spongy tissue of the penis. It is worth noting that the membranous urethra is clogged and its length almost equal to that of the prostatic urethra.

around the membranous urethra. Sphincterotomy is probably never indicated in the female.

THE URETHRA

EMBRYOLOGIC ORIGIN

The urethra develops from the caudal end of the urogenital sinus after its complete separation from the cloaca. In the male, the urethral segment of the urogenital sinus will form the prostatic and membranous urethra; in the female, it will form the entire urethra as well as the vaginal vestibule.

THE MALE URETHRA

The male urethra, which acts as the conduit for both urinary and genital systems, extends from the internal orifice in the urinary bladder to the external opening of the external meatus at the tip of the glans penis. It is divided into three regional segments: prostatic, membranous, and penile.

The Prostatic Urethra (Fig. 1–69). This segment is the widest, most distensible part of the urethra. In the average male it is about 3 cm long, traversing the substance of the pros-

tate, with relatively acute angulation at the level of the verumontanum. It is closer to the anterior surface than to the posterior surface of the prostate. Cross section shows a median longitudinal ridge posteriorly, formed by an elevation of the mucous membrane and the adjacent tissue, the crista urethralis; this represents a continuation of the superficial trigone into the prostatic urethra. There is the elevation of the verumontanum, and the vesicula seminalis. At the tip is the slitlike orifice of the prostatic utricle and on each side the small opening of the ejaculatory duct. The prostatic utricle is a cul-de-sac, a few millimeters deep, running upward and backward in the substance of the prostate. It is a remnant of the müllerian duct system. On both sides of the crista urethralis are shallow depressions called the prostatic sinus, on the floor of which are the orifices of the prostatic ducts.

The Membranous Urethra (Figs. 1–67, 1–70 to 1–72). This is the thickest segment of the urethra as it passes through the genitourinary diaphragm. It is wrongly believed that it is a very short segment; in reality, it is about 2.0 to 2.5 cm long and curves as it descends with a ventral concavity (Fig. 1–67). The membranous urethra is a muscular organ, with both smooth and skeletal musculature; the latter constitutes the external (or voluntary) urinary sphincter. The latter forms almost a complete ring around the urethra but is partially deficient in the midline posteriorly, so that it extends as an omega-shaped structure from the apex of the prostate to the bulb of the penis. In the front, the deep dorsal vein of the penis enters the pelvis between the transverse perineal ligament and the arcuate ligament of the pubis. On either side is

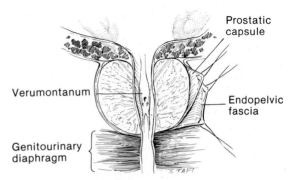

Figure 1–69. Section of the prostate gland shows the prostatic urethra, verumontanum, and crista urethralis, in addition to the opening of the prostatic utricle and the two ejaculatory ducts in the midline. Note that the prostate is surrounded by the prostatic capsule, which is covered by another prostatic sheath derived from the endopelvic fascia. The prostate is resting on the genitourinary diaphragm.

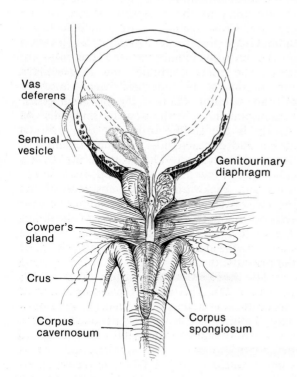

Vas
deferens

Seminal
vesicle

Cowper's
gland

Crus

Corpus
cavernosum

Genitourinary
diaphragm

Corpus
spongiosum

Figure 1–70. Anatomic relationship of the bladder, prostate, prostatomembranous urethra, and root of the penis. The prostate, situated just below the bladder base, has its apex resting on the genitourinary diaphragm, within which Cowper's glands, with their ducts extending distally, open into the bulbous part of the urethra, which is surrounded by the corpus spongiosum. Two corpora cavernosa diverge at this point, each one gaining fixation to the pubic arch.

Figure 1–71. Oblique dorsolateral view of the back of the bladder, prostate and genitourinary diaphragm. Note the back of the bladder and the vas deferens as well as the seminal vesicles joining to form the ejaculatory duct, which perforates the base of the prostate, to open at the level of the verumontanum. The ureter passes lateral to the vas deferens. The urethra is seen within the conical prostate, the apex of which rests on the genitourinary diaphragm; within it are Cowper's glands, opening into the bulbous part of the urethra.

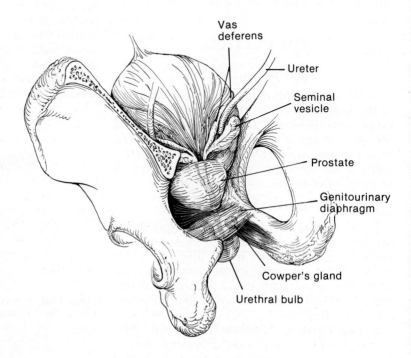

Vas
deferens

Ureter

Seminal
vesicle

Prostate

Genitourinary
diaphragm

Cowper's gland

Urethral bulb

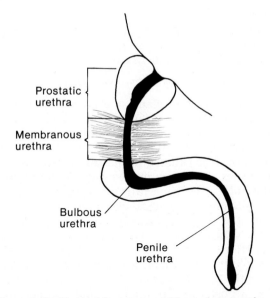

Figure 1–72. Urethral lumen, prostatic urethra, membranous urethra, bulbous urethra, and pendulous urethra, which opens into the external meatus after fusiform dilatation of the navicular fossa.

Prostatic urethra

Membranous urethra

Bulbous urethra

Penile urethra

one bulbourethral gland, the duct of which proceeds caudally to open into the bulbous urethra; on each side, at about the 3 and 9 o'clock positions, pass the cavernous nerves before they proceed to penetrate the crura of the penis.

The Penile Urethra. This segment, the longest, is contained in the corpus spongiosum. About 15 cm in length in the adult male, it extends from the end of the membranous urethra to the external meatus. It has a ventral concave curve in its proximal segment, which is continuous with the membranous urethra until it reaches the lowest level of the symphysis pubis, when it continues into the free part of the penis as the pendulous urethra. The very proximal part of the penile urethra is the widest segment and shows fusiform expansion; it is named the bulb of the urethra and is surrounded by the bulb of the penis and the bulbous spongiosus muscle. In its terminal part, as it enters the glans penis, is another minimal expansion, the fossa navicularis; then it narrows down to open at the external meatus, the narrowest point in the entire canal (Fig. 1–72).

The epithelial lining of the urethra is continuous with that of the bladder; its proximal end is transitional epithelium in nature until the level of the verumontanum. Distal to this point, it is composed of patches of pseudostratified columnar and stratified epithelium. Numerous mucous glands open into the urethra. The urethra has a rich submucosal layer, which is quite vascular and erectile.

THE FEMALE URETHRA

The female urethra is about 4 cm in length and about 6 mm in diameter. It begins at the internal meatus, approximately opposite the middle of the symphysis pubis, and runs anteriorferiorly behind the symphysis with a gentle ventral curvature firmly adherent to the anterior wall of the vagina (See Figs. 1–59 and 1–65). It traverses the perineal membrane and ends at the external urethral orifice, which is a vertical slit with prominent margins situated directly anterior to the opening of the vagina and about 2.5 cm behind the glans clitoris. Except during the passage of urine, the urethral lumen is stellate in shape and completely occluded. The epithelial lining is thrown into longitudinal folds, with many small mucous urethral glands opening throughout the entire length of the urethra. This glandular structure becomes prominent toward its distal end. Some of the glands are usually grouped together and open into one duct, the paraurethral duct, which opens at the lateral margin of the external urethral meatus. These glands are considered to be the homolog of the male prostate, and the term "female prostate" is sometimes applied to them, but they never acquire the complexity of the prostatic gland. Developmentally, the female urethra corresponds to the supramontanal part of the prostatic urethra.

The female urethra, as discussed earlier, represents the entire sphincteric mechanism for the bladder; it has a strong muscular wall, composed primarily of two coats—an inner longitudinal coat continuous with the detrusor inner longitudinal musculature, and an outer semicircular coat continuous with the detrusor outer longitudinal coat. At the middle urethral third, there is dense condensation of striated muscle fibers in the form of a ring; these fibers are partially deficient in the midline posteriorly, where they fuse into the urethrovaginal septum. Again, the urethral mucous membrane is transitional epithelium, becoming stratified squamous epithelium toward the external meatus, with a few islands of pseudostratified columnar epithelium. The submucosa is very vascular. The entire urethra is rich in elastic and collagen fibers. The female urethra is much more readily dilatable than that of the male.

INNERVATION

The muscular element of the prostatomembranous urethra in the male and the entire urethra in the female receive innervation from both divisions of the autonomic nervous system and from the somatic system. Parasympathetic cholinergic nerve endings as well as adrenergic nerve endings, especially alpha-adrenergic, are noted throughout the entire length of the urethra. Somatic fibers coming from the pudendal nerve supply the striated external urinary sphincter in both sexes.

RADIOGRAPHIC ANATOMY

The normal female urethra, well visualized during good voiding cystourethrography, is a uniform, smooth, wide, tubular structure with gentle ventral curvature, adequate lumen throughout, and relative narrowing right at the meatus.

The male urethra can be visualized readily either by retrograde studies or by voiding films. Delineation of its three main segments can be easily made radiologically.

AUXILIARY GENITAL GLANDS IN THE MALE

The auxiliary genital glands in the male consist of the seminal vesicles, the prostate, and the bulbous urethral glands, whose secretory products contribute to the seminal fluid.

The Prostate Gland

EMBRYOLOGIC ORIGIN

The prostate starts to develop at the twelfth week of embryonic life under the influence of androgenic hormones from the fetal testes. Numerous epithelial outpouchings from the urethra develop (See Fig. 1–57A). At that time, the urethra, which is the distal part of the urogenital sinus, has already acquired its own mesenchyme; this mesenchyme will later differentiate to a fibromuscular wall. This epithelial budding occurs both above and below the level of the müllerian tubercle and the adjacent opening of the ejaculatory duct. The incorporation of a wolffian element into this segment of the urogenital sinus could be a factor in the future development and differentiation of the adult prostate, as will be discussed later. The outpouching of these buds branches and rebranches to form the racemose glandular element; between them is entangled the fibromuscular tissue originally continuous with the bladder and now the prostatic stroma proper, the function of which is primarily sphincteric. All these urethral

buds will become confluent and constitute one muscular glandular organ, which will acquire an outside capsule formed from the condensation of this fibromuscular tissue.

ANATOMIC RELATIONSHIPS

The prostate gland is classically described as a compressed inverted cone. It is a firm, partly glandular, and partly fibromuscular body surrounding the very beginning of the male urethra. It is situated in the true pelvis, behind the inferior border of the symphysis pubis and the pubic arch lying in front of the ampulla of the rectum. The conical gland has its continuity with the neck of the urinary bladder (Fig. 1–73), while its apex is inferior, lying on the superior aspect of the superior fascia of the urogenital diaphragm, which is itself continuous with the fascial sheath of the prostate. The gland has a posterior, an anterior, and two inferolateral surfaces. The posterior surface is flattened transversely and vertically is convex. It lies in front of the ampulla of the rectum, separated from it by its own capsule and by Denonvilliers' fascia. The upper border of the posterior surface is the vesicoprostatic junction. The anterior surface is relatively narrow and convex and extends from the apex to the base. It is about 2.0 cm behind the pubic symphysis, separated

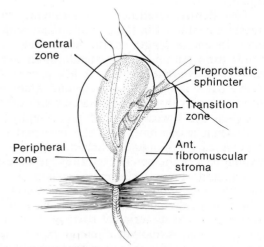

Figure 1–73. Prostate gland (anatomy adapted from McNeal's description). Note the conical configuration and the acute curvature of the urethra as it passes through the gland and the division of the prostate into a peripheral zone, a central zone, and an anterior fibromuscular stroma joining the former anteriorly. The ejaculatory ducts pass through the substance of the prostate to open at the level of the verumontanum. Just cranial to this point is the concentration of the preprostatic sphincter, and at that level also there is a transition zone that is assumed to be the site of benign prostatic hyperplasia. (Adapted from McNeal, J.E.: UICC Monographs, *48*:24, 1979.)

from it by a rich plexus of veins and some loose adipose tissue. Near its upper limit, it is connected to the pubic bone by the puboprostatic ligament. The urethra traverses the substance of the prostate and emerges a little anterosuperior to the apex of the prostate. The inferolateral surfaces are prominent and are related to the anterior part of the levator ani muscles, which are separated from the gland by a rich plexus of veins embedded in fibrous tissue forming the lateral part of the prostatic sheath.

The prostate measures about 3.5 cm transversely at its base and about 2.5 cm in its vertical and anteroposterior dimensions. Its normal weight is about 18 gm. It has a fibromuscular stroma directly continuous with the fibromuscular element of the gland itself, which, in turn, is directly continuous with the muscular element of the smooth musculature of the bladder neck. This fibromuscular stroma condenses on the periphery of the gland to form the prostatic capsule proper. The prostate is also surrounded by another fascia called the prostatic sheath, made up primarily of fibrous tissue in which a rich plexus of veins is embedded. Anteriorly the sheath is continuous with the puboprostatic ligament, and inferiorly it blends with the fascia on the deep surface of the transversus perinei. Posteriorly it is fused with the obliterated rectovesical peritoneal pouch, which at the embryologic stage extended downward to the pelvic floor but which now forms a dense layer known as the fascia of Denonvilliers, separating the rectum from the posterior of the prostate as well as the seminal vesicles and the bladder base.

STRUCTURE

The prostate gland is a musculoglandular structure. Approximately 30 per cent of its weight is a muscular mass, while the rest is a glandular epithelial element. The ducts and acini of the glandular element are lined by columnar epithelium; they gather to drain into the posterior aspect of the prostatic urethra on either side of the median elevation, as the prostatic ducts. The glandular element is primarily in the posterior and lateral parts, while the anterior segment is mainly fibromuscular.

Former classification divided the prostate gland into five lobes: anterior lobe, posterior lobe, median lobe, and two lateral lobes, as the glandular element relates to the three ducts passing through it—the prostatic urethra and the two ejaculatory ducts—which meet at the level of the verumontanum. The median lobe would be the segment trapped in the triangle between the urethra anteriorly and the plane of the ejaculatory ducts posteriorly. The posterior lobe would be behind the plane of the ejaculatory ducts and in contact with the inframontanal part of the prostatic urethra. The lateral lobes would be on each side of the urethra, whereas the anterior lobe would be a purely fibromuscular commissure joining the two lateral lobes anterior to the urethra. This classification, based on the work of Lowsley, considered that the prostate originates from five separate groups of glandular embryonic elements that later fuse as one uniform gland.

However, recent understanding of the development and structure of the prostate shows that separating the gland into five lobes does not describe any anatomic reality. After detailed anatomic and histologic study of the adult prostate, McNeal (1970) established a different nomenclature for its various parts and divided the glandular elements into two main units, the central zone and the much larger peripheral zone. Together, these two zones constitute about 95 per cent of the whole glandular structure. The remaining 5 per cent forms the transition zone, located right outside the supramontanal muscular segment of the urethra; it is assumed that this is the site of origin of all prostatic hyperplasia. The glandular tissue of this transition zone is identical to that of the peripheral zone, yet it is known that the transition zone is never the site of malignancy, whereas the peripheral zone is a common site of prostatic carcinoma. It is worth noting that the peripheral zone and the transition zone as well as the periurethral glands form an anatomic and histologic continuum, probably reflecting their common embryonic origin—the urogenital sinus. On the other hand, the central zone is morphologically distinctive; it is conceivable that its origin is embryonic wolffian duct tissue incorporated into the prostatic gland (McNeal's) (Fig. 1–73).

Condensation of smooth muscular elements in the supramontanal segment of the urethra adds to the sphincteric mechanism. From our experimental studies we were able to suggest that this muscular condensation may be considered as a genital sphincter in the male, since no counterpart exists in the female. It is probably mesonephric in origin, and its primary function may be to occlude the lumen, thus preventing retrograde ejaculation.

LIGAMENTS AND ATTACHMENTS

The prostate is well fixed in its place. Its apex rests on the superior aspect of the genitourinary diaphragm and is attached to the back of the pubic bone by the dense avascular puboprostatic ligament. It is firmly adherent to the base of the bladder superiorly and confined within the prostatic sheath, which is a reflection from the endopelvic fascia; it is well supported posteriorly by the obliterated peritoneal pouch forming the fascia of Denonvilliers.

BLOOD SUPPLY

Arterial Supply. The main blood supply to the prostate is from the inferior vesical artery, which, in turn, is a branch of the anterior division of the hypogastric artery. The vesical artery supplies branches to the lower ureter and seminal vesicle and then penetrates the substance of the prostate at the prostatovesical junction at about the 8 and 4 o'clock positions. The main trunk of the prostatic artery divides into two main branches—a peripheral one and a central branch. The central branch goes toward the urethra, supplying the urethral wall and the periurethral prostatic glands, while the peripheral branch supplies the main bulk of the prostate.

Venous Drainage. Although there are veins accompanying these arteries, the veins of the prostate are numerous; they join to form a very rich venous plexus, situated between the prostate and the prostatic sheath. The rich venous plexus of the prostate has free communication with the inferior hypogastric venous system as well as the presacral prevertebral venous plexus.

LYMPHATIC DRAINAGE

The primary lymphatic drainage from the prostatic gland goes to the external and internal iliac groups as well as to the obturator lymph nodes. Lymphatics from all these sites congregate and join the common iliac lymph nodes and then the preaortic lymph nodes.

NERVE SUPPLY

The prostate receives a rich nerve supply from both divisions of the autonomic nervous system. The sympathetic supply is probably all secretory and pervades the glandular element, but some of it may also innervate the preprostatic sphincteric unit (genital sphincter). The parasympathetic element supplies most of the muscular stroma of the prostate, which, as indicated earlier, is directly continuous with the musculature of the bladder and constitutes the main urinary sphincteric function for the prostatic urethra.

STRUCTURAL CHANGES WITH AGE

The prostate undergoes very little structural change until the age of puberty (around the tenth year). At that time, there is a significant hyperplasia of the duct epithelium and the formation of site buds, leading to an elaboration of the duct system; this development is accompanied by continuous slow increase of the size and mass of the prostate. At puberty, presumably in response to increased testosterone secretion, these changes accelerate and the prepubertal gland rapidly grows to more than twice its size, mainly from the development of acini and follicles. There is also an increase in stroma condensation. In the third decade, the complexity of the glandular element increases, with considerable infolding of the epithelium in the lumen of the follicles. The prostate remains constant in size until about the age of 45 or 50 years, when the infolding of the epithelial lumen tends to disappear: This indicates the beginning of prostatic involution. This is the time when benign prostatic hyperplasia may originate, usually in the periurethral glands or the transition zone; as it progresses, benign prostatic hyperplasia leads to compression atrophy of the original central and peripheral zones of the prostate.

The Seminal Vesicles

EMBRYOLOGIC ORIGIN

This paired organ arises as an outpouching of the terminal end of the ductus deferens. It is a highly convoluted glandular sac, about 2 inches long and not more than 1 cm wide. The seminal vesicles lie lateral to the ductus deferens on the posterior surface of the bladder base. Their coiled, membranous pouches secrete a fluid that is important to the survival of spermatozoa. The seminal vesicles were formerly thought to be storage compartments for sperm, but this has proved not to be true. However, they have a considerable luminal storage capacity, an average of 4 ml. The seminal vesicles are not palpable on rectal examination unless they are distended, inflamed, or obstructed.

MICROSCOPIC STRUCTURE

The mucous lining of the seminal vesicles, which is made up of many folds and usually is of pseudostratified columnar epithelium, contains some goblet cells whose secretions contribute to the bulk of the seminal fluid. The muscular wall is quite thin, essentially of one layer.

The Bulbourethral Glands

The bulbourethral glands, or Cowper's glands, are located in the deep perineal compartment, which will be discussed later. They lie on each side of the membranous urethra between the fascial layers of the urogenital diaphragm. Their ducts, however, run distally for about 3 or 4 mm into the corpus spongiosum of the penile bulb before they open into the bulbous urethra. They add a mucoid secretion to the seminal fluid.

THE SCROTUM

CONFIGURATION

The scrotal pouch is situated below the penis and the pubic symphysis. It is partitioned into two sacs by a partial median septum. Each compartment contains the male gonad, or testis, and its associated epididymis as well as the lower portion of the spermatic cord with its coverings.

The scrotal sac consists of (1) skin; (2) dartos muscle, which largely replaces superficial fat and Colles' fascia; (3) a thin lamina of external spermatic fascia; (4) slips of cremasteric muscle; (5) the internal spermatic fascia; and (6) an inner lining of parietal peritoneum (tunica vaginalis).

Dartos Muscle. The dartos muscle is a smooth muscle whose strands are imbedded in a bit of loose areolar tissue. When this muscle contracts, as when it is cold or during sexual stimulation, the size of the scrotum appears to shrink and its skin becomes wrinkled like that of a dried prune. A warm environment relaxes the scrotum, thus allowing more space and sagging for its contents.

External Spermatic Fascia. The external spermatic fascia is a continuation of the external oblique aponeurosis. A few slips of skeletal muscle derived from the internal oblique muscle constitute the cremasteric muscle, which adds to the scrotal wall in its upper part.

Internal Spermatic Fascia. The internal spermatic fascia is a continuation of the transversalis fascia. The transversus abdominis itself contributes nothing to the cord covering or to the scrotum, as it does not extend to the inguinal region, except as an aponeurotic slip behind the superficial ring.

Tunica Vaginalis. The peritoneal tunica vaginalis, once continuous with the peritoneal cavity but cut off from it by the obliteration of the processus vaginalis, provides the covering for the testis. It reflects as a visceral tunica over the testis and the epididymis.

BLOOD SUPPLY

The anterior scrotum derives its blood supply from the external pudendal artery, which is a branch of the femoral artery anteriorly. Posteriorly, branches of the internal pudendal artery reach the scrotum. Additional supply comes to it from the cremasteric and testicular arteries, which traverse the spermatic cord.

The ilioinguinal and genitofemoral nerves supply continuous branches to the anterior wall. The posterior scrotal nerve branches of the perineal division of the pudendal nerve supply the posterior wall. The posterior femoral cutaneous nerves help to innervate the scrotal skin.

LYMPHATIC DRAINAGE

The lymphatic drainage of the scrotum is to the superficial inguinal nodes.

Scrotal Contents: Embryologic Origin

Although sex is determined at the time of fertilization, the sex glands or gonads do not differentiate as male or female structures until the seventh week of intrauterine life. They appear as an indifferent gonad early in the fifth week. The genital ridge appears at the fourth week of embryonic life; however, its cellular element does not appear until the sixth week. The inner aspect of this epithelial mass becomes subdivided into sex cords, which are connected to the superficial germinal epithelium from which they grow. They migrate along the dorsal mesentery of the hindgut to enter the area of the genital ridge at about the sixth week. In the genital ridge are the undifferentiated gonads; they start to differentiate into testes by the seventh week. The sex cords, at first lacking a lumen, are actually of three types: (1) those near the mesorchium, forming a network, the rete testes; (2) short tubules radiating from the rete as tubule recti and connecting with (3) the longest aspect of the cord, the convoluted part that later canalizes, becoming convoluted (or seminiferous) tubules. The lumina are not acquired until puberty. In these cords are found the primary germ cells—the spermatogonia, the supporting cells that later become the Sertoli cells when the testis matures at puberty. In the mesenchyme between the cords or future tubules, the interstitial (Leydig) cells are the endocrine secretors of testosterone; they make their appearance as early as the fourth or fifth month of development in utero.

The male genital ducts are paired tubes known as the wolffian ducts. The cranial portion of the wolffian duct in both sexes is used as the secretory element, while its caudal stretch becomes associated with the developing gonad (sex cords), which unite with some of the degenerating mesonephric tubules. In the male, these tubules of the old nephric kidney become the efferent ducts of the epididymis. Part of the mesonephric duct, in which such tubules empty, becomes the duct of the epididymis, and its more caudal part becomes the ductus deferens, or vas deferens. The latter will lose its contact with the ureteral bud to empty alone into the urethra below the level of the bladder on either side of the müllerian tubercle, and will be known as the ejaculatory ducts. It is from this terminal part that the outpouching of the seminal vesicles as a blind diverticulum takes place. Some of the degenerating tubules that fail to become efferent ductules persist as rudimentary structures; they are known as the paradidymis, the cranial and caudal aberrant ductules. The blind cranial end of the upper part of the mesonephric duct remains attached to the epididymis as the appendix epididymis, while the appendix testes is a mesonephric or wolffian duct derivative.

THE TESTES

The testes are the male reproductive organs. Their glandular structure is about 4 to 5 cm in length and 2 to 3 cm in thickness. They lie within the scrotal sac, suspended by the spermatic cords. The tunica vaginalis, as visceral peritoneum, covers the testis everywhere except where it attaches to the epididymis and the spermatic cord. A capsule on the outside and numerous septa divide the testes into various compartments; these compartments converge toward the upper pole at the mediastinum region, which contains the rete testis. The septa compartmentalize the testes into as many as 400 lobules, each of which is occupied by two or more highly convoluted seminiferous tubules; if a tubule were stretched to full length, it would extend to 2 feet. It is from the epithelial lining of the tubule that spermatozoa are formed (Fig. 1–74). These tubules converge toward the rete network, where they connect by straight tubular recti, which join to open into the head of the epididymis. Most of the lining cells of the straight tubules consist of Sertoli cell elements, so that little spermatogenesis occurs at this level. The straight tubules can be considered as the first segment of the duct system.

Blood Supply. The blood supply to the testis is closely associated with that to the kidney because of their common embryologic origin.

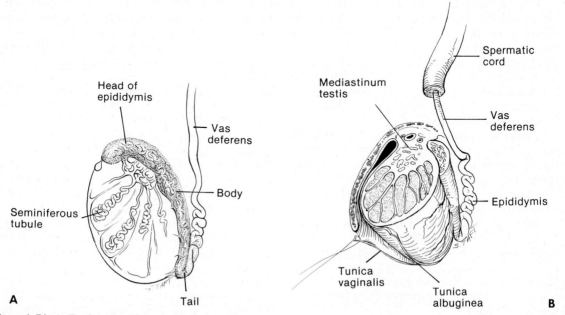

A, Head of epididymis — Vas deferens — Body — Seminiferous tubule — Tail

B, Mediastinum testis — Spermatic cord — Vas deferens — Epididymis — Tunica vaginalis — Tunica albuginea

Figure 1–74. *A*, Testis and epididymis. Note the numerous compartments of the testis, filled with the seminiferous tubules gathering into the rete testis; they join to form a markedly convoluted tubule, which becomes the epididymis that leads to the vas deferens. *B*, Cross sections of the testis show the several compartments and the mediastinum testis, as well as the coverings of the testis, with the tunica albuginea firmly adherent to its substance and the potential space surrounded by the tunica vaginalis. The epididymis attaches to the dorsomedial aspect of the testis, and the vas deferens joins the other structures of the spermatic cord.

ARTERIAL SUPPLY. The arterial supply to the testis is derived from the internal spermatics, which arise from the aorta just below the renal arteries and course through the spermatic cord to the testis, where they anastomose with the cremasterics and the arteries of the vas branching off from the hypogastric artery. All contribute to the blood supply to the testis.

VENOUS RETURN. The blood from the testis returns to the pampiniform plexus of the spermatic cord at the internal inguinal ring. The pampiniform plexus forms the spermatic veins. The right spermatic vein enters the vena cava just below the right renal vein, while the left spermatic vein empties into the left renal vein.

Lymphatics. The lymphatic drainage from the testes passes to the lumbar lymph nodes, which, in turn, are connected to the mediastinal lymph nodes.

EPIDIDYMIS

The epididymis is usually divided into three segments: a head, a body, and a tail. The head is situated at the upper pole of the testis, the body lies behind the testis on its posterior aspect, and the tail is attached to the inferior extremity. It is important to note that the body and tail of the epididymis are actually one single tube.

The straight seminiferous tubules enter the fibrous tissue of the mediastinum testes and pass upward and backward, forming at their ascent a close network of anastomosing tubules lined by flattened epithelium. This network is named the rete testis. The upper end of the mediastinum testis forms 12 to 20 ducts termed the efferent ductules, which perforate the tunica vaginalis and pass from the testis to the epididymis. The efferent ductules have at first a straight course; they then become enlarged and exceedingly convoluted, forming a series of conical masses known as the lobules of the epididymis, which together form its head. Each lobule consists of a single convoluted duct about 15 to 20 cm long. All ducts open into one, the duct of the epididymis, with complex convolutions, forming the body of the epididymis. This convoluted tubule, if stretched, will be 6 meters in length. It increases in diameter and thickness as it approaches the tail of the epididymis, where it becomes the ductus deferens. The convolutions are held together by fine areolar tissue and by bands of fibrous tissue.

DUCTUS (VAS) DEFERENS

This is a very thick, muscular duct 2 to 3 mm in diameter and about 18 inches long. Because of its heavy muscular coat it can be easily palpated through the scrotum and through the soft tissues of the spermatic cord. It travels through the spermatic cord and the inguinal canal, in company with the fascia and the cremasteric muscle of the cord, as well as the testicular artery, the pampiniform plexus, the lymphatics and nerves, and the epididymis of the testis. The vas deferens, however, has its own arterial supply, which is known as the artery of the vas deferens; it usually is a branch of the umbilical or internal iliac artery.

Leaving the cord, the ductus deferens loops over the origin of the inferior epigastric artery and passes extraperitoneally, caudally, and laterally in the pelvic wall. It passes medial to the distal end of the ureter, bends caudally to reach the midline, and lies on the posterior wall of the bladder, just medial to the seminal vesicle (Figs. 1–70 to 1–72). It terminates in a dilated, spindle-shaped ampulla, which lies between the base of the bladder and the rectum, from which it is separated by the rectovesical fascia; it finally passes downward to the base of the prostate, where it is joined at an acute angle by the duct of the seminal vesicle to form the ejaculatory duct.

Ejaculatory Duct. This is the short (about 2 cm), slender termination of the vas deferens after it has joined the duct of the seminal vesicle. It traverses the glandular tissue of the prostate to open into the prostatic urethra at the crista urethralis on either side of the prostatic utricle. The walls of the ejaculatory duct are thin, containing an outer fibrous layer and a thin layer of muscular fibers, which has an outer circular and an inner longitudinal layer. The mucous membrane is columnar epithelium.

SPERMATIC CORD AND ITS COVERING

When the testis descends into the scrotum, passing through the abdominal wall, it carries with it its vessels, its nerve supply, and its lymphatics as well as the ductus deferens. All these structures meet at the deep inguinal ring and together form the spermatic cord, which then suspends the testes in the scrotum and extends from the deep inguinal ring to the posterior border of the testes. The spermatic cord traverses the inguinal canal, having the walls of the canal as its boundary, with the ilioinguinal nerve lying in the floor of the canal. In passing through the canal it acquires covering from the layers of the abdominal wall. These coverings extend downward into the wall of the scrotum and are named the internal spermatic, cremasteric, and external spermatic fasciae. The internal spermatic fascia is a thin layer that loosely invests the spermatic cord and is derived from the transversalis fascia. The cremasteric fascia consists of a number of fasciculi united to one another by areolar tissue and continuous with the internal oblique muscle. The external spermatic fascia is a continuation of the aponeurosis of the external oblique muscle and descends from the crura of the superficial ring.

Blood and Lymph Supply. The spermatic cord is composed of arteries, veins, lymph vessels, nerves, and vas deferens; all of these are connected by areolar tissues. The arteries of the spermatic cord are the testicular artery, the cremasteric artery, and the artery of the vas. The testicular veins form the pampiniform plexus. The lymph vessels are those of the testes, which ascend to the lumbar lymphatics. The nerves are the genital branch of the genitofemoral nerve and the testicular plexus and of the sympathetic hypogastric plexus, which is joined by filaments from the pelvic plexus.

THE PENIS

EMBRYOLOGIC ORIGIN

The penis has two separate origins for its three erectile bodies. When the paired genital tubercles meet in the midline, they are responsible for the formation of the paired corpora cavernosa and their crura, which are attached to the bony pelvis. The development of the caudal end of the urogenital sinus and the paired urethral folds are responsible for the development of the bulbous and penile urethra, with the surrounding spongy tissue, which expands distally to form the glans penis.

GROSS ANATOMY

The penis is divided into three portions: the root, the body, and the glans. The root lies in the superficial perineal pouch and provides fixation and stability. The body, which constitutes the major part, is composed of three spongy erectile tissues completely covered by skin (Fig. 1–75). The glans is the distal expansion of the corpus spongiosum; it is conical and normally covered by the loose skin of the prepuce.

The two cavernous bodies lie on the dorsum of the penis and are surrounded by a double layer of dense fibrous connective tissue named Buck's fascia (tunica albuginea). They are incompletely separated by a layer of the same tissue, the septum penis, through the major part of the penile body; approaching the perineum, the corpora diverge from each other to form the crura. Each crus penis diverges from its fellow, undergoes some enlargement, and gains attachment to the pubic arch all the way down to the tuberosity of the ischia, where it has a bluntly pointed process. Each crus is firmly adherent to the ramus of the ischia and pubis and is surrounded by the fibers of the ischiocavernosus muscles. The corpus spongiosum of the penis is an erectile mass similar to that of the corpus cavernosum, but of finer construction. It surrounds the urethra, is central in position, and lies in the ventral aspect of the penis. Its midportion is of uniform thickness and forms a part of the penile shaft. However, its posterior end is bulbous (the bulbous penis); surrounded by

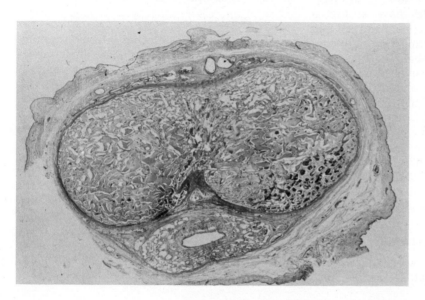

Figure 75. Histologic cross section of the adult male penis shows the main three spongy units—the two corpora cavernosa in the dorsum, and the corpus spongiosum with the urethra in its center. In the ventral portion, note the incomplete septum separating the two corpora cavernosa and the tunica albuginea as well as Buck's fascia surrounding the body of the penis.

the bulbospongiosus muscle, it lies in the superficial perineal pouch. The anterior end of the corpus spongiosum is expanded and forms the glans penis, which fits closely over the blunt rounded end of the corpus cavernosum; its raised, rounded, conical end-shape terminates the body of the penis. The urethra opens by a vertical slit at the end of the glans.

The three elongated masses of erectile tissue constituting the body of the penis are capable of considerable enlargement when they are engorged with blood during erection. When flaccid, the body of the penis is cylindrical; when erect, it approaches the form of a triangular prism with rounded angles. This erectile tissue is of spongelike meshwork of endothelium-lined spaces, surrounded by smooth muscle tissue. The skin covering the penis is remarkable for its thinness, its dark color, and its looseness of connection with the fascial sheath of the organ.

The skin of the penis is folded upon itself to form the prepuce or foreskin, which overlaps the glans for a considerable distance. The internal layer of the prepuce is confluent along the line of the neck with the thin skin that covers and adheres firmly to the glans and is continuous with the mucous membrane of the urethra at the external meatus. The prepuce is separated from the glans penis by a potential space or cleft, the preputial sac. Again, there is a superficial fascia, remarkable for the lack of any fat and consisting of loosely arranged areolar tissue into which a few fibers of the dartos muscle extend from the scrotum.

The penis is supported and suspended by two ligaments; both are continuous with the fascia of the penis and are mainly of elastic fibers. The fundiform ligament is continuous with the lower end of the linea alba; then it splits into lamina that surround the body of the penis and unite underneath it and fuse with the septa of the scrotum. The suspensory ligament, which is deep to the fundiform ligament, is triangular and attached above the front of the pubic symphysis; below, it blends with the fascia of the penis on each side of the organ.

BLOOD SUPPLY

Arterial Supply. The penis is a highly vascular organ. Most of its blood supply is from the internal pudendal artery, a branch of the hypogastric artery. This provides three main branches: the deep artery of the penis, the bulbal artery, and the urethral artery (Fig. 1–76). The deep artery of the penis runs through the entire corpus cavernosum and enters the crus toward its proximal end, at its inferomedial aspect. It supplies the entire corpus cavernosum. The urethral artery supplies branches to the corpus spongiosum, while the bulbal artery supplies the bulbous urethra as well as the bulbous spongiosus. There is also the deep dorsal artery of the penis, which runs below the transversus pubic ligament, to proceed forward to the dorsum of the penis between the layers of the suspensory ligament; it lies between the two dorsal veins and the dorsal nerves of the penis, below the penile Buck's fascia. This artery continues to supply the glans penis.

Venous Drainage. The venous return is again through three main channels: the cavernous veins and the deep and superficial dorsal veins. The cavernous vein is responsible for the venous drainage from the corpus cavernosum. The circumflex veins join the deep dorsal vein of the penis, while the superficial dorsal veins lie outside Buck's fascia and drain the prepuce and the skin of the penis and empty into the external pudendal vein. The dorsal vein drains the glans penis, as well as a good share of the

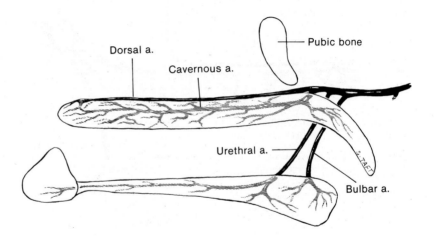

Figure 1–76. Arterial blood supply to the penis, where the two corpora cavernosa are separated from the corpus spongiosum. Note that the pudendal artery branches into the deep cavernous artery; also, it will give two other main branches, the bulbar artery and the urethral artery. The latter will supply the corpus spongiosum and the glans penis. The dorsal artery of the penis also sends blood supply to the glans penis.

Dorsal a.

Cavernous a.

Pubic bone

Urethral a.

Bulbar a.

cavernous spaces of the corpus cavernosum, and proceeds to pass between the suspensory ligament of the penis to enter the urogenital diaphragm between the arcuate and transversus pubic ligament (Fig. 1–77). It empties into the prostatic plexus.

NERVE SUPPLY

The nerve supply of the penis is primarily from the pelvic plexus, which is formed by the parasympathetic component coming from S_2–S_4, as well as a sympathetic contribution from the hypogastric plexus. A portion of the pelvic plexus, known as the prostatic plexus, lies in the cleft between the prostate and the rectum. From the prostatic plexus, a few branches proceed toward the apex of the prostate and enter dorsolaterally, perforating the genitourinary diaphragm and lying lateral to the membranous urethra and then entering the crura to be the main nerve supply to the corpus cavernosum. It is assumed that these cavernous nerves are responsible for the process of erection.

LYMPHATIC DRAINAGE

The superficial and deep inguinal lymph nodes drain to the external and common iliac nodes.

THE PERINEUM

General Description

The perineum is the most inferior end of the trunk. It is a diamond-shaped area lying between the thighs and the buttocks. It is bounded anteriorly by the pubic symphysis, laterally by the ischial tuberosity, and posteriorly by the coccyx. A line passing transversely between the ischial tuberosity through the central part of the perineum will divide the latter into an anterior urogenital triangle and a posterior anal triangle. The central part of the perineum, located between the anus and the urethral bulb in the male and between the anus and the vestibule in the female, overlies the perineal body. In the male, a median ridge, the perineal raphe, passes from the anus to become the median raphe of the scrotum and the ventral raphe of the penis.

THE ANAL TRIANGLE

The anatomy of the anal triangle is the same in both sexes. If the skin is removed, a fatty fascial layer is found, the same as the superficial fascia of the abdominal wall. It is also continuous with a similar fatty fascial layer in the urogenital triangle. In the center of the anal triangle is the opening of the anal canal. On both sides is the ischiorectal fossa, which is bounded by the ischial tuberosity as well as the sloping surface of the levator ani. Traversing the ischiorectal fossa are the inferior rectal arteries and nerves, the pudendal nerve, and the internal pudendal artery, which course through the pudendal canal, or Alcock's canal. The anal canal is surrounded by the anal sphincter, which has three divisions—subcutaneous, superficial, and deep. The subcutaneous part completely encircles the anus and is just deep to the skin. The superficial portion of the external sphincter is attached posteriorly to the coccygeal ligament and the coccyx and anteriorly

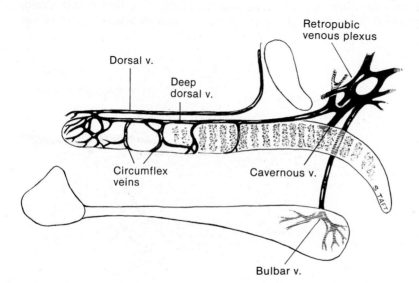

Dorsal v.

Deep
dorsal v.

Circumflex
veins

Cavernous v.

Bulbar v.

Retropubic
venous plexus

Figure 1–77. Venous drainage of the penis. Note that the cavernous spaces accumulate into one main vein, the cavernous vein, which is shown as a distinct body (in reality it is a very short segment) before it is joined by the deep dorsal vein, collecting all the circumflex veins; these two veins join the bulbar vein; together they branch out into the dense retropubic venous plexus.

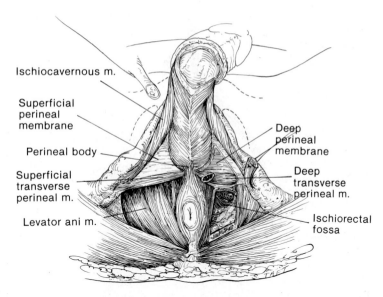

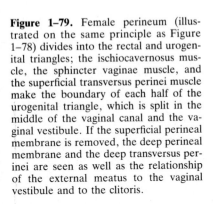

Figure 1–79. Female perineum (illustrated on the same principle as Figure 1–78) divides into the rectal and urogenital triangles; the ischiocavernosus muscle, the sphincter vaginae muscle, and the superficial transversus perinei muscle make the boundary of each half of the urogenital triangle, which is split in the middle of the vaginal canal and the vaginal vestibule. If the superficial perineal membrane is removed, the deep perineal membrane and the deep transversus perinei are seen as well as the relationship of the external meatus to the vaginal vestibule and to the clitoris.

to the perineal body. The deep portion completely encircles the anal canal; this portion is intimately fused with the sling portion of the levator ani muscle. The last two portions, the superficial and deep parts of the external sphincter, are just outside the internal anal sphincter, which is constituted primarily of the smooth musculature of the anal canal itself.

THE UROGENITAL TRIANGLE

The urogenital triangle is much more complex than the anal triangle and is different in male and female.

The Skin and Fatty Layer. If the superficial fascia is removed from the urogenital triangle

of the perineum, a membranous layer of the superficial fascia (Colles' fascia) can be seen. It will be attached posteriorly along the line that divides the urogenital triangle from the anal triangle and laterally to the pubic rami and the deep fascia on the side. This is a continuation of a membranous layer of the superficial fascia of the abdominal wall. It is also the same fascial layer that forms the dartos muscle of the scrotum; this same fascia is continuous over the penis. The attachment of this layer of fascia is quite important in relation to urinary extravasation associated with extrapelvic urethral rupture.

If the fascia is removed, the contents of the

Figure 1–79. Female perineum (illustrated on the same principle as Figure 1–78) divides into the rectal and urogenital triangles; the ischiocavernosus muscle, the sphincter vaginae muscle, and the superficial transversus perinei muscle make the boundary of each half of the urogenital triangle, which is split in the middle of the vaginal canal and the vaginal vestibule. If the superficial perineal membrane is removed, the deep perineal membrane and the deep transversus perinei are seen as well as the relationship of the external meatus to the vaginal vestibule and to the clitoris.

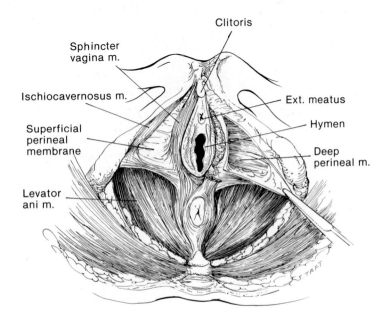

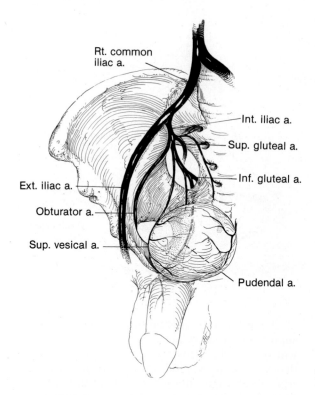

Rt. common
iliac a.

Int. iliac a.

Sup. gluteal a.

Inf. gluteal a.

Ext. iliac a.

Obturator a.

Sup. vesical a.

Pudendal a.

Figure 1–80. The arterial supply of the pelvic organs.

superficial space of the perineum are exposed. In the male, the bulbospongiosus muscle can be seen in the midline, where it covers the bulb of the penis. On either side is the ischiocavernosus muscle covering the two crura of the penis, as they are attached to the ischial and pubic arches. Two small muscles run transversely from the perineal body to the inferior pubic rami—the superficial transversus perinei muscles (Fig. 1–78). In the female, the urogenital triangle, al-

Figure 1–81. Same view as Figure 1–80 with superimposition of the nervous system, defining the sacral roots, the superior hypogastric plexus, the pelvic plexus, the prostatic nerves, the cavernous nerve, the pudendal nerve, and the obturator nerve.

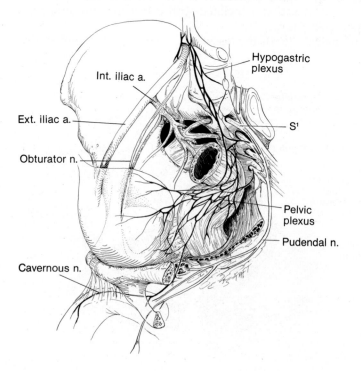

Hypogastric
plexus

Int. iliac a.

Ext. iliac a.

S¹

Obturator n.

Pelvic
plexus

Pudendal n.

Cavernous n.

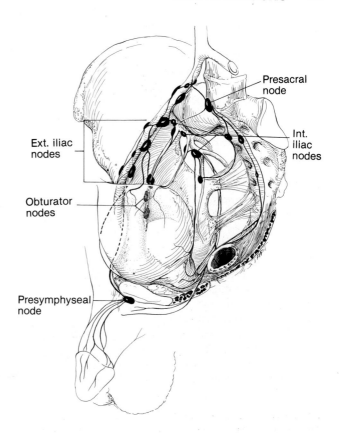

Figure 1–82. Same view as Figure 1–80, with the lymphatic system superimposed.

though different, can be considered similar if one visualizes the bulb of the penis as having been split into two halves by the vagina (Fig. 1–79).

If the contents of the superficial space are removed in the male or the female, the perineal membrane is seen. In the female, in addition to the urethra, there is a larger opening in the perineal membrane for the vagina. If this deep perineal membrane is removed, the contents of the deep space are revealed. Deep to this layer will be the thin sheet of muscle, which in the male is divided into two parts—the anterior part, surrounding the urethra and forming the sphincter urethrae; and the posterior part, the deep transversus perinei. The former muscle, which surrounds the membranous urethra and forms the external sphincter, is under voluntary control. Two glands are also found in the deep pouch of the male—Cowper's glands (the bulbourethral glands). In the female, this arrangement is essentially the same, except that there are also striated muscle fibers surrounding the vaginal canal to form the sphincter vaginae. If the muscles in the deep space are removed, a layer of deep fascia is found, which is continuous with the fascia over the obturator internus mus-

cle; if this fascial layer is removed, one reaches the inferior aspect of the levator ani muscles.

It should be re-emphasized that the only difference between the male and female anatomy in the urogenital triangle is the presence of the vaginal canal separating the midline structures into two parts. The bulbourethral glands in the male are located in the deep space, whereas the corresponding glands in the female (the greater vestibular glands) are located in the superficial space. The layers of the urogenital diaphragm are therefore: (1) the skin; (2 and 3) the fatty and membranous layers of the superficial fascia; (4) the muscular layer in the superficial space; (5) the perineal membrane; (6) the muscular layer in the deep space; and (7) the deep fascial layer. The superficial space is the space enclosing the membranous layer of the superficial fascia and the perineal membrane. The deep space is between the perineal membrane and the deep fascia on the superior side of the deep perineal muscles. This is usually what is referred to as the urogenital diaphragm.

Blood Supply. The internal pudendal artery is the main vessel for the perineum. It follows the course of the pudendal nerve. The vessel is a branch of the anterior division of the hypogastric internal iliac artery. It leaves Alcock's canal, with the pudendal artery giving its branches to the anal triangle, the inferior hemorrhoidal or rectal artery. The artery then divides into deep and superficial branches to enter the perineal pouches or compartments. The superficial branch, entering the superficial pouch as the perineal artery to supply its muscles, moves forward through the superficial compartment as the posterior labial artery or posterior scrotal artery in the male. The deep branches pierce the free posterior edge of the urogenital diaphragm to run between the perineal membrane and deep fascia in the deep compartment to supply the urethral and vaginal sphincter. One branch becomes the artery of the bulb, also called the vestibular artery.

Figures 1–80 to 1–82 represent the essential surgical, anatomic distribution of the arterial blood supply in the pelvis and the complex somatic and parasympathetic neural plexus as well as the lymphatic drainage and lymphatic chains in the pelvis. An attempt is made to relate each to important bony and ligamentous and visceral landmarks for the purpose of clarification and surgical relevance.

References

Becker, R. F., Wilson, J. W., and Gehweiler, J. A.: The perineum and pelvis. *In* Becker, R. F., et al. (Eds): The Anatomical Basis of Medical Practice. Baltimore, The Williams & Wilkins Co., 1971, pp. 637–691.

Bruschini, H., Schmidt, R. A., and Tanagho, E. A.: Studies on the neurophysiology of the vas deferens. Invest. Urol., *15*:112, 1977.

Christensen, J. B., and Telford, I. R.: Perineum and pelvis. *In* Christensen, J. B., and Telford, I. R. (Eds.): Synopsis of Gross Anatomy. 2nd ed. New York, Harper & Row, 1978, pp. 154–183.

Crafts, R. C.: Abdominopelvic cavity and perineum. *In* Crafts, R. C. (Ed.): A Textbook of Human Anatomy. 2nd ed. New York, John Wiley & Sons, 1979, pp. 269–327.

Crouch, J. E.: The urinary system. *In* Crouch, J. E. (Ed.): Functional Human Anatomy. 2nd ed. Philadelphia, Lea & Febiger, 1972, pp. 424–429.

Crouch, J. E.: The reproductive system. *In* Crouch, J. E. (Ed.): Functional Human Anatomy. 2nd ed. Philadelphia, Lea & Febiger, 1972, pp. 430–447.

Droes, J. T. P. M.: Observations on the musculature of the urinary bladder and the urethra in the human foetus. Br. J. Urol., *46*:179, 1974.

Droes, J. T. P. M., van Ulden, B. M., Donker, P. J., and Landsmeer, J. W. F.: Studies of the urethral musculature in the human foetus, newborn and adult. Urol. Int., *29*:231, 1974.

Elbadawi, A.: Anatomy and function of the ureteral sheath. J. Urol., *107*:224, 1972.

Elbadawi, A., and Schenk, E. A.: New theory of innervation of bladder musculature. Part 4. Innervation of vesicourethral junction and external urethral sphincter. J. Urol., *111*:613, 1974.

Elias, H., Pauly, J. E., and Burns, E. R.: Reproductive system. *In* Elias, H., et al. (Eds.): Histology and Human Microanatomy. 4th ed. New York, John Wiley & Sons, 1978, pp. 475–532.

Fletcher, T. F., and Bradley, W. E.: Neuroanatomy of the bladder-urethra. J. Urol., *119*:153, 1978.

Gosling, J. A., and Dixon, J. S.: The structure and innervation of smooth muscle in the wall of the bladder neck and proximal urethra. Br. J. Urol., *47*:549, 1975.

Hodges, C. V.: Surgical anatomy of the urinary bladder and pelvic ureter. Surg. Clin. North Am., *44*:1327, 1964.

Hutch, J. A.: Anatomy and Physiology of the Bladder, Trigone and Urethra. New York, Appleton-Century-Crofts, 1972.

Jonas, U., and Tanagho, E. A.: Studies on vesicourethral reflexes. I. Urethral sphincteric responses to detrusor stretch. Invest. Urol., *12*:357, 1975.

Jonas, U. and Tanagho, E. A.: Studies on vesicourethral reflexes. II. Urethral sphincteric responses to spinal cord stimulation. Invest. Urol., *13*:278, 1976.

McNeal, J. E.: The prostate and prostatic urethra: A morphologic study. J. Urol., *104*:443, 1970.

Romanes, G. J.: The pelvis and perineum. *In* Romanes, G. J. (Ed.): Cunningham's Manual of Practical Anatomy. 14th ed. Vol. 2: Thorax and Abdomen. New York, Oxford University Press, 1977, pp. 160–208.

Tanagho, E. A.: The anatomy and physiology of micturition. Clin. Obstet. Gynecol., *5*:3, 1978.

Tanagho, E. A.: Anatomy of the genitourinary tract. *In* Smith, D. R. (Ed.): General Urology. 10th ed. Los Altos, Calif., Lange Medical Publications, 1981, pp. 1–12.

Tanagho, E. A., and Miller, E. R.: Functional considerations of urethral sphincteric dynamics. J. Urol., *109*:273, 1973.

Tanagho, E. A., Miller, E. R., Meyers, F. H., and Corbett, R. K.: Observations on the dynamics of the bladder neck. Br. J. Urol., *38*:72, 1966.

Tanagho, E. A., and Pugh, R. C. B.: The anatomy and function of the ureterovesical junction. Br. J. Urol., *35*:151, 1963.

Tanagho, E. A., Schmidt, R. A., and de Araujo, C. G.: Urinary striated sphincter. What is its nerve supply? Urology, *20*:415, 1982.

Tanagho, E. A., and Smith, D. R.: The anatomy and function of the bladder neck. Br. J. Urol., *38*:54, 1966.

Waldeyer, W.: Über die Insel des Gehirns der Anthropoiden. Korrespondenzblatt der Deutschen Gessellschaft für Anthropologie, Ethnologie und Urgeschichte, *22*(10):110, 1891.

Warwick, R., and Williams, P. L.: The urogenital system. *In* Warwick, R., and Williams, P. L. (Eds.): Gray's Anatomy, 35th British ed. Philadelphia, W. B. Saunders Co., 1973, pp. 1314–1351.

Wesson, M. B.: Anatomical, embryological and physiological studies of the trigone and neck of the bladder. J. Urol., *4*:279, 1920.

Woodburn, R. T.: Anatomy of ureterovesical junction. J. Urol., *92*:431, 1964.

CHAPTER 2

Normal Renal Physiology

BRUCE R. LESLIE, M.D.
E. DARRACOTT VAUGHAN, JR., M.D.

The kidneys receive 20 per cent of the cardiac output while constituting only one-half of 1 per cent of the total body mass. The 180 liters of glomerular filtrate produced each day are finely processed to maintain the internal milieu with exquisite precision by mechanisms that continue to intrigue physiologists, nephrologists, and urologists alike.

This summary will attempt to review validated concepts of normal renal physiology as well as newer hypotheses. The urologist needs a firm understanding of renal physiology, essential in the care of patients with both normal and impaired renal function.

RENAL HEMODYNAMICS

Functional Organization of the Renal Circulation

The renal circulation is designed to simultaneously accomplish bulk filtration and reabsorption and precise selective regulation of the constituents of normal urine (Fig. 2–1). From an enormous blood flow of about a liter per minute only about 1 ml of urine per minute is formed. The energy requirement is about 10 per cent of basal oxygen consumption (Beeuwkes et al., 1981), yet the efficiency of the kidney is reflected in its low arteriovenous oxygen difference.

Originally, the renal circulation was quantified by clearance techniques measuring total renal blood flow. More recently, micropuncture and microangiographic techniques have advanced the understanding of the renal microcirculation (Barger and Mead, 1973; Bookstein and Clark, 1980). The kidney is not composed of a single homogeneous circulation but of several distinct microvascular networks. These include the glomerular microcirculation, the cortical peritubular microcirculation, and the microcirculations that nourish and drain the inner and outer medulla (Beeuwkes, 1981) (Fig. 2–1).

The gross anatomy of the renal vasculature has previously been described. The interlobular arteries taper as they pass through almost the entire cortex, and each gives rise to about 20 afferent glomerular arterioles supplying one or more of the 1.5 million glomeruli of the human kidney. The vascular pathways in the glomerulus change under different physiologic conditions. Hence there is intermittent flow within glomeruli, which may play a role in regulation of glomerular filtration rate (GFR). The discovery that the glomerular mesangium contains contractile elements that respond to angiotension II (AII) and other vasoactive substances supports this hypothesis (Brenner et al., 1980). Beyond the glomerulus the efferent arterioles either form dense peritubular capillary plexuses that nourish the proximal or distal convoluted tubules situated in the cortex or pass into the medulla (especially from juxtamedullary glomeruli) and divide into bundles of vasa recta that parallel medullary rays (Bookstein and Clark, 1980). Microdissection and injection studies recently have shown that except for the initial portion of the peritubular capillaries in the outer cortex, the efferent peritubular capillary network and the nephron arising from each glomerulus are dissociated (Beeuwkes, 1979). There are distinct outer and inner medullary capillary networks. In the inner medulla, the

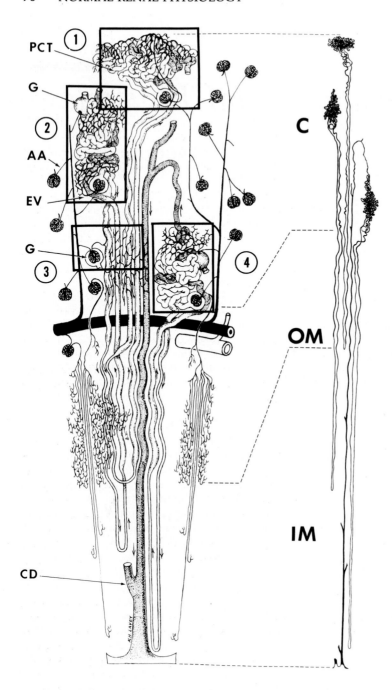

Figure 2–1. Diagram showing the vascular and tubular organization of the kidney in the dog. In the right-hand portion of the figure, nephrons arising from glomeruli in outer, middle, and inner cortex are shown to scale. Cortex (C), outer medulla (OM), and inner medulla (IM) are indicated. The left-hand portion of the figure illustrates the pattern of glomeruli (G) arising from afferent arterioles (AA). The efferent vessels (EV) from these glomeruli divide to form the peritubular capillaries. At the kidney surface, proximal convoluted tubules (PCT) are associated with a dense capillary network arising from division of superficial efferent arterioles (rectangle 1). In the middle and inner cortex, convoluted tubule segments are located close to interlobular arteries and are perfused by a complex peritubular capillary network usually derived from the efferent vessels of many glomeruli (rectangles 2 and 4). Midway between interlobular vessels, loops of Henle are grouped together with collecting ducts (CD). The peritubular capillary network of this region, derived from mid-cortical efferent arterioles, is largely oriented parallel to the tubular structures of the medullary ray (rectangle 3). In the inner or juxtamedullary cortex, glomeruli have efferent arterioles that extend downward and divide to form outer medullary vascular bundles (rectangle 4). A dense outer medullary capillary network arises from these bundles. Only thin limbs of Henle extend with collecting ducts to the papillary tip. These are accompanied by vasa recta extending from the cores of the vascular bundles. For simplicity, venous vessels have not been shown. (Modified from Beeuwkes, R., and Bonventre, J.V.: Am. J. Physiol., *229*:695, 1975.)

degree of organization of vascular-tubular relations correlates with concentrating ability (Kaissling et al., 1975).

The major changes in hydraulic pressure across the renal vascular bed are shown in Figure 2–2. The role of physical factors in the regulation of GFR will be discussed later.

MEASUREMENT OF RENAL BLOOD FLOW

The clearance of organic iodides, Diodrast, and para-aminohippurate (PAH) is used to estimate renal blood flow (RBF) and is based upon application of the Fick principle. These substances, at low plasma concentrations, are almost totally secreted by the renal tubules and there is no extrarenal metabolism, storage, or production. Accurate utilization of this technique requires normal renal function and extraction and assumes a renal venous concentration approaching zero. Since extraction is probably never complete, the term "effective renal plasma flow" (ERPF) has been used. In

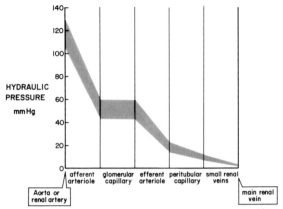

Figure 2–2. Diagram showing changes in the magnitude of intravascular hydraulic pressure from renal artery to renal vein in the Munich-Wistar rat. The steepest axial hydraulic pressure drops occur along the afferent and efferent arterioles. No significant pressure drop has been detected along glomerular capillary vessels. Thus, the cortical capillary exchange beds of the glomerular and peritubular networks operate at markedly different hydraulic pressures. Since the transglomerular hydraulic pressure difference exceeds the local oncotic pressure difference, fluid is lost from these capillaries by filtration. In the peritubular network, the transcapillary oncotic pressure difference exceeds the prevailing hydraulic pressure difference, thereby favoring fluid absorption into these capillaries.

disease states, venous sampling with actual determination of PAH extraction (E_{PAH}) is required to calculate true renal plasma flow.

Accordingly, C_{PAH} is calculated by the formula

$$U_i \times Q_u = (A_i - V_i) \times RPF$$

where

U_i = concentration of indicator in urine
Q_u = urine flow rate
A_i = concentration of indicator in arterial plasma
V_i = concentration of indicator in venous plasma
RPF = renal plasma flow rate

Rewriting this equation,

$$RPF = \frac{U_i Q_u}{A_i - V_i}$$

Since extraction is assumed to be almost complete in the clinical setting and A_i is kept constant, the equation for C_{PAH} becomes

$$RPF = \frac{U_i Q_u}{A_i} \text{ or } \frac{U_{PAH} \times V}{P_{PAH}}$$

P = Plasma concentration of PAH

The conversion of renal plasma flow rate to blood flow is achieved by dividing RPF by the plasma fraction of whole blood as estimated by the hematocrit.

$$RBF = \frac{RPF}{1 - HCT}$$

The complexity of determination of RBF by the C_{PAH} technique and the requirement of normal renal function have led to a search for alternative techniques. The use of a single-injection technique of a variety of radionuclides followed by measuring the rate of disappearance of the isotope tag from the blood or by noninvasive monitoring is discussed elsewhere (Chapter 7). The radionuclide monitoring techniques also allow calculation of differential RBF from each kidney, which is often the critical information desired in the clinical setting.

The renewed interest in a renal venous thermodilution sensor and catheter may allow the determination of differential RBF that can be coupled to renal venous sampling. In this fashion the actual determination of renal secretion of various substances, renin for example, may soon be clinically feasible (Magrini and Tarazi, 1977).

DISTRIBUTION OF RENAL BLOOD FLOW

Total RBF estimated by C_{PAH} technique is 1200 ml/min/1.73 m^2, a value that has been confirmed by a variety of methods. In infants up to 1 year of age, RBF is about one half of the adult flow; it reaches the adult level at about 3 years of age (McCrory, 1972). It should be remembered that RBF falls after age 30 and is about one half of maximum at age 90 (Davies and Shock, 1950). When related to renal mass, RBF is remarkably similar in various species, being about 4 ml/gm/min.

Although it is well documented that the perfusion rate in different regions of the kidney is not uniform, there remains considerable disagreement about regional blood flow measurement obtained by different methods under differing experimental conditions. Moreover, no clear correlation exists between distribution of renal blood flow and renal function. The utilization of inert gas washout, radioactive microspheres, or nondiffusible indicators is beyond the scope of this review (Beeuwkes, 1981; Barger and Herd, 1973). This area remains under investigation and may be relevant to our understanding of the pathophysiology of acute renal failure (Brenner and Stein, 1980). The attractive hypothesis that there is a causal relationship between the distribution of RBF and sodium handling awaits confirmation.

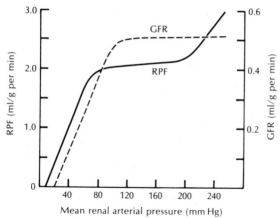

Figure 2–3. Autoregulation of renal plasma flow (RPF) and stability of glomerular filtration rate (GFR) over a similar range of mean arterial pressures. (Adapted from Shipley, R.E., and Study, R.S.: Am. J. Physiol., *167*:676, 1951.)

The renal cortex receives about 90 per cent of the total renal blood flow (5 to 6 ml/min in outer cortex), while outer medullary flow is only about 1 ml/min. However, this medullary flow, considered "sluggish" relative to the cortex, is still greater per gram than flow to the liver, brain, or resting muscle.

AUTOREGULATION OF RENAL BLOOD FLOW

The phenomenon of autoregulation of RBF is illustrated in Figure 2–3. Note that over a wide range of perfusion pressure, from 80 to 180 mm Hg, there is less than 10 per cent change in RBF or GFR. This phenomenon was described as early as 1947 (Forster and Maes, 1947) and appears to be a critical mechanism controlling renal homeostasis.

Autoregulation is not unique to the kidney but is most efficient in the renal and cerebral circulations. Since it is present in innervated, denervated, and isolated kidneys it is assumed to be mediated by events intrinsic to the kidney—hence the term "autoregulation." At present it appears that more than one proposed mechanism of autoregulation —myogenic, metabolic, tubuloglomerular feedback, and humoral—may operate. There is particular interest in the juxtaglomerular apparatus playing a critical role, although experiments utilizing a variety of angiotensin and prostaglandin blockers are conflicting (Thurau and Schnermann, 1982).

TABLE 2–1. SUMMARY OF SITE AND TRANSPORT MECHANISMS FOR NEPHRON HANDLING OF SOLUTES

Solute	Principal Sites of Nephron Handling	Mechanism and Hormonal Influences
Na⁺	Proximal tubule	Reabsorption—active
	Loop of Henle	Reabsorption—?passive
	Distal tubule	Reabsorption—active (aldosterone)
	Collecting duct	Reabsorption—active (aldosterone; ?natriuretic hormone)
K⁺	Proximal tubule	Reabsorption—active
	Loop of Henle	Reabsorption
	Distal tubule	Secretion—passive (aldosterone)
Cl⁻	Proximal tubule	Reabsorption—passive
	Loop of Henle	Reabsorption—?active
HCO₃⁻	Proximal tubule	Reabsorption—active (indirect, via H⁺ secretion)
	Distal tubule	(same)
H⁺	Collecting duct	Secretion—active
Ca⁺⁺	Proximal tubule	Reabsorption—active (PTH inhibits)
	Loop of Henle	Reabsorption—active (PTH)
Mg⁺⁺	Loop of Henle	Reabsorption—active (PTH)
	Proximal tubule	Reabsorption—active
Phosphate	Proximal tubule	Reabsorption—active
Urea	Proximal tubule	Reabsorption—passive
	Collecting duct	Reabsorption—passive (ADH)
Uric acid	Proximal tubule	Bidirectional reabsorption and secretion—active
Glucose	Proximal tubule	Reabsorption—active
Amino acids	Proximal tubule	Bidirectional reabsorption and secretion—active
Citrate	Proximal tubule	Reabsorption—active

Glomerular Filtration Rate

The elaboration of urine begins at the glomerulus with the formation of a nearly protein-free ultrafiltrate of plasma, which enters Bowman's space. As the filtrate passes through the tubules, substances may be removed (reabsorption) or added (secretion). Clearance is "a quantitative description of the rate at which the kidney excretes various substances relative to their concentration in plasma" (Smith, 1951). It is calculated as follows:

U_x = concentration of x in a timed urine collection (mg/ml)

V = volume of urine per unit time (ml/min)

P_x = concentration of x in plasma (mg/ml)

U_xV = rate of urinary excretion of x (mg/min)

C_x = U_xV/P_x = the (plasma) clearance of x (ml/min)

C_x is the volume of plasma containing x that would have to be completely cleared of x per unit time to supply an amount of x for urinary excretion at the measured rate. A summary of site and transport mechanisms for nephron handling of solutes is presented in Table 2–1. Clearance does not necessarily mean that an actual volume of plasma is, in fact, completely cleared of x. Rather, it refers to a "virtual volume" of plasma that would provide the measured amount of x.

A substance that is freely filtered and undergoes neither reabsorption nor secretion will have a clearance equal to the GFR. The clearance of inulin, a carbohydrate polymer of fructose, measured during a constant infusion, is the standard for measurement of GFR. A clearance greater than that of inulin indicates that a substance also undergoes tubular secretion; a clearance less than that of inulin implies tubular reabsorption.

Because of the difficulty in performing inulin clearance, the clearance of endogenous creatinine is used for clinical purposes as an estimate of GFR. Its plasma concentration remains stable during a 24-hour period, and its rate of excretion does not vary with urine flow. Thus, creatinine clearance (C_{cr}) can be calculated during a 24-hour collection of urine, with a plasma sample obtained at any time during the collection period. In normal man, filtered creatinine does not undergo tubular reabsorption; some tubular secretion does occur. At the plasma creatinine concentration that prevails at normal GFR, the ratio of $C_{creatinine}/C_{inulin}$ is close to 1, implying negligible secretion. At progressively lower GFR's, however, tubular secretion plays an increasingly important part in creatinine excretion. At GFR's below 30 ml/min, $C_{creatinine}$ may overestimate C_{inulin} by 50 to 80 per cent. Because this represents small absolute differences at low GFR's, $C_{creatinine}$ is satisfactory as an estimate of GFR in chronic renal insufficiency.

Kidney weight correlates better with body surface area than with either height or weight. In order to compare renal function in persons of different sizes, GFR is frequently described per standard unit of body surface area, 1.73 square meters (Smith, 1951).

FACTORS AFFECTING GLOMERULAR FILTRATION

Micropuncture studies of individual nephrons in the Munich-Wistar rat and the squirrel monkey, which possess glomeruli on the renal cortical surface, have permitted direct measurement of the factors that determine single-nephron glomerular filtration rate (SNGFR) (Brenner and Humes, 1977; Tucker and Blantz, 1977; Osgood et al., 1982). Assuming that all nephrons behave in a manner similar to those accessible to micropuncture, the regulation of whole-kidney GFR can be understood in terms of changes in one or more of the forces that regulate SNGFR. The symbols designating these forces, used in the following discussion, are summarized in Table 2–2.

The principal driving force for glomerular filtration is the hydrostatic pressure at the glomerular capillary (P_{GC}). It is a consequence of the forces that maintain systemic blood pressure—cardiac output and systemic vascular resistance. The P_{GC}, which favors ultrafiltration, is opposed by the hydrostatic pressure in Bow-

TABLE 2–2. FACTORS GOVERNING SNGFR

P_{GC}	Hydrostatic pressure in the glomerular capillary
P_T	Hydrostatic pressure in the tubule (and its proximal extension, Bowman's space)
ΔP	Net transglomerular hydrostatic pressure
π_{GC}	Oncotic pressure of glomerular capillary plasma
π_T	Oncotic pressure of tubular fluid
$\Delta\pi$	Net transglomerular oncotic pressure
P_{UF}	Effective ultrafiltration pressure ($\Delta P - \Delta\pi$)
k_f or L_p	Hydraulic permeability of glomerular capillary
A	Glomerular surface area available for ultrafiltration
K_f or L_pA	Glomerular ultrafiltration coefficient

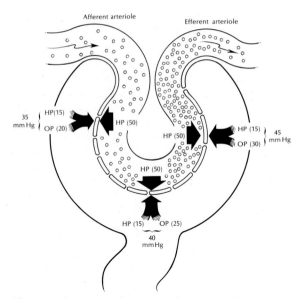

Figure 2–4. Starling forces regulating glomerular filtration. Net filtration pressure (Δ P) is the result of opposing hydrostatic pressure (HP) in the glomerular capillary and of the sum of hydrostatic pressure in Bowman's space and plasma oncotic pressure (OP). Net filtration pressure is maximal at the afferent arteriolar site of the capillary and approaches zero toward the efferent arteriolar site, because of increasing plasma oncotic pressure as a direct consequence of ultrafiltration.

man's space of the renal tubule (P_T). The difference between these values is the transmembrane hydraulic pressure gradient (Δ P):

$$\Delta P = P_{GC} - P_T \quad \text{(Fig. 2–4)}$$

Complementing these hydrostatic forces are the osmotic pressures exerted by plasma proteins, known as colloid osmotic pressure or oncotic pressure. The oncotic pressure of glomerular capillary plasma (π_{GC}) tends to oppose transcapillary fluid movement; the oncotic pressure of tubular fluid (π_T) tends to favor it. The difference between these two forces at any point is the transmembrane oncotic pressure ($\Delta\pi$):

$$\Delta\pi = \pi_{GC} - \pi_T$$

Under normal circumstances, filtration of plasma proteins is negligible and π_T is essentially zero.

At any point along the length of the capillary, the effective filtration pressure (P_{UF}) can be calculated as follows:

$$P_{UF} = \Delta P - \Delta\pi$$

As filtration proceeds along the length of the glomerular capillary, the concentration of protein, and hence π_{GC}, rises. In plasma reaching the efferent arteriole, π_{GC} has risen to a

value equal to ΔP. This local equality of ΔP and π_{GC} is known as filtration pressure equilibrium (FPE). Precisely where along the length of the capillary FPE occurs cannot be determined, but at this point SNGFR becomes zero. FPE occurs in the surface glomeruli of the Munich-Wistar rat under hydropenic conditions. Whether FPE occurs in human glomeruli remains uncertain.

In addition to P_{UF}, SNGFR is determined by both the hydraulic permeability of the glomerular capillary (k_f or L_p) and the total surface area available for ultrafiltration (A). The hydraulic permeability of the glomerular capillary is much greater than that of capillaries in nonrenal tissues. Because k_f and A cannot at present be independently measured, they are considered together as their product, the glomerular ultrafiltration coefficient, K_f or L_pA:

$$K_f = k_f \times A$$

The factors that determine SNGFR can thus be summarized by any of the following equations:

$$SNGFR = K_f(P_{UF})$$
$$SNGFR = K_f(\Delta P - \Delta\pi)$$
$$SNGFR = K_f[(P_{GC} - P_T) - (\pi_{GC} - \pi_T)]$$

The actions of these forces are illustrated in Figure 2–4.

Changes in any of the foregoing variables in health or disease will have predictable effects on SNGFR (Dworkin et al., 1983; Fried and Stein, 1983).

AUTOREGULATION OF GLOMERULAR FILTRATION RATE

Autoregulation of GFR is believed to occur mainly through variations in afferent arteriolar resistance. In response to changes in arterial pressure, this results in parallel regulation of GFR and RBF (Fig. 2–3). Only at very low arterial perfusion pressure does an increase in efferent arteriolar resistance contribute to the maintenance of P_{GC}, sustaining SNGFR at reduced RBF (Blythe, 1983).

The mechanism of autoregulation remains incompletely defined. Evidence from micropuncture studies supports the hypothesis that changes in the rate of fluid flow in the distal tubule elicit changes in glomerular arteriolar resistance. This phenomenon is known as distal tubule–glomerular feedback. The morphologic association of the macula densa portion of the distal tubule and the afferent arteriole of the same nephron suggests that these structures are involved in the autoregulatory response. Considerable controversy persists, however, over (1) what aspect of distal tubular flow is perceived as the signal that engages autoregulation and (2) what are the mechanisms and sites of changes in arteriolar resistance. The leading candidate for the signal appears to be tubular fluid chloride and its reabsorptive transport by cells of the macula densa (Wright and Briggs, 1977).

An alternative theory explains autoregulation as a consequence of variations in afferent arteriolar tone that occur as a direct result of changes in arterial blood pressure. An increase in pressure, which stretches the arteriolar smooth muscle, elicits contraction of the muscle layer, thus increasing afferent arteriolar resistance (Fried and Stein, 1983).

Glomerular Permeability

The fluid entering Bowman's space is nearly free of albumin and larger molecules. Restriction to glomerular filtration of certain molecules is known as glomerular permselectivity. The determinants of glomerular permselectivity include effective glomerular "pore" size and the electrostatic charge on the glomerular filtration barrier. The degree of filtration of a molecule is thus determined by its size, shape, and charge. Filtration of macromolecules such as albumin may also be affected by renal hemodynamics.

The filtration of molecules larger than inulin (molecular radius = 14 Å) is progressively restricted, approaching zero at molecular radii of about 40 Å (Brenner et al., 1977). The molecular radius of albumin is 36 Å.

The glomerular filtration barrier is covered by sialoproteins that bear fixed negative charges. Albumin is a polyanion at physiologic pH. Hence, it is also restricted from glomerular filtration by the interaction of these similar electrostatic charges. Neutral dextran, with a molecular radius equal to that of albumin but without a net negative charge, is filtered more than 100 times as easily as albumin (Brenner et al., 1977). In certain forms of renal disease, diminution in the glomerular charge barrier may increase glomerular permeability to albumin, resulting in proteinuria.

The glomerular filtration of albumin may also be increased by a reduction in renal plasma flow unaccompanied by a change in glomerular filtration rate. Such an increase in "filtration fraction" (the ratio of GFR/RPF) may lead to increases in the concentration of albumin in the glomerular capillary and thereby augment the gradient favoring albumin diffusion into the filtrate.

Sodium and Water

Sodium (Na) and its associated anions (mostly chloride and bicarbonate) are confined to the extracellular fluid (ECF) compartment and are the principle determinants of ECF osmolality. Because water moves freely across cell membranes, and because the osmolality of ECF is kept constant, it follows that the volume of ECF is directly related to the total body content of Na. Renal tubular reabsorption of the Na and water preserves ECF volume despite glomerular filtration of large volumes of plasma. Changes in tubular Na reabsorption defend ECF volume against changes in the filtered Na load produced by changes in GFR. In addition, changes in Na excretion maintain Na balance at varying levels of Na intake. The handling of Na by the nephron is summarized in Figure 2–5.

The reabsorption of Na ion takes place against electrical and chemical (concentration) gradients and requires expenditure of metabolic energy. Such a process is described as active transport. The energy for the bulk of Na reabsorption derives from aerobic metabolism. There is a direct, linear relationship between the rate of Na reabsorption and oxygen consumption by the kidney (Lassen et al., 1961).

The exact mechanisms of Na transport throughout the nephron continue to be investi-

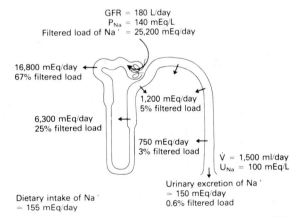

Figure 2–5. Daily renal turnover of Na^+ in a normal adult human. The diagram of the nephron represents the composite of the roughly 2 million nephrons of both kidneys. In the steady (equilibrium) state, the organism is by definition in "balance." For Na^+ this means that the daily output of Na^+ equals the daily intake. Obviously, Na^+ is excreted mainly by the kidneys; the difference between the rate of urinary excretion of Na^+ and the daily intake is made up by extrarenal routes, such as sweat, saliva, and other gastrointestinal secretions. Under normal circumstances, the extrarenal losses of Na^+ are negligible. GFR = glomerular filtration rate; P_{Na} and U_{Na} = plasma and urinary concentration of sodium, respectively.

gated. In the proximal tubule, Na in the tubular lumen travels down its concentration gradient, across the luminal (apical) membrane, into the tubular epithelial cell. Within the cell, the Na concentration is kept low by pumps in the basal and lateral membranes that extrude Na into the peritubular space, from which it can enter the peritubular capillaries. These pumps, involving the enzyme Na,K-ATPase, represent the "active" (energy-consuming) component of Na transport. For the most part, Cl reabsorption follows Na as a consequence of the negative luminal potential created by outward Na movement.

Water is reabsorbed "passively," by moving down a gradient of osmolality between tubular fluid (lower) and peritubular fluid (higher). This gradient is established by the reabsorption of Na and its attendant anions. Because the water permeability of the proximal tubule is high, only a small osmotic gradient is required to effect water movement.

Similar Na reabsorptive processes probably operate in the distal tubule and collecting ducts. Unlike these other segments, however, the thick ascending limb of the loop of Henle has a positive luminal potential. Among the mechanisms proposed to account for this is active transport of Cl with secondary, passive Na reabsorption (Burg and Green, 1973; Warnock and Eveloff, 1982).

REGULATION OF Na EXCRETION

Defense mechanisms ensure that the bulk of filtered Na is reabsorbed in the proximal nephron segments. Renal autoregulation keeps GFR, and hence the filtered Na load, constant. Should a hemodynamic disturbance occur that does change GFR, the filtered load of Na would change. The proximal tubule alters its absolute rate of Na reabsorption in parallel, so that the fractional Na reabsorption remains constant. This phenomenon, termed glomerular-tubular balance, prevents loss or accumulation of large amounts of Na. The mechanism by which glomerular-tubular balance is achieved remains uncertain. One hypothesis stresses the importance of physical factors (Brenner and Troy, 1971). Because the transglomerular passage of plasma protein is restricted, a change of GFR produces a parallel change in the protein concentration in the glomerular capillary. This fluid passes into the efferent arteriole and thence to the peritubular capillaries. Thus, a rise in GFR would result in an increase in peritubular oncotic pressure. This tends to favor net Na reabsorption. Decrements in peritubular oncotic pressure

would have the opposite effect. The importance of peritubular protein concentration in the regulation of proximal Na reabsorption has been challenged (Knox et al., 1983). An alternative theory suggests that the glomerular filtrate itself contains a substance that stimulates its own reabsorption (de Wardener, 1978). The identity of this substance is unknown.

Comparatively small changes in Na intake, as with chronic dietary changes, produce changes in urinary Na excretion via changes in the handling of Na by the collecting ducts. Except with extreme changes in ECF volume, such as can be produced by parenteral infusions, chronic Na loading is usually not associated with changes in proximal Na reabsorption. Na reabsorption by the collecting ducts is stimulated by aldosterone. Aldosterone secretion is regulated in part by ECF volume through the activity of the renin-angiotensin system. Other humoral factors may also regulate Na excretion. These include substances whose production in the kidney is related to the state of Na balance, including prostaglandins, angiotensin II, dopamine, and bradykinin. The existence of one or more "natriuretic hormones" produced in the central nervous system or at other sites in response to Na loading has also been proposed (de Wardener and Clarkson, 1982; Genest, 1983). Natriuretic hormone may act on the collecting duct to inhibit Na reabsorption, perhaps by inhibition of Na,K-ATPase.

Changes in peritubular hydrostatic pressure in the renal interstitium can alter Na handling by the loop of Henle and possibly by the collecting duct (Knox et al., 1983). An increase in interstitial pressure resulting from a rise in arterial pressure or renal vasodilation can increase renal Na excretion acutely. Whether such physical factors influence tubular function directly or through resultant changes in the levels of intrarenal hormones remains undetermined. Stimulation of the adrenergic innervation to the kidney increases tubular Na reabsorption, independent of changes in GFR or renal plasma flow (DiBona, 1977). The site at which sympathetic stimulation acts appears to be the proximal tubule.

URINARY DILUTION AND CONCENTRATION

In the proximal tubule, where some two thirds of the glomerular filtrate is reabsorbed, water follows NaCl reabsorption, and the tubular fluid remains isotonic to plasma (normally 270 to 285 mOsm/kg). Separation of NaCl from water reabsorption occurs in the loop of Henle. This mechanism generates tubular fluid that is

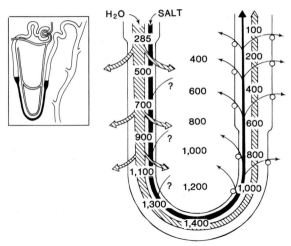

Figure 2–6. The loop of Henle, the "countercurrent multiplier." The numbers indicate the osmotic concentration in mOsm/kg H_2O of the tubular fluid and the interstitial fluid. The active transport of salt without water out of the ascending limb increases the osmotic concentration of the medullary interstitium. The small horizontal gradient is multiplied vertically by countercurrent flow. Water is reabsorbed from the descending limb by this osmotic force. Note that tubular fluid flows out of the loop at an osmotic concentration lower than that of the entering fluid. Fractionally more solute than water has been lost to the medullary interstitium.

hypotonic (dilute) compared with plasma. In the absence of vasopressin (ADH), the final urine remains dilute, permitting the excretion of a water load. The loop of Henle also helps generate a hypertonic medullary interstitium. Under conditions of water deprivation (hydropenia), ADH causes fluid in the collecting ducts to equilibrate osmotically with the medullary interstitium. This results in a hypertonic (concentrated) urine, conserving water. Urine osmolality may vary normally from 50 mOsm/kg to 1200 mOsm/kg (Fig. 2–6).

The excretion of water relative to solute may be described quantitatively as free water clearance (C_{H_2O}). Not a true clearance in the sense of inulin or creatinine, C_{H_2O} is the difference between the measured urine flow rate and the "osmolar clearance," i.e., the rate of urine formation that would be necessary to excrete the measured urinary osmolar load at a tonicity equal to that of plasma. The calculation of C_{H_2O} is summarized below.

$C_{H_2O} = V - C_{osm}$
V = urine flow rate (ml/min)
C_{osm} = osmolar clearance
       = $(U_{osm} \times V)/P_{osm}$
U_{osm} = urine osmolality (mOsm/kg)
P_{osm} = plasma osmolality (mOsm/kg)
$U_{osm} \times V$ = urinary osmolar load (mOsm/min)
$C_{H_2O} = V - [(U_{osm} \times V)/P_{osm}]$
$C_{H_2O} = V [1 - (U_{osm}/P_{osm})]$ (ml/min)

When dilute urine is produced, $U_{osm} < P_{osm}$ and C_{H_2O} is positive, implying net free water excretion. When concentrated urine is produced, $U_{osm} > P_{osm}$, and C_{H_2O} has a negative value, implying net free water conservation. Negative free water clearance ($-C_{H_2O}$) is symbolized as $T^c_{H_2O}$.

The formation of hypotonic tubular fluid occurs in the ascending thick limb of the loop of Henle. This segment is impermeable to water. The reabsorption of Cl and Na separates solute from water and reduces the osmolality of fluid leaving this segment to approximately 100 mOsm/kg. This process occurs irrespective of external water balance. Administration of a water load reduces systemic extracellular fluid tonicity and inhibits ADH secretion. In the absence of ADH, the cortical and medullary portions of the collecting duct remain impermeable to water. Because NaCl reabsorption can continue in these segments, urine osmolality may be further reduced to the minimum of 50 mOsm/kg. The excretion of dilute urine maintains ECF tonicity in response to a water load.

Concentrated urine is elaborated in response to hydropenia, which raises ECF osmolality and stimulates ADH secretion. In man, ADH binds to receptors on the basolateral membrane of collecting duct epithelial cells. This activates the enzyme adenylate cyclase, which catalyzes intracellular cyclic AMP (cAMP) formation. cAMP, via a cAMP-dependent protein kinase, facilitates phosphorylation of a component of the apical membrane. Through a process that also involves cellular microtubules, this increases the permeability of the collecting tubule to water. In the medullary portion, urea permeability is also increased. Most water reabsorption during hydropenia occurs in the cortical collecting tubule, where hypotonic luminal fluid leaving the loop of Henle equilibrates with the isotonic interstitium of the cortex. The isotonic fluid in the cortical collecting tubule subsequently becomes hypertonic in the medullary collecting duct, by osmotic equilibration with the hypertonic medullary interstitium.

The kidney generates medullary hypertonicity by means of the loops of Henle. According to the "countercurrent hypothesis," reabsorption of NaCl without water in the ascending limb, and its deposition in the interstitium, creates a local (horizontal) osmotic gradient. The increase in medullary tonicity causes water to leave the descending limb, raising its tonicity. The proximity of the descending and ascending limbs of the same tubules (arranged in hairpin curves) causes a constant gradient of tonicity at any given horizontal level to be multiplied along the vertical axis, creating high tonicities at the bend of the loop. This creates the progressive gradient of medullary tissue osmolality from corticomedullary junction to papillary tip (Fig. 2–6). Modification of the countercurrent hypothesis has been proposed to account for the importance of urea in augmenting urinary concentration (Kokko and Rector, 1972; Jamison and Robertson, 1979). According to the modified hypothesis, the process of urinary concentration begins with active chloride transport in the ascending thick limb. Urea and water, to which this segment is impermeable, remain behind in the hypotonic fluid. In the cortical and outer medullary collecting tubules, ADH augments water but not urea permeability. Water leaves these segments, raising the luminal concentration of urea. In the inner medullary collecting duct, ADH enhances urea permeability as well. Urea thus leaves the tubule and accumulates in the interstitium. This action raises medullary tonicity and causes water to leave the descending limb of Henle's loop, which is permeable to water but not to NaCl or urea. This raises the NaCl concentration of fluid reaching the hairpin turn. The ascending thin limb is impermeable to water but not to NaCl or urea. In this segment, NaCl diffuses down its concentration gradient, into the interstitium. Urea diffuses in, but at a slower rate, leading to progressive reduction of luminal tonicity in this segment. The osmotic gradients that are established are multiplied by the countercurrent mechanism. An additional effect of this mechanism is to cause some urea to remain in the medulla, where it recycles between the collecting duct, the interstitium, and the loop of Henle. This mechanism is summarized in Figure 2–7.

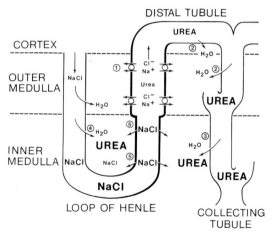

Figure 2–7. Recent modifications of the countercurrent hypothesis by Stephenson and Kokko and Rector. Both the thin ascending limb in the inner medulla and the thick ascending limb in the outer medulla, as well as the first part of the distal tubule, are impermeable to water, as indicated by the thickened lining. In the thick ascending limb, active chloride reabsorption, accompanied by passive sodium movement (1), renders the tubule fluid dilute and the outer medullary interstitium hyperosmotic. In the last part of the distal tubule and in the collecting tubule in the cortex and outer medulla, water is reabsorbed down its osmotic gradient (2), increasing the concentration of urea that remains behind. In the inner medulla both water and urea are reabsorbed from the collecting duct (3). Some urea re-enters the loop of Henle (not shown). This medullary recycling of urea, in addition to trapping of urea by countercurrent exchange in the vasa recta (not shown), causes urea to accumulate in large quantities in the medullary interstitium (indicated by large type), where it osmotically extracts water from the descending limb (4) and thereby concentrates sodium chloride in descending limb fluid. When the fluid rich in sodium chloride enters the sodium chloride–permeable (but water-impermeable) thin ascending limb, sodium chloride moves passively down its concentration gradient (5), rendering the tubule fluid relatively hypo-osmotic to the surrounding interstitium.

Acid-Base Balance

The kidney maintains the pH of the ECF by regulating the plasma bicarbonate (HCO_3^-) concentration. It does so by two processes: (1) reclamation of filtered HCO_3^- and (2) generation of new HCO_3^- by means of net acid excretion.

The normal filtered load of HCO_3^- is about 4500 mEq per day. Less than 0.1 per cent of filtered HCO_3^- appears in the final urine. Approximately 80 per cent of filtered HCO_3^- is reclaimed by the proximal tubule. Although the net result of this process is referred to as HCO_3^- reabsorption, the HCO_3^- in tubular fluid is not directly reabsorbed as such. Instead, the tubular

epithelial cells add HCO_3^- to peritubular blood as a consequence of proton (H^+) secretion. The enzyme carbonic anhydrase within the tubular epithelial cells catalyzes the hydration of carbon dioxide (CO_2) to form carbonic acid (H_2CO_3). Dissociation of H_2CO_3 yields H^+ and HCO_3^-. The H^+ is secreted into the tubular lumen, where it combines with filtered HCO_3^- to form H_2CO_3. Carbonic anhydrase is also present in the brush border, where it catalyzes the dehydration of luminal H_2CO_3 to CO_2 and water. The CO_2 can diffuse back into the cell, where it may be hydrated to form additional H_2CO_3. The HCO_3^- generated within the cell diffuses into peritubular blood, possibly via specific pathways (Warnock and Rector, 1979). The bulk of H^+ secretion by the proximal tubule appears to be coupled to Na reabsorption in a

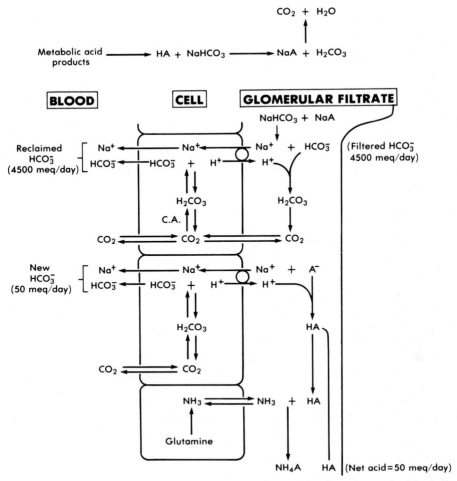

Figure 2–8. Summary of normal urinary acidification processes. (From Sebastian, A., et al.: Metabolic alkalosis. *In* Brenner, B.M., and Stein, J.H. (eds.): Acid-Base and Potassium Homeostasis. Contemporary Issues in Nephrology. Vol. 2. New York, Churchill Livingstone, 1978, p. 108.)

direct exchange mechanism (Fig. 2–8) (Warnock and Rector, 1979).

The factors that can affect proximal HCO_3^- reabsorption include (1) extracellular fluid volume—decrements in absolute or effective volume enhance HCO_3^- reabsorption, whereas increments have the opposite effect; (2) arterial P_{CO_2}—hypercapnia stimulates HCO_3^- reabsorption, whereas hypocapnia inhibits; (3) body K stores—there is a slight stimulation of proximal HCO_3^- reabsorption by prior K depletion; (4) parathormone—inhibits reabsorption; and (5) phosphate depletion—inhibits reabsorption.

The kidney adds new HCO_3^- to blood by secreting H^+ in excess of that which is necessary to reclaim filtered HCO_3. This process results in net acid excretion. Under normal circumstances, net acid excretion replaces the HCO_3^- consumed in buffering the strong acid by-products of metabolism, mainly sulfuric and phos-

phoric acids. Depending on diet, some 40 to 70 mEq of H^+ derived from such acids are produced daily. Net acid excretion may also increase in response to the addition of ketoacids or lactic acid in disease states, or to compensate for hypercapnia. The secreted H^+ is taken up by urinary buffers, principally monohydrogen phosphate ($HPO_4^=$) and ammonia (NH_3), which are converted to $H_2PO_4^-$ and NH_4^+. Net acid excretion is equal to the sum of $H_2PO_4^-$ and NH_4^+ excretion, minus any HCO_3^- that escapes reabsorption. The $H_2PO_4^-$ is also referred to as titratable acid. This term denotes the amount of strong base required to titrate urine back to pH 7.4. A comparatively small proportion of secreted H^+ is unbound to buffers, and it is this component that can result in a minimum urinary pH of about 4.4.

Most net acid excretion occurs in the collecting ducts, where H^+ is secreted by pumps that are not directly coupled to Na reabsorption. This process also depends on intracellular carbonic anhydrase. There is no brush border carbonic anhydrase in the collecting ducts. The rate of net acid excretion can be modified by (1) the electrical gradient between the tubule cell and the lumen—Na^+ reabsorption in the collecting duct creates a negative intraluminal potential; this favors H^+ secretion. The gradient is augmented by increased Na delivery and reabsorption, especially when Na^+ is accompanied by a poorly reabsorbed anion. This enhancement of H^+ secretion by Na^+ reabsorption brings about an indirect coupling of these processes; (2) mineralocorticoids—aldosterone can directly stimulate the capacity of the H^+ pump (Al-Awqati et al., 1976). In addition, by stimulating Na^+ reabsorption in the collecting duct, aldosterone enhances the electrical gradient that favors H^+ secretion; (3) buffer availability—NH_3 is produced in the kidney from glutamine. It gains access to the tubular fluid in both the proximal and the distal nephron by nonionic diffusion. Acidosis increases renal NH_3 production. Increased buffer availability, by taking up free H^+, reduces the chemical gradient against which H^+ is pumped and thus stimulates H^+ secretion. The mechanism by which a change in systemic pH affects ammoniagenesis remains undefined. Ammoniagenesis can also be stimulated by K depletion and inhibited by K loading. An adaptive increase in ammoniagenesis is the principal mechanism for the excretion of increased acid loads (Tennen, 1978).

Potassium

Over 90 per cent of plasma K undergoes glomerular filtration. Most of it is reabsorbed in the proximal tubule and the loop of Henle. The bulk of K in the final urine is added to tubular fluid by secretion in the late distal tubule and cortical collecting duct. Tubular epithelial cells in these segments take up K from peritubular fluid by a mechanism involving Na,K-ATPase (Wright and Giebisch, 1978). This gives rise to an intracellular transport pool of K. Potassium secretion is favored by the negative intratubular potential created by distal Na reabsorption, and by the concentration gradient between intracellular K and tubular fluid. In addition to these passive forces that influence K secretion, an active transport mechanism may exist (Giebisch and Stanton, 1979). There is no evidence either for a coupled exhange between Na^+ absorption and K^+ secretion or for competition between

intracellular K^+ and H^+ for tubular secretory pathways.

Potassium excretion is augmented by an increase in distal tubular fluid flow rate (as with saline or osmotic diuresis, diuretic drugs, or postobstructive diuresis). This promotes K secretion by maintaining a steep K concentration gradient between the cell and the tubular fluid. In addition, increased quantities of Na are presented to distal reabsorptive sites. The negative intratubular potential created by increased Na reabsorption also promotes K secretion.

Mineralocorticoids stimulate K secretion, possibly by stimulating Na,K-ATPase in the basolateral membrane (Giebisch and Stanton, 1979). This would increase K uptake and raise intracellular K concentration, thereby enhancing K secretion.

Calcium

Only that portion of plasma calcium which is not bound to plasma proteins is filtered at the glomerulus. Ultrafilterable calcium represents about 60 per cent of total plasma calcium. There is subsequent tubular reabsorption of 96 to 98 per cent of this filtered load. The bulk of calcium reabsorption occurs in the proximal tubule and the ascending thick limb of the loop of Henle. Additional reabsorption occurs in the distal convoluted tubule and cortical collecting duct (Sutton, 1983).

Calcium reabsorption in the proximal tubule occurs in parallel with sodium reabsorption, with a component of calcium absorption being directly sodium-dependent (Suki, 1979). Ca reabsorption in the proximal tubule is inhibited by PTH, cyclic AMP, acetazolamide, exogenous Na loading, and phosphate depletion. The effect on urinary Ca, however, depends on the behavior of more distal nephron sites. In the loop of Henle (as well as the distal convoluted tubule and collecting duct), Ca reabsorption is stimulated by PTH. This accounts for the hypocalciuric effect of this hormone despite its inhibition of proximal Ca absorption. Ca reabsorption in the loop of Henle is inhibited by furosemide. When diuretic-induced extracellular volume depletion is prevented by replacement of salt and water losses, furosemide causes an increase in urinary Ca excretion. This accounts for the efficacy of furosemide in the emergency treatment of hypercalcemia. Final modulation of urinary Ca excretion occurs in the distal tubule and collecting ducts. In these segments, active transport of Ca occurs, which can be dissociated from Na reabsorption. Thus, chlorothiazide, which inhibits distal tubular Na transport, also directly stimulates Ca absorption in this segment (Costanzo and Windhager, 1978). This may be the major explanation for the reduction in urinary Ca excretion with chronic administration of thiazides. An additional hypocalciuric effect of thiazide diuretics may result from extracellular fluid volume contraction, with consequent stimulation of Ca reabsorption in the proximal tubule.

Other factors that stimulate Ca reabsorption between the late proximal tubule and the early distal convoluted tubule include hypocalcemia, metabolic alkalosis (increased tubular HCO_3^-), vitamin D, and phosphate loading. Reabsorption is inhibited by hypercalcemia, metabolic acidosis, hypermagnesemia, and phosphate depletion (Sutton, 1983).

Phosphate

Plasma inorganic phosphate, existing as a mixture of $HPO_4^=$ and $H_2PO_4^-$, is 80 to 90 per cent ultrafilterable at the glomerulus. Of the filtered load, 80 to 97 per cent is reabsorbed. The tubular reabsorption of phosphate can increase to nearly 100 per cent in response to phosphorus deprivation. Most phosphate reabsorption occurs in the proximal tubule. The existence of a distal site of phosphate transport is also suspected (Knox et al., 1977; Dennis et al., 1979). PTH inhibits phosphate reabsorption in the proximal tubule and increases urinary phosphate. This effect is associated with increased urinary excretion of nephrogenous cyclic AMP.

EXCRETION OF ORGANIC SOLUTES

Urea

Urea is the major end product of protein catabolism in man. It is freely filtered at the glomerulus. Water reabsorption increases the urea concentration in tubular fluid, with subsequent urea diffusion out of the tubule. At typical urine flow rates of 1 ml/min, 30 to 40 per cent of filtered urea is reabsorbed in the proximal tubule. The medullary collecting ducts are also permeable to urea, and their permeability is enhanced by vasopression. Reabsorption of urea in the collecting duct is enhanced by antidiuresis and inhibited by water diuresis. Urea reabsorbed in the collecting ducts contributes to the hypertonicity of medullary interstitial fluid and plays an important role in urinary concentration.

The rate of urea reabsorption is inversely related to tubular fluid flow rate. At urine flow rates of about 2 ml/min, during water diuresis, 60 to 70 per cent of filtered urea is excreted, i.e., urea clearance is 60 to 70 per cent of the glomerular filtration rate. At low urine flow rates, during antidiuresis or reductions in renal blood flow, urea clearance may fall to 10 to 20 per cent of the glomerular filtration rate. This accounts for the disproportionate increase in BUN compared with serum creatinine in states of "prerenal azotemia."

Uric Acid

Uric acid is the end product of purine catabolism in man. On a low-purine diet, uric acid production from endogenous sources is about 700 mg per day. Two thirds of the uric acid load is excreted by the kidneys. Intestinal excretion, with degradation by bacterial enzymes, accounts for the rest. Because of its low pKa (5.75), it exists in plasma almost entirely as urate. The low pH attained in urine in the distal nephron favors the formation of uric acid, which is of limited solubility in water.

Current evidence favors a four-component model for renal handling of urate (Levinson and Sorensen, 1980): (1) Plasma urate is freely filtered at the glomerulus; (2) filtered urate undergoes nearly complete tubular reabsorption; (3) approximately 50 per cent of this reabsorbed urate is secreted into tubular fluid; and (4) postsecretory reabsorption reclaims about 80 per cent of the secreted urate. Antiuricosuric agents such as pyrazinoic acid (the metabolite of the antituberculous agent pyrazinamide) inhibit the tubular secretory mechanism. Probenecid, a uricosuric agent, acts by inhibiting postsecretory reabsorption (Fanelli, 1977). The majority of patients with gout appear to have an impairment in renal uric acid excretion, which is incompletely characterized (Rieselbach and Steele, 1974).

Urate secretion is accomplished by organic anion secretory mechanisms located in the proximal tubule. A variety of other substances share and mutually compete for this mechanism. They include oxalate, lactate, hippurate, penicillins, cephalosporins, thiazides, furosemide, and ethacrynic acid. A separate organic cation secretory mechanism also exists. Among the substances transported by this system are creatinine, cimetidine, and trimethoprim.

Glucose

Although glucose is freely filtered at the glomerulus, it undergoes essentially complete reabsorption in the early portion of the proximal tubule, so that urine is normally glucose-free. With progressively higher filtered loads (at higher plasma glucose concentrations), reabsorption increases until a tubular maximum glucose reabsorption rate (TmG) is attained. Filtered glucose in excess of the TmG appears in the urine (Smith, 1951).

Glucose transport is linked to proximal Na reabsorption. When the latter is inhibited, as by ECF volume expansion, the TmG falls. These observations have given rise to the following model: Glucose in tubular fluid interacts with a carrier mechanism in the luminal membrane of the tubular epithelial cell. This carrier, which exhibits saturation kinetics, facilitates the entry of glucose into the tubular epithelial cell. Na is required for glucose-carrier interaction. Once transported into the cell, glucose may diffuse down its own concentration gradient from tubular epithelial cell to peritubular blood.

Amino Acids

Circulating amino acids readily cross the glomerular filter and undergo nearly complete reabsorption by proximal tubular cells. This occurs via mechanisms in the brush border membrane. As in the case of glucose, this process appears to be carrier-mediated, Na-dependent, and energy-requiring (Schafer and Barfuss, 1980). Separate transport mechanisms in the basolateral membrane also mediate cellular uptake of amino acids from peritubular fluids.

Much attention has been focused on the tubular transport mechanisms for cystine and the cationic (dibasic) amino acids arginine, lysine, and ornithine. Reabsorption of these amino acids is defective in classic cystinuria. Because of the insolubility of cystine, urinary stones are formed. A model for tubular handling of these amino acids must account for the following observations: (1) Whereas patients with classic cystinuria have excessive excretion of all four amino acids, patients have been described with either isolated cystinuria or hyperdibasic aminoaciduria (arginine, lysine, ornithine) without cystinuria. (2) In cystinuric patients, the clearance of cystine can exceed creatinine clearance, implying tubular secretion of cystine. (3) Renal cortical tissue slices from cystinuric patients may show no defect in taking up cystine from the

bathing medium, compared with slices from normal subjects.

According to the currently favored model, there are separate transport systems in the basolateral and brush border membranes. In the basolateral membrane are two uptake mechanisms—one for cystine and another for arginine, lysine, and ornithine together. Amino acids that accumulate within the cell may be secreted into tubular fluid. In the brush border are three separate reabsorptive mechanisms. One is shared by all four amino acids; the second is for arginine, ornithine, and lysine only; and the third is for cystine alone (Broadus and Thier, 1979).

Citrate

Urinary citrate may help prevent calcium nephrolithiasis by chelating urinary calcium. Plasma citrate, present at concentrations of 0.05 mM to 0.3 mM, undergoes glomerular filtration and subsequent proximal tubular reabsorption. Citrate excretion in man ranges between 10 per cent and 35 per cent of the filtered load (Simpson, 1983). In addition, some of the citrate that escapes filtration is taken up by the tubular cells from postglomerular blood. Citrate that enters the cell is metabolized via the citric acid cycle to CO_2 and water.

Citrate excretion is profoundly influenced by systemic acid-base balance, through consequent changes in tubular cell pH. Metabolic alkalosis increases citrate excretion. A rise in cell pH inhibits citrate metabolism, leading to a rise in intracellular citrate concentration. The latter tends to inhibit citrate reabsorption. Metabolic acidosis has the opposite effect.

Distal renal tubular acidosis and administration of acetazolamide are associated with hypocitruria and relatively alkaline urine. Both conditions predispose to calcium nephrolithiasis and nephrocalcinosis.

ENDOCRINE FUNCTION OF THE KIDNEY

The kidney is recognized as an important endocrine organ, complementing and often interacting with its excretory functions. The major systems include renin-angiotensin, prostaglandin, kallikrein-kinin, erythropoietin, and vitamin D–metabolizing enzymes. These systems are involved in numerous aspects of renal function, including blood flow, salt and water bal-

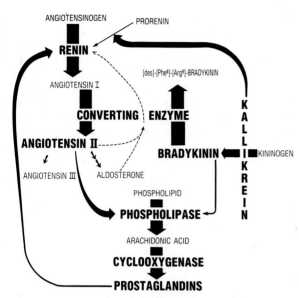

Figure 2–9. Interactions of renal hormones. Major components of the renin-angiotensin, prostaglandin and kallikrein-kinin systems are shown. Major components are shown in bold face type. Activators are indicated by solid arrows (→); inhibitors are indicated by dashed arrows (--→).

ance, renin release, red blood cell formation, and calcium metabolism (Felsen and Vaughan, 1983).

The interactions are complex and as yet incompletely understood. In some cases one system directly antagonizes another, whereas in other cases one system may actually mediate the effects of another (Fig. 2–9).

Renin-Angiotensin-Aldosterone System

The system best understood is the renin-angiotensin-aldosterone (RAAS) cascade, which is one of the major renal hormonal systems involved in the regulation of systemic blood pressure, sodium and potassium balance, and regional blood flow (Laragh and Sealey, 1981) (Fig. 2–10). Its role in the pathogenesis of renovascular hypertension is reviewed fully in Chapter 58. However, it is equally important to recognize the major role the RAAS plays day to day in normal homeostasis (Vaughan,

Figure 2–10. The renin-angiotensin-aldosterone system.

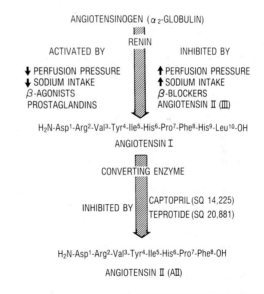

1983). Renin is secreted in response to factors that reduce arterial blood pressure or renal perfusion, such as hemorrhage, sodium depletion, or heart failure (Keeton and Campbell, 1980). The system reacts immediately to acute stimuli with the generation of the intense vasoconstrictor angiotension II (AII) to restore blood pressure. Following chronic stimulation, such as sodium depletion, homeostasis is achieved by AII stimulation of the adrenal zona glomerulosa to secrete aldosterone, which mediates distal tubular sodium retention. Eventually, if effective fluid volume and tissue perfusion are restored the further release of renin is shut off. Hence, in normal subjects, plasma renin activity (PRA) rises in response to sodium depletion and falls with sodium loading (Laragh and Sealey, 1981). Accordingly, if a normal subject exhibits a high PRA, then, by definition, he is sodium-depleted. Clinically, the PRA can be utilized as an index of sodium or volume status. Further implications of the role of AII in sodium depletion have been derived from the administration of AII antagonists to sodium-depleted animals and man. Angiotensin II blockade with saralasin or captopril in sodium-depleted normotensive rats results in a fall in blood pressure (Gavras et al., 1973; Levens et al., 1981). Similar AII dependency of blood pressure has been shown in normotensive human subjects (Streeton, 1976).

The effect of elevated PRA and AII on renal function during sodium depletion is of potentially greater clinical importance. In addition to the systemic vasoconstriction and aldosterone biosynthesis induced by AII during sodium depletion, homeostasis is ensured further by a direct effect on renal function to retard sodium and water loss. Kimbrough and coworkers first showed this effect by giving intrarenal saralasin or teprotide to sodium-depleted and -repleted animals (Kimbrough et al., 1977). AII inhibition or blockade resulted in an increase in renal blood flow, glomerular filtration rate, and sodium excretion only in the sodium-depleted animals. The primary antidiuretic effect of AII is more complex. AII modulates water excretion in both sodium-depleted and sodium-repleted animals (Levens et al., 1981).

Taken all together, the RAAS plays a major role in protecting against sodium depletion, at the expense, however, of systemic vasoconstriction and decreased organ perfusion. It is easy to envision an additive stress such as intraoperative hemorrhage or hypotension leading to further renal insult and the potential of acute renal failure in the setting of pre-existing sodium depletion.

Renal Prostaglandins

The prostaglandin cascade is complex, and numerous putative roles for the system in the kidney remain to be validated (Felsen and Vaughan, 1983). The metabolism of arachidonic acid (AA) to its products is shown in Figure 2–11. In addition, there exists a second pathway in the kidney involving the action of lipoxygenase to produce hydroxylated derivatives of AA, including 12-hydroxyeicosatetranoic acid (12-HETE) and 15-HETE (Winokur and Morrison, 1981). The role of these leukotrienes in the kidney is unknown, and investigation in this area should be a fertile field for future research.

Prostaglandin (PG) synthesis occurs in both renal cortex and medulla (Felsen and Vaughan, 1983), with the medulla having the greater synthetic capacity. Among the actions in which PG's may be involved are the following: (1) PG's play both a direct and an indirect role in renin release (Keeton and Campbell, 1980). (2) PG's oppose the action of vasopressin (AVP) (Zusman, 1981). (3) The majority of data supports a natriuretic role for PG's, but the mechanism is controversial (McGiff, 1981; Stokes, 1981). One of the more confusing areas is the role of PG's in renal blood flow (RBF) regulation. Arachidonic acid infusions increase RBF and the effect can be blocked by indomethacin (Chang et al., 1974). PGH_2 (endoperoxide) and thromboxane A_2, however, are intense renal vasoconstrictors (Morrison et al., 1977). This area of controversy is particularly important to urologists in the investigation of the increased renovascular resistance that accompanies ureteral obstruction (see Chapter 9).

Kallikrein-Kinin

The renal system least well understood in terms of its physiologic role is the kallikrein-kinin system (Fig. 2–12). Investigators have been limited by numerous methodological problems, and it is still unclear which component reflects accurately the action of the system (Felsen and Vaughan, 1983). Bradykinin is a renal vasodilator. As it also stimulates PG release (Fig. 2–9), some or perhaps all of its action may be mediated by PG's (McGiff et al., 1975). Finally, kallikrein activates the conversion of prorenin to renin *in vitro* (Sealey et al., 1982).

Other Hormonal Systems

The kidney is the major site of conversion of 25-hydroxy-vitamin D_3 [25(OH)D_3] to the

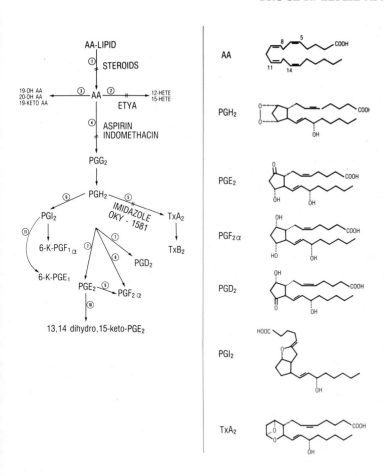

Figure 2–11. The metabolism of arachidonic acid to products is indicated. The following abbreviations are used: AA, arachidonic acid; HETE, hydroxyeicosatetraenoic acid; Tx, thromboxane; 6K-PGF$_{1\alpha}$, 6-keto-PGF$_{1\alpha}$. The circled numbers represent the following enzymes, whose corresponding inhibitors are shown in the figure as 11: 1, phospholipase; 2, lipoxygenase; 3, mixed-function oxidase; 4, cyclooxygenase; 5, thromboxane synthetase; 6, prostacyclin synthetase; 7, PG endoperoxide isomerase; 8, PG endoperoxide reductase; 9, PG 9-keto-reductase; 10, 13,14-dihydro PG reductase-15, keto PG dehydrogenase; 11, 9-PG-dehydrogenase. Structures of AA and the major renal PGs are shown on the right.

highly active 1,25(OH)$_2$D$_3$ by the mitochondrial enzyme 25-hydroxycholecalciferol-1-α-hydroxylase (Lee et al., 1981). The control of 1,25(OH$_2$)D$_3$ production and its mechanism of action to stimulate active absorption of both calcium and phosphate in the intestine are discussed in reference to urinary lithiasis (Chapter 25).

The kidney is also the major site of production of erythropoietin. This hormone is secreted in response to decreased tissue oxygen tension within the kidney. It induces primitive marrow cells to differentiate into pronormoblasts, eventually increasing red cell mass and thereby increasing tissue oxygen tension (Wintrobe et al., 1981). The location of erythropoietin secretion within the kidney may be either glomerular or juxtaglomerular. Current studies suggest active renal synthesis of erythropoietin rather than the reaction of a renal enzyme, called erythrogenin, with a plasma substrate, erythropoietinogen, as has been suggested.

References

Al-Awqati, Q., Norby, L. H., Mueller, A., and Steinmetz, P. R.: Characteristics of stimulation of H transport by aldosterone in turtle urinary bladder. J. Clin. Invest., *58*:351, 1976.

Barger, A. C., and Herd, J. A.: Renal vascular anatomy and distribution of renal blood flow. *In* Orloff, J., and Berliner, R. W. (eds.): Handbook of Physiology. Chapter 10, Section 8. Washington, D.C., Renal Physiology American Physiological Society, 1973.

Beeuwkes, R., III: Vascular-tubular relationship in the human kidney. *In* Leaf, A., and Giebisch, G. (eds.): Renal Pathophysiology—Recent Advances. New York, Raven Press, 1979, p. 155.

Beeuwkes, R., III, Ichikawa, I., and Brenner, B. M.: The

KININOGEN

← KALLIKREIN

H$_2$N-Lys-Arg-Pro-Pro-Gly-Phe-Ser-Pro-Phe-Arg-OH   KALLIDIN

← AMINOPEPTIDASE

H$_2$N-Arg-Pro-Pro-Gly-Phe-Ser-Pro-Phe-Arg-OH   **BRADYKININ**

KININASE I   KININASE II
                              (CONVERTING ENZYME)

H$_2$N-Arg-Pro-Pro-Gly-Phe-Ser-Pro-Phe-OH   H$_2$N-Arg-Pro-Pro-Gly-Phe-Ser-Pro-OH

Figure 2–12. Kallikrein-kinin system.

renal circulation. *In* Brenner, B. M., and Rector, F. C., Jr. (eds.): The Kidney. Philadelphia, W. B. Saunders Co., 1981.

Blythe, W. B.: Captopril and renal autoregulation. N. Engl. J. Med., 308:390, 1983.

Bookstein, J. J., and Clark, R. I.: Renal Microvascular Disease: Angiographic-Microangiographic Correlates. Boston, Little, Brown & Co., 1980.

Brenner, B. M., and Humes, H. D.: Mechanics of glomerular ultrafiltration. N. Engl. J. Med., 297:148, 1977.

Brenner, B. M., and Stein, J. H. (eds.): Acute renal failure. *In* Contemporary Issues in Nephrology. Vol. 6. New York, Churchill Livingstone, 1980.

Brenner, B. M., and Troy, J. L.: Post-glomerular vascular protein concentration: Evidence for a causal role in governing fluid reabsorption and glomerular balance by the renal proximal tubule. J. Clin. Invest., 50:336, 1971.

Brenner, B. M., Badr, K. F., Schor, N., and Ichikawa, I.: Humoral influences on glomerular filtration. Mineral Electrolyte Metab., 4:49, 1980.

Brenner, B. M., Bohrer, M. P., Baylis, C., and Deen, W. M.: Determinants of glomerular permselectivity: Insights derived from observations *in vivo*. Kidney Int., 12:229, 1977.

Broadus, A. E., and Thier, S. O.: Metabolic basis of renal-stone disease. N. Engl. J. Med., 300:839, 1979.

Burg, M. D., and Green, N.: Function of the thick ascending limb of Henle's loop. Am. J. Physiol., 224:659, 1973.

Costanzo, L. S., and Windhager, E. E.: Calcium and sodium transport by the distal convoluted tubule of the rat. Am. J. Physiol., 235:F492, 1978.

Davies, D. F., and Shock, N. W.: Age changes in glomerular filtration rate; effective renal plasma flow and tubular excretory capacity in adult males. J. Clin. Invest., 29:496, 1950.

Dennis, V. W., Stead, W. W., and Myers, J. L.: Renal handling of phosphate and calcium. Annu. Rev. Physiol., 41:257, 1979.

De Wardener, H. E.: The control of sodium excretion. Am. J. Physiol., 235:F163, 1978.

De Wardener, H. E., and Clarkson, E. M.: The natriuretic hormone: Recent developments. Clin. Sci., 63:415, 1982.

DiBona, G. F.: Neurogenic regulation of renal tubular sodium reabsorption. Am. J. Physiol., 233:F73, 1977.

Dworkin, L. D., Ichikawa, I., and Brenner, B. M.: Hormonal modulation of glomerular function. Am. J. Physiol., 244:F95, 1983.

Fanelli, G. M., Jr.: Urate excretion. Annu. Rev. Med., 28:349, 1977.

Felsen, D., and Vaughan, E. D., Jr.: Endocrine function of the renal parenchyma. *In* Rajfer, J. (ed.): Urologic Endocrinology. Philadelphia, W. B. Saunders Co., 1983.

Forster, R. P., and Maes, J. P.: Effect of experimental neurogenic hypertension on renal blood flow and glomerular filtration rate in intact denervated kidneys of unanesthetized rabbits with adrenal glands demedullated. Am. J. Physiol., 150:534, 1947.

Fried, T. A., and Stein, J. H.: Glomerular dynamics. Arch. Intern. Med., 143:787, 1983.

Gavras, H., Brunner, H. R., Vaughan, E. D., Jr., and Laragh, J. H.: Angiotensin-sodium interaction of blood pressure maintenance of renal hypertensive and normotensive rats. Science, 180:1369, 1973.

Genest, J.: Volume hormones and blood pressure. Ann. Intern. Med., 98(2):744, 1983.

Giebisch, G., and Stanton, B.: Potassium transport in the nephron. Annu. Rev. Physiol., 41:241, 1979.

Jamison, R. L., and Robertson, C. R.: Recent formulations of the urinary concentrating mechanism: A status report. Kidney Int., 16:537, 1979.

Kaissling, B., deRouffignac, C., Barrett, J. M., and Kriz, W.: The structural organization of the kidney of the desert rodent *Psammomys obesus*. Anat. Embryol., 148:121, 1975.

Keeton, K. T., and Campbell, W. B.: The pharmacologic alteration of renin release. Pharmacol. Rev., 32:81, 1980.

Kimbrough, H. M., Jr., Vaughan, E. D., Jr., Carey, R. M., and Ayers, C. R.: Effect of intrarenal angiotensin II blockade on renal function in conscious dogs. Circ. Res., 40:174, 1977.

Knox, F. G., Mertz, J. I., Burnett, J. C., Jr., and Haramati, A.: Role of hydrostatic and oncotic pressures in renal sodium reabsorption. Circ. Res., 52:491, 1983.

Knox, F. G., Osswald, H., Marchand, G. R., Spielman, W. S., Haas, J. A., Berndt, T., and Youngberg, S. P.: Phosphate transport along the nephron. Am. J. Physiol., 233:F261, 1977.

Kokko, J. P., and Rector, F. C., Jr.: Countercurrent multiplication system without active transport in inner medulla. Kidney Int., 2:214, 1972.

Laragh, J. H., and Sealey, J. E.: The renin-aldosterone axis for blood pressure electrolyte homeostasis and diagnosis of high blood pressure. *In* Williams, R. M. (ed.): Textbook of Endocrinology. 6th ed. Philadelphia, W. B. Saunders Co., 1981.

Lassen, N. A., Munck, O., and Thaysen, J. H.: Oxygen consumption and sodium reabsorption in the kidney. Acta Physiol. Scand., 51:371, 1961.

Lee, D. B. N., Brautbar, N., and Massry, S. G.: Renal production and biologic actions of vitamin D metabolites. Semin. Nephrol., 1:335, 1981.

Levens, N. R., Peach, M. J., Vaughan, E. D., Jr., and Carey, R. M.: Demonstration of a primary anti-diuretic action of angiotensin II: Effect of intrarenal converting enzyme inhibition in the conscious dog. Endocrinology, 108:318, 1981.

Levens, N. R., Peach, M. J., Vaughan, E. D., Jr., Weed, W. C., and Carey, R. M.: Response of blood pressure and angiotensin converting enzyme activity to acute captopril administration in normotensive and hypertensive rats. Endocrinology, 108:536, 1981.

Levinson, D. J., and Sorensen, L. B.: Renal handling of uric acid in normal and gouty subjects: Evidence for a 4-component system. Ann. Rheum. Dis., 39:173, 1980.

Magrini, F., and Tarazi, R. C.: New approach to local thermodilution: Use of pig tail catheters to avoid basic difficulties. Cardiovasc. Res., 11:576, 1977.

McCrory, W. W.: Developmental nephrology. Cambridge, Harvard University Press, 1972.

McGiff, J. C.: Prostaglandins, prostacyclin and thromboxanes. Annu. Rev. Pharmacol. Toxicol., 21:479, 1981.

McGiff, J. C., Itskowitz, M. D., and Terragno, N. A.: The action of bradykinin and eledoisin in the canine isolated kidney: Relationship to prostaglandins. Clin. Sci. Mol. Med., 49:125, 1975.

Morrison, A. R., Nishikawa, K., and Needleman, P.: Unmasking of thromboxane A_2 synthesis by ureteral obstruction in the rabbit kidney. Nature, 267:259, 1977.

Osgood, R. W., Reineck, H. J., and Stein, J. H.: Methodologic considerations in the study of glomerular ultrafiltration. Am. J. Physiol., *242*:F1, 1982.

Rieselbach, R. E., and Steele, T. H.: Influence of the kidney upon urate homeostasis in health and disease. Am. J. Med., *56*:665, 1974.

Schafer, J. A., and Barfuss, D. W.: Membrane mechanisms for transepithelial amino acid absorption and secretion. Am. J. Physiol., *238*:F335, 1980.

Sealey, J. E., Atlas, S. A., and Laragh, J. H.: Plasma prorenin: physiological and biochemical characteristics. Clin. Sci., *63*:133s, 1982.

Simpson, D. P.: Citrate excretion: A window on renal metabolism. Am. J. Physiol., *224*:F223, 1983.

Smith, H. W.: The Kidney: Structure and Function in Health and Disease. New York, Oxford University Press, 1951.

Stokes, J. B.: Integrated actions of renal medullary prostaglandins in the control of water secretion. Am. J. Physiol., *240*:F471, 1981.

Streeton, D. H. P., Anderson, G. H., and Dalakos, T. G.: Angiotensin blockade: Its clinical significance. Am. J. Med., *60*:817, 1976.

Suki, W. N.: Calcium transport in the nephron. Am. J. Physiol., *237*:F1, 1979.

Sutton, R. A. L.: Disorders of renal calcium excretion. Kidney Int., *23*:665, 1983.

Tannen, R. L.: Ammonia metabolism. Am. J. Physiol., *235*:F265, 1978.

Thurau, K., and Schnermann, J. (eds.): The juxtaglomerular apparatus. Kidney Int., Suppl. 12, 1982.

Tucker, B. J., and Blantz, R. C.: An analysis of the determinants of nephron filtration rate. Am. J. Physiol., *232*:F477, 1977.

Vaughan, E. D., Jr.: Renal hypertension. *In* Rajfer, J. (ed.): Urologic Endocrinology. Philadelphia, W. B. Saunders Co., 1983.

Warnock, D. G., and Eveloff, J.: NaCl entry mechanisms in the luminal membrane of the renal tubule. Am. J. Physiol., *242*:F561, 1982.

Warnock, D. G., and Rector, F. C., Jr.: Proton secretion by the kidney. Annu. Rev. Physiol., *41*:197, 1979.

Winokur, T. S., and Morrison, A. R.: Regional synthesis of monohydroxyeicosanoids by the kidney. J. Biol. Chem., *256*:10221, 1981.

Wintrobe, M. M., Lee, G. R., Boggs, D. R., Bithell, T. C., Forster, J., Athens, J. W., and Lukens. J. N.: Clinical Hematology. Philadelphia, Lea & Febiger, 1981.

Wright, F. S., And Briggs, J. P.: Feedback regulation of glomerular filtration rate. Am. J. Physiol., *233*:F1, 1977.

Wright, F. S., and Giebisch, G.: Renal potassium transport: Contributions of individual nephron segments and populations. Am. J. Physiol., *235*:F515, 1978.

Zusman, R. M.: Prostaglandins, vasopressin and renal water reabsorption. Med. Clin. North Am., *65*:919, 1981.

CHAPTER 3

Physiology and Pharmacology of the Renal Pelvis and Ureter*

ROBERT M. WEISS, M.D.

The function of the ureter is to transport urine from the kidney to the bladder. Under normal conditions, ureteral peristalsis originates with electrical activity at pacemaker sites located in the proximal portion of the urinary collecting system (Bozler, 1942; Weiss et al., 1967; Gosling and Dixon, 1974; Constantinou, 1974; Shiratori and Kinoshita, 1961a; Tsuchida and Yamaguchi, 1977). The electrical activity is then propagated distally and gives rise to the mechanical event of peristalsis, ureteral contraction, which propels the bolus of urine distally. Efficient propulsion of the urinary bolus is dependent on the ureter's ability to completely coapt its walls (Woodburne and Lapides, 1972). Urine passes into the bladder via the ureterovesical junction, which under normal conditions permits urine to pass from the ureter into the bladder but not from the bladder into the ureter.

CELLULAR ANATOMY

The primary functional anatomic unit of the ureter is the ureteral smooth muscle cell. The cell is extremely small, approximately 250 to 400 μ in length and 5 to 7 μ in diameter. The nucleus, which is separated from the remainder of the cell by a nuclear membrane, is ellipsoid

in shape and contains a darkly staining body, the nucleolus, and the genetic material of the cell. Surrounding the nucleus is the cytoplasm or sarcoplasm, which contains the structures involved in cell function. In the cytoplasm, frequently in close relation to the nucleus, are mitochondria that perform many of the nutritive functions of the cell.

Dispersed in the sarcoplasm are the contractile proteins actin and myosin that interact, depending upon the local calcium (Ca^{++}) concentration, to produce contraction or relaxation. The actin is dispersed throughout the sarcoplasm in hexagonal clumps and is interspersed with the less numerous clumps of the more deeply staining myosin. Any process that leads to an increase in Ca^{++} concentration in the region of the contractile proteins results in contraction, and, conversely, any process that decreases the Ca^{++} concentration in the region of the contractile proteins results in relaxation. Along the cell surface are dark bands referred to as attachment plaques, which, along with dense bodies dispersed in the cytoplasm, serve as attachment devices for the actin.

Around the periphery of the cell are numerous cavitary structures, some of which open to the outside of the cell, referred to as caveolae or pinocytic vesicles. Their exact function is not known, although they may serve a role in the nutritive functions of the cell or in the transport of ions across the cell membrane. A double-layer cell membrane surrounds the cell. The

*The original work was supported in part by Public Health Service Grant AG-00112 from The National Institute of Aging.

inner plasma membrane surrounds the entire cell, whereas the outer basement membrane is absent at areas of close cell-to-cell contact, referred to as intermediate junctions.

ELECTRICAL ACTIVITY

The electrical properties of all excitable tissues depend on the distribution of ions on both the inside and the outside of the cell membrane and on the relative permeability of the cell membrane to these ions (Hodgkin, 1958). The ionic basis for electrical activity in ureteral smooth muscle has not been fully described; however, many of its properties probably resemble those in other excitable tissues.

Resting Potential

When a ureteral muscle cell is in a nonexcited or resting state, the electrical potential difference across the cell membrane, transmembrane potential, is referred to as the resting membrane potential (RMP). The RMP is determined primarily by the distribution of potassium ions (K^+) across the cell membrane and by the permeability of the membrane to potassium (Washizu, 1966; Bennett and Burnstock, 1966; Hendrickx et al., 1975). In the resting state, the potassium concentration on the inside of the cell is greater than that on the outside of the cell, $[K^+]_i > [K^+]_o$, and the membrane is preferentially permeable to potassium. Because of the tendency for the positively charged K^+ ions to diffuse from the inside of the cell, where they are more concentrated, to the outside of the cell, where they are less concentrated, an electrical gradient is created, with the inside of the cell membrane being more negative than the outside (Figure 3–1A). The electrical gradient that is formed tends to oppose the further movement of K^+ ions outward across the cell membrane along its concentration gradient, and an equilibrium is reached. There is a greater concentration of K^+ on the inside of the membrane than on the outside, with the inside of the cell membrane being negative with respect to the outside of the cell membrane.

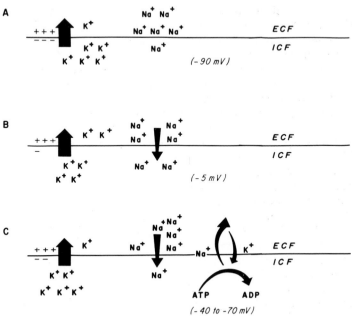

Figure 3–1. Ionic basis for resting membrane potential (RMP) in smooth muscle. In resting state, $[K^+]_i > [K^+]_o$ and $[Na^+]_o > [Na^+]_i$. A, Electrochemical changes that would occur if the membrane were solely permeable to potassium. K^+ would diffuse from the inside of the cell, where it is more concentrated, to the outside of the cell, where it is less concentrated. The outward movement of the positively charged K^+ ions would make the inside of the cell membrane negative with respect to the outside of the cell membrane. B, Electrochemical changes that would occur if the resting membrane were also permeable to sodium (Na^+). An inward movement of Na^+ along its concentration gradient would make the inside of the cell membrane less negative with respect to the outside of the cell membrane than is depicted in A. C, Pump mechanism for extruding Na^+ from within the cell against a concentration and electrochemical gradient. Inward movement of K^+ is coupled with an outward movement of Na^+. This mechanism helps maintain a steady state of ion distribution across the cell membrane and a stable RMP. ECF = extracellular fluid; ICS = intracellular fluid. (From Weiss, R. M.: Urology, *12*:114, 1978. Used by permission.)

If the membrane in the resting state was exclusively permeable to K^+, then the measured RMP of the ureteral smooth muscle cell should approximate -90 mV, the potassium equilibrium potential, as predicted by the Nernst equation

$$E_k = - \frac{RT}{nF} \ln \frac{[K^+]i}{[K^+]o}$$

where E_k is the potential difference attributable to the concentration difference of K^+, R is the molar gas constant, T is the absolute temperature, n is the number of moles and F is the faraday (Nernst, 1908). However, in the ureter and in other smooth muscles, the RMP is considerably less than the potassium equilibrium potential, with values of -33 to -70 mV, the inside of the cell being negative with respect to the outside (Washizu, 1966; Kobayashi, 1969). Thus, although the RMP of smooth muscle is primarily related to K^+, other ions probably also contribute.

One such ion that could account for the relatively low RMP of the ureter and other smooth muscles is sodium (Na^+) (Kuriyama, 1963). In the resting state, the sodium concentration on the outside of the cell membrane is greater than that on the inside, $[Na^+]_o > [Na^+]_i$. If the resting membrane were somewhat permeable to Na^+, both the concentration and the electrical gradient would support an inward movement of sodium across the cell membrane, with a resultant decrease in the electronegativity of the inner surface of the cell membrane (Fig. 3–1B).

If such an inward movement of Na^+ went unchecked, the RMP would be expected to decrease to a level lower than that actually observed, and the concentration gradient for Na^+ might become reversed. In order to maintain a steady-state ion distribution across the cell membrane with $[K^+]_o < [K^+]_i$ and $[Na^+]_o > [Na^+]_i$ and to prevent the transmembrane potential from becoming lower than the measured ureteral RMP, an active mechanism capable of extruding sodium from within the cell against a concentration and electrochemical gradient is required (Figure 3–1C). Although such an outward Na^+ pump that is coupled with an inward movement of K^+ has not been demonstrated in the ureter, it has been demonstrated in other smooth muscles and derives its energy requirements from the dephosphorylation of adenosine triphosphate (ATP) (Casteels, 1970).

The dynamic processes illustrated in Figure 3–1 enable the ureter in its resting state to maintain a constant, relatively low RMP. In addition to the mechanisms described, the distribution of chloride (Cl^-) ions across the cell membrane and the relative permeability of the membrane to Cl^- may be factors in the maintenance of the RMP in the ureter and other smooth muscles (Washizu, 1966; Kuriyama, 1963).

Action Potential

The transmembrane potential of an inactive or resting ureteral cell remains stable until it is excited by an external stimulus, whether it be electrical, mechanical (stretch), or chemical or by conduction of electrical activity (action potential) from an already excited adjacent cell. When a ureteral cell is stimulated, depolarization occurs, with the inside of the cell membrane becoming less negative than it was prior to stimulation. If a sufficient area of the cell membrane is depolarized rapidly enough to reach a critical level of transmembrane potential referred to as the threshold potential, a regenerative depolarization, action potential, is initiated (Weidmann, 1951).

The changes that occur are diagrammatically depicted in Figure 3–2. If a stimulus is very weak, as shown by arrow a, the transmembrane potential may remain unchanged. A slightly stronger, but yet subthreshold, stimulus may result in an abortive displacement of the transmembrane potential but not to such a degree that an action potential is generated (arrow b). If the stimulus is of sufficient strength to decrease the transmembrane potential to the

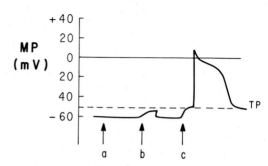

Figure 3–2. Response of ureteral transmembrane potential to stimuli. TP is threshold potential. At arrow a, weak stimulus is applied that does not alter RMP. At arrow b, stimulus is applied that decreases transmembrane potential but not to the level of TP (subthreshold stimulus). At arrow c, stimulus is applied that decreases the transmembrane potential to TP and an action potential is initiated (suprathreshold stimulus). (From Weiss, R. M.: Urology, *12*:114, 1978. Used by permission.)

threshold potential, the cell becomes excited and develops an action potential (arrow *c*). The action potential, which is the primary event in the conduction of the peristaltic impulse, has the capability to act as the stimulus for excitation of adjacent quiescent cells and through a complicated chain of events gives rise to the ureteral contraction.

When the ureteral cell is excited, its membrane loses its preferential permeability to K^+ and becomes more permeable to Na^+ and Ca^{++} ions, which move inward across the cell membrane and give rise to the upstroke of the action potential (Kobayashi, 1965; Vereecken et al., 1975 a and b; Kobayashi and Irisawa, 1964). As the positively charged Na^+ and Ca^{++} ions move inward across the cell membrane, the inside of the membrane becomes less negative with respect to the outside and may even become positive at the peak of the action potential, a state referred to as overshoot. The rate of rise of the upstroke of the ureteral action potential is relatively slow, $1.2^\pm 0.06$ V/sec in the cat (Kobayashi, 1969). This compares with a 610 V/sec rate of rise in dog cardiac Purkinje fibers (Draper and Weidmann, 1951) and a 740 V/sec rate of rise in skeletal muscle (Ferroni and Blanchi, 1965). The slowness of the rate of rise of the upstroke of the ureteral action potential accounts for the slow conduction velocity in the ureter.

After reaching the peak of its action potential, the ureter maintains its potential for a period of time (plateau of the action potential) before the transmembrane potential returns to its resting level (repolarization) (Kuriyama et al., 1967). The plateau phase of the guinea pig action potential is superimposed with multiple oscillations, a phenomenon not observed in the rat, rabbit, or cat (Fig. 3–3) (Bozler, 1938a). The plateau phase appears to depend on the persistence of a high inward Na^+ conductance, and the oscillations on the plateau of the guinea pig action potential appear to depend on an inward Ca^{++} conductance (Kuriyama and Tomita, 1970). The exact ionic mechanism for repolarization is not known but appears to be related, at least in part, to an outward movement of K^+ across the cell membrane. The duration of the action potential in the cat ranges from 259 to 405 msec (Kobayashi and Irisawa, 1964).

In summary, the transmembrane potential of the resting ureteral cell (RMP) is approximately -33 to -70 mV and is determined primarily by the distribution of K^+ ions across the cell membrane and the relatively selective permeability of the resting cell membrane to potassium. When excited by a suprathreshold stimulus, the membrane becomes less permeable to K^+ and more permeable to Na^+ and $Ca^{+,+}$, which move inward across the cell membrane and provide the ionic mechanism for the development of the upstroke of the action potential. After reaching the peak of its action potential, the membrane maintains a depolarized state—plateau of the action potential—for a period of time before the membrane potential of the activated cell returns to its resting level, repolarization. The plateau appears to be related to a persisting inward Na^+ current, and repolarization of the membrane probably is re-

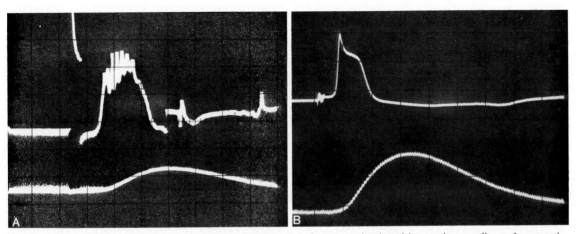

Figure 3–3. Intracellular recordings of ureteral action potentials (upper tracings) and isometric recordings of contractions (lower tracings) in response to electrical stimuli. Action potentials precede contractions. *A*, Guinea pig ureter; oscillations on plateau of action potential. *B*, Cat ureter; no oscillations on plateau of action potential. (From Weiss, R. M.: Urology, *12*:114, 1978. Used by permission.)

lated to a decrease in the membrane permeability to Na^+ and Ca^{++} and a renewed increase in permeability to potassium.

Pacemaker Potentials and Pacemaker Activity

Electrical activity arises in a cell either spontaneously or in response to an external stimulus. If the activity arises spontaneously, the cell is referred to as a pacemaker cell. Pacemaker fibers differ from nonpacemaker fibers in that their transmembrane resting potential does not remain constant but rather undergoes a slow spontaneous depolarization (Fig. 3–4). If the spontaneously changing membrane potential reaches the threshold potential, the upstroke of an action potential occurs. Changes in the frequency of action potential development may result from a change in the level of the threshold potential, a change in the rate of slow spontaneous depolarization of the resting potential, or a change in the level of the resting potential.

The ionic mechanism for pacemaker potentials in the upper collecting system or, for that matter, in other smooth muscles has not been fully determined. Several changes in ionic currents have been postulated to account for spontaneous changes in the transmembrane potential. These changes, which would make the inside of the cell less negative (that is, depolarize the membrane toward its threshold potential), include (1) a decrease in the outward K^+ current, (2) an increase in the inward Na^+ current, (3) a decrease in the pump extrusion of Na^+, or (4) an increased extrusion of Ca^{++} with resultant decrease in K^+ permeability (Tomita and Watanabe, 1973; Connor et al., 1974; Noble and Tsien, 1968).

Dixon and Gosling (Gosling and Dixon, 1971, 1974; Dixon and Gosling, 1973; Gosling, 1970) have provided morphologic evidence of specialized pacemaker tissue in the proximal portion of the urinary collecting system and have described species differences. In species with a multicalyceal system, such as the pig and man, the "pacemaker cells" are located near the pelvicalyceal border (Dixon and Gosling, 1973). Intracellular recordings have not been obtained from pacemaker cells in the upper urinary tract; however, Bozler (1942), using small extracellular surface electrodes, demonstrated the characteristic slow spontaneous depolarization of pacemaker-type fibers in the proximal portion of the isolated ureter of a unicalyceal upper collecting system. In a multicalyceal kidney, Morita and associates (1981), using extracellular electrodes, recorded low-voltage potentials that appear to be pacemaker potentials from the border of the minor calyces and the major calyx. They noted that the contraction rhythm varied in each calyx, a finding that is in accord with multiple pacemakers being present in the multicalyceal pig kidney (Constantinou et al., 1977).

At normal levels of urine output, pacemaker contractions of the calyces are frequently blocked in the renal pelvis or at the ureteropelvic junction (UPJ) (Morita et al., 1981). With increasing flow, there is a cessation of this block, and a 1:1 relationship is observed between pacemaker and ureteral contractions (Constantinou et al., 1976, 1981). In other words, at high flows, ureteric contractions occur at the same frequency as that of the calyces, whereas at lower flows, calyceal contraction frequencies are greater than those observed in the ureter.

Although the primary pacemaker for ureteral peristalsis is located in the proximal portion of the collecting system, other areas of the ureter may act as latent pacemakers. Under normal conditions, the latent pacemaker regions are dominated by activity arising at the primary pacemaker sites. When the latent pacemaker site is freed of its domination by the primary

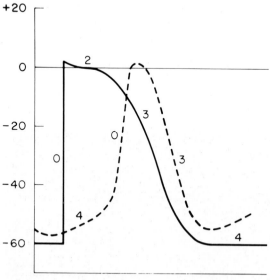

Figure 3–4. Schematic representation of pacemaker (dashed line) and nonpacemaker (solid line) action potentials: (0) upstroke or depolarization phase; (2) plateau phase; (3) repolarization phase; and (4) resting potential of nonpacemaker cell and spontaneous depolarization phase of pacemaker cell. Spontaneous decrease in transmembrane potential of pacemaker cells accounts for its spontaneous activity. (From Weiss, R. M.: Urology, 12:114, 1978. Used by permission.)

pacemaker, it, in turn, may act as a pacemaker. To demonstrate latent pacemaker sites, Shiratori and Kinoshita (1961b) transected the in vivo dog ureter at various levels. Prior to transection, peristaltic activity arose proximally from the primary pacemaker. When the ureter was transected at the UPJ, antiperistaltic waves of lower frequency than the previous normoperistaltic waves originated from the ureterovesical junction (UVJ). Division of the ureter at the UVJ did not affect the normoperistaltic waves. After division of the midureter, the normoperistaltic waves in the upper segment remained unchanged, and the lower segment demonstrated antiperistaltic waves, which originated at the UVJ at a frequency less than that of the normoperistaltic waves in the upper segment. Thus, cells at the UVJ of the dog may act as pacemaker cells when freed of control from the primary proximally located pacemaker. Latent pacemaker activity also has been demonstrated at the UVJ of the rat (Tindall, 1972), and it is possible that other regions of the ureter also may show latent pacemaker activity.

Propagation of Electrical Activity

Excitable cells possess resistive and capacitive membrane properties similar to a cable or core-conductor. The transverse resistance of the membrane is higher than the longitudinal resistance of the extracellular or intracellular fluid, allowing current resulting from a stimulus to propagate along the length of the fibers. The spread of current is referred to as electrotonic spread (Hoffman and Cranefield, 1960). The space constant (λ) determines the degree to which the electrotonic potential dissipates with increasing distance from an applied voltage. In a cable, this relationship is expressed by

$$P = P_o\, e^{-x/\lambda}$$

where x is the distance from the applied voltage, P is the displacement of the membrane potential at x, P_o is the displacement of the membrane potential at the site of the applied voltage, e is the base of the natural logarithm, and λ is the space constant. Thus, the electrotonic potential decreases by 1/e in one space constant. The space constant of the guinea pig ureter measured by extracellular stimulation is 2.5 to 3.0 mm (Kuriyama et al., 1967).

The time constant τ_m is expressed by

$$\tau_m = RC$$

where R is the membrane resistance and C is the membrane capacity. The time constant (τ_m) signifies that a small displacement of potential is decreased by 1/e of its value in one τ_m. The time constant of the guinea pig ureter measured by extracellular stimulation is 200 to 300 msec (Kuriyama et al., 1967).

The ureter acts as a functional syncytium (Bozler, 1938b). Engelmann (1869, 1870) showed that stimulation of the ureter could produce a contraction wave that propagates proximally and distally from the site of stimulation. Under normal conditions, electrical activity arises proximally and is conducted distally from one muscle cell to another across areas of close cellular apposition referred to as intermediate junctions (Uehara and Burnstock, 1970; Notley, 1970; Libertino and Weiss, 1972). The similarity of these close cellular contacts to nexuses, which have been shown to be low-resistance pathways for cell-to-cell conduction in other smooth muscles (Barr et al., 1968), suggests that a similar mechanism for conduction may be present in the ureter. Conduction velocity in the ureter is 2 to 6 cm/sec (Kuriyama et al., 1967; Ichikawa and Ikeda, 1960; Kobayashi, 1964). Conduction in the ureter is similar to that in cardiac tissue, even to the extent that the Wenckebach phenomenon (a partial conduction block) has been demonstrated in the ureter as it has in specialized cardiac fibers (Weiss et al., 1968).

CONTRACTILE ACTIVITY

The contractile event is dependent on the concentration of free sarcoplasmic Ca^{++} in the region of the contractile proteins, actin and myosin. Any process that results in an increase in Ca^{++} in the region of the contractile proteins favors the development of a contraction; any process that results in a decrease in Ca^{++} in the region of the contractile proteins favors relaxation (Fig. 3–5).

Contractile Proteins

In skeletal muscle, Ca^{++} appears to act as a derepressor. It is thought that in the relaxed state, a regulator system, consisting of the proteins troponin and tropomyosin, prevents the interaction of actin and myosin (Fig. 3–6A). In the relaxed state, the troponin that is attached to the tropomyosin is inactive, and the tropomyosin prevents the interaction between actin

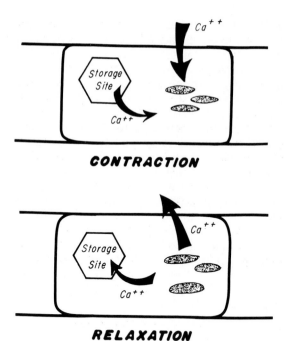

Figure 3–5. Schematic representation of calcium movements during contraction and relaxation. (From Weiss, R. M.: Urology, *12*:114, 1978. Used by permission.)

and myosin. With activation, there is an increase in the sarcoplasmic Ca^{++} concentration. The Ca^{++} binds to the troponin, producing a conformational change that results in the displacement of tropomyosin, thus allowing interaction of actin and myosin and the development of a contraction (Fig. 3–6*B*).

In smooth muscle, on the other hand, Ca^{++} appears to act as a real activator. The most widely accepted theory suggests that phosphorylation of myosin is involved in the contractile process and that a troponin-like system does not constitute the primary regulatory mechanism, as it does in skeletal muscle. With excitation, there is a transient increase in the sarcoplasmic Ca^{++} concentration from its steady-state concentration of 10^{-8} to 10^{-7} M to a concentration of 10^{-6} M or higher. At this higher concentration, Ca^{++} forms an active complex with the calcium-binding protein calmodulin (Watterson et al., 1976). Calmodulin without Ca^{++} is inactive (Fig. 3–7). The calcium-calmodulin complex activates a calmodulin-dependent enzyme, myosin light-chain kinase (Fig. 3–7). The activated myosin light-chain kinase, in turn, catalyzes the phosphorylation of the 20,000 dalton light chain of myosin (Fig. 3–8). Phosphorylation of the myosin light chain allows activation by actin of myosin Mg^{++}-ATPase activity, leading to hydrolysis of ATP and the development of smooth muscle tension or shortening (Fig. 3–9). Actin cannot activate the ATPase activity of the dephosphorylated myosin light chain.

When the Ca^{++} concentration in the region

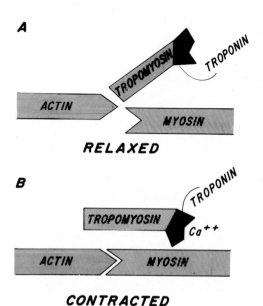

Figure 3–6. Schematic representation of contractile process in skeletal muscle. *A,* Relaxed state. *B,* Contracted state. (From Weiss, R. M.: Urology, *12*:114, 1978. Used by permission.)

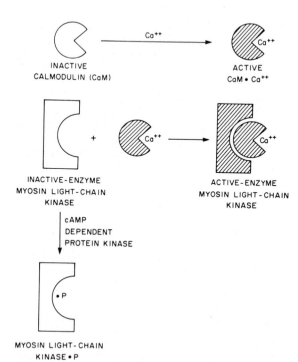

Figure 3–7. Schematic representation of contractile process in smooth muscle. Calmodulin is activated by Ca^{++}. The activated calcium-calmodulin complex activates the enzyme myosin light-chain kinase, which phosphorylates the light chain of myosin. Phosphorylation of myosin light-chain kinase decreases the rate of activation of the enzyme by the calcium-calmodulin complex.

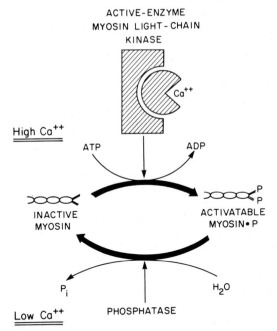

ACTIVE-ENZYME
MYOSIN LIGHT-CHAIN
KINASE

Ca^{++}

High Ca^{++}

ATP   ADP

INACTIVE
MYOSIN

ACTIVATABLE
MYOSIN•P

P$_i$ H$_2$O

Low Ca^{++} PHOSPHATASE

Figure 3–8. Schematic representation of the contractile process in smooth muscle. The activated enzyme, myosin light-chain kinase, catalyzes the phosphorylation of myosin. Myosin must be phosphorylated in order for actin to activate myosin ATPase.

of the contractile proteins is low, the myosin light-chain kinase is not active, since calmodulin requires Ca^{++} to activate the enzyme. This prevents activation of the contractile apparatus, as the myosin light chain cannot be phosphorylated, a process that must precede tension development. Furthermore, a phosphatase dephosphorylates the myosin light chain, thus preventing actin activation of myosin ATPase activity, and relaxation results. To date, there have been no studies of myosin light-chain ki-

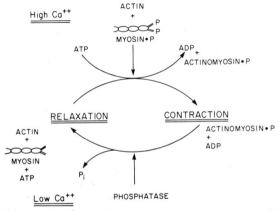

High Ca^{++}

ACTIN
+
MYOSIN•P

ATP   ADP
+
ACTINOMYOSIN•P

RELAXATION   CONTRACTION

ACTIN
+
MYOSIN
+
ATP

ACTINOMYOSIN•P
+
ADP

P$_i$

Low Ca^{++} PHOSPHATASE

Figure 3–9. Schematic representation of the contractile process in smooth muscle. Actin causes ATPase activity of phosphorylated myosin. This allows interaction of actin and myosin with the development of a contraction.

nase in the ureter, but a calcium-binding protein, presumably calmodulin, has been demonstrated (Weiss et al., 1981).

Recently, there has been evidence that phosphorylation of the enzyme myosin light-chain kinase by a cyclic AMP–dependent protein kinase decreases myosin light-chain kinase activity by decreasing the affinity of this enzyme for calmodulin (Adelstein et al., 1981). Such a process may in part account for cyclic AMP–dependent relaxation of smooth muscle.

Although most recent evidence supports the myosin phosphorylation theory of smooth muscle contractility, a minority opinion is that regulation of contraction is linked primarily to actin and that phosphorylation is not the primary mechanism. Leiotonin, a protein similar to troponin, and calmodulin are thought to be involved in the contractile process.

Calcium and Excitation-Contraction Coupling

The mechanical event of ureteral peristalsis follows an electrical event to which it is related. The calcium involved in the ureteral contraction is derived from two main sources. Since smooth muscle cells have a very small diameter, the inward movement of extracellular Ca^{++} into the cell during the upstroke of the action potential provides a significant source of sarcoplasmic calcium (see Fig. 3–5). In response to an excitatory impulse, calcium release from more tightly bound storage sites, presumably from the endoplasmic reticulum, mitochondria, and membrane-binding sites, also increases the Ca^{++} concentration in the sarcoplasm. Support for utilization of a dual source of Ca^{++} in the ureter has been provided by Vereecken and coworkers (1975a), who noted that it took approximately 45 minutes for spontaneous contractions of isolated guinea pig ureters to cease when the tissue was placed in a Ca^{++}-free medium. They interpreted this to indicate that some of the Ca^{++} involved in the contractile process is derived from tightly-bound intracellular stores. They also noted that recovery of the contractile response to electrical stimuli was almost immediate when the tissue was returned to a physiologic solution containing a normal concentration of calcium, suggesting that free extracellular Ca^{++} entering the cell during excitation also provided a source of Ca^{++} for the contractile machinery. A similar conclusion was reached by Hong and associates (1980a). Relaxation results from a decrease in the concentration of free sarcoplasmic Ca^{++} in the region of the contractile proteins. The decrease in sarcoplasmic Ca^{++} can result from uptake of Ca^{++} into intracellular storage sites or from extrusion of Ca^{++} from the cell.

Role of Cyclic Nucleotides

Although relaxation of smooth muscle may occur independently of changes in cyclic nucleotides (Vesin and Harbon, 1974), some relaxation processes are cyclic nucleotide–dependent (Triner et al., 1971). As an example of the latter mechanism, cyclic adenosine 3',5'-monophosphate (cyclic AMP, cAMP) is believed to mediate the relaxing effects of beta-adrenergic agonists in a variety of smooth muscles (Triner et al., 1971; Anderson, 1972; Kroeger and Marshall, 1974). According to this concept, the beta-adrenergic agonist isoproterenol serves as the "first messenger" and combines with a receptor on the outer surface of the cell membrane (Fig. 3–10). Isoproterenol itself does not enter the cell, but the beta-adrenergic agonist-receptor complex activates the enzyme adenylate cyclase on the inner surface of the cell membrane in close morphologic relation to the receptor. In the presence of magnesium, Mg^{++} and a guanine nucleotide, guanosine triphosphate (GTP), adenylate cyclase catalyzes the conversion within the cell of adenosine triphosphate (ATP) to cyclic AMP:

$$ATP \xrightarrow[Mg^{++},\ GTP]{adenylate\ cyclase} cAMP$$

Cyclic AMP acts as a "second" or "internal" messenger of the response elicited by the beta-adrenergic agonist. The increase in cyclic AMP through activation of an enzyme, protein kinase, and phosphorylation of proteins has been suggested to lead to the uptake of Ca^{++} into intracellular storage sites, such as the endoplasmic reticulum, with the resultant decrease of free sarcoplasmic Ca^{++} in the region of the contractile proteins (Anderson and Nilsson, 1972). The decrease in sarcoplasmic Ca^{++} in the region of the contractile proteins leads to relaxation of the smooth muscle. As previously described, the role of cyclic AMP in relaxation of smooth muscle also may be related to phosphorylation of myosin light-chain kinase by a cyclic AMP–dependent protein kinase (Adelstein et al., 1981).

There are two ways by which cyclic AMP levels may be increased within the cell. One is by increasing synthesis, which involves activation of the enzyme adenylate cyclase. The other is by decreasing degradation. The degradation of cyclic AMP involves activation of the enzyme phosphodiesterase:

$$cAMP \xrightarrow{phosphodiesterase} 5'\ AMP$$

Thus, agents that either increase adenylate cyclase activity or decrease phosphodiesterase activity may increase intracellular cAMP levels and cause smooth muscle relaxation.

Weiss and associates (1977) have demonstrated both adenylate cyclase and phosphodiesterase activities in the ureter and have shown that isoproterenol stimulates adenylate cyclase activity while theophylline inhibits phosphodiesterase activity. These two agents that relax ureteral smooth muscle would be expected to increase cyclic AMP levels, isoproterenol by increasing synthesis, theophylline by decreasing degradation. These data suggest that isoproterenol and theophylline could, at least in part, exert their ureter-relaxing effects through the cyclase-phosphodiesterase system. Further support of a role for cyclic AMP in smooth muscle

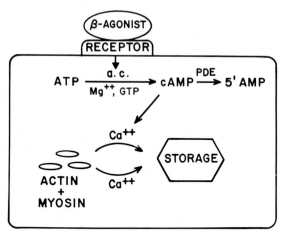

Figure 3–10. Schematic representation of the role of cyclic AMP in beta-adrenergic agonist–induced relaxation of smooth muscle. Agonist combines with receptor on the outer side of the cell membrane. The receptor-agonist complex, in turn, activates the enzyme adenylate cyclase (a.c.) on the inner surface of the cell membrane, which in the presence of magnesium (Mg^{++}) and guanosine triphosphate (GTP) results in the conversion of adenosine triphosphate (ATP) to cAMP. Cyclic AMP is postulated to cause an increased uptake of Ca^{++} into intracellular storage sites with a resultant decrease in Ca^{++} in the region of the contractile proteins, resulting in relaxation. Cyclic AMP also may have other actions not shown that inhibit the contractile process. The enzyme phosphodiesterase (PDE) degrades cAMP to 5'AMP. (From Weiss, R. M.: *In* Bergman, H. (Ed.): The Ureter. New York, Springer-Verlag, 1981, p. 137. Used by permission.)

relaxation can be derived from the finding that dibutyryl cAMP, which more readily diffuses into the intact cell and is less likely to be broken down by phosphodiesterase than is cyclic AMP, can induce relaxation of certain smooth muscles (Takago et al., 1971).

Less is known about the role of another cyclic nucleotide, guanosine 3',5'-monophosphate (cyclic GMP, cGMP) in smooth muscle function. Cyclic GMP is synthesized from guanosine triphosphate (GTP) via the enzyme guanylate cyclase and is degradated to 5'-GMP by a phosphodiesterase. To date, hormones and neurotransmitters have not been shown to activate guanylate cyclase. Phosphodiesterase activity that can degrade both cyclic AMP and cyclic GMP has been demonstrated in the canine ureter, and various inhibitors can preferentially inhibit the breakdown of one or the other cyclic nucleotide (Weiss et al., 1981). 8-Bromo cyclic GMP has been shown to cause relaxation of a number of smooth muscles (Schultz et al., 1979), and preliminary studies in our laboratories have shown that 8-bromo cyclic GMP induces relaxation of in vitro guinea pig ureteral segments. These data suggest that cyclic GMP may be involved in smooth muscle relaxation.

Intraluminal Pressures

The contractile event can be assessed clinically by measuring intraluminal pressures (Kiil, 1957). The recorded pressure complex reflects primarily pressure transmitted through the fluid column in front of the contractile wave (bolus pressure) and the pressure related to contraction and coaptation of the ureteral wall. Baseline or resting ureteral pressure is approximately 0 to 5 cm H_2O, and superimposed ureteral contractions ranging from 20 to 80 cm H_2O occur 2 to 6 times per minute (Ross et al., 1972).

Role of Nervous System in Ureteral Function

Some smooth muscles have a specific innervation of each smooth muscle fiber, whereas other syncytial-type smooth muscles lack discrete neuromuscular junctions and depend on a diffuse release of transmitter from a bundle of nerves with a subsequent spread of excitation from one muscle cell to another (Burnstock, 1970). The fact that the ureter is a syncytial type of smooth muscle without discrete neuromuscular junctions (Burnstock, 1970) has caused confusion in determining the role of the autonomic nervous system in its function.

As peristalsis may persist after transplantation (O'Conor and Dawson-Edwards, 1969) or denervation (Wharton, 1932), as spontaneous activity may occur in isolated in vitro ureteral segments (Finberg and Peart, 1970; Macht, 1916a; Malin et al., 1970), and as normal antegrade peristalsis persists after reversal of a segment of ureter in situ (Melick et al., 1961), it is apparent that ureteral peristalsis can occur without innervation. However, when analyzing the data in the literature, it is apparent that the nervous system plays at least a modulating role in ureteral peristalsis.

There is strong evidence to support the presence of excitatory alpha-adrenergic and inhibitory beta-adrenergic receptors in the ureter (Tindall, 1972; McLeod et al., 1973; Rose and Gillenwater, 1974; Weiss et al., 1978). Norepinephrine, which is primarily an alpha-adrenergic agonist although it also is able to stimulate beta-adrenergic receptors, increases the force of electrically induced ureteral contractions (Fig. 3–11) (Weiss et al., 1978). When administered in the presence of phentolamine (Regitine), an alpha-adrenergic blocking agent, norepinephrine decreases the force of ureteral contractions (Fig. 3–11) (Weiss et al., 1978). A similar reversal of action occurs in the in vivo ureter (McLeod et al., 1973; Kaplan et al., 1968) and can be explained by norepinephrine's acting primarily on inhibitory beta-adrenergic receptors when the excitatory alpha-adrenergic receptors are blocked. Propranolol (Inderal), a beta-adrenergic antagonist, potentiates the increase in contractile force induced by norepinephrine (Fig. 3–11) (Weiss et al., 1978). This can be explained by norepinephrine's acting more exclusively on excitatory alpha-adrenergic receptors when the inhibitory beta-adrenergic receptors are blocked. Furthermore, isoproterenol, a beta-adrenergic agonist, depresses contractility (Weiss et al., 1978). These data provide evidence for excitatory alpha-adrenergic and inhibitory beta-adrenergic receptors in the ureter; they are in accord with the findings of Deane (1967) and Malin and coworkers (1968) on spontaneously contracting in vitro ureteral segments and with the observations of Rose and Gillenwater (1974) and McLeod and associates (1973) on in vivo ureters. Further support for the presence of excitatory alpha-adrenergic and inhibitory beta-adrenergic receptors in the ureter includes the demonstration of adenylate cyclase activity in the ureter (Weiss et al., 1977) and the finding that when rabbits are depleted of

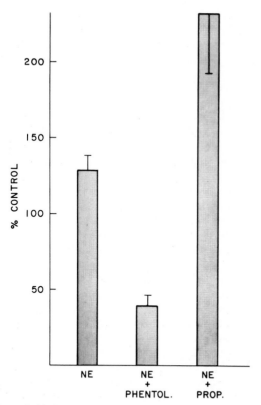

Figure 3–11. Effect of norepinephrine (NE) on electrically induced contractions of canine ureteral smooth muscle. One hundred per cent represents magnitude of control contractions. NE potentiation of contractility is inhibited by the alpha-adrenergic antagonist phentolamine (Phentol.) and activated by the beta-adrenergic antagonist propranolol (Prop.). (From Weiss, R. M.: *In* Bergman, H. (Ed.): The Ureter. New York, Springer-Verlag, 1981, p. 137. Used by permission.)

catecholamines by the administration of reserpine, their ureters undergo greater degrees of deformation when a given intraluminal pressure is applied than would result from application of the same pressure load to a ureter of a normal, non–reserpine treated animal (Weiss et al., 1974). Lastly, electrical stimulation with high-intensity, high-frequency, short-duration stimuli has been shown to release neurotransmitter, presumably from intrinsic neural tissue within the wall of the ureter (Weiss et al., 1978) and renal calyx (Longrigg, 1975).

The role of the parasympathetic nervous system in the control of ureteral function has been studied to a lesser extent. Available data suggest that cholinergic (parasympathetic) agonists potentiate ureteral contractility by directly stimulating cholinergic receptors (Vereecken, 1973) or by indirectly causing the release of catecholamines (Rose and Gillenwater, 1974).

Furthermore, DelTacca's (1978) demonstration of acetylcholine release from isolated guinea pig, rabbit, and human ureters during field stimulation, and the inhibition of this release by the neural poison tetrodotoxin, provide evidence of a role for the parasympathetic nervous system in the control of ureteral activity.

MECHANICAL PROPERTIES

Mechanical characteristics of muscle are commonly assessed by defining force-length and force-velocity relationships. Isometric force-length measurements depend on the number of linkages between the contractile proteins, actin and myosin, that are brought into action during contraction. Force-velocity relationships depend on the rate of formation and breakdown of linkages between the contractile proteins. Interventions may affect force-velocity relations, with or without affecting force-length curves (Sonnenblick, 1962). In addition to these methods of assessing mechanical properties of the ureter, the bidimensional nature of the ureter has lent itself to studies of pressure-length-diameter relations.

Force-Length Relations

Force-length relationships express the relation between the force developed by muscle when it is stimulated under isometric conditions and the resting length of the muscle at the time of stimulation. With stretching of the ureter (muscle lengthening), resting force (i.e., the tension present when the muscle is not excited) increases at a progressive rate (Weiss et al., 1972). Force developed during isometric contraction also increases with elongation until a length is reached at which maximum contractile force is achieved. With further lengthening, developed force decreases (Weiss et al., 1972). The ureter at this length is overstretched, that is, it is beyond the peak of its force-length curve. Ureteral resting tension is high at the length at which maximum contractile force is developed.

Since the ureter is a viscoelastic structure (Weiss et al., 1972), the resting or contractile force developed at any given length depends on the direction in which change in length is occurring and on the rate of length change (Weiss et al., 1972); Vereecken et al., 1973). This is referred to as hysteresis; for the ureter, at any given length, resting force is less and contractile force is greater when the ureter is allowed to shorten than when the ureter is being stretched (Fig. 3–12).

When the ureter is stretched, resting force increases. If length is kept constant at its new longer length following a stretch, changes occur that result in a decrease in resting force, i.e., stress relaxation (Fig. 3–13.) (Weiss et al., 1972). Within certain limits, when the ureter is stretched to a length beyond the peak of the force-length curve, that is, when the ureter is stretched to a length at which contractile force declines in the face of increasing muscle length, the degree of stress relaxation may be such that within a period of time, developed force no longer declines even though the increased length is kept constant (Weiss et al., 1972). Stress relaxation can thus be considered a compensatory mechanism of a viscoelastic structure to stretch.

Force-Velocity Relations

Force-velocity curves depict the relationship between the load and the velocity of short-

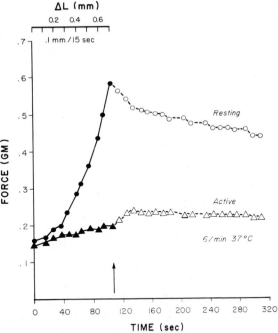

Figure 3–13. Stress relaxation. Resting and contractile (active) force of cat ureter is on the ordinate, time from onset of stretching is on the lower abscissa, and change in length (Δ L) is on the left upper corner abscissa. Muscle is stretched by a given amount and then held at a fixed length. Filled data points and solid lines show data obtained during muscle lengthening; open data points and dashed lines show data obtained after stretching has ceased (arrow) and muscle is maintained at a constant length. Resting force decreases when muscle was held at a constant length following a stretch (stress relaxation). Contractile (active) force increased during this period of time. (From Weiss, R. M., Bassett, A. L., and Hoffman, B. F.: Am. J. Physiol., *222*:388, 1972. Used by permission.)

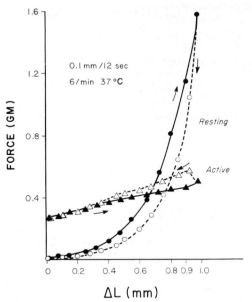

Figure 3–12. Hysteresis. Resting and contractile (active) force of cat ureter during muscle lengthening and shortening. Force is on the ordinate; change in length (Δ L) is on the abscissa. Closed data points and solid lines show data obtained during muscle lengthening. Open data points and dashed lines show data obtained during muscle shortening. Circles show resting force, and triangles show active or contractile force. Length and the direction of length change influence resting and contractile force. (From Weiss, R. M., Bassett, A. L., and Hoffman, B. F.: Am. J. Physiol., *222*:388, 1972. Used by permission.)

ening. A typical force-velocity curve as predicted by Hill's equation for muscle shortening has a hyperbolic configuration (Fig. 3–14) (Hill, 1938). From the force-velocity curve, one can extrapolate the maximum velocity of shortening, V_{max}, which represents velocity of shortening at zero load, i.e., at isotonic conditions. V_{max} is determined by the level at which the force-velocity curve crosses the ordinate. V_{max} values in the ureter are in the range of 0.5 to 0.7 lengths/second, which is in accord with observations in other smooth muscles (Aberg and Axelsson, 1965). The force-velocity curve intersects the abscissa at zero shortening, i.e., at isometric conditions where the load is great. Shortening depends on the total load lifted, with the ureter shortening to a lesser extent with heavier loads. At conditions near those of zero load, i.e., conditions of free shortening (isotonic

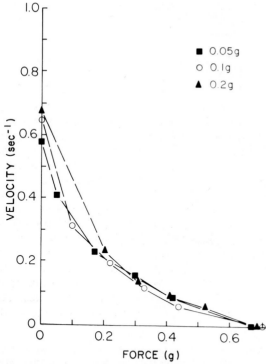

Figure legend:
- ■ 0.05g
- ○ 0.1g
- ▲ 0.2g

Figure 3–14. Force-velocity relation of guinea pig ureter. Specimens stretched by three different preloads (0.05, 0.1, and 0.2 g). The velocity of shortening on the ordinate is plotted as a function of the total load lifted on the abscissa. V_{max} is obtained by extrapolating the experimental curves to intersect the ordinate. Isometric force is given by data points where velocity equals zero. (From Biancani, P., Onyski, J. H., Zabinski, M. P., and Weiss, R. M.: J. Urol., *139*:988, 1984. Used by permission.)

conditions), the in vitro guinea pig ureter shortens by 25 to 30 per cent of its initial length.

Pressure-Length-Diameter Relations

Since ureteral muscle fibers are arranged in a longitudinal, circumferential, and spiral configuration (Tanagho, 1971), longitudinal and diametral deformation of the ureter are interrelated. Simultaneous studies of length and diameter changes in response to an intraluminal pressure load are another means of assessing the mechanical properties of a tubular structure. The ureter increases in both length and diameter after application of an intraluminal pressure, creep (Biancani et al., 1973). Deformation in response to a given intraluminal pressure load is greater in vitro than in vivo; this difference is partially negated if the in vivo preparation is pretreated with reserpine to suppress adrenergic influences (Fig. 3–15). Such data provide support for a role of the adrenergic nervous system in control of ureteral function.

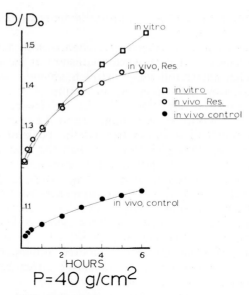

$$P = 40 \text{ g/cm}^2$$

Figure 3–15. Pressure-diameter relations. An intraluminal pressure load of 40 g/cm² was applied to rabbit ureters, and change in diameter (D/D$_o$) was measured as a function of time. Squares show data obtained from in vitro ureters. Closed circles show data obtained in vivo. Open circles show data obtained in vivo from animals previously treated with reserpine. D$_o$ = initial diameter; D = diameter during deformation.

PROPULSION OF URINARY BOLUS

The theoretical aspects of the mechanics of urinary transport within the ureter have been recently described in detail by Griffiths and Notschaele (1983) and are depicted in Figure 3–16. At normal flow rates as the renal pelvis fills,

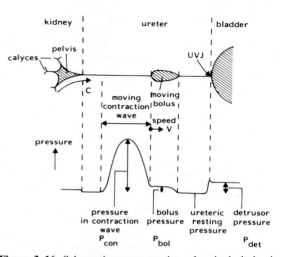

Figure 3–16. Schematic representation of a single bolus in the ureter moving away from the renal pelvis and toward the bladder. Corresponding distribution of pressure within the urinary tract is shown in the lower tracing. (From Griffiths, D. J., and Notschaele, C.: Neurol. Urodynam., *2*:155, 1963. Used by permission.)

there is a rise in renal pelvic pressure and urine is extruded into the upper ureter, which is initially in a collapsed state. Contraction waves originate in the most proximal portion of the ureter and move the urine in front of it in a distal direction. The urine that had previously entered the ureter is formed into a bolus. In order to propel the bolus of urine efficiently, the contraction wave must completely coapt the ureteral walls (Griffiths and Notschaele, 1983) and the pressure generated by this contraction wave provides the primary component of what is recorded by intraluminal pressure measurements. The bolus that is pushed in front of the contraction wave lies almost entirely in a passive, noncontracting part of the ureter (Weinberg, 1974; Fung, 1971). To enter the bladder the urine traverses the UVJ, which, when functioning properly, assures one-way transport of urine. The bolus is forced into the bladder by the advancing contraction wave, which dissipates at the ureterovesical junction.

As with any tubular structure, the ureter can transport a set maximum amount of fluid per unit time. Under normal flows, in which bolus formation occurs, the amount of urine transported per unit time is significantly less than the maximum transport capacity of the ureter. At extremely high flows, as are employed in the standard perfusion studies (Whitaker, 1973), the ureteral walls do not coapt, and a continuous column of fluid is transported rather than a series of boluses.

When transport becomes inadequate, stasis of urine occurs with resultant ureteral dilatation. Inadequate transport can result either from too much fluid entering the ureter per unit time or from too little fluid exiting the ureter per unit time. One must consider both input and output when predicting whether or not ureteral dilatation will occur. For example, a minor degree of obstruction to outflow will cause more dilatation at high-flow rates than at low-flow rates. Even a normal nonobstructed ureter will impede urine transport if the rate of flow is great enough.

Changes in ureteral dimensions that occur in pathologic states may in themselves result in inefficient urine transport, even if the contractile force of the individual fibers is unchanged. The Laplace equation expresses the relationship between the variables that affect intraluminal pressure:

$$\text{Pressure} = \frac{\text{tension} \times \text{wall thickness}}{\text{radius}}$$

An increase in ureteral diameter in itself can decrease intraluminal pressure and result in inefficient urine transport. Such dimensional changes may, at least theoretically, be deleterious (Griffiths, 1983).

Effect of Diuresis on Ureteral Function

With increasing urine flow rates, the initial response of the ureter is to increase peristaltic frequency. Maximum frequency rate increases, and then further increases in urine transport occur by means of increases in bolus volume (Briggs et al., 1972; Constantinou et al., 1974; Morales et al., 1952). At relatively low flow rates, small increases in flow result in large increases in peristaltic frequency. At higher flow rates, relatively large increases in flow result in only small increases in peristaltic frequency. As flow rate continues to increase, several of the boluses coalesce, and finally the ureter becomes filled with a column of fluid and dilates. At these high flow rates, urine transport is through an open tube.

Effects of Bladder Filling and Neurogenic Vesical Dysfunction on Ureteral Function

Ureteral dilatation can result either from an increase in fluid input or from a decrease in fluid output from the ureter. Since there is no evidence that the UVJ relaxes (Weiss and Biancani, 1983), the relationship between ureteral intraluminal pressure and intravesical pressure is important in determining the efficacy of urine passage across the UVJ into the bladder. In the case of the normal ureter under normal physiologic rates of flow, ureteral contractile pressure exceeds intravesical pressure, resulting in passage of urine into the bladder. In the dilated, poorly contracting ureter or in the normal ureter at extreme flow rates, the ureter does not coapt its walls to form boluses, and the baseline pressure in the column of urine within the ureter must exceed intravesical pressure in order for urine to pass into the bladder.

The pressure within the bladder during the storage phase is of paramount importance in determining the efficacy of urine transport across the UVJ. This is the pressure that the ureter needs to work against for the longest period of time. During filling of the normal bladder, sympathetic impulses and the viscoelastic properties of the bladder wall inhibit the magnitude of the intravesical pressure rise, i.e., the tonus limb. With filling, the normal bladder maintains a relatively low intravesical pressure (McGuire, 1983). The low intravesical pressure facilitates transport of urine across the UVJ and prevents ureteral dilatation. In the noncompliant fibrotic bladder and in some forms of neurogenic vesical dysfunction, the bladder is autonomous, and relatively small increases in bladder volume result in large increases in intravesical pressure with resultant impairment of ureteral emptying. The ureter initially responds to its decreased ability to empty by increasing its peristaltic frequency (Fredericks et al., 1972; Zimskind et al., 1969; Rosen et al., 1971). Ultimately, stasis occurs with the development of ureteral dilatation. The ureter has been shown to decompensate when intravesical pressure approaches 40 cm H_2O (McGuire et al., 1981).

PHYSIOLOGY OF THE URETEROPELVIC JUNCTION

At normal urine flows, the frequency of calyceal and renal pelvic contractions is greater than that in the upper ureter, and there is a relative block of electrical activity at the UPJ (Morita et al., 1981). At these flows, the renal pelvis fills, and as renal pelvic pressure rises, urine is extruded into the upper ureter, which is initially in a collapsed state (Griffiths and Notschaele, 1983). Ureteral contractile pressures that move the bolus of urine are higher than renal pelvic pressures, and a closed UPJ may be protective of the kidney in dissipating back-pressure from the ureter. As flow rate increases, there is cessation of the block at the UPJ and development of a 1:1 correspondence between pacemaker and ureteral contractions (Constantinou and Hrynczuk, 1976; Constantinou and Yamaguchi, 1981).

With ureteropelvic junction obstruction, there may be areas of narrowing or valvelike processes (Maizels and Stephens, 1980). In other instances, there is no gross narrowing at the UPJ, and abnormal propagation of the peristaltic impulse is a causative factor in the obstruction. In these instances, there appears to be a functional obstruction at the UPJ, since a large-caliber catheter can readily be passed through the UPJ even though urine transport is inadequate. Murnaghan (1958) related the functional abnormality to an alteration in the configuration of the muscle bundles at the UPJ, and Foote and associates (1970) observed a decrease in musculature at the UPJ. Hanna (1978), in an electron microscopic study of severe UPJ obstructions, noted abnormalities in the musculature of the renal pelvis and disruption of inter-

cellular relationships at the UPJ itself. Gosling and Dixon (1978) also observed histologic abnormalities in the dilated renal pelvis but were unable to confirm the alterations in the intercellular relationships at the UPJ. A vessel or adhesive band crossing the UPJ may potentiate the degree of dilatation in any of the forms of UJP obstruction.

The differences in the reported findings suggest a spectrum of histopathology in the group of cases referred to as ureteropelvic junction obstructions. It appears possible that, at least in some instances, disruption of cell-to-cell propagation of peristaltic activity results in impairment of urine transport across the ureteropelvic junction.

As one must consider input and output when predicting whether or not dilatation will occur, the effects of diuresis and obstruction appear to be complementary and additive with respect to the development of renal pelvic and calyceal dilatation. Some UPJ's can handle urine flow regardless of the magnitude of diuresis, others cause dilatation at even the lowest flows, and still others can handle low flows but cause massive dilatation at high flows (Fig. 3–17).

PHYSIOLOGY OF THE URETEROVESICAL JUNCTION

Griffiths (1983) has analyzed the factors involved in urine transport across the UVJ. Under normal conditions and at normal flow rates, the contraction wave, which occludes the ureteral lumen, propagates distally with the urine bolus in front of it. When the bolus reaches the UVJ, the pressure within the bolus must exceed intravesical pressure in order for the bolus of urine to pass across the UVJ into the bladder. Under these conditions, in which the contraction wave is able to coapt the ureteral wall and move the urinary bolus distally, the pressure generated by the contraction wave exceeds the pressure within the urinary bolus. The UVJ does not relax (Weiss and Biancani, 1983). Impediment of efficient bolus transfer across the UVJ into the bladder can occur when there is an obstruction at the UVJ, when intravesical pressure is excessive, or when flow rates are so high as to exceed the transport capacity of the normal UVJ. Under such conditions, in which the bolus of urine cannot pass freely into the bladder, the pressure within the bolus increases and may exceed the pressure in the contraction wave. This results in an inability of the contraction wave to completely occlude the ureter;

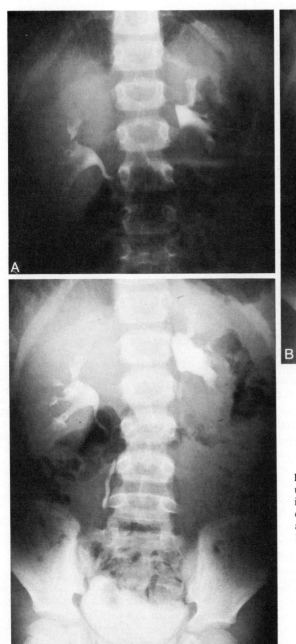
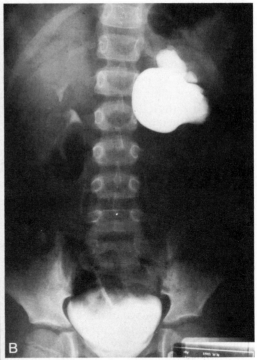

Figure 3–17. *A,* IVP shows essentially normal upper urinary tracts. *B,* Film from same child taken immediately after cardiac angiogram, which produces a massive diuresis. *C,* IVP 6 weeks after angiogram. (From Weiss, R. M.: J. Urol., *121*:401, 1979. Used by permission.)

there is retrograde flow of urine from the bolus, and only a fraction of the urinary bolus passes across the UVJ into the bladder. Griffiths (1983) has presented theoretical evidence to show that an exactly similar situation of impaired bolus transport across the UVJ would be expected if the ureter were wide or weakly contracting, even if the UVJ were perfectly normal. The wider and more weakly contracting the ureter, the lower the UVJ resistance must be in order

not to interfere with bolus transport. The resistance to flow at the UVJ has been variously attributed to forces in the trigone (Tanagho et al., 1968) and to detrusor pressure (Coolsaet et al., 1982).

The theoretical considerations outlined by Griffiths (1983) have direct clinical implications. If the UVJ were obstructed (i.e., had an abnormally high resistance to flow) or if detrusor pressure were excessive, large boluses occurring at high flow conditions would not be completely discharged into the bladder because the contraction wave pushing the bolus would be forced open, and intraureteric reflux would occur. Such obstruction at the UVJ would be detected by perfusion studies as popularized by Whitaker (1973, 1979), i.e., the Whitaker test. On the other hand, Griffiths' (1983) theory suggests that a similar breakdown of bolus discharge into the bladder can occur in the wide or weakly contracting ureter at high flow rates even if the UVJ is normal, and that such a condition would go undetected by a Whitaker test.

Effect of Obstruction on Ureteral Function

The effect of obstruction on ureteral function is dependent on the degree and duration of the obstruction, on the rate of urine flow, and on the presence or absence of infection. Following the onset of obstruction, there is a back-up of urine within the urinary collecting system with an associated increase in baseline (resting) ureteral intraluminal pressure and an increase in ureteral dimensions, i.e., length and diameter (Fig. 3–18) (Rose and Gillenwater, 1973; Biancani et al., 1976). The increase in intraluminal pressure is dependent on the continued production by the kidney of urine that cannot pass beyond the site of obstruction; the increase in ureteral dimensions results from the increased ureteral intraluminal pressure and the increased volume of urine retained within the ureter. A transient increase in the amplitude and frequency of the peristaltic contraction waves accompanies these initial dimensional and ureteral baseline (resting) pressure changes (Rose and Gillenwater, 1978). With time, as the ureter fills with urine the peristaltic contraction waves become smaller and unable to coapt the ureteral wall. Urine transport at this time becomes dependent on hydrostatic forces generated by the kidney (Rose and Gillenwater, 1973). Superimposed infection may result in a complete absence of contractions in the obstructed ureter and contributes to impairment of urine transport (Rose and Gillenwater, 1973).

Within a few hours following the onset of obstruction, intraluminal baseline ureteral pressure reaches a peak and then declines to a level only slightly higher than the normal baseline pressure. This occurs at a time in which dimensional changes remain stable (Biancani et al., 1976). The decrease in ureteral pressure can be attributed to changes in intrarenal hemody-

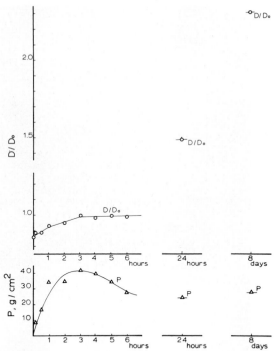

Figure 3–18. Intraluminal pressure and diameter changes subsequent to obstruction of rabbit ureter. Time from onset of obstruction is on the abscissa. Change in diameter (D/D_o) is on the upper ordinate, and intraluminal pressure is on the lower ordinate. During initial 3 hours of obstruction, intraluminal pressure increased to reach maximum and was associated with increase in diameter. Between 3 and 6 hours after onset of obstruction, pressure declined, although diametral deformation persisted. After 6 hours, pressure remained essentially unchanged, although diameter continued to increase. Each data point represents mean ± standard error of mean. D_o = initial diameter; D = diameter during deformation; P = intraluminal pressure. (Adapted from Biancani, P., Zabinski, M. P., and Weiss, R. M.: Am. J. Physiol., *231*:393, 1976.)

namics, such as a reduction in renal blood flow (Vaughan et al., 1971), with a resultant decrease in glomerular filtration rate and in intratubular hydrostatic pressure (Gottschalk and Mylle, 1956). Fluid reabsorption into the venous and lymphatic systems and a decrease in wall tension also may play a role in the reduction in baseline ureteral pressure (Rose and Gillenwater, 1978). The persistence of dimensional changes in the face of a decrease in intraluminal pressure is dependent on the hysteretic properties of the viscoelastic ureteral structure (Fig. 3–19) (Weiss et al., 1972; Vereecken et al., 1973; Biancani et al., 1973, 1976).

As the obstruction persists, there is a gradual increase in ureteral length and diameter to considerable dimensions. This occurs even though ureteral pressure remains at a relatively

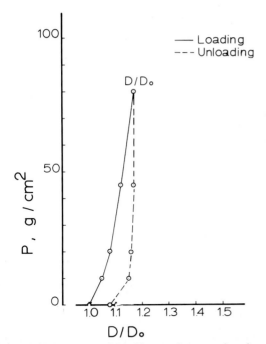

P, g / cm^2

Figure 3–19. Demonstration of hysteretic properties of ureter showing that dimensional changes are dependent on intraluminal pressure and on the direction of change of that pressure. At comparable pressures, deformations are greater during ureteral emptying than during ureteral filling. Solid line shows data obtained during loading; dashed line, data obtained during unloading. D_o = initial diameter; D = diameter during deformation; P = intraluminal pressure in g/cm^2. (Adapted from Biancani, P., Zabinski, M. P., and Weiss, R. M.: Am. J. Physiol., *231*:393, 1976.)

low and constant level. This process, observed in viscoelastic structures, is referred to as creep (Biancani et al., 1973). A continued, albeit small, urine production is required for the continuing increase in intraureteral volume. Such changes account for the relatively low intrapelvic pressures clinically observed in the massively dilated, chronically obstructed upper urinary tract (Struthers, 1969; Vela-Navarrete, 1971; Backlund et al., 1965; Djurhuus and Stage, 1976), and in experimentally produced obstruction (Schweitzer, 1973; Vaughan et al., 1970; Koff and Thrall, 1981a). One could postulate that with prolonged complete obstruction, total cessation of urine output ultimately occurs. Subsequent decrease in ureteral dimensions would depend on whether urine is reabsorbed and on the mechanical properties of the ureter at that time.

In order to determine the effect of obstruction on the contractile properties of the ureter, a rabbit model in which the ureter was totally obstructed for 2 weeks has been employed (Hausman et al., 1979; Biancani et al., 1982).

After 2 weeks of obstruction, cross-sectional muscle area increases by 250 per cent, ureteral length by 24 per cent, and ureteral outer diameter by 100 per cent. In addition to undergoing muscle hypertrophy, in vitro segments from obstructed ureters develop greater contractile forces, in both a longitudinal and a circumferential direction, than do segments from control ureters (Fig. 3–20). Determinations of stress, force per unit area of muscle, provide a means of determining whether the observed increases in developed force result from an increase in contractility or from an increase in muscle mass alone. The increases in force were associated with an increase in maximum active circumferential stress but no change in maximum active longtitudinal stress (Fig. 3–21). Since there is an increase in circumferential stress and no change in longitudinal stress, the sum of the stresses (total stress) or overall contractility increases following 2 weeks of obstruction. In order to account for these differences in longitudinal and circumferential stresses subsequent to obstruction, rotation of muscle bundles must occur; otherwise, longitudinal and circumferential stress would have increased equally. The rotation could result from the greater increase in diameter than in length following obstruction, from remodeling of the muscle fibers, or from both.

Thus, the dilated ureter following 2 weeks of obstruction is not mechanically decompensated, but rather undergoes changes that result in an increase in contractility. Despite the muscle hypertrophy and despite the increase in contractility, it is evident both clinically and experimentally that the obstructed, dilated ureter is less able than the normal ureter to generate the contractile pressures required for urine transport (Rose and Gillenwater, 1973). The decrease in the ability to generate an intraluminal pressure despite an increase in contractility results from the increase in ureteral diameter that occurs following obstruction and can be explained by the Laplace relationship:

$$\text{Pressure} = \text{stress} \times \frac{\text{wall thickness}}{\text{radius}}$$

Although contractility (stress) increases following 2 weeks of obstruction, the decrease in the wall thickness:radius ratio resulting from the marked increase in intraluminal diameter and thinning of the muscle layer accounts for the decrease in pressure. It is to be realized that a longer duration of obstruction or the presence of infection may alter these relationships.

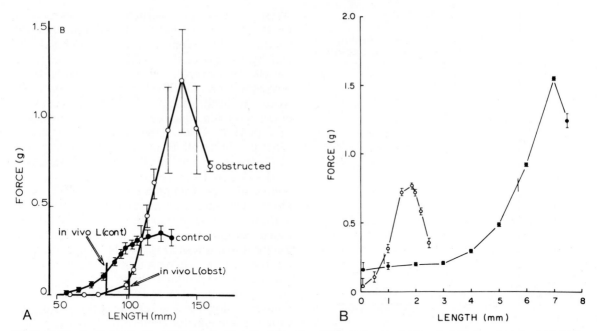

Figure 3–20. *A,* Active (contractile) longitudinal force-length relations of control (closed circles) and obstructed (open circles) rabbit ureters.

Each data point represents mean ± SEM. *B,* Active (contractile) circumferential force-length relations of obstructed (closed circles) and control (open circles) ureteral rings. Vertical bars correspond to in vivo lengths of control and obstructed segments. (*A,* From Hausman, M., Biancani, P., and Weiss, R. M.: Invest. Urol., *17:*223, 1979. *B,* From Biancani, P., Hausman, M., and Weiss, R. M.: Am. J. Physiol., *243:*F204, 1982. Used by permission.)

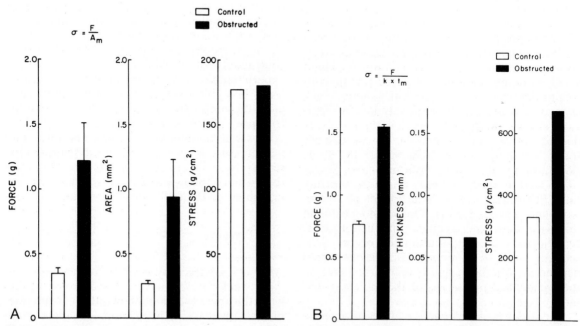

Figure 3–21. *A,* Longitudinal force, cross-sectional muscle area, and longitudinal stress at length of maximal active force development. *B,* Circumferential force, average muscle thickness, and circumferential stress at length of maximal active force development. σ = stress; F = force; A_m = cross-sectional muscle area; t_m = average thickness of muscle layer; K = a constant. (From Weiss, R. M., and Biancani, P.: Urology, *20:*482, 1982. Used by permission.)

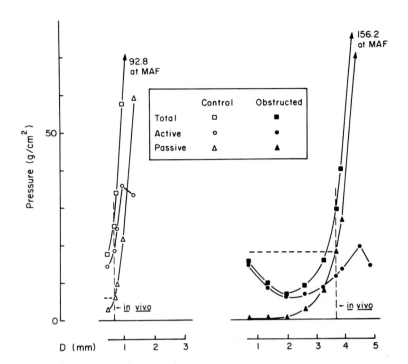

Figure 3–22. Pressure-diameter relationships of control and obstructed ureters. Calculated total, active, and passive pressures are shown as a function of intraluminal diameters (D). In vivo passive pressures are indicated by horizontal dashed lines and in vivo dimensions by vertical dashed lines. (Adapted from Biancani, P., Hausman, M., and Weiss, R. M.: Am. J. Physiol., *243*:F204, 1982.)

Estimates of intraluminal pressures as a function of diameter (pressure-diameter curves) can be calculated from in vitro circumferential force-length data (Fig. 3–22) (Biancani et al., 1982; Weiss and Biancani, 1982) and provide insight as to how obstruction interferes with urine transport. The validity of such calculations is supported by their correspondence to actual in vivo measurements (Rose and Gillenwater, 1973; Biancani et al., 1976). The obstructed ureter at in vivo dimensions has a higher resting (baseline) pressure and a lower contractile (active) pressure than do control ureters. In control ureters, the total (active + passive or resting) pressure developed at all diameters exceeds the passive pressure shown by the horizontal dotted line, and thus the generated active or contractile pressures are able to fully coapt the ureteral lumen and propel the urine bolus. In the obstructed ureter at diameters less than 3.3 mm, the passive pressure, as shown by the horizontal dotted line, exceeds the total pressure. The contraction ring therefore is incapable of contracting below this diameter, and the pressure in the whole ureter remains approximately uniform and equal to the passive pressure. The principal effect of the contraction wave in the obstructed dilated ureter is to reduce slightly the ureteral volume and thereby raise slightly the overall resting pressure. Thus, although the obstructed ureter is able to develop greater circumferential contractile forces than the control ureter, the expected intraluminal pressure generated by the obstructed ureter would be little different from baseline (resting) pressure, and the contraction wave occurring during propagation of peristalsis would be incapable of coapting the ureteral lumen and propelling the urine bolus in an effective manner.

It should be noted that the calculated active pressure in the obstructed ureter estimates the pressure that would develop if the whole ureter contracted simultaneously and uniformly throughout its whole length, rather than the pressure measured in a peristaltic contraction wave, which involves contraction of only a small segment of ureter at a given time. The fact that the calculated pressures in the obstructed ureter are, if anything, a slight overestimate of expected pressures only further supports the conclusion that the obstructed ureter is incapable of coapting its lumen and efficiently propelling the urine bolus. If, however, the urine were removed from the lumen of the ureter (for instance, by relieving the obstruction), the ureter obstructed for 2 weeks would be able to immediately coapt its lumen and produce pressures comparable to those of control ureters. This can be appreciated from Fig. 3–22, in which one can note that the total pressure in the obstructed ureter near zero diameter is comparable to the total pressure in the control ureter at a similar diameter. Thus, 2 weeks of obstruction result in an increase in ureteral contractility, but a decrease in contractile intraluminal pressures. This decrease in the ability to generate an active intraluminal pressure and to coapt the ureteral lumen impairs urine transport in the obstructed ureter.

Obstruction also has been shown to alter the hierarchic organization of the multiple coupled pacemakers that normally coordinate peristaltic activity (Constantinou and Djurhuus, 1981; Djurhuus and Constantinou, 1982). Such disruption causes discoordination of pelvic contractility with resultant incomplete emptying of the renal pelvis, which contributes to upper urinary tract dilatation.

PHYSIOLOGIC METHODOLOGIES FOR ASSESSING CLINICAL OBSTRUCTION

A variety of radiographic methodologies, the rationale for whose use is based on physiologic principles, are employed in the evaluation and differentiation of upper urinary tract dilatation and obstruction. Description of these examinations, which include diuretic urograms and diuretic radionuclide renograms, is beyond the scope of this chapter (see Chapter 7). At present, the best available methods for differentiating obstructive from nonobstructive dilatation depend on assessing the efficacy of urine transport. When transport becomes inadequate, urine stagnates and dilatation occurs. Dilatation is dependent on the compliance of the system and can result either from too much fluid entering the system per unit time or from too little fluid exiting the system per unit time. The properly functioning upper urinary tract should transport urine over the entire range of physiologically possible flow rates without undergoing marked deformational changes or increases in intraluminal pressure of a magnitude that would be deleterious to the function of the ureter, renal pelvis, or kidney.

Measurement of basal or resting intraluminal pressures does not help in differentiating obstructive from nonobstructive dilatation, since the pressures may be low even when obstruction is present (Struthers, 1969; Vela-Navarrete, 1971; Backlund et al., 1965). The values obtained vary with the state of hydration, the degree of renal function, the severity and duration of obstruction, and the compliance of the system. Perfusion studies are widely used in an attempt to differentiate dilated systems that are obstructed from those that are not obstructed (Whitaker, 1973, 1978; Reuterskiöld, 1969, 1970; Backlund and Reuterskiöld, 1969a and

b). The technique involves cannulating the dilated upper urinary tract and perfusing the system at a rate of 10 ml/min. Pressures are measured after achievement of steady-state conditions, which occurs when an equilibrium is reached between the flow into and out of the system. Fluoroscopic monitoring aids in the interpretation of the data (Coolsaet et al., 1980; Whitfield et al., 1976). The basic hypothesis in perfusion studies is that if the dilated upper urinary tract can transport 10 ml/min (a fluid load greater than it would ever be expected to handle during usual physiologic states) without an inordinate increase in pressure, then any degree of obstruction, even if present, need not be repaired. Whitaker and associates have concluded from a large clinical experience that under these flow conditions, a pressure less than 15 cm H_2O correlates with a nonobstructive state, whereas pressures greater than 22 cm H_2O invariably correlate with obstruction (Whitaker, 1978; Witherow and Whitaker, 1981). With this definition, minor degrees of obstruction could go undetected; however, the presumption is that if at high flows the hydrostatic pressure in the system is not at a level that would produce renal deterioration, then lower and more physiologic flows surely will be tolerated. The high flows are used to stress the system and thus to detect the slightest propensity to obstruction. The interpretation of data obtained by perfusion studies is schematically shown in Figure 3–23.

In order to obtain relevant information, strict adherence to detail is required in the performance of perfusion studies. One must take care to assure that an equilibrium state has been reached prior to obtaining pressure measurements. Extrinsic factors that affect resistance to flow, such as needle size, length and compliance of extrinsic tubing, viscosity of perfusion fluid, temperature, and flow rate, must be taken into account when quantitative data are obtained (Toguri and Fournier, 1982). Furthermore, the bladder needs to be continuously drained to eliminate the bladder's effect on urine transport.

When performed and interpreted properly, perfusion studies may provide clinically relevant information in selected cases. The basic problem in the interpretation of data with this and other diagnostic methods is the definition of "clinically relevant obstruction"—that is, just how much resistance to flow or increase in pressure is required to produce renal functional or anatomic deterioration as a function of time, taking into account the compliance of the system (Koff and Thrall, 1981b). Lastly, it is theoretically

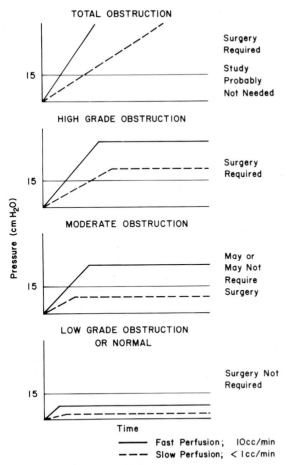

TOTAL OBSTRUCTION

Surgery Required

Study Probably Not Needed

HIGH GRADE OBSTRUCTION

Surgery Required

MODERATE OBSTRUCTION

May or May Not Require Surgery

LOW GRADE OBSTRUCTION OR NORMAL

Surgery Not Required

Time

——— Fast Perfusion; l0cc/min
– – – Slow Perfusion; < l cc/min

Pressure (cm H₂O)

Figure 3–23. Schematic representation of data that can be obtained with perfusion studies. Fast perfusion rate, 10 cc per minute, would be used in standard Whitaker test. Slow perfusion rate, < 1 cc per minute, would be closer to more physiologic rates of flow. (From Weiss, R. M.: J. Urol., *121*:401, 1979. Used by permission.)

possible that the wide or weakly contracting ureter at high flow rates may interfere with bolus transport even if the UVJ is normal (Griffiths, 1983). Such an obstructive process would not be detected by perfusion studies.

These theoretical considerations provide a rationale for ureteral tapering (Hendren, 1970), a procedure that to date has been shown to improve radiographic appearances, although questions remain as to whether it aids in preserving renal function when anatomic or functional obstruction does not exist. The Laplace relationship provides a possible explanation for anticipated improvement in function resulting from tapering. With ureteral tapering, muscle thickness and the ability of the ureteral fibers to contract (stress) remain unchanged. The decrease in radius resulting from tapering itself, according to the Laplace relationship, could

account for higher intraluminal pressures, which could improve urine transport. Thus, the tapered ureter may coapt its walls more readily and generate higher intraluminal pressure even though the material itself has not changed (Weiss and Biancani, 1982). Although the possibility of deleterious effects of the wide "nonobstructed" ureter remains controversial, one should consider such effects when interpreting data obtained with the present modalities for diagnosing obstruction and when determining management.

Relationship Between Vesicoureteral Reflux and Ureteral Function

Factors that have been implicated in the development of vesicoureteral reflux include (1) anatomic and functional abnormalities at the UVJ, (2) inordinately high intravesical pressures, and (3) impaired ureteral function. The normal intravesical ureter is approximately 1.5 cm in length and takes an oblique course through the bladder wall. It is composed of an intramural segment surrounded by detrusor muscle and a submucosal segment that lies directly under the bladder urothelium (Tanagho et al., 1968). The relationship between the length and diameter of this intravesical segment of ureter appears to be a factor in the prevention of vesicoureteral reflux (Paquin, 1959). Reflux may occur when the intravesical tunnel is destroyed. Trigonal function also may be a factor in the prevention of vesicoureteral reflux. Tanagho and associates (1965) have created vesicoureteral reflux in the cat by disruption of the trigone or by sympathectomy and, conversely, have increased the pressure within the intravesical ureter by electrical stimulation of the trigone or by administration of intravenous epinephrine. The development of vesicoureteral reflux in individuals with bladder outlet obstruction and neurogenic vesical dysfunction provides evidence that increased intravesical pressures also may be a factor in certain instances of reflux.

Although an abnormality of the UVJ is the primary etiologic factor in most cases of reflux, there is evidence to suggest that decreased ureteral peristaltic activity may be a contributory factor. This may explain why a normal ureter may not reflux even when reimplanted into a bladder without a submucosal tunnel (Debruyne et al., 1978) or why a defunctionalized refluxing ureter may cease to reflux when a proximal diversion is taken down (Teele et al., 1976;

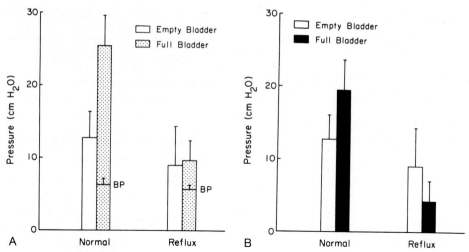

Figure 3–24. *A,* Ureterovesical junction pressures. Bladder pressure is approximately zero cm H_2O with the bladder empty and is labeled as BP with the bladder full. *B,* Pressure gradient across ureterovesical junction, obtained by subtracting bladder pressure from ureterovesical junction pressure. (From Weiss, R. M., and Biancani, P.: J. Urol., *129*:858, 1983. Used by permission.)

Weiss, 1979). The observation that vesicoureteral reflux may temporarily cease following electrical stimulation (Melick et al., 1966) further supports this possibility.

Even the mildest forms of vesicoureteral reflux are associated with a decreased frequency of ureteral peristalsis (Weiss and Biancani, 1983; Kirkland et al., 1971). Although this may offer further evidence that decreased peristaltic activity is a possible etiologic factor in the development of reflux, an alternative interpretation is that the decreased peristaltic activity reflects changes in ureteral or renal function resulting from the reflux. Lastly, the success rate of antireflux procedures is lower with poorly functioning dilated ureters; although this may be related to technical factors, decreased peristaltic activity may be a reason for failure in many instances.

Studies in normal and mildly refluxing systems have shown that there is a high-pressure zone in the distal ureter, with a resultant pressure gradient across the UVJ (Weiss and Biancani, 1983). Although the cause of the UVJ gradient is not known, the weight of the fluid within the bladder compressing the intravesical ureter may be a factor. Another causative factor may be bladder or trigonal tension that may involve myogenic or neurohumoral mechanisms. With bladder filling, there is an increase in the amplitude of the high-pressure zone that is greater in nonrefluxing than in refluxing systems. With bladder filling, the resultant UVJ-bladder pressure gradient increases in nonrefluxing systems, whereas it decreases and may

disappear in refluxing systems (Fig. 3–24) (Weiss and Biancani, 1983). This decrease in pressure gradient may correspond to the time when reflux occurs and may be related to lateralization of the ureteral orifice and shortening of the intravesical tunnel.

Effect of Infection on Ureteral Function

Infection within the upper urinary tract may impair urine transport. In 1913, Primbs showed that *Escherichia coli* and staphylococcal toxins inhibited contractions of in vitro guinea pig ureteral segments (Primbs, 1913). Subsequent studies have confirmed that bacteria and *E. coli* endotoxin can inhibit ureteral activity (Teague and Boyarsky, 1968; Grana et al., 1965; King and Cox, 1972), and pyelonephritis in the monkey has been associated with decreased peristaltic activity (Roberts, 1975). Furthermore, Rose and Gillenwater (1973) have shown that infection can potentiate the deleterious effects of obstruction on ureteral function.

In man, irregular peristaltic contractions with an often decreased amplitude have been recorded with infection, and, in the more severe cases, absence of activity has been noted (Ross et al., 1972). Furthermore, ureteral dilatation has been reported to result from retroperitoneal inflammatory processes secondary to appendicitis, regional enteritis, ulcerative colitis, or peritonitis (Makker et al., 1972). Infection also may reduce the compliance of the intravesical ureter and permit reflux to occur in situations in which the UVJ is intrinsically of marginal competence (Cook and King, 1979).

Effect of Calculi on Ureteral Function

Factors that can affect the spontaneous passage of calculi include (1) the size and shape of the stone (Ueno et al., 1977), (2) intrinsic areas of narrowing within the ureter, (3) ureteral peristalsis, (4) hydrostatic pressure of the column of urine proximal to the calculus (Sivula and Lehtonin, 1967), and (5) edema, inflammation, and spasm of the ureter at the site at which the stone is lodged (Holmlund and Hassler, 1965; Scheele, 1965).

Two factors that appear to be most useful in facilitating stone passage are an increase in hydrostatic pressure proximal to a calculus and relaxation of the ureter in the region of the stone. In support of the theory that hydrostatic pressure facilitates stone passage, artificial concretions with holes were shown to move more slowly in the rabbit and dog ureter than those without holes (Sivula and Lehtonen, 1967). Furthermore, ureteral ligation proximal to a concretion, which decreases hydrostatic pressure by decreasing urine output and which decreases peristaltic activity proximal to a stone, hampers stone passage (Sivula and Lehtonen, 1967).

With respect to the potential facilitative effect of ureteral relaxation on stone passage, the spasmolytic agents phentolamine, an alpha-adrenergic antagonist, and orciprenaline, a beta-adrenergic agonist, have been shown to dilate the ureteral lumen at the level of an artificial concretion and thus permit increased fluid flow beyond the concretion (Peters and Eckstein, 1975). Whether this spasmolytic effect would aid in stone passage has not been determined. In a study in man, renal colic was relieved by meperidine in 83 per cent of patients, by phentolamine in 63 per cent, and by propranolol, a beta-adrenergic antagonist that presumably would interfere with the beta-adrenergic inhibitory actions of catecholamines, in 0 per cent (Kubacz and Catchpole, 1972). Although these data suggest that drugs with spasmolytic effects on the ureter may relieve renal colic, whereas those with spasmogenic actions do not, no attempt was made to assess the efficacy of these agents in promoting stone passage.

Glucagon administration at the time of an excretory urogram has been suggested as a potential aid in stone passage (Lowman et al., 1977). Although this finding may be dependent on the relaxant effect of glucagon on the ureter (Boyarsky and Labay, 1969), the diuretic effects of the contrast agent, with resultant increases in hydrostatic pressure, complicate the interpretation of the clinical study.

Although the above-described pharmacologic data can be interpreted to imply that ureteral relaxation in the region of a concretion would aid in stone passage, a controlled study is not available at present. Such a study with an agent known to have strong relaxant effects on the ureter, such as theophylline (Weiss et al., 1977), would be of value, but the interpretation of the data might be difficult because of the marked variability of spontaneous stone passage in the clinical setting.

Effect of Pregnancy on Ureteral Function

Hydroureteronephrosis of pregnancy begins in the second trimester of gestation and subsides within the first month after parturition. It is more severe on the right side, and the ureteral dilatation does not occur below the pelvic brim. Roberts (1976) has presented a strong case in favor of obstruction as the etiologic factor in the development of hydroureteronephrosis of pregnancy, whereas others have suggested a hormonal mechanism for the ureteral dilatation of pregnancy (van Wagenen and Jenkins, 1939). As emphasized by Roberts (1976), (1) elevated baseline (resting) ureteral pressures consistent with obstructive changes have been recorded above the pelvic brim in pregnant women, and these pressures decrease when positional changes permit the uterus to fall away from the ureters (Sala and Rubi, 1967); (2) normal ureteral contractile pressures have been recorded during pregnancy, suggesting that hormonally induced ureteral atony is not the prime factor in ureteral dilatation of pregnancy; (3) women whose ureters do not cross the pelvic brim, i.e., those with pelvic kidneys or ileal conduits, do not develop hydronephrosis of pregnancy; (4) hydronephrosis of pregnancy usually does not occur in quadripeds, whose uterus hangs away from the ureters (Traut and Kuder, 1938); and (5) elevated ureteral pressures in the pregnant monkey return to normal when the uterus is elevated from the ureters at laparotomy or when the fetus and placenta are removed from the uterus.

Observed hormonal effects on ureteral function have been used to implicate a hormonal mechanism in the ureteral dilatation of pregnancy. Difficulties in interpretation arise from inconsistencies in the data, however. Several studies have shown an inhibitory effect of progesterone on ureteral function (Lubin et al., 1941; Hundley et al., 1942; Kumar, 1962; Padovani, 1954). Progesterone has been noted to increase the degree of ureteral dilatation during pregnancy and to retard the rate of disappearance of hydroureter in post-partum women (Lubin et al., 1941). Others, however, have failed to observe an effect of progesterone on ureteral activity in animals (Payne and Hodes, 1939; McNellis and Sherline, 1967), or in men (Schneider et al., 1953; Lapides, 1948), and still others have failed to induce changes in ureteral activity in women by the administration of estrogens, progesterone, or a mixture of these drugs (Marchant, 1972; Clayton and Roberts, 1973). Although obstruction appears to be the primary factor in the development of hydronephrosis of pregnancy, there is some evidence to suggest that a combination of hormonal and obstructive factors is involved (Fainstat, 1963).

Effect of Age on Ureteral Function

Clinically, the response of the ureter to pathologic conditions seems to vary with age. More marked degrees of ureteral dilatation are observed in the neonate and young child than in the adult. Experimental data corroborating this clinical impression can be derived from observed age-dependent differences in the response of in vitro ureteral segments to an intraluminal pressure load. The neonatal rabbit ureter undergoes a greater degree of deformation in response to an applied intraluminal pressure than does the adult rabbit ureter (Akimoto et al., 1977). Furthermore, norepinephrine decreases the diametral deformation of the neonatal rabbit ureter in response to an applied intraluminal pressure but has little effect on the deformation of the adult rabbit ureter (Fig. 3–25). Thus, the in vitro neonatal rabbit ureter appears to be more compliant and more sensitive to norepinephrine than does the adult rabbit ureter.

A progressive increase in ureteral cross-sectional muscle area is observed in the guinea pig between 3 weeks and 3 years of age. This is in accord with the findings of Cussen (1967), who noted in a human autopsy study in subjects ranging in age from 12 weeks of gestation to 12 years of age that there is a progressive increase in the population of smooth muscle cells and a small increase in the overall size of the individ-

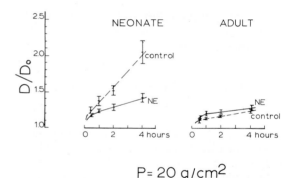

Figure 3–25. Changes in diameter of neonatal and adult rabbit ureteral segments as a function of time after application of a constant intraluminal pressure of 20 g/cm^2. Diametral deformation, D/D_o of control neonatal ureters was significantly greater than that of control adult ureters. Norepinephrine (10^{-5} M) decreased diametral deformation of neonatal ureters but had no significant effect on deformation of adult ureteral segments. D_o = initial diameter; D = diameter during deformation; P = intraluminal pressure. (From Akimoto, M., Biancani, P., and Weiss, R. M.: Invest. Urol., *14*:297, 1977. Used by permission.)

ual smooth muscle cells. In addition, an irregular increase in the number of elastic fibers was observed with increasing age.

The contractility of the ureter also is affected by age. Maximum active force of isolated guinea pig ureteral segments increases between 3 weeks and 3 years of age (Fig. 3–26) (Hong et al., 1980b). The increase in force developed between 3 weeks and 3 months of age seems to be attributable to an increase in contractility, since there is an associated increase in active stress, force per unit area of muscle. The increase in force developed between 3 months and 3 years of age can be explained by an increase in mass alone, since there is no change in active stress between these two age groups (Fig. 3–26).

Although changes in the force-length relationships of guinea pig ureter occur with age, the force-velocity relationships do not change with age (Biancani et al., 1984). Thus, although ureteral contractility increases during early development, as shown by an increase in force per unit area of muscle or stress, there appears to be no significant change in the rate of the driving reactions that control the contractile process, that is, no change in shortening, velocity, work, or power.

EFFECT OF DRUGS ON THE URETER

To assess the effect of drugs on the ureter, it is necessary to understand the anatomic, phys-

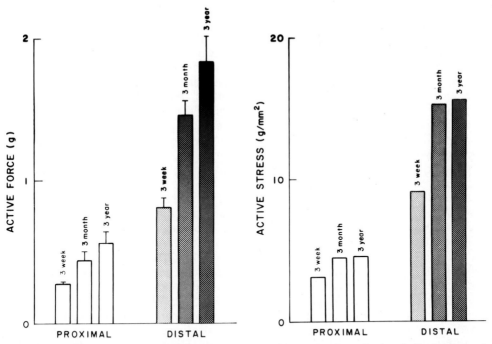

Figure 3–26. Maximal active (contractile) force and maximal active stress of proximal and distal guinea pig ureteral segments as a function of age.

iologic, and biochemical properties of the ureter, in addition to understanding the principles of drug action. For a drug to elicit a given response, it is necessary to achieve and maintain an appropriate concentration of that drug at its site of action. Factors that influence achievement of an effective concentration of drug at a site of action include the route of administration and cellular distribution of the drug; the dosage of the drug administered; the biotransformation, including metabolism and excretion, of the drug; the binding of the drug to plasma and tissue proteins; and the effects of age and disease on the absorption, distribution, metabolism, and elimination of the drug.

The literature contains considerable amounts of confusing and conflicting information concerning the effects of drugs on the ureter. To some extent, the discrepancies in the available data are due to poorly controlled experimental procedures or to attempts to compare dissimilar functional responses of the ureter to a given drug. To simplify the present section, no attempt will be made to analyze the validity of each pharmacologic study or to rationalize discrepancies in the literature; rather, an overview will be presented with an attempt to provide a consensus that at times may be prejudiced by personal bias. A recent and more complete review of drug effects on the ureter is available (Weiss, 1982).

Cholinergic Agonists

The prototypic cholinergic agonist is acetylcholine (ACh), which serves as the neurotransmitter at (1) neuromuscular junctions of somatic motor nerves (nicotinic sites); (2) preganglionic parasympathetic and sympathetic neuroeffector junctions (nicotinic sites); and (3) postganglionic parasympathetic neuroeffector sites (muscarinic sites). Acetylcholine synthesis involves

$$\text{acetyl CoA} + \text{choline} \xrightarrow[\text{acetyltransferase}]{\text{choline}} \text{ACh}$$

The acetylcholine is stored in vesicles within the synaptic terminal; its release is dependent on the influx of Ca^{++} into the terminal, which presumably causes vesicle fusion with the presynaptic terminal membrane, thereby expelling ACh into the synaptic cleft. Acetylcholine subsequently is hydrolyzed by acetylcholinesterase (AChE). The muscarinic effects of cholinergic agonists can be blocked by atropine. The effects of nicotinic agonists can be blocked by nondepolarizing ganglionic blocking agents or by high concentrations of the nicotinic agonist itself, which may cause ganglionic blockade by desensitization of receptor sites after an initial period of ganglionic stimulation.

Cholinergic agonists, which include acetylcholine, methacholine (mecholyl), carbamylcholine (carbachol), and bethanechol (Urecholine) have, in general, been observed to have an excitatory effect on ureteral function, that is, to increase the frequency and force of contractions (Rose and Gillenwater, 1974; Kaplan et al., 1968; Deane, 1967; Vereecken, 1973; Hukuhara et al., 1964; Labay et al., 1968; Barastegui, 1977; Boatman et al., 1967; Longrigg, 1974). Acetylcholine also has been shown to increase the duration of the guinea pig and rat ureteral action potential (Ichikawa and Ikeda, 1960; Prosser et al., 1955) and the number of oscillations on the plateau of the guinea pig ureteral action potential (Ichikawa and Ikeda, 1960). The excitatory effects of cholinergic agonists may be related to an indirect release of catecholamines (as supported by the finding that the excitatory effects of Urecholine can be blocked by the alpha-adrenergic blocking agent phentolamine (Rose and Gillenwater, 1974) and that the increased frequency of canine ureteral peristalsis induced by ACh can be blocked by adrenalectomy (Labay et al., 1968) or to a direct effect of the drug on muscarinic receptors. (Vereecken, 1973).

Nicotinic agonists, such as nicotine, tetramethylammonium (TMA), and dimethylphenylpiperzinium (DMPP), cause an initial stimulation of nicotinic receptors followed by desensitization of the receptor sites, with the receptor becoming unresponsive to nicotinic agonists and also to endogenous ACh, with resultant transmission blockade. Nicotine, as would be expected, has been shown to have excitatory (Boyarsky et al., 1968), biphasic (Macht, 1961a; Barastegui, 1977; Labay and Boyarsky, 1967; Santini, 1919), or inhibitory (Vereecken, 1973; Prosser et al., 1955) actions on the ureter that may be dose-dependent.

Anticholinesterases (Anti-ChE's)

Anticholinesterases prevent hydrolysis of ACh by cholinesterases and thus increase the duration and intensity of ACh action at both muscarinic and nicotinic receptor sites. With prolonged administration in high doses they can result in desensitization blockade at nicotinic sites. The effects of anticholinesterases such as physostigmine and neostigmine parallel the excitatory effects of ACh and other parasympathomimetics on the ureter (Vereecken, 1973; Prosser et al., 1955; Santini, 1919; Macht, 1916b; Slaughter et al., 1945).

Parasympathetic Blocking Agents

Atropine is a competitive antagonist of the muscarinic effects of acetylcholine. The inhibitory effects of atropine may be preceded by a transitory stimulatory effect on muscarinic receptors. Although atropine has been shown to inhibit the excitatory effects of parasympathomimetic agents (Kaplan et al., 1968; Deane, 1967; Vereecken, 1973; Barastegui, 1977; Boatman et al., 1967; Longrigg, 1974; Macht, 1916b; Gould et al., 1955) and physostigmine (Macht, 1916b) on a variety of ureteral and calyceal preparations, the majority of studies have shown that atropine itself has little direct effect on ureteral activity in a number of species (Vereecken, 1973; Boatman et al., 1967; Gould et al., 1955; Butcher et al., 1957; Mazzella and Schroeder, 1960; Reid et al., 1976; Gibbs, 1929; Washizu, 1967; Roth, 1917), including man (Kiil, 1957; Weinberg, 1962). Even when atropine has been observed to inhibit ureteral activity, its effects are frequently minimal and inconsistent (Hukuhara et al., 1964; Slaughter et al., 1945; Ross et al., 1967), thus providing little rationale for its use in the treatment of ureteral colic. Reports of the direct effects on ureteral activity of two other parasympathetic blocking agents, methantheline (Banthine) and propantheline (Pro-Banthine), have also been inconsistent (Kiil, 1957; Reid et al., 1976; Weinberg, 1962; Draper and Zargniotti, 1954; Sierp and Draper, 1964; Hanley, 1953).

Adrenergic Agonists

Norepinephrine, the chemical mediator responsible for adrenergic transmission, is synthesized in the neuron from tyrosine. Once released from the nerve terminal, some of the norepinephrine combines with receptors in the effector organ, leading to a physiologic response. The greatest percentage of the norepinephrine is actively taken up (re-uptake or neuronal uptake) into the neuron. Neuronal re-uptake regulates the duration that norepinephrine is in contact with the innervated tissue and thus regulates the magnitude and duration of the catecholamine-induced response. Agents such as cocaine and imipramine (Tofranil), which inhibit neuronal uptake, potentiate the physiologic response to norepinephrine. The enzymes monoamine oxidase (MAO) and catechol-o-methyl-transferase (COMT) provide degradative pathways for norepinephrine.

There is a general consensus that agents

that primarily activate alpha-adrenergic receptors, such as norepinephrine and phenylephrine, tend to stimulate ureteral activity (Tindall, 1972; Macht, 1916a; McLeod et al., 1973; Rose and Gillenwater, 1974; Weiss et al., 1978; Kaplan et al., 1968; Deane, 1967; Malin et al., 1968; Vereecken, 1973; Hukuhara et al., 1964; Boatman et al., 1967; Reid et al., 1976; Hannappel and Golenhofen, 1974; Casteels et al., 1971; Gruber, 1928; Ockerblad et al., 1935) and that agents that primarily activate beta-adrenergic receptors, such as isoproterenol and orciprenaline, tend to inhibit ureteral activity (Tindall, 1972; Finberg and Peart, 1970; McLeod et al., 1973; Rose and Gillenwater, 1974; Weiss et al., 1978; Deane, 1967; Malin et al., 1968; Vereecken, 1973; Reid et al., 1976; Hannappel and Golenhofen, 1974; Ancill et al., 1972; Kiil and Kjekshus, 1967). The beta-adrenergic agonist orciprenaline has been shown to dilate the ureteral lumen at the site of an artificial intraluminal concretion and has thus been suggested to have a potential role in the treatment of ureteral calculi (Peters and Eckstein, 1975). (See Effect of Calculi on Ureteral Function.) Tyramine, whose adrenergic-agonist effects are due primarily to the release of norepinephrine from adrenergic terminals, also has a stimulatory effect on the upper urinary tract (Finberg and Peart, 1970; Boyarsky and Labay, 1969; Longrigg, 1974). The reported stimulatory effects of cocaine on ureteral activity (Boyarsky and Labay, 1969) may be explained by blockage of norepinephrine re-uptake into adrenergic nerve endings, with a resultant increase in the magnitude and duration of the effect of norepinephrine.

Adrenergic Antagonists

The alpha-adrenergic antagonists phentolamine (Regitine) and phenoxybenzamine (Dibenzyline) have been shown to inhibit the stimulatory effects of norepinephrine and other alpha-adrenergic agonists in a variety of preparations (Tindall, 1972; Finberg and Peart, 1970; McLeod et al., 1973; Rose and Gillenwater, 1974; Weiss et al., 1978; Kaplan et al., 1968; Deane, 1967; Vereecken, 1973; Boatman et al., 1967; Longrigg, 1974; Hannappel and Golenhofen, 1974; Casteels et al., 1971; Gosling and Waas, 1971). Peters and Eckstein (1975) have suggested that phentolamine, because of its spasmolytic effects, might have a role in the treatment of renal colic. (See Effect of Calculi on Ureteral Function.)

The beta-adrenergic antagonist propranolol (Inderal) has been shown to block or attenuate the inhibitory effects of beta-adrenergic agonists, such as isoproterenol, in a variety of preparations (Tindall, 1972; McLeod et al., 1973; Rose and Gillenwater, 1974; Weiss et al., 1978; Vereecken, 1973; Longrigg, 1974; Reid et al., 1976; Casteels et al., 1971).

Histamine and its Antagonists

Histamine has a dual action on smooth muscle in that it may release catecholamines from sympathetic nerve endings as well as have a direct action on receptors within the smooth muscle. Excitatory effects of histamine on ureteral function have been demonstrated (Vereecken, 1973; Boatman et al., 1967; Butcher et al., 1957; Borgstedt et al., 1962; Boyarsky and Labay, 1967; Struthers, 1973; Sharkey et al., 1965), a finding that may be species-dependent (Tindall, 1972; Thackston et al., 1955). The antihistamines diphenhydramine (Benadryl) and tripelennamine (Pyribenzamine) have been shown to inhibit the effects of histamine on the ureter (Boatman et al., 1967; Butcher et al., 1957; Borgstedt et al., 1962; Sharkey et al., 1965).

Narcotic Analgesics

Morphine has been reported to increase ureteral tone or the frequency and amplitude of ureteral contractions, or both, in a variety of preparations (Vereecken, 1973; Hukuhara et al., 1964; Slaughter et al., 1945; Macht, 1916c; Gruber, 1928). Several early studies using the hydrophorograph, which was more sensitive to changes in urine flow than to changes in actual ureteral peristalsis, suggested that morphine increases ureteral activity in man (Carroll and Zingale, 1938; Ockerblad et al., 1935). However, more recent studies have failed to confirm these findings (Kiil, 1957; Weinberg and Maletta, 1961; Chen et al., 1957). The contradictory findings concerning the effect of morphine on ureteral function is further compounded by the fact that other workers have failed to observe an effect of morphine on ureteral function in various experimental preparations (Gould et al., 1955; Weinberg, 1962; Ross et al., 1967; Chen et al., 1957). Meperidine (Demerol) appears to have a similar excitatory effect on the activity of the intact dog ureter (Kaplan et al., 1968; Sharkey et al., 1968). However, Kiil (1957) failed to observe an effect of Demerol on ureteral peristalsis in man. If one considers only the effects on ureteral activity, there is no basis to preferentially favor morphine or meperidine in the treatment of renal colic. Both agents may have ureteral spasmogenic effects, which theoretically would detract from their value in the management of ureteral colic. They surely do not have potentially valuable spasmolytic actions. Their efficacy in treating colic is dependent on their central nervous system actions, which decrease the perception of pain.

Prostaglandins

Prostaglandins are derived from fatty acids and have a variety of biologic actions in various systems of the body. Their effects vary with species, type of prostaglandin, endocrine status of tissue, experimental conditions, and origin of the smooth muscle. The "primary prostaglandins," PGE_1, PGE_2, and $PGF_{2\alpha}$, are synthesized from the fatty acid arachidonic acid by enzymatic reactions that can be inhibited by indomethacin and aspirin.

Indomethacin has been employed in the management of ureteral colic (Holmlund and Sjöden, 1978). The beneficial effects probably are due to indomethacin's inhibition of the prostaglandin-mediated vasodilatation that occurs subsequent to obstruction (Allen et al., 1978, Sjöden et al., 1982). The vasodilatation theoretically would result in an increase in glomerular capillary pressure and subsequent increase in pelviureteral pressure. Indomethacin, by reducing pelviureteral pressure and thus pelviureteral wall tension, might eliminate some of the pain of renal colic that is dependent on distention of the upper urinary tract.

Prostaglandin E_1 (PGE_1) inhibits the activity of the dog ureter (Abrams and Feneley, 1976; Boyarsky et al., 1966; Wooster, 1971). Johns and Wooster (1975) suggested that the inhibitory effects of PGE_1 on ureteral activity were dependent on the sequestration of Ca^{++} at the inner surface of the cell membrane, with a resultant increase in outward potassium conductance and hyperpolarization of the membrane. In contrast to the inhibitory effects of PGE_1, prostaglandin $PGF_{2\alpha}$ ($PGF_{2\alpha}$) increases the frequency of peristalsis in the dog (Boyarsky and Labay, 1969).

Cardiac Glycosides

Ouabain, a cardiac glycoside, has an effect on ureteral activity that appears to be species-dependent. In the isolated cat ureter, ouabain produces a marked increase in contractility, which usually is followed by a late decrease in excitability (Weiss et al., 1970). In the guinea pig ureter, ouabain inhibits activity without a preliminary potentiation of contractility (Hendrickx et al., 1975; Washizu, 1968). The inhibitory effects of ouabain are accompanied by a shortening of the action potential duration, a decrease of the number of oscillations on the plateau of the guinea pig action potential, and a decrease in resting membrane potential.

Calcium Antagonists

As calcium is necessary for the development of the action potential and contraction of the ureter, agents that block the movement of Ca^{++} into the cell would be expected to depress ureteral function. The calcium channel blockers verapamil and D-600 (a methoxy-derivative of verapamil) have been shown to inhibit ureteral activity (Vereecken et al., 1975a; Golenhofen and Lammel, 1972). These inhibitory effects are accompanied by decreases in action potential duration, number of oscillations on the plateau of the guinea pig action potential, excitability, and rate of rise and amplitude of the action potential. High concentrations of verapamil and D-600 cause a complete cessation of electrical and mechanical activity.

Antibiotics

Ampicillin causes relaxation of the ureter and antagonizes the stimulatory effects of barium chloride ($BaCl_2$), histamine, serotonin, and carbachol on the ureter, suggesting that its action is directly on the smooth muscle (Benzi et al., 1970b). Chloramphenicol, the isoxazolyl penicillins, and gentamicin also have spasmolytic effects on the ureter (Benzi et al., 1970a, 1971, 1973). The tetracyclines, on the other hand, potentiate the contractile effects of $BaCl_2$ on the ureter (Benzi et al., 1973).

Hormones of Pregnancy

Progesterone inhibits ureteral activity (see Effect of Pregnancy on Ureteral Function). Although some workers have noted that estrogens increase ureteral activity (Hundley et al., 1942; Padovani, 1954), the majority of investigators have failed to observe an effect of estrogens in various animal models (Payne and Hoden, 1939;

Abramson et al., 1953) or in man (Lubin et al., 1941; Kumar, 1962; Schneider et al., 1953).

In this section, an attempt has been made to provide an assessment of the effects of the major classes of drugs on ureteral function. Many of the studies referred to were performed on animal models, and the extrapolation of the data to the intact human ureter often is difficult. In the clinical situation, the relatively sparse blood supply to the ureter limits the distribution of drug to the ureter. In addition, many drugs with potential usefulness in the management or ureteral pathology have potential untoward side effects when used in the concentrations that are required to affect the ureter. Although many drugs can influence ureteral function, their present clinical usefulness is limited.

References

Aberg, A. K. G., and Axelsson, J.: Some mechanical aspects of an intestinal smooth muscle. Acta Physiol. Scand., 64:15, 1965.

Abrams, P. H., and Feneley, R. C. L.: The actions of prostaglandins on the smooth muscle of the human urinary tract *in vitro*. Br. J. Urol., 47:909, 1976.

Abramson, D., Caton, W. L., Jr., and Roly, C. C.: The effect of relaxin on the excretion of Diodrast in the castrate hysterectomized rabbit. Am. J. Obstet. Gynecol., 65:644, 1953.

Adelstein, R. S., Pato, M. D., and Conti, M. A.: The role of phosphorylation in regulating contractile proteins. Adv. Cyclic Nucleotide Res., 14:361, 1981.

Akimoto, M., Biancani, P., and Weiss, R. M.: Comparative pressure-length-diameter relationships of neonatal and adult rabbit ureters. Invest. Urol., 14:297, 1977.

Allen, J. T., Vaughan, E. D., Jr., and Gillenwater, J. Y.: The effect of indomethacin on renal blood flow and ureteral pressure in unilateral ureteral obstruction in awake dogs. Invest. Urol., 15:324, 1978.

Ancill, R. J., Jackson, D. M., and Redfern, P. H.: The pharmacology of the rat ureter *in vivo*. Br. J. Pharmacol., 44:628, 1972.

Anderson, R. G. G.: Cyclic AMP and calcium ions in mechanical and metabolic responses of smooth muscle: Influence of some hormones and drugs. Acta Physiol. Scand. (Suppl.), 382:1, 1972.

Andersson, R., and Nilsson, K.: Cyclic AMP and calcium in relaxation in intestinal smooth muscle. Nature New Biol., 238:119, 1972.

Backlund, L., and Reuterskiöld, A. G.: Activity in the dilated dog ureter. Scand. J. Urol. Nephrol., 3:99, 1969a.

Backlund, L., and Reuterskiöld, A. G.: The abnormal ureter in children. Scand. J. Urol. Nephrol., 3:219, 1969b.

Backlund, L., Grotte, G., and Reuterskiöld, A.: Functional stenosis as a cause of pelvi-ureteric obstruction and hydronephrosis. Arch. Dis. Child., 40:203, 1965.

Barastegui, C. A.: Motility of the rat ureter *in vitro*. Responses to cholinergic drugs. Rev. Esp. Fisiol., 33:1, 1977.

Barr, L., Berger, W., and Dewey, M. M.: Electrical transmission at the nexus between smooth muscle cells. J. Gen. Physiol., 51:347, 1968.

Bennett, M. R., and Burnstock, G.: Application of the sucrose-gap method to determine the ionic basis of the membrane potential of smooth muscle. J. Physiol. (Lond.), 183:637, 1966.

Benzi, G., Arrigoni, E., and Sanguinetti, L.: Antibiotics and ureter. III: Chloramphenicol. Arch. Int. Pharmacodyn. Ther., 185:329, 1970a.

Benzi, G., Arrigoni, E., and Sanguinetti, L.: Antibiotics and ureter. V: Gentamicin. Arch. Int. Pharmacodyn. Ther., 189:303, 1971.

Benzi, G., Arrigoni, E., and Sanguinetti, L.: Effect of antibiotics on the ureter motor activity. Jpn. J. Pharmacol., 23:599, 1973.

Benzi, G., Bermudez, E., Arrigoni, E., and Berte, F.: Antibiotics and the ureter. I: Ampicillin. Arch. Int. Pharmacodyn. Ther., 183:159, 1970.

Biancani, P., Hausman, M., and Weiss, R. M.: Effect of obstruction on ureteral circumferential force-length relations. Am. J. Physiol., 243:F204, 1982.

Biancani, P., Onyski, J. H., Zabinski, M. P., and Weiss, R. M.: Force-velocity relationships of the guinea pig ureter. J. Urol. 131:988, 1984.

Biancani, P., Zabinski, M. P., and Weiss, R. M.: Bidimensional deformation of acutely obstructed in vitro rabbit ureter. Am. J. Physiol., 225:671, 1973.

Biancani, P., Zabinski, M. P., and Weiss, R. M.: Time course of ureteral changes with acute and chronic obstruction. Am. J. Physiol., 231:393, 1976.

Boatman, D. L., Lewin, M. L., Culp, D. A., and Flocks, R. H.: Pharmacologic evaluation of ureteral smooth muscle: A technique of monitoring ureteral peristalsis. Invest. Urol., 4:509, 1967.

Borgstedt, H. H., Benjamin, J. A., and Emmel, V. M.: The role of histamine in ureteral function. J. Pharmacol. Exp. Ther., 136:386, 1962.

Boyarsky, S., and Labay, P.: Histamine analog effect on the ureter. Invest. Urol., 4:351, 1967.

Boyarsky, S., and Labay, P.: Ureteral motility. Annu. Rev. Med. 20:383, 1969.

Boyarsky, S., Labay, P., and Gerber, C.: Prostaglandin inhibition of ureteral peristalsis. Invest. Urol., 4:9, 1966.

Boyarsky, S., Labay, P., and Pfautz, C. J.: The effect of nicotine upon ureteral peristalsis. South. Med. J., 61:573, 1968.

Bozler, E.: The action potentials of visceral smooth muscle. Am. J. Physiol., 124:502, 1938a.

Bozler, E.: Electric stimulation and conduction of excitation in smooth muscle. Am. J. Physiol., 122:614, 1938b.

Bozler, E.: The activity of the pacemaker previous to the discharge of a muscular impulse. Am. J. Physiol., 136:543, 1942.

Briggs, M. E., Constantinou, C. E., and Govan, D. E.: Dynamics of the upper urinary tract. The relationship of urine flow rate and rate of ureteral peristalsis. Invest. Urol., 10:56, 1972.

Burnstock, G.: Structure of smooth muscle and its innervation. *In* Bulbring, E., Brading, A. F., Jones, A. W., and Tomita, T. (Eds.): Smooth Muscle. Baltimore, The Williams & Wilkins Co., 1970, pp. 1–69.

Butcher, H. R., Jr., Sleator, W. Jr., and Schmandt, W. L.: A study of the peristaltic conduction mechanism in the canine ureter. J. Urol., 78:221, 1957.

Carroll, G., and Zingale, F. G.: A clinical and experimental study of the effect of pancreatic tissue extracts on the ureter. South. Med. J., 31:233, 1938.

Casteels, R.: The relation between the membrane potential and the ion distribution in smooth muscle cells. *In* Bulbring, E., Brading, A. F., Jones, A. W., and Tomita, T. (Eds.): Smooth Muscle. Baltimore, The Williams & Wilkins Co., 1970, pp. 70–79.

Casteels, R., Hendrickx, H., and Vereecken, R.: Effects of catecholamines on the electrical and mechanical activity of the guinea pig ureter. Br. J. Pharmacol., 43:429P, 1971.

Chen, P. S., Emmel, V. M., Benjamin, J. A., and Distefano, V.: Studies on the isolated dog ureter: The pharmacological action of histamine, levarterenol and antihistaminics. Arch. Int. Pharmacodyn. Ther., 110:131, 1957.

Clayton, J. D., and Roberts, J. A.: Radionuclide postpartum evaluation of the urinary tract during anovular therapy. Surg. Gynecol. Obstet., 137:215, 1973.

Connor, J. A., Prosser, C. L., and Weems, W. A.: A study of pace-maker activity in intestinal smooth muscle. J. Physiol. (Lond.), 240:671, 1974.

Constantinou, C. E.: Renal pelvic pacemaker control of ureteral peristaltic rate. Am. J. Physiol., 226:1413, 1974.

Constantinou, C. E., and Djurhuus, J. C.: Pyeloureteral dynamics in the intact and chronically obstructed multicalyceal kidney. Am. J. Physiol., 241: R398, 1981.

Constantinou, C. E., and Hrynczuk, J. R.: Urodynamics of the upper urinary tract. Invest. Urol., 14:233, 1976.

Constantinou, C. E., and Yamaguchi, O.: Multiple-coupled pacemaker system in renal pelvis of the unicalyceal kidney. Am. J. Physiol., 241:R412, 1981.

Constantinou, C. E., Grenato, J. J., Jr., and Govan, D. E.: Dynamics of the upper urinary tract: Accommodation in the rate and stroke volume of ureteral peristalsis as a response to transient alteration in urine flow rate. Urol. Int., 29:249, 1974.

Constantinou, C. E., Silvert, M. A., and Gosling, J.: Pacemaker system in the control of ureteral peristaltic rate in the multicalyceal kidney of the pig. Invest. Urol., 14:440, 1977.

Cook, W. A., and King, L. R.: Vesicoureteral reflux. In Harrison, J. H., Gittes, R. F., Perlmutter, A. D., Stamey, T. A., and Walsh, P. C. (Eds.): Campbell's Urology. 4th ed. Philadelphia, W. B. Saunders Co., 1979, pp. 1596–1634.

Coolsaet, B. L. R. A., Griffiths, D. J., Van Mastrigt, R., and Duyl, W. A. V.: Urodynamic investigation of the wide ureter. J. Urol., 124:666, 1980.

Coolsaet, B. L. R. A., van Venrooij, G. E. P. M., and Blok, C.: Detrusor pressure versus wall stress in relation to ureterovesical resistance. Neurourol. Urodynam., 1:105, 1982.

Cussen, L. J.: The structure of the normal human ureter in infancy and childhood. A quantitative study of the muscular and elastic tissue. Invest. Urol., 5:179, 1967.

Deane, R. F.: Functional studies of the ureter: Its behavior in the domestic pig (sus scrofa domestica) as recorded by the technique of Trendelenburg. Br. J. Urol., 39:31, 1967.

Debruyne, F. M. J., Wijdeveld, P. G. A. B., Koene, R. A. P., Chafik, M. L., Moonen, W. A., and Renders, G. A. M.: Uretero-neo-cystomy in renal transplantation. Is an antireflux mechanism mandatory? Br. J. Urol., 50:378, 1978.

DelTacca, M.: Acetylcholine content of and release from isolated pelviureteral tract. Nauyn-Schmiedebergs Arch. Pharmacol., 302:293, 1978.

Dixon, J. S., and Gosling, J. A.: The fine structure of pacemaker cells in the pig renal calices. Anat. Rec., 175:139, 1973.

Djurhuus, J. C., and Constantinou, C. E.: Chronic ureteric obstruction and its impact on the coordinating mechanisms of peristalsis (pyeloureteric pacemaker system). Urol. Res., 10:267, 1982.

Djurhuus, J. C., and Stage, P.: Percutaneous intrapelvic pressure registration in hydronephrosis during diuresis. Acta Chir. Scand., 473:43, 1976.

Draper, J. W., and Zorgniotti, A. W.: The effect of Banthine and similar agents on the urinary tract. N. Y. State J. Med., 54:77, 1954.

Draper, M. H., and Weidmann, S.: Cardiac resting and action potentials recorded with an intracellular electrode. J. Physiol. (Lond.), 115:74, 1951.

Englemann, T. W.: Zur Physiologie des Ureters. Pfluegers Arch. Gesamte Physiol. Menschen Tiere, 2:243, 1869.

Englemann, T. W.: Uber die electrische Erregung des Ureter, mit Bemerkungen uber die electrische Erregung im Allgemeinen. Pfluegers Arch. Gesamte Physiol. Menschen Tiere, 3:247, 1870.

Fainstat, T.: Ureteral dilatation in pregnancy: A review. Obstet. Gynecol. Sur., 18:845, 1963.

Ferroni, A., and Blanchi, D.: Maximum rate of depolarization of single muscle fiber in normal and low sodium solutions. J. Gen. Physiol., 49:17, 1965.

Finberg, J. P. M., and Peart, W. S.: Function of smooth muscle of the rat renal pelvis—response of the isolated pelvis muscle to angiotensin and some other substances. Br. J. Pharmacol., 39:373, 1970.

Foote, J. W., Blennerhassett, J. B., Wigglesworth, F. W., and MacKinnon, K. J.: Observations on the ureteropelvic junction. J. Urol., 104:252, 1970.

Fredericks, C. M., Anderson, G. F., and Pierce, J. M.: Electrical and mechanical responses of intact canine ureter to elevated intravesical pressure. Invest. Urol., 9:496, 1972.

Fung, Y. C.: Peristaltic pumping: A bioengineering model. In Boyarsky, S., Gottschalk, C. W., Tanagho, E. A., and Zimskind, P. D. (Eds.): Urodynamics. New York, Academic Press, 1971, pp. 177–198.

Gibbs, O. S.: The function of the fowl's ureter. Am. J. Physiol., 87:594, 1929.

Golenhofen, K., and Lammel, E.: Selective suppression of some components of spontaneous activity in various types of smooth muscle by iproveratril (verapamil). Pfluegers Arch., 331:233, 1972.

Gosling, J. A.: Atypical muscle cells in the wall of the renal calix and pelvis with a note on their possible significance. Experientia, 26:769, 1970.

Gosling, J. A., and Dixon, J. S.: Functional obstruction of the ureter and renal pelvis. A histological and electron microscopic study. Br. J. Urol., 50:145, 1978.

Gosling, J. A., and Dixon, J. S.: Morphologic evidence that the renal calyx and pelvis control ureteric activity in the rabbit. Am. J. Anat., 130:393, 1971.

Gosling, J. A., and Dixon, J. S.: Species variation in the location of upper urinary tract pacemaker cells. Invest. Urol., 11:418, 1974.

Gosling, J. A., and Waas, A. N. C. The behavior of the isolated rabbit renal calix and pelvis compared with that of the ureter. Eur. J. Pharmacol., 16:100, 1971.

Gottschalk, C. W., and Mylle, M.: Micropuncture study of pressures in proximal tubules and peritubular capillaries of the rat kidney and their relation to ureteral and renal venous pressures. Am. J. Physiol., 185:430, 1956.

Gould, D. W., Hsieh, A. C. L., and Tinckler, L. F.: Behavior of isolated water-buffalo ureter. J. Physiol. (Lond.), 129:425, 1955.

Grana, L., Kidd, J., Idriss, F., and Swenson, O.: Effects of chronic urinary tract infection on ureteral peristalsis. J. Urol., 94:652, 1965.

Griffiths, D. J.: The mechanics of urine transport in the upper urinary tract: 2. The discharge of the bolus into the bladder and dynamics at high rates of flow. Neurourol. Urodynam., 2:167, 1983.

Griffiths, D. J., and Notschaele, C.: The mechanics of urine transport in the upper urinary tract: I. The dynamics of the isolated bolus. Neurourol. Urodynam., 2:155, 1983.

Gruber, C. M.: The effect of morphine and papaverine

upon the peristaltic and antiperistaltic contractions of the ureter. J. Pharmacol. Exp. Ther., *33*:191, 1928.

Hanley, H. G.: The electro-ureterogram. Br. J. Urol., *25:*358, 1953.

Hanna, M. K.: Some observations on congenital ureteropelvic junction obstruction. Urology, *12*:151, 1978.

Hannappel, J., and Golenhofen, K.: The effect of catecholamines on ureteral peristalsis in different species (dog, guinea pig and rat). Pfluegers Arch., *55*:350, 1974.

Hausman, M., Biancani, P., and Weiss, R. M.: Obstruction induced changes in longitudinal force-length relations of rabbit ureter. Invest. Urol., *17*:223, 1979.

Hendren, W. H.: A new approach to infants with severe obstructive uropathy; early complete reconstruction. J. Pediatr. Surg., *5*:184, 1970.

Hendrickx, H., Vereecken, R. L., and Casteels, R.: The influence of potassium on the electrical and mechanical activity of the guinea pig ureter. Urol. Res., *3*:155, 1975.

Hill, A. V.: The heat of shortening and the dynamic constants of 1 muscle. Proc. R. Soc. (Ser. B), *126*:136, 1938.

Hodgkin, A. L.: Ionic movements and electrical activity in giant nerve fibres. Proc. R. Soc. Lond. (Biol.), *148*:1, 1958.

Hoffman, B. F., and Cranefield, P. F.: Electrophysiology of the Heart, New York, McGraw-Hill, 1960.

Holmlund, D., and Hassler, O.: A method of studying the ureteral reaction to artificial concrements. Acta Chir. Scand., *130*:335, 1965.

Holmlund, D., and Sjöden, J. G.: Treatment of ureteral colic with intravenous indomethacin. J. Urol., *120*:676, 1978.

Hong, K. W., Biancani, P., and Weiss, R. M.: "On" and "off" response of guinea pig ureter. Fed. Proc., *39*:711, 1980a.

Hong, K. W., Biancani, P., and Weiss, R. M.: Effect of age on contractility of guinea pig ureter. Invest. Urol., *17*:459, 1980b.

Hukuhara, T., Nanba, R., and Fukuda, H.: The effects of the stimulation of extraureteral nerves on the ureteral motility of the dog. Jpn. J. Physiol., *14*:197, 1964.

Hundley, J. M., Jr., Diehl, W. K., and Diggs, E. S.: Hormonal influences upon the ureter. Am. J. Obstet. Gynecol., *44*:858, 1942.

Ichikawa, S., and Ikeda, O.: Recovery curve and conduction of action potentials in the ureter of the guinea pig. Jpn. J. Physiol., *10*:1, 1960.

Johns, A., and Wooster, M. J.: The inhibitory effects of prostaglandin E$_1$ on guinea pig ureter. Can. J. Physiol. Pharmacol., *53*:239, 1975.

Kaplan, N., Elkin, M., and Sharkey, J.: Ureteral peristalsis and the autonomic nervous system. Invest. Urol., *5*:468, 1968.

Kiil, F.: The Function of the Ureter and Renal Pelvis. Philadelphia, W. B. Saunders Co., 1957.

Kiil, F., and Kjekshus, J.: The physiology of the ureter and renal pelvis. Proc. 3rd. Intern. Congr. Nephrol. (Washington, D. C., 1966), *2*:321, 1967.

King, W. W., and Cox, C. E.: Bacterial inhibition of ureteral smooth muscle contractility. I. The effect of common urinary pathogens and endotoxin in an in vitro system. J. Urol., *108*:700, 1972.

Kirkland, I. S., Ross, J. A., Edmond, P., and Long, W. J.: Ureteral function in vesicoureteral reflux. Br. J. Urol., *43*:289, 1971.

Kobayashi, M.: Conduction velocity in various regions of the ureter. Tohoku J. Exp. Med., *83*:220, 1964.

Kobayashi, M.: Effect of calcium on electrical activity in smooth muscle cells of cat ureter. Am. J. Physiol., *216*:1279, 1969.

Kobayashi, M.: Effects of Na and Ca on the generation and conduction of excitation in the ureter. Am. J. Physiol., *208*:715, 1965.

Kobayashi, M., and Irisawa, H.: Effect of sodium deficiency on the action potential of the smooth muscle of ureter. Am. J. Physiol., *206*:205, 1964.

Koff, S. A., and Thrall, J. H.: Diagnosis of obstruction in experimental hydroureteronephrosis. Urology, *17*:570, 1981a.

Koff, S. A., and Thrall, J. H.: The diagnosis of obstruction in experimental hydroureteronephrosis: Mechanism for progressive urinary tract dilation. Invest. Urol., *19*:85, 1981b.

Kroeger, E. A., and Marshall, J. M.: Beta-adrenergic effects on rat myometrium: role of cyclic AMP. Am. J. Physiol., *226*:1298, 1974.

Kubacz, G. J., and Catchpole, B. N.: The role of adrenergic blockade in the treatment of ureteral colic. J. Urol., *107*:949, 1972.

Kumar, D.: In vitro inhibitory effect of progesterone on extrauterine smooth muscle. Am. J. Obstet. Gynecol., *84*:1300, 1962.

Kuriyama, H.: The influence of potassium, sodium and chloride on the membrane potential of the smooth muscle of taenia coli. J. Physiol. (Lond.), *166*:15, 1963.

Kuriyama, H., and Tomita, T.: The action potential in the smooth muscle of the guinea pig taenia coli and ureter studied by the double sucrose-gap method. J. Gen. Physiol., *55*:147, 1970.

Kuriyama, H., Osa, T., and Toida, N.: Membrane properties of the smooth muscle of guinea-pig ureter. J. Physiol. (Lond.), *191*:225, 1967.

Labay, P., and Boyarsky, S.: The effect of topical nicotine on ureteral peristalsis. JAMA, *200*:209, 1967.

Labay, P. C., Boyarsky, S., and Herlong, J. H.: Relation of adrenal to ureteral function. Fed. Proc., *27*:444, 1968.

Lapides, J.: The physiology of the intact human ureter. J. Urol., *59*:501, 1948.

Libertino, J. A., and Weiss, R. M.: Ultrastructure of human ureter. J. Urol., *108*:71, 1972.

Longrigg, N.: Autonomic innervation of the renal calyx. Br. J. Urol., *46*:357, 1974.

Longrigg, N.: Minor calyces as primary pacemaker sites for ureteral activity in man. Lancet, *1*:253, 1975.

Lowman, R. M., Belleza, N. A., Goetsch, J. B., Finkelstein, H. I., Berneike, R. R., and Rosenfield, A. T.: Letter to the editor: Glucagon. J. Urol., *118*:128, 1977.

Lubin, S., Drexler, L. S., and Bilotta, W. A.: Post-partum pyelourethral changes following hormone administration. Surg. Gynecol. Obstet., *73*:391, 1941.

Macht, D. I.: On the pharmacology of the ureter. I. Action of epinephine, ergotoxine and of nicotin. J. Pharmacol. Exp. Ther., *8*:155, 1916a.

Macht, D. I.: On the pharmacology of the ureter. II. Actions of drugs affecting the sacral autonomics. J. Pharmacol. Exp. Ther., *8*:261, 1916b.

Macht, D. I.: On the pharmacology of the ureter. III. Action of the opium alkaloids. J. Pharmacol. Exp. Ther., *9*:197, 1916c.

Maizels, M., and Stephens, F. D.: Valves of the ureter as a cause of primary obstruction of the ureter: anatomic, embryologic and clinical aspects. J. Urol., *123*:742, 1980.

Makker, S. P., Tucker, A. S., Izant, R. J., Jr., and Heymann, W.: Nonobstructive hydronephrosis and hydroureter associated with peritonitis. N. Engl. J. Med., *287*:535, 1972.

Malin, J. M., Jr., Boyarsky, S., Labay, P., and Gerber, C.: In vitro isometric studies of ureteral smooth muscle. J. Urol., *99*:396, 1968.

Malin, J. M., Jr., Deane, R. F., and Boyarsky, S.: Characterization of adrenergic receptors in human ureter. Br. J. Urol., *42*:171, 1970.

Marchant, D. J.: Effects of pregnancy and progestational agents on the urinary tract. Am. J. Obstet. Gynecol. *112*:487, 1972.

Mazzella, H., and Schroeder, G.: Ureteral contractility in the dog and the influence of drugs. Arch. Int. Pharmacodyn. Ther., *128*:291, 1960.

McGuire, E. J.: Physiology of the lower urinary tract. Am. J. Kid. Dis., *2*:402, 1983.

McGuire, E. J., Woodside, J. R., Borden, T. A., and Weiss, R. M.: Prognostic value of urodynamic testing in myelodysplastic patients. J. Urol., *126*:205, 1981.

McLeod, D. G., Reynolds, D. G., and Swan, K. G.: Adrenergic mechanisms in the canine ureter. Am. J. Physiol., *224*:1054, 1973.

McNellis, D., and Sherline, D. M.: The rabbit ureter in pregnancy and after norethynodrel-mestranol administration. A radiographic and histologic study. Obstet. Gynecol. *30*:336, 1967.

Melick, W. F., Brodeur, A. E., Herbig, F., and Naryka, J. J.: Use of a ureteral pacemaker in the treatment of ureteral reflux. J. Urol., *95*:184, 1966.

Melick, W. F., Naryka, J. J., and Schmidt, J. H.: Experimental studies of ureteral peristaltic patterns in the pig. II. Myogenic activity of the pig ureter. J. Urol., *86*:46, 1961.

Morales, P. A., Crowder, C. H., Fishman, A. P., and Maxwell, M. H.: The response of the ureter and pelvis to changing urine flows. J. Urol., *67*:484, 1952.

Morita, T., Ishizuka, G., and Tsuchida, S.: Initiation and propagation of stimulus from the renal pelvic pacemaker in pig kidney. Invest. Urol., *19*:157, 1981.

Murnaghan, G. F.: The dynamics of the renal pelvis and ureter with reference to congenital hydronephrosis. Br. J. Urol., *30*:321, 1958.

Nernst, W.: Zur theorie des elektrischen reizes. Arch. f. d. ges. Physiol., *122*:275, 1908.

Noble, D., and Tsien, R. W.: The kinetics and rectifier properties of the slow potassium current in cardiac Purkinje fibres. J. Physiol. (Lond.), *195*:185, 1968.

Notley, R. G.: The musculature of the human ureter. Br. J. Urol., *42*:724, 1970.

Ockerblad, N. F., Carlson, H. E., and Simon, J. F.: The effect of morphine upon the human ureter. J. Urol., *33*:356, 1935.

O'Connor, V. J., Jr., and Dawson-Edwards, P.: Role of the ureter in renal transplantation. I: Studies of denervated ureter with particular reference to ureteroureteral anastomosis. J. Urol., *82*:566, 1969.

Padovani, E.: Ricerche urografiche ed istologiche sulle modificazioni pieloureterali indotte dagli armoni sessuali femminili. Quad. Clin. Ostet. Ginecol., *9*:67, 1954.

Paquin, A. J., Jr.: Ureterovesical anastomosis: The description and evaluation of a technique. J. Urol., *82*:573, 1959.

Payne, F. L., and Hodes, P. J.: The effect of the female hormones and of pregnancy upon the ureters of lower animals as demonstrated by intravenous urography. Am. J. Obstet. Gynecol. *37*:1024, 1939.

Peters, H. J., and Eckstein, W.: Possible pharmacological means of treating renal colic. Urol. Res., *3*:55, 1975.

Primbs, K.: Untersuchungen uber die Einwirkung von Bakterientoxinen auf der uberlebenden Meerschweinchenureter. Z. Urol. Chir., *1*:600, 1913.

Prosser, C. L., Smith, C. E., and Melton, C. E.: Conduction of action potentials in the ureter of the rat. Am. J. Physiol., *181*:651, 1955.

Reid, R. E., Herman, R., and Teng, C.: Attempts at altering ureteral activity in the unanesthetized, conditioned dog with commonly employed drugs. Invest. Urol., *12*:74, 1976.

Reuterskiöld, A. G.: Ureteric pressure variations at different flow rates and varying bladder pressures in normal dogs. Acta Soc. Med. Upsal., *74*:94, 1969.

Reuterskiöld, A. G.: The abnormal ureter in children. II. Perfusion studies on the refluxing ureter. Scand. J. Urol., Nephrol., *4*:99, 1970.

Roberts, J. A.: Experimental pyelonephritis in the monkey. III. Pathophysiology of ureteral malfunction induced by bacteria. Invest. Urol., *13*:117, 1975.

Roberts, J. A.: Hydronephrosis of pregnancy. Urology, *8*:1, 1976.

Rose, J. G., and Gillenwater, J. Y.: Pathophysiology of ureteral obstruction. Am. J. Physiol., *225*:830, 1973.

Rose, J. G., and Gillenwater, J. Y.: The effect of adrenergic and cholinergic agents and their blockers upon ureteral activity. Invest. Urol., *11*:439, 1974.

Rose, J. G., and Gillenwater, J. Y.: Effects of obstruction upon ureteral function. Urology, *12*:139, 1978.

Rosen, D. E., Constantinou, C. E., Sands, J. P., and Govan, D. E.: Dynamics of the upper urinary tract: Effects of changes in bladder pressure on ureteral peristalsis. J. Urol., *106*:209, 1971.

Ross, J. A., Edmond, P., and Griffiths, J. M.: The action of drugs on the intact human ureter. Br. J. Urol., *39*:26, 1967.

Ross, J. A., Edmond, P., and Kirkland, I. S.: Behavior of the Human Ureter in Health and Disease. Edinburgh, Churchill Livingstone, 1972.

Roth, G. B.: On the movement of the excised ureter of the dog. Am. J. Physiol., *44*:275, 1917.

Sala, N. L., and Rubi, R. A.: Ureteral function in pregnant women. II. Ureteral contractility during normal pregnancy. Am. J. Obstet. Gynecol., *99*:228, 1967.

Santani, Y.: Experimental studies of the ureter. Am. J. Physiol., *49*:474, 1919.

Scheele, K.: Die Spasmen bei Uretersteine. Z. Urol., *58*:455, 1965.

Schneider, D. H., Eichner, E., and Gordon, M. B.: An attempt at production of hydronephrosis of pregnancy, artificially induced. Am. J. Obstet. Gynecol., *65*:660, 1953.

Schultz, K., Bohme, E., Volker, A. W. K., and Schultz, G.: Relaxation of hormonally stimulated smooth muscular tissues by the 8-bromo derivative of cyclic GMP. Naunyn Schmiedebergs Arch. Pharmacol., *306*:1, 1979.

Schweitzer, F. A. W.: Intrapelvic pressure and renal function studies in experimental chronic partial ureteric obstruction. Br. J. Urol., *45*:2, 1973.

Sharkey, J., Boyarsky, S., Catacutan-Labay, P., and Martinez, J.: The *in vivo* effects of histamine and Benadryl on the peristalsis of the canine ureter and plasma potassium levels. Invest. Urol., *2*:417, 1965.

Sharkey, J., Kaplan, N., Newman, H. R., and Elkin, M.: The role of potassium in ureteral physiology and pharmacology. Invest. Urol., *6*:119, 1968.

Shiratori, T., and Kinoshita, H.: Electromyographic studies on urinary tract. II. Electromyography study on the genesis of peristaltic movement of the dog's ureters. Tohoku J. Exp. Med., *73*:103, 1961a.

Shiratori, T., and Kinoshita, H.: Electromyographic studies on urinary tract. III. Influence of pinching and cutting the ureters of dogs on their EMGs. Tohoku J. Exp. Med., *73*:159, 1961b.

Sierp, M., and Draper, J. W.: Peristalsis in the urinary tract: Experimental observations of the effect of various drugs on the musculature of the ureter. Ann. N. Y. Acad. Sci., *118*:7, 1964.

Sivula, A., and Lehtonen, T.: Spontaneous passage of artificial concretions applied in the rabbit ureter. Scand. J. Urol. Nephrol., *1*:259, 1967.

Sjödén, J. G., Wahlberg, J., and Persson, A. E. G.: The effect of indomethacin on glomerular capillary pressure and pelvic pressure during ureteral obstruction. J. Urol., *127*:1017, 1982.

Slaughter, D., Johnson, T. V., Tobalowsky, N., and VanDuzen, R.: The effect of spasmolytic drugs on the isolated ureter. Texas Rep. Biol. Med., *3*:37, 1945.

Sonnenblick, E. H.: Force-velocity relations in mammalian heart muscle. Am. J. Physiol., *202*:931, 1962.

Struthers, N. W.: The role of manometry in the investigation of pelviureteral function. Br. J. Urol., *41*:129, 1969.

Struthers, N. W.: An experimental model for evaluating drug effects on the ureter. Br. J. Urol., *45*:23, 1973.

Takago, K., Takayanagi, I., and Tomiyama, A.: Actions of dibutyryl cyclic adenosine monophosphate, papaverine and isoprenaline on intestinal smooth muscle. Jpn. J. Pharmacol., *21*:477, 1971.

Tanagho, E. A.: Ureteral embryology, developmental anatomy and myology. *In:* Boyarsky, S., et al. (Eds): Urodynamics. New York, Academic Press, 1971, pp. 3–27.

Tanagho, E. A., Hutch, J. A., Meyers, F. H., and Rambo, O. N., Jr.: Primary vesicoureteral reflux: Experimental studies of its etiology. J. Urol., *93*:165, 1965.

Tanagho, E. A., Meyers, F. H., and Smith, D. E.: The trigone: Anatomical and physiological considerations. 1. In relation to the ureterovesical junction. J. Urol., *100*:623, 1968.

Teague, N., and Boyarsky, S.: The effect of coliform bacilli upon ureteral peristalsis. Invest. Urol., *5*:423, 1968.

Teele, R. L., Lebowitz, R. L., and Colodny, A. H.: Reflux into the unused ureter. J. Urol., *115*:310, 1976.

Thackston, L. P., Price, N. C., and Richardson, A. G.: Use of antispasmotics in treatment of spastic ureteritis. J. Urol., *73*:487, 1955.

Tindall, A. R.: Preliminary observations on the mechanical and electrical activity of the rat ureter. J. Physiol. (Lond.), *223*:633, 1972.

Toguri, A. G., and Fournier, G.: Factors influencing the pressure-flow perfusion system. J. Urol., *127*:1021, 1982.

Tomita, T., and Watanabe, H.: Factors controlling myogenic activity in smooth muscle. Philos. Trans. R. Soc. Lond. (Biol. Sci.), *265*:73, 1973.

Traut, H. F., and Kuder, A.: Inflammation of the upper urinary tract complicating the reproductive period of woman. Collective review. Int. Abst. Surg., *67*:568, 1938.

Triner, L., Nahas, G. G., Vulliemoz, Y., Overweg, N.I.A., Verosky, M., Habif, D. V., and Ngai, S. H.: Cyclic AMP and smooth muscle function. Ann. N.Y. Acad. Sci., *185*:458, 1971.

Tsuchida, S., and Yamaguchi, O.: A constant electrical activity of the renal pelvis correlated to ureteral peristalsis. Tohoku J. Exp. Med., *121*:133, 1977.

Uehara, Y., and Burnstock, G.: Demonstration of "gap junctions" between smooth muscle cells. J. Cell. Biol., *44*:215, 1970.

Ueno, A., Kawamura, T., Ogawa, A., and Takayasu, H.: Relation of spontaneous passage of ureteral calculi to size. Urology, *10*:544, 1977.

van Wagenen, G., and Jenkins, R. H.: An experimental examination of factors causing ureteral dilatation of pregnancy. J. Urol., *42*:1010, 1939.

Vaughan, E. D., Jr., Shenasky, J. H., II, and Gillenwater, J. Y.: Mechanism of acute hemodynamic response to ureteral occlusion. Invest. Urol. *9*:109, 1971.

Vaughan, E. D., Jr., Sorenson, E. J., and Gillenwater, J. Y.: The renal hemodynamic response to chronic unilateral ureteral occlusion. Invest. Urol., *8*:78, 1970.

Vela-Navarrete, R.: Percutaneous intrapelvic pressure determinations in the study of hydronephrosis. Invest. Urol., *8*:526, 1971.

Vereecken, R. L.: Dynamical Aspects of Urine Transport in the Ureter. Acco, Louvain, 1973.

Vereecken, R. L., Derluyn, J., and Verduyn, H.: The viscoelastic behavior of the ureter during elongation. Urol. Res., *1*:15, 1973.

Vereecken, R. L., Hendrickx, H., and Casteels, R.: The influence of calcium on the electrical and mechanical activity of the guinea pig ureter. Urol. Res., *3*:149, 1975a.

Vereecken, R. L., Hendrickx, H., and Casteels, R.: The influence of sodium on the electrical and mechanical activity of the guinea pig ureter. Urol. Res., *3*:159, 1975b.

Vesin, M. F., and Harbon, S.: The effects of epinephrine, prostaglandins and their antagonists on adenosine cyclic 3′, 5′-monophosphate concentrations on motility on the rat uterus. Mol. Pharmacol., *10*:457, 1974.

Washizu, Y.: Grouped discharges in ureter muscle. Comp. Biochem. Physiol., *19*:713, 1966.

Washizu, Y.: Membrane potential and tension in guinea-pig ureter. J. Pharmacol. Exp. Ther., *158*:445, 1967.

Washizu, Y.: Ouabain on excitation contraction in guinea pig ureter: Fed. Proc., *27*:662, 1968.

Watterson, D. M., Harrelson, W. G., Jr., Keller, P. M., Sharief, F., and Vanaman, T. C.: Structural similarities between the Ca^{2+}-dependent regulatory proteins of 3′:5′-cyclic nucleotide phosphodiesterase and actomyosin ATPase. J. Biol. Chem., *251*:4501, 1976.

Weidmann, S.: Effect of current flow on membrane potential of cardiac muscle. J. Physiol. (Lond.), *115*:227, 1951.

Weinberg, S. R.: Ureteral function. I. Simultaneous monitoring of ureteral peristalsis. Invest. Urol., *12*:103, 1974.

Weinberg, S. R.: Application of physiologic principles to surgery of the ureter. Am. J. Surg., *103*:549, 1962.

Weinberg, S. R., and Maletta, J. J.: Measurement of peristalsis of the ureter and its relation to drugs. JAMA, *175*:109, 1961.

Weiss, R. M.: Clinical implications of ureteral physiology. J. Urol., *121*:401, 1979.

Weiss, R. M.: Pharmacology of the ureter. *In* Finkbeiner, A. E., Barbour, G. L., and Bissada, N. K., (Eds): Pharmacology of the Urinary Tract and Male Reproductive System. New York, Appleton-Century-Crofts, 1982, pp. 137–173.

Weiss, R. M., and Biancani, P.: A rationale for ureteral tapering. Urology, *20*:482, 1982.

Weiss, R. M., and Biancani, P.: Characteristics of normal and refluxing ureterovesical junctions. J. Urol., *129*:858, 1983.

Weiss, R. M., Bassett, A. L., and Hoffman, B. F.: Adrenergic innervation of the ureter. Invest. Urol., *16*:123, 1978.

Weiss, R. M., Bassett, A. L., and Hoffman, B. F.: Dynamic length-tension curves of cat ureter. Am. J. Physiol., *222*:388, 1972.

Weiss, R. M., Bassett, A. L., and Hoffman, B. F.: Effect of ouabain on contractility of the isolated ureter. Invest. Urol., *8*:161, 1970.

Weiss, R. M., Biancani, P., and Zabinski, M. P.: Adrenergic control of ureteral tonus. Invest. Urol., *12*:30, 1974.

Weiss, R. M., Hardman, J. G., and Wells, J. N.: Resistance of a separated form of canine ureteral phosphodiesterase activity to inhibition by xanthines and papaverine. Biochem. Pharmacol., *30*:2371, 1981.

Weiss, R. M., Vulliemoz, Y., Verosky, M., Rosen, M. R., and Triner, L.: Adenylate cyclase and phosphodiesterase activity in rabbit ureter. Invest. Urol., *15*:15, 1977.

Weiss, R. M., Wagner, M. L., and Hoffman, B. F.: Localization of pacemaker for peristalsis in the intact canine ureter. Invest. Urol., *5*:42, 1967.

Weiss, R. M., Wagner, M. L., and Hoffman, B. F.: Wenckebach periods of the ureter. A further note on the ubiquity of the Wenckebach phenomenon. Invest. Urol., *5*:463, 1968.

Wharton, L. R.: The innervation of the ureter, with respect to denervation. J. Urol., *28*:639, 1932.

Whitaker, R. H.: Methods of assessing obstruction in dilated ureters. Br. J. Urol., *45*:15, 1973.

Whitaker, R. H.: Clinical assessment of pelvic and ureteral function. Urology, *12*:146, 1978.

Whitaker, R. H.: The Whitaker test. Urol. Clin. North Am., *6*:529, 1979.

Whitfield, H. N., Harrison, N. W., Sherwood, T., and Williams, D. I.: Upper urinary tract obstruction: Pressure flow studies in children. Br. J. Urol., *48*:427, 1976.

Witherow, R. O'N., and Whitaker, R. H.: The predicative accuracy of antegrade pressure flow studies in equivocal upper tract obstruction. Br. J. Urol., *53*:496, 1981.

Woodburne, R. T., and Lapides, J.: The ureteral lumen during peristalsis. Am. J. Anat., *133*:255, 1972.

Wooster, M. J.: Effects of prostaglandin E_1 on the dog ureter *in vitro*. J. Physiol. (Lond.), *213*:51P, 1971.

Zimskind, P. D., Davis, D. M., and Decaestecker, J. E.: Effects of bladder filling on ureteral dynamics. J. Urol., *102*:693, 1969.

CHAPTER 4

Physiology of the Urinary Bladder

WILLIAM E. BRADLEY, M.D.

INTRODUCTION

Many changes have occurred in our understanding of urinary bladder function since the last edition of this text (Bradley and Scott, 1978; Hald and Bradley, 1983). These changes continue to result principally from animal investigation and less frequently from human studies. New techniques of tracing anatomic pathways, increased understanding of the role of neuropeptides in synaptic transmission, and insights into the neurobiology of development are perhaps the most striking developments.

Inferences drawn from animal experimentation continue to be readily applied to human physiology despite the differences between animal and human reflex development, the most important of which is the assumption of the upright biped position. However, direct knowledge of human physiology of the urinary bladder may grow more rapidly with the beginning widespread use of electrophysiologic techniques, such as evoked potential studies.

This chapter includes the following sections: (1) neuroanatomy of the central and peripheral innervation of the lower urinary tract; (2) neurophysiology of the lower urinary tract; (3) loop or reflex conceptualization of urinary bladder innervation; (4) neurouropharmacology; (5) urodynamics; (6) behavioral neurology and the urinary bladder; (7) ontogeny of urinary bladder function; and (8) description of normal voiding.

These categories represent an evident expansion of our knowledge of bladder physiology and reflect the nature of the increase in our data base in the past 10 years.

NEUROANATOMY OF CENTRAL AND PERIPHERAL INNERVATION OF THE LOWER URINARY TRACT

Introduction

Neuroanatomic studies of innervation of the lower urinary tract have benefited from the introduction of tracer methods in the experimental animal and the evoked potential technique in humans. These latter studies have been supplemented by the histologic evaluation of autopsy and biopsy material of the lower urinary tract. Older methods of tracing by inducing cell degeneration (chromatolysis) have been supplanted by other tracer techniques. The common method now consists of retrograde transport of marker substance, the principal one being horseradish peroxidase, which is transported along the axon to the cell body. The horseradish peroxidase technique depends upon retrograde axonal transport and axoplasmic flow. This method consists of injection of solutions of the enzyme into neural tissue or the immersion of pelvic nerves into such solution. The material is taken up by axons, is transported by axoplasmic flow, and appears in the neural somata in identifiable forms. The technique has been used at the light and electron microscopic level and has been employed extensively to investigate central and peripheral innervation of the detrusor muscle (DeGroat, 1975; Kuzuhara et al., 1980) and periurethral striated muscle.

The second method consists of injection of radioactive labeled substances into the neuropil, with subsequent absorption into the nerve cell and anterograde transport along its axonal pathways, followed by autoradiographic identification of the labeled compounds.

Cellular Studies

Extensive light and electron microscopic studies of cellular morphology of smooth muscle and nerve cells in the lower urinary tract have been reported (Fletcher and Bradley, 1978). These techniques have been used more extensively in the experimental animal than in humans.

Other methods for histologic investigation include the use of fluorescence histochemistry for identification of neurons that are nonadrenergic, dopaminergic, or serotonergic. These techniques have been widely utilized to investigate the innervation of the detrusor and urethra (Elbadawi and Schenk, 1966, 1968a and b, 1970; Elbadawi, 1982). Older methods include stains of neuronal and axonal degeneration after ablation (Kuru, 1965).

Other methodologies for anatomic investigation of the lower urinary tract include immunohistochemical techniques for the identification of peptide neurotransmitter substances of the lower urinary tract (Alm et al., 1977; Hokfelt et al., 1978) and evoked potential techniques.

Evoked potential techniques for the identification of reflex pathways were first utilized in the laboratory and later enjoyed wide application in the clinical investigation of neurologic disease (Starr, 1976). They have recently been used for the identification of micturition reflex pathways in the experimental animal (Bradley, 1980) and in humans (Badr et al., 1982; Haldeman et al., 1982a and b). These techniques are undoubtedly in the first phase of a long period of widespread use in the study of physiology and pathology of the lower urinary tract. The evoked potential techniques for studying the lower urinary tract consist of application of an electrical stimulus to the detrusor muscle, the periurethral striated muscle, or the pudendal nerve, with subsequent recording of a potential evoked in either the spinal cord or the cerebral cortex. The recording system includes a computer of average transients in order to select an evoked signal to be amplified that otherwise would be obscured by intercurrent neural electrical activity. These evoked potential methods address themselves exclusively to the study of afferent neural pathways.

Cerebrocortical Innervation of the Urinary Bladder (Fig. 4–1)

The cerebrocortical innervation of the urinary detrusor and periurethral striated muscle has been investigated in the experimental animal and in humans. Tracer studies of cerebral and spinal innervation have been addressed to the urinary detrusor and to the periurethral striated muscle and have employed radioactive proline and horseradish peroxidase.

The pathways for cerebral control of detrusor neurons have been investigated by the use of horseradish peroxidase (HRP) and by immunohistochemical techniques for the identification of substance P, a polypeptide transmitter agent. Specifically, these techniques have been utilized to identify the pathway of axons from the caudal portion of nucleus laterodorsalis tegmenti (TLD) in the rat to the medial frontal cortex (Sakanaka et al., 1983). Further studies have demonstrated that this pathway is exclusive for the neurons concerned with urinary bladder innervation. Moreover, these investigations showed that the projection is ipsilateral and that there is a projection to the lateral septal area. This latter area has been associated with motivational and emotional activities. This pathway was demonstrated in this study to be an ascending and descending one, since injection of HRP into the medial frontal cortex demonstrated many HRP cells in TLD. Substance P–containing fibers were observed to be of two types: (1) coarse varicose fibers in lamina II, III, and IV; and (2) fine terminals that were perineuronal in location (Fig. 4–2). The caudal portion of TLD is the nucleus of Barrington (Satoh et al., 1978a and b), which had been demonstrated many years ago to be exclusively concerned with micturition (Barrington, 1921, 1925).

In the monkey, the cerebrocortical area concerned with innervation of the periurethral striated muscle has been identified by injection of radioactive proline into area 4 (Brodmann), with subsequent radioautographic tracing of transported materials into the pudendal nucleus in the sacral spinal cord. Bilateral input was demonstrated.

In the cat, the method of the evoked potential was used to identify those cerebral areas concerned with innervation of the detrusor muscle and periurethral striated muscle (Fig. 4–3) (Bradley, 1980). These cortical areas are superimposed and are located at a site similar to those identified in tracer studies.

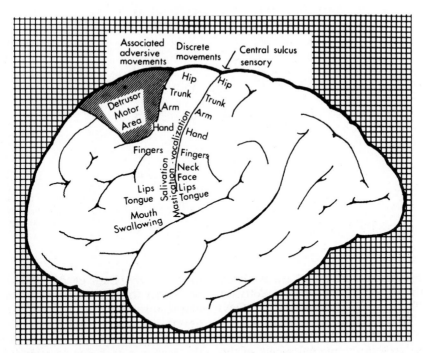

Figure 4–1. Cerebrocortical area concerned with innervation of the detrusor muscle. The cerebral location of the periurethral striated muscle is on the medial aspect of the central sulcus.

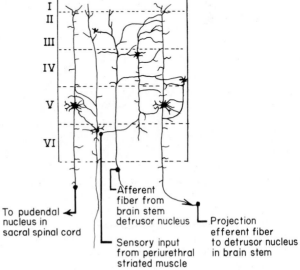

Figure 4–2. Distribution of afferent and efferent inputs to the cerebrocortical gray matter.

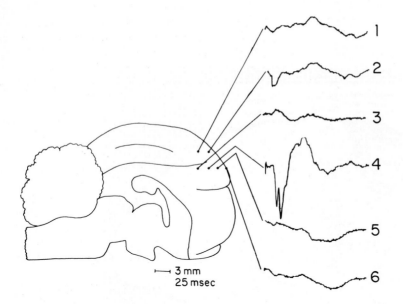

Figure 4–3. Responses evoked in cerebral cortex of cat by stimulation of detrusor urethral nerve. The diphasic cortical response is illustrated in trace 4.

In humans, cerebrocortical areas have been studied by stimulation of the urinary detrusor (Badr et al., 1982) and the pudendal nerve (Figs. 4–4 and 4–5) (Haldeman et al., 1982a and b). They have been located in the central vertex of the skull in the area of the medial aspect of the rolandic fissure. Latency times of responses have been similar for both urinary detrusor and pudendal nerve stimulation. In the urinary detrusor studies, cystoscopic introduction of stimulating electrodes was employed. The dorsal wall of the bladder just above the trigone was stimulated. Polyphasic positive-negative waves were recorded with latencies similar to those observed with pudendal nerve stimulation. The authors

of this study (Badr et al., 1982) considered the possibility that responses were obtained by stimulation of other than bladder afferents but believed that this possibility was eliminated by the use of bipolar electrodes. They concluded that the response was due to stimulation of pelvic, hypogastric, and pudendal nerves. In the pudendal nerve studies, excitation of this nerve was obtained by stimulation of the dorsal nerve of the penis. The maximum response was recorded at a location 2 cm behind the central vertex of the skull. The central transit time, measured by the latency difference between the spinal and cortical evoked responses, was observed to be longer for the pudendal nerve than

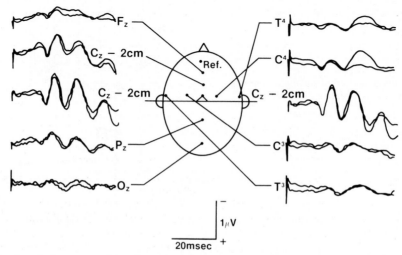

Figure 4–4. Averaged evoked responses from the scalp after stimulation of the dorsal nerve of the penis. The response is maximum in amplitude at the central vertex minus 2 cm position.

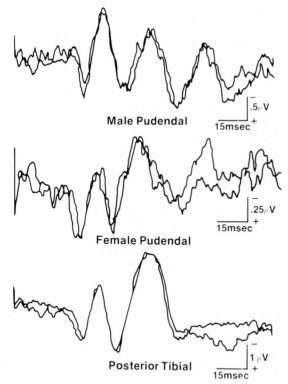

Figure 4–5. Comparison of cortical evoked responses from stimulation of the dorsal nerve of the penis (trace 1), dorsal nerve of the clitoris (trace 2), and the posterior tibial nerve (trace 3).

that obtained by stimulation of a comparable sensory nerve—the posterior tibial nerve. The reason for this difference is unknown at present.

THE THALAMUS

The thalamus is a collection of midline subcortical nuclei consisting of a rostral ventralis anterior nucleus, an intermediate ventralis lateralis nucleus, and a caudal ventralis posterior nucleus (Fig. 4–6). Essentially, these nuclei relay impulses from both autonomic and somatic peripheral sensory receptors as well as from other intracerebral nuclei, such as those of the limbic system, to specific areas of the cerebral cortex. The thalamic pathways for the urinary detrusor and periurethral striated muscle have not been precisely defined in either experimental animals or humans.

THE LIMBIC SYSTEM

The limbic lobe consists of the subcallosal and cingulate gyri as well as the hippocampal formation, amygdaloid nucleus, and dentate gyrus. The limbic system has been demonstrated in the experimental animal to be involved in somatic and visceral activities, including those

of the urinary bladder. In the cat, stimulation of the cortical areas composing the limbic system evoked either facilitation or depression of detrusor reflex contractions (Edvardsen and Ursen, 1968). The effects of limbic system function upon the urinary bladder in humans remain unexplored.

THE BASAL GANGLIA

The basal ganglia are a subcortical collection of nuclei consisting of the caudate nucleus, putamen, globus pallidus, and substantia nigra. There are many neural circuits that connect the nuclei of the basal ganglia with the cerebral cortex and other nuclei. One loop consists of the motor cortex to the caudate nucleus–putamen (striatum)–pallidum–ventralis lateralis in the thalamus–motor cortex. A second internuclear pathway is from the substantia nigra to the putamen and globus. This latter pathway transfers transmitter agent, dopamine, by axoplasmic flow from a site of synthesis in the neurons of the substantia nigra to a site of utilization in the neurons of the putamen and globus pallidus (Fig. 4–7).

The basal ganglia control muscle tone and movement. They have also been demonstrated in the experimental animal to affect detrusor reflex threshold. Hence, electrical stimulation induces depression of spontaneous detrusor reflex contractions (Porter, 1967). In Parkinson's disease, associated with a deficiency of dopamine in the neurons of the putamen and globus pallidus, there may be tremor, rigidity, bradykinesia, gait instability, and detrusor hyperreflexia. Hence, it is believed that detrusor hyperreflexia in Parkinson's disease is a sequel to the inhibitory effect of basal ganglia function. The precise anatomic relationship of the basal ganglia to the brain stem and cerebral nuclei concerned with voiding in humans is unknown.

THE BRAIN STEM

The brain stem localization of the nuclear collection first concerned with micturition was delineated by Barrington (Barrington, 1915, 1921, 1925) (Fig. 4–8). He observed that bilateral destruction of the nuclei in the brain stem by electrolytic lesions abolished voiding and suggested that the detrusor nucleus was located in the pontine-mesencephalic area. Later studies have demonstrated that this nucleus is in the caudal portion of the dorsal tegmental area of the pons rostral to the nucleus locus ceruleus (Tohyama et al., 1978). Stimulation of this area produced firing of sacral preganglionic neurons and contraction of the urinary bladder (Fig. 4–

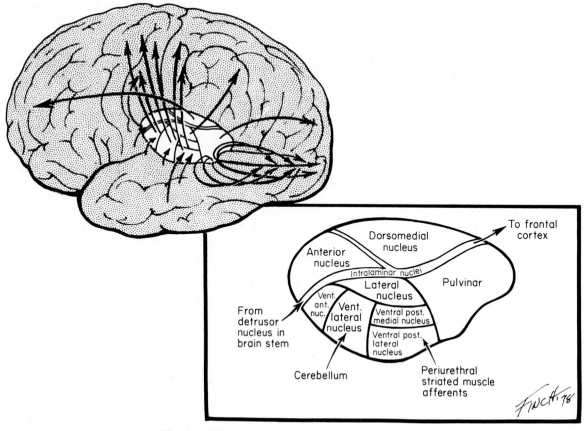

Figure 4–6. Input-output relationships of the thalamus.

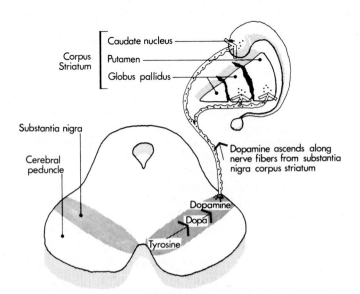

Figure 4–7. Diagram of the basal ganglia, demonstrating synthesis of dopamine in the neurons of the substantia nigra with transport to and utilization by the neurons of the putamen and globus pallidus.

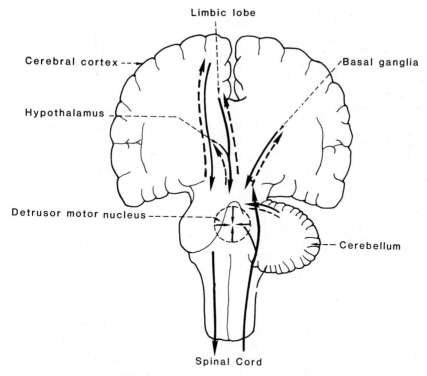

Figure 4–8. Input-output relationships of brain stem center for voiding.

9). Stimulation of afferent receptors in the urinary bladder resulted in an evoked response at the same site (Bradley and Conway, 1966).

The detrusor nucleus is composed of medium-sized, oval-shaped neurons. Two projections have been observed from this nucleus, one to the lateral hypothalamic area and one to the sacral spinal cord (Satoh et al., 1978a).

Descending projections were traced by injection of radioactive proline and leucine into the TLD region, with subsequent radioautographic examination, and into the intermediolateral cell column of the sacral spinal cord (Satoh et al., 1978a). Descending pathways traveled ventral to the vestibular nuclei to the caudal level of the medulla. Other axons radiated into the lateral portion of the reticular formation, with a substantial number terminating in the

Figure 4–9. Microelectrode electrical stimulation of brain stem center for voiding, with consequent rise in intravesical pressure.

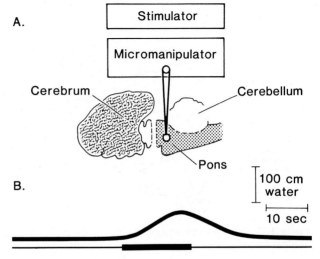

ventrolateral portion of the nucleus of the solitary tract. Descending fibers to the spinal cord traveled bilaterally, but principally ipsilaterally, to the nucleus. Examination of the ascending projections of TLD, excluding the Barrington nucleus, demonstrated a pathway to the medial frontal cortex containing the immunoreactive peptide substance P (Sakanaka et al., 1983). That the animal data are analogous to human reflex organization is suggested in a recent study (Khurona, 1982).

To date no projections have been traced from the vestibular nucleus to the conus medullaris. This nucleus has been demonstrated to have significant influence on skeletal muscle tone and movement. However, the nucleus gigantocellularis of the medulla was indicated by electrophysiologic investigation to innervate pudendal motoneurons in the sacral spinal cord (Mackel, 1979).

THE CEREBELLUM

The cerebellum is made up of gray matter consisting of neuron somata and white matter consisting of axons and is located astride the brain stem in the posterior cranial fossa. The cerebellum is a midline structure and is composed of the vermis and two lateral lobes, or hemispheres. Histologically, the cerebellum is composed of the cerebellar cortex, consisting of gray matter and an inner core of white matter. There are four pairs of intrinsic nuclei. To date,

the only nuclei demonstrated to be concerned with voiding are the fastigial nuclei. These are close to the midline in the roof of the fourth ventricle. The corticonuclear projection is from neurons in the gray matter of the anterior and posterior vermis to the fastigial nuclei.

The cerebellum is concerned with the coordination of motor activity. This may occur in one of four ways relative to the urinary bladder:

1. Maintenance of tone in somatic musculature, including the periurethral striated muscle and pelvic flow musculature.

2. Control of rate, range, and force of skeletal muscle movement, including the urinary detrusor muscle and periurethral striated muscle.

3. Suppression of motor neurons in the dorsolateral tegmental nucleus of the pons that initiate detrusor muscle contraction.

4. Possible provision of coordination between detrusor reflex muscle contraction and tightening or relaxation of the periurethral striated muscle.

Anatomic connections between the urinary bladder and the cerebellum have been established principally by the evoked potential technique (Bradley and Teague, 1969a). These studies in the experimental animal (Fig. 4–10) demonstrate midline vermian projections from stimulation of the pelvic detrusor and the pudendal urethral nerves. A diphasic, initially surface-positive response is observed. In the section

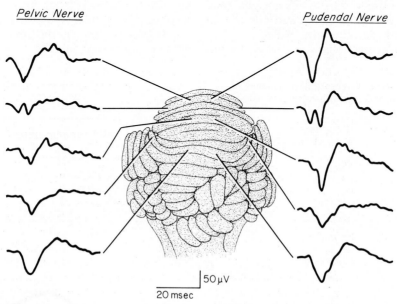

Figure 4–10. Responses evoked on anterior vermis of the cerebellum by stimulation of the pelvic detrusor and pudendal urethral nerves.

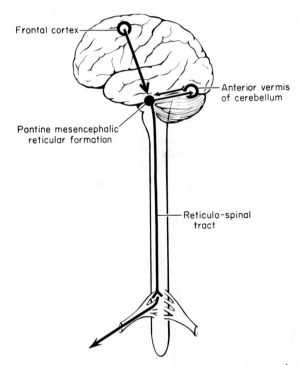

Figure 4–11. Cerebral, cerebellar, and spinal motor pathways.

on physiology of the urinary bladder it will be demonstrated that ablation of this same area in the cat evokes profound detrusor hyperreflexia. No tracer studies from the urinary bladder to the cerebellum or in the reverse direction have been reported in the experimental animal. No evoked potential studies of the cerebellum from the lower urinary tract have been reported in humans. These will be impeded for the foreseeable future by the difficulties of recording from the cerebellar surface, which is situated in a pool of electrolyte, the cerebrospinal fluid in the posterior fossa. The motor pathways from the cerebral cortex to the spinal cord include contributions from the fastigial nucleus of the cerebellum (Fig. 4–11).

Spinal Pathways of the Detrusor Muscle and the Periurethral Striated Muscle

The spinal tracts innervating the detrusor muscle and pelvic floor musculature consist of afferent and efferent pathways. These have been delineated in the experimental animal and in humans (Nathan and Smith, 1951, 1958).

The general organization of somatic reflex pathways consists of supraspinal and segmental reflex arcs (Philips et al., 1971). The segmental reflex innervation consists of afferent axons arising from tension and length receptors in skeletal muscles, which travel to synapse on motor neurons in nuclei located in the gray matter of the spinal cord. These synapses and nuclei are located at the segmental level of the spinal nerve roots innervating the skeletal muscles. Thus, pudendal sensory axons arise from muscle spindles and tendon organs in the pelvic floor musculature, including the periurethral striated muscle, and travel toward the spinal cord to enter the conus medullaris, where they divide. One group of axons enters the spinal cord to synapse on pudendal motor neurons in the gray matter of the ventral horn of the first to third sacral segments. A second group of axons courses rostrally in the dorsal columns to synapse on neurons in the cerebellum as well as passing rostrally in the medial lemniscus to synapse on neurons in the nucleus ventralis posterolateralis of the thalamus. Third-order neurons then send axons to synapse in the sensorimotor cortex. It is this pathway that has been investigated by evoked potential studies utilizing stimulation of pudendal afferent axons. From the neurons in this area of the sensorimotor cortex, axons arise that then descend in the corticospinal tracts to innervate the pudendal nuclei in the sacral gray matter (Nakagawa, 1980). They travel caudally in the lateral columns of the spinal cord to synapse on pudendal motor neurons in the conus medullaris. This pathway was defined in the primate by injection of radioactive proline into the sensorimotor cortex. There was predominant contralateral projection of the cortical pathways with lesser ipsilateral projection. The level of crossing is with the pyramidal tracts at the caudal end of the medulla.

In contrast, sensory axons from the detrusor muscle divide upon entry into the sacral spinal cord, with the bulk traveling rostrally to the dorsolateral tegmental nucleus of the pons. With application of the tracer horseradish peroxidase to the cut pelvic nerve of the cat, the tracer was detected in Lissauer's tract, the dorsal columns, the dorsolateral funiculus, and the sacral gray matter. The afferent projections included the conus medullaris and extended into the lumbar dorsal region. Afferent collaterals were arranged into two bundles: a lateral collateral pathway that conducted axons into the area of the detrusor nucleus, and a medial collateral pathway into the dorsal commissure (DeGroat et al., 1981).

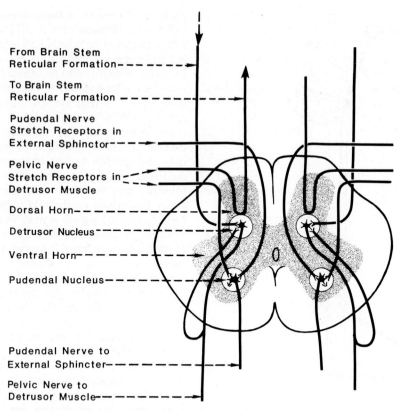

**From Brain Stem
Reticular Formation**

**To Brain Stem
Reticular Formation**

**Pudendal Nerve
Stretch Receptors in
External Sphincter**

**Pelvic Nerve
Stretch Receptors in
Detrusor Muscle**

Dorsal Horn

Detrusor Nucleus

Ventral Horn

Pudendal Nucleus

**Pudendal Nerve to
External Sphincter**

**Pelvic Nerve to
Detrusor Muscle**

Figure 4–12. Input-output relationships of conus medullaris. Recurrent inhibition pathways are observed in the pelvic motor nerves.

ANATOMY OF THE CONUS MEDULLARIS

The conus medullaris is defined as the caudal portion of the spinal cord containing sacral segments S1 to S5. The conus medullaris contains nuclear collections concerned with innervation of the smooth muscle of the urinary detrusor and the periurethral striated muscle (Fig. 4–12).

The precise location and morphology of the cell population of the detrusor and pudendal nuclei have been established by the use of tracer techniques in the experimental animal. These have been supplemented by anatomic dissection and evoked potential studies in humans (Fig. 4–13). These latter studies have also helped to define synaptic relationships.

DETRUSOR NUCLEUS (Fig. 4–14)

The sacral detrusor nucleus with its motor neurons related to innervation of the smooth muscle of the urinary detrusor and urethra is distributed over the first three sacral segments, with the principal neuronal collection at S2 in the cat (Fig. 4–15) (Morgan et al., 1979, 1981; Nadelhaft et al., 1980; DeGroat et al., 1981,

1982). In the cat, detrusor neurons were localized in the lateral band of the intramedullary afferent pathways. The neucleus has a length of 10 mm in a rostrocaudal direction over two to three segments, with approximately 74 per cent of the preganglionic population contained in S2. The cells of the detrusor nucleus of the cat were spindle-shaped and located along the gray matter in lamina V through VII. The cells are oriented in a dorsoventral direction, with the accompanying dendrites extending within the nucleus (Fig. 4–15).

The pelvic afferents to the detrusor nucleus have been studied by the techniques of evoked potential (Oliver et al., 1969) and horseradish peroxidase (Morgan et al., 1981). The latter method has demonstrated afferent endings to be densest in the area of the detrusor nucleus but to extend extensively in rostral and caudal directions (Fig. 4–15). Central afferent projections consistent with the organization of the detrusor reflex as a spinobulbospinal pathway were observed in the dorsal columns, in the dorsolateral funiculus, and in lamina I–X of the spinal gray matter. Utilizing abnormal lipid collections in autonomic neurons in Fabry's disease as a marker, Sung (Sung, 1979; Sung et al., 1979) localized detrusor motor neurons in humans from the first to the fourth sacral segments with a rostral and caudal distribution of the motor neuron cell column. Sung concluded that Onuf's nucleus was an autonomic nucleus. This has not correlated with the results of tracer studies in the experimental animal, which indicated that Onuf's nucleus innervates the periurethral striated muscle as well as other striated perineal musculature. The detrusor motor cells have also been demonstrated to contain enkephalins or opioid peptides. This finding implies that these cells utilize enkephalins as a neurotransmitter agent.

The distribution of the detrusor nuclei has also been studied by the evoked potential technique in the experimental animal and by nerve blocks in humans. In humans, asymmetry of innervation was demonstrated (Bradley et al., 1974). Asymmetry of innervation implies that there may be dominance of cerebrocortical or spinal innervation of the urinary detrusor.

THE PUDENDAL NUCLEUS

The pudendal nuclei are synonymous with Onuf's nucleus, although there is controversy concerning this conclusion. In cats and dogs, identification of the nuclei was obtained by injection of tracer substances into the striated portion of the rectal sphincter and into the periurethral striated muscle (Kuzuhara et al., 1980). The location of the nuclear portion concerned with voiding is in the ventrolateral por-

Figure 4–13. *A* and *B,* Evoked response distribution in the conus medullaris.

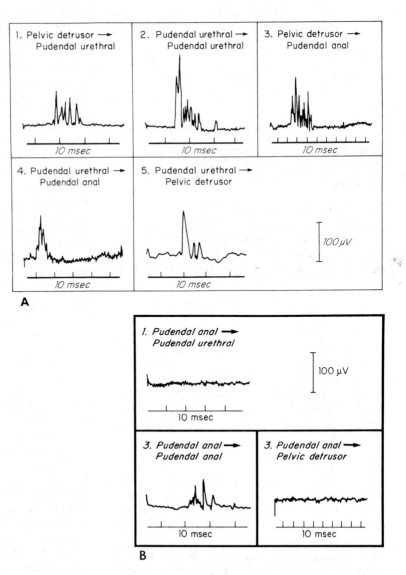

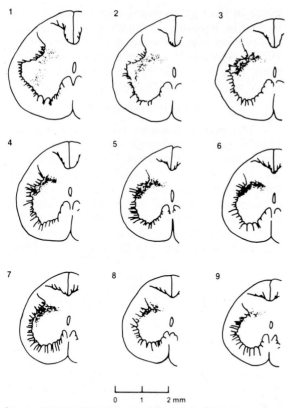

Figure 4–14. Longitudinal distribution of parasympathetic nucleus in the conus medullaris, the midportion of which is the detrusor nucleus. (From DeGroat, W. C., et al.: J. Auton. Nerv. Syst., 5:23, 1982.)

tion of the gray matter in the second sacral segment. The longitudinal distribution of the pudendal nucleus is from the caudal portion of the second sacral segment to the cranial portion of the fourth sacral segment, with the innerva-

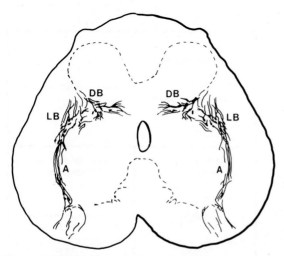

Figure 4–15. Distribution of pelvic nerve afferents in the conus medullaris, the lateral band (LB) of which distributes to the detrusor nucleus. (From DeGroat, W. C., et al.: J. Auton. Nerv. Syst., 1982.)

tion of the periurethral striated muscle at the third sacral segment and extending into the second and fourth sacral segments. This nucleus was demonstrated in radioactive proline studies to be innervated from the sensorimotor cortex and the medulla.

The anatomic connections of the pelvic and pudendal nerves and nuclei have been traced by the evoked potential technique (Figs. 4–16 to 4–18) in the experimental animal (Bradley and Teague, 1968) and in humans (Verecken et al., 1982).

THE PELVIC GANGLIA AND PELVIC PLEXUS

The pelvic nerve to the urinary detrusor and smooth muscle of the urethra contains efferent and afferent axons from the second, third, and fourth sacral segments in humans. This nerve meets with efferent sympathetic nerves descending from ganglia located along the tenth thoracic to the second lumbar vertebrae via the superior hypogastric and pelvic nerves (Fig. 4–19). The plexus contains axons and anatomic ganglia that innervate the urinary detrusor smooth muscle of the urethra and the prostate gland (Fletcher and Bradley, 1978).

The preganglionic inputs terminate synaptically on the dendrites of the neuron, axodendritic synapses, and occasionally on the cell soma of the ganglionic neurons (Fig. 4–20). There is preganglionic input from the hypogastric and pelvic nerves. These ganglia have been demonstrated in conjunction with accompanying axons as adrenergic or cholinergic. These conclusions are the result of formaldehyde fluorescence staining for catecholamines as well as histochemical methods for staining choline acetyltransferase. The finding of this enzyme, which hydrolyzes acetylcholine, has been taken by some investigators as evidence that acetylcholine is a neurotransmitter at an identified site. An additional cell, referred to as SIF (small intensely fluorescent) has also been identified in the ganglia.

Cholinergic and adrenergic presynaptic nerve terminals (Fig. 4–21) are also identifiable by electron microscopy (Feher and Vajda, 1979). There are two to three types of synaptic vesicles visible, including small, clear vesicles containing acetylcholine and dense core vesicles. The dense core vesicles may be small or large. The large dense core vesicles are believed to contain noradrenergic transmitter agent (Elbadawi and Schenk, 1970; Elbadawi, 1982). These vesicles are stainable histochemically in ultrastructural studies. The small dense core vesicles may contain a neuropeptide transmitter agent.

Ganglia can be identified in the pelvic

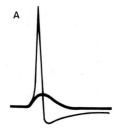

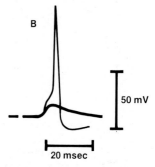

Figure 4–16. Responses evoked in pudendal motoneurons by stimulation of pudendal afferents recorded by intracellular microelectrodes.

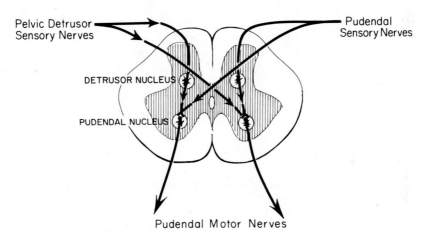

Figure 4–17. Comparison of pelvic and pudendal afferent input to pudendal nucleus in the conus medullaris.

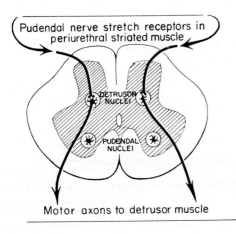

Figure 4–18. Pudendal afferent input to detrusor nucleus.

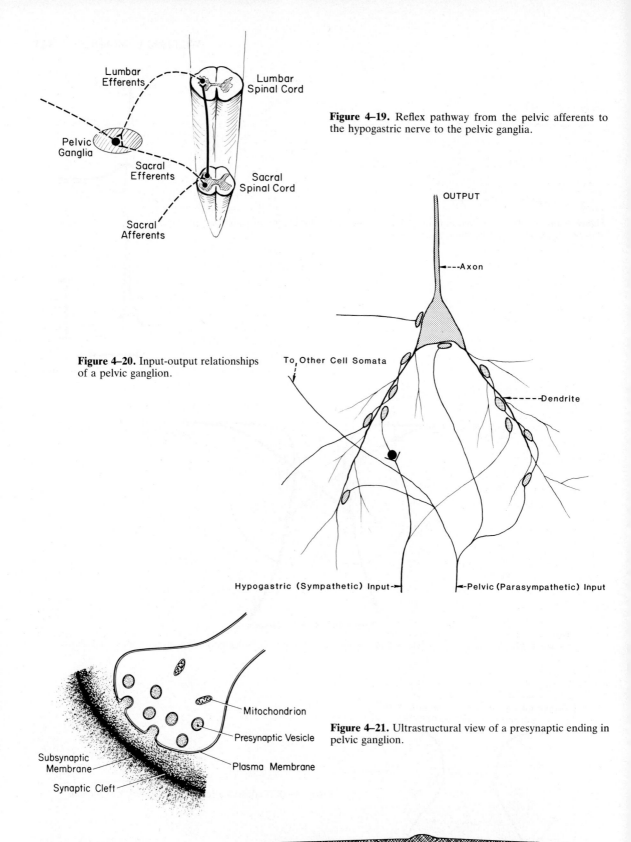

Lumbar
Efferents

Lumbar
Spinal Cord

Pelvic
Ganglia

Sacral
Efferents

Sacral
Spinal Cord

Sacral
Afferents

Figure 4–19. Reflex pathway from the pelvic afferents to the hypogastric nerve to the pelvic ganglia.

OUTPUT

Axon

To Other Cell Somata

Dendrite

Hypogastric (Sympathetic) Input

Pelvic (Parasympathetic) Input

Figure 4–20. Input-output relationships of a pelvic ganglion.

Mitochondrion

Presynaptic Vesicle

Plasma Membrane

Subsynaptic
Membrane

Synaptic Cleft

Figure 4–21. Ultrastructural view of a presynaptic ending in pelvic ganglion.

Figure 4–22. Postganglionic motor innervation. Axon varicosities (a to d) are shown.

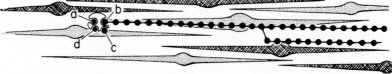

a

b

d

c

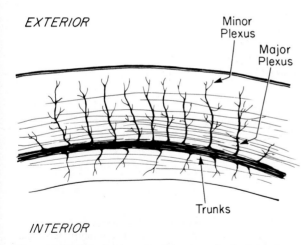

EXTERIOR

Minor Plexus

Major Plexus

Trunks

INTERIOR

Figure 4–23. Distribution of pelvic nerves in the interstices of the detrusor muscle.

plexus and in the interstices of the detrusor muscle.

The pre- and postganglionic axons consist of cholinergic and adrenergic nerves (Kluck, 1980), which course and ramify within the interstices of the detrusor muscle, principally in a lateral and posterior direction in company with the blood vessels. The axons of these bundles are either myelinated or nonmyelinated with an accompanying Schwann cell sheath (Figs. 4–22 to 4–24). It has been assumed that the myelinated axons subserve sensory function and that the nonmyelinated axons are motor in function.

No part of the vesicourethral musculature is supplied on a 1:1 basis of nerve to muscle. Rather, there is frequent nerve to muscle innervation, with adjacent cells innervated through a low-resistance extrasynaptic pathway. For example, cholinergic muscular innervation of the rat bladder is more dense in the anterior than in the posterior wall of the urinary detrusor.

The density of adrenergic neuroplexuses is low in the urinary detrusor and high in the bladder base and proximal urethra.

The innervated smooth muscle cells have frequent gap-type junctions (Fig. 4–25). Cholinergic and nonadrenergic nerve contacts with individual muscle cells are formed by axon varicosities forming passage-type contacts with individual smooth muscle cells. Cholinergic or adrenergic axons, or both, may form axoaxonal-type synapses. Recent studies of innervation demonstrate that the density of adrenergic and cholinergic innervation of the detrusor as well as physiologic and pharmacologic responses can be altered by exogenous administration of estrogen. There is both cholinergic and adrenergic innervation of the male proximal urethra. Sparse adrenergic innervation of the proximal urethra in the female has not been confirmed.

Studies of the neuromuscular contacts in the proximal urethra of humans confirm their similarity to the urinary detrusor.

URINARY DETRUSOR MUSCLE

The urinary detrusor muscle consists of smooth muscle bundles arranged in a collagen framework (Fig. 4–26). The urinary detrusor is covered on its external or intra-abdominal surface partially by peritoneum and completely by connective tissue. Lining the interior of the viscus is submucosal connective tissue and transitional epithelium referred to as urothelium. The trigone is a separate anatomic region in the base of the bladder. Its main components are small, smooth muscle fiber bundles with an almost exclusively adrenergic innervation in a rather dense collagen tissue (Gosling and Dixon, 1975; Gosling et al., 1977; Gosling, 1979). This structure represents the distal continuation of the ureters, and elements of this nature can be

Figure 4–24. Distribution of pelvic detrusor motor nerves in the smooth muscle bundles of the urinary detrusor.

Smooth Muscle Cells

Axon Varicosities

Axon Bundles

Neuro-muscular Junctions

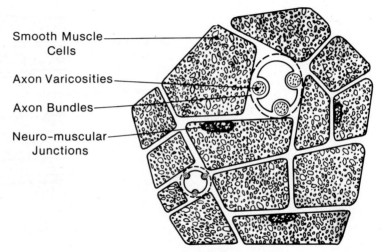

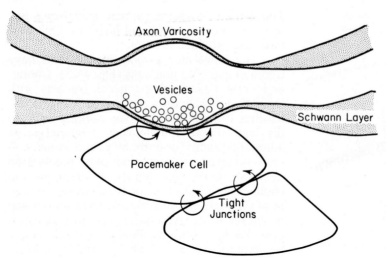

Figure 4–25. Close-contacting axon varicosity of pelvic detrusor motor nerve and a smooth muscle cell in the urinary detrusor.

traced as far down as the verumontanum of the male. It is situated internal to the so-called deep trigone, which is detrusor muscle, stretched out to envelop the distal 3 to 4 cm of the ureters as Waldeyer's sheath. Functionally, the trigone is related to the ureter, providing traction on the intravesical portion during voiding and at high bladder filling, thereby helping to prevent vesicoureteral reflux of urine. Whether it plays a part in voiding is unknown. The autonomic innervation and sensory axons are distributed in a linear longitudinal manner from rostral to caudal after appearing at the level of insertion of the ureter. Autonomic or pelvic ganglia are found in the connective tissue in close proximity to the insertion of the ureter but not in great number in the interstices of the detrusor muscle.

The architecture of the individual smooth muscle bundles in the urinary detrusor comprises randomly distributed interdigitating fibers in the bladder dome. As the bladder base is approached, these muscle bundles form arcades (Fig. 4–27). The trigonal loop or arcade intersects the detrusor loop or arcade facing in an opposite direction. When detrusor reflex excitation proceeds through the detrusor muscle at a finite coordinated conduction velocity, there is contraction of the smooth muscle arcades, producing separation at the bladder neck with consequent expulsion of intravesical content into the proximal urethra.

The individual smooth muscle cells and the smooth muscle bundles are enclosed in collagen. Within smooth muscle bundles, there is frequent fusion of the outer membranes of individual cells by a gap junction. The collagen layers are

Figure 4–26. Collagen framework of detrusor muscle.

Smooth Muscle Bundle

Smooth Muscle Interconnection

Smooth Muscle Bundle

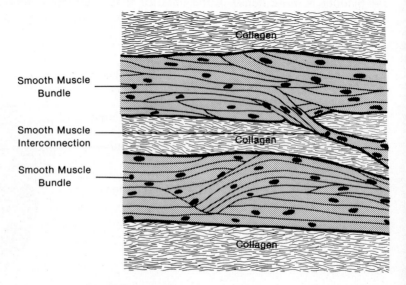

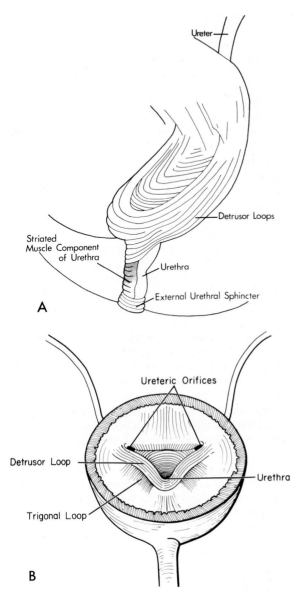

A

B

Figure 4–27. *A* and *B*, Organization of smooth muscle bundles of urinary detrusor.

Sensory Innervation of the Urinary Bladder

The sensory innervation of the urinary bladder has been investigated in the experimental animal (Fletcher and Bradley, 1970; Uemura et al., 1973, 1974, 1975) and in the human (Gosling and Dixon, 1975). Sensory nerve endings in the urinary detrusor are free and unspecialized and are distributed in the mucosa, submocosa, and interstices of the collagen compartment of the urinary detrusor (Fig. 4–28). These afferents are distributed to the hypogastric and pelvic nerves, where they conduct impulses to the spinal cord. Proprioceptive impulses are conducted to the dorsolateral tegmental nucleus of the pons and exteroceptive impulses to the thalamus.

Innervation of the Prostate Gland
(Vaalasti and Hervonew, 1980)

The human prostate is innervated by nerves staining with formaldehyde fluorescence for adrenergic nerves as well as for acetylcholinesterase. The former axons are sparse in the prostatic capsule and dense in the smooth muscle of the ducts and acini of the prostate. The acetylcholinesterase endings are more prevalent in the prostatic capsule than the adrenergic nerves but are similar in density to the adrenergic nerves in the smooth muscle of the prostatic ducts. There are many ganglia in the prostatic capsule. No direct innervation of the prostatic epithelium was observed. Whether the prostate gland is incorporated in the reflex activity of the detrusor muscle and urethra is undetermined at the present time. It is believed that the smooth muscle fibers serve to empty the gland during ejaculation.

The Urethra

The urethra can be divided into preprostatic urethra, prostatic urethra, membranous urethra, and penile urethra (Gosling and Dixon, 1975; Cullen et al., 1981).

The membranous portion of the urethra is that region which contains the principal investment of periurethral striated muscle (Andersen and Bradley, 1976; Gosling et al., 1981). The membranous portion extends from the prostate gland to the bulb of the penis (Fig. 4–29). It is indistensible and measures approximately 1 cm in length. The musculature of the pelvic floor

considerable in extent. Biochemical methods of assay utilizing hydroxyproline as an indicator of collagen content have estimated that up to 25% of the urinary bladder is composed of collagen (Swaiman and Bradley, 1967).

Since coordinated contraction of the urinary detrusor muscle has been described in the cat during detrusor reflex contraction, the possibility of an anatomic conduction system can be raised. This would consist of a structural network analogous to that in the myocardium. No such conduction system has been reported to date, suggesting that the coordination is centrally mediated.

related to the membranous urethra consists of the medial portion of the levator ani muscle. This muscle, in close proximity to the urethra, is anatomically distinct from the urethral wall. The wall of the membranous urethra consists of a thin layer of smooth muscle continuous with the prostatic urethra and a well-developed outer layer of striated muscle (Andersen and Bradley, 1976). This muscle also extends along the surface of the proximal urethra by an anterior reflection (Manley, 1966) and is anatomically distinct from the pubococcygeus portion of the levator ani. The periurethral striated muscle of the female is situated along the distal one third of the urethra and is rudimentary in form.

The muscle fibers of the periurethral striated muscle in humans have been classified from histochemical evidence as slow-twitch in type, while the adjoining pelvic floor musculature consists of fast- and slow-twitch fibers (Gosling et al., 1981). Electrophysiologic animal experiments have confirmed the presence of fast-twitch fibers. The histologic appearance is that of typical striated muscle with myofilaments with alternating dark (A) bands and light (I) bands. There is a high content of mitochondria, consistent with slow-twitch muscle.

Motor end-plates (Fig. 4–30) occur at the surface of each striated muscle cell. These have the typical appearance of a neuromuscular junction, as found in other skeletal muscle (Martin et al., 1974). However, physiologic studies have shown that these junctions are adherent to the periurethral striated muscle cells and resistant to the effects of neuromuscular blocking agents.

SENSORY INNERVATION OF THE SMOOTH MUSCLE OF THE URETHRA (Fig. 4–31)

The sensory innervation of the smooth muscle and urethelium of the urethra is similar to that of the urinary detrusor. Afferents traverse both the hypogastric and the pelvic nerves to the lumbar and sacral spinal cord. There are relatively sparse numbers of muscle spindles in the periurethral striated muscle, with an increased density in the nearly periurethral striated muscle. These spindles provide for initiation of sensory impulses from the periurethral striated muscle and closely approximated pubococcygeus (Fig. 4–32).

The sacral innervation of the periurethral striated muscle is from the S2 portion of the pudendal nucleus extending from S1 to S3 in humans (Takahashi, 1980) and the midportion of the pudendal nucleus in humans. The nucleus extends from the sixth lumbar to the first sacral segment in cats and primates (Rockswold et al., 1980a and b).

In the adult female the urethra is approximately 3 to 4 cm in length, extending from the bladder neck to the external urethral meatus. The urethra passes through the pelvic floor musculature and the anterior vaginal wall and enters the perineum. The pelvic floor musculature, specifically the pubococcygeus, lies in close proximity and consists histochemically of fast- and slow-twitch fibers.

A pair of fibromuscular ligaments anchors the anterior aspect of the female urethra to the posterior surface of the pubic symphysis (Zacharin, 1963).

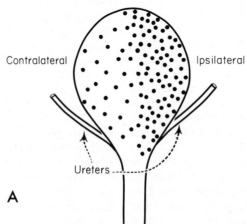

Figure 4–28. Sensory innervation of detrusor muscle. *A*, Distribution of sensory afferents. *B*, Morphology of sensory endings showing axonal coiling.

Illustration continued on opposite page

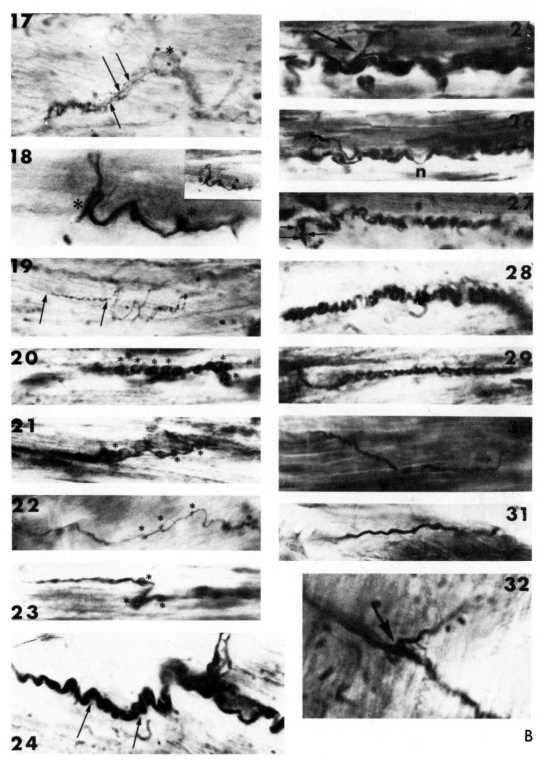

Figure 4–28 *Continued.*

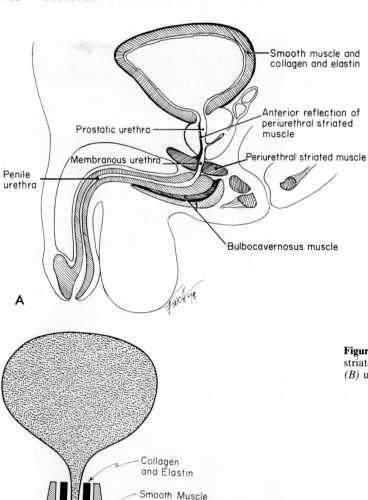

A

B

Figure 4–29. Organization of periurethral striated muscle of male *(A)* and female *(B)* urethra.

Figure 4–30. Neuromuscular junction in periurethral striated muscle.

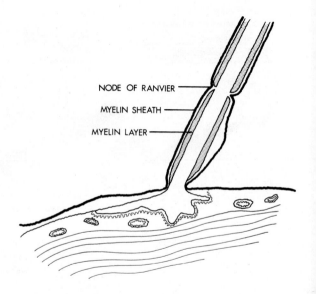

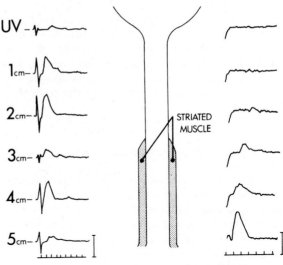

Figure 4–31. Longitudinal sensory innervation of urethra. Column on left shows responses evoked in the pelvic nerve. Column on right shows responses evoked in the pudendal nerve.

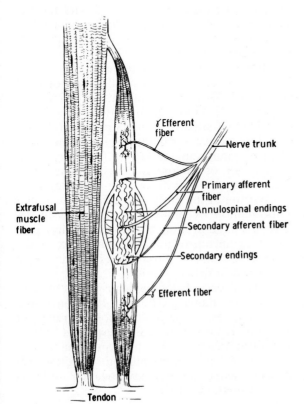

Figure 4–32. Sensory innervation of a muscle spindle (see text).

The periurethral striated muscle of the female is thinner than that of the male and consists histochemically of slow-twitch muscle fibers. There are neuromuscular junctions in the striated muscle fibers analogous to those in the male. The sacral innervation is from the second sacral segment, the midportion of the pudendal nucleus.

Summary

Knowledge of the anatomy of the urinary bladder and its connections is proceeding at an increased rate. Most of the new information is in the experimental animal, but the careful work of Takahashi in human anatomic dissections reveals what can be done. Much information may also be anticipated from clinical studies in which the results of urodynamics are combined with nuclear magnetic resonance studies of the brain and spinal cord.

NEUROPHYSIOLOGY OF THE URINARY BLADDER

INTRODUCTION

The physiology of the urinary bladder is incompletely understood. The twin functions of urine storage and expulsion are governed in part by a complex arrangement of reflex interactions. This interplay provides for coordination between the smooth and striated muscle components, resulting in voiding with low intraurethral resistance as well as voluntary control of bladder function. Most of our knowledge of urinary bladder function is based on investigation of reflex function in animals. Whether studies in the quadriped animal are freely translatable to the biped human awaits further documentation.

The physiology of the urinary bladder can be classified into the neurophysiology of reflex mechanisms and the physiology of the urinary detrusor and periurethral striated muscle.

The neurophysiology of reflex mechanisms of voiding can be further divided into the central nervous system pathways and the peripheral innervation of the urinary bladder. The specific nuclei and pathways in the central nervous system are those that clinical and experimental animal studies have demonstrated as significant in urinary bladder control. Peripheral mechanisms include the physiology of the pelvic ganglia, neuromuscular innervation of the urinary detrusor and periurethral striated muscle, and the sensory innervation of the lower urinary tract.

Classic neurophysiology consists of utilization of the two basic techniques of observing the effect of electrical stimulation and ablating the neural areas whose function is under investigation. Electrical stimulation of a portion of the nervous system may evoke peripheral effects, including contraction of the urinary bladder. However, this does not necessarily prove a direct relationship of the area stimulated to bladder control unless supplemented by studying the results of ablation. The ablation may be either surgical or pharmacologic. If ablation of a specific area produces an effect reciprocal to electrical stimulation, a physiologic relationship may be assumed. These studies can be supplemented by evoked potential investigations and by microelectrode recording techniques.

THE CEREBRAL CORTEX

Electrical stimulation of specific areas of the cerebral cortex in the animal initiates or inhibits urinary detrusor contraction (Gjone and Setekleiv, 1963). There has been no further investigation of the nature of these effects. The areas specifically studied included cerebrocortical areas associated with the limbic system as well as sensorimotor function.

Ablation of specific areas of the cerebral cortex in the experimental animal and the human results in cystometric changes, including the appearance of detrusor hyperreflexia (Langworthy et al., 1940).

Electrical stimulation of the cerebral cortex and its effect upon urinary bladder function have not been investigated in humans (Penfield and Jasper, 1954). However, the effects of ablation have been studied in patients in whom neurologic lesions of the frontal lobes have occurred (Andrew and Nathan, 1964). These revealed, as a result of cystometric observations, that destruction of a specific area of the anteroinferior portion of the prefrontal area by a vascular malformation or brain tumor (previously described in the section on neuroanatomy) produced an uncontrollable detrusor reflex or detrusor hyperreflexia. No sphincteric studies were performed in these patients.

Electroencephalographic responses to bladder filling in humans (Bradley, 1977) have suggested the role of the cerebral cortex in bladder function. However, no EEG responses specific to a given area of the cerebral cortex have been observed. The documentation of these responses awaits further investigation utilizing modern methods of EEG.

The effects of stimulation and ablation of that portion of the cerebral cortex designated as being concerned with innervation of the periurethral striated musculature have not been evaluated in the experimental animal, nor have similar studies been documented in humans.

THE THALAMUS

The thalamus is a collection of subcortical nuclei concerned with the relay of sensory impulses from peripheral receptors to the cerebral cortex. These nuclei have been demonstrated in animal and human studies to be intimately concerned with the physiology of the cerebral cortex. They can be assumed to relay ascending impulses from the urinary bladder to the cerebral cortex. However, their role in integration of these impulses is unknown, either from animal or from human studies.

THE BASAL GANGLIA

The basal ganglia have been demonstrated in both the animal and the human to influence the function of the urinary detrusor (Murnaghan, 1961; Lewin and Porter, 1965; Lewin et al., 1967; Porter, 1967). Electrical stimulation of the putamen and the globus pallidus in the cat has demonstrated suppression of detrusor reflex activity. Other studies demonstrated that basal ganglia influences were mediated through the dorsolateral tegmental nucleus of the pons, the brain stem center for detrusor reflex contractions (Porter et al., 1971).

No animal experiments have been reported in association with ablation of portions of the basal ganglia. However, patients with Parkinson's disease, which is associated with a deficiency of the neurotransmitter dopamine in the basal ganglia, have been observed to have a significant incidence of detrusor hyperreflexia or loss of voluntary control of detrusor reflex contractions (Andersen and Bradley, 1976). No documentation of the effects of the basal ganglia on the function of the periurethral striated muscle has been reported in the experimental animal. Studies in Parkinson patients have demonstrated abnormal sphincter responses (Pavlakis et al., 1983).

THE LIMBIC SYSTEM

The role of the limbic system is that of control of emotional response by integration of autonomic and somatic influences. Electrical stimulation of portions of the limbic system has revealed suppression and facilitation of urinary detrusor function (Edvardsen and Ursin, 1968). However, abnormalities of bladder function

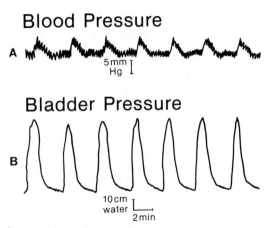

Figure 4–33. Effect of cerebellar ablation in the experimental animal, demonstrating continuous episodes of detrusor hyperreflexia.

have not been reported in patients with unilateral or bilateral temporal lobectomy (Falconer, 1974) or in patients with temporal lobe epilepsy. Further work remains on this interesting aspect of urinary bladder function. Similarly, the role of the hypothalamus in control of the urinary bladder awaits further investigation.

THE CEREBELLUM

The cerebellum regulates muscle tone and coordinates movement. Precisely how this is accomplished to secure coordinated contraction of the detrusor muscle with reciprocal relaxation of the periurethral striated muscle during voiding is unknown. The experiments that have been concluded indicate that in the cat, stimulation of the anterior vermis of the cerebellum (Bradley and Teague, 1969a and b; Martner, 1975; Bradley and Scott, 1978; Huang et al., 1979) results in profound suppression of detrusor reflex contraction. On the other hand, ablation of the anterior vermis of the cerebellum results in continuous hyperreflexic detrusor contraction (Fig. 4–33). This effect of cerebellar function on the urinary bladder is believed to be due to activation of neurons in the fastigial nucleus that transmit inhibitory impulses to the neurons of the dorsolateral tegmental nucleus of the pons.

No studies have been reported in the experimental animal of the effects of cerebellar stimulation and ablation on the function of the periurethral striated muscle. Similarly, no reports of the effects of cerebellar stimulation on urinary bladder function in humans are available. Cerebellar lesions in humans, with consequent detrusor hyperreflexia, have been reported (Leach et al., 1982).

THE BRAIN STEM

A specialized portion of the brain stem has been defined anatomically in the experimental animal as the nucleus in which detrusor reflex contraction is organized (Barrington, 1941; Tang, 1955; Tang and Ruch, 1955; Loewy et al., 1978; Satoh, 1978a and b). This nucleus has been designated as the caudal portion of the dorsolateral tegmental nucleus of the pons and is distinct from the nucleus locus ceruleus (Leger and Hernandez-Nicaise, 1980). Whether the same designation applies to humans awaits further study. However, the importance of this tegmentum-located nucleus was first demonstrated in 1921 by Barrington, who pointed out that when the area was ablated, the cat experienced permanent urinary retention. Later, evoked response testing by stimulation of pelvic detrusor nerve afferents and recording of responses in the pelvic detrusor motor nerves confirmed that these responses were of long latency and long duration (Bradley and Teague, 1968; DeGroat and Ryall, 1969). They were also abolished by spinal cord transection. It was concluded from these studies that the responses were "long routed" from sacral cord entry zones to the brain stem. Other studies demonstrated that there was no alteration in tone or response of the smooth muscle of the bladder wall to applied stretch after spinal cord transection (Tang and Ruch, 1955).

Long routing of bladder impulses to the multisynaptic networks of the brain stem reticular formation provided for reflex amplification (Figs. 4–34 and 4–35) and prolongation of the time course of the detrusor reflex.

A short latency response evoked in pelvic motor nerves by pelvic sensory nerve stimulation in chronic spinal animals has been interpreted as a reflex pathway "uncovered" by release of spinal cord pathways from rostral influences (DeGroat et al., 1982). It was emphasized in these studies, however, that the long routed evoked response was an event crucial for detrusor reflex contraction. The presence of the short latency pathway has been affirmed in morphologic studies in the experimental animal (Nolan and Brown, 1981). Two other nuclei in the brain stem may be implicated in voiding. One nucleus in the medulla, the nucleus gigantocellularis, has been shown to generate excitatory and inhibitory synaptic potentials in pudendal motoneurons (Mackel, 1979). The second nucleus, the vestibular nucleus, has not yet been investigated in terms of innervation of the periurethral striated muscle but will be in future studies.

THORACOLUMBAR SPINAL CORD

The neurons of the intermediolateral cell column of the thoracolumbar spinal cord receive sensory impulses from two sources: (1) bladder afferent impulses routing over sacral afferent pathways and a spinal cord pathway; (2) bladder afferent impulses traveling in afferent axons in the hypogastric nerve.

The precise role of these afferents is undefined, but two possibilities have been suggested: (1) That these afferent impulses to thoracolumbar neurons generate motor impulses in the hypogastric nerve. These impulses relay to the pelvic ganglia, where they inhibit pelvic nerve transmission through the ganglia. (2) That hypogastric nerve afferent impulses travel to the thoracolumbar spinal cord. Neurons in the intermediolateral cell column initiate impulses that produce either contraction of the smooth muscle of the proximal urethra by stimulation of alpha-adrenoreceptors or relaxation by stimulation of beta-adrenoreceptors.

THE CONUS MEDULLARIS

The physiologic responses of the neurons of the gray matter of the conus medullaris are a function of the output of the neurons of the detrusor nuclei and the output of the neurons of the pudendal nuclei.

The detrusor nuclei in the conus medullaris are located in a matrix of neurons concerned with micturition, defecation, and sexual function (DeGroat and Ryall, 1969). Specific detrusor neurons have been investigated in the cat, where they are located in the midportion of the lon-

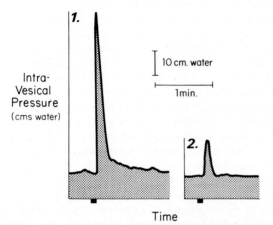

Intra-
Vesical
Pressure
(cms water)

10 cm. water

1min.

Time

Figure 4–34. Following spinal cord transection in the experimental animal, there is marked reduction in the detrusor contractile response evoked by sacral dorsal root stimulation. *1,* Intact animal. *2,* After spinal cord transection.

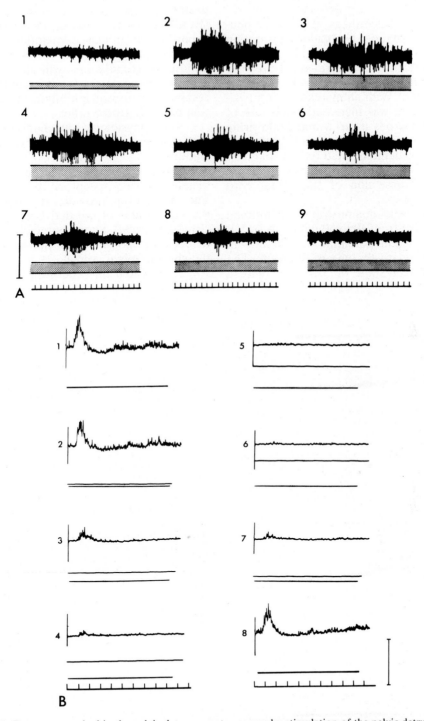

Figure 4–35. *A,* Responses evoked in the pelvic detrusor motor nerves by stimulation of the pelvic detrusor afferents. The amplitude of the response can be observed to be accentuated by increases in intravesical pressure illustrated by separation of two horizontal lines. *B,* Effect of increase in intravesical pressure on amplitude of responses evoked in pudendal nerves. With increase in intravesical pressure, illustrated by separation of two horizontal lines, there is diminution in amplitude of the pudendal evoked responses.

gitudinal cell column constituting the autonomic nucleus. The detrusor nuclei neurons have been investigated by intra- and extracellular micro-electrode studies. Recordings of detrusor neurons showed excitation by bladder distention and inhibition by colonic distention. The neurons were quiescent when intravesical pressure was below that which would evoke detrusor reflex contraction. With an increase in intravesical pressure there was increased firing rate of detrusor motoneurons up to a maximum firing frequency of 60 impulses per second. In the cat, the response was demonstrated to be evoked by A delta afferents routed by a pathway to the rostral pons. Transection of the spinal cord blocked the response.

Individual cells demonstrated membrane potentials ranging from 40 to 60 millivolts (mV). The neuronal action potential was 90 mV in amplitude and relatively long in duration. The duration was an average of 5.7 msec, with a subsequent 80 msec period of hyperpolarization. Detrusor neurons have been verified as demonstrating recurrent or Renshaw inhibition (Bradley, 1969b; DeGroat, 1976). Hence, in the experimental animal, stimulation of the pelvic nerves in the direction of the detrusor nuclei—antidromic stimulation—will alternate or abort a spontaneous detrusor reflex contraction. The results of recurrent inhibition include termination of the detrusor reflex.

The physiologic mechanisms associated with afferent input to the detrusor nuclei include:

1. Long routing of afferent impulses from bladder tension receptors to the brain stem. This mechanism provides for amplification of the time course of the detrusor reflex response (Bradley, 1969a). Short routed afferent impulses to detrusor motoneurons can be seen only in the chronic spinal animal.

2. Pudendal and other somatic (McPherson,

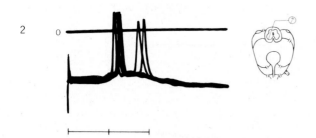

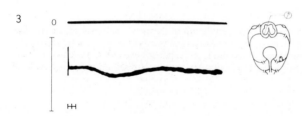

Figure 4–36. Responses evoked in pudendal motoneurons by stimulation of pudendal afferents in traces 1 and 2. In trace 3, pelvic detrusor afferent nerve stimulation resulted in low-amplitude inhibitory postsynaptic potential generation.

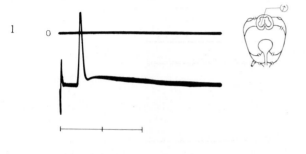

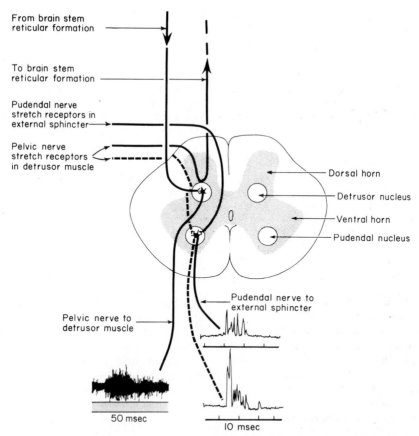

From brain stem reticular formation

To brain stem reticular formation

Pudendal nerve stretch receptors in external sphincter

Pelvic nerve stretch receptors in detrusor muscle

- Dorsal horn
- Detrusor nucleus
- Ventral horn
- Pudendal nucleus

Pudendal nerve to external sphincter

Pelvic nerve to detrusor muscle

50 msec

10 msec

Figure 4–37. The difference in amplitude, duration, and configuration between responses evoked by stimulation of pelvic detrusor afferents and pudendal afferents.

1966; Soto et al., 1980) impulses are also conducted to detrusor motoneurons. These provide for excitation and/or inhibition of detrusor motoneurons (Bradley and Teague, 1972).

3. Gating of input. Recent demonstration of the requirement of bladder distention to facilitate the appearance of the spinobulbo-evoked response affirmed earlier studies (Floyd et al., 1982; McMahon and Morrison, 1982a, b, c). This effect was attributed to activation of interneurons in the sacral spinal cord; this activation or inactivation of interneurons controls the excitation of the long routed axons to the brain stem (Fig. 4–35).

The pudendal nuclei located in the lateral portion of the ventral gray matter of the sacral spinal cord have been studied with intra- and extracellular microelectrodes in the cat. Responses evoked in pudendal motor axons by stimulation of pudendal afferents are associated with excitatory postsynaptic potentials in pudendal motoneurons (Fig. 4–36) (Bradley and Teague, 1972, 1977). On the other hand, stimulation of pelvic detrusor afferents in the cat

produces exclusive inhibitory postsynaptic action potentials in pudendal motoneurons. Hence, the effect of bladder distention is to inhibit pudendal motoneuron activity at the segmental level.

Stimulation of pudendal urethral sensory nerves and recording from pudendal urethral motor nerves demonstrated a bimodal response with short and long latency components. This differs from stimulation of pelvic detrusor afferents (Fig. 4–37). Inferred from this observation is the conclusion that pudendal afferents reorganize with segmental and supraspinal routing of afferent impulses. This is analogous to other skeletal muscle afferents. Stimulation of the supraspinal innervation of pudendal motoneurons in the cat evoked excitatory and inhibitory postsynaptic potentials in sacral pudendal motoneurons. The motoneuron action potential in the pudendal nerve is an integral part of supraspinal and segmental inputs (Fig. 4–38).

Two further characteristics of pudendal motoneurons are: (1) Primary afferent depolarization, producing presynaptic inhibition of sensory

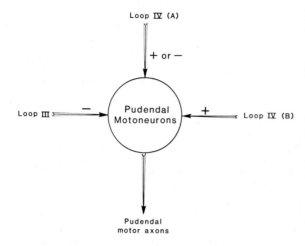

Figure 4–38. Integration of supraspinal and segmental influences on pudendal motoneurons.

input (Wojcik et al., 1983); and (2) correlation between motoneuron size and muscle fiber types in the periurethral striated muscle (Henneman, 1957, 1981; Henneman and Olson, 1965; Henneman et al., 1965). The morphologic studies of the pudendal nucleus up to the present have not included measurement of neuronal size. However, studies of motoneuronal innervation of other skeletal muscles suggest that with the stretching of muscle and the stimulation of sensory receptors there is recruitment first of the smallest pudendal motoneurons and that with increased intensity of stretch, successively larger pudendal motoneurons are recruited. Tonic or smaller motoneurons innervate smaller motor units in which the individual striated muscle cells have slow contraction speed, low maximal tension, and high resistance to fatigue. The larger motor units have fast-twitch response, high maximal tension, and low resistance to fatigue.

It is of significance that in the cat approximately 15 per cent of the composition of the sacral ventral root consists of sensory axons (Applebaum et al., 1976; Ryall and Piercy, 1970). How this affects bladder function and whether these data are applicable to humans are unknown.

PELVIC GANGLIONIC TRANSMISSION

Much of our knowledge of the physiology of the pelvic ganglia is derived from animal experimentation (Martin, 1977). There are many questions to be answered in regard to organization between ganglia. However, at present, neurophysiologic studies are addressed to organization of a single ganglion (DeGroat

and Saum, 1976; Purington et al., 1976; Booth and DeGroat, 1979; DeGroat and Booth, 1980; Griffith et al., 1980, 1981; Gallagher et al., 1982).

Input and output studies performed by stimulation of preganglionic axons and record-

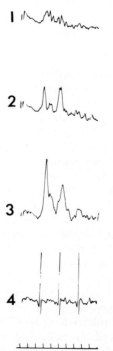

Figure 4–39. Postganglionic potentials showing progressive recruitment with increase in amplitude on repetitive preganglionic stimulation (traces 1 to 3). In trace 4, with high-frequency preganglionic stimulation there is failure of postganglionic excitation. Time marker, 1 msec.

ing from postganglionic axons in the pelvic ganglia of the cat as well as intracellular recording demonstrate a variety of effects. Excitatory transmission resulting from activation of nicotinic acetylcholine receptors suggests that the pelvic ganglion acts as a high-pass filter with maximum facilitation at a preganglionic stimulus frequency of 20 to 30 Hz (Fig. 4–39). Facilitation persists for several minutes after a train of preganglionic stimuli. Stimulation of the hypogastric nerve acts to depress pelvic ganglionic transmission, and it has been assumed that the hypogastric nerve functions as an inhibitory vesicosympathetic pathway. In the experimental animal, activation of vesical afferents in the pelvic nerve by bladder distention or electrical stimulation evoked increased unit activity in the hypogastric nerves. This results in inhibition of the detrusor muscle and inhibition of pelvic ganglionic transmission.

This inhibition was not associated with hyperpolarization of ganglion cells but was due to presynaptic depression of transmitter release. The effect is by way of excitation of alpha-receptors and may include small intensely fluorescent (SIF) cells. In a further study of neuronal activity in the pelvic ganglion, four types of cells were observed. Three types of cells had the characteristics of neurons and the fourth that of a glial or supporting cell. Neuron types 1A and 1B did not accommodate in response to direct intracellular excitation. Type 1B neuron showed spontaneous activity, which was concluded to be due to coupling with intraganglionic passage of sensory axons. All neuron types showed synaptic blockage with administration of anticholinergic agents.

NEUROMUSCULAR TRANSMISSION IN THE URINARY DETRUSOR MUSCLE
(Bennett, 1972)

Understanding of the physiology of the urinary bladder has been considerably enhanced by intracellular muscle studies of neurotransmission in the mammalian urinary bladder (Ursillo, 1961; Creed, 1971). Insertion of a microelectrode into muscle cells in different areas of the bladder, including the trigone, showed similar values of the resting membrane potential, 37.4 mV. All cells demonstrated spontaneous firing. However, there were considerable differences in the shape of the spike (Fig. 4–40). Female rabbits had differently-shaped action potentials than male rabbits. In the male, a single spike or action potential was followed by a period of hyperpolarization. In the female, smooth muscle cells demonstrated multiple action potentials superimposed on a negative de-

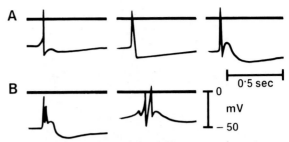

Figure 4–40. Tracings from intracellular recordings of spontaneous action potentials in detrusor muscle cells (Creed, K. E., et al., 1983). Different responses are obtained from different recording sites in the detrusor muscle.

polarization potential. Application of stimulating electrical pulses to the axonal innervation produced two episodes of depolarization. The early excitatory junction potential was unaffected by blocking agents, including atropine and guanethidine. The late potential was enhanced by administration of neostigmine and blocked by atropine. This profile of results suggests that two neurotransmitters are released at neuromuscular endings in the detrusor muscle. The first transmitter is noncholinergic and nonadrenergic in its properties, and the second is acetylcholine. These results account for the classic atropine resistance of the urinary detrusor. No inhibitory responses have been observed in the urinary detrusor muscle in response to stimulation of the motor innervation.

The mechanism of coordination of detrusor muscle contraction to produce a smooth rise in intravesical pressure (Conway and Bradley, 1969) is unknown. Stretch-induced depolarization may contribute to this response (Fig. 4–41) (Uvelus and Gabella, 1980).

PHYSIOLOGY OF THE SMOOTH MUSCLE OF THE PROXIMAL URETHRA

There are no animal or human studies of the electrophysiology of the proximal urethra. This may seem strange in view of the intense pharmacologic interest in this region as well as clinical studies of voiding dysfunction. The principal observations have been from urodynamic evaluation, roentgenographic studies of voiding, and urethral pressure profile data. These studies indicated the importance of sympathetic impulses in producing urethral dilation during detrusor contraction (McGuire and Herlihy, 1978; Woodside and McGuire, 1979; Kaneko et al., 1980; McGreer and McGreer, 1981).

PHYSIOLOGY OF THE PERIURETHRAL STRIATED MUSCLE

The periurethral striated muscle in the experimental animal contains three histochemical

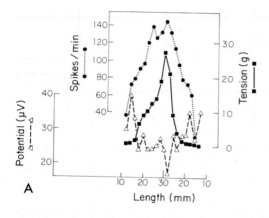

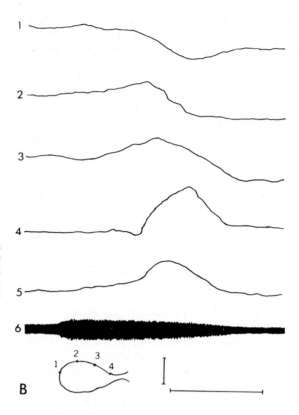

A

Figure 4–41. *A,* Effect of stretch on membrane polarization in detrusor muscle. *B,* Motility record in detrusor muscle during spontaneous detrusor reflex. Tracings 1 to 4 reflect motility changes in different areas of the detrusor muscle during pelvic motor nerve discharge (trace 5, intravesical pressure; trace 6, pelvic motor nerve discharge).

B

profiles that have been correlated with contraction force and speed as well as with resistance to fatigue (Burke et al., 1974; Critchley et al., 1980; Bazeed et al., 1982). The first group—Type II—had a pale appearance, high glycogen content, fast contraction speed, and fatigability increasing in amount in the direction of the external urinary meatus. This group constituted 35 per cent of the musculature of the periurethral striated muscle. A second group—Type I—had a small motor unit size and slow contraction speed. Type I was further divided into a fatigue-resistant and a fatigable group. The authors postulated that Type I fibers were concerned with continence at rest and Type II with phasic or rapid responses to potential urinary leakage. In humans, it was suggested from similar studies of the staining and biochemical profile of the

muscle cells that the periurethral striated muscle consisted principally of slow-twitch fibers.

Neuromuscular transmission in the periurethral striated muscle has been studied only in the cat (Fig. 4–42). Experiments consisting of intracellular recording from single muscle cells during repetitive stimulation of the pudendal motor nerves showed the process of neuromuscular transmission to be only partly cholinergic and to be resistant to total blockade by neuromuscular blocking agents (Bowen et al., 1976). This resistance has been assumed to be due to the intimate adherence of the neuromuscular junction to the striated muscle fibers. In normal animals and humans, the periurethral striated muscle and striated portion of the rectal sphincter act in concert (Bradley et al., 1974) (Fig. 4–43).

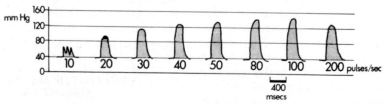

Figure 4–42. Effect of different frequencies of pudendal motor nerve stimulation on amplitude and duration of contraction of the periurethral striated muscle.

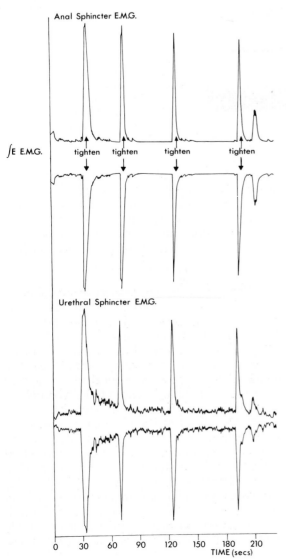

Figure 4–43. Effect of volitional tightening on sphincteric activity in the periurethral striated muscle and striated muscle of the anal sphincter in humans.

PHYSIOLOGY OF MUSCLE SPINDLES

The muscle spindles in the levator ani and periurethral striated muscle are assumed to function in a manner analogous to those in other skeletal muscle fibers. The morphology of a muscle spindle comprises two muscle groups at either end of a spindle. These muscles contract in response to action potentials in their gamma axonal innervation. When this occurs, tension is generated on the sensory endings in the equatorial region of the spindle, changing its sensitivity. With sudden applied stretch to the spindle from the surrounding skeletal muscle, impulses are generated that pass in the sensory axons to the spinal cord. The intensity of the action potential response to applied stretch is based in part upon the spindle bias produced by the axons of the gamma innervation. Further investigation of the specific muscle spindle response in the periurethral striated muscle is required. Increased activity in the gamma efferents to bladder distention has been described (Abdullah and Eldred, 1959) (Figs. 4–44 and 4–45).

SUMMARY

The physiology of the urinary bladder has undergone extensive diversification of studies and methodology since the last edition of *Campbell's Urology*. However, the studies are predominantly in the experimental animal, with few investigations being conducted in normal humans. These do indicate an order of complexity of reflex function, which may account for the difficulty in defining many clinical problems.

LOOP OR REFLEX CONCEPTUALIZATION OF URINARY BLADDER INNERVATION

INTRODUCTION

Neurologic diagnosis usually proceeds through a number of steps:

1. The first is referred to as the syndrome diagnosis, in which a careful search is made for a constellation of symptoms and signs in the history and neurologic examination suggestive of focal disease.

2. From this sifting, one proceeds to an anatomic diagnosis. This process is dependent

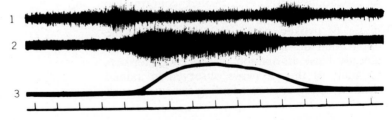

Figure 4–44. Recording on spontaneous hypogastric nerve (line 1), pelvic motor nerve (line 2), discharges and intravesical pressure (line 3) during detrusor reflex contraction.

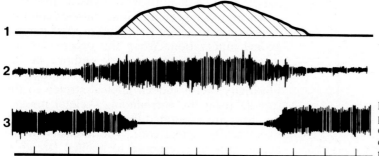

Figure 4–45. Recording of intravesical pressure (line 1), pelvic motor nerve discharge (line 2), and pudendal motor nerve discharge (line 3) during spontaneous detrusor reflex contraction.

upon knowledge of neuroanatomy and particularly of those pathways concerned with innervation of the urinary bladder. The innervation is arranged in reflex pathways, the results of whose interruption are predictable. The technique of evoked potentials defines the integrity of anatomic pathways and further refines anatomic diagnosis.

3. From a careful anatomic diagnosis and in conjunction with laboratory studies and neuroradiologic procedures, one can proceed next to a pathologic diagnosis and subsequently to an etiologic diagnosis.

When studies of bladder function in patients with overt neurologic disease are performed, they rarely stand alone but are usually subordinate to the neurologic diagnosis. When supplemented by evoked potential studies of bladder innervation, the urinary bladder dysfunction can be incorporated into the other aspects of the anatomic neurologic deficit.

From the earliest studies of bladder innervation and in concurrence with classic neurologic concepts of reflex action (Mardsen et al., 1976), there has been an accumulating body of knowledge of the reflex pathways concerned with voiding. In the experimental animal, there has been ample evidence that detrusor reflex contraction is dependent upon peripheral bladder input to the brain stem. With the use of tracer techniques there has been precise location of this nucleus. Similarly, with electrophysiologic studies of trace techniques the reflex connections of the detrusor and pudendal nuclei in the conus medullaris of the animal have been documented.

No human studies contravene these animal investigations. However, further confirmation awaits more complete utilization of the technique of evoked potential studies. With the application of the latter in humans there has already been affirmation of the characteristics of many of the pathways observed in animal studies. A key anatomic finding for evidence of

a detrusor reflex center in the brain stem awaits further investigation and confirmation (Khurona, 1982). With the demonstration of these reflex pathways in humans, assessment of neuropathic bladder involvement as well as classification of dysfunction is rendered less difficult.

LOOP I (Fig. 4–46)

This is a brain stem to cerebrocortical pathway, whose connections to subcortical nuclei include the thalamus, basal ganglia, and amygdaloid nucleus. This organization is no doubt as complex as that involved in cerebral control of voluntary motor movements (Evarts, 1973). The relationship of these subcortical nuclei as well as the lateral hemispheres of the cerebellum relaying through the superior cerebellar peduncles to the nuclei of the thalamus is unknown. In anatomic studies of the brain stem of the animal, clear direct pathways to the cerebral cortex have been shown by tracer and evoked potential studies. It can only be guessed at this time whether these are analogous to those in man. Further electrophysiologic studies, including electroencephalography, will undoubtedly contribute to this delineation. Neuropsychologic

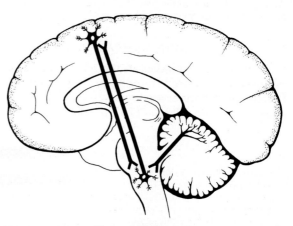

Figure 4–46. Loop I.

studies of the effect of ablation in the experimental animal on training and bladder function will also assist in this analysis. It can be postulated that cerebrocortical pathways are affected in enuresis, in incontinence in the elderly, and in other cerebral sources of detrusor hyperreflexia.

Loop I consists of to-and-fro connections from the brain stem detrusor nucleus to the medial frontal cerebral cortex. Loop I is a composite of the multiple cerebral and subcortical nuclei influencing the brain stem center for detrusor reflex control. These cerebral areas include the prefrontal cortex but may also include areas in the parietal association cortex. Whether there is cerebral asymmetry of dominance in cerebral innervation similar to that observed in language is unknown. The interrelationships of these cortical areas with the detrusor nucleus in the brain stem have similarly not been addressed. Recent studies in the rat have delineated substance P–containing pathways from the dorsolateral tegmental nucleus of the pons, excluding Barrington's nucleus, to the medial frontal cortex. The nature of these pathways for detrusor control awaits further investigation similar to that performed for other brain stem systems (Pascuzzo and Skeen, 1983).

Clearly, the nuclei of the basal ganglia have been confirmed in both animal and human studies to have an effect upon detrusor reflex control. Whether the neurons of these nuclei should be considered in series or in parallel with Loop I awaits further investigation.

LOOP II (Fig. 4–47)

Loop II consists of ascending impulses from the detrusor muscle to the brain stem detrusor nucleus and descending impulses to the sacral spinal cord. The brain stem detrusor nucleus has been clearly defined in the experimental animal by anatomic tracer studies. The importance of this nucleus was demonstrated many years ago by experimental studies in the cat (Barrington, 1931). Subsequent electrophysiologic and ablation experiments in the animal have further confirmed its importance. However, whether a similar organizational plan is present in the human biped awaits further study. Spinal cord transection results in loss of detrusor reflex control and dyssynergy between detrusor muscle contraction and relaxation of the periurethral striated muscle. The confirmation of a human brain stem detrusor nucleus would be dependent upon evoked response testing from peripheral detrusor pathways into the brain stem, a technique not feasible at present. Fur-

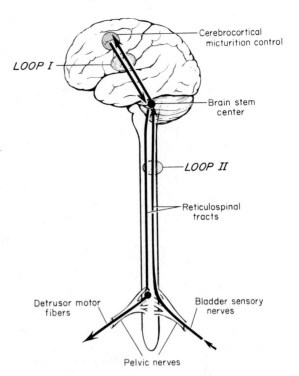

Figure 4–47. Loops I and II.

thermore, the effects of withdrawal of cerebrocortical function from the brain stem on detrusor reflex threshold have not been documented.

LOOP III (Fig. 4–48)

The afferent and efferent pathways of this reflex also have been defined in the experimental animal and are often tested in clinical evaluation of patients (Bradley et al., 1976). Whether testing of this pathway in patients can be improved to define its exclusively inhibitory role awaits further studies.

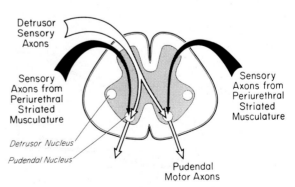

Figure 4–48. Loops III and IV B.

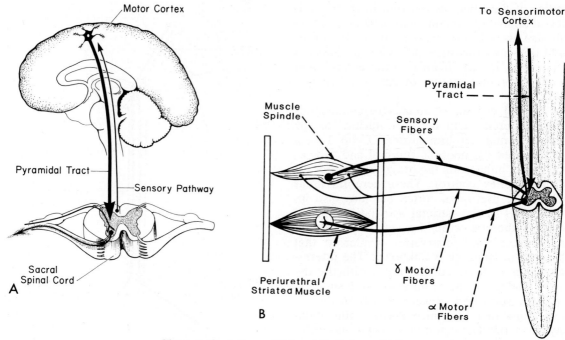

Figure 4–49. *A,* Loops IV A and B. *B,* Loop IV B.

LOOP IV (Fig. 4–49)

Loop IV consists of a supraspinal and a segmental pathway. The sum of influences from Loop III and Loop IV produces a net synaptic influence and neural output in pudendal motor axons. The exclusive inhibition in Loop III can be overridden by excitation in the supraspinal component of Loop IV. Both the segmental and the supraspinal components of Loop IV have been documented in the experimental animal and in humans. The descending portion of Loop IV has been defined by tracer studies in the primate (Nakagawa, 1980). The spinal ascending pathway has been defined by evoked potential studies in the experimental animal and in humans. The segmental portion of Loop IV has

been confirmed in the experimental animal by evoked potential studies (Oliver et al., 1970) and by tracer studies. In humans, evoked potential studies are yet to be employed to define the function of the segmental pathway.

OTHER LOOPS

Three other reflex pathways have been confirmed electrophysiologically in the experimental animal but await a demonstration by a definable methodology in humans.

These include:

1. A pathway from the proximal urethra to the detrusor muscle, providing for facilitation of detrusor reflex contraction. Abnormal excitation of this pathway has been held accountable

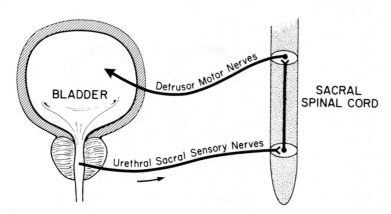

Figure 4–50. Urethra to detrusor muscle reflex pathway.

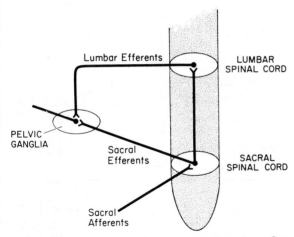

Figure 4–51. Pelvic afferent to hypogastric nerve reflex pathway.

for the detrusor hyperreflexia observed in benign prostatic hypertrophy (Fig. 4–50).

2. A pathway from the periurethral striated muscle to the urinary detrusor, producing inhibition of detrusor reflex contraction.

3. A pathway through sacral afferents to the lumbar spinal cord with excitation of lumbar efferents to the pelvic ganglia (Fig. 4–51). These pathways produce depression of synaptic transmission in the pelvic ganglia.

SUMMARY

The concept of reflex control of urinary bladder function is useful in defining anatomic diagnoses of bladder dysfunction in humans. However, before universal application of this methodology is employed further information is required.

1. More information must be acquired about cerebral control of urination and the interrelationships of subcortical nuclei. This should be facilitated by studies of cerebral control of voluntary motor movements and by research into the cognitive components of evoked potentials.

2. We need to know how to measure excitability of pudendal motoneurons. This will facilitate clinical testing of Loops III and IV.

3. We need to be able to measure downstream influences quantitatively from cerebral motor systems to the spinal cord. The use of this information in patient studies will facilitate clinical evaluation of detrusor hyperreflexia and detrusor-sphincteric dyssynergia.

NEUROUROPHARMACOLOGY

Introduction

No area of the neurosciences has been more active, exciting, and productive in the past 10 years than neuropharmacology (Hokfelt et al., 1978; Nergardh, 1980; Fried, 1981; Anderson and Marks, 1982; Bell, 1982; Gu et al., 1983; Lundberg and Hokfelt, 1983). The recent confirmation of neuropeptides as ubiquitous neurotransmitter agents and their acknowledged coexistence at presynaptic endings along with classic transmitter agents, such as acetylcholine, have dramatically altered our understanding of synaptic and neuromuscular transmission. This knowledge has been furthered by increased understanding of intracellular messengers, such as the cyclic nucleotides, inositol phospholipid, and the products of arachidonic acid.

These changes have necessarily impacted upon our comprehension of the pharmacology of the lower urinary tract. Neuropharmacology has rapidly expanded to include the identification of neuropeptides in ganglionic and neuromuscular transmission in the urinary detrusor and urethra. There are also beginning investigations of the transmitter agents in those central nervous system reflex pathways concerned with micturition.

Figure 4–52. Revised concept of synaptic transmission. Two transmitter agents are synthesized in the cell body and transported to presynaptic endings at different sites.

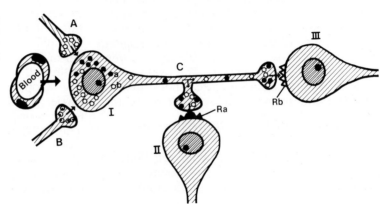

Neurotransmitter agents can be classified into amines, amino acids, and neuropeptides. ATP is in doubt as a biologic neurotransmitter agent (Dean and Downie, 1978; Choo, 1981).

Basic Aspects of Neuropharmacology

NEURONAL SYNTHESIS OF NEUROTRANSMITTER AGENTS

The cell body of the neuron is the site of synthesis of most transmitter agents. In the instance of acetylcholine the components are synthesized, and, following axoplasmic transport to the presynaptic site, there is synthesis of acetylcholine. The cell body of the neuron may synthesize amines, amino acids (McGreer and McGreer, 1981), or neuropeptides (Sotelo and Triller, 1981). Several transmitter agents may be synthesized in the same neuron (Fig. 4–52). Neurons in the central and peripheral nervous systems concerned with urinary bladder function contain acetylcholine, norepinephrine, enkephalins, substance P, and vasoactive intestinal polypeptide as well as amino acids, such as gamma-amino butyric acid and glycine.

Peptide neuronal synthesis differs from that of amines and amino acids in that recycling does not occur during postsynaptic inactivation (Snyder, 1980). Therefore, the supply of transmitter agent depends upon continuous synthesis of new transmitter agent and axonal transport to the presynaptic ending. A consequence of this arrangement is that neuropeptide replenishment at presynaptic endings is proportional to the distance of the ending from the cell body and the rate of axonal transport. The process may take hours.

On the other hand, neurons that synthesize acetylcholine produce choline acetylase and the inactivating enzyme acetylcholinesterase in the cell body for transport to the presynaptic ending. With release of the transmitter agent at the synaptic ending there is hydrolysis and reabsorption, with recycling of the transmitter agent. Similar effects occur with the release of norepinephrine and other amines. The synthesis of neurotransmitter agents in the cell body involves protein synthesis in the endoplasmic reticulum.

AXOPLASMIC TRANSPORT (Jeffrey and Austin, 1973)

The axonic connection from cell body to presynaptic ending is an active conduit, conducting proteins and enzymes synthesized in the

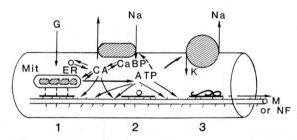

Figure 4–53. Axoplasmic transport showing conduction by bridging to neural filaments.

cell body to the synaptic ending (Fig. 4–53). There is also a return flow of materials from the synaptic endings returning to the cell body. Some of the transported material from the cell body consists of proteins and enzymes synthesized in the soma moving along neurofilaments to the synaptic ending. The enzymes transported may provide for local synthesis of transmitter agent at the synaptic ending. Neuropeptides conducted in axonal transport may be released at synaptic endings and provide for metabolic and trophic changes in cells contacted by the synaptic endings.

Hence, there are two directions of continuous axoplasmic transport: (1) anterograde from neuron cell body to presynaptic ending, and (2) retrograde from presynaptic ending to neuron soma.

Anterograde transport has been measured in the experimental animal by the injection of radioisotopes, such as C14-labeled amino acids. They are introduced by systemic injection and subsequently taken up by the cell soma. Following uptake, phospholipids, various proteins, and peptides are observed to move along the axons from the cell soma toward presynaptic endings. A fast rate of flow measured radioautographically may be up to 460 mm per day. Retrograde transport of material from presynaptic endings to cell body also occurs. Retrograde transport of acetylcholinesterase has been measured at rates of up to 200 mm per day. Retrograde transport of material is believed to be a mechanism for feedback control of protein synthesis in the cell soma.

Axoplasmic transport occurs by way of a carrier called a transport filament. The proteins to be transported are bound to transport filaments that are moved by making and breaking cross bridges using adenosine triphosphate (ATP) as an energy source. Microtubules and neurofilaments present in the axon are the basis for this mechanism.

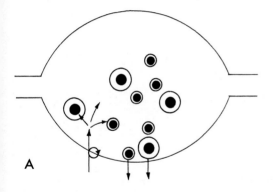

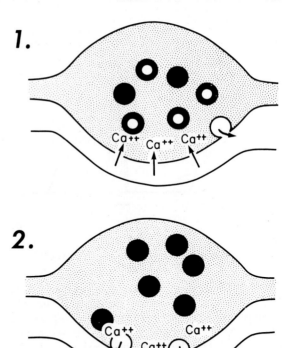

Figure 4–54. *A* and *B*, Exocytosis (see text).

EXOCYTOSIS OR NEUROTRANSMITTER RELEASE AT PRESYNAPTIC ENDING (Fig. 4–54).

Transmitter agents, including amines and peptides, are stored in synaptic vesicles in the presynaptic ending. Release of the stored transmitter agent is triggered by an action potential invading the presynaptic ending. This event is associated with calcium current flow and ingress of calcium ions. With calcium current flow there is migration of the synaptic vesicle to the cellular boundary. Fusion occurs here, with the synaptic vesicle adhering to the cellular boundary. With the occurrence of fusion there is release of transmitter agent into the intersynaptic cleft and diffusion to contact with receptors on the postsynaptic membrane. Acetylcholine and norepinephrine have been the most frequently documented transmitter agents in the peripheral innervation of the lower urinary tract. The effects of these agents, their agonists, and their antagonists are the substance of literally hundreds of publications on the subject. The other amines, dopamine and serotonin, have been implicated in central nervous system pathways concerned with voiding.

Amino acids implicated in synaptic transmission, usually in central nervous system pathways, include: (1) gamma-amino butyric acid, (2) glycine, (3) glutamate; (4) aspartate, and (5) taurine. These agents have not been demonstrated in peripheral innervation of the urinary bladder. They have most frequently been explored in synaptic transmission in the spinal cord and may be involved in those pathways concerned with micturition.

Gamma-amino butyric acid (GABA) has been found to inhibit neurocellular action. This effect is similar to that of glycine and taurine. Aspartate and glutamate have been demonstrated to be excitatory neurotransmitter agents in spinal neurons.

The evolving field of neuropeptide research continues to produce new compounds that may function as synaptic transmitter agents, neuromodulators, or hormones. These agents may act at a presynaptic or postsynaptic site. They are ubiquitous in location and include: (1) substance P, (2) cholecystokinin, (3) enkephalin, (4) vasoactive intestinal polypeptide, and (5) somatostatin.

The time course of release of amines or classic transmitter agents is considerably different from that of neuropeptides (Fig. 4–55). Since these differing classes of transmitter agents at the same presynaptic ending frequently coexist, one can observe the short time course of the amine and the long time course of the neuropeptide (Table 4–1).

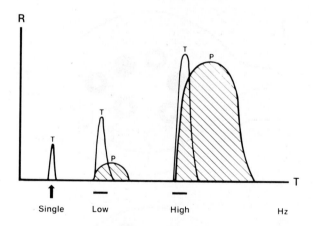

Figure 4–55. Comparison of time release of classic neurotransmitters and peptide transmitters at differing frequencies and intensities of stimulation.

RECEPTORS AND RECEPTOR-MEDIATED MEMBRANE CHANNELS

With migration of neurotransmitter agent to the postsynaptic membrane there occurs the formation of a receptor-transmitter complex and a conformational change in the postsynaptic membrane. This latter event is associated with current flow and a voltage change called the excitatory function potential.

There are specific receptor proteins in the pre- and postsynaptic membrane for each of the transmitter agents. Probably the best investigated of these is the acetylcholine receptor of the electric eel. This is a nicotinic acetylcholine receptor, with a time course shorter than that of the muscarinic receptor. This difference in time course has been ascribed to the time course of the resultant conformational protein change. The binding of two acetylcholine receptors results in the channel opening for passage of current flow. This binding is competitively blocked by D-tubocurarine.

The structure of the receptor (Fig. 4–56) is a rosette configuration, which is 8 nm in diameter with a 2-nm orifice (Hamilton, 1982). The dimension of the ion channel has been measured and is 6.5 × 6.5 A. The density of the receptor protein is increased in subsynaptic areas to

TABLE 4–1. COEXISTENCE OF CLASSIC TRANSMITTERS AND PEPTIDES

Classic Transmitter	Peptide	Tissue/Region
Dopamine	Enkephalin	Carotid body (cat)
	CCK	Ventral tegmental area
Norepinephrine	Somatostatin	Sympathetic ganglia (guinea pig)
		SIF cells (cat)
	Enkephalin	Sympathetic ganglia (rat, bovine)
		Adrenal medulla (several species)
		SIF cells (guinea pig, cat)
		Locus ceruleus (cat)
	Neurotensin	Adrenal medulla (cat)
	APP/BPP/NPY	Sympathetic ganglia (rat, cat, man)
		Medulla oblongata (rat, man)
		Locus ceruleus (rat)
Epinephrine	Enkephalin	Adrenal medulla (several species)
	APP/BPP/NPY	Medulla oblongata (rat)
5-HT	Substance P	Medulla oblongata (rat)
	TRH	Medulla oblongata (rat)
	Substance P + TRH	Medulla oblongata (rat)
	Enkephalin	Medulla oblongata (rat, cat)
ACh	VIP	Autonomic ganglia (cat)
	Enkephalin	Preganglionic nerves (cat)
		Cochlear nerves (guinea pig)
	Neurotensin	Preganglionic nerves (cat)
	LHRH	Sympathetic ganglia (bullfrog)
	Somatostatin	Heart (toad)
	Substance P + enkephalin	Ciliary ganglion (avian)
GABA	Somatostatin	Ciliary ganglion (avian)
	Motilin	Cerebellum (rat)

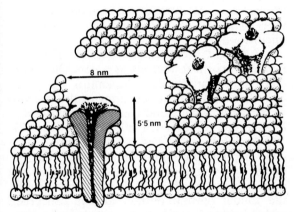

Figure 4–56. Schematic of nicotinic acetylcholine receptor (nm = nanometers [1×10^{-9} meters]).

TABLE 4–2. RECEPTOR-COUPLED INOSITOL PHOSPHOLIPID HYDROLYSIS IN NEURONAL TISSUES

Receptor Type	Location
Muscarinic cholinergic (some)	Most brain regions; superior cervical ganglion
$_1$-Adrenergic	Cerebral cortex
H$_1$-Histamine	Most brain regions
5-Hydroxytryptamine	Cerebral cortex
Substance P	Hypothalamus; striatum; substantia nigra
Neurotensin	Hypothalamus
V$_1$-Vasopressin	Hippocampus
CCK-Octapeptide	Cerebral cortex
Nerve growth factor	PC12 clonal rat cells

$10,000/\mu m^2$. The proteins composing the rosettes are glycoproteins. Other receptor proteins have been analyzed and are similar to those of the acetylcholine receptor.

VOLTAGE-DEPENDENT CHANNELS

There is a second class of ionic channels in which conformational change is not induced by complexing of transmitter agent to receptor protein but by voltage changes across the membrane. These are located at a site distant from the subsynaptic regions and in the axon.

Estrogen receptors have been demonstrated in the lower urinary tract (Caine et al., 1975; Iosif et al., 1981). Estrogen administration, in turn, may induce increases in density and distribution of cholinergic and adrenergic receptors (Levin et al., 1981).

Prostaglandins of E and F series have been demonstrated to be intracellular messengers analogous to cyclic nucleotides and inositol phospholipid of these prostaglandins. E series has been demonstrated to be the most potent in producing relaxation of the trigone, bladder neck, and proximal urethra. Its effects may be enhanced by estrogen administration.

INTRACELLULAR MESSENGERS (Downes, 1983)

The translation of conformational change in the membrane protein to intracellular changes has been ascribed to three intracellular messengers: (1) calcium, (2) inositol phospholipid, and (3) cyclic nucleotides, the most important of which is cyclic AMP.

Activation of this messenger system or of cyclic nucleotides by calcium or inositol phospholipid may trigger the activation of cellular protein kinases or the products of arachidonic acid, such as prostaglandin (Table 4–2) (Brown et al., 1980; Andersson and Sjogren, 1982).

POSTSYNAPTIC INACTIVATION

Postsynaptic inactivation of transmitter agents has been best studied for acetylcholine and adrenergic transmitter agents. Acetylcholinesterase, which is ubiquitously present in the membrane, hydrolyzes acetylcholine. There is subsequent resorption of the hydrolized products into the presynaptic endings. Catecholamines released into the synaptic cleft are inactivated principally by re-uptake into the nerve terminals that released the neurotransmitters. Those that are not taken up are inactivated by two enzymes, monoamine oxidase and catechol-O-methyltransferase (COMT).

OTHER SYNAPTIC EFFECTS (Fig. 4–57)

Other synaptic effects have been described that may be present in the neuromuscular function of the detrusor muscle and periurethral striated muscle. These include: (1) trans-synaptic inhibition, (2) autoinhibition, (3) neuromodulators (Kerizama, 1982), and (4) cell tropism.

Trans-synaptic inhibition is mediated by release of an inhibiting agent from a postsynaptic location. This transmitter agent diffuses back across the synaptic cleft to inhibit presynaptic release of a transmitter agent (Fredholm, 1981).

Autoinhibition consists of inhibition of the release of a neurotransmitter agent, initiating development of postsynaptic responses by the transmitter agent itself.

Neuromodulators are circulating agents, such as taurine, which diffusely act on presynaptic release of neurotransmitter agents.

Cell tropism consists of intracellular signal mechanisms generated by current flow in the neuronal mechanism. This receptor-coupled

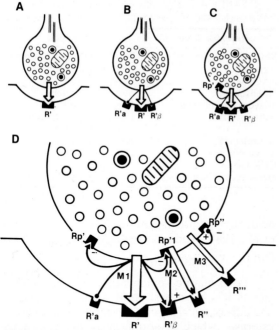

Figure 4–57. Alternative forms of chemical transmission. *A,* A single neurotransmitter acts on a single postsynaptic receptor (R'). *B,* A single neurotransmitter acts on multiple types of postsynaptic receptors. *C,* Presynaptic stimulation of a receptor Rp'. *D,* Multiple transmitter agents released from a single presynaptic ending and acting pre- and postsynaptically. (From Lundberg, J. M., and Hokfelt, T.: Trends Neurol. Sci., *6:*325, 1983.)

event may contribute to metabolic function of the neuron.

RECEPTOR ASSAYS

Receptor assays have been popularized in recent years for estimating muscarinic binding sites in detrusor muscle by utilizing QHNB (Levin et al., 1980*a*; Anderson and Marks, 1982; Klotz, 1983). The disadvantages of the techniques utilized for these data (Scatchard plots) include intense data compression at increasing concentration of ligand. Data compression may lead to a suggestion of linearity where none exists. This results in conflicting reports on the interpretation of these studies (Levin et al., 1980*a*; Anderson and Marks, 1982). As has been emphasized in discussions of Scatchard analysis and Scatchard plots, there is no substitute for data collection over a wide range of concentrations of ligand.

Pharmacology of Urinary Bladder Innervation

With the currently available data on neurotransmitter agents, we can begin to define the properties of neurotransmission in different portions of those reflex pathways concerned with micturition.

1. Loop I. Acetylcholine has been identified in cerebrocortical neurons as a generally available neurotransmitter. Dopamine has been identified as a neurotransmitter in the neurons of the basal ganglia and has been implicated in bladder control (Sillen, 1980; Sillen et al., 1979, 1980). Substance P has been confirmed as a neuropeptide transmitter in the rat from the dorsal tegmental nucleus of the pons to the medial frontal cortex. In this particular study, the caudal portion of the nucleus concerned with bladder function was excluded and must await further investigation.

2. Loop II. There are no definitive studies of the neurotransmitter composition of that portion of the dorsolateral tegmental nucleus of the pons concerned with urinary detrusor innervation. However, since substance P has been identified in other cortical pathways from more rostral portions of the same nucleus, it is a probable candidate for a similar role of neurons innervating the lower urinary tract. Gamma-amino butyric acid has also been implicated in brain stem control of micturition.

3. Loop III. The amino acid transmitter agents as well as substance P have been identified in the spinal cord. How these relate to pudendal motor pathways is currently not known.

4. Loop IV. Neurotransmitter agents have not been specifically identified in the supraspinal and segmental innervation of pudendal motoneurons.

5. Detrusor nuclei. Enkephalins have been identified in the detrusor nuclei and preganglionic axon pathways to the pelvic ganglia (Glazer and Basbaum, 1980; Kawatoni, 1983). The action of these transmitter agents in the ganglia is unknown. However, in other studies of neuronal function they have been identified as inducing suppression of neuronal activity.

6. In the pelvic ganglia, three neurotransmitter agents have been identified. These include acetylcholine, norepinephrine, and enkephalins (Kuru, 1965; Krnjevic, 1974; Khana et al., 1977; Twiddy et al., 1980). Precisely how these regulate transmission is unknown.

7. The neurotransmitter agents implicated in the urinary detrusor include acetylcholine (Brindley and Craggs, 1980), adrenergic agents and neuropeptides (Ambache and Zar, 1970; Husted et al., 1981; Krell et al., 1981; Sjogren et al., 1982). The neuropeptide receptor sites identified have been vasoactive intestinal poly-

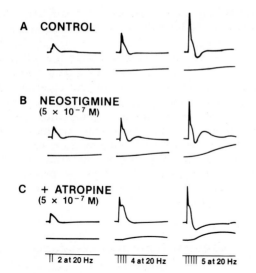

A CONTROL

B NEOSTIGMINE
$(5 \times 10^{-7}\ M)$

C + ATROPINE
$(5 \times 10^{-7}\ M)$

2 at 20 Hz   4 at 20 Hz   5 at 20 Hz

Figure 4–58. Effect of neostigmine on electrical and contractile responses in detrusor motor cells. Top trace is intracellular potential change; bottom trace is change in muscle cell tension. With addition of neostigmine to the muscle cell bath there is increase in amplitude of both components of intracellular potential change. With addition of atropine to the bath the second electrical potential is abolished, demonstrating that it is cholinergic in nature and that the first potential is noncholinergic.

peptide, somatostatin, and substance P (Fig. 4–58).

8. In the smooth muscle of the urethra, acetylcholine (Ek et al., 1977; Brindley and Craggs, 1980), norepinephrine, substance P, vasoactive intestinal polypeptide (Alumets et al., 1979), and histamine (Khana et al., 1977) have been suggested as potential transmitter agents.

9. Acetylcholine is the neurotransmitter agent in the periurethral striated muscle (Bowen et al., 1976).

10. The sensory endings in the urinary detrusor may contain acetylcholine and substance P (Pernow, 1983).

Summary

Neurouropharmacology is the most exciting aspect of current urinary bladder investigation. Undoubtedly, changes will continue to occur in our conceptualization and understanding. At the present time the principal evidence for neuropeptide transmission has been gained from experimental animal work utilizing immunoreactive identification.

Practical management of clinical problems is obviously the result of improvement in our understanding of neural transmission. This application has been facilitated by the current developments in pharmacokinetics and studies of drug metabolism.

URODYNAMICS

Introduction

Urodynamics can be defined as those studies of micturition employing the principles and laws of fluid mechanics. Urodynamics can be divided into a study of those factors concerned with urinary expulsion and urinary continence (Scott, 1973).

The factors concerned with urinary expulsion include (1) the driving pressure desired from contraction of the detrusor muscle, (2) urethral resistance, and (3) viscoelastic properties of the bladder wall.

The factors in urinary continence include (1) the bladder, (2) the bladder neck, (3) the pressure transmission factor, (4) the suspension principle, (5) levator muscle function, (6) smooth muscle of the urethra, (7) the periurethral striated muscle, (8) urethral softeners, (9) the connective tissue factor, (10) vascular and epithelial tissue, and (11) CNS factor.

Factors in Urodynamics of Voiding
(Gleason et al., 1967; Gleason and Bottacini, 1968; Griffiths, 1977; Zinner et al., 1977, 1983)

Normal urinary expulsion is in large part dependent upon the driving force developed by contraction of the detrusor muscle. A pressure build-up in the bladder is necessary to develop a pressure gradient permitting urine to flow through the urethra. In addition, intraurethral resistance is lowered during detrusor muscle contraction, reducing the energy requirement for urine expulsion.

The expulsive detrusor pressure is generated by contraction of the smooth muscle cells of the detrusor muscle. The force exerted as a result of this contraction is inversely related to the velocity of contraction (Fig. 4–59) (Sonnenblick, 1962; Berg, 1972). Increased length of the muscle cells due to increased volume results in attainment of an optimal maximal velocity of contraction and is dependent upon intraurethral resistance. More contractile units are recruited, with each unit contributing to increased force. With voiding, the load on individual muscle cells diminishes as the intravesical volume di-

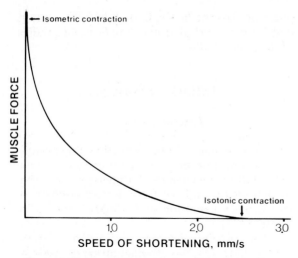

Figure 4–59. Force versus velocity of shortening diagram for muscle contraction.

minishes. As a consequence, the flow rate decreases. Whether there is coordination of this contraction by a detrusor conduction system awaits further study.

The relationship between intravesical volume, intravesical pressure, and intramural tension has been described in the Laplace equation:

$$P = R/T$$
$$P = \text{intravesical pressure}$$
$$R = \text{radius}$$
$$T = \text{intramural tension}$$

Unfortunately, this equation, which has been developed from analysis of elastic materials, has not been tested experimentally for appropriate application to biologic tissues, such as the detrusor muscle.

The rate of contraction of detrusor smooth muscle cells is considerably slower than that of striated or cardiac muscle. Prior to voiding, the intravesical pressure rises. With a closed bladder neck, energy transformation from muscle contraction to urine can be viewed as a change in potential energy of the latter. With opening of the bladder neck, about 90 per cent of the intravesical potential energy is transformed into kinetic energy of the fluid stream. Only a small portion of the potential energy is lost in friction between the urinary stream and the urethral wall. The contraction of the detrusor muscle with the bladder neck closed is isometric, and with voiding it changes to isotonic. There is also a contribution to intravesical pressure from contraction of the abdominal striated musculature. This contribution is variable, its amount being dependent upon impairment of detrusor muscle contraction. Voiding by detrusor muscle con-

traction can be viewed as more efficient than that obtained by abdominal muscle contraction.

The increased efficiency of voiding by detrusor muscle contraction is due to the following factors: (1) The bladder neck opens normally by coordinated active pull on the external urethral orifice. This process is absent in voiding by contraction of the abdominal muscles and diaphragm. In the latter, the bladder urine forces the bladder neck open by exerting a force on the circular fibers of the internal urethral orifice. (2) The intra-abdominal pressure is transferred to the urethra as well as to the intravesical space.

Urethral Flow and Resistance
(Smith, 1968)

The precise nature of urethral flow and resistance is not known. The principles of fluid mechanics indicate that urine flow is equal in all parts of the urethra once a steady state has been achieved after the initiation of voiding. This is referred to as the continuity theorem (Fig. 4–60) and is expressed by the equation

$$Q = Av$$
$$O = \text{flow rate}$$
$$A = \text{cross-sectional area}$$
$$v = \text{velocity of flow}$$

With the assumption of laminar flow, this value is the maximum velocity at the peak of a parabolic velocity profile.

Hence, since the urethra is not evenly calibrated, the velocity of urine flow varies at different levels. Where the urethra decreases in diameter, urine flow is accelerated, and where the cross-sectional area increases there is slowing of the stream. In this regard, the effective diameter of the urethra during voiding is 3 to 4 mm (10 F). The inlet configuration is important for the flow rate, with the assumption of a funnel in the normal situation.

Many applications of the principles of fluid mechanics to urine depend upon the assumption of laminar flow. However, the surface of the urethra is not smooth and may lead to turbulent flow and the production of sound during urinary flow (Bradley et al., 1977). Calculations demonstrate that the flow of urine in the male is turbulent and that the Reynolds number is in excess of 2000. (The Reynolds number is a nondimensional parameter used to determine the nature of fluid along surfaces.) Turbulence implies that fluid whirls are present and that nonlinearity of flow and energy exchanges may be present. Increased turbulence means in-

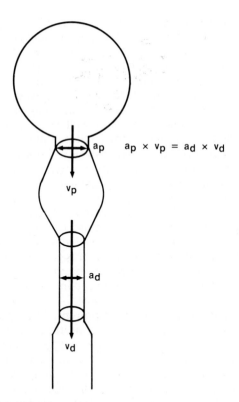

Figure 4–60. Continuity theorem of fluid flow in urethra.

creased fluid energy losses and increased resistance to flow. Abnormal states, such as diverticula and strictures, may also produce increased turbulence and resistance. During voiding the urethra behaves as an elastic conduit with an expandable capacity to accommodate a wide range of pressure and flow values.

With expulsion of urine from the external urinary meatus there is residual kinetic energy in the projected external urinary stream. The greater the value of kinetic energy, the farther the projection distance of the urinary stream. This kinetic energy can be expressed in the equation

$$K\ E\ =\ 1/2\ m\ v^{**}2$$
$$E\ =\ energy$$
$$m\ =\ mass\ of\ urinary\ stream$$
$$v\ =\ velocity\ of\ flow$$

The velocity is determined by the caliber and shape of the external urinary meatus.

In the normal male, the urinary flow rate is principally controlled by the proximal compressive zone, the membranous urethra. The external urinary meatus must be considerably narrowed before there is reduction in the flow rate of urine. In the female, flow control has been demonstrated in the distal segment.

The external urinary stream may be meas-

ured volumetrically per unit time by the use of a flowmeter (Byrne et al., 1972). The residual energy in the stream may be calculated from the equation

$$E\ =\ 1/2\ m\ v^{**}2$$
$$v\ =\ velocity\ of\ exit\ urinary\ stream$$
$$m\ =\ mass$$

Patients with urethral obstruction may have normal urinary flow rate but will have a low residual energy in the urinary stream.

Urethral resistance is difficult to quantify (Tanagho et al., 1969). The clinical finding of a normal urinary flow rate concurrent with a normal value of intravesical pressure indicates normal intraurethral resistance. Attempts to quantify urethral resistance based upon equations derived from fluid mechanics ignore the observation that the elastic characteristics of biologic tissue differ significantly from the crystalline structure of metals. The pragmatic method for expressing urethral resistance has been to plot the coordinates of volume and pressure in a diagram. A time plot of the data may also be made in order to demonstrate the variability of resistance with time. The most important measurement is that obtained at maximum flow, which provides a measurement of minimum urethral resistance.

An important observation may be the shape of the flow wave. However, it is difficult to make categorical conclusions concerning these at the present time. The inherent drawback of most pressure-flow studies is the invasive nature of the procedure. This is manifested in the use of suprapubic catheters and the exposure of the patient.

It is difficult to determine from the flow rate alone if an abnormality is present and to determine if the site of the abnormality is the propulsive (detrusor) component or the resistance (urethral) component. To define this difference, the flow studies are supplemented by cystometry, sphincter electromyography, and urethral pressure profiles. Cystometry delineates detrusor function, while the latter two procedures define urethral function.

Viscoelastic Properties of the Bladder Wall (Fig. 4–61) (Apter et al., 1972; Coolsaet et al., 1975a and b)

HOOK'S LAW

The bladder wall has elasticity and distensibility. The pressure rise is small with normal intravesical volumes. A stepwise injection of

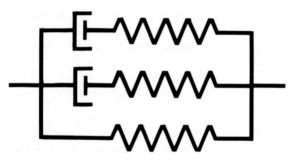

Figure 4–61. Elastic characteristics of detrusor muscle. See text for details.

fluid reveals rapid decline of pressure to preinjection levels. This rapid decline has been termed accommodation by clinicians and stress relaxation by physiologists. This latter term has been examined (Kondo and Sussett, 1974; Coolsaet et al., 1975a and b) for bladder tissue and has been found to be describable by an exponential function.

The viscoelastic properties of detrusor muscle may be defined as a combination of spring loading and pulling on the elements of a dashpot. Both are energy devices. With increase in bladder wall tension, the spring element is loaded and energy is stored. With release of bladder wall tension, energy is released by the spring and dissipated in pulling on the elements of the dashpot.

The viscoelastic properties of the bladder wall also affect the responses characteristic of the tension receptors. With increased distensibility the stimulation of these receptors may be impaired, whereas with decreased compliance the receptor sensitivity may be increased.

CONTINENCE

Urinary continence is dependent upon many different factors. Some mechanisms may be crucial, while others are contributory to normal function. Continence assumes that a positive urethral closure pressure is present, i.e., the intraurethral pressure must exceed the intravesical pressure.

Continence mechanisms may, from the urodynamic point of view, be construed as local and due to mechanical forces.

The Bladder Component. During bladder filling, the intravesical pressure is lower than the intraurethral pressure. This is the result of the distensibility of the detrusor muscle.

The Bladder Neck Component. The bladder neck factor in continence has been principally inferred from roentgenologic studies of voiding. In a normal continent individual with contrast material in the bladder, radiographic examination demonstrates that the contrast material will not pass the bladder neck despite maximal abdominal straining. The existence of a true internal sphincter accounting for this effect is in doubt. Rather, it is believed to be due to the presence of elastic and collagen tissue in the proximal urethra as well as reflex contraction of the periurethral striated muscle.

The Pressure Transmission Component. Increased intra-abdominal pressure is transmitted to the bladder and proximal urethra. The pressure rise in the proximal urethra may be higher than the intra-abdominal pressure rise and minimal in the distal third of the urethra. The pressure augmentation is due to contraction of the periurethral striated muscle. The transmission factor is determined by the location of the proximal urethra within the intra-abdominal space and upon its compliance.

The Suspension Component. The bladder neck is suspended by the pubourethral ligaments and the fascia of the pubococcygeus muscle (Zacharin, 1963). These structures anchor the bladder neck within the intra-abdominal space. With increasing laxity of the ligaments, the bladder neck is displaced. With anteroinferior displacement, there is funneling of the bladder neck during increased intra-abdominal pressure, with consequent urinary leakage. With posteroinferior displacement, there is displacement of the urethra from the intra-abdominal space. The increase in intra-abdominal pressure cannot be transferred to the proximal urethra, with resultant urinary incontinence.

The Levator Muscle Component. The levator muscles contain slow- and fast-twitch muscle fibers. The muscle contraction characteristics have been inferred from histologic and histochemical examination of the levator muscle. The muscle fibers contain a majority of slow-twitch muscle fibers (80 per cent) as well as fast-twitch fibers (20 per cent). This finding suggests that the fast-twitch fibers supply a phasic component to account for urinary continence in the presence of sudden rises in intra-abdominal pressure, the slow-twitch fibers accounting for the tonic component.

The Urethral Smooth Muscle Component. The urethral smooth muscle is under alpha-adrenergic influence either via nerve endings or by circulating alpha-adrenergic substance. Estrogen receptors have also been described in the smooth muscle of the urethra, indicating that estrogens may affect the urethral smooth muscle as well as the urothelium.

The Periurethral Striated Muscle Component. The periurethral striated muscle has a definitive role in avoidance of incontinence. The maintenance of the tonic aspects of continence has been suggested by the histologic finding that the muscle is composed of slow-twitch fibers. The phasic continence mechanism of the striated muscle can be demonstrated in combined electromyographic urethral pressure profile and by sphincter electromyography.

The tonic continence mechanism can be inferred from the resting level of sphincter EMG activity when there is low or zero bladder volume.

The Connective Tissue Component. When the contributions of striated and smooth muscle to intraurethral resistance are removed, there is residual resistance. This residual resistance has been ascribed to the collagen and elastic component of urethral tissue (Swaiman, 1967; Zinner et al., 1983).

Vascular and Epithelial Factors (Raz et al., 1972). The urethra may be conceptualized as an elastic contractile tube, in which centrally oriented forces tend to occlude the lumen during the filling phase of the bladder. To produce complete urethral occlusion the inner wall of the urethra should be soft and compressible. The inner urethral softness is provided by the epithelium and vasculature of the mucosa and submucosa. The vascular component of the urethral closure pressure profile has been estimated as approximately one third of the total measurement.

Summary

Urodynamics is a methodology employing the application of fluid mechanics to the clinical problems of voiding. The appropriateness of this application as well as its limitations will require further study and documentation.

BEHAVIORAL NEUROLOGY AND THE URINARY BLADDER

Introduction

Behavioral neurology and its effect upon urinary bladder function can truly be said to be in its infancy (Miller and Divorkin, 1977). Beginning studies of the use of biofeedback technique in the treatment of clinical voiding problems emphasize the need for fundamental neuropsychologic research in this area.

Classical Conditioning

Classical conditioning, also called pavlovian conditioning, depends upon reflex behavior where a reflex is an involuntary response that is elicited by a specific or appropriate stimulus. Hence, with bladder filling there is increasing tendency to evoke a detrusor reflex contraction at increasing volumes. Similarly, with sudden increases in intravesical pressure there is reflex contraction of the periurethral striated muscle. Classical conditioning acts to elicit a response. In pavlovian experiments, a light acting as a conditional stimulus was presented to the dog prior to the presentation of food. The dog picked up the food in its mouth and salivated—the unconditional stimulus. After several trials, the conditional stimulus—the light—evoked the salivation response. A conditional reflex continues to occur only if the conditional stimulus is occasionally presented in conjunction with the unconditional stimulus. If this does not occur, the conditional response is extinguished.

Operant conditioning consists of the attempt to modify a behavior by a system of positive and negative rewards. Biofeedback is an attempt to help the patient monitor his behavior in order to modify it.

Principles of Biofeedback

Biofeedback may be defined as the continuous feedback of external psychophysiologic data to the individual. The factors present in feedback include the following:

1. Feedback systems are closed-loop circuits.

2. Negative feedback tends to promote stability, whereas positive feedback tends to drive the reflex or circuit into oscillation—instability.

3. Feedback systems are affected by time delay.

4. Feedback systems are limited by their capacity.

5. Feedback systems have linear and nonlinear properties.

Applying the biofeedback principles to the clinical problem may employ several alternative strategies:

1. *Control of sensory input.* This may be performed by use of an environment of sensory deprivation, by use of pharmacologic agents, and by sensory overload.

2. *Control of sensory feedback.* This is performed by selective attention to a particular aspect of an overall task.

3. *Control of muscle tone.* This can be initiated either by voluntary effort or by development of sleep.

4. *Control of muscle feedback.* This consists of controlling the response to proprioceptive information from the muscles. Assisting in this process may be the audible EMG response of transformation of the cystometrogram into a visual or audible signal.

In all forms of biofeedback and behavioral modification of body function, the relationship between the patient and the therapist is of crucial significance. There should be clearly defined roles of physician or psychologist, biofeedback therapist, and biofeedback technician.

Biofeedback therapy may involve long practice sessions, which should be monitored by one of the above-named individuals. During these sessions, one or more of the team will function as a therapist.

The characteristics of the therapist should include a cheerful, positive, and encouraging attitude. This will facilitate an important component in the therapeutic relationship—the patient's desire to trust the therapist. Difficulties in attaining the therapy can be of three types: (1) breach of the therapeutic contract by therapist or patient (2) resistance by the patient in giving up his or her symptoms; or (3) the patient's lack of desire to fulfill the contract.

BIOFEEDBACK AND ALTERATION IN DETRUSOR REFLEX THRESHOLD

Numerous reports have been published on the use of urodynamic results in conjunction with visual and auditory cues to manage patients with bladder instability and detrusor-sphincter dyssynergia (Cardozo et al., 1978a and b; Schwartz, 1979; Wear, 1979; Hinman, 1980; Hafner, 1981; Husted et al., 1981; Sugar and Firlit, 1982; Milland and Oldenburg, 1983).

After initial psychologic studies, patients were instructed to keep a voiding diary consisting of the voiding and incontinence pattern for a 24-hour period. They were then instructed in the art of voiding deferment by contracting the pelvic floor, by breathing exercises, and by utilizing distraction tasks. They were then instructed to avoid voiding for a definite period of time after the first sensation. These instructions were supplemented by biofeedback consisting of cystometry, whose output was utilized to modulate an audio-oscillator as well as produce a visualized graph. The bladder was filled to capacity at each 1-hour biofeedback session. Upon the occurrence of abnormal detrusor reflex contractions, the patients used the suppression techniques they had been taught. This produced audible and visible results and caused demonstrable changes in the detrusor reflex threshold, observed in the cystometrogram as well as in the maximal amplitude of the detrusor reflex contraction. The maximum follow-up time of these patients was 2 years.

BIOFEEDBACK AND ALTERATION OF TONE AND RESPONSE OF THE PERIURETHRAL STRIATED MUSCLE

Biofeedback has also been utilized to treat patients with no evidence of neurologic disease and symptoms and signs suggestive of lower urinary tract obstruction (Pearne et al., 1977). In a group of patients managed by biofeedback there was increased striated muscle tone during voiding.

Relaxation of the periurethral striated muscle in the volitional type of sphincter dyssynergia seen in childhood has been reported to be obtained by biofeedback therapy (Manzels et al., 1979; Hinman, 1980). The child was taught to recognize an EMG pattern of dyssynergia utilizing surface EMG electrodes applied to the perianal skin. The patient was taught to identify this sound and to voluntarily suppress its appearance during voiding. Positive verbal reinforcement was used during an initial training period. The results were effective up to 19 months after an initial 24- to 48-hour training period.

Summary

Understanding of the neuropsychology of urinary bladder function is in its initial stages. Performance and measurement of effective therapy of bladder dysfunction currently employ urodynamic techniques. Utilizing these techniques in conjunction with neurophysiologic techniques may facilitate therapy.

ONTOGENY OF URINARY BLADDER FUNCTION

Introduction

Understanding of the development of urinary bladder control has progressed from initial hesitating steps to great strides. This latter has resulted from an onrush of research into the neurobiology of the developing central nervous system of the experimental animal (Hollyday, 1980; Partanin et al., 1980; Purves and Lichtman, 1980; Diamond, 1982; Fried and Lagercrantz, 1982; Purves, 1983). Concepts such as targeting and synaptic elimination have helped to point out that during a certain phase of the newborn period there is refashioning of the neural networks innervating all systems.

There have been primarily animal studies of the urogenital system, with very few human investigations to confirm the conclusions derived from the experimental animal. Future studies of development of control of the urinary bladder should address the question of whether there is restructuring of anatomic connections during the newborn period. This redistribution of anatomic arrangements will be reflected in an alteration of neuronal responses and bladder control as the individual passes from the immediate postnatal period into childhood.

The ontogeny of urinary bladder function can be reviewed in the following categories:

1. Ontogeny of detrusor reflex function (Bradley, 1967a and b; Bradley and Long, 1969).
2. Ontogeny of innervation of the periurethral striated muscle.
3. Ontogeny of the tissue elements of the bladder wall (Swaiman, 1967).
4. Ontogeny of neurouropharmacology (Levin et al., 1981; Mitolo-Cheeppa et al., 1983).

General Principles of Developmental Neurobiology

In the science of developmental neurobiology, there is consistent evidence demonstrating redistribution and restructuring of anatomic connections during the postnatal period. This is associated with the concept of a target neuron, axonal and synaptic elimination due to neuronal death, and associated alteration in physiologic responses. How these alterations occur is a matter of speculation and continuing research. Neurons may be genetically predetermined to innervate and be innervated by other sets of neurons. On the other hand, the innervation may be modulated by factors outside the neuron.

The mechanisms by which these effects occur include the secretion of a neurotrophic agent by the target cell. As a result of this arrangement, the target cell is innervated by more axons in the postnatal period than at maturity. Following restructuring, each innervating axon distributes an increasing number of synaptic endings to a smaller number of target cells. There is subsequent redistribution of inputs to a target cell. Competition between inputs ceases when a single input remains.

Encephalization implies the assumption of peripheral neural networks into the control of the central nervous system. This provides for coordinated control and the development of local sign. Local sign signifies the development of urinary bladder evacuation without concurrent defecation. This provides for selective operation of reflex function to the exclusion of others. However, this plan of operation does not provide for invulnerability to neurologic injury.

Development is also dependent upon the presence of a basic excitatory input. Depriving a cat of normal patterned visual stimulation by suturing one eye shut at birth leads to a reduction in size of the visual cortex. In brief, the extent of cerebral cortex occupied by excitatory afferents and the synapses they make can be altered by deprivation. Applied to human physiology, this suggests that the intrauterine and immediate postnatal phases of voiding are important in the establishment of normal corticoregulatory function of the urinary bladder.

Ontogeny of Detrusor Reflex Function

Ontogenic studies of detrusor reflex function were first performed utilizing cystometry and investigating the effects of ablation of the central nervous system on the occurrence or nonoccurrence of a detrusor reflex contraction. It had been demonstrated many times that spinal cord transection in the adult experimental animal abolished the detrusor reflex contraction required for normal voiding. However, in the early newborn or postnatal period, this event did not occur (Fig. 4–62). Even after suction ablation of the conus medullaris a detrusor reflex contraction could be elicited. In this period of only a vague understanding of the reshaping occurring in postnatal networks, there was no clear explanation of these effects. It was concluded, however, that a process of refashioning and reshaping of the detrusor reflex occurred in the immediate postnatal period in the rabbit. This change was reflected by the occurrence of a detrusor reflex contraction independent of and not reliant upon central neural innervation. With the maturation of the animal beyond a period of 10 to 14 days, there was encephalization or incorporation of the detrusor reflex in central neural control. With this event,

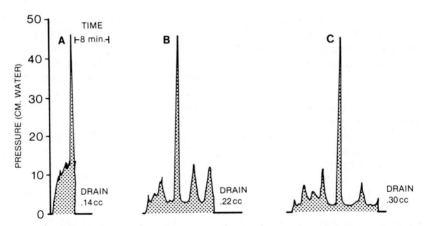

Figure 4–62. Ontogeny of the detrusor reflex. Cystometry in first week of postnatal life of the rabbit. *A,* Control. *B,* After thoracic spinal cord transection. *C,* After suction ablation of lumbosacral spinal cord.

detrusor reflex contraction became dependent upon brain stem innervation.

Subsequent studies in developmental neurobiology have suggested how these events occur. These studies have proposed a series of steps that are similar to those occurring in the developing neuromuscular junction, in autonomic ganglia, and in the central nervous system. Neurons are overproduced in early embryonic life and compete for survival. The target neuron that survives secretes a trophic factor attracting the innervating cells. There is associated neuronal death, with loss of axons and synapses. The latter has been referred to as synaptic elimination. These events have been documented in the submandibular ganglion of the rat, a parasympathetic ganglion similar to the pelvic ganglion innervating the urinary bladder. The neurons in the ganglia of the neonate are innervated by an average of five axons. As adult life is attained there is a reduction in innervation ratio of 1:1. Synaptic elimination has also been observed in other ganglia and has been correlated with reduction of norepinephrine content of the pelvic ganglion of the rat.

Ontogenic changes in urinary bladder function may also be due to changes in intensity of impulses in the somatic afferents from the perineum. Experiments from other areas in developmental neurobiology suggest that the process is an important one.

Ontogeny of Innervation of the Periurethral Striated Muscle

The ontogeny of peripheral innervation of the periurethral striated muscle has not been studied either in the experimental animal or in humans. Initial studies on the corticospinal tract in the rabbit suggest that in the immediate postnatal period there is myelination with resultant increase in conduction velocity (Bradley et al., 1969). No similar studies have been performed for the spinal innervation of the pudendal nucleus. The ontogeny of the pudendal nerve innervation of the periurethral striated muscle awaits future research.

The ontogeny of the histochemistry and pharmacologic responses of the rabbit bladder has been investigated (Levin et al., 1981). These studies demonstrated that cholinergic innervation, as measured by histochemical staining of acetylcholinesterase and response of muscle strips to bethanechol, was well developed at birth. Adrenergic innervation and tissue responsiveness to adrenergic agents was poor at birth but developed rapidly over the first 6 weeks of postnatal life. Whether similar results occur in humans awaits investigation.

The tissue elements of the bladder wall have been investigated in the postnatal rabbit (Swaiman and Bradley, 1969). These indicated changes in the collagen fraction as well as collagen to muscle protein fraction in the immediate postnatal period. These studies should be expanded and extended to humans utilizing modern biochemical techniques.

Summary

The ontogeny of the micturition reflex represents an area for intense research. To date, only initial studies have been performed in the experimental animal. These investigations indicate considerable differences between the postnatal period and adulthood. With the enormous strides in developmental neurobiology of other neural systems, application of these results to human voiding can be anticipated.

DESCRIPTION OF NORMAL VOIDING

Introduction

Normal voiding studies and investigations of the neurophysiology of voiding may be the least frequently performed procedures in a laboratory dedicated to the study of voiding dysfunction. The reasons include the practical difficulty in persuading asymptomatic individuals of all ages to undergo laboratory tests, some of which are invasive. However, this and other impediments do not lessen the urgency for data acquisition in those individuals of both sexes from childhood to old age who have no voiding complaints and who are otherwise in good health. From those studies would emerge a range of values in the different parameters similar to those reported for uroflowmetry (Von Garrelts, 1957; Backman, 1965). Clinical reports of normal voiding and continence indicate that more than one half of healthy females leak small quantities of urine during physical exercise. Normal voiding studies indicate that the individual achieves total evacuation of intravesical content with full uninterrupted urinary stream without postevacuation incontinence. More studies should be sought of normal voiding habits in asymptomatic populations, male and female, over the full span of life. The other components of these studies that have also been performed roentgenographically should include cystometry, sphincter electromyography, urethral pressure profiles, ultrasonic studies of the bladder neck (Shapeero et al., 1983) during voiding, and the newer electrophysiologic methods addressed to bladder innervation.

Normal Voiding

Normal voiding consists of a sequence of events with behavioral, neurophysiologic, and urodynamic components. The neurophysiologic events include pelvic motor nerve discharge to the detrusor muscle, with coordinated contraction of the detrusor muscle and widening and shortening of the proximal urethra. With this build-up in pelvic motor nerve discharge, there is increasing intensity of suppression of excitatory transmission in pudendal motoneurons. This produces cessation of impulse activity in the pudendal nerve, with resultant passive relaxation of the periurethral striated muscle (Fig. 4–63) (Lapides, 1958). This process has been studied in detail in the experimental animal. Urodynamic studies utilizing sphincter EMG and intravesical pressure recordings do not contravene this description. However, the interpretation of neural events in humans is inferential (Von Garrelts, 1957; Hald and Bradley, 1983).

Roentgenographic studies of normal voiding emphasize a closed bladder neck during reflex quiescence and coordinated funneling of the proximal urethra during detrusor contraction (Fig. 4–64). These studies will doubtless be considerably enhanced by the widespread application of ultrasound techniques (Siegelbaum and Tsien, 1983).

Sex differences in voiding have been studied in adults. The difference in the size of the periurethral striated investment of the female and male urethras points up the rudimentary but variable nature of this structure in the

Figure 4–63. Cystometry in 2-week-old rabbit. *A*, Control. *B*, After thoracic spinal cord transection.

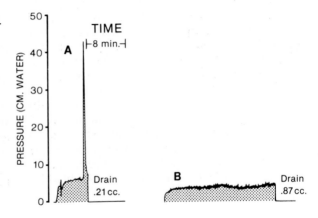

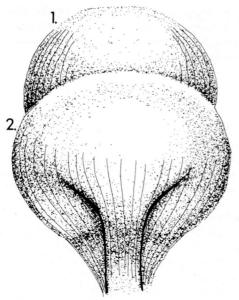

Figure 4–64. Effect of voiding is to change detrusor muscle configuration from storage organ (1) to smooth coordinate detrusor contraction with shortening and widening of the proximal urethra (2).

female. This difference may result in the common reports of the occurrence of brief episodes of urinary incontinence during physical exercise in healthy young women. With the rudimentary nature of periurethral striated muscle in females, it can be assumed that Loops III and IV, concerned with innervation of the periurethral striated muscle, are less significant.

While the electromyographic responses of the periurethral striated muscle appear to be similar in both sexes, a difference in pressures generated can be observed in the urethral pressure profile. The increased functional urethral length of the male, as demonstrated in the urethral pressure profile, in conjunction with the heavier striated muscle investment may account for greater intraurethral resistance to voiding in the male.

From birth to approximately 6 months of life, voiding is frequent and uninhibited. For the second 6-month period, voiding is less frequent and proceeds to the development of conscious bladder sensation between the ages of 1 and 2 years. From the age of 3½ to 4 years, normal filling sensation is present with both unconscious and voluntary inhibition of the desire to void. The typical sequence of acquiring bowel and bladder control in children is (1) bowel control asleep, (2) bowel control awake, (3) bladder control awake, and (4) bladder control asleep (Perlmutter, 1985).

Uroflowmetry

Uroflowmetry has been utilized as a technique for evaluation of urinary bladder dysfunction and will be described in detail in Chapter 11. However, normal values of voiding parameters have been derived from these studies (Table 4–3). Obvious sex differences occur and indicate that females void with lower intraurethral resistances than do males (Backman, 1965).

Summary

A description of normal voiding would include relaxation of the periurethral striated muscle, funneling of the bladder neck, and total evacuation of intravesical content. Clinical experience suggests this is attainable only in males as a result of a detrusor reflex contraction. In females, however, this may be possible solely as a result of straining.

Male and female differences in voiding are apparent in terms of anatomic organization and innervation. This is reflected in sphincter EMG, urethral pressure profile, uroflowmetry, and roentgenographic studies. The addition of ultrasound studies of voiding may further delineate these differences.

OVERVIEW

From this brief review of the physiology of the urinary bladder emerges a picture of what has been accomplished since the last edition of this book and part of what can be anticipated in the future.

Neuroanatomy

In neuroanatomy, it is obvious that recent research has given a clearer concept of the nuclei and neurons in the centers concerned with voiding. This work has been performed largely as the result of tracer studies in humans. There is no doubt, however, that the anatomic dissection of the pudendal plexus in humans by Takahashi represents an increase in understanding gained through persistence and scholarship. In humans, further delineation of anatomic connections has also occurred from the use of the evoked potential technique.

Future anatomic studies should be directed to three areas:

1. Increased definition of the nuclei in the

TABLE 4–3. NORMAL URODYNAMIC PARAMETERS IN ADULTS

Parameter	Men	Women
Micturition volume (ml)	450–650	320–590
Premicturition intravesicular pressure (cm H_2O)	34–50	28–42
Intravesical opening pressure (cm H_2O)	59–79	40–72
Maximum intravesical pressure (cm H_2O)	69–97	56–88
Mean intravesical pressure (cm H_2O)	61–83	46–74
Abdominal pressure contribution (%)	0–22	0–54
Opening time (sec)	5–11	5–15
Flow time (sec)	27–53	18–46
Maximum flow (ml/sec)	14–26	14–36
Mean flow (ml/sec)	11–19	11–21
Urethral resistance	0.07–0.45	0.03–0.35

brain stem and spinal cord in the experimental animal concerned with micturition. These will arise from intense use of tracer studies and the evoked potential technique.

2. A much clearer appraisal in humans of bladder innervation by the use of nuclear magnetic resonance studies of cerebral and spinal tissue performed in conjunction with urodynamic studies.

3. A more widespread use of the evoked potential technique in humans, including longer latency components concerned with cognition and voiding.

Neurophysiology

Electrophysiologic studies in the experimental animal have defined the physiology of the brain stem center for voiding as well as that of detrusor and pudendal nuclei in the sacral spinal cord. In addition, the physiology of the pelvic ganglia and detrusor muscle has undergone initial exploration. In humans, the effects of specific neurologic lesions upon voiding measured urodynamically have begun to contribute neurophysiologic data.

In the future, further definition of the function of cerebral nuclei in electrophysiologic studies can be anticipated. In humans, the joint use of nuclear magnetic resonance studies of the brain and spinal cord in conjunction with evoked potential and urodynamic studies will add to our neurophysiologic understanding.

Neuropharmacology

Neuropharmacology has undergone explosive development in the past 10 years, which has given important information on bladder function. This includes the clear definition in the urinary detrusor of at least two transmitter

agents, acetylcholine and a neuropeptide. This work promises in the future to define the central as well as the peripheral neurotransmitter processes. This will facilitate intelligent choices of pharmacologic agents in managing bladder dysfunction.

Urodynamics

Urodynamic research has initiated the process of assessing energy losses during voiding. In the future, biologic experiments should be designed to test the applicability of fluid mechanics to the voiding process. This would include experimental testing of such assumptions as the role of the Laplace theorem in assessing bladder distention. There is no doubt that measurement of the viscoelastic properties of the bladder wall will also contribute to this process.

Ontogeny of Bladder Function

The ontogeny of bladder function in the experimental animal is now being explored. What is required in the future is more aggressive investigation of human development.

Description of Normal Voiding

The description of normal voiding has been initiated with roentgenographic studies combined with urodynamic data. In the future, the use of ultrasonic evaluation of voiding directed to analysis of bladder structure without attendant roentgen exposure will facilitate a description of normal voiding.

Many exciting developments can be anticipated during the coming decade of research in bladder physiology.

References

Abdullah, A., and Eldred, E.: Activity in gamma efferent circuits induced by distension of the bladder. J. Neuropathol., *18*:590, 1959.

Alm, P., Alumets, J., Hakanson, R., and Sundler, F.: Peptidergic nerves in the genito-urinary tract. Neuroscience, *2*:751, 1977.

Alumets, J., Fahrenkrug, J., and Hakanson, R.: A rich VIP nerve supply is characteristic of sphincters. Nature, *280*:155, 1979.

Ambache, N., and Zar, M. A.: Non-cholinergic transmission by postganglionic motor neurones in the mammalian bladder. J. Physiol., *210*:761, 1970.

Andersen, J. T., and Bradley, W. E.: The urethral closure pressure profile. Br. J. Urol., *48*:341, 1976.

Anderson, G. F.: Evidence for a prostaglandin link in the purinergic activation of rabbit bladder smooth muscle. J. Pharmacol. Exp. Ther., *220*:347, 1982.

Anderson, G. F., and Marks, B. H.: Spare cholinergic receptors in the urinary bladder. J. Pharmacol. Exp. Ther., *221*:598, 1982.

Andersson, K. E., and Sjogren, C.: Aspects on the physiology and pharmacology of the bladder and urethra. Prog. Neurobiol., *19*:71, 1982.

Andrew, J., and Nathan, P. W.: Lesions of the anterior frontal lobes and disturbances of micturition and defecation. Brain, *87*:233, 1964.

Applebaum, M. L., Clifton, G. L., Coggeshall, R. E., et al.: Unmyelinated fibers in the sacral 3 and caudal 1 ventral roots of the cat. J. Physiol., *256*:557, 1976.

Apter, J. T., Mason, P., and Lang, G.: Urinary bladder wall dynamics. Invest. Urol., *9*:520, 1972.

Backman, K. A.: Urinary flow during micturition in normal women. Acta Chir. Scand., *130*:351, 1965.

Badr, G., Carlsson, D. A., Fall, M., Friberg, S., Lindstrom, L., and Ohlsson, B.: Cortical evoked potential following stimulation of the urinary bladder in man. Electroencephalogr. Clin. Neurophysiol., *54*:494, 1982.

Barrington, F. J. F.: The component reflexes of micturition in the cat. Brain, *64*:239, 1941.

Barrington, F. J. F.: The component reflexes of micturition in the cat. Parts I and II. Brain, *54*:177, 1931.

Barrington, F. J. F.: The effect of lesions of the hind and midbrain on micturition in the cat. Q. J. Exp. Physiol., *15*:181, 1925.

Barrington, F. J. F.: The relation of the hindbrain to micturition. Brain, *44*:23, 1921.

Barrington, F. J. F.: The nervous mechanism of micturition. Q. J. Exp. Physiol., *8*:33, 1915.

Bazeed, M. A., Thuroff, J. W., Schmidt, R. A., and Tanagho, E. A.: Histochemical study of urethral striated musculature in the dog. J. Urol., *128*:406, 1982.

Bell, C.: Dopamine as a postganglionic autonomic neurotransmitter. Neuroscience, *7*:1, 1982.

Bennett, M. R.: Neuromuscular Transmission in Smooth Muscle. Cambridge, Cambridge University Press, 1972.

Berg, S.: Vesical contractility I: The force-velocity relationship as an index of contractility. Invest. Urol., *9*:431, 1972.

Booth, A. M., and DeGroat, W. C.: A study of facilitation in vesical parasympathetic ganglia of the cat using intracellular recording techniques. Brain Res., *169*:388, 1979.

Bowen, J. M., Timm, G. W., and Bradley, W. E.: Some contractile and electrophysiological properties of the periurethral striated muscle of the cat. Invest. Urol., *10*:327, 1976.

Bradley, W. E.: Cerebro-cortical innervation of the urinary bladder. Tohoku J. Exp. Med., *113*:7, 1980.

Bradley, W. E.: Electroencephalography and bladder innervation. J. Urol., *118*:412, 1977.

Bradley, W. E.: Micturition reflex amplification. J. Urol., *101*:403, 1969a.

Bradley, W. E.: Regulation of the micturition reflex by negative feedback. J. Urol., *101*:400, 1969b.

Bradley, W. E.: Ontogeny of central regulation of visceral reflex activity in the rabbit. Am. J. Physiol., *212*:340, 1967a.

Bradley, W. E.: Ontogeny of central regulation of visceral reflex activity. Am. J. Physiol., *212*:340, 1967b.

Bradley, W. E., and Conway, C. J.: Bladder representation in the pontine mesencephalic reticular formation. Exp. Neurol., *16*:237, 1966.

Bradley, W. E., and Fletcher, T. F.: Innervation of the mammalian bladder. J. Urol., *101*:846, 1969.

Bradley, W. E., and Long, D. M.: Morphology of the developing mammalian bladder. Invest. Urol., *7*:66, 1969.

Bradley, W. E., and Scott, F. B.: Physiology of the urinary bladder. In Harrison, J. H., et al. (Eds.): Campbell's Urology. 4th edition. Philadelphia, W. B. Saunders Co., 1978.

Bradley, W. E., and Teague, C. T.: Synaptic events in pudendal motoneurons of the cat. Exp. Neurol., *56*:237, 1977.

Bradley, W. E., and Teague, C. T.: Electrophysiology of pelvic and pudendal nerves in the cat. Exp. Neurol., *35*:278, 1972.

Bradley, W. E., and Teague, C. T.: Cerebellar regulation of the micturition reflex. J. Urol., *101*:396, 1969a.

Bradley, W. E., and Teague, C. T.: Cerebellar control of the urinary bladder. Exp. Neurol., *23*:399, 1969b.

Bradley, W. E., and Teague, C. T.: Spinal cord organization of micturition reflex afferents. Exp. Neurol., *22*:504, 1968.

Bradley, W. E., Brackway, B. P., and Timm, G. W.: Auscultation of urinary flow. J. Urol., *118*:73, 1977.

Bradley, W. E., Conway, C. J., and Wright, F. S.: Pyramidal tract in the post natal rabbit. Electroencephalogr. Clin. Neurophysiol., *16*:565, 1969.

Bradley, W. E., Rockswold, G. L., Timm, G. W., and Scott, F. B.: Neurology of micturition. J. Urol., *115*:481, 1976.

Bradley, W. E., Scott, F. B., and Timm, G. W.: Sphincter electromyography. Urol. Clin. North Am., *1*:69, 1974.

Brindley, G. S., and Craggs, M. D.: The effect of atropine on the urinary bladder of the baboon and of man. J. Physiol., 55P, 1980.

Brooks, V. B., and Thach, W. T.: Cerebellar control of posture and movement. Handbook of Physiology, Section I. The Nervous System. Volume II, Motor Control, Part 2. Bethesda, Md., American Physiological Society, 1981.

Brown, W. W., Zenser, T. V., and Davis, B. B.: Prostaglandin E2 production by rabbit urinary bladder. Am. J. Physiol., *239*:F452, 1980.

Burke, D.: Muscle spindle function during movement. Trends Neurol. Sci., *3*:251, 1980.

Burke, R. E., Levine, D. N., Salzman, M., and Tsaires, P.: Motor units in cat soleus muscle. J. Physiol., *238*:503, 1974.

Byrne, T., Bottacini, M. R., and Gleason, D. M.: Energy loss during micturition. Invest. Urol., *10*:221, 1972.

Caine, M., Raz, S., and Zeigler, M.: Adrenergic and cholinergic receptors in the human prostate, prostatic capsule and bladder neck. Br. J. Urol., *47*:193, 1975.

Cardozo, L., Abrams, P. D., Stanton, S. L., and Feneley, R. C.: Idiopathic bladder instability treated by biofeedback. Br. J. Urol., *50*:521, 1978*a*.

Cardozo, L., Stanton, S. L., Hafner, J., and Allan, V.: Biofeedback in the treatment of detrusor instability. Br. J. Urol., *50*:250, 1978*b*.

Choo, L. K.: The effect of reactive blue, an antagonist of ATP, on the isolated urinary bladders of guinea-pig and rat. J. Pharm. Pharmacol., *33*:248, 1981.

Conway, C. J., and Bradley, W. E.: Measurement of spread of excitation in the urinary detrusor during reflex induction. J. Urol., *101*:533, 1969.

Coolsaet, B. L., van Duyl, W. A., van Mastrigt, R., et al.: Visco-elastic properties of bladder wall strips. Invest. Urol., *12*:351, 1975*a*.

Coolsaet, B. L., van Duyl, W. A., van Mastrigt, R., and Schouten, J. W.: Visco-elastic properties of the bladder wall. Urol. Int., *30*:16, 1975*b*.

Creed, K. E.: Effect of ions and drugs on the smooth muscle cell membrane of the guinea pig urinary bladder. Pflugers Arch., *326*:127, 1971.

Creed, K. E., Ishikowa, S., and Ito, Y.: Electrical and mechanical activity recorded from rabbit urinary bladder in response to nerve stimulation. J. Physiol., *338*:149, 1983.

Critchley, H. D., Dixon, J. S., and Gosling, J. A.: Comparative study of the periurethral and perianal parts of the human levator ani muscle. Urol. Int., *35*:226, 980.

Cullen, C., Fletcher, T. F., and Bradley, W. E.: Histology of the canine urethra. I. Morphometry of the male pelvic urethra. Anat. Rec., *199*:187, 1981.

Dean, D. M., and Downie, J. M.: Contribution of adrenergic and "purinergic" neurotransmission to contraction in rabbit detrusor. J. Pharmacol. Exp. Ther., *207*:431, 1978.

DeGroat, W. C.: Mechanisms underlying recurrent inhibition in the sacral parasympathetic outflow to the urinary bladder. J. Physiol., *257*:503, 1976.

DeGroat, W. C.: Nervous control of the urinary bladder of the cat. Brain Res., *87*:201, 1975.

DeGroat, W. C., and Booth, A. M.: Inhibition and facilitation in parasympathetic ganglia of the urinary bladder. Fed. Proc., *39*:2990, 1980.

DeGroat, W. C., and Ryall, R. W.: Reflexes to sacral parasympathetic neurons concerned with micturition in the cat. J. Physiol., *200*:87, 1969.

DeGroat, W. C., and Saum, W. R.: Synaptic transmission on parasympathetic ganglia in the urinary bladder of the cat. J. Physiol., *256*:137, 1976.

DeGroat, W. C., Booth, A. M., Milne, R. J., and Roppolo, M. R.: Parasympathetic preganglionic neurons in the sacral spinal cord. J. Auton. Nerv. Syst., *5*:23, 1982.

DeGroat, W. C., Nadelhaft, I., Nulne, R. J., Booth, A. M., Morgan, C., and Thor, K.: Organization of the sacral parasympathetic reflex pathways to the urinary bladder and large intestine. J. Auton. Nerv. Syst., *3*:135, 1981.

Denny-Brown, D., and Robertson, E. G.: The physiology of micturition. Brain, *56*:149, 1933.

Diamond, J.: Modeling and competition in the nervous system. Clues from the sensory innervation of skin. Cur. Top. Dev. Biol., *17*:147, 1982.

Downes, C. P.: Inositol phospholipids and neurotransmitter-receptor signalling mechanisms. Trends Neurol. Sci., *6*:313, 1983.

Edvardsen, P., and Ursin, T.: Micturition threshold in cats with amygdala lesions. Exp. Neurol., *21*:495, 1968.

Ek, A., Alm, P., Andersson, K. E., and Persson, C. G.

A.: Adrenergic and cholinergic nerves of the human urethra and urinary bladder: A histochemical study. Acta Physiol. Scand., *99*:345, 1977.

Elbadawi, A.: Ultrastructure of vesico-urethral innervation. I. Neuroeffector and cell junction in male internal sphincter. J. Urol., *128*:180, 1982.

Elbadawi, A., and Schenk, E. A.: Intra- and extraganglionic peripheral cholinergic neurons in the urogenital organs of the cat. Z. Zellforsch., *163*:26, 1970.

Elbadawi, A., and Schenk, E. A.: A new theory of innervation of bladder musculature. Part I. Morphology of the intrinsic vesical innervation apparatus. J. Urol., *99*:595, 1968*a*.

Elbadawi, A., and Schenk, E. A.: The peripheral adrenergic innervation apparatus: Intraganglionic and extraganglionic adrenergic ganglion cells. Z. Zellforsch., *87*:218, 1968*b*.

Elbadawi, A., and Schenk, E. A.: Dual innervation of the mammalian urinary bladder: A histochemical study of the distribution of cholinergic and adrenergic nerves. Am. J. Anat., *119*:405, 1966.

Evarts, E. V.: Motor cortex reflexes associated with learned movements. Science, *179*:501, 1973.

Falconer, M. A.: Mesial temporal sclerosis as a common cause of epilepsy. Lancet, *2*:767, 1974.

Fehér, E., and Vajda, J.: Interneuronal synapses in the local ganglia of the cat urinary bladder. Acta Anat., *104*:340, 1979.

Fletcher, T. F., and Bradley, W. E.: Neuro-anatomy of the bladder-urethra. J. Urol., *119*:153, 1978.

Fletcher, T. F., and Bradley, W. E.: Visceral afferent ending in the cat. Am. J. Anat., *128*:147, 1970.

Floyd, K., Hick, V. E., and Morrison, J. F. B.: The influence of visceral mechanoreceptors on sympathetic efferent discharge in the cat. J. Physiol., *323*:65, 1982.

Floyd, K., McMahon, S. B., and Morrison, J. F. B.: Inhibitory interactions between colonic and vesical afferents in the micturition reflex of the cat. J. Physiol., *322*:45, 1982.

Fredholm, B. B.: Trans-synaptic modulation of transmitter release—with special reference to adenosine. *In* Chemical Neurotransmission. New York, Academic Press, 1981.

Fried, G.: Do peptides coexist with classical transmitters in the same neuronal storage vesicles? *In* Chemical Neurotransmission. New York, Academic Press, 1981.

Fried, G., and Lagercrantz, H.: Developmental aspects of neurotransmission. *In* Klein, R. L., Lagercrantz, H., and Zimmerman, H. (Eds): Neurotransmitter Vesicles. New York, Academic Press, 1982.

Gallagher, J. P., Griffith, W. H., and Shinnick-Gallagher, P.: Cholinergic transmission in cat parasympathetic ganglia. J. Physiol., *332*:472, 1982.

Gjone, R., and Setekleiv, J.: Excitatory and inhibitory bladder responses to stimulation of the cerebral cortex in the cat. Acta Physiol. Scand., *59*:337, 1963.

Glazer, E. J., and Basbaum, A. I.: Leucine enkephalin: Localization in and axoplasmic transport by sacral parasympathetic preganglionic neurons. Science, *208*:1479, 1980.

Gleason, D. M., and Bottacini, M. R.: The vital role of the distal urethral segment in the control of urinary flow rate. J. Urol., *100*:167, 1968.

Gleason, D. M., Bottacini, M. R., Perling, D., and Lattimer, J. K.: A challenge to current urodynamic thought. J. Urol., *97*:935, 1967.

Gosling, J.: The structure of the bladder and urethra in relation to function. Urol. Clin. North Am., *6*:31, 1979.

Gosling, J. A., and Dixon, J. S.: The structure and innervation of smooth muscle in the wall of the bladder neck and proximal urethra. Br. J. Urol., *47*:549, 1975.

Gosling, J. A., and Dixon, J. S.: Sensory nerves in the mammalian urinary tract. J. Anat., *117*:133, 1974.

Gosling, J. A., Dixon, J. S., Critchley, H. O., and Thompson, S. A.: A comparative study of the human external sphincter and periurethral levator ani muscles. Br. J. Urol., *55*:35, 1981.

Gosling, J. A., Dixon, J. S., and Lendon, R. G.: The autonomic innervation of the human male and female bladder neck and proximal urethra. J. Urol., *118*:302, 1977.

Griffith, W. H., Gallagher, J. P., and Shinnick-Gallagher, P.: Sucrose-gap recordings of nerve-evoked potentials in mammalian parasympathetic ganglia. Brain Res., *209*:446, 451, 1981.

Griffith, W. H., III, Gallagher, J. P., and Shinnick-Gallagher, P.: An intracellular investigation of cat vesical pelvic ganglia. J. Neurophysiol., *43*:343, 1980.

Griffiths, D.: Urodynamic assessment of bladder function. Br. J. Urol., *49*:29, 1977.

Gu, J., Polak, J. M., and Probert, L.: Peptidergic innervation of human male genital tract. J. Urol., *130*:386, 1983.

Hafner, R. J.: Biofeedback treatment of intermittent urinary retention. Br. J. Urol., *53*:125, 1981.

Hald, T., and Bradley, W. E.: The Urinary Bladder. Baltimore, Williams & Wilkins Co., 1983.

Haldeman, S., Bradley, W. E., Bhatia, N. N., and Johnson, B. K.: Pudendal somatosensory evoked potentials. Arch. Neurol., *39*:280, 1982*a*.

Haldeman, S., Bradley, W. E., and Bhatia, N. N.: Evoked responses from pudendal nerve. J. Urol., *128*:974, 1982*b*.

Hamilton, S. L.: The Structure of the Nicotinic Acetylcholine Receptor in Proteins in the Nervous System: Structure and Function. New York, Alan R. Liss, 1982, pp. 73–85.

Henneman, E.: Recruitment of motoneurons: The size principle in motor unit types, recruitment and plasticity. *In* Desmedt Brussel, J. E. (Ed.): Health and Disease. Basel, S. Karger, 1981.

Henneman, E.: Relation between size of neurons and their susceptibility to discharge. Science, *126*:1345, 1957.

Henneman, E., and Olson, C. B.: Relations between structure and function in the design of skeletal muscles. J. Neurophysiol., *28*:581, 1965.

Henneman, E., Somjen, G., and Carpenter, D. O.: Functional significance of cell size in spinal motoneurons. J. Neurophysiol., *28*:560, 1965.

Hinman, F.: Syndromes of vesical incoordination. Urol. Clin. North Am., *7*:311, 1980.

Hokfelt, T., Schultzberg, M., Elde, R., Nilsson, G., Terenius, L., Said, S., and Goldstein, M.: Peptide neurons in peripheral tissues including the urinary tract. Immunohistochemical studies. Acta Pharmacol. Toxicol., *43*:78, 1978.

Hollyday, M.: Motoneuron histogenesis and the development of limb innervation. Curr. Top. Dev. Biol., *15*:181, 1980.

Huang, T. F., Yang, C. F., and Yang, S. L.: The role of the fastigial nucleus in bladder control. Exp. Neurol., *66*:674, 1979.

Husted, S., Sjogren, C., and Andersson, K. E.: Substance P and somatostatin and excitatory neurotransmission in rabbit urinary bladder. Arch. Int. Pharmacodyn., *252*:72, 1981.

Iosif, C. S., Batra, S., Ek, A., and Astedt, B.: Estrogen receptors in the human female lower urinary tract. Am. J. Obstet. Gynecol., *141*:817, 1981.

Jeffrey, P. O., and Austin, L.: Axoplasmic transport. Prog. Neurobiol., *2*:207, 1973.

Kaneko, S., Minami, K., Yachiker, S., and Kunta, T.: The effect of the alpha adrenergic blocking agent phentolamine on bladder neck dysfunction and a fluorescent histochemical study of bladder neck smooth muscle. Invest. Urol., *18*:212, 1980.

Kawatoni, M.: The presence of leucine-enkephalin in the sacral preganglionic pathway to the urinary bladder of the cat. Neurosci. Lett., *39*:143, 1983.

Kerizama, K.: Taurine as a neuromodulator. Fed. Proc., *39*:2680, 1982.

Khana, O. P., DeGregorio, G. J., Sample, R. G., and McMichael, R. F.: Histamine receptors in urethrovesical smooth muscle. Urology, *10*:378, 1977.

Khurona, R. K.: Autonomic dysfunction in ponto-medullary stroke. Ann. Neurol., *12*:86, 1982.

Klotz, I. M.: Ligand-receptor interactions: What we can and cannot learn from binding measurements. Trends Pharmacol. Sci., *4*:253, 1983.

Kluck, P.: The autonomic innervation of the urinary bladder, bladder neck and urethra: A histochemical study. Anat. Rec., *198*:439, 1980.

Kondo, A., and Sussett, J. G.: Viscoelastic properties of bladder. Invest. Urol., *11*:459, 1979.

Krell, R. D., McCoy, J. L., and Ridley, P. T.: Pharmacological characterization of the excitatory innervation to the guinea-pig urinary bladder in vitro: Evidence for both cholinergic and non-adrenergic, non-cholinergic neurotransmission. Br. J. Pharmacol., *74*:15, 1981.

Krnjevic, K.: Chemical nature of synaptic transmission in vertebrates. Physiol. Rev., *54*:418, 1974.

Kuru, M.: Nervous control of micturition. Physiol. Rev., *45*:425, 1965.

Kuzuhara, S., Kanazawa, I., and Nadanishi, T.: Topographical localization of the Onuf's nuclear neurons innervating the rectal and vesical striated sphincter muscle. Neurosci. Lett., *16*:125, 1980.

Langworthy, O. R., Kolb, L. C., and Lewis, L. G.: Physiology of Micturition. Baltimore, Williams & Wilkins Co., 1940.

Lapides, J.: Structure and function of the internal vesical sphincter. J. Urol., *80*:341, 1958.

Leach, G. E., Forsaii, A., Karls, P., and Raz, S.: Urodynamic manifestations of cerebellar ataxia. J. Urol., *128*:348, 1982.

Leger, L., and Hernandez-Nicaise, M.: The cat locus ceruleus. Anat. Embryol., *159*:181, 1980.

Levin, R. M., Malkowicy, B., Jacobowitz, D., and Wien, A. J.: The ontogeny of the autonomic innervation and contractile response of the rabbit urinary bladder. J. Pharmacol. Exp. Ther., *219*:250, 1981.

Levin, R. M., Shofer, F. S., and Wein, A. J.: Cholinergic, adrenergic and purinergic response of sequential strips of rabbit urinary bladder. J. Pharmacol. Exp. Ther., *212*:536, 1980*a*.

Levin, R. M., Shofer, F. S., and Wein, A. J.: Estrogen induces alterations in the autonomic responses of the rabbit urinary bladder. J. Pharmacol. Exp. Ther., *215*:614, 1980*b*.

Lewin, R. J., and Porter, R. W.: Inhibition of spontaneous bladder activity by stimulation of basal ganglia in the cat. Neurology, *15*:1049, 1965.

Lewin, R. J., Dillard, G. W., and Porter, R. W.: Extrapyramidal inhibition of the urinary bladder. Brain Res., *4*:301, 1967.

Loewy, A. D., Saper, C. B., and Baker, R. J.: Descending

projections from the pontine micturition center. Brain Res., *172*:533, 1978.

Londo, A., and Susset, J.: Viscoelastic properties of bladder. II. Comparative studies in normal studies in normal and pathologic dogs. Invest. Urol., *11*:459, 1974.

Lundberg, J. M., and Hokfelt, T.: Coexistence of peptides and classical neurotransmitters. Trends Neurol. Sci., *6*:325, 1983.

Mackel, R.: Segmental and descending control of the external urethral and anal sphincters in the cat. Physiology, *294*:105, 1979.

Manley, C. B.: The striated muscle of the prostate. J. Urol., *95*:234, 1966.

Manzels, M., King, L. R., and Firlit, C. F.: Urodynamic biofeedback: A new approach to treat vesico-sphincter dyssnyergia. J. Urol., *122*:205, 1979.

Marsden, C. D., Merton, P. A., and Morton, H. D.: Stretch reflexes and servo action in a variety of human muscles. J. Physiol., *259*:531, 1976.

Martin, A. R.: Functional transmission. II. Presynaptic mechanisms. Handbook of Physiology. Section I, The Nervous System. Volume I, Cellular Biology of Neurons, Part I. Bethesda, Md., American Physiological Society, 1977.

Martin, W. E., Fletcher, T. F., and Bradley, W. E.: Innervation of feline perineal musculature. Anat. Rec., *180*:15, 1974.

Martner, J.: Influence on the defecation and micturition reflexes by the cerebellar fastigial nucleus. Acta Physiol. Scand., *94*:1, 1975.

McGreer, P. L., and McGreer, E. G.: Amino acid neurotransmitters. *In* Siegel, G. J., and Albers, R. W. (Eds.): Basic Neurochemistry. Boston, Little, Brown & Co., 1981.

McGuire, E. J., and Herlihy, E.: Bladder and urethral responses to sympathetic stimulation. Invest. Urol., *17*:9, 1979.

McGuire, E. J., and Herlihy, E.: Bladder and urethral responses to isolated sacral motor root stimulation. Invest. Urol., *16*:219, 1978.

McMahon, S. B., and Morrison, J. F. B.: Two groups of spinal interneurones that respond to stimulation of the abnormal viscera of the cat. J. Physiol., *322*:21, 1982*a*.

McMahon, S. B., and Morrison, J. F. B.: Factors that determine the excitability of parasympathetic reflexes to the cat bladder. J. Physiol., *322*:35, 1982*b*.

McMahon, S. B., and Morrison, J. F. B.: Spinal neurons with long projections activated from the abdominal viscera of the cat. J. Physiol., *322*:1, 1982*c*.

McPherson, A.: Vesico-somatic reflexes in the chronic spinal cat. J. Physiol., *185*:197, 1966.

Milland, F. J., and Oldenburg, B. F.: Symptomatic, urodynamic and psychodynamic results of bladder re-education programs. J. Urol., *130*:715, 1983.

Miller, M. E., and Divorkin, B. R.: Effects of learning on visceral function. N. Engl. J. Med., *296*:1274, 1977.

Mitolo-Cheeppa, D., Schonauer, S., Grasso, G., Cicinelli, E., and Carratic, M. R.: Ontogenesis of autonomic receptors in detrusor muscle and bladder sphincter of human fetus. Invest. Urol., *21*:599, 1983.

Morgan, C., Nadelhaft, I., and DeGroat, W. C.: The distribution of visceral primary afferents from the pelvic nerve to Gissauer's tract and the spinal gray matter and its relationship to the sacral parasympathetic nucleus. J. Comp. Neurol., *201*:215, 1981.

Morgan, C., Nadelhaft, I., and DeGroat, W. C.: Location of bladder preganglionic neurons in the parasympathetic nucleus of the cat. Neurosci. Lett., *14*:189, 1979.

Murnaghan, G. F.: Neurogenic disorders of the bladder in Parkinsonism. Br. J. Urol., *33*:403, 1961.

Nadelhaft, I., DeGroat, W. C., and Morgan, C.: Location and morphology of parasympathetic neurons in the sacral spinal cord of the cat revealed by retrograde axonal transport of horseradish peroxidase. J. Comp. Neurol., *193*:265, 1980.

Nakagawa, S.: Onuf's nucleus of the sacral cord in a South American monkey (Saimiri): its location and bilateral cortical input from Area 4. Brain Res., *191*:337, 1980.

Nathan, P. W., and Smith, M. C.: The centrifugal pathway for micturition within the spinal cord. J. Neurol. Neurosurg. Psychiatr., *21*:177, 1958.

Nathan, P. W., and Smith, M. C.: The centripetal pathway from the bladder and urethra within the spinal cord. J. Neurol. Neurosurg. Psychiatr., *24*:262, 1951.

Nergardh, A.: Neuromuscular transmission in the corpus-fundus of the urinary bladder. Scand. J. Urol. Nephrol., *15*:103, 1980.

Nolan, M. F., and Brown, H. K.: An ultrastructural examination of dorsal root input to the sacral secondary visceral gray matter. J. Neurol. Sci., *52*:359, 1981.

Oliver, J. F., Bradley, W. E., and Fletcher, T. F.: Spinal cord distribution of the somatic innervation of the external urethral sphincter of the cat. J. Neurol. Sci., *10*:11, 1970.

Oliver, J. E., Bradley, W. E., and Fletcher, R. F.: Identification of preganglionic parasympathetic neurons in the sacral spinal cord of the cat. J. Comp. Neurol., *137*:321, 1969.

Partanin, M., Hervonen, A., and Algo, A.: Microspectrofluorimetric estimation of the formaldehyde-induced fluorescence of the developing main pelvic ganglion of the rat. Histochem. J., *12*:49, 1980.

Pascuzzo, G. J., and Skeen, L. C.: Brainstem projections to the frontal eye field in cat. Brain Res., *241*:341, 1983.

Pavlakis, A. J., Siroky, M. B., Goldstein, I., and Krane, R.: Neurourologic finding in Parkinson's disease. J. Urol., *129*:80, 1983.

Pearne, D. H., Zigelbaum, S. D., and Peyser, W. F.: Biofeedback assisted EMG relaxation for urinary retention and incontinence: A case report. Biofeedback Self Regul., *2*:213, 1977.

Penfield, W., and Jasper, H.: Epilepsy and the Functional Anatomy of the Human Brain. Boston, Little, Brown & Co., 1954.

Perlmutter, A.: Enuresis. *In* Kelalis, P. P., King, L. R., and Belman, A. B. (Eds.): Clinical Pediatric Urology. Philadelphia, W. B. Saunders Co., 1985, pp. 311–325.

Pernow, B.: Substance P. Pharmacol Rev., *35*:85, 1983.

Philips, C. G., Powell, T. P. S., and Weesendanger, M.: Projection from low threshold muscle afferents of hand and forearm to area 3A of baboon's cortex. J. Physiol., *217*:419, 1971.

Porter, R. W.: A pallidal response to detrusor contraction. Brain Res., *4*:381, 1967.

Porter, R. W., Pazo, J. H., and Dillard, G. V.: Triphasic brain stem response to detrusor contraction. Brain Res., *35*:119, 1971.

Purington, P. T., Fletcher, T. F., and Bradley, W. E.: Innervation of the pelvic viscera in the rat: Evoked potential in nerves to bladder and penis (clitoris). Invest. Urol., *14*:28, 1976.

Purves, D.: Modulation of neuronal competition by postsynaptic geometry in autonomic ganglia. Trends Neurol. Sci., *6*:10, 1983.

Purves, D., and Lichtman, J. W.: Elimination of synapses in the developing nervous system. Science, *210*:153, 1980.

Raz, S., Caine, M., and Zeigler, M.: The vascular component in the production of intraurethral pressure. J. Urol., *108*:93, 1972.

Rockswold, G. L., Bradley, W. E., and Chou, S. N.: Innervation of the urinary bladder in higher primates. J. Comp. Neurol., *193*:509, 1980*a*.

Rockswold, F. L., Bradley, W. E., and Chou, S. N.: Innervation of the external urethral and external anal sphincters in higher primates. J. Comp. Neurol. *193*:521, 1980*b*.

Ryall, R. W., and Piercy, M. F.: Visceral afferent and efferent fibers in sacral ventral roots in cats. Brain Res., *23*:57, 1970.

Sakanaka, M., Shiosaka, S., Takatsuki, K., and Tohyama, M.: Evidence for the existence of a substance P containing pathway from the nucleus laterodorsalis tegmenti (Castaldi) to the medial frontal cortex of the rat. Brain Res., *259*:123, 1983.

Satoh, K.: Descending projection of the nucleus tegmentis laterodorsalis to the spinal cord. Neurosci. Lett., *8*:9, 1978*a*.

Satoh, K.: Localization of the micturition center at dorsolateral pontine tegmentum of the rat. Neurosci. Lett., *8*:27, 1978*b*.

Schwartz, G. E.: Biofeedback and the behavioral treatment of disorders of disregulation. Yale J. Biol. Med., *52*:581, 1979.

Scott, F. B.: Correlation of flow rate profiles with diseases of the urethra in man. *In* Lutzeyer, W., and Meldhior, H. (Eds.): Urodynamics. New York, Springer Bolus, 1973, pp. 292–300.

Shapeero, L. G., Friedland, G. W., and Perkash, I.: Transrectal sonographic voiding cystourethrography: Studies in neuromuscular bladder dysfunction. Am. J. Radiol., *141*:83, 1983.

Siegelbaum, S. A., and Tsien, R. W.: Modulation of gated ion channels as a mode of transmitter action. Trends Neurol. Sci., *6*:307, 1983.

Sillen, U.: Central neurotransmitter mechanisms involved in the control of urinary bladder function. Scand. J. Urol. Nephrol. (Suppl.), *58*:1, 1980.

Sillen, U., Persson, B., and Rubenson, A.: Involvement of central GABA receptors in the regulation of the urinary bladder function of anesthetized rats. Arch. Pharmacol., *314*:195, 1980.

Sillen, U., Rubenson, A., and Hjalmas, K.: Evidence for a central monoaminergic influence of urinary bladder control mechanism. Scand. J. Urol. Nephrol. *13*:265, 1979.

Sjogren, C., Andersson, K. E., and Husted, S.: Contractile effects of some polypeptides on the isolated urinary bladder of guinea-pig, rabbit, and rat. Acta Pharmacol. Toxicol., *50*:175, 1982.

Smith, J. C.: Urethral resistance to micturition. Br. J. Urol., *40*:125, 1968.

Snyder, S. H.: Brain peptides as neurotransmitters. Science, *209*:976, 1980.

Sonnenblick, E. H.: Force-velocity relations in mammalian heart muscle. Am. J. Physiol., *202*:931, 1962.

Sotelo, C., and Triller, A.: Morphological Correlation of Electrical, Chemical and Dual Modes of Transmission in Chemical Neurotransmission. New York, Academic Press, 1981.

Soto, A., Sota, Y., and Schmidt, R. F.: Reflex bladder activity induced by electrical stimulation of hind limb somatic efferents in the cat. J. Autonom. Nerv. Syst., *1*:229, 1980.

Starr, A.: Auditory brain stem responses in brain death. Brain, *99*:543, 1976.

Sugar, E. D., and Firlit, C. F.: Urodynamic feedback: New therapeutic approach for childhood incontinence/infection. J. Urol., *128*:1253, 1982.

Sundin, T., and Dahlstrom, A.: The sympathetic innervation of the urinary bladder and urethra in the normal state and after parasympathetic denervation at the spinal root level. Scand. J. Urol. Nephrol., *7*:131, 1973.

Sung, J. H.: Autonomic neurons affected by lipid storage in the spinal cord in Fabry's disease: Distribution of autonomic neurons in the sacral cord. J. Neuropathol. Exp. Neurol., *38*:87, 1979.

Sung, J. H., Mastri, A. R., and Segal, E.: Pathology of Shy-Drager syndrome. J. Neuropathol. Exp. Neurol., *38*:353, 1979.

Swaiman, K. F.: Quantitation of collagen in the wall of the human urinary bladder. J. Appl. Physiol., *22*:122, 1967.

Swaiman, K. F., and Bradley, W. E.: Maturational biochemical changes in rabbit bladder muscle. Invest. Urol., *5*:115, 1979.

Takahashi, M.: Morphological analysis of the pudendal nerve. Acta Anat. Nippon., *55*:23, 1980.

Tanagho, E. A., Meyers, F. H., and Smith, D. R.: Urethral resistance: Its components and implications. Invest. Urol., *7*:195, 1969.

Tang, P. C.: Levels of brain stem and diencephalon controlling micturition reflex. J. Neurophysiol., *18*:583, 1955.

Tang, P. C., and Ruch, T. C.: Non-neurogenic basis of bladder tonus. Am. J. Physiol., *181*:249, 1955.

Tohyama, M., Satoh, K., and Sakaumoto, T.: Organization and projections of the neurons in the dorsal tegmental area of the rat. J. Hirnforsch., *19*:165, 1978.

Twiddy, D. A. S., Downie, J. W., and Awad, S. A.: Response of the bladder to bethanechol after acute spinal cord transection in the cat. J. Pharmacol. Exp. Ther., *215*:500, 1980.

Uemura, E., Fletcher, T. F., and Bradley, W. E.: Distribution of lumbar and sacral afferent axons in submucosa of cat urinary bladder. Anat. Rec., *183*:579, 1975.

Uemura, E., Fletcher, T. F., and Bradley, W. E.: Distribution of lumbar afferent axons in muscle coat of cat urinary bladder. Am. J. Anat., *139*:389, 1974.

Uemura, E., Fletcher, T. F., and Bradley, W. E.: Distribution of sacral afferent axons in the urinary bladder of the cat. Am. J. Anat., *136*:305, 1973.

Urry, D. W.: Molecular structures and mechanisms of transmembrane channels. *In* Haber, B., et al. (Eds.): Proteins in the Nervous System: Structure and Function. New York, Alan R. Liss, 1982, pp. 87–111.

Ursillo, R. C.: Electrical activity of the isolated nerve–urinary bladder strip preparation of the rabbit. Am. J. Physiol., *201*:408, 1961.

Uvelus, B., and Gabella, G.: Relation between cell length and force production in urinary bladder smooth muscle. Acta Physiol. Scand., *110*:357, 1980.

Vaalasti, A., and Hervonew, A.: Autonomic innervation of the human prostate. Invest. Urol., *17*:293, 1980.

Verecken, R. L., Nieirsman, M. D., Puers, B., and Van Mulders, J.: Electrophysiological exploration of the sacral conus. J. Neurol., *227*:135, 1982.

Von Garrelts, B.: Intravesical pressure and urinary flow during micturition in normal subjects. Acta Chir. Scand., *114*:49, 1957.

Wear, J. B.: Biofeedback in urology using urodynamics. J. Urol., *121*:464, 1979.

Winter, D. L.: Receptor characteristics and conduction velocities in bladder afferents. J. Psychiatr. Res., *8*:225, 1971.

Wojcik, G., Lupa, K., and Niechy, A.: Differential decerebrate control of depolarization in the central terminals of cutaneous afferents in the sacral cord. Brain Res., *266*:233, 1983.

Woodside, J. R., and McGuire, E. J.: Urethral hypotonicity after suprasacral spinal cord injury. J. Urol., *121*:783, 1979.

Zacharin, R. F.: The suspensory mechanism of the female urethra. J. Anat., *97*:423, 1963.

Zinner, N. R., Ritter, R. C., Sterling, A. M., and Danker, P.: The physical basis of some urodynamic measurements. J. Urol., *117*:682, 1977.

Zinner, N. R., Sterling, A. M., and Ritter, R. C.: Structure and forces of continence. *In* Raz, S. (Ed.): Female Urology. Philadelphia, W. B. Saunders Co., 1983.

Zinner, N. R., Sterling, A. M., and Ritter, R. C.: Role of inner urethral softness in urinary incontinence. Urology, *16*:115, 1980.

CHAPTER 5

Physiology of Male Reproduction

Hypothalamic-Pituitary Function

R. S. SWERDLOFF, M.D.

THE HYPOTHALAMIC-PITUITARY-GONADAL AXIS

The reproductive hormonal axis in men consists of five main components: (1) the extra-hypothalamic central nervous system; (2) the hypothalamus; (3) the pituitary gland; (4) the testis; and (5) the gonadal steroid-sensitive end-organs (Fig. 5–1). The components of this system function in a closely regulated manner to produce the concentrations of circulating gonadal steroids required for normal male sexual development and maintenance of sexual behavior. The reproductive axis also regulates the maturation of sperm necessary for normal fertility.

The hypothalamus is the site of production of small peptide hormone, GnRH (gonadotropin-releasing hormone), which is transported to the pituitary gland by a short portal venous system connecting the two areas. GnRH stimulates the synthesis and release of two gonadotropic hormones, LH (luteinizing hormone) and FSH (follicle-stimulating hormone). These two hormones, named after their function in females but produced in both sexes, are secreted into the general circulation and carried to the testis. In the testis they stimulate gonadal steroid secretion and are important in the maturation and maintenance of spermatogenesis. The secreted gonadal androgens, testosterone and dihydrotestosterone, act on numerous end-organs to cause development of male secondary sexual characteristics and to control (inhibit) the secre-

tion of gonadotropins. Nonsteroid secretory products of the testis may also have regulatory effects on gonadotropins.

An understanding of the reproductive axis is critical for the assessment of hypogonadism, infertility, gynecomastia, abnormal sex organ development (pseudohermaphroditism), and delayed and precocious puberty; it also may be important in the assessment and management of patients with benign hypertrophy and carcinoma of the prostate. The function and control of each of the components of the reproductive axis will be considered in detail in this and the following sections of this chapter.

Extrahypothalamic Central Nervous System

There is ample evidence in experimental animals that extrahypothalamic brain, such as the amygdala, hippocampus, and mesencephalon tissue, has both augmentary and inhibitory influences on reproductive function (Sawyer, 1974). The amygdala, a portion of the limbic system, sends signals that affect neuroendocrine function to both the anterior hypothalamic area and the ventromedial hypothalamus (VMH). The hippocampus, another portion of the limbic system, also sends projections to the VMH but through a different pathway. The midbrain connections to many areas of the hypothalamus, including the preoptic, anterior, arcuate, and medial basal hypothalamus, have been long

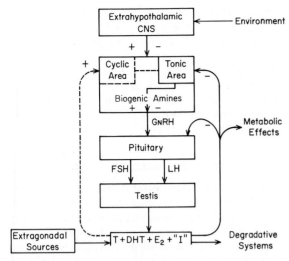

Figure 5–1. Schematic representation of the hypothalamic-pituitary-gonadal axis in the male.

established and include neurons containing the biogenic amines norepinephrine and serotonin. Although there is considerable controversy concerning the roles that the amygdala and hippocampus play in influencing gonadotropin secretion (Elendorff and Parvizi, 1980), it is clear that they are involved in conveying information from sensory systems to the hypothalamus. The sensory systems of olfaction and vision are known to have important influences on reproductive function in lower animals (Bronson, 1968; Michael, 1975; Reppert, 1980), but not all these effects have been demonstrated in humans.

In rats the diurnal rhythm of gonadotropins appears to be related to the light-dark cycle, and the effects seem to be mediated through a visual-pineal pathway influencing melatonin production. Data to support this concept include the identification of the neural pathway by which light-induced neural signals pass through the suprachiasmatic nucleus in the hypothalamus and extend to the pineal gland through noradrenergic pathways from the superior cervical ganglia (Moore, 1973). These noradrenergic signals stimulate the synthesis and activity of enzymes required for melatonin synthesis (Klein and Moore, 1979); melatonin, in turn, modulates gonadotropin secretion. Thus, light inhibits noradrenergic activity and lowers melatonin levels during the day; in the absence of light exposure, melatonin increases at night (Wilkinson et al., 1977). Levels of melatonin in the blood and urine respond rapidly to changes in photic stimulation in mammals, including nonhuman primates, producing a circadian rhythm.

Data in humans are less clear, in that diurnal changes in gonadotropins are not affected by constant light (Jimerson et al., 1977) and acute exposure to light at night does not decrease melatonin levels (Wetterberg, 1978).

While acute influences of light on gonadotropins or melatonin in humans are not significant, chronic absence or alteration in light may influence melatonin levels. Arendt and coworkers (1977) have reported a biannual melatonin rhythm in adults in Switzerland, with high values in the winter and low values in the summer. Although no definitive causal relationships between melatonin and other hormone rhythms (e.g., gonadotropins) have been established in humans, a temporal relationship between the nocturnal rise in LH in pubertal males and melatonin levels has been reported (Fevre et al., 1978). Circumstantial evidence linking visual stimuli and the reproductive system include the observations of Zacharias and Wurtman (1974) demonstrating that menarche occurs earlier in blind girls. Similar studies have not been done in boys, but blind men do not appear to have abnormal night-day patterns of blood LH, FSH, or testosterone (Bodenheimer et al., 1973).

Evidence that higher cortical function may influence reproductive function in humans includes the frequent occurrence of menstrual abnormalities in emotionally stressed women and the demonstration of depressed serum testosterone levels in mentally stressed men (Kreutz et al., 1972).

The Hypothalamus

The hypothalamus is the integrating center of the reproductive hormonal axis. It is at this level that both neural messages from the central nervous system and at least part of the humoral messages from the testis act to modulate the secretion of gonadotropin-releasing hormone, which is released into the hypophyseal-portal vessels that connect the median eminence with the adenohypophysis. Anatomically, the hypothalamus (Fig. 5–2) is bounded anteriorly by the optic chiasm, posteriorly by the mammillary bodies, laterally by the sulci formed with the temporal lobes, and superiorly by the thalamus. The most inferior portion of the hypothalamus is the median eminence, from which descends the pituitary stalk. The hypothalamus contains a large number of nuclei that are responsible for homeostatic control of many endocrine and nonendocrine systems. The anterior and ventral-medial areas of the hypothalamus are particu-

PHYSIOLOGY OF REPRODUCTION

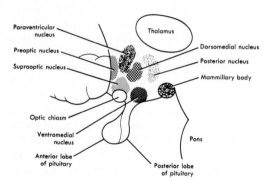

Figure 5–2. Diagrammatic representation of hypothalamic nuclei in man. (From Odell, W. D., and Moyar, D. L. *In* Physiology of Reproduction. St. Louis, C. V. Mosby Co., 1971. Used by permission.)

larly involved in control of gonadotropin secretion.

BIOGENIC AMINES

Biogenic amine secretions from nerve terminals in the hypothalamus are now believed to have important modulating influences on the secretion of GnRH. The majority of the data now available indicate that noradrenergic input (norepinephrine) augments secretion of GnRH (Barraclough and Wise, 1982; Kalra and Kalra, 1983). Dopamine has very important inhibitory effects on prolactin secretion (Yen, 1978), and while it is believed by many investigators to have inhibitory effects on GnRH secretion (Sawyer, 1975), considerable controversy exists about the latter concept (Vijayan and McCann, 1978; Kawakami et al., 1979). The influence of biogenic amines on the secretion of gonadotropins has clinical as well as physiologic importance. For instance, the well-known effects of reserpine and chlorpromazine on depression of reproductive function can now be ascribed to their inhibitory effects on norepinephrine secretion (Coppola, 1971; Barraclough and Wise, 1982) and subsequent decrease in gonadotropin secretion. Other putative neurotransmitter substances, such as endorphins and the indolamines (melatonin and serotonin) (Kalra, 1983; Rasmussen et al., 1981), may serve important regulatory functions on GnRH release from the hypothalamus. Male opiate addicts have low LH and testosterone levels and are sometimes sexually impotent (Meites et al., 1979). Administration of naloxone, a specific opiate receptor antagonist, reverses the LH inhibition produced by morphine treatment. When administered alone, naloxone increases basal LH and FSH

levels and stimulates the frequency of pulses of LH in men and women (Grossman et al., 1981). It thus appears that the site of action of opiates is at the hypothalamic level. The hypothalamus (especially the supraoptic and arcuate nuclei) has androgen and estrogen receptors and responds to differences in circulation concentrations of sex steroids by directly or indirectly changing the rate of synthesis and/or release of GnRH.

GONADOTROPIN-RELEASING HORMONE

It is now well established that a single hypothalamic decapeptide GnRH (Schally et al., 1971) has stimulatory effects on the pituitary gland that result in enhanced synthesis and release of both gonadotropic hormones, LH and FSH.

GnRH has been identified in many areas of the central nervous system but is most concentrated in the medial basal region of the hypothalamus, extending caudally and ventrally from the suprachiasmatic region to the arcuate nucleus and median eminence. GnRH is synthesized in the neurosecretory neurons and transported by axoplasmic flow to the axon terminals in the median eminence (McCann and Moss, 1975).

GnRH is released into the portal circulation in pulse, occurring at a frequency averaging one pulse every 70 to 90 minutes (Knobil, 1980; Carmel et al., 1976). GnRH has a very short half-life in the blood (approximately 2 to 5 minutes). The pituitary gland is therefore exposed to high levels of GnRH in hypophyseal-portal blood for brief periods of time. This pulsatile pattern of GnRH release appears to be essential for stimulatory effects on LH or FSH release (Belchetz et al., 1978; Wildt et al., 1981), whereas constant exposure of the gonadotropins to GnRH results in paradoxical inhibitory effects on LH and FSH release (Belchetz et al., 1978). The latter observation has been exploited by the development of long-acting GnRH analogs that suppress LH and testosterone secretion (Labrie et al., 1978; Swerdloff et al., 1983) for use as a chemical treatment of metastatic prostate cancer (Tolis et al., 1982). Variations in the pulse frequency of GnRH release may be important in determining the relative ratio of LH and FSH secreted into the peripheral circulation. Data now accumulating indicate that shortening the pulse frequency of GnRH release increases the LH to FSH ratio; lengthening the interval between GnRH pulses decreases the ratio of LH to FSH (Wildt et al., 1981). Sex steroids, neurotrans-

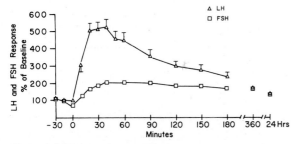

Figure 5–3. Serum LH and FSH response to a 300 μg bolus dose of LRH in normal men. A peak response of LH is seen at 20 to 40 minutes after injection. (Modified with permission from Wollesen, F., et al.: Metabolism, 25:1275, 1976.)

mitters, and pituitary gonadotropins may all modulate the pulse frequency and amplitude of GnRH secretion.

Although systems have been developed to assay GnRH in body fluids, attempts to measure this substance in the peripheral blood of animals or humans have been fraught with problems. Bioassays using large amounts of peripheral blood have been performed (Malacara et al., 1972), but these do not lend themselves well to dynamic testing; the radioimmunoassays currently available appear to be of borderline sensitivity and are adversely affected by nonspecific substances in the serum or plasma of man (Arimura et al., 1974; Ben-Jonathan et al., 1974; Keye et al., 1973; Nett et al., 1974). Clinically useful measurements of GnRH in systemic blood are not available at the present time.

GnRH has been synthesized and is available for administration in research and diagnostic studies in both experimental animals and humans. When administered intravenously, it acts rapidly, resulting in prompt release of LH and, to a much lesser extent, FSH into the blood stream (Fig. 5–3) (Wollesen et al., 1976). The response of the pituitary to GnRH is influenced by the presence of gonadal steroids (see later discussion of feedback). Testosterone hypogonadism results in an augmented response (Marshall, 1975).

Since administered GnRH should have a direct effect on the pituitary gland, it was hoped that GnRH testing would distinguish patients with hypogonadotropic hypogonadism of pituitary origin from those with hypothalamic disease. It was reasoned that those with pituitary disease would not respond to GnRH, whereas those with hypothalamic disorders would secrete LH and FSH normally after administration of GnRH. Unfortunately, a single pulse dose of GnRH is inadequate to reliably separate these

two varieties of hypogonadotropic hypogonadism (Marshall et al., 1972). One probable reason for the decreased pituitary response to GnRH in some patients with hypothalamic disorders causing hypogonadotropic hypogonadism is that the pituitary glands are chronically understimulated and have developed neither the stored reserves nor the biosynthetic machinery to respond normally to a single bolus dose of the hypothalamic hormone. This concept has been supported by evidence that repeated GnRH administration to patients with hypothalamic GnRH deficiency results in a greater response to each individual bolus dose of GnRH (Besser and Mortimer, 1974; Yoshimoto et al., 1975). This approach should be used in the attempt to separate GnRH deficiency from pituitary disease.

Pituitary

SECRETION AND MEASUREMENTS OF GONADOTROPINS (LH AND FSH)

Luteinizing hormone and follicle-stimulating hormone are glycopeptides consisting of two peptide chains (alpha and beta) (Papkoff et al., 1973; Reichert and Ward, 1974; Shome and Parlow, 1974; Ward et al., 1973). LH and FSH share a common alpha peptide chain (alpha chain) with a third pituitary hormone, TSH (thyroid-stimulating hormone), and differ from each other by the presence of a specific beta chain, the latter providing specificity of biologic action (Pierce, 1971). The function of the carbohydrate portions of the molecules is uncertain, but one important role is protection from biologic degradation (Van Hall et al., 1971).

LH and FSH are synthesized in the pituitary gland, released into the systemic blood system, and carried to the gonad, where they exert their effects. Both hormones are usually measured in the blood by radioimmunoassay techniques. Normal adult male levels of serum LH, FSH, and testosterone are presented in Table 5–1. The values determined by radioimmunoassay are fairly representative of those in the experience of other investigators. Because standards and antisera used in the assays may vary from

TABLE 5–1. SERUM LH, FSH, TESTOSTERONE, AND ESTRADIOL IN NORMAL ADULT MALES

LH	<1–15 mIU/ml
FSH	<1–15 mIU/ml
Testosterone	300–1100 ng/100 ml
Estradiol	<50 pg/ml

laboratory to laboratory, each clinician must be provided with the normal range as determined in the laboratory he is using. These radioimmunoassay techniques have replaced older bioassay methods (e.g., mouse uterine weight bioassay for total urinary gonadotropin) (Swerdloff and Odell, 1968), which were more cumbersome and often less specific in their ability to separate LH, FSH, and TSH. The LH radioimmunoassay that is generally available does not distinguish between LH and human chorionic gonadotropin (hCG). Although the latter substance is found only in pregnant women (normal and abnormal), a closely related substance is usually found in high concentrations in the blood of subjects with choriocarcinoma of the testis and may also be produced by a large number of other neoplasms (Odell, 1974). Neoplastic production of gonadotropin is best assessed by using a BhCG assay, which does not detect the normal LH levels in men. Under certain circumstances the biologic activity of LH or FSH may differ from its immunologic measurement. For this reason, radioreceptor assays (displacement of radiolabeled LH from specific LH receptors) (Leidenberger and Reichert, 1972) and in vitro bioassays (stimulation of testosterone release from Leydig cell incubates) have been developed (Dufau et al., 1974). These techniques are usually reserved for special research problems.

Because the metabolic clearance rate of LH is considerably greater than that of FSH, there is a more rapid disappearance of the former hormone from the circulation. Both hormones are secreted in an episodic fashion by the pituitary gland, but the longer survival time of FSH in the circulation is reflected by a more constant serum level of that hormone than of the more rapidly metabolized luteinizing hormone (Coble et al., 1969; Kohler et al., 1968; Marshall et al., 1973). The episodic secretion of LH and FSH results in considerable short-term variation in the serum concentrations of the two hormones. The peak-and-valley pattern of blood levels of gonadotropins is of practical clinical importance in that single measurements of circulating LH may be as much as 50 per cent above or below mean integrated hormone concentrations (Santen and Bardin, 1973) (Fig. 5–4). The amplitude of the swings in serum values produced by episodic secretion of gonadotropins is least in prepubertal children and greatest in hypogonadal patients. Significant episodic secretion of LH and FSH begins to appear in midpuberty, during which time it is specifically related to sleep (Boyar et al., 1972). As sexual maturation

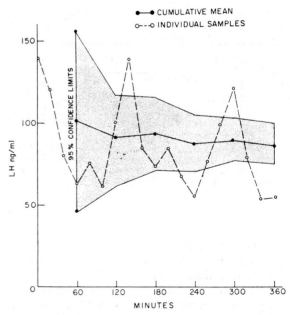

Figure 5–4. The solid line and shaded area are the cumulative mean LH level and the 95 per cent confidence limits of that mean at hourly intervals for 6 hours in a single patient. For comparison, the dotted lines and open circles represent the actual estimates of serum LH in samples obtained at 20-minute intervals. (From Santen, R. J., and Bardin, C. W.: J. Clin. Invest., 52:2617, 1973. Used by permission.)

progresses, the periodic secretion of LH becomes generalized throughout the sleep-wake cycle, and specific sleep-related elevation become less apparent. Other than these pubertal sleep-related nocturnal elevations, diurnal variations of LH and FSH do not appear to be significant in the evaluation of adult humans.

INTERRELATIONSHIP BETWEEN PROLACTIN AND GONADOTROPINS

Hyperprolactinemia is associated with disturbed reproductive functions as reflected by lowered serum testosterone levels and symptoms of hypogonadism (Carter, 1978). The mechanisms by which hyperprolactinemia induces testosterone deficiency is complex, but serum LH levels are suppressed or inappropriately low (relative to serum testosterone) in most cases, indicating that the hypothalamic-pituitary axis fails to respond to reduced testicular testosterone production. It appears that prolactin may inhibit GnRH secretion, since the pituitary responds normally to GnRH administration and the pulse frequency of LH secretion is impaired in hyperprolactinemic patients. Prompt and dramatic improvement in sexual function occurs in many hyperprolactinemic men treated with bromocriptine (dopamine agonist with prolactin-lowering activity) (Carter et al., 1978; Spark et al., 1980; Thorner et al., 1980). There is evidence to suggest that hyperprolactinemia may impair sexual function in men both by direct effect on the central nervous system and by inhibition of androgen secretion. The direct CNS effect is supported by clinical data demonstrating that androgen replacement therapy of hyperprolactinemic hypoandrogenized men did not return libido to normal as long as prolactin levels remained elevated (Carter et al., 1978). Finally, it must be recognized that some patients with prolactinomas will have hypogonadotropic hypogonadism produced by the mass lesion itself.

FEEDBACK CONTROL OF GONADOTROPINS

As depicted in Figure 5–1, the hypothalamic-pituitary-gonadal system consists of a closed-loop feedback control mechanism directed at maintaining normal reproductive function. In this system, gonadal hormones have inhibitory effects on the secretion of LH and FSH. This is easily demonstrated by the rise in serum LH and FSH that occurs after orchiectomy (Fig. 5–5) (Walsh et al., 1973). As seen in Figure 5–5, LH and FSH levels continue to rise for a long period after castration, reaching maximum levels as late as 25 to 50 days after surgery.

Although it is generally held that testosterone, the major secretory product of the testis, is the primary inhibitor of LH secretion in men, a number of testis products, including estrogens and other androgens, have the ability to inhibit LH secretion (Swerdloff et al., 1973).

Estradiol, a potent estrogen, is produced both from the testis and from peripheral conversion of androgens and androgen precursors (Longscope et al., 1969). Although the concentration of estradiol in the blood of men is relatively low compared with testosterone, it is a much more potent inhibitor of LH and FSH secretion (approximately 1000-fold) (Swerdloff and Walsh, 1973). The data indicate that estradiol in a dose equivalent to that derived from peripheral conversion of physiologic concentrations of testosterone will account for 60 per cent of the decline in LH seen with testosterone administration. This suggests that much, but not all, of the gonadotropin-regulating effects of testosterone could be mediated through estradiol. In addition to the potential direct role of estradiol in inhibition of the hypothalamic-pituitary axis, local metabolic conversion (aromatization) of testosterone or other androgen precursors to estradiol may occur in the hypothalamus, in which case estradiol inhibits GnRH production (Naftolin et al., 1971). Other mechanisms may be important, since androgens that cannot be converted to estradiol are potent inhibitors of LH and FSH (Naftolin and Feder, 1973; Stewart-Bentley et al., 1974; Swerdloff et al., 1972). In order to better define the relative role of androgens and estrogens in the control of LH secretions in intact men, attempts have been made to infuse steroids in amounts that would produce physiologic concentrations of the hormones in the blood (Sherins and Loriaux, 1973; Stewart-Bentley et al., 1974). These studies demonstrate suppression of LH levels by physiologic concentrations of both testosterone and estradiol, suggesting that both hormones may be important in LH regulation. Although it is possible that a synergistic effect of the two hormones may be responsible for physiologic

Figure 5–5. Effect of bilateral orchiectomy on serum LH and FSH concentrations in three men. (From Walsh, P. C., Swerdloff, R. S., and Odell, W. D.: Acta Endocrinol., *74*:449, 1973.)

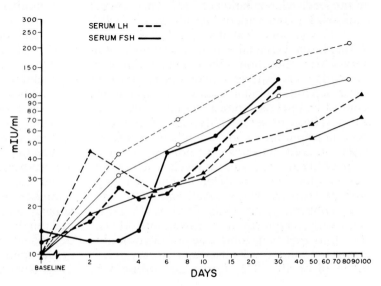

control of LH, data from experimental animals fail to demonstrate such synergism (Gay and Dever, 1971; Swerdloff and Walsh, 1973). It is of interest that patients with congenital end-organ resistance to testosterone (testicular feminization) may have a female phenotypic appearance associated with normal or above-normal serum estradiol levels and high blood LH concentrations (Faiman and Winter, 1974; Judd et al., 1972). These findings may suggest that testosterone rather than circulating estradiol is the most important physiologic controller of LH secretion.

The mechanism of feedback control of FSH secretion is even more controversial than that of LH. The rise in serum FSH after castration (Fig. 5–5) demonstrates the important role of the testis in the feedback control of FSH secretion. As for LH, both testosterone and estradiol are capable of suppressing FSH serum levels, although the relative importance of these two gonadal steroids remains undefined. In one study, Stewart-Bentley and associates (1974) infused near-physiologic amounts of testosterone and estradiol and reported suppression of LH but not FSH. Recent studies by Patterson and coworkers (1984) indicate that estradiol may have a preferential inhibitory effect on serum LH (relative to FSH) in male rats. In other studies in man, the same investigative group, Sherins and Loriaux (1973), using higher doses of steroids, reported suppression of both LH and FSH. Testosterone suppression of LH and FSH occurs even when aromatization to estradiol is blocked by testosterone (Marynick et al., 1979).

There is considerable evidence that a non-steroidal tubular factor may also be important in the feedback regulation of FSH. This concept dates back to the work of McCullagh and Walsh (1935), who suggested that a substance originating in the germinal epithelium inhibits pituitary FSH production. They named this substance inhibin. Further support for the concept of a separate tubular factor responsible for control of FSH secretion is based on evidence of elevations of serum FSH concentrations in men in whom the germinal epithelium is selectively injured, as shown by normal serum or urinary LH and testosterone levels. Circumstances in which this group of findings are seen include testis irradiation (Paulsen, 1968), antispermatogenic agents (Van Thiel et al., 1972), and early cryptorchidism (Swerdloff et al., 1971), as well as in some cases of oligospermia or azoospermia (de Kretser and Burger, 1972; Leonard et al., 1972; Rosen and Weintraub,

1971). Howard and colleagues, (1950) suggested that inhibin is secreted by the Sertoli cells. A peptide substance with selective FSH-inhibiting activities has been reported from both the semen and the testis of experimental animals (Franchimont et al., 1975; Lee et al., 1974). A number of investigators have attempted to purify these FSH-inhibitory substances from testes, follicular fluid, and seminal fluid. These reports vary greatly in the estimated molecular weight of their putative inhibin hormones (Sairam et al., 1983; de Kretser et al., 1983; Krishnan et al., 1982). It must be emphasized that even in pathologic states in which marked damage to the germinal tissue occurs, serum FSH is not elevated to castration levels unless Leydig cell function is also impaired. Both gonadal steroids and a tubular inhibitory factor thus appear to be important in maintaining normal serum FSH concentrations.

Testis

HORMONAL CONTROL OF SPERMATOGENESIS

Spermatogenesis is a complex process whereby a primitive stem cell, the Type A spermatogonium, passes a complex series of transformations to give rise to spermatozoa; in man this takes 73 days. The development of the male germ cells in the seminiferous tubule essentially consists of three phases: spermatogonial multiplication, meiosis, and spermogenesis. In the seminiferous epithelium, cells in these developmental phases are arranged in defined associations or stages. Along the seminiferous tubules, in most mammals, these stages follow one another in a regular fashion, giving rise to the wave of the seminiferous epithelium. The time interval between the appearance of the same cell association at a given point of the tubule is called the cycle of the seminiferous epithelium (Parvinen, 1982).

Although the dependence of spermatogenesis on pituitary FSH and on intratesticular testosterone has been emphasized, the precise nature of interaction between these hormones and germ cells remains poorly understood. FSH and androgens seem to have different preferential sites of action during the cycle of the seminiferous epithelium. Stages VII and VIII appear to be androgen-dependent, while maximal binding of FSH and activation of FSH-dependent enzymes occurs in Stages XIII to XV of the spermatogenic cycle (Gordeladze et al., 1982; Ritzen et al., 1981).

Steinberger (1971) demonstrated that in the hypophysectomized immature rat, testosterone alone could account for initiation of spermatogenesis and that FSH was required only for its completion (spermatid to spermatozoa). Unlike the rat, exogenous administration of testosterone to hypogonadotropic men does not induce spermatogenesis. This failure in the human is probably due to the practical limits of the dose that can be administered. By contrast, hCG administration stimulates an increase in intratesticular testosterone and promptly initiates spermatogenesis. Furthermore, in boys with precocious puberty, caused by localized Leydig cell tumors, the tubules adjacent to the androgen-producing tumors have been shown to undergo germinal maturation while the contralateral testis remains unstimulated, despite virilizing peripheral serum concentrations of testosterone. In hypogonadotropic men treated with hCG alone, maturation of the seminiferous epithelium frequently does not progress beyond the spermatid stage. In these patients, FSH alone does not initiate spermatogenesis. However, its administration to hCG-primed hypogonadal men results in completion of spermatogenesis and production of an adequate number of sperm for impregnation. Thus, both in man and in rat, FSH appears to be essential for spermiogenesis (development of spermatid into mature spermatozoa). It remains unclear, however, whether FSH is required for maintenance of spermatogenesis. In hypogonadotropic subjects primed with hCG and FSH, spermatogenesis can be maintained by hCG alone (Sherins et al., 1977).

In addition to androgens and FSH, many other proteins are secreted locally in the tubule in a cyclic fashion during the cycle of the seminiferous epithelium. The putative role of these proteins as mediators of Sertoli cell–germ cell interaction involved in the local control of spermatogenesis remains to be well characterized (Parvinen, 1982).

Changes in the Reproductive Axis with Age

CHANGES DURING SEXUAL MATURATION

The human fetal pituitary gland has the capacity not only to synthesize and store FSH and LH but also to secrete these hormones in high concentrations during gestation. Fetal serum FSH and LH levels seem to peak at midgestation (Kaplan et al., 1976). The decline during late gestation may be the result of maturation of the capacity of the hypothalamic-pituitary axis to respond to negative feedback by gonadal steroids. The same authors have noted a sex difference in fetal gonadotropins, with females having higher peak levels (particularly of FSH) than do males.

During the first years of life, serum LH and FSH levels are detectable in the blood; the concentrations of both hormones are low at birth but rise for several weeks after birth, reaching levels considerably above the lowest levels seen later between the ages of 6 and 8 years (Faiman and Winter, 1974). Figure 5–6 presents serum LH, FSH, and testosterone concentrations in boys aged 2 to 21 years (Swerdloff and Odell, 1975). There is a progressive rise from approximately age 6 to 8 years, with the increase in FSH slightly preceding the increase in LH concentrations. In contrast to the slow progressive rise in gonadotropins, there is a much steeper increase in blood testosterone, beginning at approximately age 10 to 12 years. Figure 5–7 shows the sleep-related development of the episodic secretion of LH and FSH seen in children at midpuberty (Boyar et al., 1972). As will be described in subsequent sections, LH is the primary stimulus for testosterone secretion, while both LH and FSH are important determinants of the induction and maintenance of the spermatogenic process.

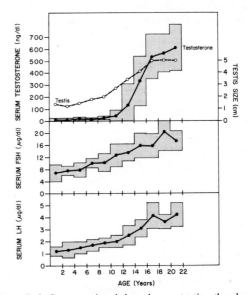

Figure 5–6. Cross-sectional data demonstrating the changes in testis size and serum LH, FSH, and testosterone during sexual maturation in boys. Not shown in this figure are the relatively higher LH and FSH levels seen in the first year of life. (From Swerdloff, R. S., and Odell, W. D.: Postgrad. Med. J., *51*:200, 1975. Used by permission.)

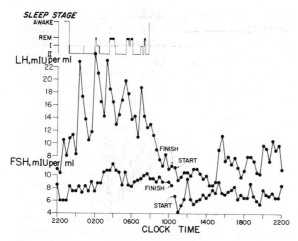

Figure 5–7. Plasma LH and FSH concentration samples every 20 minutes for 24 hours in a normal pubertal child. Gonadotropin levels are elevated during sleep. (From Boyar, R. M., et al.: N. Engl. J. Med., *289*:283, 1973. Used by permission.)

CHANGES IN OLD AGE

Decreased testicular function is frequently seen in elderly men (Swerdloff and Heber, 1982; Vermeulen et al., 1972). While there is considerable controversy as to whether this effect is a necessary concomitant of aging or reflects associated illness in aged men (Harman and Tsitouras, 1980; Sparrow et al., 1980), lowered serum testosterone levels are common in men in the seventh, eighth, and ninth decades of life (Fig. 5–8).

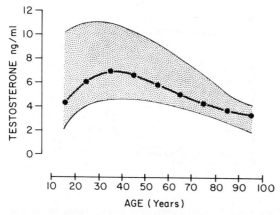

Figure 5–8. Decline with age of total testosterone. Shaded area = range of individual values. (From Baker, H. W. G., Burger, H. G., de Kretser, D. M., and Hudson, B.: Endocrinology of aging: Pituitary testicular axis. Proc. 5th Intl. Congress of Endocrinology, 1976, pp. 479–483.)

Circulating levels of both LH and FSH are increased with aging (Baker et al., 1976; Greenblatt et al., 1976; Rubens et al., 1974; Albert, 1956; Christiansen, 1972; Hashimoto et al., 1973; Haug et al., 1974; Snyder et al., 1975), providing further evidence for a primary defect at a testicular level (Fig. 5–9). Despite the wide individual variations shown in Figure 5–9, there is a consistent increase in gonadotropin levels over the age of 40. A relatively greater increase in FSH compared with LH has been reported (Christiansen, 1972), suggesting that seminiferous tubule degeneration with decreased inhibin production occurs to a greater extent than do decreases in Leydig cell function. Walsh and coworkers (1973) found that those elderly men with the greatest FSH elevations evidenced significant changes in seminiferous tubule morphology.

While the evidence for primary testicular abnormalities seems clear-cut, an additional or secondary pituitary defect has been suggested based on the observation that serum testosterone concentrations remain below normal while the testes retain the ability to respond to exogenous gonadotropin with increased testosterone secretion. Haug (1974) and Snyder and their coworkers (1975) found that both the absolute rise in gonadotropins and the ratio of stimulated to basal gonadotropins following standard GnRH testing were decreased in older men compared with younger men. Ryan (1962) found that the pituitary content of LH was increased in a group of men aged 50 to 80 compared with a group of younger men. Since the pituitary has further reserves of gonadotropin to secrete in response to lowered levels of testosterone, the question of why LH secretion is not further increased to stimulate more testosterone secretion remains unanswered.

Several explanations for decreased pituitary function with aging have been proposed. Kley and associates (1974) suggested that increased levels of estrogen and other circulating steroids would tend to inhibit gonadotropin secretion despite lowered levels of testosterone. Alternatively, centers mediating hypothalamic sensitivity to steroid feedback termed the "gonadostat" might be altered to respond to lowered levels of testosterone in aged men with inhibition of pituitary function. Such increased sensitivity to steroidal feedback occurs in prepubertal man, but there is as yet no direct evidence of such a change in feedback sensitivity in elderly men. Finally, there may be an age-related decrease in pituitary gonadotroph cellular responsiveness secondary to changes in pituitary

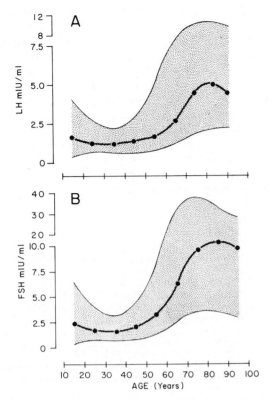

Figure 5–9. *A,* Rise in serum LH with aging. *B,* Rise in serum FSH with aging. Shaded area = range of individual values. (From Baker, H. W. G., Burger, H. G., de Kretser, D. M., and Hudson, B.: Endocrinology of aging: Pituitary testicular axis. Proc. 5th Intl. Congress of Endocrinology, 1976, pp. 479–483.)

GnRH receptor number or steps beyond receptor-binding mediating gonadotropin secretion.

In summary, a primary defect in the reproductive hormonal axis with aging occurs at a gonadal level as a result of decreased numbers of Leydig cells and degenerative seminiferous tubule changes. These changes at a testicular level result in elevations of circulating gonadotropins, but there is evidence of decreased pituitary gonadotropin secretory responses, at least to exogenous GnRH. The origins of the apparent reductions in pituitary responsiveness at a pituitary, hypothalamic, or extrahypothalamic CNS level are not clear at present and deserve further investigation.

THE HYPOTHALAMIC-PITUITARY AXIS AND THE ASSESSMENT OF HYPOGONADAL PATIENTS

Patients with under-androgenization and lowered serum testosterone levels usually fall into one of two pathophysiologic classes: primary testicular disease or a hypothalamic-pituitary disorder. These two general classes can be differentiated by the measurement of serum levels of LH and FSH.

Patients with primary Leydig cell damage have diminished feedback inhibition of gonadotropin secretion, resulting in high serum LH and FSH concentrations; this disease is therefore classified as hypergonadotropic hypogonadism. Such patients would be expected to have a diminished Leydig cell reserve and a blunted testosterone response to administered LH or to the LH-like effects of hCG (Fig. 5–10) (Paulsen et al., 1968).

The disease in patients with low serum testosterone and low or inappropriately low-normal serum LH levels is classified as hypogonadotropic hypogonadism. Such patients have an abnormality involving either the hypothalamus or the pituitary gland. This defect can be structural, such as a hypothalamic or pituitary tumor. More frequently, it is functional and is due to one of the following: (1) administration of drugs that inhibit the hypothalamic axis, such as tranquilizers, androgens (non-testosterone), or estrogens; (2) congenital inability to synthesize GnRH or LH and FSH, as in congenital hypogonadotropic hypogonadism (such patients can have isolated LH or FSH deficiency or multiple tropic hormone defects); or (3) altered hypothalamic control mechanisms, as in starvation or anorexia nervosa. The differential diagnosis and clinical evaluation of hypogonado-

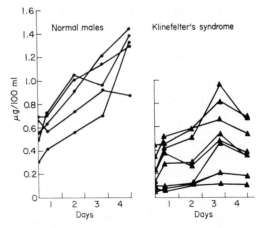

Figure 5–10. Plasma testosterone levels in normal males and in patients with Klinefelter's syndrome before and after administration of human chorionic gonadotropin (hCG). hCG was injected intramuscularly between 0800 and 0830 hours after the control plasma samples were obtained. (From Paulsen, C., Gordon, A., Carpenter, D. L., et al.: Rec. Progr. Horm. Res., *24:*321, 1973.)

tropic hypogonadism will be discussed in later chapters of this book.

In the absence of clinical or radiologic clues identifying the site of the defect, laboratory testing utilizing a single-pulse dose of GnRH may not always distinguish hypothalamic from pituitary defects. The limitations of LRH testing were discussed previously. We recommend testing such subjects with a 500 μg dose of GnRH given daily for 3 days. Serum LH should be measured before and 60 minutes after the last GnRH dose. A second test using clomiphene as the stimulus for LH and FSH secretion will be presented in detail in a later chapter. Although the mechanism of action of clomiphene is not absolutely clear, most evidence indicates that it interferes at a hypothalamic level with steroid feedback inhibition of gonadotropin secretion (Marshall, 1975). Since an intact pituitary is required for normal LH and FSH secretion, adult patients with either hypothalamic or pituitary defects will have an impaired response to clomiphene.

Difficulty also exists in separating delayed sexual maturation from incomplete hypogonadotropic hypogonadism because basal LH and FSH levels may be similarly low in both circumstances (Boyar et al., 1973). Since normal children prior to the second and third stages of puberty do not produce increased serum gonadotropins in response to administered clomiphene, this test is of little value in separating the two disorders (Marshall, 1975). GnRH testing may be of somewhat greater potential value but is limited by the smaller LH response in normal prepubertal children that can overlap with the response of patients with incomplete hypogonadotropic hypergonadism. Better resolution now seems possible by testing such patients with either chlorpromazine (Winters et al., 1982) or meteclopramide and assessing the prolactin response. Patients with delayed sexual maturation respond with an increase in serum prolactin (15 ng/ml), whereas those with hypogonadotropic hypogonadism do not. Newborns with hypogonadotropic hypogonadism may be identified by measuring the testicular volume sequentially during the first 3 months of life. Normal children will apparently double the testicular volume during this period (Cassorla et al., 1981).

Patients with severe germinal epithelial damage without concomitant loss of androgen function may have modest isolated elevation of serum FSH levels. Such a monotropic increase in FSH in patients with azoospermia or severe oligospermia is believed to be due to a decrease

of the putative germinal epithelial hormone, inhibin.

In rare instances, phenotypic male patients with clinical evidence of under-androgenization may have normal, high-normal, or elevated serum testosterone levels (Walsh et al., 1974; Wilson et al., 1974). Such patients have a partial peripheral defect in testosterone responsiveness. Classification of these disorders will be presented in Chapter 41. Serum LH levels in such patients may be either elevated or normal depending on whether hypothalamic response to testosterone is also impaired.

References

Albert, A.: Human urinary gonadotrophins. Rec. Prog. Horm. Res., 12:266, 1956.

Anton-Tay, F., and Wurtman, R.: Brain monoamines and endocrine function. In Martini, L., and Gonong, W. F. (Eds.). Frontiers in Neuroendocrinology, 1971. New York, Oxford University Press, 1971, p. 45.

Aoki, A., and Fawcett, D. W.: Is there a local feedback from the seminiferous tubules affecting activity of the Leydig cell? Biol. Reprod., 19:144, 1978.

Arendt, J., Wirtz-Justice, A., and Bradtke, J.: Annual rhythm of serum melatonin in man. Neurosci. Lett., 7:327, 1977.

Arimura, A., Kastin, A. J., and Schally, A. V.: Immunoreactive LH-releasing hormone in plasma: Midcycle elevation in women. J. Clin. Endocrinol. Metab., 38:510, 1974.

Baker, H. W. G., Burger, H. G., de Kretser, D. M., and Hudson, B.: Endocrinology of aging: Pituitary testicular axis. Proc. 5th Intl. Congress of Endocrinology, 1976, pp. 479–483.

Barraclough, C. A., and Wise, P. M.: The role of catecholamines in the regulation of pituitary luteinizing hormone and follicle-stimulating hormone secretion. Endocrine Rev., 3:91, 1982.

Belchetz, P. E., Plant, T. M., Nakai, Y., Keogh, E. J., and Knobil, E.: Hypophysial responses to continuous and intermittent delivery of hypothalamic gonadotropin releasing hormone. Science, 202:631, 1978.

Ben-Jonathan, N., Mical, R. S., and Porter, J. C.: Transport of LRF from CSF to hypophysial portal and systemic blood and the release of LH. Endocrinology, 95:18, 1974.

Besser, G. M., and Mortimer, C. H.: Effects of the gonadotropin releasing hormone in patients with hypothalamic-pituitary-gonadal diseases. Acta Fertil. Eur., 5:65, 1974.

Bhasin, S., Heber, D., Peterson, M., et al.: Partial isolation and characterization of testicular GnRH-like factors. Endocrinology, 112:1144, 1983.

Bodenheimer, S., Winter, J. S. D., and Faiman, C.: Diurnal rhythms of serum gonadotropins, testosterone, estradiol and cortisol in blind men. J. Clin. Endocrinol. Metab., 37:472, 1973.

Boyar, R., Finkelstein, J., Roffwarg, H., Kapen, S., Weitzman, E., and Hellman, L.: Synchronization of augmented luteinizing hormone secretion with sleep during puberty. N. Engl. J. Med., 287:582, 1972.

Boyar, R. M., Finkelstein, J. W., Witkin, M., Kapen, S., Weitzman, E., and Hellman, L.: Studies of endocrine function in "isolated" gonadotropin deficiency. J. Clin. Endocrinol. Metab., *36*:64, 1973.

Bronson, F. H.: Phenomenal influences on mammalian reproduction. *In* Diamond, M. (Ed.): Perspectives in Reproduction and Sexual Behavior. Bloomington, Indiana University Press, 1968, p. 341.

Brophy, P. J., and Grower, D. B.: Studies on the inhibition by 5-pregnane 3, 20-dione of the biosynthesis of 16-androstenes and dehydroepiandrosterone in boar testis preparations. Biochem. Biophys. Acta, *360*:252, 1974.

Carmel, P. W., Arani, S., and Ferin, M.: Pituitary stalk portal blood collection in rhesus monkeys: Evidence for pulsatile release of gonadotropin releasing hormone (GnRH). Endocrinology, *99*:243, 1976.

Carter, J. N., Tyson, J. E., Tolis, G., Van Vliet, S., Faiman, C., and Freesen, H. G.: Prolactin-secreting tumors and hypogonadism in 22 men. N. Engl. J. Med., *299*:847, 1978.

Cassorla, F. G., Golden, S. M., Johnsonbaugh, R. E., Heroman, W. M., et al.: Testicular volume during early infancy. J. Pediatr. *99*:742, 1981.

Chopra, I. J., Tulchinsky, D., and Greenway, F. L.: Estrogen androgen imbalance in hepatic cirrhosis. Am. J. Med., *79*:198, 1973.

Christiansen, P.: Urinary follicle-stimulating hormone and luteinizing hormone in normal adult men. Acta Endocrinol. (Copenh.), *71*:1, 1972.

Coble, Y. D., Jr., Kohler, P. O., Cargille, C. M., and Ross, G. T.: Production rates and metabolic clearance rates of human follicle-stimulating hormone in premenopausal and postmenopausal women. J. Clin. Invest., *48*:359, 1969.

Coppola, J. A.: Brain catecholamines and gonadotropin secretion. *In* Marin, L., and Ganong, W. F. (Eds.): Frontiers in Neuroendocrinology, 1971. New York, Oxford University Press, 1971.

de Kretser, D. M., and Burger, H. G.: Hormonal, histological and chromosomal studies in adult males with testicular disorders. J. Clin. Endocrinol. Metab., *35*:392, 1972.

de Kretser, D. M., Au, C. L., LeGac, F., and Robertson, D. M.: Recent studies on inhibin. *In* D'Agata, R., Lipsett, M. B., Polosa, P., et al. (Eds.): Recent advances in Male Reproduction: Molecular Basis and Clinical Implications. Vol. 7, New York, Raven Press, 1983, pp. 91–99.

Dufau, M. L., Hsueh, A. J., Agorraga, S., et al.: Inhibition of Leydig cell function through hormonal regulatory mechanisms. J. Androl., *2*:193, 1978.

Dufau, M. L., Mendelson, C., and Catt, K. J.: A highly sensitive in vitro bioassay for LH and hCG: testosterone production by dispersed Leydig cells. J. Clin. Endocrinol. Metab., *39*:610, 1974.

Ellendorff, F., and Parvizi, N.: Role of extrahypothalamic centers in neuroendocrine integration. *In* Motta, M. (Ed): The Endocrine Functions of the Brain. New York, Raven Press, 1980, pp. 297–325.

Faiman, C., and Winter, J. S. D.: The control of gonadotropin secretion in complete testicular feminization. J. Clin. Endocrinol. Metab., *39*:631, 1974.

Fevre, M., Segal, T., Marks, J. F., and Boyar, R. M.: LH and melatonin secretion patterns in pubertal boys. J. Clin. Endocrinol. Metab., *42*:1014, 1978.

Franchimont, P., Chari, S., Schellen, A. M., and Demoulin, A.: Relationship between gonadotropins, spermatogenesis, and seminal plasma. J. Steroid Biochem., *6*:1037, 1975.

Gay, V. L., and Dever, N. W.: Effects of testosterone propionate and estradiol benzoate alone or in combination on serum LH and FSH in orchidectomized rats. Endocrinology, *89*:161, 1971.

Gordeladze, J. O., Parvinen, M., Clausen, O. P. F., and Hansson, V.: Stage dependent variation in Mn^{++}-sensitive adenylyl cyclase (AC) activity in spermatids and FSH-sensitive Ac in Sertoli cells. Arch. Androl., *8*:43, 1982.

Greenblatt, R. B., Oettinger, M., and Bohler, C. S. S.: Estrogen-androgen levels in aging men and women: Therapeutic considerations. J. Am. Geriatr. Soc., *24*:173, 1976.

Grossman, A., Moult, P. J. A., Gaillard, R. C., Delitala, G., Toff, W. D., Rees, L. H., and Besser, G. M.: The opioid control of LH and FSH release: effects of a net-enkephalin analogue and naloxone. Clin. Endocrinol. *14*:41, 1981.

Harman, T. M., and Tsitouras, P. D.: Reproductive hormones in aging men. I. Measurement of sex steroids, basal luteinizing hormone and Leydig cell response to human chorionic gonadotropin. J. Clin. Endocrinol. Metab., *51*:35, 1980.

Hashimoto, T., Miyai, K., Izumi, K., and Kumahara, Y.: Gonadotrophin response to synthetic LHRH in normal subjects: Correlation between LH and FSH. J. Clin. Endocrinol. Metab., *37*:910, 1973.

Haug, E. A., Aakvaag, A., Sand, T., and Torjesen, P. A.: The gonadotropin response to synthetic GnRH in males in relation to age, dose and basal serum levels of testosterone, estradiol-17 beta and gonadotrophins. Acta Endocrinol. (Copenh.), *77*:625, 1974.

Hoffman, A. R., and Crowley, W. F., Jr.: Chronic low-dose pulsatile gonadotropin-releasing hormone treatment of idiopathic hypogonadotropic hypogonadism in men. *In* D'Agata, R., Lipsett, M. B., Polosa, P., and Van der Molen, H. (Eds.): Recent Advances in Male Reproduction: Molecular Basis and Clinical Implications. Vol. 7. New York, Raven Press: 1984, pp. 249–256.

Howard, R. P., Sniffen, R. C., Simmons, F. A., and Albright, F.: Testicular deficiency: A clinical and pathologic study. J. Clin. Endocrinol. Metab., *10*:121, 1950.

Hsu, A. V., and Troen, P.: An androgen-binding protein in the testicular cytosol of human testis. J. Clin. Invest., *61*:1611, 1978.

Hsueh, A. J., Dufau, M., and Catt, K. J.: Inhibitory effects of estrogen on Leydig cell function: Studies of FSH treated hypophysectomized rat. Endocrinology, *103*:1089, 1978.

Inano, H., and Tamaoki, B.: Bioconversion of steroids in immature rat testis in vitro. Endocrinology, *79*:579, 1966.

Jimerson, D. C., Lynch, J. J., Post, R. M., Wurtman, R. J., and Bunney, W. E.: Urinary melatonin rhythms during sleep deprivation in depressed patients and normals. Life Sci., *20*:1501, 1977.

Judd, H. L., Hamilton, C. R., Barlow, J. J., Yen, S. S. C., and Kliman, B.: Androgen and gonadotropin dynamics in testicular feminization syndrome. J. Clin. Endocrinol. Metab., *34*:229, 1972.

Kalra, S. P.: Opioid peptides—Inhibitory neuronal systems in regulation of gonadotropin secretion. *In* McCann, S. M., and Dhindsa, D. S. (Eds.): Role of Peptides and Proteins in Control of Reproduction. New York, Elsevier Biomedical, 1983, p. 63.

Kalra, S. P., and Kalra, P. S.: Neural regulation of luteinizing hormone secretion in the rat. Endocrine Rev., *4*:311, 1983.

Kaplan, S. L., Grumbach, M. M., and Aubert, M. L.: The ontogenesis of pituitary hormones and hypothalamic factors in the human fetus: Maturation of central nervous system regulation of anterior pituitary function. Rec. Prog. Horm. Res., 32:161, 1976.

Kawakami, M., Arita, J., Kimura, F., and Hayashi, R.: The stimulatory roles of catecholamines and acetylcholine in the regulation of gonadotropin release in ovariectomized estrogen-primed rats. Endocrinol. Jpn., 26:275, 1979.

Keye, W. R., Jr., Kelch, R. P., Niswender, G. D., and Jaffe, R. B.: Quantitation of endogenous and exogenous gonadotropin releasing hormone by radioimmunoassay. J. Clin. Endocrinol. Metab., 36:1263, 1973.

Klein, D. C., and Moore, R. Y.: Pineal N-acetyltransferase and hydroxyindole-O-methyltransferase: Control by the retina hypothalamic tract and the suprachiasmatic nucleus. Brain Res., 174:245, 1979.

Kley, H. K., Nieschlag, E., Bidlingmaier, F., and Kruskemper, H. L.: Possible age dependent influence of estrogens on the binding of testosterone in plasma of adult men. Horm. Metab. Res., 6:213, 1974.

Knobil, E.: The neuroendocrine control of menstrual cycle. Rec. Prog. Horm. Res., 36:53, 1980.

Knobil, E., Plant, T. M., Wildt, L., Belchetz, P. E., and Marshall, G.: Control of the rhesus monkey menstrual cycle: permissive role of hypothalamic gonadotropin releasing hormone. Science, 207:1371, 1980.

Kohler, P. O., Ross, G. T., and Odell, W. D.: Metabolic clearance and production rates of human luteinizing hormone in pre- and postmenopausal women. J. Clin. Invest., 47:38, 1968.

Kreutz, L. E., Rose, R. M., and Jennings, R.: Suppression of plasma testosterone levels and psychologic stress. Arch. Gen. Psychiatr., 26:479, 1972.

Krishnan, K. A., Panse, G. T., and Sheta, A. R.: Comparative study of inhibin from human testis, prostate and seminal plasma. Andrologia, 14:409, 1982.

Labrie, F., Auclair, C., Cusan, L., Kelly, P. A., Pelletier, G., and Ferland, L.: Inhibitory effects of LHRH and its agonists on testicular gonadotropin receptors and spermatogenesis in the rat. Int. J. Androl. (Suppl.), 2:303, 1978.

Lee, V. W. K., Keogh, E. J., deKretser, D. M., and Hudson, B.: Selective suppression of FSH by testis extracts. IRCS Med. Sci., 2:1406, 1974.

Leidenberger, F. A., and Reichert, L. E., Jr.: Evaluation of a rat testis homogenate radioligand receptor assay for human pituitary LH. Endocrinology; 91:901, 1972.

Leonard, J. M., Leach, R. B., Couture, M., and Paulsen, C. A.: Plasma and urinary follicle-stimulating hormone levels in oligospermia. J. Clin. Endocrinol. Metab., 34:209, 1972.

Longscope, C., Kato, T., and Horton, R.: The conversion of blood androgens to estrogens in normal adult men and women. J. Clin. Invest., 48:2191, 1969.

Malacara, J. M., Seyler, L. E., and Reichlin, S.: Luteinizing hormone releasing factor activity in peripheral blood from women during the midcycle luteinizing hormone ovulatory surge. J. Clin. Endocrinol. Metab., 34:271, 1972.

Marshall, J. C.: Investigative procedures. Clin. Endocrinol. Metabol. 4:545, 1975.

Marshall, J. C., Anderson, D. C., Fraser, T. R., and Harsoulis, P.: Human luteinizing hormone in man: Studies of metabolism and biological action. Endocrinology, 56:431, 1973.

Marshall, J. C., Harsoulis, P., Anderson, D. C., McNeilly, A. S., and Besser, G. M.: Isolated pituitary gonadotrophin deficiency: Gonadotrophin secretion after synthetic luteinizing hormone and follicle stimulating hormone-releasing hormone. Br. Med. J., 4:643, 1972.

Marynick, S. P., Loriaux, D. L., Sherins, R. J., Pita, J. C., Jr., and Lipsett, B.: Evidence that testosterone can suppress pituitary gonadotropin secretion independently of peripheral aromatization. J. Clin. Endocrinol. Metab., 45:296, 1979.

Matsuo, H., Baba, Y., Nair, R. M., Arimura, A., and Schally, A. V.: Structure of the porcine LH and FSH releasing hormone. I. The proposed amino acid sequence. Biochem. Biophys. Res. Commun., 43:1334, 1971.

McCann, S. M., and Moss, R. L.: Putative neurotransmitter involved in discharging gonadotropin-releasing neurohormones and the action of LH releasing hormone on the CNS. Life Sci., 16:833, 1975.

McCullagh, D. R., and Walsh, E. L.: Experimental hypertrophy and atrophy of the prostate gland. Endocrinology, 19:466, 1935.

Meites, J., Bruni, J. F., Van Vugt, D. A., and Smith, A. E.: Relation of endogenous opioid peptides and morphine to neuroendocrine functions. Life Sci., 24:1325, 1979.

Michael, R. P.: Hormonal steroids in sexual communication in primates. J. Steroid Biochem., 6:161, 1975.

Minneman, K. P., and Wurtman, R. J.: Effects of pineal compounds on mammals. Life Sci., 17:1189, 1975.

Moore, R. Y.: Retinohypothalamic projection in mammals: A comparative study. Brain Res., 49:403, 1973.

Naftolin, F., and Feder, H. H.: Suppression of luteinizing hormone secretion in male rats by 5α-androstan-17β–ol-3-one (dihydrotestosterone) propionate. J. Endocrinol., 56:155, 1973.

Naftolin, F., Ryan, K. J., and Petro, Z.: Aromatization of androstenedione by the diencephalon. J. Clin. Endocrinol. Metab., 33:368, 1971.

Nett, T. M., Akbar, A. M., and Niswender, G. D.: Serum levels of luteinizing hormone and gonadotropin-releasing hormone in cycling, castrated and anestrous ewes. Endocrinology, 94:713, 1974.

Odell, W. D.: Humoral manifestations of nonendocrine neoplasms—Ectopic hormone production. In Williams, R. H. (Ed.): Textbook of Endocrinology. 5th ed. Philadelphia, W. B. Saunders Co., 1974, p. 1105.

Ohno, H.: Major regulatory genes for mammalian sexual development. Cell, 7:315, 1976.

Papkoff, H., and Samy, T. S. A.: Isolation and partial characterization of the polypeptide chains of ovine interstitial cell-stimulating hormone. Biochem. Biophys. Acta, 147:175, 1967.

Papkoff, H., Sairam, M. R., Former, S. W., and Li, C. H.: Studies on the structure and function of interstitial-cell stimulating hormone. Rec. Prog. Horm. Res., 29:563, 1973.

Parvinen, M.: Regulation of the seminiferous epithelium. Endocrine Rev., 3:404, 1982.

Patterson, A. P., Saetor, J., Brightwell, D., Udelsman, R., Shi, Y. F., and Sherins, R. J.: Subphysiological plasma testosterone levels coupled with small doses of estradiol produce a selective elevation in FSH concentration in the adult male rat: an alternative to the inhibin hypothesis. Endocrinology. In press.

Paulsen, C. A.: Discussion. In Gonadotropins. Los Altos, Geron-X, 1968, p. 163.

Paulsen, C. A., Gordon, D. L., Carpenter, R. W., Gandy, H. M., and Drucker, W. D.: Klinefelter's syndrome and its variants: A hormonal and chromosomal study. Rec. Progr. Horm. Res., 24:321, 1968.

Payne, A. H.: Gonadal steroid sulfates and sulfatase. V. Human testicular steroid sulfatase. Partial characterization and possible regulation by free steroid. Biochem. Biophys. Acta, 258:473, 1972.

Pierce, J. G.: The subunits of pituitary thyrotropin—their relationship to other glycoprotein hormones. Endocrinology, 89:1331, 1971.

Rasmussen, D. D., Jacobs, W., Kissinger, P. T., and Malven, P. V.: Plasma luteinizing hormone in ovariectomized rats following pharmacologic manipulation of endogenous brain serotonin. Brain Res., 229:230, 1981.

Reichert, L. E., and Ward, D. N.: On the isolation and characterization of the alpha and beta subunits of human pituitary follicle-stimulating hormone. Endocrinology, 94:655, 1974.

Reppert, S. M., and Klein, D. C.: Mammalian pineal gland: basic and clinical aspects. In Motta, M. (Ed.): The Endocrine Functions of the Brain. New York, Raven Press, 1980, pp. 327–371.

Richter, C. P.: A hitherto unrecognized difference between man and other primates. Science, 154:427, 1966.

Ritzen, E. M., Hansson, V., and French, F. S.: The Sertoli cell. In Burger, H., and de Kretser, D. (Eds.): The Testis. New York, Raven Press, 1981, pp. 171–194.

Rommerts, F. F. G., Grootegold, J. A., and Van der Molen, H. J.: Physiological role for androgen binding protein steroid complex in testis? Steroids, 28:43, 1976.

Rosen, S. W., and Weintraub, B. D.: Monotropic increase of serum FSH correlated with low sperm count in young men with idiopathic oligospermia and aspermia. J. Clin. Endocrinol. Metab., 32:410, 1971.

Rubens, R., Ghont, M., and Vermeulen, A.: Further studies on Leydig cell function in old age. J. Clin. Endocrinol. Metab., 39:40, 1974.

Ryan, R. J.: The luteinizing hormone content of human pituitaries. I. Variations with sex and age. J. Clin. Endocrinol. Metab., 22:300, 1962.

Sairam, S. R., Manjunath, P., Ramasharma, K., Kato, K., and Madwharaj, H. G.: Properties of inhibin-like activity from seminal plasma and follicular fluid. In Negro-Vilar, A. (Ed.): Male Reproduction and Fertility. New York, Raven Press, 1983, pp. 149–157.

Samuels, L. T., Bussman, L., Matsumoto, K., et al.: Organization of androgen biosynthesis in the testis. J. Steroid Biochem., 6:291, 1975.

Santen, R. J., and Bardin, C. W.: Episodic luteinizing hormone secretion in man. Pulse analysis, clinical interpretation, physiologic mechanisms. J. Clin. Invest., 52:2617, 1973.

Sawyer, C. H.: Some recent developments in brain-pituitary ovarian physiology. Neuroendocrinology, 17:124, 1975.

Sawyer, C. H.: Functions of the amygdala related to feedback actions of gonadal steroids. In Eleftheriou, B. E. (Ed.): Neurobiology of Amygdala. New York, Plenum Press, 1974.

Schally, A. V., Mair, R. M. G., Arimura, A., and Redding, T. W.: Isolation of the luteinizing hormone and follicle-stimulating hormone-releasing hormone from porcine hypothalami. J. Biol. Chem., 246:7230, 1971.

Sharpe, R. M., Fraser, H. M., Cooper, I., et al.: Sertoli-Leydig cell communication via an LHRH-like factor. Nature, 290:785, 1981.

Sherins, R. H., and Loriaux, D. L.: Studies on the role of sex steroids in the feedback control of FSH concentrations in men. J. Clin. Endocrinol. Metab., 36:886, 1973.

Sherins, R. J., Winters, S. J., and Wachslicht, H.: Studies of the role of hCG and low dose FSH in initiating spermatogenesis in hypogonadotropic men (Abstract). Annual Meeting of The Endocrine Society. Chicago, June 1977.

Shome, B., and Parlow, A. F.: Human follicle stimulating hormone: First proposal for the amino acid sequence of the hormone specific subunit (hFSH). J. Clin. Endocrinol. Metab., 39:203, 1974.

Snyder, P. J., Reitano, J. F., and Utiger, R. D.: Serum LH and FSH responses to synthetic gonadotrophin releasing hormone in normal men. J. Clin. Endocrinol. Metab., 41:938, 1975.

Spark, R. F., White, R. A., and Connolly, P. B.: Impotence is not always psychogenic: newer insights into hypothalamic-pituitary-gonadal dysfunction. JAMA, 243:750, 1980.

Sparrow, D., Bosse, R., and Rowe, J. W.: The influence of age, alcohol consumption and body build on gonadal function in men. J. Clin. Endocrinol. Metab., 51:508, 1980.

Steinberger, E.: Hormonal control of mammalian spermatogenesis. Physiol. Rev., 51:1, 1971.

Stewart-Bentley, M., Odell, W. D., and Horton, R.: The feedback control of luteinizing hormone. J. Clin. Endocrinol. Metab., 38:545, 1974.

Swerdloff, R. S., and Heber, D.: Effects of aging on male reproductive function. In Korenman, S. (Ed.): The Endocrinology of Aging. New York, Elsevier, 1982.

Swerdloff, R. S., and Odell, W. D.: Hormonal mechanisms in the onset of puberty. Postgrad. Med. J., 51:200, 1975.

Swerdloff, R. S., and Odell, W. D.: Gonadotropins: Present concepts in the human. Calif. Med., 109:467, 1968.

Swerdloff, R. S., and Walsh, P. C.: Testosterone and estradiol suppression of LH and FSH in adult male rats. Duration of castration, duration of treatment and combined treatment. Acta Endocrinol., 73:11, 1973.

Swerdloff, R. S., Bhasin, S., and Heber, D.: Effect of GnRH superactive analogs (alone and combined with androgen) on testicular function in man and experimental animals. J. Steroid Biochem., 19:491, 1983.

Swerdloff, R. S., Frober, P. K., Jacobs, H. S., and Bain, J.: Search for a substance which selectively inhibits FSH-effects of steroids on prostaglandins on serum FSH and LH levels. Steroids, 21:703, 1973.

Swerdloff, R. S., Jacobs, H. S., and Odell, W. D.: Hypothalamic-pituitary-gonadal interrelations in the rat during sexual maturation. In Saxena, B. B., et al. (Eds.): Gonadotropins. New York, John Wiley & Sons, 1972, p. 546.

Swerdloff, R. S., Walsh, P. C., and Odell, W. D.: Control of LH and FSH secretion in the male: Evidence that aromatization of androgens to estradiol is not required by inhibition of gonadotropin secretion. Steroids, 20:13, 1972.

Swerdloff, R. S., Walsh, P. C., Jacobs, H. S., and Odell, W. D.: Serum LH and FSH during sexual maturation in the male rat: Effect of castration and cryptorchidism. Endocrinology, 88:120, 1971.

Thorner, M. O., Evans, W. S., MacLeod, R. M., Nunley, W. C., Jr., Rogol, A. D., Morris, J. L., and Besser, G. M.: Hypoprolactinemia: Current concepts of management including medical therapy with bromocriptine. In Goldstein, M., Lieberman, A., Cahre, D. B., and Thorner, M. O. (Eds.): Advances in Biochemical Psychopharmacology. Vol. 23, Ergot Compounds and Brain Function. Neuroendocrine and Neuropsychiatric Aspects. New York, Raven Press, 1980, pp. 165–189.

Tolis, G., Ackman, D., Stellos, A., Mehta, A., Labrie, F., Fazekas, A. T. A., Comaru-Schally, A. M., and Schally, A. V.: Tumor growth inhibition in patients with prostatic carcinoma treated with LHRH agonists. Proc. Natl. Acad. Sci. USA, 79: 1658, 1982.

Van Hall, E. V., Vaitukaitis, J. L., Ross, G. T. et al.: Immunological and biological activity of HCG following progressive desialylation. Endocrinology, 88:456, 1971.

Van Loon, G. R., Appel, N. M., and George, S. R.: Dopaminergic mechanisms regulating prolactin secretion: physiology and pathophysiology. *In* Flamigni, C., and Givens, R. J. (Eds.): The Gonadotropins: Basic Science and Clinical Aspects in Females. New York, Academic Press, 1982, pp. 327–338.

Van Thiel, D. H., Sherins, R. J., Myers, G. H., Jr., and DeVita, V. T., Jr.: Evidence for a specific seminiferous tubular factor affecting follicle-stimulating hormone secretion in man. J. Clin. Invest., *51*:1009, 1972.

Verhoeven, G., Heyns, W., and DeMoor, P.: Testosterone receptors in the prostate and other tissues. Vitam. Horm., *33*:265, 1975.

Vermeulen, A., Rubens, R., and Verdonck, L.: Testosterone secretion and metabolism in male senescence. J. Clin. Endocrinol. Metab., *34*:730, 1972.

Vijayan, E., and McCann, S. M.: Re-evaluation of the role of catecholamines in control of gonadotropin and prolactin release. Neuroendocrinology, *25*:150, 1978.

Walsh, P. C., Madden, J. D., Harrod, M. J., Goldstein, J. L., MacDonald, P. D., and Wilson, J. D.: Familial incomplete male pseudohermaphroditism, Type II. N. Engl. J. Med., *291*:944, 1974.

Walsh, P. C., Swerdloff, R. S., and Odell, W. D.: Feedback control of FSH in the male: Role of estrogen. Acta Endocrinol., *74*:449, 1973.

Ward, D. N., Reichert, L. E., Jr., Lei, W. K., Nahm, H. S., Hsia, J., Lamkin, W., and Jones, N. S.: Chemical studies of luteinizing hormone from human and ovine pituitaries. Rec. Prog. Horm. Res., *29*:533, 1973.

Wetterberg, L.: Melatonin in human physiological and clinical studies. J. Neural Transm. (Suppl.), *13*:289, 1978.

Wildt, L., Hansler, A., Marshall, G., et al.: Frequency and amplitude of gonadotropin-releasing hormone stimulation and gonadotropin secretion in the Rhesus monkey. Endocrinology, *109*:376, 1981.

Wilkinson, M., Arendt, J., and de Ziegler, D.: Determination of a dark-induced increase in pineal N-acetyltransferase activity and simultaneous radioimmunoassay of melatonin in pineal, serum, and pituitary tissue of the male rat. Endocrinology, *72*:243, 1977.

Wilson, J. D.: Metabolism of testicular androgens. *In* Hamilton, D. W., and Greep, R. D. (Eds.): Handbook of Endocrinology. Washington, D.C., American Physiological Society, 1975, pp. 431–508.

Wilson, J. D., Harrod, M. J., Goldstein, J. L., Hemsell, D. L., and MacDonald, P. C.: Familial incomplete male pseudohermaphroditism, Type I. N. Engl. J. Med., *290*:1097, 1974.

Winters, S. J., Johnsonbaugh, R. E., and Sherins, R. J.: The response of prolactin to chlorpromazine stimulation in men with hypogonadotropic hypogonadism and early pubertal boys: Relationship to sex steroid exposure. Clin. Endocrinol., *16*:321, 1982.

Wollesen, F., Swerdloff, R. S., and Odell, W. D.: LH and FSH responses to luteinizing releasing hormones in normal adult human males. Metabolism, *25*:1275, 1976.

Wollesen, F., Swerdloff, R. S., Peterson, M., and Odell, W. D.: Testosterone (T) modulation of pituitary response to LRH: Differential effects on luteinizing hormone (LH) and follicle-stimulating hormone (FSH). J. Clin. Invest., *53*:85a, 1974.

Yanaihara, T., and Troen, P.: Studies of the human testis. I. Biosynthetic pathways for androgen formation in human testicular tissue in vitro. J. Clin. Endocrinol. Metab., *34*:783, 1972.

Yen, S. S. C.: Physiology of human prolactin. *In* Yen, S. S. C., and Jaffe, R. B. (Eds.): Reproductive Endocrinology: Physiology, Pathophysiology and Clinical Management. Philadelphia, W. B. Saunders Co., 1978, pp. 152–170.

Yoshimoto, Y., Moridera, K., and Imura, H.: Restoration of normal pituitary gonadotropin reserve by administration of luteinizing hormone-releasing hormone in patients with hypogonadotropic hypogonadism. N. Engl. J. Med., *292*:242, 1975.

Zacharias, L., and Wurtman, R.: Blindness: Its relation to age of menarche. Science, *144*:1154, 1974.

The Testis, Epididymis, and Ductus Deferens*

LARRY L. EWING, Ph.D.
THOMAS S. K. CHANG, Ph.D.

INTRODUCTION

The testis and epididymis are responsible for the production and maturation, respectively, of spermatozoa, and the vas deferens for spermatozoa transport into the ejaculatory duct. The production of the male gamete requires many weeks from the initial mitotic division through the myriad changes readying it for ejaculation and fertilization. Highlights of this incredible transformation include (1) the initial mitotic divisions that produce either stem cells, which will reinitiate the spermatogenic process at a later date, or rapidly proliferating germ cells

*The authors thank Mrs. Jeanne Whitaker for her invaluable aid in the preparation of this manuscript. Preparation of this manuscript was supported, in part, by NIH Grants HD-07204, HD-15115, AM-19300, and the Henry and Marion Knott Foundation, Baltimore, Md. Special thanks to Camille Greenwald and the staff of the Population Dynamics Library, which is supported, in part, by the Population Center Grant HD-06268.

destined to become spermatozoa; (2) meiosis, which results in formation of the haploid gamete; and (3) the dramatic differentiation of the prospective gamete that results in condensation of the nuclear chromatin and formation of the acrosome, flagellum, and mitochondrial helix. Many of these later events occur as the prospective gamete is sequestered behind the blood-testis barrier and bathed in fluids rich in steroids, proteins, and other substances.

Although the spermatozoon resulting from this complex process has assumed its final shape and size, it still is incapable of progressive motility and is unable to fertilize an egg. Sometime during its epididymal sojourn, these two functions are acquired. Unfortunately, the mechanism by which the epididymis exerts these changes on the traversing spermatozoon largely is unknown. The objective of this chapter is to describe the structure and function of the human testis, epididymis, and ductus deferens. When there is paucity of information about the human systems, we will draw on our knowledge of experimental animals.

TESTIS

Gross Structure and Vascularization

The human testis is an ovoid mass that lies within the scrotum. It weighs approximately 32 gm (Harbitz, 1973a) and measures approximately 4.5 cm in length (Tishler, 1971). The testis is surrounded by a capsule made up of three layers—the outer tunica vaginalis, the middle tunica albuginea, and the innermost tunica vasculosa. The tunica albuginea contains large numbers of branching smooth muscle cells that course through the predominantly collagenous tissue (Langford and Heller, 1973). These smooth muscle cells probably impart a contractile capability to the human testicular capsule, since Rikimaru and Shirai (1972) were able to elicit contractions from the isolated human testicular capsule by electrical stimulation and specific autonomic drugs. Similar results have been reported in other species (Davis and Langford, 1969, 1970; Rikimaru and Suzuki, 1972).

The membrane immediately surrounding the seminiferous tubule is the septum of the testis. The seminiferous tubules are long V-shaped tubules, both ends of which usually terminate in the rete testis (Fig. 5–11). Lennox and Ahmad (1970) estimated that the combined length of the 600 to 1200 tubules in the human testis is approximately 250 meters. The rete testis (Roosen-Runge and Holstein, 1978) coalesces to form the ductuli efferentes, which act as conduits to carry testicular fluid and spermatozoa into the caput epididymidis (Fig. 5–11). Roosen-Runge and Holstein (1978) suggested that the rete testis topography acts as a "valve" with a built-in mechanism for activating the flow of fluid and spermatozoa toward the epididymis.

The testis has no somatic innervation but instead is innervated primarily by the intermesenteric nerves and the renal plexus (Mitchell, 1935). Baumgarten et al. (1968) found that this

Figure 5–11. Drawing of the human testis showing the seminiferous tubules, epididymis, and ductus deferens. (From Fawcett, D. W.: Perspect. Biol. Med., Winter, 1979.)

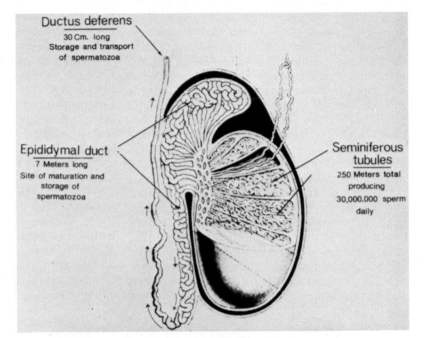

Ductus deferens
30 Cm. long
Storage and transport
of spermatozoa

Epididymal duct
7 Meters long
Site of maturation and
storage of
spermatozoa

Seminiferous
tubules
250 Meters total
producing
30,000.000 sperm
daily

adrenergic innervation is restricted primarily to small blood vessels supplying clusters of Leydig cells. Consequently, these authors concluded that the sympathetic-adrenergic innervation is of little importance for the functional integrity of the testis in man (see Hodson [1970] for a complete discussion of testicular and epididymal innervation).

The vasculature of the mammalian testis has been thoroughly discussed in three excellent reviews (Gunn and Gould, 1975; Free, 1977; Setchell, 1978). The arterial supply to the human testis-epididymis is derived from three sources: the internal spermatic artery, the deferential artery, and the external spermatic or cremasteric artery (Harrison and Barclay, 1948). Kormano and Suoranta (1971a) completed an angiographic study of the arterial pattern of 78 human autopsy testes. They observed that the spermatic artery arises from the aorta and that a single artery enters the testis in 56 per cent of cases; two branches enter in 31 per cent of cases; and three or more branches enter in 13 per cent of cases. These investigators further observed that these main branches then divide into secondary branches directed toward the rete testis; these were called centripetal branches by Hundeiker and Keller (1963).

Interestingly, many of the branches from these centripetal arteries run in the opposite direction toward the periphery of the testis and are therefore called centrifugal arteries. Kormano and Suoranta (1971b) showed that both the centripetal and the centrifugal arteries divide further and terminate in the intertubular arterioles and capillaries, which are located between the seminiferous tubules. Kormano and Suoranta (1971b) claimed that the testicular capillary network in man is similar to that in the rat. Consequently, as in the rat, the capillaries inside the columns of interstitial tissue are called the intertubular capillaries, while the rope-ladder–like capillaries running near the tunica propria of each seminiferous tubule are called the peritubular capillaries. Recently, Takayama and Tomoyoshi (1981) asserted that the capillary system in the human is more complicated than that in the rat and that the aforementioned arrangement is not always observed.

Kormano and Suoranta (1971b) suggested that the intratesticular collecting veins be called centripetal veins and those coursing in the opposite direction, centrifugal veins. Apparently, centrifugal veins drain only the peripheral part of the testis and collect into larger venous channels on the surface of the testis. Centripetal veins drain a greater part of the testis and run

directly to the region of the rete testis, where they form larger channels located around the poorly vascularized rete. These two sets of veins then intermingle with the cremasteric and differential veins to form the pampiniform plexus. Ishigami et al. (1970) stated that blood in this venous system tends to stagnate because the spermatic vein is thin-walled, is poorly muscularized, and lacks effective valves except at the inflow points into the inferior vena cava or the renal vein. This issue remains controversial.

The human testicular parenchyma is provided with approximately 9 ml of blood per 100 gm of tissue per minute (Petterson et al., 1973), which is similar to the flow rates observed in testes of numerous other species (Free, 1977; Setchell, 1978). Fritjofsson et al. (1969) claimed that in man, blood flow to the left testis varies from 1.6 to 12.4 ml/per 100 gm per minute, whereas that to the right testis ranges from 3.2 to 38.5 ml/per 100 gm per minute.

The special features of the testicular vasculature—the arrangement of a thin elongated artery coursing through a plexus of veins, the tendency of the branches of the artery to flow over the surface of the testis prior to entering the testicular parenchyma, and, finally, the centrifugal arrangement of some terminal branches of the testicular artery—are suited both to the cooling of the arterial blood through a countercurrent exchange of heat between the testicular veins and artery and to the uniform distribution of this precooled blood throughout the testis. These processes are evident in humans, since the testicular temperature is 2 to 4°C lower than rectal temperature (Agger, 1971). The obvious effects of the failure to maintain this temperature differential in the cryptorchid human testis has been discussed in detail by Marshall and Elder (1982).

The arrangement of the testicular vasculature also permits the exchange of small molecules from veins to arteries. For example, testosterone is transported from the vein to the artery via a concentration-limited, passive diffusion process in the rat (Free and Jaffe, 1975) and the human (Bayard et al., 1975). It is unknown whether this exchange of testosterone has physiologic significance.

There are prominent lymphatic ducts in the spermatic cord of the human testis (Hundeiker, 1971; Wenzel and Kellermann, 1966). The lymph capillaries that give rise to these lymph ducts originate within the intertubular spaces and do not penetrate the seminiferous tubules. Obstruction of the lymphatic ducts in the spermatic cord invariably is followed by dilatation of the interstitium but not the seminiferous tubules, suggesting that although the extracellular space of the interstitium is drained via the lymphatics, the seminiferous tubules are not.

The extracellular fluid bathing the Sertoli cells and germinal cells flows from the seminiferous tubules into the rete to form rete testis fluid, which is transported into the caput epididymidis. Originally, it was thought that the fluid probably originates both from primary secretions within the seminiferous tubules and from secretions directly into the rete (Kormano et al., 1971; Levine and Marsh, 1971; Tuck et al., 1970). However, more recently Setchell (1978) suggested that "the majority of the fluid leaving the rete, originates in the tubules." Whatever its origin, rete testis fluid is a dilute suspension of spermatozoa in a fluid isosmotic with plasma.

Rete testis fluid resembles neither plasma in the spermatic vein nor lymph in the lymphatic ducts draining the testis. Setchell and Waites (1975) reported that in the ram the ion composition and the carbohydrate, amino acid, and protein content of rete testis fluid are markedly different from those in blood plasma. They correctly pointed out that "differences in composition between the fluid inside the seminiferous tubules and excurrent ducts of the testis and

blood plasma or testicular lymph make it clear that substances do not diffuse freely into and out of tubules." Extrapolation of this idea led to the concept of a blood-testis barrier, which probably exists to a greater or lesser extent in numerous species (Setchell and Waites, 1975) including man (Koskimies et al., 1973). Setchell et al. (1969) and Setchell (1978) demonstrated this permeability barrier by measuring the entry of substances from blood plasma into rete testicular fluid and testicular lymph of rams (Fig. 5–12). Fawcett (1979) summarized these results succinctly when he stated that "a large variety of substances injected into the blood stream rapidly appeared in the testicular lymph but not in the rete testis fluid." The anatomic site of this putative barrier probably is at the tight junctions between Sertoli cell membranes. This topic is discussed in detail later in this chapter.

We can only speculate as to the consequence of such a blood-testis barrier, since the functional significance of this barrier remains to be proved. Obviously, this barrier could be important for meiosis, since the fluid bathing the germinal cells is more stable than and quite different from that in the compartments outside the barrier. In addition, the blood-testis barrier may isolate the haploid male gamete, which is

Figure 5–12. Diagram of experiments demonstrating that dyes and other substances injected intravenously rapidly appear in the lymph but not in the rete testis fluid. (From Fawcett, D. W.: Perspect. Biol. Med., Winter, 1979.)

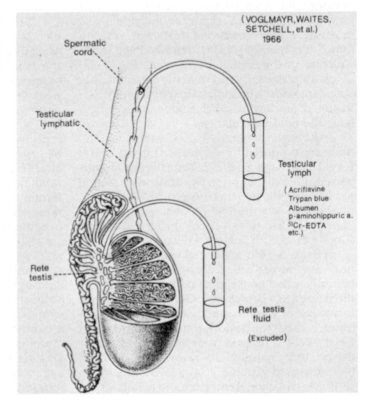

not recognized as "self" by the male immune system. A practical consideration is the possibility of differential drug access to the cells sequestered behind the barrier.

Cytoarchitecture and Function of the Testis

INTERSTITIUM

The interstitium contains blood vessels, lymph vessels, fibroblastic supporting cells, macrophages, mast cells, and Leydig cells (Fig. 5–13). The interstitium occupies about 34 per cent of the testicular volume of the human testis, of which the Leydig cells account for about 5 to 12 per cent (Christensen, 1975; Kaler and Neaves, 1978). Morphometric analysis showed the Leydig cell mass to be 0.9 gm ± SD 0.8 gm in 172 human males ranging from 40 to more than 80 years of age (Harbitz, 1973b). Stereologic analysis (Kaler and Neaves, 1978) showed that a human testis from a 20-year-old man contained approximately 700 million Leydig cells.

According to Kaler and Neaves (1978), human Leydig cells at the light microscopic level appear "as rounded or polygonal cytoplasmic profiles staining with the periodic acid–Schiff reaction and often containing a round nuclear profile with nucleolus, scattered individually or in clusters throughout the testicular interstitium." Christensen (1975) described the ultrastructure of the human Leydig cell (Fig. 5–13) as characterized by prominent mitochondria, abundant smooth endoplasmic reticulum (SER), scattered patches of rough endoplasmic reticulum, and lipid droplets.

Although numerous C_{18}, C_{19}, and C_{21} steroids are produced by the testis (Lipsett, 1974; Ewing and Brown, 1977), testosterone is purported to be the principal testicular steroid produced by the human (Lipsett, 1974). Clearly, the bulk of testosterone-producing capacity of the mammalian testis resides in the Leydig cell (Cooke et al., 1972; Hall, 1979).

Figure 5–14 is a diagrammatic representation of a Leydig cell. Cholesterol in the metabolically active pool can be derived from any of three sources (Brown and Goldstein, 1976). It is unclear at present whether the bulk of cholesterol used for testosterone biosynthesis in Leydig cells is derived from blood plasma (Anderson and Dietschy, 1977) or from de novo biosynthesis (Charreau et al., 1981). Figure 5–14 shows that cholesterol from the metabolically

active pool must be transported into the mitochondria, where the cholesterol side-chain cleavage enzyme converts it to pregnenolone and the C6 fragment isocaproaldehyde. Pregnenolone must then be transported out of the mitochondrial membrane into the smooth endoplasmic reticulum, where it is converted into testosterone. Testosterone probably then diffuses across the cell membrane and is trapped in the extracellular fluid and blood plasma by steroid-binding macromolecules.

The control of Leydig cell steroidogenesis has been reviewed exhaustively (Catt and Dufau, 1976; Christensen, 1975; Dufau and Catt, 1978; Dufau et al., 1978; Eik-Nes, 1975; Rommerts et al., 1974; Hall, 1979; Ewing, 1983). Suffice it to say that the primary, acute, regulatory effect of luteinizing hormone (LH) on testosterone production probably results in transport of cholesterol into the mitochondria or in binding of cholesterol to the cholesterol side-chain cleavage enzyme. LH probably also exerts trophic (slow) effects on Leydig cell differentiation and development (Ewing and Zirkin, 1983). Pituitary peptides other than LH (e.g., follicle-stimulating hormone, prolactin) have been shown to modify LH-stimulated Leydig cell steroidogenesis (Ewing, 1983). Finally, direct inhibition of Leydig cell steroidogenesis via estrogens and androgens may exist (Ewing, 1983).

Testosterone concentrations in peripheral blood of males, including the human, change dramatically during the life cycle. Figure 5–15 shows that a peak of testosterone occurs in the blood of the human fetus between 12 and 18 weeks of gestation. Another testosterone peak occurs at approximately 2 months of age (Fig. 5–15). Testosterone reaches a maximum concentration during the second or third decade of life, then reaches a plateau, and declines thereafter (Fig. 5–15). Additionally, annual and daily rhythms (insets A and B, Fig. 5–15) in testosterone concentration occur. Superimposed on these rhythms are irregular fluctuations in testosterone concentration in peripheral blood (inset C, Fig. 5–15). See the review by Ewing et al. (1980) for a thorough discussion of this topic.

In those species that have been studied thoroughly, the major epochs in testosterone production represent an orderly sequence of temporal signals that cause the following: first, the differentiation and development of the fetal reproductive tract; second, the neonatal organization or "marking" of androgen-dependent target tissues, assuring their appropriate response later in puberty and adulthood; third,

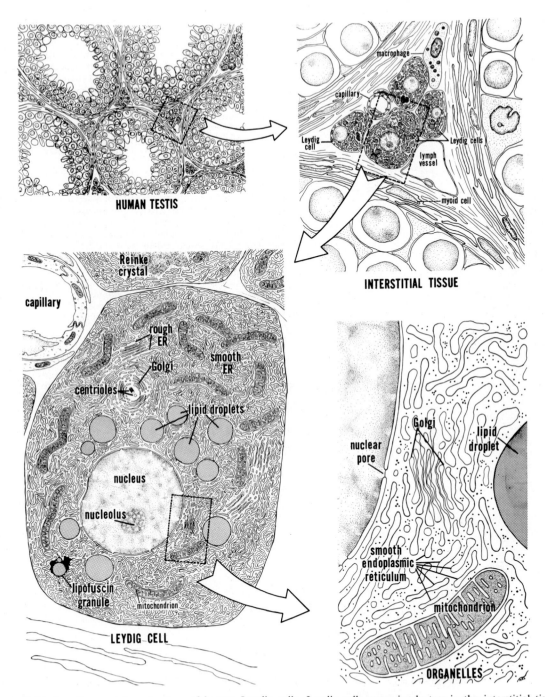

HUMAN TESTIS

INTERSTITIAL TISSUE

LEYDIG CELL

ORGANELLES

Figure 5–13. Location and fine structure of human Leydig cells. Leydig cells occur in clusters in the interstitial tissue between the seminiferous tubules (upper left). Interstitial tissue (upper right) contains macrophages and fibroblasts as well as capillaries and lymph vessels. Seminiferous tubules are surrounded by a boundary layer of myoid cells. The most abundant organelle within the cytoplasm of the Leydig cell is the smooth endoplasmic reticulum (lower left). Some of the organelles are seen in greater detail in a selected area of cytoplasm (lower right). (From Christensen, A. K.: *In* Greep, R. O., and Astwood, W. B. [Eds.]: Handbook of Physiology, Section 7. Endocrinology. Baltimore, The Williams & Wilkins Co., 1975. Copyright 1975, The American Physiological Society, Bethesda, Md.)

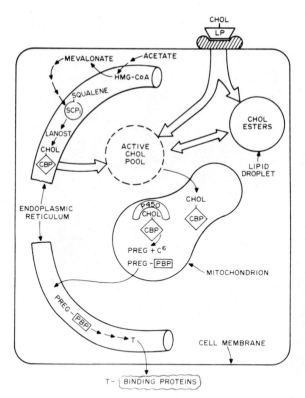

Figure 5–14. Spatial organization of the testosterone biosynthetic apparatus in a Leydig cell. Cholesterol (CHOL) in the metabolically active pool is derived from de novo synthesis, cholesterol esters in lipid droplets, or blood plasma. With the exception of HMG-CoA reductase, which resides in the endoplasmic reticulum, most early reactions in cholesterol biosynthesis take place in the cytoplasm of the cell. Squalene is the first water-insoluble intermediate in cholesterol biosynthesis. Note that squalene carrier protein (SCP₁) may be required for the conversion of squalene to lanosterol (LANOST). Other sterol carrier proteins, including cholesterol binding protein (CBP), also may exist. CBP probably transports cholesterol into the mitochondrion, where it may facilitate cholesterol binding to the P-450 component of the cholesterol side-chain cleavage enzyme. Pregnenolone (PREG) and isocaproaldehyde (C⁶) are produced by cholesterol side-chain cleavage. Pregnenolone may bind to pregnenolone-binding protein (PBP), which theoretically would aid in its transport into or within the endoplasmic reticulum. The secretion of testosterone from the Leydig cell may be facilitated by the presence of binding proteins such as albumin, androgen-binding protein, and testosterone-estradiol–binding globulin outside the Leydig cell membrane. (From Ewing, L. L., et al.: Int. Rev. Physiol., 22:41, 1980.)

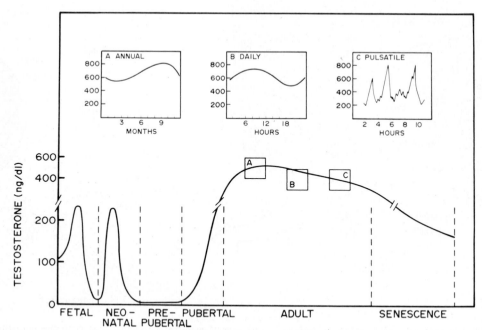

Figure 5–15. Concentration of testosterone in peripheral blood of the human male at different times of the life cycle. The peak of testosterone in the peripheral blood of the fetus occurs between 12 and 18 weeks of gestation (lower left corner; gestational age not shown). The peak of testosterone in the peripheral blood of the neonate occurs at approximately 2 months of age. Testosterone declines to low levels during the prepubertal period. The pubertal increase in testosterone concentration in peripheral blood occurs between 12 and 17 years of age. Testosterone concentration in the adult reaches its maximum during the second or third decade of life and then declines slowly through the fifth decade. Testosterone concentration in peripheral blood declines dramatically during senescence. Inset *A* shows the annual rhythm in testosterone concentration in peripheral blood of the human male. The peak and nadir occur in the fall and spring, respectively. Inset *B* shows the daily rhythm in testosterone concentration in peripheral blood of the adult human male. The peak and nadir occur in the morning and evening, respectively. Inset *C* shows the frequent and irregular fluctuations in testosterone concentration in peripheral blood of the human male. (From Ewing, L. L., et al.: Int. Rev. Physiol., 22:41, 1980.)

the masculinization of the male at puberty; and fourth, the maintenance of growth and function of androgen-dependent organs in the adult. In part, these temporal changes in testosterone production reflect a complex interaction between the pituitary gland and the testis. For a thorough discussion of this latter topic, see Faiman et al., (1981), Swerdloff and Heber (1981), DiZerga and Sherins (1981), and Santen (1981).

SEMINIFEROUS TUBULES

The seminiferous tubules contain germinal elements and supporting cells. The supporting cells include the sustentacular cells of the basement membrane and the Sertoli cells. The germinal elements comprise a population of epithelial cells, including a slowly dividing primitive stem cell population, the rapidly proliferating spermatogonia, spermatocytes undergoing meiosis, and the metamorphosing spermatids.

Sertoli Cell. The morphologic and ultrastructural characteristics of the human Sertoli cell have been described on numerous occasions (Bawa, 1963; Fawcett and Burgos, 1956; Nagano, 1966; Kerr and deKretser, 1981; Nistal et al., 1982). The Sertoli cell is a static, nonproliferating cell characterized by its irregularly shaped nucleus, prominent nucleolus, low mitotic index, Sertoli–germ cell connections, and unique tight junctional complexes between adjacent Sertoli cell membranes. The Sertoli cell rests on the basement membrane of the seminiferous tubule and extends filamentous cytoplasmic ramifications toward the lumen of the tubule (Fig. 5–16). Germinal cells are arranged between these Sertoli cell cytoplasmic projections. The undifferentiated spermatogonia are near the basement membrane of the seminiferous tubule, while the more advanced spermatocytes and spermatids are arranged at successively higher levels in the epithelial layer (Fig. 5–16).

SERTOLI-SERTOLI TIGHT JUNCTIONAL COMPLEXES. Sertoli-Sertoli junctional complexes subdivide the seminiferous epithelium into a basal compartment and adluminal compartment in many species (Flickinger and Fawcett, 1967; Dym and Fawcett, 1970), including man (deKretser and Burger, 1972; Chemes et al., 1977). This was demonstrated in two ways. First, Dym and Fawcett (1970) and Dym (1973) showed that the Sertoli-Sertoli tight junctions prevent the deep penetration of electron opaque tracers into the seminiferous epithelium from the testicular interstitium. Second, Gilula et al. (1976) perfused a rat testis with hypertonic lithium

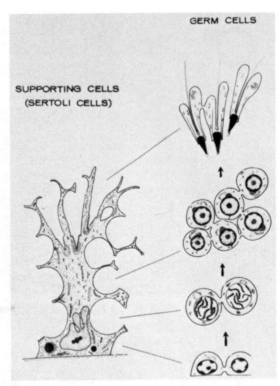

Figure 5–16. Diagrammatic representation of Sertoli and germ cells composing the seminiferous epithelium. The Sertoli cells represent a fixed population of nondividing support cells. The proliferating germ cells move upward along the sides of the Sertoli cells as they differentiate into spermatozoa. (From Fawcett, D. W.: Perspect. Biol. Med., Winter, 1979.)

chloride followed within a few minutes by an aldehyde fixative. The results of this experiment are shown in Figure 5–17. Fawcett (1979) stated that "the hypertonic solution causes immediate shrinkage and retraction of cells in the basal compartment but osmotic effects on those in the adluminal compartment are delayed by the occluding junctions." The empty spaces thus formed along the basement membrane of the seminiferous tubule represent the basal compartment of the seminiferous epithelium.

It is believed that the specialized junctional complexes between adjacent Sertoli cells form the principal site of the blood-testis barrier discussed earlier in this chapter. Apparently, spermatogonia and young spermatocytes are outside the permeability barrier in the basal compartment, whereas mature spermatocytes and spermatids are sequestered behind the permeability barrier in the adluminal compartment. It is during the extended meiotic prophase (leptotene, zygotene, pachytene) that the spermatocytes detach from the basement membrane and migrate into the adluminal compartment of

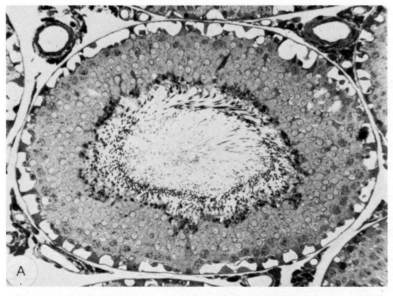

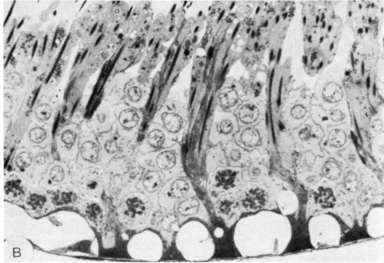

Figure 5–17. *A,* Photomicrograph of a seminiferous tubule from a rat testis perfused first with hypertonic lithium chloride, then with an aldehyde fixative. The basal compartment of the seminiferous epithelium is empty because the spermatogonia have detached from the basement lamina and have shrunk. × 350. *B,* The seminiferous epithelium from the same preparation at a higher magnification clearly shows that the basal cytoplasm of the Sertoli cell is shrunken but the cell remains attached. The spermatocytes and spermatids have been protected from the hypertonic lithium chloride by the permeability barrier. × 1200. (From Gilula, N. B., et al.: Dev. Biol., *50*:142, 1976.)

the seminiferous tubule. This migration (Fig. 5–18) was described for the rat testis by Russell (1980), who stated that "there are usually no germ cells in this specialized region of contact between Sertoli cells; however, in those stages where young spermatocytes (leptotene, zygotene) move toward the lumen, these germ cell types are noted in regions where occluding junctions exist both above and below the germ cell" (Fig. 5–18*C* to *E*). Further, Russell stated that "it has been shown that the Sertoli cell processes undermine the young spermatocytes to separate them from the basal lamina, and as the processes meet they form junctions impermeable to substances from the blood." Russell concluded that "this anatomically distinct region, having junctions both above and below the germ cell, has been termed the intermediate compartment (Fig. 5–19) and has been likened to a transit chamber in which cells may move from one compartment to another without disrupting the integrity of the blood-testis barrier."

SERTOLI–GERM CELL ASSOCIATIONS. It once was thought that there were no specialized junctions between Sertoli cells and germ cells (Fawcett, 1974). Now it is widely accepted that several Sertoli–germ cell associations exist in mammalian testes (Connell, 1974; Kaya and Harrison, 1976; Russell, 1977; Romrell and Ross, 1979; Russell and Clermont, 1976). This controversial issue has been reviewed recently by Russell (1980).

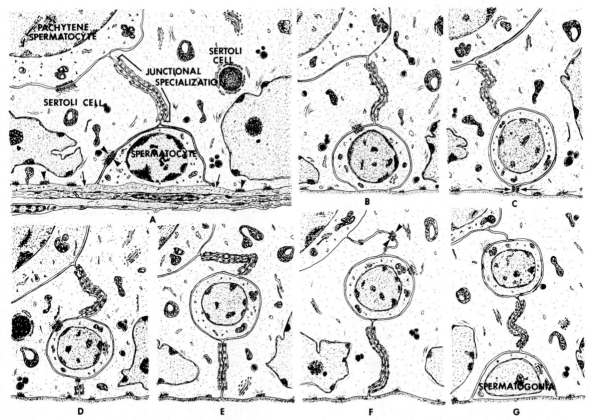

Figure 5–18. Diagram of the steps required to transfer rat primary spermatocytes from the basal to the adluminal compartment of the seminiferous tubule. Initially (*A, B*) the Sertoli cells are attached to each other above the spermatocytes by tight junctions. Next (*C to E*), Sertoli cells form new junctions below the spermatocytes, isolating the spermatocytes in an intermediate compartment, above and below which are tight junctions. The junctions above the spermatocytes then break down (*F, G*), and the spermatocytes enter the adluminal compartment. (From Russell, L.: Am. J. Anat., *148*:313, 1977.)

Figure 5–19 is a diagrammatic representation of the Sertoli cell and its configurational relationship with germ cells. Russell (1980) stated that "desmosome-like contacts function as attachment devices that maintain the integrity of the seminiferous epithelium and at the same time assure that germ cells are transported in an orderly fashion, toward the tubular lumen by virtue of configurational changes of the Sertoli cell" (Fig. 5–19). He further stated that "ectoplasmic specializations are complex surface specializations that appear to hold elongated spermatids within deep recesses of the Sertoli cell" (Fig. 5–19). Finally, he stated that "both the Sertoli cell and spermatid participate in the formation of tubulobulbar complexes which appear in the few days preceding sperm release" (Fig. 5–19). "These latter unusual structures are devices by which excess spermatid cytoplasm may be funneled from the spermatid head."

SEROTLI CELL FUNCTION. Obviously, the Sertoli cell creates a microenvironment in the adluminal compartment of the seminiferous epithelium that facilitates spermatogenesis. Unfortunately, we can only guess at the functions performed by the Sertoli cell in creating the aforementioned microenvironment in any species. This topic has been reviewed extensively (Fawcett, 1975*b*; Dym et al., 1977; Ewing et al., 1980; Ritzen et al., 1981). These functions obviously encompass physical contact with sperm cells, phagocytosis, fluid secretion, and production and secretion of a variety of molecules.

As stated earlier, physical contact of the Sertoli cell and the germ cell obviously plays some role in propelling the germ cell upward toward the lumen of the seminiferous tubule. Moreover, the intimate association between the condensing spermatid and the apical portion of the Sertoli cell during spermiogenesis is associated with the casting off of the residual cytoplasm from the developing spermatid. Lastly, the junctional complexes between adjacent Ser-

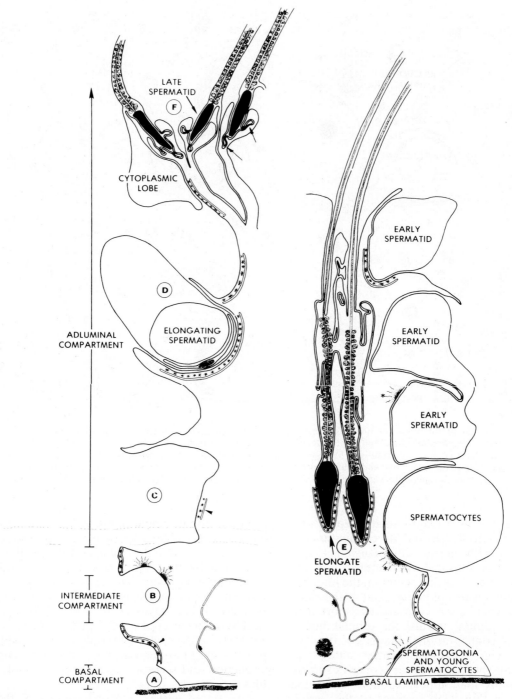

Figure 5–19. A diagrammatic representation of the tree-shaped Sertoli cell with a thickened central portion, or "trunk," and more delicate processes, or "limbs." The diagram is split vertically to allow the presentation of major configurational changes that occur during the spermatogenic cycle. Note the basal, intermediate, and adluminal compartments of the seminiferous epithelium. *A,* Spermatogonia and early spermatocytes share a position on the basal lamina and are overreached by one surface of adjacent Sertoli cells that join to form occluding junctions (site of blood-testis barrier). *B,* Sertoli cells form junctional complexes both above and below leptotene-zygotene spermatocytes in the process of being translocated from the basal to the adluminal compartment. *C,* The spermatocytes enter the adluminal compartment of the seminiferous epithelium when the higher Sertoli junctions dissociate. *D,* The elongating spermatid becomes situated within a narrow recess of the trunk of the Sertoli cell. *E,* As the spermatid elongates further, the cell becomes lodged within the body of the Sertoli cell. *F,* The advanced spermatid moves toward the lumen of the seminiferous epithelium in preparation for spermiation. Only the head region remains in intimate contact with the Sertoli cell. Specialized cell-to-cell contacts: Asterisks = desmosome–gap junction complex; arrowheads = ectoplasmic specializations; isolated arrows = tubulobulbar complexes. (From Russell, L.: Gamete Res., *3*:179, 1980.)

toli cells obviously form an important component of the blood-testis barrier with all its consequences.

Sertoli cells have been reported to actively phagocytize intratesticularly injected particulate dyes and carbon particles (Clegg and MacMillan, 1965). Russell (1980) has suggested that the bulk of cytoplasm is lost from condensing spermatids by Sertoli cell phagocytosis of tubulobulbar complexes.

The Sertoli cell functions as a polarized epithelium, its base in a plasma environment and its apex in an environment unique to the seminiferous tubule (Ewing et al., 1980). The Sertoli cell, in all probability, is the source of most of the rete testis fluid (Setchell, 1978) secreted by the mammalian testis. Therefore, the unique chemical environment of the adluminal compartment of the seminiferous tubule, in part, must be the result of Sertoli cell secretion.

Putative Sertoli cell secretory products include steroids, such as dihydrotestosterone, testosterone, androstenediols, 17β-estradiol, and numerous other C-21 steroids (Ewing et al., 1980; Mather et al., 1983). Proteins that have been identified as Sertoli cell products include ceruloplasmin, transferrin, glycoprotein 2, plasminogen activator, somatomedin-like substances, Sertoli-derived growth factor, cyclic proteins, meiosis inhibiting and promoting substances, T proteins, inhibin, and androgen-binding protein (Mather et al., 1983). The physical and chemical characterizations and specific function of most of these products remain to be fully elucidated.

Androgen-binding protein (ABP) was one of the first Sertoli cell products to be identified (Ritzen et al., 1971; Hansson and Djøseland, 1972). However, even now the function of ABP can only be surmised. It may be an intracellular carrier of androgen within the Sertoli cell. Alternatively, it may serve as a reservoir of androgenic hormones within the seminiferous tubule. Finally, it may transport testosterone from the testis into the epididymis. Nevertheless, ABP production has proven to be an excellent marker to test the hormonal regulation of Sertoli cell function.

The consensus (Means et al., 1980; Ewing et al., 1980; Ritzen et al., 1981; Davis, 1981; Mather et al., 1983) is that follicle-stimulating hormone (FSH) and testosterone play an important role in the regulation of ABP production. Mather et al. (1983) suggested that multiple agents in addition to testosterone and FSH, including progesterone, hydrocortisone, insulin, EGF, transferrin, and vitamins A and E, are required for maximal ABP secretion by Sertoli cells cultured in vitro. Unfortunately, the role of these effector molecules and the mechanism by which they regulate Sertoli cell function remain to be elucidated.

Germinal Epithelium. The epithelium of the seminiferous tubule is populated by cells that give rise to approximately 123×10^6 (range 21 to 374×10^6) spermatozoa daily in the human male (Amann and Howards, 1980). This process of sperm production is called spermatogenesis. It encompasses a proliferative phase during which spermatogonia divide either to replace their number (stem cell renewal) or to produce daughter cells committed to become spermatocytes, a meiotic phase when spermatocytes undergo reduction division, resulting in haploid spermatids; and a spermiogenic phase when spermatids undergo a dramatic metamorphosis in size and shape to form mature spermatozoa. Because of the complexity of the topic, lack of complete information regarding the human, and space limitations in this chapter, the following discussion of spermatogenesis is general in nature and references are not always made to original research. Instead, the discussion rests heavily on excellent reviews by Roosen-Runge (1969); Clermont (1972); Steinberger and Steinberger (1975); Ewing et al., 1980; Kerr and deKretser (1981); and DiZerga and Sherins (1981).

Histologic examination of the human testis with the aid of the light microscope revealed large numbers of germ cells arrayed among Sertoli cells and extending from the basement membrane to the lumen of the seminiferous tubule (Fig. 5–16). Morphologic analysis (Clermont, 1963; Heller and Clermont, 1964) revealed the presence of at least 13 recognizable germ types in the human testis. These cells were thought to represent different steps in the developmental process. Proceeding from the least to the most differentiated, they were named dark Type A spermatogonia (Ad); pale Type A spermatogonia (Ap); Type B spermatogonia (B); preleptotene primary spermatocytes (R); leptotene primary spermatocytes (L); zygotene primary spermatocytes (z); pachytene primary spermatocytes (p); secondary spermatocytes (II); and Sa, Sb1, Sb2, Sc, Sd1, and Sd2 spermatids (Fig. 5–20).

SPERMATOGONIAL PROLIFERATION AND STEM CELL RENEWAL. Pale Type A spermatogonia in the basal compartment of the seminiferous tubule formed by the overreaching Sertoli-Sertoli tight junctions divide at 16-day intervals

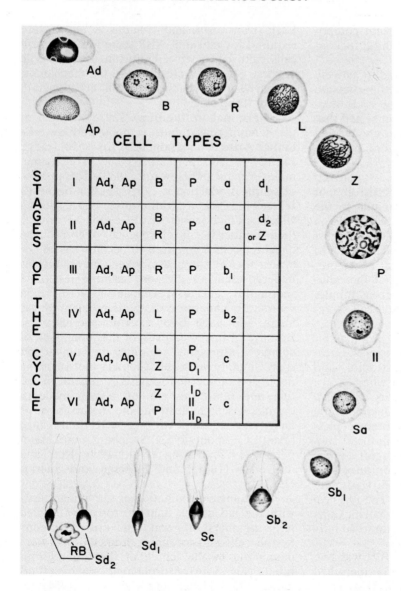

Figure 5–20. The steps of spermatogenesis in man. Ad = dark Type A spermatogonium; AP = pale Type A spermatogonium; B = Type B spermatogonium; R = resting or preleptotene primary spermatocyte; L = leptotene spermatocyte; Z = zygotene spermatocyte; P = pachytene spermatocyte; II = secondary spermatocyte; Sa(a), Sb1(b1), sb2(b2), Sc(c), Sd1(d1), Sd2(d2) = spermatids; Rb = residual body. The table shows the cells that make up the six stages of the cycle of the seminiferous epithelium (I to VI): D_1 = diakenesis; I_D and II_D = first and second maturation divisions of spermatocytes. (Modified from Clermont, Y.: Am. J. Anat. *118*:509: 1966.)

in the human (Clermont, 1972) to form B spermatogonia, which are committed to become spermatocytes. Interestingly, in the germinal epithelium the cytoplasm generally does not separate completely when the nuclei divide following mitosis. Therefore, cytoplasmic bridges are formed between adjacent spermatogonia. Evidently, this continues during meiosis, since cytoplasmic bridges have been observed between all classes of germ cells (Ewing et al., 1980). Although the functional significance of cytoplasmic bridges remains enigmatic, their presence could be important for the synchronization of cellular proliferation, differentiation, and possibly the control of gene expression in haploid cells.

Periodically the population of undifferentiated spermatogonia must be replenished (stem cell renewal). Unfortunately, the mechanism by which this is accomplished is unclear in the human (Clermont, 1972). In fact, controversy surrounds this subject in experimental animals (Bartmanska and Clermont, 1983). Suffice it to say that the division of some Type A spermatogonia gives rise to cells destined to become spermatocytes, whereas other, apparently identical, cells give rise to more stem cells.

MEIOSIS. The Type B spermatogonia interconnected by cytoplasmic bridges divide mitotically to form the primary spermatocytes that will undergo meiosis. This process has been described in general by Ewing et al. (1980) and most recently for the human by Kerr and de-Kretser (1981). Chains of interconnected mature spermatocytes are therefore found in the adluminal compartment of the seminiferous tubule behind the blood-testis barrier created by the Sertoli–Sertoli cell tight junctions. The spermatocytes complete the subsequent meiotic divisions. In most organisms a reductional division is followed by an equatorial division, resulting in the production of daughter cells with the haploid chromosome number and, as a consequence of recombination, with different genetic information. The result of this process in the human is the round Sa spermatid (Fig. 5–20).

SPERMIOGENESIS. During spermiogenesis the products of meiosis, the round Sa spermatids, metamorphose into mature spermatids (Fig. 5–20). During this metamorphosis, extensive changes occur in both the spermatid cytoplasm and the nucleus. These changes have been described in detail for the human in a recent review (Kerr and deKretser, 1981) and include migration of cytoplasmic organelles to positions characteristic of the mature spermatozoon, loss of cytoplasm, formation of the acrosome, and formation of the flagellum. If the human is similar to the rat, spermatids from a clone are connected to each other via cytoplasmic bridges and to Sertoli cells via ectoplasmic specializations.

The entire spermatogenic process in man requires approximately 64 days (Clermont, 1972). Because the human testis produces millions of spermatozoa daily, it would be grossly inefficient to wait for the entire spermatogenic process outlined above to be completed before initiating a new round of spermatogonial divisions at any given site in the seminiferous epithelium. Consequently, the proliferative phase of spermatogenesis (the differentiation of Ap to B spermatogonia) is initiated four times (every 16 days, one cycle of the seminiferous epithelium) during the approximately 64-day period required for a single Ap spermatogonium to differentiate into a spermatozoon. The result is that the seminiferous epithelium in an adult human testis is populated by one or two cohorts of spermatogonia, one or two cohorts of spermatocytes, and one or two cohorts of spermatids.

Kinetic analysis of cellular proliferation (Heller and Clermont, 1964) revealed that if spermatogenesis is viewed from a fixed point in a seminiferous tubule, six recognizable cellular associations (stages of the cycle of the seminiferous epithelium) occur one after another in a predictable and constant fashion (Fig. 5–21).

Two appearances of the same cell association span 16 days (one cycle of the seminiferous epithelium). Therefore, any one stage would appear four times during the 64 days required for an Ap spermatogonium to differentiate into a spermatozoon.

In rodents, the stages of spermatogenesis occur more or less consecutively from the first to the last stage along a given segment of the tubule in repeating sequences. One complete series of segments representing the recognized cellular associations (stages) is called the wave of the seminiferous epithelium. It has long been claimed (Roosen-Runge and Barlow, 1953; Heller and Clermont, 1964; Leidl and Waschke, 1970) that man does not exhibit a wave of the seminiferous epithelium. Instead, the stages occupy only a portion of the circumference of the tubule, thus forming a mosaic rather than a well-defined linear array of succeeding stages of spermatogenesis. This concept has been challenged by Schulze (1982), who claimed that there is an orderly sequence of stages in oblique orientation, which implies a helical arrangement of stages in the seminiferous tubule in man. This idea remains to be confirmed, however.

HORMONAL REGULATION OF SPERMATOGENESIS. Hypophysectomy results in testicular atrophy in numerous species (Steinberger, 1971), including man (Mancini et al., 1969, 1971, 1972). In the rat, "hypophysectomy apparently produces several lesions: a block in spermatid maturation, severe damage to the meiotic prophase and partial interference with the quantitative formation of type A spermatogonia" (Steinberger, 1971). Testes of hypophysectomized men are characterized by Leydig cell atrophy, peritubular hyalinization, and germinal depletion that varies from tubules containing only spermatogonia to those with scattered spermatocytes (Mancini et al., 1969).

The hormonal regimen required to restore spermatogenesis after hypophysectomy depends on whether spermatogenesis is to be maintained immediately after hypophysectomy or reinitiated after the germinal epithelium has been allowed to regress completely. Moreover, the amount of hormone required depends on the end point being measured—production of a few advanced spermatids (qualitative) or complete restoration of spermatid numbers (quantitative). Desjardins et al. (1973) showed that testosterone will maintain spermatogenesis quantitatively in rabbits treated with testosterone implants that inhibited endogenous LH production. Testosterone will also maintain spermatogenesis quantitatively in hypophysec-

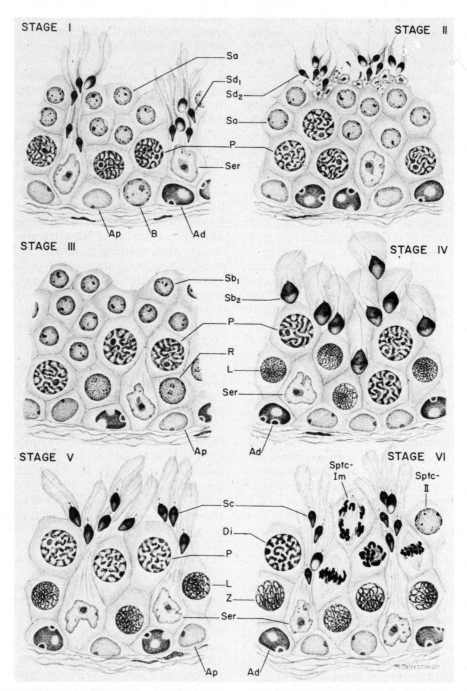

Figure 5–21. Cellular composition of the six cellular associations (Stages I to VI) found in human seminiferous tubules. Ser = Sertoli nuclei; Ad and Ap = dark and pale Type A spermatogonia; B = Type B spermatogonia; R = resting (preleptotene) primary spermatocytes; L = leptotene spermatocytes; Z = zygotene spermatocytes; P = pachytene spermatocytes; Di = diplotene spermatocytes; Sptc-Im = primary spermatocytes in division; Sptc-II = secondary spermatocytes in interphase; Sa, Sb, Sb2, Sc, Sd1, Sd2 = spermatids at various steps of spermatogenesis. (Modified from Heller, C. G., and Clermont, Y.: Rec. Prog. Horm. Res., *20*:545, 1964.)

tomized rats (Robaire and Zirkin, 1981). Finally, testosterone will initiate and maintain qualitatively spermatogenesis in humans. This was demonstrated by Steinberger et al. (1973), who reported a case of a 6-year-old boy in whom there was active spermatogenesis in the testicular tissue containing an androgen-producing Leydig cell tumor. The fact that spermatogenesis was absent in the contralateral testis, which was free of steroid-producing tumor tissue, suggested that spermatogenesis was initiated and maintained by the androgenic steroids produced by the tumor. Quantitative maintenance of spermatogenesis in the human male has not been achieved to date, probably because of the difficulty in achieving a high enough blood level of testosterone. Testosterone probably regulates spermatogenesis indirectly via the Sertoli cell (Lyon et al., 1975).

The effect of pituitary gonadotropins on spermatogenesis has been reviewed (Steinberger, 1971; Ewing et al., 1980; DiZerga and Sherins, 1981). There is little reason to suspect that luteinizing hormone (LH) acts other than by stimulating endogenous testosterone production.

The role of FSH in spermatogenesis remains more controversial. It is safe to say that FSH probably has little impact on the maintenance of spermatogenesis in intact adults (Ewing et al., 1980), including the human (Bremner et al., 1981). Instead, it has been suggested that FSH, by some poorly understood mechanism, facilitates the initiation of spermatogenesis in pubertal males and reinitiates spermatogenesis in hypophysectomized animals in which the germinal epithelium was allowed to regress post hypophysectomy (Steinberger, 1971; Ewing et al., 1980; DiZerga and Sherins, 1981). This controversial issue remains to be resolved.

Undoubtedly, other intratesticular factors, such as chalones, meiosis-inhibiting substances, meiosis-preventing substances, and as yet incompletely characterized proteins, are involved in the regulation of spermatogenesis. This topic is reviewed by Parvinen (1982).

Human spermatogenesis can be summarized as follows: Given the proper hormonal environment, a new cohort of spermatogonia (Type Ap-B) is started through spermatogenesis every 16 days at any one site in the seminiferous epithelium. At this juncture, a few primitive spermatogonia (Ap-Ap) are set aside by an equivalent mitosis to provide stem cells for a later cohort of differentiating spermatogonia. Since the first cohort of germ cells requires 64 days to differentiate into Sd2 spermatids, four cohorts of differentiating germ cells are observed in the seminiferous epithelium. The simultaneous differentiation of these different cohorts of cells over concurrent 64-day periods includes six stages of the spermatogenic cycle, which can be observed upon examination of histologic specimens of human testis.

EPIDIDYMIS

Testicular spermatozoa are not motile and are incapable of fertilizing ova. Spermatozoa become functional gametes only after they migrate through the epididymis and undergo an additional maturation process, thereby acquiring the capacities for both progressive motility and fertility. Although most studies of epididymal sperm maturation have involved laboratory and domestic animals, increasing evidence suggests that similar processes occur in man as well. The following sections describe the structures and functions of the epididymis and discuss the physiologic and biochemical events associated with sperm epididymal maturation.

Gross Structures

Anatomically, the epididymis can be divided into three regions: the caput, the corpus, and the cauda epididymidis (Figure 5–22). On the basis of histologic criteria, each of these regions can be subdivided into distinct zones separated by transition segments. The human caput epididymidis consists of 8 to 12 ductuli efferentes and the initial segment of the ductus epididymidis. The lumen of the ductuli efferentes is large and somewhat irregular in shape proximal to the testis, becoming narrow and oval near the junction with the ductus epididymidis. Distal to this junction the diameter of the duct increases slightly and thereafter remains relatively constant throughout the corpus, or body, of the epididymis. In the bulky cauda epididymidis the diameter of the duct enlarges substantially, and the lumen acquires an irregular shape. Progressing distally, the duct gradually assumes the characteristic appearance of the ductus deferens.

The entire 5 to 6 meter length of the epididymal tubule is coiled and encapsulated within a sheath of connective tissue (Lanz and Neuhäuser, 1964). Extensions from this connective tissue sheath enter the interductal spaces, forming septa that divide the duct into histologically similar regions (Kormano and Reijonen,

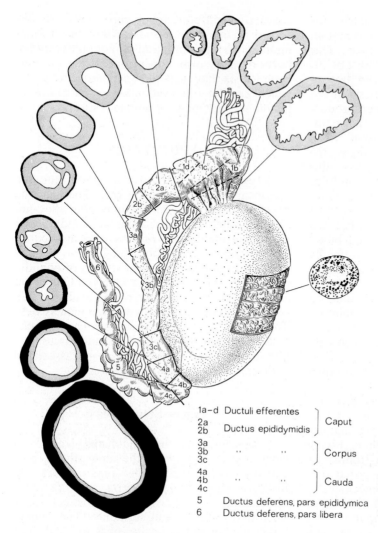

1a–d	Ductuli efferentes	
2a	Ductus epididymidis	Caput
2b		
3a		
3b	'' ''	Corpus
3c		
4a		
4b	'' ''	Cauda
4c		
5	Ductus deferens, pars epididymica	
6	Ductus deferens, pars libera	

Figure 5–22. Schematic drawing of the human epididymis showing regionalization of the ductal epithelium and muscle layer. Locations of epididymal segments shown in cross section are identified by numbers. (From Baumgarten, H. G., et al.: Z. Zellforsch. Mikrosk. Anat., *120*:37, 1971.)

1976). A loose network of tissue arises from the septa, supporting the ducts and their associated vascular supply and innervation.

CONTRACTILE TISSUE

External to the basal lamina of the ductuli efferentes and the epididymal tubule are contractile cells of varying architecture and quantity (Baumgarten et al., 1971). In the ductuli efferentes, the distal regions of the caput epididymidis, and the proximal segments of the corpus epididymidis, the contractile cells form a loose layer two to four cells deep around the tubule. These cells contain myofilaments and are connected by numerous nexus-like junctions. In the distal regions of the corpus epididymidis, other contractile cells are present. These cells are much larger than the contractile cells in the more proximal regions, have fewer nexus-like

intracellular junctions, and resemble thin smooth muscle cells. In the cauda epididymidis, the thin contractile cells decrease in number and are replaced by thick smooth muscle cells that form three layers—the outer two layers oriented longitudinally and the central layer circularly. This contractile layer increases in thickness distally and ultimately joins the ductus deferens.

INNERVATION

The innervation of the human epididymis is derived primarily from the intermediate and inferior spermatic nerves, which, in turn, arise from the superior portion of the hypogastric plexus and from the vesical plexus, respectively (Mitchell, 1935). The ductuli efferentes and the initial segments of the ductus epididymidis are sparsely innervated by sympathetic fibers (Baumgarten et al., 1968; Baumgarten and Holstein, 1967). In these regions the fibers are present in a peritubular plexus and are principally associated with blood vessels. The number of nerve fibers rises significantly at the level of the mid–corpus epididymidis and progressively increases distally along the epididymis, coincident with the appearance and proliferation of smooth muscle cells (Baumgarten et al., 1971). The differential distribution of the contractile cells and the sympathetic nerves within the epididymis may be responsible for the rhythmic peristaltic movements of the ductuli efferentes and the initial segments of the epididymis, as well as the intermittent contractile activity of the cauda epididymidis and the ductus deferens during emission and ejaculation (Risley, 1963). The significance of these physiologic events to the movement of spermatozoa through the epididymis will be discussed in a later section.

VASCULARIZATION

In humans, the caput and the corpus epididymidis receive arterial blood via a single branch from the testicular artery, which divides into the superior and inferior epididymal branches (MacMillan, 1954). The cauda epididymidis is supplied by branches from the deferential artery (artery of the vas deferens), which also communicates with the arteries of the caput epididymidis. The vasal and cremasteric arteries serve as collateral sources to the epididymis in the event that the main testicular artery is obstructed or ligated.

The arterial branches leading to the epididymis enter along the septa formed by the connective tissue sheath (Figure 5–23). Once having entered the epididymis these vessels become extensively coiled before transforming into the straight vessels of the microvascular bed (Kormano and Reijonen, 1976). The microvascularization varies significantly along the length of the ductus epididymidis, the initial segments of the caput epididymidis containing a dense subepithelial capillary network and the degree of vascularization decreasing distally along the epididymal duct.

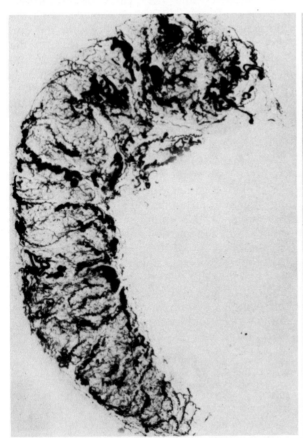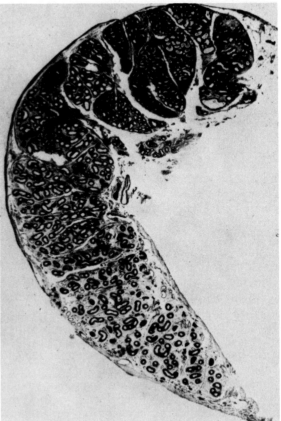

Figure 5–23. Vasculature and histology of the proximal portion of the human epididymis. Angiogram (left) shows coiled arteries entering the epididymis along connective tissue septa which, in histologic section (right), separate the epididymal tubule into distinct lobes. Magnification approximately × 3. (From Kormano, M., and Reijonen, K.: Am. J. Anat., *145*:23, 1976.)

Studies using experimental animals demonstrated that the capillary network within the epididymis is under hormonal control. For example, in rabbits, bilateral castration results in progressive deterioration and eventual disappearance of the epididymal capillary network (Clavert et al., 1981). It is not clear whether vascularization in the human epididymis is also under hormonal control.

According to MacMillan (1954), venous drainage from the corpus and cauda epididymidis join to form the vena marginalis epididymis of Haberer. The capital veins communicate with the pampiniform plexus or the vena marginalis, the latter then joining the vena marginalis testis, the pampiniform plexus, the cremasteric vein, or the deferential vein.

Lymphatic drainage of the epididymis occurs through two routes (Wenzel and Kellermann, 1966). Lymph from the caput and corpus epididymidis is removed via the same vessels draining the testis. These vessels follow the internal spermatic vein through the inguinal canal and ultimately terminate in the preaortic nodes. Lymph vessels from the cauda epididymidis join those draining the ductus deferens and terminate in the external iliac nodes.

Epithelial Histology

The epithelium of the human epididymis exhibits regional differences along the length of the duct. The junction of the rete testis and the ductuli efferentes is characterized by a distinct transition from a low to a high cuboidal epithelium. The epithelium in the ductuli efferentes consists of ciliated cells and two types of nonciliated cells (Holstein, 1969). The ciliated cells are interdispersed throughout the epithelium. Nonciliated cells with protruding apices, suggesting secretory acitivity, predominate in the proximal region of the ductuli efferentes. These cells are often present in shallow areas of the epithelium, thereby forming intraepithelial glands (Vendrely, 1981). Other nonciliated cells possessing microvilli, which suggest resorptive activity, predominate in the distal region of the ductuli efferentes. Both the nonciliated and the ciliated cells are joined apically through junctional complexes. In laboratory animals, similar junctions between epithelial cells within the caput epididymidis are thought to form a blood-epididymis barrier analogous to the blood-testis barrier (Suzuki and Nagano, 1978). The blood-epididymis barrier probably extends from the caput into the cauda epididymidis. Howards et

al. (1976) demonstrated that the barrier in the hamster cauda epididymidis is permeable to low molecular weight substances, such as water and urea, but impermeable to inulin, a compound with a molecular weight of 5000. As will be discussed later, the blood-epididymis barrier may play an important role in influencing the composition of fluid present within different segments of the epididymal lumen (Turner, 1979).

The histology of the human ductus epididymidis has been reviewed by Holstein (1969) and Vendrely (1981). The epithelium consists of two major cell types, principal cells and basal cells (Fig. 5–24). Principal cells vary in height and length of stereocilia, generally being tall (120 μm), with long stereocilia in the proximal regions of the epididymis, and small (50 μm), with short stereocilia in the more distal regions. The nuclei in these cells are elongated and often possess large clefts and one or two nucleoli. The presence of numerous micropinocytotic vesicles and multivesicular bodies near the apex of these cells suggests that they carry out resorptive processes. Basal cells are dispersed among the more numerous principal cells within the epithelium. These tear-shaped cells rest on the basal lamina and extend approximately 25 μm toward the lumen, their apices forming threads between adjacent principal cells. The morphology of basal cells remains relatively constant throughout the epididymal duct.

Functions of the Epididymis

Taken together, the observations concerning regional differences in (1) the anatomic structures of the epididymal tubule, (2) the innervation and vascularization of the duct, and (3) the histology of the epithelium support the hypothesis that the epididymis is actually a succession of different tissues (Vendrely, 1981). The following sections describe the functions of this complex system, specifically, sperm transit and storage and sperm fertility and motility maturation.

SPERM TRANSPORT

Depending on the measurements employed, sperm transport through the human male reproductive tract has been observed to require 7 to 35 days (Rowley et al., 1970). Extrapolating from daily sperm production rates, Amann (1981) observed that transit time through the epididymis varies with age and sexual activity. Sperm epididymal transit time is

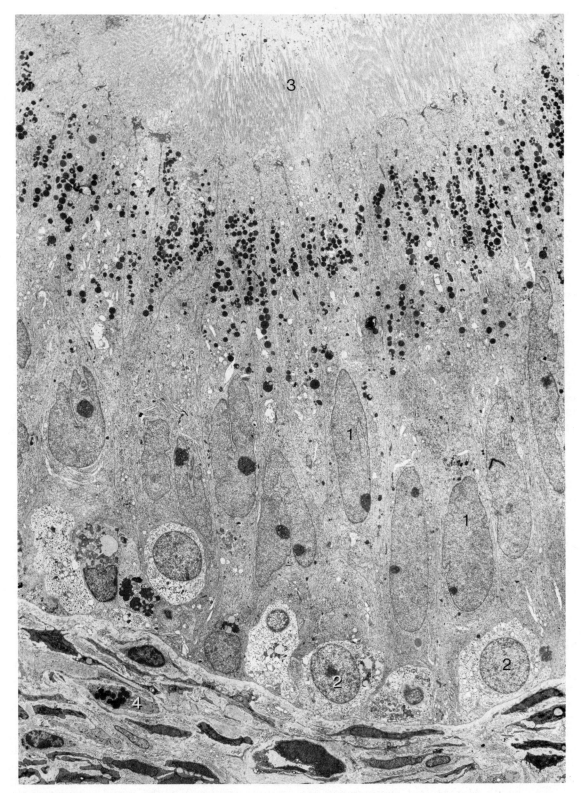

Figure 5–24. Electron micrograph of a cross section through the human ductus epididymidis. Major components of the luminal epithelium are principal cells (1), basal cells (2), stereocilia (3), and myofilaments (4). Magnification approximately × 1800. (From Holstein, A. F.: *In* Hafez, E. S. E. (Ed.): Human Semen and Fertility Regulation in Men. St. Louis, The C. V. Mosby Co., 1976. Copyright 1976, The C. V. Mosby Co., St. Louis.)

shortest in 19- to 20-year-old men, about 2.7 days. In these men, transit time through the caput–corpus epididymidis and through the cauda epididymidis is 1.7 and 1.0 days, respectively. Longest epididymal transit time is found in 16- to 18-year-old men. Epididymal passage in these individuals requires approximately 11.9 days—6.0 days for the caput–corpus epididymidis and 5.9 days for the cauda epididymidis. The variation in sperm transit time with age is attributed to differences in the daily testicular sperm production rate rather than to a direct influence of age on the epididymis. With respect to sexual activity, Amann (1981) reported that whereas sperm transit time through the caput and corpus epididymidis is not affected, "recent emissions" reduce transit time through the cauda epididymidis by 68 per cent.

Since it is generally accepted that human spermatozoa are immotile within the epididymal lumen, other mechanisms must be involved in the movement of the spermatozoa through the epididymis. These mechanisms may be inferred from the results of animal studies (Bedford, 1975; Hamilton, 1977; Courot, 1981). Initially, spermatozoa are carried into the ductuli efferentes by rete testis fluid; the flow of the fluid is facilitated by the resorption of water by ductal epithelial cells. Motile cilia in the ductuli efferentes may also assist the movement of spermatozoa into the epididymis. The principal mechanism responsible for moving spermatozoa through the epididymis is probably the spontaneous rhythmic contractions of the contractile cells surrounding the epididymal duct. The regionalization of the smooth muscle cells, and the adrenergic innervation within the epididymis described earlier, serve to optimize the ability of the epididymal duct to transport spermatozoa to the ductus deferens.

SPERM STORAGE

The number of spermatozoa present in the human epididymis is a function of age, testicular sperm production rate, and sexual activity (Amann, 1981). In men 21 to 30 years of age, the sperm reserve in each epididymis is approximately 209 million, with 57 per cent of the spermatozoa present in the cauda epididymidis. Men 31 to 55 years of age have epididymal sperm reserves of about 155 million per epididymis, of which 49 per cent are stored in the caudal region.

The length of time that spermatozoa are stored in the cauda epididymidis is not known. Studies using experimental animals demonstrated that spermatozoa can be maintained in a viable state for several weeks within the cauda epididymidis following ligation of the ductus deferens (Hammond and Asdell, 1926; Young, 1929). Other studies using animals indicated that the storage of spermatozoa within the cauda epididymidis is an active process, since hypophysectomy and castration result in the rapid passage of spermatozoa through the epididymis and the loss of sperm viability, these effects being reversible upon androgen treatment (Orgebin-Crist et al., 1976).

The fate of unejaculated epididymal spermatozoa in humans is unknown. Studies using experimental animals suggest a variety of sperm-removal mechanisms. In the rat and guinea pig, spermatozoa are lost via spontaneous seminal discharge and oral self-cleaning (Martan and Risley, 1963; Martan, 1969). Rams lose approximately 90 per cent of their daily production of 7 billion spermatozoa into urine (Lino et al., 1967), while bulls may lose about 50 per cent of the spermatozoa produced by the testis owing to resorption in the epididymis (Amann and Almquist, 1961). In humans, phagocytosis of spermatozoa by macrophages within the lumen of the epididymis is observed following ligation of the ductus deferens (Phadke, 1964; Alexander, 1972). However, removal of large numbers of spermatozoa in unvasectomized men by spermiophages, spontaneous emission, or epididymal resorption has not been reported.

MATURATION OF SPERMATOZOA

Beyond serving as a mere conduit and storage depot for spermatozoa the epididymis sustains maturation processes that result in the acquisition of progressive motility and fertility by spermatozoa. Although initial studies were conducted in laboratory and domestic animals, recent reports suggest that similar processes also occur in humans.

Sperm Motility Maturation. Human spermatozoa develop an increased capacity for progressive motility as they migrate through the epididymis (Bedford et al., 1973). The majority of spermatozoa taken from the ductuli efferentes and resuspended in culture medium are immotile or exhibit only weak tail movements. A few spermatozoa from these samples have "immature" tail movements characterized by wide-arced, "thrashing" beats that result in little forward progression (Fig. 5–25). The number of spermatozoa possessing this immature motility pattern increases in the initial segment of the epididymis. More distally, in the midcorpus region, the proportion of spermatozoa exhibiting the immature motility decreases, with a

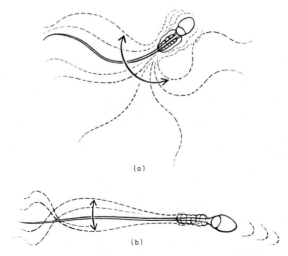

Figure 5–25. Patterns of tail movement in human epididymal spermatozoa. The pattern (a) shown by spermatozoa taken from proximal regions of the epididymis is characterized by a high-amplitude, low-frequency beat producing little forward movement. In contrast, tail movement in a large proportion of spermatozoa from the cauda epididymidis (b) is characterized by low-amplitude, rapid beats that result in forward progression. (From Bedford, J. M., et al.: J. Reprod. Fertil. (Suppl.), *18*:199, 1973.)

corresponding increase in the number of spermatozoa possessing a "mature" motility pattern characterized by high-frequency, low-amplitude beats that result in progressive motility (Fig. 5–25). In the cauda epididymidis, greater than 50 per cent of the spermatozoa possess the mature motility pattern, the remainder of the spermatozoa being immotile or having the immature motility forms observed in the proximal regions of the epididymis.

Studies involving experimental animals indicated that motility maturation may be predominantly a sperm-related process, not dependent on specific regions of the epididymis. Although hamster and rabbit spermatozoa are generally immotile in the caput epididymidis, motile spermatozoa are found in these epididymal regions following ligation of the duct at the level of the corpus epididymidis, suggesting that the development of motility is associated primarily with the intrinsic "aging" of spermatozoa within the epididymis (Horan and Bedford, 1972; Orgebin-Crist, 1969). Whether epididymal sperm motility maturation in humans is also independent of specific epididymal regions is not clear. One study reported that although the motility of ejaculated spermatozoa is initially poor following vasoepididymostomy at the level of the caput epididymidis, sperm motility improves greatly after 1½ years (Silber, 1980). Since the majority of spermatozoa from the

caput epididymidis are usually immotile, this study suggests that following vasoepididymostomy the caput epididymidis may in time undergo compensatory adaptation and acquire the ability to support sperm motility maturation (Silber, 1980). This intriguing hypothesis requires further study.

Sperm Fertility Maturation. Convincing evidence from experimental studies demonstrated that testicular spermatozoa are incapable of fertilizing eggs (Orgebin-Crist, 1969; Bedford, 1974). In most animals the ability to fertilize eggs is gradually acquired as the spermatozoa migrate into the distal regions of the epididymidis. For example, Orgebin-Crist (1969) showed that spermatozoa from the caput, corpus, and cauda epididymidis of the rabbit are able to fertilize 1 per cent, 63 per cent, and 92 per cent of exposed rabbit eggs, respectively (Fig. 5–26). Recently, evidence for epididymal sperm fertility maturation in humans was presented. Using zona pellucida–free hamster eggs to assess the fertilizing capacity of human epididymal spermatozoa, Hinrichsen and Blaquier (1980) demonstrated that while spermatozoa from the proximal regions of the epididymis are able to bind to zona-free hamster eggs, only spermatozoa from the cauda epididymidis are able to bind and penetrate the eggs. This suggests that sperm fertility maturation in humans is completed at the level of the cauda epididymidis. Other studies indicated that in humans some degree of sperm fertility maturation may occur in the caput epididymidis. Twenty-three of 121 patients initiated pregnancies after successful vasoepididymostomies at the level of the caput epididymidis (Young, 1970). In a much smaller series, one of five patients was able to successfully initiate a pregnancy 2 years following vasoepididymostomy at the level of the caput epididymis (Silber, 1980).

Although animal studies demonstrated that epididymal sperm motility maturation is in part a sperm-related and somewhat autonomous process, sperm fertility maturation appears to be dependent on exposure to specific epididymal regions. Ligation of the corpus epididymidis in the rabbit results in increased sperm motility and, to a much lesser extent, increased fertility in epididymal regions immediately proximal to the ligature. However, fertile spermatozoa are never present in the proximal regions of the caput epididymidis, indicating that the spermatozoa must undergo fertility maturation in regions distal to the proximal caput epididymidis (Orgebin-Crist, 1969; Bedford, 1967). Sperm fertility maturation in the hamster appears to

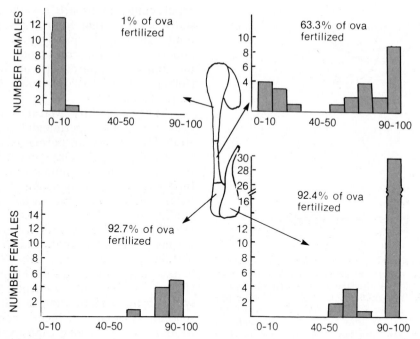

Figure 5–26. Sperm fertility maturation in the rabbit epididymis. Spermatozoa taken from distal regions of the epididymis possess higher fertilizing ability than do spermatozoa from proximal epididymal regions. (From Orgebin-Crist, M. C.: Biol. Reprod. (Suppl.), *1*:155, 1969.)

be even more dependent upon specific epididymal regions. Ligation of the corpus epididymidis does not increase the fertilizing capacity of hamster spermatozoa in any epididymal region proximal to the site of ligation (Horan and Bedford, 1972). From these animal studies it can be assumed that epididymal sperm fertility maturation in humans is also dependent on specific epididymal regions. However, it is not clear where in the human epididymis this process occurs.

Controversy exists concerning the outcome of fertilization by spermatozoa that have just acquired fertilizing capacity in the proximal regions of the epididymis. Overstreet and Bedford (1976) reported that embryonic mortality in the rabbit is not increased after fertilization with spermatozoa taken from the distal corpus epididymidis. However, other studies using rabbits (Orgebin-Crist, 1969; Orgebin-Crist and Jahad, 1977; Brackett et al., 1978), sheep (Fournier-Delpech et al., 1979), and rats (Paz et al., 1978) indicated that fertilization using immature or young spermatozoa from proximal regions of the epididymis results in a higher rate of embryonic mortality compared with fertilization using ejaculated spermatozoa or mature spermatozoa from the distal epididymidis. Because of the increasing occurrence of high vasoepididymos-

tomies using microsurgical techniques, this controversy and its relevance to humans must be resolved by future studies.

Biochemical Changes in Spermatozoa During Epididymal Maturation. Dramatic changes occur in the membranes and internal constituents of spermatozoa as they pass through the epididymis. In humans, membrane modifications during epididymal migration were studied using electron-dense ferric oxide particles (Bedford et al., 1973). Spermatozoa from the proximal regions of the epididymis do not bind these positively charged particles (Fig. 5–27). In contrast, ferric oxide particles are bound by the membrane on the tails of spermatozoa from the middle region of the corpus epididymidis and by both head and tail membranes of spermatozoa from the distal regions of the corpus epididymidis. Intense binding of particles occurs on the heads and tails of caudal epididymal spermatozoa (Fig. 5–27). The increase in ferric oxide binding indicates that as spermatozoa migrate distally within the epididymis, the surface membranes assume an increasingly negative net charge.

Studies on laboratory animals described other membrane modifications associated with sperm epididymal migration. These include alterations in sperm lectin-binding properties (Ni-

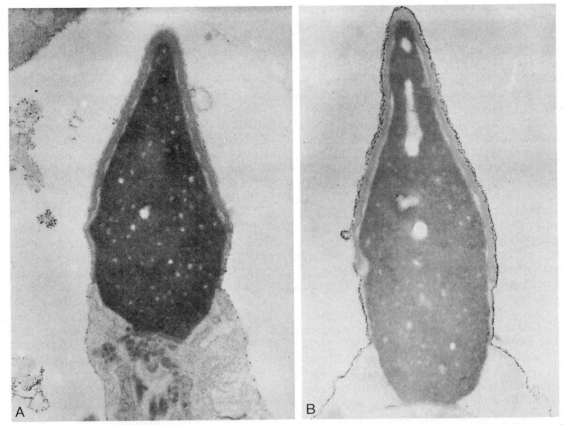

Figure 5–27. Changes in the plasma membrane of human spermatozoa during epididymal migration. Electron micrographs of human spermatozoa from the caput (*A*) and cauda (*B*) epididymidis after fixation in glutaraldehyde and exposure to a colloidal solution of ferric oxide particles at pH 8.1. Whereas the positively charged particles do not bind to caput epididymal spermatozoa, there is intense particle binding to the surface of spermatozoa from the cauda epididymidis. (From Bedford, J. M.: *In* Greep, R. O., and Astwood, E. B. (Eds.): Handbook of Physiology, Section 7. Endocrinology. Baltimore, The Williams & Wilkins Co., 1975. Copyright 1975, the American Physiological Society, Bethesda, Md.)

colson et al., 1977; Courtens and Fournier-Delpech, 1979; Olson and Danzo, 1981), glycoprotein composition (Fournier-Delpech et al., 1977; Olson and Danzo, 1981; Brown et al., 1983), immunoreactivity (Killian and Amann, 1973), and iodination characteristics (Nicolson et al., 1979; Olson and Danzo, 1981). Orgebin-Crist and Fournier-Delpech (1982) demonstrated that in the rat, sperm membrane modifications during epididymal passage result in an increased ability to adhere to the zona pellucida of the egg.

Additional biochemical changes observed in human spermatozoa during epididymal transit involve the formation of disulfide bonds within the sperm nucleus and tail (Bedford et al., 1973) and the oxidation of sperm membrane sulfhydryl groups (Reyes et al., 1976). Bedford et al., (1973) suggested that the formation of intracellular disulfide bonds may provide the sperm tail and head with the structural rigidity necessary

for progressive motility and successful penetration of eggs.

Studies using experimental animals indicated that during epididymal transit spermatozoa undergo numerous metabolic changes, including the acquisition of an increased capacity for glycolysis (Hoskins et al., 1975), modification of adenylate cyclase activity (Casillas et al., 1980), and alterations in cellular phospholipid and phospholipid-like fatty acid content (Voglmayr, 1975). Whether similar modifications occur in human spermatozoa during epididymal migration is unknown.

FACTORS INVOLVED IN EPIDIDYMAL FUNCTION

Although the mechanisms by which the epididymis carries out its functions of sperm transport, sperm maturation, and sperm storage are unclear, the consensus is that these processes are influenced by the fluids and secretions within the epididymal lumen. The constituents of this fluid have been reviewed by Turner (1979), Waites (1980), and Orgebin-Crist (1981). Studies using laboratory animals demonstrated that the biochemical composition of epididymal fluid not only differs from that of blood serum but also undergoes regional changes within the epididymis. Glycerylphosphorylcholine (GPC), carnitine, and sialic acid are present in high concentrations in epididymal fluid. In addition, epididymal fluid contains proteins that have physiologic effects on spermatozoa in vitro. Examples of these proteins are forward motility protein (Brandt et al., 1978), sperm survival factor (Morton et al., 1978), progressive motility sustaining factor (Sheth et al., 1981), and sperm motility–inhibiting factor (Turner and Giles, 1982). Other proteins are secreted into specific regions of the epididymis and subsequently become associated with spermatozoa (Orgebin-Crist, 1981; Kohane et al., 1980).

For a thorough discussion of the regionalization of epididymal fluid the reader is referred to an excellent review by Turner (1979). Suffice it to say that the osmolarity, electrolyte content, and protein composition of luminal fluid varies significantly from region to region in the epididymis. This fluid compartmentalization may reflect the multifunctional nature of the epididymis and is probably the consequence of the differential vascularization along the epididymal tubule, the semipermeability of the blood-epididymis barrier, and the selective absorption and secretion of fluid constituents by the luminal epithelium, which, as discussed earlier, undergoes dramatic changes along the length of the duct.

CONTROL OF EPIDIDYMAL FUNCTION

From animal studies it is clear that the functions of the epididymis are androgen-dependent (Orgebin-Crist et al., 1975; Turner, 1979). Bilateral castration results in the loss of epididymal weight, perturbation of luminal histology, and changes in the secretion of epididymal fluid components, including GPC, carnitine, sialic acid, and proteins. Ultimately, the epididymis loses the ability to sustain the processes of sperm motility and fertility maturation and sperm storage. Most of these degenerative processes can be reversed by androgen replacement therapy. However, the effects of androgen on the initial segments of the epididymis are thought to be mediated by androgen-binding protein and possibly other testicular factors. Thus, the consequences of androgen deprivation on the initial epididymal regions cannot be

reversed following castration or ligation of the ductuli efferentes, treatments that prevent the entrance of androgen-binding protein and testicular factors into the epididymis (Fawcett and Hoffer, 1979).

Studies using laboratory animals indicated that, compared with the accessory sex glands, the epididymis requires higher levels of androgen for maintenance of its structure and functions (Rajalakshmi et al., 1976). The regulatory effects of androgen on the epididymis appear to be mediated through dihydrotestosterone (DHT), the primary androgen in epididymal tissue extracts (Vreeburg, 1975; Pujol et al., 1976), and/or 5α-androstan-3α,17β-diol (3α-diol) (Lubicz-Nawrocki, 1973; Orgebin-Crist et al., 1975). The enzymes Δ^4-5α-reductase, which catalyzes the formation of DHT from testosterone, and 3α-hydroxysteroid dehydrogenase, which converts DHT to 3α-diol, are present in the epididymis and have been localized within the subcellular fractions of epididymal homogenates from humans (Kinoshita et al., 1980; Larminat, et al., 1980) and experimental animals (Robaire et al., 1977; Scheer and Robaire, 1983).

Studies in the rat demonstrated that epididymal functions are also influenced by temperature (Foldesy and Bedford, 1982; Wong et al., 1982). Abdominal placement of the epididymis, resulting in exposure to body temperature, causes the loss of sperm storage and electrolyte transport functions. Whether the functions of the human epididymis are similarly affected by body temperature is unknown. The potential influence of temperature on epididymal function in man may be an important consideration in investigating the relationship between varicocele and male infertility.

Spermatozoa

Mature spermatozoa stored in the cauda epididymidis and the ductus deferens are highly differentiated cells (Fig. 5–28). (See Fawcett and Bedford [1979] for reviews on sperm structure and function.) The human spermatozoon is approximately 60 μm in length (Fléchon and Hafez, 1976). The oval sperm head, about 4.5 μm long and 3 μm wide, consists principally of a nucleus, which contains the highly compacted chromatin material, and an acrosome, a membrane-bound organelle that contains the enzymes required for penetration of the outer vestments of the egg prior to fertilization (Chang and Hunter, 1975; Yanagimachi, 1978). The

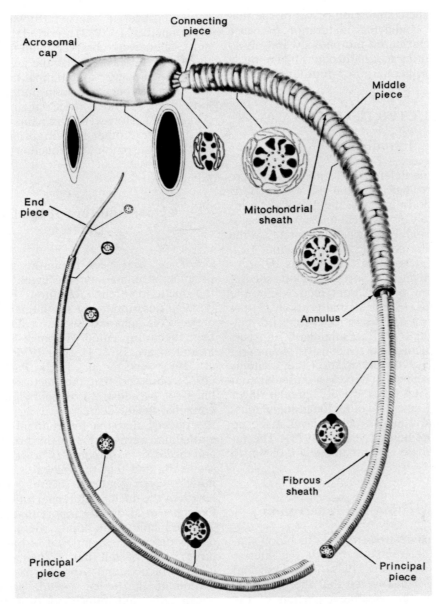

Figure 5–28. Diagram of a typical mammalian spermatozoon. The plasma membrane is omitted in order to illustrate the major components of the spermatozoon. Cross-sectional insets show the orientation of the internal cell structures. (From Fawcett, D. W.: Dev. Biol., *44*:394, 1975.)

middle piece of the spermatozoon is a highly organized segment consisting of helically arranged mitochondria surrounding a set of outer dense fibers and the characteristic 9 + 2 microtubular structure of the sperm axoneme. The mitochondria contain the enzymes required for oxidative metabolism and the production of adenosine triphosphate (ATP), the primary energy source for the cell. The outer dense fibers, rich in disulfide bonds, are thought to provide the sperm tail with the rigidity necessary for progressive motility (Bedford et al., 1973). The

sperm axoneme contains the enzymes and structural proteins necessary for transduction of the chemical energy of ATP into the mechanical movement resulting in motility. The outer dense fibers and axonemal structures present in the middle piece continue, with slight modification, through the principal piece of the spermatozoon, which is surrounded by a fibrous sheath. At the distal end of the principal piece the outer dense fibers terminate, leaving the axonemes as the primary structure in the end-piece region.

The functionally competent spermatozoon

is a result of the complex processes of spermatogenesis and epididymal maturation. Because of its highly specialized morphology and physiology the resulting spermatozoon is marvelously suited for its single purpose—reproduction.

DUCTUS DEFERENS

Introduction

The ductus deferens is a tubular structure derived embryologically from the mesonephric (wolffian) duct. In humans, the ductus deferens is approximately 30 to 35 cm in length; it begins at the cauda epididymidis and terminates in the ejaculatory duct near the prostate gland. Lich et al. (1978) stated that "the ductus deferens may be divided into five portions: (1) the sheathless epididymal portion contained within the tunica vaginalis, (2) the scrotal portion, (3) the inguinal division, (4) the retroperitoneal or pelvic portion, and (5) the ampulla." In cross section, the ductus deferens consists of an outer adventitial connective tissue sheet that contains blood vessels and small nerves, a muscular coat that is made up of a middle circular layer surrounded by inner and outer longitudinal muscle layers, and a mucosal inner layer made up of an epithelial lining (Neaves, 1975). The lumen of the tubule is approximately 0.05 cm in diameter.

Vascularization and Innervation

The ductus deferens receives its blood supply from the deferential artery via the inferior vesicle artery (Harrison, 1949). Kormano and Reijonen (1976) discovered that the microvascularization of the sheathless portion of the human ductus deferens is divided into an outer network within the adventitial layer and an inner subepithelial capillary network.

The ductus deferens of the human receives nerve fibers from both the sympathetic and the parasympathetic nervous system (Sjöstrand, 1965). The cholinergic supply is of minor importance in the motor activity of the ductus deferens (Baumgarten et al., 1975). In contrast, the human ductus deferens has a rich supply of sympathetic adrenergic nerves (Sjöstrand, 1965; Alm, 1982; McConnell et al., 1982) derived from the hypogastric nerves via the presacral nerve (Batra and Lardner, 1976). Interestingly, the ductus deferens receives a special type of

short adrenergic nerve (Sjöstrand, 1965). McConnell et al. (1982) reported that adrenergic nerve fibers were observed in all three layers of the tunica muscularis, with the greatest concentration in the outer longitudinal layer. Neurons containing other neurotransmitter substances have been identified (McConnell et al., 1982; Alm, 1982). However, it remains to be proved whether these other neurotransmitters are important in the physiologic functions of the ductus deferens.

Cytoarchitecture of the Ductus Deferens

There have been numerous studies in experimental animals on the cytoarchitecture of the ductus deferens (Hamilton, 1975). Similar detailed descriptions of the human ductus deferens at the light and electron microscopic level have been presented (Popovic et al., 1973; Friend et al., 1976; Hoffer, 1976; Paniagua et al., 1981; Riva et al., 1982). Paniagua et al. (1981) observed that the ductus deferens was lined by pseudostratified epithelium; that the epithelial height decreased along the length of the ductus; that the longitudinal folds of the epithelium were simple in the proximal region and became more complex toward the distal segments; and that the thickness of the entire muscle layer gradually decreased along the length of the ductus deferens. Hoffer (1976) and Paniagua et al. (1981) report that the pseudostratified epithelium lining the lumen of the ductus deferens is composed of basal cells and three types of tall thin columnar cells. The latter, which extend from the base of the epithelium to the lumen, include principal cells, pencil cells, and mitochondrion-rich cells. All of these cells show stereocilia and irregular convoluted nuclei. According to Paniagua et al. (1981), principal cells are the most frequent cell type in the proximal portion of the ductus deferens. In contrast, the portion of both pencil cells and mitochondrion-rich cells increases toward the distal end of the ductus deferens.

The complexity of the muscular layers, the specialized and rich adrenergic innervation, the variety of epithelial cells in the mucosal layer, and the changing structural characteristics from the proximal to the distal end suggest strongly that the ductus deferens in man is more than a passive conduit for the transport of sperm from the cauda epididymidis to the urethra.

Function of the Ductus Deferens

SPERMATOZOA TRANSPORT

There are numerous theories to explain the transport of spermatozoa through the ductus deferens in humans (Neaves, 1975; Gunha et al., 1975; Batra and Lardner, 1976). Unfortunately, data supporting these theories are fragmentary and the issue remains unresolved. However, several pertinent observations have been made. Apparently, the human ductus deferens exhibits a spontaneous motility (Ventura et al., 1973). Also, the human ductus deferens has the capacity to respond with low-amplitude peristaltic contractions when stretched (Bruschini et al., 1977). Finally, the contents of the ductus can be propelled into the urethra by strong peristaltic contractions that are elicited either by electrical stimulation of the hypogastric nerve (Bruschini et al., 1977) or by adrenergic neurotransmitters (Ventura et al., 1973; Bruschini et al., 1977; Lipshultz et al., 1981).

Prins and Zaneveld (1979, 1980a,b) have obtained interesting results regarding the transport of spermatozoa through the ductus deferens at sexual rest, after sexual stimulation, and after ejaculation. Using the rabbit as a model, they (Prins and Zaneveld, 1979) showed that "during the sexual rest, epididymal contents were transported distally through the vas deferens into the urethra in small amounts and at irregular intervals," supporting the idea that urethral disposal is a mechanism for ridding the epididymis of excess spermatozoa. Further, they (Prins and Zaneveld, 1979, 1980a,b) showed that when rabbits were sexually stimulated, spermatozoa were transported from the cauda epididymidis and proximal ductus deferens toward the distal ductus deferens. If ejaculation occurred, spermatozoa were propelled into the urethra.

After sexual stimulation and/or ejaculation, an interesting phenomenon occurred. The contents of the ductus deferens were propelled back toward the proximal epididymis and even into the cauda epididymidis because the distal portion of the ductus deferens contracted with greater amplitude, frequency, and duration than did the proximal portion of the ductus deferens (Prins and Zaneveld, 1980b). Importantly, this process was reversed upon prolonged sexual rest, and the excess cauda epididymal spermatozoa that derived from daily spermatozoa production were once again transported distally. These results were interpreted to mean that the ductus deferens of the rabbit played an important role not only in sperm transport during sexual activity but also in the maintenance of epididymal sperm reserves. It remains to be seen whether similar mechanisms are at work in sperm transport through the human ductus deferens.

ABSORPTION AND SECRETION

Based on morphologic criteria, it has been suggested that the human ductus deferens may have both absorptive and secretory functions (Hoffer, 1976; Paniagua et al., 1981). Unfortunately, we were unable to find experimental results in the human that would confirm this idea.

Hoffer (1976) and Paniagua et al. (1981) reported that the principal cells of the human ductus deferens have characteristics typical of cells that are capable of synthesizing and secreting glycoproteins. This is in keeping with reports by Gupta et al. (1974) and Bennett et al. (1974) that the rat ductus deferens synthesizes and secretes glycoproteins into the tubular lumen.

The stereocilia, apical blebbing, and primary and secondary lysosomes of principal cells in the human ductus deferens are also characteristic of cells involved in absorptive functions (Hoffer, 1976; Paniagua et al., 1981). Protein absorption from the tubular lumen of the rat ductus deferens has been observed (Friend and Farquhar, 1967). Cooper and Hamilton (1977) have shown that the terminal region and gland of the rat ductus deferens have the capacity to phagocytose and absorb spermatozoa. Whether this occurs in the human ductus deferens remains to be seen.

The structure and function of the ductus deferens probably depends on androgen stimulation because (1) the human ductus deferens converts testosterone to dihydrotestosterone (Dupuy et al., 1979); (2) castration causes atrophy of—and testosterone treatment, restoration of—monkey vas (Dinaker et al., 1977); and (3) spontaneous as well as alpha- and beta-adrenergic stimulated contractions of the rat ductus deferens are altered by castration and/or testosterone treatment (Borda et al., 1981).

References

Agger, P.: Scrotal and testicular temperature: Its relation to sperm count before and after operation for varicocele. Fertil. Steril., 22:286, 1971.

Alexander, N. J.: Vasectomy: long-term effects in the rhesus monkey. J. Reprod. Fertil., 31:399, 1972.

Alm, P.: On the autonomic innervation of the human vas deferens. Brain Res. Bull., 9:673, 1982.

Amann, R. P.: A critical review of methods for evaluation of spermatogenesis from seminal characteristics. J. Androl., 2:37, 1981.

Amann, R. P., and Almquist, J. O.: Reproductive capacity of dairy bulls. VI. Effect of unilateral vasectomy and ejaculation frequency on sperm reserves: Aspects of epididymal physiology. J. Reprod. Fertil., 3:260, 1961.

Amann, R. P., and Howards, S. S.: Daily spermatozoal production and epididymal spermatozoal reserves of the human male. J. Urol., 124:211, 1980.

Anderson, J. M., and Dietschy, J. M.: Regulation of sterol synthesis in 15 tissues of rat. II. Role of rat and human high and low density plasma lipoproteins and of rat chylomicron remnants. J. Biol. Chem., 252:3652, 1977.

Bartmanska, J., and Clermont, Y.: Renewal of type A spermatogonia in adult rats. Cell Tissue Kinet., 16:135, 1983.

Batra, S. K., and Lardner, T. J.: Sperm transport in the vas deferens. In Hafez, E. S. E. (Ed.): Human Semen and Fertility Regulation in Men. St. Louis, The C. V. Mosby Co., 1976, p. 100.

Baumgarten, H. G., and Holstein, A. F.: Catecholamine-haltige nervenfasern im hoden des menschen. Z. Zellforsch. Mikrosk. Anat., 79:389, 1967.

Baumgarten, H. G., Falck, B., Holstein, A. F., Owman, C., and Owman, T.: Adrenergic innervation of the human testis, epididymis, ductus deferens and prostate: a fluorescence microscopic and fluorimetric study. Z. Zellforsch. Mikrosk. Anat., 90:81, 1968.

Baumgarten, H. G., Holstein, A. F., and Rosengren, E.: Arrangement, ultrastructure, and adrenergic innervation of smooth musculature of the ductuli efferentes, ductus epididymidis and ductus deferens of man. Z. Zellforsch. Mikrosk. Anat., 120:37, 1971.

Baumgarten, H. G., Owan, C., and Sjöberg, N. O.: Neural mechanisms in male fertility. In Sciarra, J. J., et al. (Eds.): Control of Male Fertility, New York; Harper & Row, 1975, p. 26.

Bawa, S. R.: Fine structure of the Sertoli cell of the human testis. J. Ultrastruct. Res., 9:459, 1963.

Bayard, F., Boulard, P. Y., Huc, A., and Pontonnier, F.: Arterio-venous transfer of testosterone in the spermatic cord of man. J. Clin. Endocrinol. Metab., 40:345, 1975.

Bedford, J. M.: Effect of duct ligation on the fertilizing ability of spermatozoa from different regions of the rabbit epididymis. J. Exp. Zool., 166:271, 1967.

Bedford, J. M.: Report of a workshop. Maturation of the fertilizing ability of mammalian spermatozoa in the male and female reproductive tract. Biol. Reprod., 11:346, 1974.

Bedford, J. M.: Maturation, transport and fate of spermatozoa in the epididymis. In Greep, R. O., and Astman, E. B. (Eds.): Handbook of Physiology, Section 7. Endocrinology. Baltimore, The Williams & Wilkins Co., 1975, p. 303.

Bedford, J. M., Calvin, H. I., and Cooper, G. W.: The maturation of spermatozoa in the human epididymis. J. Reprod. Fertil. (Suppl.), 18:199, 1973.

Bennett, G., Leblond, C. P., and Haddal, A.: Migration of glycoprotein from the Golgi apparatus to the surface of various cell types as shown by autoradiography after labelled fucose injection into rats. J. Cell Biol., 60:258, 1974.

Borda, E., Agostini, M. del C., Gimeno, M. F., and Gimeno, A. L.: Castration alters the stimulatory and inhibitory adrenergic influences on isolated rat vas deferens. Pharmacol. Res. Comm., 13:981, 1981.

Brackett, B. J., Hall, J. L., and Oh, Y. K.: In vitro fertilizing ability of testicular, epididymal, and ejaculated rabbit spermatozoa. Fertil. Steril., 29:571, 1978.

Brandt, H., Acott, T. S., Johnson, D. J., and Hoskins D. D.: Evidence for an epididymal origin of bovine sperm forward motility protein. Biol. Reprod., 19:830, 1978.

Bremner, W. J., Matsumoto, A. M., Sussman, A. M., and Paulsen, C. A.: Follicle-stimulating hormone and human spermatogenesis. J. Clin. Invest., 68:1044, 1981.

Brown, C. R., von Glos, K. I., and Jones, R.: Changes in plasma membrane glycoproteins of rat spermatozoa during maturation in the epididymis. J. Cell Biol., 96:256, 1983.

Brown, M. S., and Goldstein, J. L.: Receptor mediated control of cholesterol metabolism. Science, 191:159, 1976.

Bruschini, H., Schmidt, R. A., and Janagho, E. A.: Studies on the neurophysiology of the vas deferens. Invest. Urol., 15:112, 1977.

Casillas, E. R., Elder, C. M., and Hoskins, D. D.: Adenyate cyclase activity of bovine spermatozoa during maturation in the epididymis and the activation of sperm particulate adenylate cyclase by GTP and polyamines. J. Reprod. Fertil., 59:297, 1980.

Catt, K. J., and Dufau, M. L.: Basic concepts of the mechanism of action of peptide hormones. Biol. Reprod., 14:1, 1976.

Chang, M. C., and Hunter, R. H. F.: Capacitation of mammalian sperm: biological and experimental aspects. In Greep, R. O., and Astman, E. B. (Eds.): Handbook of Physiology, Section 7. Endocrinology. Baltimore, The Williams & Wilkins Co., 1975, p. 339.

Charreau, E. H., Calvo, J. C., Nozu, K., Pignataro, O., Catt, K. J., and Dufau, M. L.: Hormonal modulation of 3-hydroxy-3-methylglutaryl coenzyme A reductase activity in gonadotropin stimulated and desensitized testicular Leydig cells. J. Biol. Chem., 256:12719, 1981.

Chemes, H., Dym, M., Fawcett, D. W., Jaradpour, N., and Sherins, R. J.: Pathophysiological observations of Sertoli cells in patients with germinal aplasia or severe germ cell depletion. Ultrastructural findings and hormone levels. Biol. Reprod., 17:108, 1977.

Christensen, A. K.: Leydig cells. In Greep, R. O., and Astwood, E. B. (Eds.): Handbook of Physiology, Section 7. Endocrinolgy. Baltimore, The Williams & Wilkins Co., 1975, p. 57.

Clavert, A., Cranz, C., and Brun, B.: Epididymal vascularization and microvascularization. In Bollack, C., and Clavert, A. (Eds.): Progress in Reproductive Biology, Vol. 8. Epididymis and Fertility: Biology and Pathology. Basel, S. Karger, 1981, p. 48.

Clegg, E. J., and MacMillan, E. W.: The uptake of vital dyes and particulate matter by the Sertoli cells of the rat testis. J. Anat., 99:219, 1965.

Clermont, Y.: The cycle of the seminiferous epithelium in man. Am. J. Anat., 112:35, 1963.

Clermont, Y.: Renewal of spermatogonia in man. Am. J. Anat., 118:509, 1966.

Clermont, Y.: Kinetics of spermatogenesis in mammals: Seminiferous epithelium cycle and spermatogonial renewal. Physiol. Rev., 52:198, 1972.

Connell, C. J.: The Sertoli cell of the sexually mature dog. Anat. Rec., 178:333, 1974.

Cooke, B. A., DeJong, F. H., van der Molen, H. J., and Rommerts, F. F. G.: Endogenous testosterone concentrations in rat testis interstitial tissue and seminiferous tubules during in vitro incubation. Nature New Biol., 237:255, 1972.

Cooper, T. G., and Hamilton, D. W.: Phagocytosis of spermatozoa in the terminal region and gland of the vas deferens of the rat. Am. J. Anat., 150:247, 1977.

Courot, M.: Transport and maturation of spermatozoa in the epididymis of mammals. In Bollack, C., and Clavert, A. (Eds.): Progress in Reproductive Biology, Vol. 8. Epididymis and Fertility: Biology and Pathology. Basel, S. Karger, 1981, p. 67.

Courtens, J. L., and Fournier-Delpech, S.: Modifications in the plasma membranes of epididymal ram spermatozoa during maturation and incubation *in utero*. J. Ultrastruct. Res., *68*:136, 1979.

Davis, A. G.: Role of FSH in the control of testicular function. Arch. Androl., *7*:97, 1981.

Davis, J. R., and Langford, G. A.: Response of the testicular capsule to acetyl choline and noradrenaline. Nature, *222*:386, 1969.

Davis, J. R., and Langford, G. A.: Response of the isolated testicular capsule of the rat to autonomic drugs. J. Reprod. Fertil., *19*:595, 1970.

deKretser, D. W., and Burger, H. G.: Ultrastructural studies of the human Sertoli cell in normal men and males with hypogonadotropic hypogonadism before and after gonadotropic treatment. *In* Saxena, B. B., et al. (Eds.): Gonadotropins. New York, Wiley Interscience, 1972, p. 640.

Desjardins, C., Ewing, L. L., and Irby, D. C.: Response of the rabbit seminiferous epithelium to testosterone administered via polydimethysiloxane capsules. Endocrinology, *93*:450, 1973.

Dinakar, R. A., Dinakar, N., and Prasad, M. R. N.: Response of the epididymis, ductus deferens and accessory glands of the castrated prepubertal rhesus monkey to exogenous administration of testosterone or 5α-dihydrotestosterone. Indian J. Exp. Biol. *15*:829, 1977.

DiZerga, G. S., and Sherins, R. J.: Endocrine control of adult testicular function. *In* Burger, H., and deKretser, D. (Eds.): The Testis. New York, Raven Press, 1981, p. 127.

Dufau, M. L., and Catt, K. J.: Gonadotrophin receptors and regulation of steroidogenesis in the testis and ovary. Vitam. Horm., *36*:461, 1978.

Dufau, M. L., Hsueh, A. J., Cigorraga, S., Bankal, A. J., and Catt, K. J.: Inhibition of Leydig cell function through hormonal regulatory mechanisms. Int. J. Androl. (Suppl.), *2*:193, 1978.

Dupuy, G. M., Boulanger, K. D., Roberts, K. D., Bleau, G., and Chapdelaine, A.: Metabolism of sex steroids in the human and canine vas deferens. Endocrinology, *104*:1553, 1979.

Dym, M.: The fine structure of the monkey Sertoli cell and its role in maintaining the blood-testis barrier. Anat. Rec., *175*:639, 1973.

Dym, M., and Fawcett, D. W.: The blood-testis barrier in the rat and the physiological compartmentation of the seminiferous epithelium. Biol. Reprod., *3*:308, 1970.

Dym, M., Raj, H. G. M., and Chemes, H. E.: Response of the testis to selective withdrawal of LH or FSH using antigonadotropic sera. *In* Troen, P., and Nankin, H. R. (Eds.): The Testis in Normal and Infertile Man. New York, Raven Press, 1977, p. 97.

Eik-Nes, K. B.: Biosynthesis and secretion of testicular steroids. *In* Greep, R. O., and Astwood, E. B. (Eds.): Handbook of Physiology, Section 7. Endocrinology. Baltimore, The Williams & Wilkins Co., 1975, p. 95.

Ewing, L. L.: Leydig cell. *In* Lipshultz, L. I., and Howards, S. (Eds.): Infertility in the Male. New York, Churchill Livingstone, 1983, p. 43.

Ewing, L. L., and Brown, B.: Testicular steroidogenesis. *In* Johnson, A. D., and Gomes, W. R. (Eds.): The Testis. Vol. 4. New York, Academic Press, 1977, p. 239.

Ewing, L. L., and Zirkin, B. R.: Leydig cell structure and steroidogenic function. Rec. Prog. Horm. Res., *39*:599, 1983.

Ewing, L. L., Davis, J. C., and Zirkin, B. R.: Regulation of testicular function: A spatial and temporal view. *In* Greep, R. O. (Ed.): International Review of Physiology, Vol. 22, Baltimore, University Park Press, 1980, p. 41.

Faiman, C., Winter, J. S. D., and Reyes, F. I.: Endocrinology of the fetal testis. *In* Burger, H., and deKretser, D. (Eds.): The Testis. New York, Raven Press, 1981, p. 81.

Fawcett, D. W.: Interactions between Sertoli cells and germ cells. *In* Mancini, R. E., and Mancini, L. (Eds.): Male Fertility and Sterility. New York, Academic Press, 1974, p. 13.

Fawcett, D. W.: The mammalian spermatozoon. Dev. Biol., *44*:394, 1975a.

Fawcett, D. W.: Ultrastructure and function of the Sertoli cell. *In* Greep, R. O., and Astwood, E. B. (Eds.): Handbook of Physiology, Section 7. Endocrinology. Baltimore, The Williams & Wilkins Co., 1975b, p. 21.

Fawcett, D. W.: The cell biology of gametogenesis in the male. Perspect. Biol. Med., Winter 1979, p. S56.

Fawcett, D. W., and Bedford, J. M. (Eds.): The Spermatozoon. Maturation, Motility, Surface Properties and Comparative Aspects. Baltimore, Urban & Schwarzenberg, 1979.

Fawcett, D. W., and Burgos, M. H.: The fine structure of Sertoli cells in human testis. Anat. Rec., *124*:401, 1956.

Fawcett, D. W., and Hoffer, A. P.: Failure of exogenous androgen to prevent regression of the initial segments of the rat epididymis after efferent duct ligation or orchidectomy. Biol. Reprod., *20*:162, 1979.

Fléchon, J. E., and Hafez, E. S. E.: Scanning electron microscopy of human spermatozoa. *In* Hafez, E. S. E. (Ed.): Human Semen and Fertility Regulation in Men. St. Louis, The C. V. Mosby Co., 1976, p. 76.

Flickinger, C., and Fawcett, D. W.: The junctional specializations of Sertoli cells in the seminiferous epithelium. Anat. Rec., *158*:207, 1967.

Foldesy, R. G., and Bedford, J. M.: Biology of the scrotum. I. Temperature and androgen as determinants of the sperm storage capacity of the rat cauda epididymis. Biol. Reprod., *26*:673, 1982.

Fournier-Delpech, S., Colas, G., Courot, M., Ortavant, R., and Brice, G.: Epididymal sperm maturation in the ram: motility, fertilizing ability, and embryonic survival after uterine artificial insemination in the ewe. Ann. Biol. Anim. Biochim. Biophys., *19*:579, 1979.

Fournier-Delpech, S., Danzo, B. J., and Orgebin-Crist, M. C.: Extraction of concanavalin A affinity material from rat testicular and epididymal spermatozoa. Ann. Biol. Anim. Biochim. Biophys., *17*:207, 1977.

Free, M. J.: Blood supply to the testis and its role in local exchange and transport of hormones. *In* Johnson, A. D., and Gomes, W. R. (Eds.): The Testis, Vol. IV. New York, Academic Press, 1977, p. 39.

Free, M. J., and Jaffe, R. A.: Dynamics of venous-arterial testosterone transfer in the pampiniform plexus of the rat. Endocrinology, *97*:169, 1975.

Friend, D. S., and Farquhar, M. G.: Functions of coated vesicles during protein absorption in the rat vas deferens. J. Cell Biol., *35*:357, 1967.

Friend, D. S., Galle, J., and Silber, S.: Fine structure of human sperm, vas deferens epithelium, and testicular biopsy specimens at the time of vasectomy reversal. Anat. Rec., *184*:584, 1976.

Fritjofsson, Å., Persson, J. E., and Pettersson, S.: Testicular blood flow in man measured with xenon-133. Scand. J. Urol. Nephrol., *3*:276, 1969.

Gilula, N. D., Fawcett, D. W., and Aoki, A.: The Sertoli cell occluding junctions and gap junctions in mature and developing mammalian testis. Dev. Biol., *50*:142, 1976.

Gunha, S. K., Kaur, H., and Ahmed, A. M.: Mechanics of spermatic fluid transport in the vas deferens. Med. Biol. Eng., *13*:518, 1975.

Gunn, S. A., and Gould, T. C.: Vasculature of the testes and adnexa. *In* Greep, R. O., and Astwood, E. B. (Eds.): Handbook of Physiology, Section 7. Endocrinology. Baltimore, The Williams & Wilkins Co., 1975, p. 117.

Gupta, G., Rajalakshmi, N., Prasad, M. R. N., and Moudgal, N. R.: Alteration of epididymal function and its relation to maturation of spermatozoa. Andrologia, *6*:35, 1974.

Hall, P. F.: Testicular hormones: Synthesis and control. *In* DeGroot, L. J., et al. (Eds.): Endocrinology, Vol. 3. New York, Grune & Stratton, 1979.

Hamilton, D. W.: Structure and function of the epithelium lining the ductuli efferentes, ductus epididymides, and ductus deferens in the rat. *In* Greep, R. O., and Astwood, E. B. (Eds.): Handbook of Physiology, Section 7. Endocrinology. Baltimore, The Williams & Wilkins Co., 1975, p. 259.

Hamilton, D. W.: The epididymis. *In* Greep, R. O., and Kablinsky, T. (Eds.): Frontiers in Reproduction and Fertility Control. Part 2. Cambridge, MIT Press, 1977, p. 411.

Hammond, J., and Asdell, S. A.: The vitality of the spermatozoa in the male and female reproductive tract. J. Exp. Biol., *4*:155, 1926.

Hansson, V., and Djøseland, O.: Preliminary characterization of the 5α-dihydrotestosterone binding protein in the epididymal cytosol fraction. *In vivo* studies. Acta Endocrinol., *71*:614, 1972.

Harbitz, T. B.: Testis weight and the histology of the prostate in elderly men. Acta Pathol. Microbiol. Scand. [A], *81*:148, 1973a.

Harbitz, T. B.: Morphometric studies of the Leydig cells in elderly men with special reference to the histology of the prostate. Acta Pathol. Microbiol. Scand. [A], *81*:301, 1973b.

Harrison, R. G.: The distribution of the vasal and cremasteric arteries to the testis and their functional importance. J. Anat., *83*:267, 1949.

Harrison, R. G., and Barclay, A. E.: The distribution of the testicular artery (internal spermatic artery) to the human testis. Br. J. Urol., *20*:5, 1948.

Heller, C. G., and Clermont, Y.: Kinetics of the germinal epithelium in man. Rec. Prog. Horm. Res., *20*:545, 1964.

Hinrichsen, M. J., and Blaquier, J. A.: Evidence supporting the existence of sperm maturation in the human epididymis. J. Reprod. Fertil., *60*:291, 1980.

Hodson, N.: The nerves of the testis, epididymis and scrotum. *In* Johnson, A. D., et al. (Eds.): The Testis. Vol. 1, New York, Academic Press, 1970, p. 47.

Hoffer, A. P.: The ultrastructure of the ductus deferens in man. Biol. Reprod., *14*:425, 1976.

Holstein, A. F.: Morphologische studien am nebenhoden des menschen. Zwanglose Abhaudl. Gebeit. Norm. Pathol. Anat., *20*:1, 1969.

Holstein, A. F.: Structure of the human epididymis. *In* Hafez, E. S. E. (Ed.): Human Semen and Fertility Regulation in Men. St. Louis, The C. V. Mosby Co., 1976, p. 23.

Horan, A. H., and Bedford, J. M.: Development of the fertilizing ability of spermatozoa in the epididymis of the Syrian hamster. J. Reprod. Fertil., *30*:417, 1972.

Hoskins, D. D., Munsterman, D., and Hall, M. L.: The control of bovine sperm glycolysis during epididymal transit. Biol. Reprod., *12*:566, 1975.

Howards, S. S., Jessee, S. J., and Johnson, A.: Micropuncture studies of the blood-seminiferous barrier. Biol. Reprod., *14*:264, 1976.

Hundeiker, M.: Lymphgefässe in parenchym des menschlichen hoden. Arch. Klin. Exp. Derm., *235*:271, 1971.

Hundeiker, M., and Keller, L.: Die gefäss architektur des menschlichen hoden. Gegenbaurs Morphol. Jahrb., *105*:26, 1963.

Ishigami, K., Yoshida, Y., Hirooka, M., and Mohri, K.: A new operation for varicocele: Use of microvascular anastomosis. Surgery, *67*:620, 1970.

Kaler, L. W., and Neaves, W. B.: Attrition of human Leydig cell population with advancing age. Anat. Rec., *192*:513, 1978.

Kaya, M., and Harrison, R. G.: The ultrastructural relationship between Sertoli cells and spermatogenic cells in the rat. J. Anat., *121*:279, 1976.

Kerr, J. B., and deKretser, D. M.: The cytology of the human testis. *In* Burger, H., and deKretser, D. (Eds.): The Testis. New York, Raven Press, 1981, p. 141.

Killian, G. J., and Amann, R. P.: Immunophoretic characterization of fluid and sperm entering and leaving the bovine epididymis. Biol. Reprod., *9*:489, 1973.

Kinoshita, Y., Hosaka, M., Nishimura, R., and Takai, S.: Partial characterization of 5α-reductase in the human epididymis. Endocrinol. Jpn., *27*:277, 1980.

Kohane, A. C., Echeverría, F. M. C. G., Piñeiro, L., and Blaquier, J. A.: Interaction of proteins of epididymal origin with spermatozoa. Biol. Reprod., *23*:737, 1980.

Kormano, M., and Reijonen, K.: Microvascular structure of the human epididymis. Am. J. Anat., *145*:23, 1976.

Kormano, M., and Suoranta, H.: An angiographic study of the arterial pattern of the human testis. Anat. Anz., *128*:69, 1971a.

Kormano, M., and Suoranta, H.: Microvascular organization of the adult human testis. Anat. Rec., *170*:31, 1971b.

Kormano, M., Koskimies, A. I., and Hunter, R. L.: The presence of specific proteins, in the absence of many serum proteins, in the rat seminiferous tubule fluid. Experientia, *27*:1461, 1971.

Koskimies, A. I., Kormano, M., and Alfthau, O.: Proteins of the seminiferous tubule fluid in man—evidence for a blood-testis barrier. J. Reprod. Fertil., *32*:79, 1973.

Langford, G. A., and Heller, C. G.: Fine structure of muscle cells of the human testicular capsule: Basis of testicular contractions. Science, *179*:573, 1973.

Lanz, T. von, and Neuhäuser, G.: Morphometrische analyse des menschlichen nebenhodens. Z. Anat. Entwicklungsgesch., *124*:126, 1964.

Larminat, M. A. de, Hinrichsen, M. J., Scorticati, C., Ghirlanda, J. M., Blaquier, J. A., and Calandra, R. S.: Uptake and metabolism of androgen by the human epididymis *in vitro*. J. Reprod. Fertil., *59*:397, 1980.

Leidl, W., and Waschke, B.: Comparative aspects of the kinetics of the spermiogenesis, *In* Holstein, A. F., and Horstmann, E. (Eds.): Morphological Aspects of Andrology. Berlin, Grosse, 1970, p. 21.

Lennox, B., and Ahmad, K. N.: The total length of tubules in the human testis. J. Anat., *107*:191, 1970.

Levine, N., and Marsh, D. J.: Micropuncture studies of the electrochemical aspects of fluid and electrolyte transport in individual seminiferous tubules, the epididymis and the vas deferens in rats. J. Physiol., *213*:557, 1971.

Lich, R., Jr., Howerton, L. W., and Amin, M.: Anatomy and surgical approach to the urogenital tract in the male. *In* Harrison, J. H., et al. (Eds.): Campbell's

Urology. Vol. 1. Philadelphia, W. B. Saunders Co., 1978, p. 3.

Lino, B. F., Braden, A. W. H., and Turnbull, K. E.: Fate of unejaculated spermatozoa. Nature, *213*:594, 1967.

Lipschultz, L. I., McConnell, J., and Benson, G. S.: Current concepts of the mechanism of ejaculation. J. Reprod. Med., *26*:499, 1981.

Lipsett, M. B.: Steroid secretion by the testis in man. *In* James, V. H., et al. (Eds.): The Endocrine Function of the Human Testis. Vol. II. New York, Academic Press, 1974.

Lubicz-Nawrocki, C. M.: The effect of metabolites of testosterone on the viability of hamster epididymal spermatozoa. J. Endocrinol., *58*:193, 1973.

Lyon, M. F., Glenister, P. H., and Lamoreux, M. L.: Normal spermatozoa from androgen-resistant germ cells of chimaeric mice and the role of androgen in spermatogenesis. Nature, *258*:620, 1975.

MacMillan, E. W.: The blood supply of the epididymis in man. Br. J. Urol., *26*:60, 1954.

Mancini, R. E., Perez Loret, A., Guitelman, A., and Ghirlanda, J.: Effect of testosterone in the recovery of spermatogenesis in hypophysectomized patients. Hormone antagonists. Gynecol. Invest., *2*:98, 1972.

Mancini, R. E., Seigner, A. C., and Perez Loret, A.: Effect of gonadotropins on the recovery of spermatogenesis in hypophysectomized patients. J. Clin. Endocrinol., *29*:467, 1969.

Mancini, R. E., Vilar, D., Donini, P., and Perez Loret, A.: Effect of human urinary FSH and LH on the recovery of spermatogenesis in hypophysectomized patients. J. Clin. Endocrinol., *33*:888, 1971.

Marshall, F. F., and Elder, J. S.: Cryptorchidism and Related Anomalies. New York, Praeger Publishers, 1982.

Martan, J.: Epididymal histochemistry and physiology. Biol. Reprod. (Suppl.), *1*:134, 1969.

Martan, J., and Risley, P. L.: The epididymis of mated and unmated rats. J. Morphol., *113*:1, 1963.

McConnell, J., Benson, G. S., and Wood, J. G.: Autonomic innervation of the urogenital system: adrenergic and cholinergic elements. Brain Res. Bull., *9*:679, 1982.

Means, A. R., Dedman, J. R., Tash, J. S., Tindall, D. J., VanSickle, M., and Welsh, M. J.: Regulation of the testis Sertoli cell by follicle stimulating hormone. Ann. Rev. Physiol., *42*:59, 1980.

Mitchell, G. A. G.: The innervation of the kidney, ureter, testicle and epididymis. J. Anat., *70*:10, 1935.

Morton, B. E., Fraser, C. F., and Sagdraca, R.: Inhibition of sperm dilution damage by purified factors from hamster cauda epididymis and by defined diluents. Fertil. Steril., *29*:695, 1978.

Nagano, T.: Some observations on the fine structure of the Sertoli cell in the human testis. Z. Zellforsch., *73*:89, 1966.

Neaves, W. B.: Biological aspects of vasectomy. *In* Greep, R. O., and Astwood, E. B. (Eds.): Handbook of Physiology, Section 7. Endocrinology. Baltimore, The Williams & Wilkins Co., 1975, p. 383.

Nicolson, G. L., Brodginski, A. B., Beattie, G., and Yanagimachi, R.: Cell surface changes in the proteins of rabbit spermatozoa during epididymal passage. Gamete Res., *2*:153, 1979.

Nicolson, G. L., Usui, N., Yanagimachi, R., Yanagimachi, H., and Smith, J. R.: Lectin-binding sites on the plasma membranes of rabbit spermatozoa. Changes in surface receptors during epididymal maturation and after ejaculation. J. Cell Biol., *74*:950, 1977.

Nistal, M., Abaurrea, M. A., and Paniagua, R.: Morphol-

ogical and histometric study on the human Sertoli cell from birth to the onset of puberty. J. Anat., *14*:351, 1982.

Olson, G. E., and Danzo, B. J.: Surface changes in rat spermatozoa during epididymal transit. Biol. Reprod., *24*:431, 1981.

Orgebin-Crist, M. C.: Studies on the function of the epididymis. Biol. Reprod. (Suppl.), *1*:155, 1969.

Orgebin-Crist, M. C.: Epididymal physiology and sperm maturation. *In* Bollack, C., and Clavert, A. (Eds.): Progress in Reproductive Biology. Vol 8. Epididymis and Fertility: Biology and Pathology. Basel, S. Karger, 1981, p. 80.

Orgebin-Crist, M. C., and Fournier-Delpech, S.: Sperm-egg interaction. Evidence for maturational changes during epididymal transit. J. Androl., *3*:429, 1982.

Orgebin-Crist, M. C., and Jahad, N.: Delayed cleavage of rabbit ova after fertilization by young epididymal spermatozoa. Biol. Reprod., *16*:358, 1977.

Orgebin-Crist, M. C., Danzo, B. J., and Cooper, T. G.: Re-examination of the dependence of epididymal sperm viability on the epididymal environment. J. Reprod. Fertil. (Suppl.), *24*:115, 1976.

Orgebin-Crist, M. C., Danzo, B. J., and Davies, J.: Endocrine control of the development and maintenance of sperm fertilizing ability in the epididymis. *In* Greep, R. O., and Astman, E. B. (Eds.): Handbook of Physiology, Section 7. Endocrinology. Baltimore, The Williams & Wilkins Co., 1975, p. 319.

Overstreet, J. W., and Bedford, J. M.: Embryonic mortality in the rabbit is not increased after fertilization by young epididymal spermatozoa. Biol. Reprod., *15*:54, 1976.

Paniagua, R., Regadera, J., Nistal, M., and Abaurrea, M. A.: Histological, histochemical and ultrastructural variations along the length of the human vas deferens before and after puberty. Acta Anat., *111*:190, 1981.

Parvinen, M.: Regulation of the seminiferous epithelium. Endocrine Rev., *3*:404, 1982.

Paz, G. F., Kaplan, R., Yedwab, G., Homonnai, Z. T., and Kraicer, P. F.: The effect of caffeine on rat epididymal spermatozoa: motility, metabolism and fertilizing capacity. Int. J. Androl., *1*:145, 1978.

Pettersson, S., Soderholm, B., Persson, J. E., Eriksson, S., and Fritjofsson, Å.: Testicular blood flow in man measured with venous occlusion plethysmography and xenon-133. Scand. J. Urol. Nephrol., *7*:115, 1973.

Phadke, A. M.: Fate of spermatozoa in cases of obstructive azoospermia and after ligation of vas deferens in man. J. Reprod. Fertil., *7*:1, 1964.

Popovic, N. A., McLeod, D. G., and Borski, A. A.: Ultrastructure of the human vas deferens. Invest. Urol., *10*:266, 1973.

Prins, G. S., and Zaneveld, L. J. D.: Distribution of spermatozoa in the rabbit vas deferens. Biol. Reprod., *21*:181, 1979.

Prins, G. S., and Zaneveld, L. J. D.: Contractions of the rabbit vas deferens following sexual activity: a mechanism for proximal transport of spermatozoa. Biol. Reprod., *23*:904, 1980*a*.

Prins, G. S., and Zaneveld, L. J. D.: Radiographic study of fluid transport in the rabbit vas deferens during sexual rest and after sexual activity. J. Reprod. Fertil., *58*:311, 1980*b*.

Pujol, A., Bayard, F., Louvet, J. P., and Boulard, C.: Testosterone and dihydrotestosterone concentrations in plasma, epididymal tissues and seminal fluid of adult rats. Endocrinology, *98*:111, 1976.

Rajalakshmi, M., Arora, R., Bose, T. K., Dinakar, N., Gupta, G., Thampan, T. N. R. V., Prasad, M. R. N.,

Kumar, T. C. A., and Moudgal, N. R.: Physiology of the epididymis and induction of functional sterility in the male. J. Reprod. Fertil., (Suppl.), *24*:71, 1976.

Reyes, A., Mercado, E., Goicoechea, B., and Rosado, A.: Participation of membrane sulfhydryl groups in the epididymal maturation of human and rabbit spermatozoa. Fertil. Steril., *27*:1452, 1976.

Rikimaru, A., and Shirai, M.: Response of the human testicular capsule to electrical stimulation and to autonomic drugs. Tohoku J. Exp. Med., *108*:303, 1972.

Rikimaru, A., and Suzuki, T.: Mechanical response of the isolated rabbit testis to electrical stimulation and autonomic drugs. Tohoku J. Exp. Med., *108*:283, 1972.

Risley, P. L.: Physiology of the male accessory organs. *In* Hartman, C. G. (Ed.): Mechanisms Concerned with Conception. New York, Pergamon Press, 1963, p. 73.

Ritzen, E. M., Hansson, V., and French, F. S.: The Sertoli cell. *In* Burger, H., and deKretser, D. (Eds.): The Testis. New York, Raven Press, 1981, p. 171.

Ritzen, E. M., Nayfeh, S. N., French, F. S., and Dobbins, M. C.: Demonstration of androgen binding components in rat epididymis cytosol and comparison with binding components in prostate and other tissues. Endocrinology, *89*:143, 1971.

Riva, A,. Testa-Riva, F., Usai, E., and Cossu, M.: The ampulla ductus deferentis in man, as viewed by SEM and TEM. Arch. Androl., *8*:157, 1982.

Robaire, B., and Zirkin, B. R.: Hypophysectomy and simultaneous testosterone replacement: effects on male reproductive tract and epididymal Δ⁴-5α reductase and 3α-hydroxysteroid dehydrogenase. Endocrinology, *109*:1225, 1981.

Robaire, B., Ewing, L. L., Zirkin, B. R., and Irby, D. C.: Steroid Δ⁴-5α-reductase and 3α-hydroxysteroid dehydrogenase in the rat epididymis. Endocrinology, *101*:1379, 1977.

Rommerts, F. F. G., Cooke, B. A., and van der Molen, H. J.: A review. The role of cyclic AMP in the regulation of steroid biosynthesis in testis tissue. J. Steroid Biochem., *5*:279, 1974.

Romrell, L. J., and Ross, M. H.: Characterization of Sertoli cell–germ cell junctional specializations in dissociated testicular cells. Anat. Rec., *193*:23, 1979.

Roosen-Runge, E. C.: Comparative aspects of spermatogenesis. Biol. Reprod., *1*:24, 1969.

Roosen-Runge, E. C., and Barlow, F. D.: Quantitative studies in human spermatogenesis. I. Spermatogonia. Am. J. Anat., *93*:143, 1953.

Roosen-Runge, E. C., and Holstein, A. F.: The human rete testis. Cell Tissue Res., *189*:409, 1978.

Rowley, M. J., Teshima, F., and Heller, C. G.: Duration of transit of spermatozoa through the human male ductular system. Fertil. Steril., *21*:390, 1970.

Russell, L.: Desmosome-like junctions between Sertoli cells and germ cells in the rat testis. Am. J. Anat., *148*:301, 1977.

Russell, L. D.: Sertoli–germ cell interactions: A review. Gamete Res., *3*:179, 1980.

Russell, L., and Clermont, Y.: Anchoring device between Sertoli cells and late spermatids in rat seminiferous tubules. Anat. Rec., *185*:259, 1976.

Santen, R. J.: Feedback control of luteinizing hormone and follicle stimulating hormone secretion by testosterone and estradiol in men: Physiologic and clinical implications. Clin. Biochem., *14*:243, 1981.

Scheer, H., and Robaire, B.: Subcellular distribution of steroid Δ⁴-5α-reductase and 3α-hydroxysteroid dehydrogenase in the rat epididymis during sexual maturation. Biol. Reprod., *29*:1, 1983.

Schulze, W.: Evidence of a wave of spermatogenesis in human testis. Andrologia, *14*:200, 1982.

Setchell, B. P.: The Mammalian Testis. Ithaca, Cornell University Press, 1978, p. 50.

Setchell, B. P., and Waites, G. M. H.: The blood-testis barrier. *In* Greep, R. O., and Astwood, E. B. (Eds.): Handbook of Physiology, Section 7. Endocrinology. Baltimore, The Williams & Wilkins Co., 1975, p. 143.

Setchell, B. P., Voglmayr, J. K., and Waites, G. M. H.: A blood-testis barrier restricting passage from blood into rete testis fluid but not into lymph. J. Physiol., *200*:73, 1969.

Sheth, A. R., Gunjikar, A. N., and Shah, G. V.: The presence of progressive motility sustaining factor (PMSF) in human epididymis. Andrologia, *13*:142, 1981.

Silber, S. J.: Vasoepididymostomy to the head of the epididymis: recovery of normal spermatozoal motility. Fertil. Steril., *34*:149, 1980.

Sjöstrand, N. O.: The adrenergic innervation of the vas deferens and the accessory male genital glands. Acta Physiol. Scand. *65*:(Suppl. 257), 5, 1965.

Steinberger, E.: Hormonal control of mammalian spermatogenesis. Physiol. Rev., *51*:1, 1971.

Steinberger, E., and Steinberger, A.: Spermatogenic function of the testis. *In* Greep, R. O., and Astwood, E. B. (Eds.): Handbook of Physiology, Section 7. Endocrinology. Baltimore, The Williams & Wilkins Co., 1975, p. 1.

Steinberger, E., Root, A., Fischer, M., and Smith, K. O.: The role of androgens in the initiation of spermatogenesis in man. J. Clin. Endocrinol. Metab., *37*:746, 1973.

Suzuki, F., and Nagano, T.: Development of tight junctions in caput epididymidal epithelium of mouse. Dev. Biol., *63*:321, 1978.

Swerdloff, R. S., and Heber, D.: Endocrine control of testicular function from birth to puberty. *In* Burger, H., and deKretser, D. (Eds.): The Testis. New York, Raven Press, 1981, p. 107.

Takayama, H., and Tomoyoshi, T.: Microvascular architecture of rat and human testes. Invest. Urol., *18*:341, 1981.

Tishler, P. V.: Diameter of testicles. N. Engl. J. Med., *285*:1489, 1971.

Tuck, R. R., Setchell, B. P., Waites, G. M. H., and Young, J. A.: The composition of fluid collected by micropuncture and catheterization from the seminiferous tubules and rete testes of rats. Eur. J. Physiol., *318*:225, 1970.

Turner, T. T.: On the epididymis and its function. Invest. Urol., *16*:311, 1979.

Turner, T. T., and Giles, R. D.: Sperm motility–inhibiting factor in rat epididymis. Am. J. Physiol., *242*:R199, 1982.

Vendrely, E.: Histology of the epididymis in the human adult. *In* Bollack, C., and Clavert, A. (Eds.): Progress in Reproductive Biology. Vol. 8. Epididymis and Fertility: Biology and Pathology. Basel, S. Karger, 1981, p. 21.

Ventura, W. P., Freund, M., Davis, J., and Pannuti, M. S.: Influence of norepinephrine on the motility of the human vas deferens: a new hypothesis of sperm transport by the vas deferens. Fertil. Steril., *24*:68, 1973.

Voglmayr, J. K.: Metabolic changes in spermatozoa during epididymal transit. *In* Greep, R. O., and Astman, E. B. (Eds.): Handbook of Physiology, Section 7. Endocrinology. Baltimore, The William & Wilkins Co., 1975, p. 437.

Vreeburg, J. T. M.: Distribution of testosterone and 5αdihydrotestosterone in rat epididymis and their concentration in efferent duct fluid. J. Endocrinol., *67*:203, 1975.

Waites, G. M. H.: Functional relationships of the mammalian testis and epididymis. Aust. J. Biol. Sci., *33*:355, 1980.

Wenzel, J., and Kellermann, P.: Vergleichende untersuchungen über das lymphgefässsystem des nebenhodens und hodens von mensch, hund und kaninchen. Z. Mikrosk. Anat. Forsch., *75*:368, 1966.

Wong, P. Y. D., Au, C. L., and Bedford, J. M.: Biology of the scrotum. II. Suppression by abdominal temperature of transepithelial ion and water transport in the cauda epididymis. Biol. Reprod., *26*:683, 1982.

Yanagimachi, R.: Sperm-egg association in mammals. *In* Moscona, A. A., and Monroy, A. (Eds.): Current Topics in Developmental Biology. Vol. 12. New York, Academic Press, 1978, p. 83.

Young, D. H.: Surgical treatment of male infertility. J. Reprod. Fertil., *23*:541, 1970.

Young, W. C.: A study of the function of the epididymis. II. The importance of an ageing process in sperm for the length of the period during which fertilizing capacity is retained by sperm isolated in the epididymis of the guinea pig. J. Morphol., *48*:475, 1929.

The Biochemistry and Physiology of the Prostate and Seminal Vesicles

DONALD S. COFFEY, Ph.D.

INTRODUCTION

The prostate represents the major organ for most of the medical and surgical problems within the field of urology. In spite of this importance, the prostate remains one of the most poorly understood glands in the human body. Even less is known about the physiology and function of the seminal vesicles; however, the seminal vesicles are almost devoid of any significant incidence of infection or abnormal growth such as benign or malignant hyperplasia. Why should the prostate be such a favored site of neoplastic growth and infections? It would appear that both glands receive the same endogenous hormones and might be subjected to the same pathologic insults by carcinogens and pathogens. Whether the marked difference in pathology of the prostate and seminal vesicles resides in intrinsic or extrinsic factors must obviously await further study and understanding (Isaacs, 1983). Because the prostate gland is central to so many major urologic problems, it will receive the major attention in this section.

What is the physiologic function of the sex accessory glands, such as the prostate, seminal vesicles, and bulbourethral (Cowper's) gland? In mammals, these glands produce a vast array of unusual and potent secretory products whose physiologic functions are all essentially unknown. The secretions of these glands constitute most of the volume and chemical components of the seminal plasma. It is still a common misconception by the layman that the testes contribute a major bulk component to the ejaculate; however, the fluid and sperm traveling directly from the testes during ejaculation compose a minute volume of less than 1 per cent of the total semen volume. What is the specific role of these sex accessory gland secretions in the fertilization process? Many investigators have even questioned the necessity for these secretions in fertilization, since in some animals it has been observed that sperm removed from the epididymis are capable of fertilizing the ovum; therefore, the sperm are capable of fertilization without even making contact with the prostatic or seminal vesicle secretions. Surgical removal of the ventral prostates or the seminal vesicles in the rat does not abolish male fertility. Although the seminal plasma may not contain factors that are absolutely essential for fertilization, the secretions may nevertheless optimize conditions for sperm motility, survival, and transport in both the male and the female reproductive tract.

In addition to a potential role in fertilization, these sex accessory secretions may also be involved in other important physiologic processes, such as protecting the genitourinary tract from pathogens and other harmful external factors gaining access through the urethra. The prostate and seminal vesicles are in a defensive position to guard the urethra at the entrance to the bladder and ejaculatory duct and to present protective biologic fluids that might hinder the progress of wayward pathogens entering these important biologic compartments. Indeed, the sex accessory tissues are active in maintaining baseline secretions (Isaacs, 1983) even in the absence of ejaculation, and this may be an essential protective function of these glands. Some clue to function might be gained in the future from studies of the evolutionary development of these sex accessory glands. Compared with other organs, there has been profound diversity in the development and comparative anatomy of the sex accessory tissue (Price and Williams-Ashman, 1961). For example, the seminal vesicles are large and prominent glands in the human and rat, but seminal vesicles are not present in the cat and dog. The presence of a prostate is universal in mammals, but between species the prostate is marked by tremendous variation in comparative anatomy, biochemistry, and pathology. The rat prostate is characterized by distinct and separate lobes with separate functions, such as the dorsal, ventral, and lateral lobes, whereas in the human and dog, these corresponding anatomic lobes are not apparent and only zones can be defined (Blacklock, 1982; McNeal 1980). Biochemical variation in the prostate between the species is also marked. In the human ejaculate the major anion is citrate, but it is chloride ion in the dog seminal plasma. There are large differences in spermidine concentrations and enzyme (such as acid phosphatase) activity, which in the human prostate is 1,000 times more abundant than in the rat prostate when compared on equal amounts of tissue. The total ejaculate volume is very variable between species, and there is no apparent biologic reason for this large variation. The ejaculate volumes of some species are: boar, 250 ml; stallion, 70 ml; dog, 9 ml; bull, 4 ml; human, 3 ml; and ram, 1 ml. In summary, no organs have such an anatomic and biochemical diversity as the sex accessory tissue. The biologic reason for this large variation, if determined, might offer insight into the functions of these mysterious glands.

We will begin with an overview of our current concepts of the organization of the human prostate gland, followed by a discussion of how we believe the growth of the prostate is regulated. Lastly, the secretory properties of the prostate and seminal vesicle glands will be discussed. Emphasis will be placed on the endocrinology and methods of regulating prostate growth, since these factors are of paramount importance in our attempts to understand the etiology and treatment of benign prostatic hyperplasia (Kimball et al., 1984; Hinman, 1983; Grayhack et al., 1975; Castor, 1974). Pertinent reviews on prostatic adenocarcinoma include those by Murphy et al., 1981; Jacobi and Hohenfellner, 1982; and Isaacs and Coffey, 1979.

For information on other important aspects of the prostate and seminal vesicle glands, the reader is directed to pertinent sections in this book (Chapters 1C, 27, 32, and 40) and to other important reviews of prostatic function by Aumuller (1983); Zaneveld and Chatterton (1982); Chisholm and Williams (1982); Murphy et al. (1981); and the classic study of Mann and Mann (1981).

ORGANIZATION AND CELL BIOLOGY

DEVELOPMENT

The prostate and seminal vesicles are very different with regard to the origin of the gland in development and the type of steroid that induces embryonic growth. The wolffian ducts develop into the seminal vesicles, epididymis, vas deferens, ampulla, and ejaculatory duct; the developmental growth of this group of glands is stimulated by fetal testosterone and not by dihydrotestosterone. The fetal growth of these glands is primarily completed by the thirteenth week. In contrast, the prostate develops from the urogenital sinus during the third month of fetal life, and growth is directed primarily by dihydrotestosterone from the conversion of fetal testosterone through the action of the enzyme 5α-reductase, which is located within the urogenital sinus. Small epithelial buds form on the posterior side of the urogenital sinus on both sides of the verumontanum, and they then invade the mesenchyme to form the prostate. The prostate develops around the urethra, the ejaculatory ducts, and the small remnants of the müllerian duct, the utriculus prostaticus, which forms the small prostatic utricle. The prostate is well differentiated by the fourth month of fetal growth.

In the embryonic development of the prostate, there is an important interaction of cellular elements within the urogenital sinus. Cunha et al. (1983) have presented convincing evidence that the target for the dihydrotestosterone-induced growth is the mesenchymal cells and not the epithelial cells. They conclude that androgen-induced prostatic epithelial morphogenesis, growth, and secretory cytodifferentiation are elicited via trophic factors emanating from androgen receptor–positive mesenchymal cells. (A more comprehensive discussion of the embryonic development of the tissue is found later in this section.)

SEX ACCESSORY GLANDS

The normal adult prostate weighs approximately 20 gm (Berry et al., 1984) and lies immediately below the base of the bladder surrounding the proximal portion of the urethra. The gland is located behind the inferior part of the symphysis pubis and rests directly above the urogenital diaphragm and in front of the rectal ampulla. The gland is composed of alveoli that are lined with tall columnar secretory epithelial cells. The acini of these alveoli drain, by a system of branching ducts and tubules, into the floor and lateral surfaces of the posterior urethra. The alveoli and ducts are embedded within a stroma of fibromuscular tissue.

The seminal vesicles develop as large paired pouches forming from the vas deferens. The glands are 4 to 5 cm long and are located directly on the posterior side of the bladder and adjacent to the rectum. The glands are composed of tubular alveoli containing viscous secretions. The seminal vesicles were so named because it was erroneously believed that they stored semen and sperm. Their secretions contribute to semen, but they do not store secretions made elsewhere, and the seminal vesicles do not store sperm. However, the ampulla at the distal end of the vas deferens does store sperm, and the seminal vesicles join the ampulla to form the beginning of the ejaculatory ducts. The ejaculatory ducts pass through the prostate and terminate below the utricle within the prostate urethra at the verumontanum.

Other minor glands complete the list of sex accessory tissues. They include Cowper's glands and the glands of Littre (Mann and Mann, 1981). The Cowper, or bulbourethral, gland is a paired, pea-sized, compound tubular gland located directly below the prostate within the urogenital sinus. This gland was named after William Cowper, who first described it in 1698. The glands empty into the urethra; the function and composition of their secretions are poorly understood. Very small urethral glands, termed glands of Littre, line the penile urethra.

All of these sex accessory tissues depend on androgens for development, growth, and maintenance of their secretory products, which contribute to the composition of the seminal plasma of the ejaculate.

PROSTATIC LOBES

For many years the prostate was believed to have a lobular structure. Prior to 1906, when Home described the middle lobe, the prostate was generally considered to be composed of two lateral lobes (LeDuc, 1939). For decades, the importance of the two or three lobes of the prostate was debated widely. However, in 1912, Lowsley proposed the existence of five prostatic lobes based upon embryologic findings: two lateral lobes, a posterior lobe, and the middle lobe. The anterior lobe, which was present in fetal material, atrophied and disappeared by the time of birth. This concept was widely adopted for the next 50 years. It is difficult to understand why this theory remained unchallenged over this period of time. Franks (1954) has emphasized that these divisions were identifiable only in the embryo and that from the last months of gestation into postnatal life no division into separate glands was possible. Furthermore, LeDuc (1939) was unable to demonstrate a posterior row of prostatic ducts, thus seriously challenging the existence of the posterior lobe of the prostate, which was given such anatomic prominence by Lowsley. In retrospect, this old concept probably arose from confusion between the anatomy of the truly normal prostate and the prostate involved by hyperplastic changes. Urologic surgeons frequently refer to midline and laterally projecting nodules of benign prostatic hyperplasia (BPH) as middle and lateral lobes, respectively. However, these "lobes" are not reference points of normal anatomy but exist only in glands with BPH.

Today the concept of a lobular structure has been replaced by a concept based on concentric zones. Many authors have suggested that the prostate could be separated into at least two independent structures, an inner and an outer zone (Young, 1926; Huggins and Webster, 1948; Franks, 1954). In more recent years the morphology of the prostate has come under intense study by several talented investigators (McNeal, 1968, 1976, 1980, 1981; Tisell and Salander, 1975; Blacklock, 1982). Of these, McNeal's work appears to be the most widely accepted. A historical and comparative analysis of McNeal's terminology to the contributions of others has been made (McNeal, 1980). Rather than dividing the prostate into arbitrary lobes, McNeal identified zones that appear to have morphologic, functional, and pathologic significance. To understand his descriptions of the prostate it is important to recognize that the prostatic urethra is not a straight tube. Rather, at the midpoint of the prostatic urethra between the apex of the prostate and the bladder neck (i.e., at the upper end of the verumontanum) the posterior wall of the urethra is kinked anteriorly in such a way that the entire proximal urethra is angled 35 degrees anterior to the course of the distal urethral segment (Fig. 5–29).

Previously, many investigators used transverse sections of the prostate taken at the level of the verumontanum for their studies. However, McNeal (1968) emphasized the need for planes other than conventional transverse sections to demonstrate differences between one part of the prostate and the other. Using sagittal, coronal, and oblique coronal sections, he divided the prostate into four distinct zones. Each zone makes contact with a specific portion of the prostatic urethra, which can be taken as the primary anatomic landmark for defining them (Fig. 5–29). The subsequent descriptions of these zones are taken directly from McNeal's many contributions (McNeal, 1968, 1976, 1980, 1981).

1. The *anterior fibromuscular stroma* is a thick sheet of connective tissue that covers the entire anterior surface of the prostate. It is a continuous sheet of smooth muscle that sur-

rounds the urethra proximally at the bladder neck, where it merges with the internal sphincter and detrusor muscle from which it originates. Near the apex, the smooth muscle merges with transverse loops of striated muscle that represent a proximal extension of the external sphincter, thus forming an incomplete sphincter along the anterior aspect of the distal urethral segment. The anterior fibromuscular stroma composes up to one third of the total bulk of the prostate. It is entirely lacking in glandular elements.

2. The *peripheral zone* is the largest anatomic subdivision of the prostate. It is a flat disc of secretory tissue, whose ducts branch out laterally from either side of the distal urethra. Laterally, some of the terminal ducts curve anteriorly to form a shallow cup around the striated sphincter and then anchor into the lateral extent of the anterior fibromuscular stroma. This zone contains 75 per cent of the total glandular tissue of the prostate. In this region, almost all carcinomas arise. Furthermore, this is the tissue sampled in most random biopsies of the prostate.

3. The *central zone* is the smaller of the two subdivisions of functioning glandular prostate, making up about 25 per cent of its mass. It contacts the urethra only at the upper end of the verumontanum, where its duct orifices open in a tight circle immediately around the ejaculatory duct orifices. The ducts branch laterally to form a flat wedge of glandular tissue with its apex at the verumontanum and its base at the base of the prostate posterior to the bladder neck. The central zone surrounds the ejaculatory ducts, completing the proximal quadrant of glandular tissue above and behind the verumontanum. McNeal distinguishes the central from the peripheral zone based on differences in architecture, and histologic features of the central zone closely resemble those of the seminal vesicle, suggesting that the central zone could be of wolffian duct origin. This possibility correlates with the uncommon occurrence of carcinoma in both the seminal vesicle and the central zone.

4. The *preprostatic tissues*, which surround the anteriorly displaced urethra proximal to the upper end of the verumontanum, is the smallest of the four regions and the most complex in its arrangement of both glandular and nonglandular elements. This term has been applied to this zone because of its sphincteric function at the time of ejaculation to prevent the reflux of seminal fluid into the bladder. Its main component is a cylindrical smooth muscle sphincter

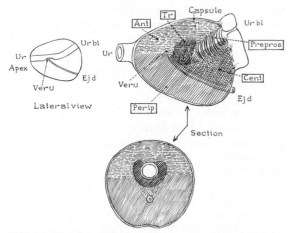

Figure 5–29. Diagrammatic representation of prostatic anatomy as described by McNeal (see text). *Upper left,* The path of the urethra (Ur) as it courses from the apex of the prostate to the bladder (bl). *Upper right,* Sagittal view illustrating the four zones of the prostate and their relationship to the ejaculatory ducts (Ejd): (1) anterior fibromuscular stroma (Ant); (2) peripheral zone (Perip); (3) central zone (Cent); (4) preprostatic tissue (Prepros); and (5) transition zone (Tr). *Bottom,* The relationship of the zones in a transverse section.

surrounding the entire preprostatic urethra. Inside this cylinder of smooth muscle are the tiny periurethral glands, which constitute less than 1 per cent of the mass of the glandular prostate. They do not possess their own periglandular musculature and are confined in their extent to the immediate periurethral stroma. Because the smooth muscle cylinder limits the expansion of the glands laterally away from the urethra, these glands grow proximally toward the bladder neck. However, at the distal margin of the smooth muscle sphincter, some ducts escape below the most distal rings of the smooth muscle sleeve, thus enabling them to develop outside its confines.

5. The *transition zone* is a small group of ducts, arising at a single point at the junction of the proximal and distal urethral segments. The ducts in this region, which compose less than 5 per cent of the mass of the normal glandular prostate, demonstrate more branching and acinar proliferation than do the other periurethral ducts. Though insignificant in size and functional importance, the transition zone and the other periurethral glands are the exclusive site of origin of benign prostatic hyperplasia (see Chapter 27).

CELLULAR COMPONENTS AND THE STROMAL MATRIX

The organization of the prostate is analogous to a bunch of grapes immersed in a fibrous gelatin. Each of these grapes would be equivalent to the alveoli, which are lined with tall columnar secretory epithelial cells that coat the periphery of acini and that drain by a system of branching ducts and tubules into the prostatic urethra. This permits the secretions of the prostate to be added to other seminal plasma components arriving through the ejaculatory ducts, which bring spermatozoa and secretions from the testes, epididymis, ampulla, and seminal vesicles. The ejaculatory ducts pass through the prostate posteriorly to the bladder neck and enter the prostatic urethra in the regions known as the verumontanum. The acini and ducts of the prostate are embedded in a tissue matrix composed of stromal components, including fibromuscular, vascular, and connective tissues.

Epithelial Cells. The prostatic epithelium is composed of three types of cells: the secretory epithelial cells, the basal cells, and/or the stem cells (see Fig. 5–30). It is not yet proved, but is believed, that the basal cells may be the stem cells. In any cell-renewing population there is the flow of cells from reserve quiescent stem cells to a more rapidly dividing transient prolif-

erating population and finally to the formation of nondividing terminally differentiated secretory cells. In the prostate the most common tall columnar epithelial secretory cells are terminally differentiated and are easily distinguished by their morphology and abundant secretory granules and enzymes that stain with acid phosphatase and other enzymes, such as leucine amino peptidase. These tall columnar (20 μ in height) secretory cells appear like rows of a picket fence resting on a basement membrane with their round nuclei located at their base. Above the nucleus is a clear zone of abundant Golgi apparatus, and the upper cellular periphery is rich in secretory granules and enzymes. The apical plasma membrane facing the lumen possesses a microvilli formation. The morphology, characteristics, and ultrastructure of these secretory cells have been described in detail by Brandes et al. (1974, 1964) and discussed by Aumuller (1983).

Basal Cells. Much smaller and less abundant are the basal cells, which are present in less than 10 per cent of the number of secretory epithelial cells. These small cells are not columnar and are rounder, with little cytoplasm and large irregular-shaped nuclei (Brandes et al., 1974). They are less differentiated and are almost devoid of secretory products, such as acid phosphatase. These basal cells appear wedged between the bases of adjacent columnar epithelial cells and are always resting on the basement membrane. They are rich in cellular tonofilaments and stain brightly with fluorescent antibodies to cytokeratin filaments of the cytoskeleton (Isaacs, 1984). It was once mistakenly thought that these cells were myoepithelial, but they are not, since they are not rich in actin or myosin. It is believed that these undifferentiated basal cells give rise to secretory epithelial cells and, as such, function as a type of stem cell (Merk et al., 1982). The importance of understanding the biology of these basal cells is clear because of the growing evidence that many neoplasias, both benign and malignant, are really stem cell diseases.

The proper identification in the prostate of stem cells and the transient proliferating cells has not been made. Indeed, there may be several types of each of these cells as well as several types of secretory cells. Good functional and immunologic markers are needed, and only currently are these studies being described (Isaacs, 1984).

The Stroma and the Prostatic Tissue Matrix. The noncellular stroma and connective tissue elements of the prostate compose what is termed the *extracellular matrix* (Fig. 5–30). The extracellular matrix has long been recognized as one of the important inductive components during normal development of many different types of cells (Bissell et al., 1982). A matrix system is defined as a biologic scaffolding or residual skeleton structure that organizes cells as well as subcellular particles. The cellular matrix system is one of the most active areas of modern cell biology (i.e., extracellular matrix, cytoskeleton, and nuclear matrix). The extracellular matrix is far more than a supporting scaffolding because it has been shown to play a central role in the development and control of cellular function (Hay, 1981). It now appears that the extracellular matrix is just one of the three major matrix systems that interact and form the overall tissue matrix system of the prostate (Isaacs et al., 1981). In this concept the epithelial cell rests upon the basement membrane, which is connected by an extracellular matrix to the stromal cells. It is believed that phase shifts and communication through these structural matrix elements may play a central role in controlling prostatic development and function (Isaacs et al., 1981; Bissell et al., 1982; Hay, 1981).

It is now established that all cells are composed of a cytomatrix or cytoskeleton network that is formed from microtubules, microfilaments, and intermediate filaments. Tubulin is ubiquitous in all cells as a microtubular protein and appears to anchor many cellular structures. The microfilaments are primarily actin, one of the major proteins in all cells. Actin has the ability to polymerize and depolymerize and, as such, makes one of the important structural chemomechanical systems that is involved in a central way with transport of particles and components within the cell.

The intermediate filaments of the cytomatrix are extremely important because they vary with differentiation and appear to define the various cell types within the body. For example, one of the intermediate filaments, called desmin, is a central component of all muscle cells, while the intermediate filament vimentin is found in all fibroblasts. Surprisingly, the intermediate filament keratin is universal as a major component of the tonofilaments of all epithelial cells. There is usually just one type of vimentin and desmin in the fibroblast or muscle cells; in contrast, in the epithelial cells the keratins represent 20 different molecular types that vary with the state of cellular differentiation and with the types of epithelial cells, ranging from stratified squamous to simple epithelial cells (Tseng et al., 1982).

The cytomatrix (cell skeleton) just described terminates in the center of the cell by direct attachment to the nuclear matrix (nuclear skeleton). The nuclear matrix is the residual scaffolding of the nucleus and contains an organizing center for many of the important nuclear functions, such as DNA replication, transcription, and steroid hormone interaction (Barrack and Coffey, 1982). The prostatic epithelial cell, therefore, has direct structural linkage via the matrix systems from the DNA to the plasma membrane. The cytomatrix then makes direct contact with the basement membrane and extracellular matrix of the stroma. This entire interlocking superstructure is termed the tissue matrix (Isaacs et al., 1981).

The epithelial cell is anchored to the base-

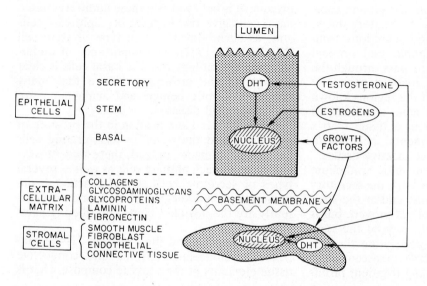

Figure 5–30. Schematic of the interaction of the epithelial and stromal components from the prostate, indicating effects of testosterone, estrogens, and growth factors on both types of cells.

ment membrane or basement lamina by an extracellular matrix protein called laminin. The laminin proteins mediate attachment of cells to the collagen Type IV of the basement membrane. Laminin is produced by epithelial cells, but not by fibroblasts, and is a large molecule with molecular domains that interact with the Type IV collagen of the basement membrane and with the cell surface glycocalyx of the epithelial cell. The basement membrane is not a membrane but a complex structure containing collagen Type IV, glycosaminoglycans, complex polysaccharides, and glycolipids. The basement membrane forms the interface with the stroma.

A second type of important prostatic glycoprotein that is involved in cell adherence in the extracellular matrix is fibronectin. Fibronectin is secreted by prostatic fibroblasts and forms an adhesive material, binding mesenchymal and epithelial cells to various types of collagen and proteoglycans. This important protein has been proposed to play a key role in morphogenesis and control of cell growth.

The connective tissue of the prostate is primarily collagen of Types I and III, which form the interstitial collagen (Bartsch et al., 1984), while Types IV and V are found primarily in the basement membrane. Woven through the stroma and connective tissue of the extracellular matrix is a complex network of glycosaminoglycans and complex polysaccharides. These polymers have long been proposed to play an important role in prostate growth (Arcade, 1954). Recently, DeKlerk (1983) isolated these impor-

tant glycosaminoglycans (GAGs) from the normal and BPH human prostates and reported that dermatan sulfate is the predominant (40 per cent) GAG, followed by heparin (20 per cent), chondroitin (16 per cent), and hyaluronic acid (20 per cent). Fetal prostates are devoid of dermatan, and chondroitin sulfate increases with BPH. GAGs are large, negatively charged polymers (polyanions) that have proved to be critical factors in the signaling of extracellular matrix events in many different tissues (Hay, 1981). It will be of interest to determine their role in prostatic function.

A clearer understanding of the control of prostate function will revolve around the question of how all of these tissue matrix components interact. There have been several recent important studies (Isaacs, 1984; Thornton et al., 1984; DeKlerk, 1983; Isaacs et al., 1981; Chung and Cunha, 1983) that all point to the importance of these structural elements. Of particular importance is the work of Isaacs (1984), who has shown the localization of keratins, laminin, fibronectin, and actin within the various cell types of the prostate by utilizing immunofluorescent studies, and the studies of Bartsch et al. (1984) and Thornton et al. (1984) on the collagens of the prostate.

MORPHOMETRICS—QUANTITATIVE HISTOLOGY

Morphometrics and sterology are the quantitative assessment of tissue components that

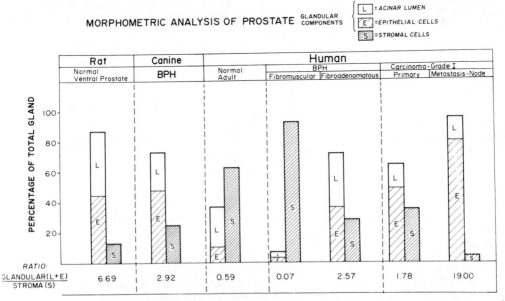

Figure 5–31. Morphometric analysis of the prostate gland from several species, showing the quantitative composition of epithelial (E), luminal (L), and stromal (S) components. The higher the glandular/stromal ratio, the more sensitive is the prostate tissue to androgen deprivation. (Adapted from Coffey, D. S., et al., 1977.)

express the per cent volume of a prostate gland occupied by a particular prostate element, such as epithelial cell, lumen, or stroma (Fig. 5–31). With electron micrograph samples it is also possible to extend these measurements to include subcellular compartments, such as total nuclear or mitochondrial volume. With light microscopy, morphometric techniques involve point-counting of ocular grids superimposed on microscopic sections to determine the per cent of total section area occupied by the tissue elements being counted. Morphometrics was first applied by Bartsch and Rohr (1975, 1977) and DeKlerk, Heston, and Coffey (1976) to study the rat prostate. Coffey, DeKlerk, and Walsh (1976) (see Fig. 5–31) and Bartsch et al. (1979) reported the first morphometric studies on normal and BPH human prostate.

In 1975, Scott and Coffey proposed that the stromal elements of the prostate might be less sensitive to androgen deprivation, possibly accounting for the differential effects of antiandrogen treatments on human BPH when compared with other animal models. This was confirmed by comparison of hormonal effects on stromal and epithelial elements of animal prostates (DeKlerk et al., 1976; Coffey et al., 1976).

SUMMARY

This first section on the anatomy and cell biology of the prostate has focused on the organization of the prostate gland, beginning with development and a description of the prostate zones proposed by McNeal. The properties of various types of cells within the prostate and the organization of the stroma and extracellular matrix were discussed. Very recent developments in cell biology point to a tissue matrix system as an important organ control system, and our knowledge has been briefly summarized (Table 5–2). For additional information on this topic, consult *The Prostatic Cell: Structure and Function*, Parts A and B, edited by G. P. Murphy, A. A. Sandberg, and J. P. Karr.

STROMAL-EPITHELIAL INTERACTIONS

There has been increasing interest in the role of the stroma in the prostate ever since the early suggestion of Franks in 1970 that epithelia require stroma for their growth, and the classic experiments of Cunha et al. (1983) that have shown the importance of the mesenchyme in the induction of the differentiation of the prostate epithelial cells. McNeal's (1978) proposal

TABLE 5–2. Summary of the Anatomy and Cell Biology of the Prostate Gland

Components	Properties
DEVELOPMENT	
Seminal vesicles	From wolffian ducts via testosterone stimulation
Prostate	From urogenital sinus via DHT stimulation
PROSTATE ZONES	
Anterior fibromuscular	30% of prostate mass, no glandular elements, smooth muscle
Peripheral	Largest zone, 75% of prostate glandular elements, site of carcinomas
Central	25% of prostate glandular elements, surrounds ejaculatory ducts, may be of wolffian duct origin, seminal vesicle–like
Preprostatic	Smallest, surround upper urethra, complex, sphincter
Transition	5% of prostate glandular elements, site of BPH
	15–30% of prostate volume
EPITHELIAL CELLS	
Basal	Reserve stem cells, small undifferentiated, keratin-rich, pluripotent, very few
Transient proliferating	Incorporate thymidine
Columnar secretory	Terminal differentiated, nondividing, rich in acid phosphatase, 20 μ tall, most abundant
	40–60% of prostate volume
STROMA CELLS	
Smooth muscle	Actin-rich
Fibroblast	Vimentin-rich and associated with fibronectin
Endothelial	Associated with fibronectin, alkaline phosphatase–positive
TISSUE MATRIX	
Extracellular	
Basement membrane	Type IV collagen, laminin-rich, fibronectin
Connective tissue	Type I and Type III collagen, elastin
Glycosaminoglycans	Sulfates of dermatan, chondroitin, and heparin; hyaluronic acid
Cytomatrix	Tubulin, actin, and intermediate filaments
Nuclear matrix	DNA tight-binding proteins, RNP (residual nuclear proteins)

that stroma may be reactivated in adult life to an embryonic state, thus stimulating the epithelial growth, has generated a great deal of interest and an effort to understand these tissue components of the prostate. We described earlier the composition of the stroma, and here we will discuss the evidence that the stroma regulates prostatic epithelial growth.

The classic experiments of Cunha et al. (1983) and Chung and Cunha (1983) demonstrated that the mesenchyme of the urogenital sinus may have the director's role in inducing the growth and cytodifferentiation of the prostate epithelial cells. They have shown that when heterografting mesenchyme with epithelial cells, the mesenchyme dictates what the epithelial cell will become. For instance, placing bladder epithelium on urogenital sinus develops prostatic epithelial cells. More surprising, using bladder epithelium from androgen-insensitive (Tfm) mice explanted to normal mesenchyme develops normal prostatic epithelial cells. In addition, the number of mesenchymal cells determines the total size of the prostate, and the epithelial cells grow out until they cover the surface of the available mesenchyme. The opposite, an excess of cells, will not cause a concomitant growth of mesenchyme. In fact, Cunha and colleagues believe the major target for androgen stimulation in the urogenital sinus is the mesenchyme and not the epithelial cells.

Recently, Chung et al. (1984) transplanted a fetal urogenital sinus into an adult rat prostate and induced a large overgrowth of adult prostatic tissue, apparently stimulated by the presence of the fetal tissue. This has raised the question of whether direct contact with an insoluble embryonic extracellular matrix or a soluble factor is responsible for these observations. Muntzing (1980) proposed that collagen of the prostate might limit prostatic growth. Mariotti and Mawhinney (1981) and Thornton et al. (1984) have provided evidence that collagen synthesis and degradation can be important events and may accompany limitation on prostate growth in animals. At present, a clear cause and effect of collagens on prostate growth has not been fully established.

The stroma of animals does contain steroid receptors and does appear to respond to estrogens (Mariotti and Mawhinney, 1981). Attempts to correlate enzyme levels with stroma composition (Bartsch et al., 1984) also indicate that stroma has androgen-metabolizing ability almost equal to that of epithelium. Efforts to separate stroma and epithelia by mechanical means and to study the isolated components have supported these conclusions (Krieg et al., 1981; Cowan et al., 1977). It is still most difficult to obtain pure viable separation of high yield of stromal and epithelial components from the human prostate.

PROSTATIC GROWTH FACTORS

A search is under way by Chung and his associates to identify a soluble prostatic growth factor that is associated with the urogenital sinus mesenchyme. Since the normal adult prostate is not growing rapidly, one would not anticipate an abundance of growth factors in the normal steady state of growth. However, many adult tissues have growth factors that can be demonstrated in in vitro assay systems. In 1979, Jacobs et al. demonstrated a growth factor in crude extracts of normal, BPH, and cancerous human prostates. Efforts are under way to identify and isolate these factors (Storey et al., 1983, 1984; Parrish et al., 1984; Lawson et al., 1981). Much work will be required to pursue these potentially important observations and to eliminate contamination of other known growth factors and protease enzymes. There is little doubt that most tissues are susceptible to growth factors and chalones, and it will be very important to unravel these cellular growth factors in normal and abnormal growth of the prostate.

STEROID IMPRINTING OF PROSTATIC GROWTH

In animal studies it appears that the presence of steroids at certain times in the life of the animal permanently marks subsequent responsiveness of the prostate to androgen-induced growth (Chung and McFadden, 1980; Rajfer and Coffey, 1979a,b; Higgins et al., 1981). This phenomenon, commonly referred to as imprinting, is dramatic in the rat. For example, if a neonate male rat is subjected to estrogens at days 1 to 5, the prostate becomes essentially inert to treatment with androgens in adult life. Under these conditions of estrogen imprinting in the neonatal period, the prostate remains diminutive even when large dosages of androgens are administered in adulthood. In contrast, treating male rats with estrogens at the weaning period produces a prostate that is oversensitive to androgen-induced growth in adult life (Rajfer and Coffey, 1979a,b). What determines these responses to imprinting in animals is unknown, but it does indicate the need for more awareness of the possibility of similar events occurring in human growth and development.

THE ENDOCRINOLOGY OF PROSTATIC GROWTH

Overview. The prostate is stimulated to grow primarily by the presence of serum testosterone. This is depicted in the schematic in Figure 5–32, in which the hypothalamus releases a decapeptide referred to as LHRH (for luteinizing hormone–releasing hormone), also called GnRH (for gonadotropin-releasing hormone). The pituitary releases the luteinizing hormone (LH) that acts directly on the testes to stimulate the steroid synthesis of testosterone, which is the major androgen stimulating prostatic growth. Most of the estrogen in the male is derived from peripheral conversion of testosterone to estrogens through an enzymatic pathway of aromatization. The direct effects of estrogens on the prostate is to *stimulate* growth in the presence of androgen and not to block androgen action. The ability of estrogens to diminish prostatic growth is not a direct effect but an indirect effect, through blocking pituitary function and decreasing LH. This is an effective "chemical castration," meaning the essential abolition of circulatory androgen by estrogen administration. Other factors stimulating prostate growth include adrenal androgens, through androstenedione. This is not a major pathway, since in animals and humans castration leads to almost complete involution of the prostate, meaning that insufficient adrenal androgens are present to stimulate any meaningful growth of the prostate.

Prolactin has often been postulated to enhance androgen-induced growth (Grayhack et al., 1955); however, several decades of study have failed to indicate the mechanism of this action, and it does not appear to be a major or direct way of regulating prostatic growth.

TESTICULAR ANDROGENS

In the normal male, the major circulating androgen is testosterone, which is almost exclusively (more than 95 per cent) of testicular origin. Under normal physiologic conditions the Leydig cells of the testis are the major source of the testicular androgens. The Leydig cells are stimulated by the gonadotropins (primarily the luteinizing hormone [LH]) to synthesize testosterone from acetate and cholesterol. The spermatic vein concentration of testosterone is 40 to 50 μg per dl and is approximately 75 times more concentrated than the level detected in the peripheral venous serum, which is approximately 600 ng of testosterone per dl. Other androgens also leave the testes by the spermatic vein; these include androstanediol, androstenedione, and dehydroepiandrosterone; however, the concentrations of these androgens are much lower than those of testosterone.

Testosterone in the plasma is primarily that synthesized by the testes, and although other steroids, such as androstenedione, can be converted by peripheral metabolism to testosterone, they probably account for less than 5 per cent of the overall production of plasma testos-

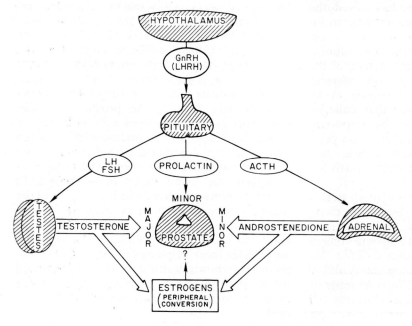

Figure 5–32. Endocrinology of the prostate. Luteinizing hormone-releasing hormone (LHRH), also termed gonadotropin-releasing hormone (GnRH), stimulates the pituitary to release the gonadotropins LH and FSH, which stimulate the testes to synthesize testosterone serum, that which is the major serum androgen stimulating prostatic growth. Peripheral conversion of the androgens by aromatization forms the main estrogen in the male. The adrenal gland is under ACTH stimulation and releases the minor androgen androstenedione, which is also converted to estrogens. Prolactin has also been shown to have a minor effect in stimulating androgen-induced prostatic growth.

terone. The total testosterone that enters the plasma is referred to as the testosterone blood production rate and is determined from the product of the metabolic clearance rate and the mean concentration of testosterone in the plasma. The average testosterone production rate in normal adult males is 6 to 7 mg per day. The mean metabolic clearance rate for testosterone is around 1000 liters per 24 hours and is related to the testosterone production rate.

The average testosterone concentration in the adult human male plasma is approximately 611 ± 186 ng per dl and is not remarkably related to age between 25 and 70 years, although it does decline gradually to approximately 500 ng per dl after 70 years of age (Table 5–3). It is recognized that plasma concentrations of testosterone can vary widely in an individual in any one day and may reflect both episodic and diurnal variations in the production rate of testosterone. In addition, longer cycles or periods have been observed if regular daily measurements are determined in the same patient for many weeks. In 12 subjects the average periodicity of the cycle varied from 8 to 30 days, with most cycles lasting 20 to 22 days (Doering et al., 1975). During these cycles the variation in the fluctuation of the testosterone level was 21 per cent.

Only the free testosterone (not protein-bound) in the plasma is available for metabolism by the liver and intestines, primarily to the 17-ketosteroids, which are secreted in the urine as the conjugates of sulfuric acid and glucuronic acid (Fig. 5–33). The total 17-ketosteroids in the urine in adult males is from 4 to 25 mg per 24 hours and is not an accurate index of testosterone production, since other steroids from the adrenals as well as nonandrogenic steroids can be metabolized to 17-ketosteroid forms. This is apparent, since the daily production rate of testosterone averages only 6 to 7 mg per 24 hours. Only small (25 to 160 μg per day) amounts of testosterone enter the urine without metabolism, and this represents less than 2 per cent of the daily testosterone production.

Although testosterone is the primary plasma androgen inducing growth of the prostate gland, it nevertheless appears to function as a prehormone, in that the active form of the androgen in the prostate is a testosterone metabolite, *dihydrotestosterone* (DHT) (Bruchovsky and Wilson, 1968a,b; Siiteri and Wilson, 1970). Dihydrotestosterone can form, in part, from peripheral conversion, which involves the reduction of the 4 double bond in testosterone through the enzymatic action of 5α-reductase. This conversion can take place directly in the prostate and seminal vesicles. Dihydrotestosterone concentration in the plasma of normal men is very low, 56 ng ± 20 per dl, in comparison with testosterone, which is 11-fold higher at approximately 611 ng/dl (see Table 5–3). In summary, although dihydrotestosterone is a potent androgen (1.5 to 2.5 times as potent as testosterone in most bioassay systems), its low plasma concentration and tight binding to plasma proteins diminish its direct importance as a circulating androgen affecting prostate and seminal vesicle growth. In contrast, dihydrotestosterone is of paramount importance within the sex accessory tissue, where it is formed from

TABLE 5–3. PLASMA LEVELS OF STEROIDS IN HEALTHY HUMAN MALES

| Common Name | Chemical Name | Plasma Concentration | | | Blood Production Rate (mg/day) | Relative Androgenicity Rat V.P. Assay |
		NG/DL	MOLARITY	RELATIVE MOLARITY		
Testosterone	17β-hydroxy-4-androstene-3-one	611 ± 186	2.1×10^{-8}	100	6.6 ± 0.5	100
Dihydrotestosterone (DHT; Stanolone)	17β-hydroxy-5α-androstan-3-one	56 ± 20	1.9×10^{-9}	9	0.3 ± 0.06	181
5α-Androstane-3α,17β-diol (3α-androstanediol)	5α-androstan-3α,17β-diol	14 ± 4	4.8×10^{-10}	2	0.2 ± 0.03	126
5α-Androstane-3β,17β-diol (3β-androstanediol)	5α-androstan-3β,17β-diol	<2	$<7 \times 10^{-11}$	<0.3		18
Androstenediol	5-androstene-3β,17β-diol	161 ± 52	5.6×10^{-9}	26		0.21
Androsterone	3α-hydroxy-5α-androstan-17-one	54 ± 32	1.9×10^{-9}	9	0.28	53
Androstenedione	4-androstene-3,17 dione	150 ± 54	5.2×10^{-9}	25	1.4	39
Dehydroepiandrosterone (DHA)	3β-hydroxy-5-androstene-17-one	501 ± 98	1.7×10^{-8}	81 ⎰	29	15
Dehydroepiandrosterone sulfate (DHAS)	17-oxo-5-androstene-3β-γl-sulfate	135,925 ± 48,000	3.7×10^{-6}	17,619 ⎱		<1
Progesterone	4-pregnene-3,20-dione	30	9.5×10^{-10}	4.5	0.75	
17β-Estradiol (E₂)	1,3,5(10)-estratriene-3,17β-diol	2.5 ± 0.8	9.2×10^{-11}	0.4	0.045	
Estrone	3-hydroxyl-1,3,5(10)-estratriene-17-one	4.6	1.7×10^{-10}	0.8		

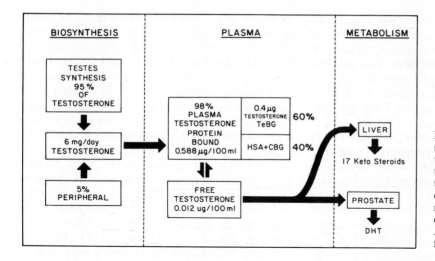

Figure 5–33. A quantitative assessment of the testicular production, plasma transport, and metabolism of testosterone. Plasma testosterone is bound to testosterone-binding globulin (TeBG), human serum albumin (HSA), and cortisol-binding globulin (CBG). All numbers are average values for the normal adult male.

testosterone. In sex accessory tissues, dihydrotestosterone binds to critical receptors and becomes the major androgen regulating the cellular events of growth and differentiation.

The plasma levels of some important steroids are summarized in Table 5–3. These values are derived as averages from several combined sources (Breuer et al., 1976; Dorfman, 1962; Frieden, 1976; Vida, 1969). The complete biologic importance of many of the different steroids circulating in the plasma has not been resolved. In addition, the steroid conjugates could function as more than dead-end metabolites.

ADRENAL ANDROGENS

There is ample biologic evidence that, under some conditions, steroids secreted from the adrenal cortex can have an influence on the growth of the prostate gland. Virilism has been observed in humans with hyperfunction of the adrenal cortex associated with neoplasia or hyperplasia of the adrenal gland. However, the effect of adrenal androgens on the prostate in noncastrated adult male rats may not be significant, since adrenalectomy has very little effect on gland size, DNA, or morphology of the sex accessory tissue (Arvola, 1961; Mobbs et al., 1973). Furthermore, following castration in animals, the prostate diminishes to a very small size (90 per cent reduction) without concomitant adrenalectomy. The very small ventral prostate (9 mg) of the castrated cat can be reduced further (7.7 mg) by performing adrenalectomy (Tisell, 1970). However, these changes are insignificant compared with the massive regression that follows castration. It has been concluded, similarly, that the prostate of man does not restore itself following castration, indicating that

adrenal androgens are insufficient to compensate for the loss of testicular function. While the androgens from the adrenal gland in castrated animals do not restore the size of the prostate gland, it is clear that administration of ACTH to castrated animals does significantly increase the growth of sex accessory tissue (Arvola, 1961; Tisell, 1970; Tullner, 1963; Walsh and Gittes, 1970). This ACTH stimulation of prostatic growth has been observed in both castrated and castrated-hypophysectomized animals but did not occur if the animals had had an adrenalectomy (Tullner, 1963). Thus, in castrated animals adrenal stimulation can cause prostatic growth.

The adrenal androgens dehydroepiandrosterone, dehydroepiandrosterone sulfate, and androstenedione are primary C_{19} steroids synthesized from acetate and cholesterol (Fig. 5–34) and are secreted by the normal human adrenal gland; these steroids can be identified in the adrenal venous blood. Essentially all of the dehydroepiandrosterone in the plasma is of adrenal cortex origin, and the production rate in man is 10 to 30 mg per day. Less than 1 per cent of the testosterone in the plasma is derived from dehydroepiandrosterone (Horton, 1976; Wieland et al., 1965).

The prostate tissue has the ability to hydrolyze the steroid glucuronide and sulfate conjugates. The prostate and seminal vesicles of the rat (Gill and Chen, 1970) and the human prostate (Farnsworth, 1975) can slowly hydrolyze dehydroepiandrosterone (DHEAS) to free steroids by a sulfatase enzymatic activity. A considerable portion of the labeled androstenedione appears as epiandrosterone and androsterone, but DHEAS and androstenedione produce only small amounts of the potent androgen 5α-reduced metabolites, such as dihydrotestosterone.

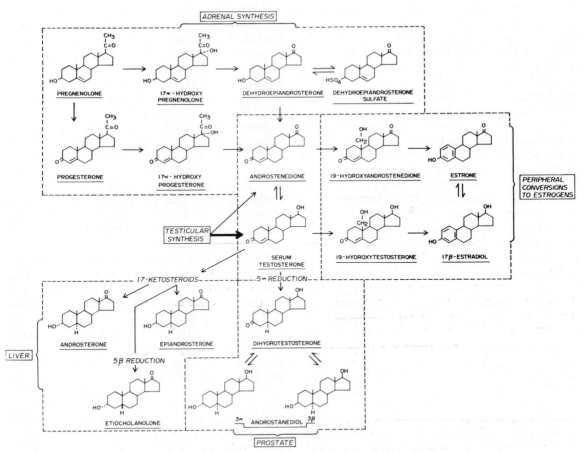

Figure 5–34. Overall synthesis and metabolism of testosterone in four body compartments: (1) adrenal synthesis of androstenedione; (2) peripheral conversion of androgens (androstenedione and testosterone) to estrogen; (3) formation of active dihydrotestosterone within the prostate; and (4) inactivation in the liver of testosterone to three types of 17-ketosteroids.

In summary, the potential for conversion of DHEAS to active metabolites exists, but the degree of 5α-conversion may be low, thereby explaining why DHEAS is not a very potent androgen.

A second adrenal androgen is androstenedione, and the plasma concentration in adult males is approximately 150 ± 54 ng per dl (Table 5–3). The blood production rate of androstenedione in human males is about 2 mg per day, with approximately 20 per cent of the androstenedione being generated by peripheral metabolism of other steroids. An important role for androstenedione in the male may be its peripheral conversion to estrogens (see Fig. 5–34). In addition, the adrenal gland produces progesterone. The plasma production rate of 0.75 mg per day is low, producing a low plasma progesterone concentration of 30 ng per dl. Although progesterone exhibits slight androgenic activity, it is not significant at the low concentrations present in normal male plasma.

In summary, under normal conditions the adrenals do not support significant growth of prostatic tissue. Attempts in the past to cure prostate cancers relapsing to castration by adrenalectomy or hypophysectomy have met with failure.

ESTROGEN PRODUCTION IN MEN

Approximately 75 to 90 per cent of the estrogens in the plasma of young healthy males is derived from the peripheral conversion of androstenedione and testosterone to estrone and estradiol (Horton, 1976; MacDonald, 1976). The pathways for synthesis of the estrogens are depicted in Figure 5–34. They involve converting these androgenic C_{19} steroids (testosterone and androstenedione) to the estrogenic C_{18} steroids by removal of the 19-methyl group and the subsequent formation of an aromatic or phenolic steroid A ring (aromatase reaction), which is present in both estradiol and estrone. Estradiol is formed from testosterone and estrone from androstenedione. These two estrogens are then interconvertible. The daily production of estradiol in the male is about 40 to 50 μg, and only 5 to 10 μg (10 to 25 per cent) of this production can be accounted for by direct testicular secretion (Horton et al., 1973; MacDonald, 1976; Siiteri and MacDonald, 1973). The dynamics of the synthesis of estrogens in human males have been quantitated by Siiteri and MacDonald (1973), who showed that of the total of 7.0 mg of testosterone produced in man each day, 0.35 per cent was converted directly to estradiol, forming 24 μg per day. Of the 2.5 mg of androstenedione produced per day, 1.7 per cent was converted to estrone, producing 42 μg per day. The interconversion of estrone and estradiol yielded a final total peripheral production of approximately 40 μg of estradiol per day. The exact location in the periphery where estrogen production occurs has not been elucidated on a quantitative basis, but it is believed that most of the daily production may involve adipose tissue. The small amount of estrogens secreted directly from the testes may originate in part from the Sertoli cells, since in culture these cells respond to FHS stimulation by producing small amounts of estradiol (Dorrington and Armstrong, 1975).

Men over 50 years of age have an increase in total plasma estradiol levels of approximately 50 per cent, with minimal change (less than 10 per cent) in the free estradiol levels because of increases in binding of the estradiol by elevated testosterone-estrogen–binding globulin (TeBG) levels, which are also age-related (Vermeulen, 1976). An age-related decrease in the plasma free testosterone level while the free estradiol level is maintained produces a 40 per cent increase in the value for the ratio of free estradiol/free testosterone (Vermeulen, 1976).

BINDING OF STEROIDS TO PLASMA PROTEINS

Less than 2 per cent of the total testosterone in human plasma is free or unbound, and the remaining 98 per cent is bound to several different types of plasma proteins (Fig. 5–33 and Table 5–4). The plasma proteins that can bind steroids include human serum albumin, testosterone-estrogen–binding protein (denoted TeBG or SBG, steroid-binding globulin), corticosteroid-binding globulin (CBG, also termed transcortin), progesterone-binding globulin (PBG), and, to a lesser extent, the alpha-acid glycoprotein (AAG). The total amount of testosterone bound to PBG and AAG is not large and is usually ignored.

The total amount of steroid bound depends on two factors: (1) the *affinity* of the steroid to bind to the protein, and (2) the *capacity*, which is the maximal potential binding when all of the protein is saturated with bound steroid; the capacity is governed by the amount of protein in the plasma. Serum albumin has a relatively low affinity for testosterone, but because of its high concentration it can bind appreciable quantities of testosterone. Therefore, albumin is a low-affinity, high-capacity binding protein. In contrast, a steroid-binding globulin (SBG or TeBG) that has been isolated from plasma has a high affinity, but the protein is present in relatively low concentrations; however, the plasma molarity of each binding protein exceeds the plasma molarity for total testosterone concentration. The majority of the testosterone bound to plasma protein is associated with TeBG protein (Vermeulen et al., 1969). For example, Vermeulen (1973) has calculated that in the normal human male, 57 per cent of the testosterone in the plasma is bound to TeBG and 40 per cent is bound to human serum albumin. Less than 1 per cent is bound to CBG, and only 2 per cent of the total testosterone is free (see Table 5–4). The normal plasma free testosterone level is therefore 12.1 $\pm$ 3.7 ng per dl or 4.2×10^{-10} M; this non-protein–bound testosterone is available to diffuse into the prostate and liver cells. In addition, a large percentage of the TeBG is saturated, whereas only a small fraction of the total capacity of CBG and albumin is utilized under normal conditions. As testosterone levels increase in the plasma, the order of increasing saturation of the plasma proteins proceeds from TeBG to CBG to albumin.

The total plasma levels of TeBG can be altered by hormone therapy. Administration of testosterone decreases TeBG levels in the plasma, while estrogen therapy stimulates TeBG levels (August et al., 1969; Burton and Westphal, 1972; Forest et al., 1968; Vermeulen et al., 1969). Estrogen also competes with testosterone for binding to TeBG, but estrogen has only one-third the binding affinity of testosterone. Therefore, administration of small amounts of estrogen increases the total concentration of TeBG, and this effectively increases the binding of testosterone and thus lowers the free testosterone plasma concentration.

Studies indicate that testosterone enters the prostate cell in the free form and that binding of testosterone to plasma proteins inhibits the uptake into the prostate (Lasnitzki and Franklin, 1972). It is apparent that effective androgen

TABLE 5–4. Properties of Plasma Proteins that Bind Testosterone in the Normal Human Male

Plasma Protein	Affinity for Testosterone			Capacity—Total Concentration in Plasma			Disposition of Testosterone in Normal Blood		
	Molecular Weight	Association Constant (M^{-1})	Relative Affinity	Amount (MG/L)	Molarity (10^{-8} M)	Relative to Testosterone Molarity	% of Plasma T Bound	Amount of Plasma T Bound (NG/100 ML)	% of Protein Capacity Utilized (% Saturated)
Albumin (HSA)	69,000	4×10^4	0.00005	38,000	55,500	26,400	40	244	0.0003
Cortisone-binding globulin; transcortin (CBG)	52,000	3×10^7	0.04	42	80	38	1	6	3
Testone-binding globulin (TeBG)	98,000	8×10^8	1.0	3.4	3.5	1.7	57	348	34
Plasma testosterone (T)	288	—	—	0.006 (total)	2.1 (total)	1 (total)	2 (free)	12 (free)	—

activity can be regulated by the extent of binding of the androgen to the steroid-binding proteins in the plasma. Indeed, Anderson et al. (1972) have postulated that altered testosterone binding to plasma proteins might produce amplified changes in free estrogen and androgen levels, and this could be an important factor in inducing gynecomastia and impotence.

The exact physiologic function of TeBG in man is not known, although the plasma concentration is inversely related to the rate of testosterone metabolism (metabolic clearance rate [MCR]); this is because free testosterone is the form metabolized by the liver (Bardin and Lipsett, 1967). In addition, estrogen therapy increases the level of TeBG and lowers the MCR of testosterone (Bardin and Mahoudeau, 1970). This may be explained by the fact that estrogen treatment increases the amount of TeBG and thus the percentage of plasma testosterone that is protein bound; therefore, there is a reduction in the amount of free testosterone in the plasma that is available either to the liver for metabolism or to the prostate for androgenic stimulation.

Castration. Since the testes normally produce approximately 95 per cent of the testosterone in the human male, it is not surprising that bilateral orchiectomy results in a reduction of approximately 93 per cent in the plasma testosterone levels. The value for plasma testosterone following bilateral orchiectomy from six different studies averaged 43 ± 32 ng per dl (Conti et al., 1975; Kent et al., 1973; Mackler et al., 1972; Robinson and Thomas, 1971; Sciarra et al., 1973; Shearer et al., 1973; Young and Kent, 1968). This postcastration level of testosterone in the castrated male is almost identical to the average testosterone level of 45 ± 16 ng per dl for the normal nonpregnant female reported in four studies. (See studies in Breuer et al., 1976.) There is also no significant difference between the low plasma level of testosterone in prepubertal boys (6.62 ± 2.46 ng per dl) or girls (6.58 ± 2.48 ng per dl) (Forest et al., 1973). In summary, the average testosterone levels in the human male are: normal adult, 611 ng per dl; castrated adult, 43 ng per dl; prepubertal male, 6.6 ng per dl.

The normal human plasma levels of androstenedione are approximately the same in both men (120 ng ± 30 per dl) and women (170 ng ± 40 per dl) (Bardin and Lipsett, 1967), and the androstenedione levels do not increase appreciably following castration of the male (Conti et al., 1975; Sciarra et al., 1973; Walsh and Siiteri, 1975).

GONADOTROPINS

The amount of testosterone produced by Leydig cells in the testes is controlled in part by the plasma levels of the luteinizing hormone (LH) released from the anterior pituitary gland. In turn, testosterone is involved in a negative feedback regulation of the pituitary. When animals are castrated, thus eliminating the major source of androgens, there is a dramatic increase in the plasma levels of both LH and FHS. After castration, specific alterations are observed in the morphology of the pituitary, in which "castration cells" are observed. The formation of these cells can be prevented by the administration of exogenous androgens. Testosterone can inhibit the synthesis of LH and the release of FHS in castrated male and female rats, but it is less effective than estrogen.

Testosterone treatment (50 mg) of intact and castrated adult males results in a marked suppression of pituitary LH release and of plasma LH levels. With increasing doses of testosterone (100 mg), the FSH plasma level is also lowered. In contrast, estrogen administered to human males causes a decrease in both LH and FSH levels. Therefore, testosterone preferentially suppresses serum LH relative to serum FSH, whereas estradiol produces parallel inhibition of both LH and FSH.

The negative feedback centers sensitive to testosterone appear to be located not only in the hypothalamus but also in the pituitary. Testosterone implants placed in the median eminence will inhibit gonadotropin secretion, and many experiments have established that the basal medial hypothalamic region is one of the major sites of negative feedback by androgens. In addition, other studies indicate that androgen can act directly on the pituitary gland, resulting in some negative feedback.

Injected ^{3}H-testosterone or ^{3}H-estradiol both have been demonstrated to be concentrated in the hypothalamus. The major androgen in the pituitary, following injection of ^{3}H-testosterone, has been identified as ^{3}H-dihydrotestosterone (DHT). Recent studies indicate that the 4α-metabolites of testosterone may be more effective than testosterone in suppressing LH plasma levels in the rat. Radioautography studies indicate that the labeled androgens concentrate in the basophil cells of the pituitary, while labeled estradiol is concentrated in the acidophils, basophils, and chromophobes.

It is now apparent that at least part of the negative feedback by steroids on the function of the pituitary is mediated by inhibiting the secretion of the LH-releasing hormone

(LHRH), which originates as a neurohumoral factor in the hypothalamus and is carried to the anterior pituitary via the hypophyseal portal blood supply. The secretion of these neurohumoral hypothalamic-releasing factors is in part under the influence of the central nervous system.

Although the initial implication of releasing hormones involved indirect methods, such as hypothalamic lesions, pituitary stalk sectioning, and pituitary transplantation, it is now possible to isolate or synthesize these releasing hormones, which are small decapeptides, and to demonstrate their effect on pituitary secretion of LH and FSH both in vivo and in vitro. It was at first surprising that LHRH stimulated the anterior pituitary to release not only LH but also FSH. This led to renaming LHRH as GnRH. This concept was intriguing but left open the question of how sex steroids would change the ratio of LH and FSH in the plasma, particularly if only one distinct releasing factor (GnRH) were indeed responsible for the regulation of both these gonadotropins. It now appears that sex steroids may also produce a direct modulation of the response by the pituitary to releasing hormones; this may partly explain the apparent paradox.

PROLACTIN

In hypophysectomized rats, exogenous androgens were not capable of restoring full prostatic growth unless these animals were given supplements of exogenous prolactin (Grayhack et al., 1955). This observation has now been confirmed in numerous animal experiments, in which prolactin was shown to be synergistic with androgens on growth (Danutra et al., 1973). In addition, prolactin increases zinc uptake in the tissue (Moger and Geschwind, 1972), alters androgen uptake and metabolism (Lloyd et al., 1973; Manandhar and Thomas, 1976), and regulates citric acid and fructose levels. Prolactin receptors have been identified in prostatic tissue (Aragona and Friesen, 1975).

The accumulated evidence that prolactin affects prostatic growth in animals has led to much speculation about a similar role in humans. Prolactin levels in human blood are elevated with estrogens, some tranquilizing drugs, and stress and can be decreased by L-dopa and ergot derivatives. At present, with improved assays, the levels are being monitored in patients of advanced age and in those with benign prostatic hyperplasia, but no clear correlation of cause and effect is yet apparent (Aragona and Friesen, 1976; Birkoff et al., 1974).

INSULIN

Like prolactin, insulin has been reported to have synergistic or permissive effects on prostatic growth, but these data have been obtained previously in rodents and often in tissue or organ culture. Angervall et al. (1967) and Sufrin and Prutkin (1974) have demonstrated that diabetic castrated rats have a diminished response to exogenous androgens that can be restored with supplements of insulin; these findings support the earlier conclusions of Calame and Lostroh (1964) and Lostroh (1971), who found that insulin was required for androgen response of the rat prostate in organ culture. There is little information on the possible role of insulin in the growth of the human prostate.

REGULATION OF PROSTATIC GROWTH AT THE CELLULAR LEVEL

Overview. It appears that cell-cell communication is at the forefront of biologic regulation. This is usually accomplished by several mechanisms as depicted in part in Figure 5–30. These include (1) long-range signals such as serum hormones, including steroid-like testosterone, estrogens and serum polypeptide hormone–like prolactin, and insulin; (2) soluble tissue growth factors that stimulate or inhibit (chalones) growth, which are elaborated over short ranges within the tissue compartment; and (3) direct structural contact between cells occurring through membrane junctions on intramembrane proteins attaching to the extracellular matrix. These interacting structural components form the important tissue matrix system discussed earlier and also reviewed by Isaacs et al. (1981). Of these systems the best understood has been the steroid regulation of prostatic growth via changes in serum testosterone levels. The steroid is bound to the steroid-binding globulins as depicted in the schematic in Figure 5–35. When the free testosterone enters the prostate cell by diffusion it is subjected to a variety of metabolic steps that appear to regulate the disposition and activity of the steroid hormone. The most important is the formation of dihydrotestosterone (DHT) and the 3α- and 3β-diols and the 6α- and 7α-triols. The most important of these biologic transformations involves steroid metabolism to DHT and the subsequent binding of the DHT to high-affinity and specific receptors in the cytoplasm, and the activation of the receptor to be translocated into the nucleus, where the steroid receptor ultimately binds to the acceptor that is believed to be DNA or the nuclear matrix structure for the steroid (see Fig. 5–35). As we

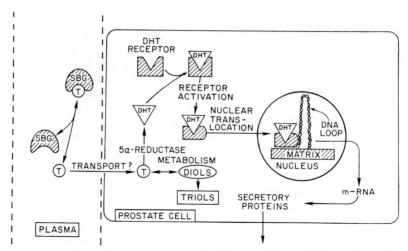

Figure 5–35. A schematic of the effects of testosterone in inducing growth in an epithelial cell. In the plasma, testosterone is bound to serum-binding globulins (SBG), such as testosterone-binding globulin and albumin. Unbound testosterone is transported by diffusion into the prostate, where it is enzymatically converted to dihydrotestosterone (DHT) through the action of 5α-reductase and further metabolized to diols (3α or 3β) and irreversibly metabolized into the inactive triols (6α or 7α). Dihydrotestosterone binds to a cytoplasmic receptor (which may actually be nuclear; see text), which is then activated and translocated to the nucleus. There the DHT receptors interact with the acceptors on the nuclear matrix and with DNA. This nuclear binding of the receptor brings about a stimulation of specific messenger RNA synthesis that is translated at the ribosomes in the cytoplasm to form secretory proteins.

follow the steps for steroid transport from the cell periphery to the DNA, the mechanisms become more vague but are nonetheless important. In summary, the intracellular events for the steroid are (1) uptake; (2) metabolism; (3) binding to receptor; (4) binding of steroid receptor to the nucleus, nuclear matrix, and specific sequences of DNA; (5) changes in DNA structure and function; and (6) expression and regulation of specific steroid-controlled genes. These steroid-induced cellular events take place in both the epithelial and stromal cells, as depicted in Figure 5–30, and occur for both testosterone and estrogens. For simplicity, these steps will be discussed in relation to the epithelial cells because differences between the steroid target cell types, such as stroma, have not been clearly resolved. It appears that estrogens may have more effect on the stromal cells, but this is not fully established at the present time. We now will discuss these aforementioned steroid-related events in more detail.

Steroid Metabolism. After the free testosterone in the plasma has entered the prostatic epithelial cell through diffusion, it is rapidly metabolized to other steroid forms by a series of prostatic enzymes (Isaacs and Coffey, 1979, 1981a,b; Berry and Isaacs, 1984). Over 90 per cent of the testosterone is *irreversibly* converted to dihydrotestosterone (DHT) (Fig. 5–36) through the action of NADPH and the enzyme 5α-reductase, located on the endoplasmic retic-

ulum and on the nuclear membrane. The enzyme 5α-reductase reduces the unsaturated bond in the testosterone between the 4 and 5 positions to form the 5α–reduced DHT (Bruchovsky, 1971; Isaacs and Coffey, 1981a,b; Anderson and Liao, 1968; Bruchovsky and Wilson, 1968a; Farnsworth and Brown, 1963; Shimazaki et al., 1965a,b). After the DHT is formed, it is subjected to a series of reversible reactions to form 3α-diol (5α-androstane 3α, 17β-diol) and 3β-diol (5α-androstane 3β, 17β-diol). The enzymes that perform this transformation are 3α- or 3β-hydroxysteroid dehydrogenase (3α-HSH or 3β-HSD). These enzymes, like 5α-reductase, utilize NADP as a cofactor, but in contrast to 5α-reductase, they can also utilize NAD. The equilibrium for the metabolism of DHT favors the formation of DHT, that is, the oxidation of the 3-hydroxy group of 3α- and 3β-diol to the 3-ketone that is present in DHT. It is known that 3α-diol is an effective androgen because of its rapid conversion to the effective DHT. On the other hand, 3β-diol is not very effective as an androgen because it is rapidly and irreversibly converted to the triol form by hydroxylation in the 6α- or 7α-position (see Fig. 5–36). The triols are very inactive as androgens and cannot reform DHT. In summary, testosterone is irreversibly metabolized to DHT that is in equilibrium with other reduced steroids primarily through oxidation and reduction at the 3-position. The steroids are inactivated by being irreversibly hydroxylated to the inactive triols. For more details on these specific reactions and their magnitude of activities in the prostates of man, dog, and rat, see Berry and Isaacs (1984) and Isaacs and Coffey (1981*a*).

Steroid Receptors. The prostate is similar to other steroid hormone target tissues in containing steroid-specific, high-affinity (10^{-9} to 10^{-10}K≡), saturable (100–1000 fmol/mg DNA equivalents of tissue) hormone receptors that appear to be translocated into the nucleus and bind to specific nuclear acceptors. (For a complete review of the general topic of the mechanism of all steroid hormone action, consult the recent review by Clark and O'Malley [1984].) Liao et al. (1974) have reviewed the general molecular mechanism associated with the functions of androgen receptors in the prostate.

The problem in assessing the level of androgen receptors in the prostate is a methodological one, because there are many binding globulins and plasma proteins that can interfere with the assay, and the labeled steroids that are used for these binding studies are often metabolized or transformed. To avoid many of these pitfalls, methyltrienolone R-1881, a synthetic androgen, has been utilized in many receptor studies as the labeled androgen. R-1881 does not bind well to many of the interfering proteins and is not actively metabolized. Another problem is that even highly specific steroid-binding ligands, such as R-1881, can also cross bind to

some extent to other steroid receptors in the prostate, such as the progesterone receptor. Care must be taken to assure investigators that their receptor assay is both biochemically and kinetically correct. The prostate is rich in protease enzymes that can rapidly degrade many enzymes and receptors, and the prostatic connective tissue prevents the disruption of many cells. Many investigators have focused their attention on the cytoplasmic receptor instead of the nuclear compartment where the androgen action is believed to occur. In fact, the cytoplasmic receptor that appears soluble in a homogenate may prove to be an artifact of cell disruption, and all steroid receptors may reside primarily within the nucleus (King and Greene, 1984; Welshons et al., 1984). For years it has been believed that steroids diffuse into the cell, where they bind specific cytoplasmic receptors; then, by a temperature-sensitive step, these cytoplasmic receptors are activated and are translocated into the nucleus, where they bind to a mysterious nuclear acceptor protein. Recent studies suggest that all of the receptor is in the nucleus and that this cytoplasmic receptor is only an artifact of their having been extracted during the homogenization technique. If this proves true, the standard schematics representing this process, as shown in Figure 5–35, must be altered to have the cytoplasmic receptor reside within the nucleus. Indeed, even within the nucleus, there appear to be several com-

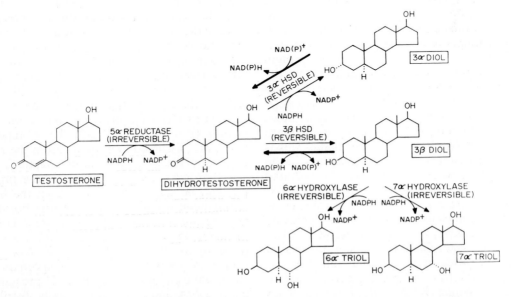

Figure 5–36. Metabolic pathways for testosterone within the prostate. Testosterone is irreversibly metabolized to the active androgen dihydrotestosterone (DHT), which is then reversibly converted into 3α- and 3β-diols. The 3β-diol is irreversibly inactivated to the more soluble 6α- and 7α-triols.

partments that can be assayed, including those that can be extracted in salt concentrations of 0.4 to 0.6 M and those that resist the salt extraction, termed salt-resistant receptors. These salt-resistant receptors appear to be a reflection of receptor associated with the nuclear skeleton or nuclear matrix component of the nucleus (Barrack and Coffey, 1980, 1982). Barrack has recently shown that the nuclear matrix may contain the acceptor site, which is defined as the nuclear proteins that specifically bind steroid receptors within target tissues (Barrack, 1983). The most careful and informative studies carried out on receptor levels in normal, benign, and cancerous human prostates have been those of Walsh and his colleagues (Barrack et al., 1983). They have given careful attention to the development of highly specific receptor assay methods and have applied them to all of the known compartments of the cell, including cytoplasmic, nuclear salt-extractable, and salt-resistant binding. These considerations are of the utmost importance, since the use of steroid receptor assays has been proposed to correlate with the hormone responsiveness of the prostate (Trachtenberg and Walsh, 1982; Murphy et al., 1981).

At present, it is not known to what the steroid receptors bind within the nucleus. Besides the possibility of the nuclear matrix (Barrack and Coffey, 1982), it appears that they may bind to specific sequences of the DNA (Clark and O'Malley, 1984). In this concept it is visualized that very specific nucleotide sequences within target tissues may directly bind steroid receptors and thus activate the genes to be expressed. The DNA appears to have topologic constraints placed upon it by proteins and topoisomerase action, which winds the protein into supercoiled loops. It is visualized that the presence of cytoplasmic receptors somehow alters the chromatin and DNA conformation so that the DNA is in a new state that is more susceptible to being copied and transcribed into messenger RNA. In many target tissues this is measured by an increase in the sensitivity of the gene to DNase activity when it is in the activated state. Once the DNA is transcribed into RNA, the RNA is processed before it is transferred out of the nucleus. This involves removing pieces of the RNA that will not become part of the final message. The action of steroids sets off a complex series of orderly and timed events starting with an increase in a protein initiation factor, messenger RNA and ribosomal RNA synthesis, cellular protein synthesis, and finally, DNA synthesis and cell replication. These events are specific for all steroid target tissues

that have been studied (Clark and O'Malley, 1984; DeKlerk et al., 1976; Liao et al., 1976).

In addition to the well-known androgen receptor, the prostate contains estrogen receptors (Ekman et al., 1983) and progesterone receptors (Ekman et al., 1982; Gustaffson et al., 1978). It is important to realize that these receptors may be distributed in various types of tissues within the prostate; indeed, the estradiol concentration appears to be highest in the nuclei of stroma in human benign prostatic hyperplasia (Kozak et al., 1982). Many of these steroid receptors may have multiple binding sites; the high-affinity, low-capacity binding has usually been referred to as Type I sites, whereas the moderate-affinity and higher-capacity binding has been termed Type II sites (Ekman et al., 1982; Clark and O'Malley, 1984).

Steroid Levels in the Prostate. Following the classic experiments of Bruchovsky and Wilson (1968a,b) and Anderson and Liao (1968) showing that dihydrotestosterone is the major intracellular androgen, there has been a flurry of activity to determine its role in abnormal growth. Siiteri and Wilson (1970) showed that dihydrotestosterone was raised 3 to 4 fold in BPH in comparison with the normal prostate. This was followed by a series of studies confirming this very important observation (Krieg et al., 1979; Meikle et al., 1978; Hammond, 1978; Geller et al., 1976). In all these studies it appeared that the DHT in BPH tissue was approximately 4 to 6 ng per gm tissue, whereas in the normal prostate the levels were much lower at 1 to 2 ng per gm tissue. More recent work has cast serious doubt on this interpretation, and more careful collection of the normal prostate from nonautopsy specimens indicates that there is no significant difference in the DHT levels between normal and BPH tissues (Walsh et al., 1983; Walsh, 1984). Although DHT may not be elevated in the prostate, the receptor content of DHT is significantly increased in the nucleus (Barrack et al., 1983). These important issues are discussed in more detail in the recent review by Walsh (1984) and in Chapter 27.

Estrogens are also present in the prostate and can be sequestered there from the blood. It has been proposed that prostatic fibroblasts are capable of converting androstenedione to estradiol through the aromatization reaction (Schweikert et al., 1983). Regardless of its source, it appears that there is approximately 50 to 100 fmol of estrogen in BPH prostate per mg of DNA and that this is equally distributed between estradiol and estrone (Kozak et al., 1982). The concentration in stroma is approximately three times that present in the epithelium. Several investigators have attempted to measure the levels of estrogen in the prostate (Ghanadian, 1982; Belis, 1983). This is an important area that requires more attention. The levels of estrogen must be correlated with the receptor levels and serum concentrations; since estrogens can be metabolized and conjugated to a variety of products, it is important that a comprehensive study be performed. The estrogen receptor in the prostate has been a controversial issue, probably because of the variations in methodology. Ekman et al. (1983) have reviewed this problem and have pointed out the evidence for multiple estrogen-binding sites in the human prostate.

Progesterone is not measurable in the prostate, although there is a progesterone receptor at concentrations approaching that of the androgen receptor; in contrast, the progesterone receptor is present only in the cytoplasm (Ekman et al., 1982). Progesterone levels are extremely low in the plasma and are not believed to be concentrated appreciably in the prostate, but progesterone can bring about changes in the prostates of animals (Belis et al., 1984). The role of progesterone is intriguing because it is a better substrate for 5α-reductase than is testosterone, and many progesterone analogs, such as cyproterone acetate, are very effective in blocking androgen binding to the receptor.

Estrogen-Androgen Synergism in Prostate Growth. Estrogens do not block androgen-induced growth of the prostate but, on the contrary, can synergize androgen effects. This has been well documented in the canine from the first work of Walsh and Wilson (1976) and subsequently by DeKlerk et al. (1979). In the aforementioned studies, the administration of estradiol to castrated dogs receiving 5α-androstane metabolites, such as DHT or 3α-diol, had a tremendous enhancement on the growth of the prostate. The presence of estrogens almost doubled the androgen-induced growth, and this was associated with the development of a glandular hyperplasia. This type of estrogen synergism could not be observed with testosterone, and the mechanism is not understood. It has been shown that estrogens increase the androgen receptor in the prostate, and this could be an important factor in this phenomenon (Trachtenberg et al., 1980; Moore et al., 1979). For more details on the estrogen-androgen changes associated with benign prostatic hyperplasia, consult the review of Walsh (1984) and Chapter 27.

DRUGS AFFECTING PROSTATE GROWTH

The classic way to control prostate growth has been through castration and androgen ablation. The major drugs used in treatment of the prostate have been estrogens, primarily diethylstilbestrol (DES), which inhibits prostate growth primarily through inhibiting the hypothalamic-pituitary-gonadal axis to block testicular synthesis of testosterone and thus lower the plasma testosterone level. As mentioned earlier, it is a misconception that estrogens block androgen actions on the prostate. When estrogens do exert a direct effect on the prostate, it is usually by stimulation of a metaplastic growth in the cells of the collecting ducts. In general, however, the estrogens lower LH levels and essentially bring about a "chemical castration." As opposed to castration, estrogen does often produce an increase in serum prolactin levels and a high incidence of gynecomastia as well as adverse cardiovascular side effects (Altwein, 1983). This has led to the search for other, more benign ways to lower plasma testosterone besides castration and estrogen therapy. Attention is currently being directed toward the use of LHRH analogs to block the hypothalamic-pituitary axis (Bergquist et al., 1979; Labrie et al., 1979, 1983).

Antiandrogens are defined as substances that can block the effects of androgens at the target tissue level and not primarily through disturbing the hypothalamic-pituitary axis. These compounds appear to interfere with the binding of DHT to its receptor and have been proposed as therapeutic agents since the early work of Scott and Wade (1969) and Geller et al. (1969, 1981). The most common antiandrogens are cyproterone acetate, flutamide, and megestrol acetate. Each of these compounds is a potent inhibitor of DHT binding to the steroid receptor in the prostate gland and to the accumulation of DHT in the nucleus (Bruchovsky, 1983; Schroder, 1983; Bartsch and Rohr, 1983; Neumann, 1983).

A wide variety of other substances have been proposed for interfering with prostatic growth, including agents to block prolactin secretion, polyenemacrolides that are believed to interfere with cholesterol metabolism, and antiestrogens as well as a host of ill-defined natural products, such as bark or pumpkin seed extracts. These compounds have proved to be ineffective and will not be discussed.

SEX ACCESSORY GLAND SECRETIONS

The normal human ejaculate has an average volume of 3 ml (range 1.5 to 6 ml) and is composed of two components, spermatozoa and the seminal plasma fluid, which can be separated easily by centrifugation. The spermatozoa are present in the range of 50 to 150 million per ml, but because of the small volume of sperm (approximately 10 μm per sperm) the volume of the spermatozoa component is insignificant, being less than 1 per cent of the volume of the total ejaculate. The seminal plasma is formed primarily from the secretions of the sex accessory tissues, which include the epididymis, vas deferens, ampullae, seminal vesicles, prostate, Cowper's (bulbourethral) gland, and glands of Littre. In an average ejaculate volume of 3.5 ml, the major contribution to the volume of the seminal plasma comes from the seminal vesicles, 1.5 to 2 ml; from the prostate, 0.5 ml; and from Cowper's gland and glands of Littre, 0.1 to 0.2 ml (Mann and Mann, 1981; Zaneveld and Chatterton, 1982). During ejaculation the secretions of these glands are released in a sequential manner (Mann and Mann, 1981; Amelar and Hotchkiss, 1965; Tauber et al., 1975). Table 5–5 shows the typical results of splitting the ejaculate into three sequential collections for analysis.

The first fractions of the ejaculate are rich in sperm and components from the prostatic secretion, such as citric acid (Mann and Mann, 1981). The concentration of fructose represents a major secretory product from the seminal vesicles and is elevated in the later fractions of the ejaculate.

The overall chemical composition of the normal human seminal plasma has been studied by many laboratories, and the results have been summarized in many excellent reviews (Aumuller, 1983; Isaacs, 1983). The book by Thaddeus Mann (1981), *The Biochemistry of Semen and of the Male Reproductive Tract,* is the most scholarly treatise on this subject. The review of physiologic studies of prostatic function by Huggins in the Harvey Lectures in 1947 is an early classic reference in this field. More concepts may be found in *Human Semen and Fertility*

Regulation in Men (1976), edited by E.S.E. Hafez, and in *The Biochemistry of Mammalian Reproduction,* edited by L.J.D. Zaneveld and R.T. Chatterton (1982).

In relation to other body fluids, the seminal plasma is unusual because of its high concentrations of potassium, zinc, citric acid, fructose, phosphorylcholine, spermine, free amino acids, prostaglandins, and enzymes (most notably acid phosphatase, diamine oxidase, β-glucuronidase, lactic dehydrogenase, α-amylase, and seminal proteinase). The normal concentrations of the biochemical components of the human seminal plasma are presented in Table 5–6.

ZINC

The very high level of zinc in human seminal plasma (15 mg per dl) appears to originate primarily from secretions of the prostate gland (Tisell and Leissner, 1984; Habib et al., 1979). In 1921 Bertrand and Vladesco reported that the human prostate had the highest concentration of zinc (50 mg per 100 gm dry weight) of any organ tested. In 1962, Mackenzie et al. reported that human seminal plasma contained 310 mg zinc per 100 gm dry weight and that spermatozoa contained 200 mg per 100 gm dry weight. In comparison, prostatic secretions from eight normal subjects had 720 mg zinc per 100 gm dry weight. Animal studies on many species have confirmed these general observations as well as the high level of tissue uptake of administered radioactive zinc-65. Many of the early experiments and concepts related to zinc in the reproductive tract have been reviewed in detail by Byar (1974).

Other investigators extended the studies with zinc to human BPH and prostatic adenocarcinoma (Gyorkey et al., 1967; Grant et al., 1975; Chandler et al., 1981; Prout et al., 1959; Schrodt et al., 1964; Whitmore, 1963; Habib et al., 1979; Tisell and Leissner, 1984). In general, these studies have reported that zinc levels are elevated or stable in BPH, whereas a marked decrease in zinc content is associated with prostatic adenocarcinoma.

The localization of zinc in the human prostate by radioautography appears to be within the epithelial cells; however, in the lateral prostate of the rat, large quantities of zinc were also associated with the stroma and particularly with the basal membrane and the elastin protein component (Chandler et al., 1977).

Many physiologic roles have been postulated for zinc since the classic studies of Gunn and Gould (1956) and Gunn et al. (1965), who correlated endocrine effects on zinc uptake and

TABLE 5–5. COMPOSITION OF HUMAN EJACULATE SPLIT INTO THREE SEQUENTIAL COLLECTIONS

Ejaculate	Volume (ml)	Sperm Concentration ($\times 10^6$/ml)	Fructose Concentration (mg/ml)
Fraction I	0.64	203	1.32
Fraction II	0.90	132	2.56
Fraction III	1.35	55	4.14
Total	2.89	111	3.02

*Adapted from data of Mann and Mann (1981) and Tauber et al. (1975).

TABLE 5–6. COMPONENTS OF HUMAN SEMINAL PLASMA*

Component	Mean Level	Range of Values	Primary Source
ELECTROLYTES (mg/dl)			
Sodium	281	240–319	
Potassium	112	56–202	
Calcium	28		Prostate
Magnesium	11		
Zinc	14	5–23	
Citric acid	376	96–1430	Prostate
Chloride	155	100–203	Prostate
CARBOHYDRATES (mg/dl)			
Fructose	222	40–638	Seminal vesicles
Inositol	50	54–63	
Ascorbic acid	13		
Sorbitol	10		
Glucose	7	0–99	
NITROGENOUS COMPOUNDS (mg/dl)			
Phosphorylcholine	315	250–380	
Spermine	273	50–350	Prostate
Urea	72		
Glycerylphosphorylcholine	66		Epididymis
Creatine	20		
Uric acid	6		
Ammonia	2		
PROSTAGLANDINS (μg/ml)			
PGE	145		Seminal vesicles
PGA	40		Seminal vesicles
PGB	21		Seminal vesicles
PGF	6		Seminal vesicles
OTHERS (mg/dl)			
Cholesterol	103	70–120	Prostate?
Sialic acid	124	64–219	
Glutathione	30		
ENZYMES			
Acid phosphatase			Prostate
King-Armstrong units/ml	340	272–408	
Sigma U/ml	66	49–72	
Alkaline phosphatase			
Sigma U/ml	6	1–12	
Diamine oxidase			Prostate
nmoles/ml/30 min	208		
β-Glucuronidase			
Fishman U/ml	39	26–42	
Lactic dehydrogenase			
Sigma U/ml	3908		
Leucine aminopeptidase			
Sigma U/ml	1173		Prostate
α-Amylase			
Street-Close U/dl/15 min	9	3–25	Prostate
Seminal proteinase			
(seminin, "fibrinolysin")			
μg% trypsin equivalent	30	20–50	Prostate
TOTAL PROTEIN (mg/dl)	4000	3500–5500	
FREE AMINO ACIDS (mg/dl)			
Neutral amino acids	638		
Basic amino acids	340		
Acidic amino acids	280		
Total	1258		

*Data compiled from Beyler et al., 1982; Mann and Mann, 1981; Polakowski and Kopta, 1982. For original references and additional detail consult these three reviews.

concentration in the prostate of the rodent. There are many important zinc-containing metalloenzymes, but the concentration of zinc in the prostate probably exceeds that present in zinc-associated enzymes (Fischer et al., 1955; Vallee, 1959; Habib et al., 1979). Zinc is known to bind many proteins, but there is also a large amount of free zinc in the seminal plasma. In 1969, Johnson et al. characterized zinc-binding protein in the prostatic secretion of the dog that contained only eight types of amino acids upon hydrolysis. Heathcote and Washington (1973) described a zinc-binding protein in human BPH that was rich in histidine and alanine. There have been other studies on zinc-binding proteins from the prostate (Fair and Wehner, 1976; Reed and Stitch, 1973), and additional information on these interesting proteins is needed. Recently, Parrish et al. (1983) suggested that, contrary to previous reports, zinc and pilocarpine-stimulated canine prostatic secretion was not bound to an 8-amino acid peptide, but rather behaved chromatographically like free zinc. It is apparent that free zinc may be the important physiologic factor.

An important role for zinc in the prostatic secretion has been suggested in the studies of Fair and Wehner (1976). (For review, see Fair and Parrish [1981].) These investigators present data that show the direct role of zinc as a prostate-derived antibacterial factor. It had been known that the prostatic secretion contained antibacterial factors (Fair et al., 1973; Stamey et al., 1968; Youmans et al., 1938). One of the important factors has now been related to the zinc concentration in expressed prostatic fluid (Fair and Wehner, 1976). In their study of 36 normal men free from bacterial prostatic infections, the mean value of zinc in the prostatic secretion was approximately 350 μg per ml, with a wide range of 150 to 1000 μg per ml. In comparison, the prostatic fluid obtained from 61 specimens collected from 15 patients with documented chronic bacterial prostatitis averaged only 50 μg per ml, with a range of 0 to 139 μg per ml. These authors propose a lower limit of normal at 150 μg per ml. In addition, in vitro studies of zinc at concentrations normally found in prostatic fluid have confirmed the bactericidal activity of zinc against a variety of gram-positive and gram-negative bacteria (Fair and Wehner, 1976).

The concentration of zinc in normal human seminal plasma (mean, 140 μg per ml) is less than half of that in the normal prostatic secretion. Earlier reports have commented on the association of decreased levels of zinc in seminal plasma with prostatitis (Bostrom and Anderson, 1971; Eliasson, 1968). It has also been observed that zinc levels in the human prostate may be decreased with chronic infections and other disease states (Hoare et al., 1956; Mawson and Fischer, 1952; Schrodt et al., 1964; Fair and Wehner, 1976; Tisell and Leissner, 1984). Although cause and effect are always difficult to resolve, the antibacterial properties of the zinc ion at physiologic concentrations suggest one possible role for high levels of zinc in the prostate gland and its secretions.

CITRIC ACID

Citrate in prostatic fluid (75 mM) is 615 times as high as that of serum (0.12 mM) (Isaacs, 1983). Therefore, the major anion in the human seminal plasma is citrate (mean, 376 mg per dl) in the range of 20 mM or 60 mEq per liter. This is compared with the chloride ion (155 mg per dl) at 40 mM. Citrate is important in maintaining the osmotic equilibrium of the prostate (Mann and Mann, 1981). Citrate is a potent binder of metal ions, and the seminal plasma concentration of citrate, 20 mM, is comparable to that of the total divalent metals, 13.6 mM (calcium, 7 mM; magnesium, 4.5 mM; zinc, 2.1 mM). Citric acid is localized in different sex accessory tissues according to species (Mann and Mann, 1981; Costello et al., 1978). However, in the human the prostate is the major source for citric acid that is present in the semen. This observation is based on the studies of Huggins and Neal (1942), who studied nine samples of human prostatic secretion and recorded values ranging from 480 to 2688 mg citric acid per dl. The values for two samples of seminal vesicle secretions were only 15 and 22 mg citric acid per dl, respectively. Assays of tissue levels of citric acid also implicate the prostate as the source of citric acid in the seminal plasma. Citric acid and acid phosphatase levels in semen have often been used as chemical indicators of prostatic function; however, citric acid seminal plasma levels cannot be equated directly with plasma levels of testosterone.

FRUCTOSE

The main sugar in semen is fructose, not glucose (Zaneveld and Chatterton, 1982; Mann and Mann, 1981). The source of fructose in human seminal plasma is the seminal vesicles (Mann and Mann, 1981). Patients with congenital absence of the seminal vesicles also have an associated absence of fructose in their ejaculates (Phadke et al., 1973). The seminal vesicle secretion contains smaller amounts of other free sugars, such as glucose, sorbitol, ribose, and fucose, and these sugars usually amount to less than 10 mg per dl. In comparison, the concentration of the reducing sugar, fructose, is approximately 300 mg per dl in human seminal secretion and has a level of 200 mg per dl in seminal plasma. These levels of fructose are under androgenic regulation, but many factors, such as storage, frequency of ejaculation, blood glucose levels, and nutritional status, can also affect the seminal plasma concentration (Mann and Mann, 1981); these considerations may account for the wide variations encountered in different semen samples from the same patient. Furthermore, plasma levels of androgens do not always correlate with seminal plasma fructose levels (Moon et al., 1970), and these levels are therefore not a reliable index of the androgenic state of the subject.

The source of fructose in seminal vesicles appears to proceed from glucose by aldose reduction to sorbitol and a ketone reduction to form fructose. These pathways have been characterized primarily by Williams-Ashman and his colleagues and are reviewed in more detail by Price and Williams-Ashman (1961), Mann and Mann (1981), and Zaneveld and Chatterton (1982). The fructose of the seminal plasma appears to provide an anaerobic and aerobic source of energy for the spermatozoa (Zaneveld and Chatterton, 1982; Mann and Mann, 1981). The cervical mucus has high concentrations of glucose and very low levels of fructose, and the sperm are capable of utilizing both types of sugars (Peterson and Freund, 1971).

CHOLINE COMPOUNDS

Of all fluids in the body, semen is the richest in choline [$(CH_3)_3 - N^+ - (CH_2)_2 - OH$]. Choline can be in the form of lecithin (phosphatidyl choline), cephalin (glycerol phosphorylethanolamine), or glycerophosphorylcholine. In man, phosphorylcholine predominates, whereas in most other species much higher levels of alpha-glycerylphosphorylcholine are present, often exceeding 1 gm per dl of seminal plasma (Mann and Mann, 1981; Price and Williams-Ashman, 1961). Seligman et al. (1975) have demonstrated that phosphorylcholine is a highly specific substrate for prostatic acid phosphatase, which is also very active in seminal plasma. The result of this enzymatic activity is the rapid formation of free choline in the first ejaculate. In contrast, glycerylphosphorylcholine is secreted primarily in the epididymis and is not readily hydrolyzed by acid phosphatase. For these reasons, Mann and Mann (1981) sug-

gested that the level of glycerylphosphorylcholine can be used as an index for assessing the contribution of the epididymal secretion to the ejaculate. The secretion from the epididymis is also under androgenic control (Dawson et al., 1957). The function of these choline compounds is unknown; it appears that they are not metabolized by spermatozoa, nor do they affect the respiration of the sperm (Dawson et al., 1957).

POLYAMINES-SPERMINE

A very reactive group of polyamines present in the seminal plasma are spermine and spermidine (Mann and Mann, 1981). Spermine levels predominate, ranging in the normal human seminal plasma from 50 to 350 mg per dl, and originating primarily from the prostate gland, which is the richest source of spermine in the body. Spermine [$NH_2 - (CH_2)_3 - NH - (CH_2)_4 - (CH_2)_4 - NH - (CH_2)_3 - NH_2$] is a very basic aliphatic polyamine. Because of its four positive charges it binds strongly to acidic or negatively charged molecules, such as phosphate ions, nucleic acid, or phospholipids. When semen is allowed to stand at room temperature, acid phosphatase enzymatically hydrolyzes seminal phosphorylcholine to form free inorganic phosphate ions, which then interact with the positively charged spermine and precipitate as large translucent yellow salt crystals of spermine phosphate. There has been much interest in spermine and other related polyamines, such as spermidine and putrescine, because of the rapid and dramatic changes in levels and ratios associated with many types of cells that have been induced into growth. Because polyamine metabolism is correlated with growth and because the potential of polyamines for interacting with DNA is documented, much speculation has resulted, but at present the biologic role of these polyamines has not been resolved (McKeehan et al., 1982; Bachrach, 1973).

Relationships between spermine levels in seminal plasma and sperm count and motility have also been suggested (Fair et al., 1973). Williams-Ashman and his colleagues have investigated in detail the biosynthesis and regulation of polyamines in the male reproductive tract and have characterized the enzymatic reactions that progress from ornithine to putrescine to spermidine to spermine (Williams-Ashman et al., 1969, 1972, 1975). The polyamines are oxidized enzymatically by diamine oxidase (present in the seminal plasma) to form very reactive aldehyde compounds that can be toxic to both sperm and bacteria (Janne et al., 1973; Zeller, 1941). The formation of these aldehyde products produces the characteristic odor of semen. It is also possible that these very toxic aldehydes or reactive polyamines themselves may protect the genitourinary tract from infective agents.

Williams-Ashman has shown that amide bonds can form between polyamines and carboxylic residues on the amino acids of proteins. Polyamines can form these adducts to protein through transglutaminase reactions (Falk et al., 1980).

PROSTAGLANDINS

Some of the most physiologically reactive small molecules in animals are the prostaglandins. These compounds can produce drastic vasoconstriction or vasodilation, depending on type and concentration. The role of prostaglandins in prostatic function has been reviewed by Farnsworth (1981). The richest sources of prostaglandins in the human are the seminal vesicles, and they appear in seminal plasma at a total concentration of approximately 100 to 300 μg per ml. For a discussion of the role of prostaglandins, see Klein and Stoff (1983). The pharmacologic effects of ingested or injected seminal fluid have been observed or suggested since ancient times. In more recent times, Goldblatt (1933, 1935) and von Euler (1934) independently reported the stimulatory effects of extracts of human seminal plasma on smooth muscle. In 1936, von Euler proposed the name "prostaglandins" for the active components, in the belief that they originated from the prostate gland. Although Eliasson (1959) established that the primary source of prostaglandin was not the prostate but the seminal vesicles, the original name has remained. Prostaglandins have a wide distribution in mammalian tissues but at much lower concentrations. Bergstrom and his colleagues recognized that there were many types of prostaglandins, and they purified and determined many of these chemical structures (Bergstrom et al., 1968). There are 15 different prostaglandins present in human semen, and they are all 20-carbon hydroxy fatty acids with a cyclopentane ring with two side chains; as such they are derivatives of prostanoic acid (Cenedella, 1975). The 15 types of prostaglandins are divided into four major groups, designated A, B, E, and F according to the structure of the five-membered cyclopentane ring, and each of these groups is further subdivided according to the position and number of double bonds in the side chain (therefore, PGE_3 indicates prosta-

glandins of E type with three double bonds in the side chain). The E group of prostaglandins is the major component in the male reproductive tract, while the F group predominates in the female system (Fuchs and Chantharaski, 1976). Fuchs and Chantharaski (1976) have summarized the reported levels of human seminal plasma prostaglandins and report the following mean values (μg per ml): PGE_1, 20; PGE_2, 15; $(PGE_1 + E_2) - 19$ OH, 100; $PGA_1 + A_2$, 9; $(PGA_1 + A_2) - 19$ OH, 31; $PGB_1 + B_2$, 18; $(PGB_1 + B_2) - 19$ OH, 3; PGF_{1a}, 3; and PGF_{2a}, 4. These compounds are very potent pharmacologic agents that have been implicated in a wide variety of biologic events in the male, including erection, ejaculation, sperm motility and transport, and testicular and penile contractions. In addition, prostaglandins from seminal fluid deposited in the vagina have been reported to affect cervical mucus, vaginal secretion, and sperm transport in the female genital tract. Not all of these effects have been established in a compelling manner, and the evidence has been reviewed in detail by Karim (1975) and by Fuchs and Chantharaski (1976). The prostaglandin type, the tissue, or the species can determine the biologic properties of prostaglandins, and limited information is available on the human male reproductive tract (Klein and Stoff, 1983). Bygdeman et al. (1970) reported that the semen of infertile men contained less PGE than normal. The cause and effect relationship for this observation has not been established.

Aspirin is a well-known inhibitor of prostaglandin synthesis, and Collier and Flower (1971) reported that therapeutic doses of aspirin given for 7 days lower PGE and PGF levels by approximately 50 per cent in the semen of healthy males. Horton et al. (1973) also have reported that high doses of aspirin reversibly lower semen prostaglandin levels. This could be of potential interest, but at present it is not known whether aspirin at any dose can affect human reproductive functions. Indomethacin is more potent than aspirin as an inhibitor of prostaglandin synthetase; it has been tested in male rats, in which it has some marginal effects on fertility (Fuchs and Chantharaski, 1976). Klein and Stoff (1983) have suggested that prostaglandins may have an important role in the etiology of BPH, but this has not been established.

LIPIDS AND CHOLESTEROL

One of the highest concentrations of lipids in the prostate is cholesterol. The importance of all this cholesterol is unknown, but Schaffner

(1983) has proposed that it is important in the etiology of BPH and has discussed how to pharmacologically regulate the level in the prostate. Scott (1945) reported that human seminal plasma contained 185 mg per dl of total lipids, 103 mg per dl of cholesterol, and 83 mg per dl of phospholipids. In comparison, prostatic secretion contained the following: total lipids, 186 mg per dl; cholesterol, 80 mg per dl; and phospholipids, 180 mg per dl. More recently, the lipids of the semen have been further described (White et al., 1976); the phospholipids of the seminal plasma are composed of 44 per cent sphingomyelin, 12.3 per cent ethanolamine plasmalogen, and 11.2 per cent phosphatidyl serine (Poulos and White, 1973). The reported levels of cholesterol in seminal plasma have varied considerably from 11 to 103 mg per dl (Eliasson, 1966; Scott, 1945; White et al., 1976). White et al. (1976) believe that the ratio of cholesterol to phospholipid in the seminal plasma stabilizes the sperm against temperature and environmental shock.

Schaffner (1983) and Goldstein (1976) studied the synthesis of cholesterol by the human prostate and reported higher levels of cholesterol in benign prostatic hyperplasia; they theorized that problems in cholesterol metabolism or blocked secretion of cholesterol may be an important etiologic factor in BPH, although this has not been established.

About two thirds of patients with prostatic adenocarcinoma (Acevedo et al., 1973; Chu et al., 1975) are reported to have elevated urinary cholesterol levels. The source of urinary cholesterol has not been determined, and it remains to be established whether this elevated urinary cholesterol is unique to prostatic cancer.

COAGULATION AND LIQUEFACTION OF SEMEN

The semen of many species clots upon ejaculation or even forms highly insoluble plugs, as is observed in rodents (Zaneveld and Chatterton, 1982; Mann and Mann, 1981). Williams-Ashman et al. (1977) have shown that these plugs are highly cross-linked by transamination reactions. Human semen coagulates into a semisolid gel within 5 minutes following ejaculation; upon further standing, the clot spontaneously liquefies within a 5- to 20-minute period to form a viscous liquid (Huggins and Neal, 1942; Mann and Mann, 1981). Calcium-binding substances, such as sodium citrate and heparin, do not inhibit the coagulation process, nor are prothrombin, fibrinogen, or factor XII required, since they are absent in seminal plasma (Mann

and Mann, 1981; Tauber and Zaneveld, 1976). The seminal clot is formed of fibers 0.15 to 10 μm in width, and its morphology differs from that of a blood fibrin clot (Huggins and Neal, 1942; Oettle, 1954; Tauber and Zaneveld, 1976; Williams-Ashman et al., 1977; Mann and Mann, 1981). From these observations and others, it appears that the coagulation of human semen is different from that of blood. In addition, factors affecting blood coagulation do not regulate semen viscosity (Amelar, 1962).

Examination of split human ejaculates indicates that the first fraction, originating primarily from Cowper's gland and the prostate, contains the liquefaction factors, and the final fraction, which is enriched by seminal vesicle secretions, is responsible for the coagulation of the ejaculate.

It has long been known that prostatic fluid has a dramatic fibrinolytic-like activity and that 2 ml of this secretion can liquefy 100 ml of clotted blood in 18 hours at 37°C (Huggins and Neal, 1942; Mann and Mann, 1981). The factors involved in such proteolytic activity in semen are being resolved (Syner et al., 1975; Tauber and Zaneveld, 1976; Zaneveld et al., 1974). Two types of seminal plasma proteolytic enzymes appear to be major factors in the liquefaction process—plasminogen activators and seminin.

Two plasminogen activators have been isolated from seminal plasma; they have molecular weights of 70,000 and 74,000 and appear to be related to urokinase (Propping et al., 1974). It is believed that the plasminogen activators originate from the prostatic secretions.

Seminin is a proteolytic enzyme (molecular weight, 30,000) that appears in the first fraction of split ejaculates and is therefore believed to originate from the prostate glands (Fritz et al., 1972; Lundquist et al., 1955; Syner et al., 1975; Propping et al., 1974; Tauber et al., 1976; Mann and Mann, 1981). This seminal proteinase was first thought to have chymotrypsin-like properties, but this was proved incorrect upon further purification and characterization; furthermore, seminin does not have true fibrinolytic activity (Syner et al., 1975).

The seminal plasma contains a variety of other proteolytic enzymes, including pepsinogen, lysozyme, alpha-amylase, and hyaluronidase. In addition, human semen inhibits the activity of the proteolytic enzyme trypsin, and this is due to the presence in the seminal plasma of such proteinase inhibitors as alpha$_1$-antitrypsin and alpha$_1$-antichymotrypsin. Isaacs (1984) has shown that the canine ejaculate contains one major protein (10 mg per ml) that is an enzyme. This protein is an esteroprotease that binds tightly to ejaculated sperm.

In summary, it appears that seminal plasma coagulation and liquefaction are under enzymatic control, but the biologic purpose of this process has not been resolved. Enzymes and proteins of the seminal vesicles and prostate glands are involved in this system. There have been reports that some infertile men may have impairment of the liquefaction process (Amelar, 1962; Bunge, 1970; Bunge and Sherman, 1954; Moon and Bunge, 1971).

Coagulation and liquefaction vary in different species. For example, the semen of the bull or dog does not coagulate, whereas the semen of rodents, such as the rat and guinea pig, is ejaculated as a firm pellet that does not appear to liquefy (Tauber and Zaneveld, 1976). In rodents, the plugs form through the action of an enzyme called vesiculase, which comes from the anterior lobe of the prostate and reacts with seminal vesicle secretions. Because of this action, the anterior lobe of the rodent prostate is also called the coagulating gland. Vesiculase is not identical with thrombin, since it does not coagulate fibrinogen, nor does thrombin clot the secretions of the seminal vesicles. Williams-Ashman et al. (1972) have established that vesiculase has transamidase activity, catalyzing the formation of gamma-glutamyl-e-lysine cross links in a clottable protein derived from the seminal vesicles. This seminal vesicle protein, which serves as a substrate for vesiculase, is a very basic substance with a molecular weight of 17,900; it has been characterized in regard to its physical properties by Notides and Williams-Ashman (1967).

There are obvious species differences in these processes. For example, in the boar, the clot appears to result from a sialomucoprotein from the bulbourethral (Cowper's) gland interacting with two proteins secreted by the seminal vesicle (Boursnell et al., 1970). These species differences make it difficult to extrapolate mechanisms in animals to the human situation.

ALBUMIN AND IMMUNOGLOBULINS

Albumin is present at 4000 mg per dl in serum but only 50 mg per ml in seminal plasma. There are many reports establishing the presence of immunoglobulins in human seminal plasma (Zaneveld and Chatterton, 1982; Friberg and Tilly-Friberg, 1976). It is possible to measure levels of IgG from 7 to 22 mg per dl and IgA from 0 to 6 mg per dl; however, no IgM has been detected (Friberg and Tilly-Friberg,

1976). The source of these antibodies is not known, although under certain conditions it appears that they are produced in the sex tissues. They are usually found at lower levels in seminal plasma than in blood, but the possibility of diffusion across the "blood–seminal plasma barrier" has not been eliminated (Mann and Mann, 1981; Friberg and Tilly-Friberg, 1976).

ACID PHOSPHATASE

One of the most important enzymes in the prostate is acid phosphatase. Its enzymatic (Lin et al., 1980) and immunologic (Choe et al., 1980) properties are often discussed in relation to its use as a clinical marker for prostatic cancer (Prellwitz and Ehrenthall, 1982; Yam, 1974). Human semen contains a high activity of acid phosphatase enzymes that originate from the secretions of the prostate gland (Kutchner and Wolberg, 1935). When prostatic cancer cells metastasize, they often continue to secrete acid phosphatases into the serum, producing elevated levels that are an important diagnostic aid in monitoring prostatic adenocarcinoma (Gutman and Gutman, 1938; Huggins and Hodges, 1941). Several factors complicate this diagnostic index: (1) Only two thirds of patients with advanced metastatic prostatic cancer have elevated serum acid phosphatase values. (2) Acid phosphatase enzymes are ubiquitous in all tissues and have particularly high concentrations in erythrocytes, platelets, osteoclasts, and bile. Other diseases, such as Gaucher's disease, Paget's disease, and hyperthyroidism, manifest moderate elevations of these enzymes. (3) The stability of prostatic acid phosphatase in the serum in vivo and in vitro can be variable, and there are several natural inhibitors of the enzyme. (4) Many different enzyme substrates have been proposed and utilized to detect prostatic acid phosphatase; these have also been used with a variety of enzyme inhibitors to improve on the differentiating capabilities of the assay system. (5) Serum levels can be elevated transiently by rectal or surgical manipulation of a normal prostate.

Enzyme Assay. Phosphatase enzymes hydrolyze many types of organic monophosphate esters to yield inorganic phosphate ions and alcohol by the following reaction:

$$R - O - PO_3H_3 + H_2O \rightarrow ROH + H_3PO_4$$

Many phosphatase enzymes exhibit optimal activity in vitro in the acid (pH 4 to 6) or alkaline (pH 8 to 11) ranges and thus may be classified broadly as either acid or alkaline phosphatase.

Both types of phosphatase appear to be ubiquitous in animal tissues.

Acid phosphatases may be further defined by factors that inhibit their enzymatic activity. For example, erythrocyte acid phosphatase is particularly sensitive to 0.5 per cent formaldehyde or copper ions (0.2 mM), while prostate acid phosphatase activity is far more sensitive to inhibition by fluoride ions (1 mM) or L-tartrate (1 mM). These inhibitors have been utilized to improve the specificity of the assay, and the differential tartrate inhibition is often used to indicate the specific prostatic acid phosphatase fraction. This is often helpful in distinguishing the serum erythrocyte acid phosphatase that leaks from damaged or hemolyzed cells because the erythrocyte enzyme is not inhibited by tartrate. Osteoclasts are also a rich source of acid phosphatase that is tartrate-insensitive; this fact is useful because of the minor elevation in serum acid phosphatase levels that accompany Paget's disease, osteoporosis, nonprostatic bone metastasis, and other conditions of increased bone resorption. Platelets may also be a source of acid phosphatase, which, like the prostate enzyme, is also sensitive to tartrate ions; thus, tartrate inhibition is not entirely specific for prostatic acid phosphatase.

Studies have been made of the enzyme kinetics of the reaction of prostatic acid phosphatase with a variety of substrates (Lin et al., 1980). It is also important to note that the enzyme in the serum is sensitive to body temperature; serum values often decrease when fever is present and may be elevated by hypothermia (Tsuboi and Hudson, 1955). Many aspects of the assay and interpretation of acid phosphatase serum levels have been reviewed in detail (Prellwitz and Ehrenthall, 1982; Lin et al., 1980; Choe et al., 1980; Bodansky, 1972; Li et al., 1973; Moncure, 1977; Sodeman and Batsakis, 1977; Yam, 1974).

Substrates. All acid phosphatases hydrolyze a wide range of natural and synthetic phosphomonoesters, and this has provided a wide variety of assay systems and the expression of many different units of activity (Table 5–7). These synthetic substrates include, in part: phenylphosphate (Gutman and Gutman, 1938); phenolphthalein phosphate (Huggins and Talalay, 1945); paranitrophenyl phosphate, also called Sigma 104 (Bessey et al., 1946; Modder, 1973); beta-naphthyl phosphate (Seligman et al., 1951); alpha-naphthyl phosphate (Babson and Read, 1959); beta-glycerophosphate (Woodward, 1959); naphthol AS-B1 phosphate (Vaughan et al., 1971); and thymolphthalein phosphate (Roy et al., 1971). The specificity of these substrates varies with the type and source of acid phosphatase; it appears that thymolphthalein phosphate may be the most specific substrate for assaying serum levels of prostatic acid phosphatase because it is a very poor substrate for the erythrocyte enzyme that is often present as a contaminant in the serum (Roy et al., 1971). It should be emphasized, however, that activity with this substrate can be found with acid phosphatase from other tissues; therefore, although it is not entirely specific for the prostate enzyme, it is still the substrate of choice for serum assays. At present there is no agreed upon standard method of assaying prostatic acid phosphatase or even of expressing the values.

The natural substrate for prostatic acid phosphatase may be phosphorylcholine phosphate (see earlier), which is rapidly hydrolyzed in the semen. Seligman and his associates have compared phosphorylcholine phosphate as a substrate for human acid phosphatase from both the prostate and the kidney and have shown that this substrate has a 1000-fold greater specificity for the prostate enzyme (Seligman et al., 1975). The biologic functions of this enzyme and its reactions are not known.

Isoenzymes. Many tissues contain several forms of acid phosphatase that can be resolved by electrophoretic techniques (Moncure, 1977). Some of these enzyme forms can be separated by subfractionation of the tissue and may be

TABLE 5–7. DEFINITION OF ACID PHOSPHATASE UNITS

Substrate	Units	Activity	C°	pH	
				ACID	ALKALINE
β-Glycerophosphate	Bodanski	mg PO₄/hr/dl	37.5	5.0	10.8
Phenyl phosphate	King-Armstrong	mg phenol/hr/dl	37.5	5.0	9.3
Phenolphthalein phosphate	Huggins-Talalay	0.1 mg phenolphth./hr/dl	37	5.4	9.7
p-Nitrophenyl phosphate	Sigma	1 μmole p-nitrophenol/hr	37	4.8	10.5
Any substrate	International unit (U or IU)	1 μmole substrate/min		As defined	

associated primarily with the lysosomes, secretions, or particular membrane fractions. Starch gel electrophoresis of prostate tissue extracts revealed 13 bands of activity, but only a single band was observed in seminal plasma (Sur et al., 1962). This observation suggested that these might be multiple forms of a common enzyme in various states of being processed for secretion. This was later supported by the observation that neuraminidase treatment, which removes sialic acid residues from the glycoprotein enzyme, converted the 13 bands to a single entity and that assay of the multiple forms could be accounted for by different amounts of sialic acid (Chu et al., 1975; Ostrowski et al., 1970; Smith and Whitby, 1968).

Human prostatic acid phosphatase is a glycoprotein of 102,000 molecular weight and contains about 7 per cent by weight of carbohydrate, which is composed of 15 residues per mole of neutral sugars (fucose, galactose, and mannose); 6 residues per mole of sialic acid; and 13 residues of N-acetylglucosamine (Chu et al., 1975). The protein can be dissociated into two subunits. In summary, many secretory proteins and enzymes are glycosylated after they have been synthesized, and it appears that this accounts for some of the isoenzyme patterns of prostatic acid phosphatase. The secretory enzyme is probably the major form, and the lysosomal acid phosphatase may be similar to that found in other tissue lysosomes.

The foregoing discussion has pertained to human prostatic acid phosphatase. It is important to note that this high enzymatic activity is not characteristic of accessory tissues in many other species, as shown in Table 5–8. Seligman et al. (1975) observed a decrease in activity from man to primates to rodents.

Serum Assays. For an excellent discussion of the details, advantages, and disadvantages of acid phosphatase as a clinical marker for prostatic cancer, consult the review of Prellwitz and Ehrenthall (1982). Circadian variations in serum acid phosphatase levels occur in patients with prostatic carcinoma, and peak levels do not occur at predictable times of the day; furthermore, these variations also occur in patients who have been castrated (Sodeman and Batsakis, 1977). More than one serum sample, taken at different times, is required to increase the probability of correct diagnostic interpretation.

Once serum is collected, it should be chilled immediately because the enzyme rapidly loses activity even at room temperature; however, it is essentially stable for days at 0°C. In addition, the loss of carbon dioxide from serum is critical because the pH may drop to alkaline ranges where the enzyme is unstable (Daniel, 1954; Yam, 1974). Therefore, buffering the collected serum with disodium hydrogen citrate to between pH 6.2 and 6.6 will help protect stored serum samples from the enzymatic inactivation that occurs in the alkaline range (Sodeman and Batsakis, 1977).

The following statement of Sodeman and Batsakis (1977) emphasizes the need for careful control in determining serum levels: "In the practice of clinical laboratory medicine, it is nearly axiomatic that of all the enzymes measured in the laboratory, acid phosphatase suffers the most from instability."

The following suggestions can be used to improve the accuracy of the determination of prostatic acid phosphatase:

1. Store samples in stoppered tubes and chill immediately.

2. If assays are delayed, add citrate buffer to between pH 6.2 and 6.6.

3. Utilize sodium thymolphthalein phosphate as the substrate at pH 6.0 in citrate buffer, incubated for 30 minutes at 37°C, as described by Roy et al. (1971). An assay requires approximately 0.2 ml of serum.

4. Report the serum levels as IU/L (International units per liter of serum; μmoles thymolphthalein phosphate hydrolyzed per minute per liter of serum).

5. To improve interpretation, obtain multiple serum samples at different times of day because of variations and circadian changes.

6. Avoid assays of serum samples that contain hemolysis, have been taken from patients

TABLE 5–8. RELATIVE AMOUNTS OF PROSTATIC ACID PHOSPHATASE ACTIVITY IN SEVERAL SPECIES*

Species	Relative Activity (per mg)
Man	1200
Baboon	1100
Rhesus monkey	130
Dog	60
Guinea pig	2.1
Squirrel monkey	1.5
Cat	1.5
Rat	1.0
Rabbit	0.25
Mouse	0.20
Hamster	0.02

*Substrate, phosphorylcholine; pH 4.8, per mg of prostatic tissue; activity relative to that in the rat.

From Paul, B. D., et al.: Ca Treatment Rep., *61*:259, 1977.

with fever, or have been taken within 24 hours of prostatic massage or transurethral resection.

The average normal value of serum acid phosphatase using the thymolphthalein phosphate method is 0.28 ± 0.09 IU/L, with a range of 0.11 to 0.60 (Roy et al., 1971).

Immunoassays. Shulman et al. (1964) first developed antibodies against human prostatic acid phosphatase. Several studies have increased the purity of the acid phosphatase enzyme (antigen), and monoclonal antibodies provided significant improvement of the resolution of immunologic assays (Prellwitz and Ehrenthall, 1982; Choe et al., 1980, 1977; Chu et al., 1977; Foti et al., 1975; Milisaukas and Rose, 1972; Moncure, 1975; Moncure and Prout, 1970; Ostrowski et al., 1970; Shulman and Ferber, 1966). These immunologic assays appeared to have great potential as a specific new diagnostic test for human prostatic acid phosphatase in serum, metastatic lesions, and isolated cells and cultures. The aforementioned assays employ double antibody radioimmunoassays (RIA), solid phase radioimmunoassays, immunofluorescent antibodies (IF), and counterimmunoelectrophoresis (CIEP). Many of these immunologic assays are so sensitive that they can detect a nanogram of enzyme protein in 0.1 ml of serum or less. The results of Choe et al. (1977), using the double antibody radioimmunoassay, were as follows (all values are given in nanograms of prostatic acid phosphatase in 0.1 ml of serum): in 162 normal men, 1.6 ± 0.8; in 10 men with nonprostatic cancer, 1.8 ± 0.6; in 22 men with localized prostatic cancer, 1.8 to 2.5; and in 21 men with metastatic prostatic cancer, 5.5 to 100. Although immunoassays are more specific, they have not yet proved to be more effective in detecting early prostatic cancer than have the more standard enzyme assays. The final advantages are not yet realized, and these problems are discussed in more detail in Chapter 32.

LEUCINE AMINOPEPTIDASE

Aminopeptidases are proteases that hydrolyze the N-terminal amino acid residue from small polypeptides. Leucine aminopeptidases are particularly active against the substrate L-leucyl-glycine, and some of these enzymes are referred to as arylamidases because the optimal substrate is L-leucyl-β-naphthylamine. The prostate is rich in the latter arylamidase type of leucine aminopeptidase (Mattila, 1969). Mattila demonstrated two forms of the enzyme in human prostatic tissue (molecular weights, 107,000 and 305,000), only one of which was similar to that of the kidney. The kidney is one of the richest sources of leucine aminopeptidases, but the tissue-specific nature of any of these isoenzymes so far has not been established.

Leucine aminopeptidase is a product of the epithelial cells of the prostate (Niemi et al., 1963) and is secreted into the lumen of the acini (Kirchheim et al., 1964). The histochemical assay of leucine aminopeptidase markedly decreases in prostatic cancer lesions even if they remain highly differentiated; this is not the case for acid phosphatase, which remains at normal histochemical levels (Kirchheim et al., 1964). The distribution of other prostatic enzymes in human prostatic cancer has been studied (Muntzing and Nilsson, 1972); Brandes and Kirchheim (1977) have reviewed the histochemical aspects.

β-GLUCURONIDASE

The enzyme β-glucuronidase hydrolyzes conjugates of glucuronic acid; the level of this enzyme in prostatic tissue remains the same or increases in prostatic cancer and BPH (Kirchheim et al., 1964; Nilsson et al., 1973). The elevation of β-glucuronidase activity in other human cancers has also been analyzed (Bartalos and Gyorkey, 1963; Fishman and Anylan, 1947). This enzyme has also been proposed as a marker for prostatic epithelial cells (Nilsson et al., 1973); however, recent studies have questioned this specific localization through stromal-epithelial separation (Cowan et al., 1977).

LACTIC DEHYDROGENASE

Lactic dehydrogenase (LDH) (molecular weight, 150,000) is composed of four subunits made from two dimers. Each subunit of 35,000 molecular weight is one of two different types of proteins (denoted M or H, which stands for muscle or heart). The LDH of muscle has four M units and that of heart has four H units. Five isoenzymes of LDH can be found in tissues with a four-subunit composition as follows: LDH I, MMMM; LDH II, MMMH; LDH III, MMHH; LDH IV, MHHH; and LDH V, HHHH). The M and H subunits appear to be the same in all tissues, but the amounts of LDH I to V can vary. There have been reports that LDH isoenzyme patterns change in cancer tissues, such as malignancy of the stomach, cervix, colon, brain, and lung (Nissen and Bohn, 1975; Moncure, 1977). Denis and Prout (1963) observed increased levels of LDH IV and V in prostatic cancer tissue. Several investigators have observed elevated ratios of LDH V/LDH I in human prostatic cancer (Elhilali et al., 1968; Flocks and Schmidt, 1972; Oliver et al., 1970).

Belitsky and his coworkers (1970) measured serum levels of LDH V/LDH I after prostatic massage and believe this may be of diagnostic value. Assay of human prostatic fluid or semen for the isoenzyme ratio has been proposed as a diagnostic tool (Elhilali et al., 1968; Grayhack et al., 1977; Hein et al., 1975; Oliver et al., 1970). Of 30 patients with prostatic adenocarcinoma, the ratio of LDH V/LDH I was elevated in 85 per cent, whereas only 12 per cent of 57 BPH patients had an elevated ratio. The values of the ratios were: normal, 0.48 ± 0.09; BPH, 1.36 ± 0.17; and prostatic cancers, 5.21 ± 0.79 (Grayhack et al., 1977). Granulocytes are rich in LDH V, and the prostate must be devoid of inflammation to avoid leukocyte contamination. An increase in the ratio above 2, in the absence of inflammation, indicates a high risk of prostatic cancer (Grayhack et al., 1977).

SEMINAL PLASMA ANALYSIS IN FERTILITY DISORDERS

There have been several reviews related to semen analysis and fertility (Amelar and Dubin, 1977; Eliasson, 1973, 1977; Freund and Peterson, 1976; Walsh and Amelar, 1977). Eliasson (1973) emphasizes that decreased secretory function of the accessory genital glands is a common finding in men with acute and chronic infection or inflammation of the prostate or seminal vesicles, and further states that a decreased secretory capacity of the male sex accessory glands is not in itself a factor in infertility. Chemical alterations in the seminal plasma, however, may indicate abnormalities. Since seminal fructose is a secretory product of the seminal vesicles, it is often used as an index of the function of this gland. Fructose is absent from the semen in three conditions (Amelar and Dubin, 1977):

1. Azoospermic males with congenital bilateral absence of the vas deferens and seminal vesicles. Embryologically, the seminal vesicles develop from the vas deferens. Therefore, when the vas deferens is absent, no fructose is present in the semen and the ejaculate also does not coagulate.

2. Obstruction of both ejaculatory ducts.

3. An unusual type of retrograde ejaculation.

Fructose analysis of the semen is a simple test and should be performed routinely in every case of azoospermia (Amelar and Dubin, 1977). For additional details on obstructive occlusions in the reproductive tract and diagnostic approaches, see the review of Marina et al. (1976).

Fructose levels may also be lowered in

TABLE 5–9. EVALUATION OF SEX ACCESSORY GLAND FUNCTION IN HUMANS*

Classification	Ejaculate Volume (ml)	Prostatic Acid Phosphatase (IU × 10^{-2}/ml)	Zinc (μg/ml)	Seminal Fructose (mg/dl)
Normal	2.5–6.0	250–600	>90	>150
Doubtful	2.0–2.4	200–249	80–90	100–150
Decreased	1.0–2.0	100–190	50–79	50–99
Severely decreased	<1.0	<100	<50	<50

*From Eliasson, R.: *In* Hafez, E. S. E., and Evans, T. N. (Eds.): Human Reproduction: Conception and Contraception. New York, Harper & Row, 1973.

vesiculitis. In addition, many authors have proposed the use of fructose levels in semen as a measurement of androgenic function, but there are serious limitations in such correlations (see earlier discussion of fructose). Moon and Bunge (1971) have also discussed these limitations.

It seems probable that the sex accessory tissue secretions may enhance or protect functional properties of the sperm, but at present we do not know how these secretions interact with sperm under either normal or abnormal conditions.

Evaluation of the individual secretory components of the sex accessory glands is important in correlating glandular activity with fertility. Eliasson (1973, 1977) has proposed biochemical standards for ascertaining secretory function of the sex accessory tissues in human semen (Table 5–9).

TRANSPORT OF MATERIALS INTO THE SEMEN

Isaacs (1983) has reviewed the active and basal secretions of the prostate. The basal prostate secretion has the following concentrations of substances that are increased several fold over concentrations in the serum: citrate, 75 mM (625 times); zinc, 0.77 mM (39 times); magnesium, 20 mM (12 times), and potassium, 48 mM (12 times). Sodium, 153 mM and bicarbonate, 20 mM, however, are essentially the same concentration in both serum and basal prostatic secretions. In contrast, other compounds are reduced in concentration in prostatic fluid in comparison with serum: glucose, 164 μg/ml (0.2 times); total lipid, 2.9 mg/ml (0.47 times), and chloride, 38 mM (0.38 times). This indicates that the prostate actively secretes and blocks the transport of specific substances. Similar differences are also observed for the comparison of seminal plasma and blood concentrations. Several natural products, such as ergothioneine and other amino acids, appear to be more highly concentrated in seminal plasma than in blood plasma (Mann and Mann, 1981). Some of these amino acids may have physiologic roles, such as the conversion of arginine to ornithine by the action of the enzyme arginase. Ornithine then becomes the precursor for polyamines such as spermine and spermidine. Arginase is found at high concentrations in human prostatic tissues (Yamanaka et al., 1972). Some of the amino acids may originate from proteolytic hydrolysis, but it seems apparent that a large portion is actually concentrated in the seminal plasma by an unknown mechanism. Other compounds are capable of entering the semen by simple diffusion, including ethanol (Farrell, 1938), iodine (Mroveth, 1971), and antibiotics (Reeves, 1976).

Compounds entering prostatic fluid may be of interest for three reasons: (1) for supplying antibiotics to treat prostatitis; (2) to account for the pathologic presence of prostatic carcinoma because carcinogens are actively sequestered into the lumen; and (3) to be utilized in the future as a means of regulating fertility by altering semen quality. Evidence exists only for the first two mechanisms. Smith and Hagopian (1981) have shown that eight carcinogens given to dogs and rats can be excreted into prostatic fluid and that the final concentrations may exceed plasma levels by over three fold. This important study has been discussed by Isaacs (1983) in relation to its potential bearing on prostatic carcinogenesis. Drugs entering prostatic secretions have been of interest because of the prevalence of prostatitis and the need for new modalities of chemotherapy. Stamey and his colleagues have made extensive studies of the ability of chemotherapeutic agents to concentrate in the prostate fluid of humans and dogs (Hessl and Stamey, 1971; Stamey et al., 1973; Winningham et al., 1968; Winningham and Stamey, 1970), and other laboratories have contributed to this knowledge (Fowle and Bye, 1972; Madsen et al., 1968; Nielsen and Hansen, 1972; Reeves et al., 1973). Although few drugs reach concentrations in the prostatic secretion that approach or surpass their concentrations in blood, some exceptions are the basic macrolides erythromycin and oleandomycin; sulfonamides; chloramphenicol; tetracycline; clindamycin; and trimethoprim (Isaacs, 1983; Reeves, 1976). In general, these drugs are assumed to pass across the membrane by nonionic diffusion, possibly by lipid solubility through the membrane; when they reach the more acidic prostatic fluid, they are protonated and acquire a more positive charge, thus becoming relatively trapped in the prostatic secretions. Several factors are critical, including the pK' of the drug and the pH of the prostatic secretions as well as the drug-binding to proteins in each compartment. Basic drugs would be more ionized in acidic prostatic fluid than in blood. Slight changes in pH can have large effects on this nonionic diffusion. The pH of the prostatic secretion in the dog may be more acidic than in man and may decrease with successive fractions during prostatic secretion collection under pilocarpine stimulation (Stamey et al., 1973). Samples of prostatic secretions from humans varied widely in pH from 6 to 8 with a mean value of 6.6; however, with prostatic inflammation the pH tended to be 7 or greater (White, 1975). Studies designed to avoid urine contamination that utilize trimethoprim distribution agree in general with these values (Fowle and Bye, 1972; Nielsen and Hansen, 1972). Studies tend to indicate that nonionic diffusion may be the most critical factor in these processes (Stamey et al., 1973). It should be realized that although prostatic secretions are slightly acidic, the pH of freshly ejaculated human semen is slightly alkaline (pH 7.3 to 7.7); on standing, semen first becomes more alkaline with the loss of carbon dioxide and then later acidic owing to accumulation of lactic acid. The therapeutic implications of the pH of the prostate fluid have been discussed in an excellent review by Fair and Parrish (1981). For excellent reviews of the diffusion of chemotherapeutic agents in prostatic tissue compartment that consider the degree of protein-binding, lipid solubility, pH, and molecular size, consult the references of Stamey (1980), Baumueller et al. (1977), Madsen et al. (1976), and Meares (1975).

In any study of transport, it is essential to study the concentration of the drug in prostatic secretion, interstitial fluid, prostatic tissue, urine, and serum, and this is best done by perfusion techniques. For a good example of how these are performed, consult the work on metioprim-sulfadiazine distribution in the canine prostate by Iversen et al. (1981) and Madsen et al. (1978).

It is apparent that much more information is required to understand the transport of materials into and out of the glands and fluids of the sex accessory tissues. This may be of prime importance in understanding normal physiology as well as the reasons for the high rate of prostatic cancer.

References

Acevedo, H. F., Campbell, E. A., Saier, E. L., et al.: Urinary cholesterol. V. Its excretion in men with testicular and prostatic neoplasms. Cancer, *32*:169, 1973.

Altwein, J. E.: Cardiovascular side effects of endocrine management of prostatic carcinoma. *In* Schroder, F. H. (Ed.): Androgens and Antiandrogens. Weesp, The Netherlands, Schering, 1983, p. 133.

Amelar, R. D.: Coagulation, liquefaction and viscosity of human semen. J. Urol., *87*:187, 1962.

Amelar, R. D., and Dubin, L.: Semen analysis. *In* Amelar, R. D., Dubin, L., and Walsh, P. C. (Eds.): Male Infertility. Philadelphia, W. B. Saunders Co., 1977.

Amelar, R. D., and Hotchkiss, R. S.: The split ejaculate: Its uses in the management of male infertility. Fertil. Steril., *16*:46, 1965.

Anderson, D. C., Marshall, J. C., Galuao-Teles, A., et al.: Gynaecomastia and impotence associated with testosterone binding. Proc. R. Soc. Med., *65*:787, 1972.

Anderson, K. M., and Liao, S.: Selective retention of dihydrotestosterone by prostatic nuclei. Nature, *219*:277, 1968.

Angervall, L., Hesselsjo, R., Nilsson, S., and Tissel, L. E.: Action of testosterone on ventral prostate, dorsolateral prostate, coagulating glands, and seminal vesicles of castrated alloxan-diabetic rats. Diabetologia, *3*:395, 1967.

Aragona, C., and Friesen, H. G.: Prolactin and aging. *In* Grayhack, J. T., Wilson, J. D., and Scherbenske, M. J. (Eds.): Benign Prostatic Hyperplasia. Proceedings of a workshop sponsored by the Kidney Disease and Urology Program of the NIAMDD, pp. 165–172. Washington, D.C., U.S. Govt. Printing Office, 1976.

Aragona, C., and Friesen, H. G.: Specific prolactin binding sites in the prostate and testis of rat. Endocrinology, *97*:677, 1975.

Arcadi, J. A.: Role of ground substance in atrophy of normal and malignant prostatic tissue following estrogen administration in orchiectomy. J. Clin. Endocrinol. Metab., *14*:1113, 1954.

Arvola, I.: The hormonal control of the amounts of the tissue components of the prostate. Ann. Chir. Gynaecol. Fenn. (Suppl.), *50*:102:1, 1961.

August, G. P., Tkachuk, M., and Grumbach, M. M.: Plasma testosterone-binding affinity and testosterone in umbilical cord plasma, late pregnancy, prepubertal children, and adults. J. Clin. Endocrinol. Metab., *29*:981, 1969.

Aumuller, G.: Morphology and endocrine aspects of prostatic function. Prostate, *4*:195, 1983.

Babson, A. L., and Read, P. A.: A new assay for prostatic acid phosphatase in serum. Am. J. Clin. Pathol., *32*:88, 1959.

Bachrach, U.: Function of naturally occurring polyamines. New York, Academic Press, 1973.

Bardin, C. W., and Lipsett, M. B.: Estimation of testosterone and androstenedione in human peripheral plasma. Steroids, *9*:71, 1967.

Bardin, C. W., and Mahoudeau, J. A.: Dynamics of androgen metabolism in women with hirsutism. Ann. Clin. Res., *2*:251, 1970.

Barrack, E. R.: The nuclear matrix of the prostate contains acceptor sites for nuclear matrix: Steroid hormone binding. Recent Prog. Horm. Res., *38*:133, 1982.

Barrack, E. R., Bujnovszky, P., and Walsh, P. C.: Subcellular distribution of androgen receptors in human normal, benign hyperplastic, and malignant prostatic tissues: Characterization of nuclear salt-resistant receptors. Cancer Res., *43*:1107, 1983.

Bartalos, M., and Gyorkey, F.: β-Glucuronidases: Their significance and relation to cancer. J. Am. Geriatr. Soc., *11*:21, 1963.

Bartsch, G., and Rohr, H. P.: Ultrastructural stereology: A new approach to the study of prostatic function. Invest. Urol., *14*:301, 1977.

Bartsch, G., and Rohr, H. P.: Endocrinological basis and clinical experience in conservative therapy in benign prostatic hyperplasia. *In* Schroeder, F. H. (Ed.): Androgens and Antiandrogens. Weesp, The Netherlands, Schering, 1983.

Bartsch, G., Brungger, A., Schweikert, U., Hinter, H., Stanzlu, J., Marth, C., Daxenbichler, G., and Rohr, H. P.: The importance of stromal tissue in benign prostatic hyperplasia: Morphological, immunofluorescence and endocrinological investigations. *In* Kimball, F. A., Buhl, A. E., and Carter, D. B. (Eds.): New Approaches to the Study of Benign Prostatic Hyperplasia. New York, Alan R. Liss, 1984, p. 179.

Bartsch, G., Fischer, E., and Rohr, H. P.: Ultrastructural morphometric analysis of the rat prostate (ventral lobe). Urol. Res., *3*:1, 1975.

Bartsch, G., Muller, H. R., Oberholzer, M., and Rohr, H. P.: Light microscopic stereological analysis of the normal human prostate in benign prostatic hyperplasia. J. Urol., *122*:487, 1979.

Baumueller, A., Hoyme, U., and Madsen, P. O.: Bacterial prostatitis, therapeutic considerations. Dtsch. Urol., *70*:589, 1977.

Belis, J. A., Adelstein, L. B., and Terry, W. F.: Influence of estradiol on accessory reproductive organs in the castrated male rat. J. Androl., *4*:144, 1983.

Belis, J. A., Lizza, E. S., and Terry, W. F.: Progesterone receptors in the prostate. *In* Kimball, F. A., et al. (Eds.): New Approaches to the Study of Benign Prostatic Hyperplasia. New York, Alan R. Liss, 1984, p. 345.

Belitsky, P., Elhilali, M. M., and Oliver, J. A.: The effect of stilbestrol on the isoenzymes of lactic dehydrogenase in benign and malignant prostatic tissue. J. Urol., *104*:453, 1970.

Bergquist, C., Nillius, S. J., Berg, H. T., Skaring, J., and Widel, H.: Inhibitory effects on gonadotropin secretion and gonadal function in men during chronic treatment with a potent stimulating luteinizing hormone releasing hormone analog. Acta Endocrinol., *91*:601, 1979.

Bergstrom, S., Carlson, L. A., and Wecks, L. R.: The prostaglandins: A family of biologically active lipids. Pharmacol. Rev., *20*:1, 1968.

Berry, S. J., and Isaacs, J. T.: Comparative aspects of prostatic growth and androgen metabolism with aging in the dog *versus* the rat. Endocrinology, *114*:511, 1984.

Berry, S. J., Coffey, D. S., Walsh, P. C., and Ewing, L. L.: Development of benign prostatic hyperplasia with age. J. Urol., *132*:474, 1984.

Bertrand, G., and Vladesco, R.: Prostatic zinc concentration. C. R. Acad. Sci., *173*:176, 1921.

Bessey, O. A., Lowry, O. H., and Brock, M. J.: A method for the rapid determination of alkaline phosphatase with five cubic millimeters of serum. J. Biol. Chem., *164*:321, 1946.

Beyler, S. A., and Zaneveld, L. J. D.: The male accessory sex glands. *In* Zaneveld, L. J. D., and Chatterton, R. T. (Eds.): Biochemistry of Mammalian Reproduction. New York, John Wiley & Sons, 1982, p. 65.

Birkoff, J. D., Lattimer, J. K., and Frantz, A. G.: Role of prolactin in benign prostatic hyperplasia. Urology, *4*:557, 1974.

Bissell, M. J., Hall, G. H., and Perry, G.: How does the extracellular matrix direct gene expression? J. Theor. Biol., *99*:31, 1982.

Blacklock, N. J.: Surgical anatomy. *In* Chisholm, G. D., and Williams, D. I. (Eds.): Scientific Foundations of Urology. 2nd ed. London, W. Heinemann, 1982, p. 43.

Bodansky, O.: Acid phosphatase. Adv. Clin. Chem., *15*:43, 1972.

Bostrom, K., and Anderson, L.: Creatinine phosphokinase relative to acid phosphatase, lactate dehydrogenase, zinc and fructose in human semen with special reference to chronic prostatitis. Scand. J. Urol. Nephrol., *5*:123, 1971.

Boursnell, J. C., Hartree, E. F., and Briggs, P. A.: Studies on the bulbourethral (Cowper's)–gland mucin and seminal gel of the boar. Biochem. J., *117*:981, 1970.

Brandes, D. (Ed.): Male Accessory Sex Organs: Structure and Function in Mammals. New York, Academic Press, 1974.

Brandes, D., and Kirchheim, D.: Histochemistry of the prostate. *In* Tannenbaum, M. (Ed.): Urologic Pathology: The Prostate. Philadelphia, Lea & Febiger, 1977, pp. 99–128.

Brandes, D., Kirchheim, D., and Scott, W. W.: Ultrastructure of the human prostate: Normal and neoplastic. Lab. Invest., *13*:1541, 1964.

Breuer, H., Hamel, D., and Kruskemper, H. L.: Methods of Hormone Analysis. New York, John Wiley & Sons, 1976.

Bruchovsky, N.: Rationale for the use of antihormones and drug combinations as a treatment for prostatic carcinoma. *In* Schroeder, F. H. (Ed.): Androgens and Antiandrogens. Weesp, The Netherlands, Schering, 1983, p. 35.

Bruchovsky, N.: Comparison of the metabolites formed in rat prostate following the in vivo administration of seven natural androgens. Endocrinology, *89*:1212, 1971.

Bruchovsky, N., and Wilson, J. D.: The conversion of testosterone to 5-androstan-17β-ol-3-one by rat prostate in vivo and in vitro. J. Biol. Chem., *243*:2012, 1968*a*.

Bruchovsky, N., and Wilson, J. D.: The intranuclear binding of testosterone and 5-androstan-17β-ol-3-one by rat prostate. J. Biol. Chem., *243*:5953, 1968*b*.

Bunge, R. G.: Some observations on the male ejaculate. Fertil. Steril., *21*:639, 1970.

Bunge, R. G., and Sherman, J. K.: Liquefaction of human semen by alpha-amylase. Fertil. Steril., *5*:353, 1954.

Burton, R. M., and Westphal, U.: Steroid hormone binding proteins in blood plasma. Metabolism, *21*:253, 1972.

Byar, D. P.: Zinc in male sex accessory organs: Distribution and hormonal response. *In* Brandes, D. (Ed.): Male Sex Accessory Organs: Structure and Function in Mammals. New York, Academic Press, 1974, pp. 161–171.

Bygdeman, M., Fredericson, B., Svanborg, K., and Samuelsson, B.: The relation between fertility and prostaglandin content of seminal fluid in man. Fertil. Steril., *21*:622, 1970.

Calame, S. S., and Lostroh, A. J.: Effect of insulin and lack of effect of testosterone on the protein of ventral prostate from castrate mice maintained as organ cultures. Endocrinology, *75*:451, 1964.

Castor, J. E.: The Treatment of Prostate Hypertrophy and Neoplasia. Baltimore, University Park Press, 1974.

Cenedella, R. J.: Prostaglandin and male reproductive physiology. *In* Thomas, J. A., and Singhal, R. L. (Eds.): Molecular Mechanisms of Gonadal Hormone Action. Baltimore, University Park Press, 1975.

Chandler, J. A., Timms, B. G., and Battersby, S.: Prostate development in zinc deficient rats. *In* Murphy, G. P., Sandberg, A. A., and Karr, J. P. (Eds.): Prostatic Cell: Structure and Function. Part A. New York, Alan R. Liss, 1981, p. 475.

Chandler, J. A., Timms, B. G., and Morton, M. S.: Subcellular distribution of zinc in rat prostate studied by x-ray microanalysis. I. Normal prostate. Histochem. J., *9*:103, 1977.

Chisholm, G. D., and Williams, D. I.: Scientific Foundations of Urology. 2nd ed. London, W. Heinemann, 1982.

Choe, B. K., Pontes, J. E., Killchoj, H. S., and Rose, N. R.: Immunohistological approaches to human prostatic epithelial cells. Prostate, *1*:383, 1980.

Choe, B. K., Pontes, E. J., McDonald, I., and Rose, N. R.: Immunochemical studies of prostatic acid phosphatase. Cancer Treat. Rep., *61*:201, 1977.

Chu, T. M., Shukia, S. K., Mittelman, A., and Murphy, G. P.: Comparative evaluation of serum acid phosphatase, urinary cholesterol, and androgensin diagnosis of prostatic cancer. Urology, *6*:291, 1975.

Chu, T. M., Wang, M. C., Kuciel, L., Valenzuela, L., and Murphy, G. P.: Enzyme markers in human prostatic carcinoma. Cancer Treat. Rep., *61*:193, 1977.

Chung, L. W. K., and Cunha, G. R. Stromal-epithelial interactions: II. Regulation of prostatic growth by embryonic urogenital sinus mesenchyme. Prostate, *4*:503, 1983.

Chung, L. W. K., and McFadden, D. K.: Sex steroid imprinting and prostatic growth. Invest. Urol., *17*:337, 1980.

Chung, L. W. K., Matsuura, J., Rocco, A. K., Thompson, T. C., Miller, G. J., and Runner, M. N.: A new mouse model for prostatic hyperplasia: Induction of adult prostatic overgrowth of fetal urogenital sinus implants. *In* Kimball, F. A., Buhl, A. E., and Carter, D. B. (Eds.): New Approaches to the Study of Benign Prostatic Hyperplasia. New York, Alan R. Liss, 1984.

Clark, J., and O'Malley, B.: Mechanisms of steroid hormone action. *In* Wilson, J. D., and Foster, D. W. (Eds.): Williams Textbook of Endocrinology. Philadelphia, W. B. Saunders Co., 1985.

Coffey, D. S., DeKlerk, D. P., and Walsh, P. C.: Benign prostatic hyperplasia: Current concepts. *In* James, V. H. T. (Ed.): Excerpta Medica Int. Congress Series #403, Endocrinology. Proceedings of the Vth Int. Congress of Endocrinology. Hamburg, July 18–24, 1976. Vol. 2. Amsterdam, Excerpta Medica, 1977.

Collier, J. G., and Flower, R. J.: Effect of aspirin on human seminal prostaglandins. Lancet, *2*:852, 1971.

Conti, C., Sciarra, F., and Sorcini, G.: Androgen Sources. *In* Bracci, N., and Di Silverio, F. (Eds.): Hormonal Therapy of Prostatic Cancer. Rome, Cofese Publishers, 1975, p. 59.

Costello, L. C., Littleton, G. K., and Franklin, R. B.: Regulation of citrate-related metabolism in normal and neoplastic prostate. *In* Sharma, R. K., and Criss, W. E. (Eds.): Endocrine Control in Neoplasia. New York, Raven Press, 1978, pp. 303–314.

Cowan, R. A., Cowan, S. K., Grant, J. K., and Elder, H. Y.: Biochemical investigations of separated epithelium and stroma from benign hyperplastic prostatic tissues. J. Endocrinol., *74*:111, 1977.

Cunha, G. R., Chung, L. W. K., Shannon, J. M., Toguchi, O., and Fujii, H.: Hormonal induced morphogenesis and growth: Role of the mesenchymal-epithelial interactions. Recent Prog. Horm. Res., *39*:559, 1983.

Daniel, O.: The stability of acid phosphatase in blood and other fluids. Br. J. Urol., *26*:156, 1954.

Danutra, V., Harper, M. E., Boyns, A. K., Cole, E. N., Brownsey, B. G., and Griffith, K.: The effect of certain stilbestrol analogues on plasma prolactin and testosterone in the rat. J. Endocrinol., *57*:207, 1973.

Dawson, R. M. C., Mann, T., and White, L. G.: Glycerophosphorylcholine and phosphorylcholine in semen and their relationship to choline. Biochemistry, 65:627, 1957.

DeKlerk, D. P.: Glycosoaminoglycans of benign prostatic hyperplasia. Prostate, 4:73, 1983.

DeKlerk, D. P., Coffey, D. S., Ewing, L. L., McDermott, I. R., Reiner, W. G., Robinson, C. H., Scott, W. W., Strandberg, J. D., Talalay, P., Walsh, P. C., Wheaton, L. G., and Zirkin, B. R.: Comparison of spontaneously and experimentally induced canine prostatic hyperplasia. J. Clin. Invest., 64:842, 1979.

DeKlerk, D. P., Heston, W. D. W., and Coffey, D. S.: Studies on the role of macromolecular synthesis in the growth of the prostate. In Grayhack, J. T., Wilson, J. D., and Scherbenske, M. J. (Eds.): Benign Prostatic Hyperplasia. Proceedings of a workshop sponsored by the Kidney Disease and Urology Program of the NIAMDD. Washington, D.C., U.S. Govt. Printing Office, 1976, pp. 43–51.

Denis, L. J., and Prout, G. R., Jr.: Lactic dehydrogenase in prostatic cancer. Invest. Urol., 1:101, 1963.

Doering, C. H., Kraemer, H. C., Brodie, K. H., and Hamburg, D. A.: A cycle of plasma testosterone in the human male. J. Clin. Endocrinol. Metab., 40:492, 1975.

Dorfman, R. I.: Methods in Hormone Research. Vol. II. Bioassay. New York, Academic Press, 1962.

Dorrington, J. H., and Armstrong, D. T.: Follicle stimulating hormone stimulates estradiol-17β synthesis in cultured Sertoli cells. Proc. Natl. Acad. Sci. U.S.A., 72:2677, 1975.

Ekman, P., Barrack, E. R., and Walsh, P. C.: Simultaneous measurement of progesterone and androgen receptors in human prostate: A microassay. J. Clin. Endocrinol. Metab., 55:1089, 1982.

Ekman, P., Barrack, E. R., Greene, G. L., Jensen, E. V., and Walsh, P. C.: Estrogen receptors in human prostate: Evidence for multiple binding sites. J. Clin. Endocrinol. Metab., 57:166, 1983.

Eliasson, R.: Seminal plasma accessory genital glands and infertility. In Cockett, A. T. K., and Urry, R. L. (Eds.): Male Infertility: Workup, Treatment and Research. New York, Grune & Stratton, 1977, pp. 189–204.

Eliasson, R.: Parameters of male infertility. In Hafez, E. S. E., and Evans, T. N. (Eds.): Human Reproductive Conception and Contraception. New York, Harper & Row, 1973.

Eliasson, R.: Biochemical analyses of human semen in the study of the physiology and pathophysiology of the male accessory genital glands. Fertil. Steril., 19:344, 1968.

Eliasson, R.: Cholesterol in human semen. Biochem. J., 98:242, 1966.

Eliasson, R.: Studies on prostaglandins. Occurrence, formation, and biological actions. Acta Physiol. Scand. (Suppl. 46) 158:1, 1959.

Elhilali, M. M., et al.: Lactate dehydrogenase isoenzymes in hyperplasia and carcinoma of the prostate: A clinical study. J. Urol., 98:686, 1968.

Fair, W. R., and Parrish, R. T.: Antibacterial substance in prostatic fluid. In Murphy, G. P., Sandberg, A. A., and Karr, J. P. (Eds.): Prostatic Cell: Structure and Function. Part A. New York, Alan R. Liss, 1981, pp. 247–264.

Fair, W. R., and Wehner, N.: The prostatic antibacterial factor: Identity and significance. In Marberger, H., et al. (Eds.): Prostatic Disease. Vol. 6. New York, Alan R. Liss, 1976.

Fair, W. R., Couch, J., and Wehner, N.: The purification and assay of the prostatic antibacterial factor (PAF). Biochem. Med., 8:329, 1973.

Falk, J. E., Park, M. H., Chung, S. I., et al.: Polyamines as physiological substrates for transglutaminases. J. Biol. Chem., 255:3695, 1980.

Farnsworth, W. E.: Human prostatic dehydroepiandrosterone sulfate sulfatase. In Goland, M. (Ed.): Normal and Abnormal Growth of the Prostate. Springfield, Ill., Charles C Thomas, 1975.

Farnsworth, W. E.: Physiological role of prostaglandin F2A in prostatic function. In Murphy, G. P., Sandberg, A. A., and Karr, J. P. (Eds.): Progress in Clinical and Biological Research. Vol. 75A. New York, Alan R. Liss, 1981.

Farnsworth, W. E., and Brown, J. R.: Testosterone metabolism in the prostate. In Vollmer, E. P. (Ed.): Biology of the Prostate and Related Tissues. National Cancer Institute Monograph 12. Bethesda, Md., National Cancer Institute, 1963, pp. 323–329.

Farrell, J. L.: The secretion of alcohol by the genital tract. J. Urol., 40:62, 1938.

Fischer, M. I., Tikkala, A. O., and Mawson, C. A.: Zinc, carbonic anhydrase and phosphatase in the prostate glands of the cat. Can. J. Biochem. Physiol., 33:181, 1955.

Fishman, W. H., and Anylan, A. J.: β-Glucuronidase activity in human tissues. Cancer, 7:808, 1947.

Flocks, R. H., and Schmidt, J. D.: Lactate dehydrogenase isoenzyme patterns of prostatic cancer and hyperplasia. J. Surg. Oncol., 4:161, 1972.

Forest, M. G., Cathiard, A. M., and Bertrand, J. A.: Total and unbound testosterone levels in the newborn and in normal and hypogonadal children: Use of a sensitive radioimmunoassay for testosterone. J. Clin. Endocrinol. Metab., 36:1132, 1973.

Forest, M. G., Rivarola, M. A., and Migeon, C. J.: Percentage binding of testosterone, androstenedione and dehydroisoandrosterone in human plasma. Steroids, 12:323, 1968.

Foti, A. G., Herschman, H., and Cooper, J. F.: A solid-phase radioimmunoassay for human prostatic acid phosphatase. Cancer Res., 35:2416, 1975.

Fowle, A. S. E., and Bye, A.: Concentrations of trimethoprim and sulfamethoxazole in human prostatic fluid. In Hejzlar, M. (Ed.): Advances in Antimicrobial and Antineoplastic Chemotherapy. Munich, Urban & Schwarzenberg, 1972, p. 1289.

Franks, L. M.: Benign nodular hyperplasia of the prostate: A review. Ann. R. Coll. Surg., 14:92, 1954.

Franks, L. M., Riddle, P. N., Carbonell, A. W., and Gey, G. O.: A comparative study of the ultrastructure and lack of growth capacity of adult human prostate epithelium mechanically separated from its stroma. J. Pathol., 100:113, 1970.

Freund, M., and Peterson, R. N.: Semen evaluation and fertility. In Hafez, E. S. E. (Ed.): Human Semen and Fertility Regulation in Men. St. Louis, C. V. Mosby Co., 1976.

Friberg, J., and Tilly-Friberg, I.: Antibodies in human seminal fluid. In Hafez, E. S. E. (Ed.): Human Semen and Fertility Regulation in Men. St. Louis, C. V. Mosby Co., 1976.

Frieden, E. H.: Chemical Endocrinology. New York, Academic Press, 1976.

Fritz, H., Arnhold, M., Forg-Brey, B., Zaneveld, L. J. D., and Schumacher, G. F. B.: Verhalten der chymotrypsin-ahnlichen Proteinase aus Humansperma gegenuber Protein-Proteinase-Inhibitoren. Hoppe-Seylers Z. Physiol. Chem., 353:1651, 1972.

Fuchs, A. R., and Chantharaski, U.: Prostaglandins and male fertility. In Hafez, E. S. E. (Ed.): Human Semen and Fertility Regulation in Men. St. Louis, C. V. Mosby Co., 1976.

Geller, J., Albert, J., Lopez, D., Geller, A., and Niwa-yama, G.: Comparison of androgen metabolites in benign prostatic hypertrophy in normal prostate. J. Endocrinol., *43*:686, 1976.

Geller, J., Albert, J., Yen, S. S. C., Geller, S., and Loza, Z. D.: Medical castration of males with megestrol acetate and small doses of diethylstilbestrol. J. Clin. Endocrinol. Metab., *52*:576, 1981.

Geller, J., Angrist, A., Nakao, K., and Newman, H.: Therapy with progestational agents in advanced prostatic hypertrophy. JAMA, *210*:1421, 1969.

Ghanadian, R.: Mechanism of action of androgens. *In* Chisholm, G. D., and Williams, D. I. (Eds.): Scientific Foundations of Urology. 2nd ed., London, W. Heinemann, 1982, p. 491.

Gill, W., and Chen, C.: Dehydroepiandrosterone sulfatase in the prostate and seminal vesicles of the rat. Biochim. Biophys. Acta, *218*:148, 1970.

Gloyna, R. E., Siiteri, P. K., and Wilson, J. D.: Dihydrotestosterone in prostatic hypertrophy. II. The formation and content of dihydrotestosterone in the hypertrophic canine prostate and the effect of dihydrotestosterone on prostate growth in the dog. J. Clin. Invest., *49*:1746, 1970.

Goland, M. (Ed.): Normal and Abnormal Growth of the Prostate. Springfield, Ill., Charles C Thomas, 1975.

Goldblatt, M. W.: Properties of human seminal plasma. J. Physiol. (Lond.), *84*:202, 1935.

Goldblatt, M. W.: A depressor substance in seminal fluid. J. Soc. Chem. Ind. (Lond.), *52*:1056, 1933.

Goldstein, N. L.: Cholesterol synthesis in the prostate gland and its relationship to benign prostatic hyperplasia. Ph.D. thesis, Rutgers University, 1976.

Grant, J. K., Fell, G. S., and Manguell, J.: Zinc in the prostate in man. *In* Goland, M. (Ed.): Normal and Abnormal Growth in the Prostate. Springfield, Ill., Charles C Thomas, 1975, p. 494.

Grayhack, J. T., Bunce, P. L., Kearns, J. W., and Scott, W. W.: Influence of the pituitary on prostatic response to androgen in the rat. Bull. Johns Hopkins Hosp., *96*:154, 1955.

Grayhack, J. T., Wendel, E. F., Lee, C., Oliver, L., and Choen, E.: Lactate dehydrogenase isoenzymes in human prostatic fluid: An aid in recognition of malignancy. J. Urol., *118*:204, 1977.

Grayhack, J. T., Wilson, J. D., and Scherbenske, M. J. (Eds.): Benign Prostatic Hyperplasia. Proceedings of a workshop sponsored by the Kidney Disease and Urology Program of the NIAMDD. Washington, D.C., U.S. Govt. Printing Office, 1975.

Gunn, S. A., and Gould, T. C.: The relative importance of androgen and estrogen in the selective uptake of Zn 65 by the dorsolateral prostate of the rat. Endocrinology, *58*:443, 1956.

Gunn, S. A., Gould, T. C., and Anderson, W. A.: The effect of growth hormone and prolactin preparations on the control by interstitial cell-stimulating hormone of uptake of 65-Zn by the rat dorsolateral prostate. J. Endocrinol., *32*:205, 1965.

Gustaffson, J. A., Ekman, P., Pousette, A., Snochowski, M., and Hogberg, B.: Demonstration of progesterone receptor in human benign prostatic hyperplasia and prostatic carcinoma. Invest. Urol., *15*:361, 1978.

Gutman, A. B., and Gutman, E. B.: An acid phosphatase occurring in serum of patients with metastasizing carcinoma of the prostate gland. J. Clin. Invest., *17*:473, 1938.

Gyorkey, F., Kyung-Wham, J., Huff, J. A., and Gyorkey, P.: Zinc and magnesium in human prostate gland: Normal, hyperplastic and neoplastic. Cancer Res., *27*:1348, 1967.

Habib, F. K., Mason, M. K., Smith, P. H., and Stitch, S. R.: Cancer of the prostate: Early diagnosis by zinc and hormone analysis. Br. J. Cancer, *39*:700, 1979.

Hammond, G. L.: Endogenous steroid levels in the human prostate from birth to old age: A comparison of normal and diseased states. J. Endocrinol., *78*:7, 1978.

Hay, E. D. (Ed.): The Cell Biology of the Extracellular Matrix. New York, Plenum Press, 1981.

Heathcote, J. G., and Washington, R. J.: Analysis of the zinc-binding protein derived from the human benign hypertrophic prostate. J. Endocrinol., *58*:421, 1973.

Hein, R. C., Grayhack, J. T., and Loldberg, E.: Prostatic fluid–lactic dehydrogenase isoenzyme patterns of prostatic cancer and hyperplasia. J. Urol., *113*:511, 1975.

Hessl, J. M., and Stamey, T. A.: The passage of tetracyclines across epithelial membranes with special reference to prostatic epithelium. J. Urol., *106*:253, 1971.

Higgins, S. J., Brooks, D. E., Fuller, F. M., Jackson, P. J., and Smith, F. E.: Function development of sex accessory organs of the male rat. Biochem. J., *194*:895, 1981.

Hinman, F., Jr. (Ed.): Benign Prostatic Hypertrophy, New York, Springer-Verlag, 1983.

Hoare, R., Delory, G. E., and Penner, D. W.: Zinc and acid phosphatase in the human prostate. Cancer, *9*:721, 1956.

Horton, E. W., Jones, R. L., and Marr, C. G.: Effects of aspirin on prostaglandin and fructose levels in human semen. J. Reprod. Fertil., *33*:385, 1973.

Horton, R. J.: Androgen hormones and prehormones in young and elderly men. *In* Grayhack, J. T., Wilson, J. D., and Scherbenske, M. J. (Eds.): Benign Prostatic Hyperplasia. Proceedings of a workshop sponsored by the Kidney Disease and Urology Program of the NIAMDD. Washington, D.C., U.S. Govt. Printing Office, 1976, pp. 183–188.

Huggins, C., and Hodges, C. V.: Studies on prostatic cancer. I. The effect of castration, of estrogen and of androgen injection on serum phosphatases in metastatic carcinoma of the prostate. Cancer Res., *1*:293, 1941.

Huggins, C., and Neal, W.: Coagulation and liquefaction of semen. Proteolytic enzymes and citrate in prostatic fluid. J. Exp. Med., *76*:527, 1942.

Huggins, C., and Talalay, P.: Sodium phenolphthalein phosphate as a substrate for phosphatase tests. J. Biol. Chem., *159*:399, 1945.

Huggins, C., and Webster, W. O.: Duality of human prostate in response to estrogen. J. Urol., *59*:258, 1948.

Isaacs, J. T.: Prostatic structure and function in relation to the etiology of prostate cancer. Prostate, *4*:351, 1983.

Isaacs, J. T., and Coffey, D. S.: Changes in dihydrotestosterone metabolism associated with the development of canine benign prostatic hyperplasia. Endocrinology, *108*:445, 1981*a*.

Isaacs, J. T., and Coffey, D. S.: Androgen metabolism of the prostate: New concepts related to normal and abnormal growth. *In* Everett, J. E., Altwein, G., Bartsch, G., and Jacoby, G. H. (Eds.): Antihormones. Bedeutung in der Urologie. Munchen, W. Zuckschwerdt Verlag, 1981*b*.

Isaacs, J. T., and Coffey, D. S.: Prostatic Cancer. UICC Technical Reports, Series 48, Report #9. Geneva, Int. Union Against Cancer, 1979.

Isaacs, J. T., Barrack, E. R., Isaacs, W. B., and Coffey, D. S.: The relationship of cellular structure and function: The matrix system. *In* Murphy, G. P., Sandberg, A. A., and Karr, J. P. (Eds.): The Prostate: Cell Structure and Function. Part A. New York, Alan R. Liss, 1981, p. 1.

Isaacs, W. B.: Structural and functional components in normal and hyperplastic prostate. *In* Kimball, F. A.,

Buhl, A. E., and Carter, D. B. (Eds.): New Approaches to the Study of Benign Prostatic Hyperplasia. New York, Alan R. Liss, 1984, p. 307.

Iversen, P., Nielssen, O. S., Vergin, H., and Madsen, P. O.: Metioprim-sulfadiazine distribution in the canine prostate. Prostate, 2:327, 1981.

Jacobi, G. H., and Hohenfellner, R.: Prostate Cancer. International Perspectives in Urology. Vol. 3. Baltimore, The Williams & Wilkins Co., 1982.

Jacobs, S. C., Pikna, D., and Lawson, R. K.: Prostatic osteoblastic factor. Invest. Urol., 17:195, 1979.

Janne, J., Holtta, E., Haaranen, P., and Elfving, K.: Polyamines and polyamine metabolizing enzyme activities in human semen. Clin. Chim. Acta, 48:393, 1973.

Johnson, L., Wickstrom, S., and Nylander, G.: The vehicle for zinc in the prostatic secretion of dogs. Scand. J. Urol. Nephrol., 3:9, 1969.

Karim, S. M. M.: Advances in prostaglandin research. In Karim, S. M. M. (Ed.): Prostaglandins and Reproduction. Baltimore, University Park Press, 1975.

Kent, J. R., Bischoft, A. J., Arduino, L. J., et al.: Estrogen dosage and suppression of testosterone levels in patients with prostatic carcinoma. J. Urol., 109:858, 1973.

Kimball, F. A., Buhl, A. E., and Carter, D. B. (Eds.): New Approaches to the Study of Benign Prostatic Hyperplasia, New York, Alan R. Liss, 1984.

King, W. J., and Greene, G. L.: Monoclonal antibodies localize oestrogen receptor in the nuclei of target cells. Nature, 307:745, 1984.

Kirchheim, D., Gyorkey, F., Brandes, D., and Scott, W. W.: Histochemistry of the normal hyperplastic and neoplastic human prostate gland. Invest. Urol., 4:403, 1964.

Klein, L. A., and Stoff, J. S.: Prostaglandins and the prostate: an hypothesis on the etiology of benign prostatic hyperplasia. Prostate, 4:247, 1983.

Kozak, I., Bartsch, W., Krieg, M., and Voigt, K.: Nuclei stroma: Site of highest estrogen concentration in human benign prostatic hyperplasia. Prostate, 3:433, 1982.

Krieg, M., Bartsch, W., Jenssen, W., and Voigt, K. D.: A comparative study of the binding of metabolism and endogenous levels of androgens in normal, hyperplastic and carcinomatous human prostate. J. Steroid Biochem., 11:615, 1979.

Krieg, M., Klotzl, G., Kaufmann, J., and Voigt, K. D.: Stroma of human benign prostatic hyperplasia: Preferential tissues for androgen metabolism and estrogen binding. Acta Endocrinol., 96:422, 1981.

Kutchner, W., and Wolberg, H.: Prostataphosphatase. Z. Physiol. Chem., 236:237, 1935.

Labrie, F., Auclair, C., Cusan, L., Kelly, P. A., Pelletier, G., and Ferland, L.: Inhibitory effects of LHRH and its agonists on testicular gonadotropin receptors and spermatogenesis in the rat. Int. J. Androl. (Suppl. 2), 303:1, 1979.

Labrie, F., Dupont, A., Belanger, A., et al.: New approach in the treatment of prostate cancer: Complete instead of only partial removal of androgen. Prostate, 4:579, 1983.

Lasnitzki, I., and Franklin, H. R.: The influence of serum of uptake, conversion and action of testosterone in rat prostate glands in organ culture. J. Endocrinol., 54:333, 1972.

Lawson, R. K., Storey, M. T., and Jacobs, S. C.: A growth factor in extracts of human prostatic tissue. In Murphy, G. P., et al. (Eds.): Prostatic Cell: Structure and Function. Part A. New York, Alan R. Liss, 1981, p. 325.

LeDuc, I. E.: The anatomy of the prostate and the pathology of early benign prostatic hypertrophy. J. Urol., 42:1217, 1939.

Li, C. Y., et al.: Acid phosphatases in human plasma. J. Lab. Clin. Med., 82:446, 1973.

Liao, S., Castaneda, E., Chudzinski, P. A., Tangen, L. M., and Liang, T.: Biochemical aspects of androgen receptors and cell stimulation of the prostate. In Grayhack, J. T., Wilson, J. D., and Scherbenske, M. J. (Eds): Benign Prostatic Hyperplasia. Proceedings of a workshop sponsored by the Kidney Disease and Urology Program of the NIAMDD, Feb. 20–21, 1975. Washington, D.C., U.S. Govt. Printing Office, 1976, pp. 33–40.

Liao, S., Fang, S., Tymoczki, J. L., and Liang, T.: Androgen receptors, antiandrogens and uptake and retention of androgens in male sex accessory organs. In Brandes, D. (Ed.): Male Sex Accessory Organs: Structure and Function in Mammals. New York, Academic Press, 1974.

Liao, S., Liang, T., Fang, S., Castaneda, E., and Shao, T. C.: Steroid structure and androgen activity. Specificities involved in the receptor binding and nuclear retention of various androgens. J. Biol. Chem., 248:6154, 1973.

Lin, M. F., Lee, J. W., Wojcieszyn, J., Wang, M. C., Valenzuela, L. A., Murphy, G. P., and Chu, T. M.: Fundamental biochemical and immunological aspects of prostatic acid phosphatase. Prostate, 1:415, 1980.

Lloyd, J. W., Thomas, J. A., and Mawhinney, M. G.: A difference in the in vitro accumulation and metabolism by the rat prostate gland with prolactin. Steroids. 22:473, 1973.

Lostroh, A. J.: Effect of testosterone and insulin in vitro on maintenance and repair of the secretory epithelium of the mouse prostate. Endocrinology, 88:500, 1971.

Lundquist, F., Thorsteinsson, T., and Buus, O.: Purification and properties of some enzymes in human seminal plasma. Biochem. J., 56:69, 1955.

MacDonald, P. C.: Origin of estrogen in men. In Grayhack, J. T., Wilson, J. D., and Scherbenske, M. J. (Eds.): Benign Prostatic Hyperplasia. Proceedings of a workshop sponsored by the Kidney Disease and Urology Program of the NIAMDD, Feb. 20–21, 1975. Washington, D.C., U.S. Govt. Printing Office, 1976, pp. 191–192.

Mackenzie, A. R., Hall, T., and Whitmore, W. F., Jr.: Zinc content of expressed human prostatic fluid. Nature, 193:72, 1962.

Mackler, M. A., Liberti, J. P., Smith, M. J. V., et al.: The effect of orchiectomy and various doses of stilbestrol on plasma testosterone levels in patients with carcinoma of the prostate. Invest. Urol., 9:423, 1972.

Madsen, P. O., Baumueller, A., and Hoyne, U.: Experimental models for determination of antimicrobials in prostatic tissue, interstitial fluid and secretion. Scand. J. Infect. Dis. (Suppl.) 14:145, 1978.

Madsen, P. O., Kjaert, B., Baumueller, A., and Mellin, H. E.: Antimicrobial agents in prostatic fluid and tissue. Infection, 4:154, 1976.

Madsen, P. O., Wolf, H., Barquin, O. P., and Rhodes, P.: The nitrofurantoin concentration in prostatic fluid of humans and dogs. J. Urol., 100:54, 1968.

Manandhar, M. S. P., and Thomas, J. A.: Effect of prolactin on the metabolism of androgens by the rat ventral prostate. Invest. Urol., 14:20, 1976.

Mann, T., and Mann, C. L.: Male Reproductive Function and Semen. New York, Springer-Verlag, 1981.

Marina, S., Pomerlo, J. M., and Zungri, E. R.: Occlusions

in the male reproductive tract. Diagnostic radiology. *In* Hafez, E. S. E. (Ed.): Human Semen and Fertility Regulation in Men. St. Louis, C. V. Mosby Co., 1976.

Mariotti, J., and Mawhinney, M. G.: Hormonal control of accessory sex organ fibromuscular stroma. Prostate, *2*:397, 1981.

Mattila, S.: Further studies on the prostatic tissue antigens. Separation of two molecular forms of aminopeptidase. Invest. Urol., 1:969.

Mawson, C. A., and Fischer, M. I.: The occurrence of zinc in the human prostate gland. Can. J. Med. Sci., *30*:336, 1952.

McKeehan, W. L., Glass, H. A., Rosser, M. P., and Adams, P. S.: Prostatic binding proteins, polyamines and DNA synthesis in rat ventral prostate. Prostate, *3*:231, 1982.

McNeal, J. E.: Regional morphology and pathology of the prostate. Am. J. Clin. Pathol., *49*:347, 1968.

McNeal, J. E.: Developmental and comparative anatomy of the prostate. *In* Grayhack, J. T., Wilson, J. D., and Scherbenske, M. J. (Eds.): Benign Prostatic Hyperplasia. Proceedings of a workshop sponsored by the Kidney Disease and Urology Program of the NIAMDD, Feb. 20–21, 1975. Washington, D.C., U.S. Govt. Printing Office, 1976, pp. 1–6.

McNeal, J. E.: Origin and evolution of benign prostatic enlargement. Invest. Urol., *15*:340, 1978.

McNeal, J. E.: Anatomy of the prostate: an historical survey of divergent views. Prostate, *1*:3, 1980.

McNeal, J. E.: The zonal anatomy of the prostate. Prostate, *1*:35, 1981.

Meares, E., Jr.: Prostatitis: A review. Urol. Clin. North Am., *2*:3, 1975.

Meikle, A. W., Stringham, J. D., and Olsen, D. C.: Subnormal tissue 3-androstane diol and androsterone in prostatic hyperplasia. J. Clin. Endocrinol., *47*:909, 1978.

Merk, F. B., Ofner, P., Qwann, P. W. L., Leav, I., and Vena, R. L.: Ultrastructral and biochemical expression of divergent differentiation in prostates of castrated dogs treated with estrogens and androgens. Lab. Invest., *47*:437, 1982.

Milisaukas, V., and Rose, N. R.: Immunochemical quantitation of prostatic phosphatase. Clin. Chem., *18*:1529, 1972.

Mobbs, B. J., Johnson, L. E., and Connolly, J. G.: Influence of the adrenal gland on prostatic activity in adult rats. J. Endocrinol., *59*:335, 1973.

Modder, C. P.: Investigations on acid phosphatase activity in human plasma and serum. Clin. Chim. Acta, *43*:205, 1973.

Moger, W. H., and Geschwind, L. L.: The action of prolactin on the sex accessory glands of the male rat. Proc. Soc. Exp. Biol. Med., *141*:1017, 1972.

Moncure, C. W.: Isoenzymes in prostatic carcinoma. *In* Tannenbaum, M. (Ed.): Urologic Pathology: The Prostate. Philadelphia, Lea & Febiger, 1977, pp. 141–156.

Moncure, C. W.: Investigation of specific antigens in prostatic cancer. National Prostatic Cancer Project Workshop, 1975. Cancer Chemother. Rep., *59*(1):105, 1975.

Moncure, C. W., and Prout, G. R., Jr.: Antigenicity of human prostatic acid phosphatase. Cancer, *25*:463, 1970.

Moon, K. H., and Bunge, R. G.: Seminal fructose as an indicator of androgenic activity: Critical analysis. Invest. Urol., *8*:373, 1971.

Moon, K. H., Osborn, R. H., Yannone, M. E., and Bunge, R. G.: Relationship of testosterone to human seminal fructose. Invest. Urol., *7*:478, 1970.

Moore, R. J., Gazak, J. M., Quebbeman, J. F.; and Wilson, J. D.: Concentration of dihydrotestosterone in 3-androstanediol in naturally occurring and androgen induced prostatic hyperplasia in the dog. J. Clin. Invest., *64*:1003, 1979.

Mroveth, A. M.: The excretion of radioiodine in human semen. Invest. Urol., *22*:61, 1971.

Muntzing, J.: Androgen and collagen as growth regulators of the rat ventral prostate. Prostate, *1*:71, 1980.

Muntzing, J., and Nilsson, T.: Enzyme activity and distribution in hyperplastic cancerous human prostates. Scand. J. Urol. Nephrol., *6*:107, 1972.

Murphy, G. P., Sandberg, A. A., and Karr, J. P. (Eds.): Prostatic Cell: Structure and Function. Part A and Part B, New York, Alan R. Liss, 1981.

Neumann, F.: Different principles of androgen deprivation for palliative treatment of prostatic cancer. *In* Schroder, F. H. (Ed.): Androgens and Antiandrogens. Weesp, The Netherlands, Schering, 1983.

Nielsen, M. L., and Hansen, I.: Trimethoprim in human prostatic tissue and prostatic fluid. Scand. J. Urol. Nephrol., *6*:244, 1972.

Niemi, M., Harkonen, M., and Larmi, T. K. L.: Enzymic histochemistry of human prostate. Arch. Pathol., *75*:528, 1963.

Nilsson, T., Schueller, E., and Staubitz, W.: Beta-glucuronidase activity of the epithelial cells and stromal cells in prostatic hyperplasia. Invest. Urol., *11*:145, 1973.

Nissen, N. I., and Bohn, L.: Patterns of lactic acid dehydrogenase isoenzymes in normal and malignant human tissues. Eur. J. Cancer, *1*:217, 1975.

Notides, A. C., and Williams-Ashman, H. G.: The basic protein responsible for clotting of guinea pig semen. Proc. Natl. Acad. Sci. U.S.A., *58*:1991, 1967.

Oettle, A. G.: Morphologic changes in normal human semen after ejaculation. Fertil. Steril., *5*:227, 1954.

Oliver, J. A., et al.: LDH isoenzymes in benign and malignant prostate tissue. The LDH/VI ratio as an index of malignancy. Cancer, *25*:863, 1970.

Ostrowski, W., et al.: The role of neuraminic acid in the heterogeneity of acid phosphomonoesterase from the human prostate gland. Biochim. Biophys. Acta, *221*:297, 1970.

Parrish, R. F., Heston, W. D. W., Pletscher, L. F., Tackett, R., and Fair, W. R.: Prostate-derived growth factors. *In* Kimball, F. A., Buehl, A. E., and Carter, D. B. (Eds.): New Approaches to the Study of Benign Prostatic Hyperplasia. New York, Alan R. Liss, 1984, p. 181.

Parrish, R. F., Perinetti, E. P., and Fair, W. R.: Evidence against a zinc binding peptide in pilocarpine stimulated canine prostatic secretion. Prostate, *4*:189, 1983.

Peterson, R. N., and Freund, M.: Factors affecting fructose utilization and lactic acid formation by human semen. The role of glucose and pyruvic acid. Fertil. Steril., *22*:639, 1971.

Phadke, A. M., Samant, N. R., and Deval, S. P.: Significance of seminal fructose studies in male fertility. Fertil. Steril., *24*:894, 1973.

Polakoski, K. L., and Kopta, M.: Seminal plasma. *In* Zaneveld, L. J. D., and Chatterton, R. T. (eds.): Biochemistry of Mammalian Reproduction. New York, John Wiley & Sons, 1982, p. 89.

Poulos, A., and White, L. G.: Phospholipids of human spermatozoa and seminal plasma. J. Reprod. Fertil., *35*:265, 1973.

Prellwitz, W., and Ehrenthall, W.: Serum and bone marrow acid phosphatase in prostatic carcinoma patients. *In* Jacobi, G. H., and Hohenfellner, R. (Eds.): Interna-

tional Perspectives in Urology. Vol. 3. Prostate Cancer. Baltimore, The Williams & Wilkins Co., 1982, p. 129.

Price, D., and Williams-Ashman, H. G.: The accessory reproductive glands of mammals. *In* Young, W. C. (Ed.): Sex and Internal Secretions. 3rd ed. Baltimore, The Williams & Wilkins Co., 1961, pp. 366–448.

Propping, D., Tauber, P. F., Zaneveld, L. J. D., and Schumacher, G. F. B.: Purification and characterization of two plasminogen activators from human seminal plasma. Fed. Proc., *33*:289, 1974.

Prout, G. R., Jr., Sierp, M., and Whitmore, W. F.: Radioactive zinc in the prostate: Some influencing concentrations in dogs and men. JAMA, *69*:1703, 1959.

Rajfer, J., and Coffey, D. S.: Sex steroid imprinting of the immature prostate: Long term effects. Invest. Urol., *16*:186, 1979*a*.

Rajfer, J., and Coffey, D. S.: Effects of neonatal steroids on male sex tissues. Invest. Urol., *17*:3, 1979*b*.

Reed, M. J., and Stitch, S. R.: The uptake of testosterone and zinc *in vitro* by the human benign hypertrophic prostate. J. Endocrinol., *58*:405, 1973.

Reeves, D. S.: Pharmacology of the prostate. *In* Williams, D. I. (Ed.): Scientific Foundations of Urology. Vol. II. Chicago, Year Book Medical Publishers, 1976.

Reeves, D. S., Rowe, R. C. G., Snell, M. E., and Thomas, A. B. W.: Further studies on the secretion of antibiotics in the prostatic fluid of the dog. *In* Brumfitt, W., and Asscher, A. W. (Eds.): Urinary Tract Infection. London, Oxford University Press, 1973, p. 197.

Robinson, M. R. G., and Thomas, B. S.: Effect of hormonal therapy on plasma testosterone levels in prostatic carcinoma. Br. Med. J., *4*:391, 1971.

Roy, A. V., et al.: Sodium thymolphthalein monophosphate: A new acid phosphatase substrate with greater specificity for the prostatic enzyme in serum. Clin. Chem., *17*:1093, 1971.

Schaffner, C. P.: Effects of cholesterol-lowering agents. *In* Hinman, F., Jr. (Ed.): Benign Prostatic Hypertrophy. New York, Springer-Verlag, 1983, p. 280.

Schriefers, H.: Factors affecting the metabolism of steroids. Vitam. Horm., *25*:271, 1967.

Schroder, F.: Androgens and Antiandrogens. Weesp, The Netherlands, Schering, 1983.

Schrodt, G. R., Hall, T., and Whitmore, W. F., Jr.: The concentration of zinc in diseased human prostate glands. Cancer, *17*:1555, 1964.

Schweikert, H. U., Bartsch, G., Totzauer, P., and Rohr, H. P.: Testosterone metabolism in the epithelium and stroma of normal human prostates of benign prostatic hyperplasia. In press.

Sciarra, F., Sorcini, G., DiSilverio, F., and Gagliardi, V.: Plasma testosterone and androstenedione after orchiectomy in prostatic adenocarcinoma. Clin. Endocrinol., *2*:110, 1973.

Scott, W. W.: The lipids of the prostatic fluid, seminal plasma and enlarged prostate gland of man. J. Urol., *53*:712, 1945.

Scott, W. W., and Wade, J. C.: Effects of cyproterone acetate on the prostate. J. Urol., *101*:81, 1969.

Seligman, A. M., et al.: Design of spindle poisons activated specifically by prostatic acid phosphatase (PAP) and new methods for PAP cytochemistry. Cancer Chemother. Rep., *59*:233, 1975.

Seligman, A. M., et al.: The colorimetric determination of phosphatases in human serum. J. Biol. Chem., *190*:7, 1951.

Shearer, R. J., Hendry, W. F., Sommerville, I. F., and

Ferguson, J. D.: Plasma testosterone: An accurate monitor of hormone treatment in prostatic cancer. Br. J. Urol., *45*:668, 1973.

Shimazaki, J., Kurihara, H., Ito, Y., and Shida, K.: Metabolism of testosterone in prostate. Separation of prostatic 17β-ol-dehydrogenase and 5-reductase. Gunma J. Med. Sci., *14*:326, 1965*a*.

Shimazaki, J., Kurihara, H., Ito, Y., and Shida, K.: Testosterone metabolism in prostate. Formation of androstane-17β-ol-3-one and androst-4-ene-3,17-dione, and inhibitory effect of natural and synthetic estrogens. Gunma J. Med. Sci., *14*:313, 1965*b*.

Shulman, S., and Ferber, J. M.: Multiple forms of prostatic acid phosphatase. J. Reprod. Fertil., *11*:295, 1966.

Shulman, S., Mamrod, L., Gonder, M. J., et al.: The detection of prostatic acid phosphatase by antibody reactions in gel diffusion. J. Immunol., *93*:474, 1964.

Siiteri, P. K., and MacDonald, P. C.: Role of extraglandular estrogen in human endocrinology. *In* Greep, R. O., and Astwood, E. B. (Eds.): Handbook of Physiology, Section 7. Endocrinology, Vol. II. Baltimore, The Williams & Wilkins Co., 1973, pp. 615–629.

Siiteri, P. K., and Wilson, J. D.: Dihydrotestosterone in prostatic hypertrophy. I. The formation and content of dihydrotestosterone in the hypertrophic prostate of man. J. Clin. Invest., *49*:1737, 1970.

Smith, E. R., and Hagopian, M.: Uptake in secretion of carcinogenic chemicals by the dog and rat prostate. *In* Murphy, G. P., Sandberg, A. A., and Karr, J. P. (Eds.): Prostatic Cell: Structure and Function. Part B. New York, Alan R. Liss, 1981, p. 131.

Smith, J. K., and Whitby, L. G.: The heterogeneity of prostatic acid phosphatase. Biochim. Biophys. Acta, *151*:607, 1968.

Sodeman, T. M., and Batsakis, J. G.: Acid phosphatase. *In* Tannenbaum, M. (Ed.): Urologic Pathology: The Prostate. Philadelphia, Lea & Febiger, 1977, p. 129.

Stamey, T. A.: Pathogenesis and Treatment of Urinary Tract Infections. Baltimore, The Williams & Wilkins Co., 1980, pp. 389–397.

Stamey, T. A., Bushby, S. R. M., and Bragonje, J.: The concentration of trimethoprim in prostatic fluid: Nonionic diffusion or active transport? J. Infect. Dis. (Suppl.), *128*:686, 1973.

Stamey, T. A., Fair, W. R., Timothy, M. M., et al.: Antibacterial nature of prostatic fluid. Nature, *218*:444, 1968.

Storey, M. T., Jacobs, S. C., and Lawson, R. K.: Epidermal growth factor is not the major growth-promoting agent in extracts of prostatic tissues. J. Urol., *130*:175, 1983.

Storey, M. T., Jacobs, S. C., and Lawson, R. K.: Preliminary characterization and evaluation of techniques for the isolation of prostate-derived growth factor. *In* Kimball, F. A., Buehl, A. E., and Carter, D. B. (Eds.): New Approaches to the Study of Benign Prostatic Hyperplasia. New York, Alan R. Liss, 1984, p. 197.

Sufrin, G., and Prutkin, L.: Experimental diabetes and the response of the sex accessory organs on the castrate male rat to testosterone propionate. Invest. Urol., *11*:361, 1974.

Sur, B. K., et al.: Apparent heterogeneity of prostatic acid phosphatase. Biochem. J., *84*:55P, 1962.

Syner, F. N., Moghissi, K. S., and Yanez, J.: Isolation of a factor from normal human semen that accelerates dissolution of abnormally liquefying semen. Fertil. Steril., *26*:1064, 1975.

Tauber, P. F., and Zaneveld, L. J. D.: Coagulation and

liquefaction of human semen. *In* Hafez, E. S. E. (Ed.): Human Semen and Fertility Regulation in Men. St. Louis, C. V. Mosby Co., 1976.

Tauber, P. F., Zaneveld, L. J. D., Propping, D., and Schumacher, G. F. B.: Components of human split ejaculates. II. Enzymes and proteinase inhibitors. J. Reprod. Fertil., *46*:165, 1976.

Tauber, P. F., Zaneveld, L. J. D., Propping, D., and Schumacher, G. F. B.: Components of human split ejaculate. J. Reprod. Fertil., *43*:249, 1975.

Tesar, C., and Scott, W. W.: A search for inhibitors of prostatic growth stimulators. Invest. Urol., *1*:482, 1966.

Thornton, M. O., Frederickson, R., Matal, J., and Mawhinney, M.: Preliminary studies on the relationship between collagen and the growth of the male accessory sex organ epithelial cells. *In* Kimball, F. A., Buehl, A. E., and Carter, D. P. (Eds.): New Approaches to the Study of Benign Prostatic Hyperplasia. New York, Alan R. Liss, 1984, p. 143.

Tisell, L. E.: Effect of cortisone on the growth of the ventral prostate, the dorsolateral prostate, the coagulating gland and the seminal vesicles in castrated adrenalectomized and in castrated non-adrenalectomized rats. Acta Endocrinol., *64*:637, 1970.

Tisell, L. E., and Leissner, K. H.: Prostatic weight and zinc concentration. *In* Kimball, F. A., Buehl, A. E., and Carter, D. P. (Eds.): New Approaches to the Study of Benign Prostatic Hyperplasia. New York, Alan R. Liss, 1984.

Tisell, L. E., and Salander, H.: The lobes of the human prostate. Scand. J. Urol. Nephrol., *9*:185, 1975.

Trachtenberg, J., and Walsh, P. C.: Correlation of prostatic nuclear androgen receptor content with duration of response and survival following hormonal therapy in advanced prostatic cancer. J. Urol., *127*:466, 1982.

Trachtenberg, J., Hicks, L. L., and Walsh, P. C.: Androgen and estrogen receptor content in spontaneous and experimentally induced canine prostatic hyperplasia. J. Clin. Invest., *65*:1051, 1980.

Tseng, S. C. G., Jarvinen, M. J., Nelson, W. G., Huang, J. W., Woodcock-Mitchell, J., and Sun, T.-T.: Correlations of specific keratins with different types of epithelial differentiation: Monoclonal antibody studies. Cell, *30*:361, 1982.

Tsuboi, K. K., and Hudson, P. B.: Acid phosphatase. III. Specific kinetic properties of highly purified prostatic phosphomonoesterases. Arch. Biophys., *55*:191, 1955.

Tullner, W. W.: Hormonal factors in the adrenal dependent growth of the rat ventral prostate. *In* Vollmer, E. P. (Ed.): Biology of the Prostate and Related Tissues. National Cancer Institute Monograph 12. Bethesda, Md., National Cancer Institute, 1963, p. 211.

Vallee, B. L.: The biochemistry, physiology, and pharmacology of zinc. Physiol. Rev., *39*:443, 1959.

Vaughan, A., et al.: Fluorometric methods for analysis of acid and alkaline phosphatase. Anal. Chem., *43*:721, 1971.

Vermeulen, A.: The physical state of testosterone in plasma. *In* James, V. H. T., Serio, M., and Maratini, L. (Eds.): The Endocrine Function of the Human Testis. Vol. I. New York, Academic Press, 1973, pp. 157–170.

Vermeulen, A.: Testicular hormonal secretion and aging in males. *In* Grayhack, J. T., Wilson, J. D., and Scherbenske, M. J. (Eds.): Benign Prostatic Hyperplasia. Proceedings of a workshop sponsored by the Kidney Disease and Urology Program of the NIAMDD, Feb. 20–21, 1975. Washington, D.C., U.S. Govt. Printing Office, 1976, p. 177.

Vermeulen, A., Verdonck, L., Van der Straeten, M., and Orie, N.: Capacity of the TeBG in human plasma and influence of specific binding of testosterone on its metabolic clearance rate. J. Clin. Endocrinol., *29*:1470, 1969.

Vida, J. A.: Androgens and Anabolic Agents. New York, Academic Press, 1969.

von Euler, U. S.: Zur Kenntnis der pharmakologischen Wirkungen von Natirsekreten und Extrackten mannlicher accessorischer Geschlechtsdrusen. Arch. Pathol. Pharmakol., *175*:78, 1934.

Walsh, P. C.: Human benign prostatic hyperplasia: Etiological considerations. *In* Kimball, F. A., et al. (Eds.): New Approaches to the Study of Benign Prostatic Hyperplasia. New York, Alan R. Liss, 1984, p. 1.

Walsh, P. C., and Amelar, R.: Embryology, anatomy and physiology of the male reproductive system. *In* Amelar, R., et al. (Eds.): Male Infertility. Philadelphia, W. B. Saunders Co., 1977.

Walsh, P. C., and Gittes, R. F.: Inhibition of extratesticular stimuli to prostatic growth in the castrate rat by antiandrogens. Endocrinology, *87*:624, 1970.

Walsh, P. C., and Siiteri, P. K.: Suppression of plasma androgens by spironolactone in castrated men with carcinoma of the prostate. J. Urol., *114*:254, 1975.

Walsh, P. C., and Wilson, J. D.: The induction of prostatic hypertrophy in the dog with androstanediol. J. Clin. Invest., *57*:1093, 1976.

Walsh, P. C., Hutchins, G. M., and Ewing, L. L.: Tissue content of dihydrotestosterone in human prostatic hyperplasia is not supranormal. J. Clin. Invest., *72*:1772, 1983.

Welshons, W. V., Lieberman, M. E., and Gorski, J.: Nuclear localization of unoccupied oestrogen receptors. Nature, *307*:747, 1984.

White, I. G., Darin-Bennett, A., and Poulos, A.: Lipids of human semen. *In* Hafez, E. S. E. (Ed.): Human Semen and Fertility Regulation in Men. St. Louis, C. V. Mosby Co., 1976.

White, M. A.: Changes in pH of expressed prostatic secretion during the course of prostatitis. Proc. R. Soc. Med., *68*:511, 1975.

Whitmore, W. F., Jr.: Comments on zinc in the human and canine prostates. *In* Vollmer, E. P. (Ed.): Biology of the Prostate and Related Tissues. National Cancer Institute Monograph 12. Bethesda, Md., National Cancer Institute, 1963, p. 337.

Wieland, R. G., Courcy, C. D., Levy, R. P., et al.: $C_{19}O_2$ steroids and some of their precursors in blood from normal adrenals. J. Clin. Invest., *44*:159, 1965.

Williams-Ashman, H. G., Corti, A., and Sheth, A. R.: Formation and functions of aliphatic polyamines in the prostate gland and its secretions. *In* Goland, M. (Ed.): Normal and Abnormal Growth of the Prostate. Springfield, Ill., Charles C Thomas, 1975, p. 222.

Williams-Ashman, H. G., Janne, J., Coppoc, G. C., Geroch, M. E., and Schenone, A.: New aspects of polyamine biosynthesis in eukaryotic organisms. Adv. Enzyme Regul., *10*:225, 1972.

Williams-Ashman, H. G., Pegg, A. E., and Lockwood, D. H.: Mechanisms and regulation of polyamine and putrescine biosynthesis in male genital glands and other tissues of mammals. Adv. Enzyme Regul., *7*:291, 1969.

Williams-Ashman, H. G., Wilson, J., Beil, R., et al.: Transglutaminase reactions associated with the rat semen clotting system. Biochem. Biophys. Res. Commun., *79*:1192, 1977.

Winningham, D. G., and Stamey, T. A.: Diffusion of

sulfonamides from plasma into prostatic fluid. J. Urol., *104*:559, 1970.

Winningham, D. G., Nemoy, N. J., and Stamey, T. A.: Diffusion of antibiotics from plasma into prostatic fluid. Nature, *219*:139, 1968.

Woodward, H. O.: The clinical significance of serum acid phosphatase. Am. J. Med., *27*:902, 1959.

Yam, L. T.: Clinical significance of the human acid phosphatases. A review. Am. J. Med., *56*:604, 1974.

Yamanaka, H., et al.: Arginase in human urogenital tumors. Gann, *63*:693, 1972.

Youmans, G. P., Liebling, J., and Lyman, R. Y.: The bactericidal action of prostatic fluid in dogs. J. Infect. Dis., *63*:117, 1938.

Young, H. H.: Young's Practice of Urology. Vol. I. Philadelphia, W. B. Saunders Co., 1926, p. 419.

Young, H. H. II, and Kent, J. R.: Plasma testosterone levels in patients with prostatic carcinoma before and after treatment. J. Urol., *99*:788, 1968.

Zaneveld, L. J. D., and Chatterton, R. T.: Biochemistry of Mammalian Reproduction. New York, John Wiley & Sons, 1982.

Zaneveld, L. J. D., Schumacher, G. F. B., Tauber, P. F., and Propping, D.: Proteinases and proteinase inhibitors of human semen. *In* Fritz, H., Tschesche, H., Greene, L. J., and Truscheit, E. (Eds.): Proteinasea. Helv. Chim. Acta, *24*:117, 1941.

THE UROLOGIC EXAMINATION AND DIAGNOSTIC TECHNIQUES

Initial Evaluation, Including History, Physical Examination, and Urinalysis

C. EUGENE CARLTON, JR., M.D.
PETER T. SCARDINO, M.D.

Urology is the special branch of medicine that deals with diseases and abnormalities of the genitourinary system of both sexes. Its study encompasses the definition and preservation of the normal and the recognition and correction of the abnormal. A unique advantage enjoyed by the urologist is the ability either to observe or palpate the lesions he is called upon to treat or to demonstrate them graphically through use of refined radiographic techniques, the ultrasonic probe, the uroflowmeter and cystometer, and the cystoscope, ureteroscope, and nephroscope. The intelligent sequential use of these techniques minimizes the chance for erroneous diagnosis.

THE HISTORY

An adequately detailed history is an essential requirement for the success of the investigational and therapeutic efforts to follow. The history should elicit all the facts about conditions that have affected the patient medically during his life and, most importantly, should include an account of those symptoms that have prompted him to seek advice. It must be remembered that in eliciting a history, one is dealing with the subjective manifestations of disease, which are altered by the capacity of patient to observe and describe them. The man-

ner in which a physician obtains a history communicates to the patient his sincere and sympathetic interest, establishing the basis for a successful physician-patient relationship.

The history logically falls into three divisions: (1) the chief complaint; (2) the past history, which should include consideration of possible familial disease related to the patient's illness; and (3) the history of the present illness, which must include information about coexisting diseases, whether or not they seem related to the patient's chief complaint.

CHIEF COMPLAINT

This is usually a definite statement by the patient of his reason for consulting the physician. It is, after all, the problem for which he is seeking relief, and it is on this basis that the patient ultimately appraises the efforts of the physician on his behalf. The patient should be allowed to indicate in his own words the nature of the trouble. Thereafter, the physician, by incisive and thorough questioning, expands on this statement with respect to the duration and severity of the complaint, its periodicity, and the degree of disability produced. A rambling exposition by the patient of his complaints may suggest to the physician that they are possibly exaggerated, that they are largely functional in nature, or that the patient is of only limited intelligence. Such conclusions should not be drawn hastily or without the benefit of supportive evidence. The physician must always be careful not to use medical terminology in his questioning, thereupon mistaking for stupidity the patient's inability to understand him. Persistent and pointed questioning may be necessary to preserve relevancy. A common example is the patient presenting with a symptom complex of prostatism who denies "trouble voiding" and states that his trouble is just the opposite—that he voids "too freely" (frequency). Another example is the necessity of specific questioning in order to differentiate the nocturia of obstruction or infection from the nocturia resulting from nocturnal diuresis of varying etiology.

PRESENT ILLNESS

Careful delineation of the evolution of the patient's present illness is of critical importance, in that it is during this questioning that the physician most often arrives at his initial impression concerning the diagnosis. It is this impression that governs subsequent diagnostic studies, and it is therefore critical to the eventual establishment of the correct diagnosis. Certain symptom complexes are so classic as to lead to an accurate diagnosis in and of themselves, i.e., prostatism, ureteral colic. All too often the inexperienced physician jumps to an initial diagnosis based on the chief complaint alone and fails to develop a lucid and sequential evolution of the present illness, thereby missing the subtle clues that would lead to the correct, although perhaps more obscure, diagnosis. A classic example is the elderly male who is referred to the urologist because of his complaints—the typical symptoms of prostatic obstruction—and who, indeed, has a large prostate and a poor stream. If one fails to elicit by careful questioning the additional symptoms of urinary urgency, frequency, and precipitancy that may accompany a coexistent uninhibited neurogenic bladder secondary to cerebrovascular insufficiency, he may have the unpleasant surprise of a patient with severe urgency incontinence and precipitancy following transurethral resection of his obstructing prostate. Eliciting such symptoms in the development of the present illness in this routine urologic problem would have led the discerning physician to the documentation of the neurologic state of the patient's bladder, allowing him to prevent the disturbing manifestations of the uninhibited neurogenic bladder by use of appropriate neuromuscular blocking agents.

The present illness is best determined by enlarging upon the patient's chief complaint, making note of the date of onset of the earliest symptoms and the onset of corollary symptoms, together with their change and severity. With the passage of time and increasing experience, the careful physician usually develops a routine of his own for listing the present illness, which he modifies or amplifies according to the problem under consideration.

PAST MEDICAL HISTORY

It is important to include all pertinent past illnesses or medical conditions in order to completely evaluate the medical status of the patient and to elicit those diseases that might have a causal relationship to the present illness. Obviously, any past illnesses that might bear upon the patient's tolerance to prospective surgery must be carefully evaluated. Sequelae of past illnesses or of concomitant disease, such as diabetes, hypertension, blood dyscrasias, or neoplasm, may call for a significant modification of both the subsequent investigative efforts and the contemplated treatment.

Careful questioning regarding the family history is of obvious importance. Numerous disease processes or pathologic states of familial incidence or genetic determination involve the urinary tract. Questioning about the patient's family history may give clues valuable to their discovery.

KEY SYMPTOMS

The following list of key symptoms defines and describes the most common symptoms found in patients who consult a urologist.

Chyluria. Passage of lymphatic fluid or chyle in the urine indicates an intrarenal urinary-lymphatic fistula, usually due to a mechanical obstruction of the lymphatics above the kidney, resulting in a spontaneous forniceal rupture. The milky urine is pathognomonic. The classic cause, rarely seen in North America, is filariasis, but retroperitoneal tumors, trauma, and tuberculosis have also been responsible. Chyluria should not be confused with cloudy urine due to infection, phosphate crystals, and the like.

Constitutional Symptoms. Weight loss, fatigue, and anorexia may be the only presenting symptoms of genitourinary disorders, particularly in children. These symptoms are often seen in patients with uremia or metastatic tumors but may simply reflect acute pyelonephritis or hydronephrosis.

Dysuria. Painful or difficult urination is usually related to inflammation of the lower genitourinary tract. Common causes include urinary tract infection, calculus, carcinoma, carcinoma in situ, and interstitial cystitis. Pain at the beginning of urination suggests a urethral cause, whereas pain after voiding suggests an etiology within the bladder. Dysuria is often accompanied by frequency and urgency in a constellation of symptoms often referred to as lower tract irritative symptoms.

Enuresis. Strictly speaking, enuresis indicates involuntary discharge of urine, but the term is commonly used to mean bedwetting, or the involuntary discharge of urine during sleep (nocturnal enuresis). Repeated, unintentional, unconscious, complete voiding at night occurs in 10 to 15 per cent of children between the ages of 4 and 12 years. It is important to note whether the symptom is continuous or intermittent and whether symptoms occur during the day as well. Few patients with enuresis will have significant pathology, but all deserve a careful office evaluation. If the history, physical examination, urinalysis, and concentrating capacity are normal, further investigation is not usually justified.

Fever and Chills. Fever, chills, and flank pain are classic symptoms of pyelonephritis.

Frequency. Urinary frequency is one of the most common urologic symptoms. The normal adult urinates five to six times a day and no more than once a night, with an average volume of 300 ml. Frequent urination may be due to an increased volume of urine (polyuria) or to a decreased capacity of the bladder. Common causes of the latter include bladder outlet obstruction, resulting in residual urine and decreased functional capacity; inflammatory conditions that increase bladder sensitivity; neurogenic bladder; pressure from extrinsic masses; and anxiety.

Hematospermia. The presence of blood in the semen is usually not an indication of significant pathology. Nevertheless, this symptom does warrant a complete history and physical examination and urinalysis. If these preliminary studies are normal, no further investigation is necessary.

Hematuria. Hematuria indicates an abnormal number of red blood cells in the urine. Greater than 2 RBC's per high-power field is considered abnormal. Dilute or alkaline urine may lyse red cells, but the dipstick test will show hemoglobinuria. Urinary casts or proteinuria indicate renal parenchymal disease. Hematuria should be characterized as gross or microscopic; initial, terminal, or total; and painful or painless (see under Key Signs). Bright red urine suggests a bladder source and dark brown urine an upper tract source. Passage of wormlike clots suggests

bleeding from the ureter. Where there are no other symptoms, the more probable diagnoses include bladder tumor, calculus, sickle cell trait, renal cell carcinoma, trauma, and exercise-induced injury. When hematuria is accompanied by urinary symptoms, the presence of calculi, infection, or bladder tumor is more likely, but BPH, renal infarction, and congenital anomalies should be considered. With systemic symptoms, one should consider renal cell carcinoma, glomerulonephritis, renal vein thrombosis, and sickle cell disease.

Hesitancy. Delay in the initiation of urination is termed hesitancy and suggests bladder outlet obstruction. The most common causes are prostatic obstruction and urethral stricture.

Incontinence. Incontinence literally means the inability to refrain from yielding to the normal urge to urinate, but it is generally used to mean failure of voluntary control of urination, with constant or frequent involuntary passage of urine. Useful classifications designate several types of incontinence. Continuous incontinence suggests a vesicovaginal fistula, ectopic ureter, or complete loss of sphincteric activity. Active incontinence indicates intermittent, unpredictable leakage, with complete but involuntary emptying of the bladder at intervals, without warning but in a normal way.

Urgency incontinence indicates a strong sudden desire to void before the patient is able to reach the bathroom. The patient is usually aware of the loss of urine. Cystitis, neurogenic bladder, bladder tumor, and recent prostatectomy are common causes.

Overflow incontinence is due to pressure of retained urine in the bladder. Urine typically dribbles out from a bladder that is greatly distended as a result of obstruction at the bladder neck or urethra. Both enuresis and stress incontinence can occur with urinary retention whenever an increase in intra-abdominal pressure causes the intravesical pressure to rise above the threshold of urethral resistance.

Stress incontinence is the sudden leakage of a small amount of urine with rapid increases in intravesical pressure due to coughing, sneezing, bending, and so forth. The incontinence is not continuous and does not occur when the patient is recumbent. Residual urine is minimal and intravesical pressures are normal, but there is a decrease in sphincter competency owing to poor muscular support.

Intermittency. Intermittent voiding is a symptom of bladder outlet obstruction and is usually accompanied by hesitancy, decrease in the size and force of the urinary stream, and postvoid dribbling. Common causes include

BPH, prostatic carcinoma, and urethral stricture, but neurogenic bladder should also be considered.

Nocturia. Excessive urination at night may be due to an increase in the amount of urine formed at night (diuretics, congestive heart failure) or a decrease in the functional capacity of the bladder (see under Hesitancy). Although often assumed to be a common symptom of prostatism, nocturia is more often unrelated to bladder function per se, and it rarely improves after prostatectomy performed primarily for nocturia.

Pain. Pain is the most common reason for seeking urologic consultation. Pain within the urinary tract is generally due either to distention or to inflammation. The severity of pain is directly related to the rapidity rather than the degree of distention.

Flank pain may be due to sudden distention of the renal capsule (hematoma, acute pyelonephritis, acute obstruction) or renal ischemia (infarction from an embolus or thrombus). Associated gastrointestinal symptoms are not uncommon because of reflex phenomena and the proximity of the pancreas, duodenum, and colon to the kidney.

Renal or ureteral colic is generally due to acute ureteral obstruction, most often from a calculus. It may be steady or spasmodic, but it rarely disappears completely between episodes. Upper ureteral pain may be referred to the ipsilateral testis or labia; midureteral pain to the flank, lower abdomen, or inguinal area; and lower ureteral pain to the suprapubic area or distal urethra.

Perineal pain in men often has its origin in the prostate or bladder. Prostatitis, prostatic carcinoma, cystitis, and bladder cancer may cause perineal, perianal, sacral, or suprapubic pain.

Pain in the Abdomen. Common urologic causes of lower abdominal pain include a distended or inflamed bladder. Pain accompanying urinary retention is associated with an extreme desire to void; pain from cystitis is associated with burning and pain on urination.

Painful Scrotum. Pain in the scrotal area may be referred from the upper ureter or from the trigone or bladder neck, or it may be local. There will be no local tenderness with referred pain. When the problem resides in the bladder, there are usually accompanying voiding symptoms, such as frequency, urgency, and dysuria. Pain of intrascrotal cause, such as from epididymitis, torsion, or tumor, is usually continuous, well localized, and more severe, but referral to the inguinal and lower abdominal areas may

occur and mimic pain of intra-abdominal causes, such as appendicitis or diverticulitis.

Painful Erection. Priapism, or persistent painful erection, indicates a prolonged persistent erection without sexual desire. The glans penis remains flaccid despite a rigid erection of the corpora cavernosa. Most causes are idiopathic, but sickle cell disease, malignant infiltration, and clotting disorders must be considered.

Pneumaturia. Passage of gas in the urine indicates a fistula between the urinary and gastrointestinal tracts, an infection due to gas-forming organisms (often in diabetics), or recent instrumentation of the urinary tract with iatrogenic instillation of air.

Polyuria. Passage of a large volume of urine in a given time must be distinguished from urinary frequency. Common causes include renal disease with decreased concentrating ability, diabetes mellitus, diabetes insipidus, and psychogenic water drinking.

Slow or Weak Stream. A decrease in the size and force of the urinary stream is a common symptom of outlet obstruction and is often accompanied by hesitancy, intermittency, and postvoid dribbling, to form a constellation of symptoms termed lower tract obstructive symptoms. In men, one should consider prostatic obstruction and urethral stricture as common causes.

Urgency. A sudden strong desire to urinate, which can be controlled at least temporarily, constitutes urinary urgency. Along with frequency and dysuria, urgency indicates inflammation of the urinary tract, often involving the trigone or urethra. Common causes include urinary tract infection, lower ureteral calculus, bladder cancer (especially carcinoma in situ), and neurogenic bladder dysfunction.

Urinary Retention. The inability to void is termed urinary retention. If acute, it is often painful, but if chronic, it may not be. The patient passes no urine or dribbles with overflow or stress incontinence. Retention is most often due to prostatic obstruction or neurogenic bladder, but occasionally urethral stricture may be the only etiology. In a child, posterior urethral valves should be considered.

PHYSICAL EXAMINATION

A complete physical examination competently performed is mandatory for any patient who is to undergo instrumentation under anesthesia or a urologic surgical procedure. This general examination will most commonly be carried out by the referring physician or the consulting internist, but the urologist must assure himself that a thorough and complete examination has been performed prior to assuming responsibility for surgical procedures.

During their years of preliminary training, all medical students are taught a system that includes the important features of the patient's physical examination, and this routine will always be followed, regardless of whether the student ultimately practices medicine, surgery, or one of the specialties. There are, however, some points in the physical examination that have an important bearing on the diagnosis of urologic disease, and these are worthy of restatement.

GENERAL OBSERVATION

Inspection of the patient's face frequently reveals much to the physician, permitting some important early generalizations regarding the authenticity and severity of his complaint. The agitated, the apprehensive, and the guilt-ridden are readily identifiable. Genuine pain and suffering are undeniably reflected in the patient's features, whereas the paradoxical serenity of the face of the patient who is relating a story of great suffering suggests that the complaints are psychogenic in origin.

The skin should be inspected for evidence of jaundice or pallor, which might suggest malignancy. Rough, dry, atonic skin is suggestive of renal failure. Skin striae and the presence of a buffalo hump over the upper thoracic spine are suggestive of hyperadrenocorticism. Gynecomastia indicates a possible endocrinopathy, perhaps associated with adrenal tumor, testicular tumor, or pituitary disorder. In the aging male, gynecomastia may well indicate portal cirrhosis or may indicate estrogen therapy for carcinoma of the prostate of which the patient may be unaware. Edema of the lower extremities suggests cardiac decompensation, venous insufficiency, or lymphatic obstruction that possibly results from metastatic genitourinary carcinoma. Atrophic hairless skin of the lower extremities may signal peripheral vascular insufficiency.

EXAMINATION OF THE KIDNEY

A kidney that is grossly enlarged by tumor, cysts, or hydronephrosis may give a fullness to the flank or may cause a rounded elevation of the abdomen. A perinephric abscess will often cause a lagging of the respiratory movement of the affected side and also may result in a bulging appearance on the affected side when compared with the opposite flank. This bulging is most noticeable when the patient sits up and leans forward.

Edema of the skin of the flank is not uncommon with perinephric abscess. An abscess adjacent to the psoas muscle will result in scoliosis with the convexity away from the involved kidney.

The kidneys are usually not palpable in adults because of their location in the uppermost portion of the abdominal cavity beneath the lower ribs. This palpation is rendered even more difficult in the presence of good muscular development or obesity. The right kidney is characteristically lower than the left kidney, particularly in thin females, and therefore somewhat more easily palpable. The most successful method of renal palpation is carried out with the patient lying supine on a hard surface (Fig. 6–1). The kidney is lifted in one hand in the costovertebral angle. On deep inspiration the kidney moves downward, and when it is lowest, the other hand is pushed firmly and deeply beneath the costal margin in an effort to trap the kidney below that point. If this is successful, the anterior hand can palpate the size, shape,

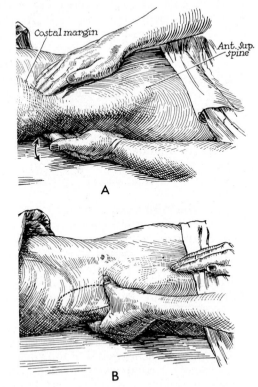

Figure 6–1. Renal palpation. *A*, By ballottement, in which the kidney is gently thrown upward by the under hand. *B*, By manual compression, with one hand as shown here (infants), or bimanually, as indicated in *A*.

and consistency of the organ as it slips back into its normal position.

Auscultation of the costovertebral area in the upper abdominal quadrant during deep expiration may reveal a systolic bruit associated with stenosis or aneurysm of the renal artery. A bruit may also be present in a large arteriovenous fistula or malformation, which may have resulted in the patient's presentation with hematuria.

Transillumination is of value primarily in neonates or small children with palpable abdominal masses. The child should be placed in a completely dark room, and when the examiner's eyes have been accustomed to darkness, a fiberoptic light source is applied to the posterior flank. Fluid-filled masses, such as hydronephroses or cysts, will result in a dull red glow in the anterior abdomen overlying the mass.

EXAMINATION OF THE BLADDER

The normal bladder cannot be palpated or percussed until it contains in excess of 150 ml of fluid. When the bladder contains more than 500 ml of fluid, it may be identified as a bulge in the suprapubic area when the patient lies supine on the examining table.

Percussion of the lower abdomen will delineate the dome of the bladder if it contains in excess of 150 ml of urine. Percussion is perhaps the most reliable way to detect a distended bladder in the obese patient. The distended bladder may be palpated as a firm, round, movable mass rising out of the pelvis, and on bimanual examination, the bladder can be palpated or percussed between the two examining hands. Careful bimanual examination should be carried out, preferably under anesthesia, in patients suspected or known to have bladder carcinoma. Unsuspected fixation of the bladder to the lateral pelvic wall obviously alters the therapeutic approach in bladder carcinoma.

EXAMINATION OF THE PENIS

If the patient has not been circumcised, the foreskin should be retracted to rule out tumor or balanitis. Dorsal slitting or circumcision is indicated in the presence of a swelling, tenderness, or discharge from beneath the foreskin that prevents its retraction.

The urethral meatus should be inspected, and its normal size and location should be documented. The meatus should be separated by the thumb and forefinger in a search for neoplastic or inflammatory lesions within the fossa navicularis. Discharge from the urethral meatus should be noted, and appropriate bacteriologic studies should be carried out on the material.

Palpation of the shaft of the penis may reveal a fibrous plaque involving the fascial coverings of the corpora cavernosa, typical of Peyronie's disease. Tender areas of induration palpated along the urethra may signify periurethritis secondary to urethral stricture. Nontender induration of the urethra suggests stricture, and a nontender mass along the course of the urethra suggests urethral carcinoma.

EXAMINATION OF THE SCROTUM AND ITS CONTENTS

Infections and inflammations of the skin of the scrotum are uncommon, but sebaceous cysts of the scrotal skin are frequent. Malignant tumors are rare, occurring primarily in chimney sweeps.

The testes should be carefully palpated between the thumb and the first two fingers. The consistency of the testes should be noted. The normal testis is quite firm, almost hard, and freely mobile. Abnormally soft testes suggest dysgenesis or endocrinopathy. A firm or hard area within the substance of the testis must be considered neoplastic until this possibility is ruled out by surgical exploration. The relative weights of the two testes should be estimated by the examiner—the tumor-bearing testis is invariably heavier than its normal mate.

The epididymis should be carefully palpated between the thumb and forefinger along its entire course. Nodular induration of the epididymis may indicate tuberculosis. A mass that is demonstrable on transillumination usually represents spermatocele, whereas a solid mass that does not transilluminate probably represents adenomatoid tumor.

A cystic mass seen around the testis on transillumination is diagnostic of a hydrocele; if this mass prevents adequate palpation of the testis, the hydrocele should be aspirated, ultrasonography performed, or the testis explored. Approximately 10 per cent of testicular tumors present with a reactive hydrocele.

The spermatic cord structure should be rolled between thumb and forefinger, and the vas deferens should be palpated along its entire course below the inguinal canal. Absence of the vas deferens is of obvious importance in the infertile male. A gravity-dependent varicocele can be seen with the patient in the upright position. A less obvious varicocele can be confirmed by the palpation of a "pulse" in the varicocele during cough or Valsalva maneuver.

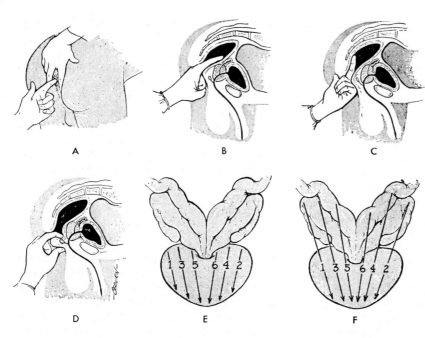

A

B

C

D

E

F

Figure 6–2. Rectal examination. *A*, Introduction of protected, well-lubricated finger. *B*, Palpation of prostate and seminal vesicles, lateral view. *C*, Palpation of anterior surface of sacrum and coccyx. *D*, Palpation of Cowper's gland. *E*, Massage of prostate for specimen collection or treatment; order of "strokes" is indicated, gradually working toward the center (verumontanum). *F*, Massage of seminal vesicles and prostate. (From Campbell, M. F.: Principles of Urology. Philadelphia, W. B. Saunders Co., 1957.)

EXAMINATION OF THE PROSTATE

During the course of their clinical training, medical students are repeatedly admonished that no physical examination is complete if it does not include a careful digital examination of the rectum, regardless of the age or sex of the patient (Fig. 6–2). Despite this fact, it is altogether amazing how often this important study is omitted or "deferred" indefinitely. Possibly a combination of two factors is responsible: (1) the physician's lack of confidence in his ability to interpret the findings correctly, and (2) his reluctance to subject the patient to a procedure that the latter regards with aversion as being undignified. The urologist works in a field that precludes his right to have qualms about either. The need for a careful, thorough palpation of the rectum to as high a level as the examining finger can reach is even more important in the aged patient.

Current statistics indicate that carcinoma of the colon is one of the two most common cancers in the elderly male in the United States, and the urologist has a unique opportunity to discover these lesions in patients who suffer prostatic symptoms. All too often, however, this opportunity is missed if the urologist fails to probe the entire interior of the rectum and focuses his attention on the examination of the prostate. If the examiner consistently follows a routine in performing the digital rectal examination, there is considerably less likelihood of serious diagnostic error. In order, the following

should be described: the tonicity of the rectal sphincter; the rectal ampulla; and the size, shape, and consistency of the prostate together with observations concerning nodules, cysts, asymmetry, induration, and fixation. The lateral sulci and the median furrow of the prostate are carefully palpated, and the size, shape, and consistency of the seminal vesicles are noted. The physician should then swing his finger in a 360 degree sweep of the interior of the rectum to search for mass lesions.

The position the patient assumes for the digital rectal examination is a matter of the examiner's preference. Most examiners prefer to have the patient stand with his toes pointed inward and bent over the end of an examining table. In aged or sick patients, it may be necessary to perform the examination with the patient in the dorsal or lateral recumbent position.

If the patient complains of severe pain on the attempted introduction of the examining finger into the rectum and if the sphincter remains tight, then a fistula in the anus or severe cryptitis may exist. A relaxed or dilated rectal sphincter suggests similar changes in the urinary sphincter and may be a clue to the diagnosis of neurogenic disease. In the adult male, the normal prostate is approximately the size of a quarter, but its shape is usually described as approximating that of a chestnut. Its lateral margins are discrete, and a moderate degree of mobility is felt when the index finger is hooked over the upper border of the gland and pushed up and down. It is of some importance to remember that only the lateral lobes of the prostate are palpable on digital rectal examination and that these are felt through the posterior lobe, which is usually a thin lamellation extending upward from the prostatic apex. The anterior lobe cannot be felt, and very rarely is the median lobe palpable. Only if the patient is very thin and has a flaccid abdominal wall can a markedly enlarged median lobe protruding intravesically be discerned. The consistency of the normal adult prostate is firm and elastic, and it offers the resiliency of a rubber ball to the examining finger. A shallow median furrow is usually palpable. This is accentuated in early prostatic hyperplasia of the lateral lobes but may become obliterated as the hyperplasia becomes more prominent. The prostate may be mushy if it is congested, owing to a lack of intercourse or to chronic infection with impaired drainage. It may be indurated because of chronic infection or may be stony hard, owing to carcinoma or calculous disease. The boggy prostate, the crepitant calculus-containing prostate, and the obvious hard carcinoma of the prostate are easily categorized. Considerable difficulty may arise for even the most experienced examiner in the differentiation of fibrosis from nonspecific infection, granulomatous prostatitis, nodulation from tuberculous infection, and firm areas due to prostatic calculi or early carcinoma. If any induration of the prostate persists following treatment of infection and the exclusion of prostatic calculi with appropriate radiography, prostatic biopsy should be carried out.

The technique of prostatic massage is indicated in Figure 6–2. If this technique is followed, a specimen of prostatic fluid can almost invariably be produced. Microscopic examination of the prostatic fluid should be carried out under low-power magnification. Normal secretions contain numerous lecithin bodies, which are similar to but much smaller than refractile-like red blood cells. Only an occasional white blood cell is present in normal prostatic secretion. An occasional epithelial cell and corpora amylacea may be seen. The presence of large numbers of pus cells is pathologic and establishes the diagnosis of prostatitis. Specimens of prostatic fluid for postmassage urine specimen should be submitted to the laboratory for appropriate bacteriologic study.

The normal seminal vesicles are rarely palpable, since their consistency is much the same as that of surrounding tissue. When distended with retained secretions, they may be felt easily, and their consistency may be boggy or almost fluctuant. Depression of these distended vesicles may yield quantities of clear secretion that usually contains only a few white blood cells. Vesicles may be so large that they obscure the outlines of the underlying prostate, and a common error is to mistake them for the prostate. Their upward lateral extension usually aids in their identification. If involved by carcinomatous extension from the prostate, they are stony hard. If involved by tuberculosis, they may be nodular.

KEY SIGNS

In this section, the most common signs of urologic disorders are defined and described, and the method of evaluation and differential diagnosis is mentioned when appropriate.

Anuria. Anuria refers to the excretion of less than 100 ml of urine in 24 hours, and severe oliguria indicates less than 600 ml in 24 hours (in the adult). The urologist is often called upon to see such a patient to rule out a postrenal cause for severe oliguria. Attention should be directed to the lower abdomen to see if the urinary bladder is distended. Careful inspection, percussion, and palpation may identify the problem. The physician also should inspect any drainage tubes. If a urethral catheter is present, it should be irrigated and any kinks straightened. If the bladder is not catheterized, a urethral catheter should be passed. If only a small amount of urine is obtained, obstruction above the level of the ureterovesical junction can be ruled out with a renal ultrasound study or retrograde pyelograms.

Bruit. Auscultation over the epigastrium may reveal the murmur associated with renal arterial stenosis in a patient with hypertension. A continuous bruit, heard over the flank, indicates a renal arteriovenous fistula.

Costovertebral Angle Tenderness. Tenderness to palpation or percussion over the flank or costovertebral angle (CVA) may indicate inflammation of the kidney from acute pyelonephritis or hydronephrosis, renal trauma, or tumor.

Edema. Edema of the genitalia may be due to local conditions, such as trauma, urinary extravasation, or pelvic or lower abdominal surgery or radiotherapy. But genital edema also arises from systemic conditions, such as congestive heart failure, renal insufficiency, hepatic failure, or hypoalbuminemia, especially in the bedridden patient. If the patient is ambulatory, the lower extremities are usually edematous as well.

Flank or Abdominal Mass. A kidney is not normally palpable except in very thin women or those with nephroptosis. The knee–elbow position or deep inspiration often helps. Bimanual palpation, with one hand lifting anteriorly in the soft tissue of the CVA and the other pressing firmly just beneath the costal margin, is particularly useful for detecting a renal mass (see Fig. 6–1). If the mass involves the kidney itself, it will often be ballotable. In children, abdominal masses are more often genitourinary than gastrointestinal in origin, with hydronephrosis, multicystic dysplastic kidney, polycystic kidney, Wilms' tumor, and nephroblastoma being the most common.

Hematuria and Pseudohematuria. Hematuria refers to passage of blood in the urine. It should be characterized as occurring at the beginning of urination (initial), throughout (total), or at the end (terminal). Initial hematuria suggests a source in the urethra, while terminal suggests the bladder neck or prostate. Total hematuria indicates a source within the bladder or above. If there is accompanying pain with voiding, this suggests cystitis or urethritis. If the pain is colicky and in the flank or abdomen, this suggests passage of clots from a renal or ureteral tumor or calculus; painless, gross total hematuria, however, suggests a bladder tumor. Even a single episode of hematuria requires a complete urologic investigation.

Pseudohematuria refers to reddish discoloration of the urine caused by pigments other than blood. Examples include medications such as Pyridium, foods such as beets, vegetable dyes, urate crystals, and porphyria.

Hypertension. When the blood pressure is persistently elevated (diastolic greater than 90), hypertension becomes a serious risk factor for the development of morbid cardiovascular complications and requires treatment. It is the urologist's role to identify hypertensive patients and to initiate an evaluation for treatable causes, when appropriate. Surgically treatable causes include renovascular and renal parenchymal diseases as well as certain adrenal tumors, such as pheochromocytoma, hyperaldosteronism, and Cushing's syndrome.

Hypospadias. This is a developmental anomaly in which the urethra opens on the underside of the penis or on the perineum in the male, or into the vagina in the female.

Inguinal Lymph Nodes. Enlarged or tender inguinal nodes may indicate inflammatory or malignant conditions of the glans penis, shaft of the penis, urethra, or scrotum in the male and the vulva, introitus, vagina, or urethra in the female.

Mass Within the Scrotum. An intrascrotal mass may be painful or painless, acute or chronic. The common painless masses include hydrocele and spermatocele, which feel cystic and transilluminate easily; scrotal hernia, which does not transilluminate but palpably extends above the neck of the scrotum into the external ring; and varicocele, palpable as a "bag of worms," usually on the left side, which enlarges when the patient stands or performs the Valsalva maneuver. A testicular tumor is usually not painful and is palpable as a mass within the tunica albuginea; it is distinguishable as a nodular, firm, irregular area in contrast to the smooth, rounded, even consistency of the normal testis.

Painful intrascrotal masses are commonly caused by epididymitis, testicular torsion, and tumors (which are painful in 20 per cent of cases). Epididymitis usually occurs after puberty; is very common; may be associated with fever, urinary infection, or urethral discharge; and can be distinguished by exquisite tenderness and induration of the epididymis itself, often extending along the vas into the spermatic cord. Torsion often causes the most severe pain; may be very sudden in onset; is not associated with infection or pyuria; and is common before puberty. In torsion, the testis may not be palpably distinct from the epididymis. With gentle elevation of the involved testicle, there is usually some relief of pain with epididymitis but not with torsion.

Paraphimosis. This condition produces tightness of the foreskin such that when retracted it cannot be reduced and acts as a constricting tourniquet, causing progressive edema of the glans.

Pelvic Mass. The most common urologic cause of a pelvic mass is a distended bladder. The bladder is not normally palpable unless it contains greater than 500 ml, at which point it begins to distend the lower abdomen. Careful inspection of the contour of the lower abdomen will suggest the diagnosis by a characteristic bulge of the full bladder. The nature of the mass can be confirmed by dullness to percussion, by an urge to void with sharp percussion, and by the disappearance of the mass with urethral catheterization. Other causes might be a distended colon, malignant tumor of the bladder, and seminal vesicle cyst in the male; in the female, a gravid uterus, fibroids, and ovarian cyst or tumor.

Penile Plaques. The firm fibrous plaques palpable on the dorsa of the corpora cavernosa over the shaft of the penis are the plastic induration of Peyronie's disease. This idiopathic disorder may cause chordee, painful erections, and impotence.

Phimosis. This condition causes tightness of the foreskin, making it difficult to retract back over the glans penis. This is usually due to chronic infections and inflammation, but it may be congenital. Serious obstruction to voiding may occur but is uncommon. A dorsal slit or circumcision may be necessary to expose the tip of the penis to rule out tumors and to allow proper hygiene.

Proteinuria. The excretion of more than 150 mg protein in 24 hours is considered abnormal. Transient proteinuria may be due to heavy exercise, fever, or congestive heart failure. Orthostatic proteinuria occurs only with standing and is associated with no increased risk for development of renal disease. Persistent proteinuria, detected by dipstick and confirmed by 24-hour urinary protein determination, indicates renal disease. A false positive dipstick reading occurs with very alkaline urine, by contamination by prostatic fluid or hemoglobin, and with certain drugs, such as penicillin and tolbutamide.

Pyuria. Pyuria is the presence of pus in the urine, usually defined as greater than 2 to 5 WBC's per high-power field of spun urinary sediment. Common causes include urinary tract infection (bacteriuria), calculi, tumors, and tuberculosis.

Undescended Testis. The testis that is not found within the scrotum may be ectopic or undescended. The ectopic testis may be at the base of the penis, in the inguinal area outside the inguinal canal, or in the femoral area of the medial thigh. The undescended or cryptorchid testis may lie at the external ring, within the inguinal canal, or in the retroperitoneum above the internal ring. Cryptorchidism is a developmental defect characterized by failure of the testis to descend into the scrotum. It can be distinguished from the far more common retractile testis in children by having the child squat or by placing him in a warm tub, allowing the cremasteric muscle to relax.

Urethral Discharge. Discharge of fluid from the urethra, either spontaneously or after manual external stripping, indicates urethritis. The most common causes are gonorrhea and nongonococcal urethritis. Gram stain and culture of the fluid are indicated.

Urinalysis

R. W. KINDRACHUK, M.D.
T. A. STAMEY, M.D.*

Many diagnostic procedures are available for the work-up of the patient with urinary tract disease. In spite of complex imaging techniques and functional measurements, a careful history and examination of the urine remain the foundation of a thorough urologic evaluation. Great attention to detail, however, must be given to all steps in the urinalysis: collection of specimens, culture of the urines, analysis of the supernatant, and microscopic examination of the urinary sediment.

COLLECTION OF SPECIMENS FOR URINALYSIS AND CULTURE

The urine should be collected in an effort to segment the voided stream into its diagnostic parts, as described in Chapter 14. In brief, the well-hydrated male initiates voiding after the foreskin is retracted and cleansed; the first few milliliters represent the urethral aliquot (VB_1, for voided bladder 1). Any volume greater than 5 to 8 ml in the VB_1 serves only to dilute the cells and bacteria from the prostatic, bulbar, and distal urethra. After the voiding of 200 to 300 ml, a second specimen, the VB_2 (voided bladder 2), is collected, which represents bladder, ureteral, and renal urine. The patient then stops voiding, residual urine is removed from the bulbar and distal urethra, and expressed prostatic secretion (EPS) is collected under sterile conditions. The EPS should appear at the urethral meatus as pure opalescent prostatic

*All of the figures and much of the text for this subsection are taken from Stamey, T. A., and Kindrachuk, R. W.: Urinary Sediment and Urinalysis: A Practical Guide for the Health Science Professional. Philadelphia, W. B. Saunders Co., 1985.

fluid, without any yellow tint of urine. Because EPS crosses the urethra, however, contamination with urethral bacteria occurs. Once the prostatic massage is completed, the patient again voids his first few milliliters of urine into a culture tube (VB_3, for voided bladder 3); this specimen will include prostatic fluid as well, but it will also be contaminated by urethral components. Because EPS collects large numbers of indigenous urethral bacteria, especially *Staphylococcus epidermidis* and diphtheroids, gram-positive prostatitis should be diagnosed only when the colony counts of the VB_3 exceed the VB_1 by ten times or more (Stamey, 1981).

In the female, the urine is collected in a similar segmented fashion, which allows localization of disease to the mucosa of the vaginal introitus, the urethra, and the bladder or kidney (Stamey, 1980). After placing the patient on the edge of a table in a semi-sitting position with the legs in stirrups, the nurse spreads the labia and swabs the vaginal introitus with two sterile cotton applicator sticks at the level of the hymenal ring. The sticks are then placed in a test tube containing 5 ml of sterile saline or transport broth. This fluid represents a semi-quantitative estimate of the bacteria and cells on the vaginal introitus, both at this level and throughout the vagina. Next, the nurse spreads the labia and carefully collects the first voided few milliliters by holding a culture tube 1 cm from the urethral meatus. This aliquot, representative of the cells and bacteria on the urethral mucosa, is labeled VB_1, similar to the male urethral aliquot. As the patient continues to void, the midstream aliquot (VB_2) is collected as late as possible in the voided stream to minimize urethral contamination and to more accurately reflect the status of bladder urine.

Whenever vaginal contamination cannot be avoided, suprapubic needle aspiration of the bladder (SPA) should always be performed. It is especially helpful in small infants who are diapered and who have extensive perineal contamination. If SPA is not feasible, and the female patient cannot void with the nurse separating the labia, direct urethral catheterization remains the best technique available to obtain an uncontaminated bladder specimen. Since the catheter will carry some organisms into the bladder, whenever possible, several hundred milliliters of bladder urine should flow through the catheter before a representative bladder aliquot is collected. Because bacteria are always carried by the catheter into the bladder, 24 hours of an oral antimicrobial agent should be given as prophylaxis in case the bladder urine is

sterile. Owing to the effective washout of urethral cells and bacteria by a clean bladder urine in the male, there is no excuse to catheterize a male for a bladder specimen if he is able to void for a midstream collection.

EXAMINATION OF THE SUPERNATANT URINE

Routine chemical analysis of the urine should be performed only on the supernatant of the centrifuged specimen because uroepithelial cells as well as inflammatory cells can give a false positive sulfosalicylic acid test for protein. This potential artifact can be avoided by centrifuging 10 to 15 ml of the midstream voided, aspirated, or catheterized urine. Glucose and pH are determined using the appropriate paper indicators. Protein is detected by pouring off 2.5 ml of supernatant urine into a Kingsbury-Clark sulfosalicylic acid test tube, to which is added 7.5 ml of 3 per cent sulfosalicylic acid.* *Any* precipitate is indicative of proteinuria and represents an abnormal finding whose cause is worth pursuing. Even 18-hour dehydrated, supernatant urine specimens from patients with normal kidneys will not show turbidity with 3 per cent sulfosalicylic acid. Normal supernatant urines contain no detectable protein with this method; thus, the presence of any turbidity constitutes a definite abnormality. False positive results may be caused by some radiographic contrast agents, massive amounts of penicillin, para-aminosalicylic acid, and tolbutamide metabolites.

Two hundred mg of urinary protein per 24 hours is often accepted as the upper limit of normal for protein excretion in healthy adults, based upon 24-hour collections of the total voided urine; 24-hour urines, however, contain millions of epithelial cells, leukocytes, red blood cells, vaginal secretions, and so forth. More recent studies on urinary protein excretion have used highly sensitive and specific radioimmunoassays (Peterson and Berggard, 1971; Mogensen, et al., 1979). They show that the healthy adult excretes only about 9 mg of albumin, 2 mg of IgA, 3 mg of IgG, and 3.3 mg of free light chains per 24 hours, suggesting that the upper limit of normal for 24-hour urinary pro-

---

*In actual practice, any clear test tube with a mark at the 2.5 ml and 10.0 ml levels will serve for detecting turbidity. Since any precipitate is pathologic, the exact amount is of little importance—which negates the need for albumin-formaldehyde standards, which are available from 10 to 100 mg per dl.

tein excretion in the supernatant is about 20 mg, not 200 mg. These data confirm the clinical observations of why sensitivity of the 3 per cent sulfosalicylic acid is uniquely useful as a routine test for urinary protein: 5 mg per dl (in a representative 1200 ml of 24-hour urine), which 3 per cent sulfosalicylic acid can just detect, is 60 mg per 24 hours—a value that is three times the normal excretion. When the 3 per cent sulfosalicylic acid test is positive on the supernatant of the centrifuged urine, more exact quantitation of the amount of protein loss can be measured by collecting a 24-hour urine, if clinically indicated. The advantages, then, of the 3 per cent sulfosalicylic acid test are (1) its greater accuracy and sensitivity over the dipstick methods, (2) its ability to detect Bence Jones protein (unlike the dipstick technique), and (3) its ease of use in determining the presence or absence of significant proteinuria.

The detection of a positive glucose test is obviously useful in diagnosing diabetes with glucosuria. The determination of pH, however, is helpful only if the urine is acid, since hydrated urines tend to be more alkaline. If the pH of the urine is important, the patient should be given pH paper (Nitrazine is adequate) to record the acidity of each voided urine throughout 24-hour periods for a more intelligent assessment. The determination of specific gravity on a hydrated urine is useless and is not performed on the supernatant. If urine concentrating ability is important to the physician, a proper dehydration test should be carried out. For routine work, examination of the supernatant is limited to the pH, the detection of glucose, and the determination of protein by the 3 per cent sulfosalicylic acid test. The last test is by far the most rewarding.

URINARY SEDIMENT

We have presented elsewhere a detailed manual, *Urinary Sediment and Urinalysis* (Stamey and Kindrachuk, 1985); it is a practical guide that medical students or house staff officers can carry in their coat pockets. The interested reader may find this manual useful.

Because 0.01 to 0.02 ml is the maximum volume that will fit comfortably under a 22 mm^2 coverglass, and because the diagnostic sediment in a grossly clear urine may be compacted into a thin, almost invisible line at the bottom of the centrifuge tube, the major error in examination of the urinary sediment is *failure to get the diagnostic sediment under the coverglass for mi-*

croscopic examination. The correct procedure is to turn the centrifuge tube upside down, discarding all the visible supernatant. If the centrifuge tube is plastic (which has poor wetting quality compared with glass), about 0.02 ml of supernatant will run down the sides of the tube to the bottom of the sediment when the tube is returned to the upright position. The tube must then be agitated either by tapping the bottom of the tube against the back of the hand, or, more directly, by vigorously tapping the tube against a tabletop. This will assure resuspension of an almost invisible sediment into a small volume of about 0.02 ml, which can then be tapped onto a microscopic glass slide and covered with a 22 mm^2 coverglass. This seemingly insignificant, but important, maneuver is the only way to get the sediment under the coverglass.

Low-Power Field Examination

With the potentially diagnostic urinary sediment now under the coverglass, the entire 22 mm^2 coverglass is scanned with the low-power field. A specific search for the six subjects listed in Table 6–1 should be systematically undertaken. Three of these six—red blood cell (RBC) casts, trichomonads, and cystine crystals—are diagnostic of specific diseases: glomerulonephritis, *Trichomonas vaginalis* infestation, and cystinuria, respectively.

When casts are encountered, whether RBC casts or cellular-granular casts, the objective should be immediately changed to the high-power field ($\times$ 400) in order to determine whether they contain RBC or not. Tamm-Horsfall mucoprotein, the basic matrix of renal casts (McQueen and Sidney, 1966), is always present in the urine and originates from the tubular epithelial cells. A cast is formed when these proteins precipitate, effected by electrolyte concentration increases and a decrease in urinary pH (one should bear in mind that as a precipitate, casts can and will dissolve, especially with an increase in pH). Hyaline casts, composed

TABLE 6–1. SIX OBJECTS OF DIAGNOSTIC IMPORTANCE: LOW-POWER FIELD (100 $\times$)

1. Red blood cell (RBC) casts
2. Cellular-granular casts
3. Oval fat macrophages
4. Trichomonads
5. Clumps of white blood cells (WBC)
6. Cystine crystals

only of this mucoprotein matrix, can occur normally in small numbers. When cellular elements are present in the renal tubular lumina, they can be entrapped by precipitation of this Tamm-Horsfall mucoprotein. This forms a mold that effectively preserves these elements and acts to localize their source for the observer.

RED BLOOD CELL (RBC) CASTS

Casts with entrapped erythrocytes, or red blood cell casts, are diagnostic of glomerular bleeding (Figs. 6–3 to 6–5). It is essential that red cell membranes be sharply defined in at least part of the cast matrix. Occasionally, it may be difficult to visualize the characteristic hyaline matrix. Fibrinogen, which enters the tubule from damaged glomeruli along with red blood cells, is probably converted to fibrin and may form the majority of the matrix in RBC casts. In those patients with more significant microscopic hematuria, hemoglobin casts are frequently seen as densely packed, reddish brown casts (Figs. 6–6 to 6–9). They represent degenerated erythrocytes and hemoglobin pigment. The presence of red blood cells or hemoglobin in a cast is an indication of bleeding within the glomerulus and, for all practical purposes, represents glomerulonephritis. This therefore indicates renal disease and may require nephrologic investigation as to the specific form of glomerulonephritis, especially if the patient is azotemic.

CELLULAR-GRANULAR CASTS

Cellular-granular casts (Figs. 6–10 and 6–57) are usually derived from renal tubular epithelial cells sloughed into the lumen and entrapped in the mucoprotein matrix. True white blood cell (WBC) casts are rarely seen, even in acute clinical pyelonephritis; when present, they require a peroxidase stain to identify the characteristic enzyme of polymorphonuclear leukocytes. Cellular-granular casts nearly always indicate tubular damage from some form of nephron disease.

The descriptive terms "coarsely granular" and "finely granular" are frequently used. It has been suggested that as degeneration progresses, coarsely granular casts demonstrate increasingly finer cellular debris and become more homogeneous. Waxy casts (Fig. 6–58), with their distinctive homogeneous smooth appearance, represent the final stage in cellular breakdown. As they require time to degenerate, they probably form as a result of prolonged nephron obstruction and oliguria. They are commonly found in patients with end-stage renal disease. In the elderly patient with nephrosclerosis, cellular-granular casts are quite frequent even in the absence of proteinuria. A variation of the cellular-granular cast is the fatty cast, which contains cholesterol bodies that appear doubly refractive with black borders when the low-power adjustment is moved finely up and down (Fig. 6–11). Their presence has the same significance as the finding of oval fat macrophages. It indicates that lipid is being lost into the nephron, either directly or as the result of renal tubular degeneration. Fatty casts are commonly found in diseases causing the nephrotic syndrome.

False casts may occur as a result of the "alkaline tide," which commonly precipitates amorphous phosphates in normal urine. The lack of a protein matrix border characteristic of pathologic casts and the presence of similar-appearing, indiscriminate precipitates scattered throughout the sediment distinguish normal phosphate casts from those characteristic of renal disease.

OVAL FAT MACROPHAGES

Histiocytes, laden with fat droplets, appear as oval brown bodies under the low-power field

---

Figure 6–3. *A,* Low-power view of a red blood cell cast. Note the distinct borders of the hyaline matrix. *B,* Same cast at high power demonstrates sharply defined red cell membranes. Berger's disease.

Figure 6–4. *A,* Red blood cell cast from a patient with biopsy-proven Berger's disease (low-power view). *B,* High-power view of same cast. Again, note well-defined matrix and sharp red cell membranes.

Figure 6–5. Sediment from postexercise urine specimen in same patient as in Figure 6–3. Presence of red blood cell cast confirms diagnosis of glomerulonephritis.

Figure 6–6. A hemoglobin cast in the same urinary sediment as Figures 6–3 and 6–4.

Figure 6–7. *A,* Hemoglobin cast at low power in unstained urinary sediment with characteristic reddish brown coloration. *B,* At high-power view an occasional red cell membrane can be faintly seen among the degenerating RBC's in a fibrin matrix. Notice lack of clear matrix border.

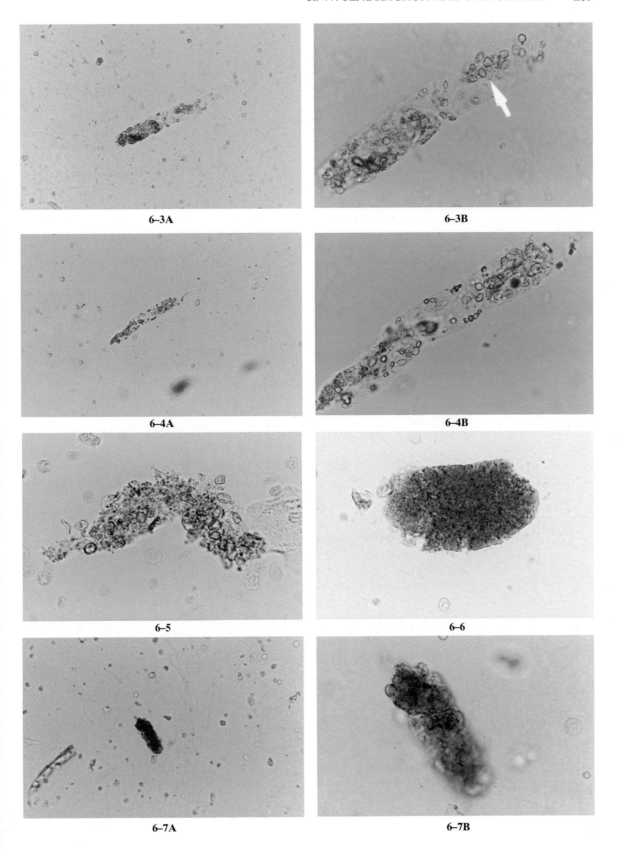

6–3A

6–3B

6–4A

6–4B

6–5

6–6

6–7A

6–7B

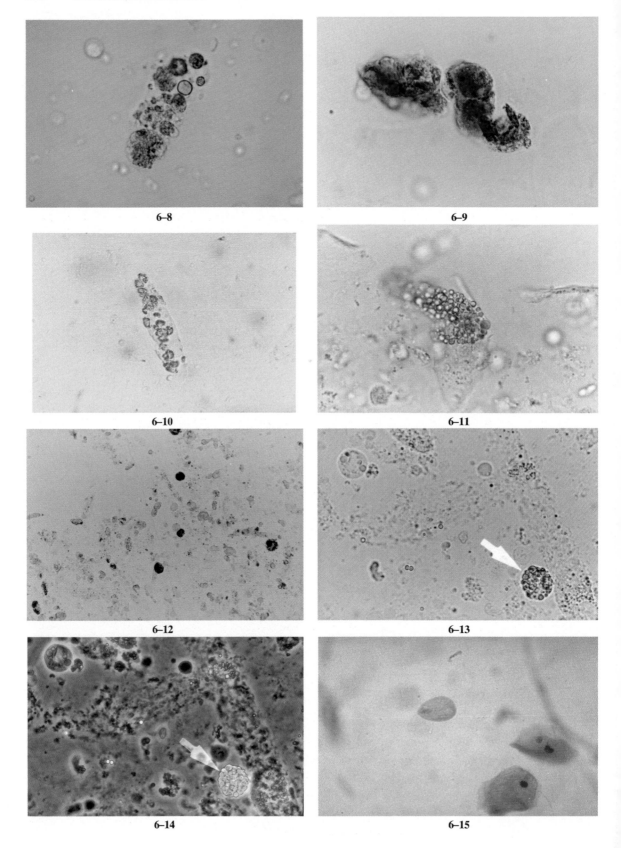

6–8

6–9

6–10

6–11

6–12

6–13

6–14

6–15

(Figs. 6–12 to 6–14). The term "oval fat macrophage" is descriptive because these histiocytes phagocytize fat droplets, similar to those seen in fatty casts. These droplets show the doubly refractile borders characteristic of fat. Oval fat macrophages have been found in a wide variety of nephropathies and indicate extensive tubular degeneration. Sediment from patients with the nephrotic syndrome commonly demonstrate these macrophages.

TRICHOMONADS

Trichomonads are most easily detected under the low-power field (Fig. 6–15). Owing to the accompanying pyuria and large numbers of contaminating squamous epithelial cells, their identification is best accomplished by seeking out sudden, jerky movements of these larger adjacent cells. Motion of their flagella is necessary to prove the presence of trichomonads. Thus, unusual, sudden motion of single leukocytes or epithelial cells nearly always signifies a trichomonad beside the cell, whose flagella can be identified by its rapid, characteristic motion when viewed with the high-power objective.

WHITE BLOOD CELLS (WBC)

While scanning with the low-power field it is valuable to note the presence of clumps of inflammatory cells, as opposed to individual ones, since this probably indicates a more severe inflammatory response.

CYSTINE CRYSTALS

The last diagnostic structure identifiable under the low-power field is a cystine crystal,

TABLE 6–2. Six Objects of Diagnostic Importance: High-Power Field (400×)

1. Bacilli
2. Streptococci
3. Staphylococci
4. Yeasts (distinction from red blood cells and biconcave oval calcium oxalate crystals)
5. Elucidation of casts
6. Types of WBC and RBC

signifying cystinuria (Fig. 6–59). The perfect "benzene ring" structure is characteristic of cystinuria. Since calcium oxalate, calcium phosphate, and urate crystals appear in normal urines with about the same frequency as in urines of stone formers, the benzene rings of cystine stones represent the only truly diagnostic crystal observed in the urine.

High-Power Field Examination

BACTERIA AND YEASTS

After complete scanning with the low-power field for the six microscopic structures listed in Table 6–1, one is now ready to study the urinary sediment with the high-power objective (Table 6–2). The single most important structure to be observed under the high-power field—indicative of a definitive diagnosis—is bacteria or yeast, *provided that the urine specimen is uncontaminated by urethral or vaginal organisms.* The volume of urine we view within one high-power field (hpf) when 0.02 ml is under the coverslip is approximately 1/20,000 to

Text continued on page 305

Figure 6–8. A combined red blood cell and hemoglobin cast with the formed cells seen only at the upper end of the cast.

Figure 6–9. Hemoglobin cast, Berger's disease. Notice characteristic reddish brown coloration.

Figure 6–10. Cellular cast. Note the hyaline matrix and the entrapped cells. Special stains would be required to identify their cellular origin.

Figure 6–11. Typical fatty cast with doubly refractile fat droplets in a patient with nephrotic syndrome due to amyloidosis. This cast still demonstrates a sharp matrix, best appreciated by finely adjusting the microscope focus up and down.

Figure 6–12. Low-power view demonstrates the classic, large, brown appearance of the oval fat macrophage in a patient with mesangial proliferative glomerulonephritis.

Figure 6–13. Higher power confirms the characteristic doubly refractile fat particles in these oval fat macrophages.

Figure 6–14. Phase-contrast illumination of the same sediment as Figure 6–13. Note the brilliance of the doubly refractile fat droplets in the oval fat macrophage.

Figure 6–15. Trichomonad. Notice the ovoid shape and motile flagella. Trichomonads are best identified under the low power by the jerky movement they impart to surrounding epithelial cells.

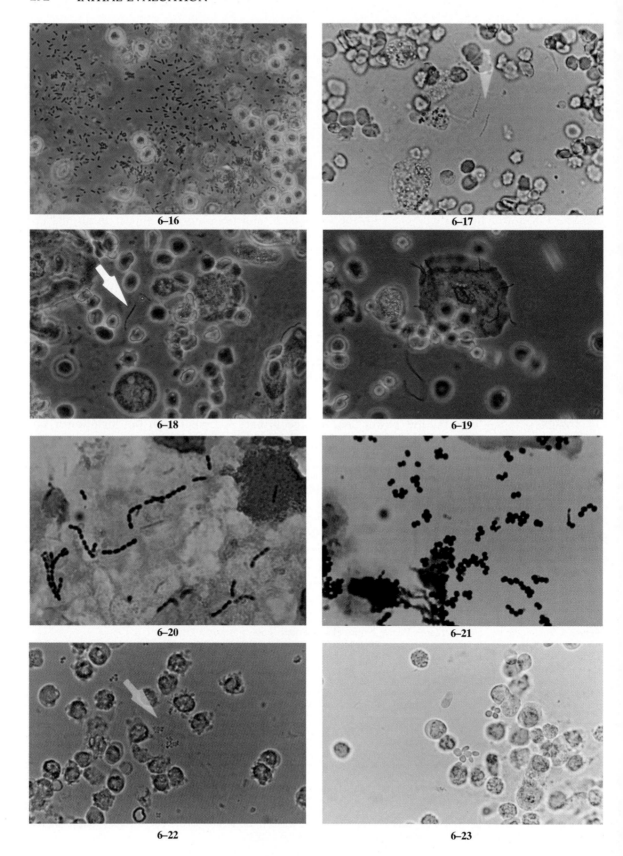

6–16

6–17

6–18

6–19

6–20

6–21

6–22

6–23

Figure 6–16. *E. coli* cystitis under the phase objective microscope.

Figure 6–17. Alpha-streptococcus urinary tract infection in a male patient with a large necrotic bladder tumor. Note the typical chaining.

Figure 6–18. Alpha-streptococci under phase microscopy. Same sediment as Figure 6–17.

Figure 6–19. Alpha-streptococci. Notice the bacterial adherence to the epithelial cell (phase objective).

Figure 6–20. Alpha-streptococci. Gram stain confirms gram-positive cocci in chains.

Figure 6–21. *Staphylococcus epidermidis*, confirmed as gram-positive cocci in clumps (oil-immersion objective).

Figure 6–22. *Staphylococcus aureus*, $>10^5$ cocci per ml, in a 78-year-old male with bilateral calcium oxalate stones.

Figure 6–23. *Candida albicans* in budding form in a patient with yeast cystitis. Note marked pyuria.

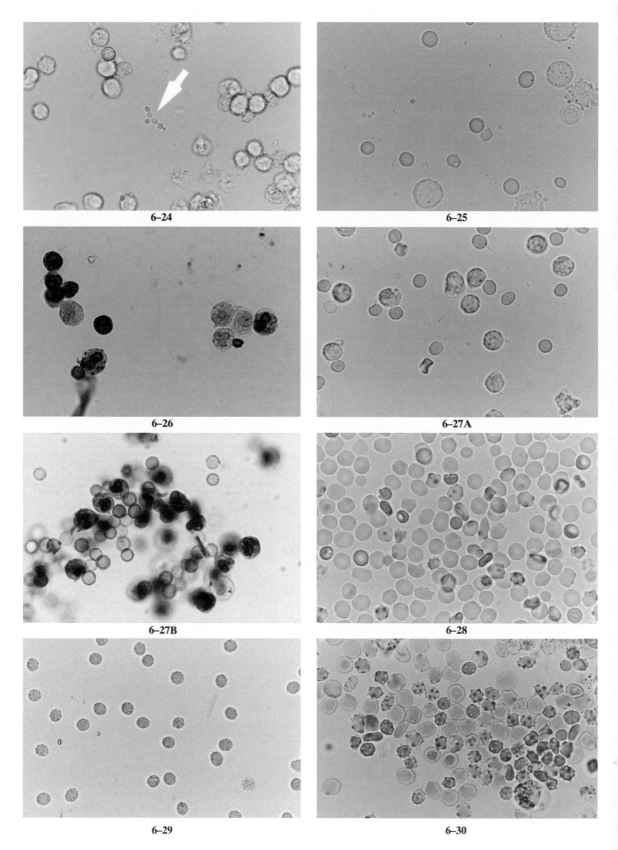

6–24

6–25

6–26

6–27A

6–27B

6–28

6–29

6–30

Figure 6–24. *Candida albicans.*

Figure 6–25. Fresh "glitter cells" in a patient with aspirin-induced pyuria. Under the high-power objective microscope, the glitter-like movement of the cytoplasmic granules was easily seen. Note also the fresh red blood cells.

Figure 6–26. Fresh white blood cells, both glittering and nonglittering, take up vital stain poorly, if at all. Drs. Sternheimer and Malbin referred to these as "pale" cells. Note the "old" WBC's (upper left-hand corner) that absorb the stain.

Figure 6–27. *A,* Old leukocytes in a patient with a *Proteus* infection and staghorn calculi. *B,* Sternheimer-Malbin stain identifies them as polymorphonuclear in origin.

Figure 6–28. Red blood cells in a sediment from a patient with an indwelling ureteral catheter. These smoothly rounded and mildly crenated red blood cells are typical of epithelial RBC's.

Figure 6–29. Red blood cells found in a postprostatic massage urine. Cystoscopy confirmed bleeding from blood vessels in the prostatic fossa. Note that cells are crenated but that there is little cell-to-cell variation.

Figure 6–30. Red blood cells in a sediment from a patient with a large necrotic bladder tumor. Both crenated and round, sometimes swollen cells are often seen in the same sediment—both types are filled with hemoglobin and show little cell-to-cell variation.

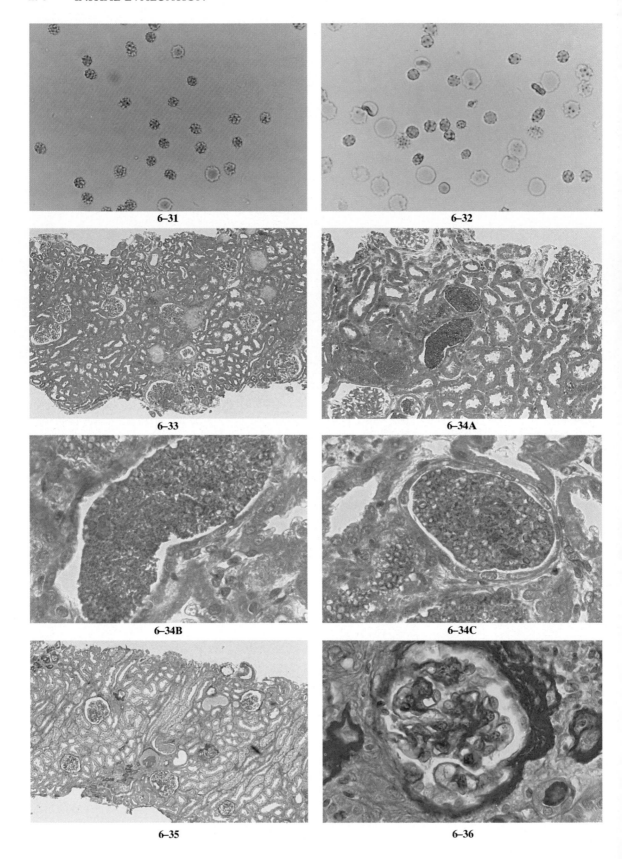

6–31

6–32

6–33

6–34A

6–34B

6–34C

6–35

6–36

Figure 6–31. Red blood cells obtained during cystoscopy in a patient with interstitial cystitis, collected in saline.

Figure 6–32. Red blood cells from a patient with interstitial cystitis; voided specimen.

Figure 6–33. Low-power view of renal biopsy in Berger's disease (hematoxylin and eosin stain). Most glomeruli demonstrate mesangial thickening; some fields show substantial number of hyalinized glomeruli.

Figure 6–34. Red blood cell cast from same needle biopsy as Figure 6–33 (hematoxylin and eosin stain). *A*, Low-power view. *B*, High-power field shows red blood cells within proximal tubule. *C*, High-power view suggests that some red blood cells already appear dysmorphic.

Figure 6–35. Periodic acid–Schiff (PAS) stain of renal biopsy (Fig. 6–33) demonstrates extent of glomerular involvement (low-power).

Figure 6–36. Higher power examination of same specimen as Figure 6–35 reveals mesangial proliferation and beginning of crescent formation.

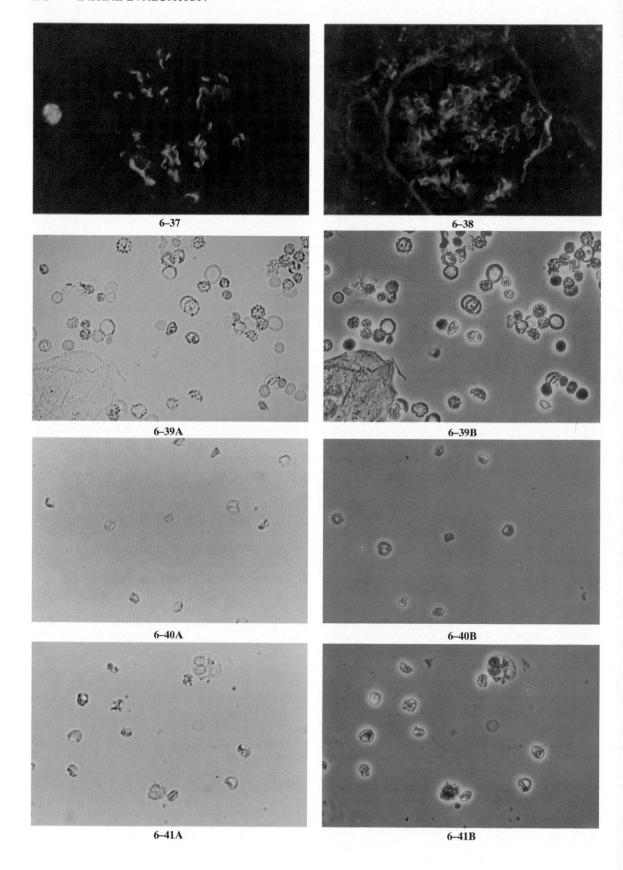

6–37

6–38

6–39A

6–39B

6–40A

6–40B

6–41A

6–41B

Figure 6–37. Immunohistochemical stain for IgA demonstrates characteristic deposits of Berger's disease.

Figure 6–38. IgG fluorescence reveals even more extensive deposits than IgA in this case.

Figure 6–39. *A,* Red blood cells from a patient with biopsy-proven Berger's disease. Observe the multitude of membrane variations characteristic of dysmorphic red blood cells. While the "crenated" forms may appear similar to the examples of epithelial bleeding, a closer look suggests that these cells are irregularly "crenated," showing asymmetric wrinkling and obvious areas of membrane loss. *B,* Same field under phase-contrast illumination. Compare the membrane irregularities with the bright-field illuminations in *A.* Note that all the diagnostic hallmarks can be recognized with standard light microscopy.

Figure 6–40. Dysmorphic red blood cells in a patient with glomerulonephritis. Same microscopic field seen under bright-field high-power *(A)* and phase high-power *(B)* microscopy. Compare these red blood cells with those seen earlier in the examples of epithelial bleeding. Note the membrane distortions and uneven distribution of the cytoplasm within the cell. Comparison between bright-field and phase objective microscopy shows easy identification of these characteristic cells with either form of illumination.

Figure 6–41. Dysmorphic red blood cells in a urinary sediment from a patient with renal involvement from Wegener's granulomatosis (biopsy showed focal and segmental glomerulonephritis), seen under bright-field *(A)* and phase *(B)* illumination. Note the irregular deposits of dense cytoplasmic material around the cell membrane.

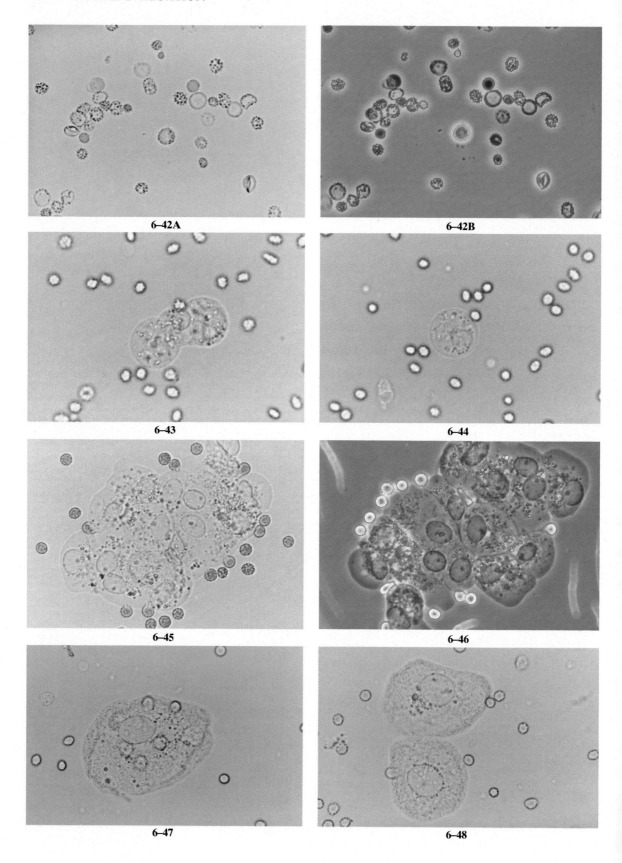

6–42A

6–42B

6–43

6–44

6–45

6–46

6–47

6–48

Figure 6–42. *A,* Initial urinary sediment seen in a young woman with microscopic hematuria (biopsy-proven Berger's disease). Note obvious dysmorphic red blood cells, with great cell-to-cell variation, consisting of both membrane irregularities and uneven cytoplasmic distributions. *B,* Same field seen under phase illumination.

Figure 6–43. Transitional epithelial cells from the bladder, scraped off the mucosa during open surgery for retropubic prostatectomy. Note the larger cytoplasmic inclusions.

Figure 6–44. Transitional epithelial cells from the bladder. Note the greater nucleus to cytoplasm ratio as compared with squamous cells.

Figure 6–45. Sheet of transitional epithelial cells scraped from the bladder during open surgery. Again, note the larger cytoplasmic granules, the large nuclei, and the prominent nucleoli. Numerous epithelial red blood cells are also present.

Figure 6–46. Same microscopic field as Figure 6–45 under phase illumination.

Figure 6–47. Transitional epithelial cells in saline lavaged from a normal bladder during cystoscopy.

Figure 6–48. Transitional epithelial cells obtained during bladder lavage with saline.

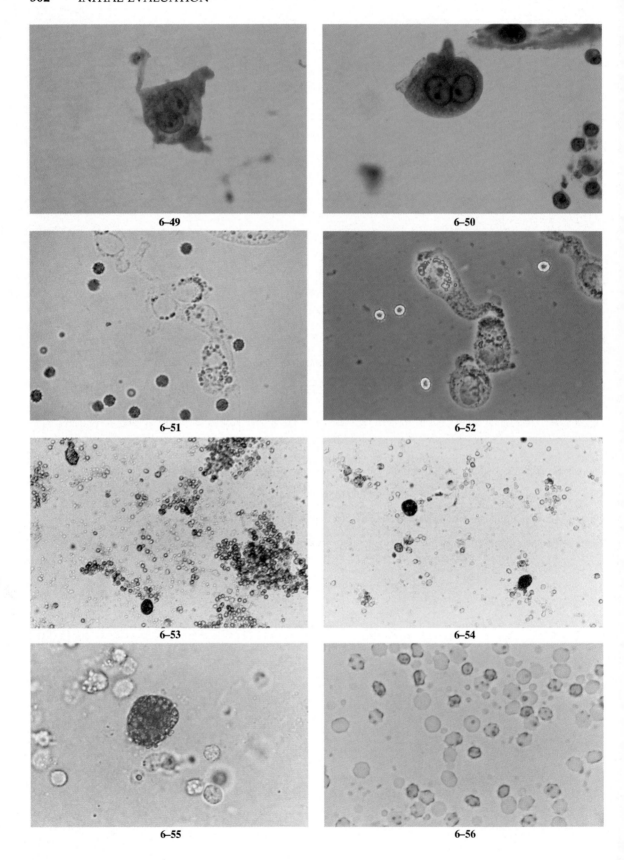

6–49

6–50

6–51

6–52

6–53

6–54

6–55

6–56

Figure 6–49. Multinucleated transitional epithelial cell, stained with Sternheimer-Malbin stain. Urine specimen was spontaneously voided in a patient with interstitial cystitis.

Figure 6–50. Transitional (bladder) epithelial cells; same sediment as Figure 6–49. Note the normal nucleoli.

Figure 6–51. Ureteral transitional cells. These caudate, or "kitelike," cells are variants with a long cytoplasmic tail. Often considered classic ureteral cells, they are not the most common ureteral epithelial cell. Observe the epithelial red blood cells secondary to scraping of the ureter.

Figure 6–52. Caudate ureteral epithelial cell under phase illumination, demonstrating large cytoplasmic granules.

Figure 6–53. Oval fat macrophages and clumps of white blood cells (low-power field) from the prostatic fluid of a patient with chronic *E. coli* bacterial prostatitis. Note the characteristic brown color of the macrophages, sometimes referred to as oval brown bodies. Background of normal secretory granules is characteristic of prostatic fluid.

Figure 6–54. Oval fat macrophages in prostatic fluid, low-power field.

Figure 6–55. Oval fat macrophage, high-power field. Note fine secretory granules found normally in prostatic fluid.

Figure 6–56. Prostatic fluid (high-power field) demonstrates epithelial red blood cells secondary to prostatic massage.

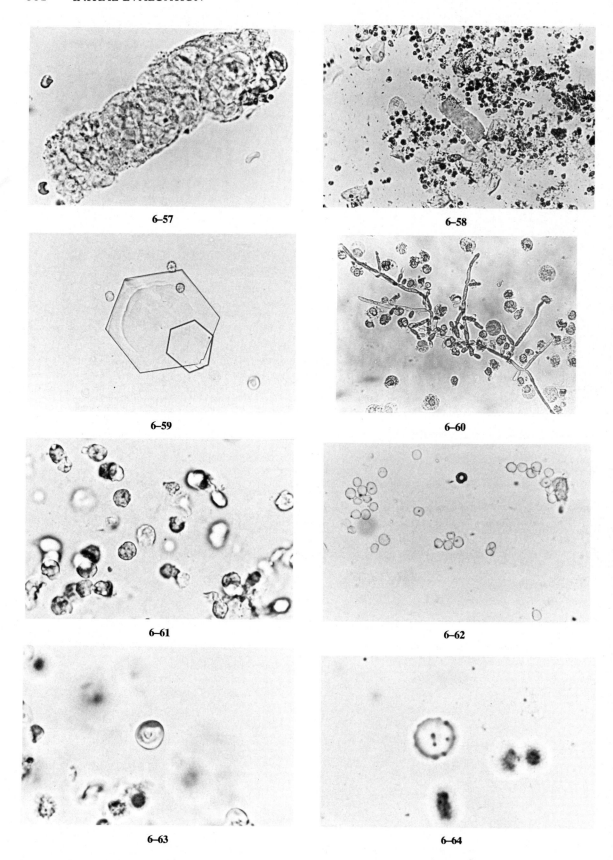

6–57

6–58

6–59

6–60

6–61

6–62

6–63

6–64

1/50,000 of a milliliter. Therefore, the bacterial count of one organism per high-power field is at least 20,000 bacteria per ml, a number that cannot be secondary to contamination by urethral or vaginal bacteria when the urine is properly collected. Thus, the finding of a single bacillus, even as rare as one every few high-power fields, is diagnostic of bacteriuria provided that the specimen (1) has been obtained by suprapubic needle aspiration of the bladder; (2) is a late midstream urine specimen from a male with the foreskin retracted; (3) is a late catheterized specimen from a female with a full bladder; or (4) is a late midstream urine from a female, collected by the nurse with the patient on an examining table as described earlier.

Gram-negative bacterial rods demonstrate a characteristic bacillary shape (Fig. 6–16). Streptococci (Figs. 6–17 to 6–20) are readily identified by standard bright-field illumination as typical beaded chains in the unstained sediment. Staphylococcal bacteriuria, especially with S. saprophyticus and S. epidermidis, is a common cause of urinary tract infections (Fig. 6–21). It must be recognized that staphylococcal bacteriuria can be diagnosed only when the staphylococci are growing in clumps (Fig. 6–22), because single, coccus-sized particles are commonly present in the urine as secretory granules from many different parts of the urinary tract. When staphylococci are present, their duplication and geometric growth produce floating colonies. Staphylococcal bacteriuria must *never* be diagnosed on the basis of single, coccus-like particles.

Yeast cells, usually from *Candida albicans*, are readily identified in the wet, unstained urine sediment by their budding and clumplike forms (Figs. 6–23 and 6–24). Yeasts can be confused with the biconcave oval form of calcium oxalate crystals and red blood cells. However, biconcave crystals are insoluble in acids and alkali and fail to show the budding typical of yeast cells. Furthermore, yeasts can be differentiated from red blood cells by their failure to stain with eosin. The pseudomycelial form (Fig. 6–60) of candiduria—which urine encourages because it supports *Candida* germination—is less common than the budding form. Often, it indicates tissue infection.

TWO TYPES OF WHITE BLOOD CELLS (WBC)

The urologist should distinguish between "old" and "fresh" white blood cells (Table 6–3). One cannot be sure of the cell line from which "old" leukocytes come, and, therefore, their significance is uncertain. They appear as small wrinkled cells with indistinct nuclear features (Fig. 6–61). These cells may be disintegrating leukocytes, but they are commonly seen in vaginal secretions of normal women and often contaminate the midstream voided specimen; presumably they represent leukocytes that migrated into the genital tract during menstruation.

"Fresh" leukocytes are large cells with abundant cytoplasmic granules; careful focusing on the nucleus will usually show that it is polymorphonuclear (Fig. 6–25). Unlike the "old" WBC's, these fresh WBC's come from a known

---

Figure 6–57. Cellular-granular cast from a patient with focal glomerulonephritis demonstrates cellular constituents and coarse granularity.

Figure 6–58. Broad waxy cast under low power shows characteristic homogeneous, brittle appearance, blunted ends, and sharp margins. As evidence of brittleness, cracks are often seen along the lateral margins. Amyloidosis.

Figure 6–59. Cystine crystal, diagnostic of cystinuria. Note perfect hexagonal ("benzene") ring. This patient presented with an undiagnosed renal calculus and hematuria.

Figure 6–60. Mycelial form of *Candida albicans* with characteristic pseudohyphae from a urine specimen obtained by suprapubic needle aspiration of the bladder. This patient had pyelonephritis and papillary necrosis. The mycelial form of *Candida albicans* usually indicates tissue invasion.

Figure 6–61. Old white blood cells. This patient has a renal calculus and *Staphylococcus aureus* urinary tract infection. One cannot be sure of the cell line from which these cells originated; they could be epithelial cells that have lost their cytoplasm, but they are probably leukocytes.

Figure 6–62. Red blood cells in a sediment from a patient with a noninfected, asymptomatic, renal pelvic calculus. Note that cells are faded but show no membrane irregularities.

Figure 6–63. Glomerular red blood cells. The red blood cell in the middle of the field demonstrates a bleb of cytoplasm extending in the direction of the observer (oil immersion).

Figure 6–64. Glomerular red blood cell showing peripheral cytoplasmic deposition (oil immersion).

TABLE 6–3. Two Types of White Blood Cells

1. "Old" = ? cell-line = ? significance

2. "Fresh" = leukocyte cell line = injury

    a. "glitter" cells
        ≤ 1.019 sp. gravity   "pale" cells
                         Sternheimer-Malbin
    b. "nonglittering"   stain
       granules

(Note: Value of suprapubic needle aspiration of the bladder and ureteral catheterization)

cell line. The significance of these cells is that a normal urinary tract *never* sheds a fresh polymorphonuclear leukocyte in the urine. The presence of even one of these cells per high-power field in the centrifuged urine sediment indicates an injury to the urinary tract, whether it be infection, a sterile renal stone irritating the pelvic mucosa, acute glomerulonephritis, or interstitial cystitis.

When the specific gravity of the urine is approximately 1.019 or less, the granules in the cytoplasm of these fresh polymorphonuclear leukocytes show great activity. With careful fine focusing of the high-power objective, the granules show a glitter-like movement, accounting for the descriptive term "glitter cells." In urines of specific gravity greater than 1.019, these granules fail to show the glittering phenomenon, but the fresh nature of these nonglittering polymorphonuclear cells with abundant granules in their cytoplasm is equally as significant as the glittering activity. Both types of fresh polymorphonuclear leukocytes historically represent the "pale cells" of Sternheimer and Malbin (1951) (Fig. 6–26).

Occasionally, in white blood cells that are neither severely disintegrated nor fresh, the Sternheimer-Malbin stain (a mixture of crystal violet and safranin marketed under the commercial name of Sedi-Stain), is useful for identifying the nucleus as polymorphonuclear (Fig. 6–27).

TWO TYPES OF RED BLOOD CELLS (RBC)

As in the case of white blood cells, there are two types of red blood cells—dysmorphic (or glomerular) and epithelial (or nonglomerular). Epithelial red blood cells are usually loaded with an even distribution of hemoglobin and have round or crenated contours. Occasionally, they may be ringlike—red cells that have lost their hemoglobin but retain intact round or slightly wrinkled cell membranes (Fig. 6–62). Dysmorphic red blood cells are irregularly

shaped cells with peculiar cellular membrane configurations (Figs. 6–63 to 6–68). Furthermore, they often have minimal hemoglobin or an uneven heterogeneous distribution of their cytoplasm. They often are so bizarre as to be passed over as noncellular by the microscopist. Indeed, Thomas Addis (1926) commented that care [during urinalysis] was necessary to avoid passing over fragmented or partially lysed red blood cells.

It was, however, Dr. Kenneth Fairley at the University of Melbourne in Australia who first showed in 1979 that these "dysmorphic" red blood cells, identified with a phase microscope, were characteristic of glomerulonephritis (Birch and Fairley, 1979). He (Fairley and Birch, 1982) and others have prospectively confirmed these findings; Fassett et al. (1982), in a series of 303 patients, demonstrated a high sensitivity (96 per cent) and specificity of these distinct phase microscopic findings. These distinctions, however, do not require the phase microscope. The qualitative difference between glomerular and nonglomerular red blood cells is readily made with the standard bright-field microscope using the high-power objective.

Bleeding from epithelial sites from the renal calyces to the urethral meatus demonstrates epithelial, nonglomerular red blood cells (Figs. 6–28 to 6–32; Fig. 6–62). Urines from patients with documented sources of hematuria—urethral, prostatic, ureteral, and renal pelvic as well as post prostatectomy—have been carefully examined using bright-field microscopy (Stamey and Kindrachuk, 1985). All clearly demonstrate the previously described regular, hemoglobin-laden red blood cells with smooth, rounded, or crenated cell membranes, or the empty, ringlike blood cells that have lost their hemoglobin.

Glomerular (Dysmorphic) Red Blood Cells. Because of the possibility of occult cancer of the urinary tract, it is important to identify the cause of red blood cells in the urinary sediment. However, many patients with glomerulonephritis present with microscopic hematuria without proteinuria in the supernatant and with no other symptoms or signs of renal disease. This is especially true of Berger's disease (IgA or IgG deposits, or both, in the mesangium of the glomerulus), in which one third of patients present with only microscopic hematuria (Clarkson et al., 1984). Since most of these patients will not have red blood cell casts in the outpatient, hydrated urine specimens, it is critical to know whether their red blood cells are characteristic of glomerulonephritis. Since Berger's disease is probably the most common cause of microscopic hematuria in patients without urinary tract stones, tumors, or infections, the problem of unnecessary and repetitive urologic examinations to seek the source of microscopic hematuria is clearly substantial.

Berger's disease, or IgA nephropathy, has assumed increasing importance in the differential diagnosis of microscopic hematuria since it was first described 15 years ago. It is now recognized as the most common form of glomerulonephritis and occurs in 18 to 30 per cent of all renal biopsies (Clarkson et al., 1984). There appears to be some geographic variation in its frequency. Although no reliable estimate now exists for the world or North American population, one study from Singapore (which examined all National Service trainees) demonstrated an incidence of between 1 and 2 per cent in the population (Sinniah et al., 1976).

IgA glomerulopathy is a disease of young people, with the peak age being 15 to 30 years, and it is approximately four times more common in males than females. While one third of patients present with manifestations of renal disease (nephritis, nephrotic syndrome, renal failure, or hypertension), an equal number present with microscopic hematuria and minimal proteinuria. More impressive, however, is the fact that at least 20 per cent of this latter group have no proteinuria (Clarkson et al., 1977, 1984). One third present with classic *macroscopic* hematuria, often coinciding with an upper respiratory tract or gastrointestinal infection.

Initially, IgA nephropathy was thought to be benign. Long-term longitudinal studies, however, indicate that 10 to 20 per cent of patients progress to renal failure and that a large number develop hypertension (Jennette and Wall, 1983). Serial serum creatinine values, frequent blood pressure readings, and urinary protein determinations constitute minimal follow-up studies.

Pathologically, the lesions demonstrate a mesangial and endothelial cell proliferation (Figs. 6–33 to 6–36). Electron microscopy shows small, granular deposits between mesangial cells and the axial basement membrane. These usually consist of IgA, often accompanied by C3, although IgG, IgM, and fibrinogen deposits may also occur (Figs. 6–37 and 6–38).

Classic glomerular red blood cells are found in this disease as well as in glomerulonephritis of all causes. Under ordinary bright-field microscopy one sees markedly irregular cellular membranes with varied configurations—blebs, targets, buds, and focal membrane loss. Furthermore, the cytoplasm demonstrates a heter-ogeneous distribution of dense hemoglobin. There is a tendency for this material to clump eccentrically at the periphery of the cell membrane. While it can be argued that the phase contrast allows more definitive discrimination of the delicate membrane changes, a comparison cell-for-cell convincingly demonstrates that these diagnostic discriminations are readily seen under ordinary bright-field illumination (Figs. 6–39 to 6–42).

We have found that not all the red blood cells in our patients with proven glomerular disease are dysmorphic, although all patients did have a majority of these cells in their urinary sediment. The transformation of normal red blood cells to dysmorphic ones is probably due to the osmotic and physical changes encountered in passage through the nephron. Differential rates of bleeding, urine flow, and osmotic change probably account for the presence of both "normal" and glomerular red blood cells in the same sediment of the patient with proven glomerular disease.

Quantification of WBC and RBC

For greater precision in clinical studies, especially when the methods of collecting the voided urine are much less precise than those advocated here, quantitative estimates of the number of cells per ml of urine become an absolute necessity for meaningful research data. However, if the physician and the laboratory technician become familiar with the qualitative distinctions between fresh and "old" leukocytes, and between epithelial and glomerular RBC's, quantitative characterization of these cells does not increase the diagnostic accuracy achieved by a careful and intelligent examination of the centrifuged urinary sediment.

Quantitative analysis of RBC's, especially the establishment of normal values, is important because of the classic teaching that no matter how few the number of RBC's per high-power field, a complete urologic workup is necessary, with at least a cystoscopy and an intravenous urogram; this urologic dictum has been justified on the basis that occult cancer of the urinary tract should be detected at an early stage when it is potentially curable. But dipstick urine screening of asymptomatic populations, an increased use of urinalysis in annual medical examinations, and better recognition now of RBC membrane fragments have led to an increase in the number of patients presenting with low numbers of RBC's in their urine.

Are RBC's normally excreted into the urine? Thomas Addis (1926) of Stanford University was the pioneer in quantitating the formed elements in the urine. He observed that normal men excreted as many as 1,200,000 RBC's every 24 hours, an observation confirmed by many later investigators. Allowing 1200 ml of urine as an average volume for 24 hours, each ml of urine should contain about 1000 RBC's as a rough approximation of the upper limits of normal; indeed, several investigators as recently as the past 5 years have reported between 500 (Kesson et al., 1978) and 8000 RBC's per ml of voided urine (Kincaid-Smith, 1982; Larcom and Carter, 1948) as their upper limits (the latter figure depends upon recognizing glomerular RBC's). Taking 1000 RBC's per ml, assume that every RBC in 15 ml of centrifuged urine is compacted into a final sediment volume of 0.02 ml. Since each high-power field of the microscope views a volume of about 1/30,000 of a milliliter, the microscopist should see 0.5 RBC per hpf or one cell every two high-power fields.* Since 1000 RBC per ml is near the upper limits of normal, and since office centrifuges are too slow to completely sediment all the RBC's, and since great care would be required to limit the volume of the supernatant resuspension to 0.02 ml, it is surely obvious why RBC's are rarely seen in the centrifuged urine sediment from healthy subjects. It is also obvious why the finding of even one or two RBC's per hpf is traditionally viewed with justifiable concern for the possibility of significant disease, such as an unsuspected tumor or stone.

Birch and Fairley (1979) reported that the RBC's found in the urine of healthy subjects

---

*1000 RBC/ml $\times$ 15 ml $\times$ 1/30,000 ml = 0.5 RBC/ml.

were glomerular, not epithelial, in origin. Indeed, later studies have shown that exercise-related hematuria is glomerular in origin as well (Fassett et al., 1982; Kincaid-Smith, 1982). These significant observations add substantial leverage to the interpretation of the occasional RBC that the microscopist should expect to find in most centrifuged urine sediments. If one learns to recognize the distortions of glomerular RBC's, he will be rewarded by easily identifying these glomerular RBC's in many otherwise "negative" urinary sediments. Conversely, the presence of epithelial RBC's, even one or two per hpf, should continue to be of substantial concern, even though it will prove to be of importance for only the occasional patient.

Epithelial Cells of the Urinary Sediment

The urologic surgeon has an unprecedented opportunity to know the appearance of every epithelial cell in the urinary tract from the renal calyx to the urethral meatus (Table 6–4). All he needs to do is to scrape the mucosa of these different uroepithelial surfaces with a knife blade at the time of open surgery; to release the blade into 5 ml of saline; and, after surgery, to observe the specific epithelial cells under the microscope.

The squamous epithelial cell, which covers the vagina, urethra, and much of the trigone of every postpubertal female, is readily recognized in Figure 6–69. It is a cell with a tight nucleus, fine granularity, and only an occasional large cystoplasmic granule.

Bladder epithelial cells (Figs. 6–43 to 6–50) demonstrate larger cytoplasmic inclusions and a

---

Figure 6–65. Glomerular red blood cell (oil immersion). Note three-dimensional asymmetry.

Figure 6–66. Glomerular red blood cell (oil immersion), showing irregular deposition of its cytoplasm at the periphery of the cell.

Figure 6–67. Glomerular red blood cells (oil immersion) demonstrate small extruded blebs of cytoplasmic material, "doughnut" cells, and irregularly crenated cells.

Figure 6–68. Compare the two dysmorphic cells with the epithelial red blood cell on the left (oil immersion).

Figure 6–69. Squamous epithelial cell demonstrating a small nucleus to cytoplasm ratio as well as fine granularity of the cytoplasm. Similar cells are found in the terminal male urethra.

Figure 6–70. Renal pelvic transitional cell demonstrating at least two nuciei.

Figure 6–71. Normal vaginal smear, low power. Note the clumps of old white blood cells and the squamous epithelial cells.

Figure 6–72. Normal prostatic fluid (high-power field), demonstrating numerous secretory granules.

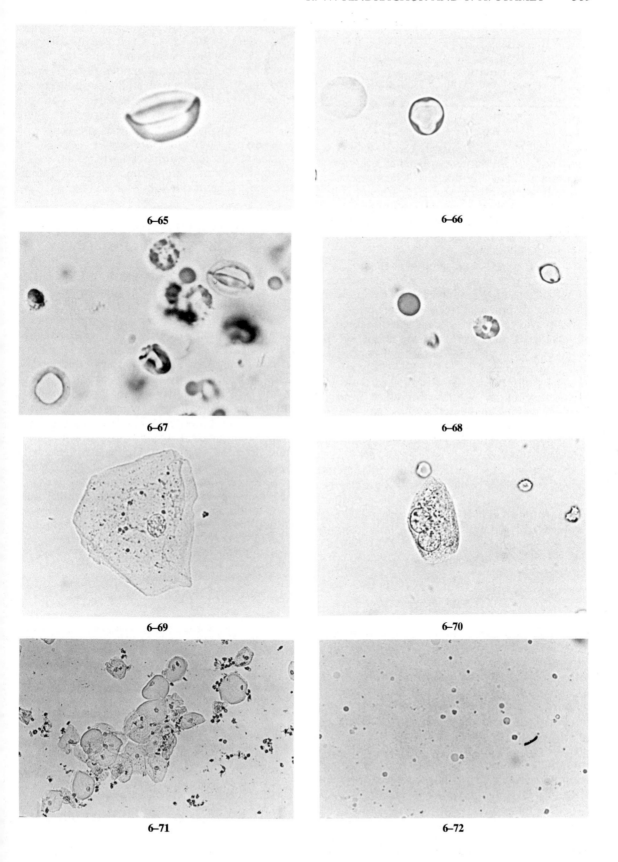

6–65

6–66

6–67

6–68

6–69

6–70

6–71

6–72

TABLE 6–4. EPITHELIAL CELLS OF URINARY SEDIMENT

1. Squamous
2. Bladder
3. Ureteral
4. Renal pelvic
        Ureteral catheter

larger nucleus to cytoplasm ratio. There is a tendency for the large cytoplasmic granules to accumulate near the nucleus. The presence of multiple nuclei in transitional epithelial cells is a normal finding; it is due mostly to the number of cells shed (or removed) and the effort taken to look for them. By themselves, they do not indicate malignancy.

Ureteral cells can demonstrate the classic "kitelike" appearance illustrated in textbooks (Figs. 6–51 and 6–52), but by no means is this the most common ureteral epithelial cell. The renal pelvic cell (Fig. 6–70) is the epithelial cell all urologists need to recognize, as it is encountered every time a ureteral catheter is passed to the renal calyces.

Few differences are observed in the transitional epithelium as one progresses from the bladder to the renal calyces. Most morphologic variation is probably dependent upon the mucosal depth of the uroepithelial cells. The only consistent finding is that as one advances up the urinary tract, the uroepithelial cells contain larger cytoplasmic granules with a greater perinuclear distribution. These granules probably represent mitochondria, which may indicate differences in function and metabolic requirements.

EXAMINATION OF THE VAGINAL SMEAR

As emphasized earlier, two cotton applicator sticks are placed in 5 ml of saline or transport broth after swabbing of the vaginal mucosa in the area of the hymenal ring. One of these cotton sticks can be removed from the culture tube, the fluid expressed onto a slide and covered with the standard coverslip. This wet preparation under the low-power field allows examination for trichomonads, mycelia (which will rarely be seen in the vagina), and clumps of leukocytes in the case of vaginitis (Fig. 6–71).

Examination with the high-power field should include a search for yeast, for fresh white blood cells (which would indicate a true inflammatory vaginitis), and for the effect of estrogen on squamous epithelium.

Many vaginal epithelial cells will be found with adherent bacteria, which will usually represent normal lactobacilli, and anaerobes, which make up the major endogenous flora. If squamous epithelial cells with indistinct borders are found covered from surface to surface with very small, rodlike organisms packed together, there is some evidence that these cells correlate with a positive culture for Gardnerella vaginalis, an organism that in combination with anaerobes is thought to cause "nonspecific vaginitis" (Vontver and Eschenbach, 1981).

EXAMINATION OF EXPRESSED PROSTATIC SECRETIONS

Once a drop of prostatic fluid is placed on a microscopic slide with a coverslip, low-power field examination should include a search for oval fat macrophages and an estimate of the number of clumps of white blood cells per low-power field as a possible indicator of the severity of inflammation. Prostatic fluid obtained in patients with acute bacterial prostatitis (chills, fever, and obstructive voiding) usually shows early macrophages. A few weeks later, the more mature and cholesterol-packed oval fat macrophages characterize the postinfection prostatic fluid (Figs. 6–53 to 6–55). Under the high-power field, examination of the prostatic fluid should include an estimate of the number of leukocytes per high-power field. Normal prostatic fluid should contain few or no white blood cells but should be loaded with innumerable secretory granules of all sizes (Fig. 6–72). Rarely, one may find RBC's in the prostatic fluid (Fig. 6–56).

References

Addis, T.: The number of formed elements in the urinary sediment of normal individuals. J. Clin. Invest., *2*:409, 1926.

Birch, D. F., and Fairley, K. F.: Haematuria: Glomerular or non-glomerular? Lancet, *2*:845, 1979.

Clarkson, A. R., Seymour, A. E., Thompson, J. A., et al.: IgA nephropathy: A syndrome of uniform morphology, diverse clinical features and uncertain prognosis. Clin. Nephrol., *8*:459, 1977.

Clarkson, A. R., Woodroffe, K. M., Bannister, J. D., et al.: The syndrome of IgA nephropathy. Clin. Nephrol., *21*:7, 1984.

Fairley, K. F., and Birch, D. F.: Hematuria: A simple method of identifying glomerular bleeding. Kidney Int., *21*:105, 1982.

Fassett, R. G., Horgan, B. A., and Mathew, T. H.: Detection of glomerular bleeding by phase-contrast microscopy. Lancet, *1*:1432, 1982.

Fassett, R. G., Owen, J. E., Fairley, J., et al.: Urinary red-cell morphology during exercise. Br. Med. J., *285*:1455, 1982.

Jennette, J. C., and Wall, S. D.: The clinical and pathologic heterogeneity of IgA nephropathy. The Kidney (National Kidney Foundation), *16*:17, 1983.

Kesson, A. M., Talbott, J. M., and Gyory, A. Z.: Microscopic examination of urine. Lancet, *2*:809, 1978.

Kincaid-Smith, P.: Haematuria and exercise-related haematuria. Br. Med. J., *285*:1595, 1982.

Kingsbury, F. B., Clark, C. P., Williams, G., et al.: Laboratory methods. The rapid determination of albumin in urine. J. Lab. Clin. Med., *11*:981, 1926.

Larcom, R. C. Jr., and Carter, G. H.: Laboratory methods. Erythrocytes in urinary sediment: Identification and normal limits. J. Lab. Clin. Med., *33*:875, 1948.

McQueen, E. G., and Sidney, M.: Composition of urinary casts. Lancet, *1*:397, 1966.

Mogensen, C. E., Vittinghus, E., and Solling, K.: Abnormal albumin excretion after two provocative renal tests in diabetes: Physical exercise and lysine injection. Kidney Int., *16*:385, 1979.

Peterson, P. A., and Berggard, I.: Urinary immunoglobulin components in normal, tubular, and glomerular proteinuria: Quantities and characteristics of free light chains, IgG, IgA, and Feγ fragment. Eur. J. Clin. Invest., *1*:255, 1971.

Sinniah, R., Pwee, H. S., and Lim, C. H.: Glomerular lesions in asymptomatic microscopic hematuria discovered on routine medical examination. Clin. Nephrol., *5*:216, 1976.

Stamey, T. A.: Pathogenesis and Treatment of Urinary Tract Infections. Baltimore, The Williams & Wilkins Co., 1980.

Stamey, T. A.: Prostatitis. Monogr. Urol., *2*:131, 1981.

Stamey, T. A., and Kindrachuk, R. W.: Urinary Sediment and Urinalysis: A Practical Guide for the Health Science Professional. Philadelphia, W. B. Saunders Co., 1985.

Sternheimer, R., and Malbin, B.: Clinical recognition of pyelonephritis with a new stain for urinary sediments. Am. J. Med., *11*:312, 1951.

Vontver, L. A., and Eschenbach, D. A.: The role of *Gardnerella vaginalis* in nonspecific vaginitis. Clin. Obstet. Gynecol., *24*:439, 1981.

CHAPTER 7

Radiology of the Urinary Tract
Urography and Cystourethrography

HARRY Z. MELLINS, M.D.

INTRODUCTION

Of all the body systems, the urinary tract is among the most amenable to accurate and extensive radiologic investigation. Modern contrast media and refined examination methods yield a high degree of sensitivity and specificity in uroradiologic diagnosis. In many large departments of radiology, a radiologist who is particularly interested in the urinary system and is informed about the salient clinical details for each patient supervises the performance and interpretation of all examinations. Although it is not always possible for each department to have a subspecialist in urologic radiology, it is important that the radiologist supervising the examination see all the radiographs as they are made and adjust the number and type of views in accordance wih the clinical problem and the ongoing radiographic findings. All portions of the anatomy should be well demonstrated, using whatever special views are necessary and helpful.

It is good practice to begin every uroradiologic examination with a plain film of the urinary tract or at least the portion of it under investigation. This is often known as a KUB radiograph, indicating that it surveys the region of the kidneys, ureters, and bladder. It is properly exposed when the film densities representing water density structures, such as kidneys and muscles, are easily distinguishable from the surrounding fat and when small calcifications

are readily outlined against soft tissues and are detectable when projected over bones. Respiratory motion and excessive radiographic kilovoltage greatly increase the difficulty of recognizing small calcifications. Radiographic apparatus capable of generating high currents should be employed so that relatively low levels of kilovoltage and short exposures can be utilized. The area from the top of the adrenals to the bottom of the prostate gland and from one lateral abdominal wall to the other should be surveyed. Often this will require the use of two films, but in smaller individuals a single film may suffice. Although plain films of the urinary tract may be sufficient when the findings establish a radiologic diagnosis, the absence of abnormal findings does not exclude abnormality. In most cases, therefore, it is more economical and more expeditious to combine the plain film with a more definitive examination, such as excretion urography, rather than to perform two separate examinations.

EXCRETION UROGRAPHY

Indications and Contraindications

Excretion urography is a highly versatile examination that can be used to demonstrate the renal parenchyma, pelvocalyceal systems, ureters, urinary bladder, and urethra. It is the basic radiologic examination of the urinary tract and requires excellent radiographic equipment, sufficient contrast medium, adequate numbers of films, and the constant supervision of a concerned physician. It can be modified and shortened when minimal radiation exposure or minimal manipulation is in the best interest of the patient.

Conditions or diseases that may constitute contraindications can be grouped under three headings: (1) risk of nephrotoxicity, (2) risk of cardiovascular toxicity, and (3) risk of idiosyncratic reaction.

NEPHROTOXICITY

It is probable that the concentration of iodinated contrast medium in the glomerular filtrate, peritubular interstitial space, and tubular cells is an important determinant of potential nephrotoxicity. The concentration levels are related to the amount of contrast medium injected and the volume of the extracellular fluid. No controlled clinical study of the effects of different dosage levels exists, but many factors suggest that nephrotoxicity is dose-related. Byrd and Sherman (1979) report an incidence of renal failure after urography of 0.16 per cent; after computed tomography of 0.14 per cent; and after angiography of a variety of organs (in which the doses are commonly considerably higher) of 0.53 per cent. Of 13 juvenile-onset diabetes patients undergoing coronary arteriography, only one did not develop acute renal failure and he received less than half the mean dose. Only three of those who developed renal failure were not oliguric, and they received the lowest volumes of radiocontrast medium (Weinrauch and Healy, 1977). Other clinical evidence of a similar nature exists. Except under special circumstances, it is wise to limit the urographic contrast dose to 0.30 mg of iodine for each kg of body weight. This is equal to 0.5 ml per lb of standard-strength contrast medium.

Dehydration, whether fortuitous or intended, decreases the volume of the extracellular fluid and is known to increase the risk of acute renal failure. The patient should be well hydrated on the day before the urographic examination. Dehydration of the patient by the use of strong laxatives should be avoided. Overnight restriction of fluid is common practice, and in previously well-hydrated patients it would appear to be entirely safe. On the other hand, adequate urograms can be made of patients who have not been given fluid intravenously or by mouth for only 2 hours—sufficient time for the period of maximum diuresis to have passed.

Multiple myeloma was formerly believed to be a contraindication because urographic contrast media, excreted in the urine as chemical salts, precipitated urinary proteins and produced obstructive casts. If the patient is well hydrated, however, this danger is virtually eliminated (Cwynarski and Saxton, 1969). In addition, modern triiodinated contrast media probably are less likely to precipitate myeloma proteins than were older contrast media.

Nephrosclerosis and other microcirculatory diseases of the renal vessels are considered to be risk factors for nephrotoxicity, probably on the basis of the decrease in renal blood flow.

It has been affirmed by many that impaired renal function predisposes to radiocontrast-induced acute renal failure. Rahimi and coworkers (1981) were concerned about this point of view, since "loss of urography and other x-ray procedures entailing the use of contrast media in patients with renal impairment would be a serious restriction in nephrology." A prospective study was made of 15 patients with varying degrees of chronic renal failure from glomerulonephritis, nephrosclerosis, obstructive uropathy, analgesic nephropathy, chronic pyelonephritis, and scleroderma, in which the fluid state of these patients was carefully monitored for 3 days before and after excretion urography. No significant changes occurred in endogenous creatinine and 51 Cr-EDTA clearances or in the plasma creatinine and urea concentrations. There was no change in the urinary activity of N-acetyl-beta-D-glucosaminidase, a highly sensitive indicator of renal tubular damage. These investigators concluded that with an appropriate state of hydration and the proper choice of amount of contrast medium, renal insufficiency is not a contraindication to contrast examination in the absence of diabetes or profound vascular disease.

Age has been considered to be a risk factor for two reasons: The incidence of microcirculatory disease is increased, and the renal reserve is probably decreased. Congestive heart failure decreases renal perfusion and thus increases the risk of renal damage.

Diabetes mellitus associated with renal insufficiency (creatinine over 1.5 mg/dl) is a strong risk factor. Hydration does not prevent the occurrence of acute renal failure, but the evidence indicates that it probably decreases the number of irreversible cases. An increase in the degree of renal failure has been recorded in diabetes patients with renal insufficiency who receive doses as low as those we recommend for the normal patient, but, in the absence of renal insufficiency, diabetes does not increase vulnerability to contrast nephrotoxicity.

CARDIOVASCULAR TOXICITY

The hypertonicity and direct chemotoxicity of ionic urographic contrast media cause varying degrees of systemic vasodilation, hypervolemia-hemodilution, altered cardiac function, and increased vascular permeability (Pfister, 1975). These changes pose a greater risk for patients who are in congestive heart failure or who have coronary artery disease than they do for normal patients.

DRUG IDIOSYNCRASY

A history of allergic diseases, such as hay fever or asthma, or previous circulatory or respiratory reactions to a urographic contast medium should dictate prudence in requesting as well as in performing the examination but does not constitute a contraindication. Most radiologists examine patients with allergic diseases without premedication but with antidotes immediately at hand (unless the diseases are severe). In the presence of a previous reaction to contrast medium more serious than urticaria or if the patient has severe asthma, premedication with corticosteroids is widely used (see *Side Effects and Reactions*). This may take the form of 100 mg of hydrocortisone administered by slow intravenous infusion 3 to 4 hours before the examination or 30 mg of prednisone daily for 3 days, including the day of the examination. A national controlled trial of corticosteroid premedication is currently in progress.

A different approach was proposed by Lalli (1974), who believes that anxiety is the most important factor in idiosyncratic reactions to urographic contrast media. He proposes that nothing should be done that might suggest the procedure has risks, such as premedication of the patient or interrogation about allergic diseases or previous reactions. If the patient raises any questions, they should be discussed forthrightly with him. Every attempt should be made to act in a calm, reassuring manner. Until it can be proved that one of these approaches is clearly more effective, an eclectic approach is probably most prudent.

Contrast Media

Since 1950, the media used in urography have been salts of triiodinated benzoic acid. The cations are either sodium or methylglucamine. Sodium salts are excreted in slightly higher concentrations and are less viscous when injected. The incidence of side effects may be slightly less with the methylglucamine salts. Excellent urography with a high degree of safety can be achieved using either type of contrast medium.

The optimum dose of contrast medium depends upon the glomerular filtation rate and the concentrating power of the kidney. It is best to select an amount of contrast medium that will produce a good nephrogram as well as a good pyelogram. Fifty ml of the commonly used agents will do this in young adults with normally functioning kidneys. Following Ettinger's experience, we have used 0.5 ml per pound of body weight for most adult patients (Ettinger, 1965). Studies by Benness (1967), Doyle et al. (1967), and Sherwood et al. (1968) indicate that up to a dose of about 300 mg I per kg, urinary iodine concentration increases. Above this level, increased osmotic diuresis causes decreased urinary contrast concentration. Since current standard-strength urographic contrast media contain between 280 and 300 mg I per ml, a dose of 1 ml per kg or 0.5 ml per lb is highly satisfactory.

The contrast medium may be injected by hand as rapidly as possible. An alternative method of injection is the drip-infusion technique, in which usually 300 ml of half-strength conventional contrast medium is introduced rapidly through an 18-gauge needle. It is generally agreed by proponents of both methods that the most important consideration is the quantity of contrast medium received by the patient. Proponents of the drip-infusion method believe that it is the most convenient way of introducing a large amount of contrast agent, while proponents of direct injection believe that it is simpler and requires a smaller amount of contrast material, on the average.

Side Effects and Reactions

Nausea and vomiting, circumoral and perirectal warmth, flushing, and transient pain in the injected arm are frequent side effects that usually have no clinical significance or relation to more serious contrast reactions. Of the idiosyncratic reactions, the most common is urticaria. Less common is conjunctivitis, rhinitis, or edema of the face or glottis. Decidedly less common is respiratory difficulty or cardiovascular collapse.

The incidence of death has generally been estimated at 1 in 40,000 examinations. In 1975, on the basis of multi-institutional data, Shehadi calculated it to be 1 in 14,000 examinations.

The experience at many large institutions tends to favor the lower incidence. In a series of 300,000 consecutive patients who underwent excretory urography at the Mayo Clinic between 1968 and 1982, there were four deaths—a mortality rate of 1 in 75,000 (Hartman et al., 1982). For comparison, these authors cited published data about the risk of a fatal reaction to an injection of penicillin, approximately 1 in 50,000. They estimated that on the basis of their experience, 24 of 25 patients with life-threatening reactions to urographic contrast media will recover if given adequate treatment. The mechanism of these contrast medium reactions is not known.

Although numerous tests of sensitivity to contrast media have been developed (including oral, ocular, intradermal, and intravenous injections of small amounts of the contrast medium to be used), none has proved effective. Individuals who have had no reaction to the intravenous injection of 0.5 to 1 ml of contrast medium have subsequently had serious reactions to the conventional dose, and the converse is also true. For many years, radiologists persisted in using the intravenous testing dose on the grounds that it was prudent medicolegally. Because of widespread agreement that the test was not of predictive value, most radiologists have now abandoned its use. Premedication with antihistaminic drugs was thought to prevent reactions, but this failed to be the experience of many investigators who conducted extensive clinical trials. The majority of radiologists no longer regularly employ premedication with antihistamines.

Treatment of Reactions

The majority of serious contrast reactions occur immediately or within 5 minutes after the injection. Occasionally, reactions will occur at 10 minutes or later. Whenever excretion urography is performed, a physician must be in attendance. Prompt recognition of a reaction and immediate treatment may be critical in saving a life. In hospitals, arrangements should be made between the departments of anesthesiology and radiology so that the radiologist can notify the department of anesthesiology instantly when resuscitation or other care of a patient is required. The use of a needle catheter (butterfly needle) that is left in place for 5 to 10 minutes after the injection of contrast medium facilitates intravenous therapy should this be necessary.

Before a urographic contrast medium is injected, the radiologist should have on hand an intravenous infusion set, a reservoir bag and face mask for oxygen inhalation, assorted needles and syringes, and a small supply of drugs. Individuals with much experience in resuscitation and emergency medicine will vary in their choice of drugs. A selection that has been found useful includes epinephrine (1:1000), aminophylline, diphenhydramine, levarterenol, hydrocortisone sodium succinate, isotonic saline solution, and 5 per cent glucose in water solution.

The mucocutaneous reactions include erythema, urticaria, and angioneurotic edema. Urticaria often does not require treatment. It usually responds promptly to 50 mg of diphenhydramine (Benadryl) given intramuscularly. Severe urticaria and angioneurotic edema can be treated by subcutaneous injection of 0.3 to 0.5 mg of epinephrine (1:1000).

Of the respiratory tract reactions, sneezing and rhinitis are minor symptoms and usually require no treatment. If they are troublesome, 50 mg of diphenhydramine (Benadryl) can be given intramuscularly. All other ventilatory or respiratory symptoms are more serious and require careful evaluation. If there is difficulty in breathing with burning or tightness of the throat, or alteration in the voice, laryngeal edema is probably present and should be treated by the subcutaneous administration of 0.3 to 0.5 mg of epinephrine. It has been emphasized by Plant and Lichtenstein (1974) that epinephrine should be given *immediately,* "before trying for an intravenous injection or even before establishing an airway." They contend that an anaphylactoid reaction treated with epinephrine in the first seconds of the reaction may be reversed within minutes, whereas after 5 minutes, epinephrine may not reverse the reaction for hours. If there is any question of an anaphylactoid reaction, epinephrine should be used. If effective, it will reverse cutaneous and upper airway edema and bronchospasm. The improved oxygenation, as well as some modest vasopressor activity, may reverse hypotension. Although vasconstrictors may precipitate ventricular arrhythmias in the presence of hypoxia or myocardial disease, the risk of using small doses of epinephrine subcutaneously is very small compared with the risk of not treating laryngeal edema.

If advanced obstruction is present, a needle tracheostomy can be performed, using a 14- or 15-gauge needle inserted percutaneously into the trachea just below the cricoid cartilage. Air is injected through a plastic connector using a 50-ml syringe. As soon as possible, an endotracheal tube can be placed. Bronchospasm with asthma is a serious symptom, often producing cyanosis. Treatment consists of subcutaneous injection of 0.3 to 0.5 mg of epinephrine (1:1000) and administration of 500 mg of aminophylline through the indwelling intravenous needle over a 10-minute period.

Pulmonary edema may occur in patients with heart failure when intravenous injection of hypertonic contrast solution produces marked expansion of the intravascular volume and overload of the left side of the heart. Intravenous injection of 20 mg of furosemide (Lasix) is indicated.

Apnea is clearly the most serious respiratory reaction, and treatment requires assisted ventilation. After removal of dentures, a nasal or oral airway should be inserted, or, if possible, an endotracheal tube should be placed. If necessary, a tracheostomy should be performed. Once an airway is established, oxygen by mask is the treatment of choice but mouth-to-mouth artificial respiration should be carried out if oxygen is not immediately availabe.

For severe hypotension, 4 mg of levarterenol in 500 ml of a 5 per cent glucose solution can be infused. Cardiac asystole should be treated immediately by closed-chest cardiac massage until the arrival of the resuscitation team.

The neurologic reactions most often encountered are headache and convulsions. Headache is generally considered to be a minor reaction. Convulsions are of two types: those that represent an exacerbation of a latent tendency to epilepsy and those that result from hypotensive collapse, cardiac arrest, or contrast medium overdosage. The former will not have concomitant cardiovascular findings and require no treatment. The latter requires cardiovascular treatment.

Physiology of Opaque Excretion

There are two major capillary beds in the kidney—the peritubular capillaries and the glomerular capillaries. Tubular cell secretion and glomerular cell filtration are the two potential avenues for elimination of contrast medium by the kidney. The former requires cellular work, and there is a maximum amount of opaque excretion that can occur in this way in any unit of time despite the level of contrast medium in the blood. Glomerular filtration, on the other hand, is directly responsible to the level of contrast in the blood. All currently employed urographic media are almost entirely excreted by glomerular filtration, although tubular secretion is a potential channel.

The amount of opaque excretion depends upon the level of contrast medium in the blood and the glomerular filtration rate. The level of contrast medium in the blood is determined by the volume injected, rate of injection, and equilibration of the contrast within both the intravascular and the extravascular spaces. The glomerular filtration rate depends upon the number and quality of functioning glomeruli and the pressure and flow rate within the glomerular capillaries. Except for remediable hypotension, the only factor accessible to the radiologist is the concentration of contrast medium in the circulating blood. Since this relates to the number of iodine-containing molecules in the nephrons, it is an important determinant of the density of the nephrogram. The contrast medium concentration of the urine filtrate in the nephron is essentially independent of the state of hydration of the patient or the ability of the patient to produce a concentrated urine. A nephrogram adequate for evaluation of renal size and shape can be produced in patients with normal renal function, and, even with standard contrast doses, in some patients with renal insufficiency (Fig. 7–1).

Factors predisposing to slow urine flow through the kidney (such as decreased renal blood flow or lowered intraglomerular blood pressure) will increase the time the urine filtrate remains in the nephron and collecting tubules, and this will lead to increased concentration of the filtrate and a dense nephrogram. About 25 per cent of the urine concentration occurs in the distal convoluted tubules and the collecting tubules and ducts. It is related to antidiuretic hormone formation and reflects the patient's state of hydration. If small doses of contrast medium are used, preliminary dehydration of the patient results in denser opacification of the urine and an improved urogram. Larger doses of contrast medium make preliminary dehydration unnecessary.

Procedure for the Urogram

At bedtime the evening before the examinataion, the patient should take a laxative with as much water as desired. Nothing else should be taken by mouth until the examination is completed the next morning. (For afternoon examinations, the preparation is adjusted accordingly.) Cleansing enemas are not helpful and may make bowel preparation worse by introducing more air into the colon.

Before performing the urographic examination the radiologist should be familiar with the patient's clinical status and with the ques-

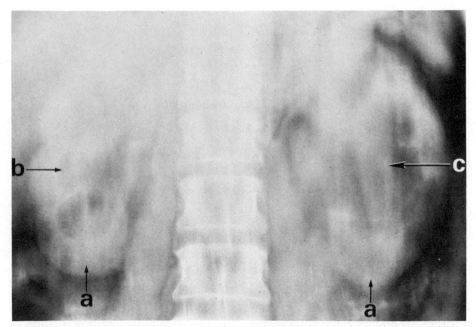

Figure 7–1. Negative pyelogram in hydronephrosis. Tomographic 1-minute film of excretory urogram: *a,* opacified parenchyma; *b,* unopacified urine in hydronephrotic calyx; *c,* unopacified urine in hydronephrotic pelvis.

tions the patient's physician would like illuminated. In the presence of renal colic, the use of compression should be avoided, and both the patient and the radiologist must be prepared for the possibility that delayed films will be needed, thus prolonging the total examination time. In the presence of lower urinary tract symptoms, a somewhat larger dose of contrast material may be used so that an excretory urethrogram can be done if it is indicated as the examination progresses. If the patient has bronchial asthma or hay fever, special care in observing the patient for the early signs of a contrast reaction is indicated. If the patient has had evidence of decreased cardiac reserve, the possibility that the injection of a large dose of a hyperosmolar substance may be sufficient to cause volume overload of the heart with pulmonary edema should be considered, and if necessary, the examination should be postponed. In patients with epilepsy, the contrast agent may precipitate a seizure. Premedication with an antiepileptic drug is a wise precaution.

Preliminary plain films of the urinary tract should cover the entire area from the superior border of the adrenal gland to the inferior border of the prostate gland in the male and the distal urethra in the female. Both flanks should be visible in the preliminary films but may be excluded by careful coning in later films in order to improve film contrast. A single 14- × 17-inch film is often adequate for this purpose in small and medium-sized adults. The use of two horizontal 10- × 12-inch films, one for the upper portion of the abdomen and the other for the lower portion, has much to recommend it (Fig. 7–2). With careful coning, the volume dose for each smaller film is less than that for the larger film, and the amount of scattered radiation is smaller, enhancing film contrast.

A preliminary plain tomogram is made to determine the proper levels for the tomograms that will be made during the nephrogram phase of the examination. If the anteroposterior diameter of the abdomen is measured at the level of the lower costal margin, the average tomographic level above the table top for midcoronal sections of the kidney can be predicted with accuracy in most cases (adapted from Newberg and Mindell, 1976):

AP Measurement (cm)	Tomographic Level (cm)
14–17	7
18–22	8
23–26	9
27–29	10
30+	11
Iliac fossa transplant	14,15

The midcoronal plane of the kidney is usually at the level of the pedicles or posterior surface of the body of L2 vertebra.

The supervising physician should inspect the preliminary films as soon as they are made, suggest ways of improving film quality, and request additional radiographs, such as oblique views, to establish whether any calcifications are

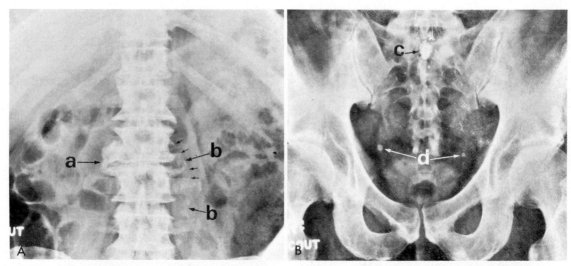

Figure 7–2. Plain roentgenograms of upper *(A)* and lower *(B)* portions of the abdomen: *a,* hypertrophic lipping; *b,* calcified aortic aneurysm (arrows); *c,* residual myelographic contrast medium; *d,* phleboliths.

likely to be within the urinary tract. If there are clinical reasons to suspect the presence of renal calculi, plain tomograms may detect stones too small to be seen on plain roentgenograms.

When the preliminary films are satisfactory, the contrast medium is injected. At Brigham and Women's Hospital all routine urographic examinations are performed by injecting a bolus of 0.5 ml per pound of body weight of a diatrizoate salt. The injection is made as fast as possible by hand, usually taking between 15 and 30 seconds, through a 19-gauge needle catheter (butterfly needle), which is left in the arm vein

for 5 to 10 minutes. Although some radiologists prefer to begin making the tomographic nephrograms 30 seconds after the onset of injection, we prefer 1 minute (Fig. 7–3). The earlier nephrogram often still demonstrates denser opacification of the cortex than the medulla, in all likelihood as a consequence of the richer blood supply. By 1 minute, nephrographic opacification of parenchyma is usually uniform, and mass lesions are more readily recognized. An exception to this rule is an ectopic lobe (lobar dysmorphism, "prominent column of Bertin"), in which a very early nephrogram demonstrates

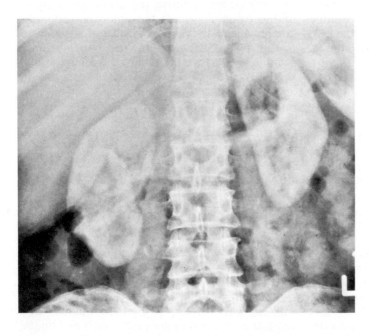

Figure 7–3. One-minute nephrogram. The apparent segmentation of the right kidney into two ovoids is normal.

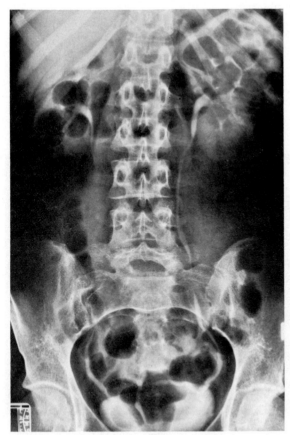

Figure 7–4. Five-minute excretion urogram. Portions of the calyces, infundibula, and ureters are unfilled because of normal systolic contraction.

the abnormal position of the cortex and medulla. Three tomographic nephrograms are made, each 1 cm apart, with the middle one at the previously determined midcoronal level. Careful selection of exposure factors is critical in assuring good tomographic nephrograms. Low-kilovoltage, fast-intensifying screens, and linear tube arcs of 25 to 40 degrees are recommended.

A 14- × 17-inch exposure is made at 5 minutes (Fig. 7–4), and ureteral compression is applied unless it is contraindicated by the presence of ureteral calculi, an abdominal aortic aneurysm, or recent abdominal operative procedures. After the 5-minute film is checked, the decision can be made whether to proceed in the usual fashion with anterior and both oblique views of the kidney with ureteral compression at 10 minutes (Fig. 7–5) or to delay filming.

It is an important principle of urography that the calyces, pelves, and ureters should, on one or another of the films, be well filled with opacified urine in order that anatomic abnormalities can be either excluded or delineated. Muscular contractions occur at every level of the upper collecting system, and an area in systole can harbor an undisclosed abnormality. The effects of systolic emptying can be prevented either by compression of the ureter or by markedly diuretic doses of contrast medium, such as those used in drip-infusion urography. With the latter approach, large volumes of urine cause the collecting system to be well filled on most exposures.

Ureteral compression, when properly applied, is a remarkable effective method of producing excellent filling of the upper collecting system. Two small rubber bladders are placed on the abdomen at the level of the fifth lumbar vertebra on either side of the midline, and a cloth band is fastened around the trunk to hold them in place. The bladders are then inflated to a degree that partly or completely occludes the ureters without producing undue discomfort for the patient. If the site of compression is too caudal, it is difficult or impossible to occlude the ureters. When the 10-minute films have been judged to show well all portions of the calyces, pelves, and upper ureters, a release film is made. This is accomplished by exposing a 14- × 17-inch film of the abdomen a few seconds after the release of abdominal compression so that the lower halves of both ureters are seen throughout their extent by the drainage from the recently obstructed upper ureters (Fig. 7–6). At 20 minutes a prone film is exposed to show the bladder (Fig. 7–7). In males over 45 and in females with signs or symptoms suggesting a urethral diverticulum, a postvoiding film of the bladder is made (Figs. 7–8 and 7–9).

Radiographic screening for renovascular hypertension by means of rapid-sequence excretory urography with films at 2, 3, 5, and 10 minutes is an inefficient method. At best, it reveals only 60 to 80 per cent of patients with renovascular lesions, and it produces many false positive results. Digital subtraction angiography is currently considered by many to be the screening method of choice. If it is not available and rapid-sequence urography is requested, false positive findings can be virtually eliminated by relying solely on the presence of delayed calyceal opacification on the involved side. It is easier to evaluate than unilateral hyperconcentration, and it is rarely the result of parenchymal disease (Fig. 7–10). The sensitivity will be only slightly less.

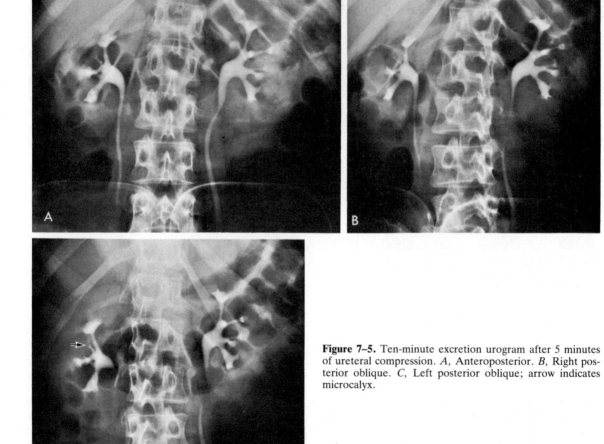

Figure 7–5. Ten-minute excretion urogram after 5 minutes of ureteral compression. *A*, Anteroposterior. *B*, Right posterior oblique. *C*, Left posterior oblique; arrow indicates microcalyx.

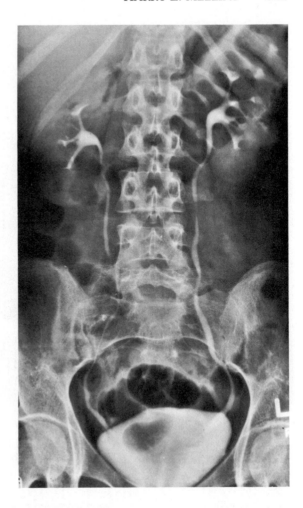

Figure 7–6. Fifteen-minute excretion urogram immediately after release of ureteral compression shows both ureters.

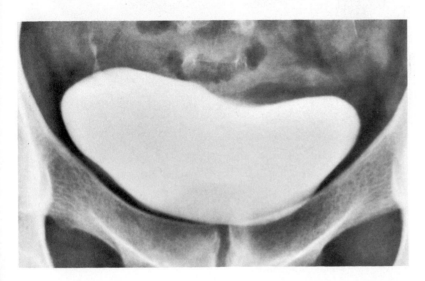

Figure 7–7. Twenty-minute excretion urogram. Supine view of bladder.

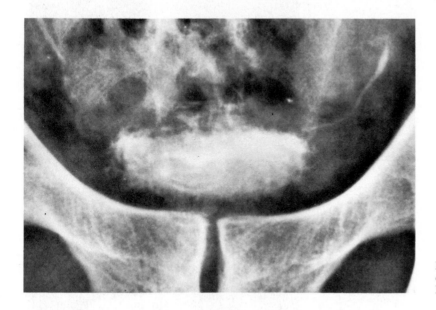

Figure 7–8. Postvoiding film of excretion urogram in man aged 45. Normal bladder emptying.

Figure 7–9. Postvoiding film of excretion urogram in woman aged 26. Round opaque collection below bladder represents urethral diverticulum. Same patient as in Figure 7–7.

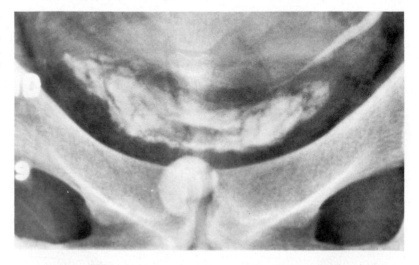

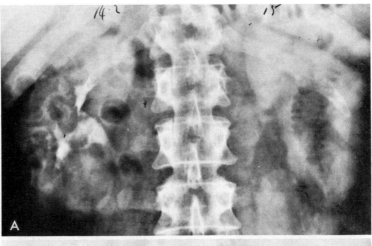

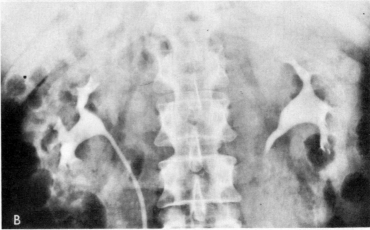

Figure 7–10. Renovascular hypertension. Excretion urogram. *A,* Delayed calyceal opacification on the left at 3 minutes. Both kidneys are normal in size and nephrographic density. *B,* Both pelves are normal in volume and density at 10 minutes.

Examination of Children

The radiologist who does urographic examinations of children should be sensitive to the needs of children and aware of how their responses to this examination differ from those of adults.

1. Fear of the procedures should be anticipated, and every attempt should be made to be gentle, reassuring, quick, and skillful.

2. The rate of opaque excretion is slower in infants than in older children and adults.

3. Severe idiosyncratic reactions to contrast media are rare in childhood.

4. The risk of inducing dehydration by the injection of contrast medium is greater than in adults.

5. Swallowed air in the small intestine is always present up to the age of 2, usually present to the age of 5, and occasionally present to the age of 7.

6. Total body opacification will occur.

7. Radiation dose is essentially cumulative.

GENERAL OUTLINE OF TECHNIQUE
(Lebowitz, 1984)

1. Use a polyethylene fused needle-catheter in an accessible arm or foot vein. A scalp vein can be used in infants.

2. Relate dose of conventional urographic contrast medium to the size of the child:
less than 12 pounds: 2 ml per pound
12 to 25 pounds: 25 ml
25 to 50 pounds: 1 ml per pound
50 to 100 pounds: 50 ml
more than 100 pounds: 0.5 ml per pound

3. Generally, no bowel preparation, fluid restriction, or compression is necessary.

4. Select the necessary exposures for each patient and avoid a routine filming schedule. A preliminary plain radiograph, 3-minute radiograph of the kidneys, and 15-minute radiograph of the kidneys, ureters, and bladder often suffice for an initial study, while a single 15-minute radiograph of the entire urinary tract may be sufficient for a follow-up study (Fig. 7–11). Prone views may be necessary to displace over-

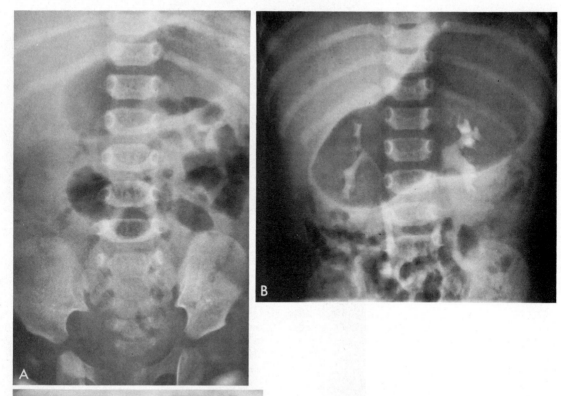

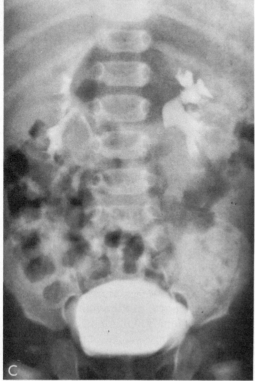

Figure 7–11. Excretory urogram of an infant. *A*, Preliminary supine plain film. *B*, Three-minute supine film. *C*, Fifteen-minute supine film. (Courtesy of Dr. Robert Lebowitz.)

lying gas shadows. Tomography is often very helpful. A lateral view often helps in localizing masses or demonstrating defects in the vertebral column. In the absence of early opaque excretion, avoid films at too frequent intervals and skip usually to 2 to 4 hours. Ultrasound examination is complementary and may eliminate the need for prolonged roentgenologic examination.

5. Shield gonads whenever feasible.

RETROGRADE PYELOGRAPHY

Indications and Contraindications

With the marked improvement in quality of excretory urography over the past 30 years, the number of retrograde pyelograms has steadily decreased. A major indication for this examination is inadequate visualization of the collecting systems by excretion urography. This is usually caused by poor renal function but may result from inability to fill all parts of the collecting system, especially the ureters. Contraindications to retrograde pyelography include some types of urinary stasis. It is better not to inject contrast medium above a ureteric obstruction because untoward reactions, such as chills and fever or cessation of urine flow, may result.

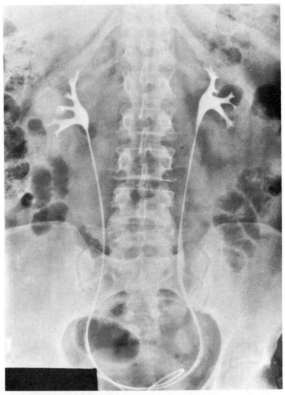

Figure 7–12. Retrograde pyelogram after injection of 4 ml of contrast medium shows calyces and pelves.

Technique

After cystoscopic examination of the bladder, one or both ureters are catheterized, usually with an opaque catheter of 5 French caliber. Catheterization is done with great care in order to avoid irritation of the ureter and consequent ureteral spasm.

The technical details of the procedure and the specific radiographs that are made depend upon the particular problem under study and the approach of the urologist. A preliminary plain film of the urinary tract is usually followed by a film showing the ureteral catheters in position. These will demonstrate the position of the ureters and the relationship of any opacities in the region of the kidneys and ureters. Oblique and lateral films, as needed, can be made to demonstrate the precise relationship of the opacities and the catheters.

A syringe can be connected to the distal end of each catheter by means of a close-fitting needle or special rubber adaptor and the renal pelvis can be emptied by aspiration. Four or 5 ml of contrast medium is slowly injected into the renal pelvis, unless it is clear from previous

urographic examinations or aspiration that there is a considerably larger capacity (Fig. 7–12). Any of the conventional urographic contrast media may be used at half strength or less. Some urologists prefer to add an antibiotic such as neomycin. Retrografin, a commercially available contrast medium, consists of 30 per cent Renografin and a 2.5 per cent concentration of neomycin. Since the examination is often done under anesthesia, the patient cannot indicate pain from overdistention of the collecting system. Infrequently, the force or volume of injection is greater than a particular collecting system can tolerate and extravasation from the calyces occurs. Reflux into the collecting ducts is not truly an extravasation. Except in the presence of urinary tract infection, extravasations have no lasting significance, although the patient may have discomfort for a few days. On rare occasions, extravasation of infected urine with venous or lymphatic uptake can lead to sepsis.

Diagnostically, extravasations and reflux into collecting tubules may obscure fine calyceal detail. Examination of the first filled radiograph after contrast injection will determine whether filling is adequate and details are clear. Addi-

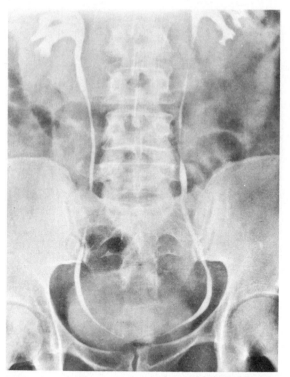

Figure 7–13. Retrograde pyelogram after ureteral filling and removal of catheters.

evaluated, an additional 2 ml of contrast medium is injected into the pelvis. As the catheter is slowly withdrawn, additional contrast medium is injected to outline the ureter, and another radiographic exposure is made (Fig. 7–13). If the withdrawal radiograph does not show an adequately filled ureter, ureteropyelograms should be made, using a catheter with an expanded tip placed against the ureteral orifice in the bladder. The bulb, acorn-tipped, or Woodruff catheter is used for this purpose. Ten minutes or longer after removal of ureteral catheters, a delayed film (drainage film, trap film) can be made for evidence of stasis. This is most often valuable in ureteropelvic junction lesions.

Intrapelvic lesions, such as nonopaque stones, may sometimes be obscured by opaque contrast medium and air may be a valuable contrast substance (Fig. 7–14). With the patient in a moderate Fowler position, about 2 ml of air is injected into the pelvis through the ureteral

tional films, as needed, can be made after injection of more contrast medium. Fixation of the kidneys as a result of perinephric inflammation or suppuration may be investigated by means of an exposure in deep inspiration superimposed on an exposure in deep expiration. Three-quarters of the usual quantity of radiation is used for each exposure. If there is a perinephric inflammatory or suppurative process, the ipsilateral kidney often remains fixed in position and a single, sharp outline of the collecting system results. On the normal side, respiratory excursion of the kidney creates two renal pelvic outlines separated by approximately 2 cm. Renal or perinephric abscess or renal tumor may displace the kidney up or down or from side to side, and these shifts are usually recognized easily on frontal views. Anterior displacement of the kidney or rotation of the kidney on its transverse axis may be difficult to detect on an anteroposterior radiograph, and a true lateral pyelogram may be the only way to identify the mass. Usually the renal pelvis is superimposed on the vertebral bodies, and its axis runs downward and anteriorly. In the presence of masses, either pole or the entire kidney may be displaced anteriorly.

After radiographs of the renal pelvis are

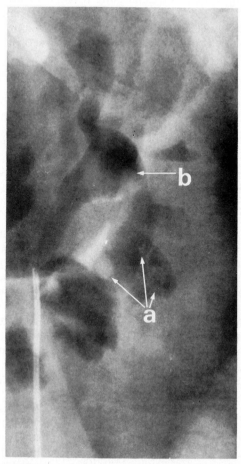

Figure 7–14. Pneumopyelogram: *a,* low-opacity calculi in the lower pole calyces are outlined by injected air; *b,* pelvis.

catheter. If this is done immediately after opaque pyelography, a double-contrast study may sometimes be achieved. Removal of the injected air may prevent the mild ureteral colic that sometimes occurs.

ANTEGRADE PYELOGRAPHY AND PERCUTANEOUS NEPHROPYELOSTOMY

Occasionally a kidney with very poor opaque excretion cannot be examined by retrograde pyelography because the ureter is impassable from below or because a cystoscopic procedure is clinically contraindicated. Percutaneous needle puncture of the renal pelvis or a calyx, with or without catheter replacement of the needle, is a safe and effective way to opacify an upper collecting system (Fig. 7–15). Percutaneous nephropyelostomy employs a

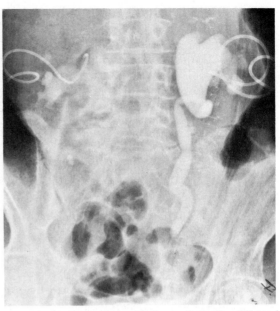

Figure 7–16. Percutaneous nephropyelostomies. Bilateral distal ureteral obstruction resulting from complications of colon carcinoma.

technique similar to that used in antegrade pyelography to place a Teflon or polyethylene catheter in the renal pelvis for temporary urinary tract drainage (Jonsson et al., 1972) (Fig. 7–16). Specific indications include: (1) localization of ureteral obstruction caused by stricture, nonopaque stone, or tumor; (2) evaluation of ureteral obstruction after urinary diversion operations; (3) hydronephrosis in a child with poor opaque excretion to identify ureteropelvic and ureterovesical obstructions; and (4) as the basic preliminary step before percutaneous lithotripsy and stone removal.

Technique

With the patient in the prone position and suspending respiration, the renal pelvis is localized either by sonographic visualization or by fluoroscopy after intravenous injection of contrast medium. The overlying skin is marked and prepared. Under local anesthesia, the skin is incised, and a 1.5-inch, 14-gauge needle with stylet is inserted its full length toward the renal pelvis. With the patient suspending respiration, a 20-gauge, thin-walled biopsy needle with stylet is advanced through the needle into the lumen of the renal pelvis. Flexible tubing connects the syringe to the needle to aspirate urine; half-strength urographic contrast medium, or full strength if needed, is injected to outline the

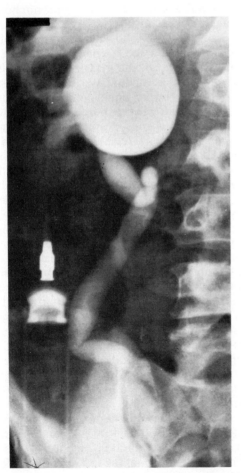

Figure 7–15. Antegrade pyelogram after sonographically guided percutaneous needle puncture and catheter substitution. (Courtesy of Dr. Edward Smith.)

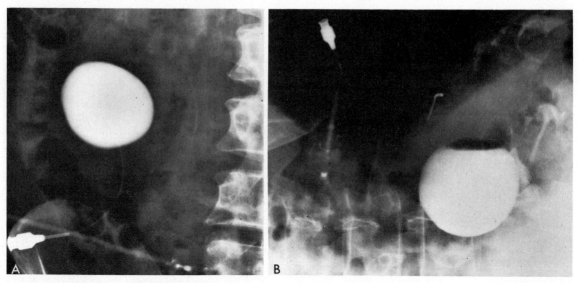

Figure 7–17. Renal cyst puncture with contrast injection. *A,* Anteroposterior view. *B,* Left lateral decubitus view.

upper collecting system to the point of obstruction. Posteroanterior, oblique, and anteroposterior radiographs are exposed to delineate the involved area. Antibiotic drugs are recommended for several days because of instrumentation above ureteral obstruction. The technique described is used by Lalli (1972) and has been notably effective and safe. In children the appropriate anesthesia or sedation for age is chosen, and a single 22-gauge spinal needle is used (Lebowitz, 1984).

RENAL CYST PUNCTURE

Sonography and computed tomography are the best methods for determining whether a renal mass is a simple cyst. Either may be used without risk of overlooking a malignancy provided that strict diagnostic criteria are used. On rare occasions, when the radiologic evidence is equivocal, renal cyst puncture with gross and microscopic examination of the fluid will permit a firm diagnosis.

The procedure can be done under either fluoroscopic or sonographic control. Under fluoroscopic control, intravenous injection of a conventional dose of urographic contrast medium is used to identify the lesion; the skin of the back is then marked to guide needle insertion. After the injection of a small amount of Xylocaine to anesthetize the skin, a 20-gauge 3.5- to 5-inch thin-walled needle connected to flexible tubing is inserted. The patient should suspend respiration while the needle traverses

the cyst wall and until the operator is not holding the needle. Usually the resistance of the renal fascia can be felt, followed by entrance of the needle into the cyst. If the fluid is clear and colorless or yellow, the mass is in all likelihood a simple cyst. Cyst fluid is carefully aspirated and replaced by an equal volume of contrast medium and air. The needle is removed while the patient suspends respiration, and radiographs are made in recumbent, erect, and decubitus positions to demonstrate the entire inner surface of the cyst (Fig. 7–17). It should be smooth throughout, and its size and shape should be the same as the nephrographic defect on similarly positioned radiographic views. This size-and-shape test will decrease or eliminate the chance of missing a tumor adjacent to a cyst (Lang, 1966). The most common cause of difficulty in interpretation is removal of much more fluid than is replaced by contrast media, with consequent inward bulging of a portion of the cyst wall. This artifact can usually be recognized by its complete smoothness and peculiar angularity. Hemorrhagic benign renal cysts are difficult to distinguish radiologically from cystic lesions caused by or associated with malignant tumors; as a rule, surgical exploration is required for such lesions.

Complications of cyst puncture are rare and consist essentially of intrarenal and perirenal hemorrhage. It is common practice to observe patients in the hospital for 12 hours for evidence of bleeding. One should be alert to the danger of puncturing an unsuspected uncalcified intrarenal arterial aneurysm, a well-circumscribed abscess, or an echinococcal cyst. If these lesions are kept in mind during the preliminary evaluation of intrarenal masses, later difficulties should be easily averted.

EXCRETORY CYSTOGRAPHY

A confident opinion about the bladder usually cannot be rendered after review of the conventional excretory urogram for several reasons. Multiple views of the bladder to display all surfaces and borders are usually not made, and the examination is limited to one or two anteroposterior views. Since it is not possible to determine, from a frontal view, whether the bladder contains unopacified urine floating on the heavier, opacified urine, one cannot be confident that even the available image is reliable. To further complicate matters, filling of a large hollow viscus with opaque contrast medium may hide as many lesions as it demonstrates. In addition, superimposed gas and feces in the small intestine and rectosigmoid colon may produce images that simulate intraluminal bladder lesions. It is probable that more effort is not directed to overcoming these difficulties and limitations because the bladder is so accessible to effective examination by cystoscopy and to a lesser degree by manual palpation. It is easy, however, for the person monitoring the urogram to predict from the clinical information which patients are likely to have intrinsic or extrinsic involvement of the bladder. By expanding the urographic examination of these patients to include good excretory cystograms, valuable information can be secured without extending or complicating all urographic examinations.

Indications

1. Pelvic fractures and other trauma to the lower abdomen and pelvis. In the presence of hematuria after pelvic or abdominal trauma, excretory urography is indicated to demonstrate or exclude injury or pre-existing abnormality of the upper tracts. If excretory cystograms show a high-riding bladder (craniad displacement of the bladder), avulsion of the urethra is highly likely, and cystostomy drainage will probably be undertaken without urethral instrumentation or retrograde urethrocystography. Bladder lacerations and compression of the bladder from below or from the side are often demonstrated, but failure to demonstrate a laceration does not exclude it, and retrograde urethrography and cystography are required if clinical suspicion of uethral or bladder injury persists.

2. After renal transplantation, for demonstration of bladder compression by lymphoceles or uriniferous pseudocysts (urinomas) (Fig. 7–18).

Figure 7–18. Excretory cystogram after renal transplantation. Displacement of the bladder to the left represents large lymphocele. The superolateral concavity represents proximity of normal lower renal pole.

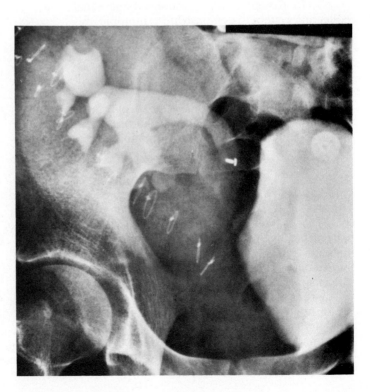

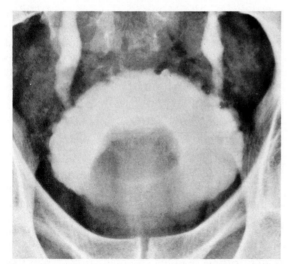

Figure 7–19. Excretory cystogram shows median prostatic lobe hypertrophy.

3. In patients with regional enteritis, colonic diverticulitis, or endometriosis, when involvement of the bladder wall is suspected.

4. In acquired disorders of micturition, when used in conjunction with excretory voiding urethrography, to determine whether the cause is (1) an organic obstructive lesion; (2) a neurogenic failure of bladder contraction as a result of a sensory defect (as in diabetes); or (3) failure of external sphincter relaxation following nerve transection during pelvic operations.

5. In patients with a nonopacifying renal collecting system to demonstrate orthotopic ureteroceles or ectopic ureteroceles.

6. For evidence of median prostatic lobe hypertrophy in patients with symptoms of prostatism and insufficient evidence of prostatic enlargement by palpation (Fig. 7–19).

7. In patients with unexplained pyuria or hematuria after excretory urography of the upper tracts, cystography is also sometimes helpful.

Techniques

The bladder is emptied before the examination begins. One ml of urographic contrast medium per pound of body weight up to a maximum of 150 ml is injected at the onset of the examination. If it is decided to do excretory cystography afer the completion of a standard-dose urogram, the original dose of contrast medium should be reinjected. After urographic examination of the kidneys, ureters, and bladder is completed, the patient is asked to drink as many glasses of water as possible in 30 to 60

minutes. Films made 1 to 1.5 hours after the onset of the urographic examination will ordinarily show a well-filled bladder. Three views of the filled bladder in the posteroanterior and both posterior oblique positions and an anteroposterior postvoiding radiograph constitute an acceptable basic examination of the bladder. Penetration of the films should be sufficient to visualize the sacrum through the bladder shadow. Occasionally a superoinferior view of the bladder with the patient sitting and leaning forward ("squat shot") will furnish useful information about herniation, diverticula, and the relationships of the lowermost portions of the ureters.

RETROGRADE CYSTOGRAPHY

Indications

Retrograde cystography can be used for all indications listed under excretory cystography. The retrograde approach is particularly valuable under certain circumstances:

1. When bladder injury is suspected and urethral injury has been excluded. Both the presence and the location of bladder rupture can be determined with the highest accuracy. It is most important to determine whether the 11rupture is intraperitoneal or extraperitoneal.

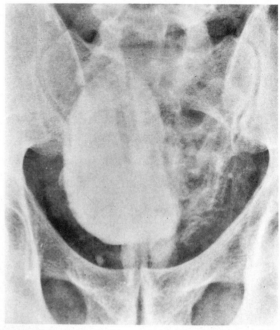

Figure 7–20. Retrograde cystogram. The indentation along the left lateral wall, containing streaks of contrast medium, represents an extraperitoneal collection.

The former will usually require laparotomy and closure of the laceration, while urethral drainage by catheter may be the procedure of choice for the latter (Fig. 7–20).

2. When cystoscopic examination of the bladder is difficult (as in some male infants or in adults with elongation or rigidity of the prostatic urethra resulting from tumor or benign prostatic enlargement).

3. To determine the size of vesical diverticula and the presence of malignant tumors or stones within them.

Technique

After catheterization of the bladder under sterile conditions, the bladder is filled with 200 to 300 ml of a 25 or 30 per cent solution of any standard urographic medium. Filling can be achieved by gravity or by careful syringe injection. Films should be made in the anteroposterior and both posterior oblique views. If the patient's condition permits, a posteroanterior view is valuable, but this may be difficult to achieve. If a mass is seen within the bladder and further views are desired, 100 to 300 ml of air can be introduced carefully into the bladder after the opaque contrast medium has been removed. Such double-contrast cystograms may clarify the extent of a bladder tumor.

If it is desired to determine whether vesicoureteral reflux occurs, voiding cystourethrography is more accurate and will demonstrate both high- and low-pressure reflux. Static retrograde cystography is less accurate and generally reveals only low-pressure reflux.

In patients with lower abdominal or pelvic trauma in whom urethral or bladder injury may be present, it is often possible to diagnose complete transection of the urethra by determining the position of the bladder on excretory cystograpy. If not, and the possibility of urethral injury remains, as in patients with straddle injuries, it is safer to proceed with retrograde urethrography under fluoroscopic control. If the urethra is normal, the Foley balloon in the fossa navicularis can be emptied and the catheter advanced into the bladder for the performance of retrograde cystography.

If the patient with pelvic fracture has had a self-retaining catheter inserted in the emergency room before a radiologic examination of the lower urinary tract, retrograde urethrography should be done by the second catheter technique of McLaughlin and Pfister (1974). A 16-gauge polyethylene catheter is inserted into the fossa navicularis next to the Foley catheter.

While manual compression is applied to the glans penis to close the urethral lumen distally, retrograde urethrography under fluoroscopic control is carried out through the polyethylene catheter. If the urethra is normal, retrograde cystography can follow.

VOIDING CYSTOURETHROGRAPHY

Voiding cystourethrography is most often performed after instillation of contrast medium into the bladder by urethral catheterization. Occasionally, if the urethral catheterization is difficult, as in some newborn infants, suprapubic bladder puncture is required. Although voiding cystourethrography can be performed after intravenous injection of urographic contrast medium, to do so compromises recognition of small degrees of vesicoureteral reflux. Ureteric filling by continuing renal excretion of opaque urine complicates identification of ureteric filling by vesicoureteral reflux.

Indications

1. Urinary infection in children and recurrent or persistent urinary infections in adults (Fig. 7–21).

2. Investigation of the cause of scarred or

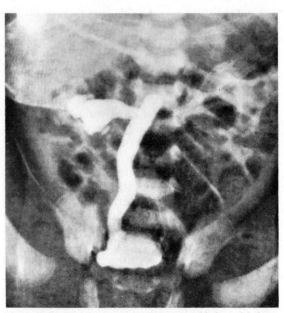

Figure 7–21. Voiding cystourethrogram of infant girl showing reflux into a lower duplicated right ureter. Only the upper member was visualized by excretion urography. (Courtesy of Dr. Robert Lebowitz.)

small kidneys, especially in children but also in some adults.

3. Evaluation of narrowing of the uretero-pelvic junction, especially if associated with dilated ureters, to identify those lesions produced by ureterovesical reflux.

4. Bilateral upper urinary tract dilatation and other signs of infravesical obstruction in boys.

5. Neurogenic lesions of the bladder and urethra in children and adults.

Technique

Since even minimal trauma to the urethra will lead to pain upon voiding, catheterization should be done with extreme gentleness. The use of plastic feeding tubes as catheters for small children is advised. It is helpful to instill a small amount of water-souble anesthetic lubricating jelly into the urethra prior to catheterization. All of these approaches will help to render the voiding phase of the examination painless and therefore uninterrupted and vigorous. This will eliminate artifacts resulting from muscle spasm or incomplete sphincteric relaxation.

Using a standard infusion set, a 15 per cent concentration of a conventional urographic contrast medium is instilled into the bladder by gravity drip from a height of 45 cm above the level of the bladder. The quantity required varies from 35 to 50 ml for a newborn infant to 200 ml or more for a child old enough to be continent through the night. It is best to fill the bladder to the verge of discomfort in older children and adults or until flow into bladder stops or slows down appreciably.

Recording of the examination may be done by fluoroscopic spot filming or by overhead radiographs. The radiation dose from cinefluorography performed by most radiologists is excessive, while the detail in tape recording is often inadequate. When fluoroscopic spot filming is used, it is important to limit fluoroscopic exposure to the absolute minimum. A spot film of the bladder and kidney area when the bladder is well filled is followed by small, well-coned spot films of the urethra during voiding. Four exposures on one film usually suffice to document the size and shape of the urethra throughout its length. The area of the trigone is scanned for evidence of reflux into the ureters during voiding; this is documented on spot films. A simpler and very effective method that eliminates fluoroscopic observation uses only one or two large films (14 × 17 inches or smaller).

With the patient in the right or left posterior oblique position, an exposure of the area from the urethra to the upper poles of the kidneys, made when voiding is well and strongly under way, is a very satisfactory method for demonstrating urethral lesions and vesicoureteral reflux. If the exposure factors do not permit delineation of both ureters on a single oblique view, both oblique views are necessary, and the patient is asked to suspend voiding after the first exposure and resume for the second. This is usually easily accomplished by older children and adults. Films of the best technical quality are usually made in the recumbent position, but if a patient finds voiding difficult in this position, upright films should be made. Gonadal shielding should be used for boys and young men but cannot be employed for girls and women because the urinary tract will be obscured.

Combined voiding cystourethrography and retrograde urethrography is the most valuable radiologic examination of the lower urinary tract in paraplegic patients with neurogenic bladders of the reflex or autonomous types. It is described in the section on retrograde urethrography.

EXCRETORY URETHROGRAPHY

Although excretory urethrography has been described for many years, it has not been generally applied. Excellent urethrographic films can be made at the end of an excretory urogram.

Indications

1. Complaints of hesitancy, urgency, or dysuria.

2. Sensation of incomplete voiding following pelvic operations or recurrent symptoms after transurethral prostatectomy.

3. Urographic evidence of bladder diverticula or saccule formation suggesting infravesical obstruction.

4. Hematuria unexplained by excretory urography.

5. Recurrent urinary infection.

Technique
(Fitts et al., 1977a)

The bladder is emptied before the examination begins. One ml of urographic contrast medium per pound of body weight to a maximum of 150 ml is injected. After the urographic examination of the kidneys, ureters, and bladder is completed, the patient is asked to drink as many glasses of water as he can until he experiences the urge to void. After scout films of the urethra in the right posterior oblique view are made with the patient recumbent, a penile (Zipser) clamp is placed on the penis just proximal to the glans, as described by Boltuch and Lalli (1975). The patient is asked to void past the clamp into a urinal, and a film is made while the patient is maintaining a good urinary stream. If desired, the patient can cease voiding after the first film and resume for a second exposure. In most cases, distal urethral compression causes adequate distention of the urethra throughout its length (Fig. 7–22). Even in the presence of significant urethral narrowing, adequate distal filling of the urethra can be achieved (Fitts et al., 1977b).

RETROGRADE URETHROGRAPHY

While this is an excellent method of demonstrating the penile, bulbar, and membranous portions of the urethra, it is usually not satisfactory for demonstrating the prostatic urethra because the urethral and vesical sphincters are closed. If a complete study of the urethra is desired, the retrograde urethrogram must be supplemented by a voiding cystourethrogram. Retrograde urethrography in women, using a double-balloon catheter that occludes the internal meatus from above and the external meatus from below, has been recommended for demonstration of urethral diverticula. Equally effective visualization of urethral diverticula in women can be accomplished by excretory voiding urethrography or voiding cystourethrography.

Technique (Males)

The simplest and probably most effective urethrographic device is a Foley catheter. The balloon should be tested by inflation and deflation several times before insertion so that it will inflate easily. Water should be injected into the balloon in 1-ml increments before catheterization so that the size of the inflated balloon can be compared with the expected size of the fossa navicularis. The tip should not be lubricated with a jelly but may be dipped into sterile water before being inserted. The catheter is inserted until the base of the balloon is no longer seen. Between 1 and 2 ml of water are carefully injected into the balloon. Resistance to very gentle traction on the catheter will indicate adequate distention. The patient will experience a sense of fullness but should not experience pain.

Conventional urographic contrast media, at half strength, are excellent for urethrography. Media containing thickening agents should not be used because venous intravasation can occur during any urethrographic procedure. A 50-ml syringe is used with an adapter for the Foley catheter. The catheter should be filled with

Figure 7–22. Excretory urethrogram of normal man with partial distal urethral occlusion by penile clamp: *a,* internal urethral meatus; *b,* verumontanum; *c,* membranous urethra; *d,* bulbar urethra; *e,* suspensory ligament; *f,* pendulous urethra; *g,* penile clamp.

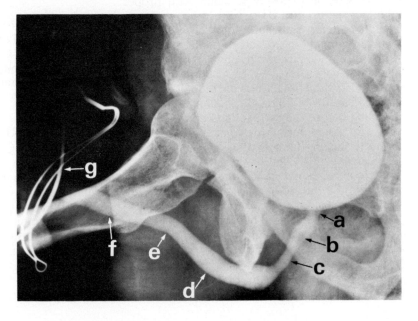

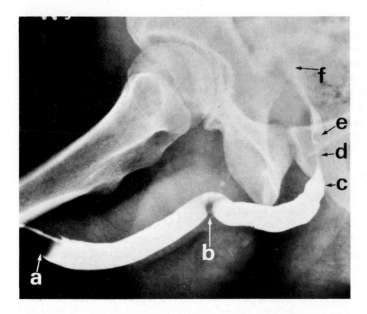

Figure 7–23. Retrograde urethrogram: *a*, balloon catheter in fossa navicularis; *b*, gas bubble (artifact) at penoscrotal junction; *c*, normal cone-shaped proximal bulbar portion; *d*, membranous portion; *e*, colliculus seminalis; *f*, intravesical protrusion of enlarged prostate gland.

contrast medium before insertion in order to eliminate air bubbles.

With the patient in the right posterior oblique position, the right thigh is drawn up to a 90 degree angle. The left thigh is extended and the penis is placed along the axis of the right thigh. The contrast material is slowly and steadily injected. When three quarters of the syringe has been emptied, the exposure is made while the injection continues. Filming can be done under fluoroscopic visualization or by the overhead tube. We do not ordinarily use fluoroscopic control except in the evaluation of urethral injury and neurogenic bladder and have no difficulty in exposing the film with proper filling of the urethra (Fig. 7–23.)

In patients with neurologic disease of the bladder, voiding cystourethrography combined with retrograde urethrography is proposed as the method of choice by McCallum and Colapinto (1976). The barrel of the 50-ml glass syringe, used for filling the bladder, is dipped in saline before the syringe is filled and is kept wet with saline during the injection in order to prevent sticking later in the examination. The bladder is gently filled to the point of overflow incontinence. Between 150 and 450 ml are usually required, but sometimes as much as 750 ml is needed. Voiding will occur through the catheter into the syringe. The procedure is monitored fluoroscopically, and spot films are made to document persistent narrowing of the urethra by prostatic enlargement and the degree of external sphincter spasm. Low-pressure reflux during bladder filling and high-pressure reflux during voiding can be observed fluoroscopically and filmed. Complications of the procedure are not frequent but include intrarenal reflux (possibly leading to acute pyelonephritis, septicemia, or septic shock) and autonomic dysreflexia with precipitous elevation of the blood pressure. If the examiner is prepared to treat these complications immediately, this valuable method of assessing paraplegic dysfunction in the lower urinary tract can be carried out safely (McCallum and Colapinto, 1976).

ADRENAL RADIOGRAPHY

Computed tomography is the primary noninvasive method of evaluating the adrenal gland. Rarely, in the case of very small lesions, or when the computed tomographic findings are equivocal, adrenal angiography may be of value.

RETROGRADE ILEOSTOURETEROGRAPHY

After diversion of the urinary stream by ureteroileostomy and formation of an ileal conduit, the excretory urogram is the follow-up examination of first choice (Fig. 7–24). If a previously normal upper urinary tract has become dilated or if a previously dilated upper tract has progressed following the surgical procedure, further radiologic examination is indicated (Lebowitz, 1984).

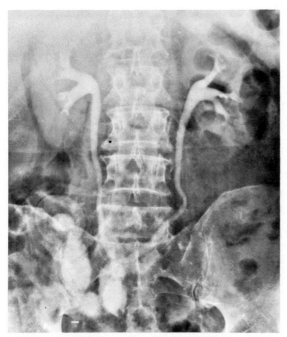

Figure 7–24. Normal excretion urogram after bilateral ureteroileostomy. The upper collecting systems and ileal conduit are of normal caliber.

Indications

In the presence of increasing dilatation of the upper urinary tracts following diversion, retrograde ileostoureterography is indicated.

Contraindications

The examination should not be performed in the presence of acute infection.

Technique

A Foley balloon catheter is tested by inflation and deflation until the balloon opens easily. After wetting with sterile water but not lubricating jelly, it is inserted into the ileostomy. About 3 to 4 ml of water in children or a larger quantity in adults is carefully injected into the balloon, and the ability to move the catheter is repeatedly tested. When the wall of the balloon appears to be snug against the intestinal wall, half-strength conventional urographic contrast medium is instilled by gravity drip from a height of 70 cm. The ileal conduit is filled under fluoroscopic control and filmed in two projections. Ileal peristalsis should be expected; absence suggests atony caused by obstruction or

infection. Free reflux up both ureters should always occur. The amount of contrast medium injected should be carefully monitored and should be kept as small as is consistent with excluding obstruction in the ileal conduit, the ureteroileal anastomoses, or the ureters themselves. When spot filming is complete, the balloon is deflated and removed (Fig. 7–25).

A progress film is made in 20 minutes to determine whether there is retention behind a previously demonstrated area of narrowing or at the stoma. Normally the entire system should be empty in 20 minutes. Occasionally there may be transient spasm of the ileal segment during the infusion (Lebowitz, 1984).

SEMINAL VESICULOGRAPHY AND EPIDIDYMOGRAPHY

These examinations have been used for evaluation of chronic inflammatory disease of the prostate gland and the seminiferous structures, diagnosis of carcinoma of the prostate, and recognition and localization of ductal causes of infertility. The studies require either a mod-

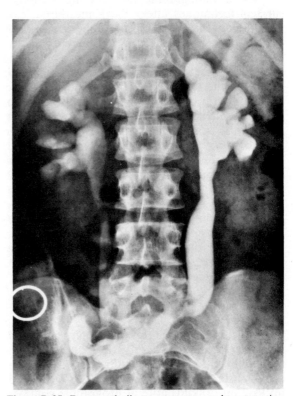

Figure 7–25. Retrograde ileostoureterogram demonstrating bilateral parenchymal atrophy, greater on the left. The ileal conduit is normal in contour. The ureteral reflux is normal, but the hydronephrosis is not.

erately difficult catheterization of the ejaculatory ducts through a urethroscope or a minor surgical procedure on the scrotum for direct instillation of contrast medium into the vas deferens. Incision into or needling of the vas deferens is not without risk of injury or stricture formation.

Indications

Recognition and localization of anatomic lesions in the seminiferous ducts.

Contraindications

The procedures should be avoided in the presence of acute infection or inflammation.

Technique

VASOSEMINAL VESICULOGRAPHY AND VASOEPIDIDYMOGRAPHY

On a radiographic table, using standard surgical techniques under local anesthesia, the vas deferens is exposed in the upper portion of the scrotal sac. Either by needle puncture or by vasotomy, a short-bevel 20-gauge needle is inserted in the direction of either the seminal vesicle or the epididymis. To eliminate the risk of further trauma to the vas deferens, fixation of the needle is not used. A urographic contrast medium in standard strength is carefully injected, using a very low capacity syringe and minimal pressure. About 1 ml suffices for vasoepididymography, and no more than 2 ml is necessary for vasoseminal vesiculography (Fig. 7–26). Anteroposterior radiographs usually suffice, and the procedure may be done bilaterally. If great detail in the region of the epididymis is desired, a single exposure using fast film and a cardboard holder in direct contact with the scrotum is useful.

EJACULATORY DUCT SEMINAL VESICULOGRAPHY

A 3 or 4 French ureteral catheter is inserted into the ejaculatory duct orifice on the verumontanum through a panendoscope. The catheter is inserted for a distance of 1 to 2 cm, and up to 2 ml of conventional urographic contrast medium is carefully injected. An anteroposterior film centered to the symphysis pubis is usually sufficient.

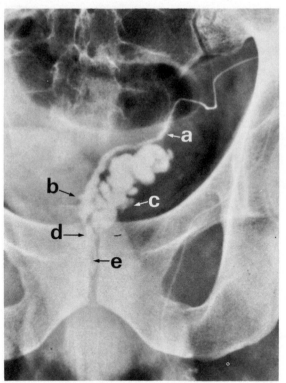

Figure 7–26. Vasoseminal vesiculogram demonstrating mild seminal vesiculitis: *a,* vas deferens; *b,* ampulla; *c,* seminal vesicle; *d,* ejaculatory duct; *e,* verumontanum. The ampulla and seminal vesicle are dilated and irregular.

CHAIN CYSTOURETHROGRAPHY

Chain cystourethrography is used in the evaluation of vesicourethral relationships in patients with stress incontinence. Many gynecologists consider it useful in deciding whether a patient can be treated surgically using a simple vaginal approach or whether the more complicated abdominal approach is needed. Interpretation of the radiologic findings is discussed briefly in the section on radiologic anatomy of the female urethra.

Technique
(Stolz and Fogel, 1972)

A 12-cm long segment of a No. 18 French straight rubber catheter is modified for use in inserting the chain. It is slit longitudinally, the front end is cut across obliquely, and the tip may be softened by sandpapering. A 20-cm long beaded metal chain (electric light pull-chain) is placed in the prepared sheath with a little of the chain protruding in front.

The urethra is catheterized, 30 ml of half-strength conventional urographic contrast medium is instilled into the bladder, and the catheter is removed. (Alternatively, the bladder could be opacified by intravenous injection or as part of an excretory urogram.)

The sterile lubricated chain-sheath assembly is introduced into the bladder. The outside end of the chain is grasped by a hemostat, and the sheath is carefully pulled off the chain and out of the urethra, leaving the chain in the bladder and urethra. The hemostat is removed, and the outside end of the chain is taped to the skin of the thigh. While the patient stands with her feet 12 inches apart (to prevent splinting of the bladder and urethra) and strains to increase intra-abdominal pressure, a fluoroscopic spot film is made in the anteroposterior position and another in the true lateral position, centered over the urethrovesical junction (Fig. 7–27).

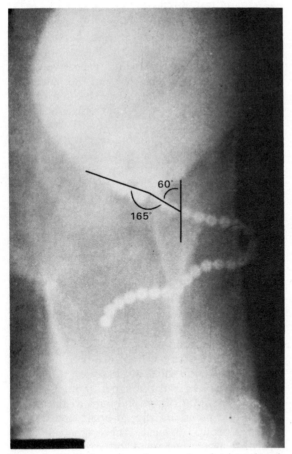

Figure 7–27. Chain cystourethrogram in erect lateral position with patient straining. The posterior urethrovesical angle (PUV) is 165 degrees and the upper urethral axis angle (UUA) is 70 degrees, indicating a Type II abnormality.

RADIOLOGIC ANATOMY OF THE NORMAL URINARY TRACT AND ITS VARIATIONS

Renal Size

Evaluation of kidney size is clearly helpful in the recognition of renal abnormality. Experience has shown that it is easier than one would think to miss differences of 1.5 cm in length between the two kidneys by simple inspection of the roentgenogram. Measurement of kidney length has been clinically worthwhile for us and is usually easier to do on the nephrogram than on the preliminary film. Because of the hyperosmolar effects of the contrast medium, kidney size is slightly larger on the nephrogram than on the plain film but this does not diminish the value of the measurement. Indeed, normal kidneys will enlarge more than ischemic kidneys, improving the chance that a significant difference in size will be recognized. Length measurements can be used either to compare one side with the other or to compare each side with a normal standard. Normal values for kidney length at all ages and over the entire range of adult heights were derived by Hodson et al. (1962) and Moell (1961).

Ordinarily the left kidney is 0.5 cm larger than the right, and the kidneys in men are an average of 0.5 cm larger than those in women. In women, kidney sizes of between 11.0 and 14.0 cm are considered normal; in men, the normal size is between 11.5 and 14.5 cm. If these limits are taken as general guidelines rather than as exact limits, they will serve as a useful screen for small and large kidneys. Comparison of kidney length with the length of a vertebral body or a vertebral body and one disc has been advocated in order to eliminate errors of magnification and to include a factor representing the patient's habitus. The ratio of renal length to the height of the posterior margins of L2 is 3.7 ± 0.37, and the statistical range of normal values is 3.0 to 4.4. The ratio of renal length to the height of the posterior margins of L2 and the L2–L3 disc is 3.1 ± 0.27, and the range of normal values is 2.6 to 3.6 (Simon, 1974). This method is probably useful if measurements are compared but is less valuable if visual estimations alone are made. Recording of linear measurements on the film has particular value when comparing examinations made at different times. Kidney length and width are not always reliable indices of renal parenchymal mass, largely because the size of the renal sinus differs from patient to patient. Nephrotomo-

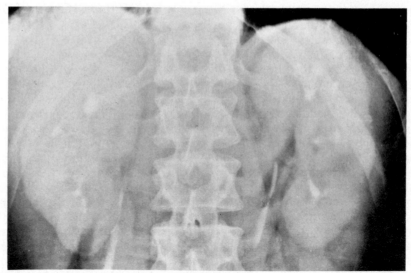

Figure 7–28. Normal variations in renal outline. Prominent right sulcus interpartialis inferior. Left renal lobation. A normal left upper pole is often bulbous when the spleen is not overriding.

grams, because they outline the functioning renal parenchyma and depict the renal sinus, give a better estimate of the volume of functioning renal tissue.

Shape

Each pyramid and the cortical tissue that surrounds it constitute an independently functioning renal lobe emptying into a calyx. A basic pattern consists of seven anterior lobes and seven posterior lobes. Rarely, the number of papillae and calyces may be greater than 14 if branching of the pelvocalyceal system is greater than usual. More commonly, the number of papillae is less than 14 because several pyramids fuse at their tips to form a single papilla. The surface of the kidney may show furrows demarcating the extent of each lobe. When seen in profile on an anteroposterior exposure, the grooves will appear as small notches along the surface of the kidney, placed roughly midway between the underlying calyces. This was formerly called *fetal lobulation* but is now more properly termed *renal lobation* because it designates a renal lobe (a pyramid and the surrounding cortex) and not a lobule (a medullary ray and the surrounding glomeruli) (Fig. 7–28).

Pyelonephritic scarring, if focal, can be distinguished from lobation because it is located on the radial axis of the underlying calyx. The area of the surface of the kidney involved by an infarct is usually more extensive than the sharp indentation of an interlobar groove. Especially

prominent interlobar grooves may be seen at roughly the junction between the upper and middle thirds and the junction between the middle and lower thirds of the lateral border of the kidney. These represent, respectively, the sulcus interpartialis superior and the sulcus interpartialis inferior and are the residua of segmental divisions in the renal substance that occurred during development (Fig. 7–28). They are without clinical importance but may be confused with fibrotic scarring. Sometimes segmentation of this type may be associated with a bifid or duplicated renal pelvis.

The lateral border of the left kidney sometimes takes the shape of two flat surfaces extending from the apices to form a rather prominent angle in about the midportion of the lateral border. This has been termed the *dromedary hump* by Frimann-Dahl. Opacification of the spleen indicates that the upper pole of the spleen is closely applied to the upper-outer border of the kidney in these cases, and the hilus of the spleen is opposite the angular portion of the lateral renal border (Fig. 7–29).

A bulge in the outline of either kidney is sometimes seen in the space between the lateral upper pole calyx and the superior middle pole calyx. Frequently the infundibula to the upper and middle poles are spread apart and appear to curve around a mass. These changes often represent an ectopic renal lobe, rotated almost 90 degrees from its usual location, with its central axis now anteroposterior in orientation (Fig. 7–30). The condition is known as lobar dysmorphism. When first observed, it was

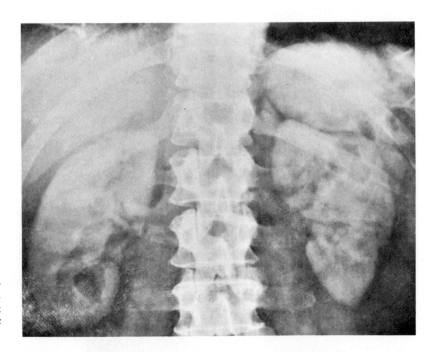

Figure 7–29. Splenic impression. Upper outer border of left kidney is concave where indented by upper pole of spleen and convex where it bulges into the splenic hilus.

thought to represent a rest of cortical tissue or an enlargement of the septum of renal cortical tissue, which normally separates two pyramids (column of Bertin). It is usually associated with a small, compressed, and slightly displaced calyx arising in the neighborhood of the fork between the major upper and middle pole infundibula. To exclude a tumor mass and confirm the presence of a normal variant, a nephrotomogram should be made soon after the intravenous injection of a large amount of contrast material while the distinction between the cortex and medulla is still clear. This film will show a thick-walled square representing the base of the lobe with the less dense center representing the medullary tissue, as seen from the base of the pyramid looking toward the apex. Tissue densities will appear normal, and no tumor masses will be visible.

Position

The abdominal level at which the kidneys lie varies with the habitus of the patient. The hilus of the right kidney generally lies at the level of the second right lumbar transverse process. The left kidney is usually 1 to 2 cm higher than the right, but in at least 10 per cent of normal individuals it is lower than the right kidney. Usually the long axes of the kidneys follow the outer border of the psoas muscle. In individuals with considerable perinephric fat,

the long axes may be vertical, and the medial borders of the kidneys no longer reach the lateral borders of the psoas muscles. The location of the kidneys varies with respiration, and it is customary to expose urographic films in expiration, thus depicting the kidneys in their highest normal position.

When a urographic examination reveals one or both kidneys to be in an unexpected position or location, the possible causes include variations related to the patient's habitus, developmental failures of ascent or rotation, and displacement by masses or other acquired disease. Evaluation should include careful consideration of the appearance of the pelvicalyceal systems and ureters. Depression of one or both kidneys for a distance of one or two vertebral bodies with evidence of ureters of normal length and without radiologic signs of a mass lesion in all likelihood represents lack of the usual retroperitoneal support. This condition, renal ptosis, must be considered a normal variant unless clear evidence of ureteropelvic obstruction attributable to the position of the kidney can be demonstrated. Kidneys that are low in position because of incomplete ascent usually show failure of complete rotation so that the renal pelvis is more anterior in location than usual. The ureteral length is shorter than usual but compatible with the position of the kidney. Displacement of the kidney by an adjacent enlarged organ or mass will usually alter the axis as well as the position of the kidney. The diagnosis

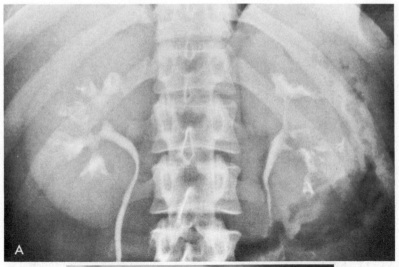

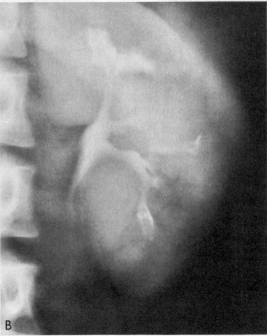

Figure 7–30. Ectopic lobe. *A,* Left upper middle pole calyx is short, and adjacent infundibula seem to curve around a mass. *B,* Nephrotomogram reveals normal tissue density in involved area.

must always be confirmed by demonstration of the offending structure.

Axial rotation of the kidney can involve the vertical, anteroposterior, or transverse axes. While rotation on the vertical axis can result from adjacent masses, such rotation accompanied by a low position of the kidney almost certainly represents a failure of normal development. Rotation on the transverse axis of the kidney can be normal when the lower pole is displaced anteriorly, usually by a large amount of perinephric fat. The renal pelvis will be foreshortened, and a film made with a 30-degree caudal inclination of the radiographic tube (Imray et al., 1977) will demonstrate a kidney of normal size and pyelocalyceal structure. Rotation on the anteroposterior axis of the kidney may be normal when the lower pole is displaced laterally, especially if this is bilateral and the patient is obese. Lateral displacement of the upper pole may be the result of extrinsic masses, but the possibility of a nonfuctioning upper pole duplication should be investigated.

Calyces

The number and distribution of calyces have been discussed in part in the previous section. The shape of the end of the calyx is

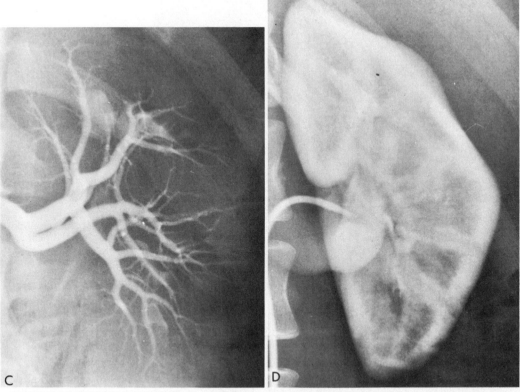

Figure 7–30 *Continued C,* Blood vessels are intrinsically normal but displaced. *D,* Vascular nephrogram shows intact cortex and medulla in abnormal orientation.

determined by the number, size, and shape of the papillae that empty into it. Calyces in the middle third of the kidney usually are supplied by a single papilla, which may be large or small. Absence of a papillary indentation usually represents atrophy or destruction of the papilla and should initiate investigation of the cause. The upper and lower pole calyces are frequently supplied by more than one papilla. These compound calyces can usually be identified by their smooth outlines and frequently by their bilateral symmetry. Occasionally, calyceal branching produces a very small calyx designated as a microcalyx (see Fig. 7–5) usually at the side of a normal-sized calyx. A small diverticular outpouching often arises from the region of the calyceal fornix, the angle between the calyx and the papilla. These are usually simple diverticula (Fig. 7–31), but occasionally they represent a variation of the microcalyx and drain a small pyramid. The lateral surfaces of the calyces are in contact with the blood vessels and fat of the renal sinus. Occasionally there may be a large amount of renal sinus fat either because the individual is obese or in response to renal atrophy. This condition, renal sinus lipomatosis (Fig. 7–32), produces changes in the calyces that

are usually characteristic. The side walls of the calyx have increased concavity while the end of the calyx may appear flattened or even convex.

The densest portion of the normal calyx is not at the very end. Because the papilla normally indents the end of the calyx, the amount of contrast material traversed in cross section by the x-ray beam is less at the level of the fornices than it is immediately proximal to the tip of the papilla. If the end of the calyx is the densest portion, it must be presumed that the papilla is not protruding into the calyx, and the cause should be sought.

Although large calyces are most often the result of acquired obstructive disease, there is an interesting congenital condition that has frequently been presumed to be an acquired obstruction, with unfortunate results for the patient. *Congenital megacalyces* (Fig. 7–33) is a condition characterized by ectatic large calyces, polygonal in contour. While the infundibula are short and broad, the renal pelvis and ureter are of normal size. The cortex is normal in thickness, neither scarred nor atrophic. The medullary pyramids are underdeveloped, the calyces are often increased in number, and there is frequently an associated non-obstructive pri-

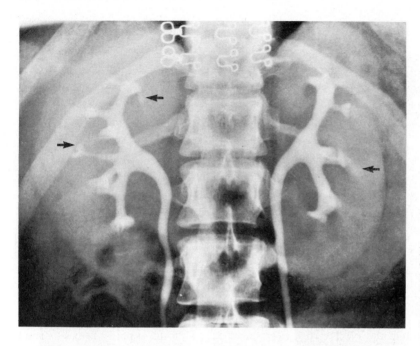

Figure 7–31. Calyceal diverticula originate from the right medial upper pole fornix and the right superior middle pole calyx. The medial portions of all pyramids are diffusely opacified, best seen in left middle calyceal group.

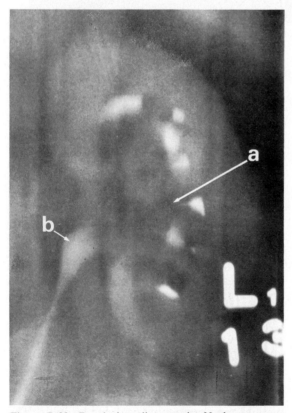

Figure 7–32. Renal sinus lipomatosis. Nephrotomogram shows a large amount of fat in large renal sinus *(a)*, a small renal pelvis *(b)*, and compressed infundibula.

mary megaureter. The only functional defect is a deficit in maximal concentrating ability. Failure to recognize this condition often has resulted in unnecessary operations and has complicated the management of the infections and renal calculi to which this condition predisposes.

The precise shapes of the fornices and calyx probably change from moment to moment depending upon the amount of urine they contain. Narath has postulated that there is a diastolic and systolic alternation. While the calyx fills the fornices are relaxed, and the sphincter at the infundibulum of the calyx is contracted. While the calyx empties the sphincter at the infundibulum of the calyx relaxes, and the side walls of the fornices contract against the papilla, possibly helping to prevent intrarenal reflux (Narath, 1940).

The infundibula of the major or minor calyces may be indented from one side by an adjacent artery or vein. Anteroposterior exposures, in which the infundibulum is superimposed on the vessel, reveal a bandlike shadow of diminished density crossing the infundibulum (Fig. 7–34). Oblique or lateral films of the infundibulum will clearly demonstrate a rounded indentation along one wall. In commonly involved locations, such as the base of the upper pole infundibulum and obliquely across the outer third of the renal pelvis, this

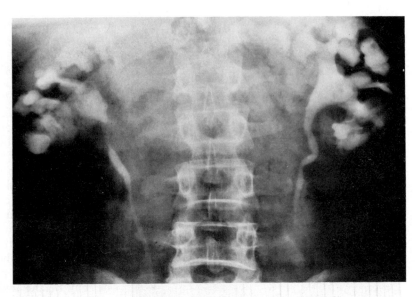

Figure 7–33. Congenital mega-calyces. The calyces are large and polygonal in contour. The pelves and ureters are not enlarged.

appearance generally makes the diagnosis a simple one.

Since the urine in the collecting tubules is reaching its final concentration and a large proportion of the volume of the papillae is occupied by collecting tubules and ducts, the papillae are often opacified on the 5-minute film and thereafter. If the opacification is homogeneous, it is a normal finding and does not represent either stasis or pyelorenal backflow (see Fig. 7–31). If the appearance is not homogeneous but consists of vertical striations with proximal convergence, the appearance represents collecting tubule ectasia or cystic dilatation of the collecting ducts (Fig. 7–35).

Pyelorenal backflow of various types may

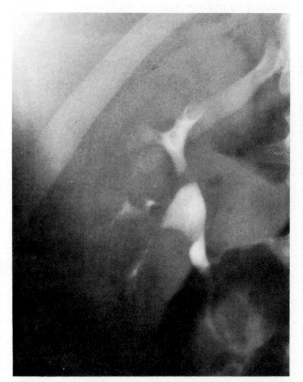

Figure 7–34. Impression on right upper major infundibulum by renal artery branch.

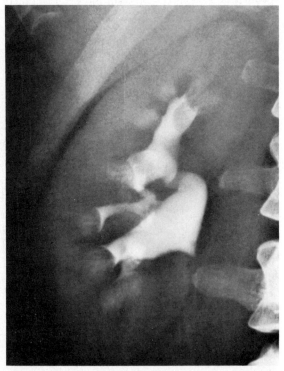

Figure 7–35. Medullary sponge kidney. Opaque longitudinal streaks in the pyramids represent dilated collecting tubules.

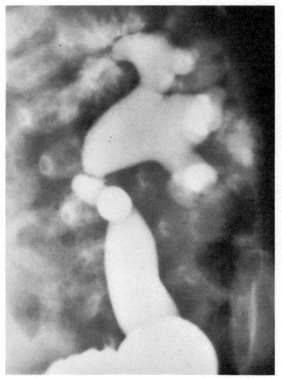

Figure 7–36. Intrarenal reflux during voiding cystourethrography. Vertically striated contrast densities, best seen in the upper pole, represent reflux filling of the collecting tubules. (Courtesy of Dr. Robert Lebowitz.)

occur during retrograde pyelography, during excretion urography if ureteral compression is used, and during voiding cystourethrography if there is vesicoureteral and pelvicalyceal reflux (Fig. 7–36). In all three circumstances there is increased intrapelvic hydrostatic pressure. Several types of pyelorenal backflow have been described: (1) pyelotubular, (2) pyelosinous, (3) pyelolymphatic, (4) pyelovenous, and (5) pyelointerstitial (Fig. 7–37).

Pyelotubular reflux can occur in the presence of increased pelvic hydrostatic pressure if the factors that normally protect the papillary duct openings fail to operate. These include (1) normal apposition of the papillary duct openings and (2) contraction of the side walls of the fornices against the papilla.

Pyelosinous backflow may occur by itself or may be the underlying process that leads to either pyelovenous or pyelolymphatic backflow. It is generally agreed that rupture of the fornix will permit urine to enter the sinus. In addition, Narath (1940) believes that in the presence of increased intracalyceal hydrostatic pressure, the mucosa of the fornix can directly absorb fluid, which will then enter the closed renal sinus ("transflow"). In either case, the fluid may then be absorbed by the lymphatics in the sinus, leading to pyelolymphatic backflow. If an injury

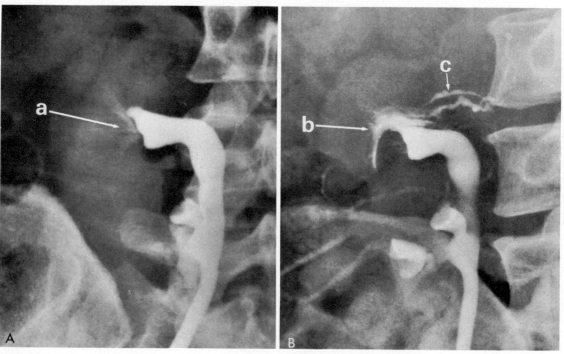

Figure 7–37. Pyelorenal backflow (*A* and *B*): *a,* pyelotubular backflow; *b,* pyelosinus backflow; *c,* pyelolymphatic backflow.

that causes rupture of the fornix also lacerates the adjacent arcuate veins, pyelovenous backflow may occur. Pyelointerstitial backflow occurs when there has been a direct laceration involving the calyx and the pyramid. It may occur from direct penetration of the papilla during retrograde ureteral catheterization, especially in patients with acute pyelonephritis.

Pelvis

When the blind upper end of the developing ureter meets the caudal end of the urogenital ridge, it widens to form the pelvis of the ureter (renal pelvis) and divides into the calyces and collecting tubules. The latter connect with the distal ends of the nephrons. There are innumerable normal shapes of the renal pelvis. An extrarenal pelvis is one in which expansion of the ureter began caudal to the renal hilus. Lack of surrounding renal tissue eliminates a constraint to the growth of the pelvis and also allows freer distention of this portion of the pelvis under increased intraureteric pressure.

The accidents of greater or lesser degrees of branching produce an infinite variety of shapes. The problem in daily radiologic practice is to determine whether the pelvis is normally large or abnormally enlarged and, if the latter, whether the point of obstruction is at the ureteropelvic junction. The tendency toward bilateral symmetry is helpful because symmetry favors a diagnosis of normality. In the presence of a questionably large pelvis, the absence of enlargement of the calyces favors the diagnosis of a normal structure. The degree of distention of the upper collecting systems is related to the volume of urine excreted. Radiographs of normal individuals made after injection of very large doses of contrast medium (for example, after angiocardiography) will show "pseudohydronephrosis."

In distinguishing between normally large and enlarged renal pelves, it is important to determine whether there is an abrupt transition between the size of the pelvis and the size of the ureter or whether there is smooth tapering. Since the image of a large renal pelvis is often superimposed upon the image of the upper ureter on anteroposterior views, it is important that oblique or lateral views that project the ureteropelvic junction parallel to the plane of the film be carefully made. As in other parts of the urinary and gastrointestinal systems, an apparent narrowing of the lumen should not be considered to represent a point of obstruction

unless there is evidence of distention above and diminished filling below. If the ureteropelvic junction appears to be narrow, but the pelvis is large and the ureter has a greater than normal caliber, the possibility of a refluxing lesion at the ureterovesical junction should be carefully considered.

Extrinsic indentations of the renal pelvis by closely applied normal arterial branches are a common normal variation. The most frequently seen indentation runs downward and outward near the lateral border of the renal pelvis (Fig. 7–38). The tubular indentation often tapers as it descends. Diverticula of the pelvis probably represent abortive attempts at branching. If duplication does occur, the upper pelvis almost always contains only the upper pole calyces, and the lower pelvis holds the middle and lower pole calyces. Very rarely, the lower pelvis is smaller. In triplication of the pelvis, which is exceedingly rare, the uppermost pelvis usually consists of a single calyx.

The psoas muscle lies on the fronts of the

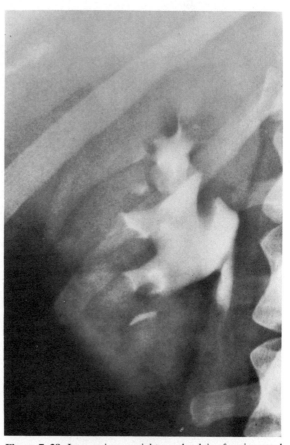

Figure 7–38. Impression on right renal pelvis of major renal artery branch. The indentation often extends completely across the pelvis and often is more shallow.

transverse processes and against the sides of the vertebral bodies. It extends posterior and medial to the renal pelves and may be responsible for the straight medial border of the pelvis that is sometimes seen. The main renal arteries and veins are anterior to the renal pelves. The second portion of the duodenum is anterior to the right renal pelvis, while the pancreas and sometimes the duodenojejunal flexure are anterior to the left renal pelvis.

Ureter

The ureter descends parallel to the midline on the anterior surface of the psoas muscle.

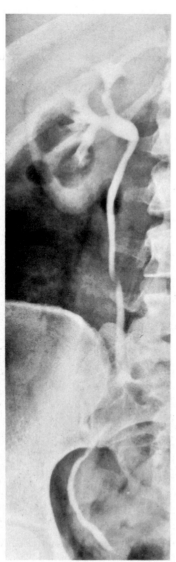

Figure 7–39. Indentation of right ureter by ovarian artery and vein at interspace between L3 and L4.

Between the L3 and L5 vertebral levels, it is crossed and often indented anteriorly and obliquely by the testicular or ovarian artery and vein (Fig. 7–39). While the ureters usually overlie the transverse processes of the vertebrae, 18 per cent of normal ureters, almost always on the right, overlie or are medial to the pedicles of the spine at the L5 and S1 levels. The right ureter often approaches the midline, particularly in young adults. No significant sex difference is apparent (Saldino and Palubinskas, 1972).

Hypertrophy of the psoas muscles can displace the ureters laterally below the renal pelves (Haines and Kyaw, 1971). The ureters turn medially with varying degrees of acuteness and descend along the anteromedial surfaces of the psoas muscles. The ureters are often closer to the midline than usual, especially at the L5–S1 vertebral level and below, because of the muscle hypertrophy (Fig. 7–40) (Bree et al., 1976).

The ureters may also be displaced by developmental variations in the cardinal vein system. Usually the posterior component (supracardinal vein) forms the infrarenal portion of

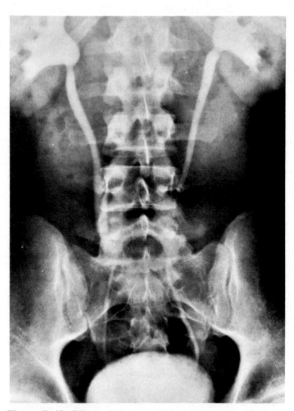

Figure 7–40. Bilateral psoas muscle hypertrophy displaces both ureters medially in the lower abdomen and pelvis and mildly compresses ureters at pelvic brim, causing slight proximal dilatation.

the inferior vena cava, and the right ureter runs lateral to it. If the anterior component of the cardinal system (subcardinal vein) persists and forms the infrarenal portion of the vena cava, the ureter runs medially behind the vena cava at the level of the body of L3 and then returns to its usual lateral position. A retrocaval ureter may be distended above the site of abnormal displacement (Fig. 7–41).

The normal areas of narrowing in the ureter are at the ureteropelvic junction, the pelvic brim, and the ureterovesical junction. The segments between them are the abdominal and pelvic portions of the ureter. Because of their shapes, they have been termed the abdominal

and pelvic spindles. The abdominal spindles are the portions predominantly involved in the ureteral dilatation that occurs in pregnancy (Fig. 7–42). The right side is more affected than the left. The more acute angle made by the right ureter as it bends posteriorly and crosses the pelvic brim, as compared with the left ureter, is believed to render it more likely to be compressed during pregnancy. Some degree of dilatation probably occurs in all pregnancies, and although residual structural changes in the ureters are said always to persist, they may not be sufficient to cause urographic changes. If infection supervenes during pregnancy, more marked and persistent dilatation occurs, and this may be the only residual evidence of that infection (Dure-Smith, 1970).

Roentgenograms will show other areas of narrowing that represent peristaltic changes. During excretion urography with normal urine output, usually not all portions of the ureter are

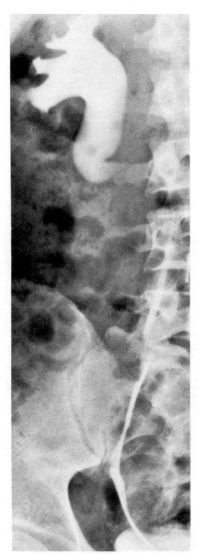

Figure 7–41. Retrocaval ureter with characteristic sharp medial angulation in the midlumbar area and medial course in the lower abdomen returns to normal position in the pelvis. The dilated renal pelvis is usually present.

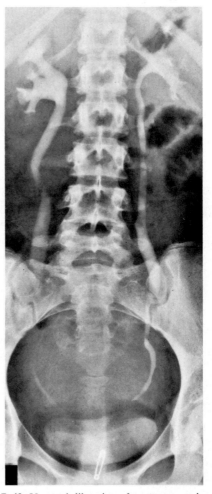

Figure 7–42. Ureteral dilatation of pregnancy ends typically at pelvic brim. Roentgenogram made 2 weeks after delivery.

seen in the filled state, and the exclusion of abnormality under these circumstances might be difficult. This difficulty can be overcome either by ureteral compression or by the diuresis produced by infusion urography. During retrograde pyelography the ureter may not be seen throughout its length if there has been trauma to the ureter, however slight. This can usually be prevented by careful technique or by ureteral catheterization using a bulb-tipped catheter. A diagnosis of ureteral stricture should not be made without consistent evidence of localized narrowing on multiple films. In almost all cases one should expect to see dilatation proximal to the area of narrowing and diminished filling below. The normal ureteral diameter is very variable and may be as high as 8 mm or more. A diagnosis of dilatation secondary to obstruction should be validated by demonstration of the point of obstruction. Dilatation resulting from infection or the use of various pharmaceuticals such as contraceptives and antidepressant medications may be more difficult to prove.

The ureter enters the bony pelvis by crossing the common iliac artery at the origin of the external iliac artery. The artery may produce either an oblique indentation or, occasionally in older individuals, a prominent medially convex curve in the course of the ureter. From a position anterior to the lower half of the sacroiliac joint, the ureter follows the inner margins of the iliac bone in an arc that is convex posteriorly and laterally. At the level of the ischial spine, it turns anteriorly and medially to reach the base of the bladder, where the ureteral orifices are about 2 cm apart. If one or both ureters deviate from this course, displacement by extrinsic pressure must be considered.

A normal variant seen in women is straightening or medial deviation of the pelvic portion of the right ureter (Fig. 7–43). The uterus is more often tilted to the left in these women. The horizontal distance from the lateral pelvic brim to the ureter ordinarily varies less than 0.5 cm between the two sides, but the normal variant group shows a difference of over 1.4 cm. Even in women with known retroperitoneal disease, medial deviation of the right ureter of this degree is not necessarily a sign of disease (Kabakian et al., 1976).

After anterior resection of the rectum, the sacroiliac portions of the ureters may be drawn together (Fig. 7–44). A similar appearance may sometimes be seen following pelvic exenteration for widespread neoplastic disease in the female pelvis. In pelvic lipomatosis, the pelvic portions of both ureters may proceed downward in a vertical line rather than in a convex outward direction. The large pelvic deposit of fat may straighten the pelvic portions of the ureters and

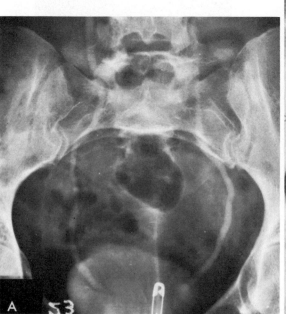 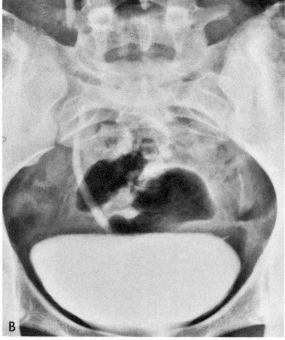

Figure 7–43. Asymmetry of pelvic ureters in normal females. *A,* Medially situated, laterally concave right ureter. *B,* Medially situated, laterally convex right ureter.

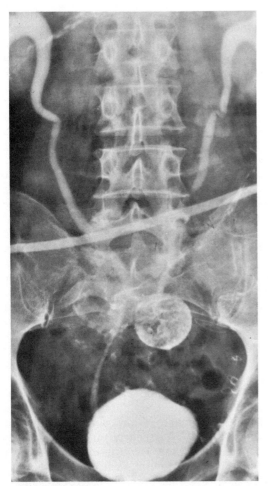

Figure 7–44. The sacroiliac portions of the ureters are medially retracted following anterior resection of the rectum.

convert the bladder to a more vertical orientation (Figs. 7–45 and 10–22).

Bladder

The shape of the empty adult bladder approaches a pyramid with four surfaces—a triangular base and three sides. The base faces posteroinferiorly; the apex points anteriorly; one of the sides faces superiorly; and the other two sides face inferiorly and laterally. Anatomically these parts of the bladder are the base or fundus, which contains the trigone; the apex, from which the urachus extends; the superior surface, which is covered by peritoneum; and the side walls, which converge with the base to form the most dependent part, the neck, where the internal urethral orifice is located.

The superior surface of the bladder may be in contact with or extrinsically indented by loops of the small intestine, the sigmoid colon, and the body of the uterus when the bladder content is small. The thickness of the bladder walls superiorly is sometimes outlined by the contrast medium internally and the extravesical fat externally. Normal values are not sharply defined, and wall thickness varies with the extent of bladder filling. Asymmetric thickening of a portion of the bladder wall should lead one to suspect infiltration by neoplasm. In men the peritoneum dips down posteriorly between the upper portion of the base of the bladder and rectum to form the rectovesical pouch. The lower portion of the base of the bladder is

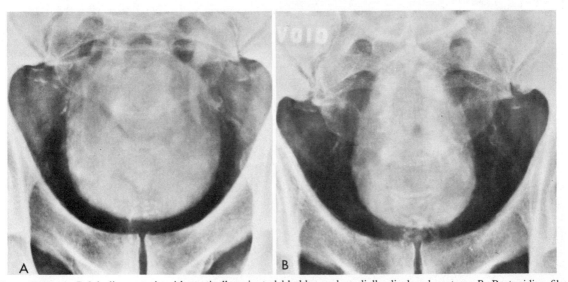

Figure 7–45. *A,* Pelvic lipomatosis with vertically oriented bladder and medially displaced ureters. *B,* Postvoiding film shows pelvic fat deposits. The enlarged prostate gland contains calculi.

related laterally to the seminal vesicles, more medially to the ampulla of the vas deferens, and centrally to the rectum. Enlargement of these structures may indent the base of the bladder, and rectovesical fistulas can occur there.

In women a narrow recess, the uterovesical pouch, occurs between the uterus and the upper surface of the bladder. The base of the bladder is adjacent to the supravaginal part of the cervix above and to the anterior vaginal wall below. Extension of carcinoma of the uterine cervix into the bladder is best sought in this area, as are vesicovaginal fistulas, which are best demonstrated in the true lateral position during cystography.

The anterior portions of the inferolateral surfaces are in contact with the retropubic space, which contains the retropubic fat pad. The space extends upward toward the umbilicus between the medial umbilical ligaments (obliterated umbilical arteries) and contains the median umbilical ligament (a remnant of the urachus). A conical upward extension of the apex of the bladder usually represents the vestigial shape of the portion of the bladder that extended to the urachus (Fig. 7–46). Anterior laceration of the urinary bladder permits extravasation into the retropubic space.

Abdominal herniation can affect the position of the bladder and ureters in two ways: Either the bladder or ureters protrude into the hernial orifice, or the bowel that protrudes into the hernial orifice displaces the bladder or ureters.

In some infants with wide inguinal rings, the inferolateral walls of the bladder may protrude on one or both sides. These so-called *bladder ears* are not significant unless a hernia operation is performed, and they usually disappear with time (Fig. 7–47) (Allen and Condon, 1961). In adults, bladder herniation occurs in 1 to 3 per cent of inguinal hernias and can occur in femoral and other hernias. On the supine film lateral placement of the opacified bladder suggests herniation on the side to which the bladder is shifted. The herniated portion of the bladder may not fill with opaque urine until delayed or prone views are made (Fig. 7–48) (Becker, 1965).

Inguinal herniation of bowel may produce extrinsic compression of the inferolateral surface of the bladder on the ipsilateral side (Fig. 7–49). If the bowel herniates on the side of the abdomen opposite its origin (e.g., sigmoid colon through right inguinal ring or ileum and cecum through left inguinal ring), the pelvic ureter on the side on which the bowel originates is displaced toward the midline, and the contralateral side of the bladder is indented (Goldin and Rosen, 1975).

An adequately penetrated roentgenogram will demonstrate the contrast-filled ureters through the image of the contrast-containing bladder. The ureters curve medially and end symmetrically about 1 cm on either side of the midline at the ureteral orifices. Between the orifices is the interureteric ridge, a band of diminished density that is concave upward, pro-

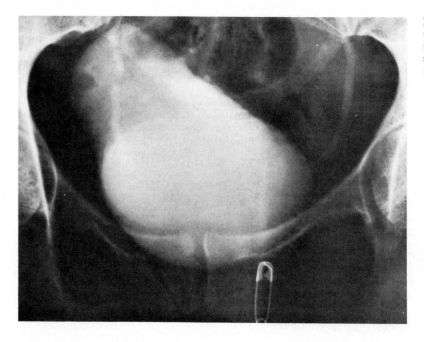

Figure 7–46. Upward extension of the bladder apex is a normal variant. Low position of bladder base suggested cystocele. Right ureter is medially situated.

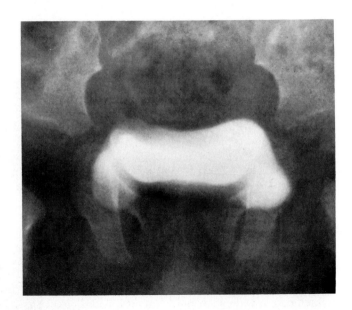

Figure 7–47. Bladder ears. Extraperitoneal protrusions of the bladder into the inguinal rings. (Courtesy of Dr. Robert Lebowitz.)

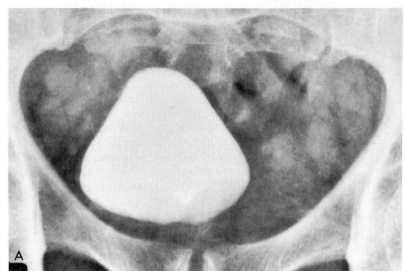

Figure 7–48. *A,* Supine view shows displacement of the bladder to the right. *B,* Erect view reveals large right bladder hernia.

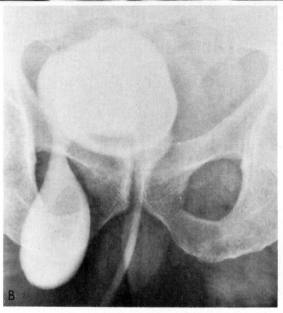

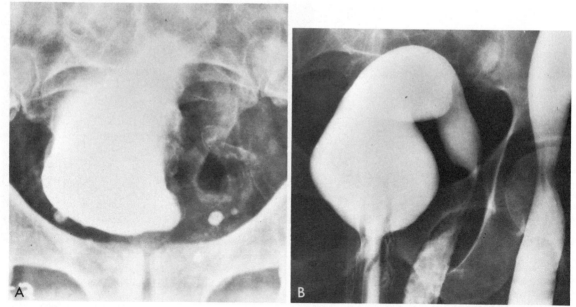

Figure 7–49. Left inguinal hernia containing sigmoid colon. *A,* Large rounded filling defect in left side of bladder. End-on view of gas-containing bowel is superimposed on bladder filling defect. *B,* Barium enema identifies sigmoid colon as the extrinsic cause.

duced by the muscle fibers that demarcate the superior border of the trigone. The region above and behind the trigone often bulges backward to form the retroureteric fossa, seen radiologically as a horizontal oval collection of contrast medium. The lumina of the intravesical ureters are separated from the retroureteric fossa by the thickness of tissue representing the ureteric wall and the overlying layers of the bladder wall (Fig. 7–50). Edema caused by inflammation or tumor results in thickening and asymmetry of the interureteric ridge.

During the early phase of bladder filling or on the postevacuation film, when there is only a small amount of contrast medium in the inferior portion of the bladder, a small midline fleck

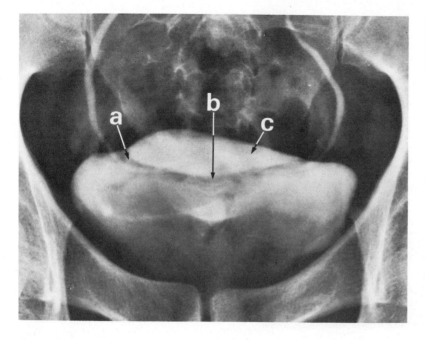

Figure 7–50. Vesicoureteral relations: *a,* combined thickness of ureteral wall and bladder mucosa; *b,* interureteric ridge; *c,* retroureteric fossa (retrotrigonal recess).

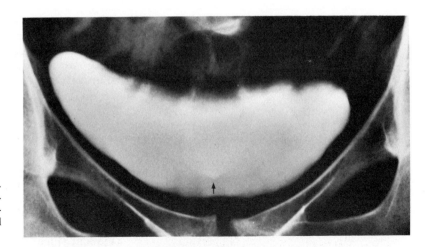

Figure 7–51. Area of increased contrast density (arrow) directed downward indicates convergence of bladder walls to internal urethral meatus.

of contrast is often seen 1 to 2 cm inferior to the ureteric orifices, demarcating the lower end of the trigone and representing the internal urethral meatus (Fig. 7–51).

Occasionally, a narrow oblique band of increased density can be seen to extend medially from one or both ureteral orifices on urographic exposures made during the early phase of bladder opacification. It has been called the ureteral jet phenomenon, which suggests an increase in the pressure of ureteral expulsion. More simply perhaps, it can be explained as streaming of the opacified urine from the ureteral orifices through the unopacified urine already in the bladder. There is no evidence that the finding has clinical importance (Fig. 7–52).

With the central ray of the x-ray beam perpendicular to the film at the level of the pubis, the base of the bladder is projected at or slightly below the superior border of the symphysis pubis. The bladder is usually symmetric on both sides of the midline, but its axis may

be slightly tilted. The mucosal lining of the filled bladder is imaged radiologically as a smooth contour. The partly filled or almost empty bladder has a redundant mucosa that appears crenulated and may easily be mistaken for trabeculation. Many false positive diagnoses of bladder changes secondary to obstruction can be avoided if clear evidence of saccules or diverticula is required for a diagnosis of trabeculation (and hence, obstruction) rather than minimal irregularities. Occasionally, urine-filled diverticula of the bladder do not fill with opaque urine during urography; this produces extrinsic indentations upon the opacified portion of the bladder that are suggestive of extrinsic masses.

Many calcifications projected over the bladder area must be differentiated from opaque bladder calculi. Phleboliths (calcified thrombi in pelvic veins) are small, rounded, and usually bilateral; they frequently contain tiny round radiolucencies that probably represent recanalizations of the thrombus. Calcified arteries cast

Figure 7–52. Streaming of opacified urine from both ureteral orifices through accumulated unopacified urine in bladder.

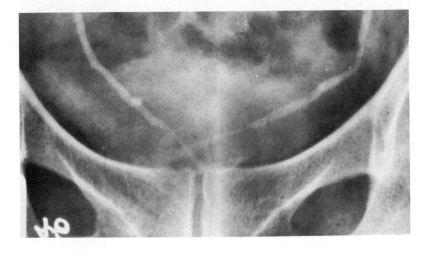

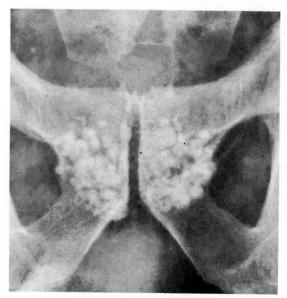

Figure 7–53. Prostatic calculi.

tubelike shadows of calcific density. Calcific lymph nodes are often mulberry-like in shape. Calcified uterine fibromyomas are often stippled and can easily be projected outside the expected location of the bladder. Calcified appendices epiploicae produce a faint, spherical, eggshell type of calcification.

Calcification in the prostate gland is paramedian and bilateral in location. Radiographically it is superimposed on the pubic bones or projected superior to them. It is stippled and, if extensive, conforms to the shape of the prostate gland (Fig. 7–53).

Overlying gas and fecal shadows remain the most significant impediment to recognition of

filling defects in the opacified bladder. Intestinal gas shadows can often be confidently differentiated from intravesical filling defects because they are surrounded by a rim of increased density representing the intestinal wall (Fig. 7–54).

Male Urethra

The posterior urethra extends from the internal urethral meatus to the inferior aspect of the urogenital diaphragm (Figs. 7–22 and 7–55). Just below the internal meatus, the urethra widens slightly. The urethral crest is a median ridge along the posterior wall that appears as a vertical filling defect. Inferiorly the crest ends as two fine diverging mucosal folds, the plicae colliculi. The crest contains an ovoid enlargement, the verumontanum (colliculus seminalis), depicted as a hemispherical filling defect. It contains the prostatic utricle, a tiny diverticulum of müllerian duct origin that on rare occasions fills during urethrography. The inferior aspect of the verumontanum is the borderline between the prostatic and membranous parts of the urethra. The ejaculatory ducts empty on each side of the verumontanum, and most of the prostatic ducts open to either side of the urethral crest. During or following infection, reflux into any of these ducts may occur. The membranous part of the urethra, 1 cm long, is the narrowest and least distensible portion. Immediately below the urogenital diaphragm, the posterior aspect of the urethra comes immediately into contact with the bulb of the penis.

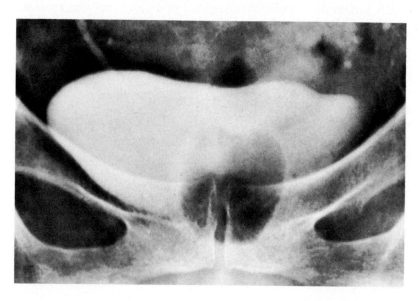

Figure 7–54. Radiolucency projected over bladder has rim of increased density (best seen on left) representing bowel wall around intestinal gas.

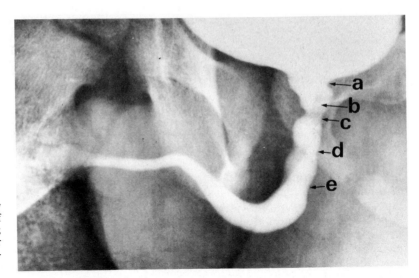

Figure 7–55. Normal urethra in boy during voiding; *a,* posterior lip of internal meatus; *b,* verumontanum; *c,* intermuscular incisura; *d,* levator ani; *e,* urogenital diaphragm. (Courtesy of Dr. Robert Lebowitz.)

A short segment of the anterior wall of the urethra is not covered by the bulb; it is called the pars nuda or bare area. In this area the urethra is crossed by the compressor nudae muscle, which is a muscular sling extending from the ischial tuberosities. The compressor nudae muscle is often contracted on retrograde studies because the patient tenses the pelvic floor. It is never contracted on voiding films, thus permitting the differentiation between this normal finding and a stricture in the area. The anterior urethra extends from the inferior portion of the urogenital diaphragm to the external urethral meatus. It is wide posteriorly in its bulbar portion. The suspensory ligament of the penis extends downward to the urethra from the symphysis pubis at the level of the penoscrotal junction. Anterior to this attachment, the pendulous portion of the urethra begins.

Just proximal to the external meatus the urethra widens again to form the fossa navicularis. Two small bulbourethral glands (Cowper's glands) are located on both sides of the midline within the urogenital diaphragm. Their ducts descend on either side of the urethra and open on the ventral surface of the bulbar urethra, usually in the proximal portion but not always. Normally they may show slight filling during retrograde urethrography but are more likely to fill if there has been a constriction beyond the ostia of the ducts (Fig. 7–56). All along the length of the anterior urethra are small mucous glands (glands of Littré), which ordinarily do not fill during urethrography but may fill if they have been infected and are dilated (Fig. 7–57).

Female Urethra

The female urethra is about 4 cm long and is normally characterized by marked distensibility (Fig. 7–58). It is narrowest just proximal to its termination, where it passes through the

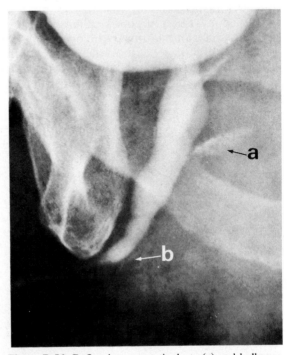

Figure 7–56. Reflux into prostatic ducts (*a*) and bulbourethral (Cowper's) duct (*b*) in gonorrheal stricture of the bulbar urethra.

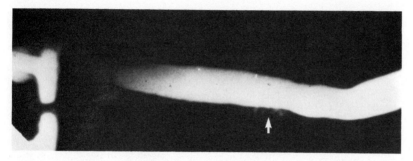

Figure 7–57. Reflux filling of dilated mucous glands on dorsal surface of pendulous urethra (arrow).

urogenital diaphragm (distal urethral segment). It is important to recognize that during forcible voiding the normal urethra may distend markedly between the internal meatus and the distal urethral segment, assuming the shape of an acorn or a spinning top. In the past this shape was thought to be associated with either constriction at the vesical neck or distal urethral stenosis. In support of a diagnosis of vesical neck obstruction, the "spinning top deformity" was said to represent poststenotic dilatation. In support of a diagnosis of distal urethral stenosis, this "deformity" was thought to represent prestenotic dilatation. There is no evidence to show that its presence denotes either abnormality. Primary bladder neck obstruction is now generally believed to be an exceedingly rare condition. The diagnosis cannot be made by radiologic examination because the internal urethral meatus is almost never the narrowest portion of the urethra. Distal urethral stenosis must be identified by direct urethral calibration. It is difficult to establish normal radiologic values for distal urethral size because the width of the opaque column in the distal segment varies from moment to moment with the expulsive force

(Shopfner, 1967). Because bulging of the urethral side walls occurs normally, it cannot be used as evidence of distal stenosis.

The axis of the urethra in relation to the plane of the bladder base has some importance in determining the surgical approach to stress incontinence (Fig. 7–27) (Stolz and Fogel, 1972). Although there is not complete agreement upon the significance of the x-ray findings, the normal posterior urethrovesical angle is 100 degrees or less, and the tilt of the upper urethra away from the vertical should be 30 degrees or less. Both of these measurements are made on upright films. The descent of the bladder should not be more than 2.5 cm below the upper margin of the symphysis pubis on upright anteroposterior radiographs. In mild cases the posterior urethrovesical angle is greater than 100 degrees, but the upper urethral angle is normal, and there is minimal descent of the bladder. In more severe cases the posterior urethrovesical angle exceeds 100 degrees, the upper urethral angle exceeds 30 degrees, and the descent of the bladder exceeds 2.5 cm. Excessive descent of the bladder by itself is not related to stress incontinence, but it does indicate a cystocele.

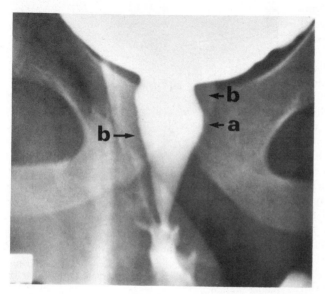

Figure 7–58. During voiding, wide distention of the normal female urethra *(a)* and vaginal filling *(b)* both are common.

Adrenal Glands

The adrenal glands have approximately the same height as the adjacent vertebral body. They are situated on the superomedial aspect of the anterior surface of each kidney. The right adrenal is roughly pyramidal in shape, with the base against the kidney, the medial surface to the right of the inferior vena cava and behind it, the posterior surface against the diaphragm, and the anterior surface against the bare area of the liver and the posterior parietal peritoneum. The left adrenal gland is roughly semicircular as seen from the front, with the convex border medially. Of its two surfaces, the posterior surface lies against the diaphragm, and the anterior surface lies against the posterior wall of the lesser sac, the splenic artery, and the body of the pancreas. The left adrenal gland is usually slightly larger than the right.

Except for the medial border of the left adrenal gland, the borders of the adrenal glands appear gently concave radiologically. Both adrenals are usually not in the same anteroposterior plane. The adrenal glands are attached to the renal fasciae, which are fused above the glands and attached to the diaphragm. They do not descend with the kidneys when the patient is in the vertical posture but are displaced, like the kidneys, by diaphragmatic movements.

Plain films of the abdomen and excretion urography without tomography can, at best, demonstrate half the adrenal tumors (excluding aldosteronomas) because of the calcification of the tumor or displacement of the kidney. Because the adrenal glands are very richly supplied with blood, excretion urography with tomography can demonstrate 70 per cent of non–aldosterone producing tumors. Computed tomography of the adrenal gland is indicated to confirm urographic findings or to localize lesions diagnosed by chemical tests.

The adrenal gland may be ectopic in location, often just above or anterior to the renal pelvis. Pheochromocytomas may occur anywhere along the sympathetic nervous chain and in the urinary bladder wall.

References

Allen, R. P., and Condon, V. R.: Transitory extraperitoneal hernia of the bladder in infants (bladder ears). Radiology, 77:979, 1961.

Becker, J.: A hernia of the urinary bladder. Radiology, 84:270, 1965.

Benness, G. T.: Urographic excretion study—dehydration and dose. Australas. Radiol., 11:261, 1967.

Boltuch, R. L., and Lalli, A. F.: A new technique for urethrography. Radiology, 115:736, 1975.

Bree, R. L., Green, B., Keiller, D. L., and Genet, E. F.: Medial deviation of the ureters secondary to psoas muscle hypertrophy. Radiology, 118:691, 1976.

Byrd, L., and Sherman, R. L.: Radiocontrast-induced acute renal failure. Medicine, 58:270, 1979.

Cwynarski, M. T., and Saxton, H. M.: Urography in myelomatosis. Br. Med. J., 1:486, 1969.

Doyle, F. H., Sherwood, T., Steiner, R. E., Breckenridge, A., and Dollery, C. T.: Large dose urography. Is there an optimum dose? Lancet, 2:964, 1967.

Dure-Smith, P.: Pregnancy dilatation of the urinary tract; the iliac sign and its significance. Radiology, 96:545, 1970.

Ettinger, A.: Personal communication, 1965.

Evans, J. A., Dubilier, W., Jr., and Monteith, J. C.: Nephrotomography: A preliminary report. Am. J. Roentgenol., 71:213, 1954.

Fitts, F. B., Jr., Herbert, S. G., and Mellins, H. Z.: Criteria for examination of the urethra during excretory urography. Radiology, 125:47, 1977a.

Fitts, F. B., Jr., Mascatello, V. G., and Mellins, H. Z.: The value of compression during excretion voiding urethrography. Radiology, 125:53, 1977b.

Gittes, R. F., and Talner, L. B.: Congenital megacalyces vs. obstruction hydronephrosis. J. Urol., 108:833, 1972.

Goldin, R. R., and Rosen, R. A.: Effects of inguinal hernias upon the bladder and ureters. Radiology, 115:55, 1975.

Haines, J. O., and Kyaw, M. M.: Anterolateral deviation of ureters by psoas muscle hypertrophy. J. Urol., 106:831, 1971.

Hartman, G. W., Hattery, R. R., Witten, D. M., and Williamson, B.: Mortality during excretory urography: Mayo Clinic experience. Am. J. Roentgenol., 139:919, 1982.

Hodson, C. J., Drewe, J. A., Karn, M. N., and King, A.: Renal size in normal children. Arch. Dis. Child., 37:616, 1962.

Hollenberg, N. K.: Renal Disease. In Wells, R. (Ed.) Microcirculation in Clinical Medicine. New York, Academic Press, 1973, pp. 61–80.

Imray, T. J., Terry, D. W., and Dodds, W. J.: The caudal angle view: A helpful adjunct in excretory urography. Radiology, 253:254, 1977.

Jonsson, M., Lindberg, B., and Risholm, C.: Percutaneous nephropyelostomy in cases of ureteral obstruction. Scand. J. Urol. Nephrol., 6:51, 1972.

Kabakian, H. A., Armenian, H. K., Deeb, Z. L., and Rizk, G. K.: Asymmetry of the pelvic ureters in normal females. Am. J. Roentgenol., 127:723, 1976.

Lalli, A. F.: Urographic contrast media reactions and anxiety. Radiology, 112:267, 1974.

Lalli, A. F.: The direct fluoroscopically guided approach to renal, thoracic and skeletal lesions. Curr. Probl. Radiol., 2:1, 1972.

Lang, E. K.: Differential diagnosis of renal cysts and tumors. Cyst puncture, aspiration and analysis of cyst content for fat as diagnostic criteria for renal cyst. Radiology, 87:883, 1966.

Lebowitz, R.: Personal communication, 1984.

McCallum, R. W., and Colapinto, V.: Urological Radiology of the Adult Male Lower Urinary Tract. Springfield, Ill., Charles C Thomas, 1976.

McLaughlin, A. P., III, and Pfister, R. C.: Double catheter technique for evaluation of urethral injury and differentiating urethral from bladder rupture. Radiology, 110:716, 1974.

Moell, H.: Kidney size and its deviation from normal in acute renal failure: A roentgen diagnostic study. Acta Radiol. Suppl. 206, 1961.

Narath, P.: The hydromechanics of the calyx renalis. J. Urol., *43*:145, 1940.

Newberg, A. H., and Mindell, H. J.: Predicting tomographic levels for urography. Radiology, *118*:460, 1976.

Pfister, R. C.: Reactions to urographic contrast media. *In* Syllabus for Categorical Course in Genitourinary Radiology. Radiological Society of North America, 1975, pp. 65–91.

Pickering, R. S., Hartman, G. W., Weeks, R. E., Sheps, S. G., and Hattery, R. R.: Excretory urographic localization of adrenal cortical tumors and pheochromocytomas. Radiology, *114*:345, 1975.

Plaut, M., and Lichtenstein, L.: Treatment of immediate hypersensitivity reactions to drugs. Ration. Drug. Ther. *8*, 1974.

Rahimi, B., Edmondson R. P., and Jones, J. F.: Effect of radiocontrast media on kidneys of patients with renal disease. Br. Med. J., *282*:1194, 1981.

Saldino, R. M., and Palubinskas, A. J.: Medial placement of ureter: A normal variant which may simulate retroperitoneal fibrosis. J. Urol., *107*:582, 1972.

Shehadi, W. H.: Adverse reactions to intravascularly administered contrast media. Am. J. Roentgenol., *124*:145, 1975.

Sherwood, T., Doyle, F. H., Breckenridge A., Dollery, D. T., and Steiner, R. E.: Intravenous urography and renal function. Clin. Radiol., *19*:296, 1968.

Shopfner, C. E.: Roentgenological evaluation of distal urethral obstruction. Radiology, *88*:222, 1967.

Simon, A. L.: Normal renal size: An absolute criterion. Radiology, *92*:270, 1974.

Stolz, J. L., and Fogel, E. J.: The chain cystourethrogram. Radiology, *103*:204, 1972.

Weinrauch, L. A., and Healy, R. W.: Coronary angiopathy and acute renal failure in diabetic azotemic nephropathy. Ann. Intern. Med., *86*:56, 1977.

Witten, D. M., Greene, L. F., and Emmett, J. L.: An evaluation of nephrotomography in urologic diagnosis. Am. J. Roentgenol., *90*:115, 1963.

Witten, D. M., Hirsch, F. D., and Hartman, G. W.: Acute reactions to urographic contrast medium. Am. J. Roentgenol., *119*:832, 1973.

Radionuclides in Genitourinary Disorders

SABAH S. TUMEH, M.D.
SALVATOR TREVES, M.D.
S. JAMES ADELSTEIN, M.D., Ph.D.

INTRODUCTION

Nuclear medicine examinations of the genitourinary system have changed dramatically during the past decade. The availability of new radiopharmaceuticals, especially technetium-99m (Tc-99m) chelates, along with improvements in instrumentation, has made possible the production of images with good anatomic detail and has extended the range of functional measurements. The introduction of computers into nuclear medicine has markedly improved our ability to quantify renal functions and to obtain dynamic examinations of the kidneys, bladder, and testes. In addition, the advent of computed tomography and ultrasonography has defined more precisely the role of radionuclides in the workup of genitourinary disorders. As a result, the main emphasis of genitourinary examinations in nuclear medicine has shifted toward the assessment of physiologic parameters and functions in various disease states. Radionuclide and radiographic examinations are generally complementary, providing different sets of data.

The equipment required to perform most of the procedures described in this chapter is an Anger scintillation camera, preferably with a large field-of-view crystal that can include both kidneys on the same image. The camera should be interfaced to a computer with software dedicated to nuclear medicine applications. The computer allows the operator to quantitate relative renal function, regional blood flow, transit time, and vesicoureteral reflux.

RADIOPHARMACEUTICALS

The most commonly used radiopharmaceuticals in genitourinary imaging are Tc-99m chelates and iodine-131 (I-131) ortho-iodohippurate. A comprehensive understanding of the different physiologic properties of these compounds is essential for their appropriate use and application in different clinical settings.

Tc-99m DTPA (diethylenetriamine pentaacetic acid) is principally excreted in urine by glomerular filtration. A small portion of the injected dose (3 to 5 per cent) is protein-bound and therefore is not available for filtration. This causes an inherent error of about the same magnitude when Tc-99m DTPA is used to measure the glomerular filtration rate (GFR). The plasma clearance of this radiopharmaceutical is triphasic, with an overall effective half-time of 1.4 hours. It reaches a peak concentration in the kidneys at 3 to 5 minutes. The main uses of Tc-99m DTPA are the assessment of blood flow to the kidneys, the computation of the GFR (Gates, 1982), and the study of the morphologic physiology of the pelvocalyceal system (Joekes, 1974; Thrall et al., 1981).

Tc-99m DMSA (dimercaptosuccinic acid) is 90 to 95 per cent bound to plasma proteins; hence, it is not available for filtration and is not useful for evaluation of the collecting system. However, it is bound to the basement membrane of the proximal renal tubular cells, and about 54 per cent of the dose remains in the renal cortex at 6 hours (Daly et al., 1978; Taylor, 1980). When imaging is performed with magnification or pinhole collimators, the outline of the renal cortex is very clearly visualized. This technique is very helpful in determining functional renal mass (Daly et al., 1978) and in the evaluation of pseudotumors (Parker et al., 1976), cortical scarring (Enlander et al., 1974), and renal trauma (Berg, 1982).

Tc-99m GHA (glucoheptonate) is excreted in part quickly by glomerular filtration (20 per cent) and slowly by tubular secretion (80 per cent). It is also bound to tubular cells, with about 19 per cent remaining in the cortex for several hours, thus allowing adequate imaging of the renal cortex. Early images delineate the collecting system, and later ones delineate the cortical mass. It is mainly employed in the assessment of renal flow, trauma, and thromboembolic disease (Berg, 1982).

Tc-99m pertechnetate is used primarily in flow studies of the kidneys and testes as well as in the assessment of vesicoureteral reflux. It is poorly concentrated in the kidney and therefore does not produce adequate renal images.

Tc-99m CO_2-DADS-A (N,N'-bis (mercaptoacetyl)-2,3-diaminopropanoate, Component A) has been recently introduced (Klingensmith et al., 1984). It is handled by the kidney in a fashion similar to ortho-iodohippurate. In time, it, or a similar compound, may replace the latter because of the superior physical characteristics of Tc-99m and the correspondingly lower radiation dose.

I-131 OIH (Ortho-iodohippurate or hippuran) is excreted in urine by glomerular filtration (20 per cent) and tubular secretion (80 per cent). Its renal extraction is extremely high, similar to that of para-aminohippurate (PAH), and definitely higher than the classic Tc-99m compounds, thus making it more effective in the evaluation of renal failure. However, because of the high radiation dose resulting from the emission of beta particles, the clinical dose is substantially smaller than that of the Tc-99m chelates. Furthermore, I-131 has a high gamma energy (364 keV), which makes it less favorable for imaging with the Anger scintillation camera.

Ga-67 citrate in serum is mostly bound to proteins (lactoferrin and transferrin) and to polymorphonuclear cells. It is excreted in urine initially and in the gastrointestinal tract later. It is mainly employed to visualize inflammatory lesions and sometimes tumors.

Tc-99m antimony colloid is an investigational pharmaceutical used to evaluate the ileopelvic lymph nodes.

TESTS AND MEASUREMENTS

Effective renal plasma flow (ERPF) can be determined by single-bolus or continuous intravenous infusion of I-131 OIH (Bianchi and Toni, 1962; Blaufox et al., 1967). Approximately 90 per cent of the dose is removed from circulation during a single passage through the kidney. The method tends to underestimate the ERPF by about 15 per cent as determined by matched PAH measurements. This inherent underestimation is probably due to different plasma-protein binding characteristics, tubular handling, or even the presence of a small fraction of free iodine in the OIH preparation. For the details of the performance of these methods, the reader is referred to the reviews by Cohen, 1974; Burbank et al., 1961; and Schwartz and Madeloff, 1961.

Perfusion can be assessed by using Tc-99m compounds (DTPA, GHA, pertechnetate) or OIH. A large-field-of-view gamma camera is placed against the back of the patient and 10 to 15 mc of one of the technetium compounds or 200 to 300 μC of OIH are injected intravenously as a bolus. Data are routinely collected and analyzed by computer assistance. In addition, analog images of each study are obtained. Each study is then assessed in two ways:

1. The first way is qualitatively, by inspecting the pictures visually, looking for early appearance of radioactivity in the kidneys, time of appearance of maximum radioactivity (which should coincide with that of the abdominal

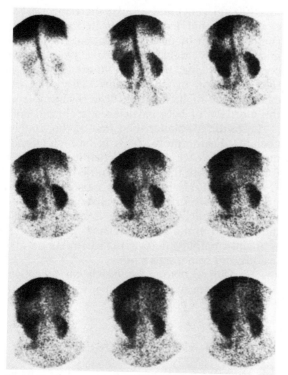

Figure 7–59. Normal dynamic scan of the kidneys in the posterior projection obtained with Tc-99m DTPA. Note that the appearance and intensity of radioactivity are similar in both kidneys and coincide with that of the abdominal aorta.

aorta), and the pattern of washout of the radiotracer from both sides (Fig. 7–59).

2. The second way is quantitatively (the radionuclide renogram), by displaying the study on the computer screen and plotting regions of interest around each kidney and over a segment of the abdominal aorta. After appropriate correction for background activity, a graph representing the change in radioactivity in each kid-

ney and aorta as a function of time can be generated. The curves are then compared for time of appearance, peaking, and washout of radioactivity from the kidneys. The renographic curve has three phases (Fig. 7–60). The first, which represents the early appearance of radioactivity in the renal vessels and perirenal tissue and uptake in the renal tubular cells, particularly in the case of OIH, usually lasts for about 40 to 50 seconds. The second phase, which shows a more gradual accumulation of radioactivity, is achieved in around 3 to 5 minutes, when radioactivity reaches the renal tubules. This phase is determined by blood flow, intrinsic renal function, urine flow rates, and, to a lesser extent, the degree of hydration of the patient (Wedeen et al., 1963). The third phase, which is seen about 5 to 8 minutes later, usually shows a gradual decrease in radioactivity in the normal kidneys. This phase represents the washout or delivery of radioactivity into the collecting systems of the kidneys. It depends, among other things, on the rate of urine production and urine flow in the collecting tubules and collecting systems.

This technique is very useful in the assessment of renal perfusion as well as in the quantitative evaluation of renal function and the presence or absence of obstruction to urine flow when it is used along with furosemide (Thrall et al., 1981).

Regional blood flow (specific blood flow in millimeters per minutes per gram of tissue) can be measured by intra-arterial injection of a bolus of radioxenon (Xe-133) dissolved in saline and it can be externally detected by the gamma scintillation camera-computer system (Grunfeld et al., 1974). Radioxenon is generally injected through a catheter placed in one of the renal arteries. Krypton-85 (Kr-85) can also be used. The washout curve can be divided into three

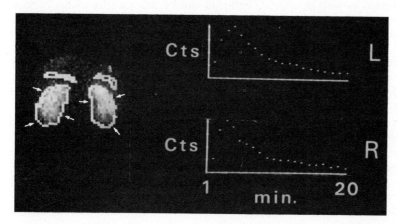

Figure 7–60. Normal renogram obtained with I-131 ortho-iodohippuran. On the left is a computer picture of the kidneys with regions of interest manually drawn around them (arrows). The small areas above the kidneys represent regions selected to correct for background activity. On the right are two curves representing radioactivity (CTS) in the kidneys (L, left; R, right) as a function of time (1 to 20 minutes). Both kidneys take up and clear radioactivity symmetrically (peak 3 to 4 minutes).

components: (1) rapid washout, which represents cortical flow; (2) renal medullary flow; and (3) slowest washout, which represents blood flow to renal and perinephric fat. In normal subjects, cortical blood flow is approximately 3.5 ml per gm per minute, and medullary flow is 0.75 ml per gm per minute. This method, though precise, has the obvious disadvantage of requiring arterial catheterization, and consequently it is applied only in selected instances when a scintillation camera is available in the arteriographic facility.

Glomerular filtration rate (GFR) can be quantified by a single injection or continuous intravenous infusion of I-125 iothalamate, which is handled by the kidney in a fashion similar to inulin (Blaufox and Cohen, 1970; Eberstadt et al., 1968; Ott and Wilson, 1975; Sigman et al., 1965). Subcutaneous injection of iothalamate has also been used successfully. Recently, Tc-99m DTPA, a gamma camera, and a computer have been employed to measure the GFR (Gates, 1982). The method described is easy, noninvasive, and requires about 15 minutes to perform. Excellent correlation has been found between the estimated GFR and the creatinine clearance at different levels of renal function. Moreover, this method can quantitate the GFR in each kidney separately. It should be noted, however, that the method depends on accurate measurement of the injected dose as well as meticulous determination of background activity.

Differential (split) renal function can now be assessed by a noninvasive method. Often, unilateral disease is disguised behind normal total renal function. In addition to shedding light on the pathophysiology of unilateral disease, the determination of unilateral renal function can have important therapeutic implications. It is often helpful to have an estimate of function in the contralateral kidney before surgery is attempted on one side. Inulin and PAH clearance methods require ureteral catheterization and are not very useful for serial determinations. Three other noninvasive methods are now available for the determination of split renal function.

1. *GFR.* As already mentioned, Tc-99m DTPA, with the aid of a gamma camera and a computer, can be used to determine the individual contribution of each kidney to the total GFR by determining renal activity at 1 to 3 minutes (Gates, 1982).

2. *Functional renal mass.* Since Tc-99m DMSA is actively taken up by the renal tubular cells, its relative uptake can be used as an index

of functioning cortical renal mass (Daly et al., 1978). Care should be exercised when performing this procedure, because the renal uptake of Tc-99m DMSA has been shown to be affected by common physiologic and biochemical changes, such as acid-base balance and hydration (Yee et al., 1981).

3. *The renogram.* The second portion of the renogram curve (see earlier section on the renogram) can be used as a crude estimate of renal function. The relative slope of that portion obtained from each kidney may be used as an index of the contribution of that kidney to the total renal function (Taplin et al., 1963).

CLINICAL APPLICATIONS

Vascular Disorders. Radionuclide techniques can be very helpful in the evaluation of renal vascular disorders. They have been used in detecting renovascular hypertension (Farmelant et al., 1970; Rosenthall, 1974; Gruenewald and Collins, 1983); in assessing the effects of trauma on renal circulation (Koenigsberg et al., 1974; Berg, 1982); and in determining compromise to the renal circulation in abdominal aortic disease, thromboembolic disease (Fig. 7–61), and renal transplants (Dossetor et al., 1970; Branch et al., 1971; zum Winkel et al., 1974; Hilson et al., 1978).

The detection of a renovascular etiology for hypertension can be achieved with the radionuclide angiogram (Farmelant et al., 1970; Rosenthall, 1974; McNeil et al., 1975). This technique discloses about 80 per cent of the cases. Unfortunately, 10 per cent of patients with essential hypertension will also have a positive test (McNeil et al., 1975). Moreover, the test cannot differentiate renovascular hypertension from other causes of unilateral renal disease. Recently, deconvolution techniques have been used to estimate a renal perfusion slope ratio and a parenchymal transit time, which, when considered along with GFR values, correlated very well with angiography with respect to site and severity of disease (Gruenewald and Collins, 1983). This method has the potential for becoming a screening test as well as a reliable, noninvasive procedure for follow-up after treatment.

Unlike arterial disorders, renal vein thrombosis cannot accurately be detected by nuclear medicine techniques. The findings are usually variable and nonspecific.

Trauma. Radiopharmaceuticals may be very useful in defining urinary tract involvement

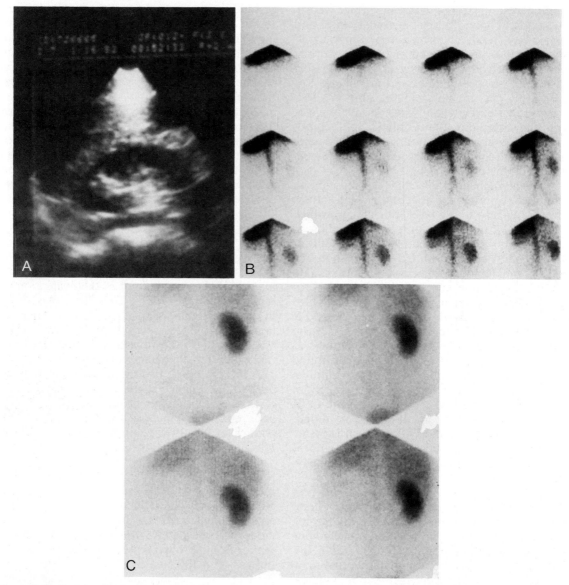

Figure 7–61. Patient with rheumatic heart disease and sudden onset of left flank pain and hematuria. *A,* An ultrasonogram of the left kidney shows normal morphology. *B,* A flow study of the kidneys obtained in the posterior projection, following intravenous injection of Tc-99m glucoheptonate. There is no perfusion of the left kidney. *C,* Delayed images of the kidneys show no uptake in the region of the left renal bed. The uptake in the right kidney is normal. In the proper clinical setting, this constellation of ultrasonographic and radionuclide findings is diagnostic of embolization into the left renal artery.

in trauma. The status of renal blood supply, the presence of renal parenchymal contusions with or without extravasation, and the integrity of the urinary bladder can all be accurately evaluated (Chopp et al., 1980; Berg, 1982).

We recommend the use of Tc-99m glucoheptonate for the workup of trauma, because the relatively high photon yield, as well as the renal handling of this radiotracer, allow evaluation of blood supply, collecting systems, and the urinary bladder. In addition, enough of the

dose is taken up by the renal tubules to permit adequate assessment of the parenchyma on delayed views.

Cortical Imaging. Technetium-99m DMSA can be used in two very important clinical settings.

1. It can be used in evaluating functioning masses (fetal lobulation, septa of Bertin) usually discovered incidentally on intravenous pyelography (IVP) or as an echogenic mass on ultrasound (Fig. 7–62). A Tc-99m DMSA scan will

show normal or increased uptake in those cases (Mazer and Quaife, 1979). Conversely, space-occupying lesions (tumors, cysts, abscesses) show decreased or lack of uptake of radioactivity (Fig. 7–63). We find magnification views, particularly with pinhole collimators, extremely helpful (Parker et al., 1976).

2. Technetium-99m DMSA can also be used in the assessment of cortical scars. This application can prove helpful in following high-risk patients, for example, those with vesico-ureteral reflux with or without recurrent upper urinary tract infections. The test is particularly attractive because of its relatively low radiation dose when compared with urography.

Obstructive Uropathy. The evaluation of renal function in postobstructive dilatation of the pelvocalyceal system can be difficult. Radio-nuclide examinations may be useful in solving this difficulty (O'Reilly et al., 1978; Thrall et al., 1981). The diuretic renogram is used to differentiate residual obstruction from postob-structive dilatation. We employ Tc-99m DTPA followed by an intravenous injection of furose-mide (20 mg) for this purpose. The data are collected and analyzed by computer. Three pat-

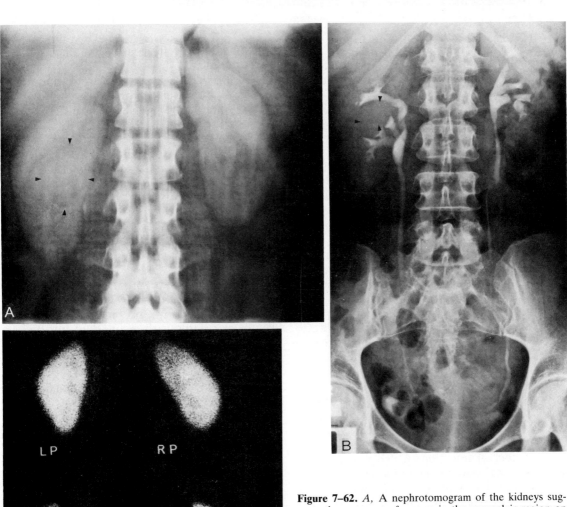

Figure 7–62. *A,* A nephrotomogram of the kidneys suggests the presence of a mass in the parapelvic region on the right (arrowheads), which is as opaque as the rest of the kidney on that side. *B,* A later film from the same IVP suggests the presence of a right parapelvic mass associated with short calyces. *C,* A Tc-99m DMSA scan of the same patient shows normal uptake in both kidneys. The constellation of urographic and radionuclide findings is pathognomonic of a displaced septum of Bertin.

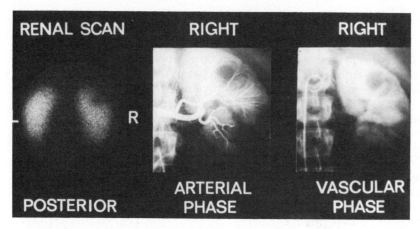

Figure 7–63. A Tc-99m DMSA scan on the left demonstrates a focal defect in the upper pole of the right kidney corresponding to the simple cyst seen on the arteriogram on the right side.

terns are seen. First, in normal patients, a rapid rise of radioactivity is followed by a rapid fall after furosemide administration. Second, in patients with nonobstructive dilatation, there is a gradual rise and a rapid fall in activity in response to furosemide (Fig. 7–64). Third, in patients with obstruction, there is a slow rise in activity and no response to furosemide (Fig. 7–65). Moreover, the radionuclide examination may help decide whether to remove a chronically obstructed kidney or to try to decompress it (Fig. 7–66). I-131 has been similarly used, but we reserve this agent for patients with poor renal function.

Inflammatory Lesions. In complicated cases, the use of radionuclides may be helpful in identifying pyelonephritis and nephric or perinephric abscesses. The most commonly used radiotracer is gallium-67 (Ga-67) citrate injected intravenously in a dose of 3 to 6 mc. We prefer to wait 48 to 72 hours before imaging because of significant normal excretion by the kidneys at earlier times. Ga-67 has been used in the diagnosis of acute pyelonephritis with an accuracy of 86 per cent (Kessler et al., 1974; Hurwitz et al., 1976) (Fig. 7–67). Two main difficulties are encountered with Ga-67 scanning. The first is its inability to differentiate intrarenal from perirenal foci of infection, which is caused by relatively poor spatial resolution. The second is its nonspecificity, that is, other inflammatory processes, such as acute tubular necrosis and vasculitis, will also lead to the concentration of gallium (Kumar and Coleman, 1976).

Renal cortical imaging with Tc-99m DMSA has been recently used in conjunction with Ga-67 for the same purpose (Handmaker, 1982) (Fig. 7–68). The technetium agent shows cortical defects that may disappear following appropriate therapy. Because of its lower radiation dose,

Tc-99m DMSA can be used to follow patients after treatment.

Acute Renal Failure. Renal scintigraphy may be helpful in clarifying the etiology of acute renal failure and in predicting recovery of function.

Of the many causes of acute renal failure, arterial occlusion secondary to trauma, aortic dissection, or thromboembolic disease is particularly amenable to diagnosis by renoscintigraphy. Lack of perfusion with no delayed uptake is the hallmark of the test (see Fig. 7–61). Acute tubular necrosis (ATN) usually shows normal perfusion and early uptake of radiotracers with no excretion and very slow washout from the kidneys. Lack of uptake of OIH in patients with ATN carries a grave prognosis (Schoutens et al., 1972; Staab et al., 1973), whereas visualization of the kidneys, no matter how slight, is usually associated with recovery of function.

Renal Transplant Evaluation. Three major parameters can be assessed with renal scintigraphy.

First, perfusion can be well evaluated using Tc-99m DTPA or Tc-99m GHA. Qualitative evaluation of transplant perfusion includes visual inspection of serial static images. Peak radioactivity usually coincides with that of the femoral artery and exceeds it in intensity in the normally perfused transplant (Fig. 7–69). Quantitative indices have been developed to express the degree of perfusion numerically. Time activity curves from the kidney and femoral artery are generated by computer assistance (Hilson et al., 1978). Although numerical indices seem to decrease subjectivity in the evaluation of transplant perfusion, it should be noted that reliability depends on careful and meticulous analysis. The lack of perfusion and absence of radionuclide uptake are indicative of transplant is-

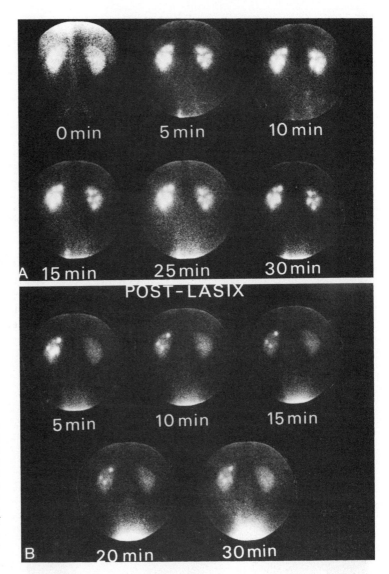

Figure 7–64. *A,* Sequential images obtained in the posterior projection following the intravenous administration of Tc-99m DTPA in a patient who had surgery for ureteropelvic stenosis on the left side. Both collecting systems are visualized. There is a collection of radioactivity in the left pelvis. *B,* Following the intravenous administration of furosemide, prompt washout of radioactivity from the left pelvis is noted. These findings are very suggestive of nonobstructive pelvicalycectasis.

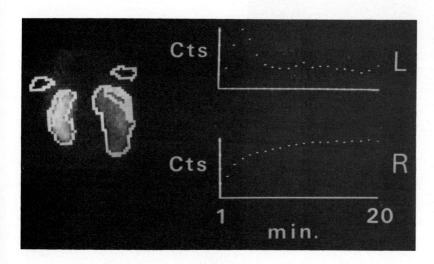

Figure 7–65. A renogram obtained with I-131 OIH. On the left is a computer picture of the kidneys with regions of interest around them. On the right are computer-produced curves representing radioactivity (Cts) as a function of time (L, left; R, right). Note that the time-activity curve on the right slowly reaches a plateau instead of dipping down as does the curve on the left, suggesting the presence of an obstructive lesion on the right side.

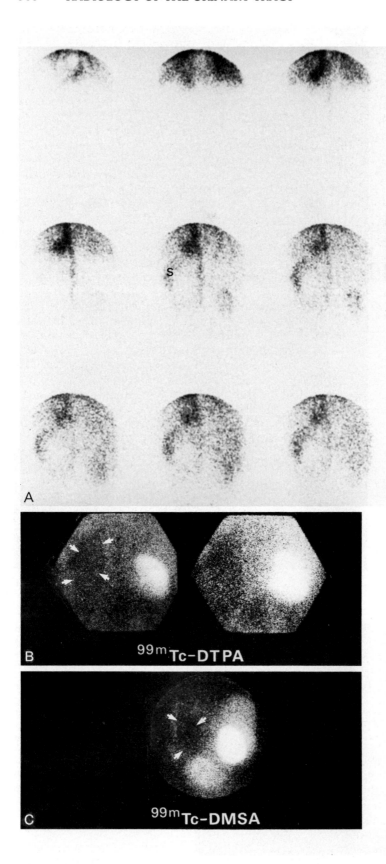

Figure 7–66. In an attempt to estimate renal function on the left side of a patient who had chronic obstruction on that side, this renal scan was obtained. *A,* Flow study obtained with Tc-99m DTPA (S, spleen). There is no activity in the left renal bed. *B,* A delayed (30 minutes) posterior picture from the same Tc-99m DTPA study. *C,* A delayed (4 hours) posterior picture from a Tc-99m DMSA study. The amount of radioactivity in the left renal bed is much less than background (arrows), indicating that this kidney is not salvageable.

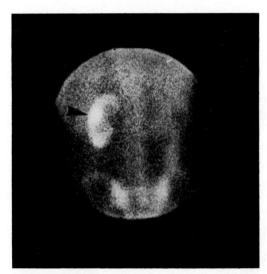

Figure 7–67. A 72-hour gallium-67 scan in the posterior projection shows radioactivity in the left kidney with a region of intense focal uptake (arrowhead). On exploration, the patient was found to have a renal carbuncle.

chemia (Fig. 7–70). However, they do not help differentiate complete arterial from venous occlusion, nor do they separate these occurrences from hyperacute rejection.

Second, the function of the transplant can be closely monitored by serial scintiscans. Deterioration of function due to parenchymal processes, such as ATN, is usually associated with preserved perfusion, no excretion, and slow washout, manifested as gradual decrease in the renal:background ratio. Slow improvement in function is usually seen in 2 to 3 weeks (Fig. 7–71). Allograft rejection, which does not usually occur before the end of the first week, is associated with more pronounced depression of perfusion. Definitive differentiation of ATN from rejection is not possible on the basis of the renal scan alone (Kirchner and Rosenthall, 1982).

Third, the assessment of integrity of the collecting system, ureter, and bladder can be evaluated by Tc-99m DTPA. Delayed views are essential, especially when leakage into a closed space is present (Fig. 7–72).

Vesicoureteral Reflux. The diagnosis of vesicoureteral reflux is traditionally made by radiographic cystography (Conway et al., 1972; Nasrallah et al., 1978; Willi and Treves, 1983). Although the anatomic definition of this technique is exquisite and far superior to radionuclide cystography, the latter has several advantages over the former. The radiation dose to the bladder and gonads is much smaller (about 1/100) for the radionuclide examination. This is very important, especially in children, and particularly so when frequent follow-up examinations are required. Radionuclide cystography is a dynamic examination, collected during the bladder filling and emptying phases. Quantification of reflux and of the bladder volume at which it occurs is possible with computer assistance. The nature of reflux, that is, whether it is continuous or intermittent, as well as the time of its occurrence with regard to bladder dynamics, can be demonstrated (Fig. 7–73).

At our institution we initially study the patient with a radiographic voiding cystogram for a clear evaluation of anatomy. The degree of reflux is then measured and is followed by radionuclide examinations.

Testicular Scanning. The main purpose of scrotal scintigraphy is to differentiate torsion from nonsurgical causes of scrotal pain, the most common of which is epididymo-orchitis. The scan is performed in the supine position. A gamma camera, interphased with a computer, collects a dynamic study over the scrotum following an intravenous injection of 0.2 mc per kg Tc-99m pertechnetate. The appearance of radionuclide in each hemiscrotum is a direct function of its blood supply. Static images are obtained at the end of the dynamic phase.

In both phases, a normal scan demonstrates symmetric activity bilaterally similar to that of the adjacent thigh.

In acute torsion, there is decreased flow to the symptomatic side initially, associated with a central area of photon deficiency on the delayed images. Missed torsion usually shows increased flow in addition to a rim of increased radionuclide due to reactive hyperemia in the scrotum whose blood supply from the pudendal artery is usually not involved (Fig. 7–74).

Inflammatory processes such as epididymo-orchitis demonstrate increased flow during the dynamic phase, as well as delayed accumulation of radionuclide on the affected side (Fig. 7–75). If this process is associated with a related (abscess) or unrelated (hydrocele) space-occupying lesion, the scintigraphic differentiation from missed torsion becomes very difficult. Scrotal scintigraphy is not very helpful in the diagnosis of torsion of the appendix testis. Uptake of radioactivity may be normal or slightly increased.

Data from Boston's Children's Hospital combined with that of two other series (Holder et al., 1977; Kogan et al., 1979) indicate that scrotal scanning has a sensitivity of 95 per cent and a specificity of 100 per cent in distinguishing

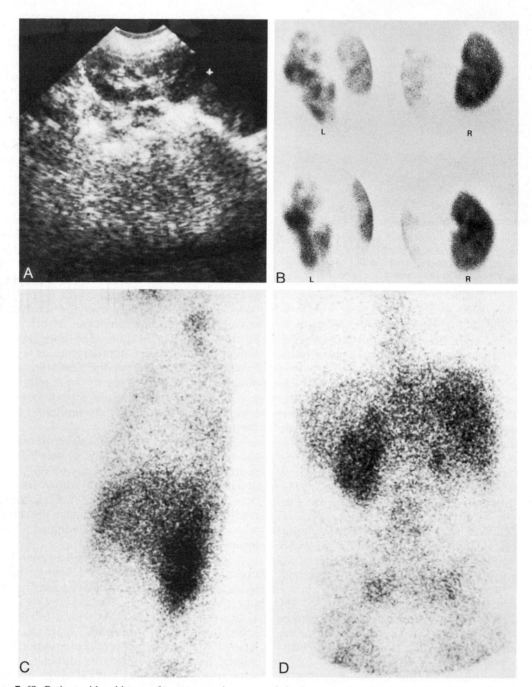

Figure 7–68. Patient with a history of recurrent urinary tract infections. *A,* An ultrasonogram of the left kidney shows normal morphology. The results of an IVP were normal. *B,* A Tc-99m DMSA scan obtained with the pinhole collimator shows multiple defects in the left kidney and normal distribution of activity in the right (L, left kidney; R, right kidney). *C* and *D,* Posterior and left lateral views from a gallium-67 scan of the same patient show intense uptake of radioactivity in the left kidney. These findings are very suggestive of pyelonephritis with multiple small abscesses.

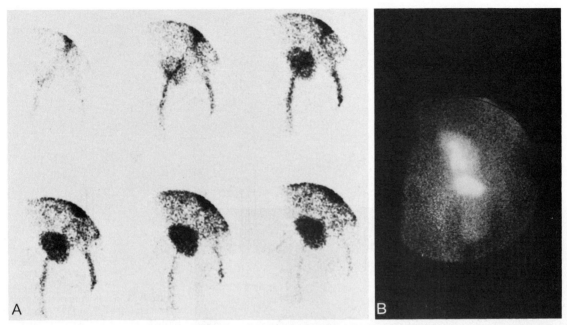

Figure 7–69. Evaluation of right renal transplant. *A,* Views of the transplanted kidney in the anterior projection following intravenous administration of Tc-99m DTPA show good perfusion of the kidney; normal peak activity coincides with the peak of radioactivity in the femoral artery on that side. *B,* A delayed picture from the same study shows excellent excretion and outline of the collecting system and urinary bladder.

Figure 7–70. Perfusion scans of a transplanted right kidney obtained on days 1 and 13 following the transplantation. *Day 1:* There is normal perfusion of the transplanted kidney. *Day 13:* No perfusion of the transplanted kidney is demonstrated. This is indicative of transplant ischemia.

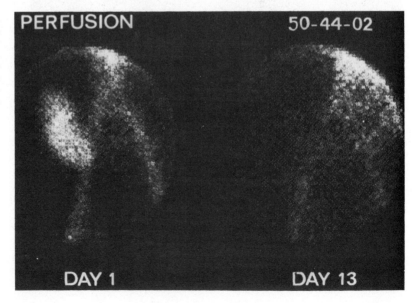

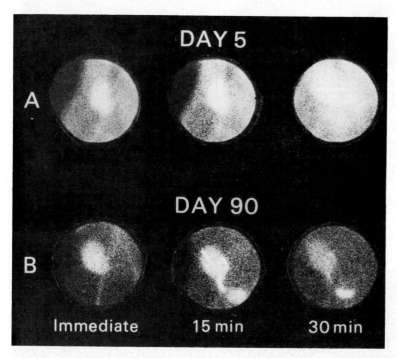

Figure 7–71. Evaluation of transplanted right kidney. Tc-99m DTPA scan performed on the fifth postoperative day *(A)* shows prompt uptake of radioactivity, with no excretion into the collecting system. The bladder is not visualized and background activity increases with time. This is indicative of acute tubular necrosis (ATN). Tc-99m DTPA scan on the ninetieth postoperative day *(B)* shows good uptake and excretion. The bladder is well seen and background activity decreases with time, indicating recovery from ATN.

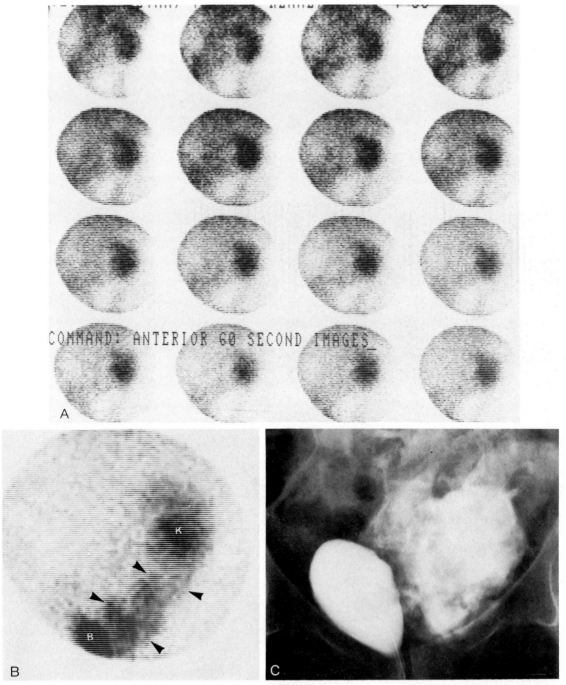

Figure 7–72. A patient with deteriorating renal function following left kidney transplantation. *A,* Flow study obtained in the anterior projection demonstrates good perfusion and uptake of radioactivity in the transplanted kidney. *B,* A 1 hour 15 minute delayed picture from the same study shows extravasation of radioactivity (arrowheads) (K, kidney; B, bladder). *C,* A cystogram confirms the presence of extravasation.

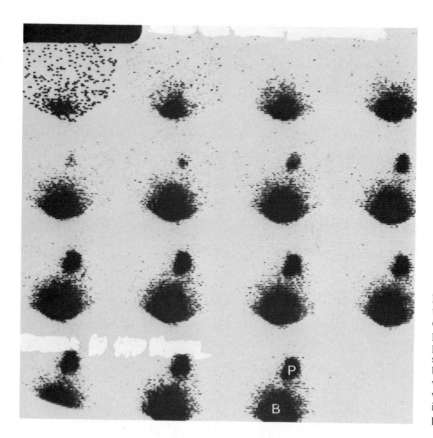

Figure 7–73. A radionuclide cystogram for the evaluation of vesicoureteral reflux. Sequential computer images obtained in the posterior projection during the instillation of radioactivity into the bladder (B). There is evidence of vesicoureteral reflux on the right with a large amount of radioactivity accumulating in the right renal pelvis (P).

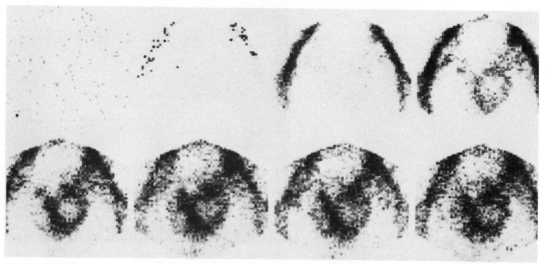

Figure 7–74. Missed testicular torsion. Patient presented with left testicular pain of 1 week's duration. Sequential computer images of the scrotum in the anterior projection demonstrate increased flow of radioactivity into the left hemiscrotum with a large central area of poor uptake of radioactivity. These findings are consistent with the diagnosis of missed testicular torsion. However, other entities, such as a testicular abscess, may present the same findings.

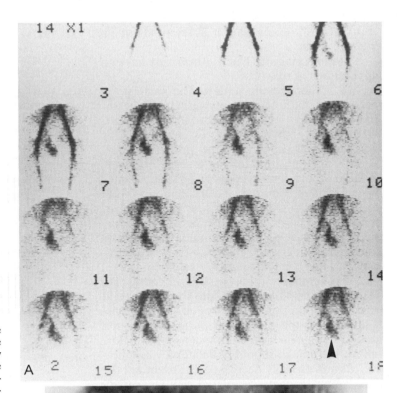

Figure 7–75. Inflammatory lesion of the scrotum. *A*, Patient presented with acute testicular pain on the right. A flow study with sequential computer images of the scrotum in the anterior projection demonstrates marked increased flow of radioactivity into the right hemiscrotum (arrowhead). *B*, A delayed image indicates markedly increased uptake in the region of the epididymis (E). There is some uptake of radioactivity in the right testicle (T), which is surrounded by a rim of decreased uptake representing a hydrocele (H).

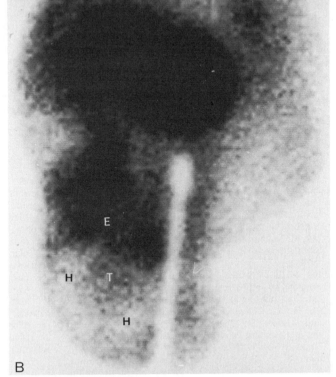

acute testicular torsion from other processes. It must be emphasized that the test should be carried out with meticulous attention to detail and that clinical correlation is essential for its interpretation.

Tumor Imaging. Nuclear medicine has two applications in this field:

1. Tumor-seeking studies. The greatest experience in this field has been with Ga-67 citrate. In a cooperative study (Sauerbrunn et al., 1978), Ga-67 uptake showed very low sensitivity for demonstrating the site of the primary tumor. Results were positive for metastases, however, in 50 to 75 per cent of cases when osseous sites were excluded. Embryonal cell carcinoma of the testicle showed Ga-67 uptake in 74 per cent of metastatic foci. It should be noted, however, that the impact of new technology, especially emission tomography and high-dose scintigraphy, has not been adequately evaluated.

2. Lymphoscintigraphy. By injecting Tc-99m antimony colloid both into the ischiorectal fossae and intradermally between the toes, visualization of the pelvic and para-aortic lymph nodes can be achieved (Kaplan, 1983). Normally, the uptake should be bilaterally symmetric. Asymmetrically decreased or absent uptake in a lymphatic chain correlated well (sensitivity 0.89; specificity 0.83) with tumor involvement in patients with testicular malignancy (Kaplan et al., 1983). The validity of this examination in other genitourinary tumor metastases awaits further clinical trials.

References

Berg, B. C., Jr.: Nuclear medicine and complementary modalities in renal trauma. Semin. Nucl. Med. *12*:280, 1982.

Bianchi, C., and Toni, P.: Possibilita di impiego dello o-iodo-ippurato di sodio (hippuran), marcato con ^{131}I, per la valutazione della portata renale plasmatica. Minerva Nucl., *6*:34, 1962.

Blaufox, M. D., and Cohen, A.: Single-injection clearances of iothalamate-^{131}I in the rat. Am. J. Physiol., *218*:542, 1970.

Blaufox, M. D., Potchen, E. J., and Merrill, J. P.: Measurement of effective renal plasma flow in man by external counting methods. J. Nucl. Med., *8*:77, 1967.

Branch, R. A., Coles, G. A., Eynon, A., Jones, G. R., and Lowder, E.: The use of radioactive hippuran in the management of cadaveric renal transplants. Br. J. Radiol., *44*:697, 1971.

Burbank, M. K., Tauxe, W. N., Maher, F. T., and Hunt, J. C.: Evaluation of radioiodinated hippuran for the estimation of renal plasma flow. Proc. Staff Meet. Mayo Clin., *36*:372, 1961.

Chopp, R. T., Hekmat-Ravan, H., and Mendez, R.: Technetium-99m glucoheptonate renal scan in diagnosis of acute renal injury. Urology, *15*:201, 1980.

Cohen M. L.: Radionuclide clearance techniques. Semin. Nucl. Med., *4*:23, 1974.

Conway, J. J., Belman, A. B., and King, L. R.: Direct and indirect radionuclide cystography. Semin. Nucl. Med., *4*:197, 1974.

Conway, J. J., King, L. R., Belman, A. B., and Thorson, T.: Detection of vesicoureteral reflux with radionuclide cystography. Am. J. Roentgenol. Rad. Ther. Nucl. Med., *115*:720, 1972.

Daly, M. J., Milutinovic, J., Rudd, T. G., Phillips, L. A., and Fialkow, P. J.: The normal ^{99m}Tc-DMSA renal image. Radiology, *128*:701, 1978.

Dossetor, J. B., Zweig, S. M., Treves, S., and Ross, W. M.: The ^{131}I ortho-iodohippurate photoscan in human renal allografts. Can. Med. Assoc. J., *102*:1373, 1970.

Eberstadt, P., Alvarez, J., and Ungay, F. A.: Simplified method for determining glomerular filtration rate with ^{131}I-sodium iothalamate. J. Nucl. Med., *9*:582, 1968.

Enlander, D., Weber, P. M., and dos Remedios, L. V.: Renal cortical imaging in 35 patients: Superior quality with ^{99m}Tc-DMSA. J. Nucl. Med., *15*:743, 1974.

Farmelant, M. H., Sachs, C., and Burrows, B. A.: Prognostic value of radioisotopic renal function studies for selecting patients with renal arterial stenosis for surgery. J. Nucl. Med., *11*:734, 1970.

Gates, G. F.: Glomerular filtration rate: Estimation from fractional renal accumulation of DTPA (stannous). A.J.R., *138*:565, 1982.

Gruenewald, S. M., and Collins, L. T.: Renovascular hypertension: Quantitative renography as a screening test. Radiology, *149*:287, 1983.

Grunfeld, J.-P., Sabto, J., Bankir, L., and Funck-Brentano, J.-L.: Methods for measurement of renal blood flow in man. Semin. Nucl. Med., *4*:39, 1974.

Handmaker, H.: Nuclear renal imaging in acute pyelonephritis. Semin. Nucl. Med., *12*:246, 1982.

Hilson, A. J. W., Maisey, M. N., Brown, C. B., Ogg, C. S., and Bewick, M. S.: Dynamic renal transplant imaging with Tc-99m DTPA (Sn) supplemented by a transplant perfusion index in the management of renal transplants. J. Nucl. Med., *19*:994, 1978.

Holder, L. E., Martire, J. R., Holmes, E. R., III, and Wagner, H. N., Jr.: Testicular radionuclide angiography and static imaging: Anatomy, scintigraphic interpretation and clinical indications. Radiology, *125*:739, 1977.

Hurwitz, S. R., Kessler, W. O., Alazraki, N. P., and Ashburn, W. L.: Gallium-67 imaging to localize urinary-tract infections. Br. J. Radiol., *49*:156, 1976.

Joekes, A. M.: Obstructive uropathy. Semin. Nucl. Med., *4*:187, 1974.

Kaplan, W. D.: Iliopelvic lymphoscintigraphy. Semin. Nucl. Med., *13*:42, 1983.

Kaplan, W. D., Garnick, M. B., and Richie, J. P.: Iliopelvic radionuclide lymphoscintigraphy in patients with testicular cancer. Radiology, *147*:231, 1983.

Kawamura, J., Hosokawa, S., Yoshida, O., Fujita, T., Ishii, Y., and Torizuka, K.: Validity of ^{99m}Tc dimercaptosuccinic acid renal uptake for an assessment of individual kidney function. J. Urol., *119*:305, 1978.

Kessler, W. O., Gittes, R. F., and Hurwitz, S. R.: Gallium-67 scans in the diagnosis of pyelonephritis. West. J. Med., *121*:91, 1974.

Kirchner, P. T., and Rosenthall, L.: Renal transplant evaluation. Semin. Nucl. Med., *12*:370, 1982.

Klingensmith, W. C., III, Fritzberg, A. R., Spitzer, V. M., Johnson, D. L., Kuni, C. C., Williamson, M. R., Washer, G., and Weill, R., III: Clinical evaluation of Tc-99m N,N'-bis (mercaptoacetyl)-2,3-diaminopropanoate as a replacement for I-131 hippurate: Concise communication. J. Nucl. Med., *25*:42, 1984.

Koenigsberg, M., Blaufox, M. D., and Freeman, L. M.: Traumatic injuries of the renal vasculature and parenchyma. Semin. Nucl. Med., 4:117, 1974.

Kogan, S. J., Lutzker, L. G., Perez, L. A., Novich, I., Schneider, K. M., Hanna, M. K., and Levitt, S. B.: The value of the negative radionuclide scrotal scan in the management of the acutely inflamed scrotum in children. J. Urol., 122:223, 1979.

Kumar, B., and Coleman, R. E.: Significance of delayed ^{67}Ga localization in the kidneys. J. Nucl. Med., 17:872, 1976.

Mazer, M. J., and Quaife, M. A.: Hypertrophied column of Bertin pseudotumor: Radionuclide investigation (letter). Urology, 14:210, 1979.

McNeil, B. J., Varady, P. V., Burrows, B. A., and Adelstein, S. J.: Cost effectiveness calculations in the diagnosis and treatment of hypertensive renovascular disease. N. Engl. J. Med., 293:216, 1975.

Nasrallah, P. F., Conway, J. J., King, L. R., Belman, A. B., and Weiss, S.: Quantitative nuclear cystogram: Aid in determining spontaneous resolution of vesicoureteral reflux. Urology. 12:654, 1978.

O'Reilly, P. H., Testa, H. J., Lawson, R. S., Farrar, D. J., and Edwards, E. C.: Diuresis renography in equivocal urinary tract obstruction. Br. J. Urol., 50:76, 1978.

Ott, N. T., and Wilson, D. M.: A simple technique for estimating glomerular filtration rate with subcutaneous injection of ^{125}I]iothalamate. Mayo Clin. Proc., 50:664, 1975.

Parker, J. A., Lebowitz, R., Mascatello, V., and Treves, S.: Magnification renal scintigraphy in the differential diagnosis of septa of Bertin. Pediatr. Radiol., 4:157, 1976.

Rosenthall, L.: Radiotechnetium renography and serial radiohippurate imaging for screening renovascular hypertension. Semin. Nucl. Med., 4:97, 1974.

Rosenthall, L., and Reid, E. C.: Radionuclide distinction of vascular and non-vascular lesions of the kidney. Can. Med. Assoc. J., 98:1165, 1968.

Sauerbrunn, B. J. L., Andrews, G. A., and Hübner, K. F.: Ga-67 imaging in tumors of the genito-urinary tract: Report of cooperative study. J. Nucl. Med., 19:470, 1978.

Schoutens, A., Dupuis, F., and Toussaint, C.: ^{131}I-hippuran scanning in severe renal failure. Nephron, 9:275, 1972.

Schwartz, F. D., and Madeloff, M. S.: Simultaneous renal clearances of radiohippuran and PAH in man (abstract). Clin. Res., 9:208, 1961.

Sigman, E. M., Elwood, C. M., and Knox, R.: The measurement of glomerular filtration rate in man with sodium iothalamate [131]I (Conroy). J. Nucl. Med., 7:60, 1965.

Staab, E. V., Hopkins, J., Patton, D. D., Hanchett, J., and Stone, W. J.: The use of radionuclide studies in the prediction of function in renal failure. Radiology, 106:141, 1973.

Taplin, G. V., Dore, E. K., and Johnson, D. E.: The quantitative radiorenogram for total and differential renal blood flow measurements. J. Nucl. Med., 4:404, 1963.

Taylor, A. T.: Quantitative renal function scanning: A historical and current status report on renal radiopharmaceuticals. In Freeman, L. M., and Weissman, H. S. (Eds.): Nuclear Medicine Annual 1980. New York, Raven Press, 1980, pp. 303–340.

Thrall, J. H., Koff, S. A., and Keyes, J. W., Jr.: Diuretic radionuclide renography and scintigraphy in the differential diagnosis of hydroureteronephrosis. Semin. Nucl. Med., 11:89, 1981.

Wedeen, R. P., Goldstein, M. H., and Levitt, M. F.: The radioisotope renogram in normal subjects. Am. J. Med., 34:765, 1963.

Willi, U., and Treves, S.: Radionuclide voiding cystography. Urol. Radiol., 5:161, 1983.

Yee, C. A., Lee, H. B., and Blaufox, M. D.: Tc-99m DMSA renal uptake: Influence of biochemical and physiologic factors. J. Nucl. Med., 22:1054, 1981.

zum Winkel, K., Harbst, H., Das, K. B., and Newiger, T.: Applications of radionuclides in renal transplantation. Semin. Nucl. Med., 4:169, 1974.

Ultrasound

EDWARD H. SMITH, M.D.
VASSILIOS RAPTOPOULOS, M.D.

Despite the many recent advances in medical technology, ultrasound remains one of the most significant modalities for the diagnosis of genitourinary tract disorders. Recent developments in ultrasound technology have led to such significant improvement in gray-scale imaging that histopathologic characterization of an organ or lesion is possible (Hricak et al., 1982). Digitalization of equipment has allowed greater consistency in producing satisfactory images. Improvement in transducer technology and electronics has significantly improved both spatial and contrast resolution. Dynamic scanners with excellent resolution are now widely available and allow production of excellent-quality images in any plane; this instrumentation has significantly reduced required operator skill and lessened examination time. It also allows complete portability so that studies can easily be carried out at the bedside, in the emergency room, or even in the operating room. In addition, visualization of structures in "real time" allows appreciation of organ movement, permitting better three-dimensional conceptualization. As a result, many studies are carried out solely with dynamic scanners, though the static images produced by articulated arm scanners allow easier orientation for the clinician who has not actually performed the study.

CLINICAL APPLICATIONS

Normal Kidneys

With improved contrast resolution, the internal architecture of the kidney can be quite satisfactorily displayed (Fig. 7–76) (Cook et al., 1977). The renal capsule is sharply outlined and is surrounded by variable amounts of perirenal fat. The cortex is relatively homogeneous with moderately high-amplitude echoes surrounding the echo-poor renal pyramids, which contrast with the strong, centrally located echo grouping representing the pelvicalyceal–sinus fat echo complex. The relatively constant position, large size, and characteristic configuration of the normal kidney permit ready ultrasound identification of renal abnormalities.

Congenital Anomalies

RENAL APLASIA AND HYPOPLASIA

When the kidney is congenitally absent, no reniform structure can be identified on that side, but the abnormally located colon in this situation may cause some confusion (Teele et al., 1977). A corroborative finding is enlargement of the opposite kidney resulting from compen-

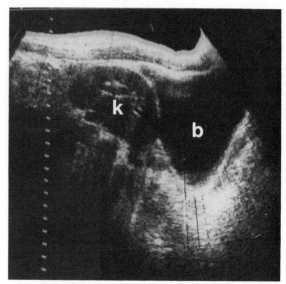

Figure 7–77. Supine scan of the true pelvis reveals an ectopic pelvic kidney (k) indenting the dome of the urine-filled bladder (b).

satory hypertrophy. When this finding is not present, it is imperative to scan the entire abdomen carefully, searching for an ectopic kidney, which is most often located in the true pelvis (Fig. 7–77). The more commonly occurring hypoplastic kidney, which is often considerably distorted and scarred, may be difficult to identify definitively with ultrasound. It is impossible to differentiate ultrasonically (or in any other way) between the congenitally small kidney and the acquired atrophied one.

HORSESHOE KIDNEYS

Horseshoe kidneys may be difficult to identify ultrasonically but may be suspected when the long axes of the kidneys converge inferiorly; this appearance may be difficult to appreciate because of the "tomographic" mode of imaging. A more reliable sign is the visualization of a variable amount of renal tissue in the midline anterior to the aorta and vertebral body.

MISCELLANEOUS CONGENITAL ABNORMALITIES

Duplex kidneys may be suspected when discontinuity of the pelvicalyceal–sinus fat echo pattern is present after carefully scanning the kidney from its lateral to medial border. The involved kidney is usually long and thin. Obstruction of an ectopic ureter (usually with hydronephrosis of the upper pole of the kidney) may be readily detected (Fig. 7–78). In order to distinguish this condition from a simple cyst, it

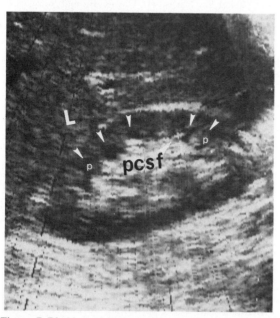

Figure 7–76. Normal kidney with sharply outlined renal capsule. The renal pyramids (p and arrowheads) are relatively sonolucent as compared with the surrounding cortex, which, in turn, is less echogenic than the adjacent liver (L) or spleen. The highly echogenic central grouping represents the pelvicalyceal–sinus fat echo complex (pcsf).

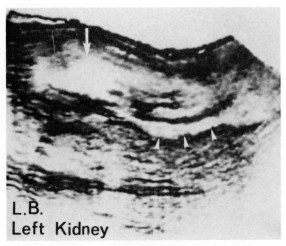

Figure 7–78. Prone longitudinal scan of hydronephrotic upper pole (arrow) and normal lower pole with dilated ectopic ureter (arrowheads) draining the upper pole. The normal ureter is not visible.

is important to identify the dilated ureter as well. If the dilated ureter is followed distally to the bladder, it may be possible to visualize a ureterocele if present (see Fig. 7–88) (Mascatello et al., 1977; Wyly et al., 1984).

POLYCYSTIC KIDNEY DISEASE

In polycystic kidney disease, ultrasound examination usually reveals both kidneys to be grossly enlarged and filled with innumerable cysts of various sizes (Fig. 7–79) (Lawson et al.,

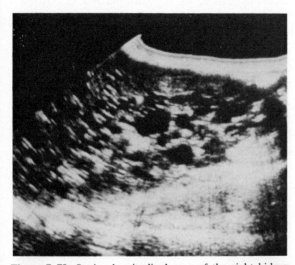

Figure 7–79. Supine longitudinal scan of the right kidney and adjacent liver. Practically the entire renal parenchyma is replaced by cysts of various sizes (black areas). The borders of the kidney are indistinct and merge with the adjacent liver, which is also severely involved by the same process.

1978). If the cysts are sufficiently large, the diagnosis is often made using intravenous urography, provided that renal function is sufficiently preserved. However, with ultrasound, the diagnosis may be made earlier in the course of the disease, and family screening in the asymptomatic patient with adult polycystic disease has been possible (Rosenfield et al., 1980). When the cysts are quite small (5 to 6 mm or less) they may be difficult to detect, but their presence may be suspected when focal strong linear reflections are present in the cortex, representing portions of the walls of the cysts. Ultrasound is also useful in investigating the symptomatic patient with polycystic disease. An infected or hemorrhagic cyst may be identified by its echogenicity or fluid-debris level, or rarely a coexistent neoplastic lesion may be found. Ultrasonically guided aspiration or drainage can then be carried out when indicated. In addition to being useful for evaluation of the kidneys, ultrasound is able to easily detect hepatic cysts and, less commonly, cysts within the pancreas and other organs (Fig. 7–79).

OTHER CYSTIC DISEASES

Ultrasound can be extremely useful in helping to sort out and classify various cystic conditions involving the kidneys by identifying the number, size, and location of the cysts; the character of the solid tissue between the cysts; the presence of calcification; and the preservation, if any, of normal renal tissue. Often a specific diagnosis can be reached on the basis of ultrasound alone, but in many cases there is considerable overlap in the ultrasonic appearance, and many other factors must be considered. The subject is beyond the scope of this chapter, and the reader is referred elsewhere for detailed discussion (Bearman et al., 1976; Grossman et al., 1983; Rego et al., 1983; Sanders and Hartman, 1984; Vela-Navarrete and Robledo, 1983).

Inflammatory Conditions

ACUTE FOCAL BACTERIAL NEPHRITIS AND RENAL ABSCESS

In acute pyelonephritis the ultrasound findings may be normal or the kidney may be diffusely enlarged. However, when acute focal pyelonephritis is present, the ultrasound examination may reveal only localized enlargement of a portion of the kidney early in the course of the disease (Fig. 7–80). Although relatively poorly defined, this mass is seen with serial

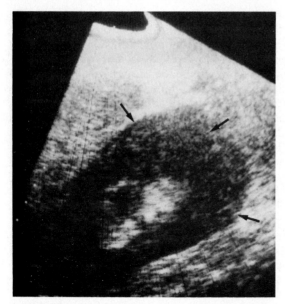

Figure 7–80. Longitudinal scan demonstrates focal enlargement of the lower pole (arrows) early in the course of acute focal pyelonephritis.

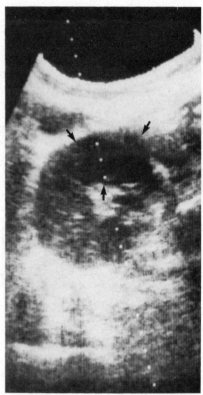

Figure 7–81. Transverse scan through the kidney reveals a localized area of decreased echoes (arrows) in a patient with acute focal pyelonephritis.

studies to contain lower amplitude echoes than the normal surrounding renal cortex (Fig. 7–81). Often, with institution of treatment, serial scans will show complete resolution of the lesion, with reconstitution of the normal renal architecture. If untreated or inadequately treated, this lesion may progress to a frank abscess, becoming better delineated with the development of a thick, irregular wall, with the central echoes being of even lower amplitude than with acute focal bacterial nephritis (Fig. 7–82) (Morehouse et al., 1984). If the lesion progresses to a frank abscess, catheter drainage under ultrasound guidance may be curative. It is important to realize, however, that small, echo-free areas early in the course of antibiotic treatment may resolve with further conservative treatment (Lee et al., 1980; Rosenfield et al., 1979).

Gas may form within a renal abscess, giving rise to a characteristic ultrasonic appearance with focal areas of increased echogenicity with shadowing. However, if gas is present throughout the kidney (emphysematous pyelonephritis), the kidney may not be recognized and may be mistaken for gas-containing bowel. Ultrasound is helpful in detecting extension of the infection outside the confines of the kidney with the development of a perinephric collection. These fluid collections usually contain low-level echoes, unless gas formation occurs (Fig. 7–83) (Kuligowska et al., 1983; Schneider et al., 1976).

Ultrasound appears to be quite accurate in

distinguishing between pyonephrosis and simple hydronephrosis. In the latter, the dilated collecting system is echo-free, whereas in a high percentage of cases of pyonephrosis, persistent, dependent echoes are present with a urine-

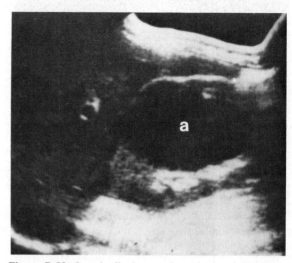

Figure 7–82. Longitudinal scan through the right kidney with echo-poor abscess (a). A fluid-debris level is present but is not visible on this image.

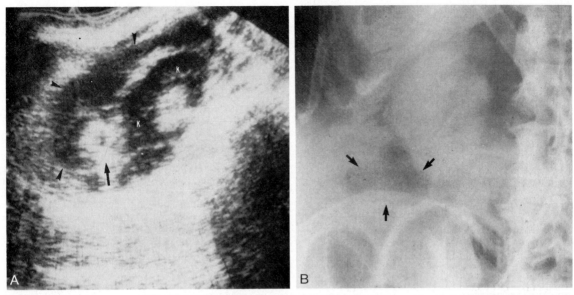

Figure 7–83. *A,* Oblique transverse view through the kidney (K) shows a large perinephric collection (arrowheads) containing a strongly echogenic focus (arrow) due to gas formation within the abscess. *B,* Ultrasound findings were confirmed by a radiograph of the area (arrows).

debris level; however, hemorrhage in a hydronephrotic kidney may present with identical findings (Fig. 7–84) (Coleman et al., 1981; Subramanyam et al., 1983).

CHRONIC INFLAMMATORY DISEASE

In chronic atrophic pyelonephritis, the ultrasound examination usually reveals a small kidney with focal loss of parenchyma and increased echogenicity in the involved area due to fibrosis. These areas may be adjacent to normal renal parenchyma. The pelvicalyceal–sinus fat echo complex may extend to the area of scarring as a linear echogenic band representing the retracted calyx (Kay et al., 1979). This appearance may be indistinguishable from renal tuberculosis or papillary necrosis. The latter conditions may, in addition, demonstrate areas of increased echogenicity with shadowing if calcifications are present (Schaffer et al., 1983).

XANTHOGRANULOMATOUS PYELONEPHRITIS

Xanthogranulomatous pyelonephritis may be suggested by the ultrasonic findings of an enlarged kidney with multiple peripheral anechoic structures caused by a dilated collecting system and a large, central, strongly echogenic focus as a result of an obstructing calculus. However, it may be difficult to distinguish this condition ultrasonically from simple hydronephrosis secondary to an obstructing calculus (Fig. 7–85). Not all cases of xanthogranulomatous pyelonephritis affect the entire kidney, nor do they all have obstructing calculi (Van Kirk et al., 1980).

Calcifications

Renal calculi may be present anywhere within the collecting system, giving rise to a characteristic ultrasound appearance with highly

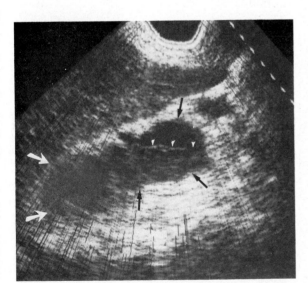

Figure 7–84. Longitudinal scan through a pyonephrotic kidney with marked dilatation of the collecting system (black and white arrows) with fluid-debris level (arrowheads).

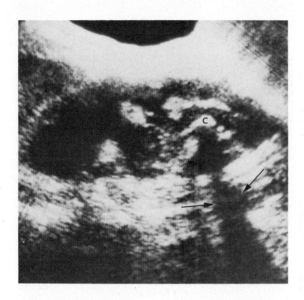

Figure 7–85. Longitudinal scan through kidney with xanthogranulomatous pyelonephritis. The kidney is enlarged, the collecting system is dilated, and there is an echogenic focus (c) with shadowing (arrows) due to an obstructing calculus. The distorted internal architecture of the kidney should differentiate this condition from simple hydronephrosis secondary to an obstructing calculus.

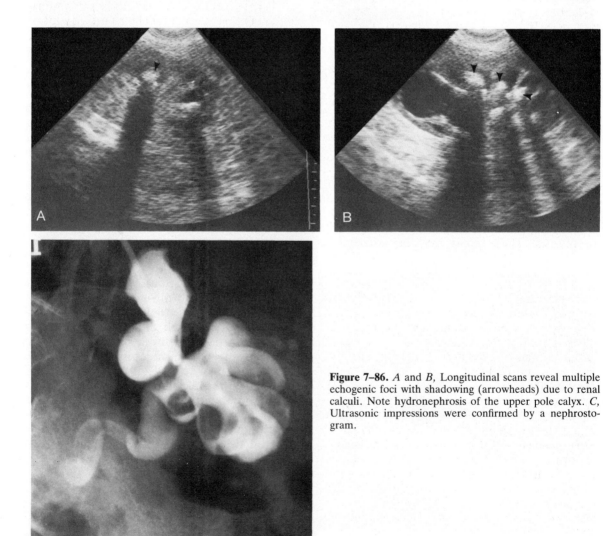

Figure 7–86. *A* and *B,* Longitudinal scans reveal multiple echogenic foci with shadowing (arrowheads) due to renal calculi. Note hydronephrosis of the upper pole calyx. *C,* Ultrasonic impressions were confirmed by a nephrostogram.

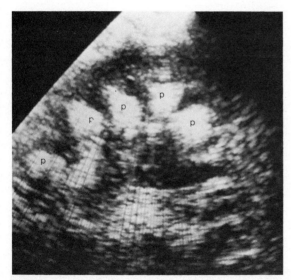

Figure 7–87. Longitudinal scan through a kidney with nephrocalcinosis. Highly echogenic foci are present in the renal pyramids (p).

echogenic foci with sharply defined shadowing (Fig. 7–86).

Nephrocalcinosis has an almost pathognomonic ultrasound appearance, with highly echogenic foci in the area of the renal pyramids, representing reversal of the normal internal sonographic architecture of the kidney in which the cortex is more echogenic than the renal pyramids. The sonographic findings may be quite striking, even when the plain radiograph is nondiagnostic (Fig. 7–87) (Cacciarelli et al., 1978).

Hydronephrosis

The ultrasonic pattern of advanced hydronephrosis is easily recognizable, with splaying of the pelvicalyceal–sinus fat echo complex. The pelvis is greatly enlarged and may present as a large, central, anechoic mass compressing the renal cortex. With proper angulation of the transducer, the parasagittal sections reveal communication of cystic finger-like projections joining the distended renal pelvis (Fig. 7–88). In mild hydronephrosis, only slight splitting of the sinus echoes may be present. With current equipment, even mild hydronephrosis can be detected; however, mild to even moderate pelvicalyceal dilatation is not infrequently secondary to overhydration or a distended bladder (Fig. 7–89), and a repeat examination after bladder emptying or fluid restriction may reveal a collecting system that appears completely normal. When findings suggestive of hydrone-

phrosis are present, it is important to carefully follow the ureter to the point of obstruction (see Fig. 7–88). This investigation may reveal an obstructing calculus, as manifested by an echogenic structure with discrete shadowing, an abdominal or pelvic mass, or other abnormality.

Series comparing the efficacy of ultrasound with intravenous urography in the detection of hydronephrosis reveal ultrasound to be quite accurate, but care must be taken to distinguish hydronephrosis from other conditions, including peripelvic cysts (Figs. 7–90 and 7–91) (Amis et al., 1982; Malave et al., 1980; Talner et al., 1981; Vela-Navarrete and Robledo, 1983).

Renal Failure

The ill patient presenting with genitourinary symptoms is traditionally studied by intravenous urography. However, not infrequently, renal function will be impaired so that evaluation by this modality is inadequate. Under these circumstances, ultrasound may provide invaluable information without resorting to the injection of contrast material, which may further impair renal function. In general, the ultrasonic appearance of the kidneys in renal failure is nonspecific; the cortex becomes more echogenic, equal to or greater than the liver or spleen, and the renal pyramids become quite apparent in contrast (Figs. 7–92 and 7–93). With increasing severity, the cortex atrophies and the sinus fat increases (Fig. 7–94) (Hricak et al., 1982; Rosenfield and Siegel, 1981). Even when a specific diagnosis is not possible, the information provided may help determine the appropriate sequence of diagnostic studies.

A specific cause of renal failure that may be detected by ultrasound is bilateral hydronephrotic kidneys, as described previously. Examination may provide further information as to the site of obstruction and possibly its cause. Polycystic renal disease, renal neoplasm with vascular involvement, severe nephrocalcinosis, and acute cortical necrosis may all have characteristic ultrasound appearances, many of which have been described earlier in the chapter (see Figs. 7–79, 7–87, and 7–88) (Cacciarelli et al., 1978; Finberg et al., 1980; Sanders and Jeck, 1976; Sefczek et al., 1984).

Ultrasound is useful in monitoring patients on chronic renal dialysis, who often develop renal cysts as well as adenomas and renal cell carcinomas. The kidneys are frequently enlarged, and spontaneous hemorrhage may occur (Andersen et al., 1983; Levine et al., 1984).

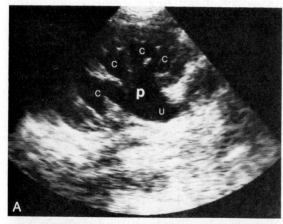

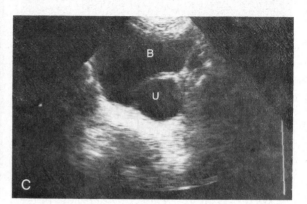

Figure 7–88. *A,* Prone longitudinal scan through hydronephrotic kidney with dilatation of the calyces (c), the pelvis (p), and the proximal ureter (u). When the ureter is followed to the pelvis, longitudinal *(B)* and transverse *(C)* scans reveal it to end in a ureterocele (U) (B, bladder). This represents an unusual example of a solitary ureter ending in an ectopic ureterocele with hydronephrosis. The more common situaton is illustrated in Figure 7–78.

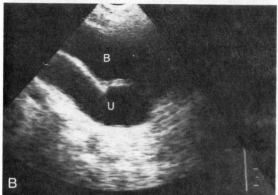

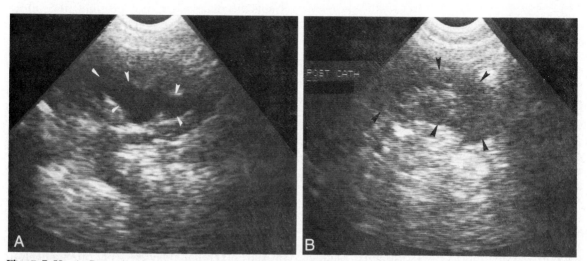

Figure 7–89. *A,* Prone longitudinal scan reveals moderate dilatation of the collecting system (arrowheads). *B,* After catheterization of a markedly distended bladder, repeat longitudinal scan reveals the dilatation to no longer be present (the renal outline is delineated by arrowheads).

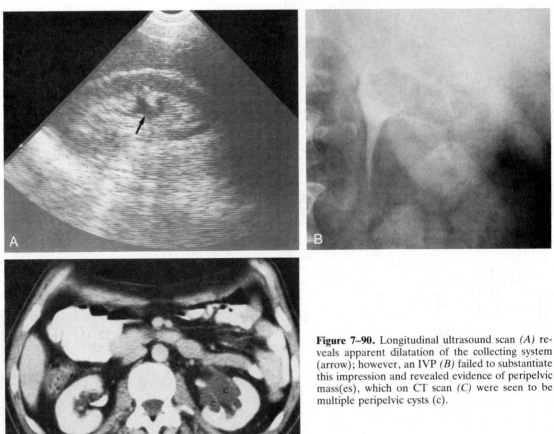

Figure 7–90. Longitudinal ultrasound scan *(A)* reveals apparent dilatation of the collecting system (arrow); however, an IVP *(B)* failed to substantiate this impression and revealed evidence of peripelvic mass(es), which on CT scan *(C)* were seen to be multiple peripelvic cysts (c).

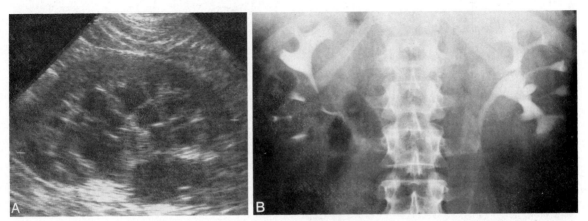

Figure 7–91. Longitudinal scan *(A)* of the kidney reveals what appear to be a dilated renal pelvis and calyces; however, an IVP *(B)* failed to substantiate this impression. This may represent polycystic disease of the renal sinus.

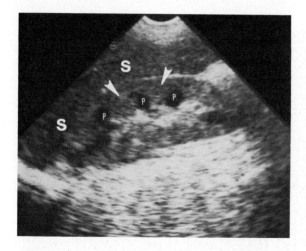

Figure 7–92. Longitudinal scan through left kidney in a patient with renal failure. The renal pyramids (p) appear to be unduly prominent owing to the increased echogenicity of the surrounding cortex (arrowheads), which appears to be equal to that of the adjacent spleen (s). Normally, the renal cortex is less echogenic than the liver or spleen.

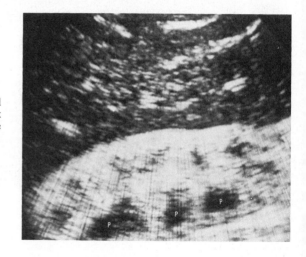

Figure 7–93. Longitudinal scan through a kidney with renal failure secondary to leukemic infiltration. The renal cortex is markedly echogenic, but the renal pyramids (p) are normal in size and echogenicity.

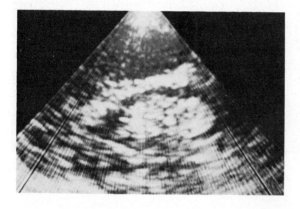

Figure 7–94. Marked cortical atrophy with compensatory increase in the renal sinus fat.

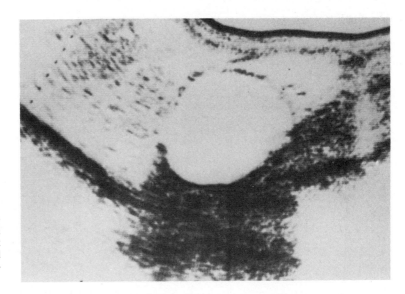

Figure 7–95. Supine longitudinal section through liver and right kidney with a large cyst in the upper pole. The cyst is echo-free, has smooth walls, and demonstrates excellent through-transmission.

Renal Masses

Masses greater than 1 cm can usually be delineated by ultrasonography. If the lesion disrupts the normal contour of the kidney or if its echogenicity is quite different from the surrounding normal renal tissue, lesions smaller than 1 cm can be detected as well. Simple renal cysts are characterized ultrasonically by a sharply outlined, usually circular structure in which there is complete absence of internal echoes, though artifactual reverberation echoes may be encountered. There should be excellent delineation of the far wall of the cyst with increased through-transmission resulting from lack of attenuation by the homogeneous fluid-filled cyst (Fig. 7–95). It is important to choose the proper frequency transducer, taking into consideration the size and depth of the lesion.

Cysts may become infected or undergo hemorrhage and subsequently can become calcified. When infected, the cyst may be ultrasonically indistinguishable from a simple cyst or may have a fluid-debris level that will vary with change in the patient's position. Bleeding into a cyst is not unusual (Jackman and Stevens, 1974). The blood may be mixed uniformly throughout the cyst fluid, and layering may be present or linear echoes may traverse the cyst, producing a septate appearance (Fig. 7–96). Complex masses may be present, resulting from clot formation. In these circumstances it is important to search for a mural tumor, though this condition is extremely rare. Mural calcification occurs in a small percentage of simple cysts and may be due to previous hemorrhage or infection. When the calcification is circumferential,

the ultrasound appearance may be confusing because of reflection of the sound beam simulating a solid lesion, and correlation with an abdominal radiograph or intravenous urogram should be undertaken. When a cystic lesion does not completely satisfy the ultrasonic criteria for a cyst as already described, further studies, including ultrasonically guided percutaneous needle aspiration, should be carried out.

Rarely, a complex cystic mass may occur, which is characterized ultrasonically by multiple noncommunicating cysts, separated by highly echogenic septa often with calcification—the so-called multilocular cyst (Banner et al., 1981).

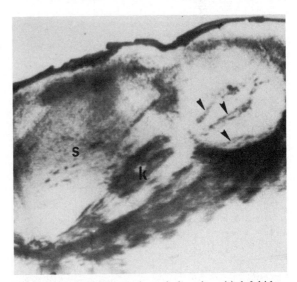

Figure 7–96. Coronal scan through the spleen (s), left kidney (k), and cystic mass inferior to the lower pole of the kidney. Multiple strands (arrowheads) through the cyst give it a septate appearance.

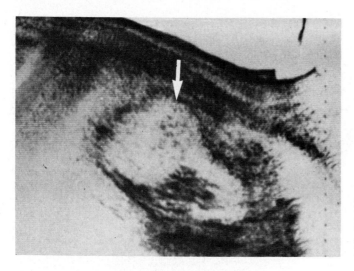

Figure 7–97. Prone longitudinal scan through large upper pole mass (arrow) containing internal echoes with poor through-transmission indicative of a solid mass, renal carcinoma (compare with Fig. 7–95).

The entity is poorly understood, and its ultrasonic appearance may be indistinguishable from that of a cystic carcinoma (Feldberg and van Waes, 1982).

Solid masses are frequently irregular, usually contain multiple internal echoes, and have relatively poor far-wall delineation. The latter characteristic is extremely important in differentiating a homogeneous solid mass from a cystic one. Because of the inhomogeneity of a solid mass, the sound beam passing through it is attenuated, resulting in a decreased echo arising from the far wall of the mass (Figs. 7–97 and 7–98). Even when disruption of the normal contour does not occur, a renal mass may be detected on the basis of displacement or inter-

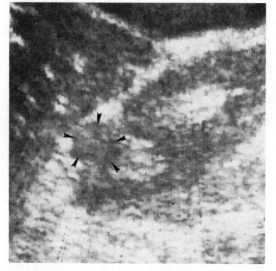

Figure 7–98. Longitudinal scan through the kidney reveals a small, solid mass (arrowheads) distorting the normal renal contour. At surgery this was found to be renal carcinoma.

ruption of the normal pelvicalyceal–sinus fat echo pattern or by the difference in its echo characteristics from the surrounding normal parenchyma. The echo pattern in renal adenocarcinomas is variable, depending on the homogeneity of the lesion and on whether areas of necrosis, hemorrhage, or cyst formation are present (Maklad et al., 1977). Areas of calcification may be present with resultant shadowing.

Most papillary cystadenocarcinomas are less echogenic then the surrounding normal parenchyma, as are most lymphomas. Occasionally these lesions may be mistaken for cysts, but attention must be paid to the far-wall echo as well as to the degree of through transmission. Most transitional cell carcinomas of the renal collecting system are difficult to detect ultrasonically because of their small size, since they often become symptomatic early in their course. If sufficiently large, however, they may cause hydronephrosis or disrupt a portion of the pelvicalyceal–sinus fat echo pattern (Fig. 7–99) (Arger et al., 1979; Subramanyam et al., 1982). This latter appearance may be indistinguishable from a renal pseudotumor (or prominent septum of Bertin), but the latter diagnosis should be suggested by a characteristic appearance on excretory urography and uptake of the isotope by the "mass" on radionuclide examination (Fig. 7–100) (Hodson and Mariani, 1982).

Lymphomatous involvement of the kidney may be either focal or diffusely infiltrating (Fig. 7–101) (Carroll, 1982; Kaude and Lacy, 1978). In the latter situation the kidneys may merely appear enlarged without evidence of a mass or abnormal internal architecture. Although the focal mass is often echo-poor, as already mentioned, any degree of echogenicity may be pres-

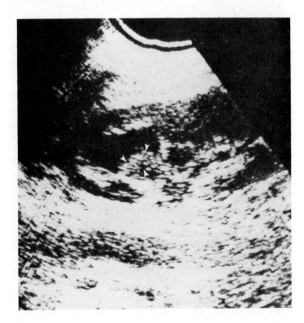

Figure 7–99. Longitudinal scan through the kidney reveals an echogenic mass (arrowheads) protruding into and obstructing the upper pole collecting system. At surgery this was identified as transitional cell carcinoma.

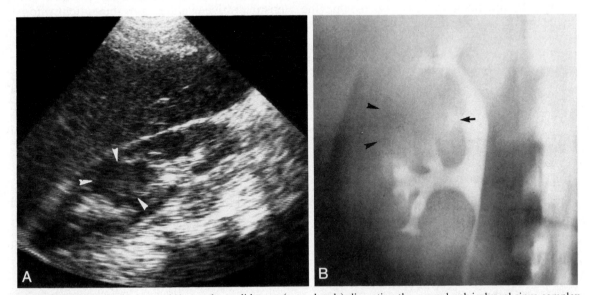

Figure 7–100. Longitudinal scan (A) reveals a solid mass (arrowheads) disrupting the normal pelvicalyceal-sinus complex. Transitional cell carcinoma is a strong consideration. However, intravenous urogram (B) reveals the typical appearance of a renal pseudotumor or septum of Bertin with an apparent mass (arrowheads) in an incomplete duplex kidney and a calyx coming directly off the renal pelvis (arrow).

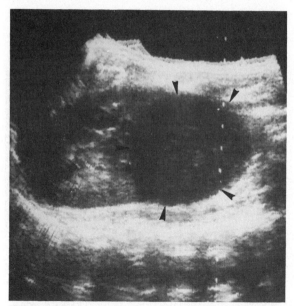

Figure 7–101. Longitudinal scan reveals a large echo-poor mass (arrowheads), due to lymphoma, occupying the inferior half of the kidney.

ent and as a result may resemble a renal carcinoma.

Metastases to the kidney from primary malignancies elsewhere are commonly found at autopsy but are rarely clinically evident. Usually they have the same ultrasonic appearance as a primary lesion, but they may also assume the distinctive characteristics of the primary site (Figs. 7–102 and 7–103).

Most benign solid masses are indistinguishable from their malignant counterparts ultrasonically. An exception to this statement is a renal angiomyolipoma, which may have a characteristic ultrasonic appearance. Because of their inhomogeneity and their high fat content, angiomyolipomas may be strikingly echogenic (Fig. 7–104). However, not all angiomyolipomas have this ultrasonic appearance, and on occasion, renal cell carcinoma will be highly echogenic because of its high fat content (Fig. 7–105) (Hartman et al., 1981). When multiple bilateral highly echogenic lesions are present in the kidneys, tuberous sclerosis should be suspected (Fig. 7–106).

When a solid renal mass is detected and carcinoma is suspected, the ultrasound examination must also include a search for liver metastases, regional adenopathy, involvement of the other kidney, and spread of tumor to the renal vein and inferior vena cava (Figs. 7–107 and 7–108) (Thomas and Bernardino, 1981). Although ultrasound can be satisfactorily used for the staging of renal carcinoma, computed tomography appears to be more accurate in that invasion of perinephric fat and adjacent tissue planes can be detected and a diagnostic study can be obtained in a higher percentage of cases (Cronan et al., 1982; Levine et al., 1980).

Ultrasonography may also be helpful in the postoperative evaluation of the patient who has undergone nephrectomy (Bernardino et al., 1978).

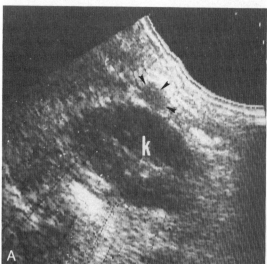
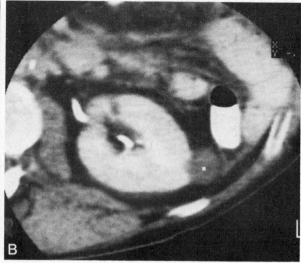

Figure 7–102. *A*, Prone, angled longitudinal scan through left kidney (k) with small, solid mass (arrowheads) arising from dorsal lateral surface of the kidney in a patient with gastric carcinoma. *B*, On CT scan, a small rectangular cursor marks the center of the mass, which represents a metastasis from the gastric carcinoma.

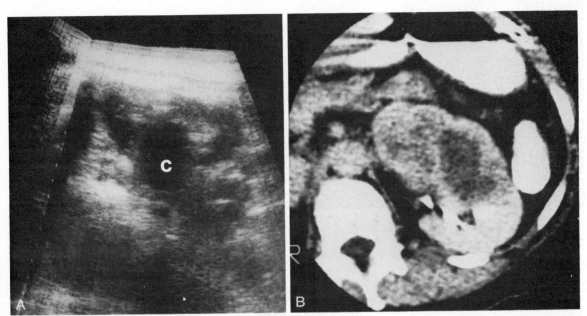

Figure 7–103. *A,* Prone longitudinal scan through the left kidney reveals a cystic-appearing mass (c) arising from the central portion of the kidney. *B,* CT scan of the left kidney reveals a complex cystic mass in the same location, representing a cystic metastasis from an ovarian cystadenocarcinoma.

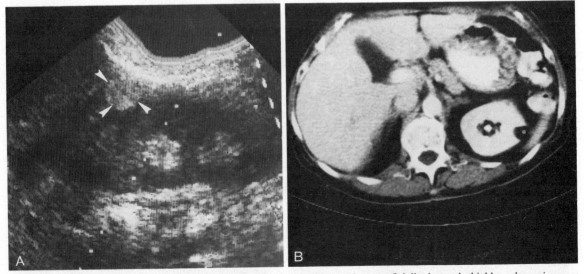

Figure 7–104. *A,* Angled longitudinal scan through left kidney reveals superficially located, highly echogenic mass (arrowheads) characteristic of an angiomyolipoma. *B,* CT scan with cursor through the lesion with a reading of -69 Hounsfield units, diagnostic of a fat-containing mass.

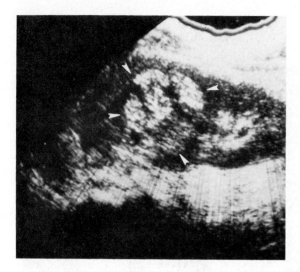

Figure 7–105. Prone longitudinal scan through the left kidney revealing a highly echogenic solid mass (arrowheads) due to a renal carcinoma containing abundant fat. This lesion could be mistaken ultrasonically for an angiomyolipoma.

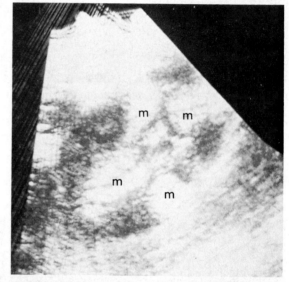

Figure 7–106. Oblique transverse view through the kidney with multiple, highly echogenic masses (m) due to multiple angiomyolipomas. The opposite kidney was similarly affected in this patient with tuberous sclerosis.

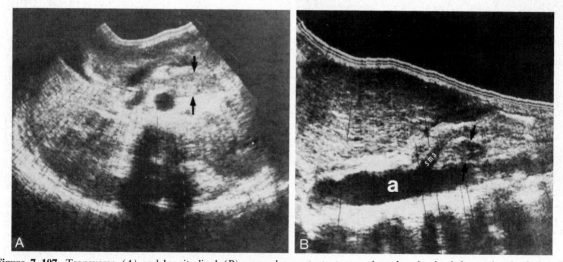

Figure 7–107. Transverse *(A)* and longitudinal *(B)* scans demonstrate tumor thrombus in the left renal vein (arrows), which is situated between the aorta (a) and the superior mesenteric artery (sma); this condition was secondary to carcinoma of the left kidney (not shown).

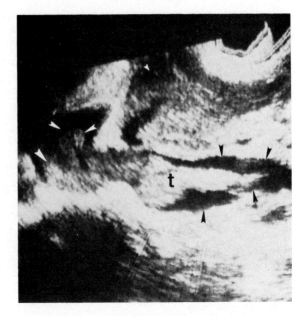

Figure 7–108. Longitudinal scan revealing tumor thrombus (t) within the inferior vena cava (black arrowheads) with extension into right atrium (white arrowheads). Patient with renal carcinoma (not shown).

Juxtarenal Masses

A mass in close proximity may displace the kidney and masquerade clinically as an intrinsic renal lesion. It is usually easy to differentiate ultrasonically between renal and juxtarenal masses and to direct further investigation more efficiently.

Adrenal lesions are ultrasonically detectable if sufficiently large (Fig. 7–109). If the examination is performed with optimal technique, even small lesions may be seen (Gunther et al.,

1984). Adrenal masses not infrequently lie superior and anterior to the kidney and may extend to the renal hilum (Fig. 7–110). Right-sided adrenal masses are often posterior to the inferior vena cava (Fig. 7–111).

Retroperitoneal masses, including primary lesions and lymphadenopathy, usually are relatively echo-poor. Perinephric fluid collections such as hematomas are readily detected and may be followed by serial examinations. Rarely, an occult renal neoplasm will present with a subcapsular bleed or perinephric hematoma.

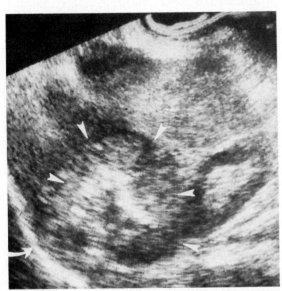

Figure 7–109. Longitudinal scan through the right upper quadrant demonstrates a large solid mass (arrowheads) representing an adrenal carcinoma displacing the right kidney inferiorly and extending to the right hemidiaphragm (arrow).

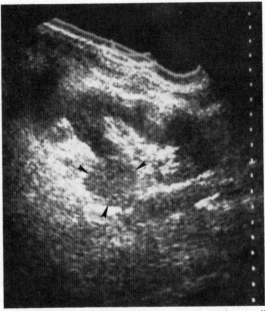

Figure 7–110. Prone longitudinal scan demonstrating a solid mass (arrowheads) ventral to the left kidney due to an adrenal pheochromocytoma.

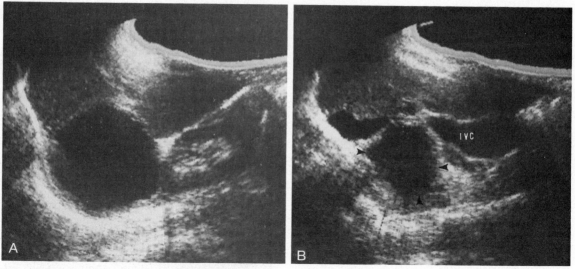

Figure 7–111. *A,* Longitudinal scan through a large cystic adrenal pheochromocytoma that displaces the right kidney inferiorly. *B,* A more medial longitudinal scan demonstrates a large, more solid retrocaval component (arrowheads) (IVC = inferior vena cava).

When such a collection occurs, it is important to search for a primary renal lesion (Watnick et al., 1972). Renal abscesses can break through the capsule of the kidney with extension into the pararenal spaces and are accurately depicted by ultrasound (see Fig. 7–83).

After a retroperitoneal lymph node dissection, a routine postoperative ultrasound examination may reveal a retroperitoneal cystic collection, usually caused by a lymphocele; however, this condition must be differentiated from a hematoma or abscess, both of which frequently, but not invariably, demonstrate internal echoes.

After trauma, ultrasound may be valuable in detecting a renal fracture, a perinephric hematoma, or a urinoma (Figs. 7–112 and 7–113) (Afschrift et al., 1982; Kay et al., 1980). If the patient is hypertensive immediately after trauma, an ultrasound examination may reveal perinephric hematoma formation consistent with the Page kidney phenomenon (Conrad et

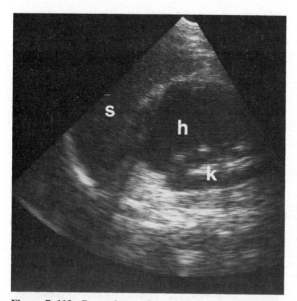

Figure 7–112. Coronal scan through spleen (s), left kidney (k), and large perinephric hematoma (h) following abdominal trauma.

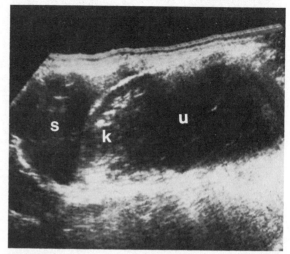

Figure 7–113. Longitudinal scan through the spleen (s), left kidney (k), and large retrorenal urinoma (u), which displaces the kidney anterosuperiorly. The urinoma was a consequence of a traumatic retrograde pyelogram.

al., 1976). If hypertension develops later on, ultrasound may demonstrate atrophy of the entire kidney or of a portion of the kidney.

Renal Transplantation

Renal transplants are particularly well suited for ultrasonic investigation, since the allograft is superficially located, with no intervening bowel gas or bony structures to interfere with the investigating sound beam (Smith, 1981). Additionally, the urine-filled bladder can act as a window, facilitating the examination. Anatomic detail is excellent, since a high-frequency transducer can be used, and visualization of the internal renal architecture is optimal (Fig. 7–114). The usual clinical dilemma is that of differentiating rejection of the renal transplant from mechanical obstruction or acute tubular necrosis. A large, tender kidney with diminishing urinary output is often so compromised that the excretory urogram is of little value.

An ultrasound examination can easily differentiate an enlarged, edematous, rejected kidney with a compressed pelvicalyceal–sinus fat echo complex from a hydronephrotic kidney with wide splaying of the pelvicalyceal system. Several ultrasonic findings suggest the diagnosis of rejection. The kidney is usually enlarged from edema, and the renal pyramids may be prominent and increased in size (this may be more apparent than real because of edema of the

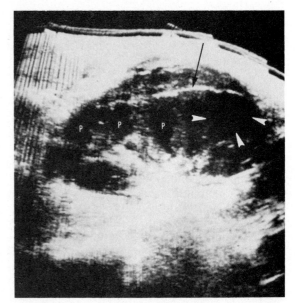

Figure 7–115. Longitudinal scan through renal allograft undergoing rejection, with prominent pyramids (P) and large sonolucent area (arrowheads) in the cortex. Hematoma following renal biopsy clearly outlines the renal capsule (arrow).

cortex immediately surrounding the pyramids). The presence of sonolucent areas in the renal cortex, secondary to edema, hemorrhage, or necrosis, also points to ongoing rejection (Fig. 7–115) (Hricak et al., 1981). Other signs include an indistinct corticomedullary junction and progressive loss of the central renal–sinus fat echo complex caused by the rejection process involv-

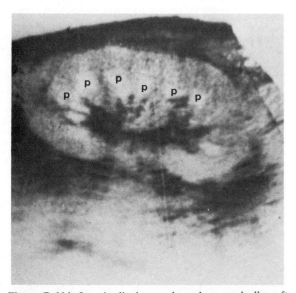

Figure 7–114. Longitudinal scan through a renal allograft with the renal pyramids (p) clearly separable from the renal cortex and pelvicalyceal echo complex.

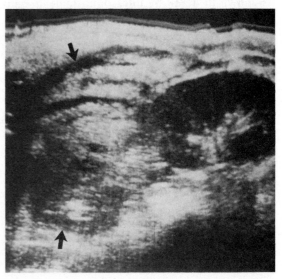

Figure 7–116. Longitudinal scan through renal allograft with large hematoma (arrows) secondary to acute rejection and spontaneous bleed.

ing the sinus fat (Hricak et al., 1981). Spontaneous rupture of the severely edematous kidney undergoing rejection may occur with resultant hematoma formation (Fig. 7–116).

COMPLICATIONS OF RENAL TRANSPLANTATION

Complications of renal transplantation include ureteral obstruction due to ureteral ischemic necrosis or rejection with hydronephrosis, or both, and the development of pararenal fluid collections including lymphocele, urinoma, hematoma, and abscess formation (Fig. 7–117). If strategically placed, these collections may mimic acute rejection. In one series of 107 renal allograft recipients who were referred for ultrasound examination with a clinical diagnosis of rejection, 14 cases of pararenal fluid collection and 14 cases of ureteral obstruction were diagnosed (Petrek et al., 1977). In order to exclude these other abnormalities, ultrasound has become the diagnostic method of choice for evaluating the renal allograft suspected of undergoing rejection.

Bladder and Prostate

When distended with urine, the bladder is easily imaged transabdominally, and calculi are readily delineated (Fig. 7–118). Residual urinary volumes may be calculated by ultrasonic means with a reasonable degree of accuracy. In addition, the narrow-necked bladder diverticulum, which is difficult to evaluate cystoscopically, can be shown in detail by ultrasound, and its emp-

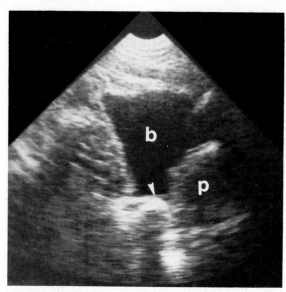

Figure 7–118. Longitudinal scan through the pelvis with an enlarged prostate gland (p) indenting the floor of the urine-filled bladder (b), with a strongly echogenic focus with shadowing (arrowhead) due to a bladder calculus.

tying characteristics can be investigated (Fig. 7–119).

A neoplasm protruding into the bladder lumen can be identified if it is sufficiently large (Fig. 7–120). Focal lesions, though highly suggestive of neoplasia, can, however, be due to benign disease (Rifkin et al., 1983). Invasion of the bladder wall may on occasion be detected ultrasonically, but the method is not sensitive enough for accurate tumor staging, because

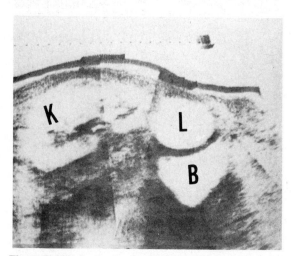

Figure 7–117. Supine longitudinal scan through renal allograft (K) with anterior inferior lymphocele (L) compressing the bladder (B).

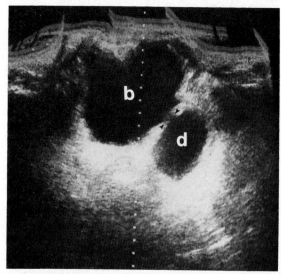

Figure 7–119. Transverse scan through the bladder (b) with narrow-necked diverticulum (d) (arrowheads).

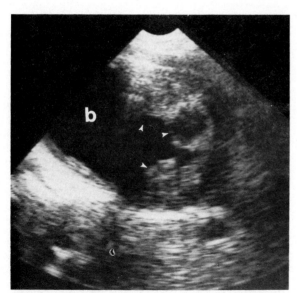

Figure 7–120. Oblique scan through the bladder demonstrating large, irregular polypoid mass (arrowheads) protruding into the bladder lumen (b), representing a transitional cell carcinoma of the bladder.

minimal to moderate extravesical extension may be missed. In contrast, exophytic growth resulting in a significant-sized mass or spread to pelvic lymph nodes may be identified. Rigidity or distortion of the bladder wall, or both, may be detected, especially with real-time ultrasound. Large extrinsic lesions may invade the bladder and at times may be confused with a primary bladder tumor.

The prostate gland can be evaluated transabdominally if careful attention to technique is employed (see Fig. 7–118). The bladder is used as a sonographic window, and the transducer is angled in a caudal direction. Size and weight can be fairly accurately estimated by this method (Abu-Yousef and Narayana, 1982). The abdominal approach can be supplemented by perineal scanning when portions of the gland are difficult to visualize. Attempts have been made to differentiate benign prostatic hypertrophy from carcinoma of the prostate by ultrasound with varying degrees of success (Greenberg et al., 1980; Greenberg et al., 1982; Resnick et al., 1978).

The "typical" appearance of benign prostatic hypertrophy reveals a sharply delineated pseudocapsule with the interior portion of the gland characterized by multiple, fine, homogeneous echoes. Small cysts and microcalculi may be present with shadowing. Conversely, carcinoma of the prostate, if large enough, may disrupt the "capsule," which appears to be asymmetric and distorted because of tumor infiltration with extension beyond the confines of the gland. Malignant nodules are usually dense and asymmetric, but at times it is difficult to distinguish malignancy from chronic prostatitis, and seemingly benign lesions are found at surgery to be malignant (Fritzsche et al., 1983). Ultrasonically guided prostatic biopsy can be quite helpful in obtaining pathologic confirmation (Holm and Gammelgaard, 1981; Fornage et al., 1983). More work has to be done in this area before the role of ultrasound in the differential diagnosis of prostatic disease is firmly established.

The recent development of transurethral and transrectal scanners holds considerable promise (Holm and Northeved, 1974; Watanabe et al., 1968). Studies have been published revealing very high-resolution ultrasound images, offering the potential for accurate staging of bladder tumors (Gammelgaard and Holm, 1980). Small lesions can be depicted, and bladder wall invasion can be visualized (Fig. 7–121). The transurethral scanner, in particular, appears very promising in this regard, whereas the transrectal scanner is more successful in demonstrating detailed anatomy of the prostate. Transurethral scanners require cystoscopic introduction, whereas transrectal scanning is far easier to perform, and its larger transducer allows for acquisition of high-resolution images of the prostate (Rifkin et al., 1983). However, bladder tumors are usually not well visualized with this technique because of the interposed gas-filled intestine.

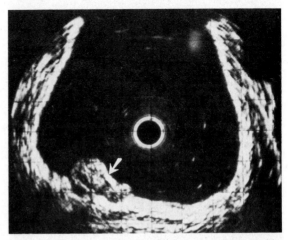

Figure 7–121. Transurethral transverse scan of the bladder shows a small polypoid bladder carcinoma (arrow) with invasion into, but not through, the bladder wall. The circle within the bladder lumen is an artifact caused by the transducer.

Scrotum

With the development of high-resolution real-time ultrasonic scanners using high-frequency transducers (5 to 10 MHz), ultrasound has become the modality of choice for detecting the pathologic condition of the scrotal contents (Arger et al., 1981; Hricak and Filly, 1983; Leopold et al., 1979). The examination can be carried out using a dedicated "small parts" real-time scanner with a built-in water bath, a high-frequency sector, or a high-frequency contact scanner. Excellent results have been achieved with each.

The normal testicular parenchyma is very homogeneous and contains medium-level echoes; the borders of the testis are usually sharply delineated and are distinguishable from surrounding structures (Fig. 7–122) (Leung et al., 1984). Along the posterior lateral border of the testis is the epididymis, with its head situated at the cranial pole of the testis. The epididymal head can be consistently identified by ultrasound; the body and tail are less consistently seen. The echogenicity of the normal epididymis is somewhat variable but is usually much coarser than the adjacent testicle. A very small amount of fluid surrounding the testis is occasionally seen and is a normal finding. Clinical examination of the scrotum can be very difficult because of painful swelling and distortion of the scrotal contents. Ultrasound has become invaluable in distinguishing testicular from extratesticular lesions and neoplastic processes from inflammatory processes. Furthermore, ultrasound is capable of differentiating benign tumors from malignant lesions with a high degree of accuracy.

Most malignant testicular tumors show decreased echogenicity or occasionally have a mixed pattern (i.e., areas of decreased and increased echogenicity as compared with the surrounding normal tissues) (Fig. 7–123). A small to moderate amount of fluid is often seen. Although echo-poor lesions within the testicle are not specific for a malignant neoplasm and may be secondary to an abscess or granuloma, malignancy is by far more common and should be considered until proved otherwise (Arger et al., 1981; Dunner et al., 1982). Conversely, most purely hyperechoic testicular lesions are benign (Vick et al., 1983).

Ultrasound is capable of detecting occult, nonpalpable testicular neoplasms in patients with proven metastatic disease as well as in patients with evidence of endocrine abnormalities or primary malignancy elsewhere (Casola et al., 1984; Emory et al., 1984; Glazer et al., 1982). In patients with disseminated germ cell tumors and clinically normal testes, focal areas of increased echogenicity in the testis may represent the residua of a "burned-out" primary testicular tumor (Shawker et al., 1983). Ultrasound examination is usually able to separate extratesticular from testicular processes. In epididymitis, the epididymis is enlarged, especially the head, with a diffuse decrease in echogenicity, presumably due to edema (Fig. 7–124). Occasionally, the echo pattern will be mixed, with a return to normal as the condition resolves with therapy. Reactive hydroceles are common with moderate to large amounts of fluid present. The testicle itself may or may not be involved in the inflammatory process.

Solid neoplasms of the epididymis are uncommon and are most often benign adenomatoid tumors (Hricak and Filly, 1983). Rarely is the epididymis involved by metastatic deposits. Epididymal cysts and spermatoceles have the appearance of cysts elsewhere in the body and cannot be differentiated ultrasonically. Although cystic, varicoceles have a tortuous course with a typical ultrasonic appearance (see Fig. 7–123). Hydroceles present as echo-free areas surrounding the testicle and occasionally may be difficult to distinguish from a large epididymal cyst. However, with a large cyst the testis is displaced anteriorly, whereas with a hydrocele the fluid usually surrounds the testicle anteriorly (Fig. 7–125). Ultrasonically, testicular torsion is

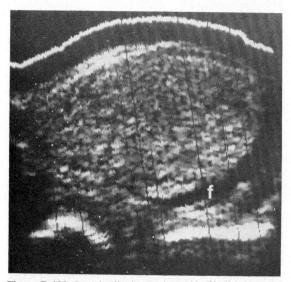

Figure 7–122. Longitudinal scan (magnified) of the normal testis demonstrates a relatively homogeneous texture. The testis is surrounded by a small amount of fluid (f). The epididymis is not well demonstrated on this scan.

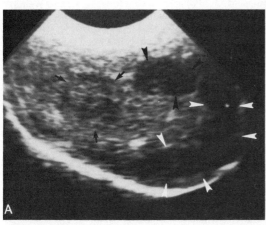 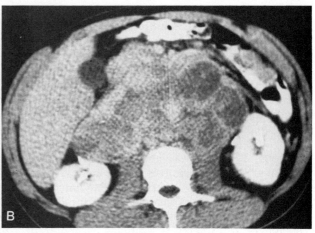

Figure 7–123. *A,* Longitudinal scan through the testis of a young man with widespread lymphadenopathy reveals two solid masses, one relatively echo-poor (black arrowheads), the other of mixed echogenicity (arrows). The epididymis was markedly enlarged and serpiginous (white arrowheads) owing to a varicocele. *B,* CT scan reveals massive lymphadenopathy, which compressed the left renal vein, giving rise to the varicocele. At surgery a mixed germ-cell tumor of the testis was found, with seminoma and embryonal cell elements present.

often difficult to distinguish from epididymo-orchitis, and occasionally problems arise in distinguishing the latter two from a testicular tumor. Most tumors do not have an associated enlargement of the epididymis, and the amount of scrotal fluid is usually much greater with torsion or inflammation than with tumor. Radionuclide flow studies can be employed in distinguishing between epididymitis and testicular torsion, since perfusion is increased in the former and decreased in the latter (Chen et al., 1983*a*; 1983*b*).

Ultrasound can also be helpful in the investigation of the undescended testis and in evaluating the extent of injury to the testis in cases of trauma (Jeffrey et al., 1983).

Ultrasonically Guided Needle Placement

Specially designed ultrasound biopsy transducers through which various-sized needles can

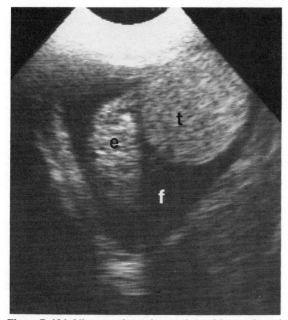

Figure 7–124. Ultrasound scan in a patient with an enlarged, tender scrotum reveals a normal testis (t) and an enlarged, coarsely echogenic epididymis (e) surrounded by a moderate amount of fluid (f). Epididymitis was diagnosed.

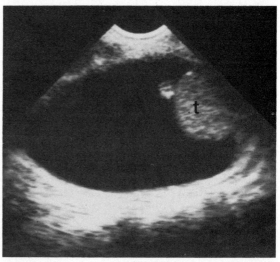

Figure 7–125. Ultrasound scan of the scrotum demonstrates a large hydrocele surrounding the anterior surface of the testis (t).

be introduced have been developed for both static and dynamic scanning (Holm et al., 1972; Saitoh et al., 1979). The real-time biopsy transducer allows the tip of the needle to be accurately positioned under direct ultrasound guidance with visualization of the needle as it traverses the tissues and enters the lesion to be sampled. This can be done rapidly and accurately and allows percutaneous aspiration biopsy of diverse lesions, including pararenal fluid collections, solid masses, and abscesses. In this manner, accurate diagnosis can be achieved and appropriate therapy instituted immediately. A thin needle (22-gauge) may be used initially and if indicated may be followed by a larger-bore needle or a catheter if drainage is required. The technique has been modified to perform percutaneous nephrostomies, either using the Seldinger technique, with a catheter placed over a guidewire, or using a specially designed sheathed needle (Baron et al., 1981; Pedersen et al., 1976; Sacks et al., 1981). Similarly, drainage of abscesses can be carried out, possibly obviating the need for formal surgery (Kuligowska et al., 1983).

In conjunction with a nephrostomy, a ureteral stent may also be introduced and positioned. In addition, ureteral strictures may be dilated by modifying the procedure to allow introduction of a balloon catheter to the point of stricture; this area is then dilated under fluoroscopic control after the injection of contrast material (Banner et al., 1983).

References

Abu-Yousef, M. M., and Narayana, A. S.: Transabdominal ultrasound in the evaluation of prostate size. J. Clin. Ultrasound, *10*:275, 1982.

Afschrift, M., de Sy, W., Voet, D., Nachtegaele, P., and Robberecht, E.: Fractured kidney and retroperitoneal hematoma diagnosed by ultrasound. J. Clin. Ultrasound, *10*:335, 1982.

Amis, E. S., Cronan, J. J., Pfister, R. C., and Yoder, I. C.: Ultrasonic inaccuracies in diagnosing renal obstruction. Urology, *19*:101, 1982.

Andersen, B. C., Curry, N. S., and Gabien, R. P.: Ultrasound useful in monitoring long-term dialysis patients for development of cysts and malignancies. Am. J. Roentgenol., *141*:1003, 1983.

Arger, P. H., Mulhern, C. B., Jr., Coleman, B. G., Pollack, H. M., Wein, A., Koss, J., Arenson, R., and Banner, M.: Prospective analysis of the value of scrotal ultrasound. Radiology, *141*:763, 1981.

Arger, P. H., Mulhern, C. B., Jr., Pollack, H. M., Banner, M. P., and Wein, A. J.: Ultrasonic assessment of renal transitional cell carcinoma: Preliminary report. Am. J. Roentgenol., *132*:407, 1979.

Banner, M. P., Pollack, H. M., Chatten, J., and Witzleben, C.: Multilocular renal cysts: Radiologic-pathologic correlation. Am. J. Roentgenol., *136*:239, 1981.

Banner, M. P., Pollack, H. M., Ring, E. J., and Wein, A. J.: Catheter dilatation of benign ureteral strictures. Radiology, *147*:427, 1983.

Baron, R. L., Lee, J. K. T., McClennan, B. L., and Melson, G. L.: Percutaneous nephrostomy using real-time sonographic guidance. Am. J. Roentgenol., *136*:1018, 1981.

Bearman, S. B., Hine, P. L., and Sanders, R. C.: Multicystic kidney: A sonographic pattern. Radiology, *118*:685, 1976.

Bernardino, M. E., Green, B., and Goldstein, H. M.: Ultrasonography in the evaluation of post-nephrectomy renal cancer patients. Radiology, *128*:455, 1978.

Cacciarelli, A. A., Young, N., and Levine, A. J.: Grayscale ultrasonic demonstration of nephrocalcinosis. Radiology, *128*:459, 1978.

Carroll, B. A.: Ultrasound of lymphoma. Semin. Ultrasound, *3*(2):114, 1982.

Casola, G., Scheible, W., and Leopold, G. R.: Neuroblastoma metastatic to the testes: Ultrasonic screening as an aid to clinical staging. Radiology, *151*:475, 1984.

Chen, D. C. P., Holder, L. E., and Melloul, M.: Radionuclide scrotal imaging: Further experience with 210 patients. Part 1: Anatomy, pathophysiology, and methods. J. Nucl. Med., *24*:735, 1983a.

Chen, D. C. P., Holder, L. E., and Melloul, M.: Radionuclide scrotal imaging: Further experience with 210 patients. Part 2: Results and discussion. J. Nucl. Med., *24*:841, 1983b.

Coleman, B. G., Arger, P. H., Mulhern, C. B., Jr., Pollack, H. M., and Banner, M. P.: Pyonephrosis: Sonography in the diagnosis and management. Am. J. Roentgenol., *137*:939, 1981.

Conrad, M. R., Freedman, M., Weiner, C., Freeman, C., and Sanders, R. C.: Sonography of the Page kidney. J. Urol., *116*:293, 1976.

Cook, J. H., III, Rosenfield, A. T., and Taylor, K. J. W.: Ultrasonic demonstration of intrarenal anatomy. Am. J. Roentgenol., *129*:831, 1977.

Cronan, J. J., Zeman, R. K., and Rosenfield, A. T.: Comparison of computerized tomography, ultrasound and angiography in staging renal cell carcinoma. J. Urol., *127*:712, 1982.

Dunner, P. S., Lipsit, E. R., and Nochomovitz, L. E.: Epididymal sperm granuloma simulating a testicular neoplasm. J. Clin. Ultrasound, *10*:353, 1982.

Emory, T. H., Charbonneau, J. W., Randall, R. V., Scheithauer, B. W., and Grantham, J. G.: Occult testicular interstitial-cell tumor in a patient with gynecomastia: Ultrasonic detection. Radiology, *151*:474, 1984.

Feldberg, M. A. M., and van Waes, P. F. G. M.: Multilocular cystic renal cell carcinoma. Am. J. Roentgenol., *138*:953, 1982.

Finberg, H. J., Hillman, B., and Smith, E. H.: Ultrasound in the evaluation of the nonfunctioning kidney. Clin. Diagn. Ultrasound, *2*:105, 1980.

Fornage, B. D., Toucle, D. H., DeGlaire, M., Faroux, M-JC.: Real-time ultrasound-guided prostatic biopsy using a new transrectal linear-array probe. Radiology, *146*:547, 1983.

Fritzsche, P. J., Axford, P. D., Ching, V. C., Rosenquist, R. W., and Moore, R. J.: Correlation of transrectal sonographic findings in patients with suspected and unsuspected prostatic disease. J. Urol., *130*:272, 1983.

Gammelgaard, J., and Holm, H. H.: Transurethral and transrectal ultrasonic scanning in urology. J. Urol., *124*:863, 1980.

Glazer, H. S., Lee, J. K. T., Melson, G. L., and McClennan, B. L.: Sonographic detection of occult testicular neoplasms. Am. J. Roentgenol., *138*:675, 1982.

Greenberg, M., Neiman, H. L., Brandt, T. D., Falkowski, W., and Carter, M.: Ultrasound of the prostate. Radiology, *141*:757, 1981.

Greenberg, M., Neiman, H. L., Vogelzang, R., and Falkowski, W.: Ultrasonographic features of prostatic carcinoma. J. Clin. Ultrasound, *10*:307, 1982.

Grossman, H., Rosenberg, E. R., Bowie, J. D., Ram, P., and Merten, D. F.: Sonographic diagnosis of renal cystic diseases. Am. J. Roentgenol., *140*:81, 1983.

Gunther, R. W., Kelbel, C., and Lenner, V.: Real-time ultrasound of normal adrenal glands and small tumors. J. Clin. Ultrasound, *12*:211, 1984.

Hartman, D. S., Goldman, S. M., Friedman, A. C., Davis, C. J., Jr., Madewell, J. E., and Sherman, J. L.: Angiomyolipoma: Ultrasonic-pathologic correlation. Radiology, *139*:451, 1981.

Hodson, C. J., and Mariani, S.: Large cloisons. Am. J. Roentgenol., *139*:327, 1982.

Holm, H. H., and Gammelgaard, J.: Ultrasonically guided precise needle placement in the prostate and seminal vesicles. J. Urol., *125*:385, 1981.

Holm, H. H., and Northeved, A.: A transurethral ultrasonic scanner. J. Urol., *111*:238, 1974.

Holm, H. H., Kristensen, J. K., Rasmussen, S. N., Northeved, A., and Barlebo, H.: Ultrasound as a guide to percutaneous puncture technique. Ultrasonics, *10*:83, 1972.

Hricak, H., and Filly, R. A.: Sonography of the scrotum. Invest. Radiol., *18*:112, 1983.

Hricak, H., Cruz, C., Eyler, W. R., Madrazo, B., Romanski, R., and Sandler, M.: Acute post-transplantation renal failure: Differential diagnosis by ultrasound. Radiology, *139*:441, 1981.

Hricak, H., Cruz, C., Romanski, R., Uniewski, M. H., Levin, N. W., Madrazo, B. L., Sandler, M. A., and Eyler, W. R.: Renal parenchymal disease: Sonographic-histologic correlation. Radiology, *144*:141, 1982.

Jackman, R. J., and Stevens, G. M.: Benign hemorrhagic renal cyst. Radiology, *110*:7, 1974.

Jeffrey, R. B., Laing, F. C., Hricak, H., and McAninch, J. W.: Sonography of testicular trauma. Am. J. Roentgenol., *141*:993, 1983.

Kaude, J. V., and Lacy, G. D.: Ultrasonography in renal lymphoma. J. Clin. Ultrasound, *6*:321, 1978.

Kay, C. J., Rosenfield, A. T., and Armm, M.: Gray-scale ultrasonography in the evaluation of renal trauma. Radiology, *134*:461, 1980.

Kay, C. J., Rosenfield, A. T., Taylor, K. J. W., and Rosenberg, M. A.: Ultrasonic characteristics of chronic atrophic pyelonephritis. Am. J. Roentgenol., *132*:47, 1979.

Kuligowska, E., Newman, B., White, S. J., and Caldarone, A.: Interventional ultrasound in detection of renal inflammatory disease. Radiology, *147*:521, 1983.

Lawson, T. L., McClennan, B. L., and Shirkhoda, A.: Adult polycystic kidney disease: Ultrasonographic and computed tomography appearance. J. Clin. Ultrasound, *6*:297, 1978.

Lee, J. K. T., McClennan, B. L., Melson, G. L., and Stanley, R. J.: Acute focal bacterial nephritis: Emphasis on gray scale sonography and computed tomography. Am. J. Roentgenol., *135*:87, 1980.

Leopold, G. R., Woo, V. L., Scheible, F. W., Nachtsheim, D., and Gosink, B. B.; High-resolution ultrasonography of scrotal pathology. Radiology, *131*:719, 1979.

Leung, M. L., Gooding, G. A. W., and Williams, R. D.: High-resolution sonography of scrotal contents in asymptomatic subjects. Am. J. Roentgenol., *143*:161, 1984.

Levine, E., Grantham, J. J., Slusher, S. L., Greathouse, J. L., and Krohn, B. P.: CT of acquired cystic kidney disease and renal tumors in long-term dialysis patients. Am. J. Roentgenol., *142*:125, 1984.

Levine, E., Maklad, N. F., Rosenthal, S. J., Lee, K. R., and Weigel, J.: Comparison of computed tomography and ultrasound in abdominal staging of renal cancer. Urology, *16*:317, 1980.

Maklad, N. F., Chuang, V. P., Doust, B. D., Cho, K. J., and Curran, J. E.: Ultrasonic characterization of solid renal lesions: Echographic and pathologic correlation. Radiology, *123*:733, 1977.

Malave, S. R., Neiman, H. L., Spies, S. M., Cisternino, S. J., and Adamo, G.: Diagnosis of hydronephrosis: Comparison of radionuclide scanning and sonography. Am. J. Roentgenol., *135*:1179, 1980.

Mascatello, V. J., Smith, E. H., Carrera, G. F., Berger, M., and Teele, R. L.: Ultrasonic evaluation of the obstructed duplex kidney. Am. J. Roentgenol., *129*:113, 1977.

Morehouse, H. T., Weiner, S. N., and Hoffman, J. C.: Imaging in inflammatory disease of the kidney. Am. J. Roentgenol., *143*:135, 1984.

Pedersen, J. F., Cowan, D. F., Kristensen, J. K., Holm, H. H., Hancke, S., and Jensen, F.: Ultrasonically guided percutaneous nephrostomy. Radiology, *119*:429, 1976.

Petrek, J., Tilney, N. L., Smith, E. H., Williams, J. S., and Vineyard, G. C.: Ultrasound in renal transplantation. Ann. Surg., *185*:441, 1977.

Rego, J. D., Jr., Laing, F. C., and Jeffrey, R. B.: Ultrasonographic diagnosis of medullary cystic disease. J. Ultrasound Med., *2*:433, 1983.

Resnick, M. I., Willard, J. W., and Boyce, W. H.: Ultrasonic evaluation of the prostatic nodule. J. Urol., *120*:86, 1978.

Rifkin, M. D., Kurtz, A. B., Choi, H. Y., and Goldberg, B. B.: Endoscopic ultrasonic evaluation of the prostate using a transrectal probe: Prospective evaluation and acoustic characterization. Radiology, *149*:265, 1983.

Rifkin, M. D., Kurtz, A. B., Pasto, M. E., and Goldberg, B. B.: Unusual presentations of cystitis. J. Ultrasound Med., *2*:25, 1983.

Rosenfield, A. T., and Siegel, N. J.: Renal parenchymal disease: Histopathologic-sonographic correlation. Am. J. Roentgenol., *137*:793, 1981.

Rosenfield, A. T., Glickman, M. G., Taylor, K. J. W., Crade, M., and Hodson, J.: Acute focal bacterial nephritis (acute lobar nephronia). Radiology, *132*:53, 1979.

Rosenfield, A. T., Lipson, M. H., Wolf, B., Taylor, K. J. W., Rosenfield, N. S., and Hendler, E.: Ultrasonography and nephrotomography in the presymptomatic diagnosis of dominantly inherited (adult-onset) polycystic kidney disease. Radiology, *135*:423, 1980.

Sacks, B. A., Palestrant, A., Vine, H., Ellison, H., Hann, L., and Ackerman, B.: Catheter/needle assembly for drainage of fluid collections. Am. J. Roentgenol., *137*:418, 1981.

Saitoh, M., Watanabe, H., Ohe, H., Tanaka, S., Itakuray, Y., and Date, S.: Ultrasonic real time guidance for percutaneous puncture. J. Clin. Ultrasound, *7*:269, 1979.

Sanders, R. C., and Hartman, D. S.: The sonographic distinction between neonatal multicystic kidney and hydronephrosis. Radiology, *151*:621, 1984.

Sanders, R. C., and Jeck, D.: B-scan ultrasound in the evaluation of renal failure. Radiology, *119*:199, 1976.

Schaffer, R., Becker, J. A., and Goodman, J.: Sonography of the tuberculous kidney. Urology, *22*:209, 1983.

Schneider, M., Becker, J. A., Staiano, S., and Campos, E.: Sonographic-radiographic correlation of renal and perirenal infections. Am. J. Roentgenol., *127*:1007, 1976.

Sefczek, R. J., Beckman, J., Lupetin, A. R., and Dash, N.: Sonography of acute renal cortical necrosis. Am. J. Roentgenol., *142*:553, 1984.

Shawker, T. H., Javadpour, N., O'Leary, T., Shapiro, E., and Krudy, A. G.: Ultrasonographic detection of "burned-out" primary testicular germ cell tumors in clinically normal testes. J. Ultrasound Med., *2*:477, 1983.

Smith, E. H.: Ultrasound in the evaluation of renal transplants. Postgrad. Radiol., *1*:3, 1981.

Subramanyam, B. R., Raghavendra, B. N., Bosniak, M. A., Lefleur, R. S., Rosen, R. J., and Horii, S. C.: Sonography of pyonephrosis: A prospective study. Am. J. Roentgenol., *140*:991, 1983.

Subramanyam, B. R., Raghavendra, B. N., and Madamba, M. R.: Renal transitional cell carcinoma: Sonographic and pathologic correlation. J. Clin. Ultrasound, *10*:203, 1982.

Talner, L. B., Scheible, W., Ellenbogen, P. H., Beck, C. H., Jr., and Gosink, B. B.: How accurate is ultrasonography in detecting hydronephrosis in azotemic patients? Urol. Radiol., *3*:1, 1981.

Teele, R. L., Rosenfield, A. T., and Freedman, G. S.: The anatomic splenic flexure: An ultrasonic renal imposter. Am. J. Roentgenol., *128*:115, 1977.

Thomas, J. L., and Bernardino, M. E.: Neoplastic-induced renal vein enlargement: Sonographic detection. Am. J. Roentgenol., *136*:75, 1981.

Van Kirk, O. C., Go, R. T., and Wedel, V. J.: Sonographic features of xanthogranulomatous pyelonephritis. Am. J. Roentgenol., *134*:1035, 1980.

Vela-Navarrete, R., and Robledo, A. G.: Polycystic disease of the renal sinus: Structural characteristics. J. Urol., *129*:700, 1983.

Vick, C. W., Bird, K. I., Rosenfield, A. T., Viscomi, G. N., and Taylor, K. J. W.: Scrotal masses with a uniformly hyperechoic pattern. Radiology, *148*:209, 1983.

Watanabe, H., Kato, H., Kato, T., Tanaka, M., and Terasawa, Y.: Diagnostic application of the ultrasono-tomography to the prostate. Jpn. J. Urol., *59*:273, 1968.

Watnick, M., Spindola-Franco, H., and Abrams, H. L.: Small hypernephroma with subcapsular hematoma and renal infarction. J. Urol., *108*:534, 1972.

Wyly, J. B., Resende, C. M. C., and Teele, R. L.: Ultrasonography of the complicated duplex kidney: Further observations. Semin. Ultrasound, CT, NMR, *5*:35, 1984.

Computed Tomography of the Kidney

STEVEN E. SELTZER, M.D.
DOMINIK J. HUBER, M.D.
HERBERT L. ABRAMS, M.D.

The purpose of this chapter is to acquaint the reader with exciting new developments in the field of high technology diagnostic imaging. Specifically, the focus is on computed tomography (CT) of the kidney, and the chapter will cover both technical and clinical topics. Technical topics include the physical principles of operation of a CT scanner and the methods for performing optimal CT of the kidney. Clinical topics include normal anatomy of the kidney and the CT appearance of a wide variety of pathologic conditions. The role of CT in the workup of common renal lesions is also presented. For additional information on CT of the entire urinary tract, the reader is referred to a recent review (Huber and Seltzer, 1983).

FEATURES OF MODERN CT SCANNERS

A CT image is produced in three steps (Christensen et al., 1978; McCullough, 1977). During the first step, multiple x-ray exposures or views of an object are obtained. The second step involves a computer-aided reconstruction of the image, and the third step entails displaying that image in various shades of gray.

Five different approaches to the task of obtaining multiple x-ray exposures of an object have been used by scanner manufacturers. Each of these approaches has employed a different configuration of x-ray tube, radiation detectors, and patient (Fig. 7–126). Every new configuration has been called a new "generation" of scanner design. In general, scanners of the third or fourth generation design are considered "state of the art." There is no definite advantage for either type. Fifth generation scanners are not widely available.

The past decade has seen a startling improvement in the quality of CT images. The ability to detect small abnormalities in the kidneys has markedly improved. Modern scanners are able to take exposures in 5 seconds or less. They have a fine spatial resolution, are capable of doing dynamic or rapid sequential scanning, and can use the computer to reconstruct images in other than the axial plane.

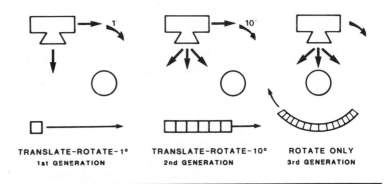

TRANSLATE-ROTATE-1°
1st GENERATION

TRANSLATE-ROTATE-10°
2nd GENERATION

ROTATE ONLY
3rd GENERATION

ROTATE TUBE-STATIONARY DETECTORS
4th GENERATION

CIRCULAR X-RAY TUBE ANODE-
STATIONARY DETECTORS
5th GENERATION

Figure 7–126. Configuration of scanners.

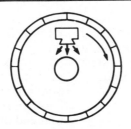

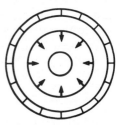

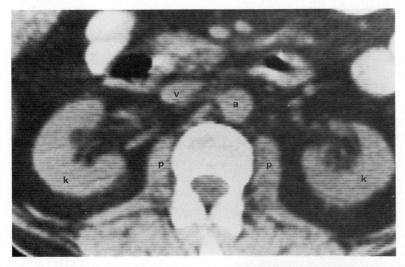

Figure 7–127. Normal kidneys (k). Without contrast enhancement, the renal parenchyma has a homogeneous density and is outlined by renal sinus and perinephric fat (p, psoas muscle; a, abdominal aorta; v, inferior vena cava). (From Huber, D. J., and Seltzer, S. E.: Postgrad. Radiol., *3*:161, 1983. Used by permission.)

Figure 7–128. Normal renal vessels. The normal renal veins are seen ventrally, and the arteries are visible dorsally.

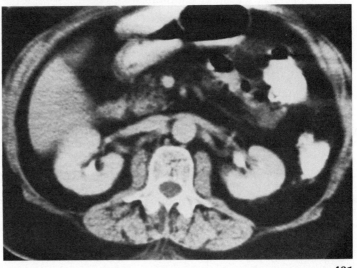

PERFORMANCE OF KIDNEY CT EXAMINATIONS

Patient Preparation

At Brigham and Women's Hospital, patients who are to undergo abdominal CT examinations generally receive oral doses of iodinated contrast material prior to scanning. The purpose of this oral contrast is to opacify the gastrointestinal tract and differentiate loops of bowel from pathologic structures. Up to 1 L of oral contrast agent is administered, starting at least 1 hour prior to the examination. Contrast agent enemas can also be given, if required.

Scanning Techniques

At most institutions, a series of contiguous, 10-mm–thick scans are performed through the kidneys prior to intravenous contrast administration. For the diagnosis of renal masses or obstructive uropathy, the value of these precontrast scans is controversial, but they are useful in detecting calcification, hemorrhage, and contrast extravasation (Engelstad et al., 1980).

Next, the patient receives an intravenous contrast bolus containing approximately 29 gm of iodine, and postcontrast scans are taken of the kidneys and other appropriate abdominal and pelvic structures. The examination can be tailored to answer specific clinical questions. For instance, if one wants to know the status of the renal veins and inferior vena cava, scans are centered on these structures and are taken as rapidly as possible following the bolus of intravenous contrast. Modern CT scanners can obtain six or more scans per minute.

Radiation Dosimetry— Complications, Precautions

The radiation dose from a CT scan slice varies with different scanners, but averages 3 rads to the skin surface (Brasch and Cann, 1982). It should be emphasized that because there is little scattered radiation, there is little additive dose from doing sequential, contiguous scans. Therefore, if the entire kidney were included in a series of nonoverlapping slices, the total dose to the kidney would equal about 3 rads.

There are few reported complications of oral contrast agents. It would be dangerous to give an oral contrast bolus to a patient who might aspirate. Complications of intravenous contrast are well known to most physicians (Shehadi and Toniolo, 1980). Major reactions, including anaphylaxis and cardiorespiratory compromise, are most feared. Minor reactions include rashes and urticaria. Nonallergic reactions include nausea and vomiting. Contrast agents' ability to induce renal failure is well known (Byrd and Sherman, 1979). Clearly, it is important to inform the radiologist if the patient has a history of prior allergy to contrast materials, iodine-containing foods, or other drugs. Similarly, it is important for the radiologist to know the adequacy of the patient's renal function and the presence of any underlying medical conditions (such as multiple myeloma, diabetes, or dehydration) that might increase the risk of development of contrast-induced renal failure.

NORMAL ANATOMY

The cross sectional anatomy of the normal kidneys is well displayed on CT scans (McClennan and Fair, 1979). The renal shape is round at the upper and lower poles, whereas the mid-kidney is oval with a central invagination caused by the renal hilum. Fat is seen commonly in the perinephric space and the renal sinus (Fig. 7–127). It is easy to distinguish all of the renal surfaces. The normal parenchyma is homogeneous and measures between 30 and 50 (HU) (Sagel et al., 1977). After administration of about 29 gm of iodine as contrast, parenchymal attenuation values rise past 100 HU.

The renal collecting system is also easily observed in cross section. Normally, it contains nonopacified urine and is visible as a water density structure outlined by peripelvic fat. After contrast, the excreted iodine fills the collecting system with high-density material. It is possible to assess the caliber of the collecting system and proximal ureter—these structures should be more densely opacified than the renal parenchyma.

The renal arteries are often seen arising from the aorta, dorsal to the renal veins (Fig. 7–128). The renal veins are larger and more ventral (Fig. 7–128). The left-sided vein is longer and curves over the ventral surface of the aorta just behind the superior mesenteric artery. The

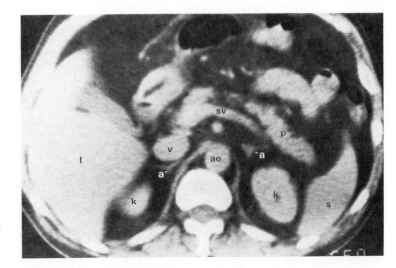

Figure 7–129. Normal anatomic relationship between the kidneys (k) and adrenals (a′), liver (l), spleen (s), IVC (v), aorta (ao), splenic vein (sv), and pancreatic tail (p). (From Huber, D. J., and Seltzer, S. E.: Postgrad. Radiol., *3*:161, 1983. Used by permission.)

right-sided vein is shorter and is often oriented obliquely.

The kidneys have important relationships to other organs (Fig. 7–129). The adrenal glands are anterior to the upper poles of the kidneys. The superior and posterior renal surfaces are near the diaphragm. The posteromedial aspects of the kidneys are close to the psoas muscles. The right kidney relates tightly to the posterior surface of the liver, and the left kidney often abuts the spleen.

Normal retroperitoneal anatomy is also easy to visualize on CT images (Love et al., 1981a; 1981b; Meyers, 1982; Parienty et al., 1981a). The kidneys are wrapped in a thin, tight-fitting renal capsule. They are then surrounded by perirenal fat that is contained within the Gerota fascia (Fig. 7–130). This fascia can be seen in up to 50 per cent of normal individuals. The Gerota fascia and its extension, the lateroconal fascia, divide the retroperitoneum into three compartments. The anterior pararenal space contains the pancreas and duodenum and the ascending and descending colons. The perirenal space contains the kidneys, adrenal glands, and ureters. The posterior pararenal space contains no normal tissues and abuts the lateral margins of the psoas muscles.

NORMAL VARIANTS AND DEVELOPMENTAL ANOMALIES

A large number of normal variants and developmental anomalies are easily visible on CT images. Urography and ultrasound play a more important role than CT in their detection

and characterization. However, it is important to recognize the appearance of these variants on CT, so as not to confuse them with pathologic structures. Prominent regions of the cortex, such as columns of Bertin, will have the same density and contrast enhancement characteristics as normal renal parenchyma. Occasionally, there is

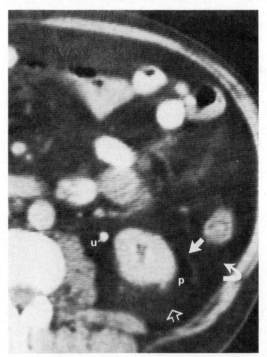

Figure 7–130. Normal retroperitoneal anatomy. The anterior (arrow) and posterior (open arrow) renal fascia surround the perirenal space (p). Lateroconal fascia (curved arrow); contrast-enhanced ureter (u′). (From Huber, D. J., and Seltzer, S. E.: Postgrad. Radiol., *3*:161, 1983. Used by permission.)

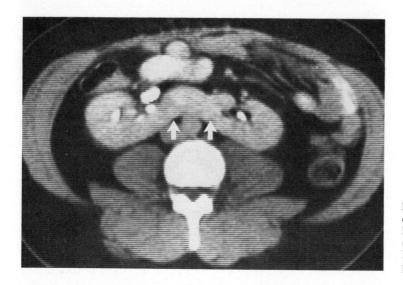

Figure 7–131. Horseshoe kidney. The contrast-enhanced "isthmus" of the fused kidneys is easily identified (arrows). (From Huber, D. J., and Seltzer, S. E.: Postgrad. Radiol., *3*:161, 1983. Used by permission.)

exuberant deposition of fat in the renal pelvis, a condition termed "sinus lipomatosis." In such cases, the renal collecting system appears splayed on a urogram, and on CT images the splaying is seen to be due to a material of fat density. The rare, extreme form of this condition, "renal replacement lipomatosis," is characterized by renal atrophy or parenchymal destruction (Thierman et al., 1983).

Renal duplications, malpositions, and fusions are also easy to visualize. On CT, horseshoe kidneys show a characteristic fusion of the lower poles across the midline (Fig. 7–131). Obstruction of the upper pole collecting system has been described—a large, tortuous, fluid-filled structure (the upper pole ureter) has been observed that connects the upper pole of the kidney with the bladder (Cramer et al., 1983). When a kidney is absent, portions of the gas-

trointestinal tract fill the renal fossa (Fig. 7–132).

Variations in venous anatomy are quite common. One can often recognize duplication of the inferior vena cava, a left-sided inferior vena cava, and circumaortic and retroaortic renal veins (Reed et al., 1982; Royal and Callen, 1979).

RENAL MASSES

CT is particularly helpful in the detection and evaluation of mass lesions because it helps differentiate between renal and extra-renal pathologic conditions, characterizes the extent and nature of lesions, and permits simultaneous assessment of neighboring structures such as renal vessels, the inferior vena cava, adjacent

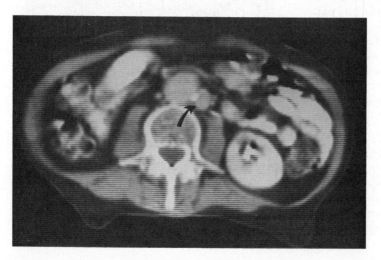

Figure 7–132. Congenital absence of the right kidney and left-sided IVC. CT scan through the level of the lower pole of the kidneys shows a normal-appearing left kidney, no right kidney, bowel in the right renal fossa, and a left-sided IVC (arrow).

fascia, and other organs. Masses are recognized on CT images when they distort the collecting system or sinus fat, or when their density differs from that of the normal parenchyma. It is easy to detect calcification, fat, or gas within a renal mass. The paragraphs that follow will describe the CT characteristics of renal cysts and tumors and their differentiation from other entities such as renal abscesses or hematomas. At the end of this section, an algorithm outlining the workup of renal masses at our hospital will be presented.

Cysts

Simple renal cysts are commonly observed incidentally on CT scans. Often they share certain characteristics: a smooth outline; homogeneous density close to that of water; no contrast enhancement; a thin wall; and smooth, sharply marginated interface with normal kidney (Fig. 7–133). McClennan et al. (1979) showed that 56 renal lesions sharing all of these characteristics proved to be benign on cyst puncture. Similarly, Sagel et al. (1977) and Magilner and Ostrum (1978) made no errors when they used these diagnostic criteria in more than 250 cases of simple renal cysts. In general, cyst puncture is not recommended if a benign-appearing cyst is discovered incidentally on a routine examination. There are some potential sources of error in the CT diagnosis of cysts. One must be certain that the lesion occupies the entire thickness of the scan slice so that density readings are reliable and do not suffer from partial-volume averaging (density of the cyst and the surrounding tissues averaged together). Also, the wall of a benign cyst may appear falsely thickened if a surrounding rim of normal renal tissue is included in the slice; this occasionally occurs at the upper or lower poles of the kidneys (Segal and Spitzer, 1979). Thickening of the wall of a benign cyst following percutaneous aspiration has also been observed (Evans et al., 1983).

Parapelvic cysts are seen as homogeneous cystic masses in the renal pelvis that distort the collecting system (Hidalgo et al., 1982; Morag et al., 1983). It is challenging to differentiate these cysts from hydronephrosis on morphologic grounds alone. Particularly when delayed scanning is used, material can be seen to accumulate in a dilated renal collecting system, whereas there will be no accumulation in a parapelvic cyst.

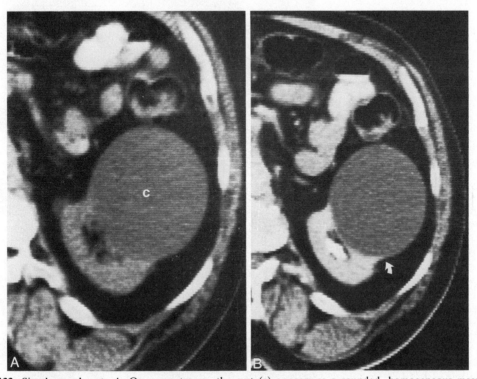

Figure 7–133. Simple renal cyst. *A,* On a scout scan, the cyst (c) appears as a rounded, homogeneous mass of water density. *B,* After administration of intravenous contrast material, the cyst shows no enhancement. The cyst wall is virtually invisible. The arrow points to the "beak" of normal renal parenchyma. (From Huber, D. J., and Seltzer, S. E.: Postgrad. Radiol., *3:*161, 1983. Used by permission.)

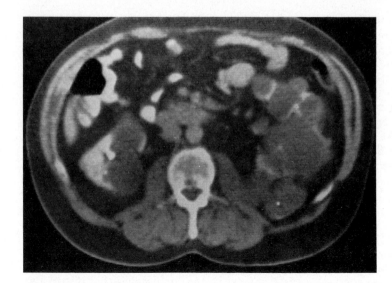

Figure 7–134. Polycystic kidneys. Both kidneys are distorted by multiple cysts. A cursor is seen over one of the left-sided cysts.

Figure 7–135. Multilocular cystic nephroma (surgically proven). *A,* Precontrast scan shows only small distortion of renal outline (arrow). *B,* Postcontrast scan shows small soft tissue mass (cursor), which enhances less than the normal renal parenchyma. (From Huber, D. J., and Seltzer, S. E.: Postgrad. Radiol., *3:*161, 1983. Used by permission.)

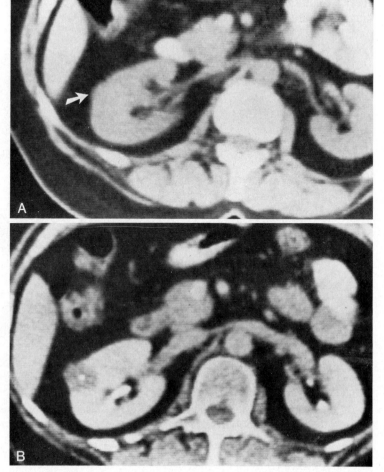

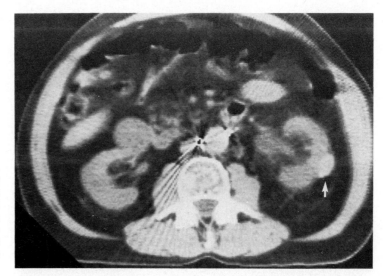

Figure 7–136. Hyperdense renal cyst. Noncontrast scan through the midportions of the kidneys shows an oval, high-density (60 HU) mass (arrow) adjacent to the lateral aspect of the left kidney. It proved to be a hemorrhagic cyst in a patient taking anticoagulants. A 4-cm diameter cyst is seen budding from the anterior surface of the right kidney.

Polycystic kidney disease can be recognized on CT images (Segal and Spataro, 1982). The kidneys are usually enlarged and distorted by multiple fluid-filled masses (Fig. 7–134). One can commonly observe cysts in other organs such as the liver, spleen, or pancreas. Cysts complicated by infection or hemorrhage have high CT densities.

Multilocular cystic nephroma is a rare lesion that is more common in childhood. The lesion can mimic a solid mass because its clustered cysts have relatively thick walls and septa (Fig. 7–135) (Parienty et al., 1981*b*).

Several investigators have described benign renal cysts that are not calcified but are denser than normal renal parenchyma (Dunnick et al., 1984; Fishman et al., 1983; Pearlstein, 1983; Sussman et al., 1984) (Figure 7–136). CT values in these lesions ranged up to 60 HU above that of normal kidneys. Most of these cysts were removed surgically and had either evidence of recent hemorrhage or a high protein content.

Benign Tumors

Sometimes a renal mass can be diagnosed confidently as a benign tumor on the basis of CT scans alone. An example of such a lesion is angiomyolipoma. Typically, the tumor is a large, fatty mass, intermixed with areas of soft tissue (Bosniak et al., 1982; Frija et al., 1980; Gentry et al., 1981; Sherman et al., 1981). CT nicely demonstrates perinephric extension and hemorrhage (Fig. 7–137). Parvey et al. (1981) pointed out that lipomas, liposarcomas, and Wilms' tumors may also contain fat.

Oncocytoma, a slow-growing tumor, has a distinct margin, a smooth contour, and a homogeneous appearance on contrast-enhanced CT (Cohan et al., 1984; Levine and Huntrakoon, 1983). Oncocytomas may calcify (Wasserman and Ewing, 1983) and may coexist with renal cell carcinomas (Cohan et al., 1984; Velasquez et al., 1984). In general, the appearance of an oncocytoma is not distinctive enough to permit discrimination from renal cell carcinoma without resorting to angiography or excision.

The CT features of mesoblastic nephroma (Bitter et al., 1982) and renal lipoma (Morgan et al., 1980) are described in isolated case reports.

Malignant Tumors

RENAL CELL CARCINOMA

CT plays a vital role in the detection, characterization, and staging of renal cell carcinomas. Generally, on precontrast scans, these tumors are equal in density to normal kidneys but have several abnormal features, including a heterogeneous core (due to the presence of necrosis or hemorrhage), thick walls, or calcifications. Following intravenous contrast, these tumors usually enhance to a lesser degree than adjacent normal renal parenchyma (see Figs. 7–138 to 7–141) (Magilner and Ostrum, 1978; Sagel et al., 1977). The accuracy of CT findings in making the precise diagnosis of hypernephroma is unknown. It is clear, for instance, that CT rarely errs in differentiating a solid from a cystic mass (Magilner and Ostrum, 1978; O'Reilly et al., 1981; Sagel et al., 1977); how-

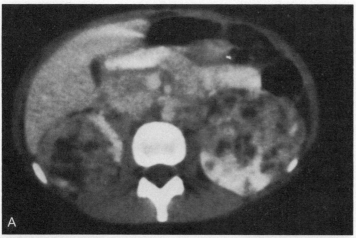

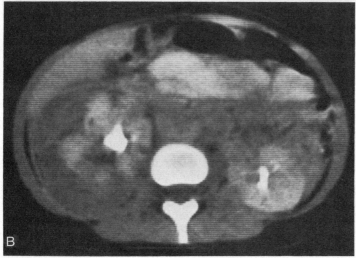

Figure 7–137. Hemorrhagic angiomyolipoma. Patient with tuberous sclerosis developed hematuria. *A,* Scan through the upper poles of the kidneys following contrast administration shows multiple fat-density areas and some preserved renal parenchyma. *B,* Several centimeters lower, a fairly homogeneous, slightly low density mass surrounds the right kidney. The findings are compatible with bilateral angiomyolipoma with bleeding and a perinephric hematoma on the right.

ever, whether that solid mass is a hypernephroma and not another type of tumor is occasionally difficult to tell. As with other solid lesions, biopsy or surgery is usually required for precise diagnosis.

Because CT can depict local extent, venous invasion, and disseminated spread of malignant renal tumors, it can be very useful in staging. Table 7–1 outlines the staging system that is

widely used for renal cell carcinoma. Stage I tumors are confined to the renal parenchyma and usually do not distort the renal outline (Fig. 7–138). Stage II tumors have extended into the perinephric space and often have irregular margins (Fig. 7–139). Tumors classified as Stage III have spread to local lymph nodes or have invaded the venous system (Fig. 7–140). Lymph node metastases are usually greater than 1.5 cm in diameter on CT. CT cannot always distinguish between hyperplastic and metastatic nodal enlargement nor can it detect tumor in normal-sized nodes. Tumor invasion into the renal vein usually enlarges the vein, and occasionally a low-density, intraluminal filling defect can be observed in the renal vein or inferior vena cava (Fig. 7–140). Stage IV tumors have grown to invade neighboring organs or have spread hematogenously (Fig. 7–141). Direct invasion of the liver by tumor is often difficult to detect; even when the fat plane between the tumor and

TABLE 7–1. STAGING RENAL CELL CARCINOMA

Stage	Findings
I	Tumor is confined to renal parenchyma; renal capsule intact
II	Tumor extends into perinephric space, but is contained within the Gerota fascia (can involve ipsilateral adrenal gland)
III	Tumor involves local lymph nodes or renal vein (with or without caval extension)
IV	Adjacent organs involved, or distant metastases present

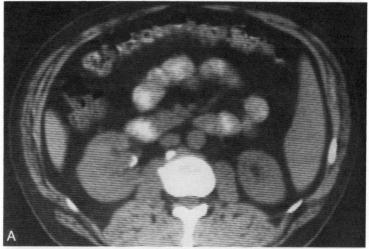

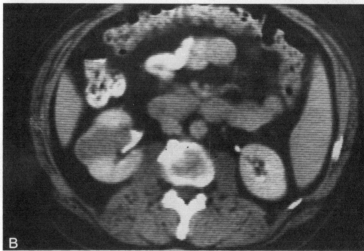

Figure 7–138. Stage I renal cell carcinoma. *A,* CT scan through the midportion of the right kidney shows a minor distortion of the right renal outline and an arc of calcification medially. *B,* Following contrast injection, the central portion of the right kidney is seen to be replaced by a soft tissue mass. At surgery, the mass was a renal cell carcinoma that distended but did not disrupt the renal capsule. The calcification was associated with the medial edge of the mass.

liver is obscured, the liver has not always been penetrated.

Many authors believe that CT does an excellent job of staging renal cell carcinomas and that it can obviate the need for routine preoperative angiography (Kothari et al., 1981; Lang, 1984; Levine et al., 1979; Love et al., 1979; Probst et al., 1981; Richie et al., 1983; Weyman et al., 1980). Table 7–2 summarizes the data from four studies that indicate the relative sensitivity and specificity of CT and angiography in this regard (Love et al., 1979; Probst et al., 1981; Richie et al., 1983; Weyman et al., 1980). CT's major limitation is its occasional inability to detect venous or caval involvement. At our institution, arteriography is performed for diagnosis or staging only when CT findings are equivocal. Vena cavography and renal venography are still commonly performed—usually when there is any uncertainty about venous invasion.

Some rare or unusual forms of renal cell carcinoma have special CT features. For example, papillary renal cell carcinoma (a slower-growing, less aggressive lesion) is noticed initially at a less advanced stage than other tumors; it is often calcified and shows less enhancement than nonpapillary tumors (Press et al., 1984). Similarly, cystic renal cell carcinomas are recognized on CT as predominantly fluid-filled lesions with a number of sinister features, that is, thick or calcified walls and inhomogeneous or septated contents (Hartman et al., 1984). It is not always possible to differentiate these cystic tumors from hemorrhagic cysts, abscesses, multilocular cystic nephromas, or cystic adenomas.

CT is a sensitive tool for monitoring the postnephrectomy space for possible tumor recurrence (Bernardino et al., 1979) (Fig. 7–142). Some of the signs of recurrence include masses in the vacant renal fossa, poor visualization of aorta or inferior vena cava, or psoas muscle

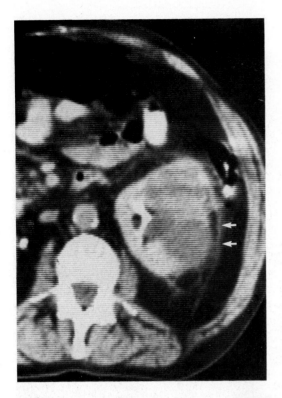

Figure 7–139. Stage II renal carcinoma, postcontrast scan. A large, irregularly enhanced mass arises from the lateral aspect of the left midkidney. Note the reactive thickening of Gerota's fascia (arrows). At surgery the tumor was seen to extend into the perinephric space but was contained within Gerota's fascia. (From Huber, D. J., and Seltzer, S. E.: Postgrad. Radiol., *3*:161, 1983.)

Figure 7–140. Stage III renal cell carcinoma. *A,* Prior to contrast administration, a soft tissue mass that sits in the region of the right renal vein is seen medially in the right kidney. *B,* Immediately following contrast injection the right renal vein is distended, and a filling defect is present within it. The defect represents tumor thrombus and involves the inferior vena cava.

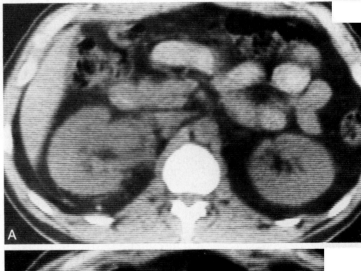

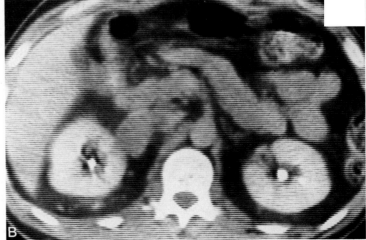

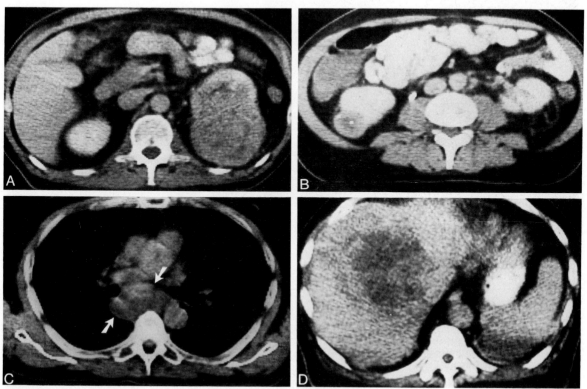

Figure 7–141. Stage IV renal cell carcinoma. *A,* CT scan through the midportion of the left kidney shows a 6-cm heterogeneous left renal cell carcinoma. *B,* Several centimeters lower, a metastasis with an area of central necrosis (cursors) is seen in the right kidney. *C,* In the lower chest, a subcarinal metastasis is observed (arrows). *D,* A scan through the liver reveals a large, lucent metastasis.

TABLE 7–2. ACCURACY OF STAGING RENAL CELL CARCINOMA

Staging	Computed Tomography		Angiography	
	SENS.	SPEC.	SENS.	SPEC.
Detection of mass	95%	?%	85%	?%
Perinephric extension	83–100	75–100	59–93	74–100
Lymph node involvement	73–90	81–100	73–90	81–100
Renal vein involvement	80–86	84–100	75–100	80–97
Inferior vena cava extension	75–100	92–100	100	100
Liver involvement	67	100	33	?

Sens. = Sensitivity or true positive rate; Spec. = Specificity or true negative rate; ? = Data not available from quoted studies.

(Adapted from Love, L. et al.: Urol. Radiol., *1*:3, 1979; Probst, P. et al.: Br. J. Radiol., *54*:744, 1981; Richie, J. P. et al.: J. Urol., *129*:1114, 1983; Weyman, P. J. et al.: Radiology, *137*:417, 1980.)

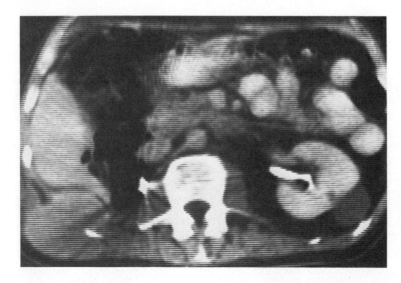

Figure 7–142. Recurrent right renal cell carcinoma. The patient had a right nephrectomy for carcinoma. Several months later, follow-up CT scan showed a mass in the right posterior abdominal wall, indicating recurrence of the tumor near its original site.

Figure 7–143. Transitional cell carcinoma. *A,* Urogram shows irregular amputation of the calyces in the lower pole of the right kidney by a large mass. *B,* CT scan through the lower pole of the right kidney shows a soft tissue mass (arrows) with a central necrotic cavity that has accumulated contrast material.

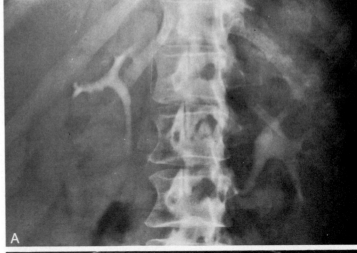

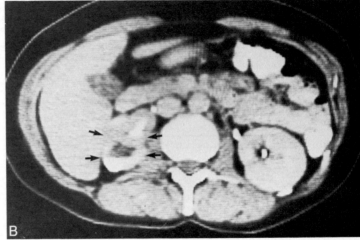

thickening. Recurrence can be simulated by scarring (Alter et al., 1979). Postoperative complications (abscess, hemorrhage, and so forth) can also be detected by CT.

TRANSITIONAL CELL CARCINOMA

Three CT patterns are typical of transitional cell carcinoma of the renal pelvis (Baron et al., 1982). These tumors may be visible as a focal, intraluminal mass; as ureteral wall thickening with luminal narrowing; or as a diffuse, infiltrating mass (Fig. 7–143). Attenuation values are similar to those of soft tissue. In Baron's series (1982), one of 22 tumors was calcified. CT proved quite accurate in staging this type of malignancy.

LYMPHOMA AND LEUKEMIA

Several studies have described the CT appearance of renal lymphoma (Chilcote and Borkowski, 1983; Hartman et al., 1982; Heiken et al., 1983; Jafri et al., 1982; Rubin, 1979). Four important patterns have been described: solitary nodules, multiple nodules, infiltration (focal or diffuse), and engulfment by contiguous retroperitoneal disease (Fig. 7–144). There is often concomitant thickening of the Gerota fascia and, occasionally, hydronephrosis.

Araki (1982) described the appearance of leukemic involvement of the kidneys in five children. He found bilaterally diffuse renal enlargement, discrete intrarenal masses, or renal hilar masses.

OTHER MALIGNANT TUMORS

The kidney is the fifth most common site for hematogenous metastases, commonly from lung, breast, or gastric primary tumors (Fig. 7–145). This kind of spread is readily observable on CT images (Bhatt et al., 1983). Interestingly, not all renal masses in patients with known nonrenal tumors are metastatic deposits. For

Figure 7–144. Renal lymphoma. Young man with diffuse histiocytic lymphoma. *A,* In June 1980, both kidneys are markedly enlarged and slightly heterogeneous secondary to infiltration by lymphoma. *B,* Three months later, after institution of chemotherapy, the kidneys have markedly decreased in size. The tip of an enlarged spleen (s) is seen on the left, posteriorly. (*A* from Huber, D. J., and Seltzer, S. E.: Postgrad. Radiol., *3*:161, 1983. Used by permission.)

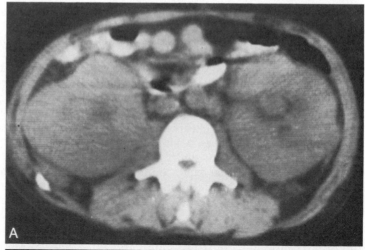

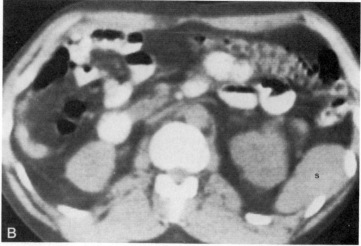

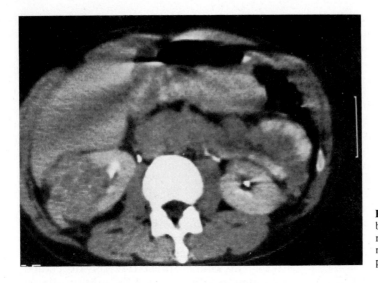

Figure 7–145. Renal metastasis. A man with bronchogenic carcinoma developed hematuria. A CT scan through the kidneys shows a nonenhancing mass in the right kidney that proved to be a metastatic deposit.

example, Pagani (1983) reviewed the pathology of seven solid renal masses that were discovered unexpectedly on CT scans of 1000 cancer patients. He found that five of the seven masses were actually renal cell carcinomas—a second primary tumor—and that only two of the seven masses were metastases. He suggested that in oncologic patients a renal mass with irregularly shaped regions of contrast enhancement should be considered a renal carcinoma, not a metastasis.

In children, Wilms' tumor is the most common renal mass—its characteristic CT appearance has been described as a large, heterogeneous cortical mass with slight contrast enhancement. About 13 per cent contain calcification and some have fat-containing areas (Fishman et al., 1983; Parvey et al., 1981).

Malignant tumors arising from other elements of the renal or perirenal stroma (e.g., rhabdomyosarcoma, fibrosarcoma, liposarcoma) are very rare but should be readily detectable on CT images.

Renal Masses with Special CT Features

FAT-CONTAINING MASSES

In an adult, a renal mass that contains only fat tissue is likely to be a lipoma. Masses that are heterogeneous but contain mature fatty elements are usually angiomyolipomas. Liposarcomas and teratomas can also have fat-containing areas. In a child, a Wilms' tumor can have mature adipose tissue within its stroma. Renal cell carcinomas do not contain mature fat and

are unlikely to masquerade as one of these fat-containing tumors on CT scans.

CALCIFIED MASSES

Most often, calcified masses in adults prove to be either a benign cyst or a renal cell carcinoma (Daniel et al., 1972). In cysts, the calcification is commonly curvilinear and peripheral, whereas in tumors it tends to be more punctate and scattered. Weyman et al. (1982) found that CT was very useful in helping to characterize calcified renal masses. They studied 21 such masses and were able to make a correct diagnosis in 18 cases. Nine renal cell carcinomas had a soft tissue mass extending beyond the calcifications. Lesions without a soft tissue mass were all benign. As they discussed, calcified malignant renal masses are most commonly renal cell carcinomas, though transitional cell carcinoma, Wilms' tumor, and metastatic tumors may also calcify. Benign renal tumors such as adenomas or angiomyolipomas can contain calcium. Benign lesions with calcifications are most often simple cysts, though calcification is also occasionally seen in multicystic or polycystic or postinfectious cystic kidneys, xanthogranulomatous pyelonephritis, vascular lesions, abscesses, hematomas, or multilocular cystic nephromas.

HIGH-DENSITY, NONCALCIFIED MASSES

The differential diagnosis of masses that are more dense than normal parenchyma but are not calcified is quite broad. Benign cysts that are complicated by bleeding (Dunnick et al., 1984; Sussman et al., 1984) or that contain viscous, proteinaceous material (Curry et al., 1982; Fishman et al., 1983b; Pearlstein, 1983) can fall into this category. Shanser (1978) reported that intravenous contrast can gradually accumulate in a benign cyst, giving the lesion an unusually high density 24 to 96 hours later. Balfe et al. (1982) described hyperdense malignant tumors.

The proper workup and treatment of these hyperdense lesions is controversial, but it is clear that they cannot be dismissed as benign. Sussman et al. (1984) stated that the benign or malignant nature of such a lesion ". . . cannot be established by CT alone" and recommended cyst puncture or surgery for diagnosis. Pearlstein (1983) recommended arteriography as the appropriate diagnostic procedure and stated, "If arteriography does not reveal tumor vessels on staining, a less aggressive surgical approach may be indicated." Balfe et al. (1982) stated that "Any seemingly simple renal cyst with high attenuation value must be regarded as suspicious." They recommended surgery for most of these lesions.

MASSES CONSIDERED INDETERMINATE ON CT IMAGES

Balfe et al. (1982) studied 60 cases in which renal lesions did not fit the criteria for either benign cyst or neoplasm. These patients were then assigned to one of three categories. In the first, termed "technically indeterminate," the masses had many characteristics of a simple cyst, but one or more features were inconsistent. For example, some of these masses were too small to have accurate CT number measurement; some were visible only on images degraded by motion artifact. All proved to be benign cysts. The second category was termed "cystlike mass without technical problem." These masses had disturbing features, including thickened wall, peripheral calcification, attenuation values higher than those typical of a benign cyst, or irregular contours. Although most turned out to be cysts complicated by bleeding or infection, several primary or metastatic malignant tumors were included in this group. The third category was termed "solid with complex features." These lesions bore some resemblance to renal neoplasms but had unusual features such as marked involvement of the perinephric space, extravasation of contrast medium, fresh hemorrhage, or a clinical presentation suggesting a nonneoplastic process. Although about half of these patients had xanthogranulomatous pyelonephritis, the other half had malignant renal tumors. Concerning the problem of indeterminate masses, Balfe and his colleagues recommended repeating CT if technical difficulty were present, possibly followed by ultrasound with needle aspiration. Angiography may reveal the classic pattern of renal cell carcinoma. If the mass resembles a cyst but has unusual features not related to technical problems, puncture is recommended, unless the mass is calcified and has an attenuation value of 40 to 60 HU, in which case surgery should be performed. If the mass has complex CT features not typical of either benign cyst or malignant tumor, surgery is recommended.

Algorithm for Workup of Renal Masses

Figures 7–146 to 7–148 present algorithms that are used to evaluate renal masses at our institution. These are followed if a renal mass is seen on the excretion urogram (Fig. 7–146) or on ultrasound (Fig. 7–147), or if it is discovered by palpation or is seen on a plain abdominal radiograph (Fig. 7–148). Although there is no single correct way to work up a renal mass, these algorithms were designed to present a cost-effective approach.

INFECTION

The spectrum of infectious diseases involving the kidneys ranges from simple pyelonephritis to renal abscess to more complicated conditions, such as xanthogranulomatous pyelonephritis. Except in some of the special circumstances detailed further on, CT is unlikely to be the primary imaging test in patients with renal infection. Urography, sonography, and scintigraphy with gallium-67 are likely to be more helpful. However, Rauschkolb et al. (1982) suggested that CT can play an important role in the evaluation of patients with renal infection or inflammatory disease. Urographic findings are often nonspecific in these patients—renal enlargement, a diminished or patchy nephrogram, or poor excretion of contrast. They felt that CT could clarify the nature of these patients' illnesses and guide the way to appropriate therapy.

To aid the diagnostician, Rauschkolb and others have described the CT findings that are characteristic of a variety of entities. For example, on CT scans, simple, acute, focal, bacterial nephritis (the so-called acute lobar nephronia) commonly creates a low-density area within the kidney in a lobar distribution. One patient with a severe infection also had air within the renal parenchyma and two others had air in the renal collecting systems. Hoffman et

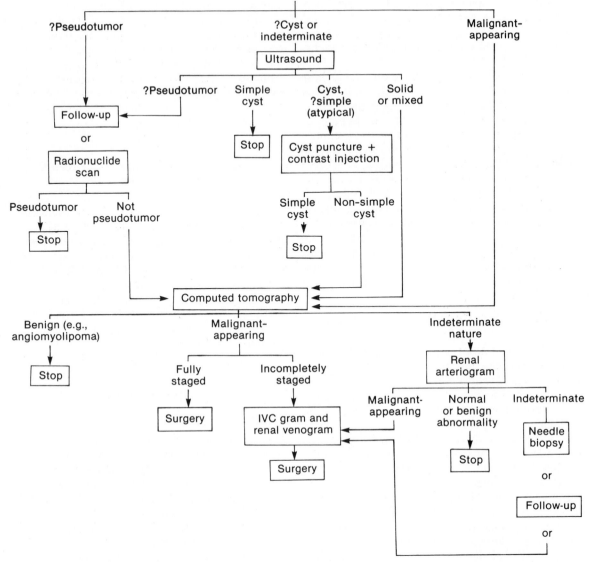

Figure 7–146. Renal mass suspected by urography.

al. (1980) described the CT findings in patients with acute pyelonephritis associated with diabetes. After contrast material was given, they noticed linear areas of low density in a striated pattern on the CT scans. We have observed this pattern in a similar case with a bilateral infection (Fig. 7–149).

Renal abscesses often demonstrate single or multiple lucencies that are rounded and nonlobar. There can be extension of the inflammatory process beyond the renal capsule (Fig. 7–150). Gas may be present within the abscess (Mendez et al., 1979). Once an abscess is detected, it may be drained percutaneously, guided by CT or another imaging technique.

Cronan et al. (1984) described successful percutaneous drainage of five renal abscesses. CT can help differentiate a renal abscess from one arising in juxtarenal tissues.

Xanthogranulomatous pyelonephritis is an uncommon form of chronic renal infection. The renal parenchyma is replaced by sheets of lipid-laden macrophages. Goldman et al. (1984) performed a clinical-radiologic-pathologic correlation study in 18 patients with xanthogranulomatous pyelonephritis. They found a diffuse form of the disease in 14 patients; characteristic CT findings included renal enlargement, parenchymal replacement by low-density areas with enhancing rims, renal pelvic calculi, and exten-

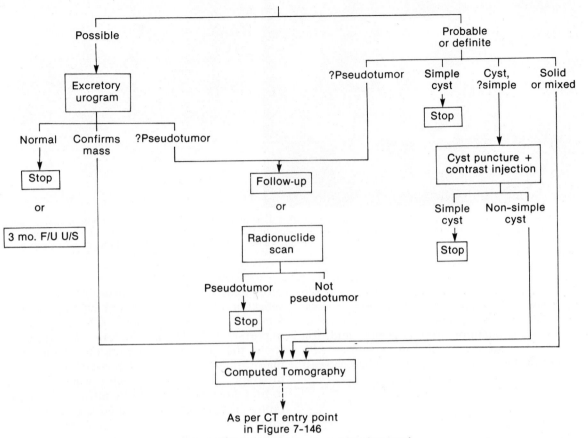

Figure 7–147. Renal mass suspected by ultrasound.

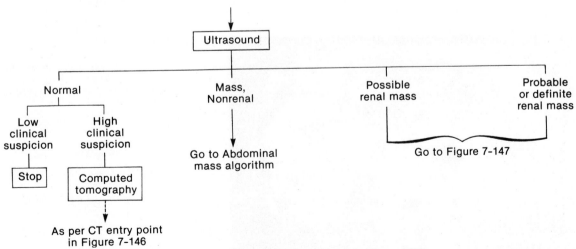

Figure 7–148. Renal mass suspected by palpation or KUB.

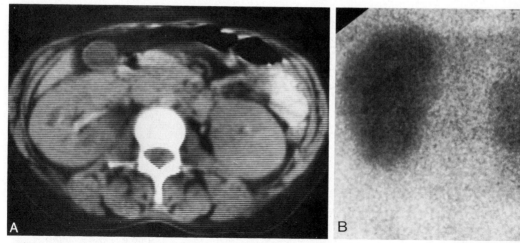

Figure 7–149. Bilateral pyelonephritis in a diabetic patient. *A,* CT scan demonstrates enlargement of both kidneys. There is diminished excretion of contrast. Streaky lucencies are seen in the renal parenchyma, particularly on the right. *B,* Gallium scan, posterior view, demonstrates intense renal uptake 48 hours after injection, confirming the diagnosis of pyelonephritis.

sion through the renal capsule to involve the perirenal or pararenal space or the psoas muscle (Fig. 7–151). Four patients had a focal form of xanthogranulomatous pyelonephritis and, on CT scans, had low-density mass lesions with enhancing rims surrounding stone-filled calyces.

TRAUMA

As pointed out by Rhyner et al. (1984) and Federle et al. (1981a), most cases of renal trauma can be evaluated adequately by clinical examination, laboratory studies, excretory urography, and angiography. At times, however, urographic findings are nonspecific and do not reflect accurately the type and extent of injury. Under these circumstances, CT can play an important role. In fact, Federle et al. (1981a) found that among 15 patients thought to have major renal trauma, CT proved superior to urography, demonstrating extravasation of urine in four cases not detected by intravenous urography. The same authors rated this technology superior for distinguishing minor from major injuries and helping select treatment. Frequently, CT allows the radiologist to determine the extent and severity of parenchymal injury and to detect perirenal hemorrhage, extravasated urine, and injuries to extraurinary structures. In complex cases, in which kidneys that

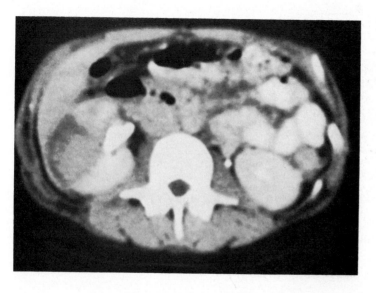

Figure 7–150. Renal abscess. CT scan shows a heterogeneous, low-density area in the right kidney laterally with some smaller lucent areas ventrally. There is some thickening of Gerota's fascia. The lesion proved to be a renal abscess.

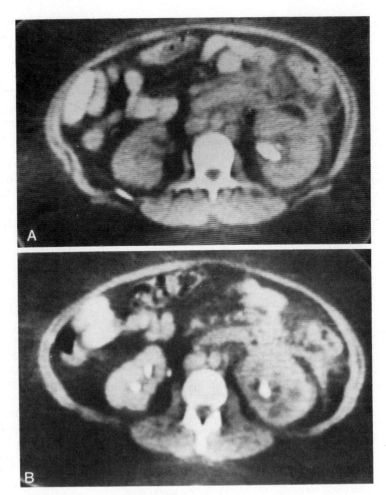

Figure 7–151. Xanthogranulomatous pyelonephritis. *A,* Precontrast CT scan shows a calculus in the central collecting system of the left kidney. The kidney is enlarged. There is thickening of Gerota's fascia, which is adherent to the kidney laterally. *B,* Following injection of contrast, the poorly functioning left kidney enhances heterogeneously.

have pre-existing congenital or acquired abnormalities are injured, CT is quite valuable for clarification of the underlying renal pathology and associated traumatic injury (Rhyner et al., 1984).

Several authors have helped offer particular insight into CT findings in cases of renal trauma (Federle et al., 1981*a*; Lang, 1983; McAninch et al., 1982; Sandler and Toombs, 1981). Renal trauma can be separated into several classes: injuries that affect mainly (1) the renal parenchyma (contusion, tear, shattered kidney, hematomas), (2) the renal artery, (3) the renal vein, (4) the renal collecting system, or (5) the ureter. Table 7–3 lists the CT findings that have been observed in these different types of injuries.

In patients with trauma, CT can be extremely valuable in detecting abnormalities in neighboring tissues or the skeleton (Federle and Brant-Zawadski, 1982).

VASCULAR LESIONS

CT plays a role that supplements clinical examination, urography, conventional angiography or digital vascular imaging in the evaluation of renal vascular lesions. On CT, normal vessels are easily observable and many pathologic conditions can be detected.

The normal renal artery and vein are commonly observable on CT scans (see Fig. 7–128). Variations in venous anatomy, such as circumaortic or retroaortic left renal veins, duplication of the inferior vena cava, or a left-sided inferior vena cava can be observed on CT images (Reed et al., 1982; Royal and Callen, 1979). The caliber of normal renal veins varies widely, but the normal left renal vein has been said never to exceed 1.5 cm (Marks et al., 1978), and the inferior vena cava never exceeds more than 3.7 cm.

TABLE 7–3. CT FINDINGS IN RENAL TRAUMA

Type of Injury	CT Findings
Parenchymal contusion	Area of decreased enhancement or extravasation of contrast. Heterogeneous enhancement with dynamic CT.
tear	Parenchymal disruption.
shattered kidney	Fracture fragments—lack of contrast enhancement indicates devitalization.
hematoma—intrarenal	Nonenhancing, intrarenal mass, with CT values of blood.
hematoma—subcapsular	Subcapsular mass, with CT values of blood.
hematoma—peri- or pararenal	Retroperitoneal mass, with CT values of blood.
Renal arterial	
tear or partial occlusion	Delayed, reduced enhancement and excretion of contrast.
complete arterial occlusion	Nonenhancement and nonexcretion of contrast.
renal artery severance with bleeding	Juxtarenal mass with CT values of blood. No enhancement of kidney.
traumatic arteriovenous fistula	Fast transit of contrast to vein.
Renal vein	
renal vein occlusion	Delayed enhancement, possibly enlarged kidney.
Collecting system disruption	Low-density juxtarenal mass corresponding to urinoma.
ureteral occlusion	Persistent nephrogram but delayed or absent excretion of contrast.

(Modified from Lang, E. K.: Radiographics, *3*:566, 1983.)

Arterial Lesions

A number of investigators have used "dynamic" CT scanning to investigate renal arterial perfusion. Both in experimental models and in patients, it has been shown that a time-dependent analysis of CT values of aorta, renal cortex, renal medulla, and renal pelvis following intravenous bolus of contrast material can help detect abnormalities in kidney blood flow (Heinz et al., 1980; Ishikawa et al., 1981; Probst et al., 1983; White et al., 1979). Normally, the density of the renal cortex increases rapidly with a slope similar to that of the aorta. Cortical density peaks, then falls gradually as contrast accumulates in the medulla. Kidneys with diminished perfusion have decreased cortical upslope or

creased peak, or both. Such a pattern is observed in cases of renal artery stenosis.

If blood flow is severely diminished, areas of ischemia develop. Visually, ischemic areas are wedge-shaped and have low density after contrast (Pazmiño et al., 1983; White et al., 1979). These lesions may be reversible if ischemia is relieved.

Irreversible or prolonged ischemia leads to infarction. Wong et al. (1984) and Glazer et al. (1983) have described the CT features of renal infarction both in patients and in experimental animals. They found that severely ischemic or infarcted areas are observable as regions of low density within 2 hours after blood flow was diminished. If the infarction is focal, these low-density areas may be wedge-shaped; if it is global, the low-density areas involve the whole kidney. Up to 47 per cent of infarcts have an enhancing rim, which is thought to be due to preserved blood flow to the periphery of the infarct via collateral vessels in the capsule. Findings that support the diagnosis of renal infarct include subcapsular fluid and thickening of the renal fascia. After healing, a focal area of scarring and parenchymal loss remains (Fig. 7–152).

An extreme form of renal injury, renal cortical necrosis, has been observed on CT and sonography (Goergen et al., 1981; Sefczek et al., 1984). Predisposing factors include complications of pregnancy (such as abruption of the placenta), trauma, sepsis, dehydration, burns, toxins, and complications of renal transplants or blood transfusions. On CT, a lucent renal cortex is seen, which is bracketed by a normal-appearing capsular area on one side and the medulla on the other. Supporting evidence for the diagnosis of renal cortical necrosis is obtained from ultrasound. The damaged cortex appears hypoechoic.

The CT appearance of the kidneys in polyarteritis nodosa has also been described (Pope et al., 1981). Multiple wedge-shaped, low-density areas were observed, which were thought to be secondary to hypoperfusion distal to microaneurysms.

Venous Lesions

Renal venous abnormalities can be observed on CT images. For example, a renal vein may appear distended. This distension may be observed in a vein that is patent or is occluded by blood clot or tumor. A patent renal vein may become distended if it is being crimped between neighboring normal structures, such as when the

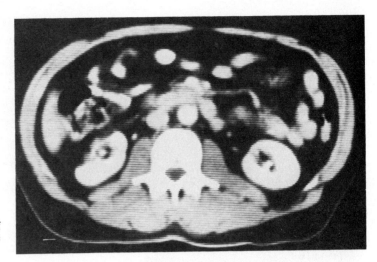

Figure 7–152. Renal infarct. Marked loss of renal parenchyma anterolaterally on the right. Normal left side.

left renal vein passes between the aorta and the superior mesenteric artery (Buschi et al., 1980) or when the vein carries extra blood flow (Thomas and Bernardino, 1981). Increased renal venous flow may be produced by kidney tumors that are hypervascular or have arteriovenous shunts. The renal vein can also carry extra blood when it serves as a collateral path to decompress the portal vein. An occluded renal vein may be distended by clot or tumor. Renal vein clots may form when renal vein flow is diminished, or they sometimes form spontaneously in patients who are severely dehydrated or have renal diseases such as glomerulonephritis. Renal vein distension by tumor is almost always caused by renal cell carcinoma. CT findings in renal vein thrombosis include enlarged kidney, a distended vein, occasional visualization of the thrombus within the vein, perirenal hemorrhage, and the so-called renal cobweb sign resulting from visualization of collateral veins (Coleman et al., 1980; Marks et al., 1978; Winfield et al., 1981). These collateral veins connect the renal vein with the azygos, gastric, adrenal, splenic, inferior phrenic, lumbar, gonadal, and ureteric veins.

NEPHROLITHIASIS AND OTHER METABOLIC ABNORMALITIES

Nephrolithiasis

As early as 1981, CT was recognized to have a unique ability to detect kidney stones that were not easily observable on conventional radiographs. Additionally, the quantitative na-

ture of CT made it possible to distinguish these relatively nonopaque calculi from other abnormalities such as soft tissue masses, blood clots, or fungus balls (Federle et al., 1981b; Pollack et al., 1981; Segal et al., 1978). Generally, even the least opaque uric acid calculus will be far more dense than other lesions in the collecting system (Fig. 7–153).

More recently, in vitro studies on urinary calculi have been performed in an effort to determine whether CT can distinguish between different kinds of stones (Hillman et al., 1984; Newhouse et al., 1984). It is important to know the chemical nature of kidney stones in order to guide selection of appropriate therapy. Hillman et al. (1984) found that CT was very accurate in separating the densities of uric acid, calcium oxalate, and struvite stones. There was, however, much overlap between the densities of other types of calculi. They concluded that "CT may prove a valuable adjunct to traditional laboratory and clinical methods in helping establish the chemical composition of calculi before selecting appropriate method of treatment." Others have found that uric acid and cystine stones could be identified because of their relatively lower densities but that several types of calcified stones could not be reliably distinguished or diagnosed (Newhouse et al., 1984).

Nephrocalcinosis

Calcification in the renal parenchyma is readily observable on CT images. Nephrocalcinosis secondary to any of the large number of causes of hypercalcemia, or structural abnor-

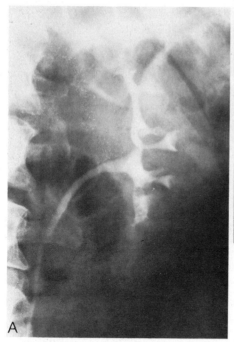

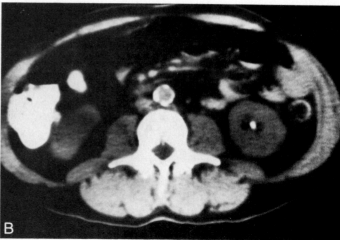

Figure 7–153. Renal calculi. *A*, Urogram shows multiple lucent filling defects in the left lower pole collecting system. *B*, CT scan through this area shows that the filling defects are due to calculi.

malities such as medullary sponge kidneys, should be readily identifiable.

Other Metabolic Abnormalities Affecting the Kidneys

The renal CT findings in congenital or acquired oxalosis have been described (Billimoria et al., 1983; Luers et al., 1980). In the congenital disease, renal cortical nephrocalcinosis has been observed. Acquired oxalosis is commonly secondary to jejunoileo-bypass surgery but may also be seen in gastrointestinal or biliary tract disorders, such as celiac disease, Crohn disease, chronic pancreatitis, biliary obstruction, or resection of the terminal ileum. CT findings include small kidneys with diffusely dense cortices (greater than 200 HU). On ultrasound, the cortex has increased echogenicity and decreased size.

Doppman et al. (1982) described the renal findings in Type I glycogen storage disease (von Gierke). Three of their eight patients showed increased density in the renal cortex (up to a maximum of 66 HU). Renal function remained normal.

Although not extensively described, renal infiltration with abnormal lipids (such as in metachromatic leukodystrophy) or amyloid may be recognizable on CT images. The CT findings

in diabetic renal disease are not well characterized, except that patients with diabetes sometimes have severe renal infections.

The role of CT in the evaluation of nephrolithiasis and other metabolic abnormalities is generally secondary to radiography, conventional tomography, urography, and ultrasound. The major role for CT will be in the differential diagnosis of renal pelvic filling defects and, possibly, in the determination of the chemical nature of renal stones.

MISCELLANEOUS ABNORMALITIES

The Juxtrarenal Spaces

The cross sectional CT anatomy of the juxtarenal spaces has been exhaustively reviewed. Several important spaces surround the kidney and they are delimited by important fascial structures (Love et al., 1981a; 1981b; Meyers, 1982; Parienty et al., 1981a; Thornbury, 1979) (Fig. 7–154). Table 7–4 lists the important juxtarenal spaces and the CT features that characterize a pathologic process in each of these regions. Subcapsular processes are delimited by the renal parenchyma and the cellophane-like renal capsule. Subcapsular processes are recognizable because they produce pressure

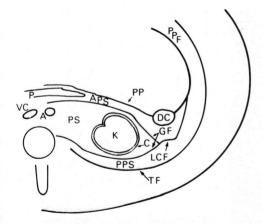

K Kidney
C Renal Capsule
PS Perirenal space
APS Anterior Pararenal space
PPS Posterior Pararenal space
PP Posterior Peritoneum
PPF Properitoneal Fat

GF Gerotas Fascia
LCF Lateroconal Fascia
TF Transversalis Fascia
P Pancreas
DC Descending Colon
A Aorta
VC Vena Cava

Figure 7–154. Diagram of juxtarenal spaces.

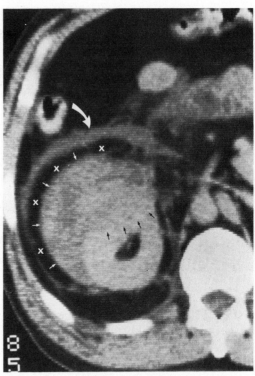

Figure 7–155. Subcapsular and pararenal hematoma. Following a percutaneous renal biopsy, the patient developed hematuria. CT scan through the midkidney shows a heterogeneous (white arrows) mass that distorts the renal outline (black arrows). The perirenal fat (x) is preserved. Gerota's fascia is thickened, and there is fluid in the anterior pararenal space (curved arrow). (From Huber, D. J., and Seltzer, S. E.: Postgrad. Radiol., *3*:161, 1983. Used by permission.)

deformity of the renal outline. Because they are enclosed by the renal capsule, they spare the perirenal fat (Fig. 7–155). Amparo and Fagan (1982) observed a subcapsular hematoma that compressed and compromised the renal parenchyma, leading to development of hypertension ("Page kidney"). Lesions in the perirenal space obscure the perirenal fat and are confined by the Gerota fascia (Fig. 7–156). Abnormalities in the anterior pararenal space preserve the perirenal fat and are confined posteriorly by the Gerota fascia and anteriorly by the posterior peritoneal lining (see Fig. 7–155). Lesions in the posterior pararenal space also preserve perirenal fat and are confined by the Gerota fascia and the transversalis fascia.

The fascia around the normal kidney can frequently be observed on CT scans. Parienty et al. (1981a) found that normal fascia was seen around both kidneys in slightly more than one half of cases and was seen on neither side in only 9 per cent of cases. With modern scanners, these fascia are seen in almost every case. The differential diagnosis of fascial thickening includes infiltration by tumor, infectious processes, inflammation (especially due to pancreatitis) (Chintapalli et al., 1982; Nicholson, 1981), or hemorrhage. Parienty et al. commented that "fascial thickening is non-specific: it is not pathognomonic of tumor, nor is it helpful in differ-

TABLE 7–4. JUXTARENAL SPACES

Space	Limiting Structures	Identifying Features
Subcapsular	Renal parenchyma Renal capsule	Pressure deformity on surface; perirenal fat preserved.
Perirenal	Renal capsule Gerota fascia	Perirenal fat obliterated.
Anterior pararenal	Gerota fascia Posterior peritoneum	Perirenal fat preserved; may reach colon or pancreas.
Posterior pararenal	Gerota fascia Transversalis fascia	Perirenal fat preserved; may reach psoas.

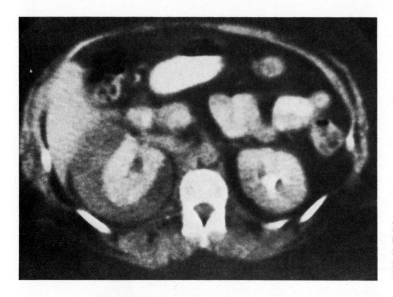

Figure 7–156. Perirenal hematoma. CT scan through the midportions of the kidneys shows a homogeneous, low-density mass in the right perirenal space. The right kidney outline is not distorted.

entiating pancreatitis from neoplasm. On the other hand, lack of fascial thickening may be helpful in ruling out renal extension of a neighboring lesion.''

Nonvisualized Kidney

The differential diagnosis of poorly or nonvisualized kidneys on intravenous urography includes abnormalities of renal arterial inflow, renal venous outflow, ureteral obstruction, intrinsic renal diseases, perinephric processes (such as abscess or other fluid collections), or congenital absence of the kidney. Several investigators have used CT to evaluate the cause of nonvisualization and found it useful for determining the size of the kidney in order to differentiate end stage renal disease from hydronephrosis. They were able to detect abnormalities indicative of mechanical ureteral obstruction, kidney stones, tumors, pyelonephritis, and perirenal abscess, and were able to observe congenital absence or hypoplasia of the kidney (Forbes et al., 1978; Karasick and Herring, 1980).

In evaluation of the poorly visualized or nonfunctioning kidney, CT appears to play a role secondary to that of ultrasound and, possibly, retrograde pyelography or radionuclide techniques.

Hydronephrosis

When a patient has mechanical ureteral obstruction, it is important to determine the cause of the blockage. Because CT can easily detect renal stones and soft tissue masses in and around the collecting system and ureter, it can make a valuable contribution to the analysis of the hydronephrotic kidney (Fig. 7–157). When the cause of obstruction is unclear on a conventional urogram, CT may explain the reason for it in up to 90 per cent of cases (Bosniak et al., 1982; Megibow et al., 1980). CT scans can give a false impression about the presence of hydronephrosis when a peripelvic cyst or subcapsular hematoma masquerades as a dilated collecting system (Amis et al., 1982).

CT certainly plays a role secondary to that of ultrasound and conventional urography in the detection of hydronephrosis and the determination of its cause. These other tests have sensitivities and specificities well over 90 per cent (Ellenbogen et al., 1978). CT is reserved for clarifying ambiguous cases.

Medical Renal Disease

Medical renal disease may be due to infectious, inflammatory, infiltrative, metabolic, or ischemic intrinsic diseases of the kidney. Because CT can estimate renal size and volume (Yokoyama et al., 1982), can depict intrinsic renal lesions, and, with the aid of contrast agents, can demonstrate renal blood flow and function, it has been employed in the investigation of medical renal disease.

Patients with medical renal disease often present with renal failure, sometimes accompanied by hypertension or an abnormal urine

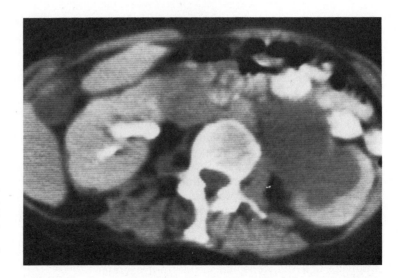

Figure 7–157. Left hydronephrosis. The nonenhanced, dilated pelvicalyceal system has the density of water. Note the dense nephrogram and the residual parenchymal thickness of the obstructed left kidney. The ureter was obstructed more distally by a pelvic mass. (From Huber, D. J., and Seltzer, S. E.: Postgrad. Radiol., *3*:161, 1983. Used by permission.)

sediment. In these patients, attention is often focused first on determining the size of the kidneys. If they are normal or small, one should consider a vascular cause for the renal failure. Radionuclide studies or conventional or digital angiography are the mainstays in this diagnosis, but dynamic CT scanning can also be used. If the kidneys are large, CT can play a supportive role to ultrasound in determining the cause of the enlargement or in staging the disease that is responsible.

Renal Transplantation

Patients who have renal transplants may develop lesions that obstruct the feeding artery, draining vein, or collecting system: they may develop peritransplant fluid collections (such as lymphocele, urinoma, abscess, hematoma, or seroma); acute tubular necrosis or transplant rejection may occur. Because CT scanning with contrast can evaluate perfusion and function of the transplanted kidney and because CT can visualize the peritransplant spaces so clearly, CT plays a role in the evaluation of failing renal allografts.

Many investigators have found that CT can demonstrate normal transplants and can detect a large variety of peritransplant fluid collections and differentiate those with lower CT densities (such as lymphocele, urinoma, and seroma) from those with higher density (abscess, hematoma) (Kittredge et al., 1978; Nakstad et al., 1982; Novick et al., 1981) (Fig. 7–158).

Fuld et al. (1984) used contrast-enhanced CT to evaluate the perfusion and function of transplanted kidneys. By performing rapid se-

Figure 7–158. Normal renal transplant. The allograft is seen in the right iliac fossa. Clips are seen on the skin and are also observed outlining the course of the transplant artery.

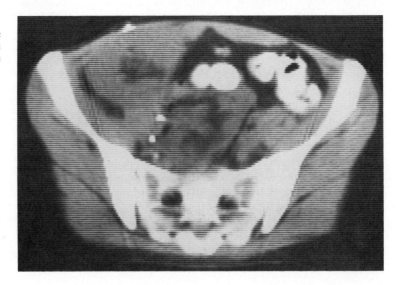

quential scans after bolus administration of contrast, they were able to measure the density of the aorta, renal cortex, and renal medulla. They plotted these densities versus time and derived several important parameters from the graphs. The corticoarterial junction time was used to assess renal perfusion, whereas the corticomedullary junction time assessed renal function. Normal patients had corticoarterial junction times that averaged less than 30 seconds, and these individuals' kidneys developed a sharp corticomedullary interface. Patients with transplant rejection had prolonged corticoarterial junction times and poorly visualized corticomedullary interfaces. In fact, the curves of the densities of the cortex and medulla did not intersect at all in 8 of 10 patients with rejection, implying that the transplants could not excrete and concentrate the contrast. The authors felt that dynamic CT scanning could help differentiate normally functioning transplants from those with acute tubular necrosis (in which perfusion would be normal but function would be decreased) or rejection (decreased perfusion as well as decreased function).

McDonald et al. (1982) used CT to study the natural history of gas trapped in the renal transplant bed. They found that 73 per cent of patients had observable gas remaining 4 days after drain removal, but only 10 per cent had such gas visible after 5 days. They concluded that gas persisting for greater than 1 week or gas that increased in amount (rather than gradually resorbing) should be considered pathologic.

Frick et al. (1984) investigated the phenomenon of postrenal transplant lymphoma. They observed six patients who developed abdominal lymphomas an average of 105 months after renal transplantation. In four of these patients, the transplant was involved with the lymphoma.

CONCLUSION

It is apparent, then, that in just over a decade, remarkable progress has been made in CT imaging of the kidney. In the future, one can look forward to increasing availability of CT scanners in hospitals of all sizes. More patients will then have access to this valuable imaging tool. Technological improvements may permit scanners to image in times as short as 50 milliseconds. Novel contrast materials are becoming available that should reduce complications related to contrast administration in CT. New knowledge based on clinical and experimental research will be accumulated that will improve our understanding of the usefulness of CT scanning in kidney diseases. One may expect that, in the future, information will become available that will clarify the roles of CT and NMR imaging in renal diseases. The horizons of diagnostic imaging of the kidney continue to expand.

References

Alter, A. J., Uehling, D. T., and Zwiebel, W. J.: Computed tomography of the retroperitoneum following nephrectomy. Radiology, *133*:663, 1979.

Amis, E. S., Jr., Cronan, J. J., and Pfister, R. C.: Pseudohydronephrosis on noncontrast computed tomography. J. Comput. Assist. Tomogr., *6*:511, 1982.

Amparo, E. G., and Fagan, C. J.: Page kidney. J. Comput. Assist. Tomogr., *6*:839, 1982.

Araki, T.: Leukemic involvement of the kidney in children: CT features. J. Comput. Assist. Tomogr., *6*:781, 1982.

Balfe, D. M., McClennan, B. L., Stanley, R. J., Weyman, P. J., and Sagel, S. S.: Evaluation of renal masses considered indeterminate on computed tomography. Radiology, *142*:421, 1982.

Baron, R. L., McClennan, B. L., Lee, J. K. T., and Lawson, T. L.: Computed tomography of transitional cell carcinoma of the renal pelvis and ureter. Radiology, *144*:125, 1982.

Bernardino, M. E., deSantos, L. A., Johnson, D. E., and Bracken, R. B.: Computed tomography in the evaluation of post-nephrectomy patients. Radiology, *130*:183, 1979.

Bhatt, G. M., Bernardino, M. E., and Graham, S. D., Jr.: CT diagnosis of renal metastases. J. Comput. Assist. Tomogr., *7*:1032, 1983.

Billimoria, P. E., Fabian, T. M., Schulz, E. E., and Chase, D. R.: Acquired renal oxalosis. J. Comput. Assist. Tomogr., *7*:158, 1983.

Bitter, J. J., Harrison, D. A., Kaplan, J., and Irwin, G. A. L.: Mesoblastic nephroma. J. Comput. Assist. Tomogr., *6*:180, 1982.

Bosniak, M. A.: Angiomyolipoma of the kidney should be diagnosed preoperatively in virtually every case. (Abstr.) Am. J. Roentgenol., *135*:209, 1980.

Bosniak, M. A., Megibow, A. J., Ambos, M. A., Mitnick, J. S., Lefleur, R. S., and Gordon, R.: Computed tomography of ureteral obstruction. Am. J. Roentgenol., *138*:1107, 1982.

Brasch, R. C., and Cann, C. E.: Computed tomographic scanning in children: II. An updated comparison of radiation dose and resolving power of commercial scanners. Am. J. Roentgenol., *138*:127, 1982.

Buschi, A. J., Harrison, R. B., Brenbridge, A. N. A. G., Williamson, B. R. J., Gentry, R. R., and Cole, R.: Distended left renal vein: CT/sonographic normal variant. Am. J. Roentgenol., *135*:339, 1980.

Byrd, L., and Sherman, R. L.: Radiocontrast-induced acute renal failure: a clinical and pathophysiologic review. Medicine, *58*:270, 1979.

Chilcote, W. A., and Borkowski, G. P.: Computed tomography in renal lymphoma. J. Comput. Assist. Tomogr., *7*:439, 1983.

Chintapalli, K., Lawson, T. L., Foley, W. D., and Berland, L. L.: Renal fascial thickening in pancreatitis. J. Comput. Assist. Tomogr., *6*:983, 1982.

Christensen, E. E., Curry, T. S., III, and Dowdey, J. E.: An Introduction to the Physics of Diagnostic Radiology. 2nd ed. Philadelphia, Lea & Febiger, 1978, pp. 329–360.

Cohan, R. H., Dunnick, N. R., Degesys, G. E., and Korobkin, M.: Computed tomography of renal oncocytoma. J. Comput. Assist. Tomogr., 8:284, 1984.

Coleman, C. C., Saxena, K. M., and Johnson, K. W.: Renal vein thrombosis in a child with the nephrotic syndrome: CT diagnosis. Am. J. Roentgenol., 135:1285, 1980.

Cramer, B. C., Twomey, B. P., and Katz, D.: CT findings in obstructed upper moieties of duplex kidneys. J. Comput. Assist. Tomogr., 7:251, 1983.

Cronan, J. J., Amis, E. S., Jr., and Dorfman, G. S.: Percutaneous drainage of renal abscesses. Am. J. Roentgenol., 142:351, 1984.

Curry, N. S., Brock, G., Metcalf, J. S., and Sens, M. A.: Hyperdense renal mass: unusual CT appearance of a benign renal cyst. Urol. Radiol., 4:33, 1982.

Daniel, W. W., Hartman, G. W., Witten, D. M., Farrow, G. M., and Kelalis, P. P.: Calcified renal masses: a review of ten years experience at the Mayo Clinic. Radiology, 103:503, 1972.

Doppman, J. L., Cornblath, M., Dwyer, A. J., Adams, A. J., Girton, M. E., and Sidbury, J.: Computed tomography of the liver and kidneys in glycogen storage disease. J. Comput. Assist. Tomogr., 6:67, 1982.

Dunnick, N. R., Korobkin, M., Silverman, P. M., and Foster, W. L., Jr.: Computed tomography of high density renal cysts. J. Comput. Assist. Tomogr., 8:458, 1984.

Ellenbogen, P. H., Scheible, F. W., Talner, L. B., and Leopold, G. R.: Sensitivity of gray scale ultrasound in detecting urinary tract obstruction. Am. J. Roentgenol., 130:731, 1978.

Engelstad, B. L., McClennan, B. L., Levitt, R. G., Stanley, R. J., and Sagel, S. S.: The role of pre-contrast images in computed tomography of the kidney. Radiology, 136:153, 1980.

Evans, D. D., Manco, L. G., and Costello, P.: Renal cyst wall thickening following percutaneous aspiration. J. Comput. Assist. Tomogr., 7:154, 1983.

Federle, M. P., and Brant-Zawadski, M. B.: Computed Tomography in the Evaluation of Trauma. Baltimore, The Williams & Wilkins Co., 1982.

Federle, M. P., Kaiser, J. A., McAninch, J. W., Jeffrey, R. B., and Mall, J. C.: The role of computed tomography in renal trauma. Radiology, 141:455, 1981a.

Federle, M. P., McAninch, J. W., Kaiser, J. A., Goodman, P. C., Roberts, J., and Mall, J. C.: Computed tomography of urinary calculi. Am. J. Roentgenol., 136:255, 1981b.

Fishman, E. K., Hartman, D. S., Goldman, S. M., and Siegelman, S. S.: The CT appearance of Wilms tumor. J. Comput. Assist. Tomogr., 7:659, 1983a.

Fishman, M. C., Pollack, H. M., Arger, P. H., and Banner, M. P.: High protein content: another cause of CT hyperdense benign renal cyst. J. Comput. Assist. Tomogr., 7:1103, 1983b.

Forbes, W. St. C., Isherwood, I., and Fawcitt, R. A.: Computed tomography in the evaluation of the solitary or unilateral nonfunctioning kidney. J. Comput. Assist. Tomogr., 2:389, 1978.

Frick, M. P., Salomonowitz, E., Hanto, D. W., and Gedgaudas-McClees, K.: CT of abdominal lymphoma after renal transplantation. Am. J. Roentgenol., 142:97, 1984.

Frija, J., Lardé, D., Belloir, C., Botto, H., Martin, N., and Vasile, N.: Computed tomography diagnosis of renal angiomyolipoma. J. Comput. Assist. Tomogr., 4:843, 1980.

Fuld, I. L., Matalon, T. A., Vogelzang, R. L., Neiman, H. L., Kowal, L. E., Hutchins, W. W., and Soper, W.: Dynamic CT in the evaluation of physiologic status of renal transplants. Am. J. Roentgenol., 142:1157, 1984.

Gentry, L. R., Gould, H. R., Alter, A. J., Wegenke, J. D., and Atwell, D. T.: Hemorrhagic angiomyolipoma: demonstration by computed tomography. J. Comput. Assist. Tomogr., 5:861, 1981.

Glazer, G. M., Francis, I. R., Brady, T. M., and Teng, S. S.: Computed tomography of renal infarction: clinical and experimental observations. Am. J. Roentgenol., 140:721, 1983.

Goergen, T. G., Lindstrom, R. R., Tan, H., and Lilley, J. J.: CT appearance of acute renal cortical necrosis. Am. J. Roentgenol., 137:176, 1981.

Goldman, S. M., Hartman, D. S., Fishman, E. K., Finizio, J. P., Gatewood, O. M. B., and Siegelman, S. S.: CT of xanthogranulomatous pyelonephritis: radiologic-pathologic correlation. Am. J. Roentgenol., 142:963, 1984.

Hartman, D. S., Davis, C. J., Jr., Goldman, S. M., Friedman, A. C., and Fritzsche, P.: Renal lymphoma: radiologic-pathologic correlation of 21 cases. Radiology, 144:759, 1982.

Hartman, D. S., Davis, C. J., Johns, T., and Goldman, S. M.: Cystic renal cell carcinoma: radiologic-pathologic correlation. (Abstr.) Am. J. Roentgenol., 142:237, 1984.

Heiken, J. P., Gold, R. P., Schnur, M. J., King, D. L., Bashist, B., and Glazer, H. S.: Computed tomography of renal lymphoma with ultrasound correlation. J. Comput. Assist. Tomogr., 7:245, 1983.

Heinz, E. R., Dubois, P. J., Drayer, B. P., and Hill, R.: A preliminary investigation of the role of dynamic computed tomography in renovascular hypertension. J. Comput. Assist. Tomogr., 4:63, 1980.

Hidalgo, H., Dunnick, N. R., Rosenberg, E. R., Ram, P. C., and Korobkin, M.: Parapelvic cysts: appearance on CT and sonography. Am. J. Roentgenol., 138:667, 1982.

Hillman, B. J., Drach, G. W., Tracey, P., and Gaines, J. A.: Computed tomographic analysis of renal calculi. Am. J. Roentgenol., 142:549, 1984.

Hoffman, E. P., Mindelzun, R. E., and Anderson, R. U.: Computed tomography in acute pyelonephritis associated with diabetes. Radiology, 135:691, 1980.

Huber, D. J., and Seltzer, S. E.: Computed tomography of the urinary tract. Postgrad. Radiol., 3:161, 1983.

Ishikawa, I., Onouchi, Z., Saito, Y., Kitada, H., Shinoda, A., Ushitani, K., Tabuchi, M., and Suzuki, M.: Renal cortex visualization and analysis of dynamic CT curves of the kidney. J. Comput. Assist. Tomogr., 5:695, 1981.

Jafri, S. Z. H., Bree, R. L., Amendola, M. A., Glazer, G. M., Schwab, R. E., Francis, I. R., and Borlaza, G.: CT of renal and perirenal non-Hodgkin lymphoma. Am. J. Roentgenol., 138:1101, 1982.

Jaschke, W., VanKaick, G., Peter, S., and Palmtag, H.: Accuracy of computed tomography in staging of kidney tumors. Acta Radiol. (Diagn.), 23:593, 1982.

Karasick, S. R., and Herring, W.: Computed tomography evaluation of the poorly or nonvisualized kidney. Comput. Tomogr., 4:39, 1980.

Kittredge, R. D., Brensilver, J., and Pierce, J. C.: Computed tomography in renal transplant problems. Radiology, 127:165, 1978.

Kothari, K., Segal, A. J., Spitzer, R. M., and Peartree, R. J.: Preoperative radiographic evaluation of hypernephroma. J. Comput. Assist. Tomogr., 5:702, 1981.

Lang, E. K.: Assessment of renal trauma by dynamic computed tomography. Radiographics, *3*:566, 1983.

Lang, E. K.: Angio-computed tomography and dynamic computed tomography in staging of renal cell carcinoma. Radiology, *151*:149, 1984.

Leopold, G. R., Tainer, L. B., Asher, W. M., Gosink, B. B., and Gittes, R. F.: Renal ultrasonography: an updated approach to the diagnosis of renal cyst. Radiology, *109*:671, 1973.

Levine, E., and Huntrakoon, M.: Computed tomography of renal oncocytoma. Am. J. Roentgenol., *141*:741, 1983.

Levine, E., Lee, K. R., and Weigel, J.: Preoperative determination of abdominal extent of renal cell carcinoma by computed tomography. Radiology, *132*:395, 1979.

Love, L., Churchill, R. J., Reynes, C. J., Moncada, R., and Demos, T.: CT of the kidney and perinephric space. Semin. Roentgenol., *16*:277, 1981*a*.

Love, L., Meyers, M. A., Churchill, R. J., Reynes, C. J., Moncada, R., and Gibson, D.: Computed tomography of extraperitoneal spaces. Am. J. Roentgenol., *136*:781, 1981*b*.

Love, L., Churchill, R. J., Reynes, C., Schuster, G. A., Moncada, R., and Berkow, A.: Computed tomography staging of renal carcinoma. Urol. Radiol., *1*:3, 1979.

Luers, P. R., Lester, P. D., and Siegler, R. L.: CT demonstration of cortical nephrocalcinosis in congenital oxalosis. Pediatr. Radiol., *10*:116, 1980.

Magilner, A. D., and Ostrum, B. J.: Computed tomography in the diagnosis of renal masses. Radiology, *126*:715, 1978.

Marks, W. M., Korobkin, M., Callen, P. W., and Kaiser, J. A.: CT diagnosis of tumor thrombosis of the renal vein and inferior vena cava. Am. J. Roentgenol., *131*:843, 1978.

McAninch, J. W., and Federle, M. P.: Evaluation of renal injuries with computerized tomography. J. Urol., *128*:456, 1982.

McClennan, B. L., and Fair, W. R.: CT scanning in urology. Urol. Clin. North Am., *6*:343, 1979.

McClennan, B. L., Stanley, R. J., Melson, G. L., Levitt, R. G., and Sagel, S. S.: CT of the renal cyst: Is cyst aspiration necessary? Am. J. Roentgenol., *133*:671, 1979.

McCullough, E. C.: Factors affecting the use of quantitative information from a CT scanner. Radiology, *124*:99, 1977.

McDonald, J. E., Lee, J. K. T., McClennan, B. L., Melzer, J. S., Sicard, G. A., Etheredge, E. E., and Anderson, C. B.: Natural history of extraperitoneal gas after renal transplantation: CT demonstration. J. Comput. Assist. Tomogr., *6*:507, 1982.

Megibow, A. J., Ambos, M. A., and Bosniak, M. A.: Computed tomographic diagnosis of ureteral obstruction secondary to aneurysmal disease. Urol. Radiol., *1*:211, 1980.

Mendez, G., Jr., Isikoff, M. B., and Morillo, G.: The role of computed tomography in the diagnosis of renal and perirenal abscesses. J. Urol., *122*:582, 1979.

Meyers, M. A.: Dynamic Radiology of the Abdomen. New York, Springer-Verlag, 1982.

Morag, B., Rubinstein, Z. J., Hertz, M., and Solomon, A.: Computed tomography in the diagnosis of renal parapelvic cysts. J. Comput. Assist. Tomogr., *7*:833, 1983.

Morgan, C. L., Reed, J. E., Calkins, R. F., and Brooks, S. D.: Renal lipoma. General Electric Ultrasound Clinics Symposium *1*:1, 1980.

Nakstad, P., Kolmannskog, F., Kolbenstvedt, A., and Sødal, G.: Computed tomography in surgical complications following renal transplantation. J. Comput. Assist. Tomogr., *6*:286, 1982.

Newhouse, J. H., Prien, E. L., Amis, E. S., Jr., Dretier, S. P., and Pfister, R. C.: Computed tomographic analysis of urinary calculi. Am. J. Roentgenol., *142*:545, 1984.

Nicholson, R. L.: Abnormalities of the perinephric fascia and fat in pancreatitis. Radiology, *139*:125, 1981.

Novick, A. C., Irish, C., Steinmuller, D., Buonocore, E., and Cohen, C.: The role of computerized tomography in renal transplant patients. J. Urol., *125*:15, 1981.

O'Reilly, P. H., Osborn, D. E., Testa, H. J., Asbury, D. L., Best, J. J. K., and Barnard, R. J.: Renal imaging: a comparison of radionuclide, ultrasound, and computed tomographic scanning in investigation of renal space-occupying lesions. Br. Med. J., *282*:943, 1981.

Pagani, J. J.: Solid renal mass in the cancer patient: second primary renal cell carcinoma versus renal metastasis. J. Comput. Assist. Tomogr., *7*:444, 1983.

Parienty, R. A., Pradel, J., Picard, J-D., Ducellier, R., Lubrano, J-M., and Smolarski, N.: Visibility and thickening of the renal fascia on computed tomograms. Radiology, *139*:119, 1981*a*.

Parienty, R. A., Pradel, J., Imbert, M-C., Picard, J-D., and Savart, P. Computed tomography of multilocular cystic nephroma. Radiology, *140*:135, 1981*b*.

Parvey, L. S., Warner, R. M., Callihan, T. R., and Magill, H. L.: CT demonstration of fat tissue in malignant renal neoplasms: atypical Wilms' tumors. J. Comput. Assist. Tomogr., *5*:851, 1981.

Pazmiño, P., Pyatt, R., Williams, E., and Bohan, L.: Computed tomography in renal ischemia. J. Comput. Assist. Tomogr., *7*:102, 1983.

Pearlstein, A. E.: Hyperdense renal cysts. J. Comput. Assist. Tomogr., *7*:1029, 1983.

Pollack, H. M., Arger, P. H., Banner, M. P., Mulhern, C. B., and Coleman, B. G.: Computed tomography of renal pelvic filling defects. Radiology, *138*:645, 1981.

Pope, T. L., Jr., Buschi, A. J., Moore, T. S., Williamson, B. R. J., and Brenbridge, A. N. A. G.: CT features of renal polyarteritis nodosa. Am. J. Roentgenol., *136*:986, 1981.

Press, G., McClennan, B. L., Melson, G. L., Weyman, P. J., Lee, J. K. T., and Mauro, M.: Papillary renal cell carcinoma—CT and ultrasound evaluation. (Abstr.) Am. J. Roentgenol., *142*:237, 1984.

Probst, P., Hoogewoud, H. M., Haertel, M., Zingg, E., and Fuchs, W. A.: Computerized tomography versus angiography in the staging of malignant renal neoplasm. Br. J. Radiol., *54*:744, 1981.

Probst, P., Mahler, F., Roesler, H., and Fuchs, W. A.: Renal artery stenosis and evaluation of the effect of endoluminal dilatation. Invest. Radiol., *18*:264, 1983.

Rauschkolb, E. N., Sandler, C. M., Patel, S., and Childs, T. L.: Computed tomography of renal inflammatory disease. J. Comput. Tomogr., *6*:502, 1982.

Reed, M. D., Friedman, A. C., and Nealey, P.: Anomalies of the left renal vein: analysis of 433 CT scans. J. Comput. Assist. Tomogr., *6*:1124, 1982.

Rhyner, P., Federle, M. P., and Jeffrey, R. B.: CT of trauma to the abnormal kidney. Am. J. Roentgenol., *142*:747, 1984.

Richie, J. P., Garnick, M. B., Seltzer, S., and Bettman, M. A.: Computerized tomography scan for diagnosis and staging of renal cell carcinoma. J. Urol., *129*:1114, 1983.

Royal, S. A., and Callen, P. W.: CT evaluation of anomalies of the inferior vena cava and left renal vein. Am. J. Roentgenol., *132*:759, 1979.

Rubin, B. E.: Computed tomography in the evaluation of

renal lymphoma. J. Comput. Assist. Tomogr., *3*:759, 1979.

Sagel, S. S., Stanley, R. J., Levitt, R. G., and Geisse, G.: Computed tomography of the kidney. Radiology, *124*:359, 1981.

Sandler, C. M., and Toombs, B. D.: Computed tomographic evaluation of blunt renal injuries. Radiology, *141*:461, 1981.

Sefczek, R. J., Beckman, I., Lupetin, A. R., and Dash, N.: Sonography of acute renal cortical necrosis. Am. J. Roentgenol., *142*:553, 1984.

Segal, A. J., and Spataro, R. F.: Computed tomography of adult polycystic disease. J. Comput. Assist. Tomogr., *6*:777, 1982.

Segal, A. J., and Spitzer, R. M.: Pseudo thick-walled renal cyst by CT. Am. J. Roentgenol., *132*:827, 1979.

Segal, A. J., Spataro, R. F., Linke, C. A., Frank, I. N., and Rabinowitz, R.: Diagnosis of nonopaque calculi by computed tomography. Radiology, *129*:447, 1978.

Shanser, J. D., Hedgcock, M. W., and Korobkin, M.: Transit of contrast material into renal cysts following urography or arteriography. (Abstr.) Am. J. Roentgenol., *130*:584, 1978.

Shehadi, W. H., and Toniolo, G.: Adverse reactions to contrast media: a report from the Committee on Safety of Contrast Media of the International Society of Radiology. Radiology, *137*:299, 1980.

Sherman, J. L., Hartman, D. S., Friedman, A. C., Madewell, J. E., Davis, C. J., and Goldman, S. M.: Angiomyolipoma: computed tomographic-pathologic correlation of 17 cases. Am. J. Roentgenol., *137*:1221, 1981.

Sussman, S., Cochran, S. T., Pagani, J. J., McArdle, C., Wong, W., Austin, R., Curry, N., and Kelly, K. M.: Hyperdense renal masses: a CT manifestation of hemorrhagic renal cysts. Radiology, *150*:207, 1984.

Thierman, D., Haaga, J. R., Anton, P., and LiPuma, J. P.: Renal replacement lipomatosis. J. Comput. Assist. Tomogr., *7*:341, 1983.

Thomas, J. L., and Bernardino, M. E.: Neoplastic-induced renal vein enlargement: sonographic detection. Am. J. Roentgenol., *136*:75, 1981.

Thornbury, J. R.: Perirenal anatomy: normal and abnormal. Radiol. Clin. North Am., *17*:321, 1979.

Velasquez, G., Glass, T. A., D'Souza, V. J., and Formanek, A. G.: Multiple oncocytomas and renal carcinoma. Am. J. Roentgenol., *142*:123, 1984.

Wasserman, N. F., and Ewing, S. L.: Calcified renal oncocytoma. Am. J. Roentgenol., *141*:747, 1983.

Weyman, P. J., McClennan, B. L., Lee, J. K. T., and Stanley, R. J.: CT of calcified renal masses. Am. J. Roentgenol., *138*:1095, 1982.

Weyman, P. J., McClennan, B. L., Stanley, R. J., Levitt, R. G., and Sagel, S. S.: Comparison of computed tomography and angiography in the evaluation of renal cell carcinoma. Radiology, *137*:417, 1980.

White, E. A., Korobkin, M., and Brito, A. C.: Computed tomography of experimental acute renal ischemia. Invest. Radiol., *14*:421, 1979.

Winfield, A. C., Gerlock, A. J., and Shaff, M. I.: Perirenal cobwebs: a CT sign of renal vein thrombosis. J. Comput. Assist. Tomogr., *5*:705, 1981.

Wong, W. S., Moss, A. A., Federle, M. P., Cochran, S. T., and London, S. S.: Renal infarction: CT diagnosis and correlation between CT findings and etiologies. Radiology, *150*:201, 1984.

Yokoyama, M., Watanabe, K., Inatsuki, S., Ochi, K., and Takeuchi, M.: Measurement of renal parenchymal volume using computed tomography. J. Comput. Assist. Tomogr., *6*:975, 1982.

Computed Tomography of the Adrenal Gland

SARWAT HUSSAIN, M.B.B.S.

In radiologic imaging of the adrenal gland, the most important goal is to differentiate cases that can be surgically or medically managed. The introduction of computed tomography (CT) in the mid-1970's has entirely changed the role of other radiologic methods. Plain film, urography, and bolus nephrotomography carry an accuracy of 70 per cent for masses greater than 2 cm in diameter (Hartman et al., 1966; Abrams et al., 1982; Pickering et al., 1975). Arteriography, venography, and venous sampling are highly accurate but hazardous techniques. Hazards include hypertensive crisis, acute adrenal rupture, and the late development of Addison disease (Abrams et al., 1982; Salz et al., 1956;

Eagen and Page, 1971; Bayliss et al., 1970). High-resolution CT is noninvasive and is able to localize the adrenal glands in up to 99 per cent of cases, demonstrating lesions as small as 5 mm in diameter (Abrams et al., 1982). CT, therefore, is now established as the initial radiologic method of choice in the work-up of adrenal disease (Abrams et al., 1983; Huebener and Treugut, 1984; Adams et al., 1983; Copeland, 1983; Hattery et al., 1981; Eghrari et al., 1980). In the majority of patients, CT provides the diagnosis, and no further radiologic investigation is necessary. In the rest of the cases, a correct diagnosis is reached by angiography.

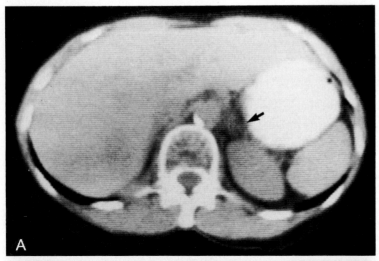

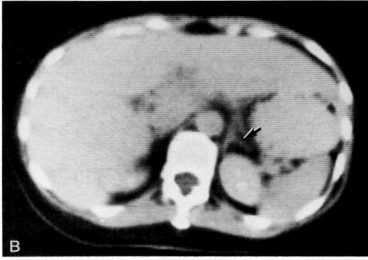

Figure 7–159. Pheochromocytoma. *A,* CT shows a small pheochromocytoma at a level (arrow) just above a normal-appearing left adrenal gland. *B,* Normal-appearing gland in the same patient (arrow).

INDICATIONS FOR CT

Candidates for CT of the adrenal gland may be divided into the following groups:

1. Those patients with signs, symptoms, or biochemical evidence of adrenal hyperfunction, or all of these.

2. Those patients with signs and symptoms of adrenal hypofunction.

3. Those patients in whom follow-up of a known adrenal mass is desired.

4. Those patients with multiple endocrine adenomatosis syndromes, types I and II, who may harbor "silent" pheochromocytomas (Moss et al., 1983).

In a small proportion of cases, angiography may be required to reach the diagnosis. One example is the patient with ectopic pheochromocytoma (Sutton, 1980). Another is the very thin patient, with a paucity of retroperitoneal fat (Moss et al., 1983); under normal circumstances, the soft tissue density of the adrenal gland stands out against the background of hypodense retroperitoneal fat. Finally, very large abdominal masses may require angiography, because CT, ultrasound, and urography may fail to differentiate adrenal from renal, hepatic, or retroperitoneal tumors (Cho, 1982).

TECHNIQUE OF CT SCANNING

Before the scanning is started, dilute iodinated contrast material (1 to 2 per cent) is administered orally to the patient to opacify the loops of the bowel. Then, 10-mm-thick contiguous sections are scanned through the upper abdomen. Once the adrenal is localized, 3- to 5-mm-thick sections are taken through the entire gland (Fig. 7–159). If a mass lesion is encountered, the adrenal scans are repeated after intravenous administration of 50 to 100 ml of 60 per cent iodinated contrast material (Moss et al., 1983). The finding of normal adrenal glands on CT when there is biochemical evidence of pheochromocytoma indicates the presence of an ectopic lesion. The CT scan must then include the lower abdomen and pelvis. If this scan is negative, a flush aortogram may be performed, followed by CT of questionable areas. If the ectopic pheochromocytoma is still undetected, selective arteriography—venography with venous sampling—is undertaken (Sutton, 1980).

CT ANATOMY

On each side of the spine, an adrenal gland is situated within the Gerota fascia in the perinephric space. The adrenal gland is firmly attached to the apex of this fascia by a fibrous band; therefore, the adrenal gland remains fixed in its location, even in the presence of renal ectopia (Abrams et al., 1982).

The right adrenal gland lies posterior to the infrahepatic portion of the inferior vena cava and the right lobe of the liver (Fig. 7–160). The right crus of the diaphragm is parallel and just medial to it. In the coronal plane, the gland is situated about 10 mm in front of the anterior vertebral tangent. On the left side, the adrenal gland lies posterior to the body and tail of the pancreas and the splenic vessels. The adjacent left crus of the diaphragm is not parallel to its

medial margin. In the coronal plane, the gland lies at the level of the aorta (Fig. 7–161). On CT (Salz et al., 1956; Eagen and Page, 1971), the length of an adrenal gland is generally 20 to 40 mm; the average cross section of the left adrenal gland is 70 to 150 mm^2, and that of the right gland is 55 to 135 mm^2 (Huebener and Treugut, 1984). Thickness has been found to be the most consistent measurement and the one most likely to vary in response to disease. The shape of the adrenal glands varies considerably on CT scans (Fig. 7–162), but the normal margins are generally straight or concave. Convex, round, or irregular margins indicate an abnormality, even when the overall size is normal.

PATHOLOGY

Adrenal disease may become apparent in a variety of ways, ranging from hypertension, electrolyte imbalance, and altered habitus to hypotension, shock, cachexia of malignancy, and sudden death. Adrenal disorders may be acute or chronic, benign or malignant. An important clinical problem is adrenal hemorrhage. This may lead to hypoadrenalism and is associated with severe septicemia, birth trauma to the newborn, renal vein thrombosis, or severe convulsions in epilepsy. For hypoadrenalism, a radiologic work-up of the adrenal glands is not commonly indicated. Patients with hyperadrenalism or with suspected adrenal mass lesions need radiologic evaluation. Adrenal masses may arise from the medulla or the cortex.

Figure 7–160. X- or K-shaped right adrenal gland. *A,* CT scan. *B,* Autopsy specimen. (From Wilms, G., et al.: J. Comput. Assist. Tomogr., *3:*467, 1979. Used by permission.)

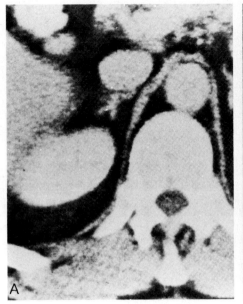
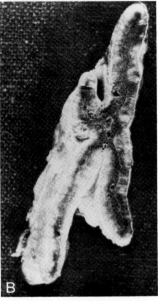

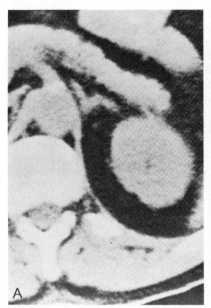
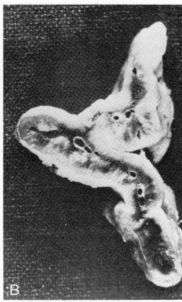

Figure 7–161. V-shaped left adrenal gland. *A,* CT scan. *B,* Autopsy specimen. (From Wilms, G., et al.: J. Comput. Assist. Tomogr., *3:*467, 1979. Used by permission.)

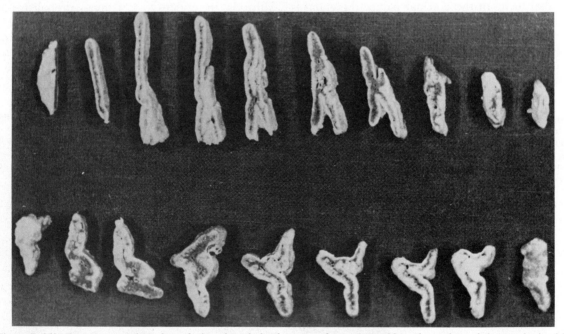

Figure 7–162. Transverse sections through the adrenal glands removed at autopsy. Note the variety of shapes obtained in this one section plane. (From Wilms, G., et al.: J. Comput. Assist. Tomogr., *3:*467, 1979. Used by permission.)

MEDULLARY ABNORMALITIES

Pheochromocytoma

Pheochromocytoma is the most common adrenal tumor. It arises from the chromaffin tissue of the adrenal medulla in 90 per cent of cases and ectopically in 10 per cent of cases (Welch et al., 1983). The most frequent ectopic location is the course of sympathetic ganglia in the para-aortic region (7 per cent); other locations include the mediastinum (1 per cent), the organ of Zuckerkandl (1 per cent), and the urinary bladder (1 per cent). As many as 10 per cent of pheochromocytomas are multicentric (Moss et al., 1983; Cho, 1982; Straube and Hodges, 1966). An increased incidence of pheochromocytoma is associated with multiple endocrine adenomatosis (MEA) syndromes, types I and II, the von Hippel–Lindau syndrome,

multiple cutaneous neuromas, and neurofibromatosis. With MEA syndromes, pheochromocytomas are intra-adrenal, bilateral, and clinically silent; sometimes they are even biochemically silent.

CT is the imaging method of choice in suspected pheochromocytoma, with an accuracy of about 95 per cent (Abrams et al., 1982; Moss et al., 1983; Tisnado et al., 1980). Most frequently, CT demonstrates a unilateral soft tissue adrenal mass between 2 and 5 cm in diameter (Welch et al., 1983). Rarely, crescentric calcification is seen. The centers of the larger tumors frequently contain areas of low attenuation, indicating the presence of hemorrhage of necrosis (Fig. 7–163). Intravenous contrast administration enhances the solid areas, thus highlighting inhomogeneity of the tumor (Moss et al., 1983; Welch et al., 1983; Tisnado et al., 1980). Ten per cent of pheochromocytomas are malig-

Figure 7–163. Large benign pheochromocytoma of the right adrenal. *A,* CT scan before contrast administration shows a homogeneous mass. *B,* Intravenous contrast highlights the solid portion of the mass.

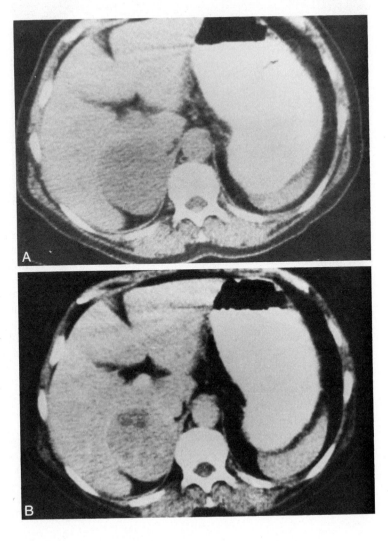

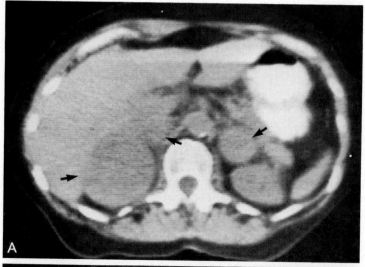

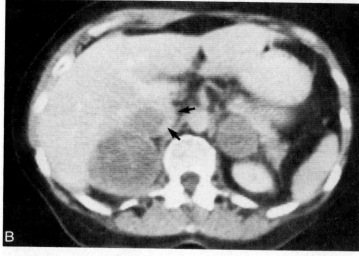

Figure 7–164. Bilateral adrenal metastases. *A*, CT scan before contrast administration shows three soft tissue masses: one mass in each adrenal and an upper pole carcinoma of the right kidney (arrows). *B*, After intravenous contrast, little enhancement of the adrenal masses is seen. The renal carcinoma shows patchy contrast enhancement. The opacified inferior vena cava is splayed around the adrenal mass (arrows).

nant and recur locally or metastasize to lymph nodes or liver. Delineation of ectopic and multiple pheochromocytomas requires angiographic evaluation when extended CT scanning of the lower abdomen and pelvis has failed to show the lesion (Sutton, 1975).

Neuroblastoma

Neuroblastoma is the most common solid tumor of childhood, occurring more often in males (MacManus, 1983). Neuroblastoma is a collective term used to describe tumors arising from the adrenal medulla and the neural crest element in the sympathetic trunk. These tumors secrete catecholamines, the metabolites of which are detectable in urine in up to 60 per cent of cases. Histologically, neuroblastomas

range from undifferentiated malignant sympathicoganglioma to benign ganglioneuroma. Hence, there is a variable clinical presentation and prognosis. In as many as 75 per cent of patients, bone, lymph node, and liver metastases are present at the time of initial diagnosis (MacManus, 1983). Spontaneous remission of the malignant variety is known to occur, especially in infants (MacManus, 1983; McLaughlin and Urich, 1977).

CT demonstrates the tumor mass, the extent of surrounding invasion, and the presence or absence of lymph node or liver metastases (Brasch et al., 1978). Administration of intravenous contrast agent usually does not lead to enhancement. Information obtained by CT contributes to initial treatment planning and to evaluation at follow-up. However, proper staging requires radiographic survey, scintigraphy, and bone marrow biopsy (MacManus, 1983).

Metastatic Disease

Because of its generous vascularity the adrenal gland is the fourth most common site of hematogenous spread of neoplastic disease (Abrams et al., 1950). Metastases to the adrenal glands are most frequently from carcinomas of the lung and breast; other malignancies are those of kidney, stomach, colon, thyroid, pancreas, and esophagus, as well as melanoma (Abrams et al., 1950). Adrenal gland metastases are asymptomatic, unless extensive parenchymal replacement of the adrenal tissue leads to hypoadrenalism. This has been most common with carcinoma of the lung (Abrams et al., 1982).

CT is the radiologic method of choice when adrenal metastatic disease is suspected and when there is need to follow known metastases (Cedermark and Ohlsen, 1981). On CT, the metastases appear most frequently as bilateral, relatively small adrenal gland masses (Fig. 7–164). However, they may be large and unilateral and may simulate a primary adrenal carcinoma (Fig. 7–165) (Dunnick et al, 1982). Large masses undergo partial necrosis and appear heterogenous. Small adrenal metastases do not enhance after intravenous contrast. Larger masses frequently enhance in a heterogenous fashion (Adams et al, 1983). Bilateral large heterogenous adrenal masses should be considered metastatic unless proved otherwise. Microscopic metastases that do not alter adrenal morphology are not detectable by radiologic means (Pagani, 1983). Rarely, direct invasion by a retroperitoneal tumor makes it difficult to identify the origin of the primary tumor (Fig. 7–166). In these instances, biopsy or angiography becomes useful (Kahn and Nickrosz, 1967).

Figure 7–165. Large left adrenal metastasis from carcinoma of lung with surrounding invasion (arrow). *A,* CT scan before contrast administration. *B,* After intravenous contrast, patchy enhancement is noted. Such metastasis can simulate primary adrenal carcinoma.

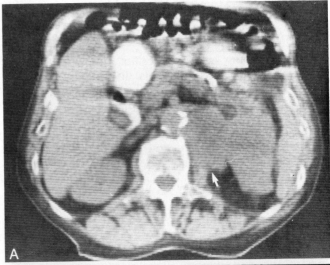

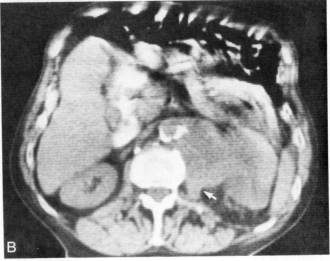

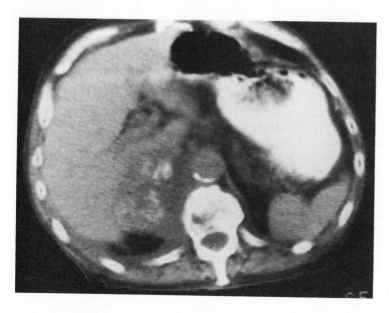

Figure 7–166. Calcific metastasis of the right adrenal from an unknown primary tumor. Note the surrounding invasion. Calcification is a rare feature of metastatic disease. It is much more common in primary adrenal carcinoma.

CORTICAL ABNORMALITIES

The Cushing Syndrome

The Cushing syndrome results from a sustained excess of glucocorticoids. In more than 80 per cent of cases, this syndrome is the result of bilateral cortical hyperplasia in response to overproduction of adrenocorticotrophic hormone (ACTH) from the anterior pituitary or, rarely, from an ectopic source. The blood ACTH levels are high. In 15 per cent of cases, the cause is an autonomous adenoma or carcinoma, in which case blood ACTH levels are low or undetectable, because ACTH secretion is suppressed by high concentrations of circulating glucocorticoids. Therefore, biochemical criteria can be used to differentiate between hyperplasia and tumors. Rarely, a tumor is ACTH-dependent, making biochemical distinction difficult. In some instances of micronodular hyperplasia, the adrenal gland may not be enlarged (Queloz et al., 1972).

CT is the initial radiologic method of choice and is usually the only study needed, because it can demonstrate enlarged glands, lateralize an adenoma, and provide a baseline study for follow-up. The most frequent CT finding in the Cushing syndrome is normal adrenal glands (Fig. 7–167). Although CT cannot exclude the diagnosis of ACTH-dependent adrenal hyperplasia, in more than 90 per cent of cases it can differentiate Cushing syndrome caused by ACTH-dependent adrenal hyperplasia from that caused by an adrenal neoplasm. Diffuse bilateral adrenal enlargement is the second most common finding. The glands are symetrically enlarged, and the borders become convex but maintain their general shape. In the remainder of patients, a mass lesion is encountered (Abrams et al., 1982; Moss et al., 1983). On CT, adrenal gland adenoma is usually seen as a 2- to 4-cm, well-defined mass, with attenuation below or equal to that of the adjacent soft tissue (Fig. 7–168). The size can range from 1 to 10 cm. Rarely, an adenoma may be cystic and may contain calcification. Adenomas seldom show contrast enhancement (Abrams et al., 1982; Adams et al., 1983; Moss et al., 1983; Sommers, 1977).

Primary Aldosteronism (the Conn Syndrome)

Primary aldosteronism results from excessive autonomous production of mineral corticoids. Seventy to 80 per cent of patients have a small, unilateral adrenal gland adenoma, which is located more frequently on the right side. The remainder have nodular cortical hyperplasia and rarely a carcinoma (Sommers, 1977).

The aim of the radiologic work-up is to differentiate adenoma from bilateral cortical hyperplasia, a distinction that is often unclear on biochemical criteria (Moss et al., 1983). Removal of the adenoma will cure hyperaldosteronism. However, bilateral adrenalectomy for hyperplasia may not be curative, and long-term medical treatment with diuretics may have to be instituted (White et al., 1980).

CT is the initial radiologic method of

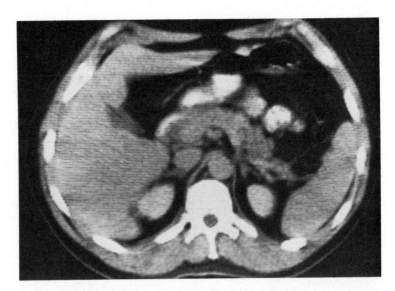

Figure 7–167. Cushing's syndrome. CT scan shows normal adrenal glands.

Figure 7–168. Cushing's syndrome: CT scan of benign left adrenal adenoma. *A*, Before contrast administration. *B*, After intravenous contrast administration, there is little enhancement. Arrow points to the remnant of the normal gland.

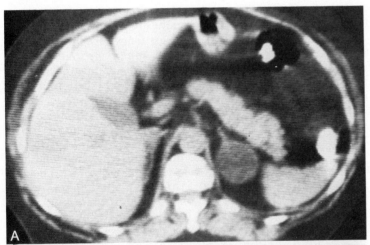

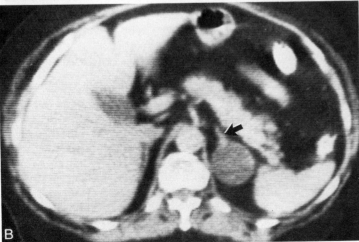

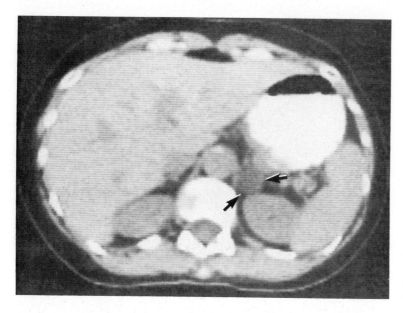

Figure 7–169. Adrenal adenoma of Conn's syndrome. Unenhanced CT scan showing a small hypodense mass of the left adrenal (arrows).

choice. In more than 90 per cent of cases, CT will correctly differentiate hyperplasia from a mass lesion. Most adenomas are small, around 1 cm in diameter, though they may range between 0.5 and 4 cm (Fig. 7–169). Using high-resolution, fast scanners, even the smaller tumors can be identified with about 85 per cent accuracy. The adenoma usually has an attenuation value lower than that of adjacent soft tissue. This is not increased by intravenous contrast administration (Adams et al., 1983; Moss et al., 1983; White et al., 1980).

Adrenal Cortical Carcinoma

Adrenal cortical carcinoma is an uncommon cancer that carries a dismal prognosis and affects all ages and both sexes. The tumor grows rapidly and, at the time of diagnosis, it is nearly always larger than 6 cm in diameter (Adams et al., 1983; Copeland, 1983; Dunnick et al., 1982). Half of all adrenal carcinomas are functioning and half are not. Functioning tumors result in the excretion of large amounts of 17-ketosteroids in the urine. Clinically, these tumors are found in patients with Cushing syndrome, adrenogenital syndrome, precocious puberty and, rarely, Conn syndrome, or any combination of these (Copeland, 1983). Nonfunctioning adrenal carcinomas are frequently discovered incidentally during radiologic work-up of unrelated disease.

The purpose of CT scanning, an imaging method of choice for this lesion, is to delineate the extent of the tumor. This is important in planning radical local surgery or in predicting prognosis for patients who do not undergo operation (Copeland, 1983; Dunnick et al., 1982). On CT, an adrenal cortical carcinoma is seen as a large mass, usually lobulated in outline and heterogenous in consistency. Enhancement of the solid areas of the tumor invariably occurs after intravenous contrast administration (Fig. 7–170). Clinically unsuspected local invasion of surrounding structures and distant metastases to lymph nodes, liver, and retroperitoneum are seen in about one third of all patients at initial evaluation (Fig. 7–171) (Copeland, 1983). Also, one third of all adrenal carcinomas will show tumor calcification at radiologic evaluation (Dunnick et al., 1982). When the tumor is very large, it may be impossible to confirm its origin by CT. In these cases, arteriography is indicated to define the vascular pedicle of the tumor (Sutton, 1975).

Adrenogenital Syndrome

Virilization in infants and children is most commonly associated with congenital bilateral cortical hyperplasia in the adrenogenital syndrome. The adrenal glands are hyperplastic as the result of an inborn error in steroid synthesis, which leads to high levels of circulating ACTH. In older children and adults, virilization or feminization is strongly suggestive of adrenal carcinoma until proved otherwise (Sommers, 1977). CT criteria for diagnosing hyperplasia and adrenal masses are applicable in these diseases.

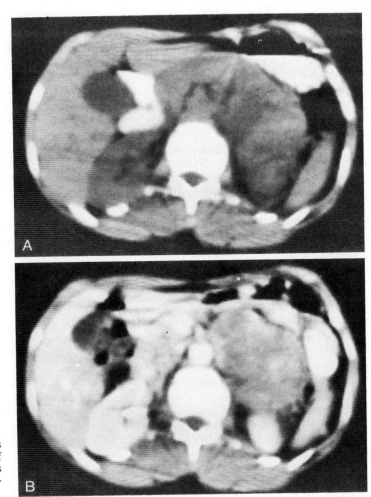

Figure 7–170. Adrenal cortical carcinoma. *A,* CT scan before contrast injection shows a large lobulated mass with displacement of surrounding viscera. *B,* After intravenous contrast administration, there is heterogeneous enhancement.

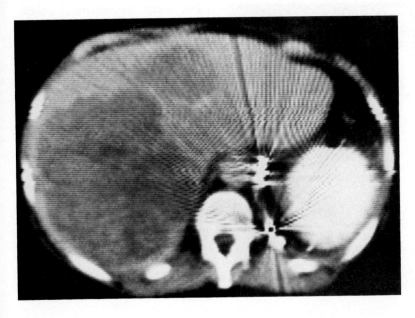

Figure 7–171. Extensive liver metastases on CT scan 3 months after the removal of the adrenal carcinoma shown in Figure 7–170.

Assessment of Tumor Pathology

Although CT is an excellent method of demonstrating morbid anatomy, a diagnosis of specific adrenal gland pathology is rarely rendered by this imaging technique alone. However, when biochemical findings are paired with radiologic observations, a correct diagnosis usually results. Clearly, it is important to be able to differentiate primary malignant from benign masses radiologically. Prognosis is greatly improved by early diagnosis and surgical removal of adrenal carcinoma (Copeland, 1983). Three CT features help to differentiate malignant from benign adrenal masses. They are (1) size, (2) contrast enhancement, and (3) heterogenous consistency of the tumor. Malignant adrenal tumors grow rapidly and are, therefore, generally larger than benign masses.

Many workers have suggested an arbitrary size threshold—3, 4, and 6 cm, for example—beyond which an adrenal mass should be considered malignant (Copeland, 1983; Prinz et al., 1982). Clearly, the size of any mass is a function of time, so this criterion alone seems unreliable for excluding the possibility of primary carcinoma. Contrast enhancement and heterogenous consistency of the mass have also been highly correlated with malignancy (Adams, et al., 1983).

Furthermore, it is important to distinguish metastatic deposits from other adrenal masses. Benign adrenal adenomas are almost never bilateral. Metastatic lesions usually are (Ceder-mark and Ohlsen, 1981). Also, CT-guided fine needle biopsy and short-term follow-up of a demonstrably enlarging lesion helps to differentiate metastatic deposits from benign ones (Copeland, 1983; Prinz et al., 1982). Sometimes, the diagnostic dilemma will persist. Pheochromocytoma, for example, can be large and heterogenous and can slow contrast enhancement. Differentiation of malignant from benign lesions is usually possible on CT, but the functional status of the tumor is currently impossible to predict.

Nonfunctioning and Incidental Adrenal Gland Masses

Adrenal gland masses can be present in patients who show no biochemical or clinical evidence of hyperadrenalism. Such lesions are encountered in up to 0.6 per cent of all abdominal CT scans and at 2 to 8 per cent of autopsies (Copeland, 1983). Nonfunctioning adrenal masses are detected more frequently by CT than by any other radiologic modality. The majority are adenomas (Fig. 7–172) (Prinz et al., 1982). Larger masses are more likely to be carcinomas, cysts, myelolipomas, hematomas, and metastases (Glazer et al., 1982). Adenomas are most common in elderly, hypertensive, and diabetic individuals, and also in patients with carcinomas of the bladder, kidney, and endometrium (Prinz et al., 1982; Glazer et al., 1982). Differentiation from metastasis may be difficult.

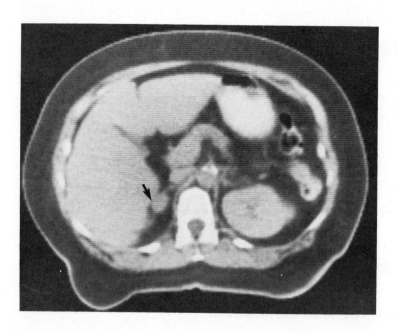

Figure 7–172. Nonfunctioning adrenal adenoma: Unenhanced CT scan shows a small soft tissue mass of the right adrenal (arrow). This mass was detected incidentally during the work-up of suspected pancreatic disease. The pancreas was normal.

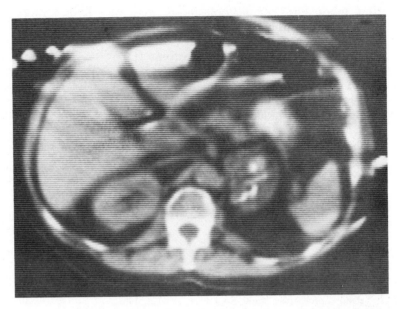

Figure 7–173. Calcific adrenal adenoma: Unenhanced CT scan showing large left adrenal mass discovered incidentally. The patient did not have any clinical or biochemical evidence of adrenal dysfunction. At surgery an unusually large benign adenoma was removed.

On CT, an adenoma appears as a well-defined soft tissue mass of 3 cm or less in diameter that does not enhance after intravenous contrast. Rarely, calcification is seen. In patients with primary nonadrenal malignancy, particularly of the lung, an adrenal mass has at least a 40 per cent chance of being metastatic (Oliver et al., 1983).

Benign incidental adrenal masses do not require excision. On CT, a myelolipoma appears as a large (up to 12 cm), hypodense mass that contains largely fat, with varying amounts of soft tissue. Fluid-filled adrenal cysts can attain large size. Adrenal hemorrhage is depicted on CT as either diffuse bilateral adrenal enlargement or as a unilateral mass. The density of the mass depends upon the age of the hematoma (Moss et al., 1983). As the hematomas grow older, the high density of acute hemorrhage and its mass effect gradually diminish. In chronic stages, adrenal hematomas lead to adrenal calcification without mass effect (Brasch et al., 1978).

Adrenal Calcification

Adrenal calcification can be seen in asymptomatic individuals (Fig. 7–173). This may be a result of childhood hemorrhage or infection without associated hypoadrenalism (Jarvis and Seaman, 1959). Addison disease that results

Figure 7–174. Wolman's disease: symmetric, punctate calcification in bilaterally enlarged adrenal glands. (From Queloz, J. M., et al: Radiology, *104*:357, 1972. Used by permission.)

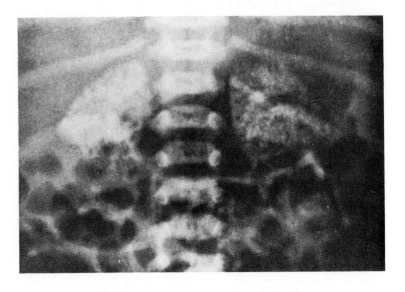

from tuberculosis or histoplasmosis may be manifested by adrenal calcification (Wilson et al., 1984). Irregular calcification is usually seen with both carcinoma and neuroblastoma (Dunnick et al., 1982; MacManus, 1983). Benign masses tend to show dense or arclike calcification. In Wolman disease, a lethal form of infantile lipoidosis, both adrenal glands are enlarged and show pathognomonic symmetric punctate calcification (Fig. 7–174) (Queloz et al., 1972). Generally, adrenal gland calcification associated with a mass lesion is more likely to be pathologically significant than a calcification without a mass.

References

Abrams, H. L., Siegelman, S. S., Adams, D. F., et al.: Computed tomography versus ultrasound of the adrenal gland: a prospective study. Radiology, *143*:121, 1982.

Abrams, H. L., Spiro, R., Goldstein, N.: Metastases in carcinoma. Analysis of 1000 autopsied cases. Cancer, *3*:74, 1950.

Adams, J. E., Johnson, R. J., Rickards, D., and Isherwood, I.: Computed tomography in adrenal disease. Clin. Radiol., *34*:39, 1983.

Bayliss, R. I., Edwards, O. M., and Starer, F.: Complications of adrenal venography. Br. J. Radiol., *43*:531, 1970.

Brasch, R. C., Korobkin, M., and Gooding, C. A.: Computed body tomography in children: evaluation of 45 patients. A.J.R., *131*:21, 1978.

Cedermark, B. J., and Ohlsen, H.: Computed tomography in the diagnosis of metastases of the adrenal glands. Surg. Gynecol. Obstet., *152*:13, 1981.

Cho, K. J.: Current role of angiography in the evaluation of adrenal disease causing hypertension. Urol. Radiol., *3*:249, 1982.

Copeland, P. M.: The incidentally discovered adrenal mass. Ann. Intern. Med., *98*:940, 1983.

Dunnick, N. R., Heaston, D., Halvorsen, R., More, A. V., and Korobkin, M.: CT appearance of adrenal cortical carcinoma. J. Comput. Assist. Tomogr. *6*:978, 1982.

Eagen, R. T., and Page, M. I.: Adrenal insufficiency following bilateral adrenal venography. J.A.M.A., *215*:115, 1971.

Eghrari, M., McLoughlin, M. J., Rosen, I. E., et al.: The role of computed tomography in assessment of tumoral pathology of the adrenal glands. J. Comput. Assist. Tomogr., *4*:71, 1980.

Glazer, H. S., Weyman, P. J., Sagel, S. S., Levitt, R. G., and McClennon, B. L.: Nonfunctioning adrenal masses: incidental discovery on computed tomography. A.J.R., *139*:81, 1982.

Goss, C. M. (ed.): Gray's Anatomy. Philadelphia, Lea & Febiger, 1973, p. 1349.

Hartman, C. W., Witton, D. M., and Weeks, R. E.: The role of nephrotomography in diagnosis of adrenal tumours. Radiology, *86*:1030, 1966.

Hattery, R. R., Sheedy, P. F., II, Stephens, D. H., and Van Heerden, J. A.: Computed tomography of the adrenal gland. Semin. Roentgenol. *16*:290, 1981.

Huebener, K. H., and Treugut, H.: Adrenal cortical dysfunction: CT findings. Radiology, *150*:195, 1984.

Jarvis, J. L., and Seaman, W. B.: Idiopathic adrenal calcification in infants and children. A.J.R., *82*:510, 1959.

Kahn, P. C., and Nickrosz, L. V.: Selective angiography of the adrenal glands. A.J.R., *101*:739, 1967.

MacManus, M.: The diagnosis and staging of neuroblastoma. Clin. Radiol., *34*:523, 1983.

McLaughlin, J. E., and Urich, H.: Maturing neuroblastoma and ganglion neuroblastoma: a study of four cases with long survival. J. Pathol., *121*:19, 1977.

Meschan, I.: Synopsis of Radiologic Anatomy with Computed Tomography. Philadelphia, W. B. Saunders Co., 1978, p. 534.

Montagne, J.-P., Kressel, H. Y., Korobkin, M., and Moss, A. A.: Computed tomography of the normal adrenal glands. A.J.R., *130*:963, 1978.

Moss, A. A., Gamsu, G., and Genant, H. K.: Computed Tomography of the Body. Philadelphia, W. B. Saunders, Co., 1983, p. 860.

Oliver, T. W., Bernardino, M. E., Miller, J., Sones, P. E., and Mansour, K.: The significance of isolated adrenal masses in the patients with non-small cell bronchogenic carcinoma (Ab). Radiology, *149*:63, 1983.

Pagani, J. J.: Normal adrenal glands in small cell lung carcinoma: CT guided biopsy. Am. J. Roentgenol., *140*:949, 1983.

Pickering, R. S., Hartman, G. W., Week, R. E., Sheps, S. G., and Hattery, R. R.: Excretory urographic localization of adrenal cortical tumors and pheochromocytomas. Radiology, *114*:345, 1975.

Prinz, R. A., Brooks, M. H., Churchill, R., et al.: Incidental asymptomatic adrenal masses detected by computed tomographic scanning: is operation required? JAMA, *248*:701, 1982.

Queloz, J. M., Capitanio, M. A., and Kirkpatrick, J. A.: Wolman's disease: Roentgen observations in 3 siblings. Radiology, *104*:357, 1972.

Salz, N. J., Luttwak, E. M., Schwarz, A., and Goldberg, G. M.: Danger of aortography in the localization of phaeochromocytoma. Ann. Surg., *144*:118, 1956.

Solomon, A., and Kreel, L.: Computed tomographic assessment of adrenal masses. Clin. Radiol., *31*:137, 1980.

Sommers, S. C.: Adrenal glands. In Anderson, W. A. D., and Kissane, J. M., (Eds.): Pathology. Vol. 2. St. Louis, The C. V. Mosby Co., 1977, p. 1658.

Straube, K. R., and Hodges, C. V.: Phaeochromocytoma and renal artery stenosis. A.J.R., *98*:222, 1966.

Sutton, D.: The radiological diagnosis of adrenal tumours. Br. J. Radiol., *48*:237, 1975.

Sutton, D.: A Textbook of Radiology and Imaging. Edinburgh, Churchill Livingstone, 1980, p. 809.

Tisnado, J., Amendola, M. A., Konerding, K. F., Shirazik, K., and Beachley, M. C.: Computed tomography versus angiography in the localization of pheochromocytoma. J. Comput. Assist. Tomogr., *4*:853, 1980.

Welch, T. J., Sheedy, P. F., Van Heerden, J. A., Sheps, S. G., Hattery, R. R., and Stephens, D. H.: Pheochromocytoma: value of computed tomography. Radiology, *148*:501, 1983.

White, E. A., Schambelan, M., Rost, C. R., Biglieri, E G., Moss, A. A., and Korobkin, M.: Use of computed tomography in diagnosing the cause of primary aldosteronism. N. Engl. J. Med., *303*:1503, 1980.

Wilms, G., Baert, A., Marchal, G., and Goddeeris, P.: CT of the normal adrenal glands: correlative study with autopsy specimens. J. Comput. Assist. Tomogr., *3*:467, 1979.

Wilson, D. A., Muchmore, H. G., Tisdal, R. G., Fahmy, A., and Pitha, J. V.: Histoplasmosis of the adrenal glands studied by CT. Radiology, *150*:779, 1984.

Renal and Adrenal Angiography*

HERBERT L. ABRAMS, M.D.
DOUGLASS F. ADAMS, M.D.

RENAL ARTERIOGRAPHY

In virtually all areas of visceral and peripheral disease, sophisticated radiology has been a requisite for proper development of a sophisticated surgical approach. This is equally true whether one is dealing with cerebral pneumography and arteriography in brain surgery, barium studies in gastrointestinal surgery, or contrast studies in renal surgery. Just 10 years after the discovery of x-rays, Voelcker and von Lichtenberg (1906) demonstrated the application of retrograde pyelography and introduced a new precision to appraisal of the renal collecting and excretory system. Not until the late 1920's, however, when Binz and Rath (1928) synthesized an organic iodine that Swick (1929) demonstrated could opacify the urinary tract on excretion, was intravenous urography introduced to the medical world. In the same year, dos Santos et al. (1929) described translumbar aortography and initiated the era of opacification of the aorta and its great abdominal branches.

During the decade of the 1940's, Doss et al. (1942) and Wagner (1946) applied translumbar aortography to the study of renal disease. A relatively blind approach to renal artery opacification, it was largely supplanted by transfemoral renal arteriography after the description by Seldinger (1953) of his ingenious method of catheter placement within the femoral artery. With the broad application of the Seldinger technique to transfemoral angiography, it was only a matter of time before selective deposition of the contrast agent in the renal artery was accomplished, initiating the modern era of high-resolution visualization of the intrarenal vascular bed. Without renal arteriography, it is inconceivable that the treatment of renovascular hypertension and the procedure of renal transplantation could possibly have reached their present status.

TECHNICAL CONSIDERATIONS

Equipment

The optimal angiographic suite requires high-powered x-ray equipment, cesium iodide image amplification, and rapid filming systems that record the radiographic image with fine detail. A description of the various types of film changers is beyond the scope of this section, but it must be emphasized that whether cassette changers, cut-film changers, or roll-film changers are employed, constant vigilance and preventive maintenance are required to sustain the quality of the examinations. There is no excuse for invasive procedures performed on ill patients that fail to yield the best radiographic information available. With 3-phase 1000-mA generators, short exposure times and low-kilovoltage techniques are available to optimize the contrast of the examinations.

Examination Technique

With few exceptions, it is essential to precede selective renal arteriography by bolus aortography. This may be accomplished by tip-occluded, straight, J-shaped, or loop catheters with multiple side holes inserted percutaneously by the Seldinger technique (Fig. 7–175). The catheter is always placed under fluoroscopic control at the level of the renal arteries, usually just below or at the L1–L2 interspace. This helps to decrease opacification of the celiac artery and the superior mesenteric artery and to reduce the number of superimposed vessels during the examination (Fig. 7–176). A useful centering point for the x-ray beam is halfway between the umbilicus and the xyphoid. Usually this will place the central ray just under the origin of the renal arteries.

A mechanical injector must be employed for the aortographic examination. Renografin 70 per cent (50 ml) is injected at a rate of 25 ml per second, and filming is accomplished at four per second for 2 seconds, two per second for 2

*This work was supported in part by USPHS grants HL11668, HL05832, and GM18674.

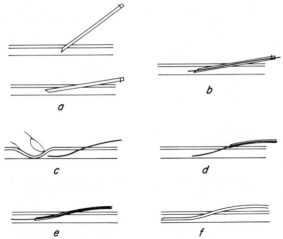

Figure 7–175. Seldinger technique of transfemoral arteriography. The needle is inserted into the artery *(a)*. A metal guidewire is passed through the needle into the artery *(b)*. The artery is compressed while the needle is removed; the metal guidewire remains in the artery *(c)*. The catheter is passed over the guidewire to the arterial wall *(d)*. The catheter is passed into the artery *(e)*. The guidewire is removed, and the catheter passed to the level of the renal arteries *(f)*.

seconds, one per second for 6 seconds, and one every 3 seconds for 15 seconds. This provides a comprehensive evaluation of the arterial, nephrographic, and venous phases of the arteriogram. In patients with rapid aortic run-off, the Valsalva maneuver will afford better opacification of the intrarenal vascular bed during aortography (Fig. 7–177) (Bergstrand and Sorensen, 1965; Abrams et al., 1967).

If the femoral pulses are absent, translumbar aortography is a simple but less desirable approach to bolus aortography. Still another method is percutaneous transaxillary catheter insertion via the left axillary artery.

The aortogram is important as a screening study to demonstrate the number, size, and condition of the main renal arteries and the relationship of the arterial origins to the aorta and to aortic disease (Figs. 7–176 and 7–177). Adequate visualization of the main renal arteries is usually obtained, and the procedure may be satisfactory for delineation of renovascular disease.

Selective arteriography is accomplished using a No. 7 thin-walled opaque polyethylene catheter with a bend somewhat greater than 90 degrees and a 2.5-cm tip (Fig. 7–178). Longer tips are difficult to introduce selectively because they cannot assume the proper angle. Long tips may also protrude too far into the renal artery and occlude it if renal artery stenosis is present. This is also true of selective injections of supplemental arteries. Free backflow is essential. It is imperative that the position of the tip of the catheter be demonstrated with a 1-ml test bolus as soon as it is placed in the artery. The catheter is then adjusted so that the tip is free and the contrast "washes out" of the artery. Failure to employ a test injection may result in subintimal injection or spasm that may be confused with an obstructing arterial lesion. Anteroposterior and oblique projections are essential, and angled views may be useful in providing more precise information about the degree and loca-

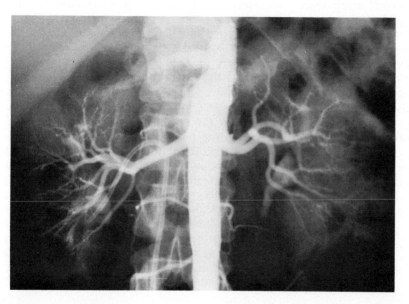

Figure 7–176. Normal renal arteriogram, aortic injection. A tip-occluded catheter has been used, and 38 ml of 76 per cent Renografin injected. The renal arterial branches are smooth and arborize normally. There is relatively little contrast material in the celiac axis and superior mesenteric artery, allowing good definition of the intrarenal branches without superimposed vessels. A catheter extends from the inferior vena cava into the right renal vein.

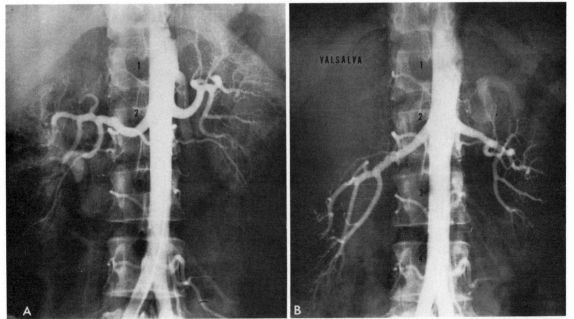

Figure 7–177. Normal renal arteriography. *A,* During expiration. The vessels arborize normally. There is minimal irregularity of the right renal artery. *B,* During the Valsalva maneuver. The kidneys are now in a position far more caudal than during the initial study. The renal arteries are stretched and uncoiled. The minimal fibromuscular hyperplasia of the right renal artery has no dynamic significance. Split function studies demonstrated equivalent renal plasma flows on both sides.

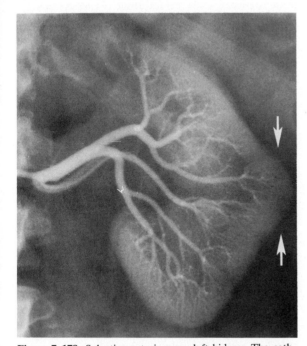

Figure 7–178. Selective arteriogram, left kidney. The catheter tip has been placed beyond the bifurcation of the main renal artery. As a consequence, there has been only flash filling of the dorsal renal arterial branch, while the ventral renal artery is well filled. The artifactual lack of opacification of the central medial portion of the kidney and the upper pole might well have been interpreted as a large area of infarction. Note the presence of a "dromedary hump" (arrows). This represents a normal variation.

tion of multiple areas of stenosis of the renal arteries (Harrington et al., 1983).

Selective renal arteriography provides optimal visualization of the intrarenal vascular bed for two reasons: There is maximal concentration of contrast agent with replacement of blood flow, and there is no superimposition of other visceral arteries such as occurs at times with aortic injections (Fig. 7–179). We prefer a catheter without side holes and an injection of 8 ml per second for 1.5 seconds (total 12 ml) of 76 per cent Renografin for selective studies. When renal carcinoma is observed, a larger volume of contrast agent (25 ml) may be injected selectively in order to evaluate the presence of renal vein involvement by tumor. There is little concern about harm to the kidney because it will be removed at surgery after demonstration of the carcinoma.

Limitations peculiar to the selective technique include failure to demonstrate the aortic origin of the arteries, tedious searching for supplemental branches, and multiple runs for each kidney. At times the catheter tip may be placed beyond a major branch, producing only partial filling of the renal vessels and a factitious appearance of infarction (Fig. 7–178). On the other hand, selective arteriography provides an optimal look at the small vessels of the kidney, particularly when combined with magnification.

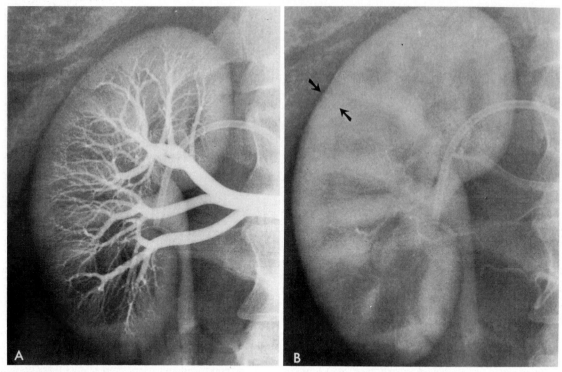

Figure 7–179. Normal renal arteriography. *A*, Arterial phase, right kidney. The main renal artery, interlobar arteries, and arcuate arteries are clearly visible. *B*, Nephrographic phase. Contrast has disappeared from the renal arteries, and there is a diffuse increase in density of the kidney. The density increase is greatest in the cortical tissue, which can now be readily measured (arrows).

There are many important details of preparation, anesthesia, needle and catheter insertion, and choice of guidewires, catheters, and needles with which the angiographer must be familiar. Further details are available in the books by Abrams (1983*a*) and Kincaid (1966) and in the report of the Inter-Society Commission on Heart Disease Resources (Judkins et al., 1976).

Contrast Agents

The popular contrast agents of two decades ago, such as Diodrast, Neoiopax, and Urokon, have long since been discarded from general use because of their toxicity. In their place, the diatrizoate agents (Hypaque and Renografin) have proved their value in many intravascular procedures, and, more recently, iothalamate (Conray) and metrizoate (Isopaque) have been widely employed.

As a means of reducing the osmotic activity of the contrast agents, which appears to be integral to their physiologic effects, interest has focused on increasing the molecular size. Almen and his coworkers have described studies with polymers such as metrizamide (Tragardh et al.,

1975). These substances obviate many of the immediate effects of the contrast agent, such as the sensation of burning at the time of injection (Almen et al., 1975). Iohexol and Iopamidol are two nonionic compounds currently under investigation (Bettmann, 1982; Mancini et al., 1983).

None of the opaque media currently in use is entirely satisfactory. The diatrizoate drugs have received very wide acceptance and are the media of choice in many institutions. We prefer Renografin, an agent that we have used for many years and with which we feel relatively comfortable. Nevertheless, the nonionic agents are very promising.

Although uncommon, reactions to contrast agents must be anticipated, and the angiographer must be aware of them. They fall into several groups: cardiovascular, respiratory, neurologic, gastrointestinal, cutaneous, and miscellaneous (Abrams, 1983*c*). It is essential that awareness of the types of reactions that may occur be coupled with careful preparation to handle the major life-threatening reactions immediately. In recent years, the effect on renal function has been emphasized, and some investigators have reported a high incidence of renal failure following arteriography (Older et al., 1976; Swartz et al., 1978). Others have reported an incidence of acute renal failure of 0.15 per cent in patients following intravenous contrast agent administration (Byrd and Sherman, 1979).

COMPLICATIONS OF RENAL ARTERIOGRAPHY

There is a small but significant risk attached to the performance of renal arteriography. Anaphylactoid reactions, renal damage, and urologic complications have received a good deal of attention in the past. The diatrizoate agents have given us a margin of safety not previously available, and the nonionic agents will increase the margin of safety. Nevertheless, as noted earlier, alterations in renal function must be anticipated in some patients. The neurologic complications observed in the past were generally associated with translumbar aortography rather than with transfemoral or selective renal arteriography.

There are significant complications associated with the insertion of the catheter, particularly at the entrance site. Local bleeding, arterial thrombosis, arterial dissection by the guidewire and the catheter, dislodgment of atheromatous plaques or thrombi, false aneurysm formation, and arteriovenous fistula have all been reported as complications of the procedure (McAfee, 1971). A recent survey (Table 7–5) indicates that there has been a significant decrease within the past decade in the incidence of complications, but it must be emphasized that there remains a small mortality and a significant morbidity. The recent use of heparin and heparinized catheters has been an important step toward the reduction of thromboembolic complications. The transaxillary and translumbar methods have a higher complication rate than the transfemoral approach.

THE NORMAL RENAL ARTERIOGRAM

Arterial Phase

The main renal arteries, although described as dorsal branches, are usually lateral or anterolateral in origin, arising from the aorta at, slightly above, or slightly below the interspace between L1 and L2. In 72 per cent of cadavers, there are single vessels of approximately equal size bilaterally (Merklin and Michaels, 1958). The diameter of the renal artery varies in normal subjects between 6 and 10 mm as measured angiographically (Edsman, 1957) and increases with advancing age. The right renal artery, arising from the aorta at or just to the right of the midline, is usually longer than the left renal artery. Supplemental renal arteries frequently pose a problem for selective angiography because they are sometimes time-consuming to find and to film and, if small, may easily be obstructed by the catheter tip. Their range of origin is wide, from T11 down to the iliac vessels. Rarely, supplemental branches may arise from visceral aortic branches (Merklin and Michaels, 1958).

The kidney may be divided into dorsal and ventral segments, and the arteries to these segments can usually be readily identified. Graves (1954) divides the kidney into five segments, recognizing two anterior and one posterior segments in the middle of the kidney and a small apical and a larger caudal segment. The orientation of the kidney is such that the dorsal arteries are usually medial; the dorsal segments and subsegments are not border-forming at the lateral margin of the kidney in the true anteroposterior projection (Boijsen, 1959). The ven-

TABLE 7–5. COMPLICATIONS OF ANGIOGRAPHY

	Femoral	Axillary	Translumbar
Number of cases	83,068	4,590	4,118
Deaths*	0.03%	0.09%	0.05%
Cardiac complications	0.29%	0.26%	0.36%
Neurologic complications (including convulsions)	0.23%	0.61%	0.02%
Local arterial obstructions*	0.14%	0.76%	0.02%
Hemorrhage*	0.27%	0.68%	0.53%
Subintimal injection* or perforation	0.44%	0.37%	1.75%
Catheter or wire breakage*	0.08%	0.02%	0.02%

*Significant differences among techniques (P<0.05).

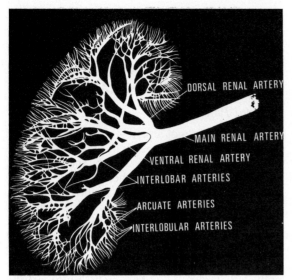

DORSAL RENAL ARTERY

MAIN RENAL ARTERY

VENTRAL RENAL ARTERY

INTERLOBAR ARTERIES

ARCUATE ARTERIES

INTERLOBULAR ARTERIES

Figure 7–180. Normal selective renal arteriogram, diagrammatic representation. Tracing demonstrates the gradual, normal diminution in size as the vessels arborize and extend out to the cortex.

tral arteries run laterally, and the ventral subsegments are border-forming along the lateral aspect of the kidney. The lower pole is usually supplied by the ventral vessel and frequently by a single arterial branch; the dorsal vessel extends cephalad to supply a variable part of the superior pole. Although the typical separation of the main renal artery into major dorsal and ventral branches is readily appreciated in most patients, there are significant differences in the branching patterns. In Figure 7–178, the ventral renal artery is visualized subserving the ventral lateral aspects of the kidney as well as the lower pole. Because the catheter tip is beyond the bifurcation, there is only flash filling of the dorsal renal artery, and the failure of filling (particularly of the dorsal segments to the middle and upper portions of the kidney) is readily appreciated.

The main branches divide at the renal hilus into proximal interlobar arteries, which subsequently divide into branch interlobar arteries (Fig. 7–180). The interlobar arteries ultimately terminate in the arcuate arteries. The interlobular arteries supplying the cortex of the kidney originate from the arcuate vessels. A careful analysis of the normal arborization of distal vessels demonstrates a reproducible, even, and regular progression to smaller and smaller vessels that have a straight or mildly curved course (Figs. 7–179 and 7–180). Normal vessels taper uniformly and evenly. With high-quality conventional radiography, the interlobular vessels

may readily be appreciated as linear parallel densities in the cortex of the kidney (Fig. 7–181). With optimal technique, failure to visualize them raises serious questions as to the presence of interlobular artery vasoconstriction. Furthermore, the interlobular arteries furnish an index of the thickness of the cortex. The linear densities that are visualized do not represent single vessels but rather summation shadows. With high-quality magnification views, particularly in animal subjects, it is possible to visualize summated shadows of glomeruli as small, dense, punctate dots in the cortex of the kidney.

Nephrographic Phase

The nephrographic phase follows the arterial phase at approximately 5 to 8 seconds and shows the distribution of the contrast agent both in the capillary bed and in the renal excretory tissue (Figs. 7–179B and 7–182B). During a brief capillary period, the nephrographic density represents the contrast in the capillary bed; in the subsequent stage of the nephrogram, contrast is mixed with urine in the tubules and collecting ducts (Edling et al., 1959). These phases overlap because of the duration of injection and the distribution of vessels. In addition to the generally increased density of the entire kidney, the cortex in the normal kidney is usually well defined and its width measurable as a dense, homogeneous band about 5 to 8 mm thick.

The nephrogram may be particularly useful when it demonstrates a local area of ischemia. Adequate nephrographic films are an integral part of every renal arteriogram. A normal nephrogram reflects a normal renal vascular bed in most instances and presents an opportunity to analyze most precisely the outlines of the kidney and to detect small cysts, infarcts, or abnormalities of contour that may not be appreciated on the urogram or on the arterial phase.

Venous Phase

About 7 to 12 seconds after injection of the contrast agent, the major renal veins become visible. Because maximal opacification may occur late, it is essential that an extended angiographic series of films be obtained (Fig. 7–182C). The renal venous anatomy is discussed in detail in the next section of this chapter, but here it must be emphasized that arteriography frequently furnishes valuable information about the integrity of the venous system. Although the failure to visualize the veins does not necessarily mean renal vein thrombosis or invasion

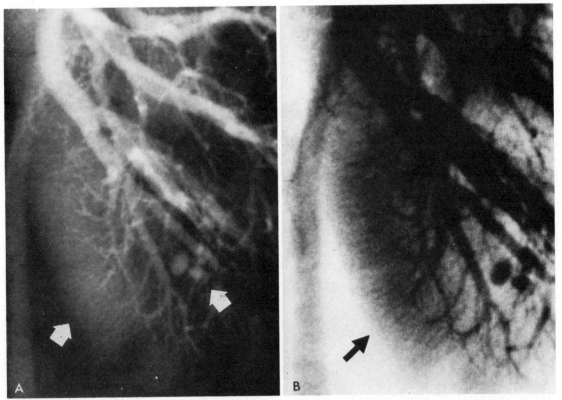

Figure 7–181. Interlobular arteries. *A* and *B,* Arteriogram and subtraction arteriogram. The linear densities to which the medial arrows point represent the interlobular vessels extending through the cortex of the kidney. These are summated shadows rather than individual interlobular arteries. Incidentally noted is an arteriovenous malformation of the kidney (lateral arrow in *A*).

by tumor, the presence of multiple collateral venous channels strongly suggests renal vein obstruction.

INDICATIONS FOR RENAL ARTERIOGRAPHY

During the past decade, the role of renal arteriography in the diagnostic evaluation of patients with renal disease has become well established. Although there are significant variations in the frequency with which it is applied to specific problems, the increased precision and decreased morbidity that have accompanied its wider application have rendered it an invaluable element in the diagnostic work-up of large groups of patients. In the sequence of radiologic diagnostic procedure, intravenous urography is almost invariably the first examination to which the patient is exposed. Depending on the nature of his problem, he may then be referred for nephrotomography, diagnostic ultrasound, com-

puted tomography, cyst puncture, or arteriography.

There are two broad echelons of indications, overlapping in character: the symptoms and signs with which the patient presents, and the suspected diagnosis based on the clinical and urographic findings. Although the symptoms and signs are usually indications for urography *per primum*, they are briefly discussed here in relationship to the ultimate likelihood of arteriography being performed.

Symptoms and Signs

Hematuria. Hematuria, unless associated with calculus and unless clearly localized to the lower urinary tract, almost invariably requires angiography. When the urogram is abnormal, arteriography lends greater precision to the diagnosis. With a normal urogram, angiography may reveal the presence of small arteriovenous malformations, renal vein varices, or small neoplasms.

Pain. Pain related to the upper urinary tract

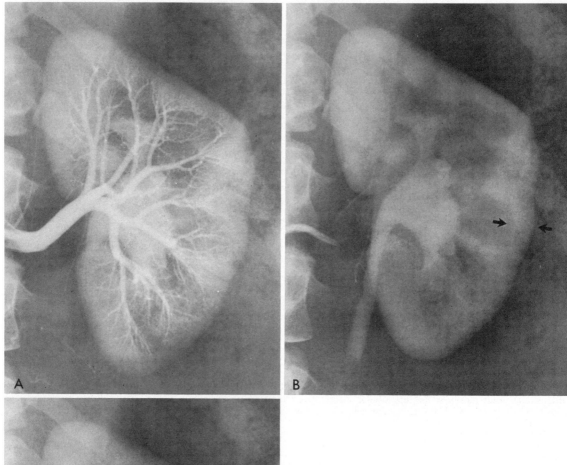

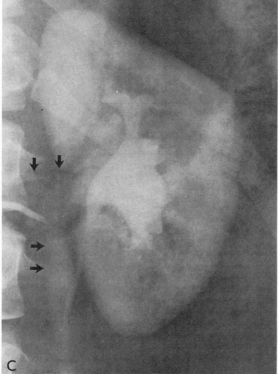

Figure 7–182. Selective renal arteriography. *A*, Arterial phase. Note the relatively distal bifurcation of the main renal arteries. The major interlobar branches drape themselves around the pyramids, the more lucent areas. *B*, Nephrographic phase (6-second film). The cortex is relatively dense (arrows) compared with the pyramids. *C*, Venous phase (112 seconds). The main renal vein is faintly opacified (upper arrows), and there is filling also of the ovarian vein, a relatively common phenomenon in renal arteriography.

is frequently localized in the flanks or lumbar region, may be sharp or dull, may simply represent a sense of discomfort, and may be intermittent or constant. Depending on the urographic findings, arteriography frequently follows.

Palpable Mass. Arteriography is commonly required to clarify the urographic findings in such patients.

Hypertension. The indication for arteriography in the presence of hypertension is most often to determine whether renal vascular disease is present. Since the urogram is normal in at least 20 per cent of individuals with significant renal artery stenosis, arteriography in such patients depends on the clinical evaluation. If the urogram is positive, arteriography is mandatory in uncontrolled hypertension. Furthermore, concomitant renal venous sampling for renin levels is essential to substantiate the causal relationship of the arterial lesion to the hypertension.

Unexplained Fever, Weight Loss, and Weakness. When the origin of these nonspecific symptoms is unclear, urography and, subsequently, arteriography may be required.

Acute Renal Failure. Patients with oliguric renal failure commonly have medical disease of the kidney. On the other hand, bilateral renal artery emboli or thrombosis, unilateral embolus in a single kidney, trauma to the kidney, rejection in a transplant, or acute renal vein thrombosis may also produce profound oliguria and renal failure. The arteriogram depicts the state of the major renal arteries and the intrarenal vascular bed.

Renal Trauma. In abdominal trauma with possible major involvement of the kidney, urography serves as a screening procedure, but frequently arteriography is required to delineate the status of both the kidney and the renal vascular bed.

Renal Transplantation. Arteriographic investigation of the donor is essential to determine whether he is a suitable candidate. The recipient who becomes oliguric also requires angiography to delineate the anastomotic site as well as the condition of the intrarenal vascular bed.

Another important indication in the patient with a kidney transplant is the presence or development of hypertension. Although this may be a part of the rejection reaction, acute tubular necrosis, or recurrence of the patient's primary disease, it may also be related to operable stenosis of the renal artery either at or near the anastomosis.

Metastasis of Unknown Origin. When bone metastases are detected without evidence of the primary site, urography and, subsequently, arteriography may be an integral part of the work-up.

Polycythemia. The presence of unexplained polycythemia, sometimes even the classic picture of polycythemia vera, may be caused by a renal neoplasm and thus require urography and arteriography.

Unexplained Hypercalcemia and Unilateral Varicocele. These as well as symptoms such as nausea, vomiting, and anorexia that have no apparent source in the gastrointestinal tract may indicate renal disease and require radiographic study, including arteriography. Left-sided varicocele occurs in carcinoma of the kidney with invasion of the renal vein and obstruction of the testicular vein.

The Postoperative Patient. Patients who have had revascularization of the kidney and in whom hypertension has not remitted usually require renal arteriography to define the status of the renal circulation.

Urographic Findings as Indications for Arteriography

As noted previously, urography is performed first when the foregoing symptoms and signs are present; it is frequently urography, therefore, that indicates the need for the special procedure. Clearly, the following urographic indications will lead to angiography in some cases but not in all. In many cases, computed tomography or ultrasound examination will fully clarify the nature of the underlying disease.

1. Renal masses.

2. Renal pseudotumors. Prominent columns of Bertin projecting into the renal sinus, renal sinus lipomatosis, the dromedary hump, focal renal hypertrophy (following infection, trauma, infarction, and obstruction and suggesting the presence of a mass)—in all of these, arteriography may help distinguish between pseudotumor and a neoplastic mass. This is particularly true when ultrasound, computed tomography, and isotope studies are inconclusive.

3. Unilateral or bilateral renal enlargement.

4. Unilateral renal nonfunction or nonvisualization.

5. A negative urogram in the presence of hematuria.

6. Abdominal trauma with an abnormal urogram.

TABLE 7–6. VASCULARITY OF RENAL CELL CARCINOMA JUDGED BY ANGIOGRAPHY*

Characteristic	Number of Cases
Avascular	6
Minimal vascularity	16
Moderate vascularity	16
Marked vascularity	62
Total	100

*After Watson, R. C., Fleming, R. J., and Evans, J. A.: Radiology, *91*:888, 1968.

7. Nonfunctioning kidneys in acute renal failure or in renal transplant.

8. A positive urogram in hypertension: disparity in renal size, appearance time, or concentration in the collecting system.

9. Calcifications in the region of the renal artery on the plain film, suggesting renal artery aneurysm.

10. Unexplained intrarenal calcifications.

APPLICATIONS OF RENAL ARTERIOGRAPHY

Renal Mass Lesions

Tumors of the Kidney. When a mass is detected by urography and the diagnosis is in doubt, renal arteriography may be extraordinarily rewarding. In addition to establishing the diagnosis, it will define the extent of the tumor, the amount of remaining parenchyma, the condition of the contralateral kidney, the presence of renal vein or caval invasion, and retroperitoneal and liver metastases. The three most common malignant tumors are renal cell carcinoma, renal pelvic tumors (transitional cell), and Wilms' tumor.

Renal cell carcinomas demonstrate abnormal vessels and are readily diagnosed by angiography in 94 to 97 per cent of cases (Table 7–6) (Meaney, 1969; Watson et al., 1968). Characteristically, the angiogram will delineate the disordered tumor vascular bed and the limits of the renal mass lesion (Figs. 7–183 and 7–184). The most common findings are as follows:

1. Hypervascularity in at least 80 per cent of cases.

2. "Random" distribution of vessels, in contrast to the uniform distribution of normal renal vessels.

3. Tortuous vessels without normal tapering.

4. Dilated vessels, with pooling of contrast material in "lakes."

5. Arteriovenous communications with early venous filling.

6. Encasement of arteries. The margins are irregular and appear fixed and unchanging during different phases of the heart cycle.

7. Staining of the tumor mass during the capillary phase.

8. Renal vein invasion with or without obstruction by tumor. Arterial tumor vessels visualized within the vein establish the presence of invasion. Failure to visualize the renal vein cannot be considered definitive evidence of tumor invasion; demonstration of a large venous collateral network is strongly suggestive (Fig. 7–184) (Simpson et al., 1974) but not conclusive (Folin, 1967).

9. Epinephrine arteriography. If 6 to 10 μg of epinephrine are injected intra-arterially 15 to 30 seconds prior to contrast injection, normal renal vessels will contract while the effect on the tumor vascular bed is less. This will allow better demarcation of the tumor mass, confirmation of the diagnosis when it is in doubt, and, at times, establishment of a positive diagnosis when the conventional arteriogram has been inconclusive (Fig. 7–185). The relative lack of responsiveness of the tumor vascular bed is probably related to the relatively lessened elements of muscular and elastic tissue in the walls of some of the tumor vessels (Abrams, 1964; Abrams et al., 1971). Within recent years, other pharmacologic agents have been employed to enhance visualization of tumor vessels. Among these, angiotensin has proved to be the effective agent (Ekelund, 1980).

10. Avascular renal cell tumors, though relatively few in number, may resemble cysts (Fig. 7–186). Cyst puncture in these patients usually demonstrates a thick, irregular wall, and aspiration of cyst fluid may reveal old blood or may be positive for renal cell carcinoma on cytologic examination (Wright and Walker, 1975).

Aside from its diagnostic usefulness, renal arteriography furnishes the surgeon with important preoperative anatomic knowledge of the renal vascular bed (Pillari et al., 1981). Furthermore, since angiography of the contralateral kidney is mandatory, the presence or absence of undetected abnormalities can also be clarified (Weyman et al., 1980). Although computed tomography is frequently adequate for preoperative diagnosis and staging of carcinoma of the kidney, many urologists find the information afforded by angiography invaluable in their preoperative assessment. A recent article by a urologist states: "The selective and bilateral

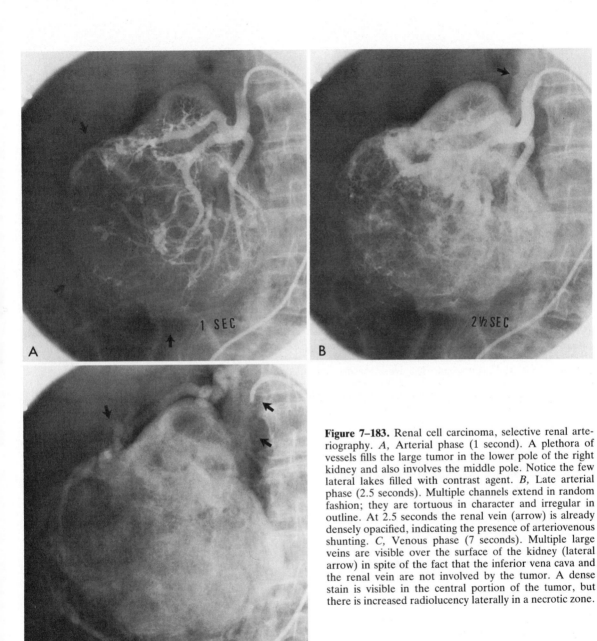

Figure 7–183. Renal cell carcinoma, selective renal arteriography. *A,* Arterial phase (1 second). A plethora of vessels fills the large tumor in the lower pole of the right kidney and also involves the middle pole. Notice the few lateral lakes filled with contrast agent. *B,* Late arterial phase (2.5 seconds). Multiple channels extend in random fashion; they are tortuous in character and irregular in outline. At 2.5 seconds the renal vein (arrow) is already densely opacified, indicating the presence of arteriovenous shunting. *C,* Venous phase (7 seconds). Multiple large veins are visible over the surface of the kidney (lateral arrow) in spite of the fact that the inferior vena cava and the renal vein are not involved by the tumor. A dense stain is visible in the central portion of the tumor, but there is increased radiolucency laterally in a necrotic zone.

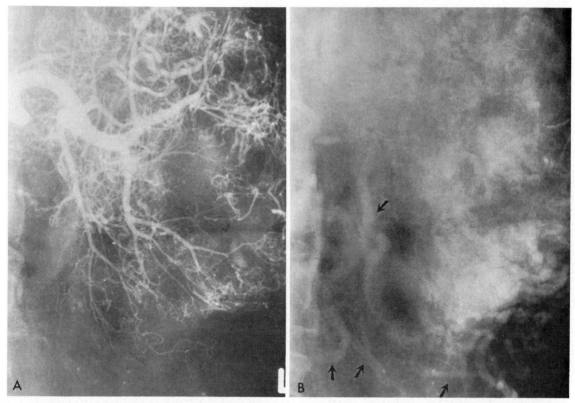

Figure 7–184. Renal cell carcinoma with renal vein involvement demonstrated during the venous phase. *A,* Arterial phase. Multiple tortuous vessels extend in random fashion virtually throughout the entire kidney. This is the classic appearance of tumor vessels. *B,* Venous phase. The dense opacification of "staining" of the renal parenchyma has no relationship to normal renal architecture. In addition multiple serpiginous channels are visible overlying, and lateral, caudal, and medial to, the kidney: All represent collateral veins. This patient had invasion and obstruction of the renal vein by renal cell carcinoma.

renal arteriogram remains the single most important test in the assessment of the primary lesion" (Jones, 1982). Furthermore, angiography may be important when a mass is solid or complex on CT scan but does not disturb the renal contour (Kam et al., 1981). The objective is not a specific diagnosis so much as the exclusion of benign vascular processes such as hemangioma, arteriovenous fistula, or aneurysm, any one of which may present as an intrarenal mass.

Renal pelvic neoplasms are usually hypovascular, but in most of them tumor vessels may be defined, particularly if magnification arteriography and epinephrine are employed. Vascular encasement and a tumor blush are relatively common, but arteriovenous shunting is never observed. In half the cases, the periureteric artery is enlarged (Rabinowitz et al., 1972) (Fig. 7–187).

In *Wilms' tumor,* arteriography, if performed, should be done bilaterally because of the known frequency of involvement of both kidneys (Fig. 7–188). Arteriography demonstrates (1) stretching of vessels, (2) narrowing of vessels, (3) displacement of vessels, (4) amputation of vessels, (5) encasement of vessels, and (6) tumor vessels. Wilms' tumor varies from relatively avascular to moderately hypervascular masses. (7) At times, metastasis to liver, retroperitoneal nodes, or other adjacent organs may be apparent.

Thus, arteriography is important not only in confirming the diagnosis but also in assessing the extent of the tumor, liver metastases, bilaterality, response to therapy, and recurrence. Angiography usually distinguishes Wilms' tumor from hydronephrosis and multicystic kidney (small, sparse vessels; no tumor vessels). Arteriography may also be helpful in the diagnosis

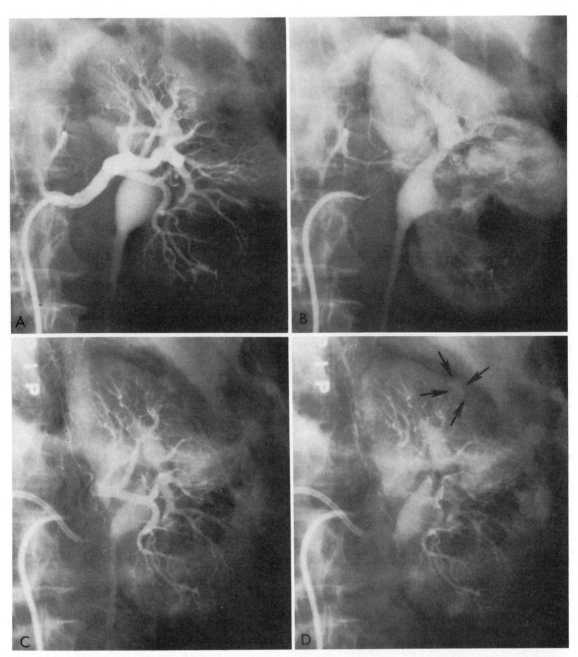

Figure 7–185. Renal cell carcinoma, epinephrine arteriography. The patient was admitted for evaluation of hematuria. The urogram suggested a cystic mass in the lower pole of the kidney. *A,* Selective renal arteriography. The vessels to the lower pole are displaced around a smooth round mass. No tumor vessels or encasement are visible. *B,* Nephrographic phase. A lucent area in the lower pole indicates the presence of a cyst. In addition, a localized invagination just above the midportion of the lateral border of the kidney suggests a prior infarct. *C,* Epinephrine arteriography (1 second). There is no filling of the vessels to the cortex of the kidney. *D,* Epinephrine arteriography (2.5 seconds). The interlobar renal arteries remain opacified, but now a small local area of increased density (arrows) extends beyond the margin of the kidney and adjacent to the upper pole. Surgical exploration revealed this lesion to be renal cell carcinoma. A benign simple cyst was present in the lower pole of the kidney. (Courtesy of Dr. Ernest Ferris.)

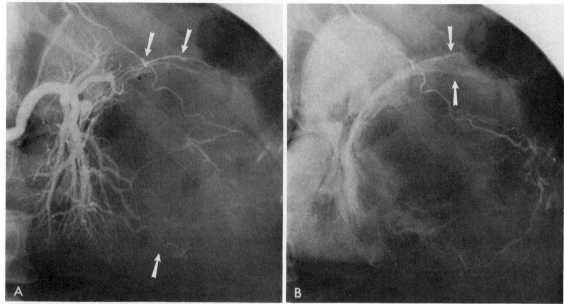

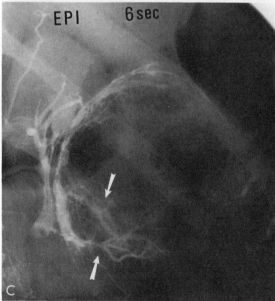

Figure 7–186. Cystic renal cell carninoma. This 46-year-old woman had a urogram because of stress incontinence. A large mass was delineated. Ultrasound indicated a cystic lesion. Puncture and aspiration revealed bloody fluid, high in LDH but with no abnormal cells. Angiography was performed. *A,* Arterial phase. The vessels are clumped together, and a large laterally placed cystic-appearing mass (arrows) has displaced blood vessels around it. A number of arteries extend toward and over the surface of this mass; some of these vessels are tortuous and beaded (arrows). *B,* Nephrographic phase (7 seconds). The normal renal parenchyma is displaced medially, particularly in the lower pole, and is relatively homogeneous in opacification. The cystic wall, opacified by contrast agent (arrows), is well beyond the limits of 1 mm in thickness at a number of sites. *C,* Epinephrine arteriogram (6 seconds). Virtually no filling of major interlobar arterial branches in the normal renal parenchyma is apparent; multiple branches (arrows) and a blush are visible in the capsule of the thick-walled cystic mass. This patient was explored surgically and found to have a cystic renal cell carcinoma with hemorrhage and tissue debris in the central cavity.

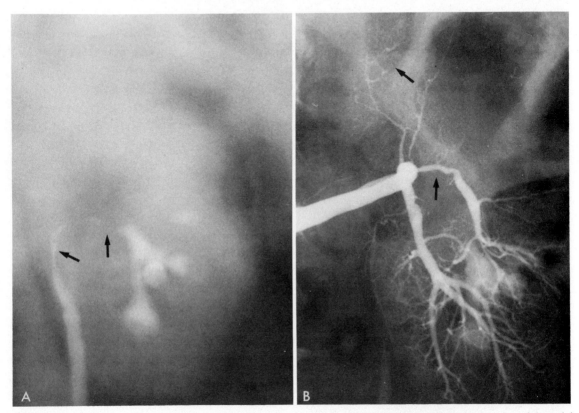

Figure 7–187. Transitional cell carcinoma of the renal pelvis. *A*, Urography, laminagram. Marked narrowing of the pelvis and the upper ureter is demonstrated (arrows). Single calyces are visible in the midportion of the kidney with no visualization of the infundibula. No calyces are visible in the upper portion of the kidney. *B*, Selective renal arteriography. Encasement of the central renal arterial branches beyond the bifurcation particularly involves the branch extending laterally from the midportion of the renal artery (lower arrow). A number of small tumor vessels are visible in the medial cephalad segment of the kidney (upper arrow). The diagnosis of transitional cell carcinoma extending into the upper and middle portions of the kidney and arising in the renal pelvis was made from the arteriograms. Nephrectomy and pathologic examination showed widespread replacement of the upper two-thirds of the kidney by the tumor, which arose in the renal pelvis.

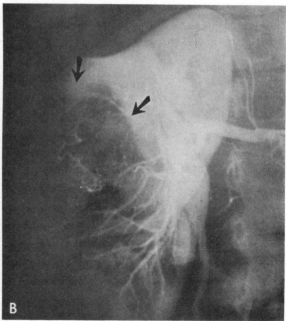

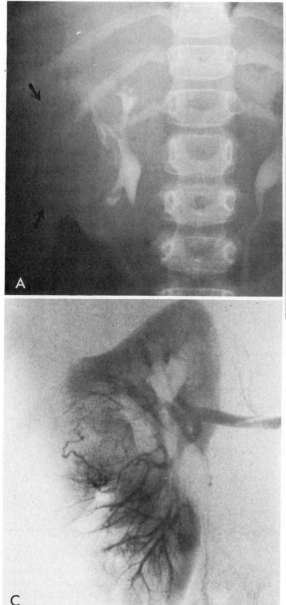

Figure 7–188. Wilms' tumor. *A,* Urogram. Displacement and distortion of the calyces to the midportion of the kidney have been produced by a large renal mass (arrows). The axis of the kidney is somewhat more vertical than normal. *B* and *C,* Selective renal arteriogram and subtraction arteriogram. Multiple tortuous and irregular vessels can be seen in the region of a mass (arrows), which obscures the lateral border of the kidney. The tumor is by no means hypervascular, but it is equally obvious that this is not an avascular mass. The tumor vessels indicate a malignant tumor; the diagnosis of Wilms' is most likely. Nephrectomy and histologic examination confirmed the diagnosis of Wilms' tumor. (Courtesy of Dr. Kenneth Fellows.)

of benign tumors such as adenomas (Vlahos et al., 1982).

Renal Cysts. When a renal mass is detected by urography, our approach is to proceed immediately to diagnostic ultrasound. If the lesion is clearly anechoic and fulfills the criteria of a simple cyst, it is usually managed conservatively. If a solid tumor, complex pattern, or atypical pattern is observed, the patient is referred for CT. Arteriography is done only if the diagnosis is uncertain.

Although cyst puncture used to be performed in most lesions over 3 cm in size, it is now generally reserved for cystic lesions of uncertain character. After cyst puncture, if there remains any question as to whether the mass is a benign cyst, arteriography may be performed with the understanding that virtually all such patients will require surgery. The angiographic criteria of simple renal cyst are well established. A radiolucent mass, sharply defined with a thin, smooth wall (1 mm in thickness) and an acute angle at the junction of cyst wall and renal cortex forming a "beak," is characteristic of a cyst (Fig. 7–189). The procedure has a high degree of accuracy but may rarely be misleading in the presence of avascular or cystic tumors. If any of the classic diagnostic criteria are lacking, epinephrine arteriography should be undertaken in order to enhance demonstration of tumor vessels. In addition, cyst puncture should be performed as the final diagnostic step if it has not yet been done.

Although polycystic kidney obviously fits within the category of "renal cysts," the urographic and arteriographic patterns are usually quite distinctive and permit a specific diagnosis in most cases (Fig. 7–190). The other types of congenital and hereditary renal cystic disease

are discussed in detail elsewhere in these volumes.

The Diagnostic Decision Tree in Solitary Renal Masses. All renal mass lesions must undergo special investigation. The stakes are reasonably high: The untreated tumor, mistakenly diagnosed as cyst, may spread locally or metastasize and move the patient into the incurable group. The benign cyst, mistakenly taken to surgery, exposes the patient to significant morbidity and mortality. A mortality rate of 1.5 to 2.4 per cent and a major morbidity rate of 30 per cent have been reported (Kropp

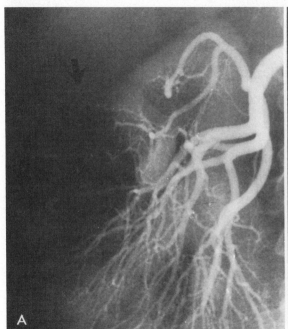

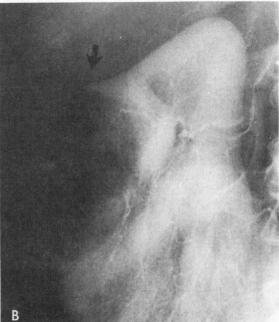

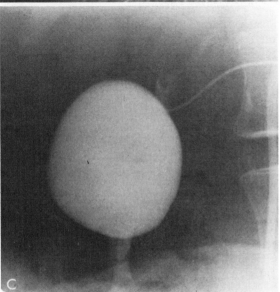

Figure 7–189. Renal cyst, selective renal arteriography. *A,* Arterial phase. The vessels to the lateral aspect of the kidney are diminished in number and displaced by a mass (arrow). *B,* Nephrographic phase. A sharp lip of cortical tissue strongly suggests the probability of benign renal cyst. No tumor vessels are apparent, nor was there any arteriovenous shunting. *C,* Cyst puncture. The wall of the cyst is smooth and accounts fully for the area of displacement of blood vessels and the absent nephrographic zone. The fluid from the cyst showed no evidence of malignant cells, and the patient was treated conservatively with observation and repeat urography 1 year later.

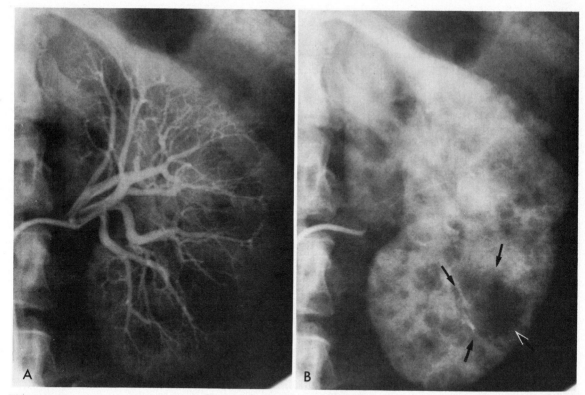

Figure 7–190. Polycystic kidney. *A,* Arterial phase. There is displacement of some peripheral renal branches, and the cortex has a mottled appearance. *B,* Nephrographic phase. Multiple small lucencies are widely disseminated throughout the entire kidney; a larger cyst (arrows) is visible in the lower pole in an area of relative lucency on both films. This is the classic appearance of polycystic disease.

et al., 1967; Plaine and Hinman, 1965). Pollack et al. (1974) have compared the biologic and economic cost associated with the radiologic versus the surgical approach to diagnosis of renal cyst (Table 7–7). Omitted from Table 7–7 is the potential cost of leaving a renal carcinoma untreated, that is, the failure to detect a carcinoma in the cyst. According to Sherwood and

TABLE 7–7. COMPARISON OF RADIOLOGIC VERSUS SURGICAL DIAGNOSIS OF RENAL CYSTS*

	Radiologic	Surgical
Diagnostic accuracy	100†	approx. 100%
Major morbidity	0%	30%
Mortality	0%	1.5%
Socioeconomic:		
Hospital days (average)	0–1	7–10
Hospital costs (average)	$130–180	$1500–2000
Lost wages (average)	1 day	27 days

*After Pollack, H. M., Goldberg, B. B., and Bogash, M.: J. Urol., *111*:326, 1974.

†Eight per cent of patients require an operation because of indeterminate status.

Trott (1975), the likelihood is less than 1 in 1000. Thus, the importance of a reasonable, systematic, and efficient approach to diagnosis requires emphasis.

Renovascular Disease

Arteriosclerosis. Arteriosclerosis is usually observed after the age of 40 and is more common in males (in contrast to dysplasia of the renal arteries). Since arteriosclerotic plaques develop most frequently at the origin or bifurcation of vessels, it is not unexpected that renal artery stenosis due to arteriosclerosis is more often than not orificial or located in the proximal third of the artery. It is frequently accompanied by aortic disease as well (Halpern et al., 1961). Aortic plaques may themselves cause stenosis or occlusion at the ostium of a renal artery.

Arteriosclerotic narrowing may vary in degree from small, insignificant plaques to complete occlusion (Figs. 7–191 and 7–192) (Abrams et al., 1967; Abrams, 1983*b*). It is usually more or less localized, may be eccentric or circumferential, and is usually irregular. The lesions may be single or multiple. In 30 to 50 per cent of

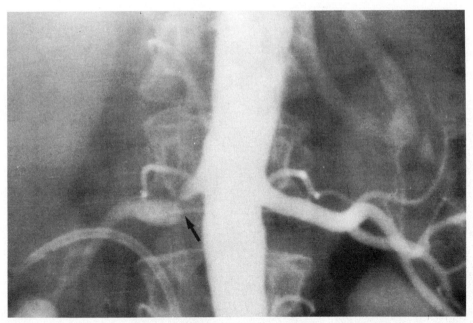

Figure 7–191. Renal artery stenosis due to arteriosclerosis. Significant eccentric narrowing of the renal artery within the first third of the blood vessel strongly suggests the arteriosclerotic etiology. Note the poststenotic dilatation.

cases they are bilateral, with one side more severely affected. Immediately beyond the stenosis a significant degree of poststenotic dilatation may be observed. This does not necessarily imply that the stenosis is dynamically important.

What is significant stenosis? When the diameter of the vessel is reduced by 80 per cent or more, the stenosis has a high chance of being causally related to the hypertension known to be present. In practice, this implies reduction to a lumen of 1 to 1.5 mm in diameter (Bookstein and Stewart, 1964). The most valuable confirmatory evidence of significant stenosis lies in demonstration of high venous renin on the side of involvement. The presence of collateral circulation usually implies a significant lesion, but significant stenosis need not be accompanied by visible collateral vessels (Abrams and Cornell, 1965).

Dysplasia of the Renal Arteries. This in-

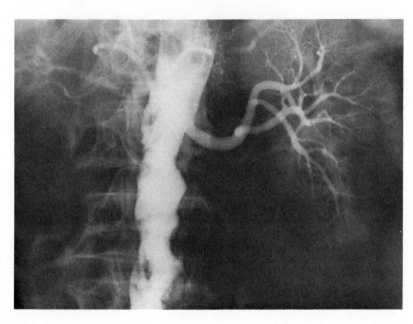

Figure 7–192. Renal artery occlusion due to arteriosclerosis. Bolus aortography demonstrates the left renal artery with normal bifurcations and multiple arteriosclerotic plaques in the aorta. The origin of the right renal artery is completely occluded by arteriosclerosis.

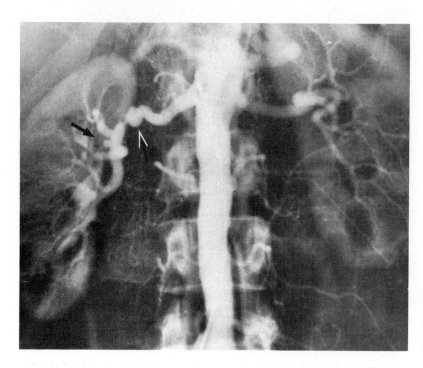

Figure 7–193. Renal artery dysplasia: mural hyperplasia with aneurysm. The middle and distal two thirds of the vessel are involved with aneurysms (arrows) and stenosis.

Figure 7–194. Renal artery dysplasia: perimedial fibroplasia. An area of severe stenosis in the middle of the relatively long segment of involvement begins at the middle third of the vessel and extends throughout the distal third. The irregular areas of narrowing are well within the apparent lumen of the vessel and do not indicate aneurysm formation. The appearance is quite typical of perimedial fibroplasia.

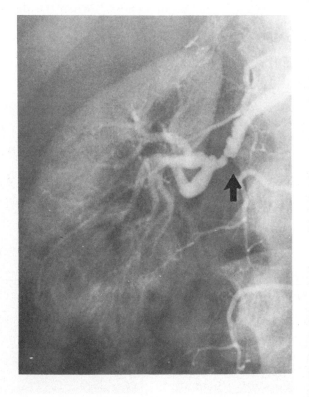

triguing lesion occurs predominantly in females, although we have seen many cases in young males as well (Ekelund et al., 1977). In about 40 to 70 per cent of cases the lesions are bilateral (Ekelund et al., 1977; Gill and Meaney, 1969; Kincaid et al., 1968). A number of different types have been described, some of which are recognizable radiologically (McCormack et al., 1966, 1967). Perhaps the most important aspect of designating the pathologic type is that the patients with so-called medial fibroplasia with aneurysms apparently show no progression of their lesions after the age of 40, whereas this is not true of the other types.

In the most common type, medial fibroplasia with aneurysm, arteriography typically reveals a "string of beads" appearance of the vessels (Fig. 7–193) with multiple concentric rings produced by the hyperplastic changes of the wall. So-called perimedial fibroplasia may produce a sausage-type appearance (Fig. 7–194), but the lumen is relatively narrowed and the more "dilated" areas are well within the projected diameter of the normal renal artery (in contrast to medial fibroplasia with aneurysm). The proximal third of the main renal artery is usually spared in both types, but the middle and distal thirds are typically involved (Abrams et al., 1967). The entire artery may be the site of disease. The process may extend into the secondary branches and produce complete occlusion. In these patients the total supply to a segment of the kidney may come via the collateral circulation. In about 40 per cent of cases the lesions are bilateral. At times, the lesions may be localized and nonrepetitive in character, as in intimal fibroplasia or in true fibromuscular hyperplasia (Fig. 7–195). The disease is not localized to the renal arteries, and other visceral branches as well as the carotid arteries may be involved (Black et al., 1978; Ekelund et al., 1977; Perry, 1972).

Branch Stenosis of the Renal Artery. Branch stenosis may be due to arteriosclerosis, dysplasia of the renal artery, thrombus, embolus, or arteritis (Fig. 7–196). In our experience, branch stenosis has been seen relatively commonly with renal artery dysplasia but not necessarily as an isolated lesion. The importance of isolated branch stenosis lies in the occasional difficulty of detecting it with conventional arteriography, although aortography may be at times highly rewarding. It is essential to study both the arteriographic and the nephrographic phases because the latter may reveal ischemic areas with great clarity. In general, selective arteriography is better adapted to demonstrating branch stenosis.

Renal Infarction. After infarction the kidney becomes smaller, with local identation due to focal loss of volume. On the urogram, the affected calyx may become distorted. The result may appear similar to focal pyelonephritis except that the loss of renal tissue appears to be excessive when compared with the degree of calyceal distortion (Abrams et al., 1967). When the whole kidney is infarcted, there is a general decrease in size and the appearance may resemble that of a congenitally hypoplastic kidney. Angiography is helpful in clarifying the cause of the abnormality. Cutoff or absence of normal vessels is associated with defects in the nephrogram. These defects may represent the infarcted tissue or the scar that has replaced it. Local increase in the circulation time is sometimes seen and may look like a tumor stain (Janower and Weber, 1965). When renal embolism causes incomplete infarction and hypertension or when segmental renal artery stenosis is associated with hypertension, deliberate therapeutic embolism may result in the infarction of the remaining viable tissue and so control hypertension (Chuang et al., 1979; Reuter et al., 1976).

Renal Artery Aneurysm. About 30 to 50 per cent of renal artery aneurysms contain calcium within their walls (Fig. 7–197). Therefore, recognition may be possible on plain films. In general, those aneurysms that calcify do not tend to rupture, whereas those without calcium are likely to rupture spontaneously.

Angiographically, the aneurysm is either *saccular* in configuration, characterized by an outpouching from the artery with an area of communication of variable width, or *fusiform* with rather uniform dilatation of the lumen over a variable distance. The fusiform type is more likely to be secondary to localized arteriosclerotic stenosis or dysplasia of the renal artery, and ít occurs as a region of poststenotic dilatation. Thus, it is also known as a "jet" aneurysm. Circulation of contrast material within the aneurysm tends to be retarded, particularly in the saccular type, whereas the remaining general circulation throughout the kidneys is normal. Hypertension has been found to accompany renal artery aneurysms in 15 per cent of cases (Boijsen and Kohler, 1963). Cure of hypertension after surgery occurs only when renal artery stenosis and the physiologic stigmata of renovascular hypertension are present (Cummings et al., 1973).

Renal Arteriovenous Fistula. Renal arteriovenous fistulas may be congenital or acquired. If acquired, trauma is the most common cause, often caused in turn by needle biopsy. Meng and Elkin (1971) demonstrated by aor-

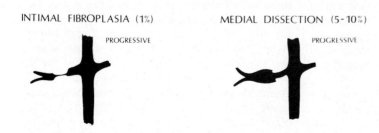

INTIMAL FIBROPLASIA (1%)

PROGRESSIVE

MEDIAL DISSECTION (5-10%)

PROGRESSIVE

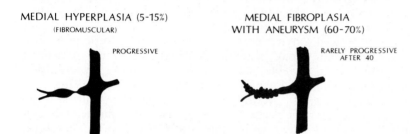

MEDIAL HYPERPLASIA (5-15%)
(FIBROMUSCULAR)

PROGRESSIVE

MEDIAL FIBROPLASIA
WITH ANEURYSM (60-70%)

RARELY PROGRESSIVE
AFTER 40

Figure 7–195. Diagram of dysplastic lesions of the renal artery. (Modified after McCormack et al., 1966, 1967, and Kincaid, 1966.)

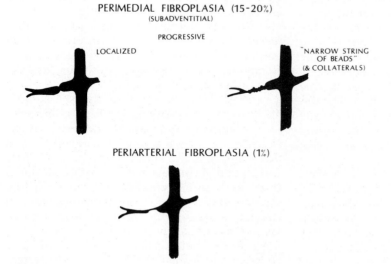

PERIMEDIAL FIBROPLASIA (15-20%)
(SUBADVENTITIAL)

PROGRESSIVE

LOCALIZED

"NARROW STRING
OF BEADS"
(& COLLATERALS)

PERIARTERIAL FIBROPLASIA (1%)

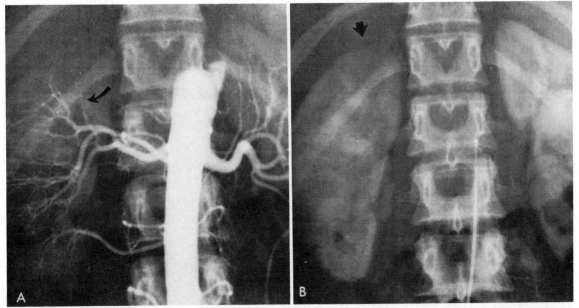

Figure 7–196. Renal artery branch stenosis. This 26-year-old woman had known hypertension of 4 years' duration. *A,* Abdominal aortogram. Three renal arteries are visible on the right. Occlusion of a small, somewhat tortuous branch to the right upper pole is visible (arrow). The peripheral small branches to the upper pole are not adequately defined. *B,* Nephrographic phase. Absence of contrast density in the upper pole of the right kidney reflects the segmental disease of the artery. The localized area of occlusion was caused by arteritis.

tography immediately following percutaneous needle biopsy that the needle tract could be visualized, that perirenal extravasation occurred commonly, that arteriovenous communication was present in about 10 per cent of patients, and that arterial occlusion, thrombus, or spasm was observed in about 20 per cent of patients.

In other series, the incidence of arteriovenous fistulas following renal biopsy has varied from 11 to 18 per cent (Bennett and Wiener, 1975; Ekelund and Lindholm, 1972; Kohler and Edgren, 1974; Lundstrom, 1974). Furthermore, it has been emphasized that ablation or nephrectomy may produce cure of hypertension associ-

Figure 7–197. Renal artery aneurysm. Selective renal arteriography demonstrates a localized, ovoid collection of contrast agent arising from the main renal artery at the bifurcation into dorsal and ventral branches. The aneurysm is associated with slight narrowing of the dorsal branch at its origin. More importantly, however, compression of the ventral renal artery (arrow) accounts for the better opacification of the branches to the lower pole and the dorsal aspect of the kidney. The ventral branches are somewhat less dense, with relatively poorer filling distally. This explains the occasional association of renovascular hypertension with renal artery aneurysm: The compression or narrowing of a major renal arterial branch may be associated with segmental ischemia and increased production of renin from the ischemic segment of the kidney.

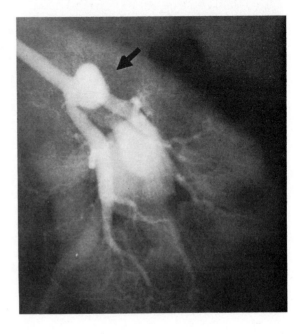

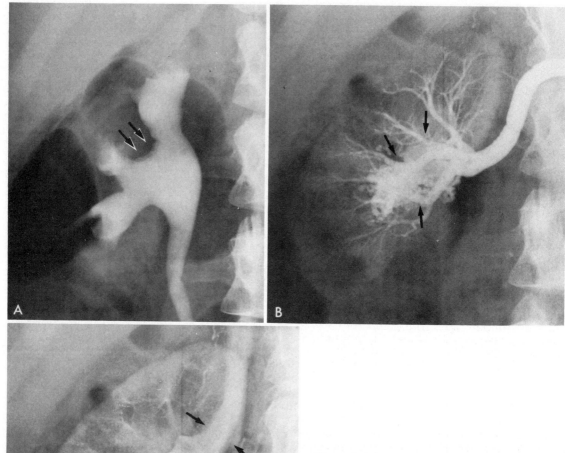

Figure 7–198. Renal arteriovenous fistula. The patient was admitted for evaluation of hematuria. *A,* Intravenous urogram. The collecting system appears normal except for an irregular serration on the lateral aspect of the pelvis between the upper and middle pole calyces. The appearance suggests a papillary tumor of the pelvis, extrinsic pressure on the pelvis from an intrarenal mass, or, possibly, vessel imprint. *B,* Selective renal arteriography. A large cluster of vessels in and adjacent to the hilus of the kidney is opacified. *C,* Nephrographic phase (4 seconds). There is early, dense filling of the renal vein and the inferior vena cava while some of the renal artery branches are still opacified. Note the absence of nephrogram in the lower pole. Double renal arteries were present.

ated with arteriovenous fistula (Jahnke et al., 1976; Moore and Phillippi, 1977; Sarramon et al., 1978). On the renal angiogram the renal artery and vein are much wider than normal, and rapid passage of contrast material directly from artery to vein can be visualized with early entry into the inferior vena cava (Fig. 7–198). When the arteriovenous fistula is smaller and more localized, enlargement and tortuosity with a serpentine appearance of the segmental arterial vessel and its branches are apparent.

Vascularity of the renal parenchyma in the area adjacent to large fistulas tends to be diminished. It may be difficult at times to differentiate multiple arteriovenous malformations from the arteriovenous shunts that occur in renal carcinoma because wide tortuous vessels and localized areas of rapid shunting to the venous system may be noted in both circumstances. In the treatment of arteriovenous fistula, transcatheter vascular occlusion is a relatively safe and effective method (Clark, 1983).

Renal Infection

In mild cases of *pyelonephritis,* no angiographic abnormality is noted. With the destruction and subsequent fibrosis of renal tissue, there is a reduced volume of renal tissue with distortion of calyces and irregularity of contour. Because the renal volume has diminished, the interlobar and arcuate vessels become crowded together, resulting in a tortuous configuration (Fig. 7–199). There may be localized areas of reduced vascularity, and scar formation (Fig. 7–199) may derange the vascular pattern so that a mottled, irregular nephrogram is produced. The renal cortex is irregular in outline, but the nephrogram may be disproportionately dense owing to crowding of the vascular bed secondary to a loss of interstitial renal tissue.

In the presence of *abscesses* or *renal inflammatory masses,* there is an increase in size and number of capsular vessels, and the abnormal intrarenal circulation is manifested by slow and diminished blood flow, stretching of interlobar branches, loss of the cortical medullary border, and loss of the kidney outline. Typical tumor vessels of hypernephroma are never observed. No arteriovenous shunts are present. Nevertheless, the distinction from hypovascular renal cell carcinoma and from large transitional cell tumors may be difficult (Koehler, 1974).

Renal Trauma

Angiographic evaluation of renal trauma has assumed greater importance in recent years (Hessel and Smith, 1974). In the presence of an abnormal urogram, many advise arteriography for clarification of the underlying abnormalities. Nonvisualization on the urogram may imply a severed renal pedicle; a profound diminution in blood flow as in shock, subcapsular hematoma, and renal vein thrombosis; or obstruction of the collecting system by clots or pre-existing disease.

The angiographic findings (Fig. 7–200) include displacement of vessels and poorly defined corticomedullary junction, suggesting an intrarenal hematoma; interruption of the renal parenchymal blush because of parenchymal laceration; extravasation of contrast material into and outside the kidney; separation of the kidney into several segments, the so-called shattered kidney; areas of poor or absent parenchymal filling with vascular occlusion indicating infarction; and small peripheral cortical defects on the nephrogram with amputation of tertiary or arcuate vessels as a reflection of peripheral vessel thrombosis with infarction.

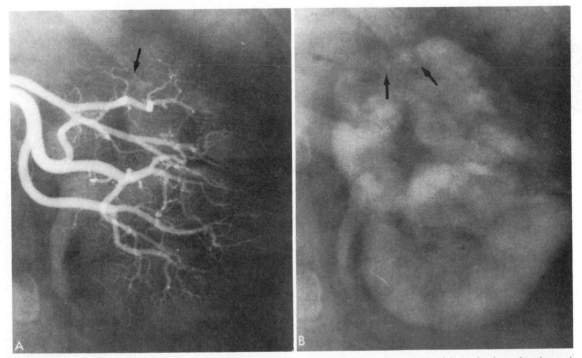

Figure 7–199. Pyelonephritis, selective renal arteriography. *A,* Arterial phase. Tortuous and irregular branches (arrow), especially in the upper pole of the kidney, are visible along with loss of the arcuate and interlobular branches to this region. The vessels to the lower pole are also tortuous but have a somewhat normal appearance. *B,* Nephrographic phase. The cortex in the upper portion of the kidney is grossly scarred and irregular, representing the fibrosis consequent to chronic infection.

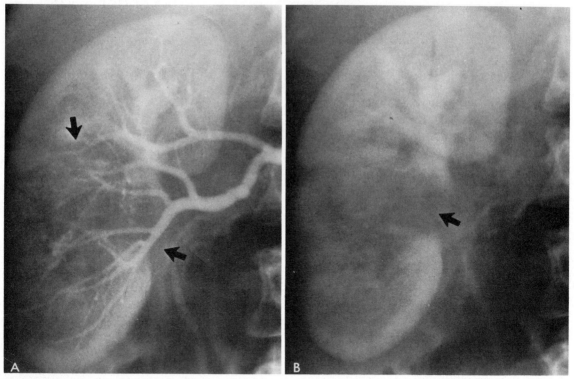

Figure 7–200. Renal trauma. *A,* Arterial phase. The vessels to the upper pole of the kidney appear relatively normal. In the midportion of the kidney and extending into the lower pole there appears to be displacement of multiple renal arterial branches and small "puddles" of contrast agent. This represents an area of intrarenal hematoma (arrows). *B,* Nephrographic phase. A large area of lucency represents the hematoma in the kidney. Notice that the cortex at the lateral aspect of the kidney is not as well marginated as in the upper and lower poles.

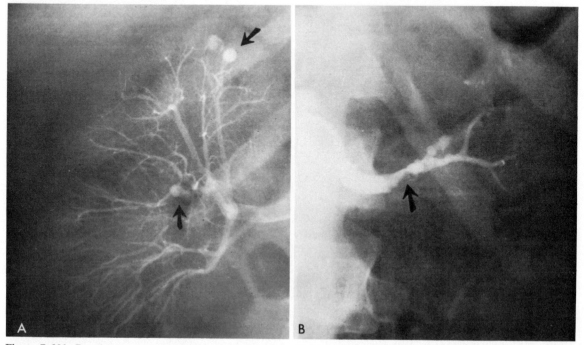

Figure 7–201. Renal trauma. *A,* Arteriogram, right kidney. Multiple small collections of contrast agent on the arterial phase represent false aneurysms caused by vessel rupture consequent to abdominal trauma in an automobile accident. This simulates the appearance sometimes seen in periarteritis nodosa. *B,* Left selective renal arteriogram. Intramural hematoma or dissection of the left renal artery (arrow) is visible, with complete obstruction to the branches of the main renal arteries beyond the bifurcation.

Renal artery occlusion is more common on the left than on the right and is an important diagnosis to establish so as to permit vascular reconstruction while the kidney is still viable (Fig. 7–201). Post-traumatic aneurysms are actually pseudoaneurysms (Fig. 7–201). *Arteriovenous fistulas* are usually caused by penetrating wounds, and surgery is indicated only when the surrounding tissue is ischemic; otherwise the fistula may heal with conservative treatment. Renal vein injuries and thromboses are uncommon and are associated with an enlarged kidney and prolonged nephrogram on urography.

Arteritis

Periarteritis nodosa is a relatively rare cause of renovascular hypertension, and only a few angiographic descriptions of this disease have been reported (Bron et al., 1965; Fleming and Stern, 1965; Halpern and Citron, 1971; Robins and Bookstein, 1972). The renal vessels are involved in about 80 per cent of cases, and the pathologic lesion, a necrotizing inflammatory process, involves primarily the arterioles and the smaller intrarenal branches of the renal artery. The intravascular inflammatory process eventually results in the formation of granulation tissue and fibrosis intermingled with areas of vessel wall destruction. Hemorrhage, thrombosis, and aneurysm formation, which is characteristic of the disease, result.

Angiographically, the demonstration of multiple aneurysms in the small and medium-sized arteries is highly suggestive, although we have seen the same appearance in lupus erythematosus. These aneurysms are of various sizes and shapes and are rather uniformly distributed through the renal parenchyma bilaterally. In addition, the medium and smaller sized intrarenal arteries may be stretched, attenuated, and diminished in number (probably as a result of thrombosis with secondary recanalization). This rather diffuse small vessel thrombosis results in variable degrees of cortical ischemia and in an irregular renal outline during the nephrographic phase owing to scattered renal infarction. Abdominal aortography may also reveal numerous small aneurysms in the splenic, hepatic, and other visceral vessels.

There are numerous types of vasculitis in which the renal vascular bed may be involved (Christian and Sergent, 1976; Halpern and Citron, 1971). Drug abuse, ergot, and serum sickness may all produce similar blood vessel abnormalities in the kidney.

Wegener's granulomatosis is associated with a destructive arteritis of blood vessels and with granuloma formation. When it involves the kidney, it usually produces a focal necrotizing glomerulonephritis, with uncommon involvement of the large arteries. At times, however, it may produce disruption of the arterial wall and pseudoaneurysms.

Arteritis may also affect multiple vessels and produce an appearance in the renal arteries similar to that in renal artery dysplasia. Together with aneurysm formation due to destruction of the media, fibrosis and cicatrix develop, and there may be profound narrowing or vascular occlusion as a result. The disease is similar to Takayasu's disease and to giant cell aortitis and arteritis of the Bantu type. Aside from the renal arteries, the aorta may be involved as well as the celiac artery, the superior mesenteric artery, and many other aortic branches.

Other Diagnostic Applications of Renal Arteriography

Many other areas in which renal arteriography may play an important role are presented in detail throughout these volumes. Impressions on the collecting system by renal artery branches may suggest significant filling defects on the urogram and can by evaluated, when suspicious, only by arteriography. Pseudotumors (real or simulated masses in the kidney that roentgenologically resemble a neoplasm but histologically consist of normal renal parenchyma) frequently present diagnostic problems. The so-called dromedary hump or splenic hump of the left kidney has frequently been mistaken for an intrarenal mass. Other pseudotumors, such as prominent columns of Bertin (Fig. 7–202), focal hypertrophy, and renal sinus lipomatosis, may be recognized by radionuclide studies (Kam et al., 1981) or computed tomography and rarely require angiography. Xanthogranulomatous pyelonephritis may mimic carcinoma, and even with the arteriographic information it is not always possible to distinguish the two. Localized hydronephrosis in a double collecting system may resemble a tumor or cyst (Fig. 7–203). Although the urographic data are usually distinctive, at times arteriography may be helpful. Similarly, the angiographic appearance of generalized hydronephrosis is quite characteristic and is useful in indicating the volume of residual functioning renal tissue (Fig. 7–204) (Aron et al., 1973).

Angiography plays a particularly important role in renal transplantation. It is an essential element in evaluating the donor and will fre-

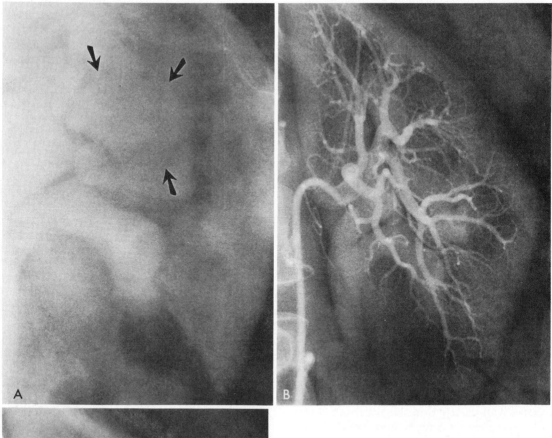

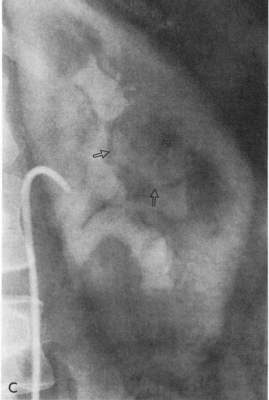

Figure 7–202. Renal pseudotumor. *A*, Urogram. Contrast material fills the collecting system. A mass (arrows) between the upper and middle portions of the kidney apparently displaces calyces and infundibula. *B*, Selective renal arteriogram. The appearance is relatively normal. A small supplementary artery to the lower pole is not filled. *C*, Nephrographic phase. At the time when the cortex is rather densely opacified, a thin round edge of cortex is also visible in the area of the apparent mass. This represents normal renal tissue, a prominent column of Bertin, rather than a significant intrarenal mass.

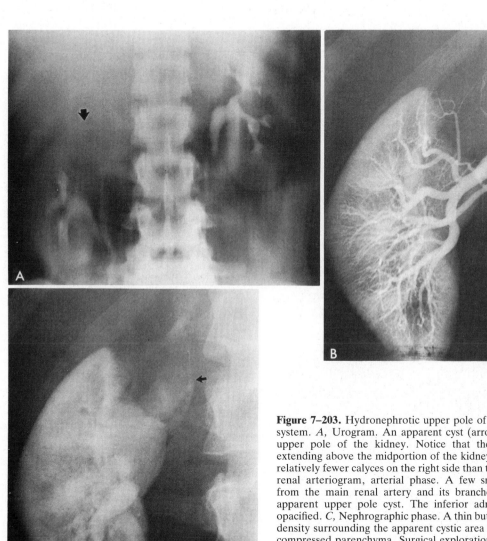

Figure 7–203. Hydronephrotic upper pole of a double collecting system. *A,* Urogram. An apparent cyst (arrow) is visible in the upper pole of the kidney. Notice that there are no calyces extending above the midportion of the kidney and that there are relatively fewer calyces on the right side than the left. *B,* Selective renal arteriogram, arterial phase. A few small vessels extend from the main renal artery and its branches to surround the apparent upper pole cyst. The inferior adrenal artery is also opacified. *C,* Nephrographic phase. A thin but definite curvilinear density surrounding the apparent cystic area medially represents compressed parenchyma. Surgical exploration revealed a hydronephrotic upper pole of a double collecting system on the right.

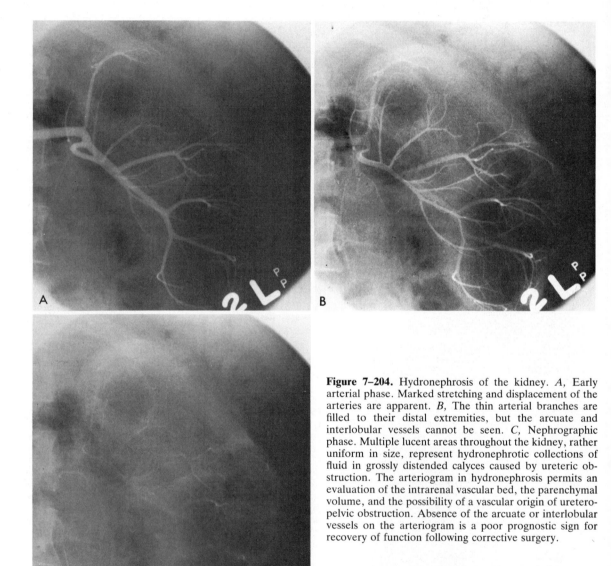

Figure 7–204. Hydronephrosis of the kidney. *A,* Early arterial phase. Marked stretching and displacement of the arteries are apparent. *B,* The thin arterial branches are filled to their distal extremities, but the arcuate and interlobular vessels cannot be seen. *C,* Nephrographic phase. Multiple lucent areas throughout the kidney, rather uniform in size, represent hydronephrotic collections of fluid in grossly distended calyces caused by ureteric obstruction. The arteriogram in hydronephrosis permits an evaluation of the intrarenal vascular bed, the parenchymal volume, and the possibility of a vascular origin of ureteropelvic obstruction. Absence of the arcuate or interlobular vessels on the arteriogram is a poor prognostic sign for recovery of function following corrective surgery.

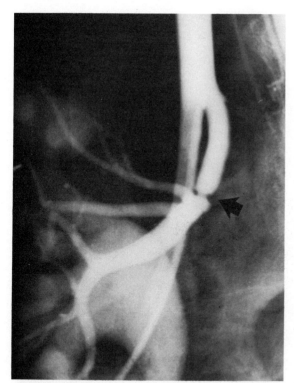

Figure 7–205. Renal artery stenosis in a transplanted kidney. Rather striking narrowing has developed at the site of anastomosis (arrow) in this patient who developed hypertension 8 months after transplantation.

quently show unsuspected abnormalities (Rabe et al., 1983). It is also frequently required in the recipient. In patients who fail to function after transplantation, in those who function initially and then experience a decrease in function, and in those who develop hypertension, angiography may clarify the underlying anatomic alterations. It is particularly useful in detecting or excluding renal artery stenosis or occlusion in the recipient (Fig. 7–205).

Applications of Renal Arteriography to Therapy

Within recent years, the selective renal catheter has become not simply a means of diagnosing disease but also one of treating it. In the presence of intrarenal bleeding, both pharmacodynamic agents and clot have been injected into the renal circulation and have caused the bleeding to cease (Fig. 7–206). With renal cell carcinoma, usually a highly vascular tumor, balloon catheters and clot or Gelfoam have been utilized to cut off blood flow to the tumor and thus to permit the surgeon to operate

in a relatively bloodless field and to diminish blood loss (Fig. 7–207). During radiation therapy, epinephrine has been infused into the kidney to produce an anoxic kidney and thereby to reduce the effect of radiation (Steckel et al., 1967).

In the presence of inoperable renal tumors, epinephrine angiography has been employed to infuse chemotherapeutic agents at high concentrations into the neoplastic mass (with relatively unresponsive vessels), while protecting the adjacent normal renal tissue (with constricted vessels). In patients with acute renal failure and widespread preglomerular arterial vasoconstriction, vasodilating agents have been infused to promote an increase of blood flow to the cortex of the kidney (Fig. 7–208).

Transcatheter thromboembolectomy with aspiration of emboli has been employed to treat acute renal artery obstruction, with successful application to uncontrollable hypertension (Millan et al., 1978). Conversely, embolization of the kidneys in patients with uncontrollable hypertension has been used successfully, although the experience is limited (Adler et al., 1978).

Because it is possible to occlude arteriovenous fistulas using such materials as cyanoacrylate (Kerber et al., 1977), some patients with hypertension associated with renal arteriovenous fistulas may be treated by this nonsurgical method in the future.

No discussion of the renal vascular bed can be complete without a consideration of the use of the catheter for the relief of renal artery obstruction. When Dotter and Judkins introduced percutaneous transluminal angioplasty (PTA) in 1964, the method was oriented exclusively toward the problem of limb ischemia. Furthermore, the catheter system was not widely accepted in this country because it was relatively cumbersome. The technology gradually improved until Grüntzig, 10 years after the introduction of PTA, devised balloons capable of being distended to a fixed diameter over a relatively long area (Grüntzig et al., 1978). The ease with which these catheters could be handled rapidly increased their use; when Grüntzig demonstrated that dilatation of renal artery stenosis was feasible, it began to be applied far more broadly to the problem.

It is unusual that a renal artery lesion cannot be approached from the femoral artery and successfully dilated. Briefly, the technique is as follows: A curved catheter is inserted into the artery through which a guidewire is passed across the stenosis. Once a catheter has been passed over this wire beyond the stenosis, the

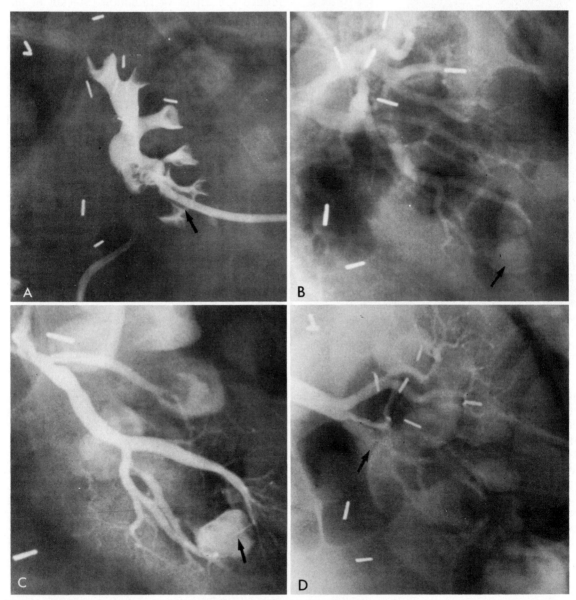

Figure 7–206. The therapeutic use of injected clot in renal artery bleeding. This patient was explored for calculous disease in the lower pole of the kidney and following surgery had persistent hematuria. *A,* The filling defect in the lower pole calyx (arrow) represents blood clot adjacent to the catheter. *B,* Aortogram. Contrast material is visible in the large lower pole calyx (arrow), but the source is not apparent. *C,* Selective renal arteriogram. A small jet of contrast agent (arrow) leaving an artery and entering the calyx of the lower pole represents a site of vessel erosion. *D,* Selective renal arteriogram after instillation of clot. No evidence of extravasation into the collecting system is now visible. The vessel to the lower pole is obstructed by clot (arrow), thus controlling the bleeding.

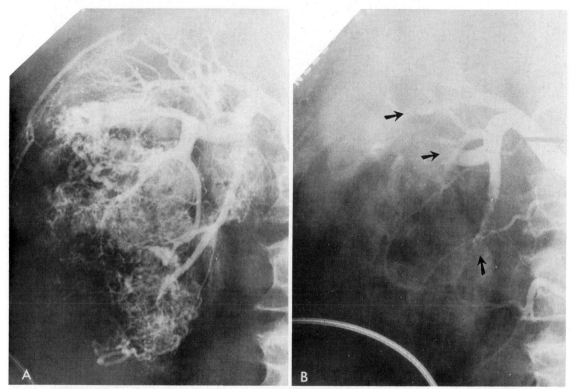

Figure 7–207. The use of injected clot to diminish vascularity of a renal cell carcinoma. *A,* Selective renal arteriogram. A large tumor mass has replaced much of the right kidney and extended into the hilar region of the right kidney and toward the spine. Grossly abnormal vessels with the classic characteristics of tumor vessels and tumor lakes are visible throughout two thirds of the kidney. *B,* Selective renal arteriogram after the instillation of clot into the main renal artery. The clot is now visible in multiple branches (arrows) of the renal artery, obstructing flow to the tumor. This approach provides a relatively bloodless field for the surgeon (if the tumor is embolized shortly before surgery) and also conserves a considerable amount of blood.

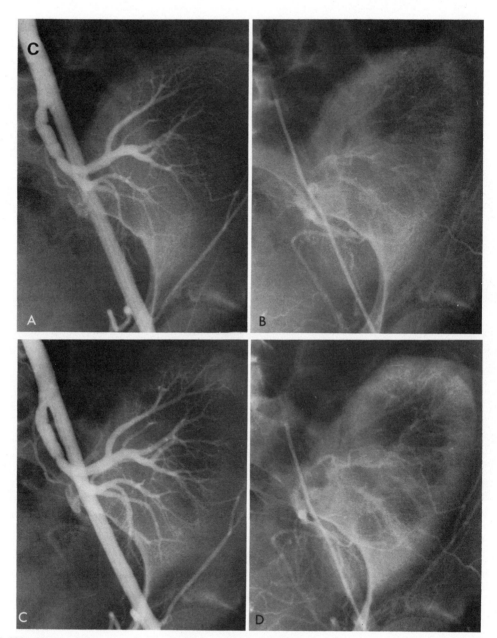

Figure 7–208. Acute tubular necrosis in a transplanted kidney. Effect of acetylcholine. *A,* The arterial phase of the arteriogram shows rapid tapering of the interlobar arteries with poor visualization of the distal vasculature. *B,* Slow transit of the contrast agent through the kidney is evident because the arteries are still visible on this 4-second film. A distinct nephrogram is visible, however. *C,* After administration of 10 mg of acetylcholine per minute for 30 minutes, the interlobular arteries and the more distal vessels are dilated. *D,* The nephrogram in this film is more dense than in the comparable control film shown in *B.* The xenon washout measurements showed a distinct increase in flow in the cortex during the acetylcholine infusion. The patient began to produce urine 14 days after the infusion of acetylcholine.

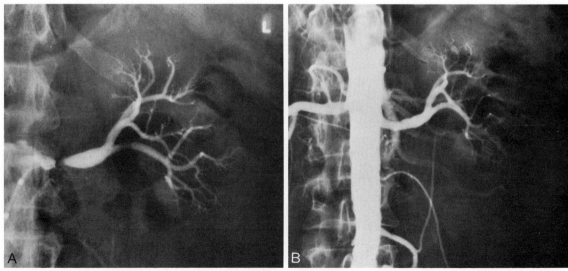

Figure 7–209. Renal angioplasty. *A*, Before. Note the severe degree of stenosis. *B*, After. A satisfactory dilatation has been achieved, with the eradication of the pressure gradient.

J-tipped guidewire remains and catheter exchange occurs with the introduction of a balloon catheter. The balloon is then dilated until a successful cosmetic result has been obtained, and until the pressure gradient demonstrates clear-cut evidence of improvement (Fig. 7–209).

Using this method, dilatation can be accomplished in between 60 and 90 per cent of patients, depending on the series, with improvement in blood pressure in 50 to 90 per cent of patients (Grim et al., 1981; Katzen et al., 1979; Mahler et al., 1982; Martin et al., 1981; Millan et al., 1979). Patients with renal artery dysplasia obtained better technical results and more gratifying responses in their blood pressure. Although there are complications of renal artery dilatation and although recurrence of stenosis may be observed, the method has proved to be an important advance in the nonoperative approach to hypertension caused by renal artery stenosis.

This section has addressed itself to the technique of renal arteriography, the normal anatomy, the indications and the applications. Clearly, it is impossible to be exhaustive within the framework of a single section, and the reader is referred to each individual subject for further elaboration on the applications of radiologic methods to evaluating and understanding diseases of the genitourinary tract.

ANGIOGRAPHY OF THE ADRENAL GLAND

While angiographic examination of the adrenal glands made preoperative localization of adrenal tumors possible in the 1960's and early 1970's (Cho et al., 1980; Ekelund and Hoevels, 1979; Hoevels and Ekelund, 1979), computed tomography has become the initial examination of choice for patients suspected of adrenal disease (Copeland, 1984; Glazer et al., 1982; Karstedt et al., 1978; Korobkin et al., 1979). In spite of successful localization of adrenal masses by computed tomography, surgeons often prefer to have a vascular "road map" prior to operation in patients with large or potentially complex masses. Adrenal hyperplasia is also more successfully recognized by arteriography than by computed tomography.

INDICATIONS

Following an initial examination by computed tomography, certain patients will be considered for angiography or venous sampling. Patients under consideration for adrenal angiography may conveniently be divided into three groups:

1. Those with or without signs, symptoms, or biochemical evidence of adrenal hyperfunction who have mass lesions in the adrenal area detected by computed tomography or conventional x-ray studies (Kuribayashi et al., 1982).

2. Those with signs, symptoms, and biochemical evidence of pheochromocytoma (Tisnado et al., 1980).

3. Those with signs, symptoms, and biochemical evidence of adrenal cortical hyperfunction without a mass detectable by computed tomography or conventional radiologic examination.

Patients in Group 1 who have large masses should be examined by arteriography so that a maximum amount of information regarding the extent of the adrenal tumor and the nature of its blood supply can be obtained. Those in Group 2 should also be studied by arteriography. This enhances the probability of detecting extra-adrenal or multiple pheochromocytomas. Adrenal radionuclide scanning looks promising for pheochromocytoma but is, at the moment, still experimental (Sisson et al., 1981). Those in Group 3 should be examined initially by adrenal phlebography, which is more likely to detect small lesions within the adrenal gland. This is particularly important when the purpose of the angiographic exploration is a search for an aldosteronoma; these lesions may be less than 0.5 cm in diameter when they present clinically.

TECHNIQUE

Adrenal Arteriography

Adrenal arteriography should begin with a mainstream aortogram performed with the tip of the catheter at the T12–L1 intervertebral disc space. This assures delivery of contrast agent to all the sites of potential arterial supply to the adrenal glands (Fig. 7–210). When the patient is being studied for possible pheochromocytoma, pelvic arteriography should be performed next with the injection of contrast agent just above the bifurcation of the aorta. For aortography and pelvic angiography we use a polyethylene pigtail No. 7 French catheter with four side holes. An injection of 25 ml per second for 2 seconds is used for aortography and 20 ml per second for 2 seconds for pelvic angiography. Serial films are obtained at the rate of two per second for 3 seconds and one per second for 7 seconds. Following aortography, selective injections of contrast agent into the renal arteries, celiac axis, phrenic arteries, and middle adrenal branches arising directly from the aorta will

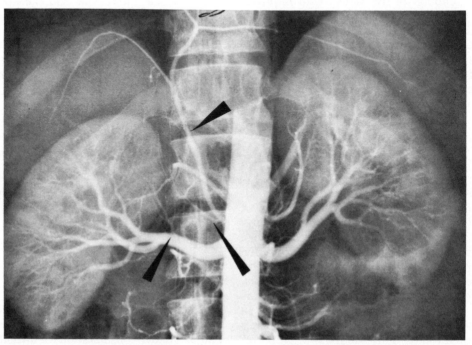

Figure 7–210. Normal aortogram demonstrating the arterial supply to the right adrenal gland (arrowheads). In this case, the inferior phrenic and the middle adrenal arteries have a common origin and the inferior adrenal artery arises from the right renal artery.

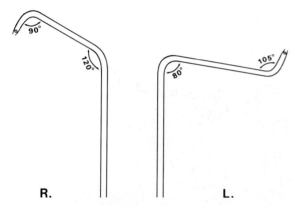

Figure 7–211. Right and left adrenal vein catheters. The tip of each catheter should measure about 1.5 cm. The segment between the primary and secondary curves of the right catheter should be about 5 cm in length, and that segment of the left catheter should be about 7 cm in length. A manipulating guide assembly is often needed to introduce the left adrenal catheter into the left renal vein.

provide dense opacification of the adrenal glands and an optimal opportunity for visualization of the tumor. A No. 7 French selective visceral catheter is used for these injections, with the rate and volume of contrast agent varying with the position of the catheter tip. The use of epinephrine (10 gm in the renal arteries and 20 gm in the celiac axis just prior to the contrast agent injection) enhances visualization of the adrenal glands in many instances (Kahn, 1971).

Adrenal Phlebography

While catheterization of the adrenal veins from the antecubital or jugular veins is possible, the most commonly used approach involves the percutaneous introduction of catheters into the femoral vein. The difference in the anatomy of the right and left adrenal veins requires that two catheters be used to facilitate entry into each adrenal vein (Fig. 7–211). Catheterization of the left adrenal vein, which drains into the cephalic surface of the left renal vein just lateral to the vertebral body, is accomplished with a left adrenal vein catheter (Fig. 7–212A). When using this catheter, a deflecting tip guide system* may be required for the initial placement of the catheter in the left renal vein. The right adrenal vein has proved more difficult to locate. It joins the right dorsal aspect of the inferior vena cava at the left of L1, but its location is less constant than is that of the left (Fig. 7–212B). In as many as 15 per cent of patients, for example, the right

---

*Cook, Inc., 925 South Curry Pike, Bloomington, Indiana 47401.

adrenal vein drains into a hepatic vein. An additional difficulty with this examination results from the similarity of appearance of an injection into a small hepatic vein and that of an injection into the right adrenal vein (Fig. 7–212C and D). The volume and rate of contrast injection vary with the site of the catheter placement and the size of the gland. Usually a rapid hand injection of less than 5 ml will suffice. Serial films may be obtained at one per second for 5 to 8 seconds. The retrograde injection of contrast agent into the adrenal veins is facilitated by the absence of valves in these veins.

Injection of contrast agents selectively into adrenal arteries or adrenal veins is accompanied by considerable discomfort. This emphasizes the need for adequate premedication for patients who are undergoing this procedure. While it is acceptable to begin the procedure with standard premedication, more should be added if the patient does not appear well sedated. The use of narcotics early in the examination will usually facilitate the procedure.

Blood samples should be obtained from each adrenal vein selectively during venography to aid in the localization of the functioning tumors.

Hazards of Angiographic Examination

Adrenal arteriography and phlebography are associated with two major hazards. In the patient with pheochromocytoma, an acute hypertensive or hypotensive episode may occasionally occur following either adrenal arteriography or phlebography. Although this is a rare event, it occurs in as many as 8 per cent of examinations (Hessel et al., 1981). This potential danger requires that an intravenous line be available in all these patients and that those practitioners examining such patients only occasionally should have the presence of an anesthesiologist during the study. Because of the urgency of prompt and appropriate therapy, an anesthesiologist should always be on call for these procedures. Many patients with pheochromocytoma now undergo angiographic examination only after the blood pressure is stabilized with phenoxybenzamine hydrochloride and propranolol hydrochloride even though there is no evidence that this controls hypertensive episodes during angiography.

The second major risk is limited to the phlebographic portion of the examination. This involves extravasation of contrast agent into the adrenal gland following a forceful retrograde contrast agent injection into the veins. This may be associated with rupture of the gland and

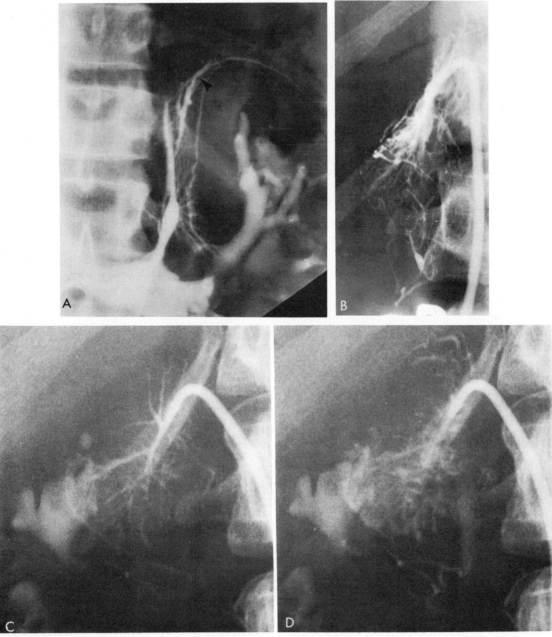

Figure 7–212. Normal adrenal venograms. *A,* The left adrenal vein drains into the cephalad surface of the renal vein. A capsular vein is seen filling (arrowhead), but the catheter tip is in the adrenal vein and fills it preferentially. Note the leaflike configuration of the intra-adrenal veins. *B,* The right adrenal vein radiates caudad from the junction of the adrenal vein and the inferior vena cava. In other patients the vein may appear more stellate because the vein joins the vena cava from the middle of the gland. *C* and *D,* Early and late films from injection into a small hepatic vein draining directly into the inferior vena cava in the region of the right adrenal vein. Note the stellate appearance of the veins, simulating a right adrenal vein. Usually the patient experiences less pain with hepatic vein injection than with adrenal vein injection, and intrahepatic branches often fill with drainage toward the hilus of the liver. In this particular case, failure of the intrahepatic branches to fill made the differentiation particularly difficult.

some degree of tissue death. While this complication was initially recognized in patients with aldosteronism, it is now commonly recognized in 8 to 10 per cent of all phlebographic examinations of the adrenal gland regardless of the indication for the study (Hessel et al., 1981). In addition to these two major hazards, all the complications of percutaneous transfemoral arteriography or inferior vena cavography may occasionally be encountered.

SPECIFIC LESIONS

Pheochromocytoma

This tumor, well known for its multiplicity and its extra-adrenal location in 10 to 20 per cent of patients, is frequently sufficiently vascular to be visualized during aortography (Fig. 7–213). Some tumors may not be apparent during the arterial phase of the aortogram or selective arteriogram, but contrast accumulation in the late capillary and venous phases may delineate the margins of the tumor.

When conventional aortography, pelvic arteriography, and selective injections into the adrenal arteries fail to demonstrate a pheochromocytoma, central venous sampling, including samples from the superior vena cava, may prove useful in establishing the level, although not the size, of the tumor (Euler et al., 1955; Harrison et al., 1968). Once the level is determined, further arteriographic studies may localize the tumor precisely. Specifically, thoracic aortography should be used to search for a mediastinal tumor when the lesion is not found in the abdomen.

Adrenal phlebography has occasionally proved useful in visualizing pheochromocytomas. It permits venous sampling, which may be useful at times but can be confusing with this particular tumor (Agee et al., 1973). Review of the literature (Agee et al., 1973; Alfidi et al., 1969; Baltaxe et al., 1973; Campbell et al., 1974; Christenson et al., 1976; Colapinto and Steed, 1971; Davidson et al., 1975; Gammill et al., 1970; Gold et al., 1972; Lanner and Rosencrantz, 1970; Levitt et al., 1975; McAlister and Lester, 1971; Nakada et al., 1973; Sutton, 1975; Zelch et al., 1974) indicates that at least 112 patients with pheochromocytoma have been examined recently by aortography and arteriography. Of these, tumors were demonstrated in 88, but in 24 patients the angiographic examination failed to detect the site of the tumor. Two false positive studies were also reported (Christenson et al., 1976). In nine patients in whom adrenal phlebography was employed, this technique failed to demonstrate the tumor in only one.

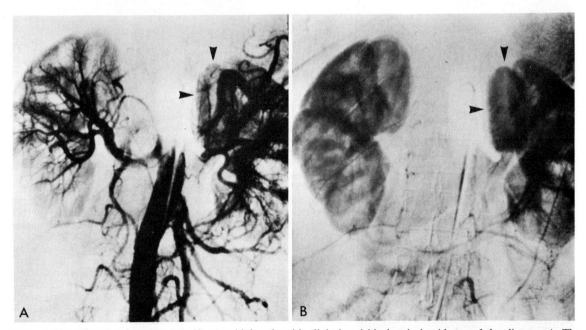

Figure 7–213. Pheochromocytoma. A 40-year-old female with clinical and biochemical evidence of the disease. *A,* The aortogram reveals a mass overlying the superior medial surface of the left kidney (arrowheads). Although there is an enlarged inferior adrenal artery arising from the left renal artery, no abnormal vessels are seen. *B,* The parenchymal blush of the pheochromocytoma can be seen (arrowheads) and is easily separated from the renal substance superimposed over its lateral surface.

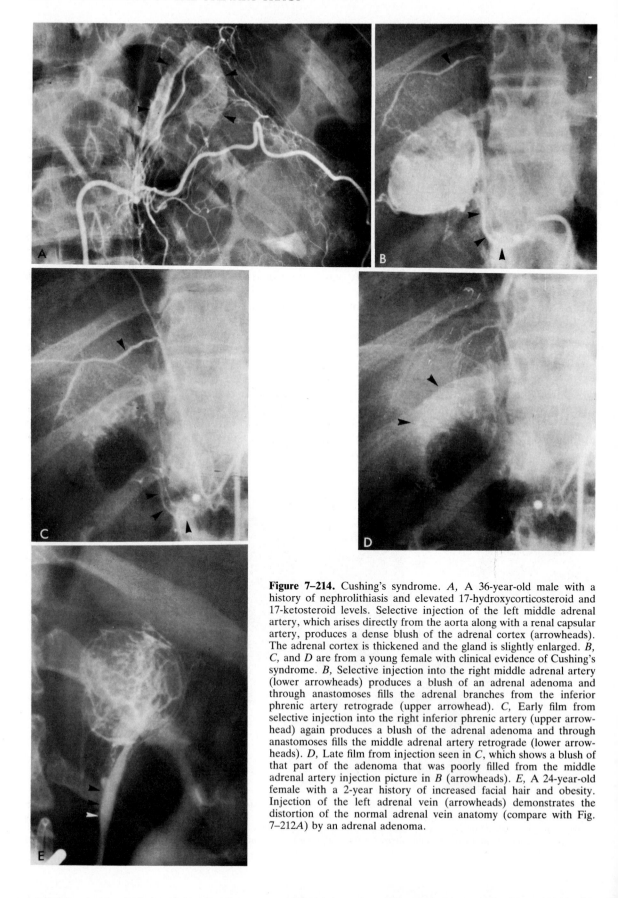

Figure 7–214. Cushing's syndrome. *A*, A 36-year-old male with a history of nephrolithiasis and elevated 17-hydroxycorticosteroid and 17-ketosteroid levels. Selective injection of the left middle adrenal artery, which arises directly from the aorta along with a renal capsular artery, produces a dense blush of the adrenal cortex (arrowheads). The adrenal cortex is thickened and the gland is slightly enlarged. *B*, *C*, and *D* are from a young female with clinical evidence of Cushing's syndrome. *B*, Selective injection into the right middle adrenal artery (lower arrowheads) produces a blush of an adrenal adenoma and through anastomoses fills the adrenal branches from the inferior phrenic artery retrograde (upper arrowhead). *C*, Early film from selective injection into the right inferior phrenic artery (upper arrowhead) again produces a blush of the adrenal adenoma and through anastomoses fills the middle adrenal artery retrograde (lower arrowheads). *D*, Late film from injection seen in *C*, which shows a blush of that part of the adenoma that was poorly filled from the middle adrenal artery injection picture in *B* (arrowheads). *E*, A 24-year-old female with a 2-year history of increased facial hair and obesity. Injection of the left adrenal vein (arrowheads) demonstrates the distortion of the normal adrenal vein anatomy (compare with Fig. 7–212*A*) by an adrenal adenoma.

Cushing's Syndrome

Patients with Cushing's syndrome require an angiographic evaluation to differentiate benign cortical adenoma from hyperplasia as the cause. Both arteriography and venography have been employed to establish the diagnosis (Fig. 7–214). In reported cases (Alfidi et al., 1969; Colapinto and Steed, 1971; Davidson et al., 1975; Lee et al., 1973; McAlister and Lester, 1971; Mitty et al., 1973; Vermess et al., 1972), 9 of 9 cases examined by arteriography were correctly diagnosed, and 30 of 32 cases studied by adrenal phlebography were correctly identified. In two venograms, tumors were discovered in normal adrenal glands. Among these cases, 14 adrenal adenomas, 20 hyperplastic glands, and 5 normal adrenal glands were correctly identified.

Aldosteronism

Hyperaldosteronism is a special problem because of the small size of aldosterone-producing adenomas. The combined approach of adrenal venography and adrenal vein sampling optimizes the retrieval of information in this group of patients (Fig. 7–215). In reported cases (Alfidi et al., 1969; Cerny et al., 1970; Colapinto and Steed, 1971; Davidson et al., 1975; Fisher et al., 1971; McAlister and Lester, 1971; Mitty et al., 1973; Nicolis et al., 1972; Sutton, 1975), 70 patients with aldosterone-producing adenomas were examined by venography; of these, 50 were correctly diagnosed. Of 12 patients examined by arteriography, 6 were correctly diagnosed.

Virilizing Syndrome

Examinations of 175 patients with virilization syndrome have been reported (Blair and Reuter, 1970; Farah et al., 1975; Gabrilove et al., 1976; Kupic and Eddy, 1970; Mitty et al., 1973; Nicolis et al., 1972). Among these patients, a virilizing adenoma was detected by arteriography in one; venography demonstrated 9 adenomas, 37 hyperplastic glands, and 1 carcinoma, with 5 false positive diagnoses of tumor. The remainder of the patients had normal venograms.

Miscellaneous Lesions

Adrenal arteriography and aortography have been utilized to study patients with adrenal cysts (Castro et al., 1975; McAlister and Lester, 1971; Wilson et al., 1972), adrenal carcinomas

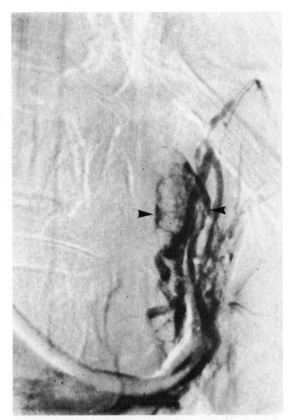

Figure 7–215. Aldosteronoma. A 46-year-old female with clinical signs of the disease. Injection into the left adrenal vein in the left posterior oblique projection outlines an aldosteronoma in the upper pole (arrowheads) of the adrenal gland. Contrast agent surrounds the tumor mass in a characteristic fashion.

(Fig. 7–216) (Alfidi et al., 1969; Colapinto and Steed, 1971; Farah et al., 1975; Lewinsky et al., 1974; McAlister and Lester, 1971), neuroblastomas (Sutton, 1975), metastases to the adrenals (Alfidi et al., 1969; Twersky and Levin, 1975; Wright, 1974), and granulomas (Kyaw, 1971). Aortography and adrenal arteriography have been highly successful in this group of patients.

CONCLUSIONS

Adrenal arteriography and phlebography should be applied in patients in whom adrenal tumors are suspected but in whom computed tomography has failed to provide adequate information. Arteriography can be, in appropriately selected cases, valuable in establishing the vascular anatomy of the gland and the presence or absence of tumor or hyperplasia.

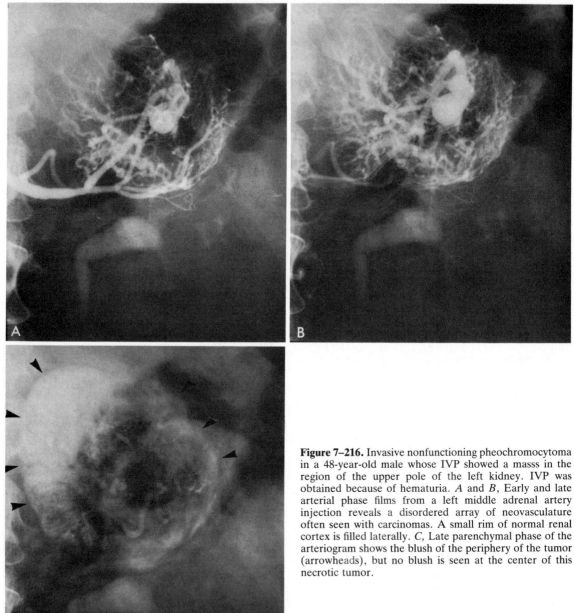

Figure 7–216. Invasive nonfunctioning pheochromocytoma in a 48-year-old male whose IVP showed a masss in the region of the upper pole of the left kidney. IVP was obtained because of hematuria. *A* and *B*, Early and late arterial phase films from a left middle adrenal artery injection reveals a disordered array of neovasculature often seen with carcinomas. A small rim of normal renal cortex is filled laterally. *C,* Late parenchymal phase of the arteriogram shows the blush of the periphery of the tumor (arrowheads), but no blush is seen at the center of this necrotic tumor.

References

Abrams, H. L. (Ed.): Angiography. 3rd ed. Boston, Little, Brown & Co., 1983*a*.

Abrams, H. L.: Renal arteriography in hypertension. *In* Abrams, H. L. (Ed.): Angiography. 3rd ed. Boston, Little, Brown & Co., 1983*b*.

Abrams, H. L.: The opaque media: physiologic effects and systemic reactions. *In* Abrams, H. L. (Ed.): Angiography. 3rd ed. Boston, Little, Brown & Co., 1983*c*.

Abrams, H. L.: The response of neoplastic renal vessels to epinephrine in man. Radiology, *82*:217, 1964.

Abrams, H. L., and Cornell, S. J.: Patterns of collateral flow in renal ischemia. Radiology, *84*:1001, 1965.

Abrams, H. L., and Obrez, I.: Epinephrine in the study of renal tumors. *In* Abrams, H. L. (Ed.): Angiography 3rd ed. Boston, Little, Brown & Co., 1983.

Abrams, H. L., Marshall, W. H., and Kupic, E. A.: The renal vascular bed in hypertension. Semin. Roentgenol., *2*:157, 1967.

Abrams, H. L., Obrez, I., Hollenberg, N. K., and Adams, D. F.: Pharmacoangiography of the renal vascular bed. Curr. Probl. Radiol., *1*:1, 1971.

Adler, J., Einhorn, R., McCarthy, J., Goodman, A., Solangi, K., Varanesi, U., and Thelmo, W.: Gelfoam embolization of the kidneys for treatment of malignant hypertension. Radiology, *128*:45, 1978.

Agee, O. F., Kaude, J., and Lepasoon, J.: Preoperative localization of pheochromocytoma. Acta Radiol. (Diagn.), *14*:545, 1973.

Alfidi, R. J., Gill, W. M., and Klein, H. J.: Arteriography of adrenal neoplasms. Am. J. Roentgenol., *106*:635, 1969.

Almen, T., Aspelan, P., and Levin, B.: Effect of ionic and non-ionic contrast medium on aortic and pulmonary arterial pressure. An angiocardiographic study in rabbits. Invest. Radiol., *10*:519, 1975.

Aron, B., Tessler, A., and Morales, P.: Angiography in hydronephrosis. Urology, *2*:231, 1973.

Baltaxe, H. A., Levin, D. C., and Imperato, J. L.: The angiographic demonstration of partially infarcted pheochromocytomas of the adrenal gland. Am. J. Roentgenol., *119*:793, 1973.

Bennett, A. R., and Wiener, S. N.: Intrarenal arteriovenous fistula and aneurysm. Am. J. Roentgenol., *95*:372, 1975.

Bergstrand, I., and Sorensen, S. E.: Renal angiography during straining. Br. J. Radiol., *38*:288, 1965.

Bettmann, M. A.: Advances in angiographic contrast agents. Am. J. Roentgenol., *139*:787, 1982.

Binz, A., and Rath, C.: Uber biochemische Eigenschaften von Derivaten des Pyridins und Chinolins. Biochem. Z., *203*:218, 1928.

Black, H. R., Glickman, M. G., Schiff, M., Jr., and Pingoud, E. G.: Renovascular hypertension: Pathophysiology, diagnosis and treatment. Yale J. Biol. Med., *51*:635, 1978.

Blair, A. J., and Reuter, S. R.: Adrenal venography in virilized women. JAMA, *213*:1623, 1970.

Boijsen, E.: Angiographic studies of the anatomy of single and multiple renal arteries. Acta Radiol. [Suppl.] (Stockh.), *183*:1, 1959.

Boijsen, E., and Kohler, R.: Renal artery aneurysms. Acta Radiol. [Diagn.] (Stockh.), *1*:1077, 1963.

Bookstein, J. J., and Stewart, B. H.: The current status of renal arteriography. Radiol. Clin. North Am., *2*:461, 1964.

Bron, K. M., Strott, C. A., and Shapiro, A. P.: The diagnostic value of angiographic observations in polyarteritis nodosa. Arch. Intern. Med., *116*:650, 1965.

Byrd, L., and Sherman, R. L.: Radiocontrast-induced acute renal failure. A clinical and pathophysiologic review. Medicine, *58*:270, 1979.

Campbell, D. R., Mason, W. F., and Manchester, J. S.: Angiography in pheochromocytomas. J. Can. Assoc. Radiol., *25*:214, 1974.

Castro, L., Schutte, H., Richardson, C., Fernandez, R. R. D., and Newman, H. R.: Adrenal cyst. Urology, *5*:574, 1975.

Cerny, J. C., Nesbit, R. M., Conn, J. W., Bookstein, J. J., Rovner, D. R., Cohen, E. L., Lucas, C. P., Warshawsky, A., and Southwell, T.: Preoperative tumor localization by adrenal venography in patients with primary aldosteronism: A comparison with operative findings. J. Urol., *103*:521, 1970.

Cho, K. J., Freier, D. T., McCormack, T. L., Nishiyama, R. H., Forrest, M. E., Kaufman, A., and Borlaza, G. S.: Adrenal medullary disease in multiple endocrine neoplasia type II. Am. J. Roentgenol., *134*:23, 1980.

Christenson, R., Smith, C. W., and Burko, H.: Arteriographic manifestations of pheochromocytoma. Am. J. Roentgenol., *126*:567, 1976.

Christian, C. L., and Sergent, J. S.: Vasculitis syndromes: Clinical and experimental models. Am. J. Med., *3*:385, 1976.

Chuang, V. P., Ernst, C. B., and Bhathena, D. B.: Evaluation of a new method for treating renal disease. Surg. Gynecol. Obstet., *148*:739, 1979.

Clark, R. A.: Angiographic management of traumatic arteriovenous fistulas: Clinical results. Radiology, *147*:9, 1983.

Colapinto, R. F., and Steed, B. L.: Arteriography of adrenal tumors. Radiology, *100*:343, 1971.

Copeland, P. C.: The incidentally discovered adrenal mass. Ann. Surg., *199*:116, 1984.

Cummings, K. B., Lecky, J. W., and Kaufman, J. J.: Renal artery aneurysms and hypertension. J. Urol., *109*:144, 1973.

Davidson, J. K., Morley, P., Hurley, G. D., and Holford, N. G. H.: Adrenal venography and ultrasound in the investigation of the adrenal gland: An analysis of 58 cases. Br. J. Radiol., *48*:435, 1975.

dos Santos, R., Lamas, A. C., and Pereira-Caldas, J.: Arteriografia da aorta e dos vasos abdominais. Med. Contemp. *47*:93, 1929.

Doss, A. K., Thomas, H. C., and Bond, T. B.: Renal arteriography: Its clinical value. Tex. Med., *38*:277, 1942.

Dotter, C. T., and Judkins, M. P.: Transluminal treatment of arteriosclerotic obstruction. Description of a new technic and a preliminary report on its application. Circulation, *30*:654, 1964.

Edling, N. P. G., Helander, C. G., Persson, F., and Asheum, A.: Renal function after selective renal angiography. Acta Radiol. [Diagn.] (Stockh.), *41*:161, 1959.

Edsman, G.: Angionephrography and suprarenal angiography. Acta Radiol. [Suppl.] (Stockh.), *155*:1, 1957.

Ekelund, L.: Pharmacoangiography of the kidney: An overview. Urol. Radiol., *2*:9, 1980.

Ekelund, L., and Hoevels, J.: Adrenal angiography in Sipple's syndrome. Acta Radiol. [Diagn.], *20*:637, 1979.

Ekelund, L., and Lindholm, T.: Arteriovenous fistulae following percutaneous renal biopsy. Acta Radiol. [Suppl.], *32*:1, 1972.

Ekelund, L., Gerlock, J., Molin, J., and Smith, C.: Roentgenologic appearance of fibromuscular dysplasia. Acta Radiol. [Diagn.] (Stockh.), *19*:433, 1977.

Euler, V., Gemsell, V. A., Strom, G., and Westman, A.: Report of a case of pheochromocytoma, with a special regard to pre-operative diagnostic problems. Acta Med. Scand., *153*:127, 1955.

Farah, J., Leach, R. B., Young, N. E., and Varley, P. F.: Adrenal venography in virilizing syndrome. Mich. Med., 7:379, 1975.

Fisher, C. E., Turner, F. A., and Horton, R.: Remission of primary hyperaldosteronism after adrenal venography. N. Engl. J. Med., *285*:334, 1971.

Fleming, R. J., and Stern, L. Z.: Multiple intraparenchymal renal aneurysms in polyarteritis nodosa. Radiology, *84*:100, 1965.

Folin, J.: Angiography in renal tumors. Its value in diagnosis and differential diagnosis as a complement to conventional methods. Acta Radiol. [Suppl.] (Stockh.), *267*:1, 1967.

Gabrilove, J. L., Nicolis, G. L., and Mitty, H. A.: Virilizing adrenocortical adenoma studied by selective adrenal venography. Am. J. Obstet. Gynecol., *125*:180, 1976.

Gammill, S., O'Neill, J., Puyay, F., and Johnson, C.: Angiography of pheochromocytomas in children. J. La. State. Med. Soc., *122*:302, 1970.

Gill, W. M., Jr., and Meaney, T. F.: Medial fibrodysplasia of the renal artery. Radiology, *92*:861, 1969.

Glazer, H. S., Weyman, P. J., Sagel, S. S., et al.: Nonfunctioning adrenal masses. Incidental discovery on computed tomography. Am. J. Roentgenol., *139*:81, 1982.

Gold, R. E., Wisinger, B. M., Geraci, A. R., and Heinz, L. M.: Hypertensive crisis as a result of adrenal venography in a patient with pheochromocytoma. Radiology, *120*:579, 1972.

Graves, F. T.: The anatomy of the intrarenal arteries and its application to segmental resection of the kidney. Br. J. Surg., *42*:132, 1954.

Grim, C. E., Luft, F. C., Yune, H. Y., Klatte, E. C., and Weinberger, M. H.: Percutaneous transluminal dilatation in the treatment of renal vascular hypertension. Ann. Intern. Med., *95*:439, 1981.

Grüntzig, A., Kuhlmann, V., Vetter, W., et al.: Treatment of renovascular hypertension with percutaneous transluminal dilatation of a renal artery stenosis. Lancet, *1*:801, 1978.

Halpern, M., and Citron, B. P.: Necrotizing angiitis associated with drug abuse. Am. J. Roentgenol., *11*:663, 1971.

Halpern, M., Finby, N., and Evans, J. A.: Percutaneous transfemoral renal arteriography in hypertension. Radiology, *77*:25, 1961.

Harrington, D. P., Levin, D. C., Garnic, J. D., Davidoff, A., Bettmann, M. A., Kuribayashi, S., and Torman, H.: Compound angulation in the angiographic evaluation of renal artery stenosis. Radiology, *146*:829, 1983.

Harrison, T. S., Bartlett, J. D., Jr., and Seaton, J. F.: Current evaluation and management of pheochromocytoma. Ann. Surg., *168*:701, 1968.

Hessel, S. J., Adams, D. F., and Abrams, H. L.: Complications of angiography. Radiology, *138*:273, 1981.

Hessel, S. J., and Smith, E. H.: Renal trauma: A comprehensive review and radiologic assessment. CRC Crit. Rev. Clin. Radiol. Nucl. Med., *5*:251, 1974.

Hoevels, J., and Ekelund, L.: Angiographic findings in adrenal masses. Acta Radiol. [Diagn.], *20*:237, 1979.

Jahnke, R. W., Messing, E. M., and Spellman, M. C.: Hypertension and post-traumatic renal arteriovenous fistula: Demonstration of unilaterally elevated renin secretion. J. Urol., *116*:646, 1976.

Janower, M. L., and Weber, A. L.: Radiologic evaluation of acute renal infarction. Am. J. Roentgenol., *95*:209, 1965.

Jones, G. W.: Renal cell carcinoma. CA, *32*:280, 1982.

Judkins, M. P., Abrams, H. L., Bristow, J. D., Carlsson, E., Criley, J. M., Elliott, L. P., Ellis, K. B., Freisinger, G. C., Greenspan, R. H., and Viamonte, M., Jr.: Report of the Inter-Society Commission for Heart Disease Resources: Optimal resources for examination of the chest and cardiovascular system. Circulation, *53*:A1, 1976.

Kahn, P. C.: Adrenal arteriography. *In* Abrams, H. L. (Ed.): Angiography. 2nd ed. Boston, Little, Brown & Co., 1971.

Kam, J., Sandler, C. M., and Benson, G. S.: Angiography in diagnosis of renal tumors: Current concepts. Urology, *18*:100, 1981.

Karstedt, N., Sagel, S. S., Stanley, R. J., et al.: Computed tomography of the adrenal gland. Radiology, *129*:723, 1978.

Katzen, B. T., Chang, J., Lukowsky, G. H., and Abramson, E. G.: Percutaneous transluminal angioplasty for treatment of renovascular hypertension. Radiology, *131*:53, 1979.

Kerber, C. W., Freeny, P. C., Cromwell, L., Margolis, M. T., and Correa, R. J., Jr.: Cyanoacrylate occlusion of a renal arteriovenous fistula. Am. J. Roentgenol., *128*:663, 1977.

Kincaid, O. W.: Renal Angiography. Chicago, Year Book Medical Publishers, 1966.

Kincaid, O. W., Davis, G. D., Hallerman, F. J., and Hunt, J. C.: Fibromuscular dysplasia of the renal arteries: Arteriographic features, classification, and observations on natural history of the disease. Am. J. Roentgenol., *104*:271, 1968.

Koehler, P. R.: The roentgen diagnosis of renal inflammatory masses—special emphasis on angiography changes. Radiology, *112*:257, 1974.

Kohler, R., and Edgren, J.: Angiographic abnormalities following percutaneous needle biopsy of the kidney. Acta Radiol. (Stockh.), *15*:514, 1974.

Korobkin, M., White, E. A., Kressel, H. Y., et al.: Computed tomography in the diagnosis of adrenal disease. Am. J. Roentgenol., *132*:231, 1979.

Kropp, K. A., Grayhack, J. T., Wendell, R. M., and Dahl, D. S.: Morbidity and mortality of renal exploration for cyst. Surg. Gynecol. Obstet., *125*:803, 1967.

Kupic, E. A., and Eddy, W. M.: Virilizing adrenal adenoma: Report of a case investigated angiographically. J. Urol., *103*:3, 1970.

Kuribayashi, S., Harrington, D. P., and Peterson, L. M.: Massive nonfunctioning adrenal cortical adenoma: Complementary roles of CT and angiography in the diagnosis. Cardiovasc. Intervent. Radiol., *5*:271, 1982.

Kyaw, M. M.: The angiographic appearance in an adrenal granuloma. J. Can. Assoc. Radiol., *22*:256, 1971.

Lanner, L. O., and Rosencrantz, M.: Arteriographic appearances of pheochromocytomas. Acta Radiol., *10*:35, 1970.

Lee, K. R., Line, F., and Sibala, J.: Adrenal adenoma and hyperplasia: The importance of arteriographic differential diagnosis. Am. J. Roentgenol., *110*:796, 1973.

Levitt, R. G., Stanley, R. J., and Dehner, L. P.: Angiography of a clinically nonfunctioning pheochromocytoma: Case report and review of the literature. JAMA, *233*:268, 1975.

Lewinsky, B. S., Grigor, K. M., Symington, T., and Neville, A. M.: The clinical and pathologic features of "nonhormonal" adrenocortical tumors: Report of twenty new cases and review of the literature. Cancer, *33*:788, 1974.

Lindvall, N., and Slezak, P.: Arteriography of the adrenals. Radiology, *92*:999, 1969.

Lundstrom, B.: Angiographic abnormalities following percutaneous needle biopsy of the kidney. Acta Radiol. (Stockh.), *15*:514, 1974.

McAfee, J. G.: Complications of abdominal aortography and arteriography. *In* Abrams, H. L. (Ed.): Angiography. 2nd ed. Boston, Little, Brown & Co., 1971.

McAlister, W. H., and Lester, P. D.: Diseases of the adrenal. Med. Radiogr. Photogr., *47*:62, 1971.

McCormack, L. J., Dustan, J. P., and Meaney, J. F.: Selected pathology of the renal artery. Semin. Roentgenol., *2*:126, 1967.

McCormack, L. J., Poutasse, E. F., Meaney, R. G., Noto, T. J., Jr., and Dustan, J. P.: A pathologic-arteriographic correlation of renal arterial disease. Am. Heart J., *72*:188, 1966.

McDonald, P.: Retroperitoneal tumors in children. *In* Abrams, H. L. (Ed.): Angiography. 3rd ed. Boston, Little, Brown & Co., 1983.

McGarity, W. C., Miles, A. E., and Hoffman, J. C.: Angiographic diagnosis and localization of endocrine tumors. Ann. Surg., *173*:583, 1971.

McLachlan, M. S. F., and Roberts, E. E.: Demonstration of the normal adrenal gland by venography and gas insufflation. Br. J. Radiol., *44*:664, 1971.

Mahler, F., Probst, P., Haertel, M., Weidman, P., and Krneta, A.: Lasting improvement of renovascular hypertension by transluminal dilatation of atherosclerotic and non-atherosclerotic renal artery stenoses: A follow-up study. Circulation, *65*:611, 1982.

Mancini, G. J. B., Bloomquist, J. N., Bhargava, V., et al.: Hemodynamic and electrocardiographic effects in man of a new, non-ionic contrast agent (Iohexol)—advantages over standard contrast agents. Am. J. Cardiol., *51*:128, 1983.

Martin, E. C., Mattern, R. F., Baer, L., Fankuchen, E. I., and Casarella, W. J.: Renal angioplasty for hypertension: Predictive factors for long-term success. Am. J. Roentgenol., *137*:921, 1981.

Meaney, T. F.: Errors in angiographic diagnosis of renal masses. Radiology, *93*:361, 1969.

Melby, J. C., Spark, R. F., Dale, S. I., Egdahl, R. J., and Kahn, P. C.: Diagnosis and localization of aldosterone-producing adenomas by percutaneous bilateral adrenal vein catheterization. Prog. Clin. Cancer, *4*:175, 1970.

Meng, C. H., and Elkin, M.: Immediate angiographic manifestations of iatrogenic renal injury due to percutaneous needle biopsy. Radiology, *100*:335, 1971.

Merklin, R. J., and Michaels, N. A.: The variant renal and suprarenal blood supply with data on the inferior phrenic ureteral and gonadal arteries. J. Int. Coll. Surg., *29*:41, 1958.

Millan, V. G., Mast, W. E., and Madias, N. E.: Nonsurgical treatment of severe hypertension due to renal artery intimal fibroplasia by percutaneous transluminal angioplasty. Med. Intell., *300*:1371, 1979.

Millan, V. G., Sher, M. H., Deterling, R. A., Jr., Packard, A., Morton, J. R., and Harrington, J. T.: Transcatheter thrombolectomy of acute renal artery occlusion. Arch. Surg., *113*:1086, 1978.

Mitty, H. A., Nicolis, G. L., and Gabrilove, J. L.: Adrenal venography: Clinical-roentgenographic correlation in 80 patients. Am. J. Roentgenol., *119*:564, 1973.

Moore, M. A., and Phillippi, P. J.: Reversible renal hypertension secondary to renal arteriovenous fistula and renal cell carcinoma. J. Urol., *117*:246, 1977.

Nakada, T., Momose, G., and Yoshida, T.: Diagnosis of adrenal hypertension. I. Selective adrenal venography and pharmacological evaluation using catheter technique for detecting pheochromocytoma. J. Urol., *109*:757, 1973.

Nicolis, G. L., Mitty, H. A., Modlinger, R. S., and Gabri-

love, J. L.: Percutaneous adrenal venography: A clinical study of 50 patients. Ann. Intern. Med., *76*:899, 1972.

Older, R. A., Miller, J. P., Jackson, D. C., Johnsrude, J. S., and Thompson, W. M.: Angiographically induced renal failure and its radiographic detection. Am. J. Roentgenol., *126*:1039, 1976.

Perry, M. O.: Fibromuscular disease of carotid artery. Surg. Gynecol. Obstet., *134*:57, 1972.

Pillari, G., Lee, W. J., and Kumari, S.: CT and angiographic correlates: Surgical image of renal mass lesions. Urology, *17*:296, 1981.

Plaine, L. I., and Hinman, F. J.: Malignancy in asymptomatic renal masses. J. Urol., *94*:342, 1965.

Pollack, H. M., Goldberg, B. B., and Bogash, M.: Changing concepts in the diagnosis and management of renal cysts. J. Urol., *111*:326, 1974.

Rabe, F. E., Smith, E. J., Yune, H. Y., Klatte, E. C., Leapman, S. B., and Filo, R. S.: Limitations of digital subtraction angiography in evaluating potential renal donors. Am. J. Roentgenol., *141*:91, 1983.

Rabinowitz, J. G., Kinkhabwala, M., Himmelfarb, E., Robinson, T., Becker, J. A., Bosniak, M., and Madayag, M. M.: Renal pelvic carcinoma: An angiographic re-evaluation. Radiology, *102*:551, 1972.

Reidbord, H. E., McCormack, L. J., and O'Duffy, J. D.: Necrotizing angiitis: II. Findings at autopsy in twenty-seven cases. Cleve. Clin. J., *32*:191, 1965.

Reuter, S. R.: Arteriography versus phlebography in the evaluation of adrenal diseases. J. Belge Radiol., *54*:575, 1971.

Reuter, S. R., Pomeroy, P. R., Chuang, V. P., and Cho, K. J.: Embolic control of hypertension caused by segmental renal artery stenosis. Am. J. Roentgenol., *127*:389, 1976.

Robins, J. M., and Bookstein, J.: Percutaneous transcaval biopsy technique in the evaluation of infarct vena cava occlusion. Radiology, *105*:451, 1972.

Sarramon, J. P., Cerene, A., Gorodetski, N., Bernadet, P., and Durand, D.: Spontaneous renal fistula and arterial hypertension—conservative treatment and healing. Eur. Urol., *4*:214, 1978.

Seldinger, S. I.: Catheter replacement of the needle in percutaneous arteriography: A new technique. Acta Radiol. (Stockh.), *39*:368, 1953.

Sherwood, T., and Trott, P. A.: Needling renal cysts and tumors: Cytology and radiology. Br. Med. J., *3*:755, 1975.

Simpson, A., Baron, M. G., and Mitty, H. A.: Angiographic patterns of venous extension of hypernephroma. J. Urol., *111*:441, 1974.

Sisson, J. C., Frager, M. S., Valk, T. W., Gross, M. D., Swanson, D. P., Wieland, D. M., Tobes, M. C., Beierwalters, W. H., and Thompson, N. W.: Scintigraphic localization of pheochromocytoma. N. Engl. J. Med., *305*:12, 1981.

Steckel, R. J., MacLowry, J. D., Holland, M. M., Paulson, D. F., and Johnson, R. E.: The Seldinger catheter in radiation therapy. Radiology, *89*:332, 1967.

Sutton, D.: The radiological diagnosis of adrenal tumors. Br. J. Radiol., *48*:237, 1975.

Swartz, R. D., Rubin, J. E., Leeming, B. W., and Silva, P.: Renal failure following major angiography. Am. J. Med., *65*:31, 1978.

Swick, N.: Darstellung der Niere und Harnwege in Rontgenbild durch intravenose Einbringung einesneuen Kontrastsoffes des Uroselectans. Klin. Wochenschr., *8*:2087, 1929.

Tisnado, J., Amandola, M. A., Konerding, K. F., Shirazi, K. K., and Beachley, M. C.: Computed tomography vs. angiography in the localization of pheochromocytoma. J. Comput. Assist. Tomogr., 4:853, 1980.

Tragardh, B., Almen, T., and Lynch, P.: Addition of calcium or other cations and of oxygen to ionic and non-ionic contrast media. Effects on cardiac function during coronary arteriography. Invest. Radiol., 10:231, 1975.

Twersky, J., and Levin, D. C.: Metastatic melanoma of the adrenal: An unusual cause of adrenal calcification. Radiology, 116:627, 1975.

Vermess, M., Schour, L., and Jaffe, E. S.: Case report: Calcification in benign non-functioning adrenal adenoma. Report of a case with selective adrenal arteriogram. Br. J. Radiol., 45:621, 1972.

Vlahos, L., Antoniou, A., Stephanopoulos, T., and Pontifex, G.: Adenoma of the kidney: Angiographic findings. Acta Urol. Belg., 50:309, 1982.

Voelcker, F., and von Lichtenberg, A.: Pyelographie (Roentgenographie des Neirenbeckens nach Killargofullung). Munch. Med. Wochenschr., 53:105, 1906.

Wagner, F. B., Jr.: Arteriography in renal diagnosis: Preliminary report and control evaluation. JAMA, 56:625, 1946.

Watson, R. C., Fleming, R. J., and Evans, J. A.: Arteriography in the diagnosis of renal carcinoma. Radiology, 91:888, 1968.

Weyman, P. J., McClennan, B. L., Stanley, R. J., Levitt, R. G., and Sagel, S. S.: Comparison of computed tomography and angiography in the evaluation of renal cell carcinoma. Radiology, 137:417, 1980.

Wilson, J. M., Woodhead, D. M., and Smith, R. B.: Adrenal cysts, diagnosis and management. Urology, 4:248, 1972.

Wright, F. W.: Adrenal metastases from renal carcinoma diagnosed by selective renal angiography. Br. J. Urol., 46:472, 1974.

Wright, F. W., and Walker, M. M.: The radiological diagnosis of "avascular" renal tumours. Br. J. Urol., 47:253, 1975.

Zelch, J. V., Meaney, T. F., and Belhobek, G. H.: Radiologic approach to the patient with suspected pheochromocytoma. Radiology, 111:279, 1974.

Renal Venography*

HERBERT L. ABRAMS, M.D.

Within the past few decades, renal venography and renal vein catheterization have been particularly useful in the study of renal vein thrombosis (Chait et al., 1968; Eisen et al., 1965; Harrison et al., 1956; Kees and Harrell, 1972; March and Halpern, 1963; Richet et al., 1965), carcinoma of the kidney (Caron et al., 1963; Kahn et al., 1968), and renovascular hypertension (Abrams et al., 1964; Fitz, 1967). Renal venography has been widely employed in physiologic studies (Bradley and Bradley, 1947; Brannon et al., 1944; Fitz, 1967; Helander et al., 1958; Kusunoki et al., 1956; Peart and Sutton, 1958) and in radiologic studies (Abrams, 1962; Abrams et al., 1964; Caron et al., 1963; Dalla Palma and Servello, 1956; Fuchs, 1961; Sorby, 1969; Steiner, 1960; Beckmann and Abrams, 1978; Beckmann and Abrams, 1979; Beckmann and Abrams, 1980). It is a relatively simple procedure technically and may be highly rewarding when employed in selected cases.

ANATOMY

The right renal vein pursues a relatively short course anterior and superior to the right renal artery and may angulate in a caudal or cephalad direction before reaching the inferior vena cava (Fig. 7–217). In 6 per cent of patients, it is joined by the right gonadal vein. Valves are present in the right renal vein in 28 to 50 per cent of autopsied cases, and in Beckmann and Abrams' study (1978) they were visualized on venography in 16 per cent of patients. In about 25 per cent of the patients we have studied, there were two or three veins on the right side (Fig. 7–218). Usually there is a major trunk and a relatively small joining vein, but at times there are two veins of equivalent size. Within the kidney the major trunks communicate freely. The two renal veins commonly join prior to entry into the inferior vena cava, but occasionally there may be independent vena caval entry. The vein has an average length of 24 mm and an average diameter of 13 mm. It usually enters the inferior vena cava at the level of the first lumbar vertebra.

The left renal vein is about three times as long as the right renal vein and pursues a much more horizontal course (Figs. 7–219 and 7–220). It varies in length between 60 and 110 mm, with an average being 84 mm. Valves are visualized on venography in 15 per cent of patients (Beckmann and Abrams, 1978). The left renal vein enters the inferior vena cava at the level of the L1-L2 interspace, most commonly with an angle

*This work was supported in part by USPHS grants HL11668, HL05832, and GM18674.

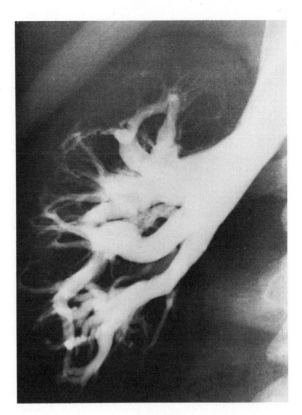

Figure 7–217. Normal right renal vein. The vein angles sharply cephalad to join the inferior vena cava.

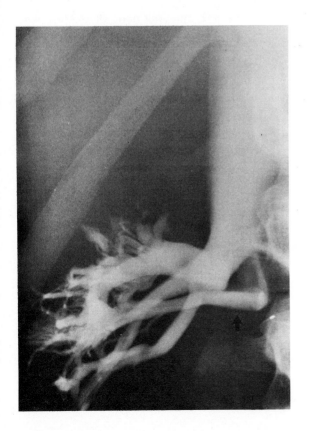

Figure 7–218. Normal right renal veins. There is a double renal vein. The more caudal vein (arrow) is horizontal, while the larger upper vein is directed cephalad.

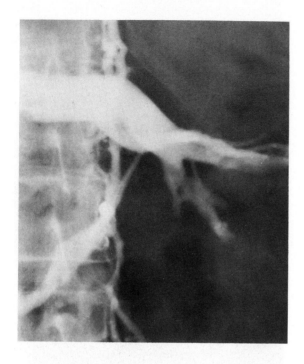

Figure 7–219. Normal left renal vein. The trans-spinal segment is horizontal. The common communication with the ascending lumbar system is opacified.

of about 90 degrees. Posteriorly it is in close contact with the third portion of the duodenum and the pancreas. Most patients have a single preaortic vein formed by a confluence of renal veins outside the renal hilum. A circumaortic venous ring was present in 7 per cent of our patients (Beckmann and Abrams, 1979) and in 16 per cent of patients in another series (Fig.

7–221) (Bosniak and Madayag, 1972). There may occasionally be two separate veins. The two segments may join prior to entry into the inferior vena cava or they may enter separately. In unusual cases, a single retroaortic vein is observed (Fig. 7–222).

On the left, the spermatic or ovarian vein empties into the renal vein consistently, and at

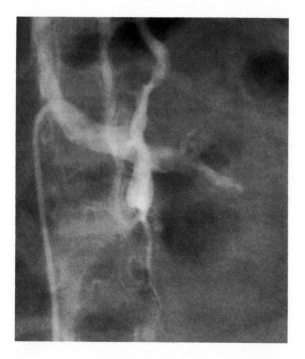

Figure 7–220. Normal left renal vein in a child. The course of the vein is more or less horizontal until close to the junction with the inferior vena cava. The ascending lumbar and vertebral veins are opacified via communicating veins.

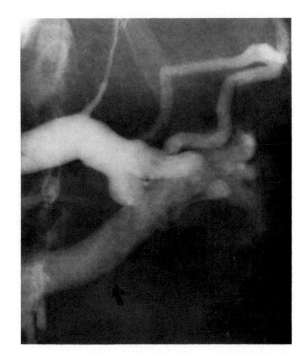

Figure 7–221. Circumaortic renal vein. The arrow points to the more caudal branch.

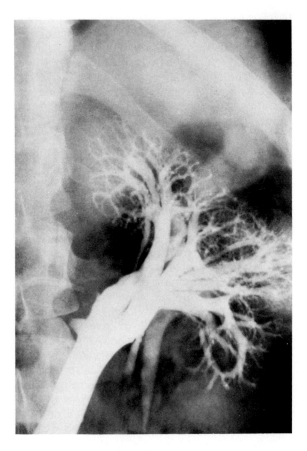

Figure 7–222. Retroaortic left renal vein. In this unusual anomaly, the left renal vein dips in a caudal direction to cross the spine dorsal to the aorta and then joins the inferior vena cava. Anatomic studies have described a single retroaortic vein in 2.4 per cent of patients.

times there may be two gonadal veins. The left adrenal vein also empties into the renal vein, but the right adrenal vein enters the inferior vena cava directly. Connections with the lumbar veins are present in a high proportion of patients (Anson et al., 1948) (see Figs. 7–219 and 7–220) and are demonstrable in about 50 per cent of cases (Abrams et al., 1964). Retrograde filling of the capsular and adrenal veins, as well as the gonadal veins, is frequently seen on the left renal venogram. In our series, the spermatic or ovarian veins were opacified in one half of the patients. In a few instances the ureteric vein was observed. The left renal vein enters the inferior vena cava in the region of the L1-L2 intervertebral space; on the right side the entry is usually slightly cephalad to that point.

The anatomy of the intrarenal veins is similar on both sides and mirrors the anatomy of the renal arterial system to a major degree. Thus, the small peripheral interlobular veins drain into arcuate veins, which join the larger interlobar veins. The interlobar veins extend directly to the major branches of the renal vein before entering the common main renal vein. All of the venous radicals are larger than their arterial counterparts.

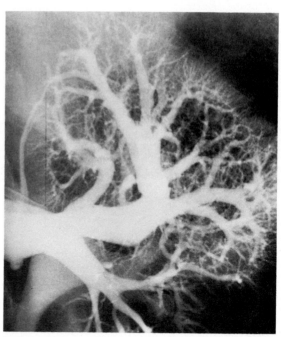

Figure 7–223. Normal left renal venogram. Epinephrine venography. Epinephrine (8 μg) was injected into the left renal artery 10 seconds prior to venography. All intrarenal branches, including the interlobular veins, are opacified.

TECHNIQUE

The catheter is passed percutaneously into the right femoral vein and is directed to the level of the renal vein. In shaping the catheter, the tip must be bent 130 degrees from its original straight shape. The length of the bent tip on the right should be about 5 cm, and on the left it should be between 9 and 10 cm. It is possible to use the right catheter for both catheterizations, though a guidance system may be necessary to help the placement in the left renal vein. The tip is extended above the renal vein and is directed to the right; with retraction, it enters the right renal vein. When the procedure has been completed, the catheter is withdrawn, is rotated to the left, and is directed into the left renal vein. It is useful to have two side holes within 1 cm of the catheter tip.

Total sustained opacification of the renal venous bed is best obtained with deliberate slowing of renal blood flow (Fig. 7–223). This is usually accomplished by injecting 6 to 10 μg of epinephrine into the renal artery followed by renal venography after 10 seconds (Abrams et al., 1962; Gyepes et al., 1969; Kahn, 1969; Olin and Reuter, 1965; Beckmann and Abrams, 1980). Renal artery catheterization is essential.

Brief catheter balloon obstruction of the renal artery accomplishes the same end. If visualization of only the main renal veins is desired, epinephrine venography is not necessarily indicated. The combination of epinephrine venography with renal vein balloon occlusion may be useful in enhancing delineation of the fine renal venous bed.

The volume of contrast agent may be varied depending on the indication for the examination. If good depiction of the intrarenal venous bed and the small veins is desired, 30 ml of 76 per cent Renografin (diatrizoate meglumine and diatrizoate sodium) should be injected within 2 seconds. If thrombus is suspected, 20 ml may be injected within 2 seconds. If invasion by carcinoma is the focus, approximately 20 ml or less may suffice. The volume should be based on a brief preliminary test injection and an assessment of whether renal venous flow is significantly diminished by occlusive disease.

Many other methods of investigating the renal veins have been described. For example, with the catheter in the inferior vena cava it is possible at times to get opacification of the mouth of the renal veins. More often, however, the dilution defects caused by the flow of nonopaque blood into the vein are visualized. Use of the Valsalva maneuver has been advocated.

By increasing the intra-abdominal pressure and diminishing the transit of contrast agent and blood from the inferior vena cava, the renal veins may be opacified (Peart and Sutton, 1958). At times this may be useful, but in our experience it has proved an inconsistent and unsatisfactory method of demonstrating the renal veins (Abrams et al., 1964). Others have noted the inefficacy of the Valsalva maneuver (Kahn, 1969). Among the more complicated approaches, balloon occlusion of the aorta and the inferior vena cava has been employed, particularly in experimental animals (Delin and Haverling, 1966; Peart and Sutton, 1958; Takaro and Kivirand, 1966). Transparietal injection (Gilsanz et al., 1965), percutaneous transrenal venography (Beres et al., 1964), and left spermatic vein injection (Gospodinow and Topalow, 1959) have all been described as methods of attaining renal venous opacification. Generally speaking, however, the more complex approaches are neither necessary nor desirable.

If renal vein thrombosis is suspected and there is a contraindication to using the femoral vein for catheter entry (such as the possibility of inferior vena caval thrombosis), an alternative technique is to pass the catheter from the antecubital vein through the right atrium into the inferior vena cava from above and then into the renal vein (Dalla Palma and Servello, 1956).

It must be emphasized that the intra-arterial injection of contrast agent is sometimes followed by relatively good renal vein opacification. Visualization is inconsistent, however, and depends to a major degree on the presence or absence of intrarenal vascular disease. If, in the presence of carcinoma of the kidney, selective renal venography is contraindicated, it is possible to inject larger volumes of contrast agent into the renal arterial bed. Once the diagnosis of carcinoma has been made and nephrectomy is anticipated, 20 or 25 ml of 76 per cent Renografin can be injected into the renal artery with a high likelihood of visualizing the renal vein. Even if this vein is occluded, the collateral circulation will usually be very well demonstrated and will indicate the presence of renal vein involvement by the neoplasm.

APPLICATIONS OF RENAL VENOGRAPHY

Renal Vein Thrombosis

Renal vein thrombosis in adults differs from that in children (Rosenmann et al., 1968). In children it is found almost exclusively in the presence of diarrhea and dehydration, and the prognosis is grave. In adults, renal vein thrombosis is often associated with underlying renal disease, including both systemic diseases, such as lupus erythematosus and amyloidosis, and primary diseases, such as nephrosclerosis, chronic glomerulonephritis, pyelonephritis, and membranous glomerulonephritis (Barclay et al., 1960; Hamilton and Tumulty, 1968; Janower, 1962). Whether renal vein thrombosis is the cause or an effect of membranous glomerulonephritis is not fully established; many authors consider it a consequence of the disease (Appel et al., 1966; Llach et al., 1975; Susin et al., 1974). In patients with the nephrotic syndrome, hypercoagulation defects (Kendall et al., 1971) may account for a high incidence of peripheral thrombophlebitis, renal vein thrombosis, and pulmonary embolism. Renal vein thrombosis may occur as an extension of thrombus within the inferior vena cava (McCarthy et al., 1963), or it may be associated with extrinsic pressure on the renal vein from an adjacent mass, such as a tumor or an aneurysm (Renert et al., 1972). Trauma is a rare cause (Chait et al., 1968; March and Halpern, 1963; Stables and Thatcher, 1973).

The response of the kidney to renal vein thrombosis depends on the rapidity and completeness of the occlusion and on the availability of collateral pathways (Hipona and Crummy, 1966; Koehler et al., 1966; Wegner et al., 1969). If the occlusion is rapid and complete, hemorrhagic infarction may occur. If the occlusion is gradual, collateral vessels may develop. The balance between the speed with which this collateral system develops and the rapidity of the occlusion determines the outcome. If the collateral system cannot accommodate the renal blood flow, the kidneys become enlarged and congested; later they may atrophy. Ligation of the renal vein may be accomplished with no long-term effects because of the collateral venous drainage, though temporary renal dysfunction may be observed (Anatkow and Kumanow, 1972).

Renal vein thrombosis is twice as common in males as in females. Clinically, it is associated with the nephrotic syndrome and frequently with hematuria (Stables and Thatcher, 1973). In addition, a third of these patients may develop pulmonary embolism; at times, this may be the presenting symptom (Stables and Thatcher, 1973). Patients with traumatic renal vein thrombosis and associated arterial occlusion do not exhibit the nephrotic syndrome but may present with recurrent pulmonary embolism (Stables and Thatcher, 1973). Autopsy examination of patients with renal vein thrombosis has shown that 24 per cent have associated inferior vena cava thrombosis, and 29 per cent have iliofemoral vein thrombosis (McCarthy et al., 1963). Of 39 patients with the nephrotic syndrome who we have examined by renal venography, only 7 had renal vein thrombosis.

Urography results may be negative in renal vein thrombosis; when they are positive, it is most often nonspecific. In the acute stage, the involved kidney is typically enlarged, with a moderate to marked reduction in function. Contrast filling of the collecting system may be significantly diminished (Fig. 7–224A), or it may be normal (Fig. 7–225A). Later, ureteral collateral vessels may produce notching of the renal pelvis and ureter (Fig. 7–225A). In the end stage, the kidney may be small and shrunken. These findings, either alone or together, are present in about one third of patients, whereas urography results are entirely normal in the others.

Renal arteriography demonstrates stretching of the intrarenal arteries in the acute stage (see Figs. 7–224B, 7–225B, and 7–226A). Transit time is protracted during the venous phase (Fig. 7–224C), the main renal vein fails to opacify, and collateral vessels may be visible (see Fig. 7–224D) (Itzchak et al., 1974; Koehler et al., 1966). If a venacavogram is performed, the usual dilution defect may be absent (Fig. 7–224E), but occasionally a clot in the renal vein may be demonstrated. Intracaval thrombus may also be visible (see Figs. 7–225C and D). Some of these findings, though highly suggestive, are not diagnostic; they may also be found in the absence of demonstrable renal vein thrombosis (Folin, 1967; Whitley et al., 1974).

An accurate diagnosis requires direct visualization of an intravascular thrombus by renal venography (Figs. 7–224F, 7–225D, 7–226B). One kidney—more commonly the left—is involved almost as often as both. Both sides, therefore, should always be examined (see Figs. 7–224 and 7–226). The renal vein may be totally occluded near the entry to the inferior vena cava or adjacent to the kidney and thus prevent opacification of the intrarenal branches (Beckmann and Abrams, 1980). In contrast to neoplastic invasion, thrombosis causes distension of the renal veins, and the central portion of the clot has a margin convex toward the inferior vena cava (Ahlberg et al., 1967). In some cases, the clot produces only partial obstruction and is seen as an intraluminal filling defect in the main renal vein (see Fig. 7–226B) or in intrarenal branches. Chronic or organized renal vein thrombus may be recognized by the demonstration of a narrow renal vein lumen with ill-defined outlines, linear bands representing synechiae, and peripheral occlusion (see Fig. 7–224F). In the transplanted kidney, oliguria, though most commonly caused by rejection, may also be associated with acute tubular necrosis, recurrence of glomerulonephritis, arterial stenosis or occlusion, renal vein thrombosis, and other causes.

Venography is the most precise method of detecting renal vein thrombosis, though computed tomography and magnetic resonance imaging may suggest the diagnosis. The early diagnosis of renal vein thrombosis is important; with appropriate anticoagulation therapy, pulmonary embolism may be prevented (Appel et al., 1966; O'Dea et al., 1976).

The renal vein may be occluded or compressed by extrinsic tumor masses or retroperitoneal fibrosis. We have studied a case in which a large tumor of the spleen in an infant displaced the kidney and caused compression of the left renal vein in association with the nephrotic syndrome (Wexler and Abrams, 1964). Once the splenic tumor was removed, the nephrotic syndrome disappeared entirely. Usually, intrarenal venous clot can be distinguished from extrinsic causes of occlusion by the intraluminal character of the filling defect.

In our experience, the risk of dislodging thrombus by the manipulation of a selective renal vein catheter is low. None of our patients developed pulmonary embolism after renal venography—an experience similar to that of other authors (O'Dea et al., 1976). This low risk is amply justified if initial or repeated pulmonary embolism can be prevented.

Renovascular Hypertension (Renal Vein Renin Determination)

Although arteriography can easily demonstrate stenosis in the renal arteries, the functional significance of the stenosis may be uncertain unless collateral vessels are present (Ernst et al., 1972). This significance and the potential surgical curability of the lesion are commonly evaluated in the light of renal vein renin activity (Bourgoignie et al., 1970; Genest and Boucher, 1971; Hunt and Strong, 1973; Korobkin et al., 1976; Schaeffer and Fair, 1974; Simmons and Michelakis, 1970; Vaughan et al., 1973). Renin,

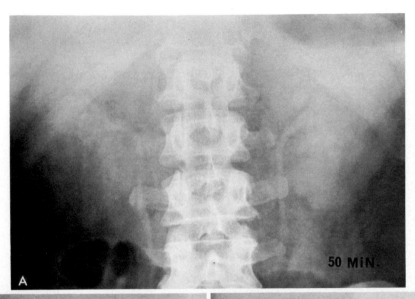

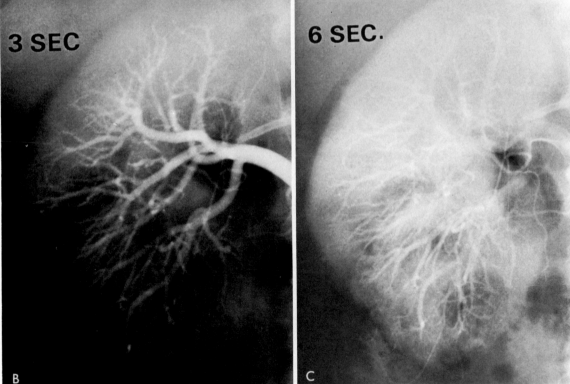

Figure 7–224. Renal vein thrombosis. *A,* Urogram. At 50 minutes there is only faint filling of the collecting system and ureters with a striking decrease in concentration. *B,* Selective renal artery arteriogram (3 seconds). Some stretching of the renal branches is visible. *C,* Selective renal arteriogram (6 seconds). There is protracted transit through the intrarenal arterial bed. *D,* Selective renal arteriogram, nephrographic phase (13 seconds). Collateral capsular veins are visible (arrows). *E,* Inferior vena cavogram. The usual dilution defect at the mouth of the renal veins, particularly on the right, is conspicuously absent. *F,* Selective right renal venogram. Extensive organized clot is present in the right renal venous system, with multiple synechiae indicating that the renal vein thrombosis is chronic. The synechiae appear as linear, thin, lucent strands intermixed with the contrast agent. Note the filling of the gonadal vein, acting as a collateral channel. Bilateral renal vein thrombosis was present.

(Illustration continued on following page)

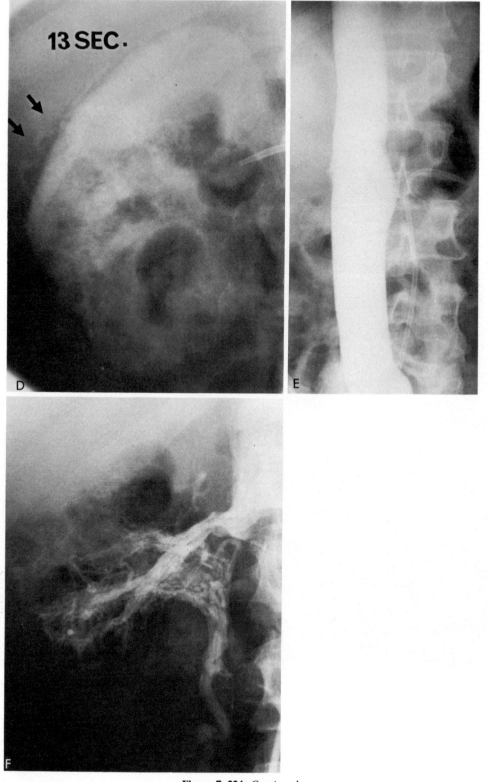

Figure 7–224. *Continued*

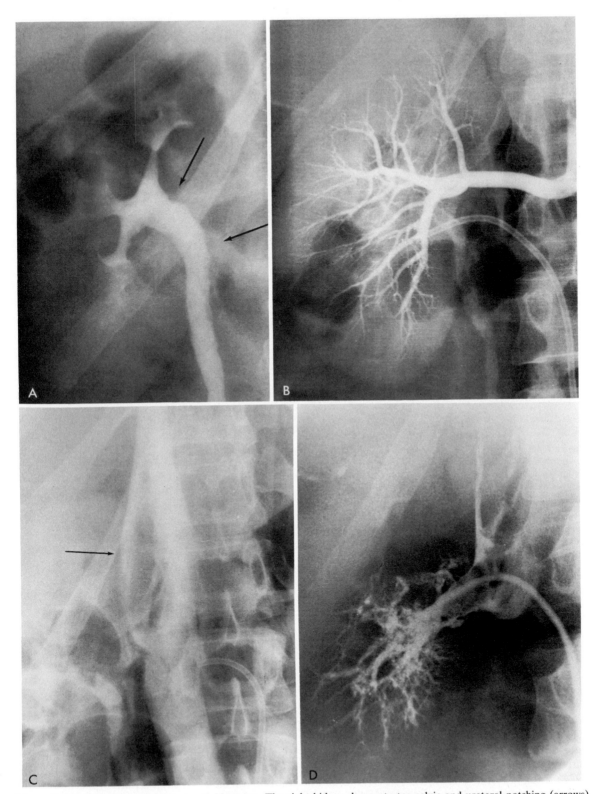

Figure 7–225. Renal vein thrombosis. *A,* Urogram. The right kidney demonstrates pelvic and ureteral notching (arrows) caused by collateral veins. The collecting system appears otherwise normal. *B,* Selective right renal arteriogram. The vessels are normal in appearance but somewhat spread because of swelling of the kidneys. *C,* Inferior vena cavogram. A large thrombus (arrow) is visible in the cava just above the right renal vein entrance. *D,* Right renal venogram. There is thrombus in the mouth of the right vein as well as in the cava. This patient also had extensive thrombus in his left renal vein.

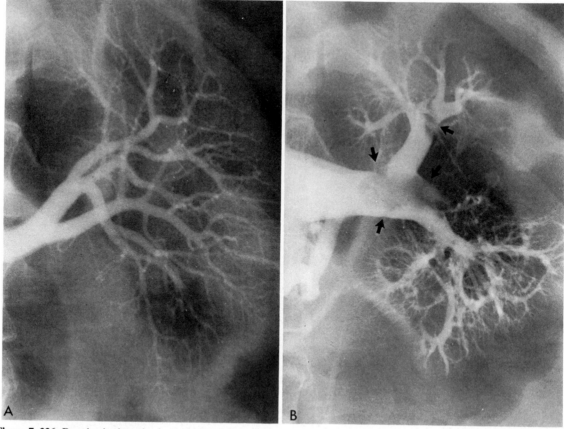

Figure 7–226. Renal vein thrombosis. *A,* Left renal arteriogram. The appearance is quite normal except for some stretching of the distal branches. Transit was prolonged. *B,* Left renal venogram. A large thrombus visible in the main renal vein extends into a number of branches (arrows). Thrombus is also present in the upper pole vein (uppermost arrow). Biopsy of the kidney showed membranous glomerulonephritis.

secreted in response to stimuli that compromise kidney perfusion, increases plasma angiotensin, which stimulates aldosterone secretion (Laragh et al., 1972). Vascular tone is regulated by an interaction between angiotensin levels and the available intravascular sodium ions. The two hormones, angiotensin and aldosterone, thus restore the sodium balance and the arterial pressure, thereby turning off renin release. The renal vein renin of the normal kidney should equal the renal artery renin. This line of reasoning supports the clinically established criteria used in diagnosing renovascular hypertension and predicting surgical curability:

1. Increased renin production of the suspect kidney: V-A/A 0.48 (V = venous renin activity; A = arterial renin activity) (Vaughan, 1974; Vaughan et al., 1973).

2. Suppression of renin secretion on the contralateral, normal side: V-A 0 (Stockigt et al., 1972; Vaughan et al., 1973).

3. A renal vein: renin ratio of 1.5:1 or

more between the involved kidney and the uninvolved kidney (Arner et al., 1965; Schaeffer and Fair, 1974; Simmons and Michelakis, 1970; Stockigt et al., 1972; Vaughan, 1974).

4. Elevated plasma renin activity (Stockigt et al., 1972).

The renin-angiotensin-aldosterone system is easily influenced by many factors in both normal patients and hypertensive patients.

Upright posture leads to increased renin production (Michelakis and Simmons, 1969). In renovascular hypertension, Michelakis and others (Michelakis and Simmons, 1969; Michelakis et al., 1969) found that the kidney with the stenotic artery produced excess renin, which led to a marked disparity in renin concentrations between the renal veins on the involved and the uninvolved sides. If such a patient changes from an upright position to a recumbent one, exaggerated renin production is not stimulated for a time, because of the high concentration of renin in the general circulation. As a result, the renal vein:renin ratio between the involved kidney and the uninvolved kidney approaches unity and briefly loses its diagnostic usefulness (Michelakis and Simmons, 1969; Michelakis et al., 1969).

Salt depletion induced by diuretics or a low dietary intake of sodium increases the renin activity. The stimulus to increased renin production affects the involved kidney more than the contralateral kidney, leading to an exaggerated renin ratio (Vermillion et al., 1969).

Antihypertensive drugs (Kuchel and Genest, 1971; Laragh et al., 1972) influence renin release in both directions. These drugs may increase renin release either by directly lowering the blood pressure or by their diuretic effect, with a consequent decrease in the blood pressure (Kuchel and Genest, 1971). The kidney with significant renal artery stenosis secretes disproportionately more renin than does the uninvolved kidney (Kaneko et al., 1967). Other drugs suppress the plasma renin activity, probably by directly interfering with the physiologic pathways of renin release (Kuchel and Genest, 1971).

Technique of Venous Sampling for Renin Assay

The same catheter used for renal venography may be employed for renin sampling. For segmental vein sampling, an additional downward deflection of 30 degrees should be incorporated in the catheter tip. At the Brigham and Women's Hospital, venous samples to be assayed for renin activity are taken from the main renal vein, the main left renal vein peripheral to the entry of the gonadal vein, and the inferior vena cava above and below the renal veins. The lower caval sample value is interchangeable with the renal artery renin concentration, since there is no low inferior vena cava–abdominal aorta pressure gradient (Vaughan et al., 1973). Correct localization of the catheter tip is essential for proper sampling (Fig. 7–227) (Paster et al., 1974). In the presence of a left circumaortic renal vein, the retroaortic vein can preferentially drain the lower poles (Korobkin et al., 1976; Paster et al., 1974; Stockigt et al., 1973). The same holds true in those rare cases of a locally circumscribed, renin-producing tumor of juxtaglomerular origin (Schambelan et al., 1973) or of a renal cyst compressing renal parenchyma and thereby creating focal ischemia. Samples should be drawn slowly to prevent aspiration from side branches (Korobkin et al., 1976; Pas-

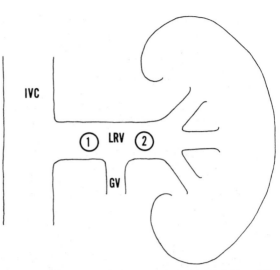

Figure 7–227. Possible errors in renal vein sampling. Diagram of left renal vein in a 50-year-old man with hypertension and embolus to the left renal artery. Initial selective renin determinations were: main right renal vein, 2034 ng per dl; main left renal vein, 2381 ng per dl. The difference was insignificant. Repeat study 3 days later demonstrated a renin value of 3138 ng per dl at site 1, compared with 14,815 ng per dl at site 2. The initial sample at site 1 was diluted by effluent from the gonadal vein.

ter et al., 1974). Simultaneous sampling of renal veins is unnecessary. Whenever arterial branch stenosis is demonstrated or suspected, selective sampling from the segmental draining vein is essential (Paster et al., 1974).

A rigid protocol should be followed for renin sampling. Samples should be obtained in hypertensive patients only after arteriographic demonstration of renal artery stenosis. This may follow abdominal aortography. Harrington et al. (1975) found no significant change in renal vein renin activity 10 minutes after aortography in a series of 56 patients. However, in a smaller series of animal experiments, other authors found an increase in renin secretion after selective renal arteriography (Katzberg et al., 1977). It is desirable, therefore, to obtain renin samples 15 to 20 minutes following selective renal arteriography. These patients should have no signs or symptoms of congestive heart failure and should preferably have received no diuretics or antihypertensive drugs (Genest and Boucher, 1971). Under standard conditions of recumbency and normal sodium intake, venous samples may then be drawn. If the results are normal or borderline, renin measurements should be repeated after stimulation by one of the following, alone or in combination:

1. Upright posture for 20 minutes (Michelakis and Simmons, 1969) to 4 hours (Genest and Boucher, 1971).

2. Sodium depletion by 3 days of severe sodium restriction at 10 mEq of furosemide per day (Genest and Boucher, 1971; Michelakis and Simmons, 1969).

3. Controlled hypotension.

Accuracy of Renin Assay

As a predictive index of the outcome of surgery in hypertensive patients with renal artery stenosis, the accuracy of renin activity varies between 70 and 95 per cent (Delin and Haverling, 1966; Genest and Boucher, 1971; Schaeffer and Fair, 1974; Simmons and Michelakis, 1970; Vaughan et al., 1973). The variability may be explained by the different criteria used and by the difference in how the patients are prepared. If the renal vein:renin ratio between the involved kidney and the uninvolved kidney is used alone, the accuracy is approximately 85 per cent. The ratios between the two sides do not take into account the occult hypersecretion of renin that takes place (though to a lesser degree) on the presumably uninvolved side (Vaughan, 1974). Such a finding suggests a nephrosclerotic kidney, and surgery might therefore be contraindicated. The additional demonstration of suppressed renin release or of an abnormally high peripheral plasma renin activity in relation to sodium excretion (indicating increased renin release) may increase the accuracy of predicting the surgical outcome to 95 per cent (Vaughan, 1974; Vaughan et al., 1973).

It is important to emphasize that absence of lateralization does not preclude a successful result from surgery; 21 per cent of such patients with renovascular disease experience amelioration of hypertension (Bourgoignie et al., 1970).

The renal venous washout time has been shown to reflect the rate of blood flow through the kidney and to be related to the renal plasma flow and to the presence of significant renal artery stenosis (Abrams et al., 1964). In the method used, contrast material was injected into the renal veins, and the washout time was determined cineangiographically. With this method, both kidneys could be evaluated and compared. With significant renal artery stenosis and reduction in the renal blood flow, the washout time was usually prolonged.

Renal Vein Varices

Pelviureteric varices are well documented as sequelae of renal vein thrombosis (Eisen et

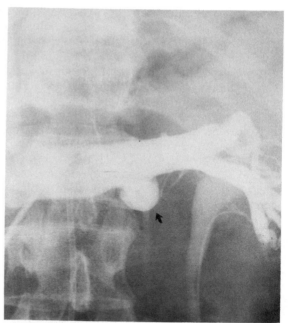

Figure 7–228. Renal vein varix. Renal venography was performed because of suspicion of renal vein thrombosis. A large varix (arrow) was observed, but its clinical significance was not apparent.

al., 1965; Weiner et al., 1974). Although there are few reports of idiopathic renal vein varices (Blaivas et al., 1977), they were found in eight (6 per cent) of the patients in the Peter Bent Brigham Hospital series. All were in the left renal venous system and consisted of either a solitary varix of the left renal vein (Fig. 7–228) or a network of veins (varicosities) adjacent to the renal pelvis. Renal vein varices are also formed in portal hypertension. They are probably more common than was previously reported, and the majority of the patients who have varices are free of symptoms. Rarely, varices may cause bleeding (Fig. 7–229). The urogram may be normal, even in cases in which varices are the source of bleeding (Jonsson, 1972; Mitty and Goldman, 1974).

Carcinoma of the Kidney

Renal venography may be an invaluable method of assessing carcinoma of the kidney (Goncharenko et al., 1979). These tumors tend to invade the renal vein and at times the inferior vena cava, and it is important preoperatively to know the extent of the tumor and whether it is operable. Knowledge of renal vein involvement also has prognostic significance (Arner et al., 1965; Crocker, 1975; Griffiths and Thackray, 1949; Hand and Broders, 1932; McDonald and

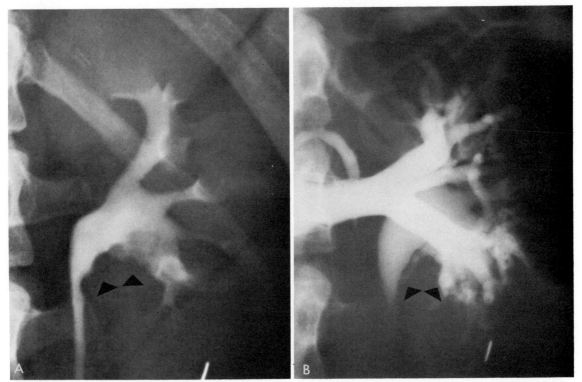

Figure 7–229. Renal vein varix. This 19-year-old girl had hematuria on the left side. Exploration was performed, and multiple varicose veins were observed in the region of the renal pelvis. She returned 2 years later with another bout of hematuria. *A,* Intravenous urogram. Notching of the undersurface of the renal pelvis and ureter is apparent (arrowheads). *B,* Retrograde renal venogram. Note filling of major veins, interlobar veins, and a tortuous vein that notches the pelvis and ureter.

Priestley, 1943; Myers et al., 1968; Riches, 1963; Riches, 1964; Riches et al., 1951) (Table 7–8). At the time of discovery, approximately one third of patients will have renal vein invasion.

If venography is required for renal vein visualization in carcinoma of the kidney, an inferior vena cavogram should be the initial step (Siminovitch et al., 1982). If the inferior vena cava is not involved, a selective renal venogram should follow (Fig. 7–230). Invasion of the renal vein by tumor is usually accompanied by a rather sharply defined, sometimes lobular, filling defect with a clearly etched edge (Fig. 7–231) (Petasnick and Patel, 1973; Watson et al., 1968); invasion can generally be distinguished from thrombus. At times, venography will establish the diagnosis after arteriography has not been helpful (Fig. 7–232) (Smith et al., 1975) or has even been misleading (Bernath et al., 1981).

Ultrasound, computed tomography, and magnetic resonance imaging may demonstrate renal vein invasion by carcinoma, but venography is the most reliable method of defining the anatomy and the extent of renal vein involvement (Weyman et al., 1980; Mauro et al., 1982). Although reservations have been expressed about renal venography in renal carcinoma (Hall, 1980), there is no evidence that it has been hazardous or has altered the course of the disease.

Nonfunctioning Kidney

In hypertensive patients, the differentiation of renal agenesis from nonfunctioning hypoplastic kidney or small, contracted kidney is clinically important. Diagnostic methods, such as abdominal aortography, cystoscopy, and retrograde pyelography, may be inconclusive and

TABLE 7–8. RENAL CELL CARCINOMA: FIVE-YEAR SURVIVAL

	Number of Patients	Number of Survivors	Percentage of Survivors
Total	1593	685	43
Without renal vein invasion	981	506	52
With renal vein invasion	612	179	29

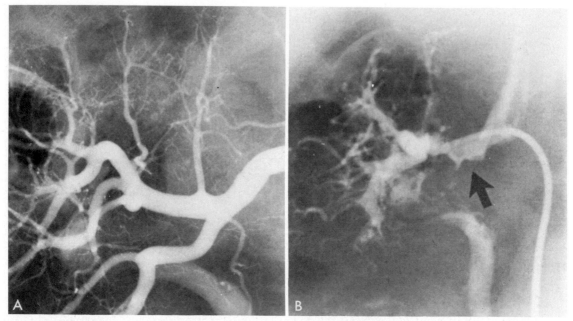

Figure 7–230. Carcinoma of the kidney. *A,* Right renal arteriogram (magnification study). There is encasement and stretching of vessels to the upper pole as well as tortuous small tumor vessels. *B,* Renal venogram (70-mm film). The right renal vein is invaded by tumor (arrow).

even misleading in these patients (Athanasoulis et al., 1973; Itzchak et al., 1974). Aortography may show the absence of a renal artery in both renal agenesis and small, shrunken kidneys (Athanasoulis et al., 1973). In addition, the presence of a ureteral orifice on cystoscopy need not imply the presence of a kidney on that side (Ney and Friedenberg, 1966).

Conversely, the absence of a renal vein on venography is pathognomonic of agenesis of the kidney (Athanasoulis et al., 1973; Braedel et

al., 1976; Itzchak et al., 1974). On the left side, the central portion of the renal vein (embryologically, the preaortic portion of the renal collar) is still present, but it drains the adrenal and the gonadal veins only, thus creating a characteristic appearance on venography (Fig. 7–233). On the right side, if the kidney does not develop there is no renal vein to catheterize.

The demonstration of a main renal vein with its lobar tributaries rules out renal agenesis. In contrast, in acquired diseases (i.e., shrunken

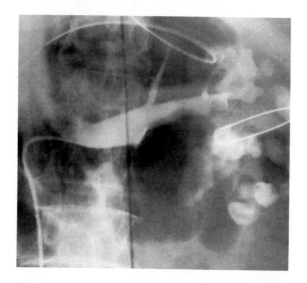

Figure 7–231. Renal vein invasion in carcinoma. Selective left renal venogram. A large filling defect protrudes into the caudal aspect of the left renal vein at the hilum of the kidney. The vein is both displaced and invaded by the neoplastic mass.

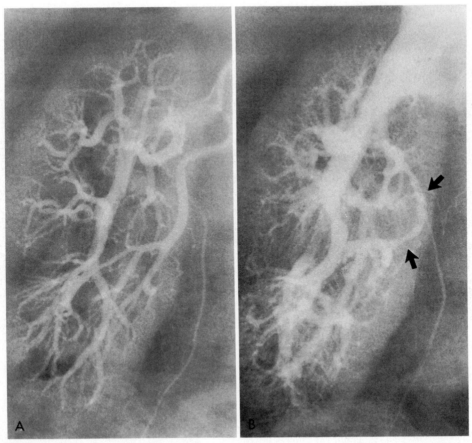

Figure 7–232. Avascular hypernephroma at the renal pelvis. *A*, Renal arteriogram. No definite abnormalities are apparent. *B*, Renal venogram. There is definite narrowing and encasement of the peripelvic renal vein (arrows). (Courtesy of Dr. Stanley Baum.)

kidneys), the main renal vein is of either normal size or only slightly diminished size, and the lobar veins are crowded and tortuous (Braedel et al., 1976; Itzchak et al., 1974). In congenital hypoplasia, the main renal vein is small, and the intrarenal veins show an otherwise normal distribution (Braedel et al., 1976). In renal dysplasia (Athanasoulis et al., 1973; Braedel et al., 1976), venography shows the presence of a disordered venous architecture.

Preoperative and Postoperative Evaluation of the Renal Veins

Prior knowledge of renal vein variations is important when retroperitoneal surgery is planned. A left circumaortic venous ring constitutes an instantaneous collateral pathway immediately after caval interruption (Beckmann and Abrams, 1978); multiple right renal veins can serve as an alternative collateral route if the inferior vena cava has been interrupted between these veins (Greweldinger et al., 1969). Therefore, a careful search for these frequent anatomic variations should be made by preoperative renal venography. If multiple right renal veins are found, or a left circumaortic venous ring is found, the caval interruption must be below the orifice of these veins in the lower lumbar region.

During retroperitoneal surgery, the surgeon may see a preaortic vein but remain unaware of an additional retroaortic component so that he tears it involuntarily while mobilizing the kidney or clamping the aorta (Mitty, 1975). Warren et al. (Warren et al., 1972; 1974) have stressed the importance of preoperative angiographic evaluation of the left renal vein in preparation for splenorenal shunts for portal hypertension. Prior knowledge of the location, appearance, and possible variations of the left renal vein allows the procedure to be tailored to the needs of each patient and therefore results in less tissue manipulation at the operating table, which

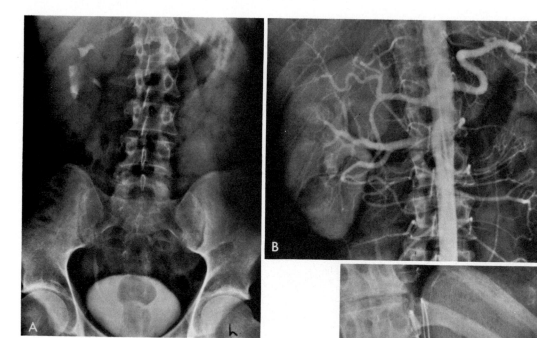

Figure 7–233. Absence of the left kidney. *A*, Intravenous urogram. The collecting system of the right kidney, the right ureter, and the bladder are opacified. There is no evidence of a left kidney. *B*, Aortogram. The hypertrophied right kidney is subserved by a single main renal artery. No left renal artery is visible. *C*, Selective left renal venogram. The catheter has entered a small vein that fills the adrenal venous system retrograde, but the film demonstrates no evidence whatsoever of normal renal venous channels. As a consequence, this represents congenital absence of the kidney rather than a small, contracted, pyelonephritic kidney. (Courtesy of Dr. R. R. Freeman, Royal Adelaide Hospital.)

is to the advantage of the patients, who often are critically ill. Postoperatively, venography is important in evaluating the patency of these shunts. Even if the left renal vein is occluded, however, the shunts might still be patent and drain into retroperitoneal collateral vessels (Sones et al., 1978).

Benign Renal Parenchymal Disease

Selective renal venography can be a useful but nonspecific method of evaluating diseases of the renal parenchyma. In *acute glomerulonephritis*, the renal venogram is normal; however, in *chronic glomerulonephritis* there may be diffuse loss of cortex, as documented by the distance between the arcuate veins and the renal surface. Similar diffuse findings may be seen in shrunken nephrosclerotic kidneys (Kahn, 1969; Rösch et al., 1975).

Localized abnormalities are characteristic of *pyelonephritis*. Areas in which the veins are tightly clustered are found in pyelonephritic scars (Kahn, 1969). Pyelonephritic pseudotumors may produce displacement of both interlobar and arcuate veins (Jonsson, 1972; Sorby, 1969).

In *hydronephrosis* (Fig. 7–234) there is spreading of the central veins, which appear narrowed, stretched, and curved (Rosch et al., 1975). The arcuate veins are irregularly filled and stretched. Rarely, anomalous renal veins may produce hydronephrosis (Gilsanz et al., 1972). In *polycystic disease*, the interlobar veins primarily are stretched, narrowed, and curved around the centrally located cysts. Typically, however, the deformed veins have smooth outlines (Rosch et al., 1975).

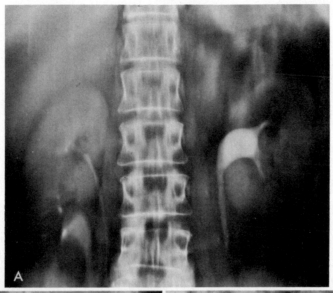

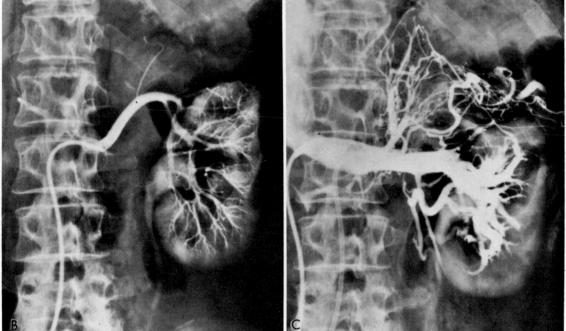

Figure 7–234. Hydronephrosis of the upper pole of a double kidney. *A,* Urogram. No calyces are filled in the medial portion of the upper pole. The right kidney has a double collecting system and double ureters. Only a single ureter is filled on the left. *B,* Selective renal arteriography. Vessels to the lower two thirds of the left kidney are well filled, but only sparse branches extend to the upper pole. The most proximal branch visualized may well be an adrenal artery or a capsular artery. *C,* Renal venography. A large cluster of veins is seen overlying the upper pole of the left kidney. Many of these appear to be adrenal veins, and the venous drainage of the mass itself cannot be clearly defined. *D,* Selective renal venography of the upper pole vein. Multiple veins extend from the upper pole vein over the surface of the upper pole mass, strongly suggesting that it is renal in origin. *E,* Percutaneous renal puncture with contrast injection. The hydronephrotic upper pole and the large dilated tortuous ureter below are opacified. (Courtesy of Dr. Iraj Hooshmand.)

Illustration continued on following page

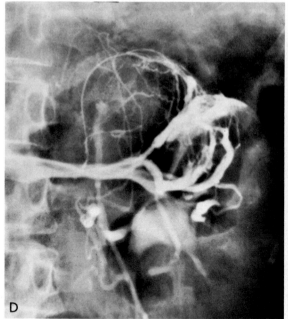

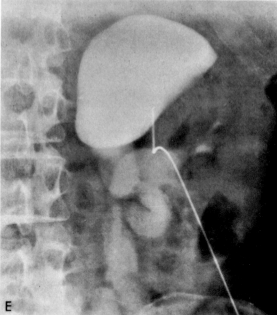

Figure 7–234. *Continued*

Renal fibrolipomatosis represents fatty replacement of destroyed or atrophic renal parenchyma. Although the urogram is frequently diagnostic when combined with tomography, the distinction from mass lesions is not always clear. The venogram may demonstrate a relatively normal distribution of venous tributaries when the urogram and the arteriogram are equivocal or suggestive of cysts or other mass lesions.

Renal venography is not required to establish the diagnosis of hydronephrosis, polycystic disease, or fibrolipomatosis. Nevertheless, when venography is indicated for other reasons (e.g., unexplained hematuria), familiarity with the venographic findings in these patients is important if the correct interpretation is to be made.

References

Abrams, H. L.: Selectivity in the study of the cardiovascular system. Calif. Med., *96*:149, 1962.

Abrams, H. L., Baum, S., and Stamey, T. A.: Renal venous washout time in renovascular hypertension. Radiology, *83*:597, 1964.

Abrams, H. L., Boijsen, E., and Borgstrom, K.-E.: Effect of epinephrine on the renal circulation. Angiographic observation. Radiology, *79*:911, 1962.

Ahlberg, N. E., Bartley, O., Chidekel, N., and Wahlquist, L.: An anatomic and roentgenographic study of the communications of the renal vein in patients with and without renal carcinoma. Scand. J. Urol. Nephrol., *1*:43, 1967.

Anatkow, J., Kumanow, C.: Selective nephro-phlebography. *In* Diethelm, L. (Ed.): Symposium of the European Association of Radiology. Mainz, Springer, 1972.

Anson, B. J., Cauldwell, E. W., Pick, J. W., and Beaton, L. E.: The anatomy of the pararenal system of veins, with comments on the renal arteries. J. Urol., *60*:714, 1948.

Appel, G. B., Williams, G. S., Meltzer, J. J., and Pirani, C. L.: Renal vein thrombosis, nephrotic syndrome and systemic lupus erythematosus. Ann. Intern. Med., *85*:310, 1966.

Arner, O., Blank, C., and Schreeb, T. B.: Analysis with references to malignancy grading and special morphological features. Acta Chir. Scand. (Suppl), *346*:1, 1965.

Assykeen, T. A., Castellino, R. A., Love, T. B., and Stamey, T. A.: Peripheral and renal vein renin activity: Effects of postural stimulation in normotensive adults. Arch. Intern. Med., *128*:378, 1971.

Athanasoulis, C. A., Brown, B., and Baum, S.: Selective renal venography in differentiation between congenitally absent and small contracted kidney. Radiology, *108*:301, 1973.

Barclay, G. P., Cameron, H. M., and Loughridge, L. W.: Amyloid disease of the kidney and renal vein thrombosis. Q. J. Med., *29*:137, 1960.

Beckmann, C. F., and Abrams, H. L.: Renal vein valves: Incidence and significance. Radiology, *127*:351, 1978.

Beckmann, C. F., and Abrams, H. L.: Circumaortic venous ring: Incidence and significance. Am. J. Roentgenol., *132*:561, 1979.

Beckmann, C. F., and Abrams, H. L.: Renal venography: Anatomy, technique, applications, analysis of 132 venograms, and a review of the literature. Cardiovasc. Intervent. Radiol., *3*:45, 1980.

Beres, J. A., Zboralske, F. F., Wilson, S. D., and Amberg, J. R.: Percutaneous transrenal venography in experimental renal vein obstruction and human renal vein thrombosis. Radiology, *83*:587, 1964.

Bernath, A. S., Addonizio, J. C., Kinkhabwala, M., and

Thelma, W.: Renal venography in diagnosis of infiltrating transitional cell carcinoma of the renal pelvis. Urology, *18*:164, 1981.

Blaivas, J. G., Previte, S. R., and Pais, V. M.: Idiopathic pelvic ureteric varices. J. Urol., *9*:207, 1977.

Bosniak, M. A., and Madayag, M.: Angiographic appearance of the circumaortic left renal vein. J. Urol., *108*:18, 1972.

Bourgoignie, J., Kurz, S., Catanzara, F. J., Serirat, P., and Perry, H. M., Jr.: Renal venous renin in hypertension. Am. J. Med., *48*:332, 1970.

Bradley, S. E., and Bradley, G. P.: The effect of increased intra-abdominal pressure on renal function in man. J. Clin. Invest., *26*:1010, 1947.

Braedel, H. U., Haage, H., Moeller, J. F., and Schindler, E.: Differential diagnostic importance in cases of unusual ectasia and renal pelvic deformity. Radiology, *119*:65, 1976.

Braedel, H. U., Schindler, E., Moeller, J. F., and Polsky, M. S.: Renal phlebography: An aid in the diagnosis of the absent or non-functioning kidney. J. Urol., *116*:703, 1976.

Brannon, E. S., Warren, J. V., and Merrill, A. J.: A method of obtaining renal venous blood in unanesthetized persons with observations on the extraction of oxygen and sodium para-amino hippurate. Science, *100*:108, 1944.

Caron, J., Bonte, G., and Ribet, M.: Technique de phlebographie renale. J. Radiol., *44*:329, 1963.

Chait, A., Stoane, L., Moskowitz, H., and Mellins, H. Z.: Renal vein thrombosis. Radiology, *90*:886, 1968.

Cope, C., and Isard, H. J.: Left renal vein entrapment. Radiology, *92*:867, 1969.

Cox, J. S., John, H. T., Bankole, M. A., and Warren, R.: Collateral circulation after renal vein occlusion. Surgery, *52*:875, 1962.

Crocker, D. W.: Renal Tumors. *In* Sommers, S. C. (Ed.): Kidney Pathology Decennial 1966–1975. New York, Appleton-Century-Crofts, 1975.

Crummy, A. B., and Hipona, F. A.: The roentgen diagnosis of renal vein thrombosis. Experimental aspects. Am. J. Roentgenol., *93*:898, 1965.

Dalla Palma, L., and Servello, M.: La phlebographie renale. Presse Med. *64*:150, 1956.

Davis, C. J., and Lundberg, G. D.: Retroaortic left renal vein. Am. J. Clin. Pathol., *50*:700, 1968.

Delin, N. A., and Haverling, M.: Renal artery and vein flow during aortic and inferior vena caval occlusion and retrograde renal phlebography. An experimental study in the pig. Invest. Radiol., *1*:148, 1966.

Dorr, R. P., Cerny, J. C., and Hoskins, P. A.: Inferior venacavograms and renal venograms in the management of renal tumors. J. Urol., *110*:280, 1973.

Dow, J. A., and Takaro, T.: Anomalous tributary of the left renal vein diagnosed by selective renal phlebography: case report. J. Urol., *98*:150, 1967.

Eisen, S., Friedenberg, M. J., and Klahr, S.: Bilateral ureteral notching and selective renal phlebography in the nephrotic syndrome due to renal vein thrombosis. J. Urol., *93*:343, 1965.

Ernst, C. B., Bookstein, J. J., Montie, J., Baumgartel, E., Boobler, S. W., and Fry, W. J.: Renal vein renin ratios and collateral vessels in renovascular hypertension. Arch. Surg., *104*:496, 1972.

Fitz, A.: Renal venous renin determinations in the diagnosis of surgically correctable hypertension. Circulation, *36*:942, 1967.

Folin, J.: Angiography in renal tumors, its value in diagnosis and differential diagnosis as a complement to conventional methods. Acta Radiol. (Suppl.) (Stockh.), *267*:30, 1967.

Fuchs, W. A.: Selective renale phlebographie. Schweiz. Med. Woschr., *91*:1, 1961.

Genest, J., and Boucher, R.: The renin-angiotensin system in human renal hypertension. *In* Onesti, G., Kim, K. E., and Moyer, J. H. (Eds.): Hypertension: Mechanism and Management. New York, Grune & Stratton, 1971.

Georgi, M., Marberger, M., Gunther, R., Orestano, F., and Halbsguth, A.; Retrograde Nierenphlebographie bei Ballonverschluss der Nierenarterie. ROEFO, *123*:341, 1975.

Gilsanz, V., Anaya, A., Estrada, R., and Toni, P.: Transparietal renal phlebography: a new method. Lancet, *1*:179, 1965.

Gilsanz, V., Estrada, R., and Malillos, E.: Transparietal renal cavophlebography. Angiology, *18*:565, 1967.

Gilsanz, V., Rabadan, M., Leiva Galvis, O., and Estrada, V.: A singular case of hydronephrosis produced by inferior left lobar renal vein demonstrated by transparietal renal phlebography. Angiology, *23*:311, 1972.

Goncharenko, V., Gerlock, A. J., Kadir, S., and Turner, B.: Incidence and distribution of venous extension in 70 hypernephromas. Am. J. Roentgenol., *133*:263, 1979.

Gospodinow, G. I., and Topalow, J. B.: Phlebography of the renal vein by way of the vena spermatica sinistra. Fortschr. Rontgenstr., *91*:664, 1959.

Greweldinger, J., Coomaraswamy, R., Luftschein, S., and Bosniak, M. A.: Collateral circulation through the kidney after inferior vena cava ligation. N. Engl. J. Med., *281*:541, 1969.

Griffiths, J. H., and Thackray, A. C.: Parenchymal carcinoma of the kidney. Br. J. Urol., *21*:128, 1949.

Gyepes, M. T., Desilets, D. T., Gray, R. K., and Katz, R. M.: Epinephrine-assisted renal venography in renal vein thrombosis: Report of two adolescents with nephritic syndrome. Radiology, *93*:793, 1969.

Hall, F. M.: Renal venography in renal cell carcinoma (letter). Am. J. Roentgenol., *34*:209, 1980.

Hamilton, C. R., and Tumulty, P. A.: Thrombosis of renal veins and inferior vena cava complicating lupus nephritis. JAMA, *206*:2315, 1968.

Hand, J. P., and Broders, A. C.: Carcinoma of kidney. J. Urol., *28*:199, 1932.

Harrington, D. P., White, R. I., Jr., Kaufman, S. L., Whelton, P. K., Russell, R. P., and Walker, W. G.: Determination of optimum method for renal venous renin sampling in suspected renovascular hypertension. Invest. Radiol., *10*:452, 1975.

Harrison, C. V., Milne, M. D., and Steiner, R. E.: Clinical aspects of renal vein thrombosis. Q. J. Med., *25*:295, 1956.

Helander, C. G., Asheim, A., and Odman, P.: A percutaneous method for catheterization of the renal vein in dogs. Acta Physiol. Scand., *45*:228, 1958.

Hipona, F. A., and Crummy, A. B.: The roentgen diagnosis of renal vein thrombosis. Clinical aspects. Am. J. Roentgenol., *98*:122, 1966.

Hollinshead, W. H., and McFarland, J. A.: The collateral venous drainage from the kidney following occlusion of the renal vein in the dog. Surg. Gynecol. Obstet., *97*:213, 1953.

Hunt, J. C., and Strong, C. G.: Renovascular hypertension. Mechanisms, natural history and treatment. Am. J. Cardiol., *32*:562, 1973.

Itzchak, Y., Adar, R., Mozes, M., and Deutsch, V.: Renal venography in the diagnosis of agenesis and small contracted kidney. Clin. Radiol., *25*:379, 1974.

Itzchak, Y., Deutsch, V., Adar, R., and Mozes, M.: Angiography of renal capsular complex in normal and pathological conditions and its diagnostic implications. C.R.C. Crit. Rev. Diagn. Imag., 5:111, 1974.

Janower, M. L.: Nephrotic syndrome secondary to renal vein thrombosis. Am. J. Roentgenol., 79:911, 1962.

Javadpour, N., Doppman, J. L., Scardino, P. T., and Bartter, F. C.: Segmental renal vein renin assay and segmental nephrectomy for correction of renal hypertension. J. Urol., 115:580, 1976.

Jonsson, K.: Renal angiography in patients with hematuria. Am. J. Roentgenol., 116:758, 1972.

Kahn, P. C.: Selective venography of the branches. In Ferris, E. (Ed.): Venography of the Inferior Vena Cava and Its Branches. Baltimore, The Williams & Wilkins Co., 1969a.

Kahn P. C.: Selective venography in renal parenchymal disease. Radiology, 92:345, 1969b.

Kahn, P. C., Wise, H. M., Jr., and Robbins, A. H.: Complete angiographic evaluation of renal cancer. JAMA, 204:753, 1968.

Kaneko, Y., Ikeda, T., Takeda, T., and Ueda, H.: Renin release during acute reduction of arterial pressure in normotensive subjects and patients with renovascular hypertension. J. Clin. Invest., 46:705, 1967.

Katzberg, R. W., Morris, T. W., Burgener, F. A., Kamm, D. E., and Fischer, H. W.: Renal renin and hemodynamic responses to selective renal artery catheterization and angiography. Invest. Radiol., 12:381, 1977.

Kees, J. C., and Harrell, R. S.: Radiographic manifestations of renal vein thrombosis. J. Urol., 108:830, 1972.

Kendall, A. G., Lohmann, R. C., and Dossetor, J. B.: Nephrotic syndrome. Arch. Intern. Med., 127:1021, 1971.

Koehler, P. R., Bowles, W. T., and McAlister, W. H.: Renal arteriography in experimental renal vein occlusion. Radiology, 86:851, 1966.

Korobkin, M., Glickman, M. G., and Schambelan, M.: Segmental renal vein sampling for renin. Radiology, 118:307, 1976.

Kuchel, O., and Genest, J.: Effect of antihypertensive drugs on renin release. In Onesti, G., Kim, K. E., and Moyer, J. H. (Eds.): Hypertension: Mechanisms and Management. New York, Grune & Stratton, 1971.

Kusunoki, T., Takayanagi, I. H., and Kobayashi, H.: A study of renal function by renal vein catheterization in the urological field. Urol. Int. 2:327, 1956.

Lang, E. K.: Arteriographic assessment and staging of renal-cell carcinoma. Radiology, 101:17, 1971.

Laragh, J. H., Baer, L. and Vaughn, E. D.: Renin, angiotensin and aldosterone system in pathogenesis and management of hypertensive vascular disease. Am. J. Med., 52:633, 1972.

Lien, H. H., and Kolbenstvedt, A.: Phlebographic appearances of the left renal and left testicular veins. Acta Radiol. (Diagn.) (Stockh.), 18:321, 1977.

Llach, F., Arieff, A. J., and Massey, S. G.: Renal vein thrombosis and nephrotic syndrome. A prospective study of 36 adult patients. Ann. Intern. Med., 83:8, 1975.

March, T. L., and Halpern, M.: Renal vein thrombosis demonstrated by selective renal phlebography. Radiology, 81:958, 1963.

Mauro, M. A., Wadsworth, D. E., Stanley, R. J., and McClennan, B. L.: Renal cell carcinoma: Angiography in the CT era. Am. J. Roentgenol., 139:1135, 1982.

McCarthy, L. J., Titus, J. L., and Daugherty, G. W.: Bilateral renal vein thrombosis and the nephrotic syndrome in adults. Ann. Intern. Med., 58:837, 1963.

McCullough, D. L., and Gittes, R. F.: Vena cava resection for renal cell carcinoma. J. Urol., 112:162, 1974.

McCullough, D. L., and Gittes, R. F.: Ligation of the renal vein in the solitary kidney: Effects on renal function. J. Urol., 113:295, 1975.

McDonald, J. R., and Priestley, J. T.: Malignant tumors of the kidney. Surg. Gynecol. Obstet., 77:295, 1943.

Michelakis, A. M., and Simmons, J.: Effect of posture on renal vein renin activity in hypertension. Its implications in the management of patients with renovascular hypertension. JAMA, 208:659, 1969.

Michelakis, A. M., Woods, J. W., Liddle, G. W., and Klatte, E. C.: A predictable error in use of renal vein renin in diagnosing hypertension. Arch. Intern. Med., 123:359, 1969.

Mitty, H. A.: Circumaortic renal collar. A potentially hazardous anomaly of the left renal vein. Am. J. Roentgenol., 125:307, 1975.

Mitty, H. A., and Goldman, H.: Angiography in unilateral renal bleeding with a negative urogram. Am. J. Roentgenol., 121:508, 1974.

Mulhern, C. V., Arger, P. U., Miller, W. T., and Chait, A.: The specificity of renal vein thrombosis. Am. J. Roentgenol., 125:291, 1975.

Myers, G. H., Fehrenbaker, L. G., and Kelalis, P. P.: Prognostic significance of renal vein invasion by hypernephroma. J. Urol., 100:420, 1968.

Ney, C., and Friedenberg, R. M.: Radiographic Atlas of the Genito-Urinary System. Philadelphia, J. B. Lippincott, 1966.

Novak, D.: Selective renal occlusion phlebography with a balloon catheter. Br. J. Radiol., 49:589, 1976.

O'Dea, M. J., Malel, R. S., Tucker, R. M., and Fulton, R. E.: Renal vein thrombosis. J. Urol., 116:410, 1976.

Olin, T. B., and Reuter, S. R.: A pharmacoangiographic method for improving nephrophlebography. Radiology, 85:1036, 1965.

Paster, S. B., Adams, D. F., and Abrams, H. L.: Errors in renal vein renin collections. Am. J. Roentgenol., 122:804, 1974.

Peart, W. S., and Sutton, D.: Renal-vein catheterization and venography, a new technique. Lancet, 2:817, 1958.

Petasnick, J. P., and Patel, S. K.: Angiographic evaluation of the nonvisualized kidney. Am. J. Roentgenol., 119:757, 1973.

Proca, E.: Technique of renal phlebography through the left spermatic vein. An aid to the management of renal carcinoma. Br. J. Urol., 38:501, 1966.

Renert, W. A., Rudin, L. J., and Casarella, W. J.: Renal vein thrombosis in carcinoma of the renal pelvis. Am. J. Roentgenol., 114:735, 1972.

Riches E.: On carcinoma of the kidney. Ann. R. Coll. Surg., 32:201, 1963.

Riches, E. W.: Analysis of patients with adenocarcinoma in a personal series. In Riches, E. W., (Ed.): Tumors of the Kidney and Ureter: Neoplastic Disease at Various Sites. Vol. 5. Baltimore, The Williams & Wilkins Co., 1964.

Riches, E. W., Griffiths, I. H., and Thackray, A. C.: New growths of the kidney and ureter. Br. J. Urol., 23:297, 1951.

Richet, G., Gillot, G., Vaysse, J., and Meyerovitch, A.: La thrombose isolee de la veine renale. J. Urol. Nephrol. (Paris), 71:758, 1965.

Rösch, J., Antonovic, R., Goldman, M. L., and Dotter, C. T.: Epinephrine renal venography. ROEFO, 126:501, 1975.

Rosenmann, E., Pollack, V. E., and Pirani, C. L.: Renal vein thrombosis in the adult: A clinical and pathologic study based on renal biopsies. Medicine, 47:269, 1968.

Royal, S. A., and Callen, P. W.: CT evaluation of anomalies of the inferior vena cava and left renal vein. Am. J. Roentgenol., 132:759, 1979.

Schaeffer, A. J., and Fair, W. R.: Comparison of split function ratios with renal vein renin ratios in patients with curable hypertension caused by unilateral renal artery stenosis. J. Urol., *112*:697, 1974.

Schambelan, M., Howes, E. L., Stockigt, J. R., Noakes, C. A., and Biglieri, E. G.: Role of renin and aldosterone in hypertension due to a renin-secreting tumor. Am. J. Med., *55*:86, 1973.

Sealey, J. E., Buhler, F. R., Laragh, J. H., and Vaughan, E. D.: The physiology of renin secretion in essential hypertension. Estimation of renin secretion rate and renal plasma flow from peripheral and renal vein renin levels. Am. J. Med., *55*:391, 1973.

Siminovitch, J. M. P., Montie, J. E., and Stratton, R. A.: Inferior venacavography in the preoperative assessment of renal adenocarcinoma. J. Urol., *128*:908, 1982.

Simmons, J. L., and Michelakis, A. M.: Renovascular hypertension: The diagnostic value of renal vein renin ratios. J. Urol., *104*:497, 1970.

Smith, J. C., Rösch, J., Athanasoulis, C. A., Baum, S., Waltman, A. C., and Goldman, M.: Renal venography in the evaluation of poorly vascularized neoplasms of the kidney. Am. J. Roentgenol., *123*:552, 1975.

Sones, P. J., Rude, J. C., Berg, D. J., and Warren, W. D.: Evaluation of the left renal vein in candidates for splenorenal shunts. Radiology, *127*:357, 1978.

Sorby, W. A.: Renal phlebography. Clin. Radiol., *20*:166, 1969.

Stables, D. P., and Thatcher, G. N.: Traumatic renal vein thrombosis associated with renal artery occlusion. Br. J. Radiol., *46*:64, 1973.

Steiner, R. E.: The renal veins and their radiologic demonstration. Bibl. Paediatr., *74*:159, 1960.

Stockigt, J. R., Hertz, P., Schambelan, M., and Biglieri, E. G.: Segmental renal-vein renin sampling for segmental renal infarction. Studies in a hypertensive patient. Ann. Intern. Med., *79*:67, 1973.

Stockigt, J. R., Noakes, C. A., Collins, R. D., and Schambelan, M.: Renal-vein renin in various forms of renal hypertension. Lancet, *1*:1194, 1972.

Susin, M., Mailloux, L., and Becker, C.: Renal vein thrombosis in patients with membraneous glomerulonephritis. Kidney Int., *6*:103A, 1974.

Takaro, T., Dow, J. A., and Kishew, S.: Selective occlusive renal phlebography in man. Radiology, *94*:589, 1970.

Takaro, T., and Kivirand, A. I.: Experimental renal phlebography. A comparison with renal arteriography. Surgery, *60*:619, 1966.

Turner, R. J., Young, W. S., and Castellino, R. A.: Dynamic continuous computed tomography: Study of retroaortic left renal vein. J. Comput. Assist. Tomogr., *4*:109, 1980.

Vaughan, E. D.: Renin sampling: Collerction and interpretation. N. Engl. J. Med., *290*:1195, 1974.

Vaughan, E. D., Buhler, F. R., Laragh, J. H., Sealey, J. E., Baer, L., Bard, R. H.: Renovascular hypertension: Renin measurements to indicate hypersecretion and contralateral suppression, estimate renal plasma flow and score for surgical curability. Am. J. Med., *55*:402, 1973.

Vermillion, S. E., Sheps, S. G., Strong, C. G., Harrison, E. G., Jr., and Hunt, J. C.: Effect of sodium depletion on renin activity of renal venous plasma in renovascular hypertension. JAMA, *208*:2302, 1969.

Warren, W. D., Salam, A. A., and Faislalo, A.: End renal vein–splenic vein shunts for total or selective portal decompression. Surgery, *72*:995, 1972.

Warren, W. D., Salam, A. A., and Hutson, D.: Selective distal splenorenal shunt. Arch. Surg., *108*:306, 1974.

Watson, R. C., Fleming, R. J., and Evans, J. A.: Arteriography in the diagnosis of renal carcinoma. Radiology, *91*:888, 1968.

Wegner, G. P., Crummy, A. B., Flaherty, T. T., and Hipona, F. A.: Renal vein thrombosis, a roentgenographic diagnosis. JAMA, *209*:1661, 1969.

Weiner, P. L., Lim, M. S., Knudson, D. H., and Semekdjian, H. S.: Retrograde pyelography in renal vein thrombosis. Radiology, *111*:77, 1974.

Wexler, L., and Abrams, H. L.: Hamartoma of the spleen: Angiographic observations. Am. J. Roentgenol., *92*:1150, 1964.

Weyman, P. B., McClennon, B. L., Stanley, R. J., Levitt, R. G., and Sagel, S. S.: Comparison of CT and angiography in the evaluation of renal cell carcinoma. Radiology, *137*:417, 1980.

Whitley, N. O., Kinkhabwala, M., and Whitley, J. E.: The collateral vein sign, a fallible sign in the staging of renal cancer. Am. J. Roentgenol., *120*:660, 1974.

CHAPTER 8

Diagnostic and Therapeutic Urologic Instrumentation

PAUL H. LANGE, M. D.

A major concern of urology is safe traversal and adequate visualization of the urinary collecting system for diagnosis and treatment. Early urologists, therefore, had to develop more than surgical skills; they also needed the skills related to endoscopy and radiographic visualization. As a result of the refinement of these skills, open surgery has rarely been necessary for the diagnosis of urologic problems. Urology is no longer unique in this regard. Rapid advances in endoscopic equipment and real-time imaging and progress in interventional radiology have enabled many surgical and medical specialties to use these noninvasive diagnostic procedures for their own concerns.

Advanced instrumentation and its skillful use are even more a part of urology today than in the past. Only a decade ago the instruments unique to urology were primarily those necessary for visualization and manipulation of the urethra and bladder: rigid endoscopic equipment for cystourethroscopy and manipulation instruments designed to pass through these endoscopes or to be introduced blindly through the urethra. Appropriately, urologic instruments were traditionally categorized under cystoscopy. However, with the recent applications of percutaneous nephrostomy and the assimilation of many techniques of interventional radiology, a new dimension and many new instruments have been added to urology. This expanded field has been given the name "endourology" (Smith et al., 1979).

Strictly speaking, endourology is defined as that discipline of urologic surgery which involves closed intervention to any part of the urinary tract for visualization or manipulation. Thus, the discipline includes both cystoscopy and percutaneous nephrostomy. Sometimes endourology is used to refer to closed interventional procedures involving only the upper urinary tract (e.g., the kidney and ureter). However, in this text we will use the word in its larger meaning.

This chapter contains information about the major instruments used in endourology. There are too many to list and describe, so an explanation of an instrument's use is included only when such a description is necessary to understand its design. In many cases, information about instrument utilization is contained in other chapters of this book. Many types of endourologic instruments are manufactured by more than one company. The functional characteristics of these instruments usually are similar, although most have their own distinguishing design. The descriptions and drawings in this chapter are intended to portray the general types of instruments, therefore, when possible the names of the specific manufacturers are omitted. With only a few exceptions, instruments used primarily for open surgical procedures in urology are not discussed.

Major instruments used by the urologist and discussed in this chapter include:

1. Urinary catheters and tools for their placement.

2. Equipment and methods for percutaneous biopsy or catheterization of the prostate, bladder, or kidney.

3. Instruments for dilation of the urethra, ureter, or percutaneous tracts.

4. Instruments for endoscopy of the urethra, bladder, ureter, and kidney.

5. Manipulative instruments for use under endoscopic or fluoroscopic guidance.

6. Real-time imaging equipment used during urologic procedures.

7. Urologic instruments that generate hydraulic waves for stone disintegration and those that transfer energy, including those used to transfer: (a) normal light for vision or laser light for tissue destruction, (b) mechanical energy for manipulation, (c) energy for diathermy, or (d) ultrasonic energy for destruction of stones.

CATHETERS

In urology, catheters are used to diagnose problems, drain urine or fluid, or maintain anatomic continuity. A variety of sizes and designs are therefore necessary to accomplish these functions. Most catheters are sized either according to the French (F scale) system or in millimeters. In both systems, the numbers refer to the outer diameter of the catheter. Often instruments are calibrated in only one scale, so urologists must be able to convert mentally from one scale to the other quickly. Each number of the F scale equals 0.33 mm, but it is easier to remember that a 30F catheter has an outer diameter of about 10 mm.

Catheter Design. Catheters have always been a major tool of urologic surgery, and, therefore, many different designs were developed over the years to suit particular requirements. Today this versatility is even greater because urology has adapted many techniques from interventional radiology and because newer biomaterials have expanded the possibilities for catheter design.

One way to categorize a catheter is by the method used to pass it into its desired location (e.g., through the urethra into the bladder) (Fig. 8–1). The first method used, and still the most common, is to pass a smooth blunt-tipped catheter directly through the passageway (e.g., urethra) into a desired area (e.g., bladder). This method works well unless the passageway is narrow or tortuous. In that case, a traditional practice is to introduce a thin filament (e.g., a filiform) through the area. This filament is first attached to a larger diameter tube, and the assembly is passed as a unit in order to dilate the tract. Progressively larger tubes are then attached to the filament and passed until the

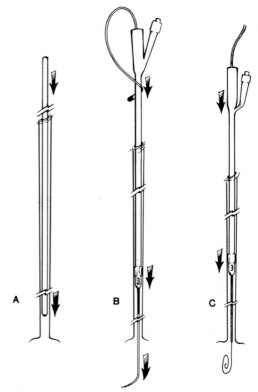

Figure 8–1. Methods of passing large-diameter catheters. *A*, Direct passage; *B*, with tapered filament passed as a unit; *C*, threaded over guidewire and tapered catheter (see Fig. 8–4).

tract is of sufficient size. At this point, a draining catheter with a hole at its tip can be attached to the filament and again passed as a unit through the tract (refer to the section on dilation). The third, and in many cases most desirable, method for passing catheters is to first negotiate a very flexible wire (a guidewire) through the passageway. Different-shaped catheters or dilators can then be threaded over this guidewire. This concept is the basis for interventional radiology. (Real-time radiographic imaging is usually required during the manipulation.) The advantages of the guidewire approach are that almost any angle or route can be negotiated and there is less chance for serious injury (White, 1976).

Catheter Size. Catheters can also be classified according to their diameter size. The traditional large-diameter catheters (14F or greater) are used primarily for transurethral bladder drainage or for tube drainage of a nephrostomy or cystostomy tract (Fig. 8–2). The curved-tip coudé catheter is sometimes more successful in negotiating the male urethra, but usually any smooth-tipped catheter will suffice.

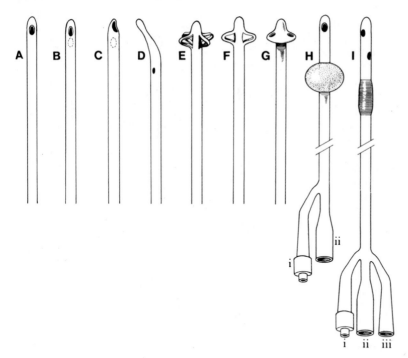

Figure 8–2. Types of large-diameter catheters. *A,* Conical tip urethral catheter, one eye; *B,* Robinson urethral catheter; *C,* Whistle-lip urethral catheter; *D,* Coudé hollow olive-tip catheter; *E,* Malecot self-retaining, four-wing urethral catheter; *F,* Malecot self-retaining, two-wing catheter; *G,* Pezzer self-retaining drain, open-end head, used for cystotomy drainage; *H,* Foley-type balloon catheter; and *I,* Foley-type three-way balloon catheter, one limb of distal end for balloon inflation (i), one for drainage (ii), and one to infuse irrigating solution to prevent clot retention within the bladder (iii).

A more important characteristic of a large-diameter catheter is its self-retaining design. Some catheters have no self-retaining characteristics and must be taped or sewn in place. The Malecot or Pezzer catheter is stretched over a stylet for insertion but has a self-retaining tip that springs into shape when released; it is especially useful for drainage when positioned in small spaces. However, the balloon-tipped, Foley catheter is the most commonly used large-diameter catheter (Figs. 8–2 and 8–3). Many of the catheters discussed are available in smaller sizes for pediatric use.

The problem with coudé, Malecot, and Foley catheters is that there is no hole at the tip for passing them over a filiform or guidewire system. The Council catheter was manufactured specifically with a hole at its tip such that it could be passed over a filiform and stylet arrangement (Fig. 8–4*A*). Today almost any catheter can be so adapted using an end-hole catheter punch that makes a smooth symmetric hole at the end of the catheter, enabling it to pass over a guidewire and tapered dilating system (Fig. 8–4,*B* and *C*). This capability is especially important in the placement of percutaneous catheters but can be important for urethral catheters also (Mazzeo et al., 1982).

The various small-diameter (less than 14F) catheters available are used primarily for retrograde catheterization of the ureter or for nephrostomy or cystostomy tubes. Traditional ureteral catheters are designed to be directed into the ureteral orifice through a cystoscope and are produced in many shapes and sizes to fit the need (Fig. 8–5). More recently, the guidewire system has been adapted for retrograde ureteral catheterization. This approach allows a guidewire introduced endoscopically to the ureteral orifice to be easily negotiated up the ureter with little risk of trauma. Catheters can be threaded over this guidewire either endoscopically or under fluoroscopic guidance alone, and great versatility in diagnostic and therapeutic procedures in the ureter and renal pelvis is achieved (Pollack, 1984). Unfortunately, almost none of the older catheters illustrated in Figure 8–5 accommodates a guidewire easily. In the past, the urologist had to use a variety of catheters traditionally made for angiographic procedures, but guidewire-accommodating catheters made especially for the ureter have been introduced recently (Fig. 8–6) (J. Vance, personal communication, 1984).

The guidewire catheters appropriate for ureteral catheterization have many uses besides drainage. For example, angiographic catheters and dilators of different shapes can be passed transurethrally retrograde into the ureter to reach almost any area of the renal collecting system (Pollack, 1984). Manipulative instruments, such as wire biopsy brushes (Fig. 8–6) (Gill et al., 1979; Lieberman et al., 1984), can then be passed through these catheters. In ad-

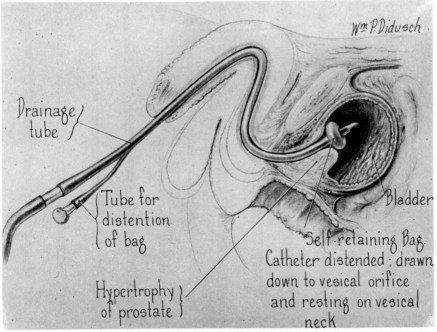

Figure 8–3. Demonstration of use of self-retaining Foley balloon catheter. (Courtesy of American Cystoscope Makers, Inc.)

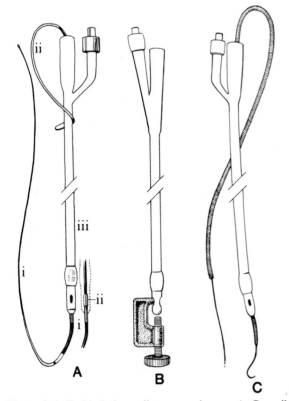

Figure 8–4. End-hole large-diameter catheters. *A,* Council catheter (iii), through which is threaded a long filiform (i) attached to a stylet (ii). Once inserted, the stylet and filiform are withdrawn through the end-hole. *B,* Foley catheter with catheter end-hole punch. *C,* Foley catheter with guidewire and tapered angiogram catheter threaded through it.

dition, balloon catheters, such as those initially designed for transluminal angioplasty (e.g., a Grüntzig balloon catheter), can be threaded over a guidewire and are especially useful for occluding or dilating the ureter (Waller et al., 1983).

The external diameter of the catheter is important when selecting one to traverse a passageway, such as a percutaneous tract or the ureter, but other catheter dimensions should also be noted. The internal diameter of the catheter is important if it is to be used for drainage. This diameter, in turn, is related to the design of the catheter and its intended purpose. For example, the inside of a Foley catheter contains the main drainage lumen but also a separate channel for balloon inflation. Consequently, this catheter has a smaller drainage channel than a nonballoon catheter (e.g., Robinson catheter) of the same F size. In addition, the internal diameter is affected by the material from which it is made.

Catheter Materials. The catheter material affects a variety of catheter characteristics, including its biocompatibility and utility. Biocompatibility is initially determined in laboratory animals by testing host tissue response and material deterioration within the host. Materials used in the urinary tract are subject to special influences, including deterioration and the propensity to precipitate urinary mucoids and crystalloids (encrustation), which can cause irrita-

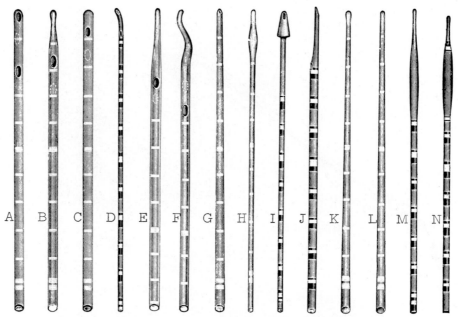

Figure 8–5. Traditional ureteral catheters and bougies. *A,* Whistle-tip ureteral catheter; *B,* olive-tip ureteral catheter; *C,* round-tip ureteral catheter; *D,* Wishard ureteral catheter; *E,* Blasucci ureteral catheter, flexible filiform tip; *F,* Blasucci ureteral catheter, flexible spiral filiform tip; *G,* Garceau ureteral catheter, graduated; *H,* Braasch bulbous ureteral catheter; *I,* Foley cone-tip catheter; *J,* Hyams double-lumen ureteral catheter; *K,* olive-tip ureteral bougie; *L,* Garceau ureteral bougie, graduated; *M,* Braasch bulbous ureteral bougie; and *N,* Dourmashkin ureteral dilator with inflatable balloon.

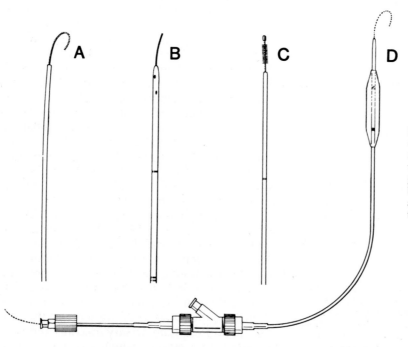

Figure 8–6. Guidewire-accommo-dating ureteral catheters. *A,* Standard angiogram catheter with guide-wire; *B,* ureteral catheter with guidewire; *C,* ureteral catheter with biopsy brush, and *D,* transluminal angioplasty catheter used for ureteral dilations or occlusions.

tion, infection, and occlusion of the catheters. The tendency to encrustation previously was determined empirically, but today it can be predicted by using scanning electron microscopy to determine surface smoothness of the material (H. K. Mardis, personal communication, 1984).

Urologic catheters are constructed of polymeric biomaterials. Polymers are complex repetitive giant molecular chains. They can occur naturally as, for example, the nucleic acids, proteins, or latex (a rubber plant by-product). There are also many synthetic polymers that have great versatility for catheter fabrication. These polymers can be classified into three groups: addition polymers (e.g., polyethylene, polyvinyl chloride, Teflon), condensation polymers (e.g., silicones and polyurethanes), and the newer block copolymers (e.g., polysiloxane modified thermoplastic elastomers).

The biomaterials used for urinary catheters have included latex, polyvinyl chloride, polyethylene, a variety of polyurethanes, some silicones, and, more recently, some of the newer block copolymers. Latex has been the standard material used for most large urethral catheters because it is soft. However, its urinary biocompatibility is not ideal and encrustation often occurs quickly. Polyvinyl chloride is a stiffer material and is used for many smaller diameter catheters, such as ureteral catheters. Its stiffness makes it easy to pass, and its strength allows small external-to-internal diameter ratios for optimal drainage. However, polyvinyl chloride causes encrustation and significant irritation to the urothelium. Polyethylene is also stiff, but, as the time it remains in the urinary tract increases, it becomes brittle. Some of the polyurethanes are better tolerated long-term and are less brittle. Currently, a variety of silicone biomaterials are best tolerated within the urinary tract in terms of mucosal irritability, encrustation, and flexibility. However, this flexibility also makes passing the catheter over a guidewire difficult, and the lack of strength of the material necessitates a large external-to-internal diameter ratio.

The assets of a biomaterial (or a catheter made from it) involve ease of device formation, strength, elasticity, and durability. The importance of these factors is related, in turn, to its intended use and method of placement. These considerations are perhaps best exemplified in the search for an ideal ureteral stent catheter.

Ureteral Stent Catheters. There are many urologic situations in which a ureteral catheter must be left in the ureter permanently or for an extended time to drain the kidney and act as a stent for healing, or to bypass a ureteral obstruction not amenable to surgical correction. These ureteral stent catheters must be (1) soft for patient comfort, (2) elastic to allow insertion percutaneously or retrograde up the ureter over guidewires, (3) resistant to encrustation and deterioration over the long term, (4) capable of forming self-retaining configurations at the tips, (5) of sufficient tensile strength to preclude breakage, and (6) of appropriate inside-outside tubing diameters to allow optimal drainage. The older ureteral catheters are ill suited to these purposes because they are too stiff, do not have sufficient self-retaining properties, and are made of polyvinyl chloride, which causes mucosal irritation and encrustation soon after insertion. Although the ideal ureteral stent has not yet been developed, catheters that can be left in the ureter for long periods now exist (Mardis, 1984).

Modern ureteral stent catheters are usually constructed of soft biocompatible materials, such as polyurethane or Silastic. Some of them have a permanent pigtail or J configuration on one or both sides, which spring into shape once a guidewire is withdrawn to make them self-retaining (Fig. 8–7). All or part of these catheters are impregnated with barium or bismuth to make them visible by x-ray. The catheters can be positioned retrograde transurethrally, antegrade through a percutaneous nephrostomy, or by a combined transurethral-transnephrostomy route.

Some of the catheters, such as the double-pigtail or double-J catheters, are meant to be truly indwelling (Fig. 8–8, *left*). The internal location decreases the risk of infection, but, if these catheters become occluded, their replacement may be difficult. Similarly, the external ureteral stent catheters may have self-retaining capacities but are designed to exit externally on one end. For example, these catheters may be placed in the kidney to exit from an enterostomy or may be positioned to drain the bladder and kidney and to exit from a percutaneous nephrostomy tract (Fig. 8–8, *right*).

The ureteral stent catheters have either a blunt tip or an open-ended tip on one or both ends. Blunt-tip varieties are usually passed with an obturator guidewire and a pusher catheter. Open-ended tips are meant to pass over a guidewire and to be advanced by a pusher catheter or by means of pushing and pulling on both ends of the catheter, as might occur when a catheter enters through a nephrostomy tract and exits out the urethral meatus. The advantage of the open-tip ureteral stent catheter is that, if it becomes plugged, a guidewire can be passed

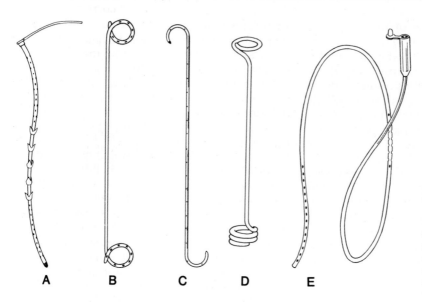

Figure 8–7. Ureteral stents. *A,* Gibbons internal ureteral stent (Heyer-Schulte); *B,* double-pigtail internal ureteral stent (VIP); *C,* double-J internal ureteral stent (Medical Engineering Corp.); *D,* double-coil catheter (Bard); *E,* universal stent (Heyer-Schulte).

through it, the tube removed, and a second catheter inserted with little difficulty (Smith, 1982).

PERCUTANEOUS INSTRUMENTS

Although a major preoccupation of urology has been to gain access to the urinary tract through the urethra, the specialty has also accumulated a variety of instruments to approach the urinary organs percutaneously. The percutaneous procedures commonly used in urology include needle biopsy of the prostate and the formation of nephrostomy or cystostomy tracts. These will be discussed in detail. Other procedures include percutaneous needle aspiration of the bladder; percutaneous needle biopsy of masses or lymph nodes located in the pelvis, abdomen, or retroperitoneum; and percutaneous biopsy or aspiration of kidney parenchyma or cysts. These latter approaches will not be discussed because the instruments used for them are not significantly different from those used in other procedures.

Needle Biopsy of the Prostate. The main method for obtaining a pathologic diagnosis

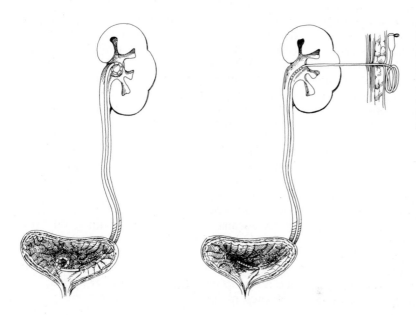

Figure 8–8. Ureteral stents. *Left,* Double-J internal ureteral stent positioned in kidney and bladder. *Right,* Universal ureteral stent positioned in kidney and bladder with exit percutaneously. Urine still drains into bladder, but catheter can be opened for percutaneous drainage and placement of a guidewire.

from a prostate that is suspected of malignancy by rectal examination is to do a needle biopsy. The three methods for biopsy are: transperineal and transrectal needle biopsy for histologic assessment, and transrectal fine-needle biopsy for cytologic examination.

For transperineal biopsy, a variety of needles are available but designs similar to the Tru-Cut* are most popular (Fig. 8–9). With the patient in the lithotomy position, the perineum is cleansed. The prostatic area to undergo biopsy is located transrectally with a finger. A needle route on either side of the midline is selected about 3 to 4 cm anterior to the rectum and infiltrated with local anesthesia. The skin is punctured with a knife blade. The biopsy needle is then passed into the prostate, with a finger in

* Travenol Laboratories, Inc., Deerfield, Illinois 60015

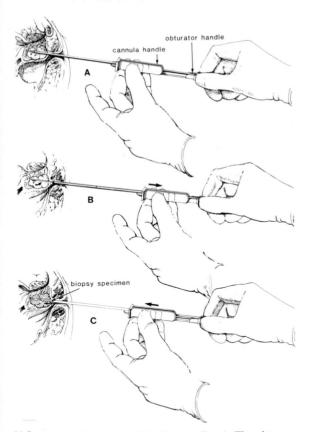

Figure 8–9. Operation of Tru-Cut needle. *A,* The obturator and cannula assembly are advanced into the area to undergo biopsy, with the obturator notch covered. *B,* The cannula handle is then pulled outward until it stops, while the obturator is held still, thus opening the specimen notch. *C,* The tissue is pressed into the notch, and the cannula assembly is advanced quickly without moving the obturator. The assembly is then withdrawn with the cannula still covering the obturator.

the rectum used as a guide, and a tissue core is obtained (Fig. 8–10).

For transrectal biopsy, the patient generally is placed on prophylactic antibiotics 24 hours before surgery, and sometimes cleansing enemas are given as well. These preparations are not as necessary for transperineal biopsy. The beveled side of a Tru-Cut needle is pressed into the pulp of the finger, and the finger and needle are passed into the rectum and guided to the appropriate prostatic area. The needle is advanced, the finger withdrawn, and a tissue core obtained (Fig. 8–11).

Fine-needle aspiration of the prostate is usually performed with a device similar to the one described by Franzen and coworkers (1960) (Fig. 8–12). The needle is connected to a syringe, placed into its cannula, and guided transrectally by a finger to the suspicious prostatic area. The syringe plunger is pulled back to create suction and the needle moved back and forth, thus aspirating cells from the suspicious prostatic area into the syringe. These cells are then prepared for cytologic analysis.

Each of the two approaches to prostatic biopsy has its advantages and disadvantages. The transrectal route has a higher incidence of infectious complications (Derlen et al., 1974), although prophylactic antibiotics have diminished this problem (Crawford et al., 1982). Transrectal biopsy also has a higher incidence of traumatic complications, such as hemorrhage or urinary retention (Derlen et al., 1974). Transperineal biopsy can sometimes be done when the lesion is first discovered. However, there may be more pain with the transperineal approach and false negative rates are higher, probably because needle placement into the desired area is more difficult perineally than it is rectally (Kaufman and Schultz, 1962). Therefore, some urologists prefer transrectal biopsy for smaller suspicious areas in the prostate. Seeding of the perineal tract has been reported, but this complication is rare (Burkholber and Kaufman, 1966).

Transrectal fine-needle aspiration of the prostate causes little discomfort, is almost without complications, and can be performed accurately on very small suspicious areas in the prostate (Epsoti, 1971). No preparation is required provided that the rectum is free of feces. However, for acceptable accuracies (>85 per cent) and no false positive results, expert cytopathologic experience in prostatic cytology is necessary. In some centers, aspiration and core prostatic biopsy are performed together for greater accuracy (Epstein, 1976).

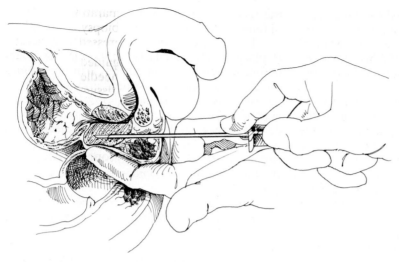

Figure 8–10. Perineal prostatic biopsy procedure.

Figure 8–11. Transrectal prostatic biopsy procedure.

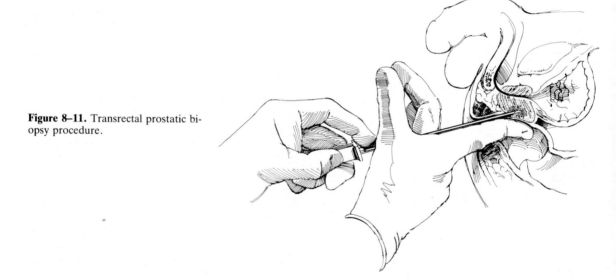

Figure 8–12. Transrectal needle aspiration biopsy procedure.

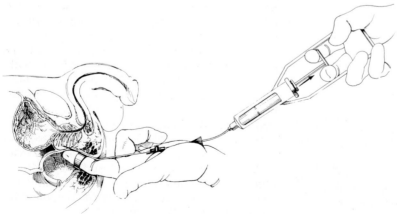

Percutaneous Nephrostomy. Percutaneous entry into the kidney has become an increasingly important procedure in urology (Stables, 1982). It is now useful for urinary diversion and as a site of entry for a variety of diagnostic and therapeutic procedures of the upper urinary tract, ranging from antegrade pyelography to percutaneous removal of ureteral or renal stones. The instruments important in percutaneous nephrostomy include real-time imaging equipment (discussed later), instruments essential for entry into the renal pelvis or calyces, tools for dilation of the percutaneous tracts, and the appropriate catheters (Fig. 8–13). Details of the percutaneous nephrostomy procedure are discussed in Chapter 9, but to understand the instruments required, one must have a rudimentary understanding of the procedure itself (Fig. 8–14).

The first requirement for percutaneous nephrostomy is to suitably visualize the upper urinary collecting system either by ultrasound or by fluoroscopy. This is accomplished by injecting contrast material intravenously, through a retrograde ureteral catheter or a thin (e.g., Chiba) needle that has been passed percutaneously directly into the renal collecting system. Once visualization is accomplished, a larger (18-gauge) beveled or diamond-tipped needle obturator with a beveled or squared-off outer Teflon cannula is placed into the renal pelvis or into an appropriate calyx. The internal needle is withdrawn, leaving the Teflon sheath through which a soft-tipped guidewire can be placed. The sheath is removed and a catheter (e.g., a 6F cobra) inserted over the guidewire, which is then manipulated so that a significant segment of the guidewire is placed into the renal pelvis or, if possible, down the ureter for support. Dilators are then placed over the wire, and the tract is expanded to the appropriate size in order to place a draining tube (e.g., a 9F pigtail catheter or a 14F Malecot catheter) or to perform other diagnostic or therapeutic maneuvers, such as removal of stones (Wickham and Miller, 1983c; Segura, et al., 1983; Clayman et al., 1984c). Methods of tract dilation will be discussed subsequently.

Percutaneous Cystostomy. Another organ approached percutaneously in urology is the bladder. Because of its hollow structure and proximity to the skin, the bladder is usually initially entered with large-caliber needles, especially when dilated. In this method, the first puncture determines the size of the tract; no guidewires are used or tract dilations performed. The most commonly used suprapubic cystos-

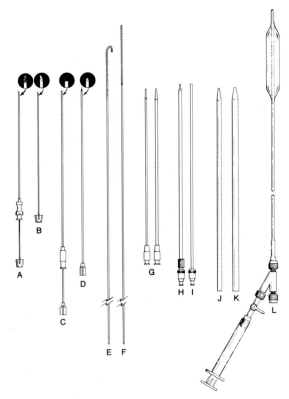

Figure 8–13. Instruments for percutaneous nephrostomy. *A* and *B*, Teflon catheter and stylet needle (beveled); *C* and *D*, Teflon catheter and stylet (diamond-tipped); *E*, J-shaped guidewire; *F*, straight guidewire; *G*, small dilators; *H*, introducer with guidewire-accommodating stylet; *I*, introducer stylet; *J* and *K*, larger dilators; and *L*, dilating balloon catheter that accommodates a guidewire. Its rugged construction allows dilation of muscle fascia, renal parenchyma, and capsule.

tomy instrument is a self-retaining catheter (e.g., Malecot, pigtail, or balloon type), which is stretched over a needle. This needle and catheter assembly punctures the skin of the abdominal wall, passing directly into the bladder from a suprapubic site. After a position within the bladder is assured by the flow of urine, the inner cannula is withdrawn and the tube secured (Fig. 8–15). Usually these tubes are 12 to 14F (Kumes and Stamey, in press).

Other suprapubic cystostomy instruments are based on the trocar principle. A trocar consists of a large pointed obturator and outer cannula, which usually is a tube with a wide, long slit (i.e., fenestration) on the end adjacent to the obturator point. The pointed obturator punctures the bladder directly and is then removed, leaving the cannula in the bladder. A catheter can then be placed through the fenestrated part of the cannula, the cannula removed and separated from the catheter, and the cath-

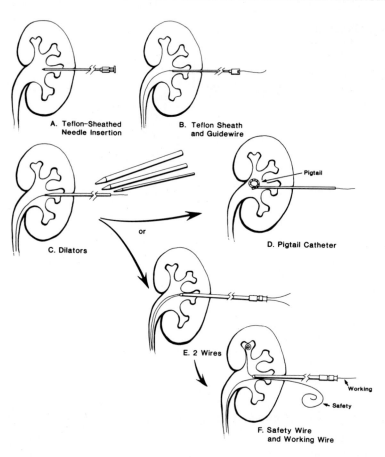

A. Teflon-Sheathed Needle Insertion

B. Teflon Sheath and Guidewire

C. Dilators

or

Pigtail

D. Pigtail Catheter

E. 2 Wires

Working

Safety

F. Safety Wire and Working Wire

Figure 8–14. Percutaneous nephroscopy procedure. *A,* Teflon stylet and needle inserted into collecting system; *B,* needle withdrawn and guidewire inserted down ureter; *C,* tract in kidney dilated with progressively larger fascial dilators; *D,* nephrostomy catheter placed in kidney over guidewire for drainage; *E,* introducer placed in kidney and second guidewire introduced; and *F,* safety guidewire (placed down ureter) secured while further dilation proceeds with "working" wire (placed here in upper pole).

eter secured to the abdominal wall (Fig. 8–16). The trocar method enables larger draining tubes (16 to 24F) to be inserted.

Percutaneous suprapubic cystostomy by the direct-puncture method may not always be appropriate. For example, if there has been previous abdominal surgery or if the bladder is small, an approach similar to that used in percutaneous nephrostomy may be more suitable (i.e., small needles, guidewires, and progressive dilation).

INSTRUMENTS FOR DILATION

Traditional Methods. Physicians have dilated urethral strictures for centuries. A traditional method, and still the most common for urethral dilation, involves directly passing a metal (often curved) instrument called a sound through the urethra (Fig. 8–17). In males with severe urethral strictures, the procedure often requires great skill. Even then trauma may occur, and re-entry through the passageway can be very difficult because no guide has preceded the dilating instrument. Accordingly, for severe

strictures the filiform and follower system was developed (Figs. 8–1, 8–4, 8–18, and 8–19). As previously discussed, filiforms are filamentous catheters of 1, 2, or 3F sizes that have a female screw tip to which is attached a large dilating catheter (bougie). In most situations, the bougie is attached to the filiform and pushed through the stricture, or sometimes a LeFort metal sound (one with a screw tip) is attached to the filiform and passed into the bladder. When an indwelling catheter is desired, the Council catheter and stylet are attached to the filiform and passed into the bladder as previously described (Fig. 8–4).

Guidewire–Sliding Catheter Dilation. The filiform and follower system, while especially useful in the urethra, has been supplanted by the guidewire–sliding catheter system for many types of dilations in urology (Figs. 8–1 and 8–20). This newer approach was developed from angiographic principles and from experience gained from dilation of percutaneous nephrostomy tracts. In this system, real-time imaging is essential. Briefly, if a tract already exists, as is the case in severe urethral strictures or in a percutaneous nephrostomy tract in which

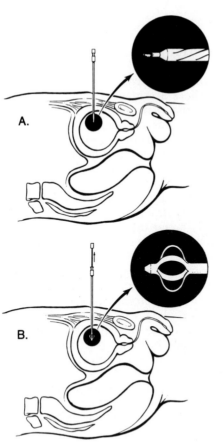

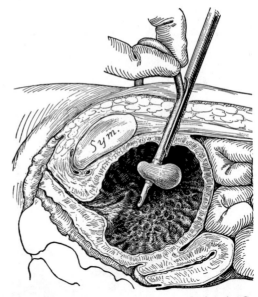

Figure 8–16. Suprapubic cystostomy employing the Campbell fenestrated trocar. After penetration of bladder with trocar, pointed obturator is removed and tube subsequently functions as a shoehorn, along the groove of which a large-diameter catheter can be introduced into the bladder. Fenestrated trocar sheath can then be removed.

Figure 8–15. Percutaneous suprapubic cystostomy. *A,* Insertion of the percutaneous catheter and stylet (Stamey type); and *B,* removal of stylet needle leaving mushroom-style catheter in bladder.

the tube has inadvertently been removed, a catheter is gently introduced as far as possible and the tract injected with radiopaque contrast material, which outlines the route. Next, a catheter and guidewire system is passed through the tract, again using real-time fluoroscopy. Dilators are used until an introducer catheter carrying

Figure 8–17. Urethral sounds and bougies. *A,* Otis bougie à boule, usually available in even sizes from 8 to 40F, used to calibrate passageways such as urethras; *B,* Van Buren urethral 40F sound; *C,* Otis urethral sound; *D,* Walther urethral sound (note tapering toward the handle); *E,* Guyon-Benique urethral sound; and *F,* LeFort urethral sound, with threaded tip for attachment of woven filiform.

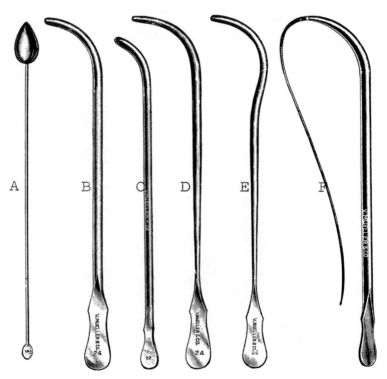

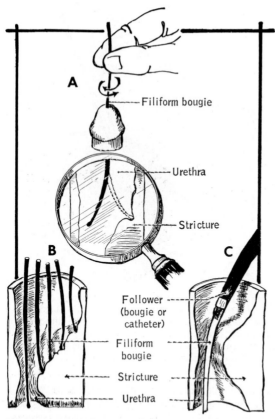

Figure 8–18. Use of filiform bougies in urethral instrumentation of stricture. As the obstruction offered by the stricture is met, the filiform is withdrawn slightly, rotated, and reintroduced as in *A*. Multiple filiforms may also be used, and as many as five or six may be used until one finally bypasses the stricture as in *B*. Inset *C* shows the attachment of the Philips follower to the filiform. The filiform passes through the stricture and guides the followers through. (Adapted from Barnes and Hadley: Urological Practice. St. Louis, C. V. Mosby Co., 1959.)

two guidewires can be passed: a stiffer guidewire for subsequent larger dilations (dilators often buckle on the guidewire, so the stiffer the guidewire the better), and a safety guidewire to assure continuity if problems with dilation are encountered. There are many guidewires and dilators available that were originally designed for anatomic situations encountered in interventional radiology. We cannot describe them all, but familiarity with all the major types is important when performing dilation.

There are several methods of guidewire dilation that are commonly used to dilate the nephrostomy tract. In the simplest system, progressively larger dilators are passed over a stiff guidewire. However, buckling and false passage are dangers of this system. To avoid buckling, another system was designed; this consists of a tapered-tip stylet catheter that passes over the guidewire to increase its stiffness, and then progressively larger dilators that are tapered to the stylet. These coaxial dilators are designed either to each fit snugly over the stylet catheter or to be telescoped onto each other (Fig. 8–20*E*). Usually the dilators are made of synthetic polymers and therefore are somewhat flexible, although rigid metal dilators that can pass over guidewires are also available and are sometimes useful in establishing tracts through scar tissue (Clayman et al., 1984c; Castaneda-Zuniga, 1984).

Balloon Dilation. Another, and usually the least traumatic, method of guidewire dilation is balloon dilation (Fig. 8–20*F*) (Clayman et al., 1983b). In this system a specially designed catheter (originally designed for transluminal angio-

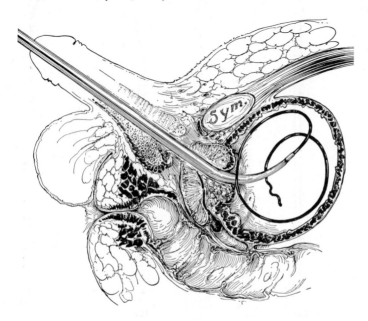

Figure 8–19. Sagittal diagrammatic view of filiform with follower attached. After the filiform has been passed into the bladder, the follower is attached and advanced into the bladder, employing the same technique as for the passage of a sound. (From Smith, D. R.: General Urology. Los Altos, Calif., Lange Medical Publications, 1959.)

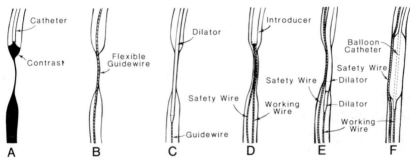

Figure 8–20. Methods of dilating a stricture or newly developed passageway. *A,* Contrast material outlines anatomy of stricture; *B,* guidewire traverses stricture or narrow passageway; *C,* low-caliber dilators pass over guidewire to expand passageway; *D,* introducer used to position second guidewire; *E,* one guidewire serves as "safety wire," and second wire is used for further dilation (larger dilators passed over small stylet dilator); *F,* alternatively, narrow passageway may be dilated with balloon catheter dilator over guidewire.

plasty) is passed over a guidewire. This catheter has a torpedo-shaped balloon at its tip, which can be inflated when desired. The balloon is so shaped to inflate to a particular rounded size and length and is made to tolerate varying degrees of pressure, depending on the structure to be dilated. These balloons come in a variety of shapes and sizes and are engineered to withstand pressures from 5 to 14 atmospheres. Balloon catheters are especially useful for dilating percutaneous nephrostomy tracts or strictures within the ureter. This system's applicability to urethral strictures is under investigation.

ENDOSCOPY

Endoscopy has been an important feature in urologic surgery since the introduction of the cystoscope during the last quarter of the nineteenth century (Khan, 1979). The instrument began as little more than a hollow tube that could be inserted transurethrally into the bladder and through which was directed reflected light. The addition of an incandescent light at the distal end of a scope and advances in miniaturization and optical technology resulted in a functional instrument for visual inspection and some manipulation in the urethra and bladder. However, these instruments were far from ideal: Illumination and clarity of vision were poor and the urologic endoscopist, while exhibiting great skill and courage, was significantly limited in what could be done. These restrictions continued into the early 1970's, when changes in the lens system and method of illumination of the cystoscope ushered in an era for urology and for all of endoscopy that today is still expanding rapidly.

The Telescopic Lens Systems. To understand the changes in the telescopic lens system, one must appreciate the basic elements of a classic cystoscopic telescope. The lens system in a rigid telescope consists of objective lenses at the distal end, a series of relay and field lenses in the middle, and ocular lenses at the eyepiece end. Objective lenses form an inverted real image of the object in a size sufficient to be assimilated into the barrel of the scope. The relay and field lenses transfer the image to the ocular lenses in a way that minimizes loss of light. The ocular lenses accomplish two purposes. Since some of the lenses in the relay system invert the image, a reverting prism is often added so the image reaches the eyepiece upright. Also, the ocular lenses magnify the last relay image.

Many changes and improvements have been made in the telescopic lens system. For example, the quality of the lenses and prisms improved because of advances in optical technology and cost of production, thus increasing the field and clarity of view. Another major change was in the relay system. Previously, this system consisted of a series of disc-like lenses separated by air spaces. These were replaced by a series of solid-rod lenses, so that light loss was reduced and the final image was brighter and had a wider field of view (Fig. 8–21*E*) (Khan, 1979; Berci, 1976a).

Another major change was the application of fiberoptic technology for illumination. Formerly, cystoscopic illumination was produced by a small incandescent bulb at the distal tip of the scope. The light was dim and unreliable and produced heat, and the arrangement significantly limited the directions that could be viewed. The fiberoptic system allowed the trans-

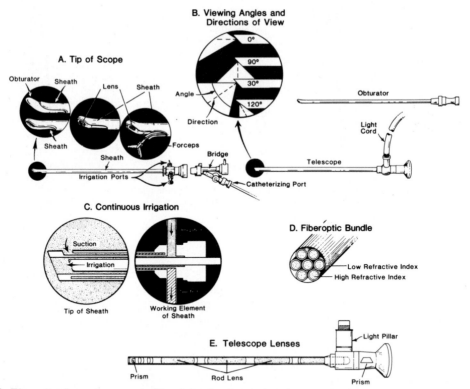

Figure 8–21. Elements of a cystoscope. *A,* Tip of the sheath may be straight or beaked. The obturator fits through the sheath and, again, may be straight or beaked. The telescope and bridge replace the obturator for viewing. *B,* Viewing angles and directions of view. *C,* Diagrammatic description of continuous irrigation. *D,* Diagrammatic illustration of fiberoptic bundle. Each fiber consists of glass of high refracted index surrounded by glass of lower refracted index. *E,* Lenses of telescope for rigid cystoscope.

mission of higher intensity light to the cystoscopic visual field. The system is composed of a cable or bundle consisting of many tiny specially designed glass fibers. Each fiber has a glass core of high refractive index, which is surrounded by glass material of lower index. Light rays that enter the fibers are thus trapped within the fiber and are transmitted down it even when the fibers are bent (Fig. 8–21 *D*). These fiberoptic bundles can also be used to transmit an optical image, provided the orientation of the fiber within the bundle is the same at the distal and proximal ends of the scope (i.e., coherent fiberoptic bundles) (Khan, 1979; Berci, 1976b; Epstein, 1980).

Fiberoptics are now used in both rigid and flexible endoscopes. In rigid endoscopes, such as a cystoscope, a flexible cord containing small fiberoptic bundles is interfaced with the rigid instrument at the "light pillar," which, in turn, is connected to other fiberoptic bundles situated in the periphery of the telescope. Flexible endoscopes, however, are different. They usually contain at least one fiberoptic bundle for light, but, in addition, instead of the rigid lens system,

flexible endoscopes have a separate coherent fiberoptic bundle for vision. Fiberoptic bundles are sensitive to heat, so that the light source, while of high intensity, must have the heat-producing region of the light spectrum dissipated or filtered out.

In the objective end of many telescopes are reflecting prisms that deviate the optical axis to the desired direction of view. The direction of view represents the relationship of the optical system to the horizontal axis of the telescope. The direction of view is also the middle of the viewing angle, which is the angle formed by the two outer visual limits of the telescopic image (Fig. 8–21*B*) and is determined by other lenses in the telescope. The directions of view that are commonly available in cystoscopic telescopes are 70 degrees or 90 degrees, 30 degrees or 12 degrees (the so-called Foroblique angle), the less common retroviewing directions of 110 degrees or 120 degrees, and 0 degrees, which needs no prism. The 20 degree or 30 degree lens is frequently used for manipulation, the 70 degree lens for a panoramic view, and the 0 degree lens for negotiation of passages such as the urethra, although the Foroblique lens also works well. The angles of view are calculated in water because the refracted indices in air or other clear fluids are different. The usual viewing angle in most telescopes is 60 to 70 degrees (Khan, 1979; Berci, 1976a). Recently, larger angles (>100 degrees) using "fish eye" lenses have become available, but the amount of peripheral distortion is greater. The physics and technology of lenses and fiberoptics are, of course, much more complicated, and the reader is referred to specialized texts for more complete descriptions (Berci, 1976a; Epstein, 1980; Hopkins, 1976a and b).

Basic Endoscopic Design. The usual cystoscope, and indeed most rigid endoscopes used in urology, has a sheath that is made in various sizes for pediatric and adult purposes and that contains ports for irrigation fluid. Through the sheath fits an obturator (for blind passage of the sheath through a tract such as the urethra) or a telescope system. The telescope system involves the actual telescope and a separate or permanently assembled "bridge" and/or "working element," which connects and positions the telescope within the sheath and itself may contain a catheterizing port for inserting a variety of manipulative instruments (Fig. 8–21).

Because of the special properties of the urinary tract, almost all urologic endoscopic instruments are constructed to use fluid for irrigation rather than air or CO_2. Irrigation is important both to distend an organ such as the bladder and to wash away debris or blood. If electrical energy is required, the irrigant must be a nonelectrolyte solution because electrolyte solutions conduct and therefore dissipate current. In these situations, iso-osmotic nonelectrolyte solutions, such as 1.5 per cent glycine, are used. Sterile water can also be used if no significant systemic absorption is anticipated, because absorption of water can cause systemic blood cell hemolysis. Finally, for maneuvers not requiring diathermy, in which there is a potential for systemic absorption of the irrigant (e.g., percutaneous nephrostomy), it is best to use irrigating solutions that are physiologic, such as normal saline.

Most urologic endoscopic instruments are constructed to use intermittent irrigation; that is, the irrigant enters and is emptied through the same lumen of the endoscope. More recently, continuous-flow systems have been developed, in which irrigating fluid enters an organ (e.g., the bladder) through an inner sheath while fluid is simultaneously sucked out through a

separate outer compartment (Fig. 8–21C). Endoscopes with this capability enable the urologist to perform procedures such as transurethral resections of the prostate or ultrasonic lithotripsy (discussed further on) without interruption for fluid evacuation (Khan, 1979).

Modern Visualization Instruments. Today, a number of rigid endoscopic instruments are available to visualize almost all areas of the urinary tract (Figs. 8–22 and 8–23). In addition to cystoscopes (both pediatric and adult) for visualization of the urethra and bladder, there are rigid ureterorenoscopes for visualization of the ureter and renal collecting system, rigid nephroscopes for visualization of the renal collecting system (usually through a percutaneous nephrostomy tract), and laparoscopes for direct visualization of the peritoneal and extraperitoneal cavities.

The rigid ureterorenoscope is about 50 cm long and usually comes in sizes ranging from 9 to 12F (Fig. 8–22F). The larger sizes have the capacity for an exchange of telescopes, thus enabling right-angle and straight viewing, and for manipulative procedures using flexible instruments inserted through a catheterizing port. In more recent models, the eyepiece is offset

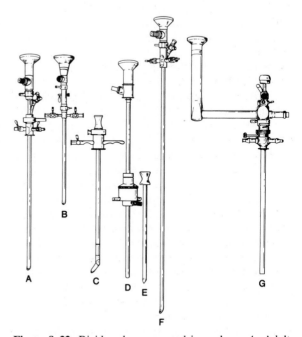

Figure 8–22. Rigid endoscopes used in urology. *A,* Adult cystoscope (telescope in sheath); *B,* pediatric cystoscope (telescope in sheath); *C,* resectoscope sheath with obturator; *D,* laparoscope cannula with telescope inserted; *E,* pointed stylet for laparoscope; *F,* ureterorenoscope with telescope in sheath (Wolf design); and *G,* universal nephroscope with telescope in sheath (Storz design).

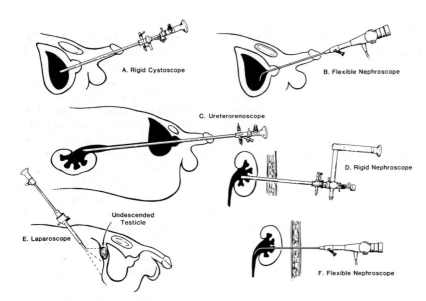

Figure 8–23. Some endoscopic instruments used in urology.

from the main sheath so that rigid manipulative instruments such as an ultrasonic probe (discussed further on) can also be passed through the scope. The ureterorenoscope is placed transurethrally through the bladder and, after ureteral dilatation, is directed (under vision) up the ureter and sometimes into the renal pelvis (Fig. 8–23C). While still relatively new, the rigid ureterorenoscope has significantly improved the urologist's ability to diagnose and treat lesions such as stones or tumors within the ureter or even the renal collecting system (Huffman et al., 1982; Ford et al., 1983).

The rigid nephroscopes originally designed for open surgery (Gittes and Williams, 1976) are now rarely used, and the most important ones are those intended for insertion through percutaneous nephrostomy tracts (Fig. 8–22G). These instruments are large-caliber (24 to 26F) and consist of a sheath and guidewire-accommodating obturator and a bridge or working element that contains a lens system and a catheterizing port. The lens eyepiece is offset so the catheterizing port can accommodate a rigid instrument, such as an ultrasonic probe. Some of the rigid nephroscopes have continuous-irrigation capacities. The instrument is usually passed fluoroscopically into the renal pelvis through a large-caliber percutaneous tract (Fig. 8–23D) and is used for extraction or disintegration of renal stones that are in a relatively straight-line orientation with the nephrostomy tract (Wickham and Miller, 1983a; Clayman, 1983).

Although they are now used extensively in other specialties, such as gastroenterology and obstetrics-gynecology, rigid laparoscopes have only recently gained a place in urology; they are used primarily for transperitoneal visualization of sexual organs, especially undescended testes (Silber and Cohen, 1980). The instrument is a trocar, which consists of a sheath or cannula through which fits a sharp-tipped obturator. The abdominal cavity is distended with CO_2 or nitrous oxide, by means of a special needle and an insufflation unit that controls gas pressure and volume, and the trocar assembly is punctured into the abdominal cavity (Fig. 8–22D and E and Fig. 8–23E). The distal end of the cannula has a side valve for the release or introduction of gas and is also fitted with an airtight lock so that the trocar can be removed and telescopes inserted without loss of gas from the abdominal cavity. Different telescopes are available that have varying directions of view or that are attached to or contain catheterizing ports for the use of manipulative instruments. Undoubtedly, other indications for laparoscopy will arise in urology, requiring urologic surgeons to become familiar with the expanding instrumentation of this field. For more information the reader is referred to reference works on laparoscopy (Boyce and Palmer, 1975).

The advent of fiberoptic technology allowed the development of flexible endoscopy, in which very small (as little as 10 μ) fiberoptic fibers were assembled into bundles, either to transmit light (noncoherent bundles) or to visualize an image (coherent bundles). Flexible endoscopic instruments also contain a port, used for irrigation or for the insertion of flexible manipulation instruments. A series of interlocking pulley-like structures within the shaft of the scope allow the tip to be bent in at least two directions. A variety of flexible endoscopes have been designed for medical disciplines, especially gastroenterology and pulmonary medicine. In urology, flexible scopes have been adapted primarily for nephroscopy. Originally, they were intended for visualization of the renal collecting system during open renal surgery. More recently, the length has been increased so that they can be used for percutaneous nephroscopy or ureteroscopy.

Several fiberoptic nephroscopes are currently available. All models are about 16F and have a 6F catheterizing port (Fig. 8–24). They have the ability to bend in at least two directions, with one arc being at least 160 degrees and a total arc being at least 250 degrees. Moreover, the total bending radius of the flexed tip is usually small enough (2 to 3 cm) to maneuver successfully within most areas of the kidney (Clayman, 1983).

Through a percutaneous nephrostomy (or at open surgery), the flexible nephroscope can directly visualize areas within the upper collecting system that are not accessible by rigid instruments (Fig. 8–23F) (Lange et al., in press). For example, this instrument can usually directly visualize most of the renal calyces and often a majority of the ureter. Recently, the flexible nephroscope has been used to perform transurethral cystoscopy and to catheterize the ureteral orifices (Fig. 8–23B) (Clayman et al., 1984a).

Flexible ureterorenoscopes have been developed to diameters as small as 7F. They are intended to be passed retrograde transurethrally up the ureter and have capabilities for irrigation and manipulation (Bush et al., 1982; Aso et al., in press). To date, these flexible instruments have not been as successful or as popular as rigid ureterorenoscopes.

Indeed, it is currently correct to generalize that for any given scope diameter, the visualization, light intensity, irrigation, catheterizing capabilities, durability, and ease of sterilization are better with rigid instruments than with flexible ones. Thus, rigid endoscopy is currently performed unless patient discomfort or the angle required for a particular procedure dictates otherwise. However, as discussed at the end of this chapter, this arrangement may be changing.

Teaching and Documentation Instruments. There are a variety of accessory attachments that can be connected to the endoscope for endoscopic teaching and documentation (Fig. 8–25). Usually these attachments are flexible and contain fiberoptic visualization bundles, an eyepiece at one end, and a special attachment at the other end that fits onto the endoscopic eyepiece and splits the visual image so that both the endoscopist and the observer can see simultaneously (Fig. 8–25A).

Still photography is accomplished using regular high-quality cameras that connect directly to the scope or the teaching attachment (Fig. 8–25B). Motion picture photography is also possible using specialized connectors. Aided by advances in solid-state electronics and miniaturization, television cameras are now available that can be connected to the fiberoptic teaching attachment or even directly to the scope itself (Fig. 8–25C and D). In this way, real-time endoscopic visualization is possible by other persons in the cystoscopy suite or by large

Figure 8–24. Flexible nephroscope (Olympus design): coherent bundle (i); light bundle (ii); catheterizing port (iii).

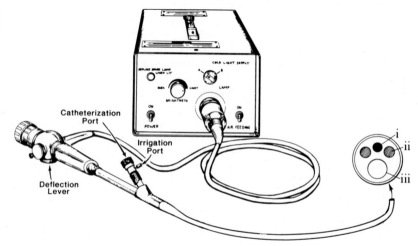

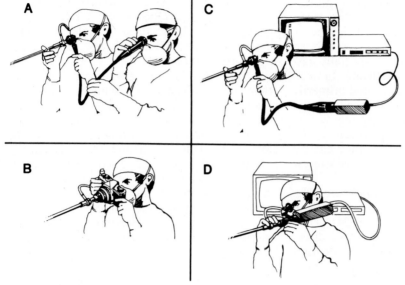

Figure 8–25. Methods of documentation and photography: *A,* Assistant looking through flexible teaching attachment. *B,* Endoscopist performing still photography through endoscope. *C,* Video recording and imaging through teaching attachment. *D,* Video recording and monitoring directly through endoscope. A side eyepiece for simultaneous endoscopic visualization is a feature of some endoscopic video cameras.

audiences in other rooms. Alternatively, the images can be stored on video tape for review later (Berci et al., 1976; Berci, 1976c).

Endoscopists in several other specialities have found TV imaging to be equal or superior to actually looking through the scope. For example, with video tape capabilities images can be reviewed or a particular image frozen during the procedure, thus increasing the speed and quality of anatomic conceptualization by the endoscopist. Also, the endoscopist is often more comfortable looking at a TV camera when performing some manipulations than when looking directly through the endoscope. For this reason many endoscopists actually perform some diagnostic and therapeutic maneuvers directly under TV guidance. In urology this approach may also have applicability. Already we have performed some percutaneous renal stone disintegrations directly under TV guidance, and it appears possible that, with some refinements, in the future other endoscopic maneuvers such as ureteroscopy, cystoscopy, and possibly even transurethral resection of the prostate may be preferable under TV guidance.

For visual documentation and teaching, powerful illumination is necessary. For example, special light sources with flash capabilities are desirable for still photography. More recently, higher intensity light sources such as those containing quartz-glass xenon arc-light bulbs have become available. These instruments greatly enhance the quality of the visual image for cinephotography, television, or video recording.

MANIPULATIVE INSTRUMENTS

Mechanical Manipulative Instruments. Urologic instruments for manipulation usually are used in association with endoscopy but are sometimes used exclusively under fluoroscopic control. These instruments are available in many sizes and shapes and are either flexible or rigid. They transfer mechanical energy or other kinds of energy from outside the body to an internal area of interest. The mechanical instruments are generally of two types: (1) those that are designed to pass through the existing catheterizing port of an endoscope; and (2) those that have a working element, such that together with a telescope (which can be inserted into it or is actually part of it), they fit into an endoscopic sheath directly. Finally, some manipulative instruments transfer nonmechanical energy, such as electrical or ultrasonic, endoscopically. Here again, these instruments are made to pass through an endoscope or are actually part of the working element of the telescope assembly.

Ureteral catheters and balloon catheters themselves are examples of transendoscopic manipulative instruments and have been discussed previously (Fig. 8–6). Some additional manipulative instruments include wire-tipped catheters arranged into baskets, snares, and loops of various configurations, all of which were originally designed to ensnare ureteral stones for transurethral removal (Fig. 8–26*A* and *B*). Recently, both the balloon and the basket concepts were combined into a single catheter for ureteral

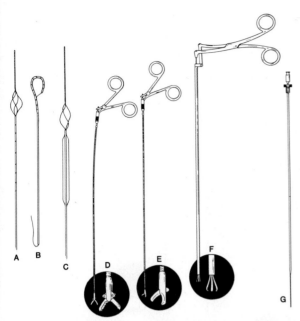

Figure 8–26. Endoscopic manipulative instruments. *A,* Ureteral stone basket (Dormia design); *B,* ureteral snare; *C,* Ruttner balloon basket; *D,* flexible alligator forceps; *E,* flexible cystoscopic scissors; *F,* rigid four-prong graspers (must be inserted through a straight catheterizing port such as is present on a rigid nephroscope); and *G,* flexible endoscopic needle.

stone removal (Figs. 8–26*C* and 8–27*B*) (Rutner and Fucilla, 1976). Moreover, nonelectrical tissue cutting can be accomplished with a flexible or rigid transendoscopic scissors (Figs. 8–26*E* and 8–27*C*). Different grasping instruments also are available, including alligator graspers of various sizes, three- or four-pronged grasping instruments, and an alligator-like grasping instrument with sharp edges, which can be used to obtain small tissue biopsies (Figs. 8–26*D* and *F* and 8–27*D*). Finally, special needles have been constructed to be inserted endoscopically for injection of drugs such as steroids (Fig. 8–26*G*).

Manipulative instruments that are a part of the working element (optical mechanical instruments) are designed to manipulate or grasp objects in ways not possible with transendoscopic instruments. An important manipulative instrument is the catheter-deflecting bridge, which facilitates ureteral catheterization transurethrally (Fig. 8–28*A*). This instrument usually fits into a cystoscopic sheath and accommodates (or has permanently attached to it) a telescope. At its proximal end, the bridge has a control system that moves a deflector at its distal tip. When a ureteral catheter has been passed

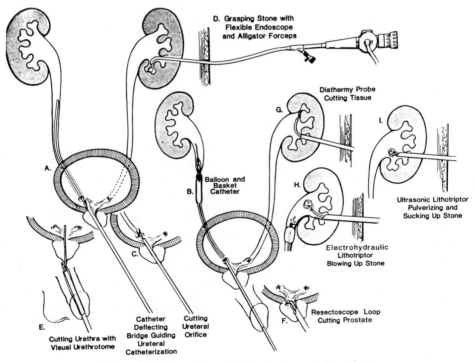

Figure 8–27. Uses of manipulative instruments in urology.

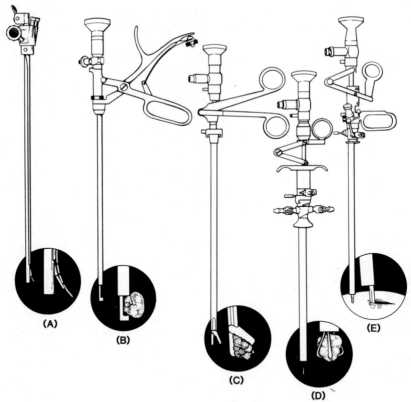

Figure 8–28. Optical mechanical instruments. *A,* Catheter-deflecting bridge, which fits into a cystoscopic sheath. In most models, a telescope fits through the bridge. Flexible instruments for ureteral intubation, such as ureteral catheters, fit through a catheterizing port on the bridge. A deflector at the tip bends the catheter and is activated by the wheel control at the proximal end of the bridge. *B,* Stone punch: A Foroblique telescope has been inserted into the instrument. This assembly fits into a large endoscopic sheath (Mauer Mayer design—Storz). *C,* Rigid alligator optical graspers. A telescope has been inserted through the optical bridge, and both have been inserted through a cystoscopic sheath. *D,* Three-pronged rigid optical grasper. The optical grasper and telescope are manufactured as one unit. It has been inserted through the sheath of a nephroscope (Storz design). *E,* Optical urethrotome. The bridge and lens assembly are manufactured as one unit. In this picture it has been inserted through a cystoscopic sheath.

through the endoscope, the deflector bends the catheter downward toward the urethral orifice (Fig. 8–27*A*).

Some other optical manipulative instruments are shown in Figure 8–28. Many of these instruments are designed to grasp or crush larger stones ($\geq$ 1.5 cm) and with greater force (Fig. 8–28*B* and *C*). These instruments fit through long ($\geq$ 24F) sheaths or are designed to pass directly through the urethra. Recently, a three-pronged optical grasper became available, which can grab objects "end-on," such as stones as large as 1.5 cm in diameter, under direct visual control. The instrument is constructed to hold the stone tighter than was possible before (Fig. 8–28*D*). This optical three-pronged grasper is designed to pass directly into the rigid nephroscope sheath and can remove large stones directly, thereby eliminating the need for ultrasonic disintegration. Finally, the visual ure-

throtome is an optical manipulative instrument designed to incise tissue, such as a urethral stricture, under direct visual guidance (Figs. 8–27*E* and 8–28*E*).

Diathermy Instruments. Among nonmechanical manipulative instruments, those that use surgical diathermy are most familiar to the urologist. Surgical diathermy is based on the principle that when a high-frequency electrical current passes through tissue, the heat that is generated at any point is directly proportional to the intensity of the current and inversely proportional to the area through which the current passes. Tissue-damaging heat is thus produced at the live or active electrode, which has a small area of contact with the tissue. The current then spreads out from the active electrode through the body to the indifferent electrode or a ground plate, which has a large area of contact with the body. If the patient is properly grounded, tissue damage occurs only at the point of contact with the live electrode.

The current generated by all diathermy units is high-frequency, so that it will not activate muscle or nerves, but the wave form of this current determines whether the tissue will vaporize (cutting) or burn and necrose (coagulation). For cutting, the wave form is continuous and of uniform amplitude. However, for coagulation, the wave form is pulsed on and off, with the current on one third to one tenth of the duration that it is off. Most surgical diathermy units are now solid-state rather than vacuum tube–spark gap. This improvement has made diathermy safer and more efficient and allows the different currents to be adjusted and even blended within the same unit. Almost all diathermy in endourology is monopolar; that is, the current flows between an active electrode and the ground plate on the patient. Increasingly, diathermy in other specialties is adapting to bipolar current — there are two active electrodes with the tissue interspaced between. Bipolar diathermy is safer and allows for finer resolution with less adjacent tissue injury. Bi-

polar diathermy will undoubtedly become more prevalent in endourology (Sittner and Fitzgerald, 1976).

The most frequently used instrument in endourology that utilizes diathermy is the resectoscope. This instrument was developed for transurethral resection of bladder and prostate tissue. Resectoscopes consist of a sheath, an obturator, a working element, a cutting electrode, and a telescope (Fig. 8–29A). Resectoscope sheaths come in varying sizes and are constructed of fiber glass or of metal with insulating material at the distal tip. The sheath may be fitted with a straight or deflecting obturator, which allows for blind passage transurethrally into the bladder (Fig. 8–22C). The working element inserts into the sheath, serves as a carriage for the telescope and the cutting electrode, provides for the diathermy wire connection to the electrode, and controls the movements of the electrode. There are many different kinds of resectoscopes, but their essential difference is in the mechanical working element by which the electrode is moved through the sheath.

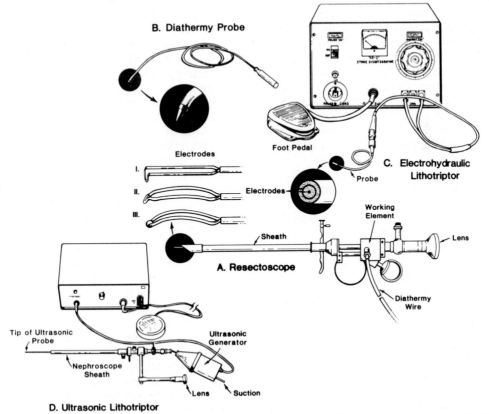

Figure 8–29. Energy-transferring manipulative and endoscopic instruments. *A,* Resectoscope: loop electrode (I); needle electrode (II); ball electrode (III). *B,* Diathermy probe. The probe is totally insulated except at its tip, which is pointed. *C,* Electrohydraulic lithotriptor (Northgate design). *D,* Ultrasonic lithotriptor (Wolf design). The ultrasonic probe has been inserted through the straight catheterizing port of the nephroscope.

Cutting electrodes are available in a variety of configurations. The loop configuration is the most popular because it is used to resect bladder or prostate tissue (Fig. 8–27F). Other electrodes include point electrodes for specific cutting and ball electrodes for fulgurating larger areas of tissue. Surgical diathermy also can be applied to an insulated wire that is passed through an endoscope (e.g., a diathermy probe) for point coagulation or cutting within the bladder, kidney, or elsewhere (Figs. 8–27G and 8–29B) (Clayman et al., 1984b).

Electrohydraulic Lithotripsy. Another instrument in urology that uses electrical energy is the electrohydraulic lithotriptor (Fig. 8–29C). First developed by Yutkin in 1950, it has evolved into an instrument of significant versatility and is produced by several manufacturers. The principle of the instrument is to use a high-capacity condenser to create a high-voltage spark between an axial and a cylindrical electrode located at the tip of the probe. In a fluid-filled organ, such as the bladder or kidney, this spark creates a hydraulic shock wave, the force of which can crack urinary stones. The instrument consists of a generator; the lithotriptor probe, which comes in sizes 5, 7, and 9F; a power cord that connects the generator to the probe; and a foot pedal for activation. The probe is flexible and can be passed through either a rigid or a flexible endoscope. The irrigant used is usually 1/6 normal saline, because stronger electrolyte solutions will not allow electrical discharge. The probe should be positioned at least several millimeters from the stone. The strength of the discharge and the pulse frequency can be varied, but the probe has a finite life span — approximately 15 to 50 total seconds of discharge. This instrument has been used to disintegrate stones in the bladder, ureter, or kidney (Fig. 8–27H). Direct visualization is essential because inadvertent discharge directly onto urothelial tissue can cause significant damage (Clayman et al., 1983a; Wickham and Miller, 1983b).

Ultrasonic Lithotripsy. The ultrasonic lithotriptor consists of a long hollow metal rod (i.e., probe), which is available in various lengths and diameters. This probe is designed to fit the straight catheterizing port of a rigid nephroscope or ureteroscope (Fig. 8–29D). The probe is connected to a transducer from which exits a cord that is connected to a high-frequency electrical generator. The generator produces specialized high-frequency electrical current, which is converted to ultrasonic vibrations by piezoceramic elements in the transducer. The vibrations are approximately 23,000 to 27,000 cycles per second (i.e., 23 to 27 kHz). With the help of acoustic resonators that determine the acoustic impedance, the ultrasonic energy is transferred into longitudinal and transverse vibrations of the probe. The probe material, length, tip, and its orientation with the crystal are constructed to produce optimal drilling when the probe is directly applied to the stone. When the power is activated by a foot pedal and the probe is applied to the stone under direct vision, the ultrasonic vibrations crack the stone and disintegrate it into small powder-like fragments that can be sucked into the rod through a port on the transducer. This suction also cools the wand to prevent overheating (Wickham and Miller, 1983b; Marberger, 1983).

Ultrasonic lithotripsy is a fast and efficient method of stone disintegration that can be used in the bladder, ureter, or kidney (Fig. 8–27I). Unlike hydraulic lithotripsy, it does not cause damage if inadvertently applied to tissue, and the stone fragments are small and usually can be sucked up rather than extracted individually. However, electrohydraulic lithotripsy is more effective on very hard stones, and because the probe is flexible it can be used with flexible endoscopy.

Extracorporeal Shock-Wave Lithotripsy. Another example of a urologic instrument that transfers nonmechanical energy is the extracorporeal shock-wave lithotriptor (ESWL) (Fig. 8–30). The principle of this modality, like that of electrohydraulic lithotripsy, centers on the generation of a hydraulic shock wave, but with ESWL the waves are produced outside the body. According to physical laws of acoustics in solids and fluids, the externally generated wave travels through the body without causing damage because there is no difference in acoustic impedance between body tissues and water. However, provided the waves are correctly focused at the tissue-stone interface, partial reflection of the waves occurs, ultimately causing short-term mechanical stress and therefore a zone of destruction at the stone site. This focusing is accomplished by the specific design of the instrument.

The theoretical considerations, design, and clinical results of ESWL have been described (Chaussey et al., 1982; Chaussey and Schmeidt, 1983). Briefly, an electrical spark is generated between two electrodes placed under water, thus creating a hydraulic shock wave (Fig. 8–31). This wave is produced within a rotationally symmetric semi-ellipsoid at its F1 focal point.

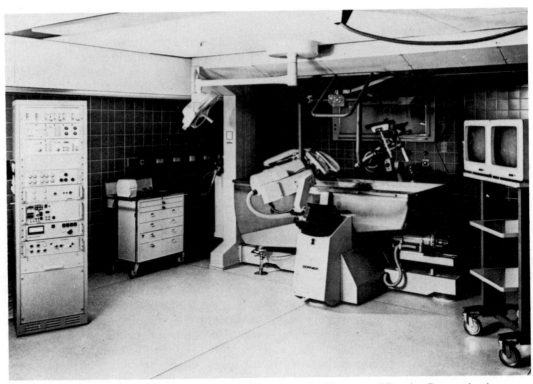

Figure 8–30. Extracorporeal shock wave lithotriptor unit. (Courtesy of Dornier Corporation.)

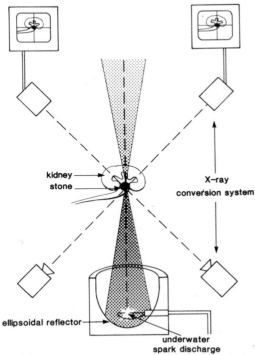

Figure 8–31. Diagrammatic representation of extracorporeal shock wave lithotripsy with two integrated x-ray conversion systems. (From Chaussey, C., et al.: J. Urol., *127*:417, 1982. Used by permission.)

The properties of an ellipse dictate that the waves are reflected off the elliptical wall and converge on a second focal point (F2).

If the patient is positioned under water so that the kidney stone is located at the F2 focal point, the stone is disintegrated by the shock waves. This positioning is accomplished by a two-plane x-ray system whose axes intersect at the F2 focus. Under fluoroscopic guidance, the patient is moved into precisely the correct position. A series of shock waves are then produced, causing the stone to be gradually disintegrated. The resultant small powder-like fragments are subsequently passed by the patient spontaneously.

ESWL has been extensively tested in the Department of Urologic Surgery at the University of Munich in Germany. Over 1000 patients with a large variety of renal stones have been successfully treated by this noninvasive method. Other urologic centers throughout the world are currently acquiring these machines. ESWL, together with the techniques and devices used for percutaneous renal and ureteral stone removal and ureterorenoscopy, has revolutionized the surgical treatment of urinary stone disease. Because of these instruments, it seems likely that open surgery will rarely be necessary for patients with urinary stones.

REAL-TIME IMAGING

Almost from the inception of the specialty, urology has required the ability to interpret roentgenograms, but the degree of participation by urologists in the actual performance of the test has varied. Certainly, for retrograde pyelography the participation has always been major: Generally, urologists insert a catheter into the ureter, inject radiographic contrast material, and then, when the time seems appropriate, instruct a radiology technician to perform a roentgenogram. Further roentgenograms are obtained based on the interpretation of the initial studies made during the procedure.

As techniques of intravenous pyelography improved, the need for retrograde pyelography decreased. This fact plus the increasing importance of angiography, ultrasonography, and computerized axial tomography for urologic diagnoses lessened the participation of the urologist in actual radiologic tests even further and, conversely, increased the role of the radiologist to the extent that urologic radiography became a subspecialty. Now this productive arrangement is changing because of the increasing need within urologic practice for real-time imaging by fluoroscopy or ultrasonography during urologic manipulations.

Fluoroscopy has become increasingly important to urology for several reasons. Accurate urodynamic assessment often requires urodynamic pressure and electromyelographic measurements together with dynamic cystography, that is, real-time radiographic imaging (i.e., fluoroscopy) and cine-fluorography or video-fluorography. Also, newer techniques, such as percutaneous nephrostomy, require fluoroscopy because they involve guidewire techniques. In addition, established manipulative procedures, such as diagnostic retrograde catheterization and blind retrograde stone basketing, now seem best performed with fluoroscopic guidance. Many of the newer endoscopic procedures, such as ureterorenoscopy or nephroscopy, often require simultaneous fluoroscopic assistance; in fact, fluoroscopy is an essential part of ESWL.

Fluoroscopy. The principles of fluoroscopy and its related safety considerations can be discussed only briefly here; for more detailed accounts the reader is referred to standard radiographic texts (Miller, 1973).

Today, a basic fluoroscopic system consists of an x-ray tube, image intensifier, video camera, and television screen. Many systems also contain specialized photographic and video recorder equipment, and sometimes equipment to obtain actual radiograms is also involved (Fig. 8–32). In all systems the x-ray tube is properly mounted so that the radiation from it strikes the fluorescent screen of the image intensifier. When the x-ray tube is activated, x-ray photons pass through the desired part of the patient. Owing to the varying attenuation coefficients of different tissues, a photon image is produced. This image is directed to the fluoroscopic screen of an image intensifier. The screen is coated with a chemical (usually cesium iodine), which converts the photon image into light scintillations.

Because the initial fluoroscopic image is of low intensity, an image intensifier is necessary to convert the image into electron beams. The beams are strengthened such that, when converted back into a fluoroscopic image, the image is brighter and therefore more easily seen. This enhanced image can then be converted into electrical signals by a black and white television camera for display on a video screen, or it can be stored by a video recording device for real-time analysis or for later review.

A permanent copy of the intensified fluorescent image can also be recorded by single-frame or cine-photography, depending on the camera. Thus, some fluoroscopic units have cameras that take single or sequential "spot" pictures of 90 to 105 mm at 1 to 20 frames per second. Other systems, designed to study motion, take cine-fluorographs of 16 or 35 mm at 30 to 60 frames per second. Finally, in some fluoroscopic systems, an x-ray film cassette can

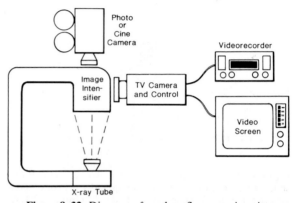

Figure 8–32. Diagram of modern fluoroscopic unit.

be interposed between the patient and the image intensifier, thus obtaining a permanent radiograph. However, the x-ray tube must emit higher amounts of radiation per unit time to produce a standard radiograph than when used for fluoroscopy.

Radiographs give the best image but, of course, cannot record real-time events as can photo- or cine-fluorography. With both these modalities, however, the film must be developed and therefore cannot be analyzed immediately, as can video imaging. The sharpness of video imaging is least ideal, but it is usually adequate for real-time viewing and manipulation.

Since most endourologic procedures require fluoroscopy in different planes, multi-axis fluoroscopy is desirable. This is achieved primarily by one of two configurations: biplane or C-arm. In the biplane configuration, two separate fluoroscopic systems operate perpendicular to each other in a fixed axis. With this arrangement, the patient must be moved to obtain oblique views, a requirement that can be difficult when the patient is under general anesthesia. However, with the C-arm or U-arm configuration, the x-ray tube and image intensifier unit can be rotated about the patient, producing an infinite variety of axes through the body. Some C-arms are also portable. Therefore, for endourologic procedures, this configuration is favored. With either configuration, the ideal x-ray table is one with a floating top that can be moved longitudinally and from side to side.

With the increasing use of fluoroscopy during urologic manipulations, it is important that urologists appreciate and practice standard radiation exposure safety principles. These include activating fluoroscopy for only short periods, keeping the image intensifier as close to the patient's body as possible, reducing the field size to the minimum necessary for manipulation, avoiding physician exposure within the field, measuring total fluoroscopy exposure time for each procedure, and wearing lead aprons and radiation-monitoring badges. In addition, there are two arrangements of the x-ray tube and image intensifier that present drastically different radiation hazards: x-ray tube beneath the table and image intensifier above the patient, and vice versa (Fig. 8–33). With the tube beneath the table, almost 99 per cent of the incidence beam intensity is absorbed by the patient's body with the operator's hands receiving only about 1 per cent. A similar but less drastic attenuation of the beam applies to the secondary radiation. The operator's eyes and thyroid are virtually completely protected by the image intensifier. The dose to the hands is also minimal. However, with the x-ray tube above the patient and the image intensifier below, the operator's hands receive significantly greater radiation. Also, the thyroid and the eyes are exposed to unattenuated secondary radiation. Because of the restrictions imposed by many standard urologic tables, the more hazardous fluoroscopic arrangement is common in cystoscopic suites. If prolonged and repeated usage is required, this arrangement can be damaging unless eye shields, protective helmets, and thyroid shields are worn (Amplatz et al., 1983).

Ultrasonography. Ultrasonic imaging has

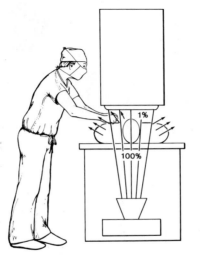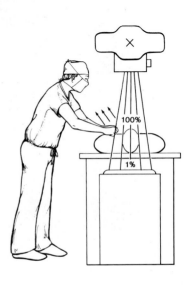

Figure 8–33. Two common fluoroscopic configurations: *A,* With x-ray tube under table, patient is effective filter, decreasing incident beam intensity to about 1 per cent; image intensifier above table protects operator's eyes and thyroid. *B,* With x-ray tube over table, operator's eyes and thyroid are exposed to unattenuated secondary radiation. (From Amplatz, K., et al.: Apple Radiol. Nov./Dec. 1983, p. 32. Used by permission.)

become an important diagnostic modality in urology, especially since the introduction of B-mode, gray-scale, and real-time capabilities. It will be discussed briefly here but is covered in more detail elsewhere in this text and in other sources (Taylor et al., 1980). Ultrasonography is important for the clinical evaluation of renal masses, and, more recently, real-time ultrasonography has assumed an increasingly important role in renal cyst puncture and percutaneous renal biopsy and nephrostomy. Also, in some centers, ultrasonography now is used to help to diagnose pathologic conditions of the scrotum. These tasks usually are performed by radiologists: Typically, the urologic surgeon rarely participated in the actual performance of the ultrasonic examination, although it is often critical for diagnosis because it is performed in real time and sonograms are obtained only at the discretion of the examiner. However, this arrangement is now changing: Urologists are becoming increasingly involved in the actual performance of the ultrasonic examination because of the availability of intracorporeal ultrasonography.

Currently, there are three types of intracorporeal ultrasonography in urology: transrectal examinations, transurethral examinations, and intraoperative examinations of the kidney. Transrectal ultrasonography was originally adapted because imaging of the prostate, seminal vesicles, and bladder is often unsatisfactory when the ultrasonic transducer is aimed through the lower abdominal wall. From this position the pelvic bones severely restrict the acoustic window through which these organs can be reached by ultrasound. Typically, in transrectal ultrasonography, a rotary real-time transducer probe is covered with a water-filled balloon (to optimize wave conduction) and positioned in the rectum. Transverse images of the structures anterior to the rectum are obtained, which quite clearly outline the prostate and seminal vesicles (Fig. 8–34). Although the ultimate utility of this modality is still to be determined, it does seem useful for judging prostatic size and for staging carcinoma of the prostate. Currently, ultrasonography cannot reliably differentiate between malignancy, chronic inflammation, and prostatic stones (Spirnak and Resnick, in press).

Recently, linear-array ultrasonic transducers have also been used transrectally to obtain real-time sagittal images of the bladder and posterior and anterior urethra during voiding (Fig. 8–34). This modality, which is called transrectal sonographic voiding cystourethrography, can be performed at the same time as other urodynamic studies, such as sphincter electromyelography and urethral or bladder pressure measurements. Such simultaneous visual imaging was previously obtained radiographically. Transrectal sonographic voiding cystourethrography appears to be equal or sometimes superior to such radiographic studies and obviates the problems of radiation exposure (Shapeero et al., 1983).

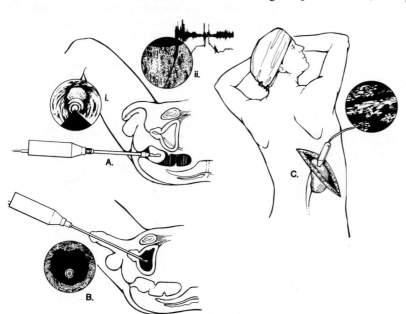

Figure 8–34. Intracorporeal ultrasound in urology. *A,* Transrectal ultrasound (water-filled balloon surrounds probe): transverse image using rotary probe (i); sagittal image of bladder and proximal urethra using linear array probe together with other urodynamic measurements (ii); *B,* transrectal ultrasonography; *C,* ultrasonic sector scan of kidney at open surgery.

Transurethral ultrasonography was developed to enhance imaging of the inside of the bladder. With the bladder filled with fluid (again, to enhance wave conduction), a rotary transducer is inserted through a cystoscopic sheath into the bladder. By altering the position of the transducer, transverse images of the entire bladder can be obtained (Fig. 8–34). This imaging appears to be particularly useful for assessing the local stages of bladder tumors (Nakamura and Niijima, 1980; Schuller et al., 1982).

Finally, ultrasonography has been applied intracorporeally to determine the location of poorly accessible calyceal stones during renal surgery. Here, a sector-scan ultrasonic transducer is moved over the surface of the kidney and the position of the stone determined by its characteristic ultrasonic image (Fig. 8–34). Small needles can then be placed through the renal parenchyma onto the stone, again using ultrasonic imaging, to guide the surgeon in an accurate and safe nephrolithotomy (Lytton, 1983).

LASERS

Details of the physics and instrumentation of light amplification by stimulated emission of radiation (LASER) are beyond the scope of this discussion, but a brief description may be useful. If a photon of a certain wavelength collides with an atom (or medium) of similar energy characteristics, an identical photon is released in the same plane and phase as the stimulating photon, thus resulting in two waves of similar length traveling in the same direction and in phase with one another. This stimulated emission of radiation is so arranged that the resultant light is amplified and has three unique properties: It is (1) of one color and wavelength (monochromicity); (2) in phase, thus forming a consistent and parallel beam (coherence); and (3) propagated with little tendency to diverge. These properties make it ideal for projection onto tissue.

This new form of light energy has been adapted for surgery. Lasers are useful because they are capable of generating an intense, almost parallel beam of electromagnetic energy that can be absorbed by tissue without contact or traction, thus causing precise local heating. This heating results in coagulation, fulguration, or vaporization, depending on the power, size, or particular wavelength of laser energy used. These capabilities and others make lasers especially applicable to endourology (Hofstetter and Frank, 1983).

There are several types of lasers, depending on which atom (i.e., medium) is used to generate energy. Each medium emits laser light of different wavelengths, and tissues react differently to different types of lasers. There are a variety of media that are capable of undergoing stimulated emission. The laser types that are most pertinent to urology are carbon dioxide (CO_2), argon, and neodymium: Yag.

The CO_2 laser uses the CO_2 molecule as the active medium and emits light with a wavelength of 10,600 μ, which is invisible. Its energy is readily absorbed by water and so most of the energy from CO_2 is absorbed within 0.01 mm of tissue, producing intense heat and vaporization at the point of impact. This allows for precise tissue removal and cutting (i.e., hemostatic light knife), but it is ineffective for deep-tissue applications. Hemostasis is good for finely vascularized tissue (i.e., vocal cords, cervix) but less useful for big vessels.

In urology, CO_2 lasers have been used primarily for nonendoscopic purposes because the energy is absorbed by water and because optic fibers for transmission of CO_2 laser light are not available for clinical use. CO_2 lasers have successfully treated external genital lesions, such as erythroplasia of Queyrat, condyloma acuminatum, and even frank carcinoma of the penis. Because healing after CO_2 laser destruction seems to occur with less scarring, the cosmetic results may be superior. For this reason, CO_2 lasers have also been used to treat urethral strictures, but the results do not demonstrate a clear advantage over other methods. These lasers have also been used as a hemostatic light knife in a variety of urologic open surgical procedures but here also seem to offer little advantage (Hall, 1982).

The argon laser emits light with a wavelength of 488 to 514 μ, which is in the green color range. Its beam is strongly absorbed by the pigments melanin and hemoglobin, therefore making it attractive for selective destruction of vascular structures. For example, it traverses the eye and coagulates retinal blood vessels. Tissue penetration is approximately 1.0 mm, and its beam is readily transmissible by optical fibers and through fluids. Argon lasers have not been tested extensively in urology. So far, no definite usefulness has been demonstrated.

The neodymium: Yag laser emits invisible light of 1060 μ wavelength. Its energy is not as readily absorbed by tissue as CO_2 or argon, so penetration can be as deep as 4 to 5 mm. The beam is easily transmitted by optical fibers and passes well through water, making it the most suitable laser for endoscopic application. Neodymium: Yag laser light seems well suited for the management of some bladder tumors because it can be readily applied endoscopically to the bladder to cause reproducible full-thickness bladder wall coagulation while maintaining bladder stability and integrity. These lasers have been used successfully for small bladder tumors and for destroying the base of larger ones after electrical resection. Tissue sloughing occurs over a period of time after the procedure, as it does following electrofulguration. Theoretical and clinical experience suggest that neodymium: Yag lasers offer advantages over conventional methods in terms of recurrence rate for bladder tumors and possibly for endoscopic treatment of limited muscle-invading tumors. Also, outpatient endoscopic surgery is more feasible with these lasers because patients experience little pain and hemostasis is often superior to that with conventional methods (Hofstetter and Frank, 1983; Hall, 1982; Smith, in press).

In summary, lasers offer definite advantages over electrical methods for endoscopic tissue destruction. With proper safeguards, destruction can be more precise and hemostasis is often superior. Finally, laser destruction lends itself to flexible endoscopy and to smaller caliber instruments. Although, to date, considerable experimental and clinical data have not demonstrated areas of urology in which lasers are clearly and practically superior to more conventional approaches, much more work is necessary to accurately determine their usefulness. For example, lasers have been used to destroy urinary stones (Watson et al., 1983), but they are not yet as effective as other methods. Also, lasers have been used to activate the endogenous photosensitizer hematoporphyrin derivative (HPD). A photosensitizer is a light-absorbing molecule capable of transferring absorbed energy to other nonabsorbing molecules. HPD is preferentially absorbed by malignant tissue after systemic administration, and this fact can be used to therapeutic advantage. For example, bladder tumors that have absorbed HPD can be detected or destroyed, or both, when exposed to laser light introduced transurethrally. This approach has been used successfully by several investigators and may be particularly appropriate to detect and treat diffuse bladder tumors or urothelial carcinoma in situ (Benson et al., 1983).

THE FUTURE

If the past can be used as an example, future progress in urologic instrumentation will be rapid. The biomedical engineering industry is aware of the needs of medicine and continues to perfect useful technology. Some believe that the next major advance in urologic surgery and, indeed, in all of surgery will be endoscopic surgery. Endoscopic instruments in urology will almost certainly undergo further miniaturization because fiberoptic design and materials are improving and becoming less expensive (Epstein, 1980). Thus, many of the rigid endoscopes will be replaced by flexible ones, and the existing flexible scopes will become smaller and more durable. Also, laser light will become more practical for tissue destruction and also as a source of illumination. Indeed, minute transistor chips will allow video cameras to be placed at the tips of catheters. In this way, images can be transmitted to the outside electronically rather than optically (Sarak and Fleischer, 1984). These advances will further decrease the caliber requirements for endoscopes, which, in turn, will allow many more endoscopic procedures to be conducted without general anesthesia.

Imaging will advance in other ways also. For example, electronic conversion of both radiographic and endoscopic visual images will allow computer manipulation for enhanced visual acuity and analysis in real time. Also in real time, stimultaneous display and processing of radiographic and endoscopic images will become increasingly common. Finally, better biocompatible materials will be developed and utilized. Already biogels (hydrophilic polymers) that shrink and swell in response to variations in surrounding fluid have demonstrated remarkable freedom from encrustation within the urinary tract during long-term implant studies. Bonding of these relatively weak gels to polymeric materials of superior strength and elasticity may offer one solution to the problem of long-term catheter tolerance (H. Mardis, personal communication, 1984).

Thus, instruments for endourology will continue to diversify and increase in sophistication. This progress will require the acquisition of new skills and knowledge by urologists and increasing support by those who provide and care for their instruments and will undoubtedly benefit the patient with urologic disease. It is important to remember, though, that now, as in the past, the art of urologic surgery entails not only tools and their skillful use but also knowledge, judgment, and compassion.

References

Amplatz, K. et al.: Percutaneous renal stone removal. Appl. Radiol., Nov./Dec.:32, 1983.

Aso, Y., et al.: Usefulness of fiber-optic hi-low ureteroscope in the diagnosis of upper urinary tract lesions. J. Urol. In press.

Benson, R. C., Jr., et al.: Treatment of transitional cell carcinoma of the bladder with hematoporphyrin derivative phototherapy. J. Urol., 130:1090, 1983.

Berci, G.: Instrumentation I: rigid endoscopes. In Berci, G. (Ed.): Endoscopy. New York, Appleton-Century-Crofts, 1976, pp. 74–112a.

Berci, G.: Instrumentation II: flexible fiber endoscopes. In Berci, G. (Ed.): Endoscopy. New York, Appleton-Century-Crofts, 1976, pp. 113–132b.

Berci, G.: Television. In Berci, G. (Ed.): Endoscopy. New York, Appleton-Century-Crofts, 1976, pp. 271–279c.

Berci, G., et al.: Permanent film records. In Berci, G. (Ed.): Endoscopy. New York, Appleton-Century-Crofts, 1976, pp. 242–270.

Boyce, H. W., Jr., and Palmer, E. D.: Laparoscopy. In Techniques of Clinical Gastroenterology. Springfield, Il., Charles C Thomas, 1975, pp. 147–177.

Burkholder, G. V., and Kaufman, J. J.: Local implantation of carcinoma of the prostate with percutaneous needle biopsy. J. Urol., 97:801, 1966.

Bush, I. M., et al.: Ureterorenoscopy. Urol. Clin. North Am., 9:131, 1982.

Castaneda-Zuniga, W.: Dilation of the nephrostomy tract. In Clayman, R. V., and Castaneda-Zuniga, W. (Eds.): Techniques in Endourology: A Guide to the Percutaneous Removal of Renal and Ureteral Calculi. Dallas, Heritage Press, 1984.

Chaussey, C., et al.: First clinical experience with extracorporeally induced destruction of kidney stones by shock waves. J. Urol., 127:417, 1982.

Chaussey, C., and Schmeidt, E.: Shock wave treatment for stones in the upper urinary tract. Urol. Clin. North Am. 10:743, 1983.

Clayman, R. V.: Percutaneous nephroscopy: a non-operative approach to the diagnosis and treatment of renal disease: Br. J. Urol. (Suppl.), 11:18, 1983.

Clayman, R. V., et al.: Flexible fiberoptic and rigid rod lens endoscopy of the lower urinary tract: a prospective controlled comparison. J. Urol., 131:715, 1984a.

Clayman, R. V., et al.: Percutaneous intrarenal electrosurgery. J. Urol., 131:864, 1984b.

Clayman, R. V., et al.: Percutaneous nephrostolithotomy: percutaneous extraction of renal and ureteral calculi from 100 patients. J. Urol., 131:868, 1984c.

Clayman, R. V., et al.: Percutaneous nephrolithotomy: an approach to branched and staghorn renal calculi. JAMA, 250:73, 1983a.

Clayman, R. V., et al.: Rapid balloon dilation of nephrostomy tract for nephrostolithotomy. Radiology, 149:884, 1983b.

Crawford, E. D., et al.: Prevention of urinary tract infection and sepsis following transrectal prostatic biopsy. J. Urol., 127:449, 1982.

Derlen, L. W., Jr., et al.: Complications of transrectal biopsy examination of the prostate gland. South. Med. J., 67:1453, 1974.

Epsoti, P. L.: Cytologic malignancy grading for prostatic carcinoma for transurethral aspiration biopsy. Scand. J. Urol. Nephrol., 5:199, 1971.

Epstein, M.: Endoscopy: developments in topical instrumentation. Science, 210:280, 1980.

Epstein, N. A.: Prostatic biopsy: a morphologic correlation of aspiration cytology with needle biopsy histology. Cancer, 39:2078, 1976.

Ford, T. F., et al.: Transurethral ureteroscopic retrieval of ureteric stones. Br. J. Urol., 55:626, 1983.

Franzen, S., et al.: Cytological diagnosis of prostatic tumors by transrectal aspiration biopsy: a preliminary report. Br. J. Urol., 32:193, 1960.

Gill, W. B., et al.: Retrograde brush biopsy of the ureter and renal pelvis. Urol. Clin. North Am., 6:573, 1979.

Gittes, R. F., and Williams, J. L.: Nephroscopy. In Berci, G. (Ed.): Endoscopy. New York, Appleton-Century-Crofts, 1976, pp. 665–676.

Hall, R. R.: Report to the Standing Committee on Urological Instruments: lasers in urology. Br. J. Urol., 54:421, 1982.

Hofstetter, A., and Frank, F.: Laser use in urology. In Dixon, J. A. (Ed.): Surgical Application of Lasers. Chicago, Year Book Medical Publishers, 1983, p. 146.

Hopkins, H. H.: Optical principles of the endoscope. In Berci, G. (Ed.): Endoscopy. New York, Appleton-Century-Crofts, 1976, pp. 3–26a.

Hopkins, H. H.: The physics of the fiberoptics endoscope. In Berci, G. (Ed.): Endoscopy. New York, Appleton-Century-Crofts, 1976, pp. 27–63b.

Huffman, J. L., et al.: Treatment of distal ureteral calculi using rigid ureteroscope. Urology, 20:574, 1982.

Kaufman, J. J., and Schultz, J. I.: Needle biopsy of the prostate: a re-evaluation. J. Urol., 87:164, 1962.

Khan, A. U.: Armamentarium in transurethral surgery. In Greene, L. F., and Segura, J. W. (Eds.): Transurethral Surgery. Philadelphia, W. B. Saunders Co., 1979, pp. 1–21.

Kumes, D. M., and Stamey, T. A.: Percutaneous suprapubic cystostomy. In Kaye, K. (Ed.): Outpatient Urologic Surgery. Philadelphia, Lea & Febiger. In press.

Lange, P. H., et al.: Percutaneous removal of calyceal and other "inaccessible" stones: instruments and techniques. J. Urol. In press.

Lieberman, R. P., Cummings, K. B., et al.: Sheathed catheter system for fluoroscopically guided retrograde catheterization, and brush and forceps biopsy of the upper urinary tract. J. Urol., 131:450, 1984.

Lytton, B.: Intraoperative ultrasound for nephrolithotomy. J. Urol., 130:213, 1983.

Marberger, M.: Disintegration of renal and ureteral calculi with ultrasound. Urol. Clin. North Am., 10:729, 1983.

Mardis, H. K.: Comparative evaluation of polymeric biomaterial devices within the urinary tract. American Urological Association (abstract). New Orleans, May 1984.

Mazzeo, V. P., Jr., et al.: A technique for percutaneous dilation of nephrostomy tracts. Radiology, 144:175, 1982.

Miller, E. R.: Equipment for the roentgenologic examination of the gastrointestinal tract. In Margulis, A. R., and Burhenne, H. J. (Eds.): Alimentary Tract Roentgenology. St. Louis, C. V. Mosby Co., 1973, pp. 18–33.

Nakamura, S., and Niijima, T.: Staging of bladder cancer by ultrasonography: a new technique by transurethral intravesicle scanning. J. Urol., *124*:341, 1980.

Pollack, H. M.: Interventional radiology. *In* Kendall, A. R., and Karafin, L. (Eds.): Urology. Vol. 1. New York, Harper & Row, 1984. In press.

Rutner, A. B., and Fucilla, I. S.: An improved helical stone basket. J. Urol., *116*:784, 1976.

Savak, M. V., and Fleischer, D. E.: Colonoscopy with a VideoEndoscope: Preliminary experience. Gastrointest. Endosc., *30*:1, 1984.

Schuller, J., et al.: Intravesicle ultrasound tomography in staging bladder cancer. J. Urol., *128*:264, 1982.

Segura, J. W., et al.: Percutaneous lithotripsy. J. Urol., *130*:1051, 1983.

Shapeero, L. G., et al.: Transrectal sonographic voiding cystourethrography: studies in neuromuscular bladder dysfunction. Am. J. Roentgenol., *141*:83, 1983.

Silber, S. J., and Cohen, R.: Laparoscopy for cryptorchidism. J. Urol., *124*:928, 1980.

Sittner, W. R., and Fitzgerald, J. K.: High-frequency electrosurgery. *In* Berci, G. (Ed.): Endoscopy. New York, Appleton-Century-Crofts, 1976, pp. 214–221.

Smith, A. D.: The universal ureteral stent. Urol. Clin. North Am., *9* (1):103, 1982.

Smith, A. D., et al.: Application of percutaneous nephrostomy: new challenges and opportunities in endourology (letter). J. Urol., *121*:382, 1979.

Smith, J. A., Jr.: Clinical experience with a neodymium: Yag laser in endoscopic surgery. J. Urol. In press.

Spirnak, J. P., and Resnick, M. I.: Transrectal ultrasonography. Urology. In press.

Stables, D. P.: Percutaneous nephrostomy: techniques, indications and results. Urol. Clin. North Am., *9*:15, 1982.

Taylor, K. J. W., et al. (Eds.): Introduction to basic principles. *In* Ultrasonography. New York, Churchill Livingstone, 1980, pp. 1–21.

Waller, R. N., III, et al.: Transluminal balloon dilation of a tuberculosis ureteral stricture. J. Urol., *129*:1225, 1983.

Watson, G. M., et al.: Laser fragmentation of renal calculi. Br. J. Urol., *55*:613, 1983.

White, R. I., Jr.: Principles of percutaneous catheterization. *In* White, R. I., Jr. (Ed.): Fundamentals of Vascular Radiology. Philadelphia, Lea & Febiger, 1976, pp. 7–16.

Wickhan, J. E. A., and Miller, R. A. (Eds.): Nephroscopy: endoscopic instruments and their accessories. *In* Percutaneous Renal Surgery. New York, Churchill Livingstone, 1983, pp. 45–74a.

Wickham, J. E. A., and Miller, R. A. (Eds.): Non-mechanical disruption of renal stones. *In* Percutaneous Renal Surgery. New York, Churchill Livingstone, 1983, pp. 75–107b.

Wickham, J. E. A., and Miller, R. A. (Eds.): Percutaneous renal access. *In* Percutaneous Renal Surgery: New York, Churchill Livingstone, 1983, pp. 17–44c.

THE PATHOPHYSIOLOGY OF URINARY OBSTRUCTION

CHAPTER 9

The Pathophysiology of Urinary Obstruction

JAY Y. GILLENWATER, M.D.

Obstructive uropathy with resultant hydronephrosis is the eventual outcome of most urologic diseases. It is well known that complete ureteral obstruction eventually destroys renal function. The postulated mechanisms are elevated ureteral pressure and decreased renal blood flow, which cause cellular atrophy and necrosis. The pathophysiologic effects of short-term complete obstructive uropathy or chronic partial obstructive uropathy can be summarized simply. All renal functions except urinary dilution are progressively impaired. The longer or more severe the obstruction, the more renal damage will result.

Thus, one can succinctly summarize the physiologic alterations in renal function that are observed in both patients and experimental animals as a result of either acute and chronic complete ureteral obstruction or chronic partial ureteral obstruction. In this chapter I will try to summarize both historical and current concepts of obstructive uropathy, including new information concerning pathophysiologic changes, mechanisms of injury, methods of determining the reversibility of damage, and methods of determining if a dilated ureter and renal pelvis have significant obstruction.

An excellent review of obstructive uropathy has been written by Wilson (1977). Other good reviews have been published by Bell (1946), Bricker (1967), Hinman (1970), Bricker and Klahr (1971), Howards and Wright (1976), and Klahr and associates (1977).

HISTORICAL ASPECTS OF HYDRONEPHROSIS

Hermann (1859) and Pfaundler (1902), in studies performed on the dog, and Allard

(1907), in a patient with exstrophy of the bladder, found that release of short-term complete unilateral ureteral obstruction was followed by diuresis with a lower concentration of chloride and urea than was seen in the opposite normal side.

In the early 1900's, studies after release of short-term complete unilateral ureteral obstruction showed a diuresis with the urine having a lower concentration of chloride and urea (Hermann, 1859; Pfaundler, 1902; Allard, 1907). Frank Hinman, Sr. carried out the first thorough systematic scientific investigation of hydronephrosis. Infection and obstruction were demonstrated to cause more rapid and severe damage (Hinman, 1919). In rats with unilateral obstruction, pathologic changes were noted as early as 1 week. Some histologic recovery after release was noted up to 60 days (Hinman, 1919). Denervation of the kidney did not affect the course of hydronephrosis (Hinman and Hepler, 1925c). Arterial or venous obstruction caused more severe damage in hydronephrosis (Hinman and Hepler, 1925a, 1925b, 1926).

Hinman studied the recovery potential after release of complete ureteral obstruction (Hinman, 1926, 1934). The studies in dogs showed that after the release of complete ureteral obstruction lasting 2 weeks and after nephrectomy of the normal kidney, function will recover to near-normal. After release of complete obstruction of 3 weeks' duration and after nephrectomy of the normal kidney, recovery of function is about 50 per cent. The animal cannot survive 4 weeks of obstruction if release of the obstruction is immediately followed by nephrectomy of the normal kidney. If nephrectomy of the normal kidney is delayed after release of the ureteral obstruction, recovery of function in the kidney obstructed 2 weeks is greater than if the opposite normal kidney is removed initially. Hinman further amplified his work in 1934. He showed that the animal did not survive complete ureteral obstruction lasting longer than 2 or 3 weeks if the opposite kidney was removed at the time of release of ureteral obstruction. Hydronephrosis lasting 3 or 4 weeks may leave sufficient function to allow survival of the animal if the opposite normal kidney is not injured for several months after release of the obstruction. The animal may survive hydronephrosis of 30 to 60 days' duration if the normal kidney is damaged gradually.

PATHOLOGY

Gross Appearances and Changes

Complete ureteral occlusion causes the renal pelvis to dilate progressively during the first few weeks. The weight of the kidney increases owing to edema, even though the renal tissue atrophies. There is perirenal and periureteral edema. After 4 to 8 weeks, there is a decrease in parenchymal weight because the atrophy of the tissue is greater than the intrarenal edema. The obstructed kidney appears dark blue with scattered areas of ischemia, wedges of congestion, necrosis, and some frank infarcts.

Microscopic Changes

Microscopic changes in progressive hydronephrosis have been demonstrated in the dog (Hinman and Morison, 1924), the rabbit (Deming, 1951; Hinman, 1945; Johnson, 1932; Sheehan and Davis, 1959; Strong, 1940), and the rat (Shimamura et al., 1966). In all the experimental animals, the progression of changes appears similar, except that there is early and fulminant papillary destruction in the rabbit (Hinman, 1945; Strong, 1940).

During the first few days of obstruction, there is flattening of the papilla with widespread dilatation of the distal nephron. The proximal tubules show a transient dilatation the first several days and then slowly atrophy. On the seventh day of obstruction, the dilated collecting tubules show some atrophy and necrosis. On the fourteenth day, there is progressive dilatation of the collecting and distal tubules, and atrophy of the proximal tubular epithelial cells is observed. By the twenty-eighth day of obstruction, there is a 50 per cent decrease in medullary thickness, with continued atrophy and dilatation of the distal and collecting tubules. The cortex is thinner, with marked atrophy of the proximal tubules. Following 8 weeks

of obstruction, only a 1-cm parenchymal strip consisting primarily of connective tissue and small oval glomeruli remains.

Pathologic changes are first noted in the glomerulus after 28 days of complete ureteral obstruction.

Proliferation of the medullary interstitial cells, which are believed to secrete prostaglandins, has been noted by the fifth day of obstruction (Sheehan and Davis, 1959; Wilson, 1972).

On microscopic examination, vascular changes consisting of numerous tears in the elastica interna in both small and large arteries have been demonstrated in rabbits (Altschul and Fedor, 1953; Sheehan and Davis, 1959) and rats (Altschul and Fedor, 1953). Rao and Heptinstall (1968) did not believe that the tears in the elastica of the vessels were impressive. Their studies also failed to identify any arterial occlusion that would account for the reduced blood flow observed in chronic hydronephrosis. An impairment in venous drainage was believed to be an important factor in nephron damage (Rao and Heptinstall, 1968).

Histochemical studies have shown a loss of the normally high alkaline phosphatase content of the proximal tubular cells after 5 days of total obstruction in rats (Wilmer, 1943). Electron microscopy of short-term obstruction and release of rat kidneys has shown cellular atrophy (with preservation of brush border) rather than dilatation in the proximal tubules. Cellular flattening and dilatation are demonstrated in the loop of Henle and the collecting tubules (Shimamura et al., 1966).

Obstruction has been noted to damage the polar regions of the kidney initially. Ransley and Risdon (1974) have shown that the openings of Bellini's ducts into the papilla are more dilated and gaping in the polar regions than in the midportion, perhaps accounting for the earlier and greater transmission of back pressure to the tubules and into the polar regions.

Recent studies (Marier et al., 1978; Dzukias et al., 1982) have shown that the distribution of Tamm-Horsfall protein casts within Bowman's space of glomeruli is pathognomonic of urinary tract obstruction or vesicoureteral reflux (which I consider a form of obstruction, since retrograde passage of urine blocks normal urine flow). Tamm-Horsfall protein is present only in the urinary tract and approximately 50 mg per day is synthesized in the ascending limb of the loops of Henle and the distal convoluted tubules. Obstruction is thought to cause reverse filtration across Bowman's capsule, although ultrafiltration across the glomerular capillary wall is also a possibility. A renal biopsy showing

Tamm-Horsfall protein within Bowman's space of the glomerulus would provide conclusive evidence that obstruction or vesicoureteral reflux was present; this evidence also has been helpful in differentiating whether the problem in some cases of renal transplants is rejection or obstruction.

Pathologic Changes in Renal Pelvis and Ureter

Urinary tract obstruction causes proximal dilatation with both functional and morphologic changes in the proximal ureter and renal pelvis. In the first phase of obstruction, muscular hypertrophy and hyperplasia occur proximal to the obstruction (Cussen and Tymms, 1972; Ladefoged and Djurhuus, 1976; Djurhuus et al., 1976a). Connective tissue consisting of collagen and elastic tissue production by the smooth muscle cells follows, with impairment of myogenic impulse transmission and disturbance of peristalsis (Gee and Kiviat, 1975; Gosling and Dixon, 1974; Djurhuus et al., 1976a; Ladefoged and Djurhuus, 1976).

The obstructing segment of the ureteropelvic junction or megaureter has an increase in collagen, which acts as an inelastic collar preventing adequate distention in the affected ureteral segment (Notley, 1971, 1972; Hanna et al., 1976).

Summary

Pathologic changes in the completely obstructed kidney correlate well with the observed physiologic changes. These histologic changes include atrophy, beginning in the first 7 days in the distal nephron. By 14 days, atrophy is noted in the cortical regions. Glomeruli are damaged last. No evidence of anatomic arterial narrowing is observed that would explain the decrease in renal blood flow in chronic hydronephrosis. The presence of Tamm-Horsfall protein casts within Bowman's space of glomeruli is pathognomonic of obstruction or vesicoureteral reflux.

ROLE OF LYMPHATICS IN HYDRONEPHROSIS

The role of renal lymphatics in normal and pathologic conditions of the kidney has not been investigated as completely as other aspects of renal function. Renal lymphatic drainage is through both hilar and capsular lymph vessels.

The first important investigation of renal lymph circulation was made in 1863 (Ludwig

and Sawarykin; cited by Rusznyák, 1960). These workers showed that ligation of the ureter was followed by dilatation of the efferent renal lymphatics. Schmidt and Hayman (1929) calculated total renal lymph flow to be between 0.31 and 3.22 ml/min. Sugarman (1942) found renal lymph volumes to be 0.25 to 0.5 ml/min in each kidney. Thus, the normal kidney produces a lymph volume similar to the volume of urine output. Murphy (1958) found that normal renal lymph flow is increased by water diuresis and ureteral obstruction. Protein is carried continuously from the renal interstitial fluid by the renal lymphatics. It is estimated that 13 to 26 gm of protein is returned daily by the renal lymphatics (Rusznyák, 1960). Acute obstruction of renal lymphatics has no significant effect on renal blood flow, glomerular filtration rate, Tm glucose, and Tm_{PAH}; however, there is an increase in excretion of sodium, chloride, and water (Rusznyák, 1960). The increased renal lymph flow with ureteral obstruction is believed to be due to elevation of intrarenal venous pressure rather than to reabsorption from the renal pelvis (Naber and Madsen, 1974).

Babics and Rényi-Vámos (1952a and b, 1950), cited by Rusznyák (1960), postulated that the preservation of renal function in hydronephrosis is due to pyelolymphatic backflow. The reabsorption of renal pelvis urine into the lymphatics allows replacement glomerular filtration to occur. They postulated that penetration of urine into the interstitial spaces induces liberation of histamine, with the resultant increase in capillary permeability and with exudation of protein-rich fluid into the interstitial space and into the lymphatics. If the lymphatics are ligated to an otherwise normal kidney, there is extensive edema of the parenchyma, the hilar fat, and even the capsule (Rusznyák, 1960). They reported that if the lymphatics alone are ligated, there is no necrosis, only a parenchymatous degeneration of the tubular cells. Ligation of both the lymphatics and the ureter produces severe renal damage with necrosis, and destruction may be seen in several days instead of several months (Földi and Romhányi, 1953a and b).

The dynamic state of hydronephrosis with reabsorption of urine from the renal pelvis and replacement glomerular filtration has been known for many years. Investigative studies have shown that various substances injected into an obstructed renal pelvis appear in the systemic circulation. The injected substances include strychnine (Tuffier, 1894), phenolsulfonphthalein (Burns and Schwartz, 1918), dye (Morison, 1929), and indigo carmine (Hinman and Lee-

Brown, 1924). Backflow of urine out of the renal pelvis was demonstrated to occur first through a rupture of the fornix (Hinman and Lee-Brown, 1924; Bird and Moise, 1926; Fuchs, 1925, cited by Olsson, 1948). Narath (1940) performed in vivo retrograde occlusion studies in animals and patients. He demonstrated pyelosinus backflow into the sinus renalis and the lymphatics without rupture into the venous system. Narath (1940) postulated that in obstructive uropathy, there is physiologic egress of fluid by pyelocanalicular and pyelosinus backflow and traumatic rupture (with higher pressures) of the calyceal fornix, and egress into both the lymphatic and the venous systems. Backflow was studied extensively in patients undergoing intravenous pyelography (Olsson, 1948); it was observed in 3.7 per cent of patients with external ureteral compression. Backflow was not observed in most of these cases until the external ureteral compression was applied. Analysis of 100 cases of backflow revealed that 89 were extravasations from ruptured fornices into the renal sinus and perirenal spaces. Eleven cases were believed to be pyelolymphatic backflow. Pyelovenous backflow was thought to be very rare.

Holmes and coworkers (1977) studied chronic unilateral obstruction in dogs for periods up to 5 weeks. Three conclusions were made: (1) The composition of renal lymph becomes similar to plasma; (2) pyelolymphatic backflow does not contribute significantly to renal lymph; and (3) there is a major diversion of hilar lymph to the capsular system.

Summary

Renal lymph volume normally approximates that of urine flow and increases with water diuresis or ureteral obstruction. Acute obstruction of renal lymphatics causes natriuresis and diuresis, with no other alteration in renal function. Ligation of both the lymphatics and the ureter is said to cause renal damage, with necrosis and destruction in several days. With ureteral obstruction, initially there is pyelocanalicular and pyelosinus backflow. With higher renal pelvis pressures, there is egress of urine into both the lymphatic and the venous systems.

TURNOVER OF RENAL PELVIS URINE IN HYDRONEPHROSIS

Numerous studies have demonstrated that various compounds placed in the totally ob-

structed renal pelvis leave by the lymphatic and venous channels (Bledsoe and Murphy, 1959; Chisholm and Calnan, 1967; Goodwin and Kaufman, 1956; Kazmin et al., 1960; Murphy et al., 1958; Myint and Murphy, 1957; Naber and Madsen, 1974, 1973a and b; Persky et al., 1957a, 1956, 1955; Tormene et al., 1963).

Naber and Madsen (1973a) found that in acute hydronephrosis, there was reabsorption of urine into the hilar lymph; the urine equaled only 0.3 per cent of the volume of the hilar lymph on calculation. The quantitiy of urine exiting from the renal pelvis in acute hydronephrosis was 0.06 ml/min. In chronic hydronephrosis of 6 to 34 days' duration, the quantity of urine exiting from the renal pelvis ranged from 0.04 to 0.16 ml/min (Naber and Madsen, 1974). Following ureteral obstruction lasting 1 week, pyelolymphatic reabsorption into hilar but not subcapsular lymph could be demonstrated. The replacement glomerular filtration rate was calculated to be 1.74 ml/min in complete ureteral obstruction of 1 week's duration and 0.4ml/min after 34 days of complete ureteral occlusion (Naber and Madsen, 1974). The "urine flow" was calculated to be 0.19 ml/min in complete ureteral occlusion. Thus, 80 to 90 per cent of the filtrate in chronic hydronephrosis is reabsorbed in the tubules and presumably exits by the renal veins. It is also believed that the majority of the fluid reabsorbed from the renal pelvis in chronic hydronephrosis exits into the renal venous system rather than into the lymphatics.

Summary

In hydronephrosis, fluid exits from the renal pelvis by (1) extravasation into the perirenal spaces, (2) pyelovenous backflow, and (3) pyelolymphatic backflow. With low pressures, much of the fluid enters the lymphatics. When the pressures are higher, fluid exits by pyelovenous backflow and extravasation. In chronic hydronephrosis, most of the urine exits into the renal venous system.

COMPENSATORY RENAL GROWTH (CURRENT CONCEPTS)

Compensatory renal growth includes both hypertrophy and hyperplasia. Exciting new work in this area concerns the renotrophic factor(s) that specifically incites or regulates compensatory renal growth. Early increase in wet and dry renal mass is noted following unilateral nephrectomy. RNA synthesis increases in 24 hours, followed by enhancement of protein and DNA synthesis. Polyamine synthesis and the rate-limiting enzyme ornithine decarboxylase may play an important role in compensatory renal growth (Preuss, 1983). Compensatory renal growth is not as great in older animals, as evidenced by sera, and tissue activators from incubating rat renal slices of younger animals show an increased thymidine incorporation into DNA (Hayslett, 1983). After unilateral renal obstruction, renal mass increases in both kidneys for the first 7 to 10 days, followed by a progressive decline in mass in the obstructed kidney. The growth in the obstructed kidney may be a local response to injury (Zelman, 1983). Recent studies have shown that the renotrophic factor stimulates the three principal forms of growth: embryonic growth, wound repair compensatory growth, and neoplastic growth (Patt, 1983). The renotrophic factor is thought to be humorally mediated and must be continually present to maintain compensatory hypertrophy. Separation of parabiotic rats shows a return of the renal mass toward baseline (Malt, 1983). Similar renotrophic factors are present in both the urine and the serum (Harris, 1983). The renotrophic factor seems to be responsible for some forms of hypertension secondary to loss of renal mass (Preuss, 1983). Renal mass and the glomerular filtration rate are increased in young insulin-dependent diabetic patients (Seyer-Hansen, 1983).

Renal tissue shows compensatory growth by undergoing hypertrophy and hyperplasia. Hypertrophy is the enlargement of cells, and hyperplasia is the replication of cells via mitosis. With loss of renal tissue, the compensatory growth of the remaining kidney tissue is mostly hypertrophic (Halliburton and Thomson, 1965; Johnson and Vera Roman, 1966; Platt, 1952).

That compensatory renal cell growth occurs by hypertrophy was concluded from morphologic findings and from the evidence of cytoplasmic enlargement because of the increases in the ratios of RNA and protein to DNA. In the repair after acute tubular necrosis, hyperplasia is believed to be dominant (Preuss and Goldin, 1975). During compensatory hypertrophy, the glomeruli do not increase in number but do increase in size, while the blood vessels increase in caliber.

The compensatory changes in renal function after release of complete ureteral obstruction of 2 weeks' duration are shown in Figure 9–1. One week after release, the CFR and Tm$_{PAH}$ are increased and the kidney shows com-

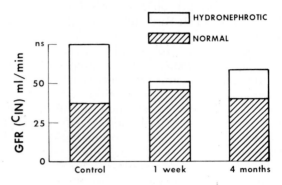

Changes in GFR after release of 14 days of unilateral ureteral obstruction

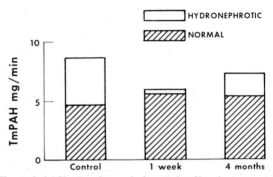

Changes in TmPAH after release of 14 days of unilateral ureteral obstruction

Figure 9–1. Changes in total glomerular filtration rate and Tm$_{PAH}$ before and after release of complete unilateral ureteral obstruction of 2 weeks' duration. The portion contributed by each kidney is depicted, showing compensatory hypertrophy of the normal kidney as well as recovery of function in the previously obstructed kidney.

pensatory hypertrophy. This hypertrophy in the normal kidney persisted at 4 months. Total renal function (GFR and Tm$_{PAH}$) is not recovered to control values, indicating that the compensatory hypertrophy in the normal kidney and the recovery of function in the previously obstructed kidney are not sufficient to restore total renal function to normal.

Effect of Dietary Protein on Kidney Disease

Brenner, Meyer, and Hostetter (1982) reviewed the effects of dietary protein on progressive kidney disease. It is postulated that continuous high protein intake causes nephron hyperperfusion and hyperfiltration, which may cause mesangial cell injury with mesangial matrix overproduction and resultant glomerular sclerosis. Addis (1917) found that excretion of urea required renal work and advocated reduced protein intake in patients with chronic renal insufficiency. Early man, in common with the animals, ate intermittent large protein meals unlike the regular high-protein meals in our society. In animals, it is clear that normally there is low renal blood flow and glomerular filtration with many of the cortical nephrons unperfused in the resting state. After ingestion of a large protein meal, some renal vasodilator mechanism combines with diet-induced extracellular fluid expansion to dramatically increase renal blood flow and the glomerular filtration rate. With regular protein intake there is sustained perfusion or hyperperfusion of the superficial and deep nephrons. Hyperperfusion of remaining nephrons is seen in diabetes, acquired renal disease, or surgical loss from renal disease. This hyperperfusion may contribute to glomerular sclerosis and the destruction of nephrons.

Summary

Loss of renal tissue causes compensatory growth by hypertrophy of the remaining tissue. This renotrophic factor is humorally mediated and has not been identified. Most studies have shown the presence of the humoral renotrophic factor in anephric animals. In the model used by Preuss and Goldin (1975), however, the renotrophic factor was not demonstrated in rats after bilateral nephrectomy. Obviously, much more work is needed in this area.

RENAL COUNTERBALANCE

The concept of renal counterbalance, with the aspects of compensatory hypertrophy and disease atrophy, was introduced by Hinman in 1919. Hinman (1943) stated, "The condition of renal counterbalance may be defined as the behavior of both kidneys up to the completion of the changes resulting from repair." Renal counterbalance ". . . is the bilateral adjustment after injury or disease is removed to a permanent condition of the division of total function."

Hinman further stated, "Experiments with the repair of hydronephrosis demonstrate that renal tissue injured by urinary back pressure has a remarkable capacity for repair; that this potency is enhanced by stimulation or the need of repair through renal insufficiency and is shown at its utmost when the demand is gradually increased; that inhibition of activity by such complicating factors as infection and imperfect relief of obstruction will affect the degree of repair and of hypertrophy as well as

their permanence; and that a repaired hydronephrosis disabled in any way by degenerative changes will atrophy progressively and total function eventually will be taken over by the healthy, more capable compensatory mate."

RENAL ATROPHY OF DISUSE (HYPOTROPHY)

Frank Hinman, Jr. (1963), stated that *"Renal counterbalance,* proposed by Hinman in 1922, implies that a damaged kidney cannot compete with its normal mate, and so it atrophies. More recent work has shown that it does not actually atrophy, but does remain in a relatively atrophic state because it is not given the stimulus to *hypertrophy."*

Hinman (1919) said, "I venture the opinion which I believe some day will be proved experimentally, that a healthy kidney, once thoroughly accustomed to doing all the work, will if let alone, continue to do it in spite of my attempt to relieve it of any part of its burden. If this is true, a crippled kidney, though potentially capable of some work, would be completely ignored when brought into competition with its big active and efficient fellow. It would have small chance to improve itself, but more likely would gradually weaken for want of proper exercise."

Hinman (1943) said that the idea of atrophy of disuse came from observing Richards' frog preparation, which showed varying rates of perfusion for groups of glomeruli, suggesting that some glomeruli were having rest periods.

If one completely believed the atrophy of disuse theory, then the assumption of Judd (cited by Hinman, 1943) "that the hydronephrotic kidney would atrophy no matter how successful the repair" would suggest that all moderately to severely hydronephrotic kidneys should be removed rather than repaired if the other kidney is normal. Hinman (1943) said that Judd made a mistake in concluding that a nephrectomy was always indicated for a well-marked hydronephrosis if the opposite kidney was sound and fully compensatory.

Hinman (1943) reported that he had overstated the case for disuse atrophy. His basic thesis that an injured kidney without stimulation (with a normal contralateral kidney) will not regain function is still accepted by some today (Anderson, 1963; Govan, 1961; Hinman, 1963). In my opinion, the damaged kidney will have some recovery with "the big active and efficient (opposite) fellow in place." There is no question that more recovery of function by the injured kidney is observed if the normal kidney is removed or damaged. Recovery of some function after release of unilateral ureteral obstruction with a normal contralateral kidney has been reported in experimental animals (Kerr, 1956; Vaughan et al., 1971) and in patients (Better et al., 1973; Edvall, 1959).

My feelings have been that the hydronephrotic kidney should be repaired if I believe that there would be enough recovery of function to sustain life, i.e., a creatinine clearance of more than 10 ml/min.

Two types of renal growth have been described by Silber: hypertrophy or compensatory renal growth and obligatory growth associated with growth of the rest of the body (Silber, 1975, 1974; Silber and Crudop, 1974, 1973; Silber and Malvin, 1974). In a series of experiments, Silber (1975) and Rist, Lee, and Gitts (1975) have studied what happens to renal function and size when additional kidneys are transplanted into normal animals. Silber states that when an additional adult kidney is transplanted into an adult, there is no decrease in size or function of any of the three kidneys (Silber, 1974; Silber and Crudop, 1974). When an additional baby kidney is transplanted into a baby rat, all three kidneys grow at a normal rate (Silber and Malvin, 1974). When a hypertrophied adult kidney is transplanted into an adult with a solitary hypertrophied kidney, however, both kidneys return to their previous size and function (Silber, 1975, 1974). Silber (1975) concludes that obligatory renal growth occurs at a predetermined standard rate regardless of the host's age or size. Rist, Lee, and Gittes (1975) transplanted two additional kidneys into male rats and followed them for 120 days. There was no change in size of either the two transplanted kidneys or the normal kidney. Thus, the animals continued to have twice the normal renal mass. The total renal blood flow and glomerular filtration rates showed no increase over normal controls. Therefore, the animal was able to modulate downward the renal functions of glomerular filtration rate and renal blood flow. In contrast, Silber (1974) found that a third kidney transplanted without a subsequent reduction in renal size occurring added 50 per cent to the host's GFR and renal blood flow.

Summary

Renal counterbalance and the concept of hypotrophy (disuse atrophy), introduced by Hinman in 1922, propose that there is a mechanism that monitors and adjusts total renal function. Thus, if one kidney is damaged, there is a stimulus for resultant hypertrophy of the remaining tissue. If recovery of total renal function to normal were achieved, then there would be no additional stimulus for the hydronephrotic kidney to recover once the obstruction is released. According to the theory of disuse atrophy, if one were to add by transplantation additional renal mass beyond what is normally needed, there should be a stimulus for hypotrophy of some of the renal tissue.

Several studies suggest that the theory of disuse atrophy is overly simplistic. It seems clear that with transplantation of additional normal kidneys into normal animals, there is no compensatory loss of renal mass. Whether renal function can be modulated downward in the animals with additional kidneys is unsettled. Two forms of renal growth have been postulated: obligatory growth, presumably under the stimulus of growth hormone, and compensatory growth, under an unknown humoral stimulus. If immature kidneys are transplanted into normal animals, obligatory renal growth of the immature kidneys continues despite the presence of renal mass greater than normal. If a kidney that has undergone compensatory hypertrophy is transplanted into an animal with a single hypertrophied kidney, however, both kidneys undergo atrophy until they reach normal size. Studies in patients and animals have shown recovery of function after release of obstruction in a hydronephrotic kidney despite the presence of the opposite hypertrophied kidney.

RETURN OF FUNCTION AFTER RELEASE OF COMPLETE URETERAL OBSTRUCTION IN HUMANS

How long can the human kidney be completely obstructed before it sustains enough damage to prevent any recovery of function after release? This is an important clinical question that must be answered with careful documentation. Although there are many accounts in the literature that report return of function after varying periods of obstruction, most are not valid, for many reasons. A valid case report should include proven complete ureteral obstruction with no proximal fistulous leak, accurate documentation of time of obstruction, and proven return of function, preferably determined with split-clearance tests. Many case reports in the literature are not sufficient, in that return of function is assumed because contrast media are seen in the kidney after intravenous injection. These same patients usually have had a straight ureteroneocystostomy that refluxes; thus, the contrast agents could have reached the kidney via reflux from the bladder. The same criticism holds true in patients with refluxing ureters who were treated by means of an ileal conduit. If at surgery the repaired ureter is intubated, the split-function studies can be performed before the catheter is pulled, proving return of function in that kidney. Also, in many of the earlier reports that described no return of function after varying lengths of time, small doses of contrast agents were used, and some of these kidneys might have functioned with the high doses of the newer contrast agents now in use. In addition, in many cases, the onset of complete obstruction is documented only by "nonfunction" demonstrated on the intravenous pyelogram.

The cases (Lewis and Pierce, 1962; Graham, 1962; Reisman et al., 1957) demonstrating return of renal function 69 and 56 days after total ureteral obstruction probably represent the longest a ureter can be obstructed with recovery of function after release of the obstruction. Return of function may well depend upon many factors other than period of obstruction, such as absence of infection, presence of an intrarenal or extrarenal pelvis in the obstructed kidney, or the degree of pyelolymphatic and pyelovenous backflow. Presumably, incomplete ureteral obstruction will destroy renal function slowly, but incomplete obstruction certainly can destroy all renal function. This loss of renal function due to partial obstruction is seen clinically with silent prostatism or ureteropelvic junction obstruction.

The urologist needs to know preoperatively whether a hydronephrotic kidney will regain function after relief of the obstruction in order to decide whether to correct the obstruction or to do a nephrectomy. Determination of recovery potential has historically been based on gross inspection or histologic evaluation at surgery or function on the preoperative intravenous urogram. Recently, renal scans with ^{99}technetium DTPA (diethylenetriaminepentaacetic acid), ^{131}I-hippuran (orthoidohippurate), and ^{99}technetium DMSA (dimercaptosuccinic acid) have been used to assess recoverability in hydronephrosis. Temporary relief of the obstruction with nephrostomy tubes followed by tests measuring renal function has been successful in determining recoverability of function in hydronephrosis.

Prediction of recoverability of function in hydronephrosis using preoperative intravenous urograms or gross and microscopic examination of the kidney has not been successful. The results of the various renal scans are conflicting on superficial examination (Table 9–1). The different agents measure different functions. ^{131}I-hippuran measures renal blood flow and correlates with the glomerular filtration rate. ^{99}Tc-DMSA accumulates in the cytoplasm of proximal tubular cells. Fifteen to 20 per cent is eliminated in urine in 24 hours and it is used to assess functioning renal cortical tissue. ^{99m}Tc-DTPA is eliminated by glomerular filtration and is used to assess the glomerular filtration rate and cortical renal blood flow. The discrepancies can be explained by the method of evaluating the scans. Scans evaluated by arbitrary mathematical analysis (Lome et al., 1979; McDougal and Flanigan, 1981; Kalika et al., 1981; Gillenwater et al., 1979; Schelfhout et al., 1983) could accurately predict the recovery potential. I have had good results using a temporary nephrostomy tube for relief of the obstruction and assessing function with creatinine clearances. In my opin-

TABLE 9–1. RESULTS OF RENAL SCAN IN PREOPERATIVELY PREDICTING RETURN OF FUNCTION FROM RELIEF OF HYDRONEPHROSIS

Agent	Accurate Prediction	Method	Author
^{99m}Tc-DTPA	Yes	Visual inspection	Lome
^{99m}Tc-DTPA	No	Visual inspection	Chibber
^{99m}Tc-DTPA	Yes	Visual inspection	Belis
^{99m}Tc-DMSA	No	Visual inspection	Chibber
^{99m}Tc-DMSA	No	Visual inspection	Chisholm
^{99m}Tc-DMSA	Yes	Quantitative	Schelfhout
^{99m}Tc-DMSA	Yes	Quantitative	McDougal
^{131}I-hippuran	Yes	Quantitative	Gillenwater
^{131}I-hippuran	Yes	Quantitative	Kalika
^{131}I-hippuran	No	Visual	Belis

ion, a temporary nephrostomy provides the most accurate method of predicting the recovery potential of a hydronephrotic kidney.

Summary

The human kidney can recover function after release of periods of obstruction longer than have been observed in experimental animals. Recovery of some function has been documented after 69 days of complete ureteral obstruction in one patient.

PATTERN OF NEPHRON RECOVERY AFTER RELEASE OF BILATERAL CHRONIC HYDRONEPHROSIS

Adequate studies of the various aspects of renal function after release of chronic hydronephrosis in patients have been done to provide insight into the integrity of renal function during obstructive uropathy. These investigations have been conducted in pediatric patients with congenital anomalies (McCrory et al., 1971; Winberg, 1959, 1958) and in adults (Berlyne, 1961; Edvall, 1959; Olbrich et al., 1957; Zetterström et al., 1958). There are also reports of some studies following the correction of partial unilateral ureteral obstruction (Better et al., 1973; Gillenwater et al., 1975; Platts and Williams, 1963). The results of these studies are not entirely comparable, but it is generally believed that the postobstructed kidney exhibits a reduction in glomerular filtration, renal blood flow, concentrating ability, hydrogen ion clearance, and phosphate excretion. Sodium reabsorption is mildly impaired, while urinary dilution is not affected.

ACUTE URETERAL OBSTRUCTION

There are few reports in the literature describing renal function after acute ureteral obstruction in patients. Bradley and Anderson (1956) studied hemodynamic changes during acute ureteral occlusion in normal subjects. They inserted large ureteral catheters up to the renal pelvis bilaterally in awake subjects; after three control periods of collection, they studied the renal blood flow by determination of clearance of para-amino-hippuric acid (PAH) after elevation of ureteral pressures from 17 to 35 mm Hg, with a mean pressure of 20 mm Hg. At this level, they found a decrease in the clearance of PAH, a decrease in the clearance

of mannitol, and an increase in the filtration fraction in the three studies. The observed decrease in PAH clearance could be due to either decreased renal blood flow or impaired proximal tubular function. Therefore, it is not possible to say whether the transient increase in renal blood flow seen with acute ureteral obstruction in the experimental animal occurs in man. These investigations would have to be performed at the operating table, with blood flow probes on the renal artery. Michaelson (1974) did percutaneous puncture of the renal pelvis to measure pressures in two patients during episodes of renal colic from ureteral stones. He found the baseline pressures to be elevated to 50 to 70 mm Hg in connection with contraction of the renal pelvis. Normal pressures were 6 mm Hg. At the time of the elevated pressure, the patient complained of severe flank pain.

CHRONIC BILATERAL URETER OBSTRUCTION

Impairment of Urinary Concentration

Impairment of urinary concentrating ability is the most consistent and probably the first derangement of physiologic function that occurs with obstructive uropathy. This has been seen in all the infants (Dorhout-Mees, 1960; Earley, 1956; Holliday et al., 1967; McCrory et al., 1971; Winberg, 1959, 1958; Zetterström et al., 1958) and adults (Berlyne, 1961; Better et al., 1973; Gillenwater et al., 1975; Muldowney et al., 1966; Olbrich et al., 1957; Platts and Williams, 1963; Vaughan et al., 1973) described in the literature. Winberg (1959) reported on a 13-year-old boy with posterior urethral valves who had a glomerular filtration rate in the normal range (mean C_{CR} of 87 ml/min/1.73 sq meters). Preoperatively, after administration of antidiuretic hormone (ADH), the urine osmolality could not achieve a level greater than 200 mOsm/kg. Five days postoperatively, the kidney was able to concentrate the urine to 500 mOsm/kg. Nine months postoperatively, a urinary osmolality concentration of 576 mOsm/kg was observed. Thus, it appears that impairment of urinary concentrating ability is one of the first signs of renal damage in hydronephrosis in humans, and this function recovers to varying extents after release of the obstruction.

Impairment of Acidification

Impairment of all phases of urinary acidification (ammonia excretion, titratable acidity, and bicarbonate absorption) due to hydronephrosis has been reported in children (Earley, 1956; McCrory et al., 1971; Winberg, 1959,

1958; Zetterström et al., 1958) and adults (Berlyne, 1961; Better et al., 1973; Gillenwater et al., 1975). This abnormality has not been as consistent a finding as the concentrating defect. The group at the Karolinska Institute in Stockholm presented four papers on acidification studies in children with hydronephrosis (Ericsson et al., 1955; Winberg, 1959, 1958; Zetterström et al., 1958). In 1955, they reported higher urine pH than expected despite low serum carbon dioxide combining power in 4 out of 4 patients. One patient had an impairment of ammonia excretion. Winberg (1958) examined five patients with hydronephrosis due to reflux. In one patient (number three), urine pH could be lowered only to 5.4, and there was impairment of ammonia excretion. Winberg (1959) reported a case of bilateral hydronephrosis in which the lowest achievable urinary pH was 5.84, with an improvement to 5.19 at 4 months and 4.9 at 9 months after surgical correction of the posterior urethral valves. Ammonia excretion was normal. McCrory and coworkers (1971) studied 15 children with chronic hydronephrosis; urine pH could be lowered to less than 6.2 in all, but in none could it be lowered to less than 5.3. These studies are difficult to evaluate because the authors state that there was an inadequate stress of acid load.

Berlyne (1961) examined seven adults with chronic bilateral hydronephrosis. Impairment of ability to acidify the urine was found in six. Two of these were able to recover some acidification; case number four had improvement of urine pH—from 5.46 to 5.30—2 months after prostatectomy, and case number seven had improvement of urine pH—from 6.10 to 5.01—1 month after prostatectomy. The ammonia excretion was abnormally decreased in five of six patients tested. The one patient whose ammonia excretion was abnormal was restudied 1 month after prostatectomy (case number four) had some return toward normal, but it was not complete (15 to 19.6 mEq/min). Titratable acidity was measured directly in two cases; it was found to be abnormal in case number five and normal in case number six (the patient in whom the urine could be acidified normally). Calculated total hydrogen excretion (NH^+ + titratable acid − HCO_3^-) was abnormally low in five of six cases.

Proximal Tubular Function

Olbrich and associates (1957) studied 32 uninfected patients with prostatism and chronic hydronephrosis. The mean maximal tubular excretion of diodone was normal. In the group that was also infected (28 patients), there was a significant decrease (44 per cent of normal) in the maximal tubular excretion of diodone. McCrory and coworkers (1971) studied Tm_{PAH} in two children with chronic hydronephrosis and impaired renal function. The Tm_{PAH} was decreased in both. In one patient, the value of Tm_{PAH} was reduced more than GFR ($\frac{C_{In}}{Tm_{PAH}} = 2.42$), indicating a greater reduction in tubular mass than in glomerular filtration. In the other patient, whose GFR was only 27 per cent of normal, the ratio of GFR to Tm_{PAH} was normal. Functioning proximal tubular mass in these two patients (with markedly reduced GFR and no ability to concentrate the urine) was still relatively preserved in proportion to the GFR.

Glomerular Filtration Rate

The glomerulus is the last portion of the kidney to show damage due to obstructive uropathy on histologic examination. Chronic hydronephrosis will significantly impair GFR if severe enough, as every clinician knows who has obtained elevated serum creatinines from these patients. This impairment has also been documented in the literature (McCrory et al., 1971; Olbrich et al., 1957; Winberg, 1958).

Renal Blood Flow

All patients studied with chronic hydronephrosis have demonstrated a decrease in renal blood flow (McCrory et al., 1971; Olbrich et al., 1957). In the patients with prostatism, the renal blood flow was decreased to about 75 per cent of normal. Renal bloodflows in three children with chronic hydronephrosis (McCrory et al., 1971) were calculated to be 380, 65.7, and 150.5 ml/min, with expected normal blood flows being 654 ml/min. The filtration fractions were increased in all the patients to greater than 0.23, with normal being 0.20. Thus, the renal blood flow decreased more than the GFR.

Summary

Abnormalities in all phases of urinary acidification (ammonia excretion, titratable acidity, and bicarbonate absorption) have been demonstrated in at least one patient with chronic bilateral hydronephrosis.

Studies in humans have demonstrated that partial obstruction impairs all measured renal functions except urinary dilution. Recovery of some function is documented after release of the obstruction.

RENAL FUNCTION AFTER RELEASE OF CHRONIC UNILATERAL HYDRONEPHROSIS IN HUMANS

Most experimental animal work on hydronephrosis has been performed with unilateral ureteral obstruction, using the contralateral kidney as a control. With unilateral obstruction, there is a normal fluid and electrolyte balance, and none of the metabolic, hormonal, or hemodynamic changes of uremia occur. Thus, in man, as in the experimental animal, split-function studies of unilateral hydronephrosis offer the best model for investigating the effects of obstruction per se on nephron function. There have been five reports in the literature describing acceptable renal function studies in patients after release of unilateral hydronephrosis (Better et al., 1973; Edvall, 1959; Gillenwater et al., 1975; Platts and Williams, 1963; Zetterström et al., 1958).

All the reported patients with unilateral hydronephrosis had impairment of glomerular filtration rate, and filtration fraction was decreased in 5 of the 6 patients studied (Better et al., 1973; Edvall, 1959; Platts and Williams, 1963), indicating more impairment of GFR than of renal blood flow. Urinary acidification was reported in three papers (Better et al., 1973; Gillenwater et al., 1975; Zetterström et al., 1958). All authors found defects in the ability of the affected kidney to lower the pH to the same degree as the normal kidney. Zetterström's patient (1958) had a relative inability to conserve bicarbonate. Better's patient (1973) had impaired excretion of titratable acidity and probably normal excretion of ammonia (if corrected for renal mass). Gillenwater and associates (1975) reported that two of the seven patients tested had impairment of urinary acidification, with defects in both absolute ammonia excretion and titratable acid excretion. One patient probably also had impairment of bicarbonate aborption. In Better's patient and in Gillenwater's case number six, fractional excretion (titratable acid and ammonia/GFR) of titratable acid and ammonia was lower in the hydronephrotic kidney, indicating greater tubular damage than glomerular damage.

Sodium reabsorption was impaired in Better's patient (1973), in all three of Platts' patients (1963), and in eight of Gillenwater's ten patients (1975). The patients had a greater fraction of filtered sodium excreted from the hydronephrotic kidney than from the normal side. This sodium-losing defect does not seem to be caused by lack of responsiveness to mineralocorticoid, since both kidneys responded with decreased sodium excretion when mineralocorticoid was administered.

All reported cases have shown an impairment in the urine concentrating ability of the hydronephrotic kidney. Gillenwater's data (1975) demonstrate that the concentrating defect is not caused by an osmotic diuresis in the hydronephrotic kidney, suggesting specific tubular damage. The concentrating defect is proportionately greater than the impairment of GFR.

Proximal tubular transport has been evaluated by measuring the secretion of PAH and the reabsorption of phosphate. Maximal tubular transport of PAH was decreased in all of the ten patients studied (Gillenwater et al., 1975). The impairment in Tm_{PAH} was not greater than the impairment in GFR. Better and coworkers (1973) reported a low excretion of phosphate because of increased tubular reabsorption in the hydronephrotic kidney. Platts and Williams (1963) had two patients with decreased phosphate excretion from the hydronephrotic kidney and one with increased phosphate excretion. Four out of nine of Gillenwater's patients (1975) had decreased phosphate excretion, but there was no significant difference in phosphate excretion between the normal and hydronephrotic patients when the group was examined as a whole. Thus, there does not seem to be a consistent pattern of abnormality in phosphate excretion in hydronephrosis.

Urinary dilution was normal in all reported cases (Better et al., 1973; Gillenwater et al., 1975).

SUMMARY

Impairment of all aspects of renal function except urinary dilution has been demonstrated in the hydronephrotic kidney of patients studied after release of unilateral ureteral obstruction.

INTRAPELVIC PRESSURES IN HUMANS

Normal

The pressure in the renal pelvis slightly exceeds the intraperitoneal and bladder pressures. Normal renal pelvic pressure measured through a ureteral catheter is 11 mm Hg (Kiil, 1970; Michaelson, 1974; Radwin et al., 1963;

Rattner et al., 1957), and it is 6.5 mm Hg with percutaneous puncture (Michaelson, 1974). The intrapelvic pressures in four normal renal pelves explored at surgery were 6 to 12 mm Hg (Underwood, 1937).

Ureteral Obstruction

Risholm (1954) experimentally obstructed the ureter in humans with a double-lumen balloon catheter and simultaneously measured pressures above the obstruction. The pressure rose to 15 to 49 mm Hg within 10 minutes. The highest pressures (31 to 77 mm Hg) were recorded within 20 to 60 minutes. Kiil (1957) found the pressures above two ureteral stones to be 40 and 50 mm Hg, respectively. The intrapelvic pressure in patients with hydronephrosis has been measured at the operating table and usually has been interpreted to be in the normal ranges (Bäcklund and Nordgren, 1966; Kiil, 1957; Melick et al., 1961; Underwood, 1937).

Two recent investigations of large numbers of patients with chronic hydronephrosis have shown elevated intrapelvic pressures in some of the cases, however (Johnston, 1969; Michaelson, 1974). Johnston (1969) measured intrapelvic pressures in children with hydronephrosis at the time of operation. In 7 of the 36 renal pelves, the pressure was 18 to 58 mm Hg; seven had a pressure of 7 to 11 mm Hg; in 9, the intrapelvic pressure was less than 7 mm Hg.

Michaelson (1974) measured intrapelvic pressures by means of percutaneous needle puncture in 84 patients who were 16 to 86 years old. Reproducible results were obtained on repeat punctures in the same patients. Mean pressure in 10 normal renal pelves during antidiuresis was 6.5 mm Hg ± 2.05. Little variation in pressure was noted with change of position, except that the pressure was 2 to 5 mm Hg higher with patient standing than with the patient supine. In two patients with ureteral calculi, baseline pressures were elevated to 20 to 25 mm Hg. These pressures increased to 50 to 70 mm Hg with contraction of the pelvis as the patients simultaneously complained of severe flank pain.

Mean pressure during antidiuresis in 41 grossly enlarged pelves with certain obstruction of urine flow was 21.2 mm Hg ± 8.7. In 12 kidneys showing nonfunction on intravenous pyelography due to obstruction, the mean pressure was 24.3 mm Hg ± 16.3. In four patients with ureteral stones, the mean intrapelvic pressure was 19.3 mm Hg (range of 10 to 24 mm Hg). These pressure elevations to above normal were statistically significant. Intrapelvic pressures decreased with increasing time of obstruction (Fig. 9–2). An average of 8 weeks later, six patients with partial obstruction had repeat percutaneous puncture done. The pressures decreased an average of 6.6 mm Hg but were still higher than the pressure in an unobstructed renal pelvis.

Summary

Renal pressure measured with percutaneous puncture in normal antidiuretic patients was 6.5 mm Hg. With ureteral obstruction due

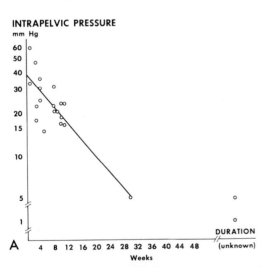

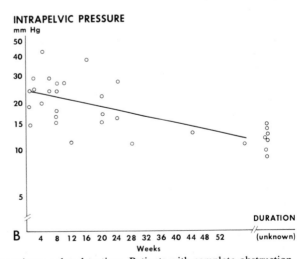

Figure 9–2. Intrapelvic pressures in enlarged renal pelves in patients, related to time. Patients with complete obstruction of flow are seen in A and those with partial obstruction of flow in B. (Data reproduced with permission from Michaelson, G.: Acta Med. Scand., [Suppl. 559]:1, 1974.)

to calculi, the baseline pressures were elevated to 20 to 25 mm Hg. During pain, the pressures had increased to 50 to 70 mm Hg. Some patients with chronic hydronephrosis also have elevated renal pelvic pressures that tend to decrease with time.

EFFECTS OF COMPLETE AND PARTIAL ACUTE OBSTRUCTION ON RENAL FUNCTION IN EXPERIMENTAL ANIMALS

Effects of ureteral obstruction on renal function are determined by the severity (complete or partial), the duration, the totality (unilateral or bilateral), and the presence or absence of infection. The discussion will be divided into acute unilateral ureteral obstruction, chronic unilateral ureteral obstruction, chronic partial ureteral obstruction, and comparison of unilateral versus bilateral ureteral obstruction. Animal experiments can be better controlled and provide information to better understand obstructive uropathy in patients.

RENAL FUNCTION DURING UNILATERAL OBSTRUCTION

Ureteral Pressure

Hydrostatic pressure of fluid proximal to the obstruction increases. The degree of elevation of pressure depends upon the rate of urine flow prior to the obstruction and the degree of ureteral muscular contraction. The maximal pressure expected without consideration of ureteral muscular contraction would be the pressure at which filtration is reduced to near zero (called "stop-flow pressure"). The stop-flow pressure is equal to the difference between glomerular capillary pressure and capillary oncotic pressure (60 mm Hg minus 25 to 30 mm Hg = 35 to 30 mm Hg). This filtration pressure is normally offset by the 15 mm Hg hydrostatic pressure in Bowman's capsule, producing a net filtration pressure of 20 to 15 mm Hg. With an increase in proximal tubular pressure due to obstruction, tubular and capsular hydrostatic pressures increase, causing a lowering of net effective filtration pressure.

Ureteral pressure increases to 50 to 70 mm Hg within a few minutes of ureteral obstruction (Obniski, 1907; Bäcklund and Nordgren, 1966; Hinman and Morison, 1924; Murphy and Scott, 1966; Taylor and Ullmann, 1961; McDonald et al., 1937). Ureteral pressure after obstruction can be further increased to 100 mm Hg by saline

or mannitol diuresis (Papadopoulou et al., 1969; Vaughan et al., 1971) (Fig. 9–3). Obstruction of 10 minutes' duration in the nondiuretic rat raises ureteral pressure only to 14 mm Hg, with no change in proximal tubular pressure (the normal is 14 mm Hg). (Gottschalk, 1950; Gottschalk and Mylle, 1956, 1957; Gottschalk, 1964). In diuretic rats, 10 to 15 minutes' obstruction is sufficient to raise both ureteral and proximal tubular pressure to maximal values of 40 mm Hg. Elevations of proximal tubular pressure were not seen when the ureteral pressure was raised to 80 mm Hg by injection of fluid. The failure of transmission of these higher ureteral pressure elevations back to the tubules is believed to be due to compression of the papillary foramina (Dominguez and Adams, 1958; Gottschalk and Mylle, 1956; Morison, 1929).

Glomerular Filtration Rate

Glomerular filtration rate decreases as tubular intraluminal pressure rises (Abbrecht and Malvin, 1960; DiBona, 1971; Papdopoulou et al., 1969; Steinhausen, 1967; Suki et al., 1966). Glomerular filtration rate decreases earlier if there is an osmotic diuresis. Without the osmotic diuresis, more reabsorption occurs, allowing glomerular filtration replacement. Glomerular filtration rates in rats with complete obstruction were 52 per cent at 4 hours, 23 per cent at 12 hours, 4 per cent at 24 hours, and 2 per cent at 48 hours (Harris and Gill, 1981; Provoost and Molenaar, 1981) (Fig. 9–4). The SNGFR is depressed in deep nephrons but not to the extent seen in cortical nephrons (Buerkert et al., 1978).

Renal Blood Flow

There is a triphasic relationship between ipsilateral renal blood flow and ureteral pressure (Fig. 9–5). The initial response is an increase in renal blood flow and ureteral pressure, suggesting preglomerular vasodilation (Finkle et al., 1968; Gilmore, 1964; Murphy and Scott, 1966; Nash and Selkurt, 1964; Navar and Baer, 1970; Persky et al., 1957a; Thurau, 1964a and b; Vaughan et al., 1971; Waugh, 1964; Wax, 1968; Winton, 1931). The initial vasodilatation is transient and lasts up to 1½ hours. Pretreatment of dogs with indomethacin, which prevents prostaglandin synthesis, inhibits the vasodilatation (Fig. 9–6).

The second phase of response occurred at 1½ to 5 hours, when the renal blood flow decreased and the ureteral pressure continued to rise. The proposed mechanism was a postglomerular rise in renal resistance that accounted for the increased ureteral pressure, presumably from filtration. During the third or

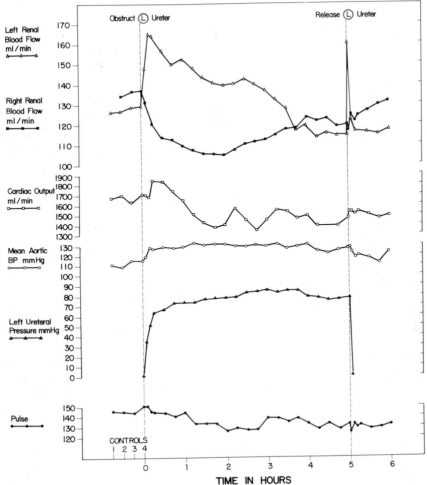

HEMODYNAMIC CHANGES DURING ACUTE TOTAL Ⓛ URETERAL OCCLUSION

Figure 9–3. Mean hemodynamic changes in eight animals with unilateral midureteral occlusion.

chronic phase (5 to 18 hours), both the renal blood flow and the ureteral pressure decreased. The proposed mechanism in the chronic phase was a preglomerular vasoconstriction. This is the same response as is seen when the tubule of a single nephron is obstructed, and preglomerular vasoconstriction was observed in only the blocked nephron (Arendshorst et al., 1974).

Tubular Function

If acute ureteral obstruction is only *partial,* urine volume decreases, osmolality increases, and urinary sodium concentration is reduced ([Hermann, 1859; Winton, 1931;] Abbrecht and Malvin, 1960; Suki et al., 1966). The more complete sodium reabsorption also raises the corticomedullary osmotic gradient, enhancing water absorption from the collecting ducts (Abbrecht and Malvin, 1960). There are minimal changes in Tm_{PAH} and Tm glucose (Abbrecht

and Malvin, 1960; Selkurt et al., 1952). If ureteral pressure is raised to 70 mm Hg, there is a 50 per cent reduction in Tm glucose and Tm_{PAH} (Malvin et al., 1964), with partial ureteral obstruction.

After acute *complete* ureteral obstruction, there is an additional decrease in glomerular filtration and in sodium concentration in the distal tubule (DiBiona, 1971).

A different pattern of tubular function is seen with *release* of acute complete ureteral obstruction. A concentrating defect after release of ureteral obstruction lasting 5 to 60 minutes at 75 to 120 mm Hg pressure has been reported (Finkle et al., 1968; Jaenike and Bray, 1960; Kessler, 1960). Renal tissue slice analysis after acute obstruction showed a decrease in the normal osmolality and in the sodium and urea gradient (Jaenike and Bray, 1960; Kessler, 1960), probably accounting for the loss of con-

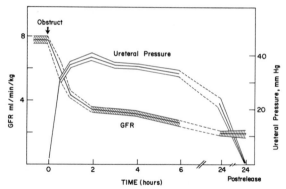

Figure 9–4. GRF and ureteral pressure in rats during ureteral obstruction, and after release of ureteral obstruction of 24 hours' duration. Mean values are connected by heavy lines, and standard errors are indicated by the shaded areas. The preobstruction values represent data from 14 rats without obstruction. (From Harris, R. H., et al.: Kidney Int., *19*:603, 1981. Reprinted with permission.)

centrating ability. Permeability to water and the absorptive capacity of the collecting duct are not altered by acute obstruction (18 hours in the rat studied after release) (Buerkert et al., 1979).

Tubular Permeability

The proximal and distal tubules have been shown to become permeable to creatinine, mannitol, and sucrose when tubular luminal pressure is doubled (Lorentz et al., 1972). This change is reversible when the increased pressure is returned to normal. The leak is believed to be through aqueous channels between tubule cells.

Summary

Ureteral pressures after acute obstruction are variable, depending upon urine flow rates. The ureteral pressure may rise to equal the filtration pressure. The first 1½ hours after complete ureteral occlusion, renal blood flow increases owing to preglomerular arterial vasodilation. After 1½ to 5 hours, there is preglomerular vasoconstriciton, causing decreased renal blood flow, but a continued rise in ureteral pressure. After 5 hours, there is preglomerular vasoconstriction, causing a reduction in both renal blood flow and ureteral pressure. The mechanism of these renal blood flow changes after ureteral occlusion is postulated to be vasodilating prostaglandins causing the initial transient vasodilation, and constrictor prostaglandins (thromboxane) causing the chronic vasoconstriction. With acute complete ureteral obstruction, glomerular filtration rate decreases,

and tubular functions are impaired. In the first few hours of partial ureteral obstruction, tubular transit time is decreased, allowing better reabsorption with a resultant decrease in urine volume, an increase in osmolality, and lowered urine sodium concentration.

EFFECTS OF CHRONIC COMPLETE UNILATERAL OBSTRUCTION OF RENAL FUNCTION IN EXPERIMENTAL ANIMALS

Ureteral and Tubular Pressures with Continuation of Obstruction

Ureteral pressures decrease within 24 hours to about 50 per cent of the peak levels (Vaughan et al., 1970) (Fig. 9–7), and ureteral pressures continue to decline gradually over the next 8 weeks despite continuation of the obstruction (Vaughan et al., 1970). After 6 to 8 weeks of obstruction, the ureteral pressure is approximately 15 mm Hg.

Measurement of proximal tubular pressures after 24 hours of ureteral obstruction shows a return to normal levels (Arendshorst et al.,

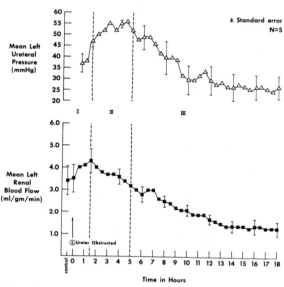

Figure 9–5. The triphasic relationship between ipsilateral renal blood flow and left ureteral pressure during 18 hours of left ureteral occlusion. The three phases are designated by roman numerals and are divided by vertical dashed lines. In Phase I, the left renal blood flow and ureteral pressure increase together. In Phase II, the left renal blood flow begins to decline, while the ureteral pressure remains elevated and, in fact, continues to rise. Phase III shows the left renal blood flow and ureteral pressure declining together.

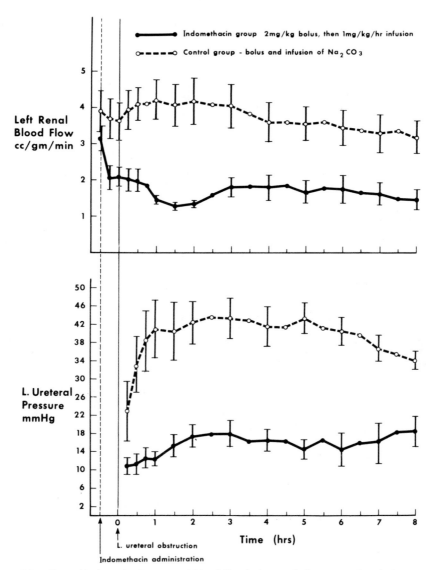

Figure 9–6. *Above*, The effect of indomethacin on renal blood flow before and after ureteral occlusion, compared with the control group renal blood flows. Indomethacin causes a prompt decrease in renal blood flow and abolishes the hyperemic response to ureteral occlusion seen in the control group. *Below*, Indomethacin markedly decreases ureteral pressure in obstructed dogs.

1974) or to levels 30 per cent below normal (Jaenike, 1970; Yarger et al., 1972). Numerous collapsed tubules are seen on the kidney surface (Jaeknike, 1970), and glomerular capillary pressure is reduced. These studies suggest that constriction of the afferent arteriole occurs.

Renal Blood Flow

A progressive chronic decrease in renal blood flow occurs, becoming 70 per cent of control at 24 hours, 50 per cent at 72 hours, 30 per cent by 6 days, 20 per cent by 2 weeks, 18 per cent at 4 and 6 weeks, and 12 per cent at 8 weeks (Moody et al., 1975; Vaughan et al., 1970) (Fig. 9–8). These studies would be com-

patible with the proposed theory of afferent arteriole constriction. Studies of intrarenal redistribution of blood flow with complete ureteral obstruction have shown, in general, that blood flow to all compartments progressively decreases over 21 days (Table 9–2) (Huland et al., 1980b). There is less decrease in the inner cortex and inner and outer medulla than in the outer cortex, causing a relative increase in total flow to the inner compartments.

Glomerular Filtration Rate

Glomerular filtration rate decreases progressively during complete ureteral obstruction. In the dog, the calculated glomerular filtration

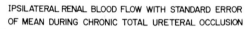

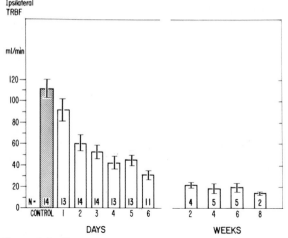

Figure 9–7. Change in ureteral pressure with chronic total ureteral occlusion.

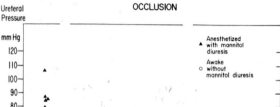

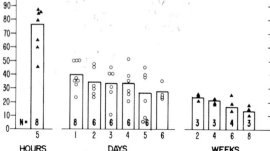

Figure 9–8. Changes in renal blood flow with chronic total ureteral occlusion in 14 dogs with chronic indwelling blood flow probes.

rate at 1 week of total occlusion was 1.74 ml/min and at 5 weeks of occlusion was 0.4 ml/min (Naber and Madsen, 1974). Filtration continues to replace fluid removed from the kidney by pyelovenous, pyelolymphatic, and pyelotubular backflows.

Glomerular filtration rates measured immediately after release of obstruction of 1 week's duration showed a mean reduction to 16 to 25 per cent of control (Kerr, 1956, 1954; Vaughan et al., 1971; Widén, 1957). Measurement of glomerular filtration immediately after release of complete ureteral obstruction of 2 weeks' duration is difficult owing to lack of urine flow immediately after release. The glomerular filtration rate is 15 per cent of control 1 week after release of complete occlusion lasting 2 weeks (Vaughan et al., 1973). Eventually, maximal recovery of GFR after the 2 weeks of obstruction reached 46 per cent of control, with the contralateral normal kidney being undisturbed.

In a single dog with 3 weeks of complete ureteral obstruction, the GFR was 6 per cent of control shortly after release. Recovery at 6 weeks was as much as 15 per cent of control (Vaughan and Gillenwater, unpublished data).

Two dogs were studied after release of total ureteral obstruction of 4 weeks' duration. Shortly after release, the GFR was 3 per cent of control. Five months later, the GFR was 35 per cent of control (Vaughan et al., 1971).

No return of function was noted after 6 weeks of total obstruction in the dog with a normal contralateral kidney.

Tubular Function

With longer periods of ureteral obstruction, there is progressive loss of tubular function. The earliest, most severe damage to tubular function occurs in the concentration of urine. Immediately after release of ureteral obstruction lasting 1 or more weeks, the kidney is unable to concentrate the urine osmolality to a level greater than that of the plasma. One week after recovery, the previously obstructed kidney concentrates the urine, but not as well as the control

TABLE 9–2. RENAL COMPARTMENT BLOOD FLOW AFTER UNILATERAL URETERAL OBSTRUCTION

	TOTAL FLOW ml/100 gm^{-1}/min	Outer Cortex			Inner Cortex Outer Medulla			Inner Medulla		
		FLOW ml/100 gm^{-1}/min	CHANGE (%)	TOTAL (%)	FLOW ml/100 gm^{-1}/min	CHANGE (%)	TOTAL (%)	FLOW ml/100 gm^{-1}/min	CHANGE (%)	TOTAL (%)
Control	565	501		89	62		11	2.3		0.3
7 Days	299	258	↓ 49	86	39	↓ 37	13	2.2	↓ 4	1
21 Days	155	128	↓ 76	83	25	↓ 60	16	1.6	↓ 31	1

Data from Huland, H., et al.: Invest. Urol., *18*:274. 1980.

(443 vs. 711 mOsm/kg). Eventually, there is complete recovery. Two weeks after release of obstruction, there is almost complete recovery (589 mOsm/kg in the obstructed kidney vs. 610 mOsm/kg in the control). With 4 weeks of obstruction, there is permanent impairment of concentrating ability.

The Tm_{PAH} 1 week after release of total obstruction of 2 weeks' duration is 13 per cent of control. There is a return of 48 per cent of control values at 4 months. Other impaired tubular functions are Tm glucose, potassium excretion, sodium reabsorption, and urinary acidification (Berlyne and Macken, 1962; Chisholm, 1964; Kerr, 1956, 1954; Vaughan et al., 1971).

Microperfusion techniques in rabbits have shown identical tubular defects in bilateral and unilateral ureteral obstruction (Hanley and Davidson, 1982). The natriuresis is due to disordered sodium reabsorption in the juxtamedullary proximal convoluted tubule, cortical proximal straight tubule, and cortical thick ascending limb of Henle's loop. Impaired concentrating ability is due to depressed function of the thick ascending limb of Henle's loop and ADH resistance of cortical collecting tubules.

Summary

Chronic complete unilateral obstruction causes impairment of all renal functions except urinary dilution. The ureteral pressures gradually decline to 15 mm Hg at 6 weeks of obstruction. Renal blood flow is reduced to 20 per cent of control by 2 weeks. The mechanism of the chronic renal vasoconstriction and the cause of tubular atrophy are unknown.

EFFECTS OF CHRONIC PARTIAL URETERAL OBSTRUCTION ON RENAL FUNCTION IN EXPERIMENTAL ANIMALS

Most studies of changes in renal function with hydronephrosis have been performed after release of the obstruction. There have been sufficient investigations of partial ureteral obstruction to allow some conclusions to be drawn (Olesen and Madsen, 1968; Stecker and Gillenwater, 1971; Suki et al., 1966; Wilson, 1972). Evaluation of renal function during partial obstruction is important. Once the obstruction is relieved, a different set of circumstances exists. These studies have shown that there is signifi-

cant impairment of renal function during mild degrees of obstruction (Stecker and Gillenwater, 1971).

Stecker and Gillenwater (1971) partially obstructed the left ureter, causing mild hydronephrosis (Fig. 9–9). Investigative work on these animals demonstrated a decrease in renal blood flow and glomerular filtration rate to 25 per cent of control (Figs. 9–10 and 9–11). Ichikawa and Brenner (1979) studied rats with 4 weeks of partial unilateral ureteral obstruction and found the SNGFR, total GFR, and initial glomerular plasma flow rate the same in both kidneys. Glomerular capillary pressure was significantly higher in the partially obstructed kidney than in the nonobstructed kidney, which served to offset the markedly reduced glomerular capillary ultrafiltration coefficient that was confined to the obstructed kidney. Humes and coworkers (1980) found in rats with hereditary hydronephrosis that filtration rates were maintained near normal because of an elevation in the mean glomerular

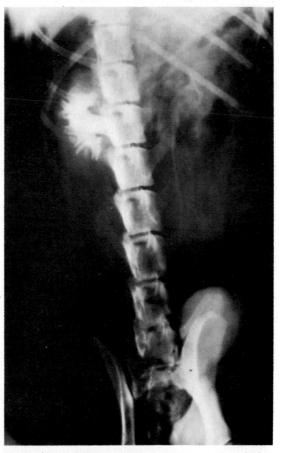

Figure 9–9. IVP in dog with partial ureteral occlusion, showing the mild obstruction. Films were obtained 3 weeks after the partial ureteral occlusion.

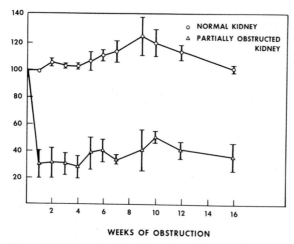

Figure 9–10. The effect of unilateral partial ureteral obstruction on glomerular filtration rate in 6 animals. Each point represents the mean ± standard deviation (SD).

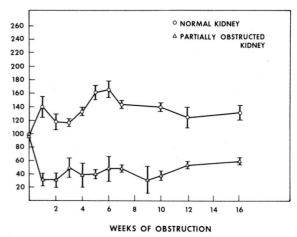

Figure 9–11. The changes occuring in the maximal para-aminohippurate transport during 4 months of unilateral partial ureteral obstruction in six animals. Each point represents the mean ± SD.

transcapillary hydraulic pressure, which effectively offsets a lower initial glomerular capillary plasma flow rate and a possible decrease in the glomerular capillary ultrafiltration coefficient relative to the hydronephrotic kidneys. There was also an impairment in hydrogen excretion and concentrating ability. Suki and colleagues (1966) found that the chronically partially obstructed kidney displayed higher urine sodium concentration as well as greater absolute and fractional sodium excretion than the control. No impairment in sodium reabsorption was noted by Olesen and Madsen (1968) or Stecker and Gillenwater (1971).

Wilson (1972) performed micropuncture studies on rats with 2 to 4 weeks of unilateral partial obstruction. The surface nephrons showed mild to moderate dilatation of the lumina of the proximal tubules. The distal tubules were more markedly dilated. The proximal intratubular pressure was slightly increased. Single nephron filtration was 76 per cent of controls. The tubular flow rate was reduced by 35 per cent, and fractional reabsorption was increased by 8 per cent. The absolute rate of fluid reabsorption in the proximal tubule was slightly, but not significantly, reduced. Fractional excretion of sodium was greater from the obstructed kidney.

Summary

Renal function studies during partial ureteral obstruction show a significant impairment of function, even with mild obstruction. The pattern of impaired function is similar to that of complete obstruction, with impairment of all aspects except urinary dilution.

DIFFERENT PHYSIOLOGIC CHANGES OF UNILATERAL AND BILATERAL URETERAL OBSTRUCTION

The most significant recent information has contrasted the physiologic changes resulting from unilateral and bilateral ureteral obstruction. The majority of these studies have utilized micropuncture techniques and have contributed to our understanding of such clinical problems as postobstructive diuresis.

Studies During Ureteral Obstruction

Proximal tubular pressure is lower than normal in unilateral ureteral obstruction but significantly increases in bilateral ureteral obstruction (Table 9–3). Distal tubule pressure is normal in unilateral ureteral obstruction but significantly increased in bilateral ureteral obstruction. Afferent arteriole pressure is significantly decreased in unilateral ureteral ob-

TABLE 9–3. DIFFERENCES IN INTRARENAL HYDROSTATIC BEFORE RELEASE OF UNILTERAL AND BILATERAL URETERAL OBSTRUCTION (24 HOURS)

	Control MM HG	Unilateral MM HG	Bilateral MM HG
Prox. tub. pressure	13.0	9.2	30.1
Distal tub. pressure	6.7	6.5	27.7
Efferent arteriole pressure	16.8	5.5	19.0

struction but increased in bilateral ureteral obstruction. The gross appearance of kidneys with unilateral ureteral obstruction differs markedly from those with bilateral ureteral obstruction. With 24 hours of unilateral ureteral obstruction there are poorly perfused and filtering nephrons with collapsed tubules (Figs. 9–12 and 9–13). Arendshorst, Finn, and Gottschalk (1974) found that blockage of a single tubule for 24 hours caused afferent arteriole constriction of *only* that nephron, causing decreased glomerular capillary pressures of *that* nephron. It was postulated that there is a feedback mechanism within each nephron. In contrast, in animals with 24 hours of bilateral ureteral obstruction most nephrons are perfused, the tubules are not collapsed, and tubular pressure is elevated (Harris and Yarger, 1974; Jaenike, 1972; McDougal

and Wright, 1972; Thirakomen et al., 1976; Walls et al., 1975; Wilson, 1974b, 1972; Yarger and Griffith, 1974).

Studies after Release of Ureteral Obstruction

The most clinically significant difference between bilateral and unilateral ureteral obstruction is the marked absolute and fractional natriuresis and diuresis after release of bilateral ureteral obstruction, whereas after unilateral ureteral obstruction only the fractional excretion of sodium and water is increased. The explanation is the greater delivery of tubular fluid out of cortical tubules because of accumulation of a natriuretic factor after bilateral ureteral obstruction.

Renal blood flow and SNGRF are 33 per

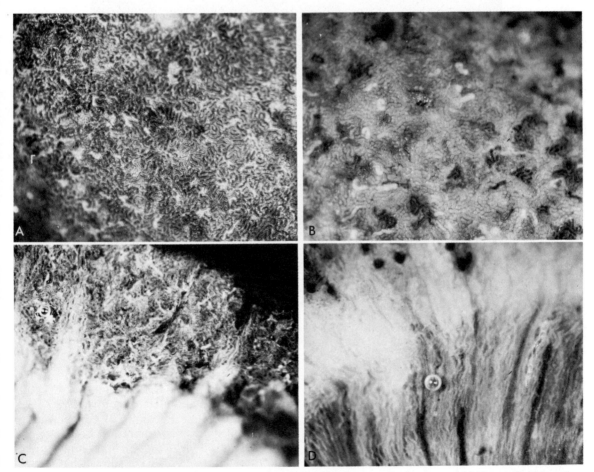

Figure 9–12. Modified Hannsen's technique. Photomicrographs comparing previously obstructed kidney with kidney from normal rat. Prussian blue (PB) is seen as black precipitate within filtering nephrons and vascular structures. *A*, Capsular surface of normal rat kidney; PB visible in nearly all superficial nephrons. *B*, Capsular surface of previously obstructed kidney, absence of PB in most tubules. *C*, Sagittal surface of normal rat kidney. Cortex is at top, medulla at bottom. PB present in nearly all nephrons and vasa recta. *D*, Sagittal surface of previously obstructed kidney; PB virtually absent in juxtamedullary nephrons, but visible in vasa recta. *C* and *D* are nonplanar fracture surfaces; hence, some areas are out of focus. (From Harris, R. H., and Yarger, W. E.: Am. J. Physiol., *227*:806, 1974.)

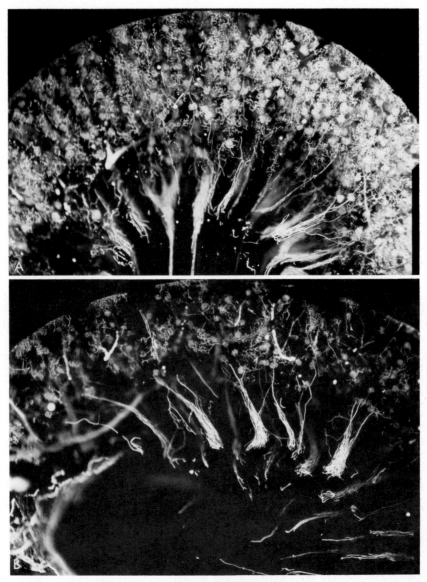

Figure 9–13. Arterial tree of untouched right kidney *(A)* and previously obstructed left kidney *(B)* injected with silicone rubber. Left kidney demonstrates multiple scattered areas of nonfilling of glomerular and peritubular capillaries in the outer cortex. Virtually no peritubular capillary filling is seen in the deep cortex and outer medulla, but filling of juxtamedullary glomerular capillaries and vasa recta is present. (From Harris, R. H., and Yarger, W. E.: Am. J. Physiol., *227:*806, 1974.)

cent of control values after release of 24 hours of bilateral and unilateral ureteral obstruction. The physiologic mechanisms are very different. The cause of the decrease in GFR is an increased tubular pressure in bilateral ureteral obstruction and an increased afferent arteriole resistance in unilateral ureteral obstruction (Tables 9–4 to 9–6). One explanation for the differences is that a vasodilating substance is retained during bilateral obstruction. The differences between bilateral and unilateral ureteral obstruction are seen despite limiting the

fluid intake of the bilateral ureteral obstruction to prevent fluid and electrolyte overload.

Distal tubular functions of concentrations and acidification are impaired in both bilateral and unilateral ureteral obstruction. Studies (Buerkert et al., 1979) have shown that permeability to water and the capacity of the collecting duct are not altered by acute obstruction. The changes that occur are due to changes in papillary blood flow, solute content of the papilla, and changes in the function of nephron segments proximal to the collecting duct. Hanley and

TABLE 9–4. Differences in Blood Flow and Filtrations after Release of Unilateral or Bilateral Ureteral Obstruction (24 Hours)

	Control	Unilateral	Bilateral
Gross appearances		Tubules collapsed	Dilated tubules
Perfusion			
Cortex		Many nonperfused areas	Mild ↓ perfusion
		Preglom. constriction	
Medulla		Glom. + vasa recta perfused	
		Agent peritub. cap. perfusion	
Distribution of blood flow		Cortical flow markedly ↓	Normal
		↑ juxtamed. flow	
RBF	10.3 ml/min/kg	33% of control	34.6% of control
Whole kid, GFR	4.23 ml/min/kg	18% of control	11.5% of control
Surface SNGFR	130 nl/min/kg	33% of control	39% of control
Juxtamedullary SNGFR	—	Markedly decreased	Decreased
Filtration in superficial nephrons	97%	40%	84%
Filtration in juxtamedullary nephrons	97%	12%	49%
Filtration fraction	0.41	0.12	0.28

Davidson (1982), using microperfusion of isolated nephrons, found that the intrinsic defects were similar in bilateral and unilateral ureteral obstruction. Natriuresis after release was due to disordered sodium reabsorption in the juxtamedullary proximal convoluted tubule, cortical proximal straight tubule, and cortical thick ascending limb of Henle's loop and ADH resistance of the cortical collecting tubule (Harris and Yarger, 1974; Walls et al., 1975; Wilson, 1974b, 1972; Yarger et al., 1972; Thirakomen et al., 1976; Jaenike, 1972; McDougal and Wright, 1972).

Summary

Significant differences have been observed in experimental animals with complete ureteral obstruction of 24 hours' duration, depending on whether the ureteral obstruction is bilateral or unilateral. The gross appearance of unilateral obstruction shows many cortical nephrons not being perfused, whereas in bilateral ureteral obstruction most nephrons are perfused. Total renal blood flow and GFR are similarly reduced

in both conditions owing to different mechanisms. In unilateral obstruction, there is vasoconstriction of the afferent arteriole, reducing blood flow and GFR. In bilateral ureteral obstruction, proximal tubular pressure and efferent arteriole resistance are increased. Natriuresis and diuresis occur after release of bilateral, but not unilateral, obstruction. This difference is noted with prevention of weight gain and fluid expansion in animals with bilateral ureteral obstruction. Blockage of a single tubule causes afferent arteriole constriction only in that single nephron, suggesting some type of feedback mechanism within each nephron.

REDISTRIBUTION OF RENAL BLOOD FLOW IN CHRONIC URETERAL OBSTRUCTION

Renal blood flow is decreased in chronic ureteral obstruction. The kidney that was obstructed chronically also showed a redistribution of cortical blood flow to the inner cortex and medulla (Bay et al., 1972; Thirakomen et al., 1976; Yarger and Griffith, 1974). Saline expan-

TABLE 9–5. Differences in Tubular Function after Release of Unilateral and Bilateral Ureteral Obstruction (24 Hours)

	Control	Unilateral	Bilateral
Postobstructive diuresis		Absent	Present
Per cent of filtration excreted (V/GFR)	1%	↓ to 0.5%	↑ to 18%
Excreted fract. filtered Na+	0.6%	↓ to 0.4%	↑ to 13%
Prox. tub. reabsorption		Decrease	Decrease
Distal tub. reabsorption			Decrease
Prox. fract. reab.	58%	74%	46%
Distal fract. reab.	12%		34%
Fract. K+ excreted	12.3%	↓ to 7%	↑ to 90%
Concentration U/P	7.6	1.35	1.47

TABLE 9–6. COMPARISON OF THE EFFECTS OF
UNILATERAL URETERAL (UUL) AND BILATERAL
URETERAL (BUL) OBSTRUCTION ON GLOMERULAR
HEMODYNAMICS

	P_T	P_G	AAPF	Ra	SNGFR
24 Hr UUL	=	↓	↓↓	↑↑	↓↓
24 Hr BUL	↑↑	=	=	=	↓↓

P_T = intratubular pressure; P_G = hydrostatic pressure gradient across glomerular capillaries; AAPF = afferent arteriole plasma flow; Ra = resistance of single afferent arteriole; SNGFR = single nephron filtration rate; UUL = unilateral ureteral ligation; BUL = bilateral ureteral ligation.

From Dal Canton, A., et al.: Kidney Int., *17*:491, 1980.

sion has also been shown to cause a similar redistribution of cortical blood flow (Blantz et al., 1971).

Silicone rubber perfusion studies of unilateral ureteral obstruction demonstrated many areas of nonperfused cortical nephrons. Perfusion of juxtamedullary glomeruli and vasa recta was maintained, while peritubular capillary perfusion in the deep cortex and outer medulla was absent (Yarger and Griffith, 1974).

Bilateral ureteral obstruction causes a decrease in renal blood flow similar to that observed in unilateral ureteral obstruction (Jaenike, 1972; McDougal and Wright, 1972; Moody et al., 1977a; Yarger et al., 1972). In contrast to unilateral ureteral obstruction, however, the distribution of blood flow between the cortex and medulla is normal (Jaenike, 1972, 1970).

POSTOBSTRUCTIVE DIURESIS

The changes in renal function after release of ureteral obstruction depend upon the duration, completeness, and extent, whether unilateral or bilateral, of the occlusion.

Unilateral Ureteral Obstruction

After release of an experimental unilateral ureteral obstruction of more than 5 hours' duration, the decreases in renal blood flow and filtration rate are associated with slightly decreased rates of solute reabsorption and a marked impairment of concentrating ability. This results in an approximately normal flow rate of dilute urine, with no tendency toward salt loss. Gillenwater and coworkers (1975) reported similar findings in 30 patients with chronic unilateral hydronephrosis. The function of the postobstructive kidney was compared with the function of the contralateral normal kidney. The first 4 days after release of the obstruction, only one kidney had significant diuresis, and this was mild (Fig. 9–14). These

postobstructive kidneys had a decrease in concentrating capacity and a slight impairment in sodium reabsorption. The filtration rate was decreased, however, to the extent that even though these kidneys excreted a higher percentage of the filtered water and sodium than the normal kidneys, the total urine volume from the former was less.

Schlossberg and Vaughan (1984) recently reported two patients with pathologic diuresis after release of unilateral ureteral obstruction. The mechanism of this unilateral postobstructive diuresis is based on the combination of preservation of glomerular filtration rate of the obstructed kidney with distal tubular damage.

Bilateral Ureteral Obstruction

Experimental Studies. Bilateral ureteral obstruction causes decreases in renal blood flow and filtration rate that are similar to those seen with unilateral obstruction (Jaenike, 1972; McDougal and Wright, 1972; Moody et al., 1975; Yarger et al., 1972). The distribution of renal blood flow is normal, as opposed to the shift from outer cortex to inner cortex and medulla that is seen with unilateral ureteral

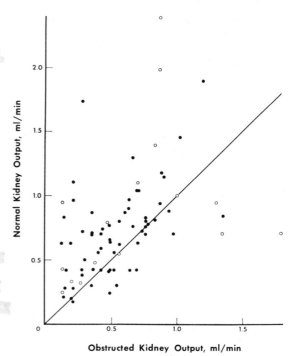

Figure 9–14. The urine flow of 30 patients during the first 4 days after correction of unilateral hydronephrosis is graphed, plotting the normal versus the previously obstructed kidney. The ten patients studied in detail are represented by open circles. The data show a lack of significant diuresis from the previously obstructed kidney. (Reproduced with permission from Gillenwater, J. Y., et al.: Kidney Int., 7:179, 1975.)

obstruction (Jaenike, 1972, 1970). After release of bilateral ureteral obstruction, a 3- to 10-fold increase in urine flow is observed, even when food and water are withheld from the animals during the period of obstruction (Feldman et al., 1974; Wilson et al., 1974). The animals have an impairment of concentrating ability and of sodium absorption that is great enough to cause diuresis and natriuresis despite the low filtration rate. Since physiologic and pathologic damages are similar in unilateral and bilateral ureteral obstruction, it would seem that a substance that is normally excreted builds up in uremia and causes the natriuresis and diuresis seen after release of bilateral ureteral obstruction. Wilson (1974a) has found that cross circulation between bilaterally obstructed uremic rats and normal rats resulted in 10-fold increases in urine flow and sodium in the normal animals. No diuresis was observed during cross circulation with unilaterally obstructed ureters.

Clinical Studies. Postobstructive diuresis was first described by Wilson and associates in 1951 and has been reviewed by Howards and Wright (1976), Howards (1973), Vaughan and Gillenwater (1973), and Goldsmith (1968). Transient increases in urine flow rates are the rule rather than the exception after release of bilateral obstruction (or of an obstruction in a solitary kidney). This diuresis usually is mild, self-limiting, and physiologic, with excretion of retained excess amounts of sodium and water. Muldowney and associates (1966) demonstrated an increase in total-body exchangeable sodium in patients with long-standing obstructive uropathy. In prospective studies, Persky and associates (1957b) found that none of six patients with urinary retention needed parenteral fluid or electrolyte replacement. One patient did remain in negative sodium (159 to 200 mEq/day) and negative water (1 to 2 L/day) balance for 4 days after relief of obstruction. Eiseman and coworkers (1955) found that 1 patient out of 24 had a large diuresis (urine volume exceeding water intake by 8 L/day).

Patients rarely have a pathologic diuresis after release of bilateral ureteral obstruction. When a postobstructive diuresis occurs, the postulated mechanisms are (1) impaired sodium reabsorption, (2) impaired urine concentrating ability, and (3) solute diuresis due to retained urea or administered glucose.

Inappropriate salt loss after release of obstruction has been reported in nine patients (Eiseman et al., 1955; Muldowney et al., 1966). Before release of the obstruction, the blood urea nitrogen ranged from 60 to 245 mg/10 ml.

The peak urine flow was 69 ml/min and averaged 30 ml/min. The glomerular filtration rates would have to be high (in the range of 70 to 100 ml/min) to produce such high urine flow rates. These high urine flow rates were an average of 32 per cent of the filtration rate. The average maximal fractional sodium excretion was 21 per cent. The duration of diuresis ranged from a few hours to 4 days. One patient died of a cerebral hemorrhage, and autopsy examination revealed normal kidneys.

Earley (1956) described one case of extreme polyuria in a 6-month-old male infant with bladder neck obstruction. The infant was not able to conserve water after dehydration or vasopressin administration. Roussak and Oleesky (1954) reported on a patient with bilateral hydronephrosis due to cancer of the prostate in whom polyuria was unresponsive to thirst or exogenous vasopressin.

Maher and associates (1963) found postobstructive diuresis due to urea in an 80-year-old patient. On the patient's admission to the hospital, the serum creatinine was 17.8 mg/100 ml, and urea was 175 mg/100 ml. During the first 8 hours, the urine volume reached a maximum of 25.8 ml/min and equaled 15.2 to 27.2 per cent of the filtration rate. Urea was the major urinary solute, representing 37 to 56 per cent of the urine osmolality during the diuresis. Homeostasis was restored within 48 hours, and the diuresis ceased.

Clinical Management. In clinical practice, a wide spectrum of responses is seen after relief of bilateral ureteral obstruction. Many patients will have mild diuresis and natriuresis, which is a physiologic excretion of retained sodium and water. Total fluid replacement is unnecessary and would only prolong this normal diuresis.

Our plan of management is to relieve the obstruction and remove the residual urine. Then the patient is weighed, blood pressures are recorded in supine and upright positions, and urine volumes are measured hourly. If the urine volume exceeds 200 ml/hr, the house officer is notified. In the alert, conscious patient, no parenteral fluids are given, and the normal thirst mechanism serves to restore fluid volume. Sodium loss can be evaluated by measuring the supine and upright blood pressure to determine whether the patient has a diminution of extracellular fluid volume. The urine can be examined for specific gravity. A low specific gravity would indicate water diuresis from fluid overload and unresponsiveness to antidiuretic hormone. A urine specific gravity of about 1.010 would suggest solute diuresis. Glucosuria can be ruled out by means of the dip stick test. If needed, measurements could be done to ascertain an excess sodium or urea loss. In the rare cases with severe pathologic loss of sodium, replacement of it may be necessary. If the patient is unconscious and has postobstructive diuresis, he or she should be followed much more closely. Certainly, it would be important to determine the cause of the diuresis. Until a specific cause is found, we usually replace 50 to 60 per cent of the output with 0.5 normal saline or Ringer's lactate solution.

Summary

Postobstructive diuresis is rare and usually occurs after release of bilateral ureteral obstruction or obstruction of a solitary kidney. The higher the initial osmotic load from retained fluids and solutes, and the higher the glomerular filtration rate, the greater the potential for polyuria. Any diuresis can be increased and prolonged with replacement therapy, which prevents a return to normal fluid and electrolyte balance. This probably will necessitate inducing a negative salt and water balance.

RECOVERABILITY OF RENAL FUNCTION AFTER RELEASE OF OBSTRUCTION

One of the fundamental principles of urologic surgery has been that relief of obstruction will prevent further deterioration of renal function. Recovery of some renal function has been assumed after relief of the obstruction. All clinicians are familiar with the patient who has silent prostatism and is admitted in urinary retention with a serum creatinine of more than 10 mg/100 ml as the result of severe bilateral hydronephrosis. Treatment with a Foley catheter will usually allow recovery of renal function after several weeks, with a serum creatinine of 2 to 4 mg/100 ml. Presumably, the ability to acidify and concentrate also increases, since the patient has an improvement in his serum CO_2 combining power and less polyuria. Improvement has been reported in glomerular filtration rate, renal blood flow, Tm diodone (Olbrich et al., 1957), concentrating ability (Berlyne, 1961; Earley, 1956; Roussak and Oleesky, 1954; Winberg, 1959), and acidification (Berlyne, 1961; Winberg, 1959) after relief of bilateral ureteral obstruction.

Kerr (1956, 1954) demonstrated how pow-

erful a stimulus contralateral nephrectomy is in causing maximal potential recovery after release of a unilaterally obstructed kidney. In experimental studies with the dog, Kerr (1956, 1954) and Vaughan and coworkers (1973) showed quite clearly that the unilaterally obstructed kidney will have a significant recovery in the presence of a normal contralateral kidney. Maximal recovery of GFR, Tm_{PAH}, and sodium and water excretion was seen 4 months after release of the obstruction.

Edvall (1959) demonstrated the recovery of renal function in a patient immediately after ureteral catheterization drainage of a constricted ureter (Fig. 9–15). He found that glomerular filtration rate and renal blood flow returned to normal levels within 2 hours. There was simultaneous loss of the compensatory hypertrophy on the opposite side. Better and coworkers (1973) reported that the creatinine clearance of a kidney that had been unilaterally obstructed increased from 2.7 to 10.2 ml/min within 1 week.

A word of caution about recoverability of function is stated by McCrory and associates (1971). They studied 15 children with complicated bilateral hydronephrosis who were hospitalized frequently and for long periods of time.

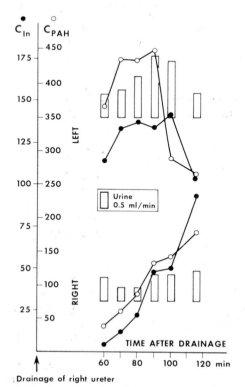

Figure 9–15. Recovery of renal function immediately after release of ureteral obstruction in a patient. (Data reproduced with permission from Edvall, C. A.: J. Appl. Physiol., *14*: 855, 1959.)

Most of these patients had nephrostomies and probably had bacteriuria. These workers state, "There was no consistent pattern of improvement in renal function after surgical treatment." There were four instances in which measurements of C_{CR}, $U_{H+}V$, and U_{mOsm}/L were repeated later; no improvement was noted in the one patient whose initial values were subnormal, and there was a decrease to subnormal levels in two. In two patients with normal values for C_{CR}, the values remained in the normal range, as did $U_{H+}V$. Data on U_{mOsm}/L were not available in one of these, but increases in U_{mOsm}/L in a subsequent study were observed in two.

Summary

Recovery of renal function occurs after release of both unilateral and bilateral ureteral obstruction. The recovery potential is dependent upon many things, most important of which are the severity of the renal injury and the presence or absence of infection. Greater recovery is seen under the stimulus of impaired function of the opposite kidney.

RENAL METABOLIC CHANGES IN HYDRONEPHROSIS

Normal Renal Metabolism

The role of renal metabolism in the body's total fuel economy and metabolism has only recently been defined. The kidneys (0.5 per cent of total body weight) receive 25 per cent of the cardiac output and consume 8 to 10 per cent of the body's oxygen. The kidneys, because of high blood flow per gram of tissue, extract only 1.5 ml of oxygen from each 100 ml of arterial blood (other organs extract 4 to 5 ml of oxygen from each 100 ml of arterial blood). The extraction of oxygen from each milliliter of blood remains constant even though blood flow is reduced, because the work load is less as a result of reduced filtration, reabsorption, and secretion. The major fraction of the energy of oxidation and decarboxylation produced in the kidney is utilized for the active reabsorption of sodium and, secondarily, of water (Gillenwater and Panko, 1971; Pitts, 1975). Renal gluconeogenesis provides as much as 50 per cent of the glucose production during starvation (Owen et al., 1969).

There is a marked difference in environment and metabolism in the different zones in the kidney (Fig. 9–16). The renal cortex is in an aerobic environment, and the major substrate used is fatty acids. The major biochemical reactions in the cortex are fatty acid oxidation, Krebs cycle oxidations, and gluconeogenesis with production of energy, CO_2, glucose, and keto-acids. The outer medulla has a mixed environment, and the major substrates used are glucose and ketoacids. The major biochemical reactions are Krebs cycle oxidations and glycolysis with production of energy, CO_2, and lactate. In contrast, the environment of the inner medulla is anaerobic, with the major substrate being glucose. The major reaction is glycolysis with production of energy and lactate. The renal cortex has a good blood supply (90 per cent of renal blood flow) with a good oxygen supply. The medulla has very low blood flow rates (3 per cent of that of the cortex) and a poor oxygen supply. The low P_{O_2} (15 to 20 mm Hg) of urine is believed to confirm the low oxygen supply to the medulla, since tubular urine oxygen rapidly equilibrates with that in the tissue in the medulla.

The substances reported to be taken up avidly by the dog kidney in vivo are free fatty acids, citric acid, lactic acid, amino acids, and the keto-acids (pyruvic and α-ketoglutaric). At higher concentrations, there is sufficient oxidation of the fatty acids to account for most of the metabolic energy of the kidney. Studies of the longer-chain fatty acids showed 15 per cent utilization of palmitic acid, 4 per cent utilization of oleic acid, and no extraction of stearic, palmitoleic, and linoleic acids. There is usually only a small renal extraction of the amino acids. In the human kidney, glutamine and proline represent most of the amino acid extraction. Alpha-ketoglutarate, citrate, lactate, and pyruvate extractions by the kidney depend upon their blood concentrations. Alpha-ketoglutarate plays a key role in the Krebs cycle, with linkage to the metabolism of fatty acids, amino acids, glucose, and so forth. Alpha-ketoglutarate infusions in the dog in vivo have shown that virtually all the alpha-ketoglutarate is removed by the liver and the kidney.

The relationship of sodium reabsorption and urine concentration to renal alpha-ketoglutarate utilization in vivo in the dog showed that it correlated in a linear fashion with T_{Na} (Stecker et al., 1973).

Renal Metabolism in Obstructive Uropathy

Levy and coworkers (1937) found that in vivo renal oxygen utilization decreased 41 per cent by the third day after ureteral occlusion.

THE METABOLISM OF KIDNEY

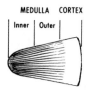

AREA	ENVIRONMENT	MAJOR SUBSTRATE(S)	MAJOR PRODUCT(S)	MAJOR REACTION(S)
Cortex	Aerobic	O_2 Fatty Acids	CO_2 Glucose Keto Acids Energy	Fatty Acid Oxidation Krebs Cycle Oxidations Gluconeogenesis
Outer Medulla	Mixed	O_2 Glucose Keto Acids	CO_2 Lactate Energy	Krebs Cycle Oxidations Glycolysis
Inner Medulla	Anaerobic	Glucose	Lactate Energy	Glycolysis

Figure 9–16. Environmental conditions and metabolic reactions in different zones of the kidney.

In 1965, Schirmer reported that renal cortical respiration was decreased by 50 per cent 48 hours after release of obstruction with further decrease to 20 per cent on the fourteenth and twentieth days of obstruction. The renal medullary tissue showed no change in its oxygen uptake. Studies of anaerobic glycolysis demonstrated a gradual increase in both cortical and medullary tissue until the eighth day, with a decrease thereafter. Schirmer and Marshall (1968) found no recovery of the depressed (33 per cent cortical respiration and increased (400 per cent) anaerobic glycolysis with release of 14 and 35 days of obstruction if the other kidney was intact.

Less oxidative mechanism is observed in the obstructed kidneys, but there is a proportionately greater increase in anaerobic glycolysis and anaerobic decarboxylation reactions (Figs. 9–17 and 9–18) (Stecker et al., 1971). Obstructed kidneys undergo an increase in DNA synthesis and in cell division (Benitez and Shaka, 1964). Increased protein, DNA, and RNA levels are found in the mouse kidney during the first 24 to 48 hours of ureteral obstruction, with decreased levels observed after 48 hours. Acute ureteral ligation did not affect renal gluconeogenesis in the rat but depressed it in the dog (Baisset et al., 1950).

The hydronephrotic kidney shows a generalized decrease in in vivo metabolic processes (Agusta et al., 1974). There is a shift from net glucose production to glucose utilization, while alpha-ketoglutarate metabolism shifts from net utilization to net production. Free fatty acid utilization is markedly decreased. No significant differences were noted between reversible injury at 2 weeks and irreversible injury at 6 weeks of total ureteral obstruction. Further in vivo renal metabolic studies (Middleton et al., 1977) showed that with 2 weeks' total ureteral obstruction there was decreased utilization of alpha-ketoglutarate, oxygen, and carbon diox-

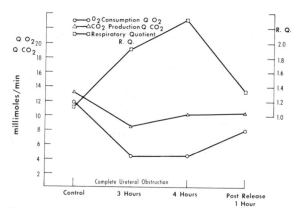

Figure 9–17. Alterations in renal O_2 consumption and CO_2 production in dogs with acute unilateral ureteral obstruction. Respiratory quotients QCO_2/QO_2 are also shown.

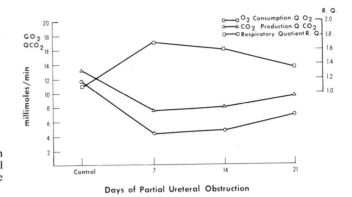

Figure 9–18. Alterations in renal O_2 consumption and CO_2 production in dogs with unilateral ureteral obstruction. Respiratory quotients QCO_2/QO_2 are also shown.

ide, decreased citrate production, and elevated respiratory quotient QCO_2/QO_2. At 6 weeks of total ureteral obstruction there was no renal alpha-ketoglutarate utilization and a marked decrease in oxygen utilization, carbon dioxide production, and citrate production. In vitro studies (Panko et al., 1978) showed that the reversibly damaged kidney (2 weeks' obstruction) could carry on certain aerobic reactions. Most aerobic metabolic reactions are inhibited in the irreversibly damaged kidney (6 weeks' obstruction). In vivo experiments showed that renal tissue ATP, ADP, and AMP fell to 50 to 70 per cent of normal at 24 hours after ureteral obstruction without further decline during ureteral obstruction of up to 7 days. Two hours after release of 24-hour obstruction, renal ATP rose to 90 to 95 per cent of normal (Nito et al., 1978). In rats' kidneys with ureteral obstruction the lactate dehydrogenase isoenzyme pattern shifts toward anaerobic metabolism in the cortex and outer medullary zones (Cestonaro et al., 1979).

Summary

Ureteral obstruction causes significant impairment of renal metabolism. There is a decrease in oxygen utilization and CO_2 production with an increase in the respiratory quotient, indicating a shift toward anaerobic metabolism. There is a significant impairment in fatty acid and alpha-ketoglutarate utilization and a loss of renal gluconeogenesis. There is an increase in the lactate to pyruvate ratio, indicating a shift toward anaerobic metabolism. With continued obstruction, progressive loss of renal metabolic function occurs until, at 6 weeks, there are marked and probably irreversible changes.

ASSOCIATION BETWEEN HYPERTENSION AND HYDRONEPHROSIS

Bilateral Hydronephrosis

Elevation of blood pressure frequently occurs in patients with chronic obstructive uropathy. The hypertension may be coincidental, from uremia, or from retained sodium and water (Muldowney et al., 1966; Vaughan and Gillenwater, 1973). In many patients, physiologic diuresis and natriuresis are seen after release of the obstruction, with return of the blood pressure to normal, which suggests a volume-dependent form of hypertension. Palmer and coworkers (1970) showed normal peripheral and renal vein renin levels in a hypertensive 16-year-old with obstruction of a solitary kidney. Postoperatively, there were natriuresis and diuresis (5 kg), with return of blood pressure to normal. This case would also seem to be one of volume-dependent hypertension. There are no data to indicate a renin-dependent mechanism for hypertension in chronic bilateral hydronephrosis in humans when there is absence of associated renal arterial stenosis.

Unilateral Hydronephrosis

Acute. Williams and associates (1938) and Beckwith (1941) found increased pressor activity in renal extracts from rats with acute unilateral ureteral ligation. Other investigators (Megibow et al., 1942; Schroeder and Neumann, 1942), however, at about the same time found less consistently elevated renal pressor activity. Vander and Miller (1964) and Vaughan and coworkers (1971) have shown significant hypertension and increased peripheral renin activity after acute unilateral ureteral occlusion in the dog.

Moody and associates (1975) have shown that intrarenal infusion of sar[1]-ala[8]-angiotensin II (P113), a competitive antagonist of angiotensin II, prevented the expected elevation in blood pressure usually observed after unilateral ureteral ligation in the dog.

Chronic. Hypertension is associated with chronic unilateral hydronephrosis but may not be caused by it. Braasch and coworkers (1940) evaluated 372 patients with hydronephrosis and found that 13.7 per cent had systolic blood pressure elevated to more than 145 mm Hg and 5.6 per cent had systolic blood pressure elevated to more than 160 mm Hg. Follow-up on 29 patients after surgical correction of the hydronephrosis demonstrated 34.4 per cent to have blood pressure returning to normal and remaining normal for 5 years. Schwartz (1969) found the incidence of hypertension with unilateral ureteral obstruction of less than 1 week's duration to be 30 per cent (9 out of 30), while that of hypertension caused by chronic unilateral ureteral obstruction was 1.35 per cent (3 out of 222). In the patients with acute ureteral obstruction (excluding concomitant renal disease), the hypertension was mild and short-lived. Chronic studies in animals with unilateral hydronephrosis (Vaughan et al., 1970) have shown that the elevated peripheral renin level returns to normal after 6 weeks.

Vaughan, Bühler, and Laragh (1974) found normal renin secretion in 13 hypertensive patients with chronic unilateral hydronephrosis. Hypertension associated with elevated renin secretion has been documented on occasion in chronic unilateral hydronephrosis, however, with return of the blood pressure and renin secretion to normal after surgical correction of the obstruction (Belman et al., 1968; Nemoy et al., 1973; Wise, 1975). There also have been many case reports describing the cure of hypertension with surgical correction of unilateral hydronephrosis, in which the underlying causes of the hypertension were undetermined (Bartels and Leadbetter, 1940; Houston, 1956; Klein et al., 1973; O'Connor, 1941). Hypertension associated with hydronephrosis may be renin-dependent and renal vein renin values are helpful in determining these incidences (Riehle and Vaughan, 1981; Weidmann et al., 1977).

Conclusions

Acute unilateral ureteral obstruction may cause hypertension owing to increased renin secretion. Chronic unilateral hydronephrosis rarely causes hypertension because of increased renin secretion. Surgical repair of the unilateral hydronephrosis solely to improve the associated hypertension must be justified by establishing proof of increased renin secretion in the absence of a renal artery obstruction. Surgical correction of hydronephrosis should usually be justified to improve renal function. Bilateral hydronephrosis is rarely associated with hypertension due to increased renin secretion. The usual relationships between hypertension and chronic hydronephrosis are coincidental or are due to volume expansion from retained sodium and water.

URINARY ASCITES

Spontaneous intraperitoneal extravasation of urine is rare but has been seen in children (France and Back, 1954; Ravitz et al., 1973) and in adults (there was an unpublished case of cancer of the prostate with urinary ascites at the University of Virginia). Urinary ascites can be produced experimentally in rats after bilateral ureteral ligation (Stoerk et al., 1970). Spontaneous extravasation into the flank is seen after acute ureteral obstruction. The point of leakage is believed to be the renal fornix. Most reported patients have been infants with obstruction from posterior urethral valves.

To prove urinary ascites, one should compare the urea or creatinine concentration of the ascitic fluid with the concentrations in the serum. Normally, the urine to plasma creatinine ratio is 30:1 to 100:1. Because of equilibration of the urine across the peritoneal membrane, the U/P ratio of fluid to plasma in urinary ascites may be as low as 2:1. Nonurine ascitic fluid would have a creatinine U/P ratio of 1:1.

ERYTHROCYTOSIS

The increased red blood cell volume associated with various disorders of the kidney (hypernephroma, renal cysts, polycystic kidney, or hydronephrosis) is more properly referred to as erythrocytosis rather than as polycythemia. In polycythemia vera, the patients have splenomegaly, leukocytosis, and thrombocytosis with erythrocytosis, whereas the patients with renal disease have only erythrocytosis, with normal oxygen saturation of the arterial blood. Jaworski and Wolan (1963) reviewed the eight previously reported cases of erythrocytosis and hydronephrosis in the literature and described an additional case. Seven of the nine patients reported had a reduction in the red blood cell volume after nephrectomy. Hirsch and Leiter (1983), report a patient with hydronephrosis and erythrocytosis. The erythropoietin blood level remained elevated after relief of the obstruction, but "follow-up 6 months later showed left hydronephrosis unchanged from the preoperative study." The postulated mechanism of the erythrocytosis is increased erythropoietin excretion by the obstructed kidney, although this is as yet unproven.

INTRAVENOUS UROGRAPHY AND HYDRONEPHROSIS

The organic compounds used as contrast media in urology are triiodide compounds derived from benzoic acid and can be divided into four groups: (1) acetrizoate, (2) diatrizoate (Hypaque, Urografin, and Renografin), (3) iothalamate (Conray), and (4) iodamide. These substances are used in the form of sodium or methylglucamine salts or in the form of a mixture. The different ways in which the COOH group of the benzoic ring is neutralized determine the pharmacologic and pharmacodynamic properties of each product, such as viscosity, toxicity, and local and systemic tolerability. The older contrast media (Diodrast, Neo-Iopax, and Urokon) are excreted by the kidneys with both glomerular filtration and small amounts of proximal tubule secretion (Woodruff et al., 1976). The more modern contrast media (Hypaque, Miokon, and Renografin) are excreted by glomerular filtration alone.

Visualization of the contrast agents in hydronephrosis is dependent upon the number of molecules of contrast agent and the total volume. With acute hydronephrosis, radiographic visualization is dependent upon the effective plasma concentration, the renal excretion, and the rate of turnover in the occluded pelvis. With acute hydronephrosis, there is a delay in appearance of both the nephrogram (opacification of the renal parenchyma by dye in the tubules and possibly in the tubular cells) and the pyelogram (appearance of contrast media at the calyces and renal pelvis), a decrease in concentration, and an increase in size of the kidney. With total acute ureteral occlusion, glomerular filtration continues at a rate of a few milliliters per minute, so that the contrast agent is still filtered into the tubules and renal pelvis. Woodruff and coworkers (1976) found poorer visualization in acute obstruction when mannitol was

given. Presumably, there is increased renal pelvic pressure from the diuresis, and the increased osmotic pressure prevents tubular reabsorption of water, with resultant replacement filtration of less contrast agent. Administration of 3 per cent NaCl intravenously was said to increase the visualization, presumably through more filtration and increased proximal tubular reabsorption of sodium and water.

Visualization in the dog with complete ureteral occlusion continues for 2 weeks and, with sporadic nephrograms, may last as long as 45 days (Woodruff et al., 1976).

In patients with hydronephrosis, a fairly good correlation exists between the ability to excrete and concentrate the contrast media and the ability to recover function after relief of the obstruction; that is, in patients with kidneys able to concentrate the contrast, we have usually seen return of function, even in dilated pelves and apparently thin cortex.

REFLEX ANURIA

Reflex anuria from neurogenic stimulation of the bladder or ureter is very rare. Stamey (1974, 1963) and Sirota and Narins (1957) clearly demonstrated that anuria after ureteral catheterization was due to edema, causing mechanical obstruction at the ureterovesical junction. Shearlock and Howards (1976) reported on the first well-documented and evaluated case of reflex anuria. They described a 32-year-old nurse who had previously undergone a right nephrectomy for retroperitoneal xanthogranulomatous disease. The patient was admitted with a 4-day history of anuria following left flank pain. Retrograde pyelography showed no ureteral obstruction, and no urine was obtained from a ureteral catheter, which was verified on radiographic studies to be in the renal pelvis. Arteriography did not show evidence of arterial obstruction. After 6 days of anuria, diuresis ensued. The initial urine osmolality was 169 mOsm/kg, and urine sodium was 11 mEq/L. These findings exclude acute tubular necrosis. Later studies revealed retroperitoneal involvement with fibroxanthogranulomatous infiltration that eventually involved the liver, the pericardium, and the bone marrow. This was successfully treated with vincristine, prednisone, and cyclophosphamide. The reflex anuria was postulated to have been initiated by transient ureteral obstruction. Hull and associates (1980) reported the short duration of anuria in a patient with a lower ureteral stone on one side. No studies were done during the anuria to define the mechanism.

Hix (1958) found that unilateral ureteral stimulation caused a 20 per cent reduction in ipsilateral renal blood flow and glomerular filtration rate. Lytton and coworkers (1969) demonstrated that bladder distention caused dogs that had undergone cutaneous ureterostomies to have a 28 per cent decrease in urine flow. Shearlock and Howards (1976) postulated that transient ureteral obstruction can initiate reflex anuria. Hauri (1983) summarizes the various pathophysiologic aspects of reflex anuria.

References

Abbrecht, P. H., and Malvin, R. L.: Flow rate of urine as a determinant of renal countercurrent multiplier system. Am. J. Physiol., 199:919, 1960.

Addis, T.: The ratio between urea content of the urine and of the blood after the administration of large quantities of urea. An approximate index of the quantity of actively functioning kidney tissue. J. Urol., 1:263, 1917.

Agusta, V. E., Panko, W. B., and Gillenwater, J. Y.: Changes in the in vivo metabolism of hydronephrotic canine kidneys. Invest. Urol., 11:379, 1974.

Allard: Arch. Exp. Pathol. Pharm., 57:241, 1907. Cited by Cushny, A. R.: The Secretion of the Urine. London, Longmans, Green and Co., 1917.

Allen, J. T., Vaughan, E. D., Jr., and Gillenwater, J. Y.: The effect of indomethacin on renal blood flow and ureteral pressure in unilateral obstruction in awake dogs. Invest. Urol., 15:324, 1978.

Altschul, R., and Fedor, S.: Vascular changes in hydronephrosis. Am. Heart J., 46:291, 1953.

Anderson, C.: Hydronephrosis. Springfield, Ill., Charles C Thomas, 1963.

Arendshorst, W. J., Finn, W. F., and Gottschalk, C. W.: Nephron stop-flow pressure response to obstruction for 24 hours in the rat kidney. J. Clin. Invest., 53:1497, 1974.

Babics, A., and Rényi-Vámos, F.: A vese üregrendszerének pathophysiologiája és mütétei (Pathophysiology and operations of the renal cavities.) (Hungarian). Akadémiai Kiadó, Budapest, 1950. Die ascendierende Pyelonephritis. Acta Med. Hung., 3:15, 1952a A vesepusztulás elmélete és klini kuma (Theory and clinical picture of renal atrophy.) (Hungarian). Akadémiai Kiadó, Budapest, 1952b. Cited in Rusznyák, I., Földi, M., and Szabó, G.: Lymphatics and Lymph Circulation. London, Pergamon Press, 1960.

Bäcklund, L., and Nordgren, L.: Pressure variations in the upper urinary tract and kidney at total ureteric occlusion. Acta Soc. Med. Ups., 71:285, 1966.

Bäcklund, L., Grotte, C., and Reuterskiöld, A.: Functional stenosis as a cause of pelvic-ureteric obstruction and hydronephrosis. Arch. Dis. Child., 40:203, 1965.

Baisset, A., Boer, A., Diaz, D., and Soula, C.: Le rein et la régulation glycémique. Rapports entre les glycémies veineuse et artérielle rénales et al sécrétion d'urine. J. Physiol. (Paris), 42:534, 1950.

Barney, J. D.: The effects of ureteral ligation, experimental and clinical. Surg. Gynecol. Obstet., 15:290, 1912.

Bartels, E. C., and Leadbetter, W. F.: Hypertension associated with unilateral noninfected hydronephrosis

treated by nephrectomy. Lahey Clinic Bull., 1:17, 1940.

Bay, W. H., Stein, J. H., Rector, J. B., Osgood, R. W., and Ferris, T. F.: Redistribution of renal cortical blood flow during elevated ureteral pressure. Am. J. Physiol., 222:33, 1972.

Beckwith, J. R.: The effect of the time factor on the amount of pressor material present in kidney after unilateral ligation of renal pedicle and after unilateral ligation of ureter. Am. J. Physiol., 132:1, 1941.

Belis, J. A., Belis, T. E., Lai, J. C. W., Goodwin, C. A., and Gabriele, D. F.: Radionuclide determination of individual kidney function in the treatment of chronic renal obstruction. J. Urol., 127:636, 1982.

Bell, E. T.: Renal Diseases. Philadelphia, Lea & Febiger, 1946.

Belman, A. B., Kropp, K. A., and Simon, N. M.: Renal-pressor hypertension secondary to unilateral hydronephrosis. N. Engl. J. Med., 278:1133, 1968.

Benitez, L., and Shaka, J. A.: Cell proliferation in experimental hydronephrosis and compensatory renal hyperplasia. Am. J. Pathol., 44:961, 1964.

Berlyne, G. M.: Distal tubular function in chronic hydronephrosis. Q. J. Med., 30:339, 1961.

Berlyne, G. M., and Macken, A.: On the mechanism of renal inability to produce a concentrated urine in chronic hydronephrosis. Clin. Sci., 22:315, 1962.

Better, O. S., Arieff, A. I., Massry, S. G., Kleeman, C. R., and Maxwell, M. H.: Studies on renal function after relief of complete unilateral ureteral obstruction of three months' duration in man. Am. J. Med., 54:234, 1973.

Bird, C. E., and Moise, T. S.: Pyelovenous backflow. JAMA, 86:661, 1926.

Blantz, R. C., Katz, M. A., Rector, F. C., Jr., and Seldin, D. W.: Measurement of intrarenal blood flow. II: Effect of saline diuresis in the dog. Am. J. Physiol., 220:1914, 1971.

Bledsoe, T., and Murphy, J. J.: The relative importance of the venous and lymphatic routes from the renal pelvis to the circulating blood. J. Urol., 81:264, 1959.

Braasch, W. F., Walters, W., and Hammer, H. J.: Hypertension and the surgical kidney. JAMA, 115:1837, 1940.

Bradford, E. R.: Observations made upon dogs to determine whether obstruction of the ureter would cause atrophy of the kidney. Br. Med. J., 2:1720, 1897.

Bradley, S. F., and Anderson, D. L.: Renal function in man during acute hydronephrosis. Bull. Univ. Maryland, 41:39, 1956.

Braun-Menendez, E.: Evidence for renotrophin as a causal factor in renal hypertension. Circulation, 17:696, 1958a.

Braun-Menendez, E.: The prophypertensive and antihypertensive actions of the kidney. Ann. Intern. Med., 49:717, 1958b.

Braun-Menendez, E.: Hypertension and the relation between body weight and kidney weight. Acta Physiol. Lat. Am., 2:2, 1952.

Brenner, B. M., Meyer, T. W., and Hostetter, T. H.: Dietary protein intake and the progressive nature of kidney disease. N. Engl. J. Med., 307:652, 1982.

Bricker, N. S.: Obstructive nephropathy. In Black, D. A. K. (Ed.): Renal Disease. Philadelphia, F. A. Davis Co., 1967.

Bricker, N. S., and Klahr, S.: Obstructive nephropathy. In Strauss, M. B., and Welt, L. G. (Eds.): Diseases of the Kidney. Boston, Little, Brown & Co., 1971.

Buerkert, J., Alexander, E., Purkerson, M. L., and Klahr, S.: On the site of decreased fluid reabsorption after release of ureteral obstruction in the rat. J. Lab. Clin. Med., 87:397, 1976.

Buerkert, J., Head, M., and Klahr, S.: Effects of acute

bilateral ureteral obstruction on deep nephron and terminal collecting duct function in the young rat. J. Clin. Invest., 59:1055, 1977.

Buerkert, J., Martin, D., and Head, M.: Effect of acute unilateral obstruction on terminal collecting duct function in the weanling rat. Am. J. Physiol., 236:F260, 1979.

Buerkert, J., Martin, D., Head, M., Prasad, J., and Klahr, S.: Deep nephron function after release of acute unilateral ureteral obstruction in the young rat. J. Clin. Invest., 62:1228, 1978.

Burns, J. E., and Scwartz, E. O.: Absorption from the renal pelvis in hydronephrosis due to permanent and complete occlusion of the ureter. J. Urol., 2:445, 1918.

Bury, H. P. R., Crane, W. A. J., and Dutta, L. P.: Cell proliferation in compensatory renal growth. Br. J. Urol., 37:201, 1965.

Carlson, D. E., and Schramm, L. P.: Interaction between neurogenic and peripheral determinants of renal vascular resistance. [Abstr.] Physiologist, 16:279, 1973.

Carlson, E. L., and Sparks, H. V.: Intrarenal distribution of blood flow during elevation of ureteral pressure in dogs. Circ. Res., 26:601, 1970.

Cestonaro, G., Emanuelli, G., Calcamuggi, G., Anfossi, G., and Gatti, G.: Renal lactate dehydrogenase (LDH) isoenzyme pattern in short-term experimental obstructive nephropathy. Invest. Urol., 17:46, 1979.

Chibber, P. J., Chisholm, G. D., Hargreave, T. B., and Merrick, M. V.: ^{99}m technetium DMSA and the prediction of recovery in obstructive uropathy. Br. J. Urol., 53:492, 1981.

Chisholm, G. D.: Bilateral renal clearance studies in experimental obstructive uropathy. Proc. R. Soc. Med., 57:571, 1964.

Chisholm, G. D., and Calnan, J. S.: Renal lymphatics and urinary tract obstruction. S. Afr. Med. J., 41:978, 1967.

Chisholm, G. D., Chibber, P. J., Wallace, D. M. A., Hargreave, T. B., and Merrick, M. V.: DMSA scan and the prediction of recovery of obstructive uropathy. Eur. Urol., 8:227, 1982.

Clausen, G., and Hope, A.: Intrarenal distribution of blood flow and glomerular filtration during chronic unilateral ureteral obstruction. Acta Physiol. Scand., 100:22, 1977.

Cohnheim, J.,and Roy, S.: Untersuchungen über die Circulation in den Nieren. Virchows Arch. [Pathol. Anat.], 92:424, 1883.

Connolly, J. G., Demelker, J., and Promislow, C.: Compensatory renal hyperplasia. Can. J. Surg., 12:236, 1969.

Cushny, A. R.: The Secretion of the Urine. London, Longmans, Green and Co., 1917.

Cussen, L. J., and Tymms, A.: Hyperplasia of ureteral muscle in response to acute obstruction of the ureter. Invest. Urol., 9:504, 1972.

Dal Canton, A., Corradi, A., Stanziale, R., Maruccio, G., and Migone, L.: Effects of 24 hour unilateral obstruction on glomerular hemodynamics in rat kidney. Kidney Int., 15:457, 1979.

Dal Canton, A., Corradi, A., Stanziale, R., Maruccio, G., and Migone, L.: Glomerular hemodynamics before and after release of 24 hour bilateral ureteral obstruction. Kidney Int., 17:491, 1980.

Dal Canton, A., Stanziale, R., Corradi, A., Andreucci, V. E., and Migone, L.: Effects of acute ureteral obstruction on glomerular hemodynamics in rat kidney. Kidney Int., 12:403, 1977.

Deming, C L.: The effects of intrarenal hydronephrosis on the components of the renal cortex. J. Urol., 65:748, 1951.

DiBona, G. F.: Effect of mannitol diuresis and ureteral occlusion on distal tubular reabsorption. Am. J. Physiol., 221:511, 1971.

Djurhuus, J. C., Nerstrom, B., Gyrd-Hansen, N., and Rask-Andersen, H.: Experimental hydronephrosis. Acta Chir. Scand., 472:17, 1976a.

Djurhuus, J. C., Dorph, S., Christiansen, L., Ladefoged, J., and Nerstrom, B.: Predictive value of renography and i.v. urography for the outcome of reconstructive surgery in patients with hydronephrosis. Acta Chir. Scand., 472:37, 1976b.

Dominguez, R., and Adams, R. B.: Renal function during and after acute hydronephrosis in the dog. Lab. Invest., 7:292, 1958.

Dorhout-Mees, E. J.: Reversible water losing state, caused by incomplete ureteric obstruction. Acta Med. Scand., 168:193, 1960.

Dzukias, L. J., Sterzel, R. B., Hodson, C. J., and Hoyer, J. R.: Renal localization of Tamm-Horsfall protein in unilateral obstructive uropathy in rats. Lab. Invest., 47:185, 1982.

Earley, L. E.: Extreme polyuria in obstructive uropathy: Report of a case of "water-losing nephritis" in an infant with a discussion of polyuria. N. Engl. J. Med., 255:600, 1956.

Edvall, C. A.: Influence of ureteral obstruction (hydronephrosis) on renal function in man. J. Appl. Physiol., 14:855, 1959.

Eiseman, B., Vivion, C., and Vivian, J.: Fluid and electrolyte changes following relief of urinary obstruction. J. Urol., 74:222, 1955.

Ericsson, N. O., Winberg, J., and Zetterstrom, R.: Renal function in infantile obstructive uropathy. Acta Paediatr., 44:444, 1955.

Feldman, R. A., Siegel, N. J., Kashgarian, M., and Hayslett, J. P.: Intrarenal hemodynamics in postobstructive diuresis. Invest. Urol., 12:172, 1974.

Finkle, A. L., Karg, S. J., and Smith, D. R.: Parameters of renal functional capacity in reversible hydroureteronephrosis in dogs. II, Effects of one hour of ureteral obstruction upon urinary volume, osmolality, TcH_2O, C_{PAH}, RBF_{kr} and pUO_2. Invest. Urol., 6:26, 1968.

Földi, M., and Romhányi, G.: A vese nyirokkeringésének jelentösége hydronephrosisban (Significance of renal lymph circulation in hydronephrosis.) Orv. Hetilap. (Hungarian), 94:315, 1953a. Untersuchungen über den Lymphstrom der Niere. Acta Med. Hung., 4:323, 1953b. Cited in Rusznyák. I., Földi, M., and Szabó, G.: Lymphatics and Lymph Circulation. London, Pergamon Press, 1960.

Földi, M., Jellinek, H., Rusznyák, I., and Szabó, G.: Eiweisspeicherung in den Endothelzellen der Lymphkapillaren. Acta Med. Hung., 7:211, 1955. Cited in Rusznyák, I., Földi, M., and Szabó, G.: Lymphatics and Lymph Circulation, p. 758. London, Pergamon Press, 1960.

France, N. E., and Back, E. H.: Neonatal ascites associated with urethral obstruction. Arch. Dis. Child., 29:565, 1954.

Fuchs, F.: Internal topography of kidney. Z. Urol. Chir., 18:164, 1925. Cited by Olsson, O.: Studies on backflow in excretion urography. Acta Radiol. [Suppl.], 70, 1948.

Gee, W. E., and Kiviat, M. D.: Ureteral response to partial obstruction: smooth muscle hyperplasia and connective tissue proliferation. Invest. Urol., 12:309, 1975.

Gillenwater, J. Y., and Panko, W. B.: Renal metabolism: Current concepts. Urol. Survey, 21:331, 1971.

Gillenwater, J. Y., Teates, D., and Marion, D. N.: Prediction of recoverability in hydronephrosis with ^{131}I-hippuran renograms. Presented at Annual Meeting, American Urological Association, New York, May 13–17, 1979.

Gillenwater, J. Y., Westervelt, F. B., Jr., Vaughan, E. D., Jr., and Howards, S. S.: Renal function after release of chronic unilateral hydronephrosis in man. Kidney Int. 7:179, 1975.

Gilmore, J. P.: Renal vascular resistance during elevated ureteral pressure. Circ. Res., 15 [Suppl.]:148, 1964.

Goldsmith, C.: Postobstructive diuresis. Kidney, 2:1, 1968.

Goodwin, W. E., and Kaufman, J. J.: Renal lymphatics. II, Preliminary experiments. J. Urol., 76:702, 1956.

Goodwin, W. E., and Kaufman, J. J.: The renal lymphatics and hydronephrosis. Surg. Forum, 6:632, 1955.

Gosling, J. A., and Dixon, J. S.: Species variation in the location of upper urinary tract pacemaker cells. Invest Urol., 11:418, 1974.

Goss, R. J., and Dittmer, J. E.: Compensatory renal hypertrophy: Problems and prospects. In Nowinski, W. W., and Goss, R. J. (Eds.): Compensatory Renal Hypertrophy, p. 299. New York, Academic Press, 1969.

Gottschalk, C. W.: Micropuncture measurements of intrarenal pressures. Circ. Res., 15[Suppl.]:110, 1964.

Gottschalk, C. W.: An experimental comparative study of renal interstitial pressure. Am. J. Physiol., 163:716, 1950.

Gottschalk, C. W., and Mylle, M.: Micropuncture study of pressures in proximal and distal tubules and peritubular capillaries of the rat kidney during osmotic diuresis. Am. J. Physiol., 189:323, 1957.

Gottschalk, C. W., and Mylle, M.: Micropuncture study of pressures in proximal tubules and peritubular capillaries of the rat kidney and their relation to ureteral and renal venous pressures. Am. J. Physiol., 185:430, 1956.

Govan, D. E.: Experimental hydronephrosis, I. J. Urol., 85:432, 1961.

Graham, J. B.: Recovery of kidney after ureteral obstruction. JAMA, 181:993, 1962.

Halliburton, I. W., and Thomson, R. Y.: Chemical aspects of compensatory renal hypertrophy. Cancer Res., 25:1882, 1965.

Hanley, M. J., and Davidson, K.: Isolated nephron segments from rabbit models of obstructive nephropathy. J. Clin. Invest., 69:165, 1982.

Hanna, M. K., Jetts, R. D., Sturgess, J. M., and Barkin, M.: Ureteral structure and ultrastructure. II. Congenital ureteropelvic junction obstruction and primary obstructive megaureter. J. Urol., 116:725, 1976.

Harris, R. H., and Gill, J. M.: Changes in glomerular filtration rate during complete ureteral obstruction in rats. Kidney Int., 19:603, 1981.

Harris, R. H., and Yarger, W. E.: Renal function after release of unilateral ureteral obstruction in rats. Am. J. Physiol., 227:806, 1974.

Harris, R. H., Hise, M. K., and Best, C. F.: Renotrophic factors in urine. Kidney Int., 23:616, 1983.

Harsing, L., Szanto, G., and Bartha, J.: Renal circulation during stopflow in the dog. Am. J. Physiol., 213:935, 1967.

Hauri, D.: Uber die reaktive oder reflexanurie. Urol. Int., 38:126, 1983.

Hayslett, J. P.: Effect of age on compensatory renal growth. Kidney Int., 23:599, 1983.

Hermann, W.: Sitzungsberichte d. k. Akad. der Wissensch. zu Wein. Math.-Naturwiss, 36:349, 1859. Cited in Cushny, A. R.: The Secretion of the Urine. London, Longmans, Green and Co., 1917.

Hinman, F.: Hydronephrosis. I, The structural change. II, The functional change. III, Hydronephrosis and hypertension. Surgery, 17:816, 1945.

Hinman, F.: The condition of renal counterbalance and the theory of renal atrophy of disuse. J. Urol., 49:392, 1943.

Hinman, F.: Pathogenesis of hydronephrosis. Surg. Gynecol. Obstet., 58:356, 1934.

Hinman, F.: Renal counterbalance. Arch. Surg., 12:1105, 1926.

Hinman, F.: Renal counterbalance: An experimental and clinical study with reference to significance of disuse atrophy. Trans. Am. Assoc. Genitourin. Surg., 15:241, 1922.

Hinman, F.: Experimental hydronephrosis: Repair following ureterocystoneostomy in white rats with complete ureteral obstruction. J. Urol., 3:147, 1919.

Hinman, F., and Hepler, A. B.: Experimental hydronephrosis: The effect of ligature of one branch of the renal artery on its rate of development. IV, Simultaneous ligation of the posterior branch of the renal artery and the ureter on the same side. Arch. Surg., 12:830, 1926.

Hinman, F., and Hepler, A. B.: Experimental hydronephrosis: The effect of changes in blood pressure and in blood flow on its rate of development, and the significance of the venous collateral system. III, Partial obstruction of the renal vein without and with ligation of all collateral veins. Arch. Surg., 11:917, 1925a.

Hinman, F., and Hepler, A. B.: Experimental hydronephrosis: The effect of changes in blood pressure and in blood flow on its rate of development. II, Partial obstruction of the renal artery: Diminished blood flow; diminished intrarenal pressure and oliguria. Arch. Surg., 11:649, 1925b.

Hinman, F., and Hepler, A. B.: Experimental hydronephrosis: The effect of changes in blood pressure and blood flow on its rate of development. I, Splanchnotomy: Increased intrarenal blood pressure and flow; diuresis. Arch. Surg., 11:578, 1925c.

Hinman, F., and Lee-Brown, R. K.: Pyelovenous backflow, its relation to pelvic reabsorption, to hydronephrosis and to accidents of pyelography. JAMA, 82:607, 1924.

Hinman, F., and Morison, D. M.: An experimental study of the circulatory changes in hydronephrosis. J. Urol., 21:435, 1924.

Hinman, F., Jr.: The pathophysiology of urinary obstruction. In Campbell, M. F., and Harrison, J. H. (Eds.): Urology. 3rd ed., p. 313. Philadelphia, W. B. Saunders Co., 1970.

Hinman, F., Jr.: The pathophysiology of urinary obstruction. Chap. 8. In Campbell, M. F. (Ed.): Urology. Vol. I. Philadelphia, W. B. Saunders Co., 1963.

Hirsch, I., and Leiter, E.: Hydronephrosis and polycythemia. Urology, 21:345, 1983.

Hix, E. L.: Uretero-renal reflex facilitating renal vasoconstrictor responses to emotional stress. Am. J. Physiol., 192:191, 1958.

Holliday, M. A., Egan, T. J., Morris, C. R., et al.: Pitressin-resistant hyposthenuria in chronic renal disease. Am. J. Med., 42:378, 1967.

Holmes, M. S., O'Morchor, P. J., and O'Morchor, C. C. C.: The role of renal lymph in hydronephrosis. Invest. Urol., 15:215, 1977.

Houston, W.: Hypertension due to hydronephrosis: Relief after nephrectomy. Br. Med. J., 2:644, 1956.

Howards, S. S.: Postobstructive diuresis: A misunderstood phenomenon. J. Urol., 110:537, 1973.

Howards, S. S., and Wright, F. S.: Obstructive injury. In Brenner, B. M., and Rector, F. C. (Eds.): The Kidney. Philadelphia, W. B. Saunders Co., 1976.

Hsu, C. H., Kurtz, T. W., Rosenzweig, J., and Weller, J.

M.: Intrarenal hemodynamics and ureteral pressure during ureteral obstruction. Invest. Urol., *14*:442, 1977.

Huland, H., and Gonnermann, D.: Pathophysiology of hydronephrotic atrophy: the cause and role of active preglomerular vasoconstriction. Urol. Int., *38*:193, 1983.

Huland, H., Leichtweiss, H. P., and Augustin, H. J.: Effect of angiotensin II agonist, alpha receptor blockage and denervation on blood flow reduction in experimental chronic hydronephrosis. Invest. Urol., *18*:203, 1980a.

Huland, H., Leichtweiss, H. P., and Augustin, H. J.: Changes in renal hemodynamics in experimental hydronephrosis. Invest. Urol., *18*:274, 1980b.

Hull, J. D., Kumar, S., and Pletka, P. G.: Reflex anuria from unilateral ureteral obstruction. J. Urol., *123*:265, 1980.

Humes, H. D., Dieppa, R. A., and Brenner, B. M.: Glomerular dynamics in rats with hereditary hydronephrosis. Invest. Urol., *18*:46, 1980.

Ibrahim, A., and Asha, H. A.: Prediction of renal recovery in hydronephrotic kidneys. Br. J. Urol., *50*:222, 1978.

Ichikawa, I., and Brenner, B. M.: Local intrarenal vasoconstrictor-vasodilator interactions in mild partial ureteral obstruction. Am. J. Physiol., *236*:F131, 1979.

Idbohrn, H.: Renal angiography in experimental hydronephrosis. Acta Radiol., [Suppl. 136]:1, 1956.

Jaenike, J. R.: The renal functional defect of postobstructive nephropathy: The effects of bilateral ureteral obstruction in the rat. J. Clin. Invest., *51*:2999, 1972.

Jaenike, J. R.: The renal response to ureteral obstruction: A model for the study of factors which influence glomerular filtration pressure. J. Lab. Clin. Med., *76*:373, 1970.

Jaenike, J. R., and Bray, G. A.: Effects of acute transitory urinary obstruction in the dog. Am. J. Physiol., *199*:1219, 1960.

Jaworski, Z. F., and Wolan, C. T.: Hydronephrosis and polycythemia: A case of erythrocytosis relieved by decompression of unilateral hydronephrosis and cured by nephrectomy. Am. J. Med., *34*:523, 1963.

Johnson, C. M.: Pathogenesis of hydronephrosis. J. Urol., *27*:279, 1932.

Johnson, H. A., and Vera Roman, J. M.: Compensatory renal enlargement: Hypertrophy vs. hyperplasia. Am. J. Pathol., *49*:1, 1966.

Johnston, J. H.: The pathogenesis of hydronephrosis in children. Br. J. Urol., *41*:724, 1969.

Kalika, V., Bard, R. H., Iloreta, A., Freeman, L. M., Heller, S., and Blaufox, M. D.: Prediction of renal functional recovery after relief of upper urinary tract obstruction. J. Urol., *126*:301, 1981.

Kazmin, M., Persky, L., and Storaasli, J. P.: Backflow patterns in experimental chronic hydronephrosis. J. Urol., *84*:10, 1960.

Kerr, W. S., Jr.: Effects of complete ureteral obstruction in dogs on kidney function. Am. J. Physiol., *184*:521, 1956.

Kerr, W. S., Jr.: Effect of complete ureteral obstruction for one week on kidney function. J. Appl. Physiol., *6*:762, 1954.

Kessler, R. H.: Acute effects of brief ureteral stasis on urinary and renal papillary chloride concentration. Am. J. Physiol., *199*:1215, 1960.

Kiil, F.: Physiology of the renal pelvis and ureter. *In* Campbell, M. F., and Harrison, J. H. (Eds.): Urology. Vol. I. 3rd ed. Philadelphia, W. B. Saunders Co., 1970.

Kiil, F.: The Function of the Ureter and Renal Pelvis. Philadelphia, W. B. Saunders Co., 1957.

Klahr, S., Buerkert, J., and Purkerson, M. L.: The kidney in obstructive uropathy. Contrib. Nephrol., *7*:220, 1977.

Klein, L. A., Lupu, A., and Brosman, S. A.: Hypertension due to traumatic ureteral occlusion. Invest. Urol., *10*:327, 1973.

Kramer, K., and Winton, F. R.: The influence of urea and of change in arterial pressure on the oxygen consumption of the isolated kidney in the dog. J. Physiol. (London), *96*:87, 1939.

Kurnick, N. B., and Lindsay, P. A.: Compensatory renal hypertrophy in parabiotic mice. Lab. Invest., *19*:45, 1968.

Ladefoged, O., and Djurhuus, J. C.: Morphology of the upper urinary tract in experimental hydronephrosis in pigs. Acta Chir. Scand., *472*:29, 1976.

Levy, S. E., Mason, M. F., Harrison, T. R., and Blalock, A.: The effects of ureteral occlusion on blood flow and oxygen consumption of the kidneys of unanesthetized dogs. Surgery, *1*:238, 1937.

Lewis, H. Y., and Pierce, J. M.: Return of function after relief of complete ureteral obstruction of 69 days' duration. J. Urol., *88*:377, 1962.

Lome, L. G., Pinsky, S., and Levy, L.: Dynamic renal scan in the non-visualizing kidney. J. Urol., *121*:148, 1979.

Lorentz, W. B., Jr., Lassiter, W. E., and Gottschalk, C. W.: Renal tubular permeability during increased intrarenal pressure. J. Clin. Invest., *51*:484, 1972.

Lowenstein, L. M., and Stern, A.: Serum factor in renal compensatory hyperplasia. Science, *142*:1479, 1963.

Ludwig, C., and Sawarykin, T.: Die Lymphwurzeln in der Niere des Säugetieres. Sitz.-Ber. Wien. Akad. Wiss., *47*:242, 1863. Cited by Rusznyák, I., Földi, M., and Szabó, G.: *In* Lymphatics and Lymph Circulation. London, Pergamon Press, 1960.

Lytton, B., Schiff, M., and Bloom, N.: Compensatory renal growth: Evidence for tissue specific factor of renal origin. J. Urol., *101*:648, 1969.

Maher, J. F., Schreiner, G. E., and Waters, T. J.: Osmotic diuresis due to retained urea after release of obstructive uropathy. N. Engl. J. Med., *268*:1099, 1963.

Malt, R. A.: Compensatory growth of the kidney. N. Engl. J. Med., *280*:1446, 1969.

Malt, R. A.: Humoral factors in regulation of compensatory renal hypertrophy. Kidney Int., *23*:611, 1983.

Malvin, R. L., Kutchai, H., and Ostermann, F.: Decreased nephron population resulting from increased ureteral pressure. Am. J. Physiol., *207*:835, 1964.

Malvin, R. L., Wilde, W. S., and Sullivan, L. P.: Localization of nephron transport by stopflow analysis. Am. J. Physiol., *194*:135, 1958.

Marier, R, Fong, E., Jansen, M., Hodson, C. J., Richards, F., and Andriole, V. T.: Antibody to Tamm-Horsfall protein in patients with urinary tract obstruction and vesicoureteral reflux. J. Infect. Dis., *138*:781, 1978.

McCrory, W. W. Shibuya, M., Leumann, E., and Karp, R.: Studies of renal function in children with chronic hydronephrosis. Pediatr. Clin. North Am., *18*:445, 1971.

McDonald, J. R., Mann, F. C., and Priestly, J. T.: The maximum intrapelvic pressure (secretory) of the kidney of the dog. J. Urol., *37*:326, 1937.

McDougal, W. S., and Flanigan, R. C.: Renal functional recovery of the hydronephrotic kidney predicted before relief of the obstruction. Invest. Urol., *18*:440, 1981.

McDougal, W. S., and Wright, F. S.: Defect in proximal and distal sodium transport in postobstructive diuresis. Kidney Int., *2*:304, 1972.

Megibow, R. S., Katz, L. N., and Rodbard, S.: The mechanism of arterial hypertension in experimental hydronephrosis. Am. J. Med. Soc., *204*:340, 1942.

Melick, W. F., Karellos, D., and Naryka, J. J.: Pressure studies of hydronephrosis in children by means of the strain gauge. J. Urol., *85*:703, 1961.

Michaelson, G.: Percutaneous puncture of the renal pelvis, intrapelvic pressure, and the concentrating capacity of the kidney in hydronephrosis. Acta Med. Scand., [Suppl. 559]:1, 1974.

Middleton, G. W., Beamon, C. R., Panko, W. B., and Gillenwater, J. Y.: Effects of ureteral obstruction on the renal metabolism of alpha-ketoglutarate and other substances in vivo. Invest. Urol., *14*:255, 1977.

Moody, T. E., Vaughan, E. D., Jr., and Gillenwater, J. Y.: Relationship between renal blood flow and ureteral pressure during 18 hours of total unilateral occlusion. Invest. Urol., *13*:246, 1975.

Moody, T. E., Vaughan, E. D., Jr., and Gillenwater, J. Y.: Comparison of the renal hemodynamic response to unilateral and bilateral ureteral obstruction. Invest. Urol., *14*:455, 1977a.

Moody, T. E., Vaughan, E. D., Jr., Wyker, A. T., and Gillenwater, J. Y.: The role of intrarenal angiotensin II in the hemodynamic response to unilateral obstructive uropathy. Invest. Urol., *14*:390, 1977b.

Morison, D. M.: Routes of absorption in hydronephrosis: Experimentation with dyes in the totally obstructed ureter. Br. J. Urol., *1*:30, 1929.

Morrison, A. R., and Benabe, J. E.: Prostaglandins and vascular tone in experimental obstructive nephropathy. Kidney Int., *19*:786, 1981.

Morrison, A. R., Thornton, F., Blumberg, A., and Vaughan, E. D., Jr.: Thromboxane A$_2$ is the major arachidonic acid metabolite of human cortical hydronephrotic tissue. Prostaglandins, *21*:471, 1981.

Muldowney, F. P., Duffy, G. J., Kelly, D. G., Duff, F. A., Harrington, C., and Freaney, R.: Sodium diuresis after relief of obstructive uropathy. N. Engl. J. Med., *274*:1294, 1966.

Murphy, G. P., and Scott, W. W.: The renal hemodynamic response to acute and chronic ureteral occlusions. J. Urol., *95*:636, 1966.

Murphy, J. J., Myint, M. K., Rattner, W. H., Klaus, R. K., and Shallow, J.: The lymphatic system of the kidney. J. Urol., *80*:1, 1958.

Myint, M. K., and Murphy, J. J.: The renal lymphatics I: The effect of diuresis and acute ureteral occlusion upon the rate of flow and composition of thoracic duct lymph. Surg. Forum, *7*:656, 1957.

Naber, K. G., and Madsen, P. O.: Renal function in chronic hydronephrosis with and without infection and the role of lymphatics: An experimental study in dogs. Urol. Res., *2*:1, 1974.

Naber, K. G., and Madsen, P. O.: Renal function during acute total ureteral occlusion and the role of lymphatics: An experimental study in dogs. J. Urol., *109*:330, 1973a.

Naber, K. G., and Madsen, P. O.: The reabsorption mechanism of substances of various molecular weights from the totally occluded renal pelvis: An experimental study in dogs. Urol. Int., *28*:256, 1973b.

Narath, P. A.: The hydromechanics of the calyx renalis. J. Urol., *43*:145, 1940.

Nash, F. D., and Selkurt, E. E.: Effects of elevated ureteral pressure on renal blood flow. Circ. Res., *15*[Suppl.]:142, 1964.

Nash, F. D., and Selkurt, E. E.: Renal hemodynamics during ureteral occlusion in the intact dog kidney. Physiologist, *6*:244, 1963.

Navar, L. G., and Baer, P. G.: Renal autoregulatory and glomerular filtration responses to gradated ureteral obstruction. Nephron, *7*:301, 1970.

Nemoy, N. J., Fichman, M. P., and Sellars, A.: Unilateral ureteral obstruction: A cause of reversible high renin content hypertension. JAMA, *225*:512, 1973.

Nishikawa, K., Morrison, A., and Needleman, P.: Exaggerated prostaglandin biosynthesis and its influence on renal resistance in the isolated hydronephrotic rabbit kidney. J. Natl. Cancer Inst., *59*:1143, 1977.

Nito, H., Descoeudres, C., Kurokawa, K., and Massry, S. G.: Effect of unilateral ureteral obstruction on renal cell metabolism and function. J. Lab. Invest., *91*:60, 1978.

Notley, R. G.: The structural basis for normal and abnormal ureteric motility. Ann. R. Coll. Surg. Engl., *49*:250, 1971.

Notley, R. G.: Electron microscopy of the primary obstructive megaureter. Br. J. Urol., *44*:229, 1972.

Nowinski, W. W.: Early history of renal hypertrophy. In Nowinski, W. W., and Goss, R. J. (Eds.): Compensatory Renal Hypertrophy. p. 1. New York, Academic Press, 1969.

Obniski: Centralbl. Physiol., *21*:548, 1907. Cited by Cushny, A.: The Secretion of the Urine. London, Longmans, Green and Co., 1917.

O'Conor, V. J.: Ureterocele with congenital solitary kidney and hypertension. Trans. Am. Assoc. Genitourin. Surg., *34*:31, 1941.

Ogawa, K., and Nowinski, W. W.: Mitosis stimulating factor in serum of unilaterally nephrectomized rats. Proc. Soc. Exp. Biol. Med., *99*:350, 1958.

Olbrich, O., Woodford-Williams, W. E., Irvine, R. E., and Webster, D.: Renal function in prostatism. Lancet, *272*:1322, 1957.

Olesen, S., and Madsen, P. O.: Renal function during experimental hydronephrosis: Function during partial obstruction following contralateral nephrectomy in the dog. J. Urol., *99*:692, 1968.

Olsson, O.: Studies on back-flow in excretion urography. Acta Radiol. [Suppl.], 70, 1948.

Orecklin, J. R., Craven, J.D., and Lecky, J. W.: Compensatory renal hypertrophy: A morphologic study in transplant donors. J. Urol., *109*:952, 1973.

Owen, O. E., Felig, P., Morgan, A. P., Wahren, J., and Cahill, C. F., Jr.: Liver and kidney metabolism during prolonged starvation. J. Clin. Invest., *48*:574, 1969.

Palmer, J. M., Zweiman, F. G., and Assaykeen. T. A.: Renal hypertension due to hydronephrosis with normal plasma renin activity. N. Engl. J. Med., *283*:1032, 1970.

Panko, W. B., Beamon, C. R., Middleton, G. W., and Gillenwater, J. Y.: Effects of obstruction on renal metabolism: renal tissue metabolite concentration after alpha-ketoglutarate infusion. Invest. Urol., *15*:331, 1978.

Papdopoulou, Z. L., Slotkoff, L. M., Eisner, G. M., et al.: Glomerular filtration during stop-glow. Proc. Soc. Exp. Biol. Med., *130*:1206, 1969.

Patt, L. M., and Houck, J. C.: Role of polypeptide growth factors in normal and abnormal growth. Kidney Int., *23*:603, 1983.

Paulson, D. F., and Fraley, E. E.: Sequential changes in bulk renal protein and polyribosomes in the acutely obstructed mouse kidney. J. Urol., *103*:257, 1970.

Persky, L., Benson, J. W., Levey, S., and Abbott, W. E.: Metabolic alterations in surgical patients. X, The benign course of the average patient with acute urinary retention. Surgery, *42*:290, 1957b.

Persky, L., Bonte, F. J., and Austen, G.: Mechanisms of hydronephrosis: Radioautographic backflow patterns. J. Urol., *75*:190, 1956.

Persky, L., Bonte, F. J., and Hubay, C. A.: Mechanisms

of hydronephrosis: The route of backflow. Surg. Forum, 7:645, 1957a.

Persky, L., Storaasli, J. P., and Austen, G.: Mechanisms of hydronephrosis: Newer investigative techniques. J. Urol., 73:740, 1955.

Pfaundler, M.: Hofmeister's Beitrage Z. Chem. Physiol., 4:336, 1902.

Pitts, R. F.: Production of CO_2 by the intact functioning kidney of the dog. Med. Clin. North Am., 59:507, 1975.

Platt, R.: Structural and functional adaptation in renal failure. Br. Med. J., 1:1313, 1952.

Platts, M. M., and Williams, J. L.: Renal function in patients with unilateral hydronephrosis. Br. Med. J., 2:1243, 1963.

Preuss, H. G.: Compensatory renal growth symposium—an introduction. Kidney Int., 23:571, 1983.

Preuss, H. G., and Goldin, H.: Humoral regulation of compensatory renal growth. Med. Clin. North Am., 59:771, 1975.

Provoost, A. P., and Molenaar, J. C.: Renal function during and after a temporary complete unilateral ureter obstruction in rats. Invest. Urol., 18:242, 1981.

Radwin, H. M., O'Dell, R. M., and Schlegel, J. V.: The renal response to acute partial obstruction. J. Urol., 90:243, 1963.

Ransley, P. G., and Risdon, R. A.: Renal papillae and intrarenal reflux in the pig. Lancet, 2:1114, 1974.

Rao, N. R., and Heptinstall, R. H.: Experimental hydronephrosis: A microangiographic study. Invest Urol., 6:183, 1968.

Rattner, W. H., Fink, S., and Murphy, J. J.: Pressure studies in the human ureter and renal pelvis. J. Urol., 78:359, 1957.

Ravitz, G. A., Kandzari, S. J., and Milam, D. F.: Neonatal urinary ascites. J. Urol., 110:141, 1973.

Ravitz, G. A., Kandzari, S. J., and Milam, D. F.: Postobstructive diuresis syndrome. W. Va. Med. J., 68:4, 1972.

Reingold, D. F., Watters, K., Holmberg, S., and Needleman, P.: Differential biosynthesis of prostaglandins by hydronephrotic rabbit and cat kidneys. J. Pharmacol. Exp. Ther., 216:510, 1981.

Reisman, D. D., Kamholz, J. H., and Kantor, H. I.: Early deligation of the ureter. J. Urol., 78:363, 1957.

Riehle, R. A., and Vaughan, E. D., Jr.: Renin participation in hypertension associated with unilateral hydronephrosis. J. Urol., 126:243, 1981.

Risholm, L.: Studies on renal colic and its treatment by posterior splanchnic block. Acta Chir. Scand., [Suppl. 184] 1, 1954.

Rist, M., Lee, S., and Gittes, R. F.: Glomerular filtration rate and effective renal plasma flow in four-kidney rats Surg. Forum, 26:577, 1975.

Roussak, N. J., and Oleesky, S.: Water-losing nephritis, a syndrome simulating diabetes insipidus. Q. J. Med., 23:147, 1954.

Rusznyák, I., Földi, M., and Szabó, G.: Lymphatics and Lymph Circulation. New York, Pergamon Press, 1960.

Schelfhout, W., Simmons, M., Oosterlinck, W., and DeSy, W. A.: Evaluation of ^{99m}Tc-dimercaptosuccinic acid renal uptake as an index of individual kidney function after acute ureteral obstruction and deobstruction: an experimental study in rats. Eur. Urol., 9:221, 1983.

Schirmer, H. K.: Renal metabolism in experimental hydronephrosis. Invest. Urol., 2:598, 1965.

Schirmer, H. K., and Marshall, R. E.: Metabolism of atrophic renal tissue following removal of complete ureteral obstruction. J. Urol., 100:596, 1968.

Schlossberg, S. M., and Vaughan, E. D., Jr.: The mechanism of unilateral post-obstructive diuresis. J. Urol., 131:534, 1984.

Schmidt, C. F., and Hayman, M., Jr.: A note upon lymph formation in the dog kidney and the effect of certain diuretics upon it. Am. J. Physiol., 91:157, 1929. Cited by Rusznyák, I., Földi, M., and Szabó, G.: Lymphatics and Lymph Circulation. New York, Pergamon Press, 1960.

Schroeder, H. A., and Neumann, C.: Arterial hypertension in rats. J. Exp. Med., 75:527, 1942.

Schwartz, D. T.: Unilateral upper urinary tract obstruction and arterial hypertension. N.Y. J. Med., 69:668, 1969.

Schwatz, M. M., Venkatachalam, M. A., and Cotran, R. S.: Reversible inner medullary vascular obstruction in acute experimental hydronephrosis. Am. J. Pathol., 86:425, 1977.

Scott, G. D.: Experimental hydronephrosis produced by complete and incomplete ligation of the ureter. Surg. Gynecol. Obstet., 15:296, 1912.

Selkurt, E. E., Brandfonbrener, M., and Geller, H. M.: Effects of ureteral pressure increase on renal hemodynamics and the handling of electrolytes and water. Am. J. Physiol., 170:61, 1952.

Seyer-Hansen, K.: Renal hypertrophy in experimental diabetes mellitus. Kidney Int., 23:643, 1983.

Shapiro, J. R., and Bennett, A. H.: Recovery of renal function after prolonged unilateral ureteral obstruction. J. Urol., 115:136, 1976.

Shearlock, K. T., and Howards, S. S.: Postobstructive anuria: A documented entity. J. Urol., 115:212, 1976.

Sheehan, H. L., and Davis, J. C.: Experimental hydronephrosis. Arch. Pathol., 68:185, 1959.

Sherman, R. A., and Blaufox, M. D.: Obstructive uropathy in patients with nonvisualization in renal scan. Nephron, 25:82, 1980.

Shimamura, T., Kissane, J. M., and Györkey, F.: Experimental hydronephrosis. Nephron dissection and electron microscopy of the kidney following obstruction of the ureter and in recovery from obstruction. Lab. Invest., 15:629, 1966.

Siegel, N. J., Feldman, R. A., Lytton, B., Hayslett, J. P., and Kashgarian, M.: Renal cortical blood flow distribution in obstructive nephropathy in rats. Circ. Res., 40:379, 1977.

Siegel, N. J., Upadhyaya, K., and Kashgarian, M.: Inhibition by indomethacin of adaptive changes in the contralateral kidney after release of unilateral ureteral obstruction. Kidney Int., 20:691, 1981.

Silber, S.: Growth of baby kidneys transplanted into adults. Surg. Forum, 26:579, 1975.

Silber, S.: Compensatory and obligatory renal growth in babies and adults. Aust. N. Z. J. Surg., 44:421, 1974.

Silber, S., and Crudop, J.: The three-kidney rat model. Invest. Urol., 11:466, 1974.

Silber, S., and Crudop, J.: Kidney transplantation in inbred rats. Am. J. Surg., 125:551, 1973.

Silber, S., and Malvin, R.: Compensatory and obligatory renal growth in rats. Am. J. Physiol., 226:114, 1974.

Silk, M. R., Homsy, G. E., and Merz, T.: Compensatory renal hyperplasia. J. Urol., 98:36, 1967.

Sirota, J. H., and Narins, L. Acute urinary suppression after ureteral catheterization: The pathogenesis of "Reflex anuria." N. Engl. J. Med., 257:1111, 1957.

Solez, K., Ponchak, S., Buono, R. H., Vernon, N., Finer, P. M., Miller, M., and Heptinstall, R. H.: Inner medullary plasma flow in the kidney with ureteral obstruction. Am. J. Physiol., 231:1315, 1976.

Stamey, T. A.: At last—a safe polyethylene ureteral catheter. Urol. Dig., 13:15, 1974.

Stamey, T. A.: Renovascular Hypertension. Baltimore, The Williams & Wilkins Co., 1963.

Stecker, J.F., Jr., and Gillenwater, J. Y.: Experimental partial ureteral obstruction. I, Alteration in renal function. Invest. Urol., 8:377, 1971.

Stecker, J. F., Jr., Panko, W. B., and Gillenwater, J. Y.: Relationship of renal substrate utilization and patterns of renal excretion. Invest. Urol., *11*:221, 1973.

Stecker, J. F., Jr., Vaughan, E. D., Jr., and Gillenwater, J. Y.: Alteration in renal metabolism occurring in ureteral obstruction in vivo. Surg. Gynecol. Obstet., *133*:846, 1971.

Steinhausen, M.: Measurement of tubular urine flows and tubular reabsorption under increased ureteral pressure. Pfluegers Arch., *298*:105, 1967.

Stoerk, H. G., Laragh, J. H., Aceto, R. M., and Budzilovich, T.: Edema and ascites following the ligation of both ureters in rats. Am. J. Pathol., *58*:51, 1970.

Strong, K. C.: Plastic studies in abnormal renal architecture. The parenchymal alterations in experimental hydronephrosis. Arch. Pathol., *29*:77, 1940.

Sugarman, J., Friedman, M., Barret, E., and Addis, T.: The distribution, flow, protein and urea content of renal lymph. Am. J. Physiol., *138*:108, 1942.

Suki, W., Eknoyan, G., Rector, F. C., Jr., and Seldin, D. W.: Patterns of nephron perfusion in acute and chronic hydronephrosis. J. Clin. Invest., *45*:122, 1966.

Taylor, M. G., and Ullmann, E.: Glomerular filtration after obstruction of the ureter. J. Physiol., *157*:38, 1961.

Thirakomen, K., Kozlov, N., Arruda, J., and Kurtzman, N.: Renal hydrogen ion secretion following the release of unilateral ureteral obstruction. Am. J. Physiol., *231*(4):1233, 1976.

Thurau, K.: Renal hemodynamics. Am. J. Med., *36*:698, 1964a.

Thurau, K. W.: Autoregulation of renal blood flow and glomerular filtration rate, including data on tubular and peritubular capillary pressures and vessel wall tension. Circ. Res., *15*[Suppl.]:132, 1964b.

Tormene, A., Millini, R., and Zangrando, O.: The role of the lymphatic system of the kidney in the physiopathology of ureteral obstruction. Urol. Int., *16*:341, 1963.

Tuffier, M.: Étude clinique et expérimentale sur l'hydronéphrose. Ann. Mal. Org. Genitourin., *12*:14, 1894. Cited by Cushny, A.: The Secretion of the Urine. London, Longmans, Green and Co., 1917.

Underwood, W. E.: Recent observations on the pathology of hydronephrosis. Proc. R. Soc. Med., *30*:817, 1937.

Vander, A. J., and Miller, R.: Control of renin secretion in the anesthetized dog. Am. J. Physiol., *207*:537, 1964.

Van Vroonhoven, T. J., Soler-Montesinos, L., and Malt, R. A.: Humoral regulation of renal mass. Surgery, *72*:300, 1972.

Vaughan, E. D., Jr., and Gillenwater, J. Y.: Unpublished data.

Vaughan, E. D., Jr., and Gillenwater, J. Y.: Diagnosis, characterization and management of postobstructive diuresis. J. Urol., *109*:286, 1973.

Vaughan, E. D., Jr., Bühler, F. R., and Laragh, J. H.: Normal renin secretion in hypertensive patients with primarily unilateral chronic hydronephrosis. J. Urol., *112*:153, 1974.

Vaughan, E. D., Jr., Shenasky, J. H., II, and Gillenwater, J. Y.: Mechanism of acute hemodynamic response to ureteral occlusion. Invest. Urol., *9*:109, 1971.

Vaughan, E. D., Jr., Sorenson, E. J., and Gillenwater, J. Y.: The renal hemodynamic response to chronic unilateral complete ureteral occlusion. Invest. Urol., *8*:78, 1970.

Vaughan, E. D., Jr., Sweet, R. E., and Gillenwater, J. Y.: Unilateral ureteral occlusion: Pattern of nephron repair and compensatory response. J. Urol., *109*:979, 1973.

Walls, J., Buerkert, J. E., Purkerson, M. L., and Klahr, S.: Nature of the acidifying defect after relief of ureteral obstruction. Kidney Int., *7*:304, 1975.

Waugh, W. H.: Circulatory autoregulation in the fully isolated kidney and in the humorally supported isolated kidney. Circ. Res., *15*[Suppl.]:156, 1964.

Wax, S. H.: Radioisotope uptake in experimental hydronephrosis. J. Urol., *99*:497, 1968.

Weidmann, P., Beretta-Piccoli, C., Hirsch, D., Reubi, F. C., and Massry, S. G.: Curable hypertension with unilateral hydronephrosis: studies on the role of circulating renin. Ann. Intern. Med., *87*:437, 1977.

Widén, T.: Restitution of kidney function after induced urinary stasis of varying duration. Acta Chir. Scand., *113*:507, 1957.

Williams, J. R., Jr., Wegria, R., and Harrison, T. R.: Relation of renal pressor substance to hypertension of hydronephrotic rats. Arch. Intern. Med., *62*:805, 1938.

Wilmer, H. A.: The disappearance of phosphatase from the hydronephrotic kidney. J. Exp. Med., *78*:225, 1943.

Wilson, B., Reisman, D. D., and Moyer, C. A.: Fluid balance in the urological patient. Disturbances in the renal regulation of the excretion of water and sodium salts following decompression of the urinary bladder. J. Urol., *66*:805, 1951.

Wilson, D. R.: Cross-circulation study of natriuretic factors in postobstructive diuresis. [Abstr.] Clin. Res., *22*:550A, 1974a.

Wilson, D. R.: The influence of volume expansion on renal function after relief of chronic unilateral ureteral obstruction. Kidney Int., *5*:402, 1974b.

Wilson, D. R.: Micropuncture study of chronic obstructive nephropathy before and after release of obstruction. Kidney Int., *2*:119, 1972.

Wilson, D. R.: Renal function during and following obstruction. Ann. Rev. Med., *28*:329, 1977.

Wilson, D. R., Honrath, U., and Sols, M.: Effect of acute and chronic renal denervation on renal function after release of unilateral ureteral obstruction in the rat. Can. J. Physiol. Pharmacol., *57*:731, 1979.

Wilson, D. R., Knox, W., Hall, E., and Sen, A. K.: Renal sodium- and potassium-activated adenosinetriphosphatase deficiency during postobstructive diuresis in the rat. Can. J. Physiol. Pharmacol., *52*:105, 1974.

Winberg, J.: Renal function in water-losing syndrome due to lower urinary tract obstruction before and after treatment. Acta Paediatr., *48*:149, 1959.

Winberg, J.: Renal function in congenital bladder neck obstruction. Acta. Chir. Scand., *116*:332, 1958.

Winton, F. R.: Influence of increase of ureteral pressure on the isolated mammalian kidney. J. Physiol., *71*:381, 1931.

Wise, H. M., Jr.: Hypertension resulting from hydronephrosis. JAMA, *231*:491, 1975.

Woodruff, M. W., Olson, H. W., and Alford, L. M.: Intravenous pyelographic visualization after complete ureteral obstruction with hypertonic solute loading. Invest. Urol., *13*:445, 1976.

Yarger, W. E., and Griffith, L. D.: Intrarenal hemodynamics following chronic unilateral ureteral obstruction in the dog. Am. J. Physiol., *227*:816, 1974.

Yarger, W. E., Aynedjian, H. S., and Bank, N.: A micropuncture study of postobstructive diuresis in the rat. J. Clin. Invest., *51*:625, 1972.

Yarger, W. E., Schocken, D. D., and Harris, R. H.: Obstructive nephropathy in the rat. J. Clin. Invest., *65*:400, 1980.

Zelman, S. J., Zenser, T. V., and Davis, B. B.: Renal growth in response to unilateral ureteral obstruction. Kidney Int., *23*:594, 1983.

Zetterström, R., Ericsson, N. O., and Winberg, J.: Separate renal function studies in predominantly unilateral hydronephrosis. Acta Paediatr., *47*:540, 1958.

CHAPTER 10

Extrinsic Obstruction of the Ureter

LESTER PERSKY, M.D.
ELROY D. KURSH, M.D.
STEWART FELDMAN, M.D.
MARTIN I. RESNICK, M.D.

The ureter is a fibromuscular conduit that traverses the retroperitoneum for a length of approximately 25 cm. Divided into abdominal and pelvic portions, the ureter relates closely to the retroperitoneal musculature, multiple visceral organs, and the vascular tree. The ureter is susceptible to the same pathologic conditions that affect the structures adjacent to it along its course. Tumors, including benign or malignant and primary or metastatic types, mass lesions such as cysts or lymphoceles, aneurysms, vascular anomalies, fluid such as blood or pus, and infectious as well as inflammatory processes may affect the ureter.

Most patients present with complaints suggesting upper urinary tract obstruction. Fever, flank pain, and gastrointestinal disturbances may appear alone or simultaneously. When the obstruction is bilateral, is slow in developing, and has been present a long time, severe renal failure with its accompanying complications may be the presenting problem. The symptom complexes associated with these conditions may mask those of ureteral obstruction. Hypertension may be the only presenting sign of unilateral obstruction. The mechanism of this is unclear, but increased renin levels have been implicated. Theories about the cause of the increased renin center on decreased renal blood flow, decreased glomerular filtration rate, and impaired tubular function (Andaloro, 1975; Strauss and Welt, 1971).

Neither the site nor the cause of the blockage may be readily apparent. The urologist, therefore, must use all his diagnostic tools to define the cause of the problem. Routine laboratory evaluations, including studies of serum electrolytes, blood urea nitrogen, serum creatinine, and creatinine clearance; urinalysis; and urine culture are all mandatory in the assessment of the obstructed patient. Excretory urography with prone, lateral, and oblique views; infusion and retrograde pyelography; barium studies; angiography; lymphangiography; and radioisotope renography are valuable radiologic procedures.

Ultrasonography and computerized tomography are very useful noninvasive techniques in the assessment of patients with ureteral obstruction (Krinsky et al., 1983). Hydronephrosis and ureteral dilatation can be accurately assessed, and the site of obstruction can often be accurately localized. Percutaneous antegrade pyelography is another technique that permits definition of the site of obstruction. An additional advantage of this invasive technique is that it can be a temporizing procedure and permit drainage of the kidney after placement of a nephrostomy tube through the needle tract. Ureteral dilatation performed through these tracts has also been reported to be of benefit in limited instances (Siegel et al., 1982). Nuclear magnetic resonance imaging is in its developmental stages, but in addition to the imaging qualities the study offers it provides physiologic information regarding renal blood flow and functional status. It is very likely that this study will provide valuable information regarding renal function that may aid the physician in choosing whether to attempt to preserve an obstructed kidney with a reconstructive procedure or whether to remove it.

There are multiple pathologic conditions that may be responsible for extrinsic obstruction of the ureter. Although extrinsic obstruction of the ureter is a relatively common finding, many of the disease entities that are responsible for this phenomenon obstruct the ureter uncommonly. The following classification was devised to allow the patient evaluation to be accomplished in an orderly, methodical fashion. The causes of obstruction are divided into these five major categories: (1) vascular lesions; (2) benign diseases of the female reproductive system; (3) diseases of the gastrointestinal tract; (4) diseases of the retroperitoneum; and (5) retroperitoneal masses. By attempting to place the cause of the ureteral obstruction under one of the five major headings, the urologist will be able to proceed with the work-up in an organized manner and avoid overlooking a major area of consideration.

VASCULAR LESIONS

Arterial Obstruction

ABDOMINAL AORTIC ANEURYSM

Ureteral obstruction may be secondary to an abdominal aortic aneurysm. Generally, an aneurysm deviates the ureter, pushing it laterally or drawing it medially. Because of its size, a large aneurysm may produce mechanical ureteral obstruction either unilaterally or bilaterally. The scarring and inflammation associated with the aneurysm can also encase and obstruct the ureter. There are two basic explanations for the development of perianeurysmic fibrosis and retroperitoneal scarring. One is that small leaks develop at the weakest points of the aneurysm. After these seal, a retroperitoneal inflammatory reaction ensues, resulting in scarring that may extend laterally to encase and obstruct the ureter. If this theory were true, the fibrous tissue should contain hemosiderin-laden macrophages, which have been conspicuously absent to date (Abbott et al., 1973). The second explanation relates to the generalized atherosclerotic process involved in the formation of the aneurysm. Atherosclerosis often has an associated desmoplastic inflammatory component that extends to involve the adventitia of the vessel and surrounding connective tissue, leading to scarring in the retroperitoneum (Abbott et al., 1973; Bainbridge and Woodward, 1982; McEntee et al., 1982).

Severe abdominal and low back pain of sudden onset is the symptom most often associated with an acute or dissecting abdominal aortic aneurysm. Patients may also complain of an abdominal mass, vague abdominal pain, and symptoms of peripheral vascular ischemia. Since an aneurysm may affect the ureter in as many as 10 per cent of cases, the urologist should be aware that these patients may seek care for urologic complaints such as flank pain, urinary tract infections, or fever. Rarely, unexplained azotemia associated with partial or complete obstruction and hydronephrosis may be the presenting problem (Abercrombie and Hendry, 1971; Labardini and Ratliff, 1967).

The diagnosis of a suspected aneurysm can generally be easily made. A pulsatile abdominal mass is almost always palpable. In addition, the examiner may find an abdominal bruit or absent femoral pulses. A plain film of the abdomen will usually demonstrate a rim of calcium outlining one wall of the aneurysm. Cross-table and true lateral x-ray films help delineate the size and position of the aneurysm. Excretory urography with lateral and oblique films establishes the presence of ureteral involvement (Fig. 10–1). Although lateral deviation of the ureter is more common, medial displacement may occur. At times, one ureter may be pushed laterally and the other drawn medially (Peck et

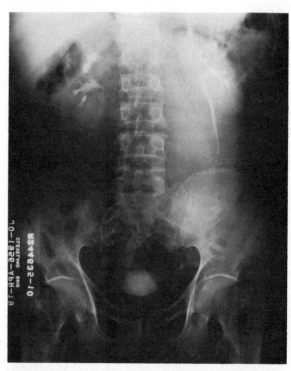

Figure 10–1. Marked deviation of the left ureter due to a large abdominal aortic aneurysm. The lower pole of the left kidney is also pushed to the left. Note the rim of calcium outlining the left wall of the aneurysm.

al., 1973). It has been suggested that ultrasonography may identify unsuspected retroperitoneal fibrosis associated with aortic aneurysms. A characteristic picture with the fibrous tissue lying anterior and anterolateral has been described (Henry et al., 1978). Although this latter picture may not be demonstrated in all cases, it is clear that ultrasound is a valuable technique in demonstrating both the aneurysm and the ureteral obstruction.

If the obstruction is severe enough to compromise kidney function, the surgeon should consider re-establishing adequate drainage of the urinary tract before resecting the aneurysm. Restoration of the best possible renal function is important, since relative renal ischemia with oliguria may be a sequela of aneurysm surgery. An effectively diuresing kidney will tolerate the ischemic insult much better than an obstructed one.

The treatment of choice of an inflammatory aneurysm with ureteral obstruction is aneurysmectomy with ureterolysis. The ureters are generally transplanted intraperitoneally or wrapped with retroperitoneal fat to prevent adherence to the residual inflammatory tissue or aneurysm wall. Care should be taken to preserve ureteral integrity when ureterolysis is performed. If urine from an obstructed, possibly infected, kidney is spilled into the retroperitoneum, the hazard of aortic graft infection is increased. Since graft infection is a possible lethal complication of aneurysm surgery, it is preferable to delay the aneurysm resection if a urine leak is suspected (Abbott et al., 1973; Bainbridge and Woodward, 1982; Wagenknecht and Madsen, 1970). An alternative to operative ureterolysis in patients who could not tolerate or who refuse surgery is the administration of steroids, which has been shown to relieve ureteral obstruction in a small number of cases (Clyne and Abercrombie, 1977).

ILIAC ARTERY ANEURYSM

Aneurysms of the internal and common iliac arteries rarely may cause ureteral obstruction. The mechanism of obstruction is the same as that described for aortic aneurysm. Operative treatment of the aneurysm usually results in relief of the obstruction (Kaufman, 1962) (Fig. 10–2).

ARTERIAL ANOMALIES

On rare occasions, a normal vessel taking a normal course and position may cause compression of the ureter (Fig. 10–3).

There are also a number of vascular anomalies that rarely may cause ureteral obstruction. Although obstruction may occur at any level, it is more frequent in the lower third of the ureter. The normal vessels may be present but with aberrant courses, or they may be rudimentary embryonic arteries that fail to disappear. The obturator (Bush, 1972), renal (Fletcher and Lecky, 1971), and common iliac arteries (Mehl, 1969) have all been reported to cause ureteral obstruction. Developmental anomalies such as a persistent umbilical artery may also cause obstruction of the ureter (Bush, 1972). The use of simultaneous pyelography and angiography is essential in making the diagnosis. Occasionally, selective angiography of the branches of the aorta is needed to delineate a small persistent embryonic vessel. Angiography done with a retrograde ureteral catheter in place is valuable to help demonstrate the point of obstruction. Treatment of a significantly obstructive vascular anomaly requires surgical exploration, at which time the surgeon must decide whether to resect the ureter or the offending vessel. When one is dealing with a rudimentary vessel, simple ligation and transection of the artery are all that is required. If major vessels are involved, transection and reanastamosis of the ureter are preferred.

OBSTRUCTIVE PHENOMENA DUE TO ARTERIAL REPAIR AND REPLACEMENT

Reconstructive vascular surgery is being performed with increasing frequency in the aged population for the treatment of peripheral and aortic vascular degenerative disease. Ureteral obstruction is a recognized complication of these procedures, but the true incidence of this problem is unknown (Antkowiak and D'Altorio, 1979; Sant et al., 1983). Retroperitoneal fibrosis secondary to the surgical procedure is the most common cause of ureteral obstruction. It is likely secondary to bleeding or excessive dissection, but other causes include direct surgical injury (ligation, ischemia) and pseudoaneurysm formation. Most patients present within 1 year following the vascular procedure, but delays up to 14 years have been reported. It is also of interest that, when evaluated, 13 per cent of the reported patients were free of symptoms and 30 per cent presented with nonurologic symptoms.

Treatment of these patients varies based on the patient's symptoms and the surgeon's experience. When contemplating repair, exact identification of the level of obstruction is essential (Fig. 10–4). In one prospective study (Heard and Hinde, 1975) of 20 patients, routine IVP's demonstrated that 20 per cent had partial

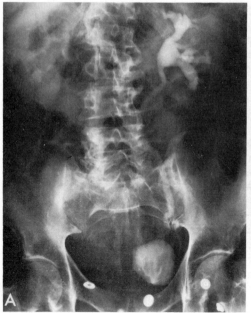
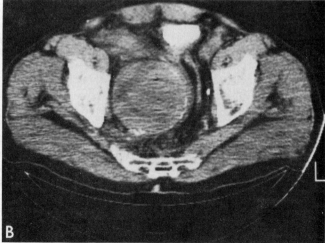
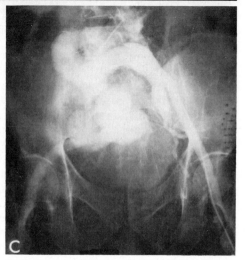

Figure 10–2. Right ureteral obstruction secondary to an aneurysm of the right hypogastric artery. *A*, Intravenous urogram demonstrating delayed visualization of right kidney and marked deviation of urinary bladder. *B*, Computerized tomographic scan demonstrating large aneurysm. Note calcification of wall. *C*, Arteriogram demonstrating extent of aneurysm.

ureteral obstruction at 2 weeks but that at 1 year resolution occurred spontaneously in half of the group. Ureterolysis is the most common repair instituted and can be performed with or without intraperitonealization. Ureteral resection and ureteroureterostomy and division and reanastomosis of the vascular graft are less frequently performed reparative procedures.

Venous Obstruction

OVARIAN VEIN SYNDROME

The ovarian veins are formed by multiple small pelvic venous channels not unlike the pampiniform plexus in the male. Joined by uterine branches, the multiple veins fuse to form single ovarian veins before crossing the pelvic brim. As the ovarian veins course over the iliac vessels, they lie only ½ inch anterior to the ureter in its midportion, crossing it to join the vena cava at the level of the third lumbar vertebra. On the left, the ovarian vein also crosses the ureter to enter the renal vein. These anatomic relationships make the ovarian veins a potential cause of ureteral obstruction (Roberts, 1970). The obstruction usually involves only the right ureter, except for conditions that cause stasis in the left renal vein with resultant enlargement of the left ovarian vein, such as encasement by carcinoma or thrombosis (Melnick and Bramwit, 1971).

In a recent article, Dure-Smith (1979) presented a convincing argument that the ovarian vein syndrome is a myth. It is questionable whether the ovarian veins have ever produced a significant obstruction at any level or whether from theoretical considerations they would ever be expected to do so. Therefore, a discussion of the ovarian vein syndrome may be of only historical interest.

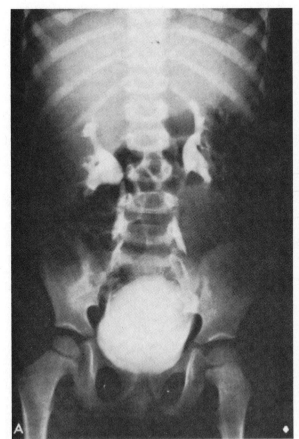 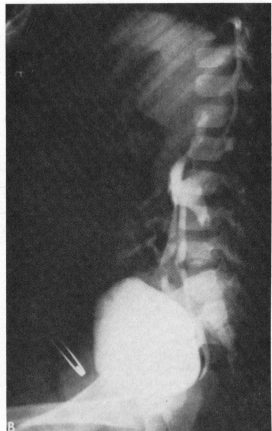

Figure 10–3. *A*, Bilateral compression of the ureters as they course over the bifurcation of the common iliac arteries in a young boy. Although there is mild dilatation of the upper ureters, the pelvocalyceal systems are normal.

B, A lateral x-ray film demonstrates the posterior relationship of the offending vessels.

Supposedly, the patient with ovarian vein syndrome usually notes the onset of symptoms during pregnancy and is multiparous, although the entity has been reported in women who have never been pregnant. The symptoms associated with recurrent urinary tract infections may also represent the presenting complaints. Most patients experience right-sided flank pain, which is generally described as a constant ache but may mimic renal colic. The pain may begin several days before menses and disappear afterward (Polse and Bobo, 1969).

Excretory urography, retrograde pyelography, and simultaneous angiography are utilized to establish the diagnosis. The obstruction most commonly occurs at the pelvic brim, where the ureter crosses the bifurcation of the common iliac artery, (Fig. 10–5) and not usually at the level of the third or fourth lumbar vertebra, where the ovarian vein crosses the ureter (Dure-Smith, 1979). Operative treatment consists of mobilization of the ureter with ligation of the offending ovarian vein. It has been emphasized that it is important to lyse the ureter well into its pelvic position to make certain that multiple areas of obstruction due to a single large ovarian vein or plexus of veins are not overlooked.

It is doubtful that the ovarian vein syndrome exists. The ureteral dilatation that is supposedly characteristic of the ovarian vein syndrome is identical to the dilatation that occurs during pregnancy. These changes may persist as unobstructed dilatation post-partum (Dure-Smith, 1979). Some of the newer diagnostic studies, such as the Lasix renogram, or percutaneous techniques, such as the Whitaker test, should be helpful in determining if the ureteral dilatation is the result of a bona fide obstruction or if it represents a persistent non-obstructed postpregnancy dilatation.

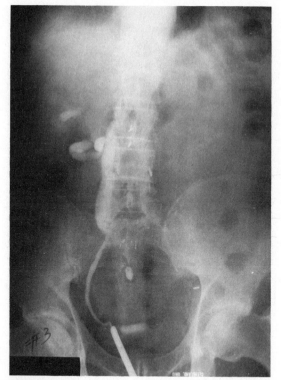

Figure 10–4. Right ureteral obstruction secondary to a vascular graft bypassing the right iliac vessels. Patient presented 2 years post surgery with complaints of dull but persistent right flank pain.

The principal differential diagnosis includes thrombosis of an adnexal mass, broad ligament hematoma with abscess formation, appendicitis, and perinephric abscess. Theoretically, treatment by anticoagulation therapy alone might suffice but so far has been used only as an adjunct to surgery. Operative treatment has consisted of ligation of both ovarian veins and usually extirpation of the veins. Ligation of the inferior vena cava has also been undertaken and is considered to be mandatory in suppurative pelvic thrombophlebitis or in the presence of pulmonary embolization.

POST-PARTUM OVARIAN VEIN THROMBOPHLEBITIS

Ovarian vein syndrome should be differentiated from post-partum ovarian vein thrombophlebitis (Dure-Smith, 1979). Post-partum thrombosis of the ovarian veins appears to be an infrequent phenomenon, but many cases may go unrecognized and some fatal post-partum pulmonary emboli may have originated from the ovarian veins.

Post-partum ovarian vein thrombophlebitis is a well-defined entity with characteristic clini-

cal features and is potentially lethal (Lynch et al., 1966; Mackler and Royster, 1968; Rosenblum et al., 1966; Mitty, 1974). Definite ureteral obstruction occurs commonly. The disease usually presents immediately post-partum. It is more common in multiparous women and involves the right side much more frequently than the left, although it may be bilateral. The patients complain of lower abdominal pain, but often the pain is in only the right lower quadrant and may radiate to the flank. There is a moderate fever and leukocytosis. A poorly defined adnexal mass may be palpable.

The etiology of the disease has been ascribed to a variety of coagulation defects that are not uncommonly associated with pregnancy and the immediate post-partum period and that lead to a hypercoagulable state. Ureteral obstruction that is common results from extension of the inflammatory process to the periureteral tissues.

RETROCAVAL URETER

The retrocaval ureter is a congenital abnormality in which the right ureter passes behind the vena cava, leading to varying degrees of ureteral compression. The etiologic factor in the syndrome is the embryologic development of the ureter (Considine, 1966). The metanephros develops in the pelvis, rising through a ring of

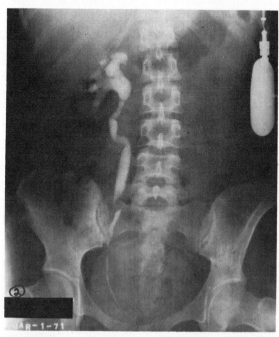

Figure 10–5. A right hydronephrosis extends to the area of the bifurcation of the common iliac artery. In the past these were thought to be consistent with ovarian vein syndrome.

embryonic venous channels as it moves to a lumbar position. The major venous channels in the very young embryo are the posterior cardinal veins. The minor venous channels, the subcardinal veins, are connected to the post-cardinal veins by numerous prominent anastomotic vessels. The supracardinal veins, which generally develop into the inferior vena cava, become apparent in the 15-mm embryo dorsal to the developing ureters. The posterior cardinal veins and the subcardinal veins lie ventral to the definitive ureteral position. Normally, the posterior cardinal vein undergoes complete regression caudal to the renal vein, allowing the ureter to assume a normal position ventral to the developing infrarenal vena cava (supracardinal vein). The subcardinal vein remains as a tributary of the inferior vena cava, the gonadal vein. Persistence of the posterior cardinal vein as the major portion of the infrarenal inferior vena cava causes medial displacement and compression of the ureter following the lateral migration of the kidney. The ureter spirals from a dorsolateral position above to a ventromedial position below around the developing inferior vena cava. Variants of the condition include duplication of the vena cava with the ureter lying beside, behind, or between the vascular limbs. The anomaly develops almost exclusively on the right side (Lepage and Baldwin, 1972; Polse and Bobo, 1969).

The onset of symptoms usually occurs during the fourth decade of life, with men predominating by a ratio of 3:1. Most patients complain of right lumbar pain, which is usually described as a dull intermittent ache but may resemble renal colic. Patients may have associated recurrent urinary tract infections or episodes suggesting recurrent acute right pyelonephritis. Symptoms may actually be attributable to calculi, the incidence of which is increased owing to stasis. Microscopic or gross hematuria is frequently present (Brito et al., 1973).

The diagnosis is made by demonstrating the characteristic changes on excretory urography. The ureter makes a typical reversed J deformity as it passes from the pelvis under the vena cava at the third or fourth lumbar vertebra. A varying degree of hydronephrosis is noted proximal to the obstruction. A right oblique x-ray film will demonstrate the close relationship of the right upper ureter to the vena cava. Retrograde pyelography may show the tortuous ureter to be in the shape of an italic S, beginning just above the pelvic brim and ending below the renal pelvis (Fig. 10–6), but it may not be possible to pass a ureteral catheter beyond the postcaval

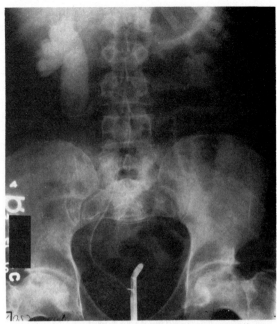

Figure 10–6. Retrograde urography shows the typical reversed-J deformity secondary to a retrocaval ureter. The retrograde catheter takes the shape of an italic S beginning just above the pelvic brim.

segment. These findings, coupled with the confirmation of the position of the ureter on an inferior venacavogram, are sufficient to make the diagnosis. It is often helpful to confirm the circumcaval route of the ureter by performing inferior venacavography with a ureteral catheter in place (Shown and Moore, 1971).

No therapy other than observation is indicated for patients without symptoms and with minimal or no caliectasis. Occasionally, nephrectomy is the procedure of choice in the presence of marked hydronephrosis and cortical atrophy if the contralateral kidney is normal. Surgery is required for the treatment of the hydronephrosis or related symptomatic problems. Harrill (1940) initially emphasized that the position of the ureter and involved structures makes transection of the pelvis with transposition and reanastomosis the most efficacious surgical treatment. The operation, therefore, is essentially a dismembered pyeloplasty. We prefer an unsplinted, unstented anastomosis with no proximal diversion. A transabdominal transperitoneal operative approach is preferred because of the ease of access to the vital structures, should the need to reach them arise. Considine (1966) suggests that the Harrill procedure should be more appropriately called the caudal division of the dilated segment, since the original ureteropelvic junction is often obliterated by the dilatation of the proximal ureter. The performance of the anastomosis as far distal on the dilated segment as possible has the advantage of preserving the blood supply of this segment, which comes from the renal artery. At times, severe adhesions make lysis of the ureter from the vena cava impossible. In this situation, the compressed segment is resected and left in situ. The ureter is then anastomosed to the proximal dilated segment anterior to the inferior vena cava. Transection with reanastomosis of the inferior vena cava has also been done but is generally not recommended.

BENIGN CONDITIONS OF THE FEMALE REPRODUCTIVE SYSTEM

Benign Pelvic Masses

PREGNANCY

Pregnancy may deleteriously affect the upper urinary tract. The cause of ureteral obstruction during pregnancy is thought to be primarily mechanical pressure from the gravid uterus. Right ureteral obstruction is more common than left. One explanation for the increased incidence of right ureteral obstruction in pregnancy is the protection of the left ureter by the interposed sigmoid colon between the ureter and the uterus. Another explanation is related to the asymmetry of the anatomic structures at the pelvic brim, particularly the iliac arteries, making the right ureter more prominent and susceptible to compression. Although rare, bilateral obstruction may also occur (Fig. 10–7) (Badr, 1973; Lapata and Adelson, 1970; D'Elia et al., 1982). Several investigators have implicated progesterone as a cause of ureteral stasis and obstruction during pregnancy. There is laboratory evidence that a large dose of progesterone decreases ureteral peristalsis, but there is no clear-cut evidence that physiologic levels of the hormone have a significant effect on the genitourinary system (Roberts and Dykhuizen, 1970; Roberts, 1971).

The symptoms of ureteral obstruction during pregnancy may be masked by the physiologic changes associated with pregnancy itself. Nausea; pain in the back, flank, and lower abdomen; dysuria; and frequency may be associated with either ureteral obstruction or pregnancy. Progression of symptoms or localization to the flank suggests the possibility of significant ureteral obstruction, particularly if there is an associated fever or urinary tract infection.

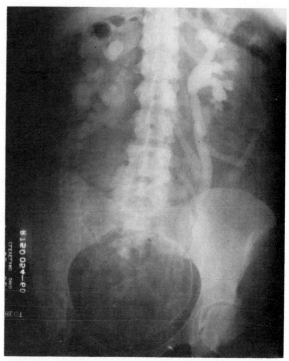

Figure 10–7. Bilateral hydronephrosis due to a gravid uterus during the third trimester. Following delivery, the hydronephrosis resolved.

If urine cultures show a persistent urinary tract infection despite appropriate antibiotic therapy, or if there is severe flank pain, further evaluation is required. Evaluation of a pregnant patient is a problem, since multiple x-ray studies cannot be safely used, especially during the first and second trimesters, because of the possibility of causing abnormal fetal development. Therefore, ultrasound is the preferred method of determining the presence of ureteral obstruction and radioisotope renography is a simple, safe means of estimating excretory function (Badr, 1973). During the first trimester, renography usually shows normal findings. Over the ensuing months, there is a progressive increase in dilatation of the urinary tract and a delay in excretion. As the pregnancy approaches term, the incidence of abnormal findings on renography approaches 70 per cent on the right side and 50 per cent on the left (Bergstrom, 1975).

If a patient is refractory to treatment, drainage of the ureter with retrograde ureteral catheterization may be necessary. This is done for a period sufficiently long to allow the infection to subside and adequate blood levels of antibiotics to be obtained. An alternative approach to long-term drainage of the upper tracts is the insertion of double J ureteral catheters. Antimicrobial therapy until the pregnancy is completed is a consideration for patients with significant obstruction and recurrent infections. Post-partum, a complete urologic investigation should be undertaken.

EXTRAUTERINE PREGNANCY

Ureteral obstruction secondary to chronic ectopic pregnancy has been reported but is apparently an extremely rare occurrence. Although ectopic pregnancy is a common problem, occurring in approximately 1 in every 1000 gravid women, the chronic ectopic pregnancy is very rare, since it is unusual for a ruptured ectopic pregnancy to seal off without causing significant clinical manifestations. Ureteral obstruction occurs from the pressure effect of the pelvic mass in association with periureteral fibrosis (Hovatanakul et al., 1971). There has also been a report of ureteral obstruction associated with another rare form of extrauterine pregnancy, the abdominal pregnancy (Levitt and Ingram, 1947).

MASS LESIONS OF THE UTERUS AND OVARY

Benign pelvic masses such as the fibroid uterus and cystic ovary may cause deviation and extrinsic obstruction of the ureter. Ureteral obstruction secondary to hydrometrocolpos has also been reported. Years ago, the reported incidence of ureteral involvement due to benign pelvic masses was as high as 50 to 65 per cent. Although the incidence may be less today, it is generally known that ureteral obstruction is a frequent finding with benign pelvic masses. The incidence increases as the size of the mass enlarges, especially if it projects above the pelvic brim.

Because of the frequency of upper urinary tract involvement, excretory urography is a mandatory part of the evaluation of all patients with pelvic masses. Ultrasonography and computerized tomography not only are valuable in determining the presence of ureteral obstruction but also provide information regarding the size, shape, and consistency of the pelvic mass. The preoperative assessment also helps prevent ureteral injury during exploratory laparotomy. The most common site of obstruction is the point where the ureter crosses the iliac vessels. Uterine fibroids most commonly affect the right side, but they may cause deviation or obstruction of the left ureter or both ureters (Fig. 10–8). As discussed in the section on pregnancy, the right ureter is involved more often because of the interposition of the sigmoid colon between the uterus and the left ureter and the increased prominence of the right ureter as it crosses the

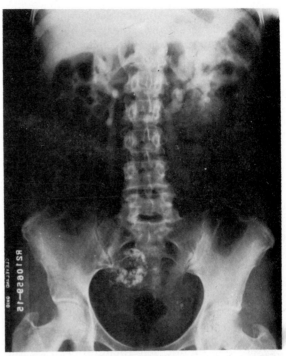

Figure 10–8. Bilateral hydronephrosis secondary to a large calcified fibroid uterus. Following a hysterectomy, the upper urinary tracts returned to normal.

right iliac artery. Generally, the ureters are deviated laterally. Ovarian cysts, which may push the ureter in a lateral or medial direction, affect the ureters less often. The ureteral obstruction and hydronephrosis are generally relieved following treatment with pelvic laparotomy and excision of the mass.

OVARIAN REMNANTS

Although rare, there have been several cases reported of obstruction of the pelvic ureter secondary to ovarian remnants (Bernie, 1972). Normally, removal of an entire ovary is a simple procedure. If the ovary and adjacent structures are involved in an extensive disease process, distorting the anatomic relationships and making the surgical dissection difficult, implantation of portions of the ovary into the exposed retroperitoneum may occur. The functioning ovarian remnant in the retroperitoneum may liberate an ovum. Rupture of an ovarian follicle is thought to be partially dependent upon the enzymatic activity of the liquor folliculi. Possibly, retroperitoneal reaction to the liquor folliculi is responsible for the extrinsic ureteral obstruction (Horowitz and Elguezabal, 1966).

Since the establishment of ureteral obstruction may depend on the liberation of an ovum, flank pain of a cyclic nature may be noted. This, in addition to a history of a previous difficult oophorectomy, suggests the possible diagnosis of an ovarian remnant (Horowitz and Elguezabal, 1966). The diagnosis is confirmed at laparotomy if a cystic retroperitoneal mass is found. Surgical treatment consists of removal of the mass, along with ureterolysis.

GARTNER'S DUCT CYST

A Gartner's duct cyst may displace the distal ureter and thus represents a theoretical cause of ureteral obstruction. The wolffian duct originally drains the embryonic pronephros and, later, the mesonephros. After the ureters have budded from its distal end, the wolffian duct atrophies in the female. The atrophic wolffian duct is known as Gartner's duct, a vestigial structure extending down the anterolateral margin of the vagina. Incomplete obliteration of the canal with subsequent epithelial secretory activity may lead to the development of retention cysts.

The diagnosis is deduced from the location of the cyst on the anterolateral wall of the vagina, usually near the upper end. No treatment is required for small asymptomatic cysts. Large cysts may protrude through the introitus and may cause local discomfort, dyspareunia, infertility, or dystocia. Transvaginal excision is the treatment for large symptomatic cysts. Rarely, a large Gartner's duct cyst may displace the distal ureter upward over the cyst wall. If this occurs, an abdominal approach has been recommended, since the cysts tend to be adherent to the bladder wall and since exposure of the ureter is improved (Rhame and Derrick, 1973).

Pelvic Inflammations

TUBO-OVARIAN ABSCESS

A patient with a tubo-ovarian abscess usually has a history of acute or chronic pelvic inflammatory disease (PID), although occasionally an abscess may develop secondary to the use of an intrauterine device in an individual who has no prior history of pelvic inflammatory disease or who has a negative gonococcal culture. Hydroureteronephrosis is frequently found in association with tubo-ovarian abscesses. Phillips (1974) reported ureteral dilation and obstruction in 17 of 45 patients with this lesion.

Abdominal pain, fever, nausea, and vomiting are the common presenting symptoms, although tubo-ovarian abscess has been reported in patients who complain of vaginal bleeding alone. The physical examination usually elicits bilateral lower abdominal pain with signs of peritoneal irritation. Pelvic examination reveals a tender adnexal mass or bilateral masses. At times, there may be a purulent exudate from the cervical os.

On roentgenologic examination, the presence of extraluminal pelvic air suggests the diagnosis of an abscess. Pelvic ultrasound is an excellent method of demonstrating the abscess. Because of the high incidence of ureteral obstruction and the risk of iatrogenic ureteral injury at the time of surgery, excretory urography or ultrasonography should be done routinely in a patient with a tubo-ovarian abscess. The ureteral blockage usually occurs at or below the pelvic brim, and in about half the patients the obstruction is bilateral. The ureter is deviated laterally in most patients, but in approximately one third, medial deviation is found. It is felt that the location of an abscess in the posterior cul-de-sac is responsible for the medial displacement. In this location, the abscess expands in an anterior direction, pushing the ureter medially. The inflammation and fibrosis associated with the abscess also function to pull the ureter medially or laterally (Phillips, 1974).

Treatment of the tubo-ovarian abscess generally consists of total abdominal hysterectomy with bilateral salpingo-oophorectomy. Aggressive surgery is recommended before the abscess perforates intraperitoneally. Although the likelihood of subsequent conception is small, a lesser procedure such as a unilateral salpingo-oophorectomy may be attempted in younger patients who desire children. This suboptimal form of surgical therapy demands careful postoperative follow-up. The deviated ureter increases the risk of ureteral injury, making the immediate preoperative placement of ureteral catheters advisable in this situation. Treatment of the abscess generally results in resolution of the ureteral obstruction.

ENDOMETRIOSIS

Endometriosis is a prevalent problem in premenopausal women, occurring in as many as 10 to 20 per cent, with a peak age incidence between 25 and 40 years. The disease is best described as the existence of normal endometrium in an ectopic location (Dick et al., 1973). Ureteral obstruction from either an extrinsic or an intrinsic endometrioma is rare, but the urologist and gynecologist must be aware of the possibility of ureteral involvement because of the high rate of unsalvageable kidneys that results (Fig. 10–9). A variable incidence of

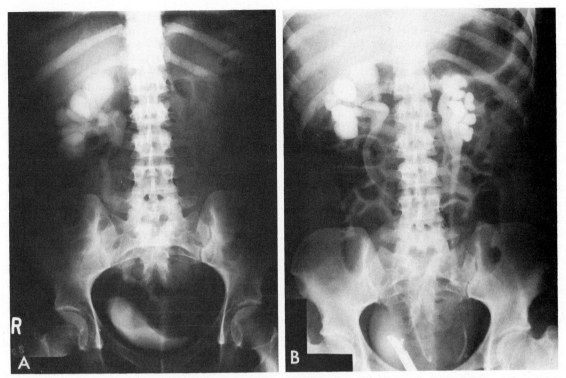

Figure 10–9. *A*, Excretory urogram reveals severe right hydroureteronephrosis and no apparent function of the right kidney in a patient with extensive endometriosis. *B*, Retrograde urography demonstrates obstruction of distal ureters. A right ureteroneocystostomy, total abdominal hysterectomy, and bilateral salpingo-oophorectomy were performed.

urinary tract involvement (ureter and bladder) of 1 to 11 per cent in women afflicted with endometriosis has been reported (Stanley et al., 1965). When the ureter is involved, the process is usually confined to the pelvic ureter. The resultant extrinsic obstruction of the ureter is primarily due to the dense adhesions associated with the endometrioma.

The symptoms associated with the condition often reflect the organs involved as well as the primary disease process itself. Patients complain of severe dysmenorrhea due to sloughing of the proliferative endometrium during menstruation. The pain and discomfort abate during pregnancy or when the women are taking progestational agents blocking ovulation and menstruation. When ureteral obstruction is present, symptoms range from mild flank pain to urosepsis and renal failure, although in most instances urologic complaints are so subtle that they go unnoticed. Intrinsic endometriomas of the ureter are even more rare than extrinsic lesions but are more likely to cause cyclic hematuria.

The diagnosis of endometriosis is established on the basis of history and pelvic examination. The finding of an adherent ovary or small, indurated, irregular, firm, and tender nodularities in the cul-de-sac or uterosacral ligaments is diagnostic of endometriosis (Gray, 1975). Since most reported cases have had a paucity of symptoms referable to the urinary tract, the diagnosis of ureteral involvement is difficult to establish unless there is a high index of suspicion. Consequently, when obstruction occurs, a nonvisualizing or severely hydronephrotic kidney is frequently encountered on the excretory urogram (Fig. 10–9). The routine use of excretory urography and/or ultrasonography in patients with pelvic endometriosis is therefore recommended in an attempt to diagnose ureteral obstruction at an earlier, salvageable stage. The radiographic findings in endometriosis of the ureter are nonspecific, at times resembling stricture or tumor of the pelvic ureter. Retrograde pyelography is helpful in delineating the lower ureter. Generally, it is impossible to pass a ureteral catheter beyond the obstruction, located most frequently 3 to 4 cm above the ureteral orifice. At pelvic laparotomy, the presence of the so-called chocolate cyst, which is an ovary filled with old retained blood, alerts the surgeon to the diagnosis of endometriosis.

Hormone therapy relieves the primary symptoms associated with endometriosis but does little to relieve the ureteral obstruction. Although there have been scattered reports of partial success with nonoperative therapy, this mode of treatment is not recommended, since the ureteral obstruction is primarily secondary to the dense adhesions associated with the endometriosis. The scarring and inflammatory reaction associated with the disease also make the surgical correction of this problem difficult and hazardous. Combined castration, total abdominal hysterectomy, and ureterolysis is the procedure of choice for patients with severe ureteral obstruction and for women who do not desire further pregnancies. A lesser procedure may be attempted if the ureteral obstruction is not too severe and the patient wishes to bear more children. The area of involvement will dictate the extent of the surgery. Extensive ovarian involvement generally necessitates a unilateral oophorectomy, with meticulous dissection and removal of the endometrioma and ureterolysis. When a more conservative operative procedure is utilized, careful follow-up is required to ensure relief of the ureteral obstruction and to ensure that the problem does not recur. During ureterolysis, careful inspection of the ureter may demonstrate associated fibrosis and stricture secondary to ureteral involvement by the endometrioma. In these instances, ureterolysis is not sufficient, and partial ureterectomy must be done with ureteroureterostomy. Nephrectomy is necessary in those patients with severe hydronephrosis, particularly if there is associated sepsis. This procedure has been done in many of the reported cases of extrinsic obstruction of the ureter by endometriosis, since the diagnosis is rarely established early.

Ureteral obstruction by extrinsic endometriosis has also recently been reported in a postmenopausal patient. The administration of conjugated estrogens to a nulliparous patient who had undergone a previous panhysterectomy apparently played an etiologic role. The ureteral obstruction was relieved after the hormones were discontinued (Brooks et al., 1969).

PERIURETERAL INFLAMMATION ASSOCIATED WITH CONTRACEPTION

Contraception has become a worldwide concern during the past few decades. Utilization of the intrauterine contraceptive device (IUD) has led to a number of complications, the most important being infection, perforation, and bleeding. There was a report of ureteral obstruction secondary to parametritis resulting from the long-term use of the IUD (Kirk et al., 1971). The incidence of pelvic inflammatory disease

associated with the IUD is approximately 1 to 1.5 per cent. Therefore, ureteral obstruction may be found more frequently if this complication is anticipated. Also, the urologist and gynecologist should consider parametritis associated with the IUD in the differential diagnosis of ureteral obstruction. Treatment with broad-spectrum antibiotics coupled with removal of the IUD has led to resolution of both the parametritis and the ureteral obstruction.

A case of ureteral injury resulting in ureteral obstruction and extravasation of urine was reported secondary to the use of the laparoscope for tubal sterilization (Stengel et al., 1974). We have seen a patient with partial ureteral obstruction without extravasation following laparoscopic sterilization (Fig. 10–10). Excessive coagulation to achieve hemostasis of the fallopian tube stumps lying against the posterior peritoneum adjacent to the ureter is probably responsible for the ureteral injury. Therefore, it is important to lift the fallopian stumps free before applying the current, and only a moderate current should be used for a short period of time.

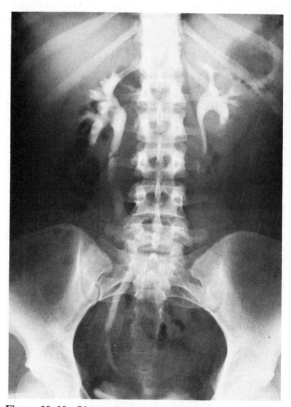

Figure 10–10. Obstruction of short segment of distal right ureter following laparoscopic sterilization. This obstruction probably resulted from excessive coagulation of the fallopian tube stumps lying against the posterior peritoneum, adjacent to the ureter.

Uterine Prolapse

The incidence of hydronephrosis associated with uterine prolapse is in the vicinity of 5 per cent. Moreover, hydroureteronephrosis occurs as often as 30 to 80 per cent of the time in patients with severe uterine prolapse. Although the mechanism is not clearly understood, there are several proposed explanations for the ureteral obstruction in women with procidentia. Obstruction of the urethra secondary to the prolapse has been ruled out as a possible cause, since large residual volumes have not been found. A bowstring effect caused by intramural stretching of the ureter has been considered a possible cause of obstruction, but radiographic and autopsy studies have failed to demonstrate the occurrence of such a phenomenon. The most reasonable explanation is the compression of the ureters outside the bladder.

As the bladder, uterus, and ureters are herniated through the weakness in the levator ani muscles, the ureters may be compressed between the uterus and the bladder, against the levators. The sections of the ueterterine arteries that cross in front of the distal ureters or the branches of the uterine vessels that form a vascular plexus surrounding the ureter may represent possible points of obstruction by acting as a sling over and around the ureter as the vessels are stretched from the procidentia. Excretory urography and autopsy examination have suggested that the point of obstruction is in the vicinity of the uterine vessels, making the second explanation more plausible.

Urinary infection, sepsis, pyonephrosis, and renal insufficiency have all been reported to be associated with uterine prolapse. Despite this and the high incidence of hydroureteronephrosis associated with uterine prolapse, urologic investigation is frequently not done preoperatively or postoperatively. In one review, excretory urography was done for less than 40 per cent of the patients with uterine prolapse admitted to a large university medical center (Lattimer, 1974). Both the gynecologist and the urologist must be aware of the need for the routine use of excretory urography or ultrasonography in the evaluation of patients with uterine prolapse.

Surgical repair of the prolapse by means of a vaginal hysterectomy and vaginoplasty is the preferred therapy. If operative therapy cannot be undertaken, a pessary may be used to reduce the uterine prolapse in an attempt to diminish the ureteral obstruction.

Ureteral Ligation

Ligation of the ureter is a form of extrinsic obstruction of the ureter that occurs iatrogenically. A surgeon may inadvertently place a suture around a ureter during abdominal or retroperitoneal surgery. Since more than 50 per cent of the cases develop during gynecologic procedures, ureteral ligation is included in this section. The incidence of ureteral damage in routine hysterectomy is less than 0.5 per cent, but alarmingly, when it occurs it is bilateral in approximately 1 out of every 6 cases (Donovan and Ragibson, 1973). Ureteral obstruction has been reported to occur following urethropexy for treatment of urinary incontinence (Kissinger et al., 1982). In these instances, sutures placed in the region of the bladder neck inadvertently pass through the bladder wall and underlying ureteral orifice. Although far less commonly than in gynecologic operations, ureteral ligation may occur during general surgical procedures such as colorectal surgery or during a difficult retrocecal appendectomy.

After its descent into the true pelvis, the ureter lies in intimate proximity to the female genital organs, making it subject to injury. The ureter is dorsal to the ovary, lateral to the infundibulopelvic ligament, and medial to the ovarian vessels. It enters the broad ligament approximately 9 or 10 cm below the iliac vessels and travels along the lateral aspect of the uterus. It then crosses the vesicovaginal space ¾ inch lateral to the uterine cervix, above the lateral fornix of the vagina. Here it is in intimate proximity to the uterine artery, which crosses above and in front, close to the ureterovesical junction. Most commonly, the ureter is damaged (1) in the ovarian fossa, during excision of large tumors or cysts; (2) in the infundibulopelvic ligament, when this is taken during hysterectomy; (3) where the ureter crosses dorsal to the uterine artery, as the artery is ligated and divided; or (4) in the vesicovaginal space, during the process of reperitonealization (Persky and Hoch, 1972).

Obviously, the best treatment for intraoperative ureteral injury is prophylaxis. In patients with pelvic masses, pelvic inflammatory disease, previous surgery adjacent to the ureter, and previous irradiation therapy, preoperative urography is indicated to ascertain the course of the ureter and the presence of ureteral obstruction. It is also advisable to obtain an excretory urogram before surgery if a difficult dissection is anticipated in the vicinity of the ureter.

The immediate preoperative placement of ureteral catheters is helpful if the surgeon expects to encounter difficulty adjacent to the ureter. If catheters are employed, they should be No. 6 French in size, since smaller catheters are difficult to palpate and larger ones may cause appreciable mucosal edema. The surgeon must not rely on the catheters for more than guidance in determining the presence of the ureter near the field of dissection. They do not prevent ureteral injury; only careful meticulous dissection in the area of the ureter can accomplish this.

When the surgeon recognizes that the ureter has been included in a ligature during an operation, the suture should be removed immediately and the injured area inspected. In most instances, nothing further is required. If the ureter appears nonviable, the area is resected and a primary anastomosis performed, or if the injury is sufficiently close to the bladder, a ureteroneocystotomy is done. Kinking of the ureter by a ligature is rectified with careful dissection (Persky and Hoch, 1972).

Unfortunately, in most instances ureteral ligation is not discovered until the postoperative period. If the patient develops flank pain, unexplained fever, leukocytosis, a paralytic ileus, or anuria, excretory urography is indicated. Retrograde pyelography is also helpful in delineating the point of obstruction. The passage of a retrograde catheter may be of therapeutic value if the obstruction is incomplete, as occurs when the ureter is kinked. If a catheter can negotiate the blocked area, further therapy is usually not required. Most patients need surgical relief of the obstruction. Formerly, a staged procedure with initial urinary diversion, such as a nephrostomy, was advised before the point of obstruction was attacked. This approach was based on the degree of anatomic distortion, the anticipated inflammatory response, and the threat of hemorrhage in the early postoperative period in the area of the ligated ureter. Reports of the successful early use of the direct approach in procedures such as ureteral deligation or ureteroneocystotomy to relieve the obstruction indicate that the staged procedure is usually no longer required (Herman et al., 1972; Hoch et al., 1975). Preliminary diversion is still advised if a marked inflammatory response or a large hematoma is anticipated in the area of the ligated ureter or if the patient is septic or a poor candidate for surgery. Today, percutaneous techniques are generally used to perform the nephrostomy.

DISEASES OF THE GASTROINTESTINAL TRACT

GRANULOMATOUS (CROHN'S) DISEASE OF THE BOWEL

The urologic complications of granulomatous (Crohn's) disease of the bowel, also known as regional enteritis or enterocolitis, include uric acid calculi, fistulae to the bladder, and the nephrotic syndrome secondary to renal amyloidosis. In addition, in the last 20 years, several reports have indicated that obstructive hydronephrosis is a frequent but seldom recognized complication. Present and associates (1963) noted a 7 per cent incidence of ureteral obstruction associated with granulomatous disease of the bowel, although they suggested that this rate may reflect the high incidence of complicated cases of this disease referred to their large center. Using radioactive renography as a more sensitive index of ureteral stasis, Schofield and associates (1968) found stasis in 50 per cent of the patients with regional enteritis.

Extrinsic compression of the ureter appears to be caused by the retroperitoneal extension of the severe inflammatory process. The periureteral fibrosis may result from the conveyance of the inflammation from the intestine and mesentery to the retroperitoneum via the lymphatics. Microintestinal perforation with accompanying inflammatory change, with or without retroperitoneal fistula and abscess, is another possible cause of ureteral obstruction (Enker and Block, 1970). Since the predominant area of involvement is the terminal ileum, the proximity of the latter to the right retroperitoneum is responsible for the occurrence of extrinsic ureteral compression on the right side in most reported cases. There have been cases of left ureteral involvement, one of which was related to significant granulomatous disease of the colon (Present et al., 1963). Bilateral ureteral obstruction has also been noted (Schofield et al., 1968).

Histologic examination of the periureteral fibrotic tissue reveals pseudomyxomatous changes with stellate cell formation similar to that seen in liposarcoma. Special stains have demonstrated collagen fibers with diffuse edema (Enker and Block, 1970).

There has been a relatively equal distribution between the sexes, and most patients with ureteral obstruction have been young, with an average age in the mid-twenties. The patients almost always have significant gastrointestinal symptoms for a protracted period of time (more than 6 months). It is noteworthy that the majority of patients have no symptoms referable to the urinary tract. Occasionally, a patient may experience frequency or dysuria. Pyuria and laboratory confirmation of a urinary tract infection have been infrequent findings. Present and associates (1963) made special note of the occurrence of pain in the hip, the anterior aspect of the thigh, or the flank, which often resulted in difficulty in walking or extending the hip joint. Several patients have had the acute onset of flank pain and fever that was felt to represent the retroperitoneal extension of the inflammatory process. Many patients have fever, but costovertebral angle tenderness is an uncommon finding. A mass may be palpable, occurring primarily in the right lower quadrant.

Moderate anemia and elevation of both the erythrocyte sedimentation rate and the white cell count are often present. Sigmoidoscopy may reveal evidence of disease, and barium studies show typical changes such as stricture and fistulization, located primarily in the terminal ileum. Excretory urography or ultrasonography confirms the presence of ureteral obstruction (Fig. 10–11). Obstruction occurs almost exclusively in the distal right ureter, usually at the level of the pelvic brim, resulting in various degrees of hydroureteronephrosis. In the early stages of obstruction, the ureter takes a normal, relatively straight, downward course, whereas in long-standing obstruction, the ureter becomes tortuous and deviated medially (Present et al., 1963). The extrinsic periureteral process generally causes symmetric tapering of the ureter. Since ureteral obstruction is generally occult, excretory urography or ultrasonography is essential to the thorough evaluation of all patients with significant involvement of the bowel by Crohn's disease, especially in patients with il-

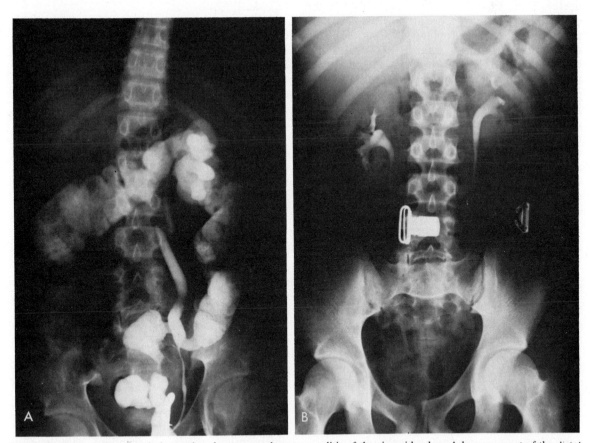

Figure 10–11. *A*, Left ureteral obstruction due to granulomatous colitis of the sigmoid colon. A long segment of the distal left ureter appears to be stenotic on this retrograde pyelogram. Residual barium from a barium enema demonstrates the inflamed sigmoid colon. This case differs from most cases of ureteral obstruction secondary to granulomatous bowel disease in that the obstruction is on the left side. *B*, Excretory urography 6 months after resection of the diseased bowel and ureterolysis shows complete resolution of the ureteral obstruction.

eocecal Crohn's disease or an abdominal mass.

The primary method of treatment for severe complicated granulomatous bowel disease is surgery. Although diversion of the involved intestinal segment was formerly done frequently, intestinal resection has become the principal form of definitive palliative surgical therapy. Ureteral obstruction is a complication of advanced inflammatory bowel disease constituting an indication for surgery. When ureteral obstruction has accompanied granulomatous bowel disease, therapy has generally been directed toward the bowel disease, without any attempts to relieve the ureter being made (Enker and Block, 1970). Enker and Block have emphasized that nearly 30 per cent of the patients treated by these means have failed to improve or have suffered significant renal loss. They reported complete and uncomplicated urinary decompression in a group of six patients treated with primary intestinal resection and ureterolysis (Enker and Block, 1970). On the other hand, Siminovitch and Fazio (1980) recently concluded in a review of 45 patients with ureteral obstruction secondary to Crohn's disease that ureterolysis is rarely indicated. Intestinal resection or staging procedures for complicated Crohn's disease were usually effective in resolving associated obstructive uropathy. Accordingly, it appears that ureterolysis is rarely required to relieve hydroureteronephrosis secondary to Crohn's disease but is indicated if there is severe associated retroperitoneal fibrosis with encasement of the ureter. If ureterolysis is contemplated, it is advisable to insert a large ureteral catheter prior to surgery.

INFLAMMATORY DISEASE OF THE APPENDIX

In the pediatric age group, appendicitis and peritonitis can cause hydroureter and hydronephrosis without evidence of mechanical obstruction. Kaplan and Keiller (1974) reported a case of a child developing azotemia and hydronephrosis requiring bilateral nephrostomy after an appendectomy for an intact inflamed appendix. Izant (1974) described three cases of hydroureteronephrosis in children with peritonitis. Although the mechanism is unclear, the obstruction subsided as the peritonitis resolved.

Appendiceal abscesses may cause both urinary tract symptoms and ureteral obstruction, primarily in the pediatric age group. The incidence of upper urinary tract obstruction secondary to an appendiceal abscess in the adult is not known, but the condition does occur and may be more frequent than is recognized. The

diagnosis of appendiceal abscess is often very difficult to establish in the pediatric patient. Dysuria and frequency may present in children 1 to 2 weeks after the onset of other gastrointestinal symptoms such as nausea, vomiting, anorexia, diarrhea, and abdominal pain. Urinary retention has also been reported in a few instances. An abdominal mass is almost always palpable. A scout film of the abdomen often shows a soft tissue shadow obliterating the right psoas margin, with displacement of the bowel gas to the left. Occasionally, a fecalith may be noted in the region of the appendix. Abdominal ultrasonography and computed tomography are useful techniques in determining the extent of the abscess. A barium enema usually shows displacement of the rectum and irregularity of the cecum. The obstruction characteristically occurs on the right side at the level of the pelvic brim but may be bilateral. The hydronephrosis resolves after surgical drainage of the abscess (Cook, 1969).

Rarely, mucocele of the appendix has also been found to be responsible for extrinsic obstruction of the ureter. This entity is usually associated with a postinflammatory appendiceal stricture, carcinoma of the appendix, or carcinoma of the cecum. A case of left ureteral obstruction secondary to a granulomatous mass that developed after appendicitis has also been reported. It was felt that the antibiotic treatment of gonococcal urethritis masked the symptoms of acute appendicitis, leading to the development of a chronic granulomatous mass (Carroll and Laughton, 1973).

DIVERTICULITIS

Diverticulitis is the most frequent complication of diverticulosis, a condition that affects approximately 5 per cent of the population. The cause of diverticulosis is unclear. A combination of factors, including diet, muscular hypertrophy, and neuromuscular dysfunction of the colon, has been implicated. Diverticulitis results when diverticula are plugged with colonic contents, leading to the establishment of an inflammatory reaction. The disease, which occurs primarily in older patients, is rarely seen in primitive and underdeveloped countries.

Urologic complications are found in approximately 20 per cent of the patients with diverticulitis, the most frequent complication being colovesical fistula. Although rare, there have been a few reports of left ureteral obstruction occurring secondary to diverticulitis (Hafner et al., 1962; Madsen and Thyboe, 1972). The probable mechanism of obstruction is the extension of an inflammatory process from the retroperitoneal perforation of diverticulitis, resulting in a retroperitoneal abscess (Bissada and Redman, 1974). The combination of ureteral obstruction and a colon lesion favors the diagnosis of malignancy, especially if there is a palpable mass, but diverticulitis should be considered in the differential diagnosis (Rees and Bolton, 1975). It has been suggested that a higher incidence of ureteral obstruction would be noted in association with diverticulitis if more patients were evaluated for this possibility. Accordingly, excretory urography or ultrasonography should be done prior to surgery to evaluate the upper tracts, to minimize the risk of ureteral injury, and to facilitate planning of the operation. Computerized tomography is also helpful in assessing the extent of disease. Placement of ureteral catheters is advisable at the time of surgical resection, especially if there is obstructive uropathy. Treatment of the ureteral obstruction associated with diverticulitis consists of treatment of the primary disease. The presence of an inflammatory diverticular mass requires a bowel resection that may be part of a two- or three-stage procedure, with preliminary colostomy.

PANCREATIC LESIONS

It is well known that pancreatic lesions occasionally produce changes in the kidney that may be confused with intrinsic renal lesions. Almost all the lesions have been in the left kidney because of the proximity of the tail of the pancreas. A pancreatic pseudocyst rarely may extend laterally into the perinephric space to displace the kidney or ureter and represents a theoretical cause of ureteral obstruction (Kiviat et al., 1971). Also, there have been several reports of ureteral obstruction being secondary to extension and metastasis from carcinoma of the pancreas (Schmidt, 1971; Wanuck et al., 1973).

DISEASES OF THE RETROPERITONEUM

Retroperitoneal Fibrosis

IDIOPATHIC

The notable French urologist Albarran is responsible for the earliest description of retroperitoneal fibrosis (as far back as 1905), but it was not until Ormond's account, first published in the English literature in 1948, that this disease became an established clinical entity. A variety of terms have been used to designate this disease, including periureteritis fibrosa, periureteritis plastica, chronic periureteritis, sclerosing retroperitoneal granuloma, and fibrous retroperitonitis. In recent years, the disease has become known as retroperitoneal fibrosis, since this term more closely describes the actual nature of the cellular response and the extent of involvement. Accordingly, to avoid confusion, the other terms should no longer be used to refer to this lesion.

Since there is now a greater awareness of this entity, the diagnosis of retroperitoneal fibrosis is being established with increasing frequency. In 1967, Utz and Moghaddam reported 56 cases of retroperitoneal fibrosis in a 6-year period at the Mayo Clinic. More recently, Lepor and Walsh (1979) provided a review of 70 cases. The disease occurs in both sexes and has been reported in an age range extending from 7 to 85 years, with a predominance in the fifth to sixth decades of life.

Pathology. Grossly, retroperitoneal fibrosis appears as an exuberant mass of tan to white, woody, fibrous tissue covering the retroperitoneal structures. The process covers the aorta, vena cava, ureters, and psoas muscles and may extend from the renal pedicle to below the pelvic brim. The center of the plaque is generally located at the level of the fourth or fifth lumbar vertebra, overlying the aortic bifurcation. It is not uncommon for the fibrous tissue to bifurcate and follow the common iliac arteries. Rarely, the fibrous process may extend into the root of the mesentery or may pass through the crura of the diaphragm to continue as fibrous mediastinitis. An association with sclerosing cholangitis has also been noted in several cases.

The fibrous process envelops the ureter, tending to drag the middle third of the ureter toward the midline. Fibrous encasement of the ureters eventually leads to hydronephrosis and varying degrees of renal failure. Although there is generally extensive involvement overlying the great vessels, significant arterial obstruction is rare. Venous obstruction is more common, apparently because of the greater compressibility of the thin-walled veins. Obstruction of the inferior vena cava or common iliac veins may cause edema of the lower extremities. In the past, it was felt that the fibrous tissue enveloped but did not invade the retroperitoneal structures. Reports have emphasized the occasional invasion of the psoas muscles and the ureters by the fibrous process (Persky and Huus, 1974; Skeel et al., 1975).

On histologic examination, the predominant finding is fibrous tissue consisting of collagen fibrils and fibroblasts. A subacute nonspecific inflammatory reaction is often present, or there may only be completely hyalinized fibrosis. The cellular infiltrate includes polymorphonuclear cells, lymphocytes, eosinophils, or plasma cells. A necrotizing arteritis has also been observed.

Etiology. There is overwhelming evidence that prolonged use of the drug methysergide (Sansert) for the treatment of migraine headaches is occasionally responsible for retroperitoneal fibrosis. Graham initially noted the occurrence of retroperitoneal fibrosis in patients taking methysergide (Graham, 1964) and later reported a 1 per cent incidence in a large number of patients taking this drug (Graham, 1966). Since that time, a number of other authors have also noted a causal relationship between methysergide therapy and retroperitoneal fibrosis. Other organ systems are also prone to fibrosis with methysergide treatment, including the heart, lungs, pleura, great vessels, and gastrointestinal tract (Kunkel, 1971). Another ergot derivative, lysergic acid diethylamide (LSD), and methyldopa (Aldomet), amphetamines, and phenacetin have been implicated as possible causes of retroperitoneal fibrosis (Aptekar, 1970; Stecker et al., 1974; Iversen et al., 1975).

The method by which ergot compounds induce retroperitoneal fibrosis is ill defined. Methysergide and LSD have similar chemical structures and belong to a class of semisynthetic derivatives of ergot alkaloids that are serotonin antagonists, acting via competitive inhibition of receptor sites. Methysergide and LSD, therefore, cause increased amounts of endogenous serotonin. Elevated serotonin levels have been associated with the fibrosis noted in carcinoid syndrome. An important relationship between increased serotonin and fibrosis has not been confirmed in the laboratory, however. The most widely accepted theory about the effect of the ergot alkaloids on the evolution of retroperitoneal fibrosis is that they act as a hapten, setting up a hypersensitivity or an autoimmune reaction (Weiss and Hinman, 1966). The associated vasculitis occasionally noted in retroperitoneal fibrosis supports this hypothesis (Jones and Alexander, 1966; Raper, 1955).

In most instances, no etiologic factor is found in patients with retroperitoneal fibrosis. Hence, the term "idiopathic retroperitoneal fibrosis" is truly applicable.

Clinical Features. Patients with retroperitoneal fibrosis generally present with a group of symptoms that help classify the disease into one of two stages. In the early stage, the signs and symptoms originate from the disease process itself, while in the advanced stage, the clinical features represent the effect of obstructive uropathy and renal failure.

A number of symptoms found in the early stage of disease are similar to those of any subacute or chronic inflammatory condition: malaise, anorexia, weight loss, and moderate pyrexia. A characteristic pain suggesting the diagnosis of retroperitoneal fibrosis occurs as often as 90 per cent of the time according to Utz and Henry (1966). This distress is insidious in onset, dull, and noncolicky. The pain has a veritable girdle distribution, since it originates in the lower aspects of the flank or lumbosacral region and extends anteriorly to both lower quadrants, the periumbilical region, or the testes. It is not altered by activity, body position, or increasing intra-abdominal pressure during bowel or bladder function. Later, the pain becomes more severe and unrelenting, suggesting a retroperitoneal lesion such as carcinoma of the pancreas or an abdominal aortic aneurysm. Oddly enough, the pain is sometimes relieved by aspirin, but not by a narcotic. Another astonishing observation is that after a simple ureterolysis without any attempts to remove the extensive fibrosis, the perverse pain is relieved. This is most surprising, since the pain is not at all characteristic of that expected with ureteral obstruction. The disease has also been reported to present as a large bowel obstruction (McCarthy et al., 1972).

There may be evidence of compression of the great vessels by the fibrotic process. Many patients exhibit mild edema of the lower extremities. More severe degrees of extrinsic obstruction of the vena cava or iliac veins may lead to the development of thrombophlebitis. Although arterial occlusion and insufficiency are rare, they do occur. The signs and symptoms of reduced circulation, including ischemic pain, may be evident in the lower extremities. Snow et al. (1977) reported a patient with severe compression of the abdominal aorta and common iliac arteries from retroperitoneal fibrosis who presented with intermittent ischemic pain in the buttocks and thighs. The pain was unusual in that the symptoms were present when the patient assumed the supine position but were relieved when the patient was sitting up or when the head of the bed was elevated. Likewise, the pedal pulses had a positional relationship, since they disappeared when the patient was lying flat. The extensive fibrotic plaque apparently caused arterial occlusion only when it was maximally stretched over the aortoiliac area.

The clinical features of the late stage are attributable to progressive ureteral occlusion. Progressive hydronephrosis may eventuate in complete ureteral obstruction and anuria. Unfortunately, the progression of disease is either very slow or silent, so that the symptoms normally present in the early stage either are not manifest or are so minimal that they are overlooked. In this situation, the patient may present with renal infection or with dull flank pain due to the increasing hydronephrosis. General deterioration, weakness, weight loss, and gastrointestinal disturbances may be the first evidence of disease secondary to progressive uremia.

Diagnosis. The diagnosis of retroperitoneal fibrosis can be made on the basis of the history and the radiologic investigation. At times, the diagnosis is not firmly established until surgical exploration. Several laboratory tests indicative of a subacute or chronic inflammatory process may be helpful, but they are not diagnostic. The erythrocyte sedimentation rate is generally increased, and there may be leukocytosis or, occasionally, eosinophilia. Anemia is generally proportionate to the degree of azotemia that is present.

Excretory urography is a beneficial study in helping establish a diagnosis in the early stage of the disease. Characteristically, there is medial deviation of the ureter, usually at the middle third, beginning at the level of the third and fourth lumbar vertebrae. Persky and Huus

(1974) emphasized that medial deviation of the ureter is not a constant finding in patients with retroperitoneal fibrosis. It has also been demonstrated that almost 20 per cent of patients with normal urograms have medial placement of the ureters (especially the right) without demonstrable evidence of pathologic change in the urinary tract (Saldino and Palubinskas, 1972). The medial displacement of the ureter in retroperitoneal fibrosis tends to extend higher than a normally deviated ureter, and the ureter often appears stiff. Varying degrees of obstruction and hydronephrosis, with tapering of the ureter as it enters the dense plaque, are almost always evident. Most retroperitoneal neoplasms displace the ureters in a lateral direction. Medial displacement of the pelvic ureters may occur after pelvic surgery such as an abdominal perineal resection or the removal of pelvic malignancy (Friedenberg et al., 1966). Other causes of medially displaced pelvic ureters include a bladder diverticulum, metastatic tumors, and aneurysms.

More recently, ultrasonography and computerized tomography have become valuable techniques for establishing a diagnosis of retroperitoneal fibrosis. The ultrasonic appearance is a smooth-bordered, relatively echo-free mass centered on the sacral promontory but extending cephalad at least to the level of the aortic bifurcation and caudad into the pelvis. Sonography can be used to follow response to therapy and detect hydronephrotic changes in the kidneys (Sanders et al., 1977). With the superior resolving power of computerized tomography the fibrosis can be shown in more detail (Fig. 10–12). Although lymphoma, metastatic carci-

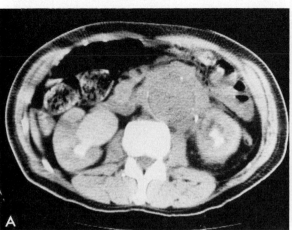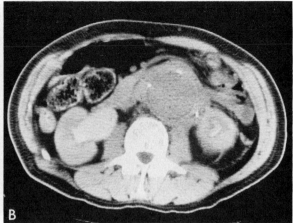

Figure 10–12. *A* and *B*, Computerized tomographic scan demonstrating extensive retroperitoneal fibrosis associated with an aneurysm of the abdominal aorta.

noma, sarcoma, and multiple myeloma may also engulf the aorta and vena cava (Sterzer et al., 1979), the symmetric distribution and geometric shape are highly suggestive of retroperitoneal fibrosis. The limits extend from the hilus superiorly to below the level of the bifurcation of the great vessels inferiorly, with the lateral borders reaching or involving the psoas muscles. The mass is confluent, with encasement of the aorta and inferior vena cava continuously, whereas lymphomas or metastatic disease may demonstrate enlarged lymph nodes separable from the great vessels (Krinsky et al., 1983). At times, needle biopsy guided by computerized tomography may help establish a correct diagnosis and avoid an exploratory laparotomy.

As wider segments of the ureter are involved, the hydronephrosis increases. Eventually, complete obstruction and anuria may develop. Retrograde urography, which is required whenever there has been inadequate demonstration of the pelvocalyceal system and ureter, again demonstrates medial deviation of the ure-

ter and varying degrees of obstruction. Oddly enough, in most instances the area of narrowing of the ureter readily permits the passage of a No. 5 or 6 French ureteral catheter (Fig. 10–13). This is considered a characteristic feature of retroperitoneal fibrosis, although Persky and Huus (1974) have emphasized that it is not a constant finding.

Ultrasonography and radioisotope renography may be helpful, particularly for anuric patients or for those in whom one side does not visualize on routine excretory urography. The curve may confirm the presence of obstructive uropathy or postrenal failure as opposed to primary renal disease. The height of the curve may also distinguish which is the better of the two kidneys when there is no visualization on either side.

Venography is helpful in delineating the area of venous obstruction and the presence of thrombosis if there is significant edema in the lower extremities. Arteriography is employed if there is evidence of arterial insufficiency.

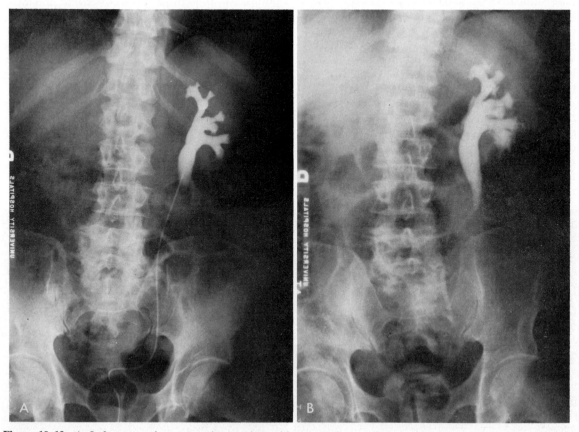

Figure 10–13. *A*, Left retrograde urogram in a patient with retroperitoneal fibrosis. Despite the obstruction, a No. 5 French ureteral catheter passes easily to the kidney. *B*, A pull-out x-ray film demonstrates a hydronephrotic left kidney with medial deviation of the ureter at the level of the fourth lumbar vertebra. Note the presence of backflow that may be secondary to ureteral obstruction.

Lymphangiography may be helpful in distinguishing retroperitoneal fibrosis from malignant causes of ureteral obstruction, especially retroperitoneal lymphoma.

Treatment. Although surgical treatment is required for most cases of retroperitoneal fibrosis, several medical measures have been found to be worthwhile. Antibiotics and external radiation have virtually no place in the treatment of this disease, in spite of reports to the contrary. If the patient has been taking methysergide, the drug should be stopped immediately. Patients with minimal obstructive changes and renal impairment may show progressive improvement within a few weeks or even days after the drug is discontinued. Of course, close follow-up with careful attention to the upper urinary tracts is mandatory. In those cases in which there has been no resolution of the mild hydronephrotic changes or in which there is evidence of progression of the disease, surgery is necessary.

Steroids have been found to be helpful in certain instances. If proper drainage of the upper tracts can be easily accomplished, steroids may be useful in preparing patients for surgery who have renal insufficiency and considerable constitutional disturbance. Operative procedures can then be done on a healthier patient on an elective as opposed to a semi-emergent basis. Patients presenting with much systemic disturbance, particularly involving the gastrointestinal tract, and laboratory evidence of active inflammation (increased erythrocyte sedimentation rate and leukocytosis) are likely to benefit from steroids (Ross and Goldsmith, 1971). In elderly patients and those debilitated from coexistent disease, the need for major surgery may possibly be averted with the aid of steroids (Ross and Goldsmith, 1971). The drugs have also been used concomitant with the discontinuation of methysergide in patients with mild hydronephrotic changes. Finally, some also advocate the use of steroids following ureterolysis. Determination of the dose of steroid remains empirical. Close observation with interval urography or ultrasonography and determinations of the erythrocyte sedimentation rate, white blood count, serum creatinine level, and creatinine clearance are necessary while the patient is taking the medication. Persistent hydronephrosis or the lack of improvement as determined from the laboratory studies indicates the need for surgical intervention.

Patients with significant renal impairment, evident from the presence of azotemia, oliguria, or anuria, benefit from a course of drainage of the upper urinary tracts. As already emphasized, despite marked hydronephrosis and significant extrinsic ureteral compression, ureteral catheters of sufficient size, or possibly double J catheters, can usually be passed to the renal pelves. This affords valuable time to allow for restoration of renal function and to improve fluid, electrolyte, and acid-base balance prior to surgery. Nephrostomy drainage is usually not required before or at the time of ureterolysis.

After the appropriate diagnostic and preoperative therapeutic measures have been instituted, surgical exploration with ureterolysis is required in most instances. Since the disease generally affects both ureters, the best approach is transabdominal, through a long midline incision. Incising the posterior peritoneum in the midline between the duodenum and the inferior mesenteric vein has been advocated (Hewitt et al., 1969). Flaps of posterior peritoneum are developed, exposing the entire retroperitoneal area and both ureters. Exposure of the individual ureters can also be achieved by mobilization of the ascending and descending colon, but this is more time-consuming. It is generally easiest to locate the ureters by exposing the parts of the dilated proximal ureters that have not been encased in the fibrous plaque. A biopsy of the fibrous tissue is taken for frozen-section analysis. Ureterolysis is usually accomplished with relative ease if the appropriate plane is found. The ureters are freed with blunt dissection immediately adjacent to the adventitia of the ureter. After the ureters are completely lysed, they are managed in several ways: They may be transplanted to an intraperitoneal position; they may be transposed laterally, interposing retroperitoneal fat between the ureters and the fibrosis; or they may be wrapped with omental fat (Tiptaft et al., 1982). On occasion, the fibrotic process may invade the ureter. Fortunately, this is usually over only a short segment of ureter. In this instance, it may be impossible to achieve satisfactory ureterolysis, necessitating both resection of a segment of ureter and ureteroureterostomy. Some advocate the use of splinting ureteral catheters during ureterolysis to facilitate dissection of the ureters and to help maintain them in a lateral position following ureterolysis.

If significant arterial encroachment is present, aorta lysis with lysis of the common iliac arteries may also be required. In most instances, a plane can be established between the fibrotic plaque and the involved vessel with relative ease. On occasion the fibrotic plaque is adherent to the vessel walls, making aorta lysis a difficult, time-consuming procedure (Snow et al., 1977). Despite this, it is possible to free most of the fibrous plaque and to restore blood flow.

Although fatalities do occur, a satisfactory outcome can generally be expected following extensive bilateral ureterolysis if renal impairment is not too severe. In those instances in which ureterolysis is done for only one ureter or over only a short segment of ureter, recurrent disease is not uncommon. Close follow-up is critically important to ensure the absence of progressive or recurrent disease. On occasion, a second operative procedure is required to extend the area of ureterolysis or to free the contralateral ureter. An opportunity for operative ingenuity is afforded in establishing satisfactory drainage of the upper tracts, such as is shown in the report of the performance of a ureteropyelostomy for recurrent disease in a duplicated system (Amar, 1970).

SECONDARY TO OTHER DISEASE PROCESSES

There are a number of diseases that cause retroperitoneal reaction, inflammation, and fibrosis that the urologist should be aware of because of the potential risk of ureteral compression. Inflammatory processes of the lower extremities with ascending lymphangitis, multiple abdominal procedures, Henoch-Schönlein purpura with hemorrhage, gonorrhea, biliary tract disease, chronic urinary tract infections, tuberculosis, and sarcoidosis have all been associated with retroperitoneal fibrosis on rare occasions. The fibrosis is most commonly found at the level of the sacral promontory and within Gerota's fascia (Scott and Cerny, 1971). Otherwise, the radiologic diagnosis and the treatment are the same as those described for idiopathic retroperitoneal fibrosis.

Methylmethacrylate is a cement commonly used for total joint replacement. A case of arterial occlusion has been reported following the use of methylmethacrylate (Hirsch et al., 1976). We have treated a patient with occlusion of the distal ureter and iliac vein secondary to the use of methylmethacrylate for total hip replacement (Fig. 10–14). Surgical exploration revealed an isolated area of marked fibrosis encasing the distal ureter and iliac vein in the

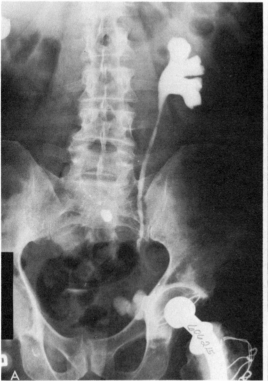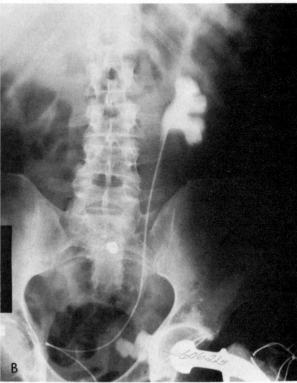

Figure 10–14. *A*, Retrograde urogram demonstrates left hydronephrosis with obstruction where the methylmethacrylate pierced the pelvis. *B*, A catheter placed in the left ureter is immediately adjacent to the methylmethacrylate. Exploration revealed encasement of the ureter in a dense mass of scar tissue, making ureterolysis impossible. A ureteroneocystostomy was performed with a psoas bladder hitch technique.

area where the methylmethacrylate pierced the pelvis. It is possible that the heat of polymerization was responsible for this reaction. Since it is not uncommon for a small amount of methylmethacrylate to penetrate through the pelvis during total hip replacement, it is anticipated that additional cases of ureteral obstruction due to the use of the cement will be noted in the future.

RADIATION-INDUCED

It has been well documented that under certain conditions radiation therapy can cause ureteral obstruction. Radiation therapy has been used extensively for the treatment of carcinoma of the cervix. Uremia is the most common cause of death in patients with carcinoma of the cervix, indicating that the distal ureters are vulnerable to obstruction. The obstruction is attributable to recurrent cancer in the vast majority of cases, but radiation-induced fibrosis may be the cause in a small number of patients (Graham and Abad, 1967; Shingleton et al., 1969). Upper urinary tract obstruction secondary to the effect of radiation is generally reported to occur in about 5 per cent of the cases with ureteral encroachment, or in less than 1 per cent of all treated patients.

The low incidence of ureteral blockage following radiation therapy, compared with the higher incidence of complications affecting the other pelvic organs such as the bladder and rectum, indicates that the ureters are relatively resistant to the effects of radiation. Significant ureteral damage can occur from fibrosis of either the periureteral tissue or the ureter itself, however. There have been several mechanisms postulated for ureteral obstruction following radiation therapy (Alfert and Gillenwater, 1972). (1) The tumor may incite a pronounced desmoplastic response in the tissue adjacent to the ureter that remains after the neoplasm has been eradicated. (2) It has been shown that infection increases the sensitivity of the ureter and periureteral tissue to radiation. Accordingly, radiation therapy is hazardous in the presence of pelvic inflammatory disease or urinary tract infection. (3) Necrosis of the tumor invading the ureteral wall may lead to fibrosis and scarring. (4) There may be direct radiation injury to the ureteral wall.

Ureteral obstruction may occur near the end of a course of radiation therapy or shortly after its completion. This type of blockage generally subsides rapidly, since it is related to edema of the pelvic tissues. The chronic ureteral obstruction that occurs 6 to 12 months or even 10 or more years following radiotherapy is related to reduced vascular supply from endarteritis obliterans and to connective tissue proliferation with contraction of fibrous tissue (Alfert and Gillenwater, 1972). Two types of ureteral blockage have been described. One is a localized stricture of the distal ureter caused by fibrosis in the parametrial tissue, and the other is a long threadlike stenosis of the pelvic portion of the ureter secondary to scarring of the pelvic connective tissue.

The late ureteral obstruction secondary to radiation therapy may be associated with urinary symptoms but more often goes unrecognized until there is severe renal damage, since it is slow and insidious in developing. For this reason, it is advisable to follow patients who have received radiotherapy with serial excretory urography, ultrasonography, or radioisotope renography (Shingleton et al., 1969). Close follow-up is mandatory in patients with pretreatment renal failure, infection, or evidence of parametritis.

Since infection may be a potent factor predisposing to ureteral damage, several prophylactic measures are advisable. Quiescent salpingitis may be exacerbated with radiotherapy (Graham and Abad, 1967). Accordingly, it is advisable to perform a preliminary bilateral salpingo-oophorectomy prior to irradiation in patients with a history or physical findings suggestive of pelvic inflammatory disease. In addition, acute infection during radiotherapy should be recognized in the closely followed patient and should be treated with bilateral salpingo-oophorectomy.

As already mentioned, the vast majority of late ureteral obstructions following radiation therapy will be secondary to recurrent cancer. In the absence of positive evidence of recurrent tumor, exploratory laparotomy is mandatory to obtain a tissue diagnosis. In a small number of cases, the obstruction will be secondary to the radiation therapy, affording an opportunity to salvage renal tissue. If the patient has a normally functioning bladder without significant radiation changes, the pelvic ureter can be lysed from the periureteral fibrotic tissue and reimplanted into the bladder. A fish-mouth type of ureteroneocystostomy without an antireflux procedure is preferable. If the pelvic ureter or bladder is badly damaged, a form of supravesical urinary diversion is required.

Retroperitoneal Abscess

The retroperitoneal space is divided into anterior and posterior compartments, with the ureters and kidneys lying in the posterior compartment (Altemeier et al., 1971). Likewise, retroperitoneal abscesses can be divided into anterior and posterior types. The posterior abscess usually results from extravasation behind a stone or renal carbuncle. Anterior abscesses are usually secondary to a gastrointestinal disease such as appendicitis, diverticulitis, and Crohn's disease. Suppurative iliac adenitis, osteomyelitis, tuberculosis, and epidural abscess represent other possible etiologic factors. A psoas abscess develops if the inflammatory process extends into the psoas muscle (Stevenson and Ozeran, 1969). Retroperitoneal inflammatory processes in either compartment may deviate or block the ureter as it courses toward the bladder.

Physical examination usually reveals fever and a tender abdominal mass. As the inflammation spreads, the patient may develop tenderness in the iliac, groin, or upper thigh areas. If the musculature is involved, the patient often lies with the hip flexed; extension elicits a positive "psoas sign." On radiographic examination, a lumbar scoliosis with the concavity toward the involved side and air along the fibers of the psoas muscle may be seen on the plain film of the abdomen. Excretory urography can be valuable in helping establish the diagnosis (Fig. 10–15). Approximately 2 per cent of all patients with retroperitoneal abscesses and 5 per cent of those with posterior abscesses have displacement or dilatation, or both, of the upper urinary tracts (Stevenson and Ozeran, 1969). Despite this low incidence of secondary involvement of the ureter, excretory urography is essential, since about 70 per cent of the posterior abscesses have a renal origin (Altemeier et al., 1971). Abdominal ultrasound and computerized tomography are excellent radiographic methods of identifying and defining the extent of the abscess.

Surgery consists of prompt extraperitoneal drainage through a large incision. Satisfactory drainage usually results in resolution of the urographic abnormalities. Since retroperitoneal scarring can conceivably cause compression of the ureter, adequate follow-up is necessary.

Retroperitoneal Hemorrhage

PRIMARY RETROPERITONEAL HEMATOMA

A retroperitoneal hematoma is usually secondary to blunt abdominal trauma, although bleeding in the retroperitoneal space may be attributable to vascular accidents, anticoagu-

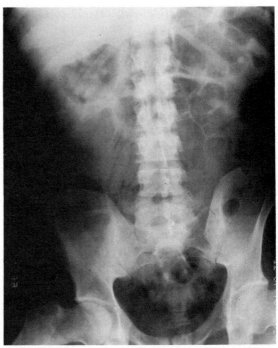

Figure 10–15. There is free retroperitoneal air along the psoas muscle caused by a psoas abscess that resulted from a perirectal infection. This delayed film of an excretory urogram shows considerable dilatation and very faint visualization of the right pelvocalyceal system and upper ureter, indicating significant ureteral obstruction.

lants, or iatrogenic causes. The physical examination may demonstrate ecchymotic flank discoloration, an adynamic ileus, and hypotension. An accumulation of blood in the retroperitoneum often causes deviation of the ureter and on rare occasions may cause obstruction. Iatrogenic hematomas or those secondary to anticoagulants generally resolve spontaneously, while large hematomas caused by abdominal trauma are usually evacuated during exploratory laparotomy.

HEMATOMA OF RECTUS ABDOMINIS MUSCLE

A hematoma of the rectus abdominis muscle may cause ureteral obstruction and vesical compression. Most of these hematomas are attributable to muscle exertion but may also be caused by degenerative muscle disease, anticoagulants, pregnancy, and direct trauma. The hematoma may extend retroperitoneally, and in a few instances, a large amount of bleeding has led to bilateral ureteral obstruction and oliguria. Rupture of the rectus abdominis muscle or the epigastric vessels, or both, leads to the acute onset of abdominal pain, tenderness, and rigidity. Immediate evacuation and ligation of the inferior epigastric vessels are essential in the treatment of this entity (Zalar and McDonald, 1969).

RETROPERITONEAL MASSES

Primary Retroperitoneal Tumors

Primary retroperitoneal tumors may arise from the neural, mesodermal, urogenital ridge, or embryonic remnant tissues. They are either benign or malignant, although the malignancies account for approximately 70 to 80 per cent of the tumors (Braasch and Mon, 1967). In general, primary retroperitoneal neoplasms are rare, the malignant lesions accounting for only 0.16 per cent of all cancers in a large county hospital during a 15-year period (Armstrong and Cohn, 1965). Lymphomas predominate, followed in frequency of occurrence by a variety of tumors, including neuroblastomas and liposarcomas. Benign growths include neurofibromas, lipomas, adenomas, and cysts. The large variety of primary tumors that occur in the retroperitoneal area is listed in Table 10–1. The prognosis is very poor for malignant neoplasms, with only 10 to 15 per cent of the patients being free of tumor at 5 years (Adams, 1974). Primary retroperitoneal tumors occasionally cause extrinsic obstruction of the ureter. There are rare case reports of ureteral obstruction found in association with such lesions as ectopic pheochromocytoma (Immergut et al., 1970), renal cysts (Evans and Coughlin, 1970), and retroperitoneal xanthogranuloma (Gup, 1972) (Fig. 10–16).

Patients most often complain of an abdominal mass and pain. Other symptoms include a wide range of gastrointestinal and genitourinary

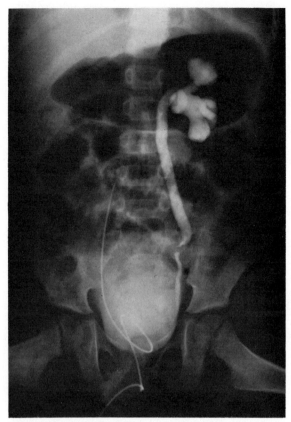

Figure 10–16. Paraganglioma causing obstruction of the midureter in an 8-year-old boy.

complaints, back pain, leg swelling, fever, anorexia, and weight loss. The abdominal mass is usually most readily palpable in the midline and has variable extensions to the pelvis and flanks. The consistency of the mass may give a clue to the type of tumor: Malignancies are hard, while benign growths tend to be soft (Adams, 1974). An abdominal mass in a child will most often

TABLE 10–1. PRIMARY RETROPERITONEAL TUMORS

Type of Tissue	Benign Neoplasms	Malignant Neoplasms
Adipose tissue	Lipoma	Liposarcoma
Fibrous tissue	Fibroma	Fibrosarcoma
Smooth muscle	Leiomyoma	Leiomyosarcoma
Striated muscle	Rhabdomyoma	Rhabdomyosarcoma
Vascular tissue	Hemangioma	Malignant hemangiopericytoma
Nerve elements	Neurilemoma	Malignant schwannoma
Lymphatic tissue	Lymphangioma	Lymphangiosarcoma
Lymph nodes		Lymphosarcoma
		Hodgkin's disease
		Reticulum cell sarcoma
Mucoid tissue	Myxoma	Myxosarcoma
Extra-adrenal chromaffin tissue	Benign pheochromocytoma	Malignant pheochromocytoma
Embryonic remnants	Nephrogenic cysts	Urogenital ridge tumor
Cell rests	Dermoid	Teratoma

be of renal or retroperitoneal origin (Raffensperger and Abousleiman, 1968).

Excretory urography, including lateral and oblique films, is the most rewarding diagnostic study. The ureter is usually displaced anteriorly and laterally. Occasionally, there may be partial or total obstruction of the ureter. The kidney is often displaced, and the renal pelvis may be distorted, flattened, or rotated (Fig. 10–17). Ultrasonography and/or computerized tomography provide invaluable information regarding the size and shape of the tumor, extent of invasion, and relationship to contiguous structures. Gastrointestinal films are necessary to rule out the intestinal tract as the primary source of the tumor. Arteriography and inferior venacavography are valuable in further delineating the extent of the tumor, particularly in the child (Tucker, 1965).

Total transperitoneal excision is the optimal operative procedure. Unfortunately, this is possible in less than 25 per cent of patients. Some retroperitoneal malignancies lend themselves to repeated attempts at removal because of their slow growth and tendency to recur locally. Radiotherapy is used as an adjunct when surgical treatment has either failed or been insufficient (Adams, 1974; Armstrong and Cohn, 1965).

Secondary Retroperitoneal Tumors

Metastases from primary malignancies anywhere in the body can spread to the retroperitoneum, leading to ureteral obstruction. Table 10–2 demonstrates the approximate incidence of the various tumors spreading to the retroperitoneum. Secondary involvement of the retroperitoneum by malignant tumors occurs in two ways: by direct extension of adjacent malignancy or by metastasis to the retroperitoneal lymph nodes. Cancers of the cervix, bladder, prostate, and colon represent the most common primary lesions extending to the retroperitoneum. Theoretically, any secondary tumor spreading to the retroperitoneum can encroach upon the ureter, leading to obstruction (Abrams et al., 1950; Kaufman and Grabstald, 1969). Although in 60 to 70 per cent of patients, ureteral obstruction occurs within 2 years of the primary diagnosis, it can present as many as 20 years later (Brin et al., 1975) (Fig. 10–18).

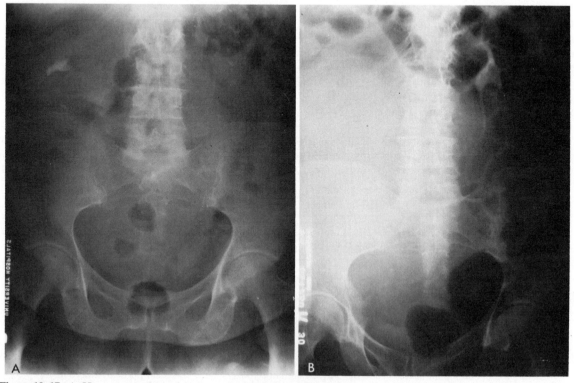

Figure 10–17. *A*, Huge retroperitoneal sarcoma causing lateral deviation of the right ureter and distortion and rotation of the kidney. *B*, Despite surgical excision, recurrent sarcoma resulted in complete obstruction and nonvisualization of the right kidney.

TABLE 10–2. SECONDARY RETROPERITONEAL
TUMORS THAT CAUSE EXTRINSIC OBSTRUCTION OF
URETER*

Cervix	
Prostate	
Bladder	Account for 70%
Colon	
Ovary, Uterus	
Stomach	
Breast	
Lymph nodes	
Pancreas	
Lung	
Gallbladder	
Testis	
Small bowel	

*Presented in order of decreasing frequency.

Ureteral obstruction can also result as a complication following surgery for treatment of these disorders (Kontturi and Kaupila, 1982).

The symptoms associated with metastatic obstruction of the ureter include a wide variety of complaints. The symptoms associated with the primary tumor and other metastases may mask those of ureteral obstruction. Flank pain, sepsis, and fever may herald extrinsic blockage of the ureter. Often, ureteral obstruction is not suspected until the patient develops oliguria or anuria and azotemia due to compression of both ureters (Norman et al., 1982). In a small number of patients, metastatic obstruction of the ureter will be the first evidence of malignancy. The obstruction is usually in the distal or pelvic ureter, although the blockage can occur anywhere along the ureter and may be at multiple sites (Fig. 10–19) as well as single ones (Fig. 10–20).

Once the diagnosis is established, the surgeon must decide whether to divert the urinary tract, especially when both ureters are obstructed. The urologist must consider the type of tumor, previous treatment, general condition of the patient, and overall prognosis before proceeding with diversion. It has been reported that 40 to 50 per cent of patients undergoing diversion for ureteral obstruction never leave the hospital, and the majority of patients live only 3 to 6 months. As a group, the patients spend approximately 60 per cent of the remainder of their lives hospitalized (Brin et al., 1975). Ulm and Klein (1960) reported on a series of patients with colon cancer in which approximately 6 per cent had ureteral obstruction secondary to metastatic disease. None of the patients survived longer than 8 months after diagnosis. On the other hand, a more recent report indicated that survival was not as dismal following palliative nephrostomy (Bodner et al., 1982). There are several groups of patients who fare better than the others: patients with carcinoma of the prostate, those with untreated carcinoma (Marks and Gallo, 1972), and patients with bilateral ureteral obstruction from direct extension of pelvic malignancy as opposed to those with bilateral ureteral obstruction from

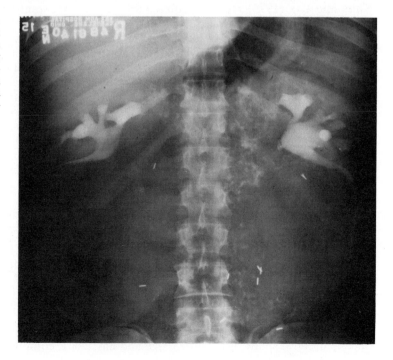

Figure 10–18. Bilateral deviation and obstruction of the ureters due to recurrent tumor involving the retroperitoneal nodes in a patient who underwent an orchiectomy for embryonal cell carcinoma 17 years earlier. The patient had been treated with radiation therapy to the periaortic area following the orchiectomy, but node dissection was not performed.

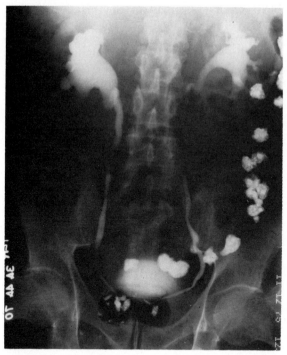

Figure 10–19. Multiple areas of bilateral ureteral obstruction secondary to retroperitoneal metastasis from pancreatic carcinoma.

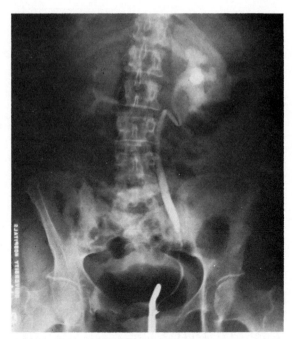

Figure 10–20. Retrograde urogram demonstrates obstruction of a small area of the lower third of the left ureter due to a retroperitoneal metastasis from gastric carcinoma.

disseminated disease originating outside the pelvis (Bodner et al., 1982). Brin and associates (1975) reported that patients with ureteral obstruction due to prostatic carcinoma spent only 30 per cent of the remainder of their lives hospitalized and had a mean survival of 1 year. Khan and Utz (1975) reported comparable figures for patients with prostatic carcinoma, citing two patients who were alive 2 and 4 years after diversion. In those patients who have never been treated for metastatic disease, the response to treatment is generally more favorable, regardless of the location or type of primary tumor.

Once the urologist decides to divert the genitourinary system, he must first decide which is the better functioning kidney. This is most effectively done with the radioisotope renogram if it is not apparent on the excretory urogram. Proximal diversion can be accomplished with either nephrostomy or cutaneous ureterostomy. Today, nephrostomy is usually achieved by utilizing percutaneous techniques. Both procedures have drawbacks. Nephrostomies have a significant incidence of associated infection and stone formation, while ureterostomies often result in stomal stenosis unless the ureter is considerably dilated. Zimskind (1967) initially described the use of the long-term indwelling silicone ureteral splint. It is nonreactive and has

a low incidence of associated infection. Its use is limited because of the technical difficulties in inserting the splint beyond the obstruction (Marmar, 1970; Orikasa et al., 1973). The double J ureteral catheter as described by Finney (1978) has become the preferred long-term ureteral stent because of the relative ease of insertion.

The lymphoproliferative disorders such as lymphoma and leukemia also obstruct the ureter by virtue of lymph node infiltration (Fig. 10–21). In a large autopsy series, 6 per cent of lymphoma patients had evidence of ureteral obstruction secondary to lymph node involvement. The genitourinary tract was involved in approximately 30 per cent of the patients. Ureteral obstruction secondary to lymphoma is, therefore, a relatively infrequent occurrence and is also a late phenomenon. Death due to urinary tract involvement accounts for only 0.5 per cent of lymphoma mortalities (Martinez Maldonado and Romirez DeArellon, 1962).

Other Mass Lesions of the Retroperitoneum

LYMPHOCELE

A lymphocele, also known as a lymphocyst, is a complication of radical pelvic surgery that

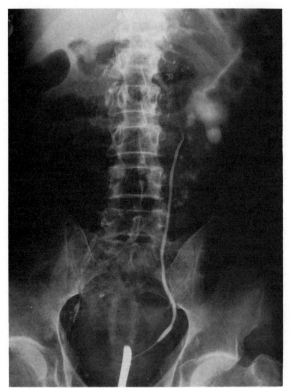

Figure 10–21. Retrograde urogram demonstrates obstruction of the upper third of the left ureter secondary to recurrent lymphoma. Ureterolysis resulted in relief of the hydronephrosis.

may lead to extrinsic obstruction of the ureter. Lymphoceles develop subsequent to pelvic lymphadenectomy and renal transplantation. A variable incidence of 12 to 24 per cent has been reported following pelvic lymphadenectomy, and significant lymphoceles develop in approximately 4 to 5 per cent of renal transplant patients (Banowsky et al., 1974; Geyer and Merrill, 1972).

Lymphoceles are believed to result from the surgical severance and inadequate closure of afferent lymphatic channels. It has been postulated that the cystic collections develop when the adjacent peritoneum becomes edematous and fibrotic, preventing the resorption of extravasated lymph. The formation of the cyst is apparently enhanced by extensive dissection, excision of large surgical specimens, the presence of tumor-bearing lymph nodes, and preoperative irradiation. Surgical preparation of the recipient kidney as well as the donor kidney may predispose to lymph leakage because many lymphatics are interrupted. In addition, factors related to the transplant state may contribute to the increased and prolonged lymph drainage. Rejection is felt to play an important role, since

it causes approximately a 20-fold increase in lymph flow, although it is uncertain whether this is from the donor lymphatics or the recipient lymphatics. Open transplant biopsy may interrupt capsular lymphatics, and ureteral obstruction is also known to increase lymphatic flow. Because the interruption of lymphatics during surgery is felt to be important in the development of lymphoceles, careful attention to the ligation of lymphatics is important to help prevent lymph pooling and cyst formation.

Eighty to 90 per cent of lymphoceles are apparent 3 weeks postoperatively. Small lymphoceles are asymptomatic. The symptoms associated with large lymphatic cysts depend on the size and location of the cyst, which may compress the ureter, the bladder, the sigmoid colon, and the iliac blood vessels. The patients may experience lower abdominal pain, frequency, and constipation. Edema of the genitalia and lower extremities is often present on the basis of both venous and lymphatic obstruction. The combination of thigh edema and groin pain may mimic thrombophlebitis. Palpation of the abdomen or bimanual pelvic or rectal examination may reveal a lower abdominal mass. At times, the mass is fluctuant, depending on the size of the cyst and the thickness of the cyst wall. Bilateral lymphoceles rarely may be responsible for oliguria and renal failure. Decreased renal function is more often seen in association with lymphoceles in kidney transplant patients.

The excretory urogram often shows anterior and medial displacement of the ureter with varying degrees of obstruction and compression of the bladder. Retrograde urography, particularly if an acorn-tip catheter is used, is often the best study for demonstrating the displacement of the lower ureter. If present, indentation of the bladder may also be displayed on a cystogram. This study is also helpful in excluding extravasation in transplant patients. Ultrasound or computerized tomography is invaluable in demonstrating and following the size of the lymphocele. Lymphangiography is a valuable adjunct if the diagnosis remains uncertain, since the puddling of contrast media in the lymphocele is demonstrated. Some also advocate aspiration of the cyst to confirm the diagnosis, although there is a danger of introducing infection.

No surgical treatment is required for most lymphoceles, since spontaneous regression usually occurs (Geyer and Merrill, 1972). Accordingly, the management consists of bed rest to reduce pain and edema, and antibiotic therapy for pelvic and urinary infections. Elastic stockings help control the edema of the lower extremities and hasten ambulation. If ureteral obstruction is present, careful observation with serial urography is necessary, and ureteral catheterization may be required to drain an infected hydronephrotic kidney. Progressive hydronephrosis and pyelonephritis, massive leg edema, or deterioration of renal function is an indication for surgery. Aspiration of the cyst is not advisable because the fluid rapidly reaccumulates. The necessity for multiple taps also increases the possibility of infection. Internal drainage appears to be the preferred surgical procedure. A transperitoneal window is made by marsupialization of the opened cyst to the peritoneum, and the sigmoid colon or cecum is anchored to the posterior wall of the cyst (Griffith and Carlton, 1970). Incision and drainage by marsupialization of the cyst to the subcutaneous and subcuticular tissue through a small skin incision, with placement of several drains and packing, have also been advocated for renal transplant patients (Banowsky et al., 1974). The latter procedure has the advantages of simplicity, rapidity of performance, lack of injury to the allograft, and prevention of recurrence. In order to reduce the chance of infection, the packing in the cyst cavity is soaked in 1 per cent neomycin solution. The packing is changed daily with a sterile technique, and antibacterial ointment is applied to the skin edges.

PELVIC LIPOMATOSIS

Pelvic lipomatosis is a proliferative process involving the mature fat of the pelvic retroperitoneal space. The proliferating adipose tissue may compress the pelvic viscera in varying degrees, including the pelvic portion of the ureters. Occasionally, marked bilateral ureteral obstruction may lead to the development of uremia.

Engels, in 1959, was the first to draw attention to this entity. Although the disease is a benign condition, it may have serious consequences and is often mistaken for a pelvic neoplasm. Pelvic lipomatosis is rare—there have been fewer than 100 cases reported—but it is probable that many recognized cases have not been included in the medical literature. There have been only four reports of pelvic lipomatosis in females (Goldstein and Vargas, 1974; Malter and Omell, 1971; Joshi and Wise, 1983) and one report in a child (Moss et al., 1972). The disease, therefore, is found almost exclusively in males in the third to sixth decades of life. An unexplained but definite predominance in the Negro race has also been noted, with about half the reported cases occurring in black patients.

The cause of pelvic lipomatosis is unknown. Some authors suggest that it represents a localized form of obesity. Rosenberg and associates (1963) described the process as a manifestation of Dercum's disease (adiposis dolorosa), an entity characterized by the presence of subcutaneous deposits of fat that are irregular and painful. Sclerosing lipogranulomatosis may have a clinical presentation similar to pelvic lipomatosis, but the pathologic findings are those of fat necrosis associated with a granulomatous response (Pallette et al., 1967). Also, involvement is often outside the pelvis, enveloping a number of organs including the aorta, vena cava, duodenum, colon, small bowel, and common bile duct. Certainly, most reported cases of pelvic lipomatosis have not been associated with the type of involvement described in Dercum's disease and sclerosing lipogranulomatosis. It is interesting to speculate about the possible connection between pelvic lipomatosis and other lipodystrophies such as mesenteric panniculitis, Whipple's mesenteric lipodystrophy, and Weber-Christian disease. Until more is known about the cause and natural history of these diseases, pelvic lipomatosis should be considered a separate entity.

On pathologic examination, the lipomatous tissue is found to be composed of mature fatty cells with or without inflammation. The inflammatory response is generally chronic and nonspecific in nature. Varying degrees of fibrosis and adhesions have been reported.

Pelvic lipomatosis is generally found in overweight patients, but most patients have not been grossly obese. Occasionally, the disease is discovered incidentally in an individual who has no presenting symptoms. When symptoms are present, they usually vary and suggest nonspecific disease referable to the pelvis or urinary tract. Symptoms include backache, suprapubic discomfort, low-grade fever, recurrent urinary tract infections, frequency, and dysuria. In a review of the literature, Barry and associates (1973) found that only half the patients had difficulty with voiding despite gross deformity of the posterior urethra and base of the bladder. Occasionally, a patient may present with the sequelae of obstructive uropathy and uremia. Gastrointestinal symptoms are minimal, with the exception of constipation in some patients. Two cases of venous obstruction with complete occlusion of the inferior vena cava and one with left external iliac vein have been reported (Schechter, 1974; Locko and Interrante, 1980).

On physical examination, a suprapubic mass may be palpable. Elevation of the prostate gland may be apparent on rectal examination.

Several authors have stressed the frequency of hypertension occuring in patients with pelvic lipomatosis (Cook et al., 1973; Moss et al., 1972), but this finding has been variable. Cystoscopy is generally difficult or impossible to perform because of elongation and elevation of the trigone and bladder neck. An increased incidence of cystitis glandularis has been noted in pelvic lipomatosis. Yalla and associates (1975) reported two cases of cystitis glandularis in patients with pelvic lipomatosis and found that six of eight patients in the literature who had undergone endoscopic evaluation were found to have variants of proliferative cystitis, notably cystitis glandularis. They suggested that the majority of patients with pelvic lipomatosis who could not be subjected to cystoscopy for technical reasons may have had proliferative cystitis. The cause of these associated proliferative changes in the bladder remains obscure.

The diagnosis of pelvic lipomatosis is established on radiographic examination. The plain film of the abdomen (KUB) shows radiolucent areas of lipomatous tissue in the bony pelvis. Albert, Herman, and Persky (1972) emphasized that the differentiation of pelvic lipomatosis from malignant neoplasm without laparotomy depends upon demonstration of the typical radiolucency surrounding the bladder and rectum. The intravenous pyelogram (IVP) usually demonstrates normal upper tracts, but on occasion there may be severe hydroureteronephrosis or, more often, mild distal ureterectasia. Elevation or vertical elongation of the bladder is seen best on a cystogram but may also be noted on the IVP (Fig. 10–22). Classically, there is also straightening and elevation of the rectosigmoid on a barium enema study. The degree of extrinsic compression may vary, but the mucosal pattern is not altered. Computerized tomography, because it can distinguish between normal fat and other soft tissue densities is ideally suited for the diagnosis of pelvic lipomatosis (Werboff et al., 1979).

Pelvic arteriography is helpful, especially if there is suspicion of pelvic malignancy. Borjsen and Nilsson (1962) state that arteriography can distinguish inflammatory disease from neoplastic disease. Inflammatory vessels are smaller (less than 0.3 mm) and the venous phase appears more rapidly in malignancy, whereas in nonmalignant conditions this phase appears 10 to 15 seconds after injection. Some also advocate double-or triple-contrast arteriography with the suprapubic perivesical injection of carbon dioxide and intravesical air. This technique demonstrates the pelvic vasculature clearly. An increased vascular supply is always noted in pelvic

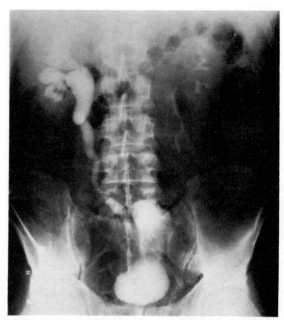

Figure 10–22. Excretory urogram demonstrates moderately severe right hydronephrosis and the classic vertical elongation of the bladder associated with pelvic lipomatosis.

lipomatosis, but the characteristic larger vessels, rapid venous filling, tumor stain, displacement, and amputation associated with malignancy are not found.

In most instances, the disease may be treated conservatively with diet control and massive weight reduction in the more obese patients. Exploratory laparotomy, which may be necessary if malignancy is suspected, demonstrates adipose tissue surrounding the bladder and rectosigmoid. Most authors have concluded that the massive amount of fat present, the adherence of the fatty tissue to the pelvic organs, and the inability to find cleavage planes preclude adequate surgical removal. In several instances, supravesical urinary diversion has been required for the treatment of marked ureteral obstruction (Pepper et al., 1971). Carpenter (1973) reported the successful removal of fatty deposits in a patient with progressive ureteral dilatation secondary to pelvic lipomatosis in whom the upper tracts returned to normal after surgery. He emphasized that the assumption that the nature of the fatty deposits precludes an adequate operation is no longer warranted. The operation was difficult and time-consuming, but with meticulous avoidance of the ureteral blood supply and preservation of a sheath of fat around the ureters, relief of ureteral obstruction was difficult and time-consuming, but with meticulous avoidance of the ureteral blood supply and preservation of a sheath of fat around the ureters, relief of ureteral obstruction was achieved. Carpenter (1973) also noted that two general clinical groups have emerged from the reported cases. The first group consists of young, stocky or obese men who have vague pelvic symptoms in whom there is a definite risk of progressive ureteral obstruction developing. The second clinical group is characterized by men more than 60 years old in whom the disease is discovered during evaluation of unrelated problems, often prostatism. There have been no serious sequelae and no significant progression of disease in this second group. Therefore, the patients who fall into the first group must be followed closely for the possibility of progressive obstruction of the upper urinary tracts occurring. Patients who demonstrate progressive ureteral obstruction may be considered for an attempt at surgical extirpation of the lipomatous tissue or, if this is not feasible, for supravesical urinary diversion.

It has already been mentioned that there is a high incidence of cystitis glandularis in patients with pelvic lipomatosis. The development of adenocarcinoma in a patient with cystitis glandularis has also been noted (Edwards et al., 1972). Based both on this and on the high incidence of adenocarcinoma of the bladder in patients with extrophy (in whom proliferative cystitis is prevalent), the diagnosis of cystitis glandularis has a definite premalignant connotation. Although no cases of adenocarcinoma have been reported associated with pelvic lipomatosis, patients with this diagnosed condition should be evaluated and followed for the possibility of cystitis glandularis and the remote possibility of adenocarcinoma developing.

SUMMARY

Extrinsic ureteral obstruction may be discovered during the evaluation of a suspected genitourinary problem or as part of the routine diagnostic work-up for other pathologic conditions that are often associated with alterations in the ureter. It is now apparent that there are multiple pathologic conditions that may be responsible for extrinsic obstruction of the ureter. When the physician encounters an extrinsic ureteral block, he must proceed methodically with the diagnostic evaluation to ascertain the cause of the obstruction. The history and physical examination must include a thorough evaluation of the vascular system, the female reproductive system, and the gastrointestinal tract. As illustrated throughout this chapter, a careful history and physical examination will often suggest a specific diagnosis. After the initial physical examination, which helps subclassify the cause of obstruction, the laboratory and radiographic studies can be done in an intelligent and orderly fashion to confirm or identify further the cause of obstruction. The urologist must constantly keep in mind the classification of the multiple entities responsible for extrinsic ureteral obstruction to avoid overlooking a possible diagnosis. Although it is not always possible to be entirely certain of the cause of obstruction until an exploratory operation is performed, an orderly evaluation will suggest the best operative approach. A thorough assessment will allow a reasonably accurate diagnosis to be made in most instances, making appropriate therapy possible.

References

Abbott, D. L., Skinner, D. G., Yalowitz, P. A., and Mulder, D.: Abdominal aortic aneurysms: An approach to management. J. Urol., *109*:987, 1973.

Abercrombie, G. F., and Hendry, W. F.: Ureteral obstruction secondary to aneurysm. Br. J. Urol., *43*:170, 1971.

Abrams, H. C., Spiro, R., and Goldstein, N.: Metastases in carcinoma. Cancer, *3*:75, 1950.

Adams, J. T.: Retroperitoneal Tumors. *In* Schwartz, S. (ed.): Principles of Surgery. New York, McGraw-Hill, 1974, p. 1339.

Albarran, J.: Retention renale per periureterite; Liberation externe de l'uretere. Assoc. Fr. Urol., *9*:511, 1905.

Albert, D. J., Herman, G. P., and Persky, L.: Pelvic lipomatosis: Report of three cases. J. Med. (Basel), *3*:282, 1972.

Alfert, H. J., and Gillenwater, J. Y.: The consequences of ureteral irradiation with special reference to subsequent ureteral injury. J. Urol., *107*:369, 1972.

Altemeier, W. A., Culbertson, W. R., and Fuller, W. D.: *In* Welch, C. E. et al.: Advances in Surgery. Vol. 5. Chicago, Year Book Medical Publishers, Inc., 1971.

Amar, A. D.: Ureteropyelostomy for relief of single ureteral obstruction due to retroperitoneal fibrosis in a patient with ureteral duplication. J. Urol., *103*:296, 1970.

Andaloro, V. A.: Mechanism of hypertension produced by ureteral obstruction. Urology, *5*:367, 1975.

Antkowiak, J. G., and D'Altorio, R. A.: Ureteral obstruction secondary to bifurcated aortic grafts. Arch. Surg., *114*:853, 1979.

Aptekar, R. G.: Possible effect of LSD. N. Engl. J. Med., *283*:765, 1970.

Armstrong, J., and Cohn, I., Jr.: Primary malignant retroperitoneal tumor. Am. J. Surg., *110*:937, 1965.

Badr, M.: Renography in normal pregnant patients. Acta Obstet. Gynecol. Scand., *52*:69, 1973.

Bainbridge, E. T., and Woodward, D. A.: Inflammatory aneurysms of the abdominal aorta with associated ureteric obstruction or medial deviation. J. Cardiovasc. Surg. (Torino) *23(5)*:365, 1982.

Banowsky, L. H., Francis, J., Braun, W. E., and Magnusson, M. O.: Renal transplantation. II. Lymphatic complications. Urology, *4*:650, 1974.

Barry, J. M., Bilbae, M. K., and Hodges, C. V.: Pelvic

lipomatosis: A rare cause of a suprapubic mass. J. Urol., *109*:592, 1973.

Beach, E. W.: Urologic complications of cancer of uterine cervix. J. Urol., *68*:178, 1952.

Bergstrom, H.: Radioisotope renography in pregnancy. Acta Obstet. Gynecol. Scand., *54*:65, 1975.

Bernie, J. E.: Ureteral obstruction secondary to ovarian remnants. J. Urol., *108*:399, 1972.

Bissada, N., and Redman, J.: Ureteral complications in diverticulitis of the colon. J. Urol., *112*:454, 1974.

Bodner, D., Kursh, E. D., and Resnick, M. I.: Palliative nephrostomy for relief of ureteral obstruction secondary to malignancy. Presented at North Central section of A.U.A. Meeting. Marco Island, Fla., Oct., 1982.

Borjsen, E., and Nilsson, J.: Angiography in the diagnosis of tumors of the urinary bladder. Acta Radiol., *57*:241, 1962.

Braasch, J. W., and Mon, A. B.: Primary retroperitoneal tumor. Surg. Clin. North Am., *47*:3, 1967.

Brewer, W. R., Caw, C. W., and Bunts, R. C.: Complete obstruction from leukemia and lymphoma. J. Urol., *98*:186, 1967.

Brin, E., Schiff, M., and Weiss, R.: Palliative urinary diversion for pelvic malignancy. J. Urol., *113*:619, 1975.

Brito, R. R., Zulian, R., Albuquerque, J., and Borges, H. J.: Retrocaval ureter. Br. J. Urol., *45*:144, 1973.

Brooks, R. J., Jr., Fraser, W. E., and Lucas, W. E.: Endometriosis involving the urinary tract. J. Urol., *102*:124, 1969.

Bush, I. M.: Obstruciton of the lower ureter by aberrant vessels in children. J. Urol., 108:340, 1972.

Carpenter, A. A.: Pelvic lipomatosis: Successful surgical treatment. J. Urol., *110*:397, 1973.

Carroll, R., and Laughton, J. W.: Obstructive uropathy due to unusual pelvic swelling. Proc. R. Soc. Med., *66*:1047, 1973.

Clyne, C.A.C., and Abercrombie, G. F.: Perianeurysmal retroperitoneal fibrosis: Two cases responding to steroids. Br. J. Urol., *49*:463, 1977.

Considine, J.: Retrocaval ureter. A review of the literature with a report on two new cases followed for fifteen years and two years, respectively. Br. J. Urol., *38*:412, 1966.

Cook, G. T.: Appendiceal abscess causing urinary obstruction. J. Urol., *101*:212, 1969.

Cook, S. A., Hayashi, K., and Lalli, A. F.: Pelvic lipomatosis. Cleveland Clin. Q., *40*:35, 1973.

D'Elia, F. L., Brennan, R. E., and Brownstein, P. K.: Acute renal failure secondary to ureteral obstruction by a gravid uterus. J. Urol., *128*:803, 1982.

Dick, A. L., Lang, R. T., Berman, B., Bhatnagar, N. S., and Seluaggi, F. P.: Post menopausal endometriosis with ureteral obstruction. Br. J. Urol., *45*:153, 1973.

Donovan, A. J., and Ragibson, R.: Identification of ureteral ligation during gynecologic operation. Am. J. Obstet. Gynecol., *116*:793, 1973.

Dure-Smith, P.: Ovarian vein syndrome: Is it a myth? Urology, *13*:355, 1979.

Edwards, D. D., Hurm, R. A., and Jaeschke, W. H.: Conversion of cystitis glandularis to adenocarcinoma. J. Urol., *108*:568, 1972.

Engels, E. P.: Sigmoid colon and urinary bladder in high fixation: Roentgen changes simulating pelvic tumor. Radiology, *72*:419, 1959.

Enker, W. E., and Block, G. E.: Occult obstructive uropathy complicating Crohn's disease. Arch. Surg., *102*:319, 1970.

Evans, A. T., and Coughlin, J. P.: Urinary obstruction due to renal cysts. J. Urol., *103*:277, 1970.

Finney, R. P.: Experience with new double J ureteral catheter stent. J. Urol., *120*:678, 1978.

Fletcher, E. W. L., and Lecky, J. W.: Retrocaval ureter obstructed by aberrant renal artery. J. Urol., *106*:184, 1971.

Friedenberg, R. M., Ney, C., Lopez, F. A., and Stachenfeld, R. A.: Clinical significance of deviations of the pelvic ureter. J. Urol., *96*:146, 1966.

Geyer, J. R., and Merrill, J. A.: Postoperative pelvic lymphocysts. J. Urol., *108*:623, 1972.

Goldstein, H. M., and Vargas, C. A.: Pelvic lipomatosis in females. J. Can. Assoc. Radiol., *25*:65, 1974.

Grabstald, H., and Mephe, M.: Nephrostomy and the cancer patient. South. Med. J., *66*:217, 1973.

Graham, J. B., and Abad, R. S.: Ureteral obstruction due to radiation. Am. J. Obstet. Gynecol., *99*:409, 1967.

Graham, J. R.: Methysergide for prevention of headache. Experiences in five hundred patients over three years. N. Engl. J. Med., *270*:67, 1964.

Graham, J. R., Suby, H. I., LeCompte, P. R., and Sadowsky, N. L.: Fibrotic disorders associated with methysergide therapy for headache. N. Engl. J. Med., *274*:359, 1966.

Gray, L. A.: The ovary and fallopian tube: Problems for the surgeon. Curr. Probl. Surg., p. 1, May 1975.

Griffth, D. P., and Carlton, C. E.: Lymphocysts: An unusual cause of ureteral obstruction. J. Urol., *103*:43, 1970.

Gup, A. J.: Retroperitoneal xanthogranuloma. J. Urol., *107*:586, 1972.

Hafner, C. D., Pontia, J. C., and Brush, B. E.: Genitourinary manifestations of diverticulitis of the colon. JAMA., *179*:76, 1962.

Harrill, H. C.: Retrocaval ureter. Report of a case with operative correction of the defect. J. Urol., *44*:450, 1940.

Heard, G., and Hinde, G.: Hydronephrosis complicating aortic reconstruction. Br. J. Surg., *62*:344, 1975.

Henry, L. G., Doust, B., Korns, M. E., and Bernhard, V. M.: Abdominal aortic aneurysm and retroperitoneal fibrosis. Ultrasonographic diagnosis and treatment. Arch. Surg., *113*:1456, 1978.

Herman, G., Guerrier, K., and Persky, L.: Delayed ureteral deligation. J. Urol., *107*:723, 1972.

Hewitt, C. B., Nitz, G. L., Kiser, W. S., Straffon, R. A., and Stewart, B. H.: Surgical treatment of retroperitoneal fibrosis. Ann. Surg., *169*:610, 1969.

Hirsch, S. A., Robertson, H., and Gorniowsky, M.: Arterial occlusion secondary to methylmethacrylate use. Arch. Surg., *111*:204, 1976.

Hoch, W. H., Kursh, E. D., and Persky, L.: Early aggressive management of intraoperative ureteral injuries. J. Urol., *114*:530, 1975.

Horowitz, M., and Elguezabal, A.: Obstruction of the ureter by recent corpus luteum located in the retroperitoneum. J. Urol., *95*:706, 1966.

Hovatanakul, P., Eachempali, U., and Cavanagh, D.: Ureteral obstruction in chronic ectopic pregnancy. Am. J. Obstet. Gynecol., *110*:311, 1971.

Immergut, M. A., Boldus, R. Kollin, C. P., and Rohif, P.: Management of ectopic pheochromocytoma producing ureteral obstruction. J. Urol., *104*:337, 1970.

Iversen, B. M., Norduke, E., and Thunold, S. L.: Retroperitoneal fibrosis during treatment with methylodopa. Lancet, *2*:302, 1975.

Izant, R., Makker, S. P., Tucker, A., and Heymann, W.: Nonobstructive hydronephrosis. N. Engl. J. Med., *287*:535, 1974.

Jones, E. A., and Alexander, M. K.: Idiopathic retroperitoneal fibrosis associated with arteritis. Ann. Rheum. Dis., 25:356, 1966.

Joshi, K. K., and Wise, H. A., II: Pelvic lipomatosis: 9-year followup in a woman. J. Urol., 129:1233, 1983.

Kaplan, G. W., and Keiller, D. L.: Ureteral obstruction after appendectomy. J. Pediatr. Surg., 9:559, 1974.

Kaplan, J., and Kudish, H.: Endometriosis obstructing the ureter. Urology, 3:225, 1974.

Kaufman, J. J.: Unusual causes of extrinsic ureteral obstruction. J. Urol., 87:319, 1962.

Kaufman, R., and Grabstald, H.: Hydronephrosis secondary to ureteral obstruction by metastatic breast cancer. J. Urol., 102:569, 1969.

Khan, A. U., and Utz, D. L.: Clinical management of cancer of prostate associated with bilateral ureteral obstruction. J. Urol., 113:816, 1975.

Kirk, R. M., Ross, G., Jr., Reddin, P. C., and Thompson, I. M.: Ureteral obstruction complicating the IUD. J.A.M.A., 215:1156, 1971.

Kirsner, J. B.: Occult obstructive uropathy complicating Crohn's disease. Arch. Surg., 101:319, 1970.

Kissinger, D. J., Beaugard, E. P., and Affuso, P. S.: Ureteral obstruction complicating urethropexy. J. Med. Soc. N. J., 79:747, 1982.

Kiviat, M. D., Miller, E. V., and Ansell, J. S.: Pseudocysts of the pancreas presenting as renal mass lesions. Br. J. Urol., 43:257, 1971.

Kontturi, M., and Kaupila, A.: Ureteric complications following treatment of gynaecological cancer. Ann. Chir. Gynaecol., 71:232, 1982.

Krinsky, S., Zieverink, S. E., Peterson, G. H., and Abaskaron, M.: Computed tomographic diagnosis of retroperitoneal fibrosis. South. Med. J., 76:517, 1983.

Kunkel, R. S.: Fibrotic syndromes with chronic use of methysergide. Headache, 11:1, 1971.

Labardini, M., and Ratliff, R.: Abdominal aortic aneurysm and the ureter. J. Urol., 98:590, 1967.

Lapata, R. E., and Adelson, B. H.: Ureteral obstruction due to compression by gravid uterus. Am. J. Obstet. Gynecol., 106:941, 1970.

Lattimer, J. K.: Obstructive uropathy associated with uterine prolapse. Urology, 4:73, 1974.

Lepage, V. R., and Baldwin, G. N.: Obstructive periureteric venous ring. Radiology, 104:313, 1972.

Lepor, H., and Walsh, P. C.: Idiopathic retroperitoneal fibrosis. J. Urol., 122:1, 1979.

Levitt, C. A., and Ingram, J. M.: Abdominal pregnancy with complete ureteral obstruction. Am. J. Obstet. Gynecol., 120:203, 1947.

Locko, R. C., and Interrante, A. L.: Pelvic lipomatosis. Case of inferior vena caval obstruction. JAMA, 244:1473, 1980.

Lynch, K. J., Screenivas, V., and Pelliccia, O.: Ovarian vein thrombophlebitis. N. Engl. J. Med., 275:1112, 1966.

Mackler, M. A., and Royster, H. P.: Right ovarian vein thrombophlebitis and ovarian arteritis. J. Urol., 100:683, 1968.

Madsen, C. M., and Thyboe, E.: Urologic complications in diverticulitis of the sigmoid colon. Acta Chir. Scand. 138:207, 1972.

Malter, I. J., and Omell, G. H.: Pelvic lipomatosis in a woman. A case report. Obstet. Gynecol., 37:63, 1971.

Marks, L. S., and Gallo, D. A.: Ureteral obstruction in patients with prostatic cancer. Br. J. Urol., 44:411, 1972.

Marmar, J. L.: The management of ureteral obstruction with silicone rubber splint catheters. J. Urol., 104:386, 1970.

Martinez Maldonado, M., and Romirez DeArellon, G.: Renal involvement in malignant lymphoma. Am. J. Med., 32:184, 1962.

McCarthy, J. G., Porter, M. R., and Veenema, R.: Retroperitoneal fibrosis and large bowel obstruction: Case report and review of the literature. Ann. Surg., 176:199, 1972.

McEntee, G. P., Smith, J. M., and Corrigan, T. P.: Renal failure from obstructive uropathy secondary to aortic aneurysm. Urology, 20:294, 1982.

Mehl, R. L.: Retroiliac artery urter. J. Urol., 102:27, 1969.

Melnick, G. S., and Bramwit, D. M.: Bilateral ovarian vein syndrome. Am. J. Roentgenol. Radium Ther. Nucl. Med., 113:509, 1971.

Mitty, H. A.: Ovarian vein septic thrombophlebitis causing ureteral obstruction. J. Urol., 112:451, 1974.

Moss, A. A., Clark, R. E., Goldberg, H. I., and Pepper, H. W.: Pelvic lipomatosis: A roentgenographic diagnosis. Am. J. Roentgenol. Radium Ther. Nucl. Med., 115:411, 1972.

Norman, R. W., Mack, F. G., Awad, S. A., Belitsky, P., Schwarz, R. D., and Lannon, S. A.: Acute renal failure secondary to bilateral ureteric obstruction: Review of 50 cases. Can. Med. Assoc. J., 127:601, 1982.

Orikasa, S., Tsuji, I., Siba, T., and Ohashi, N.: A new technique for transurethral insertion of silicone rubber tube into the obstructed ureter. J. Urol., 110:186, 1973.

Ormond, J. K.: Bilateral ureteral obstruction due to envelopment and compression by an inflammatory retroperitoneal process. J. Urol., 59:1072, 1948.

Pallette, E. M., Pattette, E. C., and Harrington, R. W.: Sclerosing lipogranulomatosis: Its several abdominal syndromes. Arch. Surg., 94:803, 1967.

Peck, D. R., Bhatt, G. M., and Lowman, R. M.: Traction displacement of the ureter: A sign of aortic aneurysm. J. Urol., 109:983, 1973.

Pepper, H. W., Clement, A. R., and Drew, J. B.: Pelvic lipomatosis causing urinary obstruction. Br. J. Radiol., 44:313, 1971.

Persky, L., and Hoch, W. H.: Genitourinary tract trauma. Curr. Probl. Surg., p. 1, Sept. 1972.

Persky, L., and Huus, J. C.: Atypical manifestations of retroperitoneal fibrosis. J. Urol., 111:340, 1974.

Phillips, J. C.: Spectrum of radiologic abnormalities due to tubo-ovarian abscess. Radiology, 110:311, 1974.

Polse, S., and Bobo, E.: Bilateral ureteral obstruction 2° to enlarged ovarian vein. J. Urol., 102:305, 1969.

Present, D. H., Rabinowitz, J. G., Banks, P. A., and Janowitz, H. D.: Obstructive hydronephrosis in regional ileitis. N. Engl. J. Med., 280:523, 1963.

Raffensperger, J., and Abousleiman, A.: Abdominal masses in children under one year of age. Surgery, 63:514, 1968.

Raper, F. P.: Bilateral symmetrical periureteric fibrosis. Proc. R. Soc. Med., 48:736, 1955.

Rees, B. I., and Bolton, P. M.: Ureteral obstruction secondary to sigmoid diverticulitis. Br. J. Surg., 62:247, 1975.

Rhame, R., and Derrick, F.: Gartner's duct cyst involving the urinary tract. J. Urol., 109:160, 1973.

Roberts, J. A.: The ovarian vein and hydronephrosis of pregnancy. Experimental studies in the rhesus monkey (Macaca multta). Invest. Urol., 8:610, 1971.

Roberts, J. A., and Dykhuizen, R. F.: The ovarian vein syndrome. Surg. Obstet. Gynecol., 130:443, 1970.

Rosenberg, B., Hurwitz, A., and Hermann, H.: Dercum's disease with unusual retroperitoneal and paravesical fatty infiltration. Surgery, 54:451, 1963.

Rosenblum, R., Derrick, F. C., Jr., and Willis, A. C.: Postpartum thrombosis of the right ovarian vein. Obstet. Gynecol., 28:121, 1966.

Ross, J. C., and Goldsmith, H. J.: The combined surgical and medical treatment of retroperitoneal fibrosis. Br. J. Surg., 58:422, 1971.

Saldino, R. M., and Palubinskas, A. J.: Medial placement of the ureter: A normal variant which may simulate retroperitoneal fibrosis. J. Urol., 107:582, 1972.

Sanders, R. C., Duffy, T., McLoughlin, M. G., and Walsh, P. C.: Sonography in the diagnosis of retroperitoneal fibrosis. J. Urol., 118:944, 1977.

Sant, G . R., Heaney, J.A., Parkhurst, E. C., and Blaivas, J. G.: Obstructive uropathy—a potentially serious complication of reconstructive vascular surgery. J. Urol., 129:16, 1983.

Schechter, L. S.: Venous obstruction in pelvic lipomatosis. J. Urol., 111:757, 1974.

Schmidt, J. D.: Bilateral ureteral obstruction due to cancer of the pancreas. J. Urol., 106:652, 1971.

Schofield, P. F., Staff, W. G., and Moose, T.: Ureteral involvement in regional ileitis. J. Urol., 99:412, 1968.

Scott, T., and Cerny, J. C.: Non-idiopathic retroperitoneal fibrosis. J. Urol., 105:49, 1971.

Shingleton, H. M., Fowler, W. C., Jr., Pepper, F. D., Jr., and Palumbo, L.: Ureteral strictures following therapy for carcinoma of the cervix. Cancer, 24:77, 1969.

Shown, T. E., and Moore, C. A.: Retrocaval ureter: Four cases. J. Urol., 105:497, 1971.

Siegel, J. H., Padula, G., Yatto, R. P., and Davis, J. E.: Combined endoscopic and percutaneous approach for the treatment of ureterocolic strictures. Radiology, 145:841, 1982.

Siminovitch, J. M. P., and Fazio, V. W.: Ureteral obstruction secondary to Crohn's disease: A need for ureterolysis. Am. J. Surg., 139:95, 1980.

Skeel, D. A., Shols, G. W., Sullivan, M. J., and Witherington, R.: Retroperitoneal fibrosis with intrinsic ureteral involvement. J. Urol., 113:166, 1975.

Snow, N., Kursh, E. D., DePalma, R. G., and Hubay, C. A.: Peripheral ischemia due to retroperitoneal fibrosis. Am. J. Surg., 133:640, 1977.

Stanley, K. E., Jr., Utz, D. C., and Dockerty, M. B.: Clinically significant endometriosis of the urinary tract. Surg. Obstet. Gynecol., 120:491, 1965.

Stecker, J. F., Jr., Rawls, H. P., Devine, C. J., and Devine, P. C.: Retroperitoneal fibrosis and ergot derivatives. J. Urol., 112:30, 1974.

Stengel, D. O., Felderman, E. S., and Zamora, D.: Ureteral injury: Complication of laparoscopic sterilization. Urology, 4:341, 1974.

Sterzer, S. K., Herr, H. W., and Mintz, I.: Idiopathic retroperitoneal fibrosis misinterpreted as lymphoma by computerized tomography. J. Urol., 122:405, 1979.

Stevenson, E., and Ozeran, R.: Retroperitoneal space abscesses. Surg. Obstet. Gynecol., 128:1202, 1969.

Strauss, M. B., and Welt, L. G.: Diseases of the kidney, 2nd ed., p. 1019. Boston, Little, Brown & Co., 1971.

Tiptaft, R. C., Costello, A. J., Paris, A. M. I., and Blandy, J. P.: The long-term follow-up of idiopathic retroperitoneal fibrosis. Br. J. Urol., 54:620, 1982.

Tucker, A. S.: The roentgenographic diagnosis of abdominal masses in children. Am. J. Roentgenol. Radium Ther. Nucl. Med., 95:76, 1965.

Ulm, A. H., and Klein, E.: Management of ureteral obstruction produced by recurrent cancer of rectosigmoid colon. Surg. Ostet. Gynecol., 110:413, 1960.

Utz, D. C., and Henry, J. D.: Retroperitoneal fibrosis. Med. Clin. North Am., 50:1091, 1966.

Utz, D. C., and Moghaddam, A.: The clinical guise of retroperitoneal fibrosis. Clin. Obstet. Gynecol., 10:238, 1967.

Wagenknecht, L. V., and Madsen, P. O.: Bilateral ureteral obstruction secondary to aortic aneurysm. J. Urol., 103:732, 1970.

Wanuck, S., Schwimmer, R., and Orkin, L.: Carcinoma of the pancreas causing ureteral obstruction. J. Urol., 110:395, 1973.

Weiss, J. M., and Hinman, F., Jr.: Reversible retroperitoneal fibrosis with ureteral obstruction associated with ingestion of Sansert. J. Urol., 95:771, 1966.

Werboff, L. H., Korobkin, M., and Klein, R. S.: Pelvic lipomatosis: diagnosis using computed tomography. J. Urol., 122:257, 1979.

Yalla, S. V., Duker, M., Burkos, H. M., and Dorey, F.: Cystitis glandularis with perivesical lipomatosis: Frequent association of two unusual proliferative conditions. Urology, 5:383, 1975.

Zalar, J. A., and McDonald, J. W.: Ureteral obstruction and vessel compression secondary to hematoma of rectus abdominis muscle. J. Urol., 102:47, 1969.

Zimskind, P. D., Fetler, T. R., and Wilkison, J. C.: Clinical use of long term indwelling silicone rubber ureteral splints inserted cystoscopically. J. Urol., 97:840, 1967.

SECTION IV

NEUROGENIC BLADDER

CHAPTER 11

Neuromuscular Dysfunction of the Lower Urinary Tract

EDWARD J. McGUIRE, M. D.

Neuromuscular dysfunction of the lower urinary tract is a common urologic problem with multiple causes. In the recent past, urologic treatment of patients with neuromuscular dysfunction was principally by the establishment of urinary drainage with catheters, by urinary diversion, or by the creation of total incontinence. Improved urodynamic testing and a better understanding of the natural history of neuromuscular dysfunction together with the use of intermittent catheterization have changed the goals of urologic treatment from the achievement of drainage at any price to preservation of low-pressure bladder urine storage and urinary continence.

LOW-PRESSURE RESERVOIR FUNCTION OF THE BLADDER

The viscoelastic properties of the bladder wall contribute to the flat pressure response to increasing bladder volumes (Kondo et al., 1972; Kondo, 1972). Abnormalities of viscoelastic properties, chiefly related to collagen deposition, result in a steep bladder pressure response to increasing volumes. Tone is an intrinsic smooth muscle response of the bladder to filling (Tang and Ruch, 1955). The increase in bladder pressure as capacity is reached is due to both tone and the viscoelastic properties of the bladder wall. Tone is probably moderated by neural factors despite some experimental evidence to the contrary (Gjone, 1966). Following complete decentralization of the bladder, the slope of the

pressure-volume curve becomes steeper (McGuire and Morrissey, 1982; McGuire and Wagner, 1977). The abnormally steep slope of the pressure-volume curve can be flattened by the administration of anticholinergic agents and by alpha-blocking agent administration, or can be increased markedly by the administration of bethanechol chloride (McGuire and Savastano, in press, a) (Fig. 11–1). The responses of the decentralized bladder to pharmacologic agents indicate both that part of the steep pressure-volume curve is due to neuromuscular activity and that reflex activity acts normally to modify tone.

Spinal Reflex Activity Involved in Low-Pressure Bladder Urine Storage

Afferent activity generated by stretch and tension receptors in the bladder wall enters the central nervous system via the dorsal root ganglia of S2–S3 and probably S4. Afferent fibers follow a long route to the brain stem, where the information is processed and spinal responses are induced (Bradley et al., 1974, 1976). Spinal responses involve increased activity of the pudendal nerve with increased external sphincter electromyogram (EMG) activity, increased urethral closing pressure, and an associated inhibition of the detrusor motor neurons in the sacral cord (McGuire et al., 1983b; Merrill et al., 1975). Thoracolumbar sympathetic activity also increases with bladder filling (Tulloch,

616

1975). The effects of sympathetic activity on the lower urinary tract include beta receptor–mediated relaxation of the detrusor smooth muscle, alpha receptor–mediated increase in urethral smooth muscle closing pressure, and an inhibitory effect at the pelvic ganglia. Norepinephrine release at the pelvic ganglia delays ganglionic transmission and bladder contraction (DeGroat and Saum, 1972). A complete intradural sacral rhizotomy or dorsal root ganglionectomy of S2–4 obviates spinal reflex responses to bladder filling (McGuire and Wagner, 1977; McGuire and Morrissey, 1982). In spinal cord–injured individuals, sacral rhizotomy prevents autonomic dysreflexia and obviates reflex detrusor contractility and the guarding reflex (McGuire and Savastano, 1984).

Supraspinal Neural Activity and Low-Pressure Storage

DeGroat (1971) demonstrated that the sensory pathway from the bladder traverses the sacral dorsal root ganglia and ascends by a long centripetal neuron to the brain stem. The concept of a brain stem center for the coordination of the neural events involved in bladder storage and in micturition is supported by urodynamic findings in patients with spinal cord lesions (Bradley et al., 1974; Krane and Siroky, 1979; McGuire and Brady, 1979). Afferent pathways from the brain stem project via the thalamus to the cerebral cortex, where they subserve cerebral appreciation of bladder events. The observed inability to inhibit reflex bladder activity in patients with supraspinal neural lesions is apparently related to functional separation of cortical and subcortical neural centers from the brain stem center (McGuire, 1978). Volitional constraint of reflex detrusor activity is a feature of normal adult life. Although all the pathways for the inhibition of detrusor activity and the imposition of volitional control over bladder reflex function are not known, one volitional pathway involves the pyramidal tract. Volitional efforts to inhibit micturition are associated with

a burst of EMG activity from the external sphincter and inhibition of detrusor motor contractility (Susset et al., 1982) (Fig. 11–2). Volitional inhibition of detrusor activity may be exerted within the brain stem, but it also appears to involve a pathway within the sacral cord (McGuire et al., 1983b; Merrill et al., 1975). Whether cortical inhibition of the detrusor motor neurons within the sacral cord by an alternative corticospinal pathway exists in man is not established (Kuru, 1965).

The basal ganglia also have an inhibitory effect on vesical contractility. Lewin and Porter (1965) recorded electrical activity from the basal ganglia that increased with bladder filling and ceased during detrusor contractility. Patients with parkinsonism often manifest uninhibited bladder activity that appears to be nonfacilitated, that is, the detrusor contraction does not continue until full vesical emptying is completed (Pavlakis et al., 1983; McGuire, 1983). The descending neural pathway for basal ganglionic influences on lower urinary tract function within the sacral cord is extrapyramidal. Lack of detrusor facilitation is seen also in patients with spinal cord injury as well as in those with lesions of the basal ganglia (Fig. 11–3).

Certain brain stem lesions are associated with permanent loss of reflex bladder activity. Spinal cord transection, which obviates brain stem influences on sacral spinal cord activity, results in low-volume, uninhibited micturition, which is associated with discoordinate external sphincter activity and is nonfacilitated (Yalla et al., 1978). The guarding reflex—the increase in external sphincter activity that is normally associated with bladder filling—is lost in patients with spinal cord injury (Blaivas, 1979). This appears to be the consequence of a lack of afferent activity reaching the brain stem. Autonomic dysreflexia—the massive sympathetic overresponse to bladder filling that occurs in patients with spinal cord injuries above the T3 level—appears to be related to a loss of supraspinal moderating influences on reflex thoracolumbar sympathetic activity evoked by bladder filling (McGuire et al., 1976b). The magnitude

Figure 11–1. Comparative cystometrograms in nonhuman primates, Ketaset sedation. *A*, Normal animal. *B*, Six weeks after complete sacral rhizotomy. *C*, Same animal as in *B*, following propantheline bromide administration. *D*, Same animal as in *B*, following propantheline bromide and phenoxybenzamine.

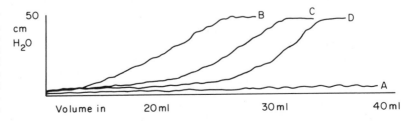

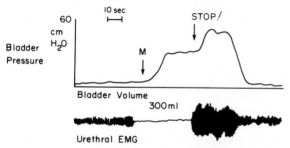

Figure 11–2. Cystometrogram with urethral sphincter EMG. Volitional micturition (M, arrow) associated with electrical silence from urethral sphincter. After voiding is in progress, the subject is asked to stop voiding, which he does by a contraction of the external sphincter, which is associated with a brief isometric rise in bladder pressure, followed by a rapid fall to baseline.

of sympathetic hyperresponse in spinal cord-injured patients suggests that ordinarily brain stem influences are involved in the moderation of the sympathetic responses.

URETHRAL RESPONSES TO BLADDER FILLING

Active components of urethral resistance include urethral smooth and skeletal muscle. The urethral smooth muscle is sympathetically innervated, and the urethral skeletal sphincter is innervated by alpha motor neurons derived from the sacral cord (Elbadawi, 1982). There is an increase in urethral smooth muscle and skeletal sphincter closing pressure during bladder filling (Fig. 11–4). There is some controversy about the precise innervation of the pelvic floor and external urethral sphincter. Donker and coworkers (1976) did not find pudendal neural fibers that innervated the "intrinsic" rhabdosphincter. The "intrinsic" rhabdosphincter consists largely of "slow-twitch" fibers, which are located entirely within the wall of the urethra (Gosling, 1979). This "intrinsic" rhabdosphincter does not take origin from, or interdigitate with, the pelvic floor proper, which is composed largely of fast-twitch fibers. Clinically, the pelvic floor and intrinsic rhabdosphincter usually operate together. With reflex detrusor activity the entire pelvic floor and intrinsic rhabdosphincter are silent electrically. The reciprocal relationship between the pelvic floor and the intrinsic rhabdosphincter and the detrusor muscle is maintained in normal states. Complete sacral rhizotomy results in loss of EMG activity, measurable from the pelvic floor and intrinsic urethral sphincter, and inability to measure peak pressures on urethral closing pressure profilo-

metry, which normally can be attributed to skeletal sphincter activity (McGuire and Savastano, 1984). In that circumstance, alpha-adrenergic blockade will obviate residual urethral closing function; that finding indicates that smooth muscle closure of the urethra is, at least partly, sympathetically mediated.

In addition to reflex increases in smooth and skeletal muscle activity during bladder filling, the urethra in normal individuals is stress-competent. An increase in intra-abdominal pressure does not typically result in urinary loss. In part, stress competence is due to reflex contractility of the external sphincter, but it is also related to the position of the urethra vis-à-vis the abdominal cavity. The proximal urethra from the bladder neck to the rhabdosphincter is, in fact, intra-abdominal. An increase in intra-abdominal pressure results in a pressure change in the bladder and proximal urethra that is equal. Provided the urethra is adequately supported and remains in an intra-abdominal posi-

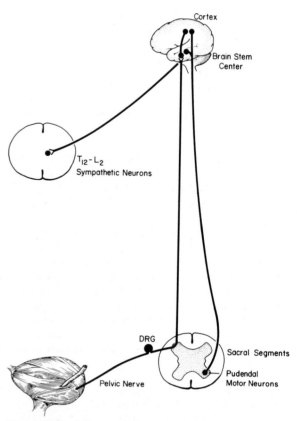

Figure 11–3. Afferent pathways and reflex responses to bladder filling. Stretch activates sensory endings that "long tract" via the sacral dorsal root ganglia to the brain stem and thence to the cortex and subcortical centers. Storage activity induced by filling includes pudendal neural firing, increased thoracolumbar sympathetic activity, and increased electrical activity recorded in the basal ganglia.

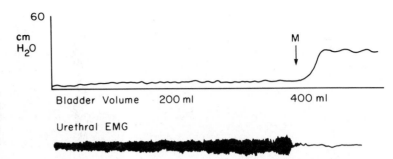

60

cm
H₂0

M

Bladder Volume   200 ml   400 ml

Urethral EMG

Figure 11–4. Cystometrogram and urethral sphincter EMG. The guarding reflex or increased EMG activity is associated with increasing bladder volumes. EMG activity ceases with volitional micturition (M).

tion, urinary leakage will not occur with an excursion in intra-abdominal pressure. On the other hand, if the smooth muscle internal sphincter mechanism, which is intra-abdominal, works poorly or not at all, the skeletal sphincter alone is incapable of resisting changes in intra-abdominal pressure with the same kind of efficiency as the smooth sphincter. In the absence of skeletal sphincter activity, provided the internal sphincter functions normally and is in a normal intra-abdominal position, the urethra will remain stress-competent (Fig. 11–5).

MICTURITION

Micturition can be defined as egress of urine from the urethra, resulting from bladder muscle contractility and urethral sphincteric relaxation.

The coordination of lower urinary tract activity involved in micturition is a brain stem function (Bradley et al., 1976). Normal micturition proceeds until complete bladder emptying is achieved and is said to be "facilitated." Continuous centripetal and centrifugal neural activity has been recorded from the spinal cord of experimental animals throughout micturition activity (Kuru, 1965). The net effect of supraspinal neural activity during micturition is facilitory.

Spinal Neural Activity and Micturition

The initial event in micturition is suppression of pudendal neural-mediated activity within the external sphincter and pelvic floor, followed by preganglionic motor discharge of the detrusor

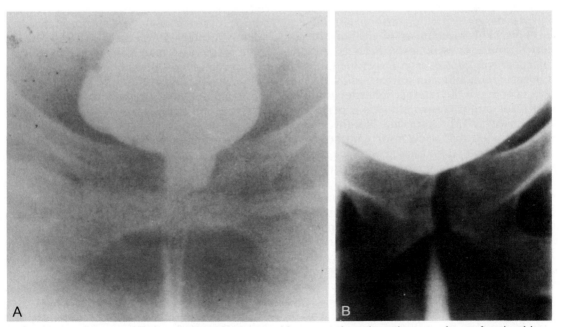

Figure 11–5. *A,* Upright cystogram in 54-year-old woman with severe urinary incontinence and a nonfunctional internal sphincter but a functional external sphincter. *B,* Upright cystogram in a male following complete intradural S1–S4 rhizotomy shows open external sphincter but closure from bladder neck distally to the open area. He is continent with intermittent catheterization.

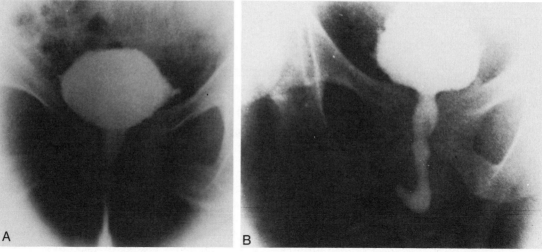

Figure 11–6. Voiding urethrogram in a male *(A)* and a female *(B)* showing patent urethra across the entire active sphincter zone.

motor neurons located in the interomedial-lateral cell bodies within the sacral 2–4 segments (Bradley et al., 1974). These preganglionic fibers leave the neural canal via the sacral foramina and join the fibers of the hypogastric nerve descending into the true pelvis as the inferior hypogastric plexus. They then course lateral to the rectum, and via a ganglionic, synapse adjacent to or in the bladder wall the postganglionic motor fibers reach the bladder muscle.

Thoracolumbar sympathetic activity is diminished during reflex micturition (Bradley et al., 1976). The mechanism of opening of the internal sphincter with micturition is still the subject of some controversy. Experimental studies in cats and nonhuman primates indicate that reflex opening of the internal sphincter is linked to detrusor motor contractility via a peripheral neural pathway (McGuire and Herlihy, 1978). The older idea that a detrusor contractile response was essential for pulling open the urethra has not been supported by experimental and clinical studies. Radiographically, the urethra opens just prior to, or at the beginning of, detrusor contractility, and the open segment of urethra encompasses the entire active sphincter zone (Fig. 11–6). Normal micturition pressures average 30 to 40 cm of water. Static lateral micturitional profile studies by Yalla and coworkers (1980) demonstrate that major stream energy loss occurs in males across the external sphincter area and averages 20 to 25 cm of water. In females, the major energy losses occur in the distal urethral segment (Gleason and Bottaccini, 1968).

Assessment of Lower Urinary Tract Function

Assessment of Storage Function. A cystometrogram, during which the pressure-volume relationships of the bladder, are measured is the standard method for the evaluation of bladder storage function. A normal bladder will fill to capacity, which in adults averages 400 to 700 ml, with a minimal rise in pressure; the mean rise being about 6 cm of water. Because information derived from simple cystometry is frequently insufficient to enable a precise diagnosis to be made or to plan management, cystometry can be combined with radiographic visualization of the bladder and urethra. That method enables the examiner to measure intravesical pressure responses to filling, and at the same time to observe the urethral sphincter mechanism.

Abnormalities of bladder storage function include decreased vesical compliance and uninhibited detrusor contractility. Since both conditions result in a bladder pressure elevation, differentiation of the two can be difficult. Radiography allows the examiner to determine whether a bladder pressure event is, in fact, a reflex contraction or poor vesical compliance. Reflex bladder contractility is associated with visible opening of the internal sphincter mechanism, whereas poor compliance is associated with an increase in intravesical pressure with no change in urethral behavior, resistance, or activity (Fig. 11–7). It is important to be able to differentiate bladder fibrosis, for example, and decreased compliance from intrinsic smooth muscle hypertonicity or bladder defunctionalization syndrome. Although differential diagnosis can be made by a bladder biopsy, a simpler method is to combine cystometry with drug administration.

Hypertonic vesical responses to filling can be moderated by the administration of anticholinergic agents or alpha-blocking agents. Hypertonic vesical responses to filling can similarly be augmented by the administration of bethanechol chloride. If the abnormal pressure-volume curve is the result of fibrosis, drugs will not influence the slope of the curve. Rapid cystometry is another method to investigate bladder compliance. The rapid infusion of a bolus of fluid into the bladder results in a sharp increase in bladder pressure with a later decline. The shape of the pressure response to filling and the slope of the curve can be related to the viscoelastic properties of the bladder wall and to "tonic," or active, factors involving smooth musculature (Susset et al., 1981).

Normal vesical storage with maintenance

of a flat pressure-volume curve is important to ureteral functional integrity (Coolsaet et al., 1982; McGuire et al., 1983a). In pigs and nonhuman primates, parallel changes in ureteral resistance to perfusion accompany changes in intravesical pressure. Assessment of ureteral function must therefore be related to bladder function. Whitaker perfusion of the ureter should be accompanied by Foley catheter drainage, to obviate the effects of intravesical pressure on ureteral resistance (Whitaker, 1979). Similarly, radioactive renograms with Lasix washout should be performed in conjunction with Foley catheter drainage of the bladder. These methods of assessment of ureteral function are relevant in patients with ureteral dilatation. A ureter that tolerates a flow of 10 ml per minute by Whitaker testing is not obstructed. However, poor bladder compliance can also be directly related to ureteral dilatation. Therefore, a study of ureteral tolerance to fluid loads is not very helpful unless bladder compliance is known to be normal. If a steep pressure-

Figure 11–7. *A,* Reflex bladder contraction with detrusor external sphincter dyssynergia in a spinally injured male. Bladder pressure rise is associated with increased EMG activity, and the cystourethrogram exposed at X – shows an open internal sphincter mechanism and a tightly closed external sphincter. Note the area of the urethra compressed by the external sphincter. *B,* Areflexic vesical dysfunction in a 9-year-old boy with myelodysplasia. Gradual bladder pressure increases with filling, with x-ray exposure made when urine leaked out the meatus. Note closure of sphincter during urinary loss and unilateral vesicoureteral reflux at the pressure required to induce urine flow. This is "autonomous voiding."

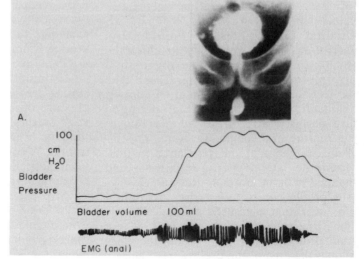

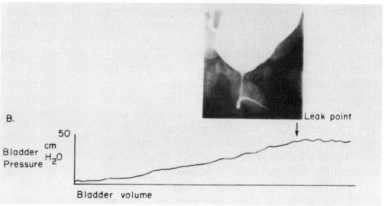

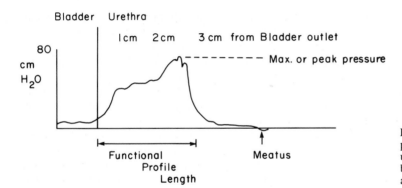

Figure 11–8. Urethral closing pressure profile in a 22-year-old woman. Positive urethral pressure deflection begins at the bladder outlet and extends distally for about 2.8 cm.

volume curve exists, there is no point in proceeding with evaluation of the ureter.

Assessment of Urethral Function And Continence

The history and physical examination are important. A person with a normal sphincteric mechanism tolerates bladder filling and changes in intra-abdominal pressure without leakage. Most individuals with urethral incompetence leak urine in the upright position when intra-abdominal pressure is increased.

Urethral Closing-Pressure Profilometry. Assessment of the forces acting to close the urethral lumen can be accomplished by urethral closing-pressure profilometry (Fig. 11–8). The original technique involved manual withdrawal of a catheter with a single lateral perfusion aperture perfused at 2 to 20 ml per minute through the urethral sphincteric zone. This allowed measurement of the resistance to fluid flow from the lateral apertures (Brown and Wickham, 1969). A normal urethral closing-pressure profile consists of a rise in urethral pressure over that measured in the bladder, beginning precisely at the bladder neck. There is a gradual increase in pressure from the bladder neck to the area of the urethra most closely associated with skeletal musculature, and then a fall-off in pressure from that area to the meatus. Measurable parameters include functional urethral length (that length of urethra manifesting a pressure higher than that of the bladder) and peak urethral closing pressure (the highest pressure measured in the urethral sphincter mechanism). In addition to water perfusion systems, CO_2 systems, membrane catheters, and microtransducer-equipped catheters have been used to study urethral function in conjunction with mechanical pullers.

All these studies provide a measure of the forces operating to close the urethra, but at present they still have limited clinical applicability. To study the components of urethral closure, urethral profilometry can be combined with EMG determinations from the external sphincter (Anderson et al., 1976). EMG activity increases as the perfusion aperture nears the area of maximal external sphincter presence. Heightened EMG responses are seen in patients with suprasacral spinal cord injury, and loss of EMG response is noted in patients with sacral or pudendal neural lesions. For a precise analysis of urethral sphincter function, urethral closing-pressure profilometry can be combined with EMG recordings and the process visualized fluoroscopically (McGuire, 1977). This permits the examiner to localize the anatomic area of the urethra from which urethral closing pressures are being recorded.

Normally, the onset of a positive urethral closing-pressure advantage over the intravesical pressure occurs precisely at the bladder neck. Peak urethral closing pressures are recorded in the area of maximal external sphincter concentration. A competent urethra is associated with manometric and radiographic closure of the proximal urethral sphincter mechanism (Fig. 11–9). Stress incontinence is associated with nonfunction of the internal sphincter mechanism from the bladder neck to the area of the intrinsic rhabdosphincter or, in females, with urethral hypermobility visible fluoroscopically (Fig. 11–10). Although urethral pressure measurements have improved our ideas of urethral dynamics, most authorities would not subscribe to any uniform explanation of urethral sphincter function at this time. It remains to be proved which urethral closing-pressure profile values are indicative in an exclusive way of continence or incontinence.

Assessment of the Control of the Micturition Reflex

A normal bladder tolerates filling without contraction. An unstable bladder does not. Normally, involuntary and voluntary control of reflex micturition result in bladder capacities consistent with 3 or 4 hours of micturition-free intervals without obtrusive symptoms. Reflex bladder contractility cannot be provoked in normal circumstances simply by filling the bladder, despite subjective discomfort. Patients with detrusor instability or a hyperreflexic bladder demonstrate reflex bladder contractility, which is provoked with little warning and without the permission of the subject studied. The term "detrusor instability" is broad and does not denote any specific neural lesion (Turner-Warwick, 1979). Unstable bladder dysfunction is common to patients with enuresis, to those with cerebral vascular disease processes, to adult females with stress incontinence, and to male patients with obstructive prostatism. The urodynamic findings in all these patient groups are similar.

There are pitfalls in the diagnosis of bladder instability both urodynamically and by history, however. In a urodynamic testing situation with an alert patient it is not unusual for a detrusor contraction not to be provoked. If the history suggests detrusor instability, it is probably best to ignore the urodynamic findings in this circumstance. Historical features that suggest detrusor instability include urgency, urge incontinence, incontinence at the sound of running water, and incontinence on the way to the toilet. On the other hand, although very rapid bladder filling may elicit an unstable bladder response, that by itself is not proof that the cause of the patient's complaint is detrusor instability. Complex urodynamic evaluation of patients with detrusor instability, including fluoroscopic observation of the bladder and urethra combined with EMG recording, has some advantages over simple cystometry in this regard. Using these methods, the first sign of reflex bladder contractility is diminished EMG activity and a decrease in urethral closing pressure. With stable bladder function, such changes in EMG and urethral closing pressure do not occur, and the guarding reflex continues to operate until the patient deliberately and volitionally attempts to initiate micturition. The observation of a decrease in EMG activity and a fall in urethral closing pressure that occurs without the subject's

Figure 11–9. *A,* Schematic diagram of the male urethral sphincter mechanism. *B,* Urethral closing pressure profile in a 22-year-old quadriplegic. Shown are normal pressures recorded from proximal and distal sphincter zones, with visible occlusion of the active sphincteric elements.

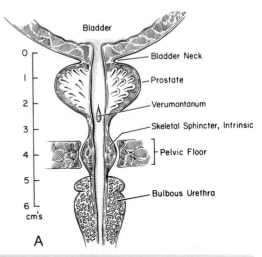

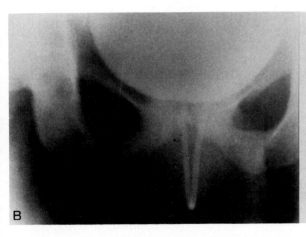

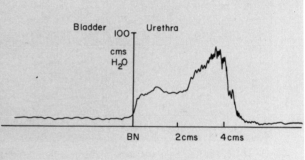

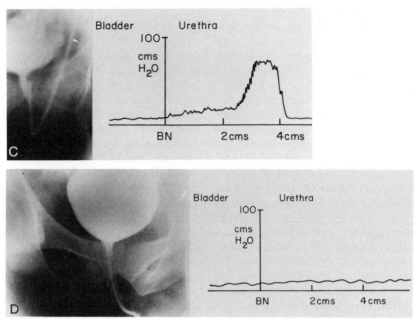

Figure 11–9 *Continued. C,* Same patient following 2 months of therapy with an alpha-blocking agent. Note open nonfunctional, no pressure internal sphincter mechanism to a level adjacent to and distal to the verumontanum. Closure is persistent monometrically and radiographically in the area of the striated sphincter. *D,* Same patient following single-plane external sphincterotomy. There is no measurable urethral pressure or radiographic closure.

knowledge and without volition enables the examiner to make the diagnosis of detrusor instability. It appears that uninhibited urethral relaxation is simply a prodromal event in reflex bladder contractility, even if the patient later becomes aware that a bladder contraction is in progress and halts it, it is likely that detrusor instability is the underlying problem.

Patients with detrusor instability show a striking lack of cerebral appreciation of bladder events (Torrens and Collins, 1975; Yeates, 1972). Since urodynamic evaluation of patients with symptoms suggestive of detrusor instability is often negative, continuous monitoring has been done by Frohneberg and coworkers (1981) and Bradley and coworkers (1982) to improve diagnostic accuracy. A continuous record of intravesical pressure made while the patient performs day-to-day activities is a much more sensitive indicator of reflex detrusor contractility as a cause of incontinence. These methods are technically demanding and expensive, but they

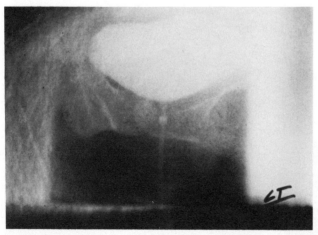
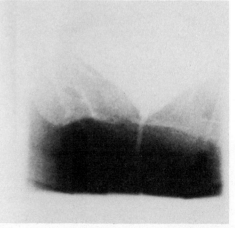

Figure 11–10. Resting right and straining left cystourethrograms in a 36-year-old woman with stress incontinence. Urethral motion and bladder base descent are associated with visible urethral urinary leakage.

demonstrate that a significant percentage of patients who do not show uninhibited bladder dysfunction on provocative cystometry will do so with less obtrusive approaches.

Assessment of Micturition

Normal micturiton involves an increase in intravesical pressure with wide opening of the urethral sphincter mechanism. Abnormal micturition may be the result of diminished or absent bladder contractility, or bladder contractility opposed by inappropriate urethral sphincteric activity, or anatomic obstruction. Accurate assessment of micturition includes definition of all the events in urinary expulsion and requires simultaneous assessment of bladder and urethral activity.

DIRECT URODYNAMIC EVALUATION

The combination of a recording of intravesical pressure with intraurethral pressure, external sphincter EMG activity, and cystourethrography enables the examiner to determine that a reflex bladder contraction has occurred and allows assessment of the interaction of the bladder and urethra throughout voiding. The "micturitional static" urethral closing-pressure profile technique involves the simultaneous recording of intravesical pressure while the urethral per-

fusion aperture of a urodynamic catheter is withdrawn through the active sphincter zone (Yalla et al., 1980). Normal individuals develop a bladder pressure of 30 to 40 cm of water at peak flow. This pressure is transmitted to the urine as stream energy and is measurable during flow along the urethra as pressure in the urethral urinary stream. In patients with anatomic or neurogenic obstruction, intravesical pressures are higher than normal, but as the urethral perfusion aperture passes the point of obstruction there is a precipitous fall-off in intraurethral pressure (Fig. 11–11). This kind of urodynamic testing requires fluoroscopy so that the examiner knows precisely the anatomic area from which the pressures are recorded.

INDIRECT METHODS

An indirect measure of the interaction of a detrusor contraction and urethral resistance is provided by flow studies (Fig. 11–12). Siroky and Krane (1983), using the data compiled by Susset and coworkers (1973), constructed a flow nomogram.

Griffiths (1973) and many others demonstrated that the relationship between flow and obstruction is relatively constant. However, in detailed studies of large patient populations with specific disorders, as, for example, benign prostatic hypertrophy, flow as an exclusive measure of micturition function has been found to be

Figure 11–11. Micturition urethral pressure profile in a quadriplegic. Once the bladder contraction has begun, the urethral pressure–sensing aperture is withdrawn out of the bladder across the sphincter zone. Bladder pressure is high (80 cm of water), but pressure in the stream is maintained at 80 cm of water through the visibly open internal sphincter. Stream pressure drops precipitously across the external sphincter area. The study shows detrusor external sphincter dyssynergia, as does the voiding cystourethrogram.

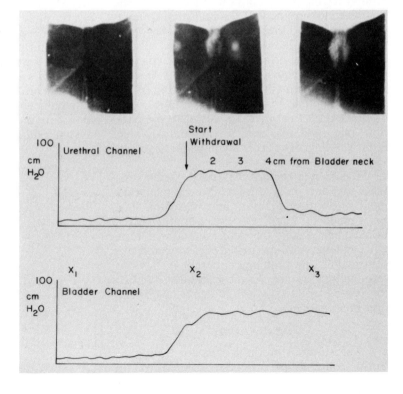

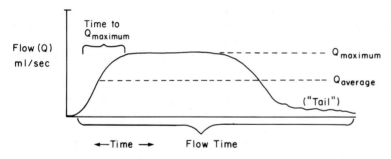

Figure 11–12. Idealized flow rate (Q) determinaton: Q max—maximum flow rate in ml per second; time to Q max—elapsed time between onset of voiding and achievement of maximum rate; Q average—total volume voided/flow time. (Flow time is adjusted to eliminate the "tail" at the end of flow.)

relatively unreliable (Coolsaet, 1983). Some patients with high flow rates are still obstructed, and some patients with low flow rates have an abnormality of detrusor contractility without obstruction. Nevertheless, flow as a screening method is a useful technique. In an effort to more accurately describe the relationship between detrusor work and flow, pressure flow studies have been performed. These methods involve intravesical pressure measurement combined with flow determinations and provide a better indication of the amount of detrusor work done to produce a given flow (Fig. 11–13). Obstruction results in an inverse relationship between bladder pressure and flow (Schafer, 1983). Measurement of intravesical pressure with an intraurethral catheter makes determined flow values inaccurate. These studies, then, from a technical viewpoint require percutaneous puncture of the bladder, which removes this kind of testing from routine clinical assessment.

The measurement of residual stream energy combined with flow determination has been described by Gleason and Bottaccini (1971). Properties of the urinary stream as it exits from the urethral meatus and impacts on a strain gauge allow the mathematical derivation of certain parameters of urethral resistance. The mathematical treatment of detrusor pressure, flow rate, and residual stream energy values improves diagnostic accuracy in patients difficult to diagnose by flow rates alone.

Resistance Factors. Efforts to assign resistance numbers derived from mathematical treatment of detrusor pressure and flow rates have been made by many workers. Although these calculations permit the determination of resistance numbers that are definitely associated with obstruction, the problems inherent in flow determinations do not permit resistance numbers to be used as unequivocal evidence of obstruction in all patients.

DRUG STUDIES

The study of urethral behavior during detrusor contractility can be enhanced by the administration of various drugs, when the effects of those drugs are measured by changes in

urinary flow. Olsson and coworkers (1977) used intravenous injection of an alpha-blocking agent with flow determinations to determine whether or not obstruction existed at the urethral smooth sphincter level. Studies indicating an increased flow rate at 1 or 2 standard deviations on a flow nomogram with the drug were indicative of proximal urethral obstruction. The studies of Abrams and coworkers (1982) and Caine and coworkers (1975), indicating that alpha receptor-mediated prostatic capsular pressure may have an influence on prostatic obstruction provide an additional experimental and clinical basis for the use of phentolamine testing in patients suspected of having obstructive prostatism. Similar studies done in patients with spinal cord injury who were suspected of having internal sphincter dyssynergia have been useful. However, the internal sphincter mechanism is normally linked to detrusor contractile behavior, and wide opening of the internal sphincter is a normal component of a bladder contraction. Therefore, although phentolamine flow testing is useful in patients with internal sphincter dyssynergia resulting from neurogenic causes and in patients with obstructive prostatism, other methods are equally applicable. Detrusor external sphincter dyssynergia is a much more common condition than detrusor internal sphincter dyssynergia, but there is no ideal pharmacologic

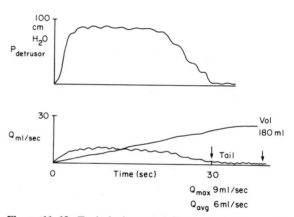

Figure 11–13. Typical obstructed flow curve with poor Q max, low Q average, high bladder pressure, and borderline voided volume.

method to immediately decrease external sphincter activity that can be used in conjunction with urodynamic testing, except for pudendal blockade.

STOP FLOW TESTING

Assessment of the detrusor muscle power and contractile speed can be done by stop flow testing (Coolsaet, 1979). Micturition with a steady flow is attained, and then the patient is asked to stop voiding. Micturition is halted by contraction of the external sphincter, and the detrusor response at precisely that moment is recorded. In normal individuals the bladder pressure rises briefly and then falls to baseline. Patients with fibrosis of the bladder wall or detrusor muscle pathology demonstrate a poor rise in intravesical pressure with stop flow, whereas patients with uninhibited detrusor dysfunction show an augmented detrusor pressure response to stop flow testing with a slow fall-off in bladder pressure. The slope and the height of the pressure curve demonstrated by an isometrically contracting detrusor allow inferences to be made about the speed of muscular shortening (velocity) and the overall power of bladder contractility. Stop flows in women with stress incontinence may be difficult to interpret because these patients may be unable to completely obstruct the urethra rapidly enough to allow an isometric bladder contraction. Coolsaet (1982) used a balloon catheter, which he snapped down to occlude the bladder neck and which allowed the development of a true isometric bladder contraction. Stop flows can also be used to assess the function of the inhibitory mechanism, which usually operates to control reflex bladder contractility. Normally, an external sphincter contraction in the face of a contracting detrusor will result in rapid inhibition of bladder activity and a fall in bladder pressure. Patients with uninhibited bladder activity demonstrate an increased isometric peak pressure with a prolonged elevation following an attempt to stop micturition. In many instances an obstructed bladder will behave in a similar manner.

CLINICAL EXPRESSION OF NEUROGENIC VESICAL DYSFUNCTION

POOR STORAGE FUNCTION RESULTING FROM ABNORMAL VISCOELASTIC PROPERTIES OF THE BLADDER WALL ASSOCIATED WITH FIBROSIS

Vesical fibrosis may result from radiation injury, chronic urinary tract infection, catheter drainage, inflammation of the bladder associated with interstitial cystitis, or carcinoma in situ. Long-standing bladder outlet obstruction may result both in the deposition of collagen and in impaired detrusor contractility. Abnormal viscoelastic bladder properties are associated with a steep pressure-volume relationship on cystometric testing. The bladder pressure may rise steeply with the first incremental volume, but, more commonly, an initial flat pressure curve is supplanted by a progressive upward deflection in intravesical pressure. The adverse effects of altered viscoelastic properties include poor micturition, residual urine, urinary tract infection, ureteral dilatation, vesicoureteral reflux, and a risk to renal function. The relationship between altered bladder storage behavior and ureteral function is linear. Intravesical pressures are paralleled by an increase in ureteral resistance to perfusion. High pressure storage function is frequently associated with febrile urinary tract infections.

Treatment. Since one of the factors contributing to intravesical pressure is maintenance of urethral resistance, which allows bladder filling to a pressure that can be deleterious, urethral resistance can be obviated, the patient made incontinent, and condom catheter drainage utilized to preserve continence. This method is not satisfactory with very small contracted bladders following chronic catheter drainage, in which case treatment must improve bladder capacity. In some cases, this may be accomplished by cyclic filling of the bladder. Although the defunctionalized bladder will respond to cyclic filling, it is not clear that all fibrotic bladders will respond in the same way. Moreover, the risks of cyclic filling in patients with chronic long-standing urinary tract infection, particularly if associated with prolonged catheter drainage, are substantial. It may be necessary to supplant the bladder as a reservoir by partially excising it and using bowel as an augmentation cystoplasty, in order to achieve satisfactory reservoir function. Supravesical diversion is the last alternative. It should be obvious that avoidance of methods of treatment (e.g., chronic catheterization in patients with neurogenic vesical dysfunction) that lead to vesical fibrosis is preferable to urinary diversion.

DISORDERS OF THE BLADDER CHARACTERIZED BY POOR STORAGE ASSOCIATED WITH MUSCULAR HYPERTONICITY

Bladder decentralization results from pelvic neural injury at the time of extirpative surgery for carcinoma of the rectum or uterus, sacral root lesions, and lesions of the sacral spinal cord itself. Decentralization, with time, is associated

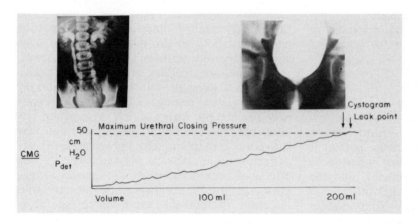

Figure 11-14. Intravenous urogram showing bilateral hydroureter in a 9-year-old myelodysplastic child. Urodynamic study shows poor bladder compliance, with leakage of urine at an intravesical pressure equal to maximum resting urethral resistance. The cystogram taken at the time of leakage shows an open bladder outlet but persistent urethral closure in the maximal pressure zone.

with the development of muscular hypertonicity (McGuire and Morrissey, 1982). The neural mechanism necessary for relaxation of the internal and external sphincter with a reflex increase in intravesical pressure requires pelvic neural integrity. Since decentralization of the bladder results from a loss of pelvic neural integrity, the hypertonic bladder faces a fixed urethral resistance. Intravesical pressure rises until urethral resistance is overcome and urine leaks (McGuire and Wagner, 1977).

Decentralization of the bladder is also often associated with neural lesions that influence sphincteric function. Patients who develop vesical decentralization following radical extirpative surgery may show an associated deficiency in urethral smooth muscle closing function (McGuire, 1975). Patients with sacral cord or sacral root lesions may demonstrate denervation of the rhabdosphincter in association with vesical decentralization. Abnormalities of urethral innervation modify urethral resistance and influence the intravesical pressure required to drive urine across the sphincter mechanism. Eighty per cent of myelodysplastic individuals demonstrate bladder decentralization in association with loss of internal urethral sphincter function (Fig. 11-14). The major impediment to urinary flow in this case is external urethral sphincter pressure. The magnitude of urethral sphincter resistance in patients with decentralized bladder dysfunction is related to upper urinary tract deterioration. If urethral resistance and, therefore, the bladder pressure required to push urine across the sphincteric mechanism is greater than 40 cm of water, the development of ureteral dilatation and vesicoureteral reflux can be expected (McGuire et al., 1983c). If urethral resistance is lower than 40 cm of water, ureteral dilatation and vesicoureteral reflux will not develop, although incontinence may be a problem.

Since prognosis with respect to upper urinary tract function can be related to urethral resistance after decentralization, and secondarily to intravesical pressure, urodynamic evaluation should include these specific variables. One method of assessment of the important factors related to prognosis involves filling the bladder via a No. 8 French tube with a measurement of intravesical pressure at the time of urinary egress across the urethra. Alternatively, one can fill the bladder under fluoroscopic control via a small urodynamic catheter and observe the behavior of the urethral sphincteric mechanism during filling. An open internal sphincter from the bladder neck to the area of the pelvic floor, without a change in intravesical pressure, is indicative of a sympathetic neural lesion resulting in urethral smooth sphincter nonfunction. Urethral smooth sphincter dysfunction can be related to severe urinary incontinence. At the time of a measurable bladder pressure event, observation of the urethral sphincter mechanism provides information that can enable the examiner to determine whether this is reflex or areflexic bladder activity. The typical events in reflex bladder contractility involve wide opening of the entire sphincter mechanism or, in those patients with neurogenic vesical dysfunction, dyssynergic activity of the external sphincter with an increase in bladder pressure. In contrast, areflexic detrusor dysfunction is associated with fixed urethral behavior in the face of a measured increase in intravesical pressure.

Following decentralization, intravesical pressures of greater than 40 cm of water at the time of urethral urinary flow are almost invariably associated with external sphincter activity. Intravesical pressures lower than 40 cm of water are generally associated with lack of external sphincter activity. Internal sphincter pressures are rarely as high as 40 cm of water, but external sphincter pressures are usually 40 cm of water or greater. Since bladder decentralization is

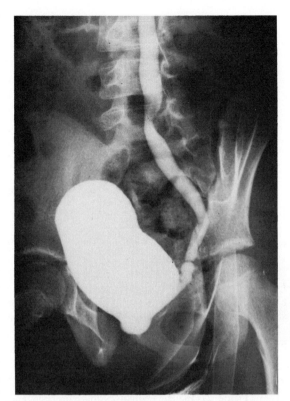

Figure 11–15. Cystourethrography in a 7-year-old child with myelodysplasia. The bladder is filled via No. 8 French urodynamic catheter. The bladder neck and proximal urethra were open at the beginning of the study. Leak point pressure (urethral opening pressure) was 52. Before contrast leaked across the external sphincter, left vesicoureteral reflux occurred.

associated with areflexic detrusor dysfunction, intermittent catheterization is a reasonable method of management (Fig. 11–15). Safe intermittent catheterization requires that those volumes recovered at the time of intermittent catheterization be associated with bladder pressures of less than 40 cm of water. If the bladder capacity is small and compliance poor, intermittent catheterization schedules must be adjusted to be frequent enough to avoid high intravesical pressures, or something must be done to improve bladder compliance.

Bladder compliance can be improved by cyclic filling combined with administration of anticholinergic agents or alpha-blocking agents, both of which are effective following decentralization (McGuire and Savastano, in press, a; Stockamp, 1975). If external sphincter function is present, however, alpha blockade will not diminish peak urethral closing pressure values significantly, although the effects of alpha-blocking agents on the proximal sphincter mechanism, which is essential for passive continence, may lead to involuntary urinary loss.

DISORDERS OF LOWER URINARY STORAGE FUNCTION ASSOCIATED WITH URETHRAL DYSFUNCTION

Abnormalities of Urethral Supporting Structures. The position of the urethra within the abdominal cavity, or of that part of the smooth sphincter mechanism from the bladder neck to the rhabdosphincter, has important consequences with respect to the ability of the urethra to resist changes in intra-abdominal pressure. Stress urinary incontinence is associated with poor urethral support and, at the time of an increase in intra-abdominal pressure, with rotational descent of the urethra into the potential space of the vagina (McGuire et al., 1976a). Abnormalities of urethral position with changes in intra-abdominal pressure need not necessarily be associated with diminished urethral closing pressure and can be diagnosed by physical examination or by radiography (Enhorning, 1961; McGuire et al., 1976a).

Urethral Dysfunction Due to Tissue Loss. Transurethral resection, excision of a urethral diverticulum, and, occasionally, childbirth injury can lead to injury to the internal sphincter mechanism associated with gross incontinence. Upright cystourethrography combined with manometric assessment of the urethral closing-pressure profile value is the most accurate method of diagnosis (Yalla et al., 1982). Males continent following prostatectomy manifest residual closing pressure from the area of the verumontanum to the area associated with the rhabdosphincter. Postprostatectomy incontinence is associated with a lack of closing pressure in this crucial zone of the urethra distal to the verumontanum, despite maintenance of respectable urethral closing pressure measured from the area of the rhabdosphincter (McGuire, 1977). The advantage of radiography combined with pressure measurements lies in the ability to detect the degree and extent of urethral urinary loss, and in the ability to precisely estimate the site of the dysfunction of the sphincter leading to that urinary loss (Fig. 11–16).

Disorders of Storage Function Associated with Urethral Denervation. While complete sacral cord injury or S1–S4 sacral rhizotomy both result in loss of external sphincter activity, the sympathetic innervation of the urethra escapes this kind of neural lesion. Internal sphincter function remains normal, and continence is usually well preserved despite the necessity for intermittent catheterization (McGuire and Wagner, 1977). Although urethral closing pressure in this circumstance is lower than in the converse

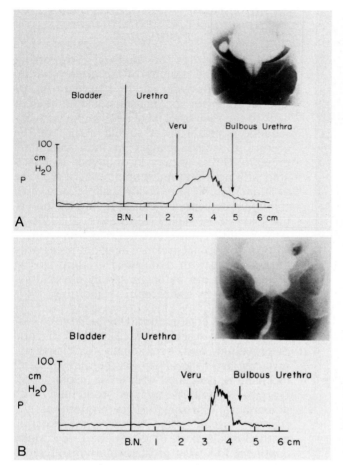

Figure 11–16. *A*, Upright cystourethrogram and urethral closing pressure profile in a 52-year-old man continent following transurethral prostatectomy. *B*, Upright cystourethrogram and urethral closing pressure profile in a 62-year-old man incontinent following prostatectomy.

situation characterized by loss of internal sphincter function and preservation of external sphincter function, continence is much better preserved. The assessment of urethral function is best accomplished by upright cystourethrography combined with urethral pressure profile measurements with an EMG recording from the intrinsic rhabdosphincter. However, an EMG is not absolutely essential, since peak urethral closing-pressure values of greater than 40 cm of water in the area typically associated with rhabdosphincter activity can be related to external sphincter function.

The ability to reflexively and volitionally contract the external sphincter can easily be ascertained radiographically and manometrically. An open nonfunctional internal sphincter from which no pressures can be recorded, and which is filled with contrast material radiographically, is diagnostic of urethral internal sphincter nonfunction (Woodside and McGuire, 1979). This is associated with severe incontinence and can be related to the loss of thoracolumbar spinal cord activity, as, for example, in myelo-

dysplastic patients or in patients who suffer spinal cord infarction. Total loss of internal sphincter function can also follow extensive pelvic extirpative surgery, as, for example, abdominoperineal resection for carcinoma of the rectum, low anterior resection for carcinoma of the rectosigmoid, and radical hysterectomy for carcinoma of the uterus or cervix. In addition, traumatic pelvic fractures can be associated with total denervation of the internal sphincter mechanism (Fig. 11–17).

Weakness of urethral closing pressure exerted by urethral smooth muscle, which also can be associated with severe incontinence, can be the result of prolonged treatment with alpha-adrenergic blocking agents or drugs used for the control of hypertension, which have alpha-blocking side effects, as well as major ataractic agents with alpha-blocking side effects (Fig. 11–18). While weakness of urethral smooth sphincter function due to tissue loss, or as a result of treatment with alpha-blocking agents, may improve with drug therapy, or the cessation of drug therapy with alpha-blocking side effects, urethral dysfunction associated with total sympathetic denervation does not respond to alpha-stimulating agents.

Augmentation of urethral resistance surgically can be achieved by a pubovaginal sling, implantation of an inflatable sphincter, or periurethral Teflon injection. Before treatment that increases urethral closing efficiency is undertaken, assessment of bladder storage function and reflex contractile ability is essential. If bladder compliance is poor and areflexic bladder function is present, increasing urethral resistance may lead to upper urinary tract deterioration (Fig. 11–19). If disorders of urethral closing pressure exist in conjunction with hyperreflexic bladder dysfunction, augmentation of urethral resistance is unlikely to be successful in controlling incontinence and may lead to

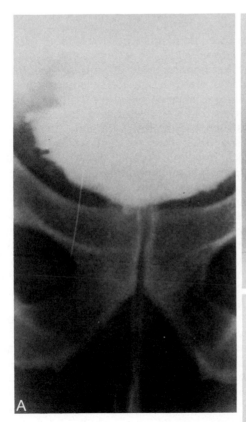

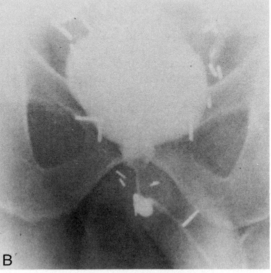

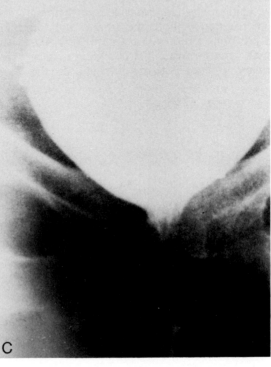

Figure 11–17. *A,* Upright cystogram in a 20-year-old paraplegic woman following complete S1–S4 sacral rhizotomy. Note normally closed internal sphincter. *B,* Upright cystogram in a 50-year-old male following abdominoperineal resection for carcinoma of the rectum. Note open nonfunctional internal sphincter that encompasses the negative shadow of the verumontanum. *C,* Upright cystogram in a 40-year-old woman following Wertheim hysterectomy. Note open internal sphincter.

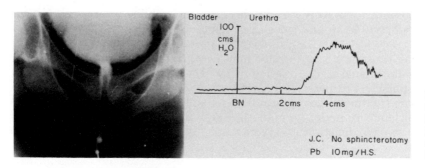

Figure 11–18. Upright cystoure-throgram and urethral profile in a 29-year-old quadriplegic treated for 30 days with an alpha-blocking agent. Note position of verumon-tanum.

upper urinary tract deterioration. Disorders of continence function associated with tissue loss are rarely associated with uncontrollable hyper-reflexic bladder dysfunction or abnormalities of bladder compliance and may be treated much more safely by artificial sphincteric implanta-tion, a Kaufman prosthesis, or Teflon injection of the urethra (Scott et al., 1973; Kaufman, 1978; Politano, 1978).

DISORDERS OF BLADDER STORAGE FUNCTION ASSOCIATED WITH UNCONTROLLABLE DETRUSOR REFLEX ACTIVITY

Unstable bladder dysfunction occurs in pa-tients with supraspinal neural or vascular dis-ease, parkinsonism, the dementias, and spinal neural disease. Idiopathic detrusor instability is a common concomitant of obstructive uropathy and of stress incontinence. The diagnosis of bladder instability is made by provocative cys-tometry, using high filling rates and performing a cystometrogram in both the supine and the upright positions (Turner-Warwick, 1979). Pa-tients with detrusor instability complain of sud-den urinary urgency with no warning. In the

advanced dementias, however, there may be no symptoms at all. It is important to determine the volume required to initiate the unstable bladder response and to measure residual urine volumes. Since detrusor instability may occur in conjunction with obstruction, the suspicion that obstructive uropathy is the underlying problem is supported by significant residual urine vol-umes. In addition, diabetic patients and patients with peripheral neural injuries may require large volumes to initiate an unstable bladder re-sponse. Although the best treatment for non-obstructive detrusor hyperreflexia is anticholi-nergic agents and timed voiding, these methods are totally inappropriate for patients with ob-structive uropathy or for those with neural le-sions associated with high-volume detrusor in-stability, who are much better treated by intermittent catheterization.

Treatment of Bladder Instability Not As-sociated with Obstruction. Delay in reflex de-trusor contractility and improved cerebral ap-preciation of bladder events can be achieved by the administration of anticholinergic agents, as, for example, oxybutynin chloride, 5 mg t.i.d.-q.i.d.; dicyclomine hydrochloride, 20 to 40 mg

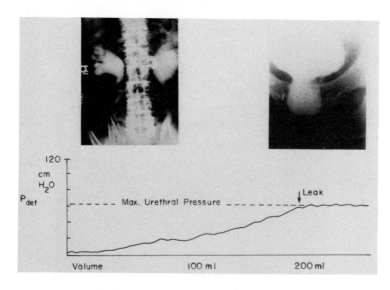

Figure 11–19. Fifty-six-year-old man with severe day and nighttime incontinence following abdominoperineal resection and transurethral prostatectomy to im-prove "voiding." Upright cystogram shows dilated prostatic urethra. Intrave-nous urogram shows hydroureter and hy-dronephrosis. Cystometrogram shows an areflexic, hypertonic bladder, which leaks urine at a pressure of 62 cm of water across the distal sphincter mechanism. This patient could be treated by external sphincterotomy and a prosthetic device, but he responded to intermittent cathe-terization and anticholinergic agents.

q.i.d.; propantheline, 15 to 30 mg, t.i.d.; or the tricyclic antidepressants, for example, imipramine hydrochloride, 10 to 75 mg q.i.d. While there are few double-blind studies of the efficacy of these agents, they can be effective. Patients who fail to improve with anticholinergic medication alone can often be treated with both a tricyclic antidepressant and an anticholinergic agent, with improved results and better tolerance of side effects. Bladder-training techniques combined with medication have also been found useful for patients with idiopathic detrusor instability (Frewen, 1979).

Detrusor instability that remains totally refractory to treatment with drugs can be treated by bladder overdistention (Pengelly, 1979), by subtrigonal neurolytic procedures (Ingelman-Sundberg, 1978), by partial rhizotomy (Torrens and Griffith, 1976), by bladder excision and reanastomosis, or by supratrigonal resection and augmentation cystoplasty (Green et al., 1983; Gittes, 1976). Diversion can be used as a treatment of last resort. In general, refractory detrusor instability occurs in patients with the demyelinating diseases, those with spinal cord injury or disease, and those who develop detrusor instability after prolonged bladder overdistention or prolonged obstruction, or both. In some instances, however, intractable detrusor instability may be a hysterical conversion reaction. It should be obvious that diversion for psychiatric disease will be an unsatisfactory method of treatment. Since some patients with bladder instability, in fact, are obstructed and develop retention with anticholinergic therapy, it is reasonable to check on urinary residuals after institution of anticholinergic therapy to be certain that complete vesical emptying is present.

SENSORY INSTABILITY OR URGENCY WITHOUT INCONTINENCE

Urgency and frequency of urination without incontinence occur in response to bladder inflammation but may be idiopathic, at least as determined by current diagnostic techniques. Traditional urologic evaluation is helpful in such patients rather than urodynamic evaluation, which usually shows only stable bladder function with poor subjective volume tolerance. Medication effective for contractile detrusor instability does not effect relief of poor volume tolerance. Poor volume tolerance can result from cystitis (bacterial, fungal, protozoal, or interstitial), and from bladder calculi, carcinoma in situ, and radiation or chemical injury. In the majority of patients, no clear etiology can be established and the symptoms are often attributed to prostatitis, urethritis, prostatodynia, or psychologic causes. As with most multifactorial symptom complexes, the majority of patients have an idiopathic condition that responds poorly to empirical treatment of obstruction, infection, or hyperreflexia. Some patients do improve as the result of bladder overdistention or DMSO instillation. If diffuse vesical scarring with collagen deposition is present, excision of the bladder, leaving only the trigone, and augmentation cystoplasty or diversion may be required as a last resort (Gittes, 1976).

ABNORMAL MICTURITION AND ANATOMIC OBSTRUCTION ASSOCIATED WITH COORDINATE BLADDER EXTERNAL SPHINCTER RELATIONSHIPS

The etiology of bladder outlet obstruction is variable. Perhaps the most common cause of bladder outlet obstruction is prostatic hypertrophy. Urinary flow rates are usually diminished, vesical pressures are usually elevated, and residual urine may be present. The diagnosis of obstructive uropathy by indirect methods, i.e., flow rates or even bladder pressure measurements, is complicated by low-pressure, low-flow states, denervation of the bladder, poor reflex function due to myogenic injury, and disorders of detrusor contractility (Coolsaet, 1983).

The initial response of the bladder to obstruction is usually compensatory, but longstanding obstruction may result in detrusor decompensation and asymptomatic urinary retention until overflow incontinence develops. In doubtful cases, endoscopic visualization is unreliable as the sole diagnostic test for obstruction, and pressure flow studies, bladder pressure with voiding cystourethrography, or static micturitional urethral closing-pressure profilometry may be necessary (Fig. 11–20). If detrusor decompensation occurs and no reflex function is present, intermittent catheterization as a temporizing measure is useful until reflex function recovers, in which case a definite diagnosis of obstructive uropathy can be made, the obstructive process localized, and appropriate surgical therapy instituted.

Detrusor Instability and Obstruction. Approximately 50 per cent of males with obstructive uropathy demonstrate detrusor instability. Treatment with anticholinergic agents of detrusor instability related to obstruction is inappropriate and often precipitates urinary retention. If obstruction is thought to be the cause of detrusor instability, pressure flow studies, bladder pressure and voiding cystourethrography, or micturitional urethral closing-pressure

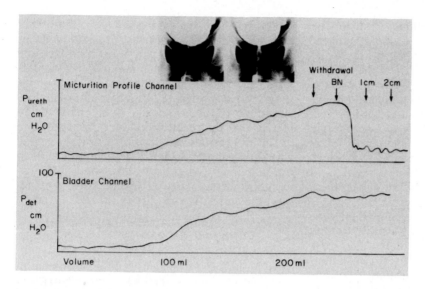

Figure 11–20. Obstructive uropathy in a 28-year-old man. Cystometrogam shows high bladder pressure during micturition. Static micturitional profile shows a large pressure drop across the bladder neck. Cystourethrogram shows poor opening of the bladder outlet.

profile testing should provide sufficient information for a clear diagnosis. The last two methods provide precise information about the actual area of obstruction. In females, bladder instability is common and does not often respond to empirical procedures for the relief of outlet obstruction. While obstructive bladder outlet disease clearly occurs in women, it is relatively rare (Gleason and Bottaccini, 1982). High-grade urethral obstruction in females is frequently associated with bladder decompensation rather than hypertrophy and increased bladder irritability.

Abnormal Micturition Associated with Discoordinate Detrusor Sphincter Syndromes. Spinal shock occurs immediately following spinal cord injury and persists for days to weeks, depending on the severity and level of the injury. Spinal shock results in loss of reflex bladder activity, but with preservation of internal sphincter closing pressures. Areflexic bladder dysfunction can be safely managed by intermittent catheterization. Urinary infection in a hospital setting should be treated with appropriate antimicrobial agents. Virtually all patients with new spinal cord injuries will develop at least one urinary tract infection during the stage of spinal shock. This is rarely associated with a febrile response and can often be managed by direct instillation of antimicrobial agents into the bladder at the time of intermittent catheterization (Rhame and Perkash, 1979; Pearman, 1974).

Recovery of reflex bladder and skeletal sphincter activity occurs weeks to months after the injury, and urodynamic evaluation should be performed at this time. The assessment of bladder storage function is particularly impor-

tant. Low-pressure bladder storage for those volumes recovered at the time of intermittent catheterization should be present (McGuire and Savastano, 1983). If not, and if reflex detrusor activity continues to occur with urinary leakage, anticholinergic medication can be given to prolong low-pressure bladder storage. If reflex detrusor activity cannot be suppressed with anticholinergic agents, and voiding pressures as a result of detrusor sphincter dyssynergia are greater than 50 cm of water, males may require external sphincterotomy, and females a neurolytic procedure to stop reflex detrusor activity.

Patients with incomplete spinal cord injury should be preferentially maintained on intermittent catheterization and vigorous anticholinergic therapy rather than subjected to any irreversible operative procedure, since the possibility for evolution into reasonably normal lower urinary tract function is good. Approximately 70 per cent of patients with complete upper motor neuron lesions will respond to anticholinergic medication and can be safely managed by intermittent catheterization indefinitely. Constant catheter drainage should be avoided in spinal cord injury patients, since 50 per cent of these so treated will eventually demonstrate upper urinary tract changes (Hackler, 1977).

Those patients who leak urine between intermittent catheterization as well as those with high voiding pressures, unsuppressible reflex detrusor activity, and a febrile urinary tract infection require treatment that stops reflex detrusor activity or diminishes outlet resistance. Males may be treated by external sphincterotomy and condom catheter drainage. Despite adequate sphincterotomy, residual urine will continue to be present postoperatively. The measure of the effect of an external sphincterotomy is related to intravesical pressure at the time of urinary flow and not the absence of residual urine. Reflex vesical activity following spinal cord injury does not continue until the bladder is empty; it is nonfacilitated. Cholinergic medication is usually ineffective in improving vesical emptying, serving to increase external sphincter activity as well as tone. The end result of cholinergic therapy is often further impairment in micturitional efficiency (Yalla et al., 1978).

Total sphincterotomy with Credé expression voiding is necessary to induce complete bladder emptying in most patients with suprasacral spinal cord injury (Perkash, 1976). That is not required, however, for maintenance of normal upper urinary tract function and freedom from febrile urinary tract infections, since these are the result of low bladder storage and micturition pressures and are unrelated to residual urine volume.

Problems in Females. Uncontrollable reflex bladder activity with detrusor sphincter dyssynergia can be associated with upper urinary tract deterioration in females, but the more common problem is urinary incontinence. Interruption of reflex pathways at the sacral root level by rhizotomy of S2–S4, or dorsal root ganglionectomy of S2–S4, or percutaneous rhizotomy can control reflex bladder activity and autonomic dysreflexia (Torrens and Griffith, 1976; McGuire and Wagner, 1977). Alternative procedures include vesical resection with augmentation cystoplasty. In quadriplegic females, continent vesicostomy using either ileum or a bladder flap can facilitate intermittent catheterization, even for those individuals with very limited hand function (Green et al., 1983).

Sacral rhizotomy induces a loss of external anal sphincter activity and rectal decentralization, which leads to constipation and even obstipation. This should be anticipated prior to rhizotomy. Although dorsal root ganglionectomy does not result in total loss of anal sphincter activity, it is associated with lack of reflex rectal emptying, which must be compensated with a vigorous "bowel program" for example, two bisacodyl tablets at night, followed by a bisacodyl suppository in the morning on an every-other-day schedule.

Sacral denervation in males is usually avoided because reflex penile erections are lost following the procedure. Although little is known about homologous sexual function in females, including clitoral erection and regression, vaginal lubrication, and labial changes, there is little reason to doubt that these reflex responses are also impaired after rhizotomy.

Autonomic Dysreflexia. This syndrome, consisting of a vigorous overresponse to afferent visceral and sometimes somatic stimuli, was described in 1917 by Head and Riddock (Head and Riddock, 1917). Typically, vesical filling, urethral instrumentation, or voiding induces the response, which consists of an increased blood pressure, piloerection, sweating, blotchy skin rash, and increased pulse pressure with a slow heart rate and a pounding occipital headache. While autonomic dysreflexia can occur with any lesion above T5, it usually occurs in patients with cervical lesions. This syndrome, if episodic and associated with increased bladder volumes, responds to measures that induce bladder urine flow, that is, sphincterotomy or an increase in frequency of intermittent catheterization. The administration of small doses of an alpha-blocking agent, for example, prazosin (1 mg, b.i.d.) or phenoxybenzamine (10 mg, h.s.), is useful.

Acute autonomic dysreflexia that is sustained can be treated by the intravenous injection of phentolamine mesylate (5 mg, IV), or by chlorpromazine administration (2 to 4 mg intravenously or 10 to 25 mg intramuscularly) (McGuire and Rossier, 1983). Intractable, sustained autonomic dysreflexia, which may occur following external sphincterotomy or in patients with pyocystis, is best treated by intravenous or intramuscular chlorpromazine administration together with oral prazosin. Autonomic dysreflexia that either does not respond or persists as a result of an irritative focus that cannot be satisfactorily treated may require sacral rhizotomy. Low spinal anesthesia for patients with the potential to develop autonomic dysreflexia who require urethral or bladder instrumentation or surgery effectively blocks dysreflexic responses.

Multiple Sclerosis. Although urodynamic findings in patients with multiple sclerosis are similar to those in patients with spinal cord injury, treatment and long-term management are complicated by the progressive nature of the disease and consequent changes in visceral and somatic function, as well as the additional problem of supraspinal neural lesions (Blaivas, 1980). Urologically, there are two broad categories of patients with multiple sclerosis. Stable MS tends to respond to treatment, and urodynamic patterns remain fixed for months to years. Most such patients suffer from simple bladder instability without detrusor sphincter dyssynergia (Thomas et al., 1981). Progressive multiple sclerosis, on the other hand, is associated with overt bladder sphincter dyssynergia, detrusor hyperreflexia, and, frequently, urinary tract infections. This kind of symptom complex does not reliably respond to anticholinergic agents and intermittent catheterization, nor is it often completely resolved by external sphincterotomy.

In a small minority of multiple sclerosis patients, bladder areflexia is present and may persist for months to years. On the other hand, bladder areflexia may gradually evolve with treatment by intermittent catheterization into a hyperreflexic dyssynergic pattern. Foley catheter drainage in patients with the demyelinating diseases should be a treatment of last resort. The complications of catheter drainage are often worse than the problem that prompted the catheter use in the first place.

CONDITIONS CHARACTERIZED BY POOR REFLEX BLADDER ACTIVITY OR NO REFLEX BLADDER ACTIVITY

Absence of bladder reflex activity may result from the neuropathy of diabetes (Ioanid et al., 1980), tabes dorsalis, pernicious anemia, posterior spinal cord lesions, and prolonged bladder overdistention. Subjective appreciation of bladder filling is poor or absent, and the bladder is usually not trabeculated. If trabeculation is present, the underlying etiology may be obstructive or neurogenic. Provided that bladder storage function is normal, intermittent catheterization is the treatment of choice; it can be used indefinitely, or until reflex activity is recovered and the underlying obstructive etiology demonstrable.

Absence of reflex activity with poor storage function, characterized by an increased slope on the cystometrogram and bladder trabeculation, usually requires some treatment to induce better bladder compliance. Cyclic bladder filling with anticholinergic agents or augmentation cystoplasty may be required to preserve continence and protect upper tract function. Bladder areflexia, poor storage, and ureteral dilatation require immediate treatment, which may be a reduction in outlet resistance by transurethral resection and external sphincterotomy, transurethral resection alone, or alpha-blockade and external sphincterotomy with the deliberate creation of incontinence. Alternatively, augmentation cystoplasty to achieve satisfactory reservoir function may be employed.

Poor Reflex Activity and Low-Pressure Low-Flow States. This condition may be the result of obstruction that is difficult to prove because detrusor pressures are poor, but it may also occur for other reasons, including idiopathic causes. If the condition is nonobstructive, operations to decrease outlet resistance are not indicated. Some patients with parkinsonism fit into this category and respond poorly to prostatectomy; unless detrusor pressures are elevated and the detrusor contraction sustained, it is better to avoid prostatectomy in patients with parkinsonism (McGuire, 1983). If bladder storage function is normal, intermittent catheterization is the method of choice rather than an empirical reduction in urethral resistance.

Psychogenic Retention. This condition is characterized by painful bladder overfilling, with persistent volitional override of detrusor contractile activity. A cystometrogram combined with an electromyogram shows increasing and sustained EMG activity despite attempts to induce micturition. These findings are not specific for a psychogenic etiology and can be seen in patients with painful operative wounds, after hemorrhoidectomy, with intervertebral disc herniation, and in many other disease states. The treatment of choice is intermittent catheterization and not a surgical decrease in outlet resistance.

References

Abrams, P. H., Shaw, P. J. R., Stone, R., and Choa, R. G.: Bladder-outflow obstruction treated with phenoxybenzamine. In Phenoxybenzamine in Disorders of Micturition. Oxford, Smith, Kline and French, 1982.

Andersen, J. T., Bourne, R. B., and Bradley, W. E.: Combined electromyography and gas urethral pressure profilometry before and after transurethral resection of the prostate. J. Urol., 116:622, 1976.

Blaivas, J. G.: A critical appraisal of specific diagnostic techniques. In Krane, R., and Siroky, M. (Eds.): Clinical Neuro-Urology. Boston, Little, Brown & Co., 1979.

Blaivas, J. G.: Management of bladder dysfunction in multiple sclerosis. Neurology, 30:12, 1980.

Bradley, W. E., Bhatia, N. and Haldeman, S.: Twenty-four hour continuous monitoring. Proceedings of the American Urological Association, 1982; abstract #113.

Bradley, W. E., Rockswold, G. L., Timm, G. W., and Scott, F. B.: Neurology of micturition. J. Urol., 115:481, 1976.

Bradley, W. E., Timm, G. W., and Scott, F. B.: Innervation of the detrusor muscle and urethra. Urol. Clin. North Am., 1:3, 1974.

Brown, M. and Wickham, J. E. A. The urethral pressure profile. Br. J. Urol., 41:211, 1969.

Caine, M., Raz, S., and Zeigler, M.: Adrenergic and cholinergic receptors in the human prostate, prostatic capsule and bladder neck. Br. J. Urol., 47:193, 1975.

Coolsaet, B. L. R. A.: Detrusor energy factors. In Hinman, F. Jr., Ed.: Benign Prostatic Hypertrophy. New York, Springer-Verlag, 1983.

Coolsaet, B. L. R. A.: Stop-test: a preoperative determination of bladder contractility. In Proceedings of IXth Annual Meeting of ICS. Rome, 1979.

Coolsaet, B. L. R. A., VanVenrooij, G. E. P. M., and Blok, C.: Detrusor pressure versus wall stress in relation to ureterovesical resistance. Neurourol. Urodyn. *1*:105, 1982.

DeGroat, W. C.: Nervous control of the urinary bladder of the cat. Brain Res *87*:201, 1971.

DeGroat, W. C., and Saum, W. R.: Sympathetic inhibition of the urinary bladder and of pelvic ganglionic transmission in the cat. J. Physiol., *220*:297, 1972.

Donker, P. J., Droes, J. T. P. M., and VanUlden, B. M.: Anatomy of the musculature and innervation of the bladder and the urethra. *In* Williams, D. I., and Chisolm, G. D. (Eds.): Scientific Foundations of Urology. Chicago, Year Book Medical Publishers, 1976.

Elbadawi, A.: Neuromorphologic basis of vesico-urethral functions. Neurourol. Urodyn., *1*:3, 1982.

Enhorning, G.: Simultaneous recording of intraurethral and intravesical pressure. Acta Chir. Scand. (Suppl.), *276*:1, 1961.

Frewen, W.: Role of bladder training in the treatment of the unstable bladder. Urol. Clin. North Am., *6*:273, 1979.

Frohneberg, D., Thuroff, J. W., Petri, E., and Jonas, U.: Telemetric urodynamic investigations in patients with intravesical obstruction. Proceedings of the American Urological Association, 1981; abstract # 216.

Gittes, R. F.: Augmentation cystoplasty. *In* Libertino, J. (Ed.): Reconstructive Surgery in Urology. Philadelphia, W. B. Saunders Co., 1976.

Gjone, R.: Peripheral autonomic influence on the motility of the urinary bladder in the cat. III. Micturition. Acta Physiol. Scand. *66*:81, 1966.

Gleason, D. M., and Bottaccini, M. R.: The vital role of the distal urethral segment in the control of urinary flow rate. J. Urol., *100*:167, 1968.

Gleason, D. M., and Bottaccini, M. R.: The voiding dynamometer. *In* Hinman, F., Jr.: (Ed.): Hydrodynamics of Micturition. Springfield, Ill., Charles C Thomas, 1971.

Gleason, D. M., and Bottaccini, M. R.: Urodynamic norms in female voiding II: the flow modulation zone and voiding dysfunction. J. Urol., *127*:495, 1982.

Gosling, J.: The structure of the bladder and urethra in relation to function. Urol. Clin. North Am., *6*:31, 1979.

Green, D., Mitcheson, H. D., and McGuire, E. J.: Management of the terrible bladder by continent vesicostomy and ileocecocystoplasty. J. Urol.,*130*:133, 1983.

Griffiths, D. J.: The mechanics of the urethra and micturition. Br. J. Urol., *45*:497, 1973.

Hackler, R. H.: A 25 year prospective mortality study in the spinal cord injured patient: comparison with the long term living paraplegic. J. Urol., *117*:486, 1977.

Head, H., and Riddock, G.: The automatic bladder, excessive sweating and some other reflex conditions in gross injuries of the spinal cord. Brain, *41*:188, 1917.

Ingelman-Sundberg, A.: Partial bladder denervation for detrusor dyssynergia. Clin. Obstet. Gynecol., *21*:797, 1978.

Ioanid, C P., Norca, N., and Pop, T.: Incidence and diagnostic aspects of bladder disorders in diabetics. Eur. Urol., *7*:211, 1980.

Kaufman, J. L.: The silicone-gel prosthesis for the treatment of male urinary incontinence. Urol. Clin North Am., *5*:393, 1978.

Kondo, A.: Visocoelastic properties of the bladder. Ph.D. thesis, Faculty of Medicine, University of Sherbrooke, Sherbrooke, Quebec; 1972.

Kondo, A., Susset, J., and Lefaivre, J.: Viscoelastic properties of bladder. I. Mechanical model and its mathematical analysis. Invest. Urol., *10*:154, 1972.

Krane, R. J., and Siroky, M. B.: Classification of neurourologic disorders. *In* Krane, R. J., and Siroky, M. B., (Eds.): Clinical Neuro-Urology. Boston, Little, Brown & Co., 1979.

Kuru, M.: Nervous control of micturition. Physiol. Rev., *45*:425, 1965.

Lewin, R. J., and Porter, R. W.: Inhibition of spontaneous bladder activity by stimulation of the globus pallidus. Neurology *15*:1049, 1965.

McGuire, E. J.: Combined radiographic and manometric assessment of urethral sphincteric function. J. Urol. *118*:626, 1977.

McGuire, E. J.: Neurogenic incontinence in males. Urol. Clin. North Am., *5*:335, 1978.

McGuire, E. J.: Observations of a part-time urodynamicist. J. Urol., *129*:102, 1983.

McGuire, E. J.: Urodynamic evaluation after abdominal-perineal resection and lumbar intravertebral disc herniation. Urology, *6*:63, 1975.

McGuire, E. J., and Brady, S.: Detrusor-sphincter dyssynergia. J. Urol., *121*:774, 1979.

McGuire, E. J., and Herlihy, E.: Bladder and urethral responses to isolated sacral motor root stimulation. J. Urol., *16*:219, 1978.

McGuire, E. J., and Morrissey, S. G.: The development of neurogenic vesical dysfunction after experimental spinal cord injury or sacral rhizotomy in non-human primates. J. Urol., *128*:1390, 1982.

McGuire, E. J., and Rossier, A. B.: Treatment of acute autonomic dysreflexia. J. Urol., *129*:1185, 1983.

McGuire, E. J., and Savastano, J. A.: Effects of alpha blockade, and anticholinergic agents on the decentralized primate bladder. Neurourol Urodyn. In press.

McGuire, E. J., and Savastano, J. A.: Long term followup of spinal cord injury patients managed by intermittent catheterization. J. Urol., *129*:775, 1983.

McGuire, E. J., and Savastano, J. A.: Urodynamic findings and clinical status following vesical denervation procedures for control of incontinence. J. Urol., *132*:87, 1984.

McGuire, E. J., and Wagner, F., Jr.: The effects of sacral denervation on bladder and urethral function, Surg. Gynecol. Obstet., *114*:343, 1977.

McGuire, E. J., Lytton, B., Pepe, V., and Kohorn, E. I.: Stress urinary incontinence. Am. J. Obstet. Gynecol., *47*:255, 1976a.

McGuire, E. J., Morrissey, S., and Savastano, J. A.: Bladder and ureteral pressure relationships in non-human primates. Invest. Urol., *130*:374, 1983a.

McGuire, E. J., Morrissey, S., Zhang, S., and Horwinski, E.: Control of reflex detrusor activity in normal and spinal injured non-human primates. J. Urol., *129*:197, 1983b.

McGuire, E. J., Wagner, F. M., and Weiss, R. M.: Treatment of autonomic dysreflexia with phenoxybenzamine. J. Urol., *115*:53, 1976b.

McGuire, E. J., Woodside, J. R., and Borden, T. A.: Upper urinary tract deterioration in patients with myelodysplasia and detrusor hypertonia: a follow up study. J. Urol., *129*:823, 1983c.

McGuire, E. J., Woodside, J. R., Borden, T. A., and Weiss, R. M.: Prognostic value of urodynamic testing in myelodysplastic patients. J. Urol., *126*:205, 1981.

Merrill, D. C., Conway, C. C., and DeWolf, W.: Urinary incontinence: treatment with electrical stimulation of the pelvic floor. Urology, *5*:67, 1975.

Olsson, C. A., Siroky, M. B., and Krane, R. J.: The phentolamine test in neurogenic bladder. J. Urol., *117*:481, 1977.

Pavlakis, A. J., Siroky, M. B., Goldstein, I., and Krane,

R. J.: Neurologic findings in Parkinson's disease. J. Urol., *129*:80, 1983.

Pearman, J. W.: The value of kanamycin-colistin bladder instillations in reducing bacteriuria during intermittent catheterization of patients with acute spinal cord injury. Br. J. Urol., *51*:367, 1974.

Pengelly, A.: Effect of prolonged bladder distention on detrusor function. Urol. Clin. North Am., *6*:279, 1979.

Perkash, I.: An attempt to understand and to treat voiding dysfunctions during rehabilitation of the bladder in spinal cord injury patients. J. Urol., *115*:36, 1976.

Politano, V. A.: Periurethral Teflon injection for urinary incontinence. Urol. Clin. North Am., *5*:415, 1978.

Rhame, F. S., and Perkash, I.: Urinary tract infections occurring in recent spinal cord injury patients on intermittent catheterization. J. Urol., *122*:669, 1979.

Schafer, W.: Detrusor as the energy source of micturition. *In* Hinman, F., Jr. (Ed.): Benign Prostatic Hypertrophy. New York, Springer-Verlag, 1983.

Scott, F. B., Bradley, W. E., and Timm, G. W.: Treatment of urinary incontinence by implantable prosthetic sphincter. Urology, *1*:252, 1973.

Siroky, M B., and Krane, R. J.: Hydrodynamic significance of flow rate determination. *In* Hinman, F., Jr. (Ed.): Benign Prostatic Hypertrophy. New York, Springer-Verlag, 1983.

Stockamp, K.: Treatment with phenoxybenzamine of upper urinary tract complications caused by intravesical obstruction. J. Urol. *113*:128, 1975.

Sundin, T., Dahlstrom, A., Norlen, Y., and Svedmyr, N.: The sympathetic innervation and adrenoceptor function of the human lower urinary tract in the normal state and after parasympathetic denervation. Invest. Urol., *14*:322, 1977.

Susset, J. G., Brissot, R. B., and Regnier, C. H.: Stop flow technique: a way to measure detrusor strength. J. Urol., *127*:489, 1982.

Susset, J. G., Ghoneim, G. M., and Regnier, C. H.: Rapid cystometry: a useful clinical test. Proceedings of the American Urological Association; New England Section, *12*:40, 1981.

Susset, J. G., Picker, P., Kretz, M., and Jorest, R.: Critical evaluation of uroflowmeters and analysis of normal curves. J. Urol., *109*:874, 1973.

Tang, P. C., and Ruch, T. C.: Non-neurogenic basis of bladder tonus. Am. J. Physiol., *181*:249, 1955.

Thomas, T. M., Karran, O. D., and Meade, T. W.: Management of urinary incontinence in patients with multiple sclerosis. J. R. Coll. Gen. Pract., *31*:296, 1981.

Torrens, M. J., and Collins, C. D.: The urodynamic assessment of adult enuresis. Br. J. Urol., *47*:433, 1975.

Torrens, M. J., and Griffith, H. B.: Management of the uninhibited bladder by selective sacral rhizotomy. J. Neurosurg., *44*:176, 1976.

Tullock, A. G.: Sympathetic activity of internal urethral sphincter in empty and partially filled bladder. Urology, *5*:353, 1975.

Turner-Warwick, R. T.: Observations on the function and dysfunction of the sphincter and detrusor mechanisms. Urol. Clin. North Am., *6*:13, 1979.

Whitaker, R. H.: The Whitaker test. Urol. Clin. North Am., *6*:529, 1979.

Woodside, J. R., and McGuire, E. J.: Detrusor hypertonicity after Wertheim's hysterectomy. J. Urol., *127*:1143, 1982.

Woodside, J. R., and McGuire, E. J.: Urethral hypotonicity following suprasacral spinal cord injury. J. Urol., *121*:783, 1979.

Yalla, S. V., Blunt, K. J., Fam, B. A., Constantinople, N. L., and Gittes, R. F.: Detrusor-urethral sphincter dyssynergia. J. Urol., *118*:1026, 1978.

Yalla, S., Karsh, L., Kearney, G., Fraser, L., Finn, D., DeFellipo, N., and Dyro, F. M.: Postprostatectomy urinary incontinence: urodynamic assessment. Neurourol. Urodyn., *1*:77, 1982.

Yalla, S. V., Sharma, G. V. R. K., and Barsamian, E. M.: Micturitional static urethral pressure profile: a method of recording urethral pressure profile during voiding and the implications. J. Urol., *124*:649, 1980.

Yeates, W. K.: Disorders of bladder function. Ann. Coll. Surg., *50*:335, 1972.

INFERTILITY

CHAPTER 12

Male Infertility

RICHARD J. SHERINS, M.D.
STUART S. HOWARDS, M.D.

Concepts regarding the evaluation and management of the infertile male have evolved since the mid-1970's primarily because of the development of new methodology. Nevertheless, the cause of male infertility is often obscure, and the clearly defined causes are infrequent or rare. This chapter outlines an approach to evaluating the infertile male and develops concepts of management based on the detection of abnormalities in testicular physiology. We emphasize the pitfalls and common errors in diagnosis to provide a rational basis for therapy.

Lack of understanding of what truly constitutes male infertility leads to the most common errors in diagnosis and treatment. Heretofore, physicians have relied primarily on semen analysis in their assessment of the male, since no mechanism is available to test the biologic fertility potential of human sperm among multiple female recipients. Thus, it is often an assumption on the part of the physician that an ejaculate is inadequate for impregnation. Errors in interpretation frequently develop because of lack of understanding of what constitutes the minimally adequate ejaculate.

The marked variability of semen analyses, usually due to differences in methods of collecting samples, contributes to this misinterpretation. In recent years, it has also become apparent that subtle gynecologic abnormalities, such as inadequate ovulatory sequences or tubo-ovarian inflammatory disease, may remain unrecognized unless rigorously excluded. These disorders contribute significantly both to misinterpretation of the fertility potential of the male and to results of treatment of such men (Sherins, 1974). Accordingly, we wish to emphasize that evaluation of the infertile male implies and demands thorough gynecologic review of the sexual partner to recognize any coexistent disease.

Finally, selection of an appropriate treatment regimen for an infertile male is often confusing and difficult because therapeutic successes are few and unpredictable. These realities re-emphasize the need for precision in diagnosis and for adoption of an attitude that the male is fertile until proved otherwise. An empirical approach to the treatment of such men is difficult to justify. In our opinion, the physician provides a great service to the infertile couple by being truthful when adequate therapy is not available. We have found that infertile couples are willing to accept alternative approaches, such as adoption or artificial insemination, when their physician has provided a thorough evaluation and discussion of the findings.

EVALUATION OF THE INFERTILE MALE

The foundation of the investigation of the infertile male is the history and physical examination. The space in this section devoted to these areas is limited only because the arts of history taking and physical examination are more appropriately discussed in different forums. On the other hand, the topic of semen evaluation is presented in great detail, since this material is not available elsewhere in this text. Of course, a complete examination includes further studies of abnormalities uncovered during the preliminary evaluation.

History

In the majority of infertile males, the history is unremarkable. Nevertheless, a careful review is necessary, since occasionally it will reveal the cause of the infertility. As outlined

640

in Table 12–1, the history should include contraceptive and coital practices, previous pregnancies, and a thorough review of the wife's gynecologic function. A few points warrant emphasis.

Occupational exposure to toxic agents such as the pesticide dibromochloropropane (DBCP) may interfere with spermatogenesis (Milby and Whorton, 1980). Excessive use of alcohol (Boiesen et al., 1979), marihuana, and perhaps tobacco (Population Information Program, Johns Hopkins University, 1979; Evans et al., 1981) also reduces semen quality. In utero exposure to diethylstilbestrol (DES) causes an increased incidence of epididymal cysts, a slightly increased frequency of cryptorchidism, but little or no effect on semen quality in those men who do not have an undescended testis.

Medical and surgical diseases and their treatments may compromise reproductive function. The vas deferens and the testicular blood supply can be easily injured during a hernia repair in an infant. Men with congenital hypogonadotropism often have associated midline defects such as anosmia, color blindness, cerebellar ataxia, harelip, and cleft palate.

Many drugs interfere with spermatogenesis, including small quantities of estrogen that are occasionally included in vitamin preparations. Cimetidine (Funder and Mercer, 1979), but not ranitidine (Knigge et al., 1983), may interfere with male reproductive function. A drug, febrile illness, allergic reaction, or other stress may injure the germinal epithelium. The effect of the insult will be seen in the ejaculate 1 to 3 months later. Smallpox is the most common cause of obstructive azoospermia in India. The sexual history may reveal that the couple does not understand the mechanics of intercourse or that they avoid coitus during the fertile period because of mittelschmerz (intense abdominal pain in the female partner at midcycle). The use of vaginal lubricants should be discouraged because they interfere with sperm motility. If they are absolutely necessary, petroleum jelly or glycerin is less detrimental than the other commercial lubricants (Goldenberg and White, 1975). (See also references under Drugs and Toxins.) The physician should determine whether the wife is ovulating (by means of a menstrual history and temperature chart) and whether she has been carefully evaluated for subtle causes of infertility.

Although it is clear that extreme heat can interfere with spermatogenesis, there is no documentation that jockey shorts cause infertility. In fact Alexander (1981) has shown that jockey shorts do not affect semen parameters whereas frequent hot baths decrease sperm motility by 10 per cent but do not affect sperm density.

TABLE 12–1. History

I. Sexual History
  Duration of sexual relations with and without birth control
  Methods of birth control
  Sexual technique: penetration, ejaculation, use of lubricants (some are spermatocidal)
  Frequency and timing of coitus. Does it coincide with ovulation?
  Past marital history of both partners, including pregnancies and miscarriages

II. Past History
  Developmental: Age of testicular descent, age of puberty, history of prepubertal obesity; gynecomastia, congenital abnormalities of urinary tract or central nervous system
  Surgical: Orchiopexy, pelvic or retroperitoneal surgery, herniorrhaphy, sympathectomy, vasectomy, injury to genitals, spinal cord injury
  Medical: Urinary infections, venereal disease (including nonspecific urethritis), mumps, renal disease, diabetes, radiotherapy, recent allergic febrile or viral illness (may affect semen quality), epididymitis, tuberculosis, smallpox (causes obstructive azoospermia) or other chronic diseases, anosmia, midline defects
  Drugs: Complete list of all past and present medications. Many drugs interfere with spermatogenesis, erection, and ejaculation
  Occupation and habits: Exposure to chemicals and heat, hot baths, steam baths, radiation, cigarettes, alcohol
  Past marital history of both partners; any offspring with other partners
  Previous infertility evaluations and treatments

III. Family History
  Testicular atrophy
  Hypogonadotropism
  Cryptorchidism
  Congenital midline defects

IV. Female Reproductive History
  Growth and development
  Menstrual history
  Temperature chart
  Galactorrhea
  Mittelschmerz
  Hirsutism

Physical Examination

Most infertile men are found to be normal on physical examination, but a careful examination should be conducted because it may reveal the cause of the infertility. Table 12–2 outlines the elements of the physical examination. The most important of these is the testis size. Since the tubules and germinal elements account for approximately 98 per cent of the

TABLE 12–2. PHYSICAL EXAMINATION

I. General: Habitus, hair distribution, breasts, secondary sexual development, height and span, upper and lower proportions, surgical scars

II. Neurologic: Visual fields, anosmia, rectal sphincter tone, perineal sensation, deep tendon reflexes

III. Genital tract: Penis, urethral meatus, urethra and corpus spongiosum, prostate, testis, epididymis, vasa, and other scrotal contents (varicocele)

testis mass, a reduction in the number of germ cells leads to testicular atrophy. In addition, Leydig cell function is almost always preserved in infertile men, and decreased virilization is very uncommon. The length or, preferably, the volume of the testis should be noted. The lower limit of normal length for a mature testis is approximately 4.0 cm. The volume can be estimated with an orchidometer, which is a commercially available series of graded sizes of plastic model testes. Table 12–3 presents the range of normal and abnormal volumes for the human testis. Testicular volume correlates well with semen quality and fertility.

Abnormalities of the vas deferens, seminal vesicles, prostate, and testicular venous drainage may cause infertility. The vas deferens and accessory ducts may be absent. The scrotum should be checked in the supine and upright positions before and during a Valsalva maneuver to rule out a varicocele. The area of the seminal vesicle along the rectum above the prostate should be examined bimanually. The normal seminal vesicle is difficult to palpate.

TABLE 12–3. COMPARISONS OF TESTICULAR DIMENSIONS (LENGTH × WIDTH) AND VOLUME FOR PREPUBERTAL, PUBERTAL, AND NORMAL ADULT MEN

Clinical Status	Volume (ml)	Length × Width (cm) (cm)
Prepubertal	1	1.6 × 1.0
	2	2.0 × 1.2
	3	2.3 × 1.4
	4	2.5 × 1.5
	5	2.7 × 1.6
	6	2.9 × 1.8
Pubertal	8	3.1 × 2.0
	10	3.4 × 2.1
	12	3.7 × 2.3
	15	4.0 × 2.5
Adult*	20	4.5 × 2.7
	25	5.0 × 3.0
	30	5.5 × 3.2

*Normal adult testicular size 24 ± 4(SD)ml. (n = 44).

The diseased seminal vesicle may be tender or firm or both. If indicated by the history, physical examination, urinalysis, or semen analysis, the prostate should be massaged in order to collect fluid for cytologic and bacteriologic study.

Laboratory Studies

Laboratory investigation in all patients should include a urinalysis and semen analysis (see following section). If the urinalysis reveals pyuria or bacteria or if there is a suggestion of urinary tract infection from the history and physical examination, the urine should be cultured. If bacterial prostatitis is suggested by the history or physical examination, a three-glass urinalysis and cultures are indicated. Three-glass tests should also be obtained if pyuria or bacteriuria is detected on the routine urinalysis. Semen cultures are uninterpretable without cultures of the first voided (urethral) urine and the bladder urine, since the normal male anterior urethra usually is colonized with bacteria (Fowler, 1981). If *Mycoplasma, Chlamydia,* or *Trichomonas* infection is a possibility, special cultures and tests can be obtained. However, a therapeutic trial of tetracycline or metronidazole (Flagyl) is inexpensive and often more practical. Chlamydial infections can cause nonspecific urethritis (Schachter, 1978) and epididymitis (Berger et al., 1978; Scheibel et al., 1983) and *Ureaplasma urealyticum* may cause nonspecific urethritis (Taylor-Robinson and McCormack, 1980). However, these infestations are uncommon in men presenting for infertility evaluation and rarely cause male infertility (Fowler, 1981).

As determined by history and physical examination, selected patients will require laboratory evaluation of their reproductive endocrine function. The ready availability of radioimmunoassays for testosterone, luteinizing hormone (LH), and follicle-stimulating hormone (FSH) have made it possible for all clinicians to evaluate the endocrine function of their patients (Table 12–4).

Elevated serum FSH and LH determinations help in distinguishing men with primary testicular failure from men who are normal. In sexually mature men with isolated germ cell depletion and no clinical evidence of hypogonadism, FSH levels are increased in proportion to the loss of testicular germ cells, whereas LH and testosterone concentrations generally remain within the normal range regardless of the etiology of the testicular injury (Fig. 12–1, Table 12–4). When germinal aplasia is present, mean

TABLE 12–4. Summary of Range of Values for Serum FSH, LH, and Testosterone in Normal Men, Men with Germinal Aplasia, and Hypogonadotropic Men

Clinical Status	FSH (mIU/ml)	LH (mIU/ml)	Testosterone (ng/100 ml)
Normal men	4–25	4–18	250–1200
Germinal aplasia	25–90	8–25	200–700
Hypogonadotropic hypogonadism	2–4	2–4	30–50

Abbreviations: FSH, Follicle-stimulating hormone; LH, luteinizing hormone.

FSH levels are increased approximately five-fold.

There has been considerable debate about the mechanism of the apparently "selective" increase in FSH levels. There appears to be specific feedback regulation of FSH secretion by the seminiferous epithelium. A nonsteroidal factor called "inhibin," produced by the seminiferous epithelium, has been suggested on the basis of numerous studies in which FSH concentrations have been found to be markedly increased when testicular germ cells are depleted (Van Thiel et al., 1971; Baker et al., 1976). Evidence is accumulating that inhibin originates in the Sertoli cell (Steinberger and Steinberger, 1976) and may be a protein (Ramasharma et al., 1984). Sex steroids also modulate FSH secretion; thus, interactions of the various hormones of the hypothalamic-pituitary-testicular axis are complex.

Some studies have demonstrated that testosterone and estradiol exert an inhibitory influence on both FSH and LH secretion (Sherins and Loriaux, 1973; Santen et al., 1975; Winters et al., 1979; Marynick et al., 1979). It should be recalled that the majority of estradiol in man is produced by conversion of testosterone in peripheral tissues. Thus, testosterone serves as a prehormone for estradiol production. Studies in the experimental animal have shown that testosterone alone can maintain both gonadotropins within the normal range in the absence of the testes, suggesting that "inhibin" may not be required to regulate FSH secretion (Sherins et al., 1982). Further, in animals a "selective" increase in FSH concentration can be induced in the castrate by lowering testosterone production and increasing estradiol production. Similar sex steroid regulation of FSH secretion in men probably also occurs: A study of men with "selective" increase in FSH levels showed that testosterone production and free testosterone levels were both reduced by 50 per cent despite the absence of clinical signs of hypogonadism or significant increase in LH concentration (Booth and Loriaux, 1983).

Serum testosterone concentration is usually low in men who have profound failure of Leydig cell function. Such men often have a history of decreased libido with impotency, and any male with such a history requires endocrine studies. However, even in men with end-stage testicular failure, such as in alcoholic cirrhosis or Klinefelter's syndrome, the total testosterone concentration can be misleading within the normal male range because of an increase in testosterone-binding globulin (TeBG) level which results from diminished androgen and elevated estrogen production in these conditions (Van Thiel et al., 1974). Thus, the diagnosis of primary

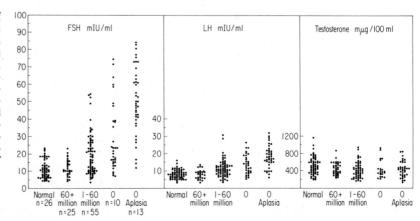

Figure 12–1. Concentration of serum FSH, LH, and testosterone in normal men and infertile men whose total sperm output is more than 60 million, 1 to 60 million, zero (azoospermic), and zero owing to germinal aplasia. FSH, Follicle-stimulating hormone; LH, luteinizing hormone. (Reproduced with permission from Wachslicht-Rodbard and Sherins: Basic Reproductive Medicine, vol. 2, Reproductive Function in Men, MIT Press, 1982.)

testicular failure is confirmed when serum FSH and LH levels are elevated in the presence of testicular atrophy.

Normal peripheral plasma levels of testosterone and dihydrotestosterone (DHT) are 250 to 1200 ng/dl and 30 to 90 ng/dl, respectively. The vast majority of the circulating DHT is not secreted directly by the Leydig cells, but rather comes from the conversion of testosterone to DHT in peripheral androgen-sensitive tissues. The circulating androgens are approximately 98 per cent bound to plasma proteins, including TeBG. The free testosterone in the blood is probably the physiologically important fraction. The serum testosterone concentration may vary by a factor of 2 or 3 from hour to hour. The vacillations occur in a predictable pattern because of its pulsatile release. Therefore, single tests that give borderline results cannot be interpreted and must be repeated.

On the other hand, serum testosterone is the best test for detecting gondadotropin deficiency. The mean serum LH and FSH concentrations are significantly lower in hypogonadotropic patients than in normal men, but there is an overlap between the values found in hypogonadotropics and those at the lower limit in normal males (Table 12–4).

The endocrine function of the testis is gradually and progressively altered during aging. Histologic changes occasionally appear as early as the third decade of life and are increasingly frequent in older men (Bishop, 1970). The most common degenerative changes are thickening of the tubule basement membrane and tunica propria, intratubular fibrosis, and reduction in number of germ cells in the seminiferous epithelium. Nevertheless, fertility has been documented in a 94-year-old man (Bishop, 1970). Mean levels of free testosterone decline in men after age 50, although total circulating testosterone is stable until at least age 70 (Stearns et al., 1974). After 60, there is also an elevation in the plasma levels of estradiol (Kley et al., 1975; Stearns et al., 1974). These normally occurring changes in senescent testis function become important in assessment of the fertility potential in older men.

Male infertility secondary to congenital adrenal hyperplasia is very rare. The indications for evaluation of adrenal function in an infertile man are:

1. A history of precocious puberty.
2. A family history of congenital adrenal hyperplasia.
3. Short stature.
4. Testicular enlargement that may be indicative of adrenal rests in the testis.

The plasma concentration of 17-hydroxyprogesterone is elevated in these patients and is the best single test for identification of men with congenital adrenal hyperplasia. If the serum concentration of 17-hydroxyprogesterone cannot be obtained, the concentration of pregnanetriol in the urine is the next best screening test and should be determined.

In summary, thyroid and adrenal function tests are almost never necessary in evaluating the male with idiopathic infertility. Since hypothyroidism never causes infertility in man, the common practice of evaluating thyroid function in infertile males is irrational. Serum testosterone values are worthwhile when there is clinical evidence of androgen deficiency, but the total testosterone level may be misleading within the normal range. Serum FSH levels are helpful in evaluating severely oligospermic or azoospermic men, since an elevated serum FSH level indicates severe germ cell depletion.

A buccal smear to detect nuclear chromatin (Barr bodies) and/or a determination of karyotype will assist in making a diagnosis of Klinefelter's syndrome and other congenital diseases associated with chromosomal abnormalities. In certain patients with mosaic karyotypes, the chromosomal abnormality can be detected only in the testicular cells and therefore may be missed on routine chromosome studies of blood or skin. Nevertheless, it is not practical to perform testicular karyotype tests routinely. Chandley et al. (1973) found 2.1 per cent of 1599 subfertile men had an abnormal karyotype compared with 0.5 per cent of 1560 control men. Kjessler (1974) found that 6.6 per cent of 1363 male patients in barren marriages exhibited major chromosome abnormalities. The incidence in men with abnormal semen is approximately 10.0 per cent. Two thirds of these patients had Klinefelter's syndrome or one of its variants. Slightly more than 1 per cent of the men had aberrations in autosomal chromosomes.

There is evidence that immune factors play a role in selective cases of male infertility (Mumford and Warner, 1983). Men with adequate sperm counts and unexplained poor sperm motility or sperm agglutination should be evaluated for antisperm antibodies. We test the serum first because it is easier to obtain a serum assay. If this is positive, we evaluate the semen. The most commonly used assays are the Kibrick macroagglutination test, the Franklin-Dukes tube-slide agglutination test, the Friberg microagglutination test, and the Isojima immobilization test. Fluorescent antibody assays are sensitive, but give many false-positive results.

Mathur et al. (1979) used a Coombs' passive hemagglutination method, and Hass et al. (1981) developed a radiolabeled-antiglobulin test that reveals the immunoglobulin species (IgM, IgG, IgA) of antisperm antibodies. There is little or no IgM antibody in the semen, and the semen levels of IgA and IgG are only about 1 per cent of the serum concentration (Mumford and Warner, 1983). IgG and IgA diffuse from the serum into the reproductive fluids. IgA may also be locally secreted into the semen.

Semen Analysis

Semen analysis is the cornerstone of the evaluation of the infertile male. Nevertheless, it is *not* a test of fertility. No one contests the diagnosis of sterility in the absence of sperm. However, there is considerable controversy and confusion regarding what constitutes the minimally adequate ejaculate.

Semen analysis is a critical part of the evaluation of the male partner of an infertile couple. Ideally, the results provide an accurate estimation of a man's sperm production and the functional capabilities of those sperm, especially regarding fertility potential. However, standard semen characteristics do not provide a strong predictive index because they are always indirect measures of sperm function. Presently, practical methods for directly assessing the fertility potential of a man are not readily available, as in animal husbandry where cross-breeding to multiple females is utilized to judge fertility. Heterologous in vitro fertilization is a step in this direction. The reliability of semen analysis can be markedly improved by utilizing proper collection technique and careful interpretation of the data.

Van Leeuwenhoek first observed sperm under the microscope in 1677. One century later, Lazzaro Spallanzani published quantitative studies on amphibian seminal fluid. Another hundred years passed before a similar analysis of human semen appeared in the English literature. Then, in 1929, Macomber and Sanders published an article entitled "The Spermatozoa Count," which launched the modern era of semen analysis. Since that time, semen analysis has become a critical step in the evaluation of the male partner of an infertile union. Clinically, the emphasis has been on evaluation of the spermatozoa. However, the noncellular components of semen may also play a role in fertilization. The biochemistry of semen has been extensively reviewed by Mann (1964). In the following paragraphs, an outline of clinical semen analysis will be presented.

COLLECTION

The authors prefer to obtain the semen specimen after 1 full day of sexual abstinence, that is, 36 to 48 hours postejaculation, because this interval does not disrupt the sexual habits of the couple. It is important for each laboratory to prescribe a standard continence period, since changes in the interval between ejaculations increases the variability of the results of semen analysis. Even with this precaution, the results of semen analysis are rather inconsistent, and therefore multiple analyses are indicated in any equivocal or difficult situation. This may require study for periods as long as 6 months.

The specimen should be placed in a clean, dry, wide-mouthed container supplied by the physician. If the patient is asked to procure the bottle, there is a risk of introducing artifacts secondary to the previous contents of the container or to the solutions used to clean it. The specimen may be obtained at home or in the physician's office, but it should be kept warm during transit. It is very unusual for a patient to object to masturbation as a form of inducing ejaculation. When there is an objection, coitus interruptus is an alternative method of obtaining the specimen. If the patient has religious objections to both masturbation and withdrawal, he can use a perforated plastic condom manufactured by the Milex Corporation of Chicago, and if he is of the Catholic faith, he may have the condom perforated by a priest. Patients should be advised not to use ordinary condoms, since they may contain spermicides, as do many vaginal lubricants. In the rare situation in which none of these methods is satisfactory to the patient, the physician will have to rely on postcoital examination of the ejaculate in the vagina. The patient should understand that an incomplete collection is not only worthless but also misleading. The time of ejaculation should be recorded.

PHYSICAL CHARACTERISTICS

Freshly ejaculated semen is a coagulum. The constituents of the semen responsible for coagulation originate in the seminal vesicles. Therefore, in patients with congenital bilateral absence of the vas deferens who have undeveloped seminal vesicles, coagulation does not occur.

The human ejaculate can be divided into several fractions (Oettle, 1957):

1. The first, or pre-ejaculatory fraction,

comes from the mucous urethral (Littre's) and bulbourethral (Cowper's) glands.

2. The fraction that follows is a low-viscosity, opalescent liquid that contains no spermatozoa and is derived from the prostate.

3. The third, or principal, fraction is a mixture of prostatic fluid, gel from the seminal vesicles, and spermatozoa from the vas deferens and distal epididymis.

4. The terminal fraction contains gel and spermatozoa from the seminal vesicles.

Liquefaction of the semen can occur as early as 3 to 5 minutes after ejaculation but may take up to 25 minutes. The seminal proteinase, seminin, is probably the enzyme primarily responsible for this phenomenon in human semen (Tauber et al., 1980). There is suggestive but inconclusive evidence that failure of the ejaculate to liquefy is a cause of human infertility. The effect of this abnormality remains unclear because semen of other species, such as the rat, never liquefies, and in the human, sperm may be found in the cervical mucus before liquefaction has occurred (Sobrero and MacLeod, 1972). Failure of liquefaction is a different problem from that of high-viscosity liquefied semen (see later discussion). Syner and associates (1975) found that seminin accelerates liquefaction of the semen of some, but not all, men with slow-liquefying ejaculates. They have suggested clinical use of seminin. Alpha amylase (Wilson and Bunge, 1975) and suputolysin (Upadhyaya et al., 1981) do facilitate liquefaction, but we feel that the efficacy of this treatment is not documented.

The concentration of the liquefying proteolytic enzymes in the ejaculate is not correlated with the eventual viscosity of the seminal fluid. The viscosity of the specimen can be evaluated while pouring the specimen from the collection bottle into a graduated cylinder to measure the volume. Semen of normal viscosity flows freely and can be poured drop by drop. Semen of higher than normal viscosity may inhibit sperm motility. Amelar (1962) suggested two methods of reducing the viscosity of such specimens. One method is to mix one or two parts of Alevaire, a detergent (Winthrop Laboratories, New York), with one part semen. The second method is to aspirate the specimen into a syringe and forcibly eject it through an 18-gauge needle three to five times. MacLeod (1965) believed that increased viscosity is of no clinical significance, since the immediate postcoital test demonstrates that sperm reach the cervical canal within 3 minutes after ejaculation, before liquefaction.

We believe that when there is a question of inhibition of sperm motility and transport secondary to slow liquefaction or increased viscosity, two additional tests should be performed. First, an aliquot of the semen should be aspirated and ejected three or four times with a syringe through an 18- or 20-gauge needle and placed on a slide, and then the sperm motility should be microscopically evaluated. Second, the postcoital motility of the vaginal sperm should be checked. If the latter test reveals satisfactory motility, there is no problem. If the slide test reveals good motility but the postcoital test demonstrates poor motility, the patient's wife should be evaluated by a gynecologist for a cervical defect. If the slide test and the postcoital examination both show poor motility, one of the above-mentioned treatments may be instigated, although their effectiveness has not been proved.

The volume of the ejaculate can be measured in a standard graduated cylinder. The normal range varies markedly, depending on the abstinence interval. In our laboratory, the mean semen volume for normal men is 3 ml (range 1 to 6 ml) when abstinence is 36 to 48 hours. The prostate and seminal vesicles provide more than 95 per cent of the total volume of the ejaculate in man. Thus, very small ejaculates reflect either partial retrograde ejaculation or an abnormality in the physiology of these organs. Men with congenital absence of the vas and seminal vesicles have a very low volume (0.2 to 0.5 ml) of noncoagulating ejaculate. A complete bilateral obstruction of the vas deferens would not noticeably decrease the volume of the ejaculate. Dubin and Amelar (1971), in their study of 1294 consecutive cases of male infertility, noted low semen volume (less than 1 ml) in 1.8 per cent of the series and high semen volume (over 4.5 ml) in 10 per cent. They recommended homologous artificial insemination (AIH) for the patients with low volumes and insemination with the first fraction of the split ejaculate or withdrawal coitus for those with high volumes. Although we have been impressed with AIH in the treatment of men with low semen volume who are otherwise normal, the efficacy of these methods remains to be documented. Many other authors would not consider volumes over 4.5 as abnormal. Of course, the abstinence interval affects the volume of the ejaculate, and therefore normal volumes must be determined for each abstinence interval.

CONCENTRATION

Freund (1968), Hotchkiss (1970), Amelar and Dubin (1973), Eliasson (1975), and a committee of the World Health Organization (1980) have all outlined standard methods for performing a semen analysis. We will describe a method similar to those used by these authors.

After liquefaction, the well-mixed specimen is aspirated into a clean, standard, white blood cell pipette to the zero point mark on the pipette stem. The pipette chamber is then filled with a saturated solution of sodium bicarbonate with 1 per cent phenol added to immobilize the spermatozoa. The loaded pipette is shaken, and the first few drops from the stem of the pipette are discarded, after which a drop of the mixture is placed onto a Neubauer standard blood cell counting chamber. Five blocks of 16 squares each, comprising a total of one fifth of the red blood cell field, are observed, and all spermatozoa within the area, including those touching the lower and right-hand (or any two) sides of each block of 16 squares, are counted. This number is multiplied by 10^6, that is, one million. The process is repeated, and the average of two determinations is the number of spermatozoa per milliliter.

The margin of error in this technique is at least 10 per cent. In samples with a low concentration of spermatozoa, a 1:10 dilution rather than a 1:20 dilution may be used. The semen is drawn to the 1 mark in the pipette, and from that point the procedure is carried out as described above, except that the count is divided by 2 before multiplying by 10^6. If the specimen has very few cells, the entire red blood cell field may be counted, that is, 400 small squares. If the 1:10 dilution has been used, the actual count is multiplied by 10^5, and this number is the sperm count per milliliter. Regardless of the method used, the total sperm count is the product of the count per milliliter times the number of milliliters in the specimen. The total sperm count is a more reliable measure of sperm output than sperm concentration because it is not affected by variations in semen volume. In laboratories performing large numbers of semen analyses, an automated counting system, utilizing an instrument such as the Coulter counter, can be employed. However, the automated method is imprecise when the sperm concentration is below 10 million per ml.

MOTILITY

The motility of the sperm should be evaluated within 2 hours after ejaculation. For accurate reproducible results, the specimen should be kept at body temperature; the sperm concentration should be 10 to 60 million sperm/ml; and the depth of the smear should be at least 8 to 10 microns, or micrometers (μm) (Amann, 1981). At least 5 μl (diluted if the concentration is greater than 60 million sperm/ml) of semen is placed on a standard microscopic slide, and a cover slip is positioned over the drop. A phase-contrast microscope, at a magnification of 250 $\times$, is ideal. One hundred successive cells are observed, and the percentage of these cells that are motile is recorded. Then multiple fields are scanned, and the percentage of motile sperm in each field is estimated. The quality of the motile sperm should also be graded on a scale of 0 to 4. Zero signifies no motility; 1, sluggish activity; 2, poor to fair motility; 3, good motion; and 4, excellent forward progression (Hotchkiss, 1970). This is an arbitrary and subjective evaluation, but with experience, it is moderately consistent. MacLeod (1965) believed that repeated determinations of motility at intervals of up to 24 hours have no rationale, since in the normal physiologic setting, sperm leave the semen and enter the cervical mucus within minutes. For this reason and also because of practical considerations, we determine motility once. Prolonged continence can artificially depress motility.

During the motility evaluation, any evidence of sperm agglutination should also be noted. Occasional clumps of agglutinated sperm are neither unusual nor abnormal. There is increased clumping in some patients with inflammatory disorders. Sperm may agglutinate head to head, tail to tail, or head to tail. Agglutination may be associated with sperm antibodies in the semen and blood. These antibodies are usually IgA or IgG immunoglobulins. If excessive agglutination is observed or if there is poor motility with normal sperm density and morphology, an immunologic evaluation may be indicated (see Immunologic Disorders).

More sophisticated methods, utilizing laser-doppler techniques (Jouannet et al., 1977), computer-aided analysis of motion pictures (Amann and Hammerstedt, 1980), videomicrography (Overstreet et al., 1981), and photon correlation spectroscopy (Frost and Cummins, 1981) have been designed to evaluate sperm motility. Cinemicrography documents that morphologically normal sperm swim faster and straighter than morphologically abnormal sperm (Katz et al., 1982). The average velocity of human sperm measured by these techniques is 48 (videomicroscopy) to 96 (light-scattering) μm per second. Although these techniques provide more accurate and detailed analysis of sperm motility, they are not widely used in clinical practice. If no spermatozoa are moving, the patient is said to have *necrospermia*. This is a misnomer, since metabolic studies reveal that these immobile spermatozoa are usually alive. Pedersen and Rebbe (1975) have shown that all of the sperm of one such patient lacked the dynein arms of the microtubules in the tail motor complex (Fig. 12–2). Since then, several different morphologic abnormalities of the axonemal complex have been associated with immotile sperm.

If inner dynein arms are absent but the remainder of the axonemal complex is normal, the spermatozoa are motile, although the velocity and beat frequency are one-half normal (Jouannet et al., 1983). Specific biochemical abnormalities have also been described in patients with necrospermia and axonemal deficiencies (Baccetti, 1981). Many patients with im-

motile sperm have morphologically normal sperm. Gagnon et al. (1982) have documented decreased activity of the enzyme protein-carboxyl methylase in patients with nonmotile sperm.

MORPHOLOGY

The human seminal cytology serves as a sensitive index of the germinal epithelium (MacLeod, 1964). Evaluation of the morphology of spermatozoa requires more patience and experience than determining concentration or motility. Nevertheless, a clinician can acquire these skills if desired. Observing unstained spermatozoa under the "high dry" objective of the microscope can yield morphologic information. However, staining the cells is definitely preferable. Hotchkiss (1970) outlines three simple staining techniques, but many researchers in the field prefer the excellent but more complicated Papanicolaou technique (MacLeod, 1964). A less complicated, acceptable alternative follows.

A portion of the specimen is spread on a dry glass slide, using a second slide or cover slip as for a differential white blood count. The specimen is allowed to air dry and is fixed with

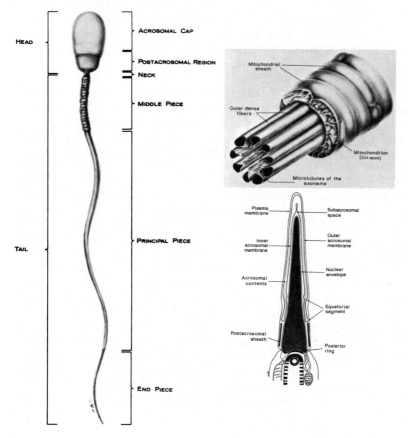

Figure 12–2. *Left,* A spermatozoon as seen with the light microscope. It is depicted without the cell membrane. *Right* (above), A segment in the middle piece of the typical mammalian spermatozoon, showing the relationship of the mitochondrial sheath, the outlet dense fibers, and the doublets of the axoneme. *Right* (lower), A diagram of a sagittal section of a primate sperm head. The posterior ring marks the junction of the head and neck. (From Fawcett, D.: Devel. Biol., *44*:394, 1975.)

10 per cent formalin for 1 minute. It is rinsed and stained with Myer's hematoxylin for 2 minutes, re-rinsed, and dried. Then 200 successive cells are evaluated, using the oil immersion objective. Alford and Rivard (1981) recommend an even simpler method. They mix 2 drops of semen with 2 drops of Sedi-stain (Clay-Adams Corp.) on a microscope slide, place a coverslip over the specimen, and examine the slide with high dry power and the oil immersion objective.

Although more than 70 variations in sperm morphology have been described, it is more practical to divide the cells into normal, immature, small, large, amorphous, and tapering forms (Fig. 12–3) (MacLeod, 1965). The normal human spermatozoon head is 3.0 to 5.0 μm long and 2.0 to 3.0 μm wide (Eliasson, 1975). MacLeod showed that the morphologic picture

of a given individual is remarkably constant, and any variation in morphologic characteristics of the semen reflects an insult to the testis, such as a viral infection, heat, or radiation. The presence of more than 2 to 3 per cent of immature forms in the ejaculate is a certain sign of stress. These cells appear in the ejaculate within 14 to 21 days of the onset of many illnesses, especially viral infections. The immature cells are usually accompanied by an increase in amorphous and tapering forms (MacLeod, 1964). Sherins et al. (1977) also found, in a carefully documented longitudinal study of the semen of 119 men, that seminal cytology is the most stable seminal parameter and predictor of fertility.

Electron microscopic studies by Fawcett (personal communication, 1975) of human

Figure 12–3. *A*, Diagrammatic representation of certain deviations in shape and size of human spermatozoa. *1*, Small form; *2*, normal size and shape; *3*, megaloform; *4*, acute tapering form; *5*, moderate taper; *6*, tendency to taper; and *7*, bicephalic.

B, *1*, Immature cell with distorted chromatin; *2–5* and *17*, various types of abnormal spermatozoa; *11–14*, immature cells of germinal line (large spermatids—note peripheral position of nuclei and partial extrusion of one nucleus); *10*, three spermatid nuclei in single cytoplasm (note vacuoles, which are present later in spermatozoa); *15* and *16*, cytoplasmic "ghosts" of spermatids, the nuclei having been extruded. (Reproduced with permission from MacLeod, J.: Fertil. Steril., *13*:29, 1962.)

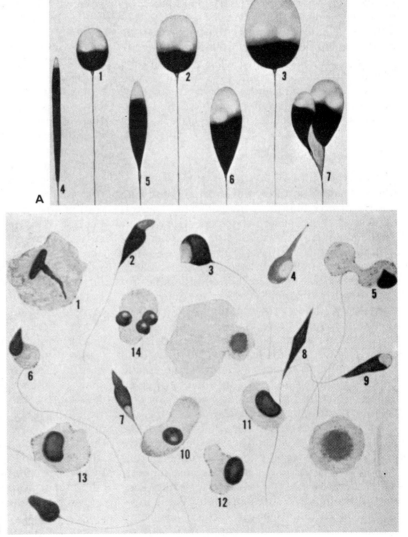

sperm suggest that the tapered forms that MacLeod has discussed may not be pathologic forms but rather normal variations and staining artifacts. The confusion may arise from the facts that the Papanicolaou technique does not stain the acrosome, that a normal sperm seen on edge looks tapered, and that extra cytoplasm present at the neck of the sperm is missed unless the scanning electron microscope is used (Fawcett, 1975). Nevertheless, the differential seminal cytology is useful in assessing semen quality. The interpretation of morphology is complicated by the enormous heterogeneity of normal human sperm. Depending upon one's methodology, a "normal" semen specimen contains 60 per cent or more normal forms and may have 2 to 3 per cent immature forms.

It is extremely difficult to distinguish immature spermatogenic cells from leukocytes with conventional staining techniques. Many laboratories erroneously report immature spermatogenic cells as leukocytes. Therefore, it is difficult to interpret reports that state that abnormal quantities of either of these forms are present. This difficulty may cause errors in the interpretation of semen analysis. Couture et al. (1976) and Nahoum and Cardozo (1980) have described a technique that facilitates the differentiation of leukocytes from immature germ cells.

NORMAL VALUES

Interpretation of the results of the standard semen analysis is often the most difficult and important task that faces the clinician. There is agreement that a semen specimen with greater than 200 million total spermatozoa, 60 per cent motility characterized as 3+ to 4, and few abnormal or immature forms is an excellent specimen. However, there is considerable debate as to the minimally adequate semen. It is important to realize that "minimally adequate" semen parameters are not the same as the "average" parameters in fertile men. It is extremely important to bear in mind that these tests are imprecise, and, in addition, the female makes a contribution to the fertility of any given couple. Therefore, it is neither possible nor wise to make dogmatic statements concerning the lower level of adequacy. It is clear that over the past several years authorities in the field have been revising downward the acceptable concentration of sperm. Studies of fertile men requesting bilateral vasectomy to achieve sterility support the contention that individuals with "low" sperm concentrations may be fertile. Nelson and Bunge (1974) found that these men had an average sperm count of 48 million per ml and that 20 per cent of these fertile men had fewer than 20 million sperm per ml in their ejaculate. Rehan et al. (1975), in a similar study of 1300 men, found that the mean sperm count was 79 million sperm per ml. Twenty-three per cent had counts below 40 million per ml, and 7 per cent had counts below 20 million per ml.

Each laboratory must establish its own normal values, since variables such as abstinence period, analytical techniques, and technician's judgment affect the results of semen analysis.

A controlled abstinence period is essential, since total sperm count increases by 87 million sperm per day between 1 and 5 days of abstinence (Schwartz et al., 1979). We feel that total sperm count is usually a more useful parameter than sperm concentration because it avoids variation in semen volume. Daily sperm production (DSP) in healthy men is 300 million and declines somewhat with age starting in the 30's (Amann, 1981). Total sperm count and daily sperm output (number of sperm ejaculated per day), in a man who ejaculates very frequently, are much lower than DSP. The reason for this discrepancy is unknown.

Criteria taken from the literature may not be appropriate in another setting. The data of Sherins et al. (1977) suggest that the minimally adequate number of specimens to define good or poor quality semen is three over a 2-month interval, although 97 per cent of men who had a good sperm concentration at the time of the first analysis continued to show a good concentration after as many as nine analyses. In equivocal cases six to nine analyses over a 4-month period were necessary to characterize the semen accurately. The frequency distribution of the various semen parameters among fertile and infertile men referred for evaluation of infertility is shown in Figure 12–4. Most men with greater than 20 million sperm per ml or 60 million total sperm after one day of abstinence are fertile, and some men with even lower counts are also fertile (Sherins et al., 1977; MacLeod, 1951). Motility is the most variable parameter in semen analysis and predicts fertility status only when consistently very good or poor. In contrast, semen morphology is rather stable in longitudinal semen studies. Sherins et al. (1977) found that the percentage of oval forms and sperm concentration correlated best with fertility and that 75 per cent of normal men had greater than 60 per cent normal oval forms.

Just as in dealing with patients with apparently terminal carcinomas, it is our feeling that except for patients with persistent azoospermia

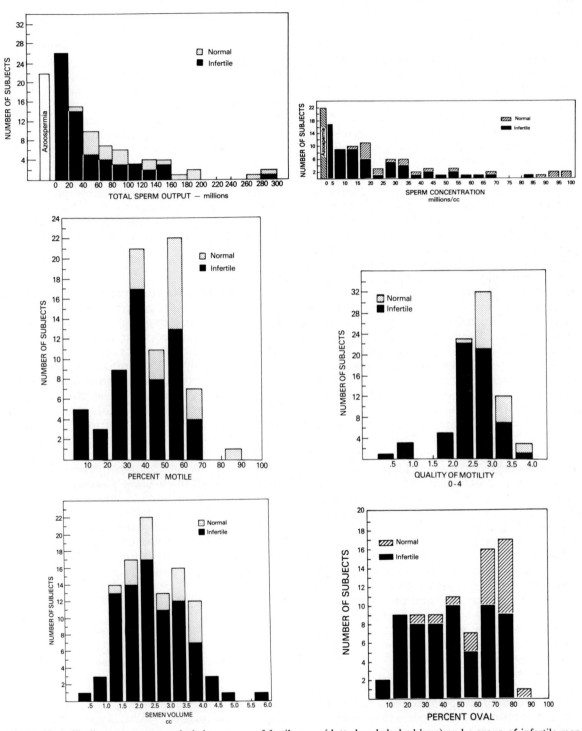

Figure 12–4. Findings on semen analysis in a group of fertile men (dotted and slashed bars) and a group of infertile men (solid bars). The distribution of the men within each group is compared. (From Sherins, R. J., et al.: *In* Troen, P., and Nankin, H. (Eds.): New Concepts of the Testis in Normal and Infertile Men: Morphology, Physiology and Pathology. New York, Raven Press, 1977.)

or severe oligospermia and elevated serum FSH, one should never give a totally negative prognosis.

ADDITIONAL PARAMETERS

Many components of normal semen are not monitored in a routine semen analysis. There has been extensive investigation of several of these factors. Thus far, few, if any, of these studies have proved to be clinically useful.

Fructose is produced in the seminal vesicles of most higher animals, and additional small amounts come from the ampullary glands in some animals. The production is an androgen-dependent process. The normal range of concentration in human semen is 120 to 450 mg/100 ml. Concentrations of below 120 mg/100 ml usually reflect underlying pathology such as inflammation of the seminal vesicles, androgen deficiency, partial obstruction of the ejaculatory ducts, or incomplete ejaculation. If the seminal vesicles are absent or the ejaculatory ducts are completely obstructed, there will be no fructose in the semen. Fructose can be detected in human seminal plasma by using a reagent composed of 50 mg of powdered resorcinol and 33 ml of concentrated hydrochloric acid diluted to 100 ml with water. The semen is mixed with the reagent in a 1:10 ratio and boiled. An orange-red color will develop within 60 seconds after the initiation of boiling if fructose is present. This test is useful in the azoospermic male, for the absence of fructose indicates either a congenital absence of the vas deferens and seminal vesicles or an obstruction. Absence of coagulation of the semen, a small volume ejaculate, and increased concentration of citric acid confirm this diagnosis.

Many investigators have examined the metabolism, membrane physiology, and biochemistry of ejaculated human spermatozoa. The respiratory rate, the ability to metabolize substrates such as fructose, and the effect of ions, pH, proteins, and osmolality on the metabolism of sperm of fertile and infertile men have been studied. Thus far, none of these metabolic tests is clinically useful.

Whereas the seminal vesicles contribute fructose and prostaglandins to the semen, the prostate secretes zinc, magnesium, dehydrogenases, aminotransferases, citric acid phosphatase, and spermine. A test for spermine derivatives is used to identify human semen in criminal investigations. Eliasson (1975) observed that the concentration of acid phosphatase in the semen is frequently depressed in men with asymptomatic prostatitis. After treatment, the levels often return to normal.

The range of pH for human seminal fluid was found by Raboch and Skachova (1965) to be 7.05 to 7.80. Thus far, no correlation has been found between pH and fertility. Similarly, there has been no correlation between the concentration of electrolytes in human seminal plasma and fertility.

Supravital staining is a technique that has been used in animal experimentation to differentiate living from dead spermatozoa. The methods used in evaluation of animal semen have not proved as reliable when used for human spermatozoon evaluation. New techniques are also available to stain and visualize the acrosome; thus far, these methods have not had useful application in clinical practice.

SPERM-CERVICAL MUCUS PENETRATION ASSAY

Sperm motility in cervical mucus can be examined in vivo (the postcoital test) or in vitro. The postcoital test involves examination of cervical mucus obtained after intercourse (Moghissi, 1976). A positive test suggests good semen and mucus quality. A poor postcoital test, in a couple with a normal semen analysis, implies a cervical factor as the cause of infertility. Unfortunately, timing is critical in this test and there is a lack of standardization resulting in many equivocal tests and misleading interpretations. If sperm-cervical mucus interaction appears abnormal, a semen-mucus cross-penetration test should be performed using patient and fertile donor control specimens (Table 12–5).

To avoid the inconvenience and variability of the postcoital and cross-penetration tests, several in vitro sperm-mucus tests have been described using preovulatory (23 days) human

TABLE 12–5. SEMEN-MUCUS CROSS-PENETRATION TEST*

Semen		Mucus		Interpretation
Patient	+	Donor	⊕	Pathology in patient
Donor	+	Patient	⊖	mucus
Patient	+	Donor	⊖	Pathology in patient
Donor	+	Patient	⊕	semen
Patient	+	Donor	⊕	Pathology specific
Donor	+	Patient	⊕	to patient couple
Patient	+	Donor	⊖	Pathology in both
Donor	+	Patient	⊖	patient semen and
				patient mucus

*Adapted from Overstreet, J. W., et al.: Fertil. Steril., *33*:534, 1980.

cervical mucus (Mumford and Warner, 1983; Kremer and Jager, 1976) or bovine cervical mucus (Alexander, 1981; Bergman et al., 1981). These examinations can be done either on a microscope slide or in a round or flat capillary tube (Mills and Katz, 1978). The capillary tube technique is more quantitative. It should be emphasized that these tests do not directly measure fertility and the results can be misleading (Matthews et al., 1980), just as the results of semen analyses may be difficult to interpret.

SPERM-OOCYTE INTERACTION

Since semen analysis and sperm penetration assays are only very rough indications of male fertility, investigators have developed tests of sperm-oocyte interaction. The basis of this work is attributed to Yanagimachi (1972), who reported that if the zona pellucida is removed from a hamster egg, cross-species fertilization with guinea pig sperm could occur. Yanagimachi et al. (1976) then demonstrated that properly incubated human sperm could also penetrate zona pellucida-free hamster eggs. Barros et al. (1978) found a rough correlation between these tests and human male fertility, and Rogers et al. (1979) reported an excellent correlation. Since that time, many groups have used this test with varying results (Chang and Albertsen, 1983). Some investigators report a large number of false-negative (fertile men labeled infertile) and/or false-positive (infertile men deemed fertile) results. No one alleges that the test is an infallible indicator of fertility status.

Fertilization requires a coordinated timed sequence of events:
1. Spermatogenesis.
2. Epididymal sperm maturation.
3. Ejaculation.
4. Sperm transport in the female.
5. Sperm capacitation.
6. Acrosome reaction.
7. Sperm binding to the zona pellucida.
8. Sperm penetration into the zona pellucida.
9. Sperm entry into the perivitelline space.
10. Sperm fusion with the vitellus.

Semen analysis gives information concerning steps 1 through 3. The mucus penetration tests give insight into step 4. Sperm-oocyte interaction tests using denuded hamster ova evaluate steps 5, 6, 9, and 10. Overstreet et al. (1980) used human ova in the assay to evaluate steps 7 and 8 and found that some individuals have a defect in either or both of these steps; these men have normal hamster egg penetration test results, but they are infertile.

The cross-species sperm-egg penetration test requires incubation of the sperm in culture media long enough for capacitation and the acrosome reaction to occur. The sperm are then incubated with a large number of zona pellucida-free eggs and viewed under a microscope. The most commonly used end point for a positive test is decondensation of the sperm nucleus in the egg cytoplasm. The test is scored by the per cent of ova penetrated and/or by the number of decondensed sperm heads per egg. Each laboratory has to establish its normal values and define criteria for positive and negative results. There is tremendous variability from laboratory to laboratory, depending on how the test is performed. At this time, the sperm-oocyte interaction assay is an interesting research tool that can be clinically useful in selected cases. However, even if the assay is skillfully done, individuals with infertility due to abnormalities of sperm transport or a postfertilization phenomenon will not be identified. These tests must be interpreted by sophisticated clinicians and are not a substitute for the traditional complete and thoughtful evaluation of the infertile couple.

X-ray

Vasography and seminal vesiculography are necessary to identify the site of obstruction in azoospermic men with normal spermatogenesis. These studies are also occasionally indicated in other patients in whom the history, physical examination, and semen analysis raise the possibility of obstruction of the ductal system. The contrast agent may be injected either into the vas deferens or into the ejaculatory ducts. Because it is often difficult to catheterize the ejaculatory duct, direct injection of the vasa is commonly used. This usually requires a scrotal incision, since percutaneous injection of the vasa is not often successful.

The small, smooth-walled, 0.5- to 1.0-mm lumen of the vas deferens dilates as it passes under the trigone of the bladder to become the 3- to 5-cm long ampulla of the vas, which is irregular and tortuous. The ampulla, in turn, joins the excretory duct of the seminal vesicle to form the 1.5- to 2.0-cm long smooth ejaculatory duct, which enters the posterior urethra 2.0 to 2.5 cm from the bladder neck just lateral to the opening of the prostatic utricle on the verumontanum (Fig. 12–5). The paired seminal vesicles arise at an angle of 50 to 60 degrees from the horizontal and extend 4.5 to 6.0 cm under the base of the bladder. They have a capacity of 3.5 ml.

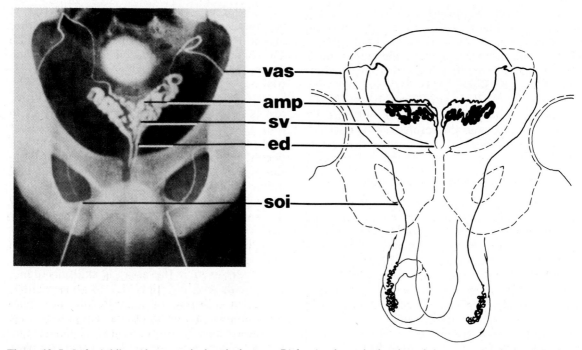

Figure 12–5. *Left,* A bilateral vasoseminal vesiculogram. *Right,* A schematic drawing of the excurrent ducts of the male reproductive system. *Vas,* Vas deferens; *amp,* ampulla of the vas deferens; *sv,* seminal vesicles; *ed,* ejaculatory duct; *soi,* site of injection.

Our technique of seminal vesiculography is as follows. After the vas has been surgically exposed, a 23-gauge needle is inserted into the lumen, pointing toward the distal end. Radiopaque contrast material suitable for intravenous pyelogram studies is diluted 1:2 with saline and 2.5 ml is injected. The needle may be reinstated pointing toward the epididymis, and 0.3 to 0.5 ml of the contrast agent is injected. This proximal study will not rule out obstruction in the proximal or mid-epididymis. Therefore, this step is often omitted, and the patency of the proximal portion of the excurrent duct system is documented by demonstrating the presence of spermatozoa at the time of surgical repair. Supine (Fig. 12–5) and oblique radiographs of the pelvis are obtained. The oblique film demonstrates the ejaculatory ducts, which may be obscured on the anteroposterior film by contrast refluxing into the bladder. The contrast will stay in the seminal vesicles for days if no ejaculation occurs. The patency of the distal portion of the ductal system can be determined without radiographic studies by injecting methylene blue and observing the color of the efflux from a urethral catheter. This method is perfectly satisfactory during vasovasostomy, but it does not yield information about the seminal vesicles or the epididymis.

Evidence of obstruction or inflammation from these studies will direct subsequent therapy. Some authors have advised against these procedures because of the possibility of stricture formation. Using the technique outlined above, rather than the method of incising the vas and utilizing modern contrast agents, we have not had any such complications nor do we anticipate a significant number of them.

Biopsy

Testicular biopsy is mandatory in azoospermic men with normal-sized testes to distinguish between ductal obstruction and spermatogenic failure as the cause of azoospermia. In men with poor semen quality or azoospermia and small testes, the results of a pathologic evaluation will rarely if ever alter therapy. However, the biopsy often assists in making a definitive diagnosis, which helps the physician in giving the patient a prognosis and avoiding unnecessary treatment in irredeemable situations. Bilateral biopsy is indicated if there is any suggestion from the history and physical examination that the patient has different lesions on each side, such as ductal obstruction and primary testicular failure.

TECHNIQUE

Testicular biopsies can be performed with local anesthesia or general anesthesia. If local anesthesia is used, either the spermatic cord or the area of the incision is infiltrated with lidocaine (Xylocaine). When vasography is also indicated, we prefer to use general anesthesia. The details of the surgical technique are presented in Chapter 84.

Electron microscopic studies are not currently of practical value in the routine clinical evaluation of infertile men; however, Chemes et al. (1977) found preliminary electron microscopic evidence suggesting that abnormalities of Sertoli cells are present in many infertile men.

Gordon et al. (1965) demonstrated a significant temporary decrease in sperm count in 22 to 42 days following bilateral testicular biopsy in 9 of 16 (45 per cent) subjects. They suggested that the suppression of spermatogenesis might be secondary to antibody formation. However, Ansbacher and Gangai (1975) found no circulating sperm-immobilizing or sperm-agglutinating antibodies up to 14 days after testicular biopsy in oligospermic men. We do not feel that Gordon's findings contraindicate biopsy in properly selected patients.

INTERPRETATION

The interpretation of the pathologic studies are complicated by the lack of a uniform system of nomenclature. The basic characteristics that should be evaluated include the number and size of seminiferous tubules, the thickness of the tubule basement membrane, the state of the germinal epithelium, the degree of fibrosis in the interstitium, and the condition of the Leydig cells. The classification scheme that follows is arbitrary but practical.

Normal (Fig. 12–6A). The normal testes are made up largely of seminiferous tubules separated by a scant loose interstitium composed of Leydig cells, blood vessels, lymphatics, and connective tissue. The androgen-producing, round to polygonal, acidophilic Leydig cells are scattered in groups and often contain crystalloids of Reinke. The thin basement membrane of seminiferous tubules separates the Sertoli and germinal cells from the vessels and lymphatics. Thus, exchange of all hormonal regulators, nutrients, and therapeutic agents on the one hand and of waste products on the other occurs across this membrane. The basement membrane is lined by Sertoli cells and spermatogonia. The more mature germ cells are intimately associated with the Sertoli cells away from the basement membrane. (See the section on spermatogenesis.) Patients with obstructive azoospermia usually have normal testicular histologic findings.

Germinal Aplasia (Fig. 12–6B). Patients with this condition, also known as the Sertoli-only syndrome, are permanently infertile. There is a striking absence of germinal cells in all or most of the seminiferous tubules. The tubules are uniform in appearance and have a slight reduction in diameter. The histologic findings are otherwise normal.

Maturation Arrest (Fig. 12–6C). Inspection of testes with the lesion reveals that generally spermatogenesis does not proceed beyond the primary spermatocyte, the secondary spermatocyte, or the spermatid. The level of the block is similar in all tubules of a given patient, but it varies from patient to patient. The causes of these lesions are unknown. However, Frajese et al. (1974) have presented data showing that the germ cells of patients with spermatocytic arrest synthesize deoxyribonucleic acid (DNA) more slowly than normals, whereas the germ cells of patients with spermatid arrest synthesize DNA more rapidly than normals. This suggests that there is a completely different defect causing these two apparently similar abnormalities.

Hypospermatogenic and Other Nonspecific Abnormalities of Spermatogenesis (Fig. 12–6D). In a significant percentage of the biopsies of testes of infertile men, all of the normal spermatogenic cells are present but in decreased numbers. The usual organization of the germinal epithelium is disrupted, and immature cells are found in the lumina of the tubules. Individual cells may have abnormal nuclei. This pathologic picture probably results from several distinct abnormalities, but to date no practical gain has been achieved by further subdividing this group.

Klinefelter's Syndrome and Other Fibrotic States (Fig. 12–6E). The testes in Klinefelter's syndrome undergo a gradual decrease in spermatogenic activity that eventually leads to the disappearance of all germ and Sertoli cells. The tubules become fibrotic and hyalinized, resulting in a small and usually firm testis. Leydig cells appear clumped, but the total number is not increased. The serum testosterone level is low or normal. A variety of insults such as infection may result in fibrosis; thus, not all sclerotic testes are caused by Klinefelter's syndrome.

Hypogonadotropic Hypogonadism (Fig. 12–6F). This testicle has not been stimulated by gonadotropins. Note the very small seminiferous tubular diameter, absence of germ cells and

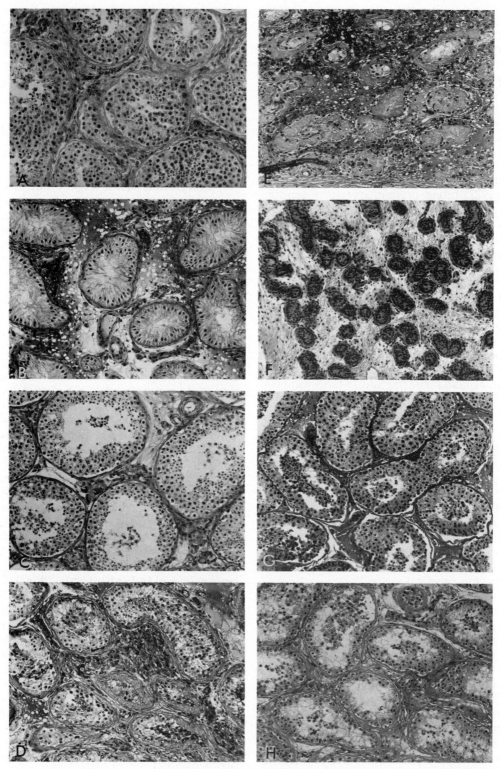

Figure 12–6. Testicular biopsies. *A,* Normal; *B,* Germinal aplasia; *C,* Maturation arrest; *D,* Hyperspermatogenesis; *E,* Klinefelter's syndrome; *F,* Hypogonadotropic hypogonadism; *G,* Fertile eunuch; *H,* Adult testis, post-hypophysectomy. Hemotoxylin and eosin staining; × 160.

Leydig cells. This biopsy is indistinguishable from that of a 7-month fetus.

Fertile Eunuch Syndrome (Fig. 12–6G). This variant of hypogonadotropic hypogonadism is due to partial gonadotropin deficiency. Notice the normal spermatogenesis but the reduced number of Leydig cells.

Posthypophysectomy Adult Male (Fig. 12–6H). Hypophysectomy in an adult male who was once sexually mature produces testicular atrophy in which there is a large seminiferous tubule with variable depletion of the germ cells and absence of Leydig cells.

Miscellaneous. A number of conditions other than those just mentioned cause abnormalities in the testicular biopsy. These include tumors, inflammatory diseases, endocrine deficiencies, myotonic muscular dystrophy, vascular disease, cryptorchidism, drugs, and irradiation.

QUANTIFICATION AND INCIDENCE

In an effort to gain more information from testicular biopsies and to correlate the histologic findings with the semen analysis, several investigators have attempted to quantitate the biopsy findings. To date these methods remain research techniques with little clinical application.

Because various authors have used different nomenclature and indications for biopsy, it is not possible to garner from the literature a uniform incidence for the lesions listed. However, the most common abnormalities found in biopsy specimens of testes of infertile men are hypospermatogenesis and maturation arrest. Germinal cell aplasia, fibrosis, and normal histology are less commonly, but not infrequently, encountered. Reviews of the subject have been published by Nelson (1950) and Wong et al. (1974; 1973a,b), among others.

CLASSIFICATION AND ETIOLOGY OF DISORDERS ASSOCIATED WITH MALE INFERTILITY

This section presents a classification of male infertility based on etiology and pathophysiology. Often, a complete understanding of the events leading to the infertile state is not possible. Nevertheless, precision in diagnosis should be emphasized, since misdiagnosis is common and may result in inappropriate treatment. Table 12–6 relates the findings on semen analysis to the etiologic classification of male infertility states that are described below.

TABLE 12–6. CLASSIFICATION OF MALE INFERTILITY STATUS BY CRITERIA OF SEMEN ANALYSIS

I. Absent Ejaculation
1. Drugs
2. Surgery
3. Vascular occlusion
4. Diabetes mellitus
5. Psychologic disturbances

II. Azoospermia
1. Seminiferous tubular sclerosis
   a. Klinefelter's syndrome
   b. Chromatin negative Klinefelter's syndrome
2. Germinal aplasia
   a. Idiopathic
   b. Drug/x-ray
   c. Klinefelter's syndrome with mosaicism
   d. XYY syndrome
3. Maturation arrest
   a. Idiopathic
   b. XYY syndrome
   c. Varicocele
4. Ductal obstrution

III. Nonmotile Spermatozoa (Necrospermia)
1. Kartagener's syndrome
2. Prolonged abstinence
3. Idiopathic

IV. Oligospermia
1. Idiopathic
2. Cryptorchidism
3. Varicocele
4. Drugs
5. Systemic infection

V. Normal But Infertile
1. Gynecologic abnormality
2. Abnormal coital habits
3. Systemic infection
4. Immunologic

Endocrine Disorders

The endocrine causes of male infertility are due primarily to states of gonadotropin deficiency. Hypogonadotropic hypogonadism may be selective, in which case pituitary secretion of other trophic hormones is normal; or it may be associated with multiple trophic hormone deficiencies, as in idiopathic panhypopituitarism or hypothalamic-pituitary tumor. The absence of LH and FSH leads to failure of sexual maturation in the prepubertal patient and to decreased libido and involution of sexual characteristics in the adult. Thus, it is essential in evaluating such subjects to have a clear understanding of normal pubertal events.

ISOLATED HYPOGONADOTROPIC HYPOGONADISM

Hypogonadotropic hypogonadism can occur as an isolated deficiency of pituitary LH and FSH secretion. The disorder is seen in both sexes and may be sporadic, or it may present as a familial defect (Biben and Gordan, 1955;

Kallman et al., 1944; Nowakowski and Lenz, 1961; Santen and Paulsen, 1973a; Sparks et al., 1968).

The disorder is usually inherited as an autosomal dominant trait with variable penetrance (Santen and Paulsen, 1973 *a*; Merriam et al., 1977), but autosomal recessive (Ewer, 1968) and X-linked transmission has also been implicated in the inheritance of the disorder. A variety of distinctive neurologic, genital, and somatic anomalies have been described in association with isolated gonadotropin deficiency (Table 12–7). The most prominent of these is anosmia (lack of sense of smell), which is due to absence of the olfactory tracts (Bardin, 1971).

The etiology of isolated hypogonadotropic hypogonadism appears to be an absence of hypothalamic gonadotropin-releasing hormone (GnRH) release, since exogenous GnRH administration stimulates normal LH and FSH secretion from the pituitary (Yoshimoto et al., 1975; Bremner et al., 1977; Hoffman and Crowley et al., 1982).

Delay in sexual maturation is the hallmark of the syndrome. Since prepubertal boys are by definition sexually immature, hypogonadotropic hypogonadism is not clinically evident until puberty. Although the alternative diagnosis of constitutionally delayed puberty can be made only in retrospect, the presence of anosmia or one of the other somatic midline defects may be a clue to the possibility that sexual maturation will not proceed spontaneously. However, demonstration of the onset of proper progression of pubertal events is ultimately required to differentiate these two states.

Testicular enlargement, which normally precedes peak height growth by 2 years (Marshall and Tanner, 1970), does not occur in boys with true hypogonadotropism. Thus, careful measurement of testicular size may be a clue to the onset of puberty prior to the establishment of other pubertal features. In addition, a family history of delayed puberty favors the diagnosis of late pubescence. Testicular biopsy typically shows totally immature seminiferous tubules and absent Leydig cells (Fig. 12–6), which are equivalent to the features of a testis of a 7-month fetus (Van Wagenen and Simpson, 1965). These features are not pathognomonic, but the normal peripubertal testis often shows a greater degree of germinal epithelial development.

Unfortunately, the measurement of serum LH and FSH per se does not easily distinguish the hypogonadotropic male, since serum gonadotropin concentrations in these subjects are within the lower limits of normal in most routine assays (Kulin, 1967; Reiter et al., 1973). Although clomiphene administration will increase serum LH and FSH in normal men and will serve as a diagnostic test of pituitary LH and FSH reserve (Bardin et al., 1967), prepubertal boys remain unresponsive to short-term clomiphene administration until midpuberty, Tanner Stage III (Kulin et al., 1971; Nankin et al., 1971). Thus, clomiphene unresponsiveness does not distinguish the hypogonadotropic from the normal boy with delayed puberty. Moreover, long-term administration of clomiphene also fails to initiate any increase in serum LH or FSH in hypogonadotropic subjects (Santen et al., 1971). It is of interest that clomiphene has been shown to increase serum LH and FSH levels in subjects with hypogonadotropic hypogonadism associated with the Prader-Willi syndrome (Hamilton et al., 1972). This suggests that the mechanism for gonadotropin deficiency in this syndrome differs from that of the others described earlier.

Gonadotropin-releasing hormone (GnRH) has become available in most medical centers for diagnostic testing. Most prepubertal children and patients with gonadotropin deficiency release LH and FSH in response to GnRH administration (Bell et al., 1973; Hashimoto et al., 1972; Roth et al., 1972; Yen et al., 1972; Zarate

TABLE 12–7. NEUROLOGIC, GENITAL, AND SOMATIC ANOMALIES ASSOCIATED WITH ISOLATED HYPOGONADOTROPIC HYPOGONADISM

Physical Feature	Reference
I. Neurologic	
(1) Anosmia—CN I.	Kallman et al., 1944
(2) CN V	de Mosier, 1954
(3) Möbius syndrome—CN III, IV, VI	
(4) Nerve deafness—CN VIII	de Gennes et al., 1970
(5) Mental retardation	Kallman et al., 1944
(6) Cerebellar ataxia	Neuhauser and Opitz, 1975
(7) Retinitis pigmentosa	Reinfrank and Nichols, 1964
II. Genital	
(1) Cryptorchidism	de Mosier, 1954
(2) Microphallus	Nowakowski and Lenz, 1961
(3) Hypospadias	
III. Somatic	
(1) Harelip	Kallman et al., 1944
(2) Cleft palate	de Mosier, 1954
(3) Short fourth metacarpals	Bardin et al., 1969
(4) Prader-Willi syndrome	Hamilton et al., 1972
(5) Congenital adrenal hypoplasia	Hay et al., 1981

Abbreviation: CN, Cranial nerve.

et al., 1973). Thus, this test does not differentiate between normal prepubertal boys and boys with gonadotropin deficiency. However, the response to GnRH suggests that the etiology of hypogonadotropic hypogonadism is due to an absence of this releasing factor.

Studies have shown that untreated subjects with isolated gonadotropin deficiency fail to increase serum prolactin levels when given a standard chlorpromazine challenge (1 mg/3 kg intramuscularly), whereas normal men increase prolactin levels more than 15 ng/ml above their baseline values (Winters et al., 1978). This apparent prolactin deficiency appears to be due to insufficient sex steroid exposure, since hypogonadotropic patients become normally responsive to chlorpromazine after they have been treated with testosterone or human chorionic gonadotropin (hCG). It is significant that untreated hypogonadotropic men can be distinguished from boys with constitutional delay of puberty by their prolactin response to chlorpromazine when other physical features of sexual maturation and standard laboratory criteria (as described above) are otherwise indistinguishable (Winters et al., 1982).

FERTILE EUNUCH SYNDROME

Very rarely, a male will present with signs of eunuchoidism and variable secondary sexual development but will have large testes (McCullagh et al., 1953; Pasqualini and Bur, 1955). Testicular biopsy shows maturation of the germinal epithelium (Fig. 12–6), but Leydig cells are absent. The ejaculate may even contain sperm. These men have been called "fertile eunuchs," and they represent a special subcategory of patients with hypogonadotropic hypogonadism.

Because of the testicular enlargement and early signs of virilization, differentiation of this type of man from one who is midpubertal may be very difficult. The patient usually presents with failure to progress through puberty, and it is the persistent incompletion of sexual maturation that suggests that this is a pathologic state. Since arrest of pubertal maturation is common in patients with pituitary tumors, the physician must exclude tumor by appropriate radiographic, ophthalmologic, and endocrine function testing. However, some men presenting with this syndrome do not have pituitary tumors and represent a variant of isolated hypogonadotropic hypogonadism.

Early reports of such cases showed that urinary and plasma FSH levels were normal but LH levels were low (Faiman et al., 1968;

McCullagh et al., 1953; Pasqualini and Bur, 1955). The cause of this disorder was attributed to a selective deficiency of LH secretion; the presence of adequate FSH permits spermatogenesis. In our opinion, since initiation of spermatogenesis requires stimulation of intratesticular testosterone, the fertile eunuch syndrome represents partial hypogonadotropic hypogonadism in which there is adequate LH to stimulate high intratesticular levels of androgen, but inadequate testosterone secretion to provide effective virilizing levels of androgen in the peripheral tissues. Accordingly, eunuchoidal proportions develop despite testicular maturation.

Although gonadotropin measurements per se are unreliable for diagnosis, plasma testosterone levels are low. Confirmation of the diagnosis, in the absence of pituitary tumor, resides in the demonstration that Leydig cell function does not progress spontaneously.

POSTPUBERTAL GONADOTROPIN DEFICIENCY

Hypogonadotropism in a sexually mature male usually results from the presence of a pituitary tumor. Not uncommonly, the only pituitary function affected is secretion of gonadotropin. Hence, such a patient may present with loss of libido, decreased potency, and reduced ejaculate volume as a consequence of decreased Leydig cell function. It should be emphasized that these symptoms may persist for years before other signs of an expanding pituitary tumor appear, i.e., headache, visual field loss, and deficiency of thyroid or adrenal trophic hormones.

Loss of secondary sexual characteristics is a late manifestation of this disease, often requiring 5 to 10 years. By contrast, the testes become small and atrophic earlier. Testicular biopsy (Fig. 12–6) shows sloughing of the germinal epithelium into the lumen of the tubule, eventually leading to complete loss of spermatogonia. The absence of mature Leydig cells is a most important finding (Albert et al., 1954). However, laboratory support of the diagnosis of gonadotropin deficiency in the adult male rests primarily with the demonstration of below normal plasma testosterone levels (250 to 1200 ng/dl, since plasma and urinary gonadotropin concentrations are difficult to distinguish from normal.

CONGENITAL ADRENAL HYPERPLASIA

It has been suggested that adrenal hyperplasia secondary to 21-hydroxylase deficiency may produce oligospermia in afflicted men when overproduction of adrenal androgens inhibits pituitary gonadotropin secretion (Wilkins and Cara, 1954). Although congenital adrenal hyperplasia is a rare disorder (1:5000), recognition of such a state associated with infertility would prompt appropriate treatment and allow reversal of gonadotropin suppression.

At least five variants of congenital adrenal hyperplasia have been recognized, each resulting in a unique clinical syndrome (Bongiovanni, 1972). The most common form of congenital adrenal hyperplasia is 21-hydroxylase deficiency. The syndrome is familial, affecting both males and females. The overproduction of adrenal androgens usually leads to precocious puberty and short stature (adrenogenital syndrome). In the absence of precocious puberty, diagnosis of congenital adrenal hyperplasia in the male can be difficult, since excess virilization of an otherwise normal sexually mature man is undetectable. Although very rare, men with mild congenital adrenal hyperplasia could remain undiagnosed until adulthood but might benefit from glucocorticoid therapy. Since there are no conclusive data to support the use of steroids in the treatment of idiopathic infertility, it behooves the physician to distinguish between these disorders.

Twenty-one hydroxylase deficiency results in impaired conversion of 17-hydroxyprogesterone to 11-desoxycortisol and of progesterone to 11-desoxycorticosterone. The former results in a decrease in cortisol synthesis, which in turn leads to increased adrenocorticotropic hormone (ACTH) secretion and adrenal hyperstimulation. Thus, 21-hydroxylase deficiency leads to overproduction of adrenal testosterone, which secondarily inhibits gonadotropin secretion. Since 21-hydroxylation does not occur in the Leydig cell, this defect does not inhibit testicular steroidogenesis; however, it affects the testis indirectly.

Careful laboratory evaluation is essential to confirm the clinical diagnosis, particularly when a mild deficiency state is suspected. Since the block in cortisol synthesis is compensated by increased ACTH secretion, plasma cortisol levels and urinary 17-hydroxycorticoid excretion levels remain in the low normal range. By contrast, the levels of 17-ketosteroids, which are derived from weak adrenal androgens other than testosterone, and pregnanetriol, the metabolic product of 17-hydroxyprogesterone, are usually increased in urine. Although elevated 17-ketosteroid and pregnanetriol levels are the classic laboratory features, they are not always elevated.

Adult onset of a mild attenuated form of 21-hydroxylase deficiency has been reported for females who present with hirsutism and oligomenorrhea, but only more recently has the disorder been reported in men (Chrousos et al., 1981), probably because signs of mild androgen excess are inapparent in men. Recent studies of a man with cryptic congenital 21-hydroxylase deficiency demonstrated that unstimulated plasma 17-hydroxyprogesterone levels are highly variable during 24-hour sampling, elevated mostly at night during sleep; however, the levels increased approximately 20-fold following ACTH stimulation, well above the response range for normal men.

Several case reports have described an increase in sperm output following glucocorticoid administration to men with congenital adrenal hyperplasia (Burke et al., 1973; Fore et al., 1972). This is in keeping with the observations of Wilkens and Cara (1954), who demonstrated prompt testicular growth and maturation after treating older boys with this syndrome. Some studies have actually documented that LH secretion is impaired in untreated boys (Boyer et al., 1973; Radfar et al., 1977) and that LH suppression is reversed following glucocorticoid administration (Radfar et al., 1977).

To our knowledge, however, there are no data on the fertility status of male patients with adult onset of the attenuated form of 21-hydroxylase deficiency. Studies of the classical form of the disease, wherein subjects present in childhood with precocious puberty and short stature, show that sperm output and fertility are preserved (Urban et al., 1978). By contrast, oligospermia is a common finding in patients with classical 21-hydroxylase deficiency whose course has been complicated by testicular adrenal rest tumors (Burke et al., 1973; Radfar et al., 1977). The mechanism for the oligospermia probably results from a combination of factors including mechanical obstruction to the outflow of sperm, destruction of the seminiferous tubule and changes in the testicular hormonal milieu. In such cases, the oligospermia may not be corrected by dexamethasone suppression of the adrenal (Burke et al., 1973; Radfar et al., 1977; Chrousos et al., 1981), but the physician should make a reasonable attempt to try to accomplish this.

Testicular tumors are occasionally seen in association with congenital adrenal hyperplasia. (Glenn and Boyce, 1963; Burke et al., 1973;

Fore et al., 1972; Radfar et al., 1977; Chrousos et al., 1981). Adrenal cells may become trapped in gonadal tissue during embryologic development in 10 per cent of normal boys (Dahl and Bahn, 1962). When ACTH secretion is increased, these cells become hyperplastic and present as testicular tumors. When the adrenal cells remain outside the testis along the epididymis and spermatic cord, the tissue usually resembles true adrenal glandular architecture (adrenal rests). Often, however, these tumors are intratesticular, and histologically they resemble true Leydig cell neoplasms. In two studies of men with "Leydig cell" tumors and congenital adrenal hyperplasia, glucocorticoid administration resulted in prompt reduction in testicular size (Fore et al., 1972; Radfar et al., 1977). In addition, increased concentration of cortisol was found in the testicular venous effluent. Thus, the apparent "Leydig cell" masses were functionally under ACTH control and were probably true adrenal cells. Since orchiectomy is appropriate treatment for Leydig cell neoplasms, the differentiation of ectopic adrenal neoplasms in men with congenital adrenal hyperplasia is critical because castration in these patients can be avoided.

Congenital Disorders Associated with Karyotype Abnormalities

With the advent of techniques that determine the chromosomal composition of cells, a variety of testicular disorders have been shown to be associated with abnormalities of the karyotype. Patients with mixed gonadal dysgenesis (streak gonad plus contralateral testis) have profound fetal testicular failure and present as male pseudohermaphrodites with female phenotypic features. The interested reader is referred to discussions presented elsewhere in this book and to classic texts on abnormalities in sexual differentiation. More commonly, karyotype abnormalities are associated with seminiferous tubular sclerosis (Klinefelter's syndrome) or varying degrees of germinal depletion (XYY syndrome). Although the precise relationship between the chromosomal abnormalities and the testicular dysfunction has not been defined, these associations emphasize the need for discovery of the biochemical causes of other tubular diseases. From recent studies, it has also become clear that men with a normal peripheral karyotype may be infertile owing to abnormalities of only the meiotic chromosomes of the testicular germ cells.

KLINEFELTER'S SYNDROME

This disorder was described in 1942 as a syndrome of hypogonadal men with small firm testes, gynecomastia, and elevated urinary gonadotropins (Klinefelter et al., 1942). This triad of signs results from sclerosis of the seminiferous tubules. With the development of techniques for analysis of sex chromatin (Plunkett and Barr, 1956) and for chromosomal analysis (Jacobs and Strong, 1959), it became apparent that many individuals with seminiferous tubular sclerosis had an extra X chromosome that was derived from nondisjunction of the meiotic chromosomes of the gametes from either parent.

The frequency of chromatin-positive buccal smears in large scale surveys has been estimated as 0.2 per cent in newborns (MacLean et al., 1964), and in noninstitutionalized men (Paulsen et al., 1964). This incidence is significantly higher among men with mental retardation (de la Chapelle, 1963; Ferguson-Smith, 1959). Thus, Klinefelter's syndrome is the most common cause of frank hypogonadism.

There has always been some uncertainty about the precise definition of the syndrome because chromosomal analysis was not available when the syndrome was first described. It has been estimated that approximately 25 per cent of men with the clinical triad will fail to demonstrate the extra X chromosome (Barr, 1966); in these men the disorder has accordingly been referred to as chromatin-negative Klinefelter's syndrome. This nomenclature stems from the lack of understanding of other causes of seminiferous tubular sclerosis as well as from technical difficulties in demonstrating the extra X chromosome in some patients with chromosomal mosaicism (Paulsen et al., 1968). Federman (1967) has suggested that Klinefelter's syndrome should be defined on the basis of the chromosomal abnormality. Thus, any man with more than one X chromosome in any cell line would be considered to have Klinefelter's syndrome.

The clinical features of the syndrome have been well reviewed (Barr, 1966; Becker et al., 1966; Paulsen et al., 1968). Although it has been reported that testis size is smaller in prepubertal boys with Klinefelter's syndrome (Laron and Hochman, 1971), a significant decrease in testicular size is not evident until pubescence begins. Virilization begins at the appropriate time. The patient usually seeks medical advice because completion of puberty is delayed, and gynecomastia, eunuchoidism, or impotence becomes apparent (Table 12–8). Occasionally, virilization is adequate and the patient does not

TABLE 12–8. COMMON CLINICAL AND LABORATORY FEATURES IN CLASSIC (XXY) KLINEFELTER'S SYNDROME*

Pathologic Feature	Frequency (%)
Histologic evidence of impaired spermatogenesis	99
Small testes	98
Azoospermia	95
Elevated urinary gonadotropin titer	83
Retarded facial hair growth	81
Impaired libido or potency	66
Gynecomastia	50
Impaired scrotal development	28
Impaired penile development	22

*Adapted from Paulsen, C. A., et al.: Recent Prog. Horm. Res., 24:321, 1968.

present until later in adult life when infertility becomes manifest. In addition to mental retardation, a wide variety of psychiatric disturbances is common (Becker et al., 1966; Theilgaard et al., 1971). Although cryptorchidism (Bergada et al., 1969), carcinoma of the breast (Harnden et al., 1971; Lynch et al., 1974; Robson et al., 1968), and hypothyroidism (Federman, 1967; Plunkett et al., 1964) have been reported in association with the syndrome, the incidences are very low and are probably similar to those observed among otherwise normal men.

The clinical syndrome results from primary testicular failure of both tubules and Leydig cells. The marked decrease in testicular mass is due to the seminiferous tubular sclerosis (Fig. 12–6). Elastic fibers in the tunica propria are characteristically absent, indicating failure of normal tubular maturation. Usually, the tubules are obliterated, but scant numbers of Sertoli cells and spermatogonia may be seen in the testis biopsy. These features result in the azoospermic ejaculate. Leydig cells are very prominent in the testis biopsy owing to the marked reduction in tubules. Although the Leydig cells appear hyperplastic, the total mass of Leydig cells per testis is normal (Ahmad et al., 1969; Dykes, 1968).

Confirmation of the diagnosis rests on the demonstration of a chromatin-positive buccal smear or the presence of an extra X chromosome following analysis of cells from blood, skin, bone marrow, or testis. It is usually not necessary to obtain a karyotype unless the buccal smear is negative or unless there are unusual features in the clinical evaluation. Assessing the gonadotropin and sex steroid levels is also helpful but occasionally may be misleading. Urinary gonadotropin and plasma FSH levels are usually markedly increased, reflecting the profound seminiferous tubular injury. Plasma testosterone, however, is within the normal range in 40 per cent of patients with Klinefelter's syndrome (Paulsen et al., 1968). This apparently "normal" value results from binding of testosterone to increased levels of TeBG in plasma, producing a spuriously high value. The true production rate of testosterone is estimated to be markedly reduced (Gabrilove et al., 1970; Lipsett et al., 1965). The increased plasma LH level (Paulsen et al., 1968) is a more reliable index of the Leydig cell failure. Of interest are the high normal levels of plasma estradiol (Ruder et al., 1974) and the increased level of urinary estradiol excretion (Gabrilove et al., 1970) in the face of marked testicular failure. This imbalance of estrogen to androgen appears to be responsible for the gynecomastia and increased TeBG levels characteristic of the syndrome (Chopra et al., 1973).

Although the 47,XXY karyotype is the most common pattern in Klinefelter's syndrome, men with 48,XXYY, 48,XXXY and 49,XXXXY karyotypes have been reported. The clinical features are generally the same in all, although skeletal abnormalities are more common in association with multiple X chromosomes (Atkins and Connelly, 1963).

By contrast, when XY/XXY chromosomal mosaicism exists, the clinical features of Klinefelter's syndrome may be less severe (Paulsen et al., 1968). In this setting the testis biopsy shows less severe fibrosis, the tubules contain more mature germ cells, and the histology may be nearly normal. A few men with Klinefelter's syndrome are fertile, probably because there is a normal clone of cells within the testis (Foss and Lewis, 1971). In general, a larger testis is in keeping with chromosomal mosaicism. Therefore, the physician should perform a karyotype analysis in men with azoospermia and maturation arrest.

XYY SYNDROME

A report of a tall man with an extra Y chromosome in his karyotype analysis first appeared in 1961 (Sandberg et al., 1961). By 1965 it was noted that individuals with the XYY karyotype appeared with unexpectedly high frequency in an institution for persons with mental defects and antisocial behavior (Jacobs et al., 1965). The large number of investigations that followed supported the contention that individuals with the XYY syndrome are found with greater frequency among subjects with behavioral abnormalities (Walzer, 1976). However, the XYY karyotype occurs in only 0.1 to 0.4

per cent of newborn infants (Balodimos et al., 1966; Price et al., 1966; Walzer, 1976), and an unequivocal association of this karyotypic abnormality and antisocial behavior has not been established. A similar association has been made between tall stature and the XYY karyotype (Hook and Kim, 1971; Sandberg, 1961), and it has been proposed that tall stature per se may predispose the individual to misbehavior rather than the chromosomal abnormality (Hook, 1973).

A number of testicular abnormalities have been reported in association with the XYY karyotype (Table 12–6). These range from varying degrees of maturation arrest of germinal elements within the seminiferous tubules (Baghdassarian et al., 1975; Skakkebaek et al., 1973) to complete germinal aplasia (Santen et al., 1970). The ejaculates from these subjects are accordingly severely oligospermic or azoospermic. However, seminiferous tubular sclerosis similar to that found in Klinefelter's syndrome (Balodimos, 1966), in male pseudohermaphroditism (Ferrier et al., 1967), in congenital adrenal hyperplasia (Iinuma et al., 1974), and in megatestis (Skakkebaek et al., 1973; Zeuthen et al., 1973) have also been reported. To confuse the issue further, XYY men may also be normal and may father children (Stenchever and MacEntyre, 1969). Thus, the XYY karyotype has many phenotypic associations, and no consistent syndrome has been described.

Measurement of plasma and urinary testosterone, LH, and FSH has generally demonstrated values within the normal male range (Ismail et al., 1968; Lundberg and Wahlstrom, 1970; Nielsen et al., 1969). Abnormalities in these laboratory parameters are associated with the more severe testicular dysfunctions found in other primary testicular disorders.

MISCELLANEOUS CHROMOSOMAL ABNORMALITIES

In addition to Klinefelter's syndrome and the XYY syndrome, male infertility with oligospermia may also be associated with abnormalities of the meiotic chromosomes of the germ cells. Testicular biopsy has demonstrated reduction in chiasma formation during meiotic prophase in several oligospermic men who were otherwise normal 46,XY males (Hulten et al., 1970; Pearson et al., 1970). Maturation arrest of the germinal elements was a common feature. In three infertile men, a small proportion of the spermatogonial cells demonstrated grossly fragmented chromosomes (Skakkebaek et al., 1973).

Male subjects with Down's syndrome provide evidence that autosomal abnormalities may also lead to significant testicular dysfunction. Swerzie et al. (1971) reported five patients with trisomy 21 in whom testicular biopsy revealed a varied pattern of seminiferous tubular pathology. In some subjects there was complete germinal aplasia and increased serum FSH, while in others there was at least a moderate degree of arrest in germ cell maturation. Although there was no seminiferous tubular sclerosis and clinically the men were sexually mature, serum LH levels were consistently elevated. Campbell et al. (1982) report testicular atrophy and increased serum FSH concentrations among 17 men with Down's syndrome and indicate that LH levels are also elevated among those subjects older than 30 years. Translocations of portions of autosomes have also been demonstrated in chromosome analysis of oligospermic men (Kjessler, 1974; Plymate et al., 1976; Sarto et al., 1976).

Interestingly, errors of both mitotic chromosomes (Kjessler, 1974) and meiotic chromosomes (Hembree et al., 1976) have been demonstrated in testicular tissue and peripheral blood of men whose wives became pregnant but in whom early abortion was frequent. These reports highlight the possibility that subtle genetic mechanisms may be responsible for otherwise unexplained infertility.

Cryptorchidism

The reported incidence of unilateral cryptorchidism varies somewhat depending on the author and on the age of the subjects surveyed. Scorer and Farrington (1971) suggest that completion of descent cannot be evaluated until after the third postnatal month and that spontaneous descent is unlikely to occur after age 1 year. The best estimates of the incidence of cryptorchidism are 1 per cent at the age of 1 year and 0.8 per cent in adult men (Scorer and Farrington, 1971); however, some authors have reported a considerably higher frequency. These overestimates probably result from the failure to differentiate between retractile testes and true undescended testes.

The incidence of infertility in men with cryptorchidism is controversial. Differences in opinion are often related to selection of patients. Abdominal testes are clearly different from those lying at the inguinal ring. Recognition of the retractile testis, which is caused by a hyperactive cremasteric reflex, is also critical. Scorer and Farrington (1971) suggest that the cryptorchid testis should be categorized as retractile, obstructed, or ectopic.

Differentiating the genesis of cryptorchidism is important in assessing the value of orchiopexy to the patient's fertility potential. While it is clear that surgical correction provided a good cosmetic result, it is not certain that such a procedure enhances fertility potential. One scrotal testis should be adequate for normal fertility. Yet, in patients with unilateral cryptorchidism, the incidence of infertility is higher than expected (Lipshultz, 1976; Lipshultz et al., 1976). Since descent of the testis into the scrotum requires normal fetal testicular function, some authors have suggested that in the truly cryptorchid patient there is dysgenesis of both testes but maldescent of only one (Charny, 1960; Johnston, 1965; Sohval, 1954).

Sixteen men who had previously undergone surgical correction for unilateral cryptorchidism, after having a unilateral vasectomy on the "normal scrotal" testis, were shown to have azoospermia or severe oligospermia (Eldrupt and Steven, 1980; Alpert and Klein, 1983). These data suggest that the previously cryptorchid testis severely impaired spermatogenesis, which was not corrected by orchidopexy. There is also evidence that a unilaterally cryptorchid testis can interfere with spermatogenesis in the contralateral normal gonad (Hoschioan, 1975; Harrison et al., 1981). Therefore, an argument can be made for orchiectomy instead of orchidopexy in boys with a unilateral undescended testis. However, at the present time, we feel that orchidopexy is the treatment of choice.

There is abundant experimental evidence in rodents that increasing the intratesticular temperature only a few degrees (42 to 43° C) for as little as 30 minutes results in damage to primary spermatocytes (Steinberger and Dixon, 1959). Similar experiments in men produce oligospermia within 3 weeks that lasts approximately 50 days (MacLeod, 1941). Experimental cryptorchidism in rats produces rapid impairment of Sertoli cell and Leydig cell function (Jégou, 1983). There is also increasing evidence that an undescended testis in a young male becomes morphologically abnormal by age 1 to 3 years (Hadziselimovic, 1977; Mininberg et al., 1982; Hedinger, 1979), although in some cases there is no dramatic alteration until puberty (Bar-Maor et al., 1979).

The evidence cited above has led many experts to recommend that orchidopexy be done very early in life. We believe that the critical question—whether or not the early morphological alterations seen in cryptorchid testes are reversed by orchidopexy—is unanswered. Therefore, we recommend early surgical intervention (at 18 to 30) months but do not feel that surgery is necessary in the first year of life.

The scrotal testis in patients with unilateral cryptorchidism has been reported to be minimally atrophic (Hoschoian, 1975; Lipshultz, 1976). These data are in contrast to the compensatory hypertrophy of the scrotal testis reported by Laron (1969). In our experience, marked contralateral hypertrophy does occur but is distinctly uncommon (5 per cent, unpublished data). Bilateral testicular atrophy is more in keeping with the apparent increase in infertility found in these patients. This finding is well reviewed by Lipshultz (1976), who compared the fertility rates from a series of studies of unilaterally cryptorchid patients with and without operation. The data demonstrate a significant reduction in fertility potential in both groups despite prophylactic orchiopexy.

Discrepancies in the fertility potential among the various studies probably represent differences in the type of cryptorchidism in the subjects. Unfortunately, there are no prospective studies that relate post-therapy semen quality to anatomic descriptions of the testes at surgery. Semen quality is very poor in most patients with bilateral cryptorchidism and is reduced in the great majority of patients with unilateral cryptorchidism despite therapy (Lipshultz, 1976; Lipshultz et al., 1976).

A review of Leydig cell function and hypothalamic pituitary gonadal interaction in men with unilateral cryptorchidism provides further insight into testicular dysfunction. Despite normal basal levels of testosterone and LH, in patients with corrected unilateral cryptorchidism the response of LH to GnRH is greater than normal, suggesting a small but compensated Leydig cell failure (Laron et al., 1975; Lipshultz, 1976). Far more striking was the increase in both basal FSH concentration and GnRH-induced FSH release. The data indicate a significant seminiferous tubular defect in feedback regulation of FSH, a point consistent with the characteristic reduced sperm output and decreased tubular germinal elements. Reduced Leydig cell function is more evident in boys with bilateral cryptorchidism, particularly in those with abdominal testes (Rivarola et al., 1970).

Varicocele

Varicocele has been recognized for some time as a relatively frequent cause of male infertility. Celsus in the first century A.D. described superficial and deep varicoceles and noted the presence of testicular atrophy on the affected side. The first reports of improvement in semen quality and pregnancy following varicocelectomy for male infertility appeared in 1929 (Macomber and Sanders) and 1937 (Wilhelm). Varicocele was not widely recognized as a correctable factor in male infertility until Tulloch's report in 1952. Subsequently, a variety of studies appeared in the literature suggesting that there was an important role for varicocelectomy among some infertile men (Table 12–9).

Despite these important clinical correlations, the etiologic relationship of varicocele to infertility remains unclear. A varicocele is an abnormal tortuosity and dilatation of the veins of the pampiniform plexus within the spermatic cord. Approximately ninety per cent of varicoceles appear on the left side. This is usually ascribed to the fact that the left testicular vein inserts into the left renal vein. Incompetence of the valvular structure in the internal spermatic vein also plays an important role (Saypol, 1981; Saypol et al., 1983).

Solitary right varicoceles are usually secondary to venous thrombosis or situs inversus with direct insertion of the right internal spermatic vein into the right renal vein (Ahlberg et al., 1966). We believe that bilateral varicocoles are uncommon.

In a study among Air Force recruits (ages 17 to 24), varicocele was identified in 151 of 1592 (9.5 per cent) men examined (Johnson et al., 1970). Of 94 subjects with varicocele, 25 per cent had reduced sperm counts and 56 per cent produced sperm with decreased motility. MacLeod (1969) similarly found that 758 of 8000 patients (9.4 per cent) had varicocele, and 50 per cent of these had impaired semen quality. These data, taken together with evidence that many men with varicocele have no difficulty in impregnating their spouses (Russell, 1953), suggest that the varicocele per se may not be a causative factor in infertility but rather a manifestation of a more fundamental testicular disorder. Certainly, many men with varicoceles are fertile.

A variety of mechanisms have been proposed to account for the abnormalities in spermatogenesis associated with varicocele. These include elevation of intrascrotal temperature due to venous dilatation (Zorgniotti and MacLeod, 1973), reflux of venous blood from the left adrenal gland to the testis, thus exposing the testis to increased concentrations of adrenal steroids and catecholamines (Comhaire and Vermuelen, 1974), and decreased testicular blood flow (Saypol, 1981). MacLeod (1969) has suggested that patients with varicocele may also have epididymal dysfunction, which produces altered sperm motility. None of these mechanisms has been convincingly proved.

We have shown that a surgically induced unilateral varicocele in rats or dogs results in bilateral increased testicular blood flow and temperature and interferes with spermatogenesis (Saypol et al., 1981). This work suggests that increase in blood flow is the initial event and is followed sequentially by elevated temperature, decreased spermatogenesis, seminiferous tubule atrophy, and finally decreased blood flow.

Although a varicocele is usually quite prominent, diagnosis often requires careful evaluation. The patient must be examined in an upright posture to avoid venous compression. To increase hydrostatic pressure and venous reflux, the patient should be asked to do a Valsalva maneuver. Occasionally, mild exercise or prolonged standing can be used to bring out a latent varicocele. When there is a high degree of suspicion for varicocele but the clinical findings are equivocal, a retrograde venogram may confirm the diagnosis. We do not aggressively pursue the diagnosis of "subclinical varicocele," since we do not feel that there is sufficient data to support repairing it. Other competent clinicians disagree.

The seminal patterns of infertile men with varicocele have been well described by MacLeod (1965, 1969). Sperm concentration was less than 20 million/ml in 65 per cent of subjects, motility was markedly diminished in 90 per cent, and the seminal cytology disclosed a prominent "stress pattern" in which tapering, amorphous, and immature cells were abundant. This seminal pattern corresponds closely to the altered testicular histologic appearance reported by Etriby et al. (1967) and by Dubin and Hotchkiss (1969); they reported that there is prominent germinal cell hypoplasia or maturation arrest and premature sloughing of spermatids into the tubular lumen. Occasionally, subjects may be azoospermic and may demonstrate severe maturation arrest or even germinal aplasia.

We believe that these alterations in semen quality and testicular histology are not specific effects of testicular injury and are not pathognomonic of varicocele. Rodriguez-Rigau et al. (1978) found that "stress pattern" was equally common among oligospermic men with and without varicocele.

We have used the Doppler stethoscope, thermography, nuclide scans, or venography to discover subclinical varicocele, but the results of these techniques are often difficult to interpret. Also, as mentioned, we are not convinced that a subclinical varicocele should be repaired.

In general, measurements of serum FSH, LH, or sex steroid concentrations are of no further diagnostic aid. Swerdloff and Walsh (1975) found that men with varicocele have normal Leydig cell function and normal FSH levels in spite of the altered seminiferous tubular function. An occasional subject may have an increased serum FSH concentration when germinal depletion is severe.

Surgical repair of a varicocele offers the most encouraging results of all the therapeutic approaches to the infertile male. (See Chapter 12.) A summary of the reported experience is shown in Table 12–9. On the average, varicocelectomy is followed by improvement in semen quality in approximately 70 per cent of cases, and the ensuing pregnancy rate varies from 30 to 55 per cent. At first glance, these results appear impressive; however, these high success rates are not invariable when a large number of urologists have been polled (Getzoff, 1973). Differences in results appear to be related both to patient selection and to the definition of success. Getzoff (1973) found that among 200 urologists, 25 per cent reported no success with varicocelectomy, and 39 per cent noted a success rate of less than 5 per cent. There is no well-controlled statistically documented study proving that varicocele repair improves fertility. One small, controlled investigation showed no increase in fertility after surgical repair of the varicocele (Nilsson et al., 1979). However, several series comparing infertile men who underwent surgical repair with individuals who elected medical treatment (Stewart, 1974; Cockett et al., 1979; Newton et al., 1980) claimed a higher fertility rate among the surgically treated men.

Because many fertile men are included in surgical series, some of the pregnancies that occur are unrelated to the treatment. Nevertheless, surgical repair probably helps a small but significant percentage of treated men.

Percutaneous occlusion of the internal spermatic vein is an alternative to surgery. The spermatic vein can be occluded with sclerosing solutions (Seyferth et al., 1981), steel coils (Gonzalez et al., 1982), or balloon catheter (Walsh and White, 1981; Riedl et al., 1981). Careful attention must be paid to the level of obstruction to avoid recurrent varicocele (Kaufman et al., 1983). This technique avoids general anesthesia and the trauma associated with open surgical repair, but it can be complicated by pulmonary embolization. If it proves to be safe and effective, it may replace surgical repair. We use the percutaneous technique only in patients with recurrent varicocele in whom we always perform a diagnostic venogram.

Regardless of the technique used, patient selection for varicocelectomy should include a rigorous gynecologic evaluation of the wife. One must exclude any subtle abnormality of tubal transport or ovulatory sequences that might cause infertility. The physician should also be cautious in offering surgery unless the patient's semen quality is suboptimal. Azoospermia is not an absolute contraindication to varicocelectomy, since some men with no sperm in the ejaculate respond to surgery (Mehan, 1976).

Ductal Obstruction

Occlusion of the excretory ducts of the testis is a reversible cause of male infertility. The incidence of ductal obstruction among infertile men has been reported as 7.4 per cent by

TABLE 12–9. CHANGES IN SEMEN QUALITY AND PREGNANCY RATE AMONG SEVERAL STUDIES EVALUATING THE ROLE OF VARICOCELECTOMY IN MALE INFERTILITY

	Number of Patients	Per Cent Improved Semen Quality	Pregnancy Rate
Davidson, 1954	12	92	41
Tulloch, 1955	30	66	30
Scott and Young, 1962	166	70	31
Hanley and Harrison, 1962	60	70	30
MacLeod, 1965	77	74	42
Brown, Dubin, and Hotchkiss, 1967	185	60	43
MacLeod, 1969	108	70	44
Brown, 1976	251	58	41
Dubin and Amelar, 1977	986	70	53
Lome and Ross, 1977	88	78	51
McFadden and Mehan, 1978	68	62	40
Cockett et al., 1979	56	Not reported	25

Dubin and Amelar (1971). The causes of ductal obstruction include congenital absence of the ductal system, ductal stricture following infection, vasectomy, and functional obstruction.

The ductal system may be congenitally absent (Amelar and Hotchkiss, 1963; Charny and Gillenwater, 1965). Usually there is an associated absence of the seminal vesicles, ampulla, vas deferens, and a major portion of the epididymis. Unilateral renal agenesis has also been noted in some affected men. The cause of this developmental anomaly is usually unknown. However, cystic fibrosis, a rare disorder of infancy, is almost always associated in males with congenital hypoplasia or absence of these excretory ducts (Kaplan et al., 1968; Taussig et al., 1972). Because of the absence of seminal vesicles, these patients have, in addition to azoospermia, a low ejaculate volume, semen that does not coagulate at the time of ejaculation, and absence of fructose in the seminal plasma. No satisfactory treatment is available for this condition.

By contrast, stricture of the excretory ducts acquired following infection of those structures may be remediable. Bilateral tuberculous epididymitis can result in epididymal occlusion and azoospermia. Prompt antibiotic therapy can maintain fertility in men with genital tuberculosis and may eliminate the need for later surgical intervention (Obrant and Lindquist, 1964). In addition, tubercle bacilli have been identified in semen and can be transmitted to the wife during coitus (Lattimer et al., 1954). Prior to the antibiotic era, gonorrheal urethritis frequently progressed to an obstructive epididymitis. Currently, gonorrhea is an unusual cause of male infertility. It is worth noting that smallpox is the most common cause of ductal obstruction in India, where the disease is still prevalent, and filariasis may lead to similar complications (Beach, 1948). Vasoepididymal anastomoses may successfully bypass the obstruction and restore normal fertility potential to men with this lesion.

Today vasectomy is the leading cause of infertility secondary to ductal obstruction. It is important to recognize that a variety of surgical procedures are available to bypass obstructions of the epididymis and vas deferens (see Chapter 84); however, pregnancies do not always follow patent reanastomoses.

The hallmark of men with obstruction of the excretory ducts is azoospermia in association with normal testicular size. The majority opinion is that testis size, Leydig cell function, and serum FSH and LH levels remain unchanged

following obstruction of the ducts (Baillie, 1962; Johnsonbaugh et al., 1975; Rosemberg et al., 1974; Smith et al., 1976). The effect of obstruction on the seminiferous epithelium is more controversial and variable. Studies by Horan (1975) suggest that the species of animal used in the experiment may be critical to the interpretation of these effects. Ligation of the ductuli efferentes directly adjacent to the testis (Harrison, 1953) invariably induces loss of germinal elements within the seminiferous tubules. Thus, men with complete, long-standing proximal obstruction may have testicular atrophy. These data do not refute the usual findings of normal testicular size and intact spermatogenesis that are present in most patients with more distal ductal obstruction. It is also interesting that incomplete occlusion of the vasa efferentia fails to produce germinal damage (Harrison, 1953).

Scorer and Farrington (1971) describe in detail congenital deformities of the epididymis and vas. They report absence of the entire vas, absence of the body and tail of the epididymis, obstruction of the distal epididymis with adjoining vas present, obstructions limited to the region between the testis and the epididymis, and cystic changes in the caput epididymidis. Lesions at the level of the caput epididymidis or rete testis might easily be missed.

Ejaculatory Problems

Certain ejaculatory disturbances can lead to "functional obstruction" of the vas. Any process that interferes with sympathetic innervation or anatomic integrity of the smooth muscle of the bladder neck can alter bladder neck contractility and result in retrograde ejaculation or more commonly failure of emission. Interruption of sympathetic innervation can also cause failure of emission. Any man who states that he has an erection and comes to a climax but sees scant semen should be suspected of having retrograde ejaculation or failure of emission. Retrograde ejaculation can be confirmed by demonstrating reduced semen volume and the presence of numerous sperm in a postejaculation urine specimen.

Retrograde ejaculation may follow transurethral or open surgical resection of the bladder neck or prostate, bilateral sympathectomy (Whitelaw and Smithwick, 1951), bilateral retroperitoneal lymphadenectomy, or extensive pelvic surgery, particularly proctectomy and colectomy. However, the syndrome may be much more subtle. It can appear spontaneously or may result from diabetic visceral neuropathy (Green and Kelalis, 1968); or it may follow the use of antihypertensive drugs that block sympathetic tone. In the diabetic it is important to note that the neuropathy may precede overt carbohydrate intolerance. Partial retrograde ejaculation has been reported in three nondiabetic men who had a low volume of semen (0.5 ml) devoid of sperm. However, the postejaculatory urine contained 100 to 300 million sperm (Keiserman et al., 1974).

When retrograde ejaculation occurs, sperm can be recovered from the bladder after ejaculation and used as an inseminate (Hotchkiss et al., 1955; Walters and Kaufman, 1959). Pregnancies result when care is taken to time the insemination precisely with ovulation, to use specimens that contain motile spermatozoa, and to wash and concentrate the sperm gently during processing from the urine. Some physicians prefer to alkalinize the urine by asking the patient to take bicarbonate of soda for a day prior to the ejaculation. The addition of 4 per cent human albumin to the retrieved sperm may increase their fertility potential (Scammell et al., 1982). Sympathomimetic drugs (Stewart and Bergant, 1974) and certain antihistamines (Andalor and Dube, 1975) and imipramine (Nijman et al., 1982) may be effective in patients with diabetic and postsurgical retrograde ejaculation or failure of emission. We have shown that 4 days of treatment with sympathomimetic drugs is more effective than 1 day (Proctor and Howards, 1983). If medical treatment results in a small ejaculate, artificial insemination may result in pregnancy. (Thiagarajah et al., 1978). Electrostimulation (Martin et al., 1983) is not yet a practical solution for failure of ejaculation in men.

Recently, Handelsman et al. (1984) reported 29 cases of men with a combination of obstructive azoospermia and chronic sinopulmonary infections, known as Young's syndrome. Men with this syndrome have apparently mild respiratory dysfunction, but show no evidence of cystic fibrosis known to cause obstructive azoospermia. Further, none of the men displayed features of Kartagener's syndrome (ultrastructural defect of the dynein arms), in which impaired ciliary motility leads to chronic respiratory infection and nonmotile sperm. The etiology of the disorder is unclear; however, the mechanism appears to involve thickened epididymal secretions. Handlesman et al. (1984) feel that the syndrome is relatively common, but we know of no prospective epidemiologic study that provides such data. Interestingly, five men were able to impregnate their wives early in the course of their marriage, suggesting that when sperm can be ejaculated, they are of normal function.

Drugs and Toxins

It has become increasingly evident that the germinal epithelium may be injured by a variety of physical and chemical agents. Not only will heat, radiation, and toxic chemicals such as pesticides (Glass et al., 1979; Lipshultz et al., 1980; Lantz et al., 1981) deplete the germ cells from the seminiferous tubules, but also many commonly used drugs such as alcohol, marihuana, and chemotherapeutic agents can induce germinal depletion that may persist and even affect androgen production from the Leydig cells. The germinal epithelium is a rapidly dividing tissue and, like the bone marrow and gastrointestinal tract, is affected by agents that interfere with cell division. It is likely that many drugs and toxic products also affect the Sertoli cells supporting germinal maturation. In view of the increasing number of toxic agents now associated with testicular germ cell depletion, one wonders about a potential role of unrecognized drug or toxin exposure in the genesis of idiopathic oligospermic infertility and azoospermia associated with maturation arrest of the germinal epithelium. While infertility usually results from an adult exposure to such agents, it is also evident that in utero exposure to such drugs as DES can result in reproductive tract anomalies and ductal obstruction.

CHEMOTHERAPY

The success of chemotherapy in treating such malignancies as lymphoma, leukemia, and testicular neoplasms has lead to increased long-term survival and new concerns for the long-term toxic effects of these therapies on normal host tissues. Although many of the acute effects of antineoplastic drugs have been well defined, comparatively little attention has been paid to gonadal dysfunction resulting from such treatment. Many, but not all, chemotherapeutic drugs have profound and long-lasting effects on gonadal function. Both germ cell production (Schilsky and Sherins, 1985) and testicular endocrine function (Booth and Loriaux, 1983) may be affected. Data from studies of animals (Auerbach, 1958; Steinberger et al., 1959; Steinberger and Nelson, 1957; Meistrich et al., 1982; Sieber and Adamson, 1975) and man (Schilsky and Sherins, 1985) indicate that toxicity varies with the drug class and combination of agents used in treatment, the total dose administered, and age and pubertal status of the patient at the time of therapy.

Testicular function in adult men is susceptible to injury by many chemotherapeutic agents. The primary lesion is one of progressive germ cell depletion. Drugs most commonly associated with germinal depletion are shown in Table 12–10. The alkylating agents are particularly noteworthy. For single-drug therapy, reversible germ cell depletion has been noted for chlorambucil (Richter et al., 1970) at doses below 400 mg, nitrogen mustard (Spitz, 1948), cyclophosphamide (Fairly et al., 1972) below 10 gm, and doxorubicin (Shamberger et al., 1981) at 500 mg/m².

Some multiagent chemotherapeutic regimens have been extensively studied such as MOPP (nitrogen mustard, vinristine, procarbazine and prednisone) used as therapy for patients with Hodgkin's disease. Such treatment renders approximately 90 per cent of men permanently sterile because of induced germinal aplasia (Van Thiel et al., 1971; Sherins and de Vita, 1973; Waxman et al., 1982; Whitehead et al., 1982; Chapman et al., 1981). By contrast, cyclophosphamide (10 gm) and doxorubicin induce permanent germinal depletion primarily in older men above 40 years (Shamberger et al., 1981b), whereas methotrexate plus vincristine has little effect on testicular function at any age (Shamberger et al., 1981a).

Evaluation of the effects of chemotherapy on gonadal function in children is particularly complex because of variables introduced by the continuum of changes occurring during puberty. Prior to the onset of puberty, the testicular germinal epithelium appears to be more resistant to moderate doses of toxic drugs than is the adult testis (Sherins et al., 1978; Pennisi et al., 1975; Blatt et al., 1981). By contrast, the adolescent testis shows increased sensitivity to chemotherapy. Prepubertal boys with Hodgkin's disease treated with MOPP show no testicular injury; however, adolescents develop not only germinal aplasia and azoospermia but also gynecomastia and Leydig cell failure at doses that in the adult appear to primarily deplete the germinal epithelium (Sherins et al., 1978). A note of caution should be voiced about the latter point, since a recent study in men with germinal aplasia and "selective" increase in FSH indicates that androgen production and free testosterone levels are reduced by 50 per cent, although total plasma testosterone concentration remains within the normal range (Booth and Loriaux, 1983).

Since the use of multiagent chemotherapy for malignant disorders continues to increase because of treatment successes, awareness of the long-term complications of these drugs is important. In addition to the depletion of germ cells, considerable interest has arisen about the potential mutagenic effects of such drugs in subjects who have return of spermatogenesis. Although irradiation and alkylating agents are known to be mutagenic and to produce self-aborting conceptuses in lower species (Auerbach, 1958), there is no conclusive evidence of their mutagenicity in man. In rodents, however, x-rays and alkylating agents have been shown to produce anatomic abnormalities of the sperm head at dosages that do not cause germinal depletion (Bruce et al., 1974; Wyrobek and Bruce, 1975). It is not known whether these altered sperm are capable of impregnation.

RADIATION THERAPY

The testis is known to be highly radiosensitive, most likely because of rapid cell division of the germinal epithelium. By comparison with a growing literature describing adverse effects of chemotherapy, there is a paucity of data documenting the effects of radiation on human testicular function (Sanderman, 1966). Until recently, there have been few useful guides to the threshold for radiation damage. Studies of single-dose x-ray exposure to normal male volunteers demonstrate a dose-dependent depletion and recovery of the germinal epithelium (Rowley et al., 1974; Paulsen, 1973; Clifton and Bremner, 1983). At 15 rad, a transient decrease in sperm output is evident, while at dosages above 50 rad aspermia appears. At 200 to 300

TABLE 12–10. Chemotherapeutic Drugs Associated with Testicular Germ Cell Depletion

Degree of Risk	Drug
Definite	Chlorambucil
	Cyclophosphamide
	Nitrogen mustard
	Busulfan
	Procarbazine
	Nitrosoureas
Probable	Doxorubicin
	Vinblastine
	Cytosine arabinoside
	cis-Platin
Unlikely	Methotrexate
	5-Fluorouracil
	6-Mercaptopurine
	Vincristine
	Bleomycin

rad, full recovery of sperm production requires approximately 3 years; at 400 to 600 rad the interval is about 5 years; and above 600 rad, sterility is generally permanent. A recent assessment of the effects of fractionated radiation on testicular function in men with Hodgkin's disease (Shapiro et al., 1984) indicates that dose-related injury is similar to that observed with single-dose exposure, but recovery appears to be prolonged (Shapiro et al., 1984; Speiser et al., 1973). At very high doses (2400 rad), as delivered directly to the testes of boys with gonadal relapse from acute lymphoblastic leukemia, profound Leydig cell failure with androgen deficiency can occur (Brauner et al., 1983).

Techniques to shield the testes from radiation have been employed when the expected testicular dose is high, but there have been few studies that accurately assess scatter radiation when the treatment beam is directed to sites other than the pelvis. Radiation scatter and leakage can be important contributors to germinal depletion, especially when the distance between the testes and the radiation field edge is less than 30 cm (Kinsella et al., 1982). A simple testicular shield has been developed that reduces testicular exposure to less than 1 per cent of the patient's prescription dose (Kinsella et al., 1982); thus, depending on the distance from the field edge to the gonads, a threefold to tenfold reduction in testicular dose can be accomplished.

ALCOHOL

Of perhaps even greater practical significance is the deleterious effect of alcohol on testicular function. Chronic alcoholism characterized by alcoholic hepatitis, fatty liver, and hepatic fibrosis and/or cirrhosis is associated with profound gonadal failure and suppression of pituitary gonadotropin release (Chopra et al., 1973; Van Thiel et al., 1974; Baker et al., 1976; Bertello et al., 1983). The hypogonadism of this syndrome is characterized by marked testicular atrophy due to depletion of the germinal cells and peritubular fibrosis. Impotence, decreased beard and pubic hair, gynecomastia, and small prostate size secondary to Leydig cell failure are also present. Plasma testosterone levels are generally lower than normal but often remain within the normal range. However, free testosterone, the active fraction at the tissue receptor sites, is reduced (Mendelson et al., 1977) because TeBG levels are markedly increased. Thus, total plasma testosterone is a misleading measurement in this syndrome. Plasma FSH and LH levels are variably elevated despite the profound

testicular failure because gonadotropin secretion is also blunted (Bertello et al., 1983). In many respects these patients resemble men with Klinefelter's syndrome.

Studies in normal men with good nutrition have demonstrated that after just 5 days of consuming large quantities of alcohol (220 ml/day), there is blunting of the episodic release of testosterone and a fall in mean testosterone levels (Gordon et al., 1976). Administration of alcohol for 4 weeks produces further reduction in plasma testosterone levels and a decrease in testosterone secretion. Studies of patients during the period of hangover after acute alcohol ingestion likewise demonstrate a reduction in plasma testosterone levels (Ylikahri et al., 1974). Studies of testicular tissue in vitro indicate that alcohol impairs testosterone synthesis (Badr et al., 1977; Gordon et al., 1980), and thus it would appear highly likely that alcohol directly alters testicular function.

MARIHUANA

In a similar fashion, there has been considerable interest in the possible adverse effects of marihuana on testicular function (Nahas, 1975; Maugh, 1975). There have been conflicting results as to whether marihuana lowers plasma testosterone levels (Kolodny et al., 1974; Mendelson et al., 1974). The differences in results may well be due to variations in the definition of "heavy use," the dosage of absorbed cannabis, and the duration of exposure. However, marihuana has been associated with development of gynecomastia (Harmon and Alapoulios, 1972). Hembree et al. (1976) presented preliminary data that demonstrate a marked fall in sperm output 4 weeks after initiation of heavy marihuana exposure. Certainly, more work in this area is required before the physician can come to a definitive conclusion. Nevertheless, cannabis is a potential hazard to testicular function.

DIETHYLSTILBESTROL

The findings of the association of sterility, cryptorchidism, cystic changes of the epididymis, and testicular atrophy in mice exposed prenatally to DES (McLachlin et al., 1975; McLachlan, 1981) are very important because they helped to focus medical attention on the potentially serious impact on reproductive function of drug exposure to the developing fetus. A synthetic estrogen, DES had been used extensively to prevent involuntary abortion in recurrently aborting women. The risk to the developing human fetus was highlighted when

Herbst et al. (1975) was able to associate DES exposure during early pregnancy with an increased incidence of vaginal adenocarcinoma, a very rare malignancy in young women of DES-treated mothers. Studies of DES-exposed male offspring (Gill et al., 1976) has disclosed an increased incidence of epididymal cysts, testicular atrophy, and cryptorchidism (Cosgrove et al., 1977; Whitehead and Leiter, 1981), but questionable effects, in our opinion, on semen quality in most of the subjects evaluated. Unlike the result in exposed female offspring, there has not been to date any evidence for an increased potential for genital tract malignancy. One wonders whether many of the congenital obstructive epididymal lesions and cryptorchidism in men may occur as a result of intrauterine drug exposure.

MISCELLANEOUS DRUGS

It is increasingly evident that a number of drugs, chemicals, and industrial products have adverse effects on male reproductive function; however, few data are available on the effects of most drugs. High doses of nitrofurantoin (Furadantin) (Nelson and Bunge, 1957; Steinberger and Nelson, 1957), sulfa drugs (Toth, 1979), cimetidine (Van Thiel et al., 1979) and amebicides (MacLeod, 1961), among others, have been shown to cause reversible germ cell depletion, but the effects of other drugs such as colchicine have not been confirmed when carefully studied by prospective analysis (Bremner and Paulsen, 1976). As mentioned earlier, occupational exposure to such toxic products as DBCP can induce germinal depletion and infertility (Glass et al., 1979; Lipshultz et al., 1980; Milby and Whorton, 1980). In view of the increasing evidence that a variety of chemicals have adverse effects on the germinal epithelium, the physician should be concerned about potential testicular injury in any patient who uses drugs chronically.

Systemic Illness

There is very little information about the effects of systemic illness on testicular function. In addition to the potential toxic side effects of drugs that might be employed to treat an underlying disease, fever, protein catabolism, and the direct influence of the disease process itself on reproductive function may be relevant. Fever has long been known to alter spermatogenesis. Abundant experimental data in rodents and some data in man clearly show that increasing the intratesticular temperature only a few degrees (to 42° C, or 107.6° F) for as little as 30 minutes results in damage to the primary spermatocytes that is evident within a few hours (Steinberger and Dixon, 1959). Similar studies in men by MacLeod and Hotchkiss (1941) show that oligospermia appears within 3 weeks after heat exposure and lasts approximately 50 days.

Changes in seminal cytology following viral and bacterial illnesses are well described by MacLeod (1964, 1966). MacLeod emphasizes that recovery of the semen may not take place for several weeks or even months following the insult. Not only may the sperm count fall to near azoospermic levels, but the seminal cytology may show a marked decrease in normal oval forms and reciprocal increases in small, tapered, and amorphous cells. Similar changes in the ejaculate can occur after allergic reactions and emotional disturbances (MacLeod, 1964). The seminal features are indistinguishable from those characteristic of varicocele; thus, the physician must review a series of ejaculates for each patient over a period of 4 to 6 months to avoid making an error in interpretation of results that are transient in nature (Sherins, 1974).

Gonadal dysfunction among uremic men is another excellent example of how systemic disease may alter reproductive function. Uremia is well known to be associated with decreased libido, impotence, and infertility (Elstein et al., 1969; Feldman and Singer, 1975; Guevara et al., 1969; Lin and Fang, 1975), and gynecomastia may be prominent (Swerdloff et al., 1970). The cause of the metabolic disturbance is unknown. Even when patients are undergoing chronic hemodialysis, there is a progressive decline in plasma testosterone and sperm output, which is associated with reciprocal increases in serum LH and FSH levels, respectively (Lin and Fang, 1975; Holdsworth et al., 1977; Chopp and Mendez, 1978). Testicular biopsy reveals maturation arrest of the germinal elements and occasionally germinal aplasia. The mechanism whereby renal failure produces testicular dysfunction is not entirely clear; however, since LH and FSH levels are both elevated and there is a subnormal testosterone response to administer hCG, chronic renal failure appears to significantly interfere with testosterone production (Holdsworth et al., 1977). This may in turn account for the reduced spermatogenesis. Following renal transplantation, improvement of Leydig cell function and sperm output occurs within 3 months of surgery despite immunosuppressive therapy to prevent rejection.

Abnormal Morphology and Sperm Function

The need to search for specific causes of poor semen quality is clearly illustrated by the findings of structural abnormalities of sperm in some men with nonmotile spermatozoa. A variety of ultrastructural anomalies have been described with the use of the electron microscope; these are not always evident with standard light microscopy. Pedersen et al. (1971) reported an infertile man with a high output of nonmotile sperm. The sperm in this condition are pear-shaped and tapered and show ultrastructural abnormalities of the subacrosomal space and mitochondrial changes in the midpiece region. The presence of round-headed sperm of the Schirren-Holstein type (Anton-Lamprecht et al., 1976) is yet another rare disorder, in which there is complete absence of the acrosomal cap and also frequent tail abnormalities of the axoneme complex. These sperm display moderately normal motility, however, and appear in adequate numbers in the ejaculate. Presumably, the infertility relates to the underlying structural abnormality.

Perhaps most interesting is the description of nonmotile sperm in men with Kartagener's syndrome (situs inversus, chronic sinusitis, and bronchiectasis). This bronchitic disorder is associated with immotile cilia in areas where there is normally mucociliary transport. Electron microscopy of sperm reveals that the dynein arms are missing from the nine microtubular filament couplets in the axoneme complex of the sperm tail (Ebasson et al., 1977; Afzelius, 1976; Pedersen and Rebbe, 1975; Pedersen et al., 1971). This ultrastructural abnormality leads to the nonmotility of the sperm which appears to be related to the immotility of cilia of the bronchial tree.

A study of subjects with nonmotile spermatozoa, encompassing men with and without Kartagener's syndrome, demonstrated that the sperm nonmotility is associated with a deficiency in the sperm tail of protein carboxylmethylase (Gagnon et al., 1982), an enzyme required for ciliary movement, and does not represent necrospermia (dead sperm). This finding of a biochemical abnormality of sperm function is conceptually important, since, as discussed in other parts of this chapter, idiopathic male infertility appears to be related more to altered sperm function than to sperm numbers per se. Although there have been no data identifying other biochemical abnormalities in sperm of men with idiopathic infertility, studies in the experimental animal offer provocative "food for thought" for the practicing physician. Protein carboxylmethylase activity is located in the sperm tail (Bouchard et al., 1980) and the methyl acceptor protein for the enzyme increases remarkably as sperm maturation progresses between the testis and cauda epididymis (Casteneda et al., 1983). A seminal plasma factor has also been found that is capable of inhibiting spermatozoal motility (de Lamirande et al., 1983) whose origin appears to be from the seminal vesicle (de Lamirande and Gagnon, 1984).

Although it is not practical to perform ultrastructural or biochemical analyses on sperm of all men with marginal or poor semen quality, these examples serve to illustrate how important it is to be precise in the diagnosis of seminal abnormalities. It is no wonder that treatment of men with poor semen quality by administering a variety of nonspecific pharmacologic agents is rarely successful.

Genital Tract Infections

Infectious diseases are known to produce infertility in man. However, most infectious processes of the male reproductive tract are uncommon. The subject is well reviewed in an article by Fowler and Kessler (1983). Some, such as gonorrhea, smallpox, and tuberculosis (Chakravarty et al., 1968), produce inflammatory changes of the ductal system and result in obstruction at the level of the epididymis or vas deferens. Others, such as mumps, result in an acute orchitis characterized by intense interstitial edema and mononuclear infiltration. (McKendrick and Nishtar, 1976). Mumps orchitis appears to have a prevalence of 30 per cent of males with mumps parotitis 10 years of age or older (Beard et al., 1977). The orchitis is bilateral in approximately 30 per cent of individuals with testicular involvement (Werner, 1950). Most prepubertal males do not develop orchitis. When the edema is marked, permanent destruction and atrophy of the seminiferous tubular epithelium may occur (Ballew and Masters, 1954; Werner, 1950). The testicular failure may be profound and in some instances lead to clinical signs of hypogonadism and gynecomastia. By contrast, syphilis may involve both testis and epididymis; however, syphilitic orchitis usually predominates, again producing diffuse interstitial inflammation with gumma formation and endarteritis.

Controversy surrounds the role of genital mycoplasma infection in infertility. Cytomegalovirus, *Chlamydia,* herpes, and *Mycoplasma* infections have been recognized in both male and female reproductive tracts (Centifano et al., 1972; Holmes et al., 1975; Lang and Kummer, 1972; Taylor-Robinson and McCormack, 1980). These organisms may reside chronically in the cervix or male ductal structures and may be transmitted venereally. Friberg and Gnarpe (1974) and Toth et al. (1983) have both suggested that the T-mycoplasma infection rate is higher among couples with idiopathic infertility (76 per cent) and that appropriate antibiotic therapy results in an improved pregnancy rate. However, De Louvois et al. (1974) examined the seminal fluid of fertile and infertile men and found no difference in the T-mycoplasma infection rate, and Harrison et al. (1975) and Ulstein et al. (1976) reported that doxycycline treatment did not improve semen quality or the conception rate among infertile couples in whom T-mycoplasma were recovered from the seminal fluid. In addition, Ulstein et al. (1976) report that T-mycoplasma and cytomegalovirus are more common in the seminal fluid and postprostatic massage urine of fertile men than of infertile patients. In a study of 205 infertile women, *Mycoplasma hominis* (but not *U. urealyticum*) was more common in women with a history of pelvic inflammatory disease, but no relationship could be determined between this finding and cervical or uterine inflammation, semen quality, pyosemia, or results of a postcoital test (Gump et al., 1984). Clearly, further studies in the area are indicated.

Although uncommon, chronic bacterial infection of semen may also be an unsuspected cause of male infertility (Fowler and Kessler, 1983). Using an improved staining technique for differentiating immature germ cells from white blood cells in seminal fluid, Couture et al. (1976) and Ulstein et al. (1976) demonstrated that coliform infection of semen or prostate may be associated with increased seminal leukocytes and sloughing of early spermatids into the ejaculate. Antibacterial treatment resulted in prompt improvement in sperm quality when infections were eradicated. These investigators stress the importance of proper collection of postprostatic massage urine and semen (Stamey, 1965) so that the site of the genital infection can be ascertained. A two-glass urine specimen excludes urethral contamination. A prostatic massage while the bladder is still partially filled, followed by urination, provides a sample with expressed prostatic secretion.

Sexual Dysfunction

Abnormalities of sexual performance are important etiologic factors in the genesis of infertility because they are potentially reversible. The spectrum of disorders confronting the physician may include decreased libido, impotence, poor coital timing, premature ejaculation, and failure of intromission. The subject is well reviewed by Levine (1976) and Geboes et al. (1975). It is important to emphasize that sexual inadequacy is usually occult when the patient first presents with the problem of infertility. We find that considerable time and effort are required on the part of the physician to uncover and corroborate that sexual inadequacy is the cause of a couple's infertility. In one large series, sexual dysfunction as a cause of infertility is reported to be 5 per cent (Dubin and Amelar, 1971).

Decreased libido and potency can be secondary to profound testicular dysfunction and may be the source of a couple's infertility. However, some men have normal testicular function but profound impotence, which results in failure to initiate an erection or to maintain the erection until ejaculation has occurred. Depression and anxiety about sexual inadequacies and fear of pregnancy are common psychologic factors. Additionally, the discovery of oligospermia or azoospermia itself may provoke feelings of sexual inadequacy in the male; it is also not uncommon for an intense infertility evaluation to create disturbances in sexual performance in both husband and wife. Although impotence results most commonly from emotional disturbances, it behooves the physician to determine whether there is an organic cause.

In some couples coitus may not occur in conjunction with ovulation. Surprisingly, some patients simply fail to comprehend that ovulation usually occurs only at midcycle. Other couples may have intercourse infrequently, thus increasing the chance that coitus may not be timed with ovulation. We have even seen couples who abstained at midcycle owing to mittelschmerz. In addition, religious and ethical considerations may be important in coital timing, as in some Orthodox Jewish couples, who abstain until 1 week following the last menstrual flow (Nida) (Gordon et al., 1975).

Failure of intravaginal ejaculation can also cause infertility. Men with premature ejaculation or severe degrees of hypospadias, chordee, or phimosis may not ejaculate into the vagina, although vaginal penetration may seem to be adequate. Functional obstruction of the ductal system, vascular insufficiency of the phallus, and alteration of sympathetic innervation can lead to impotence or retrograde ejaculation. Occasionally, a man may be able to maintain an erection but be unable to ejaculate, so-called ejaculatory incompetence (Dubin and Amelar, 1972). Less commonly, retention of an intact hymen may preclude intromission or direct the penis into the urethra or anus. Much more subtle but pertinent is the fact that there may be aberrant sexual practices (oral or anal sex, sadomasochistic fetishes) that go unrecognized.

All in all, this cluster of abnormalities emphasizes the need for the physician to obtain an accurate and detailed history of sexual performance. We have found the wife to be an excellent source for verification of sexual technique.

Immunologic Disorders

Immunologic factors may cause male infertility in selected men (Mumford and Warner, 1983). The antigenicity of sperm in an experimental setting has been known for 85 years (Metchnikoff, 1899). Studies of autoimmune infertility have been based either on experiments in which animals have been vaccinated with testicular tissue or on observations of the presence of antibodies to spermatozoa in the sera of some infertile men and women.

Allergic orchitis has been induced experimentally in a variety of species, including the guinea pig, rat, rhesus monkey, and man (Mancini et al., 1965). Histologically, the lesion consists of progressive cytolysis of germ cells, leaving behind essentially unaffected Sertoli cells and Leydig cells. The histologic lesion appears in 1 to 8 weeks and is reversible after 24 weeks. By immunofluorescence, the antibody has been localized to the acrosome of spermatozoa and spermatids, but probably all germ cells are affected. It is assumed that circulating antibodies are less important because their titers are low and inconsistent and because no strict correlation exists between their presence and the severity of the gonadal lesion. Thus, cell-mediated toxicity, which is involved in delayed hypersensitivity, may be imported (Brannen et al., 1974). Although experimental allergic aspermatogenesis serves as a useful theoretical model for male infertility, there are no data demonstrating that such a phenomenon occurs spontaneously.

Sperm antibodies in humans have been reported in approximately 3 to 7 per cent of infertile men and in 20 per cent of men with ductal obstruction (Fjallbrant, 1968; Phadke and Padukone, 1964; Rumke, 1968; Rumke and Hellinga, 1959; Haas et al., 1981).

Human semen contains at least 16 antigens. Spermatozoa have a minimum of seven, four of which are identical to those of the seminal plasma. It appears likely that sperm acquire some of these antigens during their transit through the ductal system (Hekman and Rumke, 1969), since "coating" antibodies are present in seminal plasma in which no sperm are present. Importantly, only two cases have been reported in which there is documentation of acute allergic reactions to human seminal proteins (Halpern et al., 1967; Levine et al., 1973). It is not clear why such a syndrome is not more common if the proposed theories of seminal immunization are valid. As mentioned in the Evaluation section of this chapter, men with adequate sperm counts who have poor sperm motility or sperm agglutination should be screened for serum antisperm antibodies. If these are present in high titer, the semen should also be checked for antisperm antibodies.

There is little evidence that patients with severe oligospermia or those without antisperm antibodies in the semen will respond to any treatment. There are reports, however, that men with adequate sperm counts and antibodies in the semen become fertile after treatment. High doses of systemic corticosteroids have been used by several authors with apparent partial success in selected men (Table 12–11). This treatment is experimental and may be complicated by corticosteroid side effects. Another approach to therapy is to wash the sperm and/or enrich it using artificial media (Shulman et al., 1978; Witkin, 1982; Mumford and Warner, 1983). The success rate of this treatment has not been high.

In summary, although sperm antibodies are more common among infertile men than among fertile men, there is no conclusive evidence that these antibodies cause infertility. However, there is suggestive evidence that some men with good sperm counts and antisperm antibodies in the semen respond to therapy.

MEDICAL MANAGEMENT OF TESTICULAR DYSFUNCTION

In previous sections we have presented the various disorders of the testis according to their known pathophysiology. Despite their diverse causes, treatment of many of these disorders has much in common. When Leydig cell func-

TABLE 12–11. Effect of Corticosteroid Therapy in Inducing Pregnancy

Author(s)	Drug and Dose	Pregnancies
Hendry et al., 1981	Methylprednisolone, 32 mg p.o. t.i.d.; day 21 to 28 of wife's cycle	14/45 (31%)
Mathur et al., 1981	Prednisone, 15 mg p.o. q.d., for 3 to 26 weeks	9/25 (36%)
Shulman and Shulman, 1982	Methylprednisolone, 96 mg/day; day 21 to 28 of wife's cycle	31/71 (44%)*
Hargreave and Elton, 1982	Methylprednisolone as above	5/13 (38%)*
	Betamethasone, 0.5 mg q.i.d. × 30, then tapered	6/7 (85%)*

*Because significant numbers of patients were lost to follow-up, the success rate may be spuriously high.

tion is deficient, whether due to lack of gonadotropins or primary testicular failure, androgenization is indicated. The presence of hypogonadotropism provides the opportunity to induce spermatogenesis and virilization (Table 12–12). We have chosen to organize the fundamentals of such treatment around the drug agents available.

A far more complex discussion develops in relation to the appropriate management of men with idiopathic infertility. For the physician to judge the efficacy of his or her therapy, there must be precision in diagnosis, exclusion of known irreversible testicular defects, and awareness of the potential for a subtle gynecologic abnormality in the spouse and recognition of the marked fluctuating quality of semen normally inherent in the ejaculate. Here, we have chosen to review the available data, present the current controversies, and emphasize the pitfalls that the physician must avoid in managing such patients.

Androgen Deficiency

The indications for androgen replacement therapy include those disorders in which there is either hypogonadotropic hypogonadism or primary Leydig cell failure. It should be emphasized that all patients treated with exogenous androgen will be infertile during treatment because spermatogenesis requires high levels of intratesticular testosterone plus FSH. Exogenous androgen is used only for virilization.

The distinction between hypogonadotropic hypogonadism and normal physiologic delay of puberty is often difficult in the absence of midline neurologic, genital, or somatic defects or a positive family history, as in Kallmann's syndrome. Confirmation of a diagnosis of true delayed puberty requires demonstration of normal pubertal progression at a later time in life or an appropriately large increase in prolactin levels following a chlorpromazine challenge. Because of the importance of normal psychosexual

TABLE 12–12. Summary of Clinical, Laboratory, and Management Features of Major Diagnostic Categories in Male Infertility

Testicular Size	Laboratory Values			Diagnosis	Treatment
	FSH	LH	Testosterone		
Not palpable	↑	↑	↓	Anorchia	Surgical exploration
	↑	↑	N or ↓	Bilateral cryptorchidism	Surgical exploration and orchiopexy if possible
1–4 ml	↓	↓	↓	Hypogonadotropic hypogonadism	hCG and FSH to induce spermatogenesis; testosterone to virilize only
1–3 ml	↑	↑	N or ↓	Klinefelter's syndrome	Testosterone to virilize only
8–15 ml	↑	N	N	Germinal aplasia	None
12–15 ml	N or ↑	N	N	Severe maturation arrest	None
12–20 ml	N	N	N	Mild hypospermatogenesis	Evaluate wife; varicocelectomy
20–30 ml	N	N	N	Obstructive azoospermia	Ductal anastomosis

Abbreviations: FSH, Follicle-stimulating hormone; hCG, human chorionic gonadotropin; LH, luteinizing hormone.

maturation, the physician usually needs to consider androgen therapy for most sexually immature boys by the age of 15 years. Since androgen therapy will suppress endogenous secretion of FSH and LH, testicular growth will not occur despite the onset of virilization. Because onset of spontaneous puberty may not occur until the late teens or early 20's, we suggest that the physician discontinue therapy periodically until the patient is in his mid-20's to determine whether he can maintain his own testosterone secretion and virilization.

In hypogonadotropic men, gonadotropins can always be substituted for the exogenous androgen when fertility is desired. Formerly, there had been concern that androgens would alter the subsequent response of the testis to gonadotropin administration. Fortunately, this is not the case. Hypogonadotropic men have responded to gonadotropins and fathered children following use of testosterone for as long as 9 to 12 years (Martin, 1967).

In patients with growth hormone deficiency and short stature, therapeutic decisions are more complex. Initially, it is not clear whether there is an associated lack of gonadotropin, because patients with isolated growth hormone deficiency are also sexually immature. They will achieve pubescence spontaneously after administration of growth hormone. In order to obtain maximum height, androgen administration is usually postponed until bone age reaches 12 years or until no further growth in height is achieved using growth hormone in order to avoid premature epiphyseal closure. Androgens are then administered to provide the additional growth spurt with virilization.

In men who become hypogonadotropic after they are sexually mature, androgens or gonadotropins can be effectively used to maintain normal levels of testosterone. When there is no concern about future fertility, administration of testosterone is preferred because of its lower cost and less frequent injection schedule. However, when procreation is desired, hCG should be used to stimulate Leydig cell function in preference to direct administration of testosterone. MacLeod (1970) has demonstrated that hCG, in addition to stimulating testosterone secretion, can maintain spermatogenesis in such patients. There has also been some concern that long-term exogenous androgen administration may promote testicular fibrosis in men in whom testicular maturation has already occurred. However, the data at present are not adequate to prove this point.

In men with infertility, Leydig cell function is usually preserved although in the presence of complete germ cell depletion testosterone production is decreased by 50 per cent (Booth and Loriaux, 1983). However, only 5 per cent of infertile men have profound Leydig cell failure with clinical signs of hypogonadism. Klinefelter's syndrome and related disorders involving seminiferous tubular sclerosis are the most common diseases requiring androgen replacement. However, some men with bilateral cryptorchidism, especially of the abdominal variety, may also need treatment. It is important to recognize that these patients generally have adequate Leydig cell function to enter puberty at the correct time, but their progress through puberty is very slow. They usually do not achieve complete masculinization.

Androgen is available in both oral and parenteral forms. Fluoxymesterone and 17α-methyl testosterone are the most commonly used short-acting oral preparations. Their primary usefulness is in those patients who are needle-shy. Oral androgens are less potent than parenteral forms and fail to produce complete sexual maturation in eunuchoidal men.

Long-acting testosterone esters (enanthate or cypionate) are the preparations of choice for parenteral administration. The usual dose is 200 mg intramuscularly every 2 weeks. We have found that treatment intervals of 3 to 4 weeks are inadequate to stimulate or maintain full virilization (Schulte-Beerbuhl and Nieschlag, 1980). When the physician is concerned about the need to stop androgen replacement quickly, he may wish to use testosterone propionate, a short-acting parenteral androgen. This agent is particularly useful in treating older men when there is concern of rapid prostatic enlargement or in treating men in whom androgen replacement may cause emotional disturbances.

Side effects of androgen therapy include prostatic hypertrophy, acne, priapism, gynecomastia, and erythrocytosis (Sherins and Winters, 1978). These reactions are generally dose-related and reversible. Hepatic dysfunction has been reported, particularly with 17 α-methyl testosterone; it includes bromsulphalein retention and increases in plasma transaminases, lactate dehydrogenase (LDH), and bilirubin concentrations. These changes are due to intrahepatic cholestasis and are usually reversible. Androgens in high dosages may induce hepatoma formation or development of peliosis hepatis, a cystic dilatation of the liver venules. In general, androgens are safe and are well tolerated, but adverse effects do occur and should be watched for, particularly in the subject who will receive treatment for an entire lifetime.

Gonadotropin Deficiency

Exogenous gonadotropin administration is very effective in the stimulation of spermatogenesis in men with hypogonadotropic hypogonadism. Two drug agents are available in the United States for this purpose, hCG, which is analogous to LH and stimulates the Leydig cell to secrete testosterone, which is required to initiate germinal maturation within the seminiferous tubule and human menopausal gonadotropin (Pergonal), which is used for its FSH content to complete spermatogenesis and allow sperm to appear in the ejaculate.

To initiate spermatogenesis, a high intratesticular level of androgen is required. Accordingly, exogenous administration of androgen alone or androgen with FSH is not adequate (MacLeod, 1970; Mancini, 1970) because under these conditions the intratesticular testosterone concentration is low; therefore, hCG must be used to stimulate endogenous testosterone secretion. In the sexually immature male with hypogonadotropic hypogonadism, hCG can be used as an alternative to testosterone in the initial phase of promoting virilization, or it may be substituted for testosterone later after masculinization has developed (Table 12–12).

The usual dose of hCG is 2000 IU intramuscularly three times per week. This regimen will provide normal adult levels of plasma testosterone that are indistinguishable from those achieved using parenteral androgen replacement at 200 mg every 2 weeks. Virilization is not usually completed until after approximately 4 years of either treatment. Since high cost makes chronic therapy with hCG less practical, it is generally used in conjunction with FSH when spermatogenesis is desired. The combination of hCG, 2000 IU, and FSH (Pergonal), 75 to 150 IU three times per week, will stimulate spermatogenesis in most hypogonadotropic men (MacLeod, 1970; Paulsen, 1965). Although the sperm concentration usually does not exceed 10 million/ml, impregnation of the spouse usually occurs (Paulsen et al., 1970) because these sperm are normal.

More recently, Sherins (1982) has demonstrated that when as little as 25 to 38 IU of FSH (Pergonal) is administered three times per week to hypogonadotropic men who have been virilized with hCG, spermatogenesis is completed and sperm appear in the ejaculate. These data define the minimal requirements of FSH for spermatogenesis and suggest that gonadotropin replacement can be more cost effective.

It should be noted that in patients with the fertile eunuch syndrome who are partially hypogonadotropic and show some evidence of germ cell maturation, therapy with hCG alone may produce full spermatogenesis and sufficient levels of ejaculated sperm to allow impregnation (Paulsen et al., 1970; Sherins, 1982). Moreover, in the posthypophysectomy patient or in the hypogonadotropic male who has developed good sperm output following hCG and Pergonal therapy, hCG alone may be adequate to maintain spermatogenesis (MacLeod, 1970; Mancini, 1970; Johnsen, 1978; Sherins, 1982).

In subjects with isolated hypogonadotropic hypogonadism, in which the defect is a congenital absence of hypothalamic GnRH, it is now possible to administer GnRH to stimulate endogenous gonadotropin release. Intermittent pulsatile delivery of GnRH, approximately every 2 hours, is required to stimulate gonadotropin release (Belchetz et al., 1978). Chronic low-dose pulsatile administration of GnRH using a portable infusion pump can induce puberty, complete sexual maturation and provide effective endogenous gonadotropin release to stimulate spermatogenesis (Skarin et al., 1982; Hoffman and Crowley, 1982). However, by comparison to administration of exogenous gonadotropins given intramuscularly three times per week, continuous pulsatile administration is recommended only for patients who have adequate physician and institutional support.

Idiopathic Infertility

Idiopathic infertility is an eponym for ignorance. It is no wonder that results of treatment for such individuals are so highly variable and controversial. Confusion about the efficacy of therapy is related to a variety of errors in both diagnosis and management, many of which can be avoided by an astute physician. The following list summarizes problems common to many infertility evaluations (Table 12–13).

1. Failure to consider or document adequately the reproductive potential of the spouse.
2. Improper patient selection.
   (a) Failure to exclude recognizable causes of testicular dysfunction before treatment.
   (b) Failure to recognize that substantive changes in sperm count and semen quality can occur spontaneously.

TABLE 12–13. ETIOLOGIC FACTORS THAT SHOULD BE EXCLUDED DURING EVALUATION OF THE APPARENTLY INFERTILE MALE

1. Subtle gynecologic abnormality in the coital partner
2. Improper semen analysis
   a. Abstinence interval—uncontrolled
   b. Duration of observations—too short
   c. Number of samples—too few
3. Recent fever or illness
4. Drugs/x-ray/alcohol administration
5. History of cryptorchidism
6. Abnormal karyotype
7. Venereal disease
8. Abnormal coital habits
9. Failure of erection, emission, or ejaculation

(c) Poor understanding of the minimally adequate ejaculate.

(d) Improper techniques for the collection of semen.

(e) Inadequate semen data prior to treatment.

3. Errors in management.

(a) Use of empirical therapy early in the evaluation because of patient pressure for treament.

(b) Failure to define therapeutic goals precisely.

(c) Inadequate understanding of the drug agents employed.

(d) Lack of knowledge concerning specific abnormality of sperm function.

In evaluating any man for suspected infertility consideration of the reproductive potential of the spouse is extremely important because impregnation always involves husband and wife. It is not uncommon for each partner to contribute problems that reduce the couple's fecundity. No amount of treatment of the male will improve his fertility potential unless his coital partner ovulates, the sperm can reach the ovum, and the conceptus can be imbedded and maintained in the uterus.

Failure to adequately document abnormalities of female reproductive potential is so common that it deserves special mention. In perhaps 5 per cent of cases, abnormalities in coital habits preclude pregnancy. Since this feature is difficult to extract during an initial history, a high index of suspicion should be maintained by the physician during subsequent interviews. It is often helpful to discuss this potential problem with the wife in order to corroborate the history. We have found in our interviews that there is considerable lack of understanding as to when ovulation occurs, that coitus may be surprisingly

infrequent, that couples purposely avoid coitus in the preovulatory period when chances for pregnancy are highest hoping "to save up sperm," use sperm-absorbing vaginal lubricants, douche immediately after coitus, and fail to achieve intravaginal ejaculation.

Diseases of the cervix, abnormalities of the ovulatory process, and obstruction of the oviducts must be excluded for each couple. Regardless of specialty, the nongynecologist should be prepared to obtain from the wife an appropriate reproductive history. If a woman has had a child within the past 3 to 5 years, has had no intervening pelvic infections, and continues to menstruate regularly, she is probably normal. However, subtle abnormalities of ovulation and pelvic inflammatory disease can develop. Amenorrhea reflects anovulation, and regular menses generally indicate normal ovulatory sequences. Nevertheless, some women who claim to have regular menses can have anovulation, intermittent ovulation, or cycles with inadequate corpus luteum function (Dodson et al., 1975; Jones, 1976; Rakoff, 1976; Sherman and Korenman, 1974a,b; Strott et al., 1970).

In a study of 100 "infertile" men in which the wives were re-examined with regard to their gynecologic normalcy, the incidence of abnormalities in the wives was strikingly high, despite the fact that they had been previously screened for tubal and ovarian disease (Sherins, 1974). The incidence of subtle gynecologic abnormalities was highest (50 per cent) among the wives of men whose total sperm output was greater than 60 million, and 30 per cent of these women became pregnant following appropriate treatment of their disorder. Of the men with a total sperm output of below 60 million, 15 per cent had wives with coexistent gynecologic disorders, and 6 per cent of the men were able to impregnate their spouses when therapy was directed to the wife. Analysis of the ejaculate data showed that pregnancies could occur even when the total sperm output was as low as 27 million. Thus, the data emphasize the importance of recognizing subtle gynecologic abnormalities and defining the minimally adequate ejaculate.

Proper patient selection is critical for the interpretation of any treatment regimen directed toward the male. Two types of problems exist. First, there is the unwitting inclusion of normal men and patients with spontaneously reversible dysfunction, and second, the variable inclusion of men with irreversible testicular disease that could be recognized and excluded if a more adequate work-up were provided (Table 12–13). In men with marginal ejaculates whose wives ovulate only intermittently, treatment of the husband by any modality, when followed by a pregnancy, is usually assumed to be a treatment success. In fact, a direct cause-and-effect relationship between treatment of the male and the ensuing pregnancy has not been established. The physician is merely unaware of the existing subtle gynecologic disorder. Such errors in interpretation of therapy could be avoided if there were a more careful evaluation of the wife and if all treatment regimens were properly designed.

Additionally, when the male has been inadequately evaluated before treatment, subsequent changes in his ejaculate may bear no relationship to the treatment provided. Not only can fever, illness, and drugs alter sperm output during one or two sperm cycles (74 days each) following cessation of the event, but also differences in ejaculatory frequency and reduction in emotional stress markedly alter sperm output and semen quality. Thus, pretreatment studies should be standardized to reduce errors in interpretation. We suggest as an absolute minimum the following steps:

1. Obtaining 3 to 6 appropriately collected ejaculates during a period of 4 to 6 months before instituting any pharmacologic agent.

2. Continuing treatment for at least 3 months.

3. Collecting a similar number of ejaculates during and after therapy to establish whether there is a sustained change.

However, the inherent marked variability of sperm output and semen quality demand that a clinical trial of empirical therapy contain placebo controls and be designed as a randomly assigned, double-blinded, cross-over study to avoid bias and to provide convincing evidence of drug efficacy to the practicing physician (Chalmers et al., 1983; Lavori et al., 1983; Collins et al., 1983; Louis et al., 1983).

The differences in opinion about what constitutes the minimally adequate ejaculate are of considerable importance. Unlike the situation in animal husbandry, no practical mechanism of testing the biologic fertility potential of semen among multiple female recipients is available. Therefore, it is always an assumption on the part of the physician that an ejaculate is adequate or inadequate for impregnation. In older reports, sperm concentrations of greater than 60 million/ml were considered to be normal, but subsequently the lower limit was set at 20 million/ml (MacLeod and Gold, 1951). Recent studies have further emphasized that the sperm count is not the sine qua non for male fertility (Sherins et al., 1977; Smith and Steinberger, 1977; Steinberger, 1976), since impregnation by men with sperm concentrations of only 10 to 20 million/ml can occur. The demonstration that hypogonadotropic men who have been treated with gonadotropin can impregnate their spouses with sperm concentration of only 2 to 5 million/ml further supports this hypothesis (MacLeod, 1970; Paulsen, 1965).

These findings emphasize the need to design treatment regimens more carefully. From the preceding discussion, one could ask a series of rhetorical questions that as yet have no conclusive answers. If pregnancy does not ensue following treatment of the male, should therapy be considered inadequate? In a man with a sperm concentration of greater than 20 million/ml, is any increase in sperm output physiologically important? How important is a small shift in semen quality? Should an improvement in seminal cytology without change in sperm output be considered a response? And finally, how do we predict which men with idiopathic infertility are more likely to respond to therapy?

ANDROGEN

The use of androgen in the treatment of idiopathic infertility stems in part from the knowledge that testosterone is an important requirement in normal spermatogenesis and maturation of sperm during epididymal transport. Following hypophysectomy in the rat, spermatogenesis can be reinitiated by administering very high doses of testosterone (Boccabella, 1963). This effect appears to be mediated by providing high intratesticular levels of androgen (Dvoskin, 1943). This hypothesis is supported by data in hypogonadotropic men, in whom physiologic replacement of androgen fails to induce spermatogenesis, and by data in normal men, in whom testosterone inhibits gonadotropin release and secondarily produces atrophy of the germinal epithelium (Heller et al., 1950). At physiologic levels of replacement, high intratesticular concentrations of testosterone cannot be achieved (Heller et al., 1970; Morse et al., 1973; Steinberger et al., 1973); therefore, spermatogenesis cannot occur.

Testosterone Rebound. In 1950, Heller et al. reported the first systematic study on the effects of testosterone administration on the suppression of sperm output and its subsequent recovery following cessation of treatment. Androgen administered for 10 weeks induced azoospermia, and sperm concentrations increased to pretreatment levels 6 to 18 months following cessation of therapy. In some oligospermic men, sperm counts and testicular biopsy improved following treatment. Heckel et al. (1951) reported a similar improvement in oligospermic men following testosterone administration. Subsequently, however, this modality has been reported to be variably successful (Charny, 1959; Getzoff, 1955; Joel, 1960; Lamensdorf et al., 1975; Paulsen et al., 1977; Rowley and Heller, 1972; Charny and Gordon, 1978). The most recent larger studies are summarized in Table 12–14.

In this mode of treatment, testosterone propionate, 50 mg three times per week, or testosterone enanthate (Delatestryl), 200 mg weekly, is administered for 12 to 20 weeks; it results in azoospermia in almost all of the subjects. Treatment is then stopped, and the subjects' ejaculates are followed for several years. Reappearance of sperm in the ejaculate usually occurs in 2 to 3 months. The most encouraging report (Rowley and Heller, 1972) reviews 163 patients, of whom 110 (67 per cent) went on to

TABLE 12–14. SUMMARY OF REPORTED EXPERIENCE OF TREATMENT OF IDIOPATHIC INFERTILITY

Drug	No. Patients	Improved Semen	Pregnancy	Placebo Controls	Reference
Testosterone					Getzoff, 1955
	168	34	16	–	Charny, 1959
	163	110	67	–	Rowley and Heller, 1972
	145	48	39	–	Lamensdorf et al., 1975
	21	8	9	–	Paulsen et al., 1977
	255	133	65	–	Charny and Gordon, 1978
Mesterolone	80	25	9	–	Schellen and Beek, 1972
	12	3	4	–	Barwin et al., 1973
	15	0	–	–	Giarola, 1974
	20	–	3	–	Keough et al., 1976
Human chorionic gonadotropin	9	0	0	–	Sherins, 1974
	117	13	10	–	Homonnai, 1978
	64	44	23	–	Cheval and Mehan, 1979
	47	8	3	–	Margalioth, 1983
Human menopausal gonadotropins	9	2	0	–	Troen et al., 1970
	26	0	0	–	Schirren and Toyosi, 1970
	275	74	20	–	Lunenfeld et al., 1972
	9	0	0	–	Sherins, 1974
	9	4	1	–	Paulsen, 1977
	8	4	1	–	Rosemberg, 1976
	37	8	3	–	Homonnai et al., 1978
	48	29	10	–	Schill et al., 1982
GnRH	10	3	0	–	Zarate et al., 1973
	4	1	0	–	Schwarzstein et al., 1975
Clomiphene	79	20	0	–	Jungek et al., 1964
	15	11	0	–	Mellinga and Thompson, 1966
	15	1	0	–	Mroueh et al., 1967a,b
	69	23	5	–	Palti, 1970
	114	±	19	Yes	Foss et al., 1973
	11	3	0	Yes	Wieland et al., 1972
	101	33	19	–	Schellen and Beek, 1974
	16	±	3	–	Reyes and Faiman, 1974
	22	18	0	–	Paulson et al., 1975
	10	8	9	–	Check and Rakoff, 1977
	16	10	5	–	Epstein, 1977
	32	–	13	–	Paulson, 1977
	54	4	4	–	Charny, 1979
	92	–	17	–	Newton et al., 1980
	53	35	14	–	Ross et al., 1980
	30	21	3	Yes	Ronnberg, 1980
Tamoxifen	21	15	–	–	Vermuelen and Comhaire, 1978
	9	1	1	Yes	Willis et al., 1977
	25	25	10	–	Buvat et al., 1983
Testolactone	9	8	5	–	Vigersky and Glass, 1981
	20	5	0	Yes	Clark and Sherins, 1983

produce ejaculates with at least 25 per cent greater sperm concentration; and 67 men (41 per cent) impregnated their wives. Although this report is rather encouraging, there are several problems in interpreting the data. To induce azoospermia, these investigators used norethandrolone (Nilevar), a drug that is no longer on the market. Their control data were sparse (three specimens), and in approximately one third to one half of their subjects, the sperm concentration exceeded 20 million/ml. More recently, Charny and Gordon (1978) reported a study of 255 oligospermic men given testosterone in whom approximately 50 per cent achieved twofold increases in sperm count and 25 per cent impregnated their wives after the androgen was stopped. We are concerned that some of the subjects in these studies may have been fertile prior to treatment. We note, furthermore, that pregnancy did not appear until 18 or 24 months following cessation of treatment in many couples.

Selection of patients for treatment, the sparse number of control semen specimens and lack of placebo controls are ubiquitous problems in all of the studies. In addition, the authors often conclude that an ejaculate is improved when the response may be limited to a very few ejaculates—i.e., a nonsustained result. Although the mechanism of this "rebound" effect is unknown, we find the data provocative. At present, the efficacy of this treatment should be considered inconclusive. Additional double-blind, placebo-controlled trials should be conducted.

Oral Androgens. Interest in the use of oral androgen to improve the status of the infertile male derives from the observation that epididymal sperm require androgen to fully mature their fertilizing capabilities (Lubicz-Nawrocki, 1973; Prasad et al., 1974). Although there is no evidence of Leydig cell failure among oligospermic men, a series of studies have been reported during the past few years in which oligospermic infertile men have been treated with oral androgens (methyl testosterone, mesterolone, Halotestin). Mesterolone is a derivative of dihydrotestosterone. It was originally claimed that this drug did not suppress endogenous gonadotropin secretion (Petry et al., 1968) and hence was not likely to induce testicular atrophy. Subsequently, suppression of gonadotropin secretion was shown to occur at doses of above 100 mg/day (Keough et al., 1977).

Early reports on oral androgens showed that some oligospermic men had improved sperm output and impregnated their wives when given doses of 20 to 60 mg/day for 12 weeks (Barwin et al., 1973; Schellan and Beek, 1972). However, more recent studies have been much less encouraging (Giarola, 1974; Keough et al., 1976; see also Table 12–14). Taking a different approach, Brown (1975) used fluoxymesterone (Halotestin) in an attempt to modify poor sperm motility in infertile men with high sperm output (mean concentration 66 million/ml). He reported improved sperm motility in 50 per cent of the subjects, and pregnancy occurred in 25 per cent of the couples.

In reviewing these studies we note that there was a striking absence of adequate diagnostic work-up of husband and wife, the number of control semen specimens was totally inadequate, and at best the incidence of pregnancy was low. We feel that this approach to treatment of the male with idiopathic infertility will be unrewarding in most instances.

GONADOTROPIN

During the decade from the mid-1960's to the mid-1970's, it became evident that gonadotropin replacement in hypogonadotropic men can stimulate complete spermatogenesis and induce sperm output that is adequate to allow impregnation. These results have encouraged many investigators to test whether gonadotropin administration per se or stimulation of endogenous gonadotropin release would similarly improve spermatogenesis among men with primary seminiferous tubular failure. Since the pituitary testicular axis is intact, the rationale for such treatment is pharmacologic—to increase intratesticular testosterone concentration with hCG or to supplement existing levels of endogenous FSH.

Gonadotropins. Since the first reports of the use of hCG and human menopausal gonadotropin (hMG) in the treatment of men with idiopathic infertility, a large body of literature has appeared, providing conflicting testimony about the efficacy of these forms of therapy. Lunenfeld et al. (1972) summarizes the literature on this subject (Table 12–14), and the data are discussed at length in two early reviews (Rosemberg, 1976; Steinberger, 1976). Lunenfeld reviews the reported experience in treating 275 severely oligospermic men and shows that although variable improvement in semen was reported in approximately 50 per cent of patients, pregnancy was documented in only 7.3 per cent of the couples. It had been suggested that insufficient gonadotropin had been administered in most of the early studies to establish conclusively whether this form of therapy would be of value. Subsequently, several well-planned investigations using hCG and hCG/hMG combinations were developed (Paulsen et al., 1976; Rosemberg, 1976; Sherins, 1974; Schirren and Toyosi, 1970; Troen et al., 1970). The data speak for themselves (Table 12–14). Among 52 carefully chosen subjects for whom extensive control semen data were available, administration of hMG at the high doses (up to 300 IU FSH daily) for prolonged intervals (15 to 30 weeks) failed to alter sperm output or achieve impregnation except in two instances (Paulsen et al., 1976; Rosemberg, 1976). More recent uncontrolled studies of hCG alone (Table 12–14) or hCG plus hMG show similar increases in sperm output and pregnancy rate as reported in the earlier studies.

Review of the earlier reports leads us to conclude that most of the early optimism for use of gonadotropin was based on studies in which patient selection and control semen data were totally inadequate. In some instances patients with hypogonadotropism were included in the study. This emphasizes the most important distinction in proper patient selection—that is, the need to exclude men with the fertile eunuch syndrome from those with true idiopathic infertility. In addition to the low rate of success with hMG, one must also consider that this medication is expensive and that it requires parenteral administration. The authors are unaware of any data that might aid the physician in selecting those few subjects who might benefit from hMG therapy.

Clomiphene and Tamoxifen. Following the observation that clomiphene, an antiestrogen, increases gonadotropin release, a number of investigators have studied the effect of this drug on the gonad. Unlike the induction of ovulation following clomiphene therapy in women, no such clear-cut response in spermatogenesis has been seen in men (Heller et al., 1969). A large number of studies have reported (Table 12–14) that changes in sperm output following clomiphene administration are highly variable. The drug has generally been given in dosages of 25 to 50 mg daily for 3 to 6 months. The earliest studies failed to report any pregnancy as a consequence of treatment. However more recent studies suggested that there may be an increased pregnancy rate following prolonged drug exposure.

There are several major problems in these studies, which limit interpretation of the findings. Almost all suffer from lack of adequate control and treatment data so that quantitative evaluation of sperm output is impossible. Thus, only the pregnancy rate can be analyzed with any confidence, and this assumes that patient selection was rigorous. In this regard, two of the earlier studies deserve further emphasis. Wieland et al. (1972) administered cis-clomiphene, 5 to 10 mg/day for 3 months, followed by a placebo course of equal duration. The Wieland data demonstrate that during prolonged observation, increases in sperm output do occur but in a totally unpredictable pattern. Of 11 oligospermic men, none impregnated his wife after treatment. Subsequently, Foss et al. (1973) reported an experience using clomiphene in 114 infertile men. In this double-blinded study clomiphene, 100 mg/day for 10 days each month for 3 months, was used with a placebo. Although 19 pregnancies (14 per cent) occurred, it was not possible to confirm or refute the assertion that clomiphene was the effective agent. These investigators recognized that pregnancy was more common in wives of the men with the highest pretreatment peak sperm counts, but made no mention of pregnancies that occurred in association with sustained high sperm output. This study also lacks adequate control data, but it provides a much more appropriate method for analyzing treatment of idiopathic infertility. At present, data on the efficacy of clomiphene are inconclusive.

A similar series of clinical trials in oligospermic men using tamoxifen, rather than clomiphene, has been performed (Table 12–14). Increase in sperm count and some pregnancies are reported. However, it is again noteworthy that the placebo-controlled trial of Willis et al. (1977) showed the lowest rate of improved semen quality (10 per cent) and pregnancy (10 per cent).

Aromatase Inhibitor. Vigersky and Glass (1981) reported the successful use of testolactone, an aromatase inhibitor, in the treatment of a few men with idiopathic infertility. Testolactone is a steroid that acts to inhibit the peripheral conversion of testosterone to estradiol. Its structure is similar to testosterone. A broad clinical experience has developed with the compound through its use in patients with metastatic breast carcinoma. Testolactone (Teslac) has been used in physiologic studies of normal men (Marynick et al., 1979), where at doses of 2 gm/day, peripheral estradiol concentration decreased from 30 to 10 pg/ml associated with a concomitant increase in both LH and FSH levels owing to the loss of feedback inhibition from the reduction in estradiol concentration. With the increase in gonadotropin levels, serum testosterone also increased to twice its pretreatment concentration, presumably due to the greater gonadotropin stimulation.

Studies in rodents have demonstrated an important inhibitory action of estradiol on testosterone biosynthesis within the testis, and these changes subsequently lead to testicular atrophy with loss of a significant portion of the germinal epithelium. The use of testolactone in the treatment of men with idiopathic infertility is thus based on the following principles:

1. Inhibition of estradiol formation (testolactone is an aromatase inhibitor).

2. Increase in testosterone synthesis secondary to reduction in levels of estradiol and increase in gonadotropin stimulation.

3. Change in the testosterone to estradiol ratio, which may influence the germinal content of the seminiferous epithelium.

Using testolactone at 1 gm/day orally for 6 months, Vigersky and Glass (1981) demonstrated a modest increase in sperm density in eight of nine oligospermic men in whom three were subsequently able to impregnate their wives. Although these data are provocative, this study failed to utilize placebo controls as described earlier in this section. To this point a second study using testolactone at 2 gm orally per day in men with idiopathic oligospermic infertility has been reported (Clark and Sherins, 1983) in which a randomized, placebo-controlled, double-blinded, cross-over design was utilized. Twenty patients were evaluated during a control period exceeding 4 months and who were followed frequently during a succeeding 16-month period. While the drug produced the expected endocrine changes in Leydig cell and pituitary function, mean sperm counts remained unchanged during placebo and drug periods. Three men who had taken testolactone sustained increases in sperm output above their basal range, but two men taking placebo had similar rises. Clark and Sherins, therefore, conclude that the drug had no more effect on fertility than placebo. Further, no pregnancies ensued.

Luteinizing Hormone–Releasing Hormone. GnRH increases gonadotropin release; when administered chronically by parenteral injection, it has been effective in secondarily increasing testicular maturation and sperm output in hypogonadotropic men. Accordingly, several preliminary reports have appeared in the literature on the use of this drug in oligospermic men with an intact pituitary gonadal axis (Schwarzstein et al., 1975; Zarate et al., 1973). Thus far, among the 14 reported cases (Table 12–14), there is no evidence to suggest any

advantage of this mode of therapy over direct gonadotropin administration. In addition, it lacks approval of the Food and Drug Administration (FDA) and requires multiple daily parenteral injections.

MISCELLANEOUS DRUGS

Over the years a variety of other empirical pharmacologic agents have been employed to test whether there is any benefit to men with idiopathic infertility. Foremost among these is triiodothyronine, one of the thyroid hormones. Despite its early proponents and later contradictory reports, this form of treatment is still used by some physicians. We find no evidence to support the use of this drug in men with infertility problems.

Similarly, glucocorticoids (Stewart and Montie, 1973) and arginine (Schachter et al., 1973) have their advocates. However, detailed studies fail to demonstrate that these drugs have any effectiveness in oligospermic men (Jungling and Bunge, 1976; Mancini et al., 1966). More recently, a placebo-controlled trial with bromocriptine (Hovatta et al., 1979; Montanari et al., 1978) and metergolide (Liserdol) (Masala et al., 1979) were used to suppress prolactin release, but no significant effect on sperm output or pregnancy rate was demonstrated. The list could go on, but it would be counterproductive to describe a series of empirical remedies for which there is no evidence of efficacy.

In summary, none of the medical regimens for male infertility secondary to idiopathic oligospermia has been proved to be effective. Gonadotropins, GnRH, clomiphene, tamoxifen, testolactone, and nonrebound dosages of androgen are rarely, if ever, more successful than no treatment. There is little rationale for and no conclusive evidence that arginine, thyroid hormone, corticosteroids, and miscellaneous medications effect spermatogenesis in men with idiopathic oligospermia. Therefore, we wish to re-emphasize the importance of a thorough diagnostic work-up to exclude men who could be fertile prior to treatment, and to stress, once again, that any clinical trial assessing the efficacy of a drug in treating idiopathic oligospermic infertility be properly designed to include assignment of placebo controls in a randomized, double-blinded, cross-over design.

In view of the high rate of fertility of hypogonadotropic men treated with gonadotropin replacement, who impregnate their wives with sperm counts of only 2 to 5 million per ejaculate, it seems to us that the possibilities in treating sexually mature oligospermic men successfully will rely on our ability in the future to define specific biochemical defects in sperm function.

References

Evaluation (History, Physical Examination, Laboratory Studies)

Aiman, J. and Griffin, J. E.: The frequency of androgen receptor deficiency in infertile men. Clin. Endocrinol. Metab., *54:*725, 1982.

Alexander, N. J.: Semen analysis: The method and interpretation. *In* Sciarra, J. (Ed.): Gynecology and Obstetrics. Hagerstown, Harper and Row, 1981.

Baker, H. W. G., Bremner, W. J., Burger, H. G., de Kretser, D. M., Dulmanis, A., Eddie, L. M., Hudson, B., Keough, E. J., Lee, V. W., and Rennie, G. C.: Testicular control of follicle-stimulating hormone secretion. Recent Prog. Horm. Res., *32:*429, 1976.

Berger, R. E., Alexander, E. R., Monda, G. D., Ansell, J., McCormick, G., and Holmes, K. K.: *Chlamydia trachomatis* as a cause of acute "idiopathic" epididymitis. N. Engl. J. Med., *298:*301, 1978.

Bishop, M. W. H.: Aging and reproduction in the male. J. Reprod. Fertil. (Suppl.), *12:*65, 1970.

Boiesen, P. T., Lindholm, J., Hagen, C., Bahnsen, M., and Fabricius-Bjerre, N.: Histological changes in testicular biopsies from chronic alcoholics with and without liver disease. Acta Path. Microbiol. Scand. Sect A, *87:*139, 1979.

Booth, J. D., and Loriaux, D. L.: Selective control of follicle-stimulating hormone secretion: New perspectives. *In* D'Agata, R., et al. (Eds.): Recent Advances in Male Reproduction: Molecular Basis and Clinical Implications. New York, Raven Press, 1983, pp. 269–277.

Chandley, A. C., Edmond, P. E., and Christie, S.: Cytogenetics and infertility in man. Ann. Hum. Genet. *39:*231, 1973.

Evans, H. J., Fletcher, J., Torrance, M., and Hargreave, T. B.: Sperm abnormalities and cigarette smoking. Lancet, *1:*627, 1981.

Fowler, J. E., Jr.: Infections of the male reproductive tract and infertility: A selected review. J. Androl., *3:*121, 1981.

Funder, J. W., and Mercer, J. E.: Cimetidine, a histamine H_2 receptor antagonist, occupies androgen receptors. J. Clin. Endocrinol., *48:*189, 1979.

Goldenberg, R. L., and White, R.: The effects of vaginal lubricants on sperm motility in vitro. Fertil. Steril., *26:*872, 1975.

Haas, G. G., Cines, D. B., and Schreiber, A. D.: Immunologic infertility: Identification of patients with antisperm antibody. N. Engl. J. Med., *303:*722, 1981.

Kjessler, B.: Chromosomal constitution and male reproductive failure. *In* Mancini, R. E., and Martini, L. (Eds.): Male Fertility and Sterility, New York, Academic Press, 1974, p. 231.

Kley, H. K., Nieschlag, E., and Krustemper, H. L.: Age dependence of plasma oestrogen response to HCG and ACTH in men. Acta Endocrinol., *79:*95, 1975.

Knigge, U., Dejgaard, A., Wollesen, F., Ingerslev, O., Bennett, P., and Christiansen, P. M.: The acute and long-term effect of the H_2-receptor antagonists cimetidine and ranitidine on the pituitary-gonadal axis in men. Clin. Endocrinol., *18:*307, 1983.

Marynick, S. P., Loriaux, D. L., Sherins, R. J., Pita, J. C., and Lipsett, M. B.: Evidence that testosterone acts as both an androgen and an estrogen in suppressing pituitary gonadotropin secretion in men. J. Clin. Endocrinol. Metab., *49:*396, 1979.

Mathur, S., Williamson, H. O., Landgrebe, S. G., et al.: Application of passive hemagglutination for evaluation of antisperm antibodies and modified Coombs' test for detecting male autoimmunity to sperm antigens. J. Immunol. Methods, *30:*381, 1979.

Milby, T. H., and Whorton, D.: Epidemiological assessment of occupationally related, chemically induced sperm count suppression. J. Occup. Med., *22:*77, 1980.

Mumford, D. M., and Warner, M. R.: Male fertility and immunity. *In* Lipshultz, L. I., and Howards, S. S. (Eds.): Infertility in the Male. New York, Churchill Livingstone, 1983.

Population Reports, Series L, Number 1. Population Information Program. Baltimore, Johns Hopkins University, March 1979.

Ramasharma, K., Sairam, M. R., Seidah, N. G., Chretien, M., Manjunath, P., Schiller, P. W., Yamashiro, D., and Li, C. H.: Isolation, structure and synthesis of a human seminal plasma peptide with inhibin-like activity. Science, *223:*1199, 1984.

Rumke, P., Van Amstel, N., Messer, E. N., and Bezemer, P. O.: Prognosis of fertility of men with sperm agglutinins in the serum. Fertil. Steril., *25:*393, 1974.

Santen, R. J.: Is aromatization of testosterone to estradiol required for inhibition of luteinizing hormone secretion in men? J. Clin. Invest., *56:*1555, 1975.

Schachter, J.: Medical Progress: Chlamydial infections (first of three parts). N. Engl. J. Med., *298:*428, 1978.

Scheibel, J. H., Anderson, J. T., Brandenhoff, P., Geerdesn, J. P., Bay-Neilsen, A., Schultz, B. A., and Walter, S.: *Chlamydia trachomatis* in acute epididymitis. Scand. J. Urol. Nephrol., *17:*47, 1983.

Sherins, R. J., and Loriaux, D. L.: Studies on the role of sex steroids in the feedback control of FSH concentration in men. J. Clin. Endocrinol., *36:*886, 1973.

Sherins, R. J., Patterson, A. P., Brightwell, D., Udelsman, R., and Sartor, J.: Alteration in the plasma testosterone–estradiol ratio: An alternative to the inhibin hypothesis. *In* The Cell Biology of the Testis. Ann. N. Y. Acad. Sci., *383:*295, 1982.

Stearns, E. L., MacDonnell, J. A., Kaufman, B. J., Padua, R., Lucman, T. S., Winters, J. S. D., and Faiman, C.: Declining testicular function with age: Hormonal and clinical correlates. Am. J. Med., *57:*761, 1974.

Steinberger, A., and Steinberger, E.: Secretion of an FSH inhibiting factor by cultured Sertoli cells. Endocrinology, *99:*918, 1976.

Taylor-Robinson, D., and McCormack, W. M.: Medical progress: The genital mycoplasmas (second of two parts). N. Engl. J. Med., *302:*1063, 1980.

Tyler, H. M., Saxton, C. A. P. D., and Parry, M. J.: Administration to man of UK-37,248-01, a selective inhibitor of thromboxane synthetase. Lancet, *1:*629, 1981.

Van Thiel, D. H., Lester, R., and Sherins, R. J.: Hypogonadism in alcoholic liver disease. Gastroenterology, *67:*1188, 1974.

Van Thiel, D. H., Sherins, R. J., Meyers, G. H., Jr., and DeVita, V. T., Jr.: Evidence for a specific seminiferous tubular factor affecting FSH secretion in man. J. Clin. Invest., *51:*1009, 1971.

Wall, J. R., Stedronska, J., and David, R. D.: Immunologic studies of male infertility. Fertil. Steril., *26:*1035, 1975.

Winters, S. J., Janick, J. J., Loriaux, D. L., and Sherins,

R. J.: Studies on the role of sex steroids in the feedback control of gonadotropin concentration in men II: Use of the estrogen antagonist clomiphene citrate. J. Clin. Endocrinol. Metab., *48*:222, 1979.

Semen Analysis

Alford, L.M., and Rivard, D. J.: A simple stain for differentiating semen constituents. J. Urol., *126*:609, 1981.

Amann, R. P.: A critical review of methods for evaluation of spermatogenesis from seminal characteristics. J. Androl., *2*:37, 1981.

Amann, R. P., and Hammerstedt, R. H.: Validation of a system for computerized measurements of spermatozoal velocity and percentage of motile sperm. Biol. Reprod., *23*:647, 1980.

Amelar, R. D.: Coagulation, liquefaction and viscosity of human semen. J. Urol., *87*:187, 1962.

Amelar, R. D., and Dubin, L.: Male infertility: Current diagnosis and treatment. Urology, *1*:1, 1973.

Baccetti, B., Burrini, A. G., Pallini, V., and Renieri, T.: Human dynein and sperm pathology. J. Cell Biol., *88*:102, 1981.

Belsey, M. A., Eliasson, R., Gallegos, A. J., Moghissi, K. S., Paulsen, C. A., and Prasad, M. R. N.: Laboratory manual for the examination of human semen and semen-cervical mucus interaction. Singapore, Press Concern, 1980.

Couture, M., Ulstein, M., Leonard, J. M., and Paulsen, C. A.: Improved staining method for differentiating immature germ cells from white blood cells in human seminal fluid. Andrologia, *8*:61, 1976.

Dubin, L., and Amelar, R. D.: Etiologic factors in 1244 consecutive cases of male infertility. Fertil. Steril., *22*:496, 1971.

Eliasson, R.: Analysis of semen. *In* Behrman, S. J., and Kistner, R. W. (Eds.): Progress in Infertility. Boston, Little, Brown and Co., 1975.

Freund, M.: Semen analysis. *In* Behrman, S. J. (Ed.): Progress in Infertility. Boston, Little, Brown and Co., 1968.

Frost, J., and Cummins, H. Z.: Motility assay of human sperm by photon correlation spectroscopy. Science, *212*:1520, 1981.

Gagnon, C., Sherins, R. J., Phillips, D. M., and Bardin, C. W.: Deficiency of protein-carboxyl methylase in immotile spermatozoa of infertile men. N. Engl. J. Med., *306*:821, 1982.

Hotchkiss, R. S.: Infertility in the male. *In* Campbell, M. J., and Harrison, J. H. (Eds.): Urology, 3rd ed. Philadelphia, W. B. Saunders Co., 1970.

Jouannet, P., Escalier, D., Serres, C., and David, G.: Motility of human sperm without outer dynein arms. J. Submicrosc. Cytol., *15*:67, 1983.

Jouannet, P., Volochine, B., Deguent, P., Serres, C., and David, G.: Light scattering determination of various characteristic parameters of spermatozoa motility of a series of human sperm. Andrologia, *9*:36, 1977.

Katz, D. F., Diel, L., and Overstreet, J. W.: Differences in the movement of morphologically normal and abnormal seminal spermatozoa. Biol. Reprod., *24*:566, 1982.

MacLeod, J.: The semen examination. Clin. Obstet. Gynecol., *8*:115, 1965.

MacLeod, J.: Human seminal cytology as a sensitive indicator of the germinal epithelium. Int. J. Fertil., *9*:281, 1964.

MacLeod, J.: Semen quality in one thousand men of known fertility and eight hundred cases of infertile marriage. Fertil. Steril., *2*:115, 1951.

Macomber, D., and Sanders, M. B.: The spermatozoa count. N. Engl. J. Med., *200*:981, 1929.

Mann, T.: The Biochemistry of Semen of the Male Reproductive Tract. London, Methuen and Co., 1964.

Nahoum, C. R. D., and Cardozo, D.: Staining for volumetric count of leukocytes in semen and prostatevesicular fluid. Fertil. Steril., *34*:68, 1980.

Nelson, C. M. K., and Bunge, R. G.: Semen analysis: Evidence for changing parameters of male fertility potential. Fertil. Steril., *25*:503, 1974.

Oettle, A. G.: Morphologic changes in normal human semen after ejaculation. Fertil. Steril., *5*:227, 1957.

Overstreet, J. W., Price, M. J., Blazak, W. F., Lewis, E. L., and Katz, D. F.: Simultaneous assessment of human sperm motility and morphology by videomicrography. J. Urol., *126*:357, 1981.

Pedersen, H., and Rebbe, H.: Absence of arms in the axoneme of immobile human spermatozoa. Biol. Reprod., *12*:541, 1975.

Raboch, J., and Skachova, J.: The pH of human ejaculate. Fertil. Steril., *16*:252, 1965.

Rehan, N. E., Sobrero, A. J., and Fertig, J. W.: The semen of fertile men: Statistical analysis of 1300 men. Fertil. Steril., *26*:492, 1975.

Schwartz, D., Laplanche, A., Jouannet, P., and David, G.: Within-subject variability of human semen in regard to sperm count, volume, total number of spermatozoa and length of abstinence. J. Reprod. Fertil., *57*:391, 1979.

Sherins, R. J., Brightwell, D., and Sternthal. P. M.: Longitudinal analysis of semen of fertile and infertile men. *In* Troen, P., and Nankin, H. (Eds.): New Concepts of the Testis in Normal and Infertile Men: Morphology, Physiology and Pathology, New York, Raven Press, 1977, pp. 473–488.

Sobrero, A. J., and MacLeod, J.: The immediate postcoital test. Fertil. Steril., *23*:245, 1972.

Syner, F. N., Moghissi, K. S., and Yanez, J.: Isolation of a factor from normal human semen that accelerates dissolution of abnormally liquefying semen. Fertil. Steril., *26*:1064, 1975.

Tauber, P. F., Propping, D., Schumacher, G. F. B., and Zaneveld, L. J. D.: Biochemical aspects of the coagulation and liquefaction of human semen. J. Androl., *1*:280, 1980.

Upadhyaya, M., Hibbard, B. M., and Walter, S. M.: Use of sputolysin for liquefaction of viscid human semen. Fertil. Steril., *35*:657, 1981.

Wilson, V. G., and Bunge, R. G.: Infertility and semen nonliquefaction. J. Urol., *113*:509, 1975.

Sperm–Cervical Mucus Penetration Assay

Alexander, N. J.: Evaluation of male infertility with an *in vitro* cervical mucus penetration test. Fertil. Steril., *36*:201, 1981.

Bergman, A., Amit, A., David, M. P., et al.: Penetration of human ejaculated spermatozoa into human and bovine cervical mucus: I. Correlation between penetration values. Fertil. Steril., *36*:363, 1981.

Kremer, J., and Jager, S.: The sperm-cervical mucus contact test: A preliminary report. Fertil. Steril., *27*:335, 1976.

Matthews, C. D., Makin, A. E., and Cox, L. W.: Experience with *in vitro* sperm penetration testing in infertile and fertile couples. Fertil. Steril., *33*:187, 1980.

Mills, N. R., and Katz, D.: A flat capillary tube system for assessment of sperm movement in cervical mucus. Fertil. Steril., *29*:117, 1978.

Mumford, D. M., and Warner, M. R.: Male fertility and immunity. *In* Lipshultz, L. I., and Howards, S. S.

(Eds.): Infertility in the Male. New York, Churchill Livingstone, 1983.

Moghissi, K. S.: Postcoital test: Physiologic basis, technique and interpretation. Fertil. Steril., 27:117, 1976.

Sperm-Oocyte Interaction

Barros, C., Gonzalez, J., Herrera, E., et al.: Fertilizing capacity of human spermatozoa evaluated by actual penetration of foreign eggs. Contraception, 17:87, 1978.

Chang, T. S. K., and Albertsen, P. C.: Interpretation and utilization of the zona pellucida–free hamster egg penetration test in the evaluation of the infertile male. In Howards, S. S., and Lipshultz, L. I. (Guest Eds.): Seminars in Urology, Vol. 2, No. 2, p. 124, 1984.

Overstreet, J. W., Yanagimachi, R., Katz, D. F., et al.: Penetration of human spermatozoa into the human zona pellucida and the zona-free hamster egg: A study of fertile donors and infertile patients. Fertil. Steril., 33:534, 1980.

Rogers, B. J., Van Campen, H., Ueno, M. et al.: Analysis of human spermatozoal fertilizing ability using zona-free ova. Fertil. Steril., 32:664, 1979.

Yanagimachi, R.: Penetration of guinea-pig spermatozoa into hamster eggs in vitro. J. Reprod. Fertil., 28:477, 1972.

Yanagimachi, R., Yanagimachi, H., and Rogers, B. J.: The use of zona-free animal ova as a test system for the assessment of the fertilizing capacity of human spermatozoa. Biol. Reprod., 15:471, 1976.

Biopsy

Ansbacher, R., and Gangai, M. P.: Testicular biopsy: Sperm antibodies. Fertil. Steril., 26:1239, 1975.

Chemes, H. E., Dym, M., Fawcett, D. W., Javadpour, N., and Sherins, R. J.: Pathophysiological observations of Sertoli cells in patients with germinal aplasia and severe germ cell depletion: ultrastructural findings and endocrine levels. Biol. Reprod., 17:108, 1977.

Frajese, G., Santiemma, V., and Massimo, R.: In vitro autoradiographic studies of DNA synthesis in human testis with spermatogenic arrest. Clin. Genet., 6:401, 1974.

Gordon, D. L., Barr, A. B., Herrigel, J. E., and Paulsen, C. A.: Testicular biopsy in man: I. Effect upon sperm concentration. Fertil. Steril., 16:522, 1965.

Nelson, W. O.: Testicular morphology in eunuchoidal and infertile men. Fertil. Steril., 1:477, 1950.

Wong, T. W., Straus, F. H., and Warner, N. E.: Testicular biopsy in the study of male infertility: III. Pretesticular causes of infertility. Arch. Pathol., 98:1, 1974.

Wong, T. W., Straus, F. H., and Warner, N. E.: Testicular biopsy in the study of male infertility. I. Testicular causes of infertility. Arch. Pathol., 95:151, 1973a.

Wong, T. W., Straus, F. H., and Warner, N. E.: Testicular biopsy in the study of male infertility. II. Post-testicular causes of infertility. Arch. Pathol., 95:160, 1973b.

Hypogonadotropic Hypogonadism, Fertile Eunuch Syndrome, Postpubertal Gonadotropin Deficiency

Albert, A., Underdalh, L. O., Greene, F., and Lorenz, N.: Male hypogonadism, IV: The testis in prepubertal or pubertal gonadotropic failure. Proc. Staff Meet. Mayo Clin., 29:131, 1954.

Bardin, C. W.: Hypogonadotropic hypogonadism in patients with congenital defects. Birth Defects (original article series), 7:175, 1971.

Bardin, C. W., Ross, G. T., and Lipsett, M. B.: Site of action of clomiphene citrate in men: A study of the pituitary–Leydig cell axis. J. Clin. Endocrinol., 27:1558, 1967.

Bardin, C. W., Ross, G. T., Rifkind, A. B., Cargille, C. M., and Lipsett, M. B.: Studies of the pituitary–Leydig cell axis in young men with hypogonadotropic hypogonadism and hyposmia: Comparison with normal men, prepubertal boys and hypopituitary patients. J. Clin. Invest., 48:2046, 1969.

Bell, J., Spitz, I., Slonim, A., Perlman, A., Segal, S., Palti, Z., and Rabinowitz, D.: Heterogeneity of gonadotropin response to LH-RH in hypogonadotropic hypogonadism. J. Clin. Endocrinol., 36:791, 1973.

Biben, R. L., and Gordan, G. S.: Familial hypogonadotropic eunuchoidism. J. Clin. Endocrinol., 15:931, 1955.

Bremner, W. J., Fernando, N. N., and Paulsen, C. A.: The effect of luteinizing hormone releasing hormone in hypogonadotropic eunuchoidism. Acta Endocrinol., 86:1, 1977.

de Gennes, J. L., Turpin, G., De Grouchy, J., and Pialoux, P.: Études clinique biologique histologique et genetique du syndrome de de Mosier. Ann. Endocrinol., 31:841, 1970.

de Mosier, G.: Études sur les dysraphies cranio-encephaliques. Schweiz. Arch. Neurol. Psychiatr., 74:309, 1954.

Ewer, R. W.: Familial monotropic pituitary gonadotropin insufficiency. J. Clin. Endocrinol. Metab., 28:783, 1968.

Faiman, C., Hoffman, D. L., Ryan, R. J., and Albert, A.: The "fertile eunuch" syndrome: Demonstration of isolated luteinizing hormone deficiency by radio-immunoassay technique. Proc. Staff Meet. Mayo Clin., 43:661, 1968.

Golden, M. P., Lippe, B. M., and Kaplan, S. A.: Congenital adrenal hypoplasia and hypogonadotropic hypogonadism Am. J. Dis. Child., 131:1117, 1977.

Hamilton, G. R., Scully, R. E., and Kliman, B.: Hypogonadotropinism in Prader-Willi syndrome: Induction of puberty and spermatogenesis by clomiphene citrate. Am. J. Med., 52:322, 1972.

Hashimoto, T., Miyai, K., Izunii, K., and Kumahara, Y.: Isolated gonadotropin deficiency with response to luteinizing hormone–releasing hormone. N. Engl. J. Med., 287:1059, 1972.

Hay, I. D. Smail, P. J., and Forsyth, C. C.: Familial cytomegalic adrenocortical hypoplasia: An X-linked syndrome of pubertal failure. Arch. Dis. Child., 56:715, 1981.

Hoffman, A. R., and Crowley, W. F.: Induction of puberty in men by long-term pulsatile administration of low-dose gonadotropin releasing hormone. N. Engl. J. Med., 307:1237, 1982.

Kallman, F. J., Schoenfeld, W. A., and Barrera, S. E.: The genetic aspects of primary eunuchoidism. Am. J. Ment. Defic., 48:203, 1944.

Kulin, H. E., Reiter, E. O., and Bridson, W. E.: Pubertal maturation of the gonadotropin stimulatory response to clomiphene: A case report. J. Clin. Endocrinol., 33:551, 1971.

Kulin, H. E., Rifkind, A. B., Ross, G. T., and Odell, W. D.: Total gonadotropin activity in the urine of prepubertal children. J. Clin. Endocrinol., 27:1123, 1967.

Marshall, W. A., and Tanner, J. M.: Variations in the pattern of pubertal changes in boys. Arch. Dis. Child., 45:13, 1970.

Matthews, W. B., and Rundle, A. T.: Familial cerebellar ataxia and hypogonadism. Brain, 87:463, 1964.

McCullagh, E. P., Beck, J. C., and Schaffenburg, C. A.:

A syndrome of eunuchoidism with spermatogenesis, normal urinary FSH and low or normal ICSH (fertile eunuchs). J. Clin. Endocrinol., *13*:489, 1953.

Merriam, G. R., Beitins, I. Z., and Bode, H. H.: Father-to-son transmission of hypogonadism with anosmia: Kallman's syndrome. Am. J. Dis. Child., *131*:1216, 1977.

Nankin, H. R., Yanaihara, T., and Troen, P.: Response of gonadotropins and testosterone to clomiphene stimulation in a pubertal boy. J. Clin. Endocrinol., *33*:360, 1971.

Neuhauser, G., and Opitz, J. M.: Autosomal recessive syndrome of cerebellar ataxia and hypogonadotropic hypogonadism. Clin. Genet., 7:426, 1975.

Nowakowski, H., and Lenz, W.: Genetic aspects of male hypogonadism. Recent Prog. Horm. Res., *17*:53, 1961.

Pasqualini, R. O., and Bur, G. E.: Hypoandrogenic syndrome with spermatogenesis. Fertil. Steril., *6*:144, 1955.

Reinfrank, R. F., and Nichols, F. L.: Hypogonadotropic hypogonadism in the Lawrence-Moon syndrome. J. Clin. Endocrinol. Metab. 24:48, 1964.

Reiter, E. O., Kulin, H. E., and Hamwood, S. M.: Preparation of urine containing small amounts of FSH and LH for radioimmunoassay: Comparison of the kaolin-acetone and acetone extraction techniques. J. Clin. Endocrinol., *36*:661, 1973.

Roth, J. C., Kelch, R. P., Kaplan, S. L., and Grumbach, M. M.: FSH and LH response to luteinizing hormone releasing factor in prepubertal and pubertal children, adult males and patients with hypogonadotropic and hypergonadotropic hypogonadism. J. Clin. Endocrinol., *35*:926, 1972.

Santen, R. J., Leonard, J. M., Sherins, R. J., Gandy, H. M., and Paulsen, C. A.: Short- and long-term effects of clomiphene citrate on the pituitary-testicular axis. J. Clin. Endocrinol., *33*:970, 1971.

Santen, R. J., and Paulsen, C. A.: Hypogonadotropic eunuchoidism: I. Clinical study of the mode of inheritance. J. Clin. Endocrinol., *36*:47, 1973a.

Santen, R. J., and Paulsen, C. A.: Hypogonadotropic eunuchoidism. II. Gonadal responsiveness to exogenous gonadotropins. J. Clin. Endocrinol., *36*:55, 1973b.

Sherins, R. J., Winters, S. J., and Wachslicht, H.: Studies of the role of HCG and low dose FSH in initiating spermatogenesis in hypogonadotropic men. Abstract 312, 59th Annual Meeting of the Endocrine Society, Chicago, June 8–10, 1977.

Sparkes, R. S., Simpson, R. W., and Paulsen, C. A.: Familial hypogonadotropic hypogonadism with anosmia. Arch. Intern. Med., *121*:534, 1968.

Van Wagenen, G., and Simpson, M. E.: Embryology of the Ovary and Testis *Homo sapiens and Macaca mulatta.* New Haven. Yale University Press. 1965.

Volpe, R., Metzler, W. S., and Johnston, M. W.: Familial hypogonadotropic eunuchoidism with cerebellar ataxia. J. Clin. Endocrinol., *23*:107, 1963.

Winters, S. J., Johnsonbaugh, R. E., and Sherins, R. J.: The response of prolactin to chlorpromazine stimulation in men with hypogonadotropic hypogonadism and early pubertal boys: Relationship to sex steroid exposure. Clin. Endocrinol., *16*:321, 1982.

Winters, S. J., Mecklenburg, R. S., and Sherins, R. J.: Hypothalamic function in men with hypogonadotropic hypogonadism. Clin. Endocrinol., *8*:417, 1978.

Yen, S. S. C., Rebar, R., Vandenberg, G., Naftolin, F., Ehara, Y., Engblom, S., Ryan, K. J., and Benirschke, K.: Synthetic luteinizing hormone-releasing factor. A potent stimulator of gonadotropin release in man. J. Clin. Endocrinol., *34*:1108, 1972.

Yoshimoto, Y., Moridera, K., and Imura, H.: Restoration of normal pituitary gonadotropin reserve by administration of luteinizing hormone releasing hormone in patients with hypogonadotropic hypogonadism. N. Engl. J. Med., *292*:242, 1975.

Zarate, A., Kastin, A. J., Soria, J., Canales, E. S., and Schally, A. V.: Effect of synthetic luteinizing hormone-releasing hormone (LH-RH) in two brothers with hypogonadotropic hypogonadism and anosmia. J. Clin. Endocrinol., *36*:612, 1973.

Congenital Adrenal Hyperplasia

Bongiovanni, A. M.: Disorders of adrenocortical steroid biogenesis (the adrenogenital syndrome associated with congenital adrenal hyperplasia). *In* Stanbury, J. B., Wyngaarden, J. B., and Frederickson, D. S. (Eds.): The Metabolic Basis of Inherited Disease. New York, McGraw-Hill, 1972.

Boyar, R. M., Finkelstein, J. W., David, R., Roffwerg, H., Kapen, S., Weitzman, E. D., and Hellman, C.: Twenty-four hour patterns of plasma luteinizing hormone and follicle-stimulating hormone in sexual precocity. N. Engl. J. Med., *289*:282, 1973.

Burke, E. F., Gilbert, E., and Velhing, D. T.: Adrenal rest tumors of the testis. J. Urol., *109*:649, 1973.

Chrousos, G. P., Loriaux, D. L., Mann, D. L., and Cutler, G. B.: Late-onset 21-hydroxylase deficiency mimicking idiopathic hirsutism or polycystic ovarian disease: An allelic variant of congenital virilizing adrenal hyperplasia with a milder enzymatic defect. Ann. Intern. Med., *96*:143, 1982.

Chrousos, G. P., Loriaux, D. L., Sherins, R. J., and Cutler, G. B. Unilateral testicular enlargement resulting from inapparent 21-hydroxylase deficiency. J. Urol., *126*:127, 1981.

Dahl, E., and Bahn, R. C.: Aberrant adrenal cortical tissue near the testis in human infants. Am. J. Pathol., *40*:587, 1962.

Fore, W. W., Bledsoe, T., Weber, D. M., Akers, R., and Brooks, T.: Cortisol production by testicular tumors in the adrenogenital syndrome. Arch. Intern. Med., *130*:59, 1972.

Glenn, J. F., and Boyce, W. H.: Adrenogenitalism with testicular adrenal rests simulating interstitial cell tumor. J. Urol., *89*:456, 1963.

Radfar, N., Bartter, F. C., Easley, R., Kolins, J., Javadpour, N., and Sherins, R. J.: Evidence for endogenous LH suppression in a man with bilateral testicular tumors and congenital adrenal hyperplasia. J. Clin. Endocrinol., *45*:1194, 1977.

Urban, M. D., Lee, P. A., and Migeon, C. J.: Adult height and fertility in men with congenital virilizing adrenal hyperplasia. N. Engl. J. Med., *299*:1392, 1978.

Wilkins, L., and Cara, J.: Further studies on the treatment of congenital adrenal hyperplasia with cortisone. V. Effects of cortisone therapy on testicular development. J. Clin. Endocrinol., *14*:287, 1954.

Klinefelter's Syndrome

Ahmad, K. N., Lennox, B., and Mack, W. S.: Estimation of the volume of Leydig cells in man. Lancet, 2:461, 1969.

Atkins, L., and Connelly, J. P.: XXXXY sex-chromosome abnormality. Am. J. Dis. Child., *106*:514, 1963.

Barr, M. L.: The natural history of Klinefelter's syndrome. Fertil. Steril., *17*:429, 1966.

Barr, M. L., and Carr, D. H.: Sex chromatin, sex chromosomes and sex abnormalities. Canad. Med. Assoc. J., *83*:979, 1960.

Becker, K. L., Hoffman, D. L., Albert, A., Underdahl, L. O., and Mason, H. L.: Klinefelter's syndrome. Arch. Intern. Med., *118*:314, 1966.

Bergada, C., Farias, N. E., deBehar, B. M. R., and Cullen, M.: Abnormal sex chromatin pattern in cryptorchidism, girls with short stature and other endocrine patients. Helv. Paediatr. Acta, *4*:372, 1969.

Chopra, I. J., Tulchinsky, D., and Greenway, F. L.: Estrogen-androgen imbalance in men with hepatic cirrhosis. Ann. Intern. Med., *79*:198, 1973.

de la Chapelle, A.: Sex chromosome abnormalities among the mentally defective in Finland. J. Ment. Defic. Res., *1*:129, 1963.

Dykes, J. R. W.: Histometric assessment of human testicular biopsies. J. Pathol., *97*:429, 1969.

Federman, D. D.: Abnormal Sexual Development. Philadelphia, W. B. Saunders Co., 1967.

Ferguson-Smith, M. A.: The prepubertal testicular lesion in chromatin-positive Klinefelter's syndrome (primary micro-orchidism) as seen in mentally handicapped children. Lancet, *1*:219, 1959.

Foss, G. L., and Lewis, F. J. W.: A study of four cases with Klinefelter's syndrome, showing motile spermatozoa in their ejaculates. J. Reprod. Fertil., *25*:401, 1971.

Gabrilove, J. L., Nicolis, G. L., and Hausknecht, R. U.: Urinary testosterone, oestrogen production rate and urinary oestrogen in chromatin positive Klinefelter's syndrome. Acta Endocrinol., *63*:499, 1970.

Harnden, D. C., MacLean, N., and Langlands, A. O.: Carcinoma of the breast and Klinefelter's syndrome. J. Med. Genet., *8*:460, 1971.

Jacobs, P. A., and Strong, J. A.: A case of human intersexuality having a possible XXY sex determining mechanism. Nature, *183*:302, 1959.

Klinefelter, H. G., Jr., Reifenstein, E. C., Jr., and Albright, F.: Syndrome characterized by gynecomastia, aspermatogenesis without a-Leydigism and increased secretion of follicle-stimulating hormone. J. Clin. Endocrinol., *2*:615, 1942.

Laron, Z., and Hochman, I. H.: Small testes in prepubertal boys with Klinefelter's syndrome. J. Clin. Endocrinol., *32*:671, 1971.

Lipsett, M. B., Davis, T. E., Wilson, H., and Canfield, C. J.: Testosterone production in chromatin-positive Klinefelter's syndrome. J. Clin. Endocrinol., *25*:1027, 1965.

Lynch, H. T., Kaplan, A. R., and Lynch, J. F.: Klinefelter's syndrome and cancer. A family study. J.A.M.A., *229*:809, 1974.

MacLean, N., Harnden, D. G., Bond, J., Court-Brown, W. M., and Mantle, D. J.: Sex-chromosome abnormalities in newborn babies. Lancet, *1*:286, 1964.

Paulsen, C. A., deSouza, A., Yoshizumi, T., and Lewis, B. M.: Results of a buccal smear survey in noninstitutionalized adult males. J. Clin. Endocrinol., *24*:1182, 1964.

Paulsen, C. A., Gorden, D. L., Carpenter, R. W., Gandy, H. M., and Drucker, W. D.: Klinefelter's syndrome and its variants: A hormonal and chromosomal study. Recent Prog. Horm. Res., *24*:321, 1968.

Plunkett, E. R., and Barr, M. L.: Testicular dysgenesis affecting the seminiferous tubules principally, with chromatin-positive nuclei. Lancet, *2*:853, 1956.

Plunkett, E. R., Rangecroft, G., and Heagy, F.: Thyroid function in patients with sex chromosome anomalies. J. Ment. Defic. Res., *8*:25, 1964.

Robson, M. C., Santiago, G., and Hung, T. W.: Bilateral carcinoma of the breast in a patient with Klinefelter's syndrome. J. Clin. Endocrinol., *28*:897, 1968.

Ruder, H. J., Loriaux, D. L., Sherins, R. J., and Lipsett, M. B.: Leydig cell function in men with disorders of spermatogenesis. J. Clin. Endocrinol., *33*:244, 1974.

Theilgaard, A., Nielsen, J., Sorensen, A., Froland, A., and Johnson, S. G.: A psychological-psychiatric study of patients with Klinefelter's syndrome, 47,XXY. Acta Jutlandica, *43*:1–148, 1971.

XXY Syndrome

Baghdassarian, A., Bayard, F., Borgaonkar, S., Arnold, E. A., Solez, K., and Migeon, C. J.: Testicular function in XYY men. Johns Hopk. Med. J., *136*:15, 1975.

Balodimos, M. C., Lisco, H., Irwin, I., Merrill, W., and Dingman, J. F.: XYY karyotype in a case of familial hypogonadism. J. Clin. Endocrinol., *26*:443, 1966.

Ferrier, P. E., Ferrier, S. A., Scharer, K. O., Genton, N., Hedinger, C., and Klein, D.: Multiple chromosome aberrations: XO/XY/XYY mosaicism and a translocation in the same family. Helv. Paediatr. Acta, *22*:516, 1967.

Hook, E. B.: Behavioral duplications of the human XYY genotype. Science, *179*:139, 1973.

Hook, E. B., and Kim, D. S.: Height and antisocial behavior in XY and XYY boys. Science, *172*:284, 1971.

Iinuma, K., Tanae, A., and Tanaka, G.: An XYY baby with Prader syndrome. Clin. Genet., *6*:323, 1974.

Ismail, A. A. A., Harkness, R. A., Kirkham, K. E., Loraine, J. A., Whatmore, P. B., and Brittain, R. P.: Effect of abnormal sex-chromosome complements on urinary testosterone levels. Lancet, *1*:220, 1968.

Jacobs, P. A., Brunton, M., Melville, M. M., Brittain, R. P., and McClemont, W. F.: Aggressive behavior, mental subnormality and the XYY male. Nature, *208*:1351, 1965.

Lundberg, P. O., and Wahlstrom, J.: Hormone levels in men with extra Y chromosomes. Lancet, *2*:1133, 1970.

Nielsen, J., Yde, H., and Johansen, K.: Serum growth hormone level after oral glucose load, urinary excretion of pituitary gonadotropin and 17-ketosteroids in XYY syndrome. Metabolism, *18*:993, 1969.

Price, W. H., Strong, J. A., Whatmore, P. B., and McClemont, W. F.: Criminal patients with XYY sex-chromosome complement. Lancet, *1*:565, 1966.

Price, W. H., and Van Der Molen, H. J.: Plasma testosterone levels in males with the 47,XYY karyotype. J. Endocrinol., *47*:117, 1970.

Sandberg, A. A., Kopef, G. F., Ishihara, T., and Hauschka, T. S.: An XYY human male. Lancet, *2*:488, 1961.

Santen, R. J., deKretser, D. M., Paulsen, C. A., and Vorhees, J.: Gonadotrophins and testosterone in the XYY syndrome. Lancet, *2*:371, 1970.

Skakkebaek, N. E., Zeuthen, E., Nielsen, J., and Yde, H.: Abnormal spermatogenesis in XYY males: A report on 4 cases ascertained through a population study. Fertil. Steril., *24*:390, 1973.

Stenchever, M. C., and MacIntyre, M. N.: A normal XYY man. Lancet, *1*:680, 1969.

Walzer, S., and Gerald, P. S.: Social class and frequency of XYY and XXY. Science, *190*:1228, 1976.

Zeuthen, E., Nielsen, J., and Yde, H.: XYY males found in a general male population. Hereditas, *74*:283, 1973.

Miscellaneous Chromosomal Abnormalities

Campbell, W. A., Lowther, J., McKenzie, I. and Price, W. H.: Serum gonadotropins in Down's syndrome. J. Med. Genetics, *19*:98, 1982.

Hembree, W. C., Jagiello, G., Fang, J. F., and Romas, N. A.: Male reproductive dysfunction and germ cell chromosomes (Abstract No. 291). 58th Annual Meeting of The Endocrine Society, San Francisco, June 1976.

Hulten, M., Eliasson, R., and Tillinger, K. G.: Low chiasma count and other meiotic irregularities in two infertile 46, XY men with spermatogenic arrest. Hereditas, 65:285, 1970.

Kjessler, B.: Chromosomal constitution and male reproductive failure. In Mancini, R. E., and Martini, L. (Eds.): Male Fertility and Sterility, New York, Academic Press, 1974, p. 231.

Pearson, P. L., Ellis, J. D., and Evans, H. J.: A gross reduction in chiasma formation during meiotic prophase and a defective DNA repair mechanism associated with a case of human male infertility. Cytogenetics, 9:460, 1970.

Plymate, S. R., Bremner, W. J., and Paulsen, C. A.: The association of D-group chromosomal translocations and defective spermatogenesis. Fertil. Steril., 27:139, 1976.

Sarto, G. E., and Therman, E.: Large translocation t(3q − ;4p +) as probable cause of semisterility. Fertil. Steril., 27:784, 1976.

Skakkebaek, N. E., Bryant, J. I., and Philip, J.: Studies on meiotic chromosomes in infertile men and controls with normal karyotypes. J. Reprod. Fertil., 35:23, 1973.

Swerzie, S., Hueckel, J., Hudson, B., and Paulsen, C. A.: Endocrine, histologic and genetic features of the hypogonadism in patients with Down's syndrome. Abstract 440. 51st Annual Meeting of The Endocrine Society, San Francisco, 1971.

Cryptorchidism

Alpert, F., and Klein, R. S.: Spermatogenesis in the unilateral cryptorchid testis after orchiopexy. J. Urol., 129:301, 1983.

Bar-Maor, J. A., Nissan, S., Lernau, O. Z., Oren, M., and Levy, E.: Orchidopexy in cryptorchidism assessed by clinical histologic and sperm examinations. Surg. Gynecol. Obstet., 148:855, 1979.

Charny, C. W.: The spermatogenic potential of the undescended testis before and after treatment. J. Urol., 83:697, 1960.

Eldrup J., and Steven, K.: Influence of orchidopexy for cryptorchidism on subsequent fertility. Br. J. Surg., 67:269, 1980.

Ewing, L. L., and Schanbacher, L. M.: Early effects of experimental cryptorchidism on the activity of selected enzymes in rat testis. Endocrinology. 87:129, 1970.

Hadziselimovic, F.: Cryptorchidism ultrastructure of normal and cryptorchid testis development. Adv. Anat. Embryol. Cell Biol., 53:3, 1977.

Harrison, R. G., Lewis-Jones, D. I., Moreno De Marval, M. J., and Connolly, R. C.: Mechanism of damage to the contralateral testis in rats with an ischaemic testis. Lancet, 2:723, 1981.

Hedinger, C. H. R.: Histological data in cryptorchidism: Cryptorchidism, diagnosis and treatment. Pediatr. Adolesc. Endocrinol., 6:3, 1979.

Hoschoian, J. C., and Andrada, J. A.: Androgen biosynthesis in experimental cryptorchidism. Fertil. Steril., 26:730, 1975.

Jégou, B., Risbridger, G. P., and de Kretser, D. M.: Effects of experimental cryptorchidism on testicular function in adult rats. J. Androl., 4:88, 1983.

Johnston, J. H.: The undescended testis. Arch. Dis. Child., 40:113, 1965.

Laron, Z., Dickerson, Z., Prager-Lewin, R., Keret, R., and Halabe, E.: Plasma LH and FSH response to LRH in boys with compensatory testicular hypertrophy. J. Clin. Endocrinol., 40:977, 1975.

Laron, Z., and Zilka, E.: Compensatory hypertrophy of testicle in unilateral cryptorchidism. J. Clin. Endocrinol., 29:1409, 1969.

Lipshultz, L. I.: Cryptorchidism in the subfertile male. Fertil. Steril., 27:609, 1976.

Lipshultz, L. I., Caminos-Torres, R., Greenspan, C., and Snyder, P. J.: Testicular function after unilateral orchiopexy. N. Engl. J. Med., 295:15, 1976.

MacLeod, J., and Hotchkiss, R. S.: The effect of hyperpyrexia upon spermatozoa counts in men. Endocrinology, 28:780, 1941.

Mininberg, D. T., Rodger, J. C., and Bedford, J. M.: Ultrastructural evidence of the onset of testicular pathological conditions in the cryptorchid human testis within the first year of life. J. Urol. 128:782, 1982.

Rivarola, M. A., Bergada, C., and Cullen, M.: HCG stimulation test in prepubertal boys with cryptorchidism, in bilateral anorchia and in male pseudohermaphroditism. J. Clin. Endocrinol., 31:526, 1970.

Scorer, C. G., and Farrington, G. H.: Congenital deformities of the testis and epididymis. London, Butterworth and Co., 1971.

Sohval, A. R.: Histopathology of cryptorchidism. Am. J. Med., 16:346, 1954.

Steinberger, E., and Dixon, W. J.: Some observations on the effect of heat on the testicular germinal epithelium. Fertil. Steril., 10:578, 1959.

Swerdloff, R. S., Walsh, P. C., Jacobs, H. S., and Odell, W. D.: Serum LH and FSH during sexual maturation in the male rat: Effect of castration and cryptorchidism. Endocrinology, 88:120, 1970.

Varicocele

Ahlberg, N. E., Bartley, O., Chidekel, N., and Fritjofson, A.: Phlebography in varicocele scroti. Acta Radiol., 4:517, 1966.

Brown, J. S.: Varicocelectomy in the subfertile male: a ten-year experience with 295 cases. Fertil. Steril., 27:1046, 1976.

Brown, J. S., Dubin, L., and Hotchkiss, R. S.: Venography in the subfertile male with varicocele. J. Urol., 98:388, 1967.

Cockett, A. T. K., Urry, R. L., and Dougherty, K. A.: The varicocele and semen characteristics. J. Urol., 121:435, 1979.

Comhaire, F., and Vermeulen, A.: Varicocele sterility: Cortisol and catecholamines. Fertil. Steril., 25:88, 1974.

Davidson, H. A.: Treatment of male subfertility: Testicular temperature and varicoceles. Practitioner, 173:703, 1954.

Dubin, L., and Amelar, R. D.: Varicocelectomy: 986 cases in a twelve-year study. Urology, 10:446, 1977.

Dubin, L., and Amelar, R. D.: Varicocelectomy as therapy in male infertility: A study of 504 cases. Fertil. Steril., 26:217, 1975.

Dubin, L., and Hotchkiss, R. S.: Testis biopsy in subfertile man with varicocele. Fertil. Steril., 20:50, 1969.

Etriby, A., Girgis, S. M., Hefnawy, H., and Ibrahim, A. A.: Testicular changes in subfertile males with varicocele. Fertil. Steril., 18:666, 1967.

Etriby, A., Ibrahim, A. A., Mahmoud, Z. K., and Elhaggar, S.: Subfertility and varicocele I. Venogram demonstration of anastomosis sites in subfertile men. Fertil. Steril., 26:1013, 1975.

Getzoff, P. L.: Surgical management of male infertility: Results of a survey. Fertil. Steril., 24:553, 1973.

Gonzalez, R., Narayan, P., Castaneda-Zuniga, W. R., and Amplatz, K.: Transvenous embolization of the internal spermatic veins for the treatment of varicocele scroti. Urol. Clin. North Am., 9:177, 1982.

Hanley, H. G., and Harrison, R. G.: Nature and surgical treatment of varicocele. Br. J. Surg., *50*:64, 1962.

Johnson, D. E., Pohl, D. R., and Rivera-Correa, H.: Varicocele: An innocuous condition. South. Med. J., *63*:34, 1970.

Kaufman, S. L., Kadir, S., Barth, K. H., Smyth, J. W., Walsh, P. C., and White, R. I.: Mechanisms of recurrent varicocele after balloon occlusion or surgical ligation of the internal spermatic vein. Radiology, *147*:435, 1983.

Lome, L. G., and Ross, L.: Varicocelectomy and infertility. Urology, *9*:416, 1977.

MacLeod, J.: Further observations on the role of varicocele in human male infertility. Fertil. Steril., *20*:545, 1969.

MacLeod, J.: Seminal cytology in the presence of varicocele. Fertil. Steril., *16*:735, 1965.

Macomber, D., and Sanders, M. M.: The spermatozoa count. N. Engl. J. Med., *200*:981, 1929.

McFadden, M. R., and Mehan, D. J.: Testicular biopsies in 101 cases of varicocele. J. Urol., *119*:372, 1978.

Mehan, D. J.: Results of ligation of internal spermatic vein in the treatment of infertility in azoospermic patients. Fertil. Steril., *27*:110, 1976.

Newton, R., Schinfeld, J. S., and Schiff, I.: The effect of varicocelectomy on sperm count, motility and conception rate. Fertil. Steril., *34*:250, 1980.

Nilsson, S., Edvinsson, A., and Nilsson, B.: Improvement of semen and pregnancy rate after ligation and division of the internal spermatic vein: Fact or fiction? Br. J. Urol., *51*:591, 1979.

Riedl, P., Lunglmayr, G., Stackl, W.: A new method of transfemoral testicular vein obliteration for varicocele using a balloon catheter. Radiology, *139*:323, 1981.

Rodriguez-Rigau, L. J., Weiss, D. B., Zuckerman, Z., Grotjan, H. E., Smith, K. D., and Steinberger, E.: A possible mechanism for the detrimental effect of varicocele on testicular function in man. Fertil. Steril., *30*:577, 1978.

Russell, J. K.: Varicocele in groups of fertile and subfertile men. Proc. Soc. Study Fertil., *4*:31, 1953.

Saypol, D. C.: Varicocele. J. Androl., *2*:61, 1981.

Saypol, D. C., Howards, S. S., Turner, T. T., and Miller, E. D., Jr.: Influence of surgically induced varicocele on testicular blood flow, temperature, and histology in adult rats and dogs. J. Clin. Invest., *68*:39, 1981.

Saypol, D. C., Lipshultz, L. I., and Howards, S. S.: Varicocele. *In* Lipshultz, L. I., and Howards, S. S. (Eds.): Infertility in the Male. New York, Churchill Livingstone, 1983.

Scott, L. S., and Young, D. L.: Varicocele: A combined study of its effects on human spermatogenesis and on results produced by spermatic ligation. Fertil. Steril., *13*:325, 1962.

Seyferth, W., Jecht, E., and Zeitler, E.: Percutaneous sclerotherapy of varicocele. Radiology, *139*:335, 1981.

Stewart, B. H.: Varicocele in infertility. Incidence and results of surgical therapy. J. Urol., *112*:222, 1974.

Swerdloff, R. S., and Walsh, P. C.: Pituitary and gonadal hormones in patients with varicocele. Fertil. Steril., *26*:1006, 1975.

Tulloch, W. S.: Consideration of sterility factors in light of subsequent pregnancies. Edinburgh Med. J., *59*:29, 1952.

Tulloch, W. S.: Varicocele in subfertility: results of treatment. Br. Med. J., *2*:356, 1955.

Walsh, P. C., and White, R. I., Jr.: Balloon occlusion of the internal spermatic vein for the treatment of varicoceles. J.A.M.A., *246*:1701, 1981.

Wilhelm, S. F.: Sterility in the male. *In* Burghard, F. F., and Kanavel, A. B. (Eds.): Oxford Loose Leaf Surgery. New York, Oxford University Press, 1937, p. 746.

Zorgniotti, A., and MacLeod, J.: Studies in temperature, human semen quality and varicocele. Fertil. Steril., *24*:854, 1973.

Ductal Obstruction, Ejaculatory Disturbances

Amelar, R. D., and Hotchkiss, R. S.: Congenital aplasia of the epididymides and vas deferentia: Effects on semen. Fertil. Steril., *14*:44, 1963.

Andaloro, V. A., Jr., and Dube, A.: Treatment of retrograde ejaculation with brompheniramine. Urology, *5*:520, 1975.

Baillie, A. H.: Observations comparing the effects of epididymal obstruction at various levels on the mouse testis with those of ischaemia. J. Anat., *96*:335, 1962.

Beach, E. W.: Genital manifestation in early filariasis. J. Urol., *59*:371, 1948.

Charny, C. W., and Gillenwater, J. Y.: Congenital absence of the vas deferens. J. Urol., *93*:399, 1965.

Dubin, L., and Amelar, R. D.: Etiologic factors in 1294 consecutive cases of male infertility. Fertil. Steril., *22*:496, 1971.

Green, L. F., and Kelalis, P. P.: Retrograde ejaculation of semen due to diabetic neuropathy. J. Urol. *98*:693, 1968.

Handelsman, D. J., Conway, A. J., Boylan, L. M., and Turtle, J. R.: Young's syndrome: Obstructive azoospermia and chronic sinopulmonary infections. N. Engl. J. Med., *310*:3, 1984.

Harrison, R. G.: The effect of ligation of the vasa efferentia on the rat testis. Proc. Soc. Stud. Fertil., *5*:95, 1953.

Horan, A. H.: When and why does occlusion of the vas deferens affect the testes. Fertil. Steril., *26*:317, 1975.

Hotchkiss, R. S., Pento, A. B., and Kleegman, S.: Artificial insemination with semen recovered from the bladder. Fertil. Steril., *6*:37, 1955.

Johnsonbaugh, R. E., O'Connell, K., Engel, S. B., Edson, M., and Sode, J.: Plasma testosterone, luteinizing hormone and follicle-stimulating hormone after vasectomy. Fertil. Steril., *26*:329, 1975.

Kaplan, E., Schwachman, H., Perlmutter, A. D., Rule, A., Khan, K. T., and Holschaw, D.: Reproductive failure in males with cystic fibrosis. N. Engl. J. Med. *279*:65, 1968.

Keiserman, W. M., Dubin, L., and Amelar, R. D.: A new type of retrograde ejaculation: Report of three cases. Fertil. Steril., *25*:1071, 1974.

Lattimer, J. R., Colmore, H. P., Sanger, G., Robertson, D. H., and McLellan, F. C.: Transmission of genital tuberculosis from husband to wife via semen. Am. Rev. Tuberc., *69*:618, 1954.

Martin, D. E., Warner, H., Crenshaw, T. L., Crenshaw, R. T., Shapiro, C. E., and Perkash, I.: Initiation of erection and semen release by rectal probe electrostimulation (RPE). J. Urol., *129*:637, 1983.

McLachlan, J. A., Newbold, R. R., and Bullock, B.: Reproductive tract lesions in male mice exposed prenatally to diethylstilbestrol. Science. *190*:991, 1975.

Nijman, J. M., Jager, S., Boer, P. W., Kremer, J., Oldhoff, J., and Koops, H. S.: The treatment of ejaculation disorders after retroperitoneal lymph node dissection. Cancer, *50*:2967, 1982.

Obrant, K. O., and Lindquist, S.: Fertility after chemotherapy im male patients with genital tuberculosis. Fertil. Steril., *15*:440, 1964.

Proctor, K. G., and Howards, S. S.: The effect of sympathomimetic drugs on postlymphadenectomy aspermia. J. Urol., *129*:837, 1983.

Rosemberg, E., Marks, S. G., Howard, P. J., and James, L. D.: Serum levels of follicle stimulating and luteinizing hormones before and after vasectomy in men. J. Urol., *111*:626, 1974.

Scammell, G. E., Stedronska, J., and Dempsey, A.: Successful pregnancies using human serum albumin following retrograde ejaculation: A case report. Fertil. Steril., *37*:277, 1982.

Scorer, C. G., and Farrington, G. H.: Congenital Deformities of the Testis and Epididymis. London, Butterworth and Co., 1971.

Smith, K. D., Tcholakian, R. K., Chowdury, M., and Steinberger, E.: An investigation of plasma hormone levels before and after vasectomy. Fertil. Steril., *27*:145, 1976.

Stewart, B. H., and Bergant, J. A.: Correction of retrograde ejaculation by sympathomimetic medication: Preliminary report. Fertil. Steril., *25*:1073, 1974.

Taussig, L. M., Lobeck, C. C., Di Sant'Agnese, P. A., Ackerman, D. R., and Kattwinkel, J.: Fertility in males with cystic fibrosis. N. Engl. J. Med., *287*:586, 1972.

Thiagarajah, S., Vaughan, E. D., Jr., and Kitchin, J. D., III: Retrograde ejaculation: Successful pregnancy following combined sympathomimetic medication and insemination. Fertil. Steril., *30*:96, 1978.

Walters, D., and Kaufman, M. S.: Sterility due to retrograde ejaculation of semen. Report of pregnancy by autoinsemination. Am. J. Obstet. Gynecol., *78*:274, 1959.

Whitelaw, J. P., and Smithwick, R. H.: Some secondary effects of sympathectomy with particular reference to disturbances of sexual function. N. Engl. J. Med., *245*:121, 1951.

Drugs and Toxins

Auerbach, C.: Mutagenic effects of alkylating agents. Ann. N.Y. Acad. Sci., *68*:731, 1958.

Badr, F. M., Bartke, A., Dalterio, S. et al.: Suppression of testosterone production by ethyl alcohol: Possible mode of action. Steroids, *30*:647, 1977.

Baker, H. W. G., Burger, H. G., de Kretser, D. M., et al.: A study of the endocrine manifestations of hepatic cirrhosis. Q. J. Med., *177*:145, 1976.

Bertello, P., Gurillo, L., Faggiuolo, R., Veglio, F., Tamagnone, C., and Angeli, A.: Effect of ethanol infusion on the pituitary-testicular responsiveness to gonadotropin releasing hormone and thyrotropin releasing hormone in normal males and in chronic alcoholics presenting with hypogonadism. J. Endocrinol. Invest., *6*:413, 1983.

Berthelsen, J. G., and Skakkebaek, N. E.: Gonadal function in men with testis cancer. Fertil. Steril., *39*:68, 1983.

Blatt, J., Poplack, D. G., and Sherins, R. J.: Testicular function in boys after chemotherapy for acute lymphoblastic leukemia. N. Engl. J. Med., *304*:1121, 1981.

Booth, J. D., and Loriaux, D. L.: Selective control of follicle stimulating hormone secretion: New perspectives. *In* D'Agata, R. et al. (Eds): Recent Advances in Male Reproduction: Molecular Basis and Clinical Implications. New York, Raven Press, 1983, pp. 269–277.

Brauner, R., Czernichow, P., Cramer, P., Schaison, G., and Rappaport, R.: Leydig cell function in children after direct testicular irradiation for acute lymphoblastic leukemia. N. Engl. J. Med., *309*:25, 1983.

Bremner, W. J., and Paulsen, C. A.: Colchicine and testicular function in man. N. Engl. J. Med., *295*:1384, 1976.

Bruce, W. R., Furrer, R., and Wyrobek, A. J.: Abnormalities in the shape of murine sperm after acute testicular x-irradiation. Mutat. Res., *23*:381, 1974.

Chapman, R. M., Sutcliffe, S. B., and Malpas, J. S. Male gonadal dysfunction in Hodgkin's disease. J.A.M.A., *245*:1323, 1981.

Chopra, T. J., Tulchinsky, D., and Greenway, F. L.: Estrogen-androgen imbalance in men with hepatic cirrhosis. Ann. Intern. Med., *79*:198, 1973.

Clifton, D. K., and Bremner, W. J.: The effect of testicular x-irradiation on spermatogenesis in man: A comparison with the mouse. J. Androl., *4*:387, 1983.

Cosgrove, M. D., Benton, B., and Henderson, B. E.: Male genitourinary abnormalities and maternal diethylstilbestrol. J. Urol., *117*:220, 1977.

Fairly, K. F., Barrie, J. A., and Johnson, W.: Sterility and testicular atrophy related to cyclophosphamide therapy. Lancet, *1*:568, 1972.

Gill, W. B., Schumacher, G. F. B., and Bibbo, M.: Structural and functional abnormalities in the sex organs of male offspring of mothers treated with diethylstilbestrol (DES). J. Reprod. Med., *16*:147, 1976.

Glass, R. J., Hyness, R. N., Mengle, D. C., Powell, K. E., and Kahn, E.: Sperm count depression in pesticide applicators exposed to dibromochloropropane. Am J. Epidemiol., *109*:346, 1979.

Gordon, C. G., Altman, K., Southern, A. L., Rubin, E., and Lieber, C. S.: Effect of alcohol (ethanol) administration on sex-hormone metabolism in normal men. N. Engl. J. Med., *295*:793, 1976.

Gordon, G. G., Vittek, J., Southern, A. L., Munnangi, P., and Lieber, C. S.: Effect of chronic alcohol ingestion on the biosynthesis of steroids in the rat testicular homogenate in vitro. Endocrinology, *106*:1880, 1980.

Harmon, J., and Aliapoulios, M. A.: Gynecomastia in marihuana users. N. Engl. J. Med., *287*:936, 1972.

Hembree, W. C., Zeidenberg, P., and Nahas, G.: Marihuana effects on human gonadal function. *In* Nahas, G., Poton, W. D. M., and Idanpaan-Heittila, J. (Eds.): Marihuana: Chemistry, Biochemistry and Cellular Effects. New York, Springer Verlag, Inc., 1976, pp. 521–532.

Herbst, A. L., Poskanzer, D. C., Robboy, S. J., Friedlander, L., and Schully, R. E.: Prenatal exposure to stilbestrol (a prospective comparison of exposed female offspring with unexposed controls) N. Engl. J. Med., *292*:334, 1975.

Kinsella, T. J., Fraass, B. A., and Glatstein, E.: Late effects of radiation therapy in the treatment of Hodgkin's disease. Cancer Treat. Rep. *66*:991, 1982.

Kolodny, R. C., Masters, W. H., Kolodny, R. M., and Toro, G.: Depression of plasma testosterone levels after chronic intensive marihuana use. N. Engl. J. Med., *290*:872, 1974.

Lantz, G., Cunningham, G. R., Huckins, C., et al.: Recovery from severe oligospermia after exposure to dibromochloropropane. Fertil. Steril., *35*:46, 1981.

Lipshultz, L. I., Ross, C. E., Whorton, D., et al.: Dibromochloropropane and its effects on testicular function in man. J. Urol., *124*:464, 1980.

MacLeod, J.: Studies in human spermatogenesis: The effect of certain anti-spermatogenic compounds. Anat. Rec., *139*:250, 1961.

Maugh, T. H.: Marihuana: New support for immune and reproductive hazards. Science, *190*:865, 1975.

McLachlan, J. A.: Rodent models for perinatal exposure to diethylstilbestrol and their relation to human disease in the male. *In* Herbst, A. L., and Bern, H. A. (Eds.): Developmental Effects of Diethylstilbestrol (DES) in Pregnancy. New York. Thieme-Stratton, Inc., 1981, pp. 148–157.

McLachlan, J. A., Newbold, R. R., and Bullock, B.: Reproductive tract lesions in male mice exposed prenatally to diethylstilbestrol. Science, *190*:991, 1975.

Meistrich, M. L., Finch, M., da Cunha, M. F., Hacher, U., and Au, W. W.: Damaging effects of fourteen chemotherapeutic drugs on mouse testis cells. Cancer, 42:122, 1982.

Mendelson, J. H., Kuehnle, J., Ellingboe, J., and Babor, T. F.: Plasma testosterone levels before, during and after chronic marihuana smoking. N. Engl. J. Med., 291:1051, 1974.

Mendelson, J. H., Mello, N. K., and Ellingboe, J.: Effects of acute alcohol intake on pituitary-gonadal hormones in normal human males. J. Pharmacol. Exp. Ther., 202:676, 1977.

Milby, T. H., and Whorton, D.: Epidemiological assessment of occupationally related, chemically induced sperm count suppression. J. Occup. Med., 22:77, 1980.

Nahas, G. G.: Marihuana. J.A.M.A., 233:79, 1975.

Nelson, W. O., and Bunge, R. G.: The effect of therapeutic dosages of nitrofurantoin upon spermatogenesis in man. J. Urol., 77:275, 1957.

Paulsen, C. A.: The study of radiation effects on the human testis: Including histologic, chromosomal and hormonal aspects. Final Progress Report AEC Contract AT (45-1)-2225, Task Agreement 6 RLO-2225-2, 1973.

Pennisi, A. J., Gruskin, C. M., and Lieberman, E.: Gonadal function in children with nephrosis treated with cyclophosphamide. Am. J. Dis. Child., 129:315, 1975.

Richter, P., Calamera, J. C., Morgenfeld, M. C., Kierszenbaum, A. L., Lavieri, J. C., and Mancini, R. E.: Effect of chlorambucil on spermatogenesis in the human with malignant lymphoma. Cancer, 25:1026, 1970.

Rowley, M. J., Leach, D. R., Warner, G. A., and Heller, C. G.: Effect of graded doses of ionizing radiation on the human testis. Radiat. Res., 59:665, 1974.

Sanderman, R. F.: The effects of irradiation on male human fertility. Br. J. Radiol., 39:901, 1966.

Schilsky, R. L., and Sherins, R. J.: Gonadal dysfunction. In De Vita, V., et al. (Eds.): Principles and Practice of Oncology. Philadelphia, J. B. Lippincott Co., 1985, pp. 1713–1717.

Shamberger, R. C., Rosenberg, S. A., Seipp, C. A., and Sherins, R. J.: The effects of high dose methotrexate and vincristine on ovarian and testicular functions in patients undergoing postoperative adjuvant treatment for osteosarcoma. Cancer Treat. Rep., 65:739, 1981a.

Shamberger, R. C., Sherins, R. J., and Rosenberg, S. A.: The effects of postoperative adjuvant chemotherapy and radiotherapy on testicular function in men undergoing treatment for soft-tissue sarcoma. Cancer, 47:2368, 1981b.

Shapiro, E., Kinsella, R. J., Fraass, B. A., Rosenberg, S. A., and Sherins, R. J.: The effects of fractionated irradiation on testicular function. Abstr. Am. Urol. Assoc., New Orleans, April 1984.

Sherins, R. J., and DeVita, V. T., Jr.: Effect of drug treatment for lymphoma on male reproductive capacity: Studies of men in remission after therapy. Ann. Intern. Med., 79:216, 1973.

Sherins, R. J., Olweny, C. L. M., and Ziegler, J. L.: Gynecomastia and gonadal dysfunction in adolescent boys treated with combination chemotherapy for Hodgkin's disease. N. Engl. J. Med., 299:12, 1978.

Sieber, S. M., and Adamson, R. H.: Toxicity of antineoplastic agents in man: Chromosomal aberrations, antifertility effects, congenital malformations and carcinogenic potential. Adv. Cancer Res., 22:57, 1975.

Speiser, B., Rubin, P., and Casarett, G.: Aspermia following lower truncal irradiation in Hodgkin's disease. Cancer, 32:692, 1973.

Spitz, S.: The histological effects of nitrogen mustard on human tumors and tissues. Cancer, 1:383, 1948.

Steinberger, E., et al.: A radiomimetic effect of triethylenemalamine on reproduction in the male rat. Endocrinology, 65:40, 1959.

Steinberger, E., and Nelson, W. D.: The effect of furadroxyl treatment and x-irradiation on the hyaluronidase concentration of rat testes. Endocrinology, 60:105, 1957.

Toth, A.: Reversible toxic effect of salicylazosulfapyridene on semen quality. Fertil. Steril., 31:538, 1979.

Van Thiel, D. H., Gavaler, J. S., Smith, W. J., et al.: Hypothalamic-pituitary-gonadal dysfunction in men using cimetidine. N. Engl. J. Med., 300:1012, 1979.

Van Thiel, D. H., Lester, R., and Sherins, R. J.: Hypogonadism in alcoholic liver disease: Evidence for a double defect. Gastroenterology, 67:1188, 1974.

Van Thiel, D. H., Sherins, R. J., Meyers, G. H., Jr., and DeVita, V. T., Jr.: Evidence for a specific seminiferous tubular factor affecting FSH secretion in man. J. Clin. Invest., 51:1009, 1971.

Waxman, J. H., Terry, Y. A., Wrigley, P. F. M., Maplas, J. S., Rees, L. H., Besser, G. M., and Lister, T. A.: Gonadal function in Hodgkin's disease: Long-term follow-up of chemotherapy. Br. Med. J., 285:1612, 1982.

Whitehead, E. D., and Leiter, E.: Genital abnormalities and abnormal semen analyses in male patients exposed to diethylstilbestrol in utero. J. Urol., 125:47, 1981.

Whitehead, E., Shalet, S. M., Blackledge, G., Todd, I., Crowther, D., and Beardwell, C. G.: The effects of Hodgkin's disease and combination chemotherapy on gonadal function in the adult male. Cancer, 49:418, 1982.

Wyrobek, A. J., and Bruce, W. R.: Chemical induction of sperm abnormalities in mice. Proc. Natl. Acad. Sci. U.S.A., 72:4425, 1975.

Ylikahri, R., Huttunen, M., Harkonen, M., et al.: Low plasma testosterone values in men during hangover. J. Steroid Biochem., 5:655, 1974.

Systemic Illness

Chopp, T. R., and Mendez, N.: Sexual function and hormonal abnormalities in uremic men on chronic dialysis and after renal transplantation. Fertil. Steril., 29:661, 1978.

Elstein, M., Smith, E. K. M., and Curtis, J. R.: Reproductive potential of patients treated by maintenance hemodialysis. Br. Med. J., 2:734, 1969.

Feldman, H. A., and Singer, I.: Endocrinology and metabolism in uremia and dialysis: A clinical review. Medicine, 54:345, 1975.

Guevara, A., Vidt, D., Hallberg, M. C., Zorn, E. M., Pohlman, C., and Wieland, R. G.: Serum gonadotropin and testosterone levels in uremic males undergoing intermittent dialysis. Metabolism, 18:1062, 1969.

Holdsworth, S., Atkins, R. C., and de Kretser, D. M.: The pituitary-testicular axis in men with chronic renal failure. N. Engl. J. Med., 296:1245, 1977.

Lin, V. S., and Fang, V. S.: Gonadal dysfunction in uremic men. A study of the hypothalamic-pituitary-testicular axis before and after renal transplantation. Am. J. Med., 58:655, 1975.

MacLeod, J.: Human seminal cytology as a sensitive indicator of the germinal epithelium. Int. J. Fertil., 9:281, 1964.

MacLeod, J.: The Clinical Implications of Deviations in Human Spermatogenesis as Evidenced in Seminal Cytology and the Experimental Production of These Deviations. In Proceedings of the 5th World Congress on Fertility and Sterility, Stockholm, 1966. Excerpta Medica Int. Congress Series 133. Princeton, N.J., Excerpta Medica Foundation, 1966.

MacLeod, J., and Hotchkiss, R. S.: The effect of hyperpyrexia upon spermatozoa counts in men. Endocrinology, *28*:780, 1941.

Sherins, R. J.: Clinical aspects of treatment of male infertility with gonadotropins: Testicular response of some men given hCG with and without Pergonal. *In* Mancini, R. E., and Martini, L. (Eds.): Proceedings of the Serono Symposium on Male Fertility and Sterility. Vol. 5. New York, Academic Press, 1974, pp. 545–565.

Steinberger, E., and Dixon, W. J.: Some observations on the effect of heat on the testicular germinal epithelium. Fertil. Steril., *10*:578, 1959.

Swerdloff, R. S., Kantor, G., and Korenman, S. G.: Gonadotropin dissociation in uremic gynecomastia: High plasma LH, low FSH and normal estradiol. Clin. Res., *18*:172, 1970.

Abnormal Morphology and Sperm Function

Afzelius, B. A.: A human syndrome caused by immotile cilia. Science, *193*:317, 1976.

Anton-Lamprecht, I., Kotzur, B., and Schopp, E.: Round-headed human spermatozoa. Fertil. Steril., *27*:685, 1976.

Bouchard, P., Gagnon, C., Phillips, D. M., and Bardin, C. W.: The localization of protein carboxyl methylase in sperm tails. J. Cell Biol., *86*:417, 1980.

Castaneda, E., Bouchard, P., Saling, P., Phillips, D., Gagnon, C., and Bardin, C. W.: Endogenous protein carboxyl methylation in hamster spermatozoa: Changes associated with capacitation in vitro. Int. J. Androl., *6*: 482, 1983.

de Lamirande, E., Bardin, C. W., and Gagnon, C.: Aprotinin and a seminal plasma factor inhibit the motility of demembranated reactivated rabbit spermatozoa. Biol. Reprod., *28*:788, 1983.

de Lamirande, E., and Gagnon, C.: Origin of a motility inhibitor within the male reproductive tract. J. Androl. *5*:269, 1984.

Ebasson, R., Mossberg, B., Conner, P., and Afzelius, B. A.: The immotile-cilia syndrome. A congenital ciliary abnormality as etiologic factor in chronic airway infections and male sterility. N. Engl. J. Med., *297*:1, 1977.

Gagnon, C., Sherins, R. J., Phillips, D. M., and Bardin, C. W.: Deficiency of protein carboxyl methylase in immotile spermatozoa in infertile men. N. Engl. J. Med., *306*:821, 1982.

Pederson, H., and Rebbe, H.: Absence of arms in the axoneme of immobile human spermatozoa. Biol. Reprod., *12*:541, 1975.

Pederson, H., Rebbe, H., and Hammen, R.: Human sperm fine structure in a case of severe asthenospermia-necrospermia. Fertil. Steril., *22*:156, 1971.

Genital Tract Infections

Ballew, J. W., and Masters, W. H.: Mumps: A cause of infertility. Fertil. Steril., *5*:536, 1954.

Beard, C. M., Benson, R. C., Kelalis, P. P., Elveback, L. R., and Kurland, L. T .: The incidence of mumps orchitis in Rochester, Minnesota, 1935 to 1974. Mayo Clinic Proc., *52*:3, 1977.

Centifano, V. M., Drylie, D. M., Deardourff, S. L., and Kaufman, H. E.: Herpes virus type 2 in the male genito-urinary tract. Science, *178*:318, 1972.

Chakravarty, S. C., Sirear, D. K., and Majumdar, P. R.: Genital tuberculosis in males. Seminal fluid culture and vaso-seminal vesiculography studies. J. Indian Med. Assoc., *5*:283, 1968.

Couture, M., Ulstein, M., Leonard, J. M., and Paulsen, C. A.: Improved staining method for differentiating immature germ cells from white blood cells in human seminal fluid. Andrologia, *8*:61, 1976.

De Louvois, J., Harrison, R. F., Blades, M., Hurley, R., and Stanley, V. C.: Frequency of mycoplasma in fertile and infertile couples. Lancet, *1*:1073, 1974.

Fowler, J. E., and Kessler, R.: Genital tract infections. *In* Lipshultz, L. I., and Howards, S. S. (Eds.): Infertility in the Male. New York, Churchill Livingstone, 1983, pp. 283–298.

Friberg, J., and Gnarpe, H.: Mycoplasma infections and infertility. *In* Mancini, R. E., and Martini, L. (Eds.): Male Fertility and Sterility. Proceedings of the Serono Symposia. Vol. 5, pp. 327–335. New York, Academic Press, 1974.

Gump, D. W., Gibson, M., and Ashikaga, T.: Lack of association between genital mycoplasmas and infertility. N. Engl. J. Med., *310*:937, 1984.

Harrison, R. F., De Louvois, J., Blades, M., and Hurley, R.: Doxycycline treatment and human infertility. Lancet, *1*:605, 1975.

Holmes, K. K., Handsfield, H. H., Wang, S. P., Wentworth, B. B., Turck, M., Anderson, J. B., and Alexander, E. R.: Etiology of nongonococcal urethritis. N. Engl. J. Med., *292*:199, 1975.

Lang, D. J., and Kummer, J. F.: Demonstration of cytomegalovirus in semen. N. Engl. J. Med., *287*:756, 1972.

McKendrick, G. D. W., and Nishtar, T.: Mumps orchitis and sterility. Public Health, *80*:277, 1976.

Stamey, T. A., Govan, D. E., and Palmer, J. E.: The localization and treatment of urinary tract infections: The role of bacteriocidal urine levels as opposed to serum levels. Medicine, *44*:1, 1965.

Taylor-Rubinson, D., and McComark, W. M.: Medical progress: the genital mycoplasmas (second of two parts). N. Engl. J. Med., *302*:1063, 1980.

Toth, A., Lesser, M. L., Brooks, C., and Labriola, D.: Subsequent pregnancies among 161 couples treated for T-mycoplasma genital tract infection. N. Engl. J. Med., *308*:505, 1983.

Ulstein, M., Capell, P., Holmes, K. K., and Paulsen, C. A.: Nonsymptomatic genital tract infection and male infertility. *In* Hafez, E. S. E. (Ed.): Human Semen and Fertility Regulation in Men. St. Louis, C. V. Mosby Co., 1976, pp. 355–369.

Werner, C. A.: Mumps orchitis and testicular atrophy. Ann. Intern. Med., *32*:1066, 1950.

Sexual Dysfunction

Dubin, L., and Amelar, R. D.: Etiologic factors in 1294 consecutive cases of male infertility. Fertil. Steril., *22*:469, 1971.

Dubin, L., and Amelar, R. D.: Sexual causes of male infertility. Fertil. Steril., *23*:579, 1972.

Geboes, K., Steeno, O., and DeMoor, P.: Sexual potence in man. Andrologia, *7*:217, 1975.

Gordon, J. A., Amelar, R. D., Dubin, L., and Tendler, M. D.: Infertility practice and orthodox Jewish law. Fertil. Steril., *26*:480, 1975.

Levine, S. B.: Marital sexual dysfunction: Ejaculatory disturbances. Ann. Intern. Med., *84*:575, 1976.

Immunologic Disorders

Brannen, G. E., Kwart, A. M., and Coffey, D. S.: Immunologic implications of vasectomy: I. Cell mediated immunity. Fertil. Steril., *25*:508, 1974.

Fjallbrant, B.: Interrelation between high levels of sperm antibodies, reduced penetration of cervical mucus by spermatozoa, and sterility in men. Acta Obstet. Gynecol. Scand., *47*:102, 1968.

Haas, G. G., Cines, D. B., and Schreiber, A. D.: Immunologic infertility: Identification of patients with anti-sperm antibody. N. Engl. J. Med., 303:722, 1981.

Halpern, B. N., Ky, T., and Robert, B.: Clinical and immunological study of an exceptional case of reaginic type sensitization to human seminal fluid. Immunology, 12:247, 1967.

Hargreave, T. B., and Elton, R. A.: Treatment with intermittent high dose methylprednisolone or intermittent betamethasone for antisperm antibodies: Preliminary communication. Fertil. Steril., 38:586, 1982.

Hekman, A., and Rumke, P. H.: The antigens of human seminal plasma with special reference to lactoferrin as a spermatozoa-coating antigen. Fertil. Steril., 20:312, 1969.

Hendry, W. F., Stedronska, J., Parslow, J., and Hughes, L.: The results of intermittent high dose steroid therapy for male infertility due to antisperm antibodies. Fertil. Steril., 36:351, 1981.

Levine, B. B., Siraganian, R. P., and Schenkein, I.: Allergy to human seminal plasma. N. Engl. J. Med., 288:894, 1973.

Mancini, R. E., Andrada, J. A., Seraceni, D., Bachman, A. E., Lavieri, J. C., and Nemirovsky, M.: Immunological and testicular response in man sensitized with human testicular homogenate. J. Clin. Endocrinol., 25:859, 1965.

Mathur, S., Baker, E. R., Williamson, H. O., Derrick, F. C., Teague, K. J., and Fudenberg, H. H.: Clinical significance of sperm antibodies in infertility. Fertil. Steril., 36:486, 1981.

Metchnikoff, E.: Études sur la resorption des cellules. Ann. Inst. Pasteur, 13:737, 1899.

Mumford, D. M., and Warner, M. R.: Male fertility and immunity. In Lipshultz, L. I., and Howards, S. S. (Eds.): Infertility in the Male. New York, Churchill Livingstone, 1983.

Phadke, A. M., and Padukone, K.: Presence and significance of autoantibodies against spermatozoa in the blood of men with obstructed vas deferens. J. Reprod. Fertil., 7:163, 1964.

Rumke, P.: Sperm agglutinating autoantibodies in relation to male infertility. Proc. R. Soc. Med., 61:275, 1968.

Rumke, P., and Hellinga, G.: Autoantibodies against spermatozoa in sterile men. Am. J. Clin. Pathol., 32:357, 1959.

Shulman, S., Harlin, B., Davis, P., et al.: Immune infertility and new approaches to treatment. Fertil. Steril., 29:309, 1978.

Shulman, J. F., and Shulman, S.: Methylprednisolone treatment of immunologic infertility in the male. Fertil. Steril., 38:591, 1982.

Witkin, S. S.: IgA antibodies to spermatozoa in seminal and prostatic fluids of the subfertile man. J.A.M.A. 247:1014, 1982.

Medical Management of Testicular Dysfunction (Androgen Deficiency, Gonadotropin Deficiency, Idiopathic Infertility)

Barwin, N. B., Clarke, S. D., Biggart, J. D., and Lamont, A.: Mesterolone in the treatment of male infertility. Practitioner, 211:669, 1973.

Belchetz, P. E., Plant, T. M., Nakai, Y., Keogh, E. J., and Knobil, E.: Hypophyseal responses to continuous and intermittent delivery of hypothalamic gonadotropin releasing hormone. Science, 202:631, 1978.

Bergada, C., and Mancini, R. E.: Effects of gonadotropins in the induction of spermatogenesis in human prepubertal testes. J. Clin. Endocrinol., 37:935, 1973.

Boccabella, A. V.: Reinitiation and restoration of spermatogenesis with testosterone propionate and other hormones after a long-term post-hypophysectomy regression period. Endocrinology, 72:787, 1963.

Booth, J. D., and Loriaux, D. L.: Selective control of follicle stimulating hormone secretion: new perspectives. In D'Agata, R., et al. (eds): Recent Advances in Male Reproduction: Molecular Basis and Clinical Implications. New York, Raven Press, 1983, pp. 269–277.

Brown, J. S.: The effect of orally administered androgens on sperm motility. Fertil. Steril., 26:305, 1975.

Buvat, J., Ardaens, K., Lemaire, A., Gauthier, A., Gasnault, J. P. and Buvat-Herbaut, M.: Increased sperm count in 25 cases of idiopathic normogonadotropic oligospermia following treatment with tamoxifen. Fertil. Steril., 39:700, 1983.

Chalmers, T. C., Celano, P., Sacks, H. S. and Smith, H.: Bias in treatment assignment in controlled clinical trials. N. Engl. J. Med., 309:1358, 1983.

Charny, C. W.: Clomiphene therapy in male infertility: A negative report. Fertil. Steril., 32:551, 1979.

Charny, C. W.: The use of androgens for human spermatogenesis. Fertil. Steril., 10:557, 1959.

Charny, C. W.: Treatment of male infertility with large doses of testosterone. J.A.M.A., 160:98, 1956.

Charny, C. W., and Gordon, J. A.: Testosterone rebound therapy: A neglected modality. Fertil. Steril., 29:64, 1978.

Check, J. H., and Rakoff, A. E.: Improved fertility in oligospermic males treated with clomiphene citrate. Fertil. Steril., 28:746, 1977.

Cheval, M. J., and Mehan, D. J.: Chorionic gonadotropins in the treatment of the subfertile male. Fertil. Steril., 31:666, 1979.

Clark, R. V., and Sherins, R. J.: Clinical trial of testolactone for treatment of idiopathic male infertility. (abstr.) J. Androl., 4:31, 1983.

Collins, J. A., Wrixon, W., Janes, L. B., and Wilson, E. H.: Treatment-independent pregnancy among infertile couples. N. Engl. J. Med., 309:1201, 1983.

Crooke, A. C., Davies, A. G., and Morris, R.: Treatment of eunuchoidal men with human chorionic gonadotropin and follicle stimulating hormone. J. Endocrinol., 42:441, 1968.

Dodson, K. S., MacNaughton, M. C., and Coutts, J. R. T.: Infertility in women with apparently ovulatory cycles I. Comparison of their plasma sex steroid and gonadotropin profiles with those in the normal cycle. Br. J. Obstet. Gynecol., 82:615, 1975.

Dvoskin, S.: Local maintenance of spermatogenesis in hypophysectomized rats with low dosages of testosterone from intratesticular pellets. Proc. Soc. Exp. Biol. Med., 54:111, 1943.

Epstein, J. A.: Clomiphene treatment in oligospermic infertile males. Fertil. Steril., 28:741, 1977.

Foss, G. L., Tindall, V. R., and Birkett, J. P.: The treatment of subfertile men with clomiphene citrate. J. Reprod. Fertil., 32:167, 1973.

Gattuccio, F., D'Alia, O., Bartolo, G. L., Orlando, G., Janni, A., Izzo, P., Canale, D., and Menchini-Fabris, G. R.: Gonadotropic therapy in men with hypogonadotropic hypogonadism. J. Androl., 5:106, 1984.

Gemzell, C., and Kjessler, B.: Treatment of infertility after partial hypophysectomy with human pituitary gonadotrophins. Lancet, 1:644, 1964.

Getzoff, P. L.: Clinical evaluation of testicular biopsy and the rebound phenomenon. Fertil. Steril., 6:465, 1955.

Giarola, A.: Effect of mesterolone on the spermatogenesis of infertile patients. In Mancini, R. E., and Martini, L. (Eds.): Male Fertility and Sterility. Proceedings of the Serono Symposia. Vol. 5, New York, Academic Press, 1974 pp. 479-495.

Granville, G. E.: Successful gonadotropin therapy of infertility in a hypopituitary man. Arch. Intern. Med., 125:1041, 1970.

Heckel, N. J., Rosso, W. A., and Kestel, L.: Spermatogenic rebound phenomenon after testosterone therapy. J. Clin. Endocrinol., 11:235, 1951.

Heller, C. G., Morse, H. C., Su, M., and Rowley, M. J.: The role of FSH, ICSH and testosterone during testicular suppression by exogenous testosterone in normal men. In Rosemberg, E., and Paulsen, C. A. (Eds.): The Human Testis, New York, Plenum Press, 1970, p. 249.

Heller, C. G., Nelson, W. O., Hill, I. B., Henderson, E., Maddock, W. O., Jungek, E. C., Paulsen, C. A., and Mortimore, G. E.: Improvement in spermatogenesis following depression of human testes with testosterone. Fertil. Steril., 1:415, 1950.

Heller, C. G., Rowley, M. J., and Heller, G. V.: Clomiphene citrate: A correlation of its effects on sperm concentration and morphology, total gonadotropins, ICSH, estrogen and testosterone excretion and testicular cytology in normal men. J. Clin. Endocrinol., 29:638, 1969.

Hoffman, A. R., and Crowley, W. F.: Induction of puberty in men by long-term pulsatile administration of low-dose gonadotropin releasing hormone. N. Engl. J. Med., 307:1237, 1982.

Homonnai, Z. T., Peled, M., and Paz, G. F.: Changes in semen, quality and fertility in response to endocrine treatment of subfertile men. Gynecol. Obstet. Invest., 9:244, 1978.

Hovatta, O., Koskimies, A. I., Ranta, T., Stenman, U. H., and Seppala, M.: Bromocriptine treatment of oligospermia: A double blind study. Clin. Endocrinol., 11:377, 1979.

Joel, C. A.: The spermiogenic rebound phenomenon and its clinical significance. Fertil. Steril., 11:384, 1960.

Johnsen, S. G.: A study of human testicular function by the use of human menopausal gonadotrophin and of human chorionic gonadotrophin in male hypogonadotrophic eunuchoidism and infantilism. Acta Endocrinol., 53:315, 1966.

Johnsen, S. G.: Maintenance of spermatogenesis induced by hMG treatment by means of continuous hCG treatment in hypogonadotropic men. Acta Endocrinol., 89:763, 1978.

Jones, G. S.: The luteal phase defect. Fertil. Steril., 27:351, 1976.

Jungck, E. C., Roy, S., Greenblatt, R. B., and Mahesh, V. B.: Effect of clomiphene citrate in spermatogenesis in the human. Fertil. Steril., 15:40, 1964.

Jungling, M. L., and Bunge, R. G.: The treatment of spermatogenic arrest with arginine. Fertil. Steril., 27:282, 1976.

Keough, E. J., Burger, H. G., de Kretser, D. M., and Hudson, B.: Nonsurgical management of male infertility. In Hafez. E. S. E. (Ed.): Human Semen and Fertility Regulation in Men. St. Louis, C. V. Mosby Co., 1976, pp. 452–463.

Lamensdorf, H., Compere, D., and Begley, G.: Testosterone rebound therapy in the treatment of male infertility. Fertil. Steril., 26:469, 1975.

Lavori, P. W., Louis, T. A., Bailar, J. C., and Polansky, M.: Designs for experiments—parallel comparisons of treatment. N. Engl. J. Med., 309:1291, 1983.

Louis, T. A., Lovori, P. W., Bailar, J. C., and Polansky, M.: Cross-over and self-controlled designs in clinical research. N. Engl. J. Med., 310:24, 1984.

Lubiez-Nawrocki, C. M.: The effects of metabolites of testosterone on the viability of hamster epididymal spermatozoa. J. Endocrinol., 58:193, 1973.

Lunenfeld, B., Mor, A., and Mani, M.: Treatment of male infertility: Human gonadotropins. Fertil. Steril., 18:581, 1967.

Lunenfeld, B., Insler, V., Katz, M., and Goldman, B.: Medical Treatment of Infertility. World Health Organization, International Reference Centre for Fertility-Promoting Agents. Tel-Hashomer. Israel, Chaim Sheba Medical Centre, 1972.

Lytton, B., and Kase, N.: Effects of human menopausal gonadotropin on a eunuchoidal male. N. Engl. J. Med., 274:1061, 1966.

Lytton, B., and Mroueh, A.: Treatment of oligospermia with urinary human menopausal gonadotropin: A preliminary report. Fertil. Steril., 17:696, 1966.

MacLeod, J.: The effects of urinary gonadotropin following hypophysectomy and in hypogonadotropic eunuchoidism. In Rosemberg, E., and Paulsen, C. A. (Eds.): The Human Testis. New York, Plenum Press, 1970, pp. 577–590.

MacLeod, J., and Gold, R. Z.: The male factor in fertility and infertility. II. Spermatozoon counts in 1000 men of known fertility and in 1000 cases of infertile marriage. J. Urol., 66:436, 1951.

MacLeod, J., Pazianos, A., and Ray, B.: The restoration of human spermatogenesis and of the reproductive tract with urinary gonadotropins following hypophysectomy. Fertil. Steril., 17:7, 1966.

Madsen, H., Andersen, O., and Hause, P.: Bromocriptine treatment for male infertility. Andrologia, 12:379, 1980.

Mancini, R. E.: Effects of urinary FSH and LH on the testicular function in hypogonadal patients. In Rosemberg, E., and Paulsen, C. A. (Eds.): The Human Testis. New York, Plenum Press, 1979, pp. 563–575.

Mancini, R. E., Lavieri, J. C., Muller, F., Andrada, J. A., and Saraceni, D. J.: Effect of prednisolone upon normal and pathologic human spermatogenesis. Fertil. Steril., 17:500, 1966.

Mancini, R. E., Seiguer, A. C., and Perez-Lloret, A.: Effect of gonadotropins on the recovery of spermatogenesis in hypophysectomized patients. J. Clin. Endocrinol., 29:467, 1969.

Mancini, R. E., Vilar, O., Donini, P., and Lloret, A. P.: Effect of human urinary FSH and LH on the recovery of spermatogenesis in hypophysectomized patients. J. Clin. Endocrinol., 33:888, 1971.

Margalith, E. J., Laufer, N., Persist, E., et al.: Treatment of oligospermia with human chorionic gonadotropin: hormonal profiles and results. Fertil. Steril.,39:841,1983.

Martin, F. I. R.: The stimulation and prolonged maintenance of spermatogenesis by human pituitary gonadotrophins in a patient with hypogonadotrophic hypogonadism. J. Endocrinol., 38:431, 1967.

Marynick, S. P., Loriaux, D. L., Sherins, R. J., Pita, J. C., and Lipsett, M. B.: Evidence that testosterone acts as both an androgen and an estrogen in suppressing pituitary gonadotropin secretion in men. J. Clin. Endocrinol. Metab., 49:396, 1979.

Masala, A., Delitala, G., Alagna, S., DeVilla, L., Rovasio, P. P., and Lotti, G.: Dynamic evaluation of prolactin secretion in patients with oligospermia: Effects of treatment with metergolide. Fertil. Steril., 31:63, 1979.

Mellinger, R. C., and Thompson, R. T.: The effect of clomiphene citrate in male infertility. Fertil. Steril., 17:94, 1966.

Montanari, G. D., and Volpe, A.: Bromocriptine treatment for oligospermia and asthenospermia with normal prolactin (letter). Lancet, 1:160, 1978.

Morse, H. C., Horike, N., Rowley, M., and Heller, C. G.: Testosterone concentrations in testes of normal men: Effects of testosterone propionate administration. J. Clin. Endocrinol., 37:882, 1973.

Mroueh, A., Lytton, B., and Kase, N.: Effect of clomiphene citrate on oligospermia. Am. J. Obstet. Gynecol., 98:1033, 1967a.

Mroueh, A., Lytton, B., and Kase, N.: Effects of human chorionic gonadotropin and human menopausal gonadotropin (Pergonal) in males with oligospermia. J. Clin. Endocrinol., 27:53, 1967b.

Newton, R., Schinfeld, J. S., and Schiff, I.: Clomiphene treatment of infertile men: Failure of response with idiopathic oligospermia. Fertil. Steril., 32:399, 1980.

Palti, Z.: Clomiphene therapy in defective spermatogenesis. Fertil. Steril., 21:838, 1970.

Paulsen, C. A.: The Effect of Human Menopausal Gonadotrophin on Spermatogenesis in Hypogonadotrophic Hypogonadism. In Proceedings of the Sixth Pan-American Congress of Endocrinology, Mexico City, 1965, pp. 398–407.

Paulsen, C. A., Espeland, D. H., and Michals, E. L.: Effects of HCG, HMG, HLH and HGH administration on testicular function. In Rosemberg, E., and Paulsen, C. A. (Eds.): The Human Testis. New York, Plenum Press, 1970, p. 547.

Paulsen, C. A., Plymate, S. A., and Leonard, J. M.: Current concepts in the management of male infertility. In Troen, P., and Nankin, H. (Eds.): New Concepts of the Testis in Normal and Infertile Men: Morphology, Physiology and Pathology. New York, Raven Press, 1977, p. 549.

Paulson, D. F.: Clomiphene citrate in the management of male hypofertility: Predictors for treatment selection. Fertil. Steril., 28:1226, 1977.

Paulson, D. F., Wachsman, J., Hammond, C. B., and Wiebe, H. R.: Hypofertility and clomiphene citrate therapy. Fertil. Steril., 26:982, 1975.

Petry, R., Rausch-Stroomann, J. G., Hienz, H. A., Senge, T., and Mauss, J.: Androgen treatment without inhibiting effect on hypophysis and male gonads. Acta Endocrinol., 59:497, 1968.

Polishuk, W. Z., Palti, Z., and Laufer, A.: Treatment of defective spermatogenesis with human gonadotropins. Fertil. Steril., 18:127, 1967.

Prasad, M. R. N., Rajalakshmi, M., Gupta, G., Dinakar, N., Arora, R., and Karkun, T.: Epididymal environment and maturation of spermatozoa. In Mancini, R. E., and Martini, L. (Eds.). Male Fertility and Sterility. Proceedings of the Serono Symposia. Vol. 5. New York, Academic Press, 1974, pp. 459–478.

Rakoff, A. E.: Ovulatory failure: Clinical aspects. Fertil. Steril., 27:473, 1976.

Reyes, F. I., and Faiman, C.: Long term therapy with low dose cisclomiphene in male infertility: Effects on semen, serum FSH, LH, testosterone and estradiol, and carbohydrate tolerance. Int. J. Fertil., 19:49, 1974.

Ronnberg, L.: The effect of clomiphene treatment on different sperm parameters in men with idiopathic oligozoospermia. Andrologia, 12:261, 1980.

Rosemberg, E.: Medical treatment of male infertility. Andrologia, 8:95, 1976.

Rosemberg, E.: Gonadotropin therapy of male infertility. In Hafez, E. S. E. (Ed.): Human Semen and Fertility Regulation in Men. St. Louis, C. V. Mosby Co., 1976, pp. 464–475.

Rosemberg, E., Mancini, R. E., Crigler, J. F., Jr., and Bergada, C.: Effect of human menopausal gonadotropin on prepubertal testes. In Rosemberg, E. (Ed.):

Gonadotropins, 1968. Los Angeles, Geron-X, Inc., 1968.

Ross, L. S., Kandel, G. L., Prinz, L. M., and Auletta, F.: Clomiphene treatment of the idiopathic hypofertile male: High-dose alternate-day therapy. Fertil. Steril. 33:618, 1980.

Rowley, M. J., and Heller, C. G.: The testosterone rebound phenomenon in the treatment of male infertility. Fertil. Steril., 23:498, 1972.

Sandblom, R. E., Matsumoto, A. M., Schoene, R. B., Lee, K. A., Giblin, E. C., Bremner, W. J., and Pierson, D. J.: Obstructive sleep apnea syndrome induced by testosterone administration. N. Engl. J. Med., 308:508, 1983.

Schachter, A., Goldman, J. A., and Zuckerman, Z.: Treatment of oligospermia with the amino acid arginine. J. Urol., 110:311, 1973.

Schellen, T. M. C. M.: Results with mesterolone in the treatment of disturbances of spermatogenesis. Andrologia, 2:1, 1970.

Schellen, T. M. C. M., and Beek, J. M.: The influence of high doses of mesterolone on the spermiogram. Fertil. Steril., 23:712, 1972.

Schellen, T. M. C. M., and Beek, J. M.: The use of clomiphene treatment for male sterility. Fertil. Steril., 25:407, 1974.

Schill, W. B., et al.: Combined hMG/hCG treatment in subfertile men with idiopathic normagonadotropic oligozoospermia. Int. J. Androl., 5:467, 1982.

Schirren, C., and Toyosi, J. O.: Assessment of gonadotropin therapy in male infertility. In Rosemberg, E., and Paulsen, C. A. (Eds.): The Human Testis. New York, Plenum Press, 1970, p. 605.

Schulte-Beerbuhl, M., and Nieschlag, E.: Comparison of testosterone, dihydrotestosterone, luteinizing hormone and follicle stimulating hormone in serum after injection of testosterone enanthate or testosterone cypionate. Fertil. Steril., 33:201, 1980.

Schwarzstein, L., Aparicio, N. J., Turner, D., Calamera, J. C., Mancini, R., and Schally, A. V.: Use of synthetic luteinizing hormone releasing hormone in treatment of oligospermic men: A preliminary report. Fertil. Steril., 26:331, 1975.

Sherins, R. J.: Clinical Aspects of treatment of male infertility with gonadotropins: testicular response of some men given hCG with and without Pergonal. In Mancini, R. E., and Martini, L. (Eds.): Male Fertility and Sterility. Proceedings of the Serono Symposia. Vol. 5. New York, Academic Press, 1974, pp 545–565.

Sherins, R. J.: Hypogonadotropic hypogonadism. In Garcia, C. R., et al. (Eds.): Current Therapy of Infertility. 2nd ed. St. Louis, C. V. Mosby Co., 1984, pp. 147–152.

Sherins, R. J., Brightwell, D., and Sternthal, P. M.: Longitudinal analysis of semen of fertile and infertile men. In Troen, P., and Nankin, H. (Eds.): New Concepts of the Testis in Normal and Infertile Men: Morphology, Physiology and Pathology. New York, Raven Press, 1977, pp. 473–488.

Sherins, R. J., and Winters, S. J.: Management of disorders of the testis. In Melmon, K., and Morrelli, H. P. (Eds.): Clinical Pharmacology: Basic Principles and Therapeutics. 2nd ed. New York, Macmillan, 1978, pp. 579–591.

Sherman, B. M., and Korenman, S. G.: Measurement of plasma LH, FSH, estradiol and progesterone in disorders of the human menstrual cycle: The short luteal phase. J. Clin. Endocrinol., 38:89, 1974a.

Sherman, B. M., and Korenman, S. G.: Measurement of serum LH, FSH, estradiol and progesterone in disorders of the human menstrual cycle: The inadequate luteal phase. J. Clin. Endocrinol., *39*:145, 1974*b*.

Skarin, G., Nilius, S. J., Wibell, L. and Wide, L.: Chronic pulsatile low-dose GnRH therapy for induction of testosterone production and spermatogenesis in a man with secondary hypogonadotropic hypogonadism. J. Clin. Endocrinol. Metab., *55*:723, 1982.

Smith, K. D., and Steinberger, E.: What is oligospermia? *In* Troen, P., and Nankin, H. (Eds.): New Concepts of the Testis in Normal and Infertile Men: Morphology, Physiology and Pathology. New York, Raven Press, 1977, pp. 489–504.

Snyder, P. J., and Lawrence, D. A.: Treatment of male hypogonadism with testosterone enanthate. J. Clin. Endocrinol. Metab., *51*:1335, 1980.

Steinberger, E.: Nonsurgical therapy of male infertility. Andrologia, *8*:77, 1976.

Steinberger, E., Root, A., Ficher, M., and Smith, K. D.: The role of androgens in the limitations of spermatogenesis in man. J. Clin. Endocrinol., *37*:746, 1973.

Stewart, B. H., and Montie, J. E.: Male infertility: An optimistic report. J. Urol., *110*:216, 1973.

Strott, C. A., Cargille, C. M., Ross, G. T., and Lipsett, M. B.: The short luteal phase. J. Clin. Endocrinol., *30*:246, 1970.

Troen, P., Yanaihara, T., Nankin, H., Tominaga, T., and Lever, H.: Assessment of gonadotropin therapy in infertile males. *In* Rosemberg, E., and Paulsen, C. A. (Eds.): The Human Testis. New York, Plenum Press, 1970, p. 591.

Vermuelen, A., and Comhaire, F.: Hormonal effects of an antiestrogen Tamoxifen in normal and oligospermic men. Fertil. Steril., *29*:320, 1978.

Vigersky, R. A., and Glass, A. R.: Effects of delta-1-testolactone on the pituitary-testicular axis in oligospermic men. J. Clin. Endocrinol. Metab., *52*:897, 1981.

Wieland, R. G., Ansari, A. H., Klein, D. E., Doshi, N. S., Hallberg, M. C., and Chen, J. C.: Idiopathic oligospermia: Control observations and response to cisclomiphene. Fertil. Steril., *23*:471, 1972.

Willis, K. J., London, D. R., Bevis, M. A., Butt, W. R., Lynch, S. S., and Holder, G.: Hormonal effects of tamoxifen in oligospermic men. J. Endocrinol., *73*:171, 1977.

Zarate, A., Valdes-Vallina, F., Gonzalez, A., Perez-Ubiena, C., Canales, E. S., and Shally, A. V.: Therapeutic effect of synthetic LHRH in male infertility due to idiopathic azoospermia and oligospermia. Fertil. Steril., *24*:485, 1973.

SEXUAL FUNCTION

CHAPTER 13

Sexual Function and Dysfunction

ROBERT J. KRANE, M.D.

The past decade has seen a marked increase in both clinical and research activity in the field of erectile dysfunction. In the laboratory, research concerning hemodynamics and neurophysiology has increased exponentially. Clinically, the availability of therapeutic options has led to newer and more sophisticated diagnostic techniques and to the development of multidisciplinary diagnostic centers. This chapter will first review the known physiologic mechanisms involved in erectile function, which include the vascular, neurologic, and hormonal systems. A discussion of the clinical causes of impotence will follow, and last, a review of pertinent diagnostic and therapeutic considerations will be presented.

PENILE ERECTION

The physiology of penile erection involves a complex interaction of the vascular, neurologic, and hormonal systems of the body. Although extensive basic investigation is currently being carried out, many aspects of the neurologic, hormonal, and vascular input to the penis are unclear. For example, regarding the hemodynamics of erection, what is the anatomy and physiology of the shunt mechanism that permits blood to fill the corpora cavernosa? What is the nature of the control mechanism of the venous effluent from the penis: Is it an active neurologic venoconstriction or a passive anatomic obstruction to venous outflow? Regarding the neurophysiology of erections, it is apparent that the primary nervous pathway from the spinal cord to the penis is parasympathetic in nature. However, penile erection is not a cholinergic event, and in many different laboratories, the search

for the final neurotransmitter is currently in progress. Finally, it is clear that the hormonal milieu affects male sexual function, but the exact mechanisms involved remain to be determined.

Over the past decade, we have seen a dramatic increase in basic scientific research directed toward understanding erectile physiology. This research is now beginning to bear fruit. In this section we will review our current knowledge about erectile physiology, both from basic laboratory studies and from clinical inference. When appropriate, theoretical possibilities will be entertained and clinical implications explored.

Hemodynamics

The blood supply to the penis is entirely from the internal pudendal artery, except for some minor scrotal and epigastric arterial branches (Newman, 1983) (Fig. 13–1). In about 75 per cent of individuals the internal pudendal artery arises from the lowest division of ischial pudendal trunk of the internal iliac artery. Its origin is usually at the level of the sciatic notch. This artery may arbitrarily be divided into four segments, which are termed the pelvic, gluteal, ischiorectal, and perineal segments. The pelvic segment of the internal pudendal artery is directed toward the ischial spine. The gluteal segment begins at the lower part of the greater sciatic foramen and crosses the back of the tip of the ischial spine and enters the perineum through the lesser sciatic foramen. The ischiorectal segment passes through the pudenal (Alcock's) canal in the ischiorectal fossa and then becomes the perineal segment. Since the perineal segment enters the penis, this vessel has at

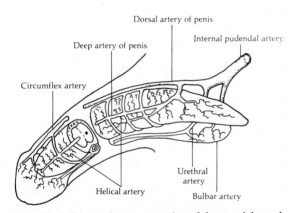

Figure 13–1. Schematic representation of the arterial supply to the penis. (From Newman, H.F.: *In* Krane, R.J., et al. (Eds.): Male Sexual Dysfunction. Boston, Little, Brown & Co., 1983.)

times been termed the penile artery. At the level of the urogenital diaphragm, the perineal segment of the internal pudendal artery divides into four terminal branches: the bulbar branch, the spongiosal branch, the cavernosal or deep penile artery, and the dorsal penile artery. The spongiosal or urethral artery penetrates the tunica of the corpus spongiosum and runs in a longitudnal direction within the spongiosal tissue. Along its route it supplies the corpus spongiosum and urethra and finally the glans penis. The dorsal penile artery enters the penis and continues distally beneath Buck's fascia just outside the tunica albuginea. The paired dorsal arteries run longitudinally alongside the unpaired dorsal vein that is between them. The arteries eventually terminate in short helical branches in the glans penis. Along their route several circumflex branches are evident and pass around the corpus cavernosum, penetrating both it and the corpus spongiosum. The dorsal artery also eventually provides blood supply to the glans penis. The cavernosal or deep penile artery is clearly the most important branch with regard to erectile physiology. These paired arteries have a common origin with the dorsal arteries as they form the most distal bifurcation just outside the tunica of the corpora cavernosa. The cavernosal arteries pass longitudinally within the corporal bodies, usually in a medial position (Golstein and Krane, in press). The main function of these arteries is to supply the corpora cavernosa. The corporal arteries give off terminal tortuous branches known as helicine arteries, which were first described in 1835 by Müller (Müller, 1835) and have been reported by numerous other investigators (Vastarini-Cresi, 1902; Clara, 1939). Each of the helical

arteries divides and arborizes into several subdivisions that eventually give rise to small end-arteries. These end-arteries pass directly into the cavernous tissue or into arteriovenous shunts that pass through the cavernous tissue directly into the cavernous venous system without the benefit of a capillary bed. Recently, the possibility of an alternative pathway for helical arterial blood flow has been described (Wagner et al., 1982). With the use of plastic casts in 47 cadavers, "shunt" arteries connecting the helical arteries of the corporal artery with arteries of the glans penis and corpus spongiosum have been described (Wagner et al., 1982). The importance of these arteries has yet to be determined.

Venous outflow from the penis proceeds via three main sets of veins: the superficial, intermediate, and deep along with multiple anastomotic venous interconnections. The superficial dorsal vein drains the skin and subcutaneous tissues superficial to Buck's fascia. In contrast, the intermediate venous system is deep to Buck's fascia but superficial to the tunica albuginea and, as its main vein, includes the deep dorsal vein of the penis. The deep dorsal vein drains the glans penis, part of the corpus spongiosum, and the corpora cavernosa. Emissary veins coming from both the spongiosal and the cavernosal tissue anastomose with the deep dorsal vein. In addition, there are superficial anastomoses between this system and the superficial dorsal vein of the penis. The third main venous system is the deep vein of the penis, which is not to be confused with the deep dorsal vein. This system provides the major drainage of blood from the corpora cavernosa. It is important to note that no muscular deep veins have ever been identified within the corpora cavernosa (Newman and Northup, 1981). The proximal portion of the corpus spongiosum drains through the bulbar veins into the deep veins of the penis. Although much disagreement has existed in the past concerning the venous drainage of specific areas of the penis, it is relatively safe to assume that the proximal portions of the corpora cavernosa and corpus spongiosum empty through the deep veins of the penis, while the distal portions of these structures drain primarily through the deep dorsal vein.

It is self-evident that, during formation of an erection, the amount of blood entering the cavernosal spaces must exceed the amount of blood leaving this tissue. The increase in blood volume within the corpora cavernosa during erection is determined by the length and circumference to which the tunica albuginea can be stretched. At the point of maximal stretch, the amount of blood entering the corpora and the amount of blood leaving the corpora again become equal. Therefore, the points of physiology to be determined are: (1) What is the mechanism that brings about preferential filling of the corporal spaces? (2) Quantitatively, what is the blood flow through the corpora in the flaccid state and how does it differ during an erection? (3) What happens to the venous drainage during the formation and maintenance of an erection? The hemodynamics of penile erection have been investigated mainly through anatomic studies and animal experiments (Watson, 1964; Ashdown and Gilanpour, 1974). Most investigators now agree that a decrease in corporal vascular resistance and a concomitant increase in arterial inflow into the corpora are mainly responsible for the phenomenon of penile erection (Holmquist and Olin, 1969; Lue et al., 1983; Shirai and Ishii, 1981). For example, Henderson and Roepke (1966) demonstrated in dogs that intracorporal pressure approached that of the aorta during an erection, while flow through the deep veins increased over that of the flaccid state by seven fold. Their conclusion was that arterial inflow overwhelmed the capacity for venous outflow. Other experiments have shown that a reduction of arterial inflow during a nerve-stimulated erection in animals prevents an erection from occurring (Goldstein and Krane, 1983). Dorr and Brody (1967) showed that during an erection created by pelvic nerve stimulation, arterial pressure within the major arteries was unchanged in comparison with the flaccid state and concluded that increased flow to the penis was secondary to a marked decrease in vascular resistance within the penis. Later, they were to show that neither dorsal vein compression nor opening of the vein to atmospheric pressure will create or alter a nerve-mediated erection in dogs. This was confirmed by others. Newman and coworkers (1964) perfused the corpora of cadavers and were able to reproduce erections only by directly infusing fluid into the corporal spaces at rates of between 20 and 50 ml per minute. Perfusion through the internal pudendal arteries in the same cadavers at rates of between 78 and 142 ml per minute resulted in only moderate distention and edema of the penis but no true erection (Newman et al., 1964). One might interpret the experiment in several ways. The fact that increases in flow through the pudendal artery did not produce an erection speaks for an active neurologic mechanism that can direct blood flow into the cor-

poral spaces during formation of an erection. The fact that an erection could be produced in a cadaver by direct perfusion of the corpora supports the theory that an erection is due to an increase in arterial inflow rather than to an active venoconstriction, as the latter would be impossible in the cadaver. The minor role of active muscular venoconstriction was also shown by Semans and Langworthy (1939), who removed the ischiocavernosus and bulbocavernosus muscles in the cat and were still able to produce nerve-stimulated erections. In addition, erections often occur in spinal cord–injured patients in whom the pelvic floor is paralyzed (Bors and Comarr, 1960). All of these observations make it unlikely that active venoconstriction is necessary for the initiation or maintenance of penile erection.

However, a passive venous occlusion may well contribute to the vascular mechanism of erection. For example, using a xenon washout technique before and during visual sexual stimulation, Wagner has shown a definite reduction in penile outflow during tumescence (Wagner, 1981). This has been interpreted as evidence for the presence of some sort of venous regulatory mechanism during the onset of erection. At the present time, the exact nature of venous outflow control is unclear.

There is little doubt, however, that arterial inflow does increase substantially. Normally, blood flow through the internal pudendal artery in man is in the area of 10 ml per minute. We have recently shown that, during a pelvic nerve–stimulated erection in the dog, flow through this artery increases by approximately five to six fold (Goldstein and Krane, in press) (Fig. 13–2). As pressure within the aorta does not change, this can be explained only by a marked reduction in the vascular resistance of the penis. This factor has been confirmed by Lue and colleagues (1983) in the primate. In this model, stimulation of the pelvic nerve is rapidly followed by increase in flow in the internal pudendal artery and shortly thereafter by increases in intracorporal pressures.

The nature of the regulatory mechanism that directs blood flow either into the efferent venous system (flaccidity) or into the trabecular spaces of the corpora cavernosa (erection) has been studied by several investigators. In 1900, Von Ebner identified in the penile arterioles intraluminal intrusions that have since been called penile pads, cushions, or polsters (Von Ebner, 1900; Ercolani, 1869). In 1921, Kiss analyzed the histology of the penile vessels and their intrusions (Kiss, 1921). In 1950, Rotter

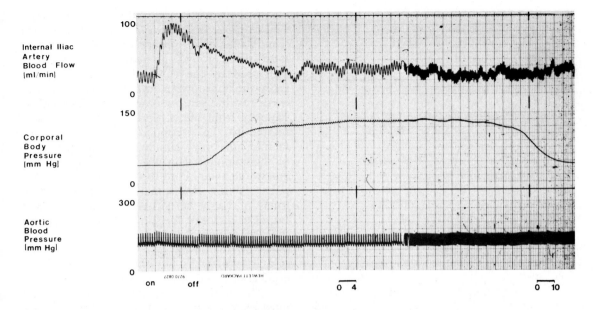

Figure 13–2. Data derived from pelvic nerve stimulation experiment in the dog. Note that after an 8-second stimulation (on-off) the first change that occurs is an increase in flow through the internal iliac artery. This is followed by a rise in intracorporeal pressure. After peak intracorporeal pressure is attained, blood flow through the internal iliac artery returns to a stable level just above normal resting blood flow. Also note the marked prolongation of intracorporeal pressure change following only an 8-second pelvic nerve stimulation. (From Siroky, M., and Krane, R.J.: *In* Krane, R.J., et al. (Eds.): Male Sexual Dysfunction. Boston, Little, Brown & Co., 1983.)

and Schurman found similar polsters in virtually all branches of the arterial and venous tree of the penis (Rotter and Schurman, 1950). All these investigators attributed to these polsters the ability to regulate penile blood flow, presuming that during polster contraction vascular resistance within the penis was lowered, and, conversely, that during polster relaxation this resistance was raised.

The microscopic anatomy of the penile vasculature was studied by Conti in 1952 (Conti, 1952) (Fig. 13–3). He again found muscular polsters (Ebner's pads) in both the afferent and the efferent vasculature of the corpora and presumed that they were able to control the amount and distribution of blood flow. Conti postulated a shunting of arterial blood to the venous return during penile flaccidity. Therefore, during active contraction of the cushions or polsters, the arteriovenous (AV) shunts would close and blood would be trapped in the cavernosus spaces. The presence of AV shunts was corroborated by Newman and coworkers, by injecting microspheres 100 μ in diameter through the pudendal artery and finding them in the pudendal veins. Larger spheres could not be passed from the arteries to the veins, and thus it was concluded that arteriovenous shunts

were, in fact, present and were, at most, 100 μ in diameter (Newman et al., 1964).

However, the role of penile polsters remains unclear. As long ago as 1939, Deysach denied the existence of penile polsters and felt that erection was produced by a series of sluice valves of the corpora cavernosa (Deysach, 1939). In addition, polsters have been found in arteries throughout the body, even in places where no regulatory mechanism is known to exist. Further arguments against a physiologic role for polsters have centered around the theory that they represent a response to stress or aging. Robertson advanced this theory on the basis that polsters were most likely to be present at branching points (Robertson, 1960). They have also been demonstrated to occur at the very places where lateral pressure drops can exert contraction force on the intima. Some feel that pulsatile stress at these points is significant (Texon, 1967). In addition, polsters have not been identified in the newborn and were also absent in a series of patients receiving massive doses of estrogen (Newman and Tschertkoff, in press). In recent studies, Benson has concluded that polsters are an early manifestation of arterial sclerotic disease (Benson et al., 1981). It is probably safe to assume that the original theo-

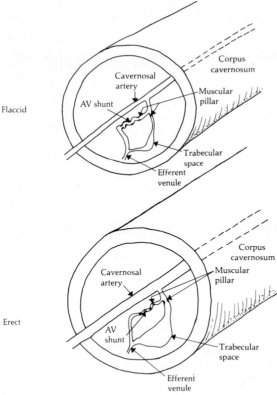

Figure 13–3. Schematic representation of Conti's concept of arteriolar-venule shunts and how they participate in appropriately directing cavernosal blood flow by muscular polsters. (From Siroky, M.B., and Krane, R.J.: *In* Krane, R.J., et al. (Eds.): Male Sexual Dysfunction. Boston, Little, Brown & Co., 1983.)

ries concerning the role of polster activity in the reorientation of blood flow into the cavernous spaces are not correct. However, an active mechanism for this reorientation must exist and appears to be under neurologic control.

Neurophysiology

After reaching the conclusion that an erection is created by an increase in blood flow to the penis and, in addition, redirection of that blood flow to the cavernous spaces, one is faced with the question of identifying the underlying neurophysiologic mechanisms that produce these effects. All levels of the central and peripheral nervous systems participate in the neural control of erection. A spinal reflex mechanism or pathway for erection is probably present in man and becomes evident following complete spinal cord injury. In the intact human, however, penile erection is a much more complicated process, which is controlled, to a great

extent, by the cerebral cortex. Clearly, there is a wide range of auditory, olfactory, and visual stimuli that may produce erection without any local stimulation of the penis. These stimuli are processed by the cerebral cortex, which then sends the appropriate output to the sacral spinal cord, resulting in penile erection. The efferent pathway from the cerebral cortex is intimately related to the preoptic hypothalamic region, median forebrain bundle, and substantia nigra of the midbrain (Siroky and Krane, 1979). It enters the spinal cord through the ventrolateral pons. Within the spinal cord itself, efferent tracts probably lie within the lateral columns. Impulses may exit the spinal cord through either the thoracolumbar sympathetic or the sacral parasympathetic nerves. This section will deal primarily with the peripheral neurophysiologic aspects of erection (Fig. 13–4).

The penis receives sensory innervation almost exclusively through the pudendal sensory nerves that enter the sacral spinal cord. The pudendal nerve is a mixed nerve that provides motor supply to the pelvic floor muscles and sensory supply to the penis itself. There are nonspecific free spray nerve endings that serve as sensory receptors in the glans penis and penile skin (Malenovsky and Sammerova, 1972). Some pacinian corpuscles are found in the deeper layers of the skin. In some animal species, e.g., the cat, sensory receptors of the glans penis have been shown to be androgen-dependent (Cooper, 1972). In animal studies, anesthesia of the glans penis or dorsal penile nerve section impairs the ability of the animal to perform sexual intercourse but does not affect its ability to achieve erection (Cooper and Aronson, 1969). Clinically, one may stimulate the penile skin and measure conduction time between the penis, the sacral cord, and the cerebral cortex. Conduction velocity of the pudendal sensory nerve to the cord is slower than conduction velocity of the tibial nerve. In addition, central conduction time between the sacral cord and the cerebral cortex (approximately 28 msec) is significantly slower than central conduction time after posterior tibial nerve stimulation (Siroky and Krane, 1983).

The major motor supply to the penis is provided by the sacral parasympathetic nerves. In 1863, Eckhardt performed a classic experiment in which he showed that electrical stimulation of the sacral parasympathetic nerve (or nervi erigentes) produced a penile erection in dogs (Eckhardt, 1863). Subsequently, the nervi erigentes were found to exit the spinal cord via the anterior routes of S2 to S4. For many years, erectile function was presumed to be entirely a parasympathetic event, and pelvic nerve stimulation continues to be used as a classic animal model for the study of erectile physiology. Many experiments clearly point to the fact that the sacral parasympathetic nerves are preganglionic. For example, a number of investigators have demonstrated little or no effect on nerve-stimulated erections in dogs, bulls, or rabbits by pretreating or simultaneously treating with atropine (Henderson and Roepke, 1966; Dzuick and Narton, 1962). Subsequently, several investigators found that pretreatment with a ganglionic blocking agent, such as nicotine or hexamethonium, did abolish the erectile response to pelvic nerve stimulation in animals (Dorr and Brody, 1967; Langley and Anderson, 1895). Several investigators have used intra-arterial injections of acetylcholine and have failed to show any penile vascular or corporal pressure responses (Dorr and Brody, 1967; Penttila, 1966). These

experiments demonstrate that the penile erection is relatively atropine-resistant, which makes it unlikely that acetylcholine is the final neurotransmitter causing vascular engorgement of the penis.

Attention was drawn to the sympathetic nervous system for the first time after the classic experiment by Root and Bard in 1947 (Root and Bard, 1947). They showed that following removal of all parasympathetic innervation by ablation of the entire sacral spinal cord, full erections were seen in male cats in the presence of estrous female cats. In the same animals, spinal cord transection above the thoracolumbar sympathetic outflow abolished erectile activity. These findings led to the concept that the thoracolumbar sympathetic nerves could serve either as the primary pathway for what was known as psychologically mediated erection or as an alternative pathway in cases in which there was ablation of the sacral parasympathetic nerves.

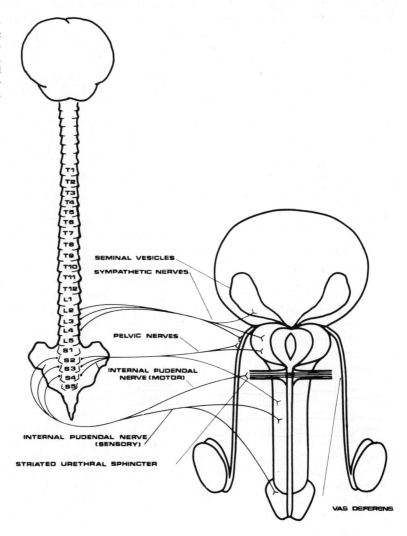

Figure 13–4. Schematic representation of the autonomic and somatic neurologic input into the lower urogenital organs. (From Siroky, M.B., and Krane, R.J.: *In* Krane, R.J., and Siroky, M.B. (Eds.): Clinical Neuro-Urology. Boston, Little, Brown & Co., 1979.)

Support for this concept was derived from the observation that close to 25 per cent of patients with complete sacral cord lesions had psychogenically mediated erections (Bors and Comarr, 1960).

More recent studies have shown that in patients with complete lesions due to spinal cord injury above thoracolumbar outflow, 82 per cent had reflex erections involving both the corpora cavernosa and the corpus spongiosum. In contrast, only 35 per cent of patients with lesions below T12 had such erections, the majority having erections involving only the corpora cavernosa (Chapelle et al., 1980). Thus, it appears that the thoracolumbar sympathetic outflow may primarily induce engorgement of the corpus spongiosum rather than the corpora cavernosa. Certainly, it does not appear that, in the neurologically intact man, the thoracolumbar sympathetic outflow plays a significant role in initiating or maintaining penile erection. A model for bilateral ablation of these tracts is provided by radical retroperitoneal node dissection for testis tumor. In that situation, emission and ejaculation may be abolished, thereby proving that sympathetic outflow has been ablated, and nonetheless there is no effect on erectile ability.

In 1969, Baumgarten and coworkers reported the presence of adrenergic fibers in the corpus cavernosum of both the cat and the monkey with a less prominent adrenergic supply to the corpus spongiosum (Baumgarten, 1969). This study led to considerable research activity centered around the possibility that the final neural transmitter involved may be adrenergic. Using glyoxylic acid histofluorescence techniques, Benson and coworkers have also shown catecholamine fluorescent fibers and terminals in both the corpora cavernosa and the corpus spongiosum (Benson et al., 1980). These fibers wind through the trabeculae and approach the walls of the cavernous spaces in the corpora cavernosa. Few of these fibers occur in the corpus spongiosum. Blood vessels of cavernosum and spongiosum demonstrate adrenergic varicosities.

Semans and Langworthy (1939) showed that stimulation of the sympathetic trunk in several experimental species would not result in penile erection and indeed caused detumescence of a pelvic nerve–induced erection. Although one might draw from this experiment the conclusion that the sympathetic or adrenergic mechanisms are, if anything, antagonistic to erection, one must remember that experimental electrical stimulation of the thoracolumbar outflow may result in unselective stimulation of vasoconstric-

tor and vasodilator fibers, whereas physiologic stimulation may result in selective stimulation of vasodilator fibers only. Dorr and Brody could not produce erections in dogs by intra-arterial injection of norepinephrine (Dorr and Brody, 1967).

Benson and associates, using acetylcholinesterase localization techniques, showed that parasympathetic nerve fibers, in contrast to the abundant adrenergic fibers, are seen infrequently in human corpora cavernosa and corpus spongiosum (Benson et al., 1980). Electron microscopic studies of human erectile tissue demonstrate no clear-cut cholingergic vesicles, whereas norepinephrine-containing vesicles are evident. In addition, large opaque vesicles that may represent either purinergic or peptidergic nerve fibers have been visualized (McConnell et al., 1979). In vitro corporal cavernosal strip experiments have shown that norepinephrine can induce contraction in these strips. This action can be blocked with phentolamine pretreatment (McConnell et al., 1979). Therefore, it appears that human penile erectile tissues do show, at least in vitro, a response to pharmacologic alpha-adrenergic stimulation. Studies of catecholamine tissue concentrations performed by Melman have demonstrated norepinephrine to be present in high concentrations in the smooth muscle of the penis (Melman and Henry, 1979). The typical tissue norepinephrine concentrations are greater than those one would expect to find in vascular smooth muscle alone. In his studies, diabetic impotent patients showed significantly reduced levels of tissue norepinephrine in their erectile tissue (Melman, 1983). Wein and coworkers have shown that the density of alpha-adrenergic receptors was nearly ten times that of beta-adrenergic receptors in human corporal cavernosal tissue (Wein et al., 1983).

Adrenergic agonists and antagonists have also been studied in vivo. Domer and associates demonstrated that the combination of alpha-adrenergic blockade and beta-adrenergic stimulation could produce pharmacologic erections in cats (Domer et al., 1978). The combination of alpha-antagonists and beta-agonists has also been shown to produce erectile activity in dogs. Siroky and Krane (1983) have shown similar responses in dogs, albeit diminished, to terbutaline (a beta-agonist). They noted that this effect was blocked by propranolol, a beta-blocking agent. In man, oral administration of large doses of alpha- and beta-adrenergic antagonists (phenoxybenzamine and propranolol) does not seem to affect erectile capabilities.

Therefore, one is left with the fact that a

completely satisfactory explanation of erection is provided neither by an exclusively cholinergic mechanism nor by an exclusively adrenergic one. For this reason, a host of other potential neutrotransmitters have been studied. At present, it appears that histamine, serotonin, prostaglandins, and various amino acids do not fulfill the criteria for the final neurotransmitter (Benson, 1983).

Based on the finding of peptidergic vesicles in ultrastructural studies, the possibility of a polypeptide's being the putative neurotransmitter has been entertained. Previously, the effects of bradykinin and substance P on rat penile artery strips had been studied, showing little or no response (Klinge and Sjostrand, 1974). The polypeptide being investigated most intensively at present is vasoactive intestinal polypeptide (VIP). VIP was originally isolated from porcine duodendum and has since been found in abundance in multiple systems (Said and Mutt, 1970). Under light microscopy, VIP has been anatomically localized in penile vasculature and corpora of both animals and man (Larsson, 1977). It has been shown to cause relaxation of the retractor penis muscle in the dog, cat, and bull (Sjostrand et al., 1981). In the cat and man, VIP has been shown to be present in the vas deferens, prostate, urethra, and penis and has been found in high concentrations in the cavernous tissue (Larsen et al., 1981). VIP is known to have a vasodilatory effect and has been shown to cause in vitro relaxation of corporal cavernosal strips in both the monkey and the rabbit (Willis et al., 1981). However, it had little effect in the same tissue in the guinea pig, dog, and cat. It is of interest that submandibular gland secretion, which is under the control of the parasympathetic nervous system, is resistant to atropine blockade. Infusion of VIP, however, causes vasodilation, while the combination of acetylcholine and VIP produces both vasodilation and secretion (Lundberg et al., 1980). These findings have led to the thought that both neurotransmitters may be relevant to the mechanism of penile erection. Recently, Goldstein and co-workers (unpublished data) have shown in dogs that VIP production rates in the corpora cavernosa increase by almost 15 fold after pelvic nerve stimulation. It remains for further research to determine the exact neurotransmitter or transmitters involved in erectile function, however.

After review of the foregoing material, it becomes apparent that a unifying theory of the neurovascular physiology of erectile function is still elusive. What is known is that (1) the parasympathetic sacral outflow acts as a preganglionic nerve; (2) there appears to be a more distal neuron involved whose neurotransmitter is yet to be determined; (3) the initiation of an erection involves an increase of blood flow to the penis, presumably secondary to a decrease in vascular resistance at the corporal level; (4) decrease in venous return during penile erection appears to be a passive rather than a neurologically mediated active event. The questions that still must be answered include: (1) What is the anatomic site or sites on which the neurotransmitters act to shunt blood flow from the arterial inflow to the cavernous spaces? (2) What is the nature of the neurotransmitter and what are its agonists and antagonists?

It was mentioned earlier that the entire process of erection in humans is under considerable control by higher centers. Extensive neurophysiologic experiments in the monkey by MacLean located positive loci for erection most rostrally in the anterior medial part of the hypothalamus (the paraventricular nucleus) (MacLean and Ploog, 1962). Fibers from this area follow the course of the median forebrain bundle. Cortical loci have been identified in the gyrus rectus and also in parts of the subcorticolimbic system concerned with vision (mammillary bodies and cingulate gyrus). Kluver and Bucy (1939) reported hypersexual activity in monkeys following bilateral temporal lobectomies. The gyrus rectus and septum pellucidum are mainly concerned with the olfactory apparatus, and the presence of positive loci for erection clearly relates this apparatus to sexual function. The mammillary bodies, thalamus (medial dorsal nucleus), and cingulate gyrus represent a system involved primarily with visual stimuli, which makes its first appearance in the mammal, reaching its ultimate development in primates. This may suggest an evolutionary shift from olfactory to visual input as the primary stimulus for erection.

Electroencephalographic studies have shown that the hippocampus also plays a role in penile erection. The hippocampus and cingulate gyrus constitute important centers in the limbic lobe of Broca ("visceral brain"), from which there are extensive connections with the thalamus and hypothalamus. Subcortical lesions in the medial preoptic region of the hypothalamus abolish sexual activity in male rats (Slimp et al., 1978). Conversely, electrical stimulation of this region of the hypothalamus (as well as nearby structures) facilitates mating activity in experimental animals. In lower animals as well as in the primate the preoptic anterior hypothalamic region is thus an important center for determining heterosexual (but not autosexual) behavior (Robinson and Mishkin, 1966).

Hormonal Considerations

The role of circulating androgens with regard to erectile physiology and sexual behavior remains somewhat unclear. It seems apparent that libido and sexual behavior in the human male depend on some threshold amount of plasma testosterone, which varies between individuals and even within the same individual. Rat castration produces a clear-cut change in sexual behavior. After castration, ejaculation is first lost, followed by intromission, and finally by cessation of mounting (Davidson, 1975). The loss of these functions always occurs in a similar sequence but with differing lag time between castration and change of function. Testosterone disappears from the circulation within a few hours after castration. However, the various aspects of sexual behavior described above may continue for weeks and months. Bilateral adrenalectomy in conjuction with castration does not change the sequence of events or the lag time. Treatment of castrated rats with exogenous testosterone will eventually restore all aspects of mating behavior. The lag time between initiation of treatment and full recovery of mating behavior is usually several weeks, but lag time will be greatly reduced if testosterone replacement is given shortly after castration. Basically, these observations demonstrate that the rat deprived of testosterone will cease to exhibit its usual sexual behavior, but that with testosterone replacement, normal behavior can be restored. Experiments have shown that the amount of circulating testosterone required to permit continued mating behavior in the castrated rat is much less than the normal level of circulating testosterone (Davidson, 1975). Several important questions remain, namely, what is the site of action of testosterone in the male rat (e.g., the genitals, the spinal cord, the brain)?

In dogs and rats that have had spinal cord sections as well as castration, exogenously administered testosterone restored responses to genital stimulation. These findings would indicate that, in the dog, testosterone probably has some spinal or peripheral action. However, the primary site of action of testosterone in controlling sexual behavior clearly appears to be in the brain, and specifically in the anterior hypothalamic preoptic area (Davidson, 1975). In rats, implanting small amounts of testosterone in various parts of the brain after castration revealed that 75 to 80 per cent of animals in which the testosterone was placed in the hypothalamic preoptic area resumed full sexual behavior. Similar hormonal implants in other parts of the brain did not significantly restore this type of behavior (Davidson, 1975).

It is difficult, of course, to extrapolate from the animal to the human experience, especially with regard to the hormonal influence on sexual behavior. To understand the role of testosterone, one must analyze indirect evidence from various situations involving either replacement therapy for hypogonadal states or castration. When castration has been performed, the resultant sexual function has ranged from complete loss of libido to normal activity (Ellis and Grayhack, 1963; Roen, 1965). Most observers agree that libido appears to be much more dependent on testosterone than on erectile ability. In a famous study by Ellis and Grayhack (1963) of 82 men with carcinoma of the prostate treated with surgical or medical castration, a surprisingly high number of patients who were potent prior to therapy remained so. It may well be that if one had followed the patients long enough, loss of libido and impotence would have eventually resulted. Thus, in this study we may be seeing those patients whose lag time between castration and ablation of sexual behavior is very long. However, the surprisingly high number of patients who may remain sexually active following castration seems to argue against this. In addition, patients may have been unwilling to admit to loss of potency. It is only by nocturnal penile tumescence testing that one can accurately determine whether or not potency has been preserved.

Studies have shown in humans that prior to, during, and following sexual relations, serum gonadotropin and prolactin levels remain unchanged (Starns et al., 1973). When testosterone levels have been correlated with frequency of coitus and orgasm, some have shown a direct correlation, while others have shown an inverse correlation (Kraemer et al., 1976). The efficacy of replacing testosterone in men with known androgen deficiency has been shown by Money (1961). Other studies have shown that testosterone replacement in hypogonadal men produced significant difference in results when compared with placebo (Skakkebach et al., 1981; Davidson et al., 1979). However, this was not the case when impotent men without androgen deficiency were treated (Benkert et al., 1979). A recent Scottish study of hypogonadal men revealed that erectile activity was preserved in most; however, their response to visual sexual stimuli was greatly reduced (Skakkebach et al., 1981). In a more recent study, erectile responses to visual sexual stimuli were similar in normal, hypogonadal, and testosterone-treated hypogonadal men (Kwan et al., 1983). However, in hypogonadal men, nocturnal erections and spontaneous daytime erections were increased in frequency after testosterone replacement. It would appear that the role of testosterone in male sexuality is primarily in the area of sexual interest and motivation.

Clearly, the incidence of impotence in men increases after the age of 50 to 55 years. This fact was originally found by Kinsey, who attributed it to the aging process and psychologic factors related to aging (Kinsey et al., 1948). However, it is known that levels of free circulating testosterone decrease with age, and, more specifically, the ratio between estradiol and free testosterone increases with age. The relationship between changes in levels of circulating hormones, age, and age-related impotence remains to be determined.

Lastly, in patients with hyperprolactinemia, more than 90 per cent will exhibit evidence of either sexual or reproductive dysfunction (Perryman and Thorner, 1981). Hyperprolactinemia is associated with low or low-normal circulating testosterone levels. The exact mechanism that leads to low testosterone levels in this disorder is not known, although suppression of gonadotropin-releasing hormone has been postulated. Replacement by exogenous testosterone to restore normal levels does not, however, reverse the erectile dysfunction (Perryman and Thorner, 1981).

EJACULATION

Ejaculation is a complex process that is composed of three phenomena: seminal emission (delivery of semen into the posterior urethra), ejaculation (propulsion of semen from posterior urethra to the outside), and bladder neck closure. These events are reflex in nature and require coordination between the autonomic and somatic nervous systems in order to achieve effective delivery of semen. The reflex involves the sensory pathway through the dorsal nerve of the penis which, as previously discussed, constitutes the sensory branch of the pudendal nerve. Sensory impulses travel along this nerve, eventually reaching the sensory cortex. The efferent limb of this reflex travels through the anterior lateral column of the spinal cord to the thoracolumbar sympathetic outflow. Stimulation of the thoracolumbar sympathetic trunks produces smooth muscle contraction of the epididymis, vas deferens, seminal vesicles, and prostate along with closure of the bladder neck (Langley and Anderson, 1895). The ability to propel the semen through the urethra is provided mainly by somatic pudendal motor efferents to the striated muscle of the pelvic floor. This interaction between the somatic and autonomic nervous systems produces the rhythmic expulsion of semen through the external urethral meatus.

Neurophysiologic Considerations

Histochemical studies have shown the presence of adrenergic as well as cholinergic nerve fibers in the epididymis, vas deferens, and seminal vesicles (see Fig. 13–4) (Sjostrand, 1965). A system of short adrenergic nerves that arise within the organ innervated has been shown to be present in these structures. These short adrenergic neurons receive presynaptic fibers from the thoracolumbar outflow of the spinal cord (Siroky and Krane, 1979). Histochemical studies have shown extensive adrenergic innervation of the human prostate. Pharmacologic studies on human tissue demonstrate that the prostatic capsule and bladder trigone respond briskly to noradrenaline, a response that may be blocked by phentolamine (Caine et al., 1975).

Langley and Anderson (1895) observed that stimulating the lumbar sympathetic outflow resulted in vas deferens and seminal vesicular contractions. These results were prevented by hypogastric nerve section. Root and Bard (1947) demonstrated that removal of the sympathetic chain below the diaphragm in the cat abolished emission. The response of the guinea pig vas deferens to hypogastric nerve stimulation may be blocked by ganglionic blocking agents, thus pointing to the fact that the long adrenergic fibers from the thoracolumbar outflow are primarily preganglionic structures that terminate on the short adrenergic nerve (Baumgarten et al., 1969).

It appears that different nerves of the thoracolumbar sympathetic outflow may have different functions. Stimulation of the lumbar sympathetic nerves has resulted in contraction of the posterior urethra in dogs, while stimulation of the lower thoracic and upper lumbar sympathetic ganglia has produced seminal emission into the posterior urethra (Kimma et al., 1975). These effects have been shown to be mediated by alpha-adrenergic receptors. Electromyographic studies in dogs have shown that during ejaculation the bladder neck undergoes rhythmic EMG activity mainly confined to its ventral portion (Koelberg et al., 1962). Electromyographic activity of the striated urethral sphincter in man has been recorded during ejaculation and has also been shown to undergo rhythmic contraction (Koraitim et al., 1977). Therefore, it may be reasonable to conclude that seminal emission and bladder neck closure to prevent retrograde ejaculation are primarily under the control of the sympathetic nervous system via thoracolumbar sympathetic outflow acting on short adrenergic nerves. The rhythmic contractions necessary to propel the semen once it has reached the posterior urethra are probably under somatic motor control (pudendal nerve) and are caused by rhythmic contractions of the bulbocavernosus and ischiocavernosus muscles.

Numerous clinical conditions may cause lack of emission or retrograde ejaculation. Close to 62 per cent of sexually active patients will report retrograde ejaculation following prostatectomy. This may also occur in patients with diabetic neuropathy. After bilateral sympathectomies at L2, inability to ejaculate has been reported in 38 per cent of patients (Whitelaw and Smithwick, 1951). In classic bilateral radical retroperitoneal node dissection for testicular cancer, close to 100 per cent of patients report lack of ejaculation. This has been shown to be due to failure of emission of sperm into the posterior urethra rather than to retrograde ejaculation (Kedia et al., 1975).

Adrenergic antagonists have been shown to produce ejaculatory failure clinically. This includes phenoxybenzamine, thioridazine, and guanethidine (Kedia and Markland, 1975). With spinal cord injury, especially in patients with complete sacral cord lesions, approximately 20 per cent will have ejaculation and orgasm. Ejaculation in the group with sacral cord injuries is usually dribbling ejaculation, as the contribution of the pelvic floor musculature is absent (Bors and Comarr, 1960).

Clinically, two primary problems with ejaculation may occur. The first is inability to ejaculate, known as ejaculatory incompetence or ejaculatory impotence. This is a rare disorder seen in approximately 0.14 per cent of the general population. Although the etiology is unknown, it is almost entirely secondary to psychologic causes and treatment should be directed toward such disorders. The second problem is premature ejaculation. Men with this problem will usually ejaculate during foreplay or as soon as an attempt at penetration is made. The cause for this dysfunction is also thought to be psychologic in a majority of patients. This condition is almost always successfully treated with contemporary sex therapy, mainly utilizing what has become known as the squeeze technique (Masters and Johnson, 1970). In cases of lack of ejaculation, one must, of course, be assured that no underlying neuropathic disease is present before psychologic therapy is considered.

SECONDARY IMPOTENCE

Classically, impotence has been thought of as being primary or secondary. Primary impotence refers to the inability to obtain an erection throughout one's life, dating back to adolescence. In contradistinction, secondary impotence refers to the loss of the ability to obtain normal erections that was present at one time in one's life. Primary impotence traditionally has been considered to be related to deep-seated psychiatric problems. More recently, newer testing techniques have shown that many patients with primary impotence have an underlying traumatic vascular injury suffered in childhood or early adolescence.

CAUSES OF IMPOTENCE

This section will detail the more common disorders that may lead to secondary impotence.

Endocrine Disoders. The true incidence of endocrine dysfunction as a cause of impotence remains unclear and is the subject of continuing dispute. Estimates ranging from 4 to 35 per cent have been made concerning the incidence of an underlying endocrinologic causation (Spark et al., 1980). As mentioned previously, the relationship between the level of testosterone and sexual behavior remains to be elucidated. Three distinct endocrinologic syndromes have been associated with erectile dysfunction. Hypogonadotrophic hypogonadism results from primary failure of LH secretion by the anterior pituitary. The second disorder (hypergonadotrophic hypogonadism) results from primary failure of testosterone secretion by the testes. Finally, hyperprolactinemia is usually the result of a prolactin-secreting pituitary tumor. Hyperprolactinemia patients have decreased or low-normal testosterone levels. Despite the use of exogenous testosterone, impotence will not be reversed solely by this means. The treatment of hyperprolactinemia is bromocriptine or surgical ablation of the pituitary tumor.

In general, if impotence is secondary to an endocrine cause, one must localize the defect to either the gonadal or the hypothalamic-pituitary level. Several caveats should be heeded prior to labeling an individual as having endocrine impotence. The presence of a low testosterone level in an impotent patient in no way establishes this diagnosis with certainty. One must remember that serum testosterone levels vary diurnally (lowest in the afternoon) and that they may be diminished by anxiety, stress, or depression. For this reason, tripooled serum samples are preferred to single testosterone determinations. Furthermore, a normal testosterone level may be found in a patient whose impotence has an endocrine etiology, as that individual may require a higher level of testosterone to function normally. Unfortunately, many physicians have treated impotent patients with low-normal or slightly depressed testosterone levels with exogenous testosterone and have seen a positive response. This has led to the erroneous assumption that a testosterone deficit is the cause of impotence in such patients. However, a response to exogenous testosterone may be mediated by heightened libido as well as a known antidepressant effect of androgens. All these effects may contribute to the return of potency in patients with situational or psychogenic impotence as well as in patients with underlying endocrine abnormalities. The true diagnosis of endocrine impotence can be made only after a reproducible abnormality in serum testosterone levels is confirmed by nocturnal penile tumescence (NPT) monitoring that reveals organic impotence. Treatment with specific hormones should produce a prompt return of sexual function as well as changing the NPT tracing.

Patients with hypothalamic-pituitary disorders producing impotence will have reduced serum testosterone levels and inappropriately low gonadotropin levels. Reduced testosterone levels would be expected to result in an increase in pituitary LH secretion if the hypothalamus and pituitary were functioning normally. Therefore, when LH levels are normal or decreased in the face of abnormally low serum testosterone levels, one must rule out the possibility of an underlying hypogonadotrophic hypogonadism. Examples of congenital syndromes that may result in this endocrinologic disorder include the Kallmann syndrome, Prader-Willi syndrome, and Laurence-Moon-Biedl syndrome. It must be remembered that most patients with congenital hypothalamic-pituitary disorders usually will first seek advice from a pediatrician or endocrinologist regarding delayed puberty rather than present to a urologist with problems of impotence. Acquired disease of the hypothalamic-pituitary system will usually be due to an underlying pituitary tumor. Examples of other hypothalamic syndromes causing hypogonadism are the idiopathic variety, various infiltrative disorders including sarcoid, tuberculosis, and eosinophilic granulomas as well as cysts within the area.

Endocrinologic impotence most commonly originates at the gonadal level and is primary gonadal failure resulting in a reduced circulating testosterone level and an appropriately elevated serum LH level. This disorder is termed hypergonadotrophic hypogonadism. The causes include Klinefelter's syndrome, chemotherapeutic agents, and radiotherapy.

Hyper- and hypothyroidism have been associated with a decrease in potency. In some series, a decrease in libido is seen in a majority of patients with hyperthyroidism (Kidd et al., 1979). An older man with hyperthyroidism may not display the obvious signs and symptoms of thyrotoxicosis but rather may merely be depressed and show loss of libido. The etiology of this decreased libido is at present unclear. Surprisingly, serum testosterone levels may often be at the upper limits of normal in hyperthyroidism. In contrast, testosterone levels may be decreased in patients with hypothyroidism, possibly owing to a shift in metabolic transformation of testosterone to etiocholanolone or to a decrease in testosterone-binding globulin. The latter decrease may actually increase free testosterone, thus making it difficult to relate impotence secondary to hypothyroidism to an androgen-deprived state.

Diabetes Mellitus. Diabetes mellitus is probably the most frequent single cause for erectile dysfunction in the United States today. Despite the discovery and use of insulin, this complication has continued and remains more common than either retinopathy or nephropathy. Approximately half of the male diabetic population in the United States complains of some degree of sexual dysfunction (Waxman, 1980).

As was mentioned earlier, erectile function is dependent upon a complex interaction of vascular, neurologic, hormonal, and psychologic factors. Any of these may be altered in a chronic disease such as diabetes. In hopes of elucidating the etiology of diabetic impotence, evidence for and against each of these variable factors will be reviewed.

Large-vessel and small-vessel disease has

been strongly associated with diabetes and has been well described. In impotent diabetics, vascular lesions have been reported in autopsy series (Ruzbarsky and Michal, 1977) as well as in arteriographic studies (Herman et al., 1978). Ruzbarsky and coworkers (1977) have shown post-mortem changes of advanced atherosclerosis in the small penile arteries in 15 impotent diabetic men. These arterial changes worsened with age. These diabetic patients were compared with nondiabetic men, and it was concluded that penile vascular disease in diabetics showed accelerated progression as compared with nondiabetics at the same age (Ruzbarsky and Michal, 1977). In our own series, we found a marked increase in vasculogenic impotence with increasing age (Goldstein et al., 1983). In most of our older non–insulin dependent diabetics, almost all impotence was secondary to vasculogenic causes.

As stated earlier, a neuropathy of the sensory portion of the pudendal nerve, the thoracolumbar sympathetic outflow, or the sacral parasympthetic outflow will result in altered erectile and ejaculatory function. Faerman and associates (1974), in a post-mortem study of impotent diabetic men, demonstrated that the corpus cavernosal tissue showed alterations in nerve fibers that were not present in potent males. Melman (1983) has demonstrated a reduction in corporal tissue norepinephrine levels in impotent diabetics as compared with normal men. Cystometrography has been performed on impotent diabetic males, and in one series 75 per cent of impotent diabetics were found to have neurogenic detrusor areflexia (Ellenberg, 1971). When sacral evoked-potential studies have been performed, they have been abnormally prolonged in 30 to 85 per cent of patients studied (Vacek and Lachman, 1977). This led to the conclusion that a large proportion of impotence in diabetics was neurologic in origin.

Earlier studies demonstrated possible endocrine etiology for diabetic impotence. Based on urinary excretion levels of pituitary gonadotropins, it was felt that hypogonadotrophic hypogonadism was a leading cause of diabetic impotence (Horstmann, 1950). However, with the recent advent of radioimmunoassay techniques, no endocrine abnormalities in significant numbers have been reported (Jensen et al., 1979).

Peyronie's Disease. Peyronie's disease is characterized by formation of a fibrous plaque intimately involved with the tunica albuginea of the penis. The plaque is most commonly on the dorsal surface of the corpora. It was first described by Peyronie in 1873 as causing an upward bend of the penis during erection (Ashworth, 1960). Most cases of this disease involve men in their fourth or fifth decade of life, although patients as young as 18 years and as old as 80 years have been reported. Patients present to the physician complaining of curvature of the penis, painful intercourse, pain and tenderness, or the presence of a hard mass on the dorsum of the penis. This disease has also been associated with other disorders, such as Dupuytren's contracture and fibrous degeneration of the external ear cartilage.

The diagnosis of this disorder is made on physical examination by palpating an indurated plaque on the dorsal surface of the penis. Corroboration can be obtained by Polaroid photographs of the erect penis showing typical upward and often lateral curvature. X-ray of the area may show calcification in up to 20 per cent of cases. An artificial erection may be created in the office by injecting saline into one corpus, thus simulating the abnormalities seen during erection.

Although several hypotheses concerning the cause of this disease have been entertained, to date no known etiology has been determined. Interestingly, histocompatibility antigen studies have shown a correlation between the presence of the B7 cross-reacting group and Peyronie's disease (Willscher et al., 1979). This group includes HLA-B7, BW22, B27, and BW42. In one group, close to 88 per cent of patients were noted to have one of these antigens (Willscher, 1983), whereas another study showed no correlation between Peyronie's disease and the B7 cross-reacting group (Leffell et al., 1982). More recently a familial form of Peyronie's disease has been reported (Nyberg et al., 1982). Inheritance appears to be on the basis of an autosomal dominant trait. However, 90 per cent of those with Peyronie's disease in this study had a B7 cross-reacting histocompatibility antigen. It is hypothesized (Bias et al., 1982) that although Peyronie's disease appears to be transmitted by an autosomal dominant gene, the disorder may be influenced or modified by other genes (e.g., the B7 cross-reacting group).

Patients have been treated with a wide variety of medical therapies, including vitamin E, cortisone, para-aminobenzoate, radiotherapy, DMSO, ultrasound, parathormone, and procarbazine (Willscher, 1983). None of these approaches appears to offer a marked advantage over any other. In addition, one must remember that there is an incidence of spontaneous regression (or lack of progression) in the natural history of this disorder.

Several surgical procedures have been advocated for the treatment of Peyronie's disease and will be discussed in greater detail in the chapter on penile surgery. The most commonly used surgical procedure involves the removal or excision of the plaque and a grafting procedure usually using a dermal patch (Wild et al., 1979). Results from this procedure have ranged from poor to excellent (Wild et al., 1979; Melman and Holland, 1978). In addition, patients with Peyronie's disease have had all types of inflatable and noninflatable penile prostheses implanted, usually with good to excellent results (Raz et al., 1977; Small, 1978). A lesser used procedure has been ventral foreshortening, whereby the ventral aspect of the corpus is foreshortened by removing part of the tunica albuginea in the region opposite the plaque. Although only a few series have been reported, results to date have been excellent (Borrelli et al., 1983) (Fig. 13–5). It is the author's feeling that the latter operation is a reasonable initial procedure, especially in men who are still able to have sexual intercourse and merely want some straightening of the upward penile curvature. It is also the author's opinion that grafting procedures or implanatation of penile devices should not be performed in patients who still maintain the ability to have sexual intercourse despite the presence of Peyronie's disease.

Drug-Induced Impotence. Drug-induced sexual dysfunction is a relatively common problem. Unfortunately, the exact mechanisms whereby many drugs alter sexual function remain poorly understood. In recent review of patients in the medical outpatient clinic, 25 per cent of the cases of impotence were believed to have an underlying drug-associated cause (Slag et al., 1983). Therefore, it seems realistic to review at least some of the broader classes of drugs that may be involved with altered sexual function.

ALCOHOL. Although small amounts of alcohol may act as a sexual stimulant or at least decrease inhibitions regarding sex, alcohol abuse may lead to impotence. Alcohol-induced impotence may be partially psychologic in origin but is most likely to be related to alcoholic neuropathy. Certainly, in patients with alcohol-induced impotence, sacral evoked-potential studies have shown prolongation consistent with the theory of this disorder's being neurogenic in origin (Krane and Siroky, 1980). In addition, there is reasonable evidence that many chronic alcoholics develop a hypoandrogenic state. Serum testosterone levels in impotent alcoholics have been lower, presumably secondary to the effect of alcohol on testosterone metabolism (Van Thiel and Lester, 1974). A more recent study demonstrated that acute alcoholic consumption in normal men decreased testosterone production and increased testosterone clearance in most subjects (Gordon et al., 1976).

MEDICATIONS. Antihypertensive medicines have long been associated with the development of impotence. Although these drugs often have quite different mechanisms of action, they may for varied reasons cause erectile dysfunction. In a recent study, the incidence of propranolol-induced impotence was 15 per cent (Penttila, 1966). This was somewhat dose-related, as patients receiving more than 120 mg a day were more likely to become impotent. A newer beta-blocking agent, metoprolol (Lopressor), has also been associated with impotence in higher dosages. Prazosin hydrochloride, which is an alpha-adrenergic blocking agent, was associated with impotence in only 0.6 per cent of patients being treated with that agent (Papadopoulos, 1980). Similarly, phenoxybenzamine appears to preserve erectile ability. Reserpine, which also acts as an adrenergic blocking agent, has long been associated with impotence, although this may well be secondary to its known depressive action. Other antihypertensive agents, such as clonidine, methyldopa, monamine oxidase inhibitors, guanethidine, and thiazides, have also been associated in varying degrees with impotence (Goldstein, 1983). Many of these drugs may act centrally rather than on the corporal vasculature itself. A recent study in animals by

Figure 13–5. The ventral foreshortening procedure to straighten the dorsal curvature secondary to Peyronie's plaque is shown. Note that the urethra is dissected free of underlying tunica albuginea. The tunica is then cut at an appropriate level and resutured to produce the desired result. (From Borrelli, M., et al.: World J. Urol., 1 (4):257, 1983.)

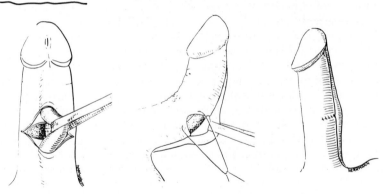

Melman shows that methyldopa appears to cause impotence in rats on the basis of central mechanisms (Melman et al., 1983).

Although some of the antihypertensives may, in fact, have peripheral and central blocking actions that lead to impotence, an alternative hypothesis should be considered. Many patients with hypertension may also have atherosclerotic changes in their pelvic vasculature and therefore some degree of pelvic vascular insufficiency. It may well be that simply treating their hypertension and decreasing the pressure head in the hypogastric artery will result in the ability to have an erection. As was mentioned before, it takes almost a five- to sixfold increase in flow through the pudendal artery to create an erection; the decrease in pressure head into an already impaired pelvic vasculature may be the real cause of impotence associated with many of the antihypertensive medications. Another possible explanation for the development of impotence in patients receiving antihypertensives that have an alpha-blocking activity (guanethidine, phenoxybenzamine, methyldopa) is that all are associated with ejaculatory incompetence. It is possible that the loss of ejaculatory ability may on some psychologic basis lead to impotence. It is interesting to note that the United States Veterans Administration Cooperative Study on Anti-Hypertensive Agents (1977) showed no significant difference in impotence regardless of treatment regimen employed. Since many of these agents have different peripheral and central actions, this may lend further credence to the hypothesis that the impotence is secondary to underlying vascular insufficiency rather than to a specific action of the drug.

A number of drugs have been associated with elevation of serum prolactin, and many of these agents have also been associated with sexual dysfunction. Prolactin is a hormone that is secreted by the pituitary and is under hypothalamic control. Secretion of prolactin can be inhibited by prolactin-inhibiting factor, which most probably is dopamine (del Pozo and Brownwell, 1979). Therefore, drugs that deplete dopamine stores or act as dopamine antagonists may increase serum prolactin. Drugs that have been associated with increases in serum prolactin and impotence include phenothiazines, tricyclic antidepressants, haloperidol, methyldopa, reserpine, meprobamate, cimetidine, amphetamines, and opiates (Goldstein, 1983).

As mentioned before, testosterone appears to have some relationship to sexual behavior and sexual function. Drugs that alter testosterone levels have also been associated with impaired libido and impotence. Cyproterone acetate, a commonly used antiandrogen, has been used in treating deviant male sexual behavior and has been shown to result in a loss of hypersexuality within 2 weeks (Laschet and Laschet, 1977). Exogenous estrogens have also been associated with impotence (Kent, 1973). Spironolactone, also used as an antihypertensive agent, has been associated with impotence. This drug causes lower testosterone and increased testosterone clearance (Rose et al., 1977). Marijuana, when used chronically, has been shown to decrease testosterone levels and has also been associated with impotence (Kolodny et al., 1974).

It is impossible to list and document every known drug that has been associated with erectile dysfunction. This discussion has highlighted the groups of drugs that have been associated with erectile failure and, when possible, described their mode of action.

IATROGENIC IMPOTENCE

This section will deal primarily with surgical manipulation that leads to impotence and also with the relationship of radiation therapy to the development of sexual dysfunction.

Arterial Procedures. Leriche (1923) first described arterial occlusive disease within the abdominal aortic bifurcation as a cause for erectile dysfunction. Since then there have been numerous studies showing that large-vessel aortoiliac disease may be the basis for pelvic vascular insufficiency in secondary impotence (May et al., 1969; Michal et al., 1974). More recently, however, attention has been drawn to the occurrence of impotence following aortoiliac or aortofemoral bypass procedures that result in a decrease in hypogastric arterial blood flow (Queral et al., 1979). Any aorto–iliac–femoral bypass procedure that reduces hypogastric blood flow may lead to impotence, especially one involving a proximal end-to-end anastomosis between the aorta and the bypass graft with a distal end-to-side anastomosis between the graft and the iliac or femoral artery. In this situation, hypogastric blood flow is totally dependent on retrograde flow from the distal iliac or femoral artery. If there is disease in the proximal external iliac artery, this blood flow is restricted, and a potent patient may be converted to an impotent patient by this type of procedure. Therefore, when preparing for reconstructive arterial procedures, one must take into account disease in the external iliac artery. Accordingly, reconstructive procedures incorporating an end-to-side proximal aortic anatomosis should be considered. In addition, endarterectomies of the external iliac or the hypogastric artery may be useful as an adjunct to the main procedure in order to enable sufficient blood to enter the pudendal artery.

Renal Transplantation. Renal transplantation is usually carried out using an end-to-end anastomosis between the host hypogastric artery and the donor renal artery. In some cases, impotence may result on the basis of severely reduced penile blood pressure. The likelihood of impotence increases when a second renal transplant is placed on the contralateral side using the same type of end-to-end anastomosis. In several reviews, an extremely high incidence of impotence has been noted following bilateral renal transplantations performed in this manner (Budin et al., 1979; Gittes and Waters, 1979). Therefore, it is recommended that when a contralateral renal transplant is required, an end-to-side anastomosis between the host external iliac artery and the donor renal artery be performed in order to preserve blood flow through the hypogastric artery.

A similar situation, in which both hypogastric arteries are ligated, may occur during radical pelvic surgery, especially radical cystectomy. Penile vascular insufficiency after radical cystectomy is clearly not the sole cause of postoperative impotence, as psychologic and neurogenic factors must also be considered.

Pelvic Irradiation. External beam irradiation to the pelvis has been used in treating bladder, prostate, and colon malignancies. Typically, patients with prostatic malignancy receive 5000 rads to the whole pelvis and a boost of 2000 rads to the prostatic area. The incidence of impotence following external beam radiation for prostate cancer ranges from 22 to 84 per cent (Bagshaw et al., 1975; Mollenkamp et al., 1975). A recent clinical study performed at Boston University showed that 63 per cent of patients had a change in erectile potency after external beam radiation therapy, whereas no patient noted this after I-125 interstitial implantation or after pelvic lymphadenectomy (Goldstein et al., 1983). Patients who received external beam irradiation for prostate cancer had normal neurologic and endocrine function, whereas in all cases in which impotence resulted, penile Doppler studies showed a reduction in penile blood pressure. Patients who noted a change in erectile capacity following irradiation had a higher incidence of both hypertension and cigarette smoking. Both animal and clinical studies support the concept of vascular damage

and restriction of blood flow through vessels that have been exposed to radiation (Sarns, 1965). Radiation-induced erectile dysfunction may well be vasculogenic in etiology, with vascular risk factors, such as hypertension and cigarette smoking, playing a supporting role.

Operations for Priapism. Impotence may result as a complication of surgical procedures to treat priapism. Most procedures used in the treatment of this disease involve effecting an increase in venous run-off from the corpora. This is accomplished by direct end-to-side anastomosis of the saphenous vein to the corpus, surgical anastomosis between the corpus cavernosum and corpus spongiosum, or percutaneous drainage of the distal corpus through the glans penis (Winter procedure). Usually, potency will be restored after a suitable postoperative period has elapsed, probably as a consequence of the spontaneous closure of the shunt that has been created. In a small proportion of patients, however, this will not occur and impotence will continue. This can be diagnosed by infusion cavernosography.

Neurologic Mechanisms. Neurosurgical procedures, especially those developed to control myoclonus, have been associated with impotence (Meyers, 1962). Spinal procedures to treat cervical spondylitis, cervical or lumbar disc disease, or tumors of the spinal cord have also been associated with impotence (Siroky et al., 1979). In addition, impotence may result from spinal cord infarction secondary to aortic aneurysm repair.

Sacral rhizotomy, which is performed occasionally in patients with severe vesical hyperreflexia, results in bilateral destruction of the anterior and posterior roots of S2–S4. As a by-product of this procedure, one would expect that erectile dysfunction would also result. Some centers have turned to differential sacral rhizotomy in which only one or two roots are sectioned in order to reduce the possibility of this complication (Rochswold et al., 1973).

The incidence of impotence after abdominal perineal resection (Miles resection) for malignant disease varies between 50 and 100 per cent (Devlin et al., 1971; Dwight et al., 1969). It is interesting to note that when this procedure is performed for benign disease, impotence is rarely produced (Yeager and Van Heerden, 1980). Surgery for benign disease of the rectum requires dissection limited to the wall of the rectosigmoid, thereby preventing destruction of the pelvic parasympathetic nerves, which are located in the pararectal space bilaterally. Obviously, when one is performing this operation for the removal of cancer, a wider resection is required and injury to these nerves often results, thereby causing the high incidence of erectile dysfunction.

Radical cystectomy and radical prostatectomy are also associated with a high incidence of postoperative impotence. As mentioned before, radical cystectomy may decrease pudendal blood flow, especially when both hypogastric arteries are ligated. In addition, the paravesical neuronal plexuses are usually sectioned during this procedure, thereby producing both neurologic and vascular insufficiency of the penis. In the case of radical prostatectomy, it appears that the resultant impotence is primarily neurologic. The periprostatic autonomic plexus is usually injured during this procedure. When care is taken to preserve this plexus, potency also is usually preserved (Walsh et al., 1983).

Transurethral external sphincterotomy, transurethral prostatic resection, and transurethral direct-vision urethrotomy have also been associated with impotence (Kiviat, 1975; Madorsky et al., 1976; McDermott et al., 1981). The exact cause of this is still being debated. It can be speculated, however, that vascular and neurologic injury may result from the coagulating current. Infusion of irrigating fluid into the corpora by inadvertent injury to the tunica albuginea may also play a role in causing impotence.

One cannot exclude psychologic factors resulting from many of these procedures, especially those in which a stoma for either stool or urine is created. There is little doubt that the changes in self-esteem and body image can easily lead to erectile dysfunction. In the case of transurethral prostatic resection in which an underlying organic cause remains indeterminate, it is most likely that the basis for impotence is mainly psychologic.

EVALUATION OF THE IMPOTENT PATIENT

The diagnostic approach to the impotent patient has changed markedly in recent years, undoubtedly as a result of the increased number of therapeutic options. In addition to the history and physical examination, a number of specialized sophisticated techniques have been developed both to differentiate between organic and psychogenic impotence and to compartmentalize the impotent patient into a vasculogenic, neurogenic, or endocrinologic etiologic category. No matter what one's particular approach to the evaluation of the impotent patient is, the evaluation itself should provide a probable etiology so that one may intelligently formulate an appropriate therapeutic plan.

The evaluation of the impotent patient is increasingly being performed in multidisciplinary or multispecialty impotence–sexual dysfunction clinics. These clinics are usually directed by either a urologist or a psychiatrist with input from other subspecialties such as neurology, psychology, vascular surgery, endocrinology, and so forth. These clinics, by virtue of their multispecialty approach, usually offer increased expertise as well as any and all types of diagnostic evaluations and therapeutic regimens.

The usual approach to the impotent patient is to attempt to distinguish whether he is suffering from psychogenic or organic impotence. Several important caveats should be mentioned in this regard. The presence of a known disorder that might produce impotence (e.g., multiple sclerosis, diabetes, and so forth) should not deter the physician from a complete evaluation in order to be sure that the impotence itself is not psychologically induced, the disorder being merely coincidental. Conversely, the identification of an important psychologic problem need not imply that this is the cause of erectile dysfunction, as it may well be the effect of organic impotence. Clearly, in both instances a complete evaluation should obviate a false diagnosis. Lastly, there are patients who suffer from a combination of psychogenic and organic impotence. The 70-year-old male with hypertension and diabetes who has recently lost his wife may indeed have a combination of psychologic and organic factors. Similarly, the 25-year-old diabetic who has recently undergone toe amputations may also have a combination of these etiologies. In the quest to obtain a specific diagnosis one must always remember that on occasion the etiology is multifactorial.

History. The first task in taking a history from the impotent patient is to determine if, indeed, he is suffering from impotence. For this purpose we define impotence as the inability to create or maintain an erection when desired and at an appropriate time. After this has been established, the patient's problem must be further defined. Important questions to be answered include: How long has the patient noticed erectile dysfunction? Did the problem begin abruptly or insidiously? Is there an associated decrease in libido? Is the problem one of inability to achieve an erection or inability to maintain an erection or both? Does position or movement alter or affect the penile tumescence or rigidity? Does the patient ever get a normal or near-normal erection (e.g., during masturbation, with other partners, or upon awakening)? Is there any change in the ejaculatory function? Lastly, what is the patient's assessment of his maximal erection? (This can be expressed in terms related to a clock face, with 6 o'clock signifying no erection and 11 o'clock signifying complete erection.)

Responses to these questions more often than not will greatly aid in determining whether the patient is suffering from psychogenic or organic impotence and may at times point to the potential diagnosis of vasculogenic impotence. Patients with underlying psychogenic impotence usually have a rather abrupt change in their erectile ability, which is often associated with an important life event (e.g., divorce, change of job, death of spouse, and so forth). In contrast, patients with organic impotence (e.g., diabetic, vascular) usually report a slow, insidious onset of progressive erectile failure. Patients with psychogenic impotence may on certain occasions have a relatively normal erection, such as upon awakening, in the middle of the night, or with other partners. A noticeable decrease in libido as a primary complaint may reflect a hormonal deficit or psychologic depression. Most often, diminished libido is secondary to the primary erectile dysfunction. In our experience, marked changes in libido are more often seen in patients with psychogenic impotence than in those with organic impotence. It is also our experience that changes in ejaculation are more often seen in patients with psychogenic impotence than in those with organic impotence (except for neurogenic impotence). The combination of diminished ejaculate and concomitant loss of libido should alert one to the diagnosis of hypogonadism.

Obviously, one should attempt to ascertain whether any of the factors that have been outlined previously pertain to the patient. Such factors include a wide variety of commonly used drugs that were discussed earlier. In particular, hypertensive patients receiving antihypertensive agents are prone to pelvic vascular insufficiency, as described previously. Certainly, patients receiving various antipsychotic agents as well as estrogens should be identified.

Patients suffering from vasculogenic impotence frequently have little or no history indicative of peripheral vascular insufficiency. However, comparing patients with vasculogenic impotence with age-matched nonimpotent patients or age-matched nonvasculogenic impotent patients, one sees an increased incidence of hypertension, claudication, and diabetes in the vasculogenic impotence group (Goldstein et al., 1982). It is not surprising that a higher incidence of these vascular risk factors exists in patients suffering from pelvic vascular insufficiency leading to impotence. It is important, therefore, that these factors be documented in the history.

Physical Examination. In general, the physical examination of the impotent patient will be unrewarding with regard to etiologic clues.

Generally, one looks for the development of normal secondary sex characteristics, as they are a gross index of androgen stimulation. One should note body and facial hair patterns, muscular development, and the presence of gynecomastia. The size and consistency of the testes should be evaluated as well as the presence of bilateral or unilateral cryptorchidism. Many patients with endocrinopathies characterized by androgen deficiency present to the pediatrician, endocrinologist, or internist because of delayed puberty. In adults, hypogonadal disorders will usually present with loss of libido.

The vascular tree may be evaluated by palpating femoral as well as dorsalis pedis pulses. In addition, the dorsal penile pulses may be palpated and their quality noted. Neurologic examination referable to the sacral dermatoses includes pinprick sensation in the perineum and the presence or absence of the bulbocavernosus reflex. This reflex is evoked by squeezing the glans penis and digitally palpating the anal sphincter area. In addition, a thorough rectal examination should be performed to rule out any neoplastic prostatic disease. The corpora cavernosa should be palpated mainly to determine the presence or absence of Peyronie's plaques.

Laboratory Tests. Prior to seeking urologic care, most patients have seen their local physicians, who have performed complete blood counts as well as tests relating to hepatic function. Fasting and 2-hour postprandial blood sugar levels have usually been determined to rule out the presence of diabetes mellitus. In addition, serum testosterone and prolactin levels should be determined. Patients with a diminished or low-normal testosterone level should undergo repeat serum testosterone studies accompanied by FSH and LH determinations. Patients with high prolactin levels are referred directly to the endocrinologist for further evaluation.

If repeat testosterone levels remain low and gonadotropin levels are not appropriately elevated, the patient is referred to an endocrinologist for evaluation of hypogonadotrophic hypogonadism. In our experience, the majority of these patients turn out to have no endocrinologic disease when more sophisticated endocrine measurements, such as testosterone production rates, are performed. Patients who have diminished testosterone levels and appropriately elevated gonadotropin levels are treated with intramuscular testosterone enanthate, 200 mg, every 3 weeks. Clearly, some of these patients will have psychogenic impotence, while others will have true hormonal impotence. In some cases it is very difficult to differentiate these groups diagnostically. It seems reasonable, therefore, to curtail testosterone administration after several treatments and to expect those patients with primarily psychogenic impotence to have continued potency despite cessation of testosterone therapy. In contrast, patients with true hormonal impotence would be expected to lose their potency rather quickly. Although this is not a foolproof test, it at least offers patients with an underlying psychogenic problem the opportunity to be properly diagnosed rather than to continue prolonged testosterone therapy unnecessarily.

Psychometric Testing. Quite a number of psychologic or psychometric tests have been applied to the diagnosis of patients with erectile dysfunction. The most popular of these has been the Minnesota Multiphasic Personality Inventory (MMPI). Other tests that are available include the Derogatis Sexual Functioning Inventory (DSFI), the Walker Sex Form (WSF), and the California Personality Inventory (CPI). At present there is considerable disagreement as to which, if any, of these tests is best able to distinguish psychogenically impotent from non–psychogenically impotent patients (Marshall et al., 1980; Schoenberg et al., 1982).

Beutler and coworkers (1976) were first to attempt to differentiate psychogenic from biologic causes of impotence by using the MMPI. Using certain decision rules based on this test, their method correctly identified 90 per cent of patients deemed psychogenically impotent by nocturnal tumescence studies. In addition, they determined that there was no clear personality type associated with either psychogenic or organic impotence. Other investigators have attempted to use decision rules similar to those developed by Beutler for the MMPI and have found them to be unable to differentiate organic from psychogenic impotence (Marshall et al., 1980). For the same reasons, the author has not found the application of psychometric testing to the evaluation of the impotent patient particularly informative or helpful.

Nocturnal Penile Tumescence Testing. The concept of nocturnal penile tumescence (NPT) was first described in infants by Halverson (1940) and in adults by Ohlmeyer (1944). By the middle of the 1960's, nocturnal penile tumescence was recognized as a naturally occurring phenomenon, and various monitoring techniques were developed by two specific groups, namely, Fisher and coworkers and Karacan and coworkers (Fisher et al., 1965; Karacan et al., 1966). It was Karacan's group that, in 1970, first suggested the use of nocturnal penile tumescence monitoring as a clinical tool for the differential diagnosis of impotence (Karacan, 1983).

In the normal male, three to five erections, each lasting 25 to 35 minutes and together accounting for 20 to 40 per cent of sleep time, will occur each night (Fisher et al., 1965) (Fig. 13–6). This is largely correlated with rapid eye movement (REM) sleep, although the two phenomena may occur independently. With increasing age, total tumescence time as well as duration of each tumescence episode gradually decreases (Karacan et al., 1975). The "morning erection" is merely a nocturnal penile erection that occurs just prior to awakening. A morning erection is therefore unrelated to a distended bladder (a belief that is held by many patients).

Nocturnal penile tumescence testing is usually done over a two- to three-night period. This is to obviate the possibility of the "first-night effect," in which poor sleep states and poor tumescence is found secondary to the measurement of tumescence itself. Simultaneously with measurement of penile circumferential change, monitoring by electroencephalogram (EEG), electro-oculogram (EOG), or electromyogram (EMG) from the bulbocavernosus muscle may be done. Penile tumescence is measured by two strain gauges that are positioned around the subcoronal region and around the base of the penis. These are both mercury-filled silicone tubing, which, when stretched, causes the mercury column inside to narrow and thereby increase electrical resistance. Therefore, small variations in circumferential change can be recorded on the accompanying chart recorder. The normal findings are three to five erectile episodes per night, each ranging from 25 to 35 minutes in duration. Normal expansile change varies from 15 to 30 mm at the distal penis to 24 mm at the proximal penis.

It should be noted at this point that a true test of the worth of nocturnal penile tumescence monitoring has not been carried out. Most data concerning the validity of this test have been of an indirect nature, in that groups of patients previously determined to have psychogenic or organic impotence are then re-evaluated by their nocturnal penile tumescence tracings.

The use of this test in impotence assessment

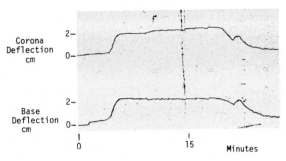

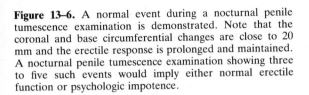

Figure 13–6. A normal event during a nocturnal penile tumescence examination is demonstrated. Note that the coronal and base circumferential changes are close to 20 mm and the erectile response is prolonged and maintained. A nocturnal penile tumescence examination showing three to five such events would imply either normal erectile function or psychologic impotence.

is based on two assumptions. The first is that the mechanism of nocturnal penile erections is similar or identical to that of an erection during sexual stimulation. Although this assumption has been questioned by some, it is more than probable that the physiologic mechanisms responsible for the development of nocturnal erection are, in fact, similar to those operative during sexual stimulation. The second assumption is that the patients with psychogenic impotence will respond in a manner similar to the patient who is not impotent. Therefore, the patient with psychogenic impotence would be expected to have the normal number of erectile episodes, each of normal duration and with appropriate circumferential changes. Conversely, the patient with nonpsychologic or organic impotence would not be expected to have the normal amount of erectile activity or the normal circumferential changes associated with it.

This second assumption has been challenged on several levels. First, the question of whether purely psychogenic factors can inhibit nocturnal penile tumescence changes has never been totally resolved. Karacan studied the relationship between dream content during REM sleep and erectile changes during those episodes

(Karacan et al., 1966). He found a significant decrease in the number of full erections when dream content was thought to have a higher anxiety score. This finding was also noted by Fisher (Fisher et al., 1965). As mentioned before, the "first-night effect" (alterations in penile response secondary to anxiety induced by the testing procedure) has been described by many. The "first-night effect" serves as a good example of psychologic inhibition of penile tumescence, which can produce an abnormal NPT in patients with purely psychogenic impotence. Both Karacan and Fisher have found a group of patients, constituting 15 to 20 per cent of all those tested, who had abnormal NPT but no recognizable organic pathology (Fisher et al., 1979; Karacan et al., 1978). Whether this group merely represents one with undetected organic pathology or whether it represents an example of psychogenic inhibition of penile tumescence changes remains unanswered.

Be that as it may, NPT testing still remains an important part of the evaluaion of the impotent patient. This is true especially when the findings on NPT testing mimic the findings described by the patient (Figs. 13–7 to 13–9). For example, when a patient describes an erection that is initially normal but poorly sustained and

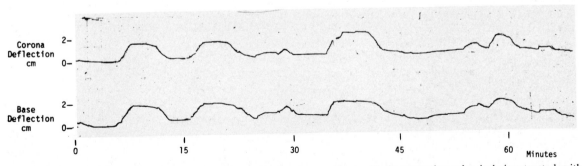

Figure 13–7. A nocturnal penile tumescence examination in a patient with hypertension who is being treated with antihypertensive medication. His complaint is poorly sustained and nonrigid erections. His nocturnal penile examination shows short unsustained erectile activity with relatively normal circumferential change. As this examination cannot test rigidity, it is entirely consistent with the patient's history. In our experience, when NPT data such as these corroborate the patient's history, one is almost always dealing with an underlying organic problem.

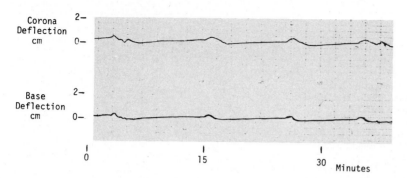

Figure 13–8. An NPT study from a patient complaining of essentially no erectile activity. In our experience, two nights of this type of minimal erectile activity is consistent with the diagnosis of impotence secondary to an underlying organic disorder.

on NPT testing demonstrates precisely the same thing, this tends to support the diagnosis of organic impotence. In addition, patients may describe only partial erections and consistently show this on NPT testing, thus corroborating their history. Lastly, in our experience with nearly 1,000 nocturnal penile tumescence examinations, we have yet to see a patient with a completely normal NPT tracing who has anything but an underlying psychogenic problem. This has also been the experience of others (Kaya et al., 1979).

Nocturnal penile tumescence testing may be carried out in the hospital (e.g., a sleep laboratory) or at home. NPT testing performed with an observer present is clearly the best way of using this examination (Van Ansdalen and Wein, 1983). The main advantage is that this meets a major objection to nocturnal penile tumescence testing, namely, that it does not measure rigidity. Between 10 and 17 per cent of patients with relatively normal circumferential change nevertheless have decreased penile rigidity, making their erection insufficient for intromission (Wein et al., 1981). With the use of an observer and an alarm that will sound at the appropriate circumferential change, one can awaken the patient and corroborate the finding of decreased rigidity more easily. At home, the

use of an NPT monitor will not suffice to determine rigidity but will show circumferential change. In addition, careful monitoring within a sleep laboratory can verify the changes that the patient describes in discussing his lack of erectile ability. On occasion a patient with psychogenic impotence, to whom one can demonstrate that his nocturnal erections are normal, may find this a therapeutic event. Lastly, studies performed within a sleep laboratory can corroborate that the characteristics of the patient's sleep are in fact normal (Van Arsdalen and Wein, 1983).

Several attempts have been made to measure penile rigidity, as this is one of the major drawbacks of nocturnal penile tumescence testing. Karacan has designed a device that measures buckling pressure; he has found that greater than 100 mg Hg buckling pressure is definitely sufficient rigidity to make intromission possible, while less than 60 mm Hg buckling pressure is inadequate for vaginal penetration (Karacan et al., 1978). In another attempt to measure rigidity, a snap gauge was developed by the Dacomed Corporation incorporating three plastic strips with varying force characteristics (Fig. 13–10). Evaluation of the snap gauge indicates that it correlates well with nocturnal penile tumescent testing in terms of circumferential

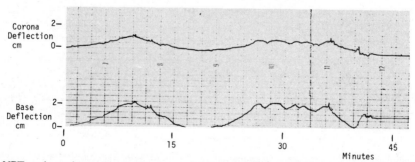

Figure 13–9. An NPT study performed on a patient complaining of inability to achieve or maintain a rigid erection. As in Figure 13–7, there is a good correlation between the NPT study and the patient's history. Note the slow onset of circumferential change, as opposed to the normal in Figure 13–6, and the inability to sustain circumferential change. In our experience, this type of NPT data is usually found in patients with underlying vasculogenic impotence.

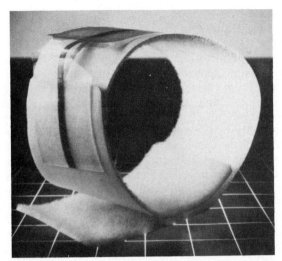

Figure 13–10. A penile snap gauge developed to measure penile rigidity. We have found an excellent correlation between the results of NPT testing and concomitant snap gauge testing. In addition, when artificially creating an erection by continuous intracorporeal saline flow, the three elements of the snap gauge break at approximately 80, 100, and 120 mm Hg of intracorporeal pressure. (Photo courtesy of DACOMED Corporation.)

change as well as in differentiating organic from psychogenic impotence (Ek et al., 1983).

Vascular Testing Techniques. Although many differential approaches have been suggested to evaluate both pressure and flow within the penis in a noninvasive manner, the most commonly used method employs a Doppler stethoscope. A special 1.2-inch inflatable cuff is applied at the base of the penis to measure systolic pressure in both the dorsal and the cavernosal arteries (Jevtich, 1980) (Fig. 13–11). The cutoff pressure is determined by inflating the cuff above systolic pressure and slowly deflating the cuff until blood flow is re-established as determined by the Doppler probe.

There are several known methods for recording systolic penile blood pressure. The earliest to be reported used a plethysmograph and was described by Britt and coworkers (1971). Again, a 1-inch pneumatic cuff was placed around the base of the penis and a circular strain gauge was placed distally and attached to a plethysmograph. Both the plethysmograph curve (representative of volume change/pulse) and penile systolic pressure could be obtained. Gaskell (1971) in his original description employed a spectroscope, in which he noted a change in color in the glans penis; he reported this as penile systolic pressure, again using a pneumatic cuff at the base of the penis. In 1975, Abelson introduced the Doppler ultrasound

method, first using a Doppler transducer within the inflatable cuff (Abelson, 1975). This later was changed to the currently used method that utilizes an inflatable 1-inch pneumatic cuff at the base of the penis and a pencil-probe Doppler placed directly over the specific artery to be tested (Fig. 13–12).

In general, penile systolic pressure is compared with brachial systolic pressure by calculating the ratio of penile to brachial systolic pressure. This ratio is termed the penile brachial index (PBI) (Queral et al., 1979). A ratio of 0.6 or less has been shown to be indicative of vasculogenic impotence. Conversely, a ratio of 0.75 or more is indicative of normal arterial inflow. It should be remembered that Engel, in his first description of the penile brachial index, found that potent individuals have average indices of greater than 0.96 (Engel et al., 1978). Our experience with approximately 1,000 penile Doppler studies indicates that a normal patient should have a penile/brachial index of greater than 0.9. Therefore PBI's of less than 0.9 are considered abnormal, although not diagnostic of vasculogenic impotence, and must be corroborated by other tests, such as nocturnal penile tumescence studies.

The penile systolic pressure has also been related to brachial pressure by the creation of a penile brachial mean pressure (PBMP). The mean brachial pressure is calculated as brachial

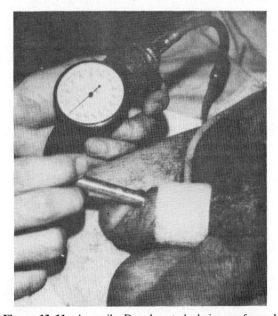

Figure 13–11. A penile Doppler study being performed. Note the small cuff at the base of the penis attached to a sphygmomanometer. A pencil-like Doppler stethoscope, as described in the text, is used and can easily distinguish both corporeal arteries.

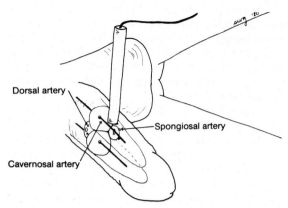

Figure 13–12. Schematic demonstration of penile Doppler study measuring the pressure in the corporeal artery. In performing a penile Doppler study, one first identifies each cavernosal artery and dorsal artery. The Doppler probe is then placed over the cavernosal artery to be measured. The penile cuff is inflated until no pulsation is noted and then slowly deflated until pulsations within the artery being studied are heard. (From Goldstein I., et al.: J. Urol., *128*:300, 1982.)

pulse pressure divided by 3 plus brachial diastolic pressure (Montague et al., 1980). A penile systolic pressure (PSP) that is less than the mean brachial pressure by 30 mm Hg or more was felt to indicate significant vascular insufficiency.

Another study to consider is the penile flow index, which measures penile artery acceleration (penile velocity divided by penile rise time) (Velcek et al., 1980). This method has not gained widespread acceptance. More recently, a dynamic penile Doppler study (known as the pelvic steal test) has been developed (Goldstein et al., 1982). In this test, PBI determinations are made on both corporal cavernosal arteries at rest and following leg and buttock exercises. A drop of PBI of greater than 0.15 after exercise is considered indicative of a vascular steal producing decreased blood flow to the penis. Patients who have difficulty maintaining erections, especially during movement, may have a "steal phenomenon" in which blood is preferentially directed toward muscles in the legs or buttocks, thereby causing insufficient flow to the pudendal artery.

Invasive vascular techniques aim at the diagnosis of arterial vascular insufficiency (pudendal arteriography) and venous vascular insufficiency (infusion cavernosography). Although large-vessel arteriography was used as early as 1963 to study vasculogenic impotence (Canning et al., 1963), it was not until 1973 that Michal performed the first pudendal arteriogram (Michal et al., 1980). Michal and his coworkers as well as Ginestié and his coworkers were the

pioneering groups involved in penile arteriography (Michal et al., 1980; Ginestié and Romien, 1976). Michal also developed the technique of phalloarteriography, which combined the pudendal arteriogram with the infusion cavernosogram (Michal and Pospichal, 1978). Michal also felt that the cavernosal infusion would increase the size of the pudendal artery, thereby simplifying the interpretation of the x-ray study.

Both these groups were instrumental in defining the procedure of penile or pudendal arteriography as well as in categorizing the abnormalities that could be diagnosed by this type of study. Small-vessel disease in the pudendal and penile arteries took the form of arteriosclerotic narrowing, stenoses, aneurysmal dilatation, and so forth. In essence, all the abnormalities in other small vessels could also be appreciated in the smaller pudendal-penile circulation. In addition, abnormal arteriovenous malformation has been reported (Zorgniotti et al., 1983).

The technique used at our institution for pudendal angiography (Miller et al., 1982) involves the use of local anesthetic, namely, xylocaine, injected with the contrast agent. We used epidural anesthesia in our initial group; however, at present no general anesthesia is required. In addition, a vasodilator, such as tolazoline HCl, is injected at the same time. A lead shield is used to protect the scrotal contents, and a Foley catheter is placed per urethra to help identify the penile vessels. Both pudendal arteries are visualized by selective bilateral hypogastric injections. Initially, a catheter is passed via the femoral artery route to the bifurcation of the aorta, and aortoiliac arteriograms are obtained. Next, with the use of a cobra C2-6 French catheter, the contralateral hypogastric artery is catheterized and pudendal arteriograms are obtained by injecting 60 ml of contrast over 20 seconds. After a 10-second delay, one film per second is taken over the next 20 seconds. The procedure is then repeated on the ipsilateral side. There is no need for superselective catheterization of the internal pudendal artery. Occasionally, because of difficulty in negotiating the aortic bifurcation with a catheter, two femoral sticks will be required.

For examining the aortoiliac vessels, the pelvis is filmed in both anterior oblique positions. For selective pudendal studies, the side injected is filmed in the anterior oblique view.

Normally, the terminal branches of the internal pudendal artery, namely, the dorsal and deep (cavernosal) penile arteries and the artery to the bulb, are visualized (Fig. 13–13). Usually,

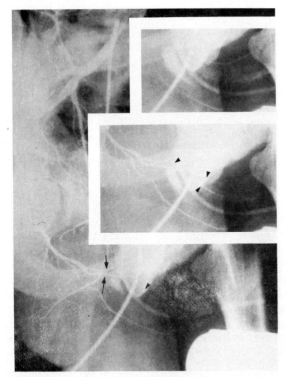

Figure 13–13. A normal pudendal arteriogram. In the large picture, the downward arrow is pointing to the bulbar branch, which distally dips caudally to form the bulbar blush. The upward arrow points to the penile artery, which will subsequently divide to the dorsal and cavernosal branches. The lower inset shows small arrows pointing to the bulbar artery and subsequently to the cavernosal and dorsal arteries of the penis. In the upper inset a dorsal artery is demonstrated by the small arrow and a blush is seen within cavernous tissue itself. Note also that a Foley catheter is within the urethra. This is always placed prior to the performance of a pudendal arteriogram and helps with anatomic localization; the bulbar blush is always proximal to the urethral catheter, while the bifurcation of the penile artery to form the dorsal and cavernosal branches is always distal to the urethral catheter.

a bulbar blush will also be seen (Fig. 13–14). An accessory pudendal artery is seen in 10 per cent of cases, and this artery may give rise to any or all of the aforementioned vessels. In our experience, localized internal pudendal disease usually has been secondary to atherosclerosis or trauma (Figs. 13–15 and 13–16).

The indications for pudendal arteriography remain somewhat unclear. In our institution, the feeling is that selective pudendal arteriography should not be considered a riskless procedure. In the performance of nearly 130 arteriograms we have had 3 cases with major complications. All involved formation of intimal dissection of the hypogastric origin, one involving the need for arterial repair. Therefore, we reserve pudendal arteriography for patients with

documented evidence of vasculogenic impotence who are considered to be candidates for vascular bypass procedures. Other patients who may be candidates for large-vessel procedures or percutaneous angioplasties might also be considered for arteriography. These particular instances will be further discussed toward the end of this chapter under vascular procedures for impotence.

The second invasive vascular procedure to be considered is infusion cavernosography (May and Hirtl, 1955). This procedure is performed simply by putting a narrow-gauge needle into the corpus cavernosum itself and directly infusing saline or contrast medium or both (Fig. 13–17). This procedure has been well described by Jevtich (1983). The indications for this procedure also remain somewhat unclear. Our feeling is that patients who have abnormal nocturnal penile tumescence testing accompanied by inability to maintain erections and normal Doppler studies are candidates for infusion cavernosography. Infusion cavernosography is essentially used to rule out abnormal cavernosal filling or anomalous venous drainage.

Terence Fitzpatrick, one of the early proponents of this technique, has been advocating this procedure since the early 1970's (Fitzpatrick, 1973). More recently, Ebbehoj and Wag-

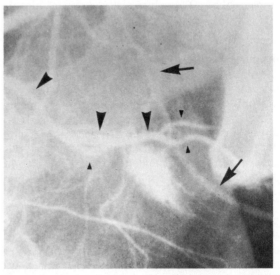

Figure 13–14. A cone-down view of the penile artery and its tributaries in a normal pudendal arteriogram. The large arrowheads point downward to the penile artery. The first small upward-pointing arrowhead indicates the bulbar branch, which, if followed distally, forms the bulbar blush, which is proximal to the urethral catheter (arrows). The two other small arrowheads that are distal to the urethral catheter mark the dorsal artery (downward-pointing) and the cavernosal artery (upward-pointing).

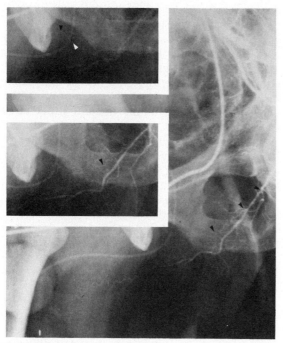

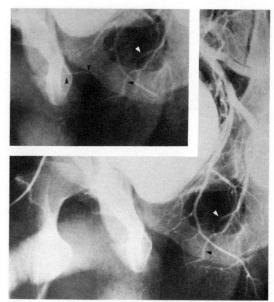

Figure 13–16. Pudendal arteriogram performed in a young male with a history of motor vehicle accident and pelvic trauma. In the large picture, one sees merely 1 to 2 cm of the proximal penile artery with a relatively normal superficial perineal artery. In the inset, one sees reconstitution of the more distal penile artery, which, in contradistinction to patients with atherosclerosis, is of normal caliber. This patient subsequently underwent microsurgical revascularization by anastomosis of the inferior epigastric artery to the dorsal artery of the penis, which was successful in restoring his potency.

Figure 13–15. A markedly abnormal pudendal arteriogram. In the large picture, the two downward-pointing arrowheads indicate severely diseased distal internal pudendal and penile arteries. The relatively normal artery seen caudally is the superficial perineal artery. In the lower inset, the arrowhead marks a more distal aspect of this diseased penile artery. In the upper inset, one sees poorly visualized bulbar and dorsal arteries after they bifurcate, as noted by small arrowheads. Both these arteries are abnormal with respect to their caliber. This arteriogram is consistent with the clinical picture of small vessel atherosclerosis.

ner (1979) have described abnormal venous drainage of the corpora due to fistulas between the distal corpus and the glans penis. It is of interest that when the surgical procedure was performed to obliterate these abnormal connections, potency was restored. As cavernosography gains more widespread acceptance and usage, perhaps both the indications for this procedure and the incidence of venous incompetence as a cause for impotence will become clearer.

Specialized Neurologic Testing. Neurogenic impotence may occur secondary to neurologic lesions in the peripheral, sacral, or suprasacral regions. Probably the most important aspect of making the diagnosis of underlying neurologic impotence is the patient's history. A past history of head trauma, intracerebral lesions, alcoholism, diabetes, spinal cord problems including cervical spondylolisthesis or trauma, or multiple sclerosis should be noted. In our experience, the finding of an occult neurologic lesion as the cause of impotence is quite rare. More commonly, one has a history

of a neurologic disease or a neurologic lesion and concomitant impotence. The issue then is to determine whether the neurologic aspect of the patient's history is causative or coincidental.

In addition to a neurologic examination, which should include a search for evidence of peripheral neuropathy, specialized neurologic examinations utilizing evoked potentials may be

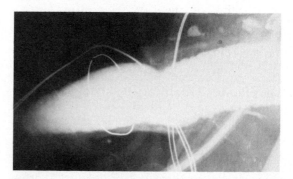

Figure 13–17. Infusion cavernosography that reveals relatively normal cavernous tissue and no abnormal venous drainage. The indentation noted on the dorsal surface represents an area where a dorsal foreshortening procedure of Nesbit had been performed. This infusion cavernosogram was carried out with nocturnal penile tumescence monitoring and continuous monitoring of intracorporeal pressure.

performed. These include determination of the dorsal penile nerve conduction velocity (Gerstenberg and Bradley, 1983), sacral evoked-potential studies (Krane and Siroky, 1980), and genitocerebral evoked-potential studies (Halderman, 1982). These examinations require sophisticated and expensive equipment, which, for the most part, will be available in specialized centers. In addition to these tests, a more recently described examination that can be performed is biothesiometry (Newman, 1970). This tests the vibratory sensation of afferent nerves emanating from the penis.

It is important to note that the neurologic tests that will be described in this chapter do not per se measure the viability or the conduction velocity in autonomic nerves that are directly responsible for the development of erection. As was mentioned previously, the "erection reflex" has the pudendal nerve as the afferent or sensory pathway and the sacral parasympathetic nerves as the efferent or motor pathway. The first half of this reflex, namely, the sensory pudendal nerve, can be measured by biothesiometry as well as by determining nerve conduction velocity in the dorsal penile nerve and sacral evoked-potential studies. Unfortunately, there is no effective means of measuring the efferent parasympathetic pathways, except indirectly, by performing cystometrography (Ryden et al., 1981). When cystometrography is performed in this setting, one should also consider bethanechol supersensitivity testing. In practice, it is quite rare to document parasympathetic nerve damage with CMG and bethanechol testing if no voiding symptoms are present.

The sacral evoked-potential study or sacral latency time is merely an electrophysiologic representation of the bulbocavernosus reflex (Krane and Siroky, 1980). It is performed by stimulating the penile skin and measuring the time (latency) required to record the first response obtained in the bulbocavernosus muscle (Fig. 13–18). Therefore, the reflex arc that is being measured is pudendal sensory to pudendal motor. One can also have a recording electrode at the base of the spine and record the time between penile stimulation and the response in the sacral spinal cord. This can provide a representation of the nerve conduction velocity of the pudendal sensory nerve. The test itself is performed by using either a block skin stimulating electrode or a ring electrode directly on the penile shaft. Square wave stimuli are delivered at a frequency of one per second, with a duration of 1 msec. The stimulation is increased to determine sensory threshold and reflex

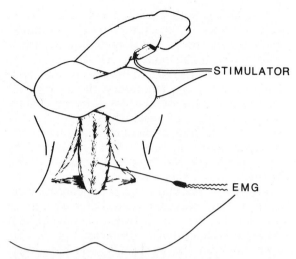

Figure 13–18. A schematic representation of the electrode placement for sacral evoked potential studies. A bar electrode is placed for stimulation of the penile skin, and a concentric needle electrode is placed for recording in the ipsilateral bulbocavernosus muscle. (From Krane, R.J., and Siroky, M.B.: J. Urol., *124*:872, 1980.)

threshold. Sensory threshold implies the first sensation of stimulation, and reflex threshold implies the onset of a consistent bulbocavernosus muscle contraction. Usually between 8 and 32 stimulations are averaged to determine a response (Fig. 13–19).

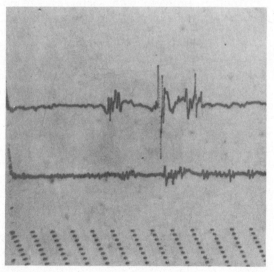

Figure 13–19. An oscilloscopic recording of an abnormal sacral evoked potential study. The upper line is the event being tested. On the left, a stimulus artifact is seen. As one proceeds along the upper line, the first and then second components of the sacral evoked potential are recorded. The first and second components begin at approximately 49 and 70 msec, respectively. The second line represents an averaged response that is beginning to be seen. This particular study was done after four stimulations. Usually 16 to 32 stimulations are required before an obvious averaged response is noted.

As this is both a crossed and an uncrossed reflex, a block electrode may be placed unilaterally on the penis and a recording electrode unilaterally in the bulbocavernosus muscle to determine the crossed and uncrossed responses, respectively. In our laboratory, the average response time for a sacral evoked-potential study is approximately 35 msec (Krane and Siroky, 1980). The determination of conduction velocity of dorsal penile nerve was first popularized by Gerstenberg (Gerstenberg and Bradley, 1983). In this study, a ring electrode is placed in the distal part of the penis and the recording electrode at the proximal part. After successive stimulations, the time between stimulation and response is determined. By measuring the distance between the electrodes, one can determine whether a normal or abnormal conduction velocity is present within this nerve.

It must be remembered that the results of these tests must be correlated with other examinations, such as nocturnal penile tumescence studies. As mentioned before, these tests merely measure somatic and not autonomic nerve function. In addition, the finding of an abnormal sacral latency time or nerve conduction velocity of the dorsal penile nerve does not necessarily establish the diagnosis of neurologic impotence, since the demonstrated nerve dysfunction may not be the cause of the erectile dysfunction.

Another problem with sacral evoked-potential studies is that they do not address the possibility of suprasacral neurologic disease as a cause of impotence. This fact led to the development of the genitocerebral evoked-potential study, in which the penis is stimulated in the same manner as previously described and EEG leads are placed at appropriate sites on the scalp (Halderman et al., 1982). In addition, active electrodes are placed over the L1 vertebra to measure response time to the sacral cord, as described earlier. Again, square wave stimuli are delivered at a frequency of 1 per second, with a duration of 0.2 msec at a constant current of 6 to 15 ma. A typical study of this type takes approximately 2 hours and usually includes 256 samplings per study. In our laboratory, the average value for total latency (penis to cerebral cortex) is 40.9 msec (Fig. 13–20). This is distributed as peripheral conduction time (penis to sacral cord), which averages 12.4 msec, and central conduction time (sacral cord to cerebral cortex), which averages 28.5 msec (Goldstein, 1983b). Therefore, using this study one can categorize patients into three distinct groups: (1) patients with abnormal peripheral conduction times and normal central conduction times;

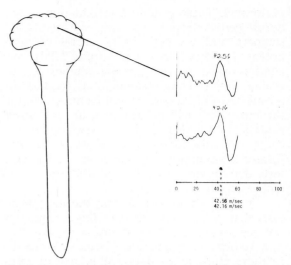

Figure 13–20. A typical somatosensory evoked response study in a normal patient. This study is carried by stimulating penile skin and recording at the cerebral level. In this particular case the latency recorded was approximately 42 msec, which, as noted, was reproducible on a subsequent study. As with the sacral evoked potential study, somatosensory evoked potential studies require multiple stimulations and a signal averager. In this case, 256 stimulations were required before the curves shown were obtained.

(2) patients with normal peripheral conduction times and abnormal central conduction times; and (3) patients with both peripheral and central delays in conduction times (Fig. 13–21). This test is the only one available that addresses the problem of diagnosing suprasacral neurologic impotence; again, it must be correlated with nocturnal penile tumescence examinations before an absolute diagnosis can be made.

Biothesiometry tests the vibratory sensation of the afferent nerves from the penis (Newman, 1970). This is a simpler examination and can be made readily available to the practitioner. It requires a device capable of sending vibratory signals to the skin that can be quantified in terms of voltage. The fingers on both hands and the toes on both feet are tested first, followed by the penile skin. In normal individuals, the same vibratory threshold will be found in the fingers, toes, and penis. Obviously, patients with some degree of sensory neuropathy of the penis will have elevated vibratory sensation threshold in this examination. As vibration sense may be one of the earliest modalities lost in peripheral neuropathy, this test may, in fact, be one of the more sensitive examinations that one can perform to test pudendal nerve sensory abnormalities (Goldstein et al., in preparation). We recommend biothesiometry as an excellent screening test for penile sensory disturbances. However, it must be emphasized that all forms

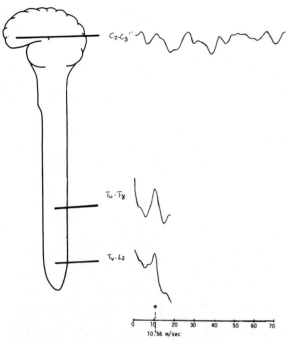

Figure 13–21. Results of penile skin stimulation and recording electrodes both at the cerebral level and at the spinal level. This study was done on a quadriplegic with a complete cervical cord transection. The latency between penile skin stimulation and the recording at L2 is approximately 10.56 msec. When a recording electrode is placed at T8 the latency is slightly longer. However, no reproducible latency could be determined by recording at the cerebral level, indicating a complete block to afferent stimulation.

of testing for neurologic impotence are incapable of testing the autonomic outflow to the penis.

As treatment options have increased and will increase in the future, the need for more specialized testing also increases. The object of any test is to compartmentalize the patient's problem with respect to its etiology. Clearly, as revascularization procedures or nerve stimulation procedures become available, it is all the more important to determine which patients will be candidates for these types of therapeutic options. As screening for all patients in whom the diagnosis is not obvious, it is recommended that, in addition to baseline serum hormone studies, one should perform some form of nocturnal penile tumescence examination and, when possible, a test of penile blood flow or pressure.

TREATMENT OF IMPOTENCE

The therapeutic options for erectile dysfunction fall under three main headings. Medical therapy usually consists of hormonal replacement, which has been described previously.

Nonhormonal medical therapy will be discussed briefly, athough little in the way of advances in this field has taken place. The psychiatric or psychologic approaches to treatment of erectile dysfunction have mainly been behavioristically oriented and patterned after the work of Masters and Johnson (1970). Surgical intervention has increased considerably over the past decade and has focused on implantable penile prostheses. More recently, surgical procedures aimed at revascularization or at decreasing venous drainage of the penis have been developed and merit discussion.

In the field of nonhormonal medical therapy, only one drug deserves mention. Yohimbine, an alpha-blocking agent, has been tried in non–double blind studies on impotent patients with reasonable response rates (about 26 per cent) (Morales et al., 1982). Obviously, further investigation and more rigid testing criteria are necessary before one can determine the exact worth of this drug.

Prior to the work of Masters and Johnson, psychologic treatment of sexual dysfunction was psychoanalytic in orientation. The view at that time was that sexual dysfunction was a manifestation of deep-seated psychologic conflict. Therefore, it was argued that treatment should be aimed not at the sexual dysfunction itself but rather at the underlying cause. This view implied the use of classic Freudian psychoanalytic methods. With the advent of Masters and Johnson and others, the concept of direct treatment of the sexual dysfunction became more widely accepted. Behavioristically oriented therapy for both erectile dysfunction and premature ejaculation has gained widespread acceptance and is now the treatment of choice for psychogenic impotence. The premise underlying the Masters and Johnson approach was that most patients with sexual dysfunction have a relatively minor psychologic problem that can be cured by brief and more direct treatment. The goals of sex therapy are basically to decrease or eliminate performance anxieties that interfere with erectile development and to ensure an adequate level of physical and psychologic stimulation, which is usually accomplished by increasing a couple's sexual repertoire. One component of therapy utilizes sensate focus exercises (Masters and Johnson, 1970). These exercises attempt to encourage the couple to sexually enjoy one another in a relaxed manner, free of inhibition and guilt. The problem of performance anxiety is dealt with by promoting a gradual increase in sexual conduct. The initial exercises focus on pleasure rather than the achievement of an erection. When erectile function develops, the patients gradually continue their exercise until coitus is possible. Because of the slow rate at which these exercises progresses, the performance anxiety is reduced to a minimum. An important element inherent in this type of therapy is the willingness of both the male and the female partner to assume mutual responsibility for sexual function.

Kaplan (1975) has emphasized the need for treatment of personal as well as interpersonal conflicts. Thus, many sex therapists currently do not practice the classic Masters and Johnson program but add, to one degree or another, some form of psychiatric or psychologic therapy. This type of approach has become known as couple's therapy (Hengeveld, 1983).

In general, this relatively nondemanding, slowly progressive, behavioristic approach has shown a 60 to 80 per cent improvement or cure rate in selected couples. However, in nonselected patient populations, these results are only in the 30 to 55 per cent range. Although only a few long-term follow-up studies have been performed, those studies that are available suggest that a fair number of patients have recurrence of their original erectile dysfunction (Hengeveld, 1983). This type of therapy is also widely used in the treatment of premature ejaculation. In this case, the relaxation exercises act to desensitize the patient, and the process becomes one of reconditioning.

Factors that reduce the chance of restoring erectile dysfunction by behavioristically oriented sex therapy include long duration of impotence (usually greater than several years), older age, low sex drive, and homosexual inclinations. In addition, patients with significant mental disorders or psychosis are clearly not good candidates for sex therapy (Cooper, 1981; Reynolds, 1977).

As mentioned previously, the surgical approach to erectile dysfunction is based mainly on implantation of a penile device. The indications, operative techniques, and results of this type of surgery are discussed in depth in Chapter 81. In this section the discussion will be concerned with operations aimed at increasing vascular supply to the corpora or at decreasing venous drainage of the corpora.

As early as 1908 Lydston performed the first vascular procedures for impotence in more than 100 cases (Lydstron, 1908). His operation consisted of ligating both the superficial and the deep dorsal veins of the penis, believing that this type of obstruction to venous outflow increases the ability to initiate an erection. In 1936, Lowsley described a procedure that consisted of plicating the ischiocavernosus muscles in addition to ligating the deep dorsal vein of the penis (Lowsley and Bray, 1936). This procedure was performed in 51 patients, with excellent results in 31. Although Leriche (1923) first published the association between thrombosis of the lower aorta and erectile dysfunction, it was not until 1972 that revascularization of the corpora cavernosa was performed by Michal (Michal et al., 1974).

Historically, penile revascularization procedures may be divided into the early procedures, which consisted of direct revascularization of the corpus achieved by anastomosing the vessel to the tunica albuginea, and later procedures, consisting of indirect revascularization using the dorsal or corporal artery itself. Direct revascularization of the corpora either by use of a saphenous vein graft between the femoral artery and the tunica albuginea or by direct anastomosis of the inferior epigastric artery to the tunic albuginea have largely been abandoned because of poor long-term results (Hawatmeh et al., 1982; LeVeen, 1978). Although these procedures did produce an early success rate of 50 to 70 per cent in several series (Michal et al., 1980; Zogniotti et al., 1980), long-term potency rates were quite poor. By 1 year postoperatively, most patients were once again impotent (LeVeen, 1978). Another problem with the direct procedures, especially when the saphenous vein was used as a bypass between the femoral artery and the corpus itself, is priapism. The best results using this procedure were realized when microvascular anastomoses were performed and anticoagulant therapy of some sort was given postoperatively. Technical difficulties ensued when a small vessel was anastomosed to a thickened tunica albuginea as well as when postoperative kinking of the anastomosis occurred. It may well be that many of the postoperative surgical failures were secondary to thrombosis of either the inferior epigastric artery or the saphenous vein because of insufficient run-off within the corpus cavernosum itself.

Indirect revascularization has generally utilized inferior epigastric artery, which may be anastomosed either to the dorsal artery of the penis or to the corporal artery itself (Michal et al., 1980; MacGregor and Konnack, 1982). In this procedure, the inferior epigastric artery is dissected out of its bed behind the rectus muscle and brought through a subcutaneous tunnel to the base of the penis. In Michal's first description of this procedure (Michal et al., 1980), an anastomosis was then made to the dorsal artery

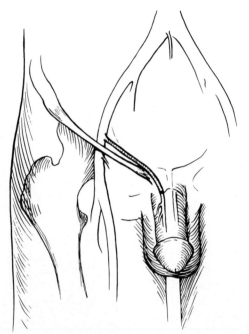

Figure 13–22. The Michal II procedure, in which the inferior epigastric artery is anastomosed to the dorsal artery of the penis in an end-to-side fashion. (From Hawatmeh, I.S., et al.: Vascular surgery for the treatment of the impotent male. *In* Krane, R.J., et al. (Eds.): Male Sexual Dysfunction. Boston, Little, Brown & Co., 1983.)

in an end-to-side manner using microsurgical techniques (Fig. 13–22). In his patients, anticoagulant therapy was given postoperatively and he reported a success rate of 60 per cent.

Indirect revascularization has several theoretical advantages over direct corporal body revascularization. The arterial anastomosis is proximal to the vasomotor control area, thus allowing for a more physiologic erection to occur. In addition, the corporal tissue is not exposed to systemic blood pressure over prolonged periods of time, thus obviating the potential for priapism and corporal fibrosis.

As stated previously, the Michal II operation involves an end-to-side microvascular anastomosis between the inferior epigastric artery and the dorsal artery of the penis. Several newer procedures that are based on this procedure have already been developed. Direct end-to-side anastomosis between the inferior epigastric artery and the corporal artery itself has been performed (MacGregor and Konnack, 1982). At our institution, we have modified the Michal II operation to perform an end-to-end anastomosis between the inferior epigastric artery and the proximal portion of the dorsal artery of the penis. This operation depends largely on the integrity and patency of the bifurcation of the

penile artery into the corporal and dorsal artery. Thus, blood flowing through the inferior epigastric artery is directed proximally through the dorsal artery of the penis into the corporal artery (Figs. 13–23 and 13–24).

The indications for these procedures remain somewhat debatable at present. Clearly, prior to undertaking a procedure of this sort, the patient must undergo all the evaluations described earlier in this chapter. There must obviously be documentation of decreased penile arterial flow or pressure by appropriate Doppler or plethysmographic evaluation. In addition, a pudendal arteriogram is imperative to document the degree and anatomic position of the arterial lesions in question. Lastly, we strongly recommend a preoperative psychologic assessment, as many of our patients have required psychologic help postoperatively, especially when the bypass surgery has been successful.

Diseases that produce vasculogenic impotence deserve some mention at this point. In a large percentage of diabetics, as described earlier, the underlying etiology for impotence is

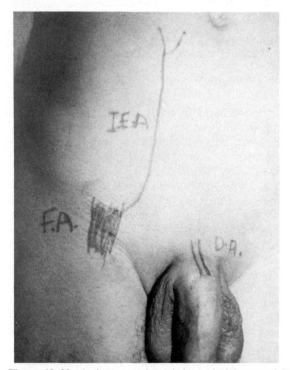

Figure 13–23. A demonstration of the underlying arterial anatomy of the inferior epigastric artery and the dorsal artery of the penis. To harvest the inferior epigastric artery, a paramedian incision is made and the rectus muscle is retracted medially. A smaller midline dorsal incision is made directly over the dorsal artery of the penis. The inferior epigastric artery is then transected at its uppermost point and brought out subcutaneously to the dorsal artery.

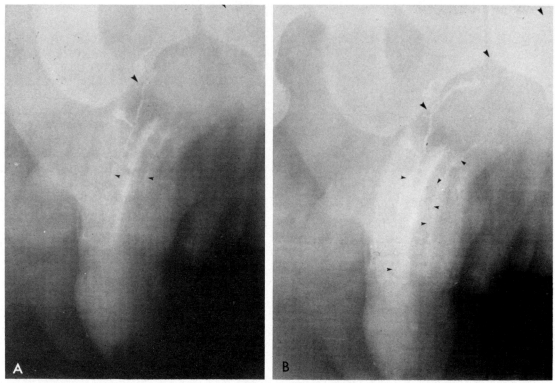

Figure 13–24. An intraoperative radiographic study in which the left proximal dorsal artery of the penis is infused with contrast medium in a retrograde manner. *A,* Following administration of 5 ml of contrast agent, one begins to see a cavernosal blush as well as the left and right corporal arteries (small central arrowheads). *B,* Following administration of 10 ml of contrast agent, one can visualize clearly both corporal arteries as well as significant bilateral corporal blush. This indicates that in this situation anastomosing the inferior epigastric artery in an end-to-end fashion to the proximal dorsal artery of the penis should result in increasing blood supply to both corporal arteries as well as to both corpora.

vasculogenic. Obviously, one must completely rule out any underlying neurogenic abnormality in these patients prior to considering revascularization. An important group of patients who may clearly benefit from this type of surgery are those who have been rendered impotent by trauma to the perineum or pelvis. This younger group will usually have abnormalities limited to the pudendal artery. Thus, they are ideal candidates for revascularization, as their dorsal and corporal arteries will usually be normal.

As our experience with impotence testing increases, some patients who heretofore were thought to have a psychologic disorder are being shown to have organic disease. Recently, we have seen several patients thought to have primary impotence who, in fact, had suffered perineal trauma in childhood, occasionally forgotten by the individual himself. Pudendal arteriography and penile Doppler studies were able to document the problem, and penile revascularization was able to cure it. Lastly, patients with hypertension are known to develop pelvic vascular insufficiency. We have used the

penile revascularization procedures on a group of hypertensive males in their 50's. The results of this surgery have not been as rewarding as those reported by others or as those in our traumatic group. It would appear that the final pathway for erectile function is the corporal artery. If the corporal artery is severely diseased, it seems that no type of revascularization procedure will give long-term cure rates. One must take this fact into account when considering the performance of such procedures on older patients with generalized atherosclerosis. It is expected that the success rates in older individuals will be decreased because of the potential for atherosclerosis in the corporal artery. In addition, even if success is possible the question will always arise as to how long it will take for further atherosclerotic changes in the corporal artery to develop. It is only with time and further experience with penile revascularization procedures that these questions will be answered.

As noted previously, the incidence and diagnosis of venous insufficiency causing impotence remain unclear. An operative approach aimed at decreasing anomalous venous drainage through cavernospongiosal fistulas has been described by Ebbehoj and Wagner (1977). Virag (1981) presented ten cases of venous insufficiency–related impotence treated by arterialization of the dorsal vein. After 1 year, eight patients were still potent. The procedure of dorsal penile vein arterialization is performed by anastomosing the epigastric artery to the dorsal vein. Virag (1982) believes that it can also be performed to correct arterial insufficiency to the penis.

This chapter on sexual function and dysfunction has attempted to update this exciting and fast-developing field. In the field of physiology, attempts at determining the neurotransmitter or neurotransmitters involved in creating an erection may some day lead to successful nonhormonal medical therapy. As our knowledge of the pharmacology of erection increases, pharmacologic tests for differentiating and diagnosing certain forms of this disorder may become available. With our increasing knowledge of the anatomic and neurologic aspects of erectile function, the potential for nerve stimulators, either external or implantable, for the treatment of impotence may come to fruition. Lastly, the development of newer and better vascular procedures may make this surgical option a more realistic one.

REFERENCES

Abelson, D.: Diagnostic value of the penile pulse and blood pressure: A Doppler study of impotence in diabetics. J. Urol., *113*:636, 1975.

Ashdown, R. R., and Gilanpour, H.: Venous drainage of the corpus cavernosum penis in impotent and normal bulls. J. Anat., *117*:159, 1974.

Ashworth, A.: Peyronie's disease. Proc. R. Soc. Med., *53*:642, 1960.

Bagshaw, M. A., Ray, G. R., Pistenma, D. A., et al.: External beam radiation therapy of primary carcinoma of the prostate. Cancer, *36*:723, 1975.

Baumgarten, H. G., Falck, B., and Lange, W.: Adrenergic nerves in the corpora cavernosa penis of some mammals. Z. Zellforsch., *95*:58, 1969.

Benkert, O., Witt, W., Adam, W., et al.: Effects of testosterone undecanoate on sexual potency and the hypothalamic–pituitary–gonadal axis of impotent males. Arch. Sex. Behav., *8*:471, 1979.

Benson, G. S.: Penile erection. In search of a neurotransmitter. World J. Urol., *1*:209, 1983.

Benson, G. S., McConnell, J., Lipschultz, L. I., et al.: Neuromorphology and neuropharmacology of the human penis. J. Clin. Invest. *65*:506, 1980.

Benson, G. S., McConnell, J. A., and Schmidt, W. A.: Penile polsters: functional structures or atherosclerotic changes? J. Urol., *125*:800, 1981.

Beutler, L. E., Scott, F. B., and Karacan, I.: Psychological screening of impotent men. J. Urol., *116*:193, 1976.

Bias, W., Nyberg, L., Hochberg, M., and Walsh, P. C.: Peyronie's disease: A newly recognized autosomal-dominant trait. Am. J. Med. Genet., *12*:227, 1982.

Borrelli, M., et al.: Surgical correction of Peyronie's disease using Nesbit's technique—an excellent way to reconstruct erectile potency. World J. Urol., *1*:257, 1983.

Bors, E., and Comarr, A. E.: Neurologic disturbance of sexual function with special reference to 529 patients with spinal cord injury. Urol. Surv., *10*:191, 1960.

Britt, D. B., Kemmerer, W. T., and Robison, J. R.: Penile blood flow determination by mercury strain gauge plethysmography. Invest. Urol., *8*:673, 1971.

Budin, J. A., et al.: Vascular-induced erectile impotence in renal transplant recipients. J. Urol., *121*:721, 1979.

Caine, M., Raz, S., and Zeigler, M.: Adrenergic and cholinergic receptors in the human prostate, prostate capsule and bladder neck. Br. J. Urol., *47*:93, 1975.

Canning, J. R., Bowers, L. M., Lloyd, F. A., et al.: Genital vascular insufficiency and impotence. Surg. Forum, *14*:298, 1963.

Chapelle, P. A., Durand, J., and Lacert, P.: Penile erection following complete spinal cord injury in man. Br. J. Urol., *52*:216, 1980.

Clara: Die Arter-venose Anastomosen. Leipzig, J. Barth, 1939.

Conti, G.: L'erection du penis humain et ses bases morphologico-vascularies. Acta Anat., *14*:217, 1952.

Cooper, A. J.: Short-term treatment in sexual dysfunction: a review. Compr. Psychiatry, *22*:206, 1981.

Cooper, K. C.: Cutaneous mechanoreceptors of the glans penis of the cat. Physiol. Behav., *8*:793, 1972.

Cooper, M. L., and Aronson, L. R.: Behavioral implications of a histological study of the sensory innervation of the penis of intact and castrated cats. Am. Zool., *9*:570, 1969.

Davidson, J. M.: Hormones and sexual behavior in the male. Hosp. Pract., September, 1975, pp. 126–132.

Davidson, J. M., Camargo, G. A., and Smith, E. R.: Effects of androgen on sexual behavior in hypogonadal men. J. Clin. Endocrinol. Metab., *48*:95, 1979.

del Pozo, E., and Brownwell, J.: Prolactin I. Mechanisms of control, peripheral actions and modification by drugs. Horm. Res., *10*:143, 1979.

Devlin, H. B., Plant, J. A., and Griffin, M.: Aftermath of surgery for anorectal cancer. Br. Med. J., *3*:413, 1971.

Deysach, L. J.: The comparative morphology of the erectile tissue of the penis with especial emphasis on the probable mechanism of erection. Am. J. Anat., *64*:111, 1939.

Domer, F. R., Wessler, G., Brown, R. L., et al.: Involvement of the sympathetic nervous system in the urinary bladder internal sphincter and in penile erection in the anesthetized cat. Invest. Urol., *15*:404, 1978.

Dorr, L. D., and Brody, M. J.: Hemodynamic mechanism of erection in the canine penis. Am. J. Physiol., *213*:1526, 1967.

Dwight, R. W., Higgins, G. A., and Keehn, R. J.: Factors influencing survival after resection in cancer of the colon and rectum. Am. J. Surg., *117*:512, 1969.

Dzuick, P. J., and Norton, H. W.: Influence of drugs affecting the autonomic system on seminal ejaculation. J. Reprod. Fertil., *4*:47, 1962.

Ebbehoj, J., and Wagner, G.: Insufficient penile erection due to abnormal drainage of cavernous bodies. Urology, *13*:507, 1979.

Eckhardt, C.: Untersuchungen uber die erektion des penis beim hund. Beitr. Anat. Phisiol., *3*:123, 1863.

Ek, A., et al.: Nocturnal penile rigidity measured by snapgauge band. J. Urol., *129*:964, 1983.

Ellenberg, M.: Impotence in diabetes: the neurologic factor. Ann. Intern. Med., *75*:213, 1971.

Ellis, W. J., and Grayhack, J. T.: Sexual function in aging males after orchiectomy and estrogen therapy. J. Urol., *89*:895, 1963.

Engel, G., Burnham, S. J., and Carter, M. F.: Penile blood pressure in the evaluation of erectile impotence. Fertil. Steril., *30*:687, 1978.

Ercolani, J. B.: Des tissues des organs erectiles. J. de l'Anat., 1869.

Faerman, I., Glocer, L., Fox, D., et al.: Impotence and diabetes: Histological studies of the autonomic nervous fibers of the corpora cavernosa in impotent diabetic males. Diabetes, *23*:971, 1974.

Fisher, C., Gorss, J., and Zuch, J.: Cycle of penile erections synchronous with dreaming (REM) sleep. Arch. Gen. Psychiatry, *12*:29, 1965.

Fisher, C., Schiavi, R. C., Edwards, A., et al.: Evaluation of nocturnal penile tumescence in the differential diagnosis of sexual impotence. Arch. Gen. Psychiatry, *36*:431, 1979.

Fitzpatrick, T. J.: Spongiosograms and cavernosograms: a study of their value in priapism. J. Urol., *109*:843, 1973.

Gaskell, P.: The importance of penile blood pressure in cases of impotence. Can. Med. Assoc. J., *105*:1047, 1971.

Gerstenberg, T. C., and Bradley, W. E.: Nerve conduction velocity measurement of dorsal nerve of penis in normal and impotent males. Urology, *21*:90, 1983.

Ginestié, J. F., and Romieu, A.: L'exporation radiologique de l'impuissance. Paris, Maloine, 1976.

Gittes, R. F., and Waters, W. B.: Sexual impotence: The overlooked complication of a second renal transplant. J. Urol., *121*:719, 1979.

Goldstein, I.: Drug-induced sexual dysfunction. World J. Urol., *1*:239, 1983a.

Goldstein, I.: Neurologic impotence. *In* Krane, R. J., Siroky, M. B., and Goldstein, I. (Eds.): Male Sexual Dysfunction. Boston, Little, Brown & Co., 1983b.

Goldstein, I., et al.: Biothesiometry. In preparation.

Goldstein, I., et al.: Radiation-associated impotence. A clinical study of its mechanism. JAMA, *251*:903, 1984.

Goldstein, I., and Krane, R. J.: Blood and lymph circulations of the penis. *In* Abramson, D. I., and Dobrin, P. B. (Eds.): Blood Vessels and Lymphatics in Organ Systems. New York, Academic Press, in press.

Goldstein, I., and Krane, R. J.: Effects of hypotension on the hemodynamics of penile erection. Surg. Forum, *34*:662, 1983.

Goldstein, I., and Krane, R. J.: Unpublished data.

Goldstein, I., Siroky, M. B., and Krane, R. J.: Impotence in diabetes mellitus. *In* Krane, R. J., Siroky, M. B., and Goldstein, I. (Eds.): Male Sexual Dysfunction. Boston, Little, Brown & Co., 1983.

Goldstein, I., Siroky, M. B., Nath, R. L., et al.: Vasculogenic impotence: role of the pelvic steal test. J. Urol., *128*:300, 1982.

Goldstein, I., et al.: The pelvic steal test: Proximal flow restriction with distal flow redistribution. AUA Annual Meeting. Kansas City, Mo., 1982, p. 174.

Gordon, G., Altmon, K., Southren, L., et al.: Effect of alcohol (ethanol) administration on sex-hormone metabolism in normal men. N. Engl. J. Med., *295*:793, 1976.

Halderman, S., et al.: Pudendal evoked responses. Arch. Neurol., *39*:280, 1982.

Halverson, H. M.: Genital and sphincter behavior of the male infant. J. Genet. Psychol., *56*:95, 1940.

Hawatmeh, I. S., et al.: Vascular surgery for the treatment of the impotent male. In Krane, R. J., Siroky, M. B., and Goldstein, I. (Eds.): Male Sexual Dysfunction. Boston, Little, Brown & Co., 1983.

Hawatmeh, I. S., Gregory, J. G., Houttuin, E., et al.: The diagnosis and surgical management of vasculogenic impotency. J. Urol., *127*:5, 1982.

Henderson, V. W., and Roepke, M. H.: On the mechanism of erection. Am. J. Physiol., *210*:257, 1966.

Hengeveld, M. W.: Erectile dysfunction: A sexological and psychiatric review. World J. Urol., *1*:227, 1983.

Herman, A., Adar, R., and Rubinstein, Z.: Vascular lesions associated with impotence in diabetic and nondiabetic arterial occlusive diabetes. Diabetes, *27*:975, 1978.

Holmquist, B., and Olin, T.: Angiography of the internal pudendal artery at electrical stimulation of the pelvic nerves and an injection of posterior pituitary hormones. Scand. J. Urol. Nephrol., *3*:291, 1969.

Horstmann, P.: The excretion of androgens in human diabetes mellitus. Acta Endocrinol., *5*:261, 1950.

Jensen, S. B., Hagen, C., Frøland, A., et al.: Sexual function and pituitary axis in insulin-treated diabetic men. Acta Med. Scand. (Suppl.):*624*:65, 1979.

Jevtich, M. J.: Experience with penile arterial pulse sounds. Proceedings of the First International Conference on Corpus Cavernosum Revascularization, *4*:31, 1980.

Jevtich, M. J., and Maxwell, D. D.: Invasive vascular procedures. *In* Krane, R. J., Siroky, M. B., and Goldstein, I. (Eds.): Male Sexual Dysfunction. Boston, Little, Brown & Co., 1983.

Kaplan, H. S.: The New Sex Therapy. New York, Brunner/Mazel, 1975.

Karacan, I.: Clinical value of nocturnal erections in the prognosis and diagnosis of impotence. Med. Asp. Hum. Sex., *4*:27, 1983.

Karacan, I., Goodenough, D. R., Shapiro, A., et al.: Erection cycle during sleep in relation to dream anxiety. Arch. Gen. Psychiatry, *15*:183, 1966.

Karacan, I., Salis, P. J., and Williams, R. L.: The role of the sleep laboratory in the diagnosis and treatment of impotence. *In* Williams, R. L., Karacan, I., and Frazier, S. H. (Eds.): Sleep Disorders, Diagnosis and Treatment. New York, John Wiley & Sons, 1978.

Karacan, I., Williams, R. L., Thornby, J. I., et al.: Sleep-related penile tumescence as a function of age. Am. J. Psychiatr., *132*:931, 1975.

Kaya, N., et al.: Nocturnal penile tumescence and its role in impotence. Psychiatr. Annu., *9*:426, 1979.

Kedia, K. R., and Markland, C.: The effect of pharmacologic agents on ejaculation. J. Urol., *114*:569, 1975.

Kedia, K. R., Markland, C., and Fraley, E. E.: Sexual function following high retroperitoneal lymphadenectomy. J. Urol., *114*:237, 1975.

Kent, J. R.: Estrogen dosage and suppression of testosterone levels in patients with prostatic carcinoma. J. Urol., *109*:858, 1973.

Kidd, G. S., Glass, A. R., and Vigersky, R. A.: The hypothalamic-pituitary-testicular axis in thyrotoxicosis. J. Clin. Endocrinol. Metab., *48*:798, 1979.

Kimma. Y., et al.: Role of adrenergic receptor mechanism in closure of the internal urethral orifice during ejaculation. Urol. Int., *30*:341, 1975.

Kinsey, A. C., Pomeroy, W. B., and Martin, C. E.: Sexual Behavior in the Human Male. Philadelphia, W. B. Saunders Co., 1948.

Kiss, F.: Anatomisch-histologische untersuchungen uber die erektion. Ztsch. F. Anat., *61*:455, 1921.

Kiviat, M. D.: Transurethral sphincterotomy: Relationship of site of incision to postoperative potency and delayed hemorrhage. J. Urol., *114*:399, 1975.

Klinge, E., and Sjostrand, N. O.: Contraction and relaxation of the retractor penis muscle and the penile artery of the bull. Acta Physiol. Scand. (Suppl.), *420*:1, 1974.

Kluver, H., and Bucy, P. C.: Preliminary analysis of functions of the temporal lobes in monkeys. Arch. Neurol. Psychiatr., *42*:979, 1939.

Koelberg, S., et al.: Preliminary results of an electromyographic study of ejaculation. Acta Clin. Scand., *123*:478, 1962.

Kolodny, R. C., Masters, W. H., Kolodner, R. M., et al.: Depression of plasma testosterone levels after chronic intensive marijuana use. N. Engl. J. Med., *290*:872, 1974.

Koraitim, M., Schafer, W., Melchior, H., et al.: Dynamic activity of bladder neck and external sphincter in ejaculation. Urology, *10*:130, 1977.

Kraemer, H. C., Becker, H. B., Brodie, H. K., et al.: Orgasmic frequency and plasma testosterone levels in normal human males. Arch. Sex. Behav., *5*:125, 1976.

Krane, R. J., and Siroky, M. B.: Studies on sacral evoked potentials. J. Urol., *124*:872, 1980.

Kwan, M., Greenleaf, W., Mann, J., et al.: The nature of androgen action on male sexuality: A combined laboratory–self-report study on hypogonadal men. J. Clin. Endocrinol. Metab., *57*:557, 1983.

Langley, J. N., and Anderson, H. K.: The innervation of the pelvic viscera and adjoining viscera. IV. The internal generative organs. J. Physiol., *19*:122, 1895.

Larsen, J. J., Ottesen, B., Fahrenkrug, J., et al.: Vasoactive intestinal polypeptide (VIP) in the male genitourinary tract. Invest. Urol., *19*:211, 1981.

Larsson, L. I.: Occurrence of nerves containing vasoactive intestinal polypeptide immunoactivity in the male genital tract. Life Sci., *21*:523, 1977.

Laschet, V., and Laschet, L.: Antiandrogens in the treatment of sexual deviations of men. J. Steroid Biochem., *6*:821, 1977.

Leffell, M., Devine, C., Horton, C., et al.: Non-association of Peyronie's disease with HLA B7 cross-reacting antigens. J. Urol., *127*:1223, 1982.

Leriche, R.: Des oblitérations artérielles hautes oblitération de la terminaison de l'aorte comme cause d'insuffisance circulatoire des membres inférieures. Bull. Soc. Chir. (Paris), *49*:1404, 1923.

LeVeen, H. H.: Vein graft for vascular impotence. Med. World News, *3*:73, 1978.

Lowsley, O. S., and Bray, J. C.: The surgical relief of impotence. JAMA, *107*:2029, 1936.

Lue, F. F., et al.: Physiology of penile erection. World J. Urol., *1*:194, 1983.

Lundberg, J. M., Anggård, A., Fahrenkrug, J., et al.: Vasoactive intestinal polypeptide in cholinergic neurons of exocrine glands: functional significance of coexisting transmitters for vasodilatation and secretion. Proc. Nat. Acad. Sci. USA, *77*:1651, 1980.

Lydston, G. F.: The surgical treatment of impotence. Am. J. Clin. Med., *15*:1571, 1908.

MacGregor, R. J., and Konnack, J. W.: Treatment of vasculogenic erectile dysfunction by direct anastomosis of inferior epigastric artery to central artery to corpus cavernosum. J. Urol., *127*:136, 1982.

MacLean, P. D., and Ploog, D. W.: Cerebral representation of penile erection. J. Neurophysiol., *25*:19, 1962.

Madorsky, M. L., Ashamalla, M.G., Schussler, I., et al.: Post-prostatectomy impotence. J. Urol., *115*:401, 1976.

Malenovsky, L., and Sammerova, J.: Sensory innervation of the clitoris and penis in the macaque. Folia Morphol., *20*:192, 1972.

Marshall, P., Surridge, D., and Delva, N.: Differentiation of organic and psychogenic impotence on the basis of MMPI decision rules. J. Consult. Clin. Psychol., *48*:407, 1980.

Masters, W. H., and Johnson, V. E.: Human Sexual Inadequacy. Boston, Little, Brown & Co., 1970.

May, F., and Hirtl, H.: Das cavernosogramm. Urol. Int., *2*:120, 1955.

May, A. G., DeWeese, J. A., and Rob, C. G.: Changes in sexual function following operation on the abdominal aorta. Surgery, *65*:41, 1969.

McConnell, J., Benson, G. S., and Wood, J.: Autonomic innervation of the penis: a histochemical and physiological study. J. Neural. Transm., *45*:227, 1979.

McDermott, D. W., Bates, R. J., Heney, N. M., et al.: Erectile impotence as complication of direct-vision cold-knife urethrotomy. Urology, *18*:467, 1981.

Melman, A.: Catecholamine levels in penile corpora. In Krane, R. J., Siroky, M. B., and Goldstein, I. (Eds.): Male Sexual Dysfunction. Boston, Little, Brown & Co., 1983.

Melman, A., and Henry, D. P.: The possible role of the catecholamines of the corpora in penile erection. J. Urol., *121*:419, 1979.

Melman, A., and Holland, T. F.: Evaluation of the dermal graft inlay technique for the surgical treatment of Peyronie's disease. J. Urol., *120*:421, 1978.

Melman, A., et al.: Effect of chronic alphamethyldopa upon sexual function in adult male rat. J. Urol., *129*:643, 1983.

Meyers, R.: Three cases of myoclonus alleviated by bilateral ansotomy, with a note on postoperative alibido and impotence. J. Neurosurg., *19*:71, 1962.

Michal, V., and Pospichal, J.: Phalloarteriography in the diagnosis of erectile impotence. World J. Surg., *2*:239, 1978.

Michal, V., et al.: Revascularization procedure of the cavernous bodies. In Zorgniotti, A. W., and Rossi, G. (Eds.): Vasculogenic Impotence. Proceedings of First International Conference on Corpus Cavernosum Revascularization. Springfield, Ill., Charles C Thomas, 1980a.

Michal, V., et al.: Vasculogenic impotence. Arteriography of the internal pudendal arteries and passive erection. In Zorgniotti, A. W., and Rossi, G. (Eds.): Vasculogenic Impotence. Proceedings of the First International Conference on Corpus Cavernosum Revascularization. Springfield, Ill., Charles C Thomas, 1980b.

Michal, V., Kramár, R., and Barták, V.: Femoro-pudendal bypass in the treatment of sexual impotence. J. Cardiovasc. Surg., *15*:356, 1974.

Miller, K., et al.: The radiology of male impotence. Radiographics, *2*:131, 1982.

Mollenkamp, J. S., Cooper, J. F., and Kagan, A. R.: Clinical experience with supervoltage radiotherapy in carcinoma of the prostate. Preliminary report. J. Urol., *113*:374, 1975.

Money, J.: Components of eroticism in men. I. The hormones in relation to sexual morphology and sexual desire. J. Nerv. Ment. Dis., *132*:239, 1961.

Montague, D. K., et al.: Diagnostic screening for vasculogenic impotence. In Rossi, G., and Zorgniotti, A. W. (Eds.): Vasculogenic Impotence. Springfield, Ill., Charles C. Thomas, 1980.

Morales, A., Surridge, D. H., Marshall, P. G., et al.: Nonhormonal pharmacological treatment of organic impotence. J. Urol., *128*:45, 1982.

Müller, J.: Entdechung der bei der erektion des mannlichen gliedes wirksamen arterien bei dem menschen und cm thieren. Arch. Anat. Physio. U. Wiss. Med., p. 202, 1835.

Newman, H. F.: Physiology of erection: anatomic considerations. In Krane, R. J., Siroky, M. B., and Goldstein, I. (Eds.): Male Sexual Dysfunction. Boston, Little, Brown & Co., 1983.

Newman, H. F.: Vibratory sensitivity of the penis. Fertil. Steril., 21:791, 1970.

Newman, H. F., and Northup, J. D.: Mechanism of human penile erection: An overview. Urology, 17:399, 1981.

Newman, H. F., and Tschertkoff, V.: Penile vascular cushions and erection. Invest. Urol. In press.

Newman, H. F., Northup, J. D., and Devlin, J.: Mechanism of human penile erection. Invest. Urol., 1:350, 1964.

Nyberg, L., Bias, W., Hochberg, M., and Walsh, P. C.: Identification of an inherited form of Peyronie's disease with autosomal dominant inheritance and association with Dupuytren's contracture and histocompatibility B7 cross reacting antigens. J. Urol., 128:48, 1982.

Ohlmeyer, P., et al.: Periodische vorgauge in schlaf. Pflugers Arch., 248:559, 1944.

Papadopoulos, C.: Cardiovascular drugs and sexuality. Arch. Intern. Med., 140:1341, 1980.

Penttila, O.: Acetycholine, biogenic anines and enzymes involved in their metabolism in penile erectile tissue. Ann. Med. Exp. Biol. Fenn. (Suppl.), 44:9, 1966.

Perryman, R. L., and Thorner, M. O.: The effects of hyperprolactinemia on sexual and reproductive function in men. J. Androl., 5:233, 1981.

Queral, L. A., Whitehouse, W. M., Jr., Flinn, W. R., et al.: Pelvic hemodynamics after aortoiliac reconstruction. Surgery, 86:799, 1979.

Raz, S., DeKernion, J. B., and Kaufman, J. J.: Surgical treatment of Peyronie's disease: A new approach. J. Urol., 117:598, 1977.

Reynolds, B. S.: Psychological treatment models and outcome results for erectile dysfunction: a critical review. Psychol. Bull., 84:1218, 1977.

Robertson, J. H.: Influence of mechanical factors on the structure of the peripheral arteries and the localization of atherosclerosis. J. Clin. Pathol., 13:199, 1960.

Robinson, B. W., and Mishkin, M.: Ejaculation evoked by stimulation of the preoptic area in the monkey. Physiol. Behav., 1:269, 1966.

Rochswold, G. L., et al.: Differential sacral rhizotomy in the treatment of neurogenic bladder dysfunction: Preliminary report of six cases. J. Neurosurg., 38:748, 1973.

Roen, P. R.: Impotence: A concise review. N.Y. State J. Med., 65:2576, 1965.

Root, W. S., and Bard, P.: The mechanism of feline erection through sympathetic pathways with some remarks on sexual behavior after de-afferentation of the genitalia. Am. J. Physiol., 150:80, 1947.

Rose, L. I., Underwood, R. H., Newmark, S. R., et al.: Pathophysiology of spironolactone-induced gynecomastia. Ann. Intern. Med., 87:398, 1977.

Rotter, W., and Schurman, R.: Die blutegefasse des menschlichen penis. Virchows Arch., 318:352, 1950.

Ruzbarsky, V., and Michal, V.: Morphologic changes in the arterial bed of the penis with aging: Relationship to the pathogenesis of impotence. Invest. Urol., 15:194, 1977.

Rydin, E., Lundberg, P. O., and Brattberg, A.: Cystometry and mictometry as tools in diagnosing neurogenic impotence. Acta Neurol. Scand., 63:181, 1981.

Said, S. I., and Mutt, V.: Polypeptide with broad biological activity: Isolation from small intestine. Science, 169:1217, 1970.

Sarns, A.: Histological changes in the larger blood vessels of the hind limb of the mouse after x-irradiation. Int. J. Radiat. Biol., 9:165, 1965.

Schoenberg, H. W., Zarins, C. K., and Segraves, R. T.: Analysis of 122 unselected impotent men subjected to multidisciplinary evaluation. J. Urol., 127:445, 1982.

Semans, J. H., and Langworthy, O. R.: Observations on the neurophysiology of sexual function in the male cat. J. Urol., 40:836, 1939.

Shirai, M., and Ishii, N.: Hemodynamics of erection in man. Arch. Androl., 6:27, 1981.

Siroky, M. B., and Krane, R. J.: Physiology of male sexual function. In Krane, R. J., and Siroky, M. B. (Eds.): Clinical Neuro-Urology. Boston, Little, Brown & Co., 1979.

Siroky, M. B., and Krane, R. J.: Neurophysiology of erection. In Krane, R. J., Siroky, M. B., and Goldstein, I. (Eds.): Male Sexual Dysfunction. Boston, Little, Brown & Co.,1983.

Siroky, M. B., Sax, D. S., and Krane, R. J.: Sacral signal tracing: The electrophysiology of the bulbocavernosus reflex. J. Urol., 122:661, 1979.

Sjöstrand, N.: The adrenergic innervation of the vas deferens and the accessory male genital glands. Acta Physiol. Scand., (Suppl.), 65:257, 1965.

Sjöstrand, N., Klinge, E., and Himberg, J. J.: Effects of VIP and other putative neurotransmitters on smooth muscle effectors of penile erection. Acta Physiol. Scand., 113:403, 1981.

Skakkebaeh, N. E., Bancroft, J., Davidson, D. W.: et al.: Androgen replacement with oral testosterone undecanoate in hypogonadal men: A double blind controlled study. Clin. Endocrinol., 14:49, 1981.

Slag, M. F., et al.: Impotence in medical clinic outpatients. JAMA, 249:1736, 1983.

Slimp, J. C., Hart, B. L., and Goy, R. W.: Heterosexual, autosexual and social behavior of adult male rhesus monkeys with medial preoptic anterior hypothalamic lesions. Brain Res., 142:105, 1978.

Small, M. P.: Peyronie's disease and penile implantation (Letter.) J. Urol., 119:579, 1978.

Spark, R. F., White, R. A., and Connolly, P. B.: Impotence is not always psychogenic. JAMA, 243:750, 1980.

Stearns, E. L., Winter, J. S., and Falman, C.: Effects of coitus on gonadotropin, prolactin and sex steroid levels in man. J. Clin. Endocrin. Metab., 37:687, 1973.

Texon, J.: Mechanical factors involved in atherosclerosis. In Brest, A. W., and Mayor, J. H. (Eds.): Atherosclerotic Vascular Disease. New York, Appleton-Century-Crofts, 1967.

Vacek, J., and Lachman, M.: Bulbocavernosus reflex in diabetes with erectile disorders. Clinical and electromyographic study. Cas. Lek. Cesk., 116:1015, 1977.

VanArsdalen, K. N., and Wein, A J.: A critical review of diagnostic test used in the evaluation of the impotent male. World J. Urol., 1:218, 1983.

Van Thiel, D. H., and Lester, R.: Sex and alcohol. N. Engl. J. Med., 291:251, 1974.

Vastarini-Cresi, G.: Communicazioni dirette tra le arterie e el vene vei maninfer. Mon. Zool. Ital., 13:136, 1902.

Velcek, D., Sniderman, K. W., Vanghan, E. D., Jr., et al.: Penile flow index utilizing a Doppler pulse wave analysis to identify penile vascular insufficiency. J. Urol., 123:669, 1980.

Veterans Administration Cooperative Study Group on Antihypertensive Agents: Propranolol in the treatment of essential hypertension. JAMA, 237:2303, 1977.

Virag, R.: Syndrome d'erection unstable per insuffisance veineuse-diagnostic et correction cliurgicale a propos de 10 cas. J. Mal. Vasc., 6:3, 1981.

Virag, R.: Revascularization of the penis. *In* Bennett, A. (Ed.): Management of Male Impotence. Baltimore, Williams & Wilkins Co., 1982.

Von Ebner, V.: Uber klappnatige vorrichtungen in der arterien der schwellkoper. Anat. Anz., 18:79, 1900.

Wagner, G., Willis, E. A., Bro-Rasmussen, F., et al.: New theory on the mechanism of erection involving hitherto undescribed vessels. Lancet, 1:416, 1982.

Wagner, G.: Erection, physiology and endocrinology. *In* Wagner, G., and Green, R. (Eds.): Impotence. New York, Plenum Press, 1981.

Walsh, P. C., Lepor, H., and Eggleston, J.: Radical prostatectomy with preservation of sexual function: anatomical and pathological considerations. Prostate, 4:473, 1983.

Watson, J. W.: Mechanism of erection and ejaculation in the bull and ram. Nature, 204:95, 1964.

Waxman, S. G.: Pathophysiology of nerve conduction: Relation to diabetic neuropathy. Ann. Intern. Med., 92:297, 1980.

Wein, A. J., Fishman, R., Carpiniello, V. L., et al.: Expansion without significant rigidity during nocturnal penile tumescence testing: a potential source of misinterpretation. J. Urol., 126:343, 1981.

Wein, A. J., Van Arsdalen, K., and Levin, R. M.: Adrenergic corporal receptors. *In* Krane, R. J., Siroky, M. B., and Goldstein, I. (Eds.): Male Sexual Dysfunction. Boston, Little, Brown & Co., 1983.

Whitelaw, G. P., and Smithwick, R. H.: Some secondary effects of sympathectomy with particular reference to disturbances of sexual function. N. Engl. J. Med., 245:121, 1951.

Wild, R. M., Devine, C. J., Jr., and Horton, C. E.: Dermal graft repair of Peyronie's disease: Survey of 50 patients. J. Urol., 121:47, 1979.

Willis, E., et al.: Vasoactive intestinal polypeptide (VIP) as a possible neurotransmitter involved in penile erection. Acta Physiol. Scand., 113:545, 1981.

Willscher, M. K.: Peyronie's disease. *In* Krane, R. J., Siroky, M. B., and Goldstein, I. (Eds.): Male Sexual Dysfunction. Boston, Little, Brown & Co., 1983.

Willscher, M. K., Cwazka, W. F., and Novick, D. E.: The association of histocompatibility antigens of the B7 cross-reacting group with Peyronie's disease. J. Urol., 122:34, 1979.

Yeager, E. S., and Van Heerden, J. A.: Sexual dysfunction following proctocolectomy and abdominoperineal resection. Ann. Surg., 191:169, 1980.

Zorgniotti, A. W., et al.: Selective arteriography for vascular impotence. World J. Urol., 1:213, 1983.

Zorgniotti, A. W., Rossi, G., Padula, G., et al.: Diagnosis and therapy of vasculogenic impotency. J. Urol., 123:674, 1980.

INFECTIONS AND INFLAMMATIONS OF THE GENITOURINARY TRACT

CHAPTER 14

Infections of the Urinary Tract: Introduction and General Principles*

LINDA M. DAIRIKI SHORTLIFFE, M.D.
THOMAS A. STAMEY, M.D.

INTRODUCTION

All urinary tract infections (UTI) accompanied by bacteriuria, regardless of their frequency or severity, can now be managed successfully by the practicing urologist; this statement could not have been made when the previous edition of *Campbell's Urology* was published. The major events of the last 20 years that have clarified our understanding and substantially contributed to the successful management of patients with UTI are the following.

● Greater accuracy in assessing the presence or absence of urinary infections. Both suprapubic needle aspiration of the bladder (SPA) and urethral catheterization avoid contamination of bladder urine with bacteria from the perineum, a contamination that is inherent in every voided urine from females. Use of these techniques has been accompanied by a greater appreciation of the serious limitations of the 100,000 bacteria per ml concept in assessing "significance" of urine cultures. Moreover, urinary infections induced by catheterization can be prevented by simple prophylaxis.

● Recognition that most recurrent urinary infections, including those that cause serious renal damage, are *reinfections* of the urinary tract.

● Recognition that susceptibility to recurrent UTI is mainly characterized by an abnormally high carriage of fecal bacteria on the vaginal and urethral mucosa, a carriage that is apparently related to increased bacterial attachment to squamous epithelial cell receptors.

● Recognition that bacteria that infect the urinary tract come from the fecal flora. Oral antimicrobial agents can adversely influence this bacterial reservoir. These antimicrobials may induce resistance in the resident fecal flora or may replace the resident flora with more pathogenic strains, thereby determining in large part the character of the next urinary infection.

● Documentation that low-dosage, prophylactic antimicrobial therapy with drugs that have minimal or no adverse effect on the fecal flora is the single most powerful clinical tool for preventing recurrent UTI. With greater accuracy in the diagnosis of recurrent infections (by use of SPA or urethral catheterization, when necessary) and better appreciation that other disease conditions such as interstitial cystitis can produce bladder irritative symptoms without infection, intelligent prophylactic management of recurrent UTI is almost 100 per cent successful in the prevention of urinary infection.

● Recognition of the few urologic abnormalities that cause bacteria to persist in the urinary tract despite adequate courses of antimicrobial therapy. We should remember that the kidney is *never* the cause of bacterial persistence in the absence of stones, necrotic papillae, congenital anomalies, or azotemia.

---

*Some passages in this chapter are reproduced with permission from Stamey, T. A.: Pathogenesis and Treatment of Urinary Tract Infections. Baltimore, Williams & Wilkins Co., 1980.

• Introduction of new antimicrobial agents with (1) broader spectrums of activity, (2) different, and sometimes advantageous, effects on the fecal flora, and (3) different pharmacokinetics (including better diffusion across epithelial membranes). These agents have increased the clinician's effectiveness in the treatment of life-threatening acute infections as well as in the prophylactic control of reinfections of the urinary tract.

• Lastly, better understanding of the natural history of both single and recurrent urinary tract infections in infants, children, and adults of all ages. This knowledge has led to more intelligent therapy because the ultimate patient risks are better known than they were 20 years ago. Thus, a more aggressive recognition of the few patient categories at risk for either serious morbidity or destruction of renal tissue is important for all clinicians who treat patients with urinary tract infections.

Because application of these eight issues has essentially solved the problem of how to manage urinary tract infections accompanied by bacteriuria—in both the prevention of morbidity and the preservation of renal function—readers should seek those details that especially relate to these pivotal points. This will ensure clinical competence in the application of these concepts to their urologic practice.

DEFINITIONS

It is useful to define a few commonly used terms that will occur repeatedly in this and subsequent chapters.

Bacteriuria—the presence of bacteria in the urine, with the specific implication that these bacteria are present in the bladder urine, i.e., they are not contaminants that have been added to a sterile bladder urine. The term includes both renal bacteriuria and bladder bacteriuria. Bacteriuria can occur with or without pyuria; it can be symptomatic or asymptomatic. When it is detected by population studies (screening surveys), "screening" bacteriuria (Sc BU) is a more precise and descriptive term than "asymptomatic" bacteriuria, especially since the latter term is clinically useful for describing the presence or absence of symptomatology in the individual patient seen in the office.

Pyelonephritis—a term that has limited usefulness for both clinician and pathologist and one that requires careful definition. It has limited histologic usefulness because a variety of renal diseases, including obstruction and infarction as well as infection, produce the same histologic picture in the renal cortex.

Clinically, the term "pyelonephritis" should be limited to a description of patients with chills, fever, and flank pain, a combination that is reasonably specific for an acute bacterial infection of the kidney. The term should not be used if flank pain is absent, a problem that causes serious difficulties in diagnosing infants and children too young to localize the site of their discomfort. We shall use the term "pyelonephritis" to mean a clinical syndrome with chills, fever, and flank pain that is almost always accompanied by bacteriuria and pyuria.

When bacterial infection of the kidney causes a focal, coarse scar in the renal cortex overlying a calyx, almost always accompanied by some calyceal distortion (Fig. 14–1), it can be detected radiographically or by gross exam-

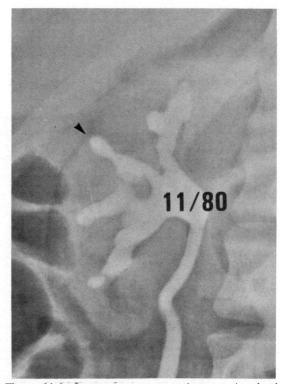

Figure 14–1. Intravenous urogram demonstrating focal, coarse scarring in the right kidney of an 18-year-old girl with a history of many recurrent fevers between 2 months and 2 years of age. Cystogram at age 2 years established an atrophic left kidney with marked reflux up to the left kidney and slight reflux up to the right kidney. Intravenous urogram at age 6 established severe atrophy of the left kidney. She had no infections between ages 6 and 15 years. Several reinfections occurred at age 15, which ceased with prophylactic therapy. Her blood pressure has remained normal, and her serum creatinine was 0.9 mg per dl at age 18. She is now 21 years old and has stopped antimicrobial prophylaxis for 18 months without infections or introital colonization with Enterobacteriaceae. Note that all calyces are blunted and that one extends to the capsule (arrow) because of atrophy of the overlying cortex.

ination of the kidney. Less commonly, renal scarring from infection can result in generalized thinning of the renal cortex with a small kidney appearing radiologically similar to post-obstructive atrophy (Fig. 14–2). These characteristic radiologic changes, when accompanied by vesicoureteral reflux (VUR), have been referred to as reflux nephropathy, emphasizing the role of reflux in the resultant scarring. But because focal, coarse scarring secondary to clinical pyelonephritis is also demonstrable in the absence of reflux, we have not used the term "reflux nephropathy" to describe the characteristic scarring of bacterial renal infection. We prefer the terms "focal, coarse renal scarring" and "atrophic pyelonephritis" to describe these two characteristic radiologic findings.

Cystitis—indicates inflammation of the bladder, whether used as a histologic, bacteriologic, cystoscopic, or clinical description of symptomatology; clinical symptoms are usually urinary frequency and dysuria, often accompanied by urgency and tenesmus. Bacterial cystitis, as opposed to nonbacterial cystitis (radiation, interstitial, and so forth), is a useful term.

Urethritis—like cystitis, refers to inflammation of the urethra and requires an adjective for modification, for example, "nongonococcal" urethritis. Symptoms arising from urethritis and cystitis are difficult, if not impossible, to distinguish in the female, but pure urethritis in the female—unlike in the male—is very rare.

Prophylactic antimicrobial therapy—refers to the prevention of reinfections of the urinary tract by the administration of drugs. When this term is used correctly in reference to the urinary tract, it is assumed that bacteria have been eliminated before prophylaxis is begun.

Suppressive antimicrobial therapy—refers to the suppression of an existing infection that the physician is unable to eradicate. This suppression may result in a sterile urine, as in the case of a small infection stone in a normal kidney or in an *Escherichia coli* bacterial prostatitis in which the organisms remain in the prostate even though the urine is maintained sterile with single-tablet, nightly dosage of an antimicrobial agent. Suppressive is also a useful term when recurrent acute symptoms are prevented in a poor-risk patient with a large stag-

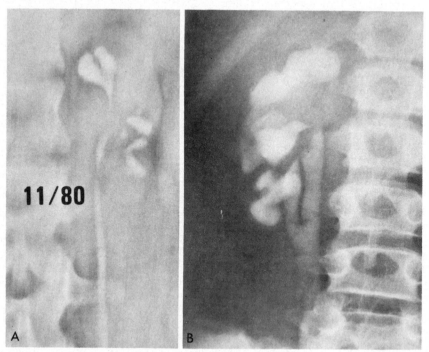

Figure 14–2. *A*, Intravenous urogram of the contralateral left kidney from the same patient as in Figure 14–1. The severe pyelonephritic atrophy, undoubtedly caused by febrile urinary infections during early infancy with reflux into different segments of the kidney, produced an irregular cortical scarring. Note how all the calyces extend to the capsule with irregular, intervening areas of cortex. *B*, Pyelonephritic atrophy, suggestive of postobstructive atrophy, in a 20-year-old female with spina bifida, neurogenic bladder, and many episodes of fever and bacteriuria in early childhood. Observe the uniform, regular atrophy of the renal cortex, suggesting reflux of bacteria simultaneously into virtually all nephrons. This type of pyelonephritic atrophy is uncommon compared with that shown in *A* and is characteristic of obstruction with superimposed infection.

horn infection calculus in whom the antimicrobial agent serves to reduce ("suppress") the bacterial numbers without achieving a sterile urine. In all instances, to resort to suppressive antimicrobial therapy is an admission of defeat (sometimes in the best interest of the patient) in the challenge of managing a difficult urinary infection.

Chronic—a poor term, since it defies a clean definition. It should be avoided in the context of urinary tract infections except for chronic bacterial prostatitis. A child who has recurrent monthly episodes of pyelonephritis, even when accompanied by renal scarring, might be considered to have a "chronic" infection, but he or she, in fact, has a series of acute reinfections with different bacterial strains.

Complicated—a term commonly used in clinical antibiotic trials in an effort to distinguish between women with simple, recurrent bacterial cystitis (almost always reinfections in patients who have a monotonous 90 per cent plus bacteriologic cure rate regardless of the antibiotic) and others who are thought to be in the trial with a "complicated" urinary tract. Complicated is as bad a term as chronic, unless the unusual circumstances of the urinary tract are presented in detail for each entry. For example, "complicated" urinary tracts with infection stones are doomed to failure regardless of the antibiotic on trial, whereas chronic bacterial prostatitis will show nearly 100 per cent successful treatment as long as follow-up is less than 30 days after completion of the drug regimen. Thus, the term "complicated" as a group designation is clearly meaningless unless the special circumstances of each individual urinary tract are broken out into meaningful subgroups, an analysis that is rarely, if ever, carried out.

Relapse—as opposed to bacterial reinfections means consecutive urinary infections caused by the same bacterial strain. It is a useful term when used in the European sense of consecutive infections regardless of the time lapse between them. Unfortunately, investigators in the United States often use the term with a 2-week or less limitation between recurrences and thereby imply that the kidney is the site of bacterial persistence. Reinfections of the urinary tract can readily recur within 2 weeks with the same bacterial strain that has remained on the vagina and urethra; the "relapse" then is from the reinfection route of the rectum to vagina to bladder and not from the kidney (Stamey, 1980). As will be seen in the next section, our classification avoids the use of the confusing term "relapse," but is widely used in the liter-

ature both old and new; the careful reader will take notice of each author's definition and his implications in using the term.

CLASSIFICATIONS

In our experience at Stanford, all infections in the urinary tract can be divided into one of four simple categories (Stamey, 1975):

I. First infections
II. Unresolved bacteriuria during therapy
III. Bacterial persistence ⎤ "Recurrent"
⎥ urinary
IV. Reinfections ⎦ infections

The term *recurrent urinary infections* obviously applies either to patients with bacterial persistence in a focus within the urinary tract or to reinfections from outside the urinary tract. It is also clear that until a bacteriuric episode is resolved with proper antimicrobial therapy, the nature of the recurrence—bacterial persistence or reinfection—cannot be classified.

First Infections. Little can be said about first infections; the biologic cause is presumably the same as that in reinfections. Initial infections in domiciliary (nonhospitalized) women are usually sensitive to all antimicrobial agents, and only about one fourth of such women will experience a recurrence in the next few years.

Unresolved Bacteriuria During Therapy. The term *unresolved bacteriuria* is useful because it emphasizes that the initial therapy has been inadequate. Sterilization of the urine during therapy is a prerequisite for successful treatment and for characterization of the nature of the recurrence. The clinician often fails to sterilize the urine during therapy and fails to recognize this problem because (1) cultures of the urine are not obtained during treatment or (2) if they are obtained, he misinterprets bacterial counts of less than 10^5 per ml as contaminants. Clearly, if *any* of the infecting strain is present in the midstream voided urine during therapy, regardless of how low the number, one cannot be certain the bacteria have been eradicated.

The causes of unresolved bacteriuria, in descending order of importance, are shown in Table 14–1.

The most common cause of unresolved bacteriuria during treatment is the presence of organisms resistant to the antimicrobial agent selected to treat the infection. The clinical setting is almost invariably one in which the patient

TABLE 14–1. CAUSES OF UNRESOLVED BACTERIURIA IN DESCENDING ORDER OF IMPORTANCE

Bacterial resistance to the drug selected for treatment
Development of resistance from initially sensitive bacteria
Bacteriuria caused by two different bacterial species with mutually exclusive sensitivities
Rapid reinfection with a new, resistant species during initial therapy for the original sensitive organism
Azotemia
Papillary necrosis from analgesic abuse
Giant staghorn calculi in which the "critical mass" of sensitive bacteria is too great for antimicrobial inhibition
Self-inflicted infections or deception in taking antimicrobial drugs (a variant of Munchausen's syndrome)

has a recent history of antimicrobial therapy, a treatment that has produced resistant organisms among the fecal flora that have reinfected the urinary tract. Tetracyclines and sulfonamides are notorious for producing resistance in the fecal bacteria. Moreover, through resistance transfer factors (R factors), a single course of treatment with one of these drugs may produce bacteria that are simultaneously resistant to several other agents such as ampicillin, cephalosporins, streptomycin, and chloramphenicol. Thus, a recent history (3 months or less) of antimicrobial therapy increases the likelihood that resistant fecal flora have colonized the vaginal introitus and produced a urinary tract infection that will require sensitivity testing to select a drug capable of sterilizing the urine.

The second, but a less common, cause of unresolved bacteriuria is the development of resistance in a previously sensitive population of organisms infecting the urinary tract. This form of resistance is easy to recognize clinically because within 48 to 72 hours of starting therapy a previously sensitive population of 10^5 or more bacteria per ml of urine is replaced by an equal population of completely resistant bacteria of the same species through selection of a resistant clone undetected in the original sensitivity testing. Selection of resistant clones from dense bacterial populations (10^8 bacteria or more) occurs in about 8 per cent of patients treated with 1 gm per day of tetracycline (Stamey et al., 1974) and about 7 per cent of patients treated with 4 gm per day of nalidixic acid (Stamey and Bragonje, 1976). These percentages are not insignificant.

The third cause of unresolved bacteriuria is the presence of a second unsuspected species that is resistant to the antimicrobial agent chosen to treat the predominant infecting organism. In these mixed infections, one of the two organisms acquires dominance over the other and often appears on culture plates as a pure culture of the dominant species. Treatment of the dominant organism unmasks the presence of the second strain. Before the advent of nalidixic acid and the cephalosporins, it was not uncommon to treat a *Klebsiella* urinary infection with colistin (Colymycin) only to find on the second or third day of therapy a *Proteus mirabilis*. With the broader spectrum antimicrobial agents, this is much less of a problem than it was 15 years ago.

The fourth cause is rapid reinfection with a new, resistant species before the completion of 5 to 10 days of therapy for the original infecting organism. Fortunately, most reinfections, even in highly susceptible females, do not recur this quickly. Nevertheless, the physician will have the urine sterile within 48 hours of starting therapy and a new, resistant strain can infect the bladder from introital carriage by the fifth to tenth day of therapy, making it appear as if the original bacteriuria were unresolved.

The fifth cause of unresolved bacteriuria is azotemia, in which the bacteriuria continues with sensitive bacteria; the urine cannot be sterilized because the antimicrobial agent cannot be delivered into the urine by the diseased kidney. Bioassay of urinary antimicrobial concentration in these cases usually shows the level of the drug to be below the minimal inhibitory concentration of the infecting organism.

The sixth cause is related to azotemia and papillary necrosis ("analgesic" nephritis), but these patients have serum creatinine concentrations greater than 2 mg per dl accompanied by severe defects in medullary concentrating capacity; they can be bacteriuric while taking an antimicrobial agent to which the organism is sensitive. Sometimes the antimicrobial agent can be switched to one with even higher urinary concentrations, with the patient encouraged *not* to force fluids, and the bacteriuria can be resolved.

The seventh cause of unresolved bacteriuria relates to those rare patients with giant staghorn calculi who have such an inordinate mass of bacteria near the surface of the stone that even urinary levels of bactericidal drugs in nonazotemic patients are inadequate to sterilize the urine. The phenomenon of a "critical density" is well known in sensitivity testing, in which it is recognized that even sensitive bacteria cannot be inhibited once they reach a certain critical density on the agar plate. Although these giant staghorn calculi are rare, and smaller calculi do not interfere with sterilization of the urine, this is the only circumstance (other than renal failure and the occasional patient with analgesic nephritis) in which sensitive bacteria can continue to cause an unresolved bacteriuria in the presence of proper antimicrobial therapy.

The last cause of unresolved bacteriuria occurs in those patients who have variants of the Munchausen syndrome. These unfortunate individuals, all females in our experience, need to be sick and use their urinary tract infections as the excuse. We have documented one patient who had learned to pass a urethral catheter first into her rectum and then her bladder. Some secretly omit their oral antibiotics while steadfastly asserting that they never miss a dose. The Munchausen syndrome presents with a horrendous clinical history and invariably a delicate collecting system on intravenous urogram without a single renal scar. Careful bacteriologic observations usually indicate the implausibility of the clinical picture.

Bacterial Persistence. Once the bacteriuria has resolved, i.e., the urine sterilized for several days and the antimicrobial agent stopped, recurrence with the same organism can arise from a site *within* the urinary tract that was excluded from the high urine concentrations of the antimicrobial agent. We have identified 13 correctable urologic abnormalities that cause bacteria to persist within the urinary tract between episodes of recurrent bacteriuria (Table 14–2). The relationship of these abnormalities to bacterial persistence as well as the documentation that surgical excision removes the infection as a source of recurrent bacteriuria is presented elsewhere in detail (Stamey, 1980). Once the urologist recognizes that the cause of the patient's recurrent bacteriuria is bacterial persistence, Table 14–2 should serve as a check list for known, correctable causes. Some of the causes

TABLE 14–2. CORRECTABLE UROLOGIC ABNORMALITIES THAT CAUSE BACTERIAL PERSISTENCE AND RECURRENT URINARY TRACT INFECTION

Infection stones
Chronic bacterial prostatitis
Unilateral infected atrophic kidneys
Vesicovaginal and vesicointestinal fistulas
Ureteral duplication and ectopic ureters
Foreign bodies
Urethral diverticula and infected paraurethral glands
Unilateral medullary sponge kidneys
Nonrefluxing, normal-appearing, infected ureteral stumps following nephrectomy
Infected urachal cysts
Infected communicating cysts of the renal calyces
Papillary necrosis in a single calyx
Paravesical abscess with fistula to bladder

are subtle, and many require cystoscopic localization of the infection with ureteral catheters to accurately define the focus of bacterial persistence.

Reinfections. Considering the relative rarity of patients with bacterial persistence (Table 14–2) and the enormous number of women and children with recurrent urinary infections, it is probably not an exaggeration to conclude that at least 99 per cent of all recurrent infections in females are reinfections of the urinary tract. It is for this reason that the biologic cause of reinfections in females is so important.

DIAGNOSIS OF BACTERIURIA

We have reviewed elsewhere the historical, theoretical, and observational basis for the diagnosis of bacteriuria (Stamey, 1980). Although most bacteria allowed to incubate for several hours in bladder urine will reach colony counts of 10^5 bacteria per ml, this statistical number is fraught with two limitations for the clinician who treats patients. The first is that 20 to 40 per cent of women with symptomatic urinary infections present to their physician with less than 10^5 bacteria per ml of urine (Stamey et al., 1965; Mabeck, 1969a; Kunz et al., 1975; Kraft and Stamey, 1977), probably because of the slow doubling time of bacteria in urine (q 30 to 45 min) combined with frequent bladder emptying (q 15 to 30 min) from irritation; these low bacterial counts, sometimes less than 1000 bacteria per ml and frequently between 1000 and 10,000 per ml, lead to underdiagnosis. Indeed, in a recent study of women presenting to a university student health center, Stamm and associates (1982) proposed that the best diagnostic criterion for culture detection in young symptomatic women with urinary frequency and dysuria is 100 bacteria or more per ml *(E. coli)*, not 100,000 per ml. Fortunately, most of these patients will have symptoms of urinary infection, most will have pyuria on urinalysis, and the informed physician will treat the patient for infection even if the colony count is 5000 *E. coli* per ml.

The second limitation of the 10^5 cutoff is one of overdiagnosis: Females susceptible to infection often carry large numbers of pathogenic bacteria on their perineum which contaminate an otherwise sterile bladder urine. In the original studies by Kass (1960), a single culture of 10^5 or more bacteria per ml had a 20 per cent chance of representing contamination. There is no statistical way to avoid these two major limitations on the interpretation of the midstream voided culture in the female; for this reason, efforts to automate the count of bacteria in the urine, no matter how sophisticated, can never help the clinician who is faced with the individual patient.

What can be done to avoid these limitations? In order of decreasing complexity, (1) the bladder urine can be aspirated suprapubically, providing the highest degree of reliability (Stamey et al., 1965); (2) the female patient can void in the lithotomy position on an examining table, after the perineum is cleaned with soap and water, while the nurse collects a midstream specimen (Stamey et al., 1965); and (3) the patient can be catheterized. Bladder aspiration, while neither painful nor dangerous, is unpleasant for the patient. Highly useful in newborn infants (Newman et al., 1967) and in patients with paraplegia, bladder aspiration should be used in any female who persists with a questionable culture. A single aspirated specimen reveals the bacteriologic status of the bladder urine without introducing urethral bacteria, which can start a new infection. We have described the second method, in which specimens are collected with the patient on a cystoscopy table, in detail (Stamey et al., 1965) and continue to use it in both the office and the hospital, but most physicians will find this too involved to use routinely. Nevertheless, when possible, the nurse should clean the perineum carefully, remove the soap, retract the labia, and collect the patient's midstream specimen herself.

While the first two techniques described above are ideal, it is easy to understand why the third—urethral catheterization—will remain an attractive alternative for many practicing physicians. Urethral catheterization of the female, however, will not prevent contamination of the catheterized sterile bladder urine by urethral bacteria. With careful technique, however, such as the one used by Marple (1941), the presence of small numbers of bacteria, even 1000 per ml, should mean the presence of a urinary infection. The objection to the catheter, of course, is that it produces a bladder bacteriuria in some patients who have sterile urine. This incidence of infection varies with the type of patient catheterized, from 1 per cent of healthy schoolgirls in the series by Turck and coworkers (1962) to 20 per cent in women hospitalized on a medical ward (Thiel and Spühler, 1965). The incidence, then, of catheter-induced urinary infections is primarily determined by the population at risk, with the lowest incidence occurring in nonhospitalized, healthy women. If antibacterial solutions are left in the bladder after catheterization, the risk of a catheter-induced infection is minimal. For example, Pearman (1971) catheterized patients with acute traumatic spinal cord injury every 6 hours until their bladder function returned. At each catheterization the urine was cultured; 150 mg of kanamycin with 30 mg of colistin sulfate in 25 ml of sterile water was left in the bladder. Of 1547 catheterizations performed in nine female patients, nine instances of bacteriuria occurred (an incidence of 1 in 172 catheterizations or 0.6 per cent); almost all the infections were caused by either enterococci or *Staphylococcus epidermidis*. An easier way to prevent catheter-induced infections in those patients thought to have sterile urine is to give one or two tablets of an oral antimicrobial agent, such as nitrofurantoin or trimethoprim-sulfamethoxazole. This has been our technique at Stanford for years, and catheter-induced infections in our outpatient population are virtually nonexistent. Ireland and associates (1982) catheterized 100 women immediately prior to abdominal hysterectomy; 50 received a single dose of 160 mg trimethoprim with 800 mg of sulfamethoxazole (TMP-SMX). Only two patients developed a postoperative urinary infection. In contrast, 35 per cent of the 50 control patients developed infections. The 4 per cent infection rate in the single-dose prophylactic group indicates impressive protection, not only from the catheter-induced bacteria but also from the exigencies of postoperative abdominal surgery.

Suprapubic needle aspiration of the bladder is rarely required in the male for the diagnosis of bacteriuria except for diagnosis of anaerobic infections. If the foreskin (of the uncircumcised male) is carefully retracted and the glans cleaned with soap, washed, and dried, or if the male is circumcised, culture of the midstream urine, especially after 200 to 300 ml of urine has washed across the urethra, is about as reliable as needle aspiration of the bladder. Unlike the female, then, it is inexcusable to catheterize a male patient for a urine culture.

OFFICE METHODS OF URINE CULTURE

If a urologist is to deal effectively and intelligently with urinary infections, he must culture the urine—and the more often, the better. Two efficient, inexpensive, and accurate techniques are available that the office nurse can easily learn to manage. The best, although slightly more expensive and troublesome to acquire, is direct surface plating on split agar, disposable plates (Fig. 14–3). One half is blood

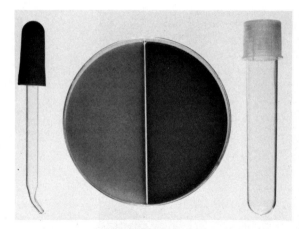

Figure 14–3. Materials required for bacteriologic culture: calibrated, curved-tip pipette, plastic disposable culture plate, and sterile disposable culture tube. (From Stamey, T. A.: J. Urol., 97:926, 1967. Copyright 1967, The Williams & Wilkins Company, Baltimore.)

agar, which grows both gram-positive and gram-negative bacteria, and the other is desoxycholate or eosin–methylene blue, which grows gram-negative bacteria, some of them, such as *E. coli*, in a very characteristic manner. Once these plates are obtained from a local hospital in which the media personnel in the bacteriology section are willing to pour them, simple curved-tip eyedroppers are sufficient to deliver about 0.1 ml of urine onto each half of the plate (Fig. 14–4). After overnight incubation in an inexpensive incubator, the number of colonies is estimated, often identified (after some experience), and multiplied by 10 to report the culture in bacteria per ml of urine. The technique has been presented elsewhere in detail (Stamey, 1980).

A simpler, but somewhat less accurate and intellectually pleasing, technique is the use of

dip-slides (Fig. 14–5). These are plastic slides attached to screw-top caps, and they have soy agar (a general nutrient agar to grow all bacteria) on one side and eosin–methylene blue or MacConkey's agar for gram-negative bacteria on the opposite side. A slide is dipped into urine, the excess allowed to drain off onto a paper towel, replaced into its plastic bottle, and incubated. The volume of urine that attaches to the slide is between 1/100 and 1/200 ml. Hence, the colony count is 100 to 200 times the number of colonies that become visible with incubation. In actual practice, the growth is compared with a visual standard and reported as such. It is more difficult to recognize the species of bacteria with this technique, but it is more than adequate.

Many other office technique are available, but there are disadvantages to them all—some in reliability (especially the chemical indices of bacteriuria), some in costs, and others in complexity.

It is to be emphasized that the urine must be refrigerated immediately upon collection and should be cultured within 24 hours of refrigeration. One advantage to the dip-slide is the ease with which the urine can be immediately cultured without the necessity of refrigeration. Indeed, patients can culture their own urine at home, keep the slide at room temperature, and bring it to the office within 48 hours. The interpretation of positive cultures, however, is limited by the technical problems already discussed. A sterile or low-count culture in the absence of urinary frequency is valid and can be very helpful.

THE ROLE OF URINALYSIS IN THE DIAGNOSIS OF BACTERIURIA

Microscopic examination of the urinary sediment adds valuable information to the di-

Figure 14–4. Curved-tip, eye-dropper technique of streaking divided agar plate with 0.1 ml (two drops) of urine. (Reproduced by permission from Stamey, T. A.: Prevention of Recurrent Urinary Infections. Science & Medicine Publishing Company, New York, 1973.)

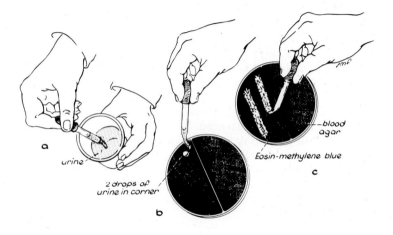

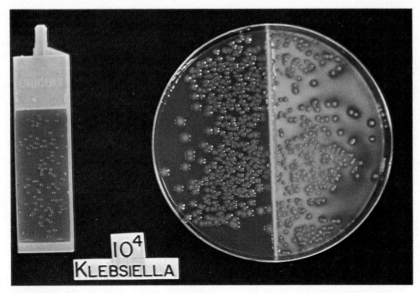

Figure 14–5. The dip-slide on the left is compared with a split-agar surface plate on the right. The urine contained 10,000 colonies of *Klebsiella* per ml (about 200 times the number of colonies on the dip-slide and 10 times the number on either side of the split-agar plate).

agnosis and evaluation of urinary tract disorders, but the microscope can be a trap for the unwary in the diagnosis and follow-up of patients with urinary infections. There are three major sources of error.

The most important error results from the limitation imposed by the microscope on the volume of urine that can be observed. If the volume of urine that can comfortably rest beneath a standard 22-mm coverglass is carefully measured (0.01 ml) and the number of high dry fields ($\times 570$ magnification) present beneath the cover glass is estimated, it is disturbingly apparent that one high dry field represents a volume of approximately 1/30,000 ml. There are excellent studies that show that the bacterial count must be approximately 30,000 per ml before bacteria can be found in the sediment, stained or unstained, spun or unspun (Sanford et al., 1956; Kunin, 1961). For these reasons, a negative urinalysis for bacteria never excludes the presence of bacteria in numbers of 30,000 per ml or less. As already pointed out, many circumstances can reduce the bacterial colony count in bladder urine to numbers less than 30,000 per ml. Those who adopt the method for office bacteriology presented in this chapter, and who not only look at spun aliquots under the microscope but also culture the urine, will convince themselves in the first week that tens of thousands of bacteria per ml can be present on the culture plate that cannot be found in the microscopic sediment.

The second error made by the examiner who relies solely on the microscope is the reverse of the first error: Bacteria are seen in the microscopic sediment but the urine culture is reported to be sterile. The voided urine from the female, even when collected on the cystoscopy table under carefully controlled conditions, can contain many thousands of lactobacilli and corynebacteria. These bacteria are readily seen under the microscope, and, although they are gram-positive, they often appear gram-negative (gram-variable) if stained. Strict anaerobes, usually gram-negative bacilli, also make up a significant mass of the normal vaginal flora (Marrie et al., 1978).

The third major error that results from relying solely on the microscope for the diagnosis of urinary infection lies in the interpretation of pyuria. There is probably no more meaningless query in the whole field of medicine than "How many white blood cells (WBC's) in the centrifuged urine are significant?" The number of WBC's seen under the microscope depends on (1) how the specimen was obtained (especially the degree of vaginal contamination in the female or urethral contamination in the male); (2) the rate of urinary production (the degree of hydration) at the time of collecting the specimen; (3) the intensity of the tissue reaction of the uroepithelial surfaces to the disease process; (4) the volume, time, and speed of centrifugation; and (5) the volume in which the physician resuspends the urinary sediment after pouring off the supernatant. Thus, the number of WBC's present in the spun sediment can vary so markedly as to be meaningless.

Moreover, many diseases of the urinary tract produce significant pyuria in the absence of bacterial infection. Whereas tuberculosis is the well-recognized example of abacterial pyuria, staghorn calculi and stones of smaller size can produce intense pyuria with clumps of WBC's in the absence of urinary infection. Almost any injury to the urinary tract, from chlamydial urethritis to glomerulonephritis and interstitial cystitis, can elicit large numbers of fresh polymorphonuclear leukocytes (glitter cells). Depending on the state of hydration, the intensity of the tissue reaction producing the cells, and the method of urine collection, any number of WBC's can be seen in the microscopic sediment in the presence of a sterile urinary tract. The presence or absence of pyuria in the centrifuged urine is the worst of all criteria for the diagnosis of a urinary infection.

Pyuria, however, can be quantitated in the uncentrifuged urine by measuring either the WBC excretion rate (in a timed urine collection) as WBC's per hour or the WBC concentration as WBC's per ml in a random, nontimed urine sample. Both methods require that a fresh, unspun sample of urine be placed in a counting chamber of exact volume, such as the Neubauer haemocytometer or the Fuchs-Rosenthal chamber, which has twice the depth (0.2 mm) and volume of the Neubauer chamber. Mabeck has advocated a timed urine collection in which the results are expressed as WBC's per hour (Mabeck, 1969b); he found that women without evidence of urinary tract disease excrete fewer than 400,000 leukocytes per hour. Gadeholt (1964, 1968), however, in a detailed and scientific analysis of the errors involved in counting cells in urine, argues for simply expressing the results as cells per mm³ of urine in nontimed specimens; he notes that the upper limit of a normal cell count is assumed to be 8 erythrocytes and 13 leukocytes plus nonsquamous epithelial cells per mm³ of urine. Any clinical investigator who wants to quantitatively count cells in the urine should study Gadeholt's investigations very carefully.

We quantitate leukocyte counts in the voided urine of our patients whom we follow closely for research purposes; we use the Fuchs-Rosenthal chamber and report the results as leukocytes per ml of urine. In a careful study of 16 control woman volunteers who had never had urinary infections, the first voided 5 to 10 ml collected by the nurse on the cystoscopy table contained 2700 ± 6300 leukocytes per ml (*n* = 116). In 123 collections in the same 16 volunteers, the midstream urine collected in the same manner contained 300 ± 700 leukocytes per ml. On the other hand, when volunteer controls collected their own urine samples by voiding from the toilet seat and cleaning their labia twice with a 4 × 4 gauze sponge wet with tap water, the first voided sample from 14 women studied 21 times contained 2300 ± 2600 leukocytes per ml of urine. Midstream samples from the same 14 women, but collected 96 times, contained 900 ± 2400 leukocytes per ml. These latter data, then, indicate that a midstream urine from a normal, premenopausal woman, collected as outlined, should contain less than 7000 leukocytes per ml in 99 per cent of individuals (900 + 2½ standard deviations). If the urine specimen is collected from the paient on the cystoscopy table, the upper limit of normal should be 2050 leukocytes per ml of urine. This latter figure, when vaginal contamination is minimized, approaches the leukocyte counts reported by Musher and associates (1976) in 49 of 51 healthy adult men who had 5000 leukocytes per ml or less in urine with a mean WBC count of 1300 per ml. Kesson and coworkers (1978) also showed that < 2000 leukocytes per ml of voided urine was characteristic of normal women without infection.

It must be emphasized, however, that as useful as quantitative WBC counts are, the physician must still centrifuge an aliquot and examine it under a good microscope in order to diagnose many diseases of the urinary tract (see Chapter 6, subsection on urinalysis). Indeed, if we were forced to make a choice and could not do both (a quantitative WBC count and a qualitative, centrifuged examination of the urinary sediment), we would choose without hesitation a careful study of the centrifuged urinary sediment.

LOCALIZATION OF THE SITE OF URINARY INFECTION

Bladder

SUPRAPUBIC NEEDLE ASPIRATION OF THE BLADDER (SPA)

Before a suprapubic needle aspiration is performed, the patient should force fluids until the bladder is full. The site of the needle puncture is in the midline, between the symphysis pubis and the umbilicus, and directly over the palpable bladder. The full bladder in the male is usually palpable because of its greater muscle tone; unfortunately, the full bladder in the female is frequently not palpable. In such patients, the physician performing the aspiration must rely on the observation that suprapubic pressure directly over the bladder produces an unmistakable desire to urinate. After determining the approximate site for needle puncture, the local area is shaved and the skin is cleansed with an alcohol sponge; a cutaneous wheal is raised with a 25-gauge needle and any local anesthetic (Fig. 14–6). A 3½-inch, spinal, 22-gauge needle is introduced through the anesthetized skin; the progress of the needle is arrested just below the skin within the anesthetized area and, with a quick plunging action, similar to any intramuscular injection, the needle is advanced into the bladder. Most patients experience more discomfort from the initial anesthetization of the skin than they feel with the second stage when the needle is advanced into the bladder. After the needle has been introduced, a 20-ml syringe is used to aspirate 5 ml of urine for culture and 15 ml of urine for centrifugation and urinalysis. The obturator is reintroduced into the needle, and both needle and obturator are withdrawn. A small dressing is placed over the needle site in the skin. If urine is not obtained with complete introduction of the needle, the patient's bladder is not full and is usually deep within the retropubic area. When no urine is obtained with the first try, it is probably wiser to desist until the bladder is full. Nevertheless, we have often made several attempts without complications, but it is uncomfortable for the patient.

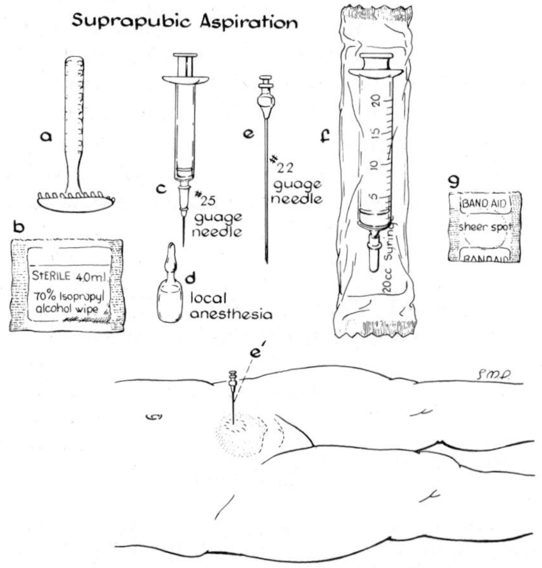

URETHRAL CATHETERIZATION IN THE FEMALE

In a remarkable study that was well ahead of its time, Philpot (1956) obtained catheterized urines from 50 volunteer normal women after washing the introitus with green soap and rinsing with potassium mercuric iodide: 66 per cent were sterile, 28 per cent had 1 to 30 bacteria per ml, and 6 per cent had 30 to 400 bacteria per ml; none of the contaminating bacteria were gram-negative bacteria or even enterococci. Regardless of the technique of catheterization, however, some sterile bladder urines will be contaminated by urethral bacteria; the consideration of a sterile urine, therefore, even with catheterization, must remain statistical. The catheter cannot offer a categorical delineation between the presence and absence of bacteria. A small, No. 10 to 14 French, soft plastic catheter should be used for catheterization after the labia and urethral meatus are cleaned with soap and water; the labia minora should be separated during the meatal washing and the catheterization. It is, of course, impossible to remove the bacteria on the distal third of the urethral mucosa.

Kidney

URETERAL CATHETER LOCALIZATION

We began in 1959 to localize the site of bacteriuria by ureteral catheterization studies, publishing the technique in 1963 (Stamey and Pfau, 1963) and the results in 1965 (Stamey et al., 1965). The technique is simple but exacting; the urologist should consult a more detailed description (Stamey, 1980) before actually performing this localization technique. The validity depends upon controlling the number of bacteria from the bladder that contaminate the ureteral catheters as they pass through the bladder into the ureteral orifices. The bladder must be thoroughly irrigated before both ureteral catheters are passed into a small volume of residual irrigating fluid. A culture is obtained through both ureteral catheters simultaneously, and then each catheter is passed into the ureter or renal pelvis. Four serial cultures are obtained from each kidney. In addition to quantitative bacterial counts on each specimen, determination of either specific gravity or urine creatinine on the

Figure 14–6. Technique of suprapubic aspiration of the bladder (SPA). (Reproduced by permission from Stamey, T. A.: Prevention of Recurrent Urinary Infections. Science & Medicine Publishing Company, New York, 1973.)

TABLE 14–3. CLINICAL EXAMPLES OF URETERAL CATHETERIZATION STUDIES IN
LOCALIZING THE SITE OF BACTERIURIA

Source*	Bladder Infection (Bacteria/ml)	Left Renal Infection (Bacteria/ml)	Right Renal Infection (Bacteria/ml)	Bilateral Renal Infection (Bacteria/ml)
CB	$>10^5$	5000	$>10^5$	4000
WB	900	300	1000	20
LK_1	20	2000	20	400
LK_2	0	2200	0	350
LK_3	0	2500	0	500
LK_4	0	2200	0	400
RK_1	10	0	10,000	260
RK_2	0	0	10,000	220
RK_3	0	0	8000	300
RK_4	0	0	12,000	250

*Abbreviations: CB = catheterized patient, cystoscopic specimen
WB = controlled, "wash bladder" specimen collected after copious irrigation of the bladder.
LK_1, LK_2, etc. = serial cultures of urine from the left kidney.
RK_1, RK_2, etc. = serial cultures of urine from the right kidney.

renal samples can be very helpful in interpreting a change in diuresis in relation to bacterial counts. The technique has been presented in detail, with several examples each of infections localized to the bladder, to one kidney, and to both kidneys (Stamey, 1980). Classic examples of each site are shown in Table 14–3.

When this technique was applied to large numbers of bacteriuric patients, 50 per cent were found to have bladder infection only; 25 per cent, unilateral renal bacteriuria; and 25 per cent, bilateral renal bacteriuria (Table 14–4) (Stamey et al., 1965). These figures have been confirmed by at least five investigators in three countries (the United States, England, and Australia) and can be taken as a good approximation for any general bacteriuric adult population. Although many patients with renal stones and other kidney abnormalities in the presence of bacteriuria can increase the proportion of renal infections, the urologist should never assume the kidney is involved if an important decision is to be made. It is mandatory that the patient be started on the appropriate antibacterial agent

TABLE 14–4. LOCALIZATION OF URINARY TRACT
INFECTIONS IN 95 FEMALES AND 26 MALES
WITH BACTERIURIA

Number and Sex	Bladder Only	Unilateral Renal Bacteriuria	Bilateral Renal Bacteriuria
95 females	38 (40%)	27 (28%)	30 (32%)
26 males	16 (62%)	6 (26%)	4 (15%)

From Stamey, T. A., Govan, D. E., and Palmer, J. M.: Medicine, *44*:1, 1965. Used by permission.

before leaving the cystoscopy room; we usually use an aminoglycoside. In several hundred localizations in the past 25 years, we have never infected a contralateral sterile kidney despite always carrying a few bacteria into the renal pelvis.

FAIRLEY BLADDER WASHOUT TEST

When Dr. Ken Fairley observed the ease with which infections localized to the bladder (Table 14–3) were washed free of bacteria by the irrigating fluid, he astutely realized this might be accomplished with a Foley catheter followed by serial cultures that would essentially represent ureteral urine. He modified his original 1967 procedure in 1971 to the following protocol (Fairley et al., 1971):

After collecting the initial specimen, the bladder is emptied through a urethral catheter and 40 ml of 0.2% neomycin, together with one ampoule of "Elase," is introduced into the bladder. After 10 minutes, the bladder is distended with 0.2% neomycin to reduce the folds in the mucosa and the catheter is clipped off for 20 minutes. The bladder is then emptied and washed out with 2 liters of sterile saline solution. Some of the saline of the final washout is collected for culture and, after emptying the bladder, a further three, timed, specimens are collected at 10-minute intervals. Bacterial counts are done on all specimens.

"Elase," a combination of two lytic enzymes—fibrinolysin and desoxyribonuclease— was apparently added to produce a cleaner bladder surface in terms of potential exudative mucosal lesions. The truth is that, except for acute hemorrhagic cystitis, almost all bacteriuric patients have a surprisingly clean and normal-appearing bladder mucosa; it is unlikely that the addition of these enzymes plays any role in changing the bladder mucosa, and we know of no studies that have demonstrated a beneficial effect of these enzymes in reducing bacteria that may be stuck to the mucosa. The neomycin, on the other hand, is probably important. In his 1971 paper, Fairley gave specific criteria for separating bladder from renal infection:

Renal infection was assumed to be present when the timed specimen collected 20–30 minutes after bladder washout contained more than 3000 bacteria/ml, and in addition this 20–30 minute specimen contained more than 5 times as many bacteria as were present in the final bladder washout specimen. Bladder infection was assumed to be present when the final timed specimen (20–30 minutes after the bladder washout) was sterile.

Using these criteria, 21 of 48 patients in this general practice study showed evidence of renal infection, 22 showed the infection was limited to the bladder, and only 5 studies were equivocal. There can be little, if any, doubt as to the validity of this procedure and these criteria. The Fairley washout test has been used widely through the world, although often with some modifications that have not always been clearly described.

ANTIBODY-COATED BACTERIA IN URINARY INFECTIONS

In 1974, Thomas, Shelokov, and Forland reported a significant advance in the diagnosis of urinary tract infections. They observed that if the bacteria in the urine of a patient with urinary infection were centrifuged, washed, and mixed with fluorescein-conjugated antihuman globulin, antibody-coating of the bacteria could be seen under a fluorescence microscope as a typical apple-green fluorescence. Thomas and her colleagues reported that 34 of 35 patients with pyelonephritis had bacteria that were fluorescent antibody–positive (FA+), while bacteria from 19 of 20 patients with cystitis were not antibody-coated (FA−). Employing Thomas' technique, Jones et al. (1974), in the same issue of the same journal, reported using the Fairley washout method to localize the site of bacterial infection in 23 of 26 patients; the antibody-coating technique correctly predicted the site of infection (18 renal, 8 bladder) in 25 of 26 patients.

Other studies in adults have confirmed the usefulness of this immunofluorescent technique in separating renal from bladder infection (Harding et al., 1978; Kohnle et al., 1975). To be sure, there are some false negative results in

renal bacteriuria when, if the bacteria are studied very early in the course of an acute infection, there has not been time to generate local antibody. It is also true that a few asymptomatic ascending infections will not stimulate local antibody formation, but these exceptions are not a great disadvantage to the test.

On the other hand, false positive findings caused by local production of bladder antibody have virtually invalidated the test in children (Hellerstein et al, 1978; Forsum et al, 1976; Scherf et al, 1978). The latter authors from Hamburg, Germany, carefully localized with a Fairley test each bacteriuric recurrence in children; they reported that 61 per cent of 75 lower tract localizations were FA+. We have observed local production of antibody in the bladder of adults, as evidenced by many submucosal lymphoid follicles at cystoscopy (Stamey, 1980).

Despite these few problems in adults, discussed elsewhere in substantial detail (Stamey, 1980), Thomas' antibody-coating test is useful, although it will not replace either ureteral catheterization or the Fairley test. By indicating that the urinary infection is severe enough to cause local antibody production (whether in the kidney or in the bladder), it adds a dimension to research on urinary infections that is not provided by direct localization techniques. For example, the observation that the bladder of children commonly produces antibody is useful information and casts some doubt on whether chills, fever, and C-reactive protein represent adequate evidence of pyelonephritis as opposed to cystitis.

C-REACTIVE PROTEIN

C-reactive protein (CRP) is a nonantibody, nonantimicrobial, acute-phase substance that appears in the serum during a variety of unrelated illnesses (infection, cancer, myocardial infarction, and so forth). It is measured by its ability to react with a group-specific polysaccharide C-substance of *S. pneumoniae*. CRP appears during the acute phase of diseases and disappears during convalescence when specific antibody begins to increase in infectious diseases.

The Göteborg group has studied CRP extensively in an effort to decide whether pyelonephritis is present in febrile infants and children (Jodal et al., 1975; Jodal and Hanson, 1976). They feel it is superior to the antibody-coating test as an indication of acute pyelonephritis (Wientzen et al., 1979), which is perhaps not surprising since CRP appears immediately whereas antibody response requires a few days. Jodal and Hanson (1976) showed that CRP returned to normal within 7 days of the onset of acute pyelonephritis if the patient was adequately treated. In a more recent pediatric study, Hellerstein and associates (1982) compared the Fairley washout test with the C-reactive protein test; CRP failed to identify over half of the girls with renal bacteriuria who did not have signs of acute pyelonephritis. CRP was elevated in symptomatic children with acute pyelonephritis.

From the therapeutic point of view, children who were CRP-positive (≥ 28 $\mu g/ml$) had the same rate of recurrent UTI, 14/42 (33 per cent), as those who were CRP-negative, 14/40 (35 per cent), when treated with 10 days of an oral cephalosporin and despite substantial differences in the clinical characteristics of the CRP-positive and negative groups (McCracken et al., 1981).

FEVER

Because many children present with fever as the only sign of bacterial or viral infection, how reliable is fever (greater than 38°C) as a sign of pyelonephritis in a patient with bacteriuria? Since the answer to this question requires localization studies, either ureteral catheterization or the Fairley test, before treatment in febrile, sick patients, it is easy to understand the paucity of data. Although fever has generally been accepted as a sign of renal infection, the observation that bladder bacteriuria in children causes production of antibody may be reason for caution in this assumption. The most challenging questions have come from the Hamburg group, whose aggressive localization studies in children and adults (Huland et al., 1982; Busch and Huland, 1984) as well as in patients with end-stage renal disease (Huland et al., 1983) have shown substantial incidences of fever and even flank pain in bacteriuric patients whose infection was localized to the bladder. Dr. Jan Winberg (1983) believes that the temporary 2 to 3 months of depressed urinary concentrating ability that he observed in febrile girls is strong evidence of kidney involvement. The issue appears unresolved and much more controversial than a few years ago.

Kidney or Bladder Localization? Does It Make any Practical Difference?

The different techniques available to decide whether a specific episode of bacteriuria involves the kidneys or is limited to the bladder have been presented in this section, but does it really make any difference? In the 99 per cent of patients whose recurrences are reinfections, we believe that it makes little difference, if any. The key to prevention is prophylaxis, which works equally well whether the bladder infections ascend to the kidneys or not. From a scientific research basis, however, in which understanding the natural history of the development of coarse renal scarring or pyelonephritic atrophy is important, these techniques may be critical. But for the practical management of the patient, we are unconvinced that it makes any important difference.

For those few patients, with bacterial persistence the causes of which are listed in Table 14–2, exact localization of the site of infection is clearly crucial to achieving a sterile urine without constant antimicrobial therapy. Ureteral catheterization, using our techniques at Stanford, not only allows separation of bacterial persistence into upper and lower urinary tracts, but also separation of the infection between one kidney and the other, and even localization of infection to ectopic ureters or to nonrefluxing ureteral stumps (by using saline irrigation) (Stamey, 1980). Indeed, since the urologist holds the key to identifying the site of bacterial persistence in the urinary tract, he needs to be thoroughly familiar with these techniques.

Lower Urinary Tract Localizations

Because it appeared by the early 1960's that almost all infections were reinfections and because Gallagher et al. (1965) showed in a general practice study that about 31 per cent of the women presenting with dysuria, frequency, and suprapubic cramps had sterile (*zero* bacteria) bladder urines, it was time to concentrate on the lower urinary tract. We began to develop techniques, based on segmenting the voided urine into sequential aliquots, which allows bacteriologic assessment of the urethra and prostate in the male and the urethra and vaginal vestibule in the female, without the artifacts and morbidity introduced by instrumentation. These techniques require multiple cultures, and the bladder urine must be sterile at the time of sampling.

MALES: URETHRA AND PROSTATE

The required aliquots are illustrated in Figure 14–7. The patient must be well hydrated with a full bladder to ensure proper collections. The foreskin is fully retracted and should be maintained in this position throughout all collections to avoid contamination. So important is this maneuver that the foreskin should be

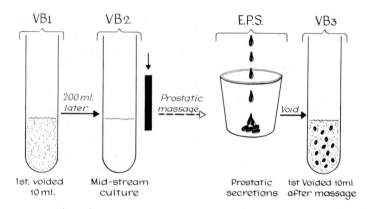

Figure 14–7. Segmented cultures of the lower urinary tract in the male. (Reproduced by permission from Meares, E. M., and Stamey, T. A.: Invest. Urol. 5:492, 1968.)

taped back in the retracted position by a loose circular strip of adhesive around the midshaft of the penis. The glans is cleaned with a detergent soap, which is removed with a wet sponge, and the glans is then dried carefully with a sterile sponge. Throughout the collections, contamination of the specimens must be prevented in the uncircumcised male; if the foreskin slips over the meatus during these collections, the results can be rendered meaningless. Thousands of gram-negative bacteria can reside beneath the uncircumcised foreskin even though it is easily retractable and seemingly clean; the presence of these foreskin bacteria can be a major source of confusion in localizing the site of infection in the lower urinary tract.

The VB_1 (the symbol for "voided bladder one") is collected by holding the sterile culture tube directly in front of the urethral meatus. As the patient initiates the urinary stream, the physician quickly removes the VB_1 tube from the stream of urine, limiting the collection to 5 to 10 ml. When the patient has voided approximately 200 ml (about one half of the bladder urine), the second culture tube, VB_2 (the symbol for "voided bladder two"), is inserted into the stream of urine for a 20-ml sample, a volume adequate to centrifuge 15 ml for urinalysis and send 5 ml for culture. The patient is instructed to immediately stop voiding. After shaking any residual urethral urine from the shaft of the penis, he places his elbows on an examining table with his legs separated but straight. The urologist should first remove any residual drops of urine from the meatus with tissue paper; it is useful to press the bulbar urethra posteriorly with blunt but gentle pressure in case further residual urine can be expressed from the urethral meatus. By sitting on a chair in a position sideways to the patient, the examiner can massage the prostate with his right hand while holding the sterile container to collect the EPS

(expressed prostatic secretion) in his left hand; in this way, drops of prostatic secretion can be observed directly to appear at the meatus and to fall uncontaminated into the sterile container. The first drop to appear should be pure opalescent prostatic fluid without any yellow tint of urine. Sometimes when there has been little or no prostatic fluid expressed, pressure with the right thumb or the back of the middle finger on the bulbar urethra will produce several drops that have accumulated in the wide part of the urethra. Sometimes a steady, increasingly firm digital pressure on one lateral lobe will empty the prostatic glands better than the standard massage from base to apex. After as many free drops of EPS as possible have been obtained, there is always a residual drop along the urethra that is used last to prepare a microscopic slide for coverslip examination. The patient is then asked to void again, and the VB_3 (the symbol for "voided bladder three") is collected in exactly the same manner as was the VB_1. Both the VB_1 and the VB_3 *must* be limited to a minimal volume in the bottom of the test tube. Equally important, all of the detergent must be removed before any of these cultures, especially the VB_1 is collected. If the patient is circumcised, it is unnecessary to cleanse the glans before collecting the cultures.

When possible, 0.1 ml or even more of EPS should always be surface-streaked onto the appropriate agar plates. Quantitative bacteriologic loops of 0.01 ml or less should be avoided because the volume cultured is too small to detect the small numbers of bacteria (100 bacteria per ml and less), which often characterize chronic bacterial prostatitis.

The critical importance of comparing the colony counts in the segmented aliquots of the VB_1 with the VB_3 or the VB_1 with the EPS in documenting the diagnosis of bacterial prostatitis, as well as limiting the volume of urine in the VB$_1$ in order to characterize urethritis, is covered in detail in Chapter 17 on prostatitis.

FEMALE: VAGINAL VESTIBULE AND URETHRA

The technique used at Stanford for the past 20 years to study the bacteria (and inflammation) of the vaginal vestibule, urethra, and midstream urine is illustrated in Figure 14–8.

Vaginal Vestibule Cultures. The female is placed on the cystoscopy table in a semi-sitting position with her legs in stirrups. The nurse, wearing sterile rubber gloves, spreads the labia and swabs the vaginal vestibule with two sterile cotton applicator sticks held together; this maneuver is performed in a circular motion covering all four quadrants at the level of the hymenal ring. The cotton tips of the applicator sticks are always in view as they thoroughly sample the mucosal surface. These applicator sticks are then place in a test tube containing 5 ml of transport broth or sterile saline and immediately refrigerated. If there is a question of vaginal irritation, the physician removes one of these cotton swab sticks, presses it onto a microscopic slide, and covers the drop of fluid with a 22-mm coverglass. Examination of this wet preparation can be diagnostic for trichomonads, yeast, or mycelial forms of fungi, and for fresh inflammatory leukocytes. The culture tube with the swab stick(s) is vigorously agitated in the laboratory, the cotton applicator stick(s) removed, 0.1 ml of fluid cultured, and the bacteria in the 5 ml of transport saline or broth are reported as bacteria per ml.

Urethral and Midstream Urine Cultures. After the vaginal specimen is obtained, the nurse spreads the labia with one hand and collects the first voided 5 to 10 ml by holding a culture tube 1 cm from the urethral meatus; this culture, representative of the urethral flora, is labeled VB$_1$. As the patient continues to void, the midstream aliquot (VB$_2$) is collected 200 ml later in a similar fashion while the nurse keeps the labia apart and obtains a reasonably uncontaminated midstream specimen. Observe that the perineum is not cleaned before or after these cultures are collected; since the labia are continuously retracted, washing the urethral meatus makes little difference because the contaminating bacteria reside inside the distal third of the urethra. These urethral and midstream aliquots are refrigerated within minutes and cultured within a few hours.

About 10 per cent of our women patients are unable to void on the cystoscopy table with a nurse in attendance. These women are carefully instructed in the collection technique and are permitted to obtain their own specimens by sitting on the back edge of the toilet seat, holding the labia apart with one hand, and collecting the specimens as described above. Without question, the latter technique produces substantial contamination compared with the specimens collected with the patient on the cystoscopy table.

The usefulness of these introital cultures of the vagina, as well as the urethral and midstream specimens, is covered in Chapter 15.

TISSUE AND STONE CULTURES

It is clinically useful to culture stones removed from the urinary tract to document that bacteria reside within their interstices. Tissue cultures are primarily useful for research information.

Using sterile technique at the operating table, the surgeon places the stone or fragment of tissue into a sterile culture tube containing 5 ml of saline; the culture is packed in ice and sent to the bacteriologic laboratory where, after agitation of the stone or tissue in the 5 ml of

Figure 14–8. Segmented cultures of the lower urinary tract in the female. (Reproduced by permission from Stamey, T. A.: Pathogenesis and Treatment of Urinary Tract Infections. Baltimore, The Williams & Wilkins Company, 1980.)

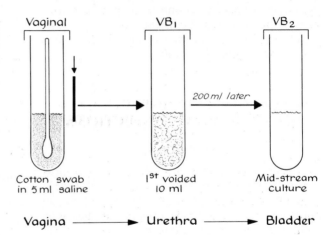

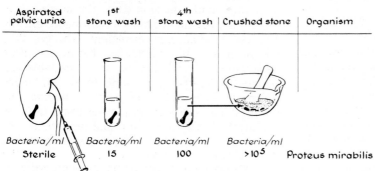

Bacteriologic Stone Culture
(P.R. – age: 46 yr. ♀)

Aspirated pelvic urine	1st stone wash	4th stone wash	Crushed stone	Organism
Bacteria/ml Sterile	Bacteria/ml 15	Bacteria/ml 100	Bacteria/ml >10⁵	Proteus mirabilis

Figure 14–9. Method of culturing stones at surgery. Urine is aspirated to assure sterility, and stone (or portion of it) is placed in 5 ml of cold saline. See text for bacteriologic techniques of washing and crushing the stone. In this example, note that the number of *P. mirabilis* is in the fourth wash increased 1000 times when the stone was crushed, clearly demonstrating that large numbers of bacteria were inside the stone. (From Nemoy, N. J., and Stamey, T. A.: JAMA, *215*:1470, 1971. Copyright 1971, American Medical Association.)

saline, 0.1 ml is surface-streaked on both blood agar and eosin–methylene blue (EMB) agar. The saline is then poured off the specimen; with sterile forceps the stone or tissue is transferred to a second 5 ml of sterile saline. After agitation to ensure a reasonable washing action, the saline is again decanted and the specimen is transferred to a third 5 ml of saline and finally to a fourth 5 ml of saline. This last saline wash is cultured quantitatively in the same manner as the first. The remainder of this fourth 5 ml of saline is poured with the stone into a sterile mortar and pestle dish. After crushing the stone (or grinding the tissue in a tissue blender) in the fourth saline wash, 0.1 ml is again cultured on both blood agar and EMB. The difference in colony counts between the first and fourth saline washes represents the washing effect of the saline transfers on the surface bacteria of the stone or tissue. The difference between the fourth saline wash before and after crushing (or grinding, for tissue) represents the difference between surface bacteria and bacteria within the specimen. An example of this method of stone culture is shown in Figure 14–9; this middle-aged female had suffered from recurrent *Proteus mirabilis* urinary infections secondary to a struvite stone in her right lower pole calyx. The figure shows the culture results of this stone after it was surgically removed.

IMAGING TECHNIQUES IN GENITOURINARY INFECTIONS

INDICATIONS

Radiologic studies are unnecessary in most simple genitourinary infections, but in certain patients they may be useful (Table 14–5). In these patients, radiologic imaging studies may determine acute infectious processes that re-

quire further intervention or may find the etiology of complicated infections.

First, radiologic procedures are needed to identify patients with genitourinary infections who require intervention in addition to their antimicrobial treatment. A urinary infection associated with possible urinary tract obstruction must be evaluated. These are patients with calculi, especially infection (struvite) stones, ureteral tumors, ureteral strictures, congenital obstructions, or previous genitourinary surgery that may have caused obstruction, such as ureteral reimplantation or urinary diversion procedures. Patients with papillary necrosis risk impacting necrotic papillae causing acute ureteral obstruction. Urologic intervention may also be needed in patients whose symptoms of acute clinical pyelonephritis persist after 5 to 6 days of appropriate antimicrobial therapy; they often have perinephric or renal abscesses. Patients with polycystic kidney disease who are on dialysis are apparently particularly prone to

TABLE 14–5. INDICATIONS FOR RADIOLOGIC INVESTIGATION IN ACUTE CLINICAL PYELONEPHRITIS

History of calculi, especially infection (struvite) stones
Potential ureteral obstruction in (e.g., ureteral strictures, tumors)
Papillary necrosis (e.g., patients with sickle cell anemia, severe diabetes mellitus, analgesic abuse)
Congenital genitourinary abnormalities, such as a ureterocele or a small nonfunctioning kidney
Neuropathic bladder
History of genitourinary surgery that predisposes to obstruction, such as ureteral reimplantation or ureteral diversion
Poor response to appropriate antimicrobial agents after 5 to 6 days of treatment
Polycystic kidneys in patients on dialysis or with severe renal insufficiency
Unusual infecting organisms, such as tuberculosis, fungus, or urea-splitting organisms (e.g., *Proteus*)
Diabetes mellitus

developing perinephric abscesses. Patients with diabetes mellitus can develop special complications from urinary infections; they may get emphysematous pyelonephritis or papillary necrosis. Finally, patients with unusual organisms such as tuberculosis, fungus, or urea-splitting bacteria (e.g., *Proteus*) should be examined for abnormalities within the urinary tract such as strictures, fungus balls, or obstructing stones.

The second reason radiologic evaluation is needed in patients with genitourinary infections is diagnostic. In patients whose bacteriuria fails to resolve after appropriate antibiotics or who have rapid recurrence of infection, abnormalities that cause bacterial persistence should be sought (Table 14–2). Several reports of females with recurrent urinary infections show, however, that excretory urograms are unnecessary for routine evaluation if women who have special risk factors are excluded (Fair et al., 1979; Engel et al., 1980; Fowler and Pulaski, 1981; Fairchild et al., 1982). (See the discussion of patients at risk of serious morbidity and/or renal scarring from recurrent bacteriuria.) In none of these studies has information useful in the management of these patients been obtained from the excretory urogram. Furthermore, excluding excretory urograms in the routine evaluation of these patients represents a substantial financial saving.

The following are useful imaging techniques in genitourinary infections.

Plain Film of the Abdomen–KUB. The plain film of the abdomen is useful for the rapid detection of radiopaque calculi and unusual gas patterns in emphysematous pyelonephritis. It may show abnormalities, such as an absent psoas or abnormal renal contour, that suggest perirenal or renal abscess, but these findings are nonspecific.

Plain Film Renal Tomograms. Plain film renal tomograms will show small or poorly calcified stones despite overlying gas and fecal shadows. Struvite and uric acid stones that contain small amounts of calcium may be seen on these films but not on routine plain films of the abdomen. Tomograms will also localize findings (calcifications or gas) to the kidney.

Excretory Urogram. The excretory urogram has been a routine examination to evaluate patients with complicated infection problems but is not required in uncomplicated infections. The radiologic features of acute clinical pyelonephritis will be discussed under that section. This study is useful to determine the exact site and extent of urinary tract obstruction but is not the best screening test for hydronephrosis, pyonephrosis, or renal abscess.

Voiding Cystourethrogram. This has been cited as the most important examination in assessing vesicoureteral reflux in children (Lebowitz, 1978). It may be used to evaluate patients with neuropathic bladders and the rare female who has a urethral diverticulum causing her persistent infections.

Renal Ultrasound. The renal ultrasound study has become an important renal imaging technique because it is noninvasive, easy to perform, and offers no radiation risk to the patient. It is particularly useful in eliminating the concern of hydronephrosis associated with urinary tract infection, pyonephrosis, and perirenal abscesses. It is also useful for following renal growth in children who have had urinary infections. A disadvantage is that the study is dependent upon the interpretative and performance skills of the examiner. Furthermore, the study may be technically poor in patients who are obese or who have dressings, drainage tubes, or open wounds overlying the area of interest.

Radionuclide Studies. Although I-131 hippuran and technetium-99 glucoheptonate scans have been used to detect focal parenchymal damage, renal function impairment, and decreased renal perfusion in acute renal infections (McAfee, 1979), these scans have not been popular at most institutions. Two radionuclides that have been used to detect renal or perirenal infections are gallium-67 and indium-111. Gallium has been used to distinguish some upper from lower tract infections (Hurwitz et al., 1976; Kessler et al., 1974; Mendez et al., 1978; Mendez et al., 1980; Patel et al., 1980), but the false negative and false positive results limit its usefulness (Hurwitz et al., 1976). This technique has also been useful in the detection of focal bacterial nephritis and infected renal cysts (Hoffer, 1980). Gallium has the disadvantage of being unable to differentiate simple inflammatory processes from pyelonephritis, pyonephrosis, perirenal abscess, or renal tumors (Hampel et al., 1980). False positive findings may be caused by the accumulation of the radionuclide in the colon and sterile healing tissues, whereas false negative findings may be caused by the normal accumulation of the substance in liver or spleen, which may obscure small pathologic accumulations. Indium-111 labeling of white blood cells has provided a more specific means of identifying areas of inflammation but requires that 30 to 40 ml of the patient's blood be obtained and the white cells labeled. Some have recommended that this study be used in conjunction with abdominal ultrasound in the detection of intra-abdominal abscesses, especially when focal signs are absent

(Carroll et al., 1981). In general, the radio-nuclide studies are helpful in cases in which an intra-abdominal abscess is suspected but localizing signs are absent, or in cases in which clinical suspicion of abscess remains high but ultrasound and computerized tomographic studies are equivocal or negative (Biello et al., 1979; Hampel et al., 1980). Furthermore, because the gallium scan is performed 48 hours after injection and the indium scan at 24 hours, there is considerable delay before the studies can be interpreted; therefore, these studies may not be useful in patients who are acutely ill.

Computerized Tomography. Computerized tomography is the radiologic modality that offers the best anatomic detail, but its cost prevents it from being a screening procedure. Computerized tomography is useful in the diagnosis of acute focal bacterial nephritis and renal and perirenal abscesses (Mendez et al., 1979; Kuhn and Berger, 1981; Mauro et al., 1982; Wadsworth et al., 1982). When used to localize renal abscesses, it improves the approach to surgical drainage and permits percutaneous approaches. Its usefulness is, however, limited in uncooperative patients.

IMMUNOLOGIC RESPONSES TO GENITOURINARY INFECTION

Although both cellular and humoral immune responses are observed in genitourinary infections, this section will focus primarily on the humoral immune response, which is better understood. The cellular response will be mentioned briefly in the section on pyelonephritis. Much research during the past 10 years has been devoted to the genitourinary immune response to bacterial infection because of the potential use of this response in diagnosing severe urinary infections. Humoral immunity is characterized by the formation of antibodies (immunoglobulins) in response to invasive bacterial antigens. These antibodies may be produced and found systemically in the blood, or locally within the genitourinary tract. New, more sensitive methods of measuring these antibodies have improved our knowledge of humoral immunity. Knowledge of the response of these antibodies to infecting bacteria (antigen-specific antibodies) is clinically useful because investigators have studied these antibodies as markers to distinguish between acute or chronic pyelonephritis and cystitis.

Direct Agglutination Tests. Bacterial agglutination is performed by mixing dilutions of serum with bacterial suspensions. The presence of serum antibodies to the bacteria (antigen-specific antibodies) is detected by agglutination of particles. Primarily multivalent antibodies, such as IgM, combine with surface bacterial antigens to cause the clumping. Since IgM is seen most commonly during the early phases of an acute infection, this method has limited use in detecting chronic infections in which IgG is more important.

Passive Agglutination Tests. Many bacterial polysaccharide and protein antigens may nonspecifically stick to the surface of red blood cells. When these red blood cells with their attached antigens are mixed with dilutions of serum, antigen-specific antibodies can be detected by measuring agglutination of the red blood cells.

Fluorescent Antibody Coating of Bacteria. As will be discussed later, it was hoped that fluorescent antibody–coating of bacteria would differentiate between upper and lower tract urinary infections. Although the test is not as specific as was originally thought, it is useful. The test is based upon the presence of antibodies that appear in the urine during urinary infection. These antigen-specific antibodies may bind to the infecting bacteria. When a fluorescein-conjugated antiserum to human immunoglobulins (either IgM, IgG, and IgA together, or individually) is mixed with the bacteria from infected urine, the fluorescein-conjugated antiserum binds to the antigen-specific antibodies that are bound to the bacteria; the fluorescent antibody–coated bacteria are seen under a fluorescence microscope. A disadvantage to this test is that observation of fluorescence may be subjective and is not quantitative.

Enzyme-Linked Immunosorbent Assays or Radioimmunoassays for Immunoglobulins. The enzyme-linked immunosorbent assays (ELISA) and radioimmunoassays (RIA) are sensitive laboratory procedures to detect and quantitate many chemicals and proteins. In the urinary tract, they have been used to detect and measure serum, urine, and prostatic fluid total immunoglobulins and antigen-specific antibodies. The tests are similar and use specially labeled antisera to the immunoglobulin heavy-chain fractions (IgM, IgG, and IgA) to detect antibody to bacteria (antigen-specific antibody). These tests measure antigen-specific antibodies belonging to any of the immunoglobulin classes (IgM, IgG, and IgA) and are more sensitive and quantitative than agglutination or hemagglutination tests.

Immunoglobulin Response in Pyelonephritis. Beginning about 20 years ago investigators discovered, in adults with acute pyelonephritis, that antibodies to the infecting bacteria could be measured in the serum. Measurements by bacterial agglutination revealed that serum antibodies (primarily IgM) against the infecting bacteria were elevated in human acute clinical pyelonephritis; these elevated titers decreased after the pyelonephritis was treated but were persistently elevated when the patient remained infected (Percival et al., 1964). Similar studies in adults with bacteriuria, proteinuria, pyuria, and radiographic findings of chronic pyelonephritis have shown that serum antigen-specific antibody titers measured by indirect immunofluorescence are persistently elevated; these patients were not, however, proven to have upper tract infections by using the techniques discussed earlier (Nimmich et al., 1976). Some investigators found that passive hemagglutination titers, which favor measurement of IgM antibodies, are not reliably elevated in patients they had defined to have chronic pyelonephritis (Nimmich et al., 1976; Scarpelli et al., 1979). Other workers, using animal models of pyelonephritis caused by direct renal injection of bacteria, have confirmed elevation of serum antigen-specific antibody (measured by agglutination) by the third day, a peak of the antibody level 6 days after infection, and then a decline in antibody production after this (Miller and North, 1971). Other studies confirm that serum antigen-specific antibodies measured by any technique are elevated more frequently, and to a greater extent, in pyelonephritis than in cystitis (Percival et al., 1964; Neter, 1975; Hanson et al., 1975; Akerlund, 1978), but it must be emphasized that serum antibodies were not always elevated in pyelonephritis.

Antigen-specific antibodies stimulated by urinary infections have also been identified in human and animal urine both directly and indirectly. Whether these urinary antibodies are filtered from the serum into the urine or whether they are produced locally has only recently been shown. Miller and North (1971) caused pyelonephritis in rats by direct inoculation of bacteria into the kidney. In this model of pyelonephritis they showed that after infection the activity of antibody-forming cells was increased, and that as the infection progressed, antibody-producing cells were found in the infected kidney. Although they detected no urinary antigen-specific antibodies when they assayed the rat urine at 4-day intervals for 40 days, they used the agglutination technique, which is too insensitive to detect antibody in the urine. Smith and associates (1974), using a more sensitive enzyme-linked immunoassay, detected urinary antibody in pyelonephritic rabbits (made pyelonephritic by the intravenous injection of *E. coli* while the right ureter was transiently obstructed). They detected urinary antigen-specific IgG and IgA antibodies 11 days after infection and urinary IgM later. Both antigen-specific IgG and IgM were present in serum by day 6. These investigators concluded that serum and local urinary antibody are produced independently and that serum antibody is not the result of antibody synthesized in the kidney (Smith et al., 1974). Later it was shown, again in experimental pyelonephritis produced in rabbits as just described, that antibody-coated bacteria appeared by the eleventh day after infection, 3 days after serum antibody is detected (Smith et al., 1977). These investigators concluded that a positive test for antibody-coated bacteria indicates that a local immune response to bacterial O-antigen has occurred. Similarly, in experimentally induced pyelonephritis in rats, antibody-coated bacteria were found in the urinary sediment in 9 of 11 rats, but disappeared in 7 of the 9 rats with antibody-coated bacteria when the pyelonephritic kidney was removed; it was later found that the two rats that continued to produce antibody-coated bacteria had bacteria in the contralateral kidney (Favaro et al., 1978). In human studies, investigators found in nine patients urinary IgA antibodies to mycoplasma 1 to 4 days after acute *Mycoplasma hominis* pyelonephritis; this was followed by urinary IgG antigen-specific antibodies (Erno and Thomsen, 1980). Furthermore, Akerlund's studies (1978) in humans with urinary infections show differences in the avidities of urinary and serum antibodies to infecting bacteria and no correlation between urine and serum IgA antibody levels—more evidence that production of antibodies occurs locally in the urinary tract.

Immunoglobulin Response in Bacterial Prostatitis. In longitudinal studies in males with acute and chronic bacterial prostatitis we have found distinct systemic and local humoral immune responses (Shortliffe et al., 1981b). Antigen-specific antibodies were measured by a sensitive and quantitative solid-phase radioimmunoassay (Shortliffe et al., 1981a). In acute bacterial prostatitis that is cured by antimicrobial therapy, serum and prostatic fluid antigen-specific IgG were both elevated immediately after infection but declined slowly over the next 6 to 12 months (Fig. 14–10*A*). In contrast, the antigen-specific IgA in the prostatic fluid was

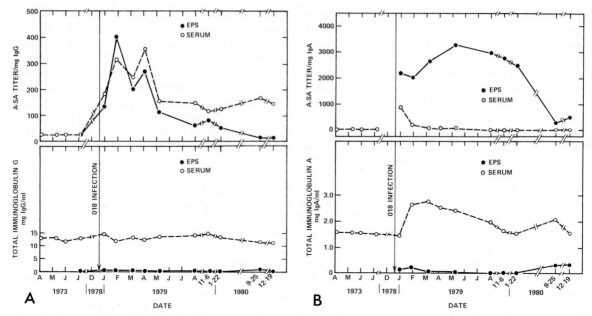

Figure 14–10. *A,* This is an example of a longitudinal study of total IgG immunoglobulin and antigen-specific responses in serum and expressed prostatic fluid (EPS) in a patient with acute bacterial prostatitis who was cured by antibiotics. In the upper portion of the figure, both serum and prostatic fluid IgG rise soon after the infection with *E. coli 018,* and then fall toward normal. The lower portion of the figure shows that total IgG immunoglobulin changes little during the infection. Antigen-specific antibodies were measured by radioimmunoassay and total immunoglobulins by radial immunodiffusion. *B,* This shows values for total IgA immunoglobulin and antigen-specific antibody in the serum and EPS for the same patient. EPS antigen-specific IgA was elevated for almost 2 years after the infection. The serum antigen-specific antibody response is negligible. (From Shortliffe, L. M. D., Wehner, N., and Stamey, T. A.: J. Urol., *125:* 509, 1981. Reproduced by permission.)

elevated after infection and began to decline only after 12 months; after a month the elevation in serum IgA was not detectable (Fig. 14–10*B*). In chronic bacterial prostatitis that is cured by antimicrobial therapy, prostatic fluid antigen-specific IgA and IgG are both elevated—antigen-specific IgA for almost 2 years and antigen-specific IgG for 6 months before returning toward normal (Fig. 14–11). In chronic bacterial prostatitis neither serum IgA nor serum IgG is substantially elevated (Fig. 14–11). Furthermore, in males with bacterial prostatitis who are refractory to treatment, prostatic fluid IgG and IgA are persistently elevated.

Diagnostic Use of Antibody Titers. Although serum or urinary antibody titers may be useful in acute urinary tract infections, they are far from diagnostic. As discussed earlier, individual patients cannot be diagnosed as having pyelonephritis or cystitis by using antibody titers of fluorescent antibody–coated bacteria tests; although patients with acute pyelonephritis *usually* have positive antibody-coating of bacteria and elevated serum or urine antigen-specific antibody titers, the results of the tests overlap with those of cystitis patients (Ratner et al.,

1981; Budde et al., 1981; Bilges et al., 1979; Hawthorne et al., 1978). Since the results of these antibody tests are dependent upon the natural history of the immune response, the tests may be negative very early in the infection or if the humoral immune system is incompletely developed, as in infancy (Pylkkanen, 1978; Wientzen et al, 1979). Furthermore, high antibody titers or positive antibody-coating of bacteria may reflect severity of disease (tissue invasion by bacteria) rather than site of disease. For these reasons, measurements of antigen-specific antibody in serum, urine, or prostatic fluid may be more useful in chronic bacterial infections than in acute infections.

PYELONEPHRITIS

Clinical Pyelonephritis

Although pyelonephritis is defined as inflammation of the kidney and renal pelvis, the diagnosis is clinical. True infection of the "upper urinary tract" can be proved by catheterization tests (ureteral catheterization or bladder wash-

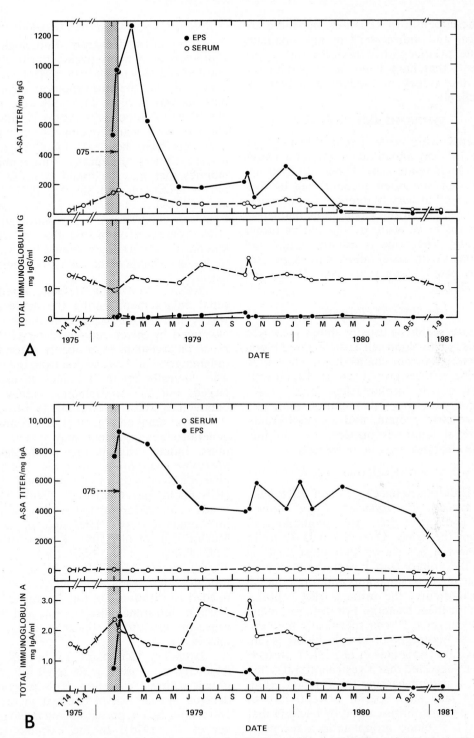

Figure 14–11. *A,* This is an example of a longitudinal study of IgG total immunoglobulins and antigen-specific antibodies in a patient with a chronic bacterial prostatitis who was cured by antimicrobial treatment. In this case the IgG antigen-specific antibodies in the serum and expressed prostatic fluid (EPS) are discrepant. The elevation in EPS antigen-specific IgG returns to normal after only a few months. Minimal elevation in serum antigen-specific IgG was measured. Again, as with acute bacterial prostatitis, serum and prostatic fluid total IgG immunoglobulins vary little over time. *B,* This shows the IgA total immunoglobulins and antigen-specific antibodies for the same patient. As with the patient with acute bacterial prostatitis, after treatment of the chronic infection only the elevation in EPS antigen-specific IgA is remarkable. This elevation persists for longer than 2 years. (From Shortliffe, L. M. D., Wehner, N., and Stamey, T. A.: J. Urol., *125*:509, 1981. Reproduced by permission.)

out) as described in this chapter, but these are impractical and unnecessary in most patients with acute pyelonephritis; none of the noninvasive tests that have been developed to tell whether the kidney or bladder is infected is totally reliable.

SYMPTOMS AND SIGNS

Patients with acute pyelonephritis have chills, fever, and unilateral or bilateral costovertebral angle tenderness. These so-called upper tract signs are often accompanied by dysuria, increased urinary frequency, and urgency; it is, however, the former symptoms that cause the diagnosis to be acute pyelonephritis rather than cystitis. The urine is usually cloudy and malodorous. Acute renal failure may be present in the rare case (Olsson et al., 1980; Richet and Mayaud, 1978).

LABORATORY FINDINGS

Urinary sediment usually shows increased white cells, white blood cell casts, and red blood cells. Bacterial rods or chains of cocci are often seen. Urine cultures grow bacteria. Blood tests may show a polymorphonuclear leukocytosis, increased erythrocyte sedimentation rate, elevated C-reactive protein, and elevated creatinine if renal failure is present. In addition, creatinine clearance may be decreased.

BACTERIOLOGY

The Enterobacteriaceae, *E. coli, Klebsiella, Proteus* species, *Enterobacter, Pseudomonas, Serratia,* and *Citrobacter,* are commonly cultured from the urine. Over the past 10 to 15 years, research has shown that most bacteria infecting the urinary tract possess fimbriae that allow attachment to squamous and uroepithelial cells. Furthermore, the urinary tract contains receptors for these bacteria. For instance, many pyelonephritogenic *E. coli* specifically bind epithelial cell receptors of the P blood group antigen system (Kallenius et al., 1981). In fact, it has been suggested that if vesicoureteral reflux is absent, a patient bearing the P blood group phenotype may have special susceptibility to recurrent pyelonephritis caused by bacteria that bind to the P blood group antigen receptors (Lomberg et al., 1983). Bacterial K antigens and endotoxins may also contribute to pathogenicity (Kaijser et al., 1977) and endotoxins. Some of these factors will be discussed in detail in Chapters 15 and 16.

Of the gram-positive organisms only *Streptococcus fecalis* and, less commonly, *Staphylococcus aureus* are important causes of pyelonephritis.

RADIOGRAPHIC FEATURES

Intravenous Urogram. Radiologic findings characteristic of acute pyelonephritis have been emphasized only recently because it was thought previously that the intravenous urogram in these patients was normal. In 24 per cent (Little et al., 1965) to 28 per cent (Silver et al., 1976) of patients with acute pyelonephritis, abnormal urograms have been attributed to the acute disease. Others confirm the radiographic abnormalities that may be found in acute pyelonephritis (Harrison and Shaffer, 1979; Richie et al., 1978; Barth et al., 1976; Teplick et al., 1978; Cameron and Azimi, 1974). Since an intravenous urogram is often performed in acute pyelonephritis, the urologist should be aware of the radiologic changes that may be seen in this disease.

RENAL ENLARGEMENT. Generalized or focal renal enlargement during the acute infection was seen in about 20 per cent of the urograms examined by Silver and associates (1976). This renal enlargement is probably caused by the inflammation and congestion from the infection. The clinically involved kidney is usually enlarged, but the contralateral kidney may be enlarged as well (Silver et al., 1976).

Focal renal enlargement, less common than generalized enlargement, may appear as a renal mass. Indeed, this finding, *focal bacterial nephritis or acute lobar nephronia,* has been emphasized as causing a renal mass only since 1978 (Rosenfield and Glickman, 1978). This mass needs to be differentiated from a neoplasm or intrarenal abscess (Sotolongo et al., 1982; McDonough et al., 1981; Konetschnik et al., 1982; Funston et al., 1982; Little et al., 1965; Teplick et al., 1978; Barth et al., 1976). Although other radiologic modalities may be needed to differentiate this lesion from a neoplasm or intrarenal abscess, time and treatment cause the mass to disappear, although scarring may occur.

IMPAIRED CONTRAST EXCRETION. Physiologic changes during acute renal infection may impair contrast excretion. This is manifest by delayed appearance of contrast in the calyces and diminished nephrogram and pyelogram (Silver et al., 1976). In the extreme case, the collecting system may not be visualized (Richie et al., 1978; Teplick et al., 1978).

NONOBSTRUCTIVE DILATION OF THE URINARY COLLECTING SYSTEM. Dilation of the ureter and renal plevis without an obstructive cause may be seen during acute pyelonephritis (Teplick et al., 1978; Kass et al., 1976; Silver et al., 1976). This may be caused by the bacterial endotoxins that paralyze the collecting system.

CORTICAL STRIATIONS IN THE NEPHRO-GRAM. In the nephrogram phase of the urogram (or arteriogram) in acute pyelonephritis, cortical striations may be seen (Davidson and Talner, 1973; Silver et al., 1976; Teplick et al., 1978). Although their etiology is unknown, they are thought to be caused by intratubular obstruction by pus or by occluded arterioles and consequent nonperfused foci (Davidson and Talner, 1973).

URETERAL STRIATIONS. Parallel lucent renal pelvic and ureteral streaks have been seen in acute pyelonephritis (Harrison and Shaffer, 1979). These are probably caused by mucosal edema.

Renal Ultrasound. Although renal ultrasound is useful to show renal size and collecting system obstruction and to delineate focal bacterial nephritis, in most infected kidneys no findings are seen on ultrasound that are not seen on the urogram.

Renal Angiogram. Angiograms are unnecessary in acute bacterial pyelonephritis, except for the diagnosis of unusual patients. Most angiograms will be normal, but they occasionally show attenuated and stretched interlobar arterial branches as well as the cortical striations seen on the urogram (Teplick et al., 1978; Barth et al., 1976).

PATHOLOGY

In acute pyelonephritis the kidney may be grossly enlarged. The capsule strips easily, and suppuration may soften areas of parenchyma. There are usually small yellow-white cortical abscesses mixed with parenchymal hyperemia. Histologically, the parenchyma shows a focal, patchy infiltrate of neutrophils. Bacteria are often in the infiltrate. Early in the inflammatory process, this infiltrate is limited to the interstitium, but later abscesses may cause tubular destruction; the glomeruli are usually spared.

Chronic Pyelonephritis

The definition of chronic pyelonephritis, is controversial. As previously noted under *Definitions,* the term "chronic pyelonephritis" has been used to refer to a variety of chronic renal lesions and has been used synonymously with interstitial nephritis, reflux nephropathy, chronic atrophic pyelonephritis, and focal coarse renal scarring. In contrast to the patient with clinical acute pyelonephritis, the patient with chronic pyelonephritis is diagnosed by radiologic and pathologic means. Even when a patient has a radiographically scarred, shrunken kidney with microscopic evidence of inflammation,

there is often no recent or remote history of urinary infection and no sign of viable bacteria. This has caused speculation that nonviable bacterial antigens and autoimmune reactions may account for scarring (Aoki et al., 1969; Cotran and Piessens, 1976). So far, however, there is little support for an autoimmune antibody-mediated injury (Cotran and Piessens, 1976). For the purposes of this discussion, when the term "chronic pyelonephritis" is used it will refer to the small, contracted, atrophic kidney or to the coarsely scarred kidney that has been produced by bacterial infection, recent or remote.

SIGNS AND SYMPTOMS

Many patients diagnosed as having chronic pyelonephritis have no urologic symptoms, and the condition is discovered incidentally. Children or pregnant women with chronic pyelonephritis may present with a urinary infection, but many are diagnosed because of symptoms that are related to the complications of chronic azotemia, such as hypertension, visual impairment, headaches, increased fatigue, polyuria, and polydipsia; these patients may have vesicoureteral reflux or recurrent urinary infections.

LABORATORY FINDINGS

Urinary sediment may show leukocytes, proteinuria, and, rarely, leukocyte casts. Studies comparing a pyelonephritic kidney with a normal contralateral one have shown that a medullary defect in the pyelonephritic kidney causes the loss of filtered water and sodium (Stamey, 1980); thus, urinary concentrating capacity is impaired. Creatinine clearance may be decreased, and serum creatinine may be increased.

RADIOLOGIC FINDINGS

Intravenous Urogram. The intravenous urogram is the best technique to diagnose chronic pyelonephritis. The involved kidneys are usually small and atrophic. Focal coarse renal scarring with clubbing of the underlying calyx is characteristic (Witten et al., 1977) (Figs. 14–1 and 14–2); since the scarring and atrophy commonly affect the renal poles, the renal parenchyma is especially thin in these areas. These findings are unilateral or bilateral. When they are unilateral, the contralateral kidney is often hypertrophied. Even localized areas of normal renal tissue within a scarred kidney may undergo compensatory hypertrophy, suggesting a renal mass (Witten et al., 1977). These pseudotumors sometimes need to be differentiated from neoplasms by other radiologic imaging techniques.

Voiding Cystourethrogram. The voiding cystourethrogram is useful, particularly in children, to show vesicoureteral reflux, which may be associated with focal renal scarring.

PATHOLOGY

In chronic pyelonephritis the gross kidney is often diffusely contracted, scarred, and pitted. The scars are U-shaped, flat, broad-based depressions with red-brown granular bases. The scarring is often polar with underlying calyceal blunting. The parenchyma is thin, and the corticomedullary demarcation is lost.

Histologic changes are patchy. There is usually an interstitial infiltrate of lymphocytes, plasma cells, and occasional polymorphonuclear cells. Portions of the parenchyma may be replaced by fibrosis, and although glomeruli may be preserved, periglomerular fibrosis is often seen. In some affected areas, glomeruli may be completely fibrosed and tubules atrophied. Leukocyte and hyalin casts are sometimes in the tubules; the latter may cause resemblance to the thyroid colloid—hence, the description "renal thyroidization" (Braude, 1973). In general, the changes are nonspecific; they may also be seen in toxic exposures, postobstructive atrophy, hematologic disorders, postirradiation nephritis, ischemic renal disease, and nephrosclerosis.

PATHOGENESIS

Bacterial Access. Although acute renal infection has been caused by the hematogenous route in animals, it is generally accepted that, in humans, acute bacterial pyelonephritis is caused by the ascending route (Kaijser and Larsson, 1982). The pathogenesis of urinary infections in females is discussed in Chapter 15. The transport of bacteria into the kidney may be assisted by the presence of P blood group antigen receptors in the collecting system and ducts (Lomberg et al., 1983), decreased ureteral peristalsis caused by bacterial endotoxins (King and Cox, 1972), vesicoureteral reflux, and bacterial adherence properties.

Since many patients with radiologic or pathologic evidence of "pyelonephritic" scarring do not have a history of urinary infection, and bacteria cannot be cultured from their renal tissue or urine, the term "abacterial pyelonephritis" or "interstitial nephritis" has been used. Work by Aoki and associates (1969) showed that bacterial antigen could be detected in the renal tissue by immunofluorescent localization in six of seven patients with abacterial pyelonephritis.

Immunologic Response to Infection. Much knowledge about the immune response to bacterial infection of the kidney has been derived from experimental animal models (Kaijser et al., 1978; Fierer et al., 1971; Bille and Glauser, 1982; Roberts et al., 1982; Glauser et al., 1978; Slotki and Asscher, 1982; Roberts et al., 1981; Shimamura, 1981; Miller and Phillips, 1981; Brooks et al., 1977). These studies have tried to relate bacterial infection and subsequent renal scarring.

In humans and animals, bacterial infection of the kidney stimulates humoral and cellular immune responses (Miller et al., 1979). In pyelonephritis the systemic humoral response is characterized by a rise in both total and anti–*E. coli* IgG. Locally, bacterial infection of the kidney stimulates total and anti–*E. coli* IgM, IgA, and IgG (Miller et al., 1979); this response does not, however, appear to be associated with the scarring seen in chronic pyelonephritis. The cause of the renal scarring that unpredictably follows infection is unclear. With a rat model of pyelonephritis that was induced by retrograde injection of *E. coli* in a partially obstructed ureter, Glauser et al. (1978) showed that maximal renal exudation and suppuration occurred 3 days after infection and lasted until the fifth day. During this period of maximal suppuration the kidneys were enlarged (renal mass increased) and had numerous cortical abscesses, but this was then followed by extensive parenchymal scarring with a 50 per cent loss of renal mass at 21 days, and a 70 per cent loss at 75 to 90 days. Similarly, Slotki and Asscher (1982) examined rat kidneys at fixed time intervals after direct bacterial infection and showed that polymorphonuclear leukocytes infiltrated the tissue as early as 6 hours after infection; mononuclear cells appeared by 16 hours when macroscopic pustules began to appear on the renal cortex. Maximal suppuration was seen at 3 to 5 days with microabscesses scattered throughout the cortex and medulla, while collagen appeared on the fifth day and cortical depressions were seen on the sixth day. Roberts et al. (1981) caused experimental pyelonephritis in monkeys by injecting *E. coli* retrograde into the kidney until pyelotubular backflow occurred. With this model they showed that mononuclear cells infiltrated the renal pelvic interstitium in a wedge toward the medulla and cortex. They also showed that similar injection with heat-killed bacteria caused a humoral immune response but no cellular response or subsequent renal scarring.

These animal studies support the theory that the leukocyte response is at least partially responsible for renal scarring. Avoiding the acute suppurative response to renal bacterial infection by using antimicrobial and other agents, several investigators have shown a decrease and ablation of scarring (Glauser et al., 1978; Slotki and Asscher, 1982; Miller and Phillips, 1981; Shimamura, 1981). Glauser et al. (1978), using 10 days of antimicrobial treatment with ampicillin and gentamicin, showed that rat kidneys were sterile at 75 to 90 days and that minimal scarring and loss of renal mass (8 per cent) were observed if antimicrobial treatment was started 28 to 30 hours after the onset of infection. If treatment was started 5 days after infection, the pyelonephritic kidneys, although sterilized, were shrunk to 30 per cent of their original mass and were indistinguishable from untreated kidneys. Similarly, Slotki and Asscher (1982) showed that treatment within 24 hours of infection (amoxicillin and gentamicin for 10 days), prevented or reduced scarring. Miller and Phillips (1981), using an experimental model of pyelonephritis caused by direct bacterial injection into the kidney, showed reduced scarring if treatment was begun within 4 days of infection (ampicillin, carbenicillin, nitrofurantoin, and cephalothin).

Other research suggests that the bactericidal activity of the neutrophils causes the initial damage to the renal tubular cells (Roberts et al., 1982). During bacterial phagocytosis, enzymes, superoxide, and oxygen radicals are released, and these investigators have shown that the addition of superoxide dismutase, which inhibits superoxide production, decreases renal inflammation and tubular damage caused by bacteria. From this they have concluded that superoxide contributes to the renal tubular cell damage seen in acute bacterial infection.

Although most of this work has been done on rats, which possess a unicalyceal system, the results support observations in humans. Children under 4 years of age with intrarenal reflux commonly have renal scarring present before they have their first documented urinary infection. If histories of undiagnosed febrile illnesses in early childhood do, indeed, represent pyelonephritis, untreated infections may be the cause of scarring in the "chronic pyelonephritic" kidney.

Association with Reflux Nephropathy. The association of the small, scarred, clubbed kidney with vesicoureteral reflux is called reflux nephropathy. The role that urinary bacterial infection plays in reflux nephropathy is controversial. Whether the small scarred kidney is secondary to urinary infection is difficult to establish because the occurrence of a bacterial pyelonephritic scar in a previously documented unscarred kidney is a rare event. Moreover, it is often difficult to distinguish a pyelonephritic kidney from a congenitally abnormal one. The question as to why all persons with vesicoureteral reflux do not develop reflux nephropathy is complicated but is partially addressed by Ransley and Risdon (1979) in experimental studies involving piglets. In their work they reported intrarenal reflux only in papillae of a particular morphology; they describe a "nonrefluxing" papilla, which is conical and has papillary ducts that close when calyceal pressure is increased, and a "refluxing" papilla, which is larger and has papillary ducts that are wide open. Furthermore, they found that renal scarring occurred only in piglet kidneys exposed to reflux with infected urine and only in those areas drained by "refluxing" papillae. Scars did not occur when the urine was sterile.

The natural history and prevalence of reflux nephropathy found incidentally in adults is unknown. If adult bacteriuric women are screened, reflux nephropathy is present in 0.6 per cent (Alwall, 1975) to 1 per cent (Kincaid-Smith and Bullen, 1965). In a nephrology clinic, Kincaid-Smith and Becker (1979) studied 55 patients with reflux nephropathy and found that most were under 30 years of age. A urinary tract infection was the diagnostic event in 80 per cent; 20 per cent had had enuresis that had never been investigated. In 27 per cent, reflux nephropathy was diagnosed during pregnancy because of urinary infection, hypertension, albuminuria, and post-partum edema. Approximately 50 per cent of the patients had elevated serum creatinine values, 38 per cent had hypertension (diastolic pressure greater than 90), and 35 per cent had proteinuria (greater than 0.2 gm in 24 hours). In half of the patients having proteinuria, renal function declined further during follow-up (a mean of 15.5 months) (Kincaid-Smith and Becker, 1979).

The importance of reflux nephropathy in children will be discussed in Chapter 16.

SEQUELAE OF PYELONEPHRITIS

Although we know that certain adults have increased risk of renal damage from bacteriuria (this subject is discussed in detail in the section *Adult Patients at Risk of Serious Morbidity and/ or Renal Scarring from Recurrent Bacteriuria*), acute clinical pyelonephritis does not cause scarring in most adults with normal urinary tracts. Most of the changes of chronic pyelonephritis seem to occur in infancy, probably because the growing kidney is most susceptible to scarring. In a review that examined the long-term effect or urinary tract infections in adults, it was concluded that renal damage is rare in nonobstructive urinary infections (Stamey, 1980), but that it does occur (Davidson and Talner, 1978; Davies et al., 1972; Bailey et al., 1969; Feldberg, 1982). In most reports of renal change after acute nonobstructive bacterial pyelonephritis, calyceal and papillary distortion similar to that occurring in papillary necrosis is seen, but focal cortical scars characteristic of chronic pyelonephritic changes are absent. Instead, the urograms showed generalized shrinkage of the kidneys after the acute infection. Two of the four patients reported by Davidson and Talner (1978) had diabetes in addition to pyelonephritis.

The natural history of patients with chronic pyelonephritis will be discussed in Chapter 16, Urinary Tract Infections in Infants and Children, under *Course and Prognosis*, since these changes are usually discovered in childhood. When discovered in the adult, a few studies have examined the prognosis. In a longitudinal study of patients with the radiologic changes of bilateral chronic pyelonephritis defined by focal parenchymal scarring and calyceal clubbing, the calculated 5-year survival rate was 95 per cent and the 10-year survival, 86 per cent (Gower, 1976). The survival rate for patients with changes of unilateral chronic pyelonephritis was 100 per cent at both 5 and 10 years. This investigator also observed that during the study period of 5 to 135 months, bacteriuria found in patients more than 20 per cent of the time could not be correlated with deteriorating renal function; infection was, however, often associated with the appearance or growth of renal calculi. The relationships of the pyelonephritic kidney with end-stage renal disease and hypertension have been examined. In one report of 161 patients with end-stage renal disease requiring dialysis, 42 (26 per cent) had "chronic pyelonephritis" with bacteriuria in the past or when studied (Huland and Busch, 1982). All of the 42 with chronic pyelonephritis and end-stage renal disease had, however, a complicating factor: 66.7 per cent had vesicoureteral reflux, 14.3 per cent had analgesic abuse, 11.9 per cent had nephrolithiasis, 4.8 per cent had pyelonephritis during pregnancy, and 2.4 per cent had hydronephrosis. The association between hypertension and the pyelonephritic kidney has been addressed by Pfau (1978), who concluded that the association of "chronic pyelonephritis" and hypertension is usually coincidental (Pfau and Rosenmann, 1978). This agrees with a study in 1973 that examined 74 women who had been admitted to the hospital some 10 to 20 years before with pyelonephritis; only 14.5 per cent

of these women had hypertension, a rate similar to that found in a random female population of the same age (Parker and Kunin, 1973).

Pyonephrosis

The rapid diagnosis and treatment of pyonephrosis are essential to avoid renal parenchymal loss and sepsis. Patients with pyonephrosis often have symptoms similar to those seen with acute pyelonephritis but have obstructive hydronephrosis in addition. On occasion these patients may have only elevated temperatures and complaints of vague gastrointestinal discomfort.

Renal ultrasound is the most useful procedure to diagnose pyonephrosis. In as many as 50 per cent of cases the obstructed pyonephrotic kidney is nonfunctioning, and many more may function poorly (Coleman et al., 1981). As a result, the intravenous urogram is often unhelpful, whereas renal ultrasound is helpful. In pyonephrosis, the renal sonogram may show one of four patterns: (1) persistent echoes from the inferior portion of the collecting system, (2) a fluid-debris level with dependent echoes that shift when the patient changes position, (3) strong echoes with acoustic shadowing from air in the collecting system, or (4) weak echoes from a dilated, poorly transonic renal collecting system (Coleman et al., 1981). In simple hydronephrosis, the dilated pelvis always shows good ultrasonic transmission. If ultrasound is nondiagnostic and the intravenous urogram shows nonfunction or poor visualization with pelvic filling defects, the retrograde pyelogram usually shows ureteral obstruction with irregular filling defects in the renal pelvis caused by purulent sediment. If it is possible to pass a ureteral catheter into the renal pelvis past the obstruction, drainage is diagnostic and therapeutic.

Once the diagnosis of pyonephrosis is made, the treatment is drainage of the infected pelvis and initiation of appropriate antimicrobial drugs. A ureteral catheter can be passed to drain the kidney, but if the obstruction prevents this, a percutaneous nephrostomy tube can be placed. Once the patient is hemodynamically stable and on appropriate antimicrobial drugs, other procedures are usually needed to identify and treat the source of the obstruction.

Xanthogranulomatous Pyelonephritis

Xanthogranulomatous pyelonephritis describes pathologic changes that accompany an unusual chronic renal infection. In this condition, gross renal examination reveals yellow nodules and pericalyceal granulation. The entity is uncommon and is found in only about 0.6 per cent (Malek et al., 1972) to 1.4 per cent (Ghosh, 1955) of patients with renal inflammation who are evaluated pathologically; its importance is, however, that it is "a great imitator" (Malek and Elder, 1978; Tolia et al., 1980). It is often misdiagnosed as a renal tumor (Malek and Elder, 1978; Tolia et al., 1981; Lorentzen and Overgaard, 1980; Anhalt et al., 1971; Flynn et al., 1979). Although the etiology of the reaction is unknown, it is almost always associated with both infection and obstruction.

Clinical Presentation. Most of the patients present with flank pain (69 per cent), fever and chills (69 per cent), and persistent bacteriuria (46 per cent) (Malek and Elder, 1978). Additional vague symptoms, such as malaise, may be present. On physical examination, 62 per cent of the patients had a flank mass, and 35 per cent had had previous calculi (Malek and Elder, 1978).

Bacteriology and Laboratory Findings. Although review of the literature shows *Proteus* to be the most common organism involved with xanthogranulomatous pyelonephritis (Anhalt et al., 1971; Tolia et al., 1981), *E. coli* is also common. The prevalence of *Proteus* may reflect its association with stone formation and subsequent chronic obstruction and irritation. In their analysis of 26 cases, Malek and Elder (1978) found that renal tissue cultures grew bacteria in 22 of 23 cases. Anaerobes have also been cultured (Malek and Elder, 1978; Winn and Hartstein, 1982).

Urinalysis usually shows pus and protein. In addition, blood tests often reveal anemia and may show hepatic dysfunction in up to 50 per cent of the patients (Malek and Elder, 1978).

Radiologic Findings. The intravenous urogram shows renal calculi in 38 per cent (Malek, 1978) to 70 per cent (Anhalt et al., 1971) of patients, lack of excretion in 27 per cent (Malek and Elder, 1978) to 80 per cent (Anhalt et al., 1971), a renal mass in 62 per cent (Malek and Elder, 1978), and calyceal deformity in 46 per cent (Malek and Elder, 1978). Renal ultrasound usually reveals an enlarged kidney with a large central echogenic area and increased parenchymal anechoic pattern (VanKirk et al., 1980). Arteriography shows hypovascular areas, but there may be some hypervascular areas (Malek and Elder, 1978; Tolia et al., 1981; VanKirk et al., 1980). Therefore, radiologic studies, although distinctive, often cannot differentiate between xanthogranulomatous pyelonephritis and renal cell carcinoma.

Pathology. The pathologic process is usu-ally unilateral, although cases of bilateral disease have been reported. Xanthogranulomatous pyelonephritis may be divided into three extents of retroperitoneal involvement: (1) kidney alone, (2) kidney and perinephric fat, and (3) kidney, perinephric fat, and extensive retroperitoneum (Malek and Elder, 1978). In addition, the disease may involve the kidney diffusely or the pericalyceal tissue alone (Tolia et al., 1980; Moller and Kristensen, 1980).

Grossly, the involved kidney usually shows yellow-white nodules, pyonephrosis, and hemorrhage (Moller and Kristensen, 1980). Foamy lipid-laden histiocytes (xanthoma cells), which simulate renal carcinoma cells, are characteristic. Necrosis and inflammation are often associated; hemosiderin is commonly in the histiocytes (Moller and Kristensen, 1980). As emphasized by Moller and Kristensen (1980), the xanthoma cells are not specific to xanthogranulomatous pyelonephritis but also appear in other conditions, such as obstructive pneumonia, in which inflammation and obstruction are associated (Moller and Kristensen, 1980). Transitional cell carcinoma of the renal pelvis has been reported with this disease (Tolia et al., 1981; McDonald, 1981).

In the majority of cases, the diagnosis is made postoperatively by the pathologist. For this reason, a test that offered the promise of preoperative diagnosis would be valuable. In a preliminary report some investigators have shown that preoperative cytologic studies of the urinary sediment in four of five patients with pathologically proved xanthogranulomatous pyelonephritis showed renal xanthoma cells (Ballesteros et al., 1980). Four other kidneys that had hydronephrosis or chronic inflammation alone had cytologic findings negative for xanthoma cells.

Treatment. The primary obstacle to the correct treatment of xanthogranulomatous pyelonephritis is incorrect diagnosis. In most patients the diagnosis is made postoperatively. In fact, in Malek's series of 26 patients (Malek, 1978) only 1 of 26 patients was correctly diagnosed preoperatively. Furthermore, because the renal abnormality is often diagnosed preoperatively as a renal tumor, nephrectomy is usually performed. If localized xanthogranulomatous pyelonephritis is diagnosed preoperatively or at exploration, it is amenable to partial nephrectomy (Malek and Elder, 1978; Tolia et al., 1980). If diffuse and extensive disease into the retroperitoneum exists, then removal of the kidney and perinephric fat may be needed. Under these circumstances the surgery may be difficult and may involve dissection of granulomatous tissue from the diaphragm, great vessels, and bowel (Flynn et al., 1979; Malek and Elder, 1978).

MALACOPLAKIA

Malacoplakia is an unusual inflammatory disease that was originally described to affect the bladder but has been found to affect the genitourinary or gastrointestinal tract, skin, lungs, bones, and mesenteric lymph nodes. In a review of 153 cases, the urinary tract was involved in 58 per cent (bladder, 40 per cent; ureter, 11 per cent; renal parenchyma, 16 per cent) and the retroperitoneum was involved in 16 per cent (Stanton and Maxted, 1981). Patients with genitourinary malacoplakia have chronic coliform bacteriuria.

Presentation. Within the urinary tract, the ratio of females to males with malacoplakia is 4 to 1, but this disparity does not occur in other body tissues (Stanton and Maxted, 1981). The patients often are debilitated, are immunosuppressed, and have other chronic diseases. The symptoms of bladder malacoplakia are bladder irritability and hematuria. Cystoscopy reveals mucosal plaques or nodules. As these lesions progress, they may become fungating, firm, sessile masses that cause filling defects of the bladder, ureter, or pelvis on intravenous urogram. The distal ureter may become strictured or stenotic and cause subsequent renal obstruction or nonfunction (Sexton et al., 1982). A typical patient with renal parenchymal disease may have one or more radiographic masses and chronic *E. coli* infections. When malacoplakia involves the testis, epididymo-orchitis is present. Malacoplakia of the prostate is rare, but when it occurs it may be confused with carcinoma clinically (Shimizu et al., 1981).

Pathology. The diagnosis is made by biopsy. The lesion is characterized by large histiocytes, known as von Hanseman cells, and small basophilic, extracytoplasmic, or intracytoplasmic calculospherules called Michaelis-Gutmann bodies, which are pathognomonic. Electron microscopy has revealed intact coliform bacteria and bacterial fragments within phagolysosomes of the foamy-appearing malacoplakic histiocytes (Lewin et al., 1976; Stanton and Maxted, 1981). In their review of the subject, Stanton and Maxted (1981) emphasize that although pathognomonic for the disease, Michaelis-Gutmann bodies may be absent in early malacoplakia and are not necessary for the diagnosis.

Pathogenesis. The pathogenesis is unknown, but several theories are popular. In 93 patients who had cultures of urine, diseased tissue, or blood, 89.4 per cent had coliform infections (Stanton and Maxted, 1981). Moreover, 40 per cent of the patients in this review had an immune deficiency syndrome, autoimmune disease, carcinoma, or another systemic disorder. This association of coliform infections and compromised health status in patients with malacoplakia is well recognized.

It is hypothesized that bacteria or bacterial fragments form the nidus for the calcium phosphate crystals that laminate the Michaelis-Gutmann bodies. Most investigations into the pathogenesis of this disease support theories that a defect in intraphagosomal bacterial digestion accounts for the unusual immunologic response that causes malacoplakia.

Treatment. Treatment of malacoplakia is treatment of the chronic bacterial infection; this subject is well reviewed by Stanton and Maxted (1981). Although multiple long-term antimicrobials have been used, including many antituberculosis agents, the sulfonamides, rifampin, and trimethoprim are thought to be especially useful because of their intracellular bactericidal activity (Maderazo et al., 1979). Other investigators have used ascorbic acid and cholinergic agents, such as bethanechol, to stimulate bactericidal activity and have reported good results. Surgical intervention may, however, be necessary if the disease progresses in spite of antimicrobial treatment.

FASTIDIOUS ORGANISMS

Anaerobes in the Urinary Tract. Although symptomatic anaerobic infections of the urinary tract are documented, they are uncommon. The distal urethra, perineum, and vagina are normally colonized by anaerobes. Whereas 1 to 10 per cent of voided urine specimens are positive for anaerobic organisms (Finegold, 1977), anaerobic organisms found in suprapubic aspirates are much more unusual (Gorbach and Bartlett, 1974). Clinically symptomatic urinary tract infections in which only anaerobic organisms are cultured are rare, but these must be suspected when a patient with bladder irritative symptoms has cocci or gram-negative rods seen on microscopic examination of the centrifuged urine (catheterized, suprapubic aspirated, or voided midstream urine), and routine quantitative aerobic cultures fail to grow organisms (Ribot et al., 1981).

Anaerobic organisms are frequently found

in suppurative infections of the genitourinary tract. In one study of suppurative genitourinary infections in males, 88 per cent of scrotal, prostatic, and perinephric abscesses included anaerobes among the infecting organisms (Bartlett and Gorbach, 1981). The organisms found are usually *Bacteroides* species including *Bacteroides fragilis, Fusobacterium* species, anaerobic cocci, and *Clostridium perfringens* (Finegold, 1977). The growth of clostridia may be associated with cystitis emphysematosa (Bromberg et al., 1982).

Mycobacterium Tuberculosis and Other Atypical Mycobacteria. These organisms may be found when cultures for acid-fast bacteria are requested; they do not grow under routine aerobic conditions and may be found during evaluation for sterile pyuria. It has been emphasized that the mere presence of the mycobacteria may not indicate tissue infection and that factors such as symptoms, endoscopic or radiologic evidence of infection, abnormal urine sediment, absence of other pathogens, repeated demonstration of the organism, and presence of granulomas be considered before therapy is instituted (Brooker and Aufderheide, 1980; Thomas et al., 1980). Mycobacterium tuberculosis is discussed in Chapter 23, Genitourinary Tuberculosis.

Chlamydia and Mycoplasma. These organisms are not routinely grown in aerobic culture but have been implicated in genitourinary infections. Their role in the urinary tract is discussed in Chapter 19, Sexually Transmitted Disease.

PERINEPHRIC ABSCESS

The high mortality rate from perinephric abscesses is in part caused by the long delay in making the diagnosis; mortality has been as high as 56 per cent (Salvatierra et al., 1967). The diagnosis is difficult to make from a patient's history and physical examination alone because the findings are nonspecific. Over the past 20 years two medical advances have improved the diagnosis and treatment of this condition: (a) new radiologic techniques to assist in the diagnosis and (b) antimicrobial agents.

Perinephric abscesses are thought to arise from hematogenous seeding from sites of infection or from renal extension of ascending urinary infections. When renal capsular infections rupture into the perirenal space, the abscess spreads. Thorley and associates (1974), in their review of perinephric abscesses, found that the literature about perinephric abscesses had changed since the introduction of antimicrobial agents in the 1940's. They reported that the percentage of cases caused by staphylococci decreased from 45 per cent before 1940 to 6 per cent after 1940, and those cases attributable to *E. coli* and *Proteus* rose from 8 to 30 per cent and 4 to 44 per cent, respectively. They think this change reflects the expeditious use of antibiotics to treat skin and wound infections since the 1940's; this use of antibiotics decreases the chance of hematogenous seeding from the infection.

Clinical Presentation. As emphasized by Thorley and associates (1974), the classic patient who has a cutaneous or urinary tract infection followed in 1 to 2 weeks by fever and unilateral flank pain is uncommon. In their group of 52 patients, 58 per cent had symptoms longer than 14 days. The most common complaints were fever, flank or abdominal pain, chills, and dysuria; physical findings showed flank or abdominal tenderness and fever (Thorley et al., 1974, Saiki et al., 1982). In Saiki's review (1982) a flank mass was present in 47 per cent of the patients.

In two series, 36 per cent (Thorley et al., 1974) to 42 per cent (Merimsky and Feldman, 1981) of patients had diabetes and 19 per cent had calculi (Thorley et al., 1974).

Bacteriology and Laboratory Findings. As discussed before, *Staphylococcus* is still cultured from perinephric abscesses, but the majority of abscesses are caused by either *E. coli* or *Proteus* (Saiki et al., 1982; Thorley et al., 1974; Merimsky and Feldman, 1981). Most patients had a white blood count greater than 10,000 (Thorley et al., 1974; Truesdale et al., 1977; Saiki et al., 1982). Surprisingly, admission urinalyses were normal in 25 per cent of the 51 patients with perinephric abscesses evaluated by Thorley and associates (1974).

Radiologic Findings. Recent radiologic imaging techniques have improved the likelihood of diagnosing a perinephric abscess preoperatively. Renal sonography and computerized tomography provide new means of diagnosis and treatment. Although the abdominal plain film has been reported normal in 40 per cent of patients with perinephric abscesses (Thorley et al., 1974), abnormalities that may be seen on the affected side are missing psoas shadows, apparent renal masses, absent renal outlines, calculi, and retroperitoneal gas. This same group reported that approximately 20 per cent of their patients had normal intravenous urograms. When abnormalities occurred they were on the side of the abscess and showed a

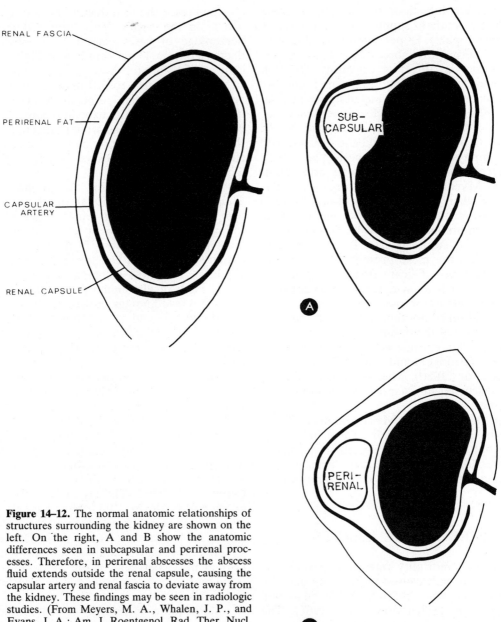

Figure 14–12. The normal anatomic relationships of structures surrounding the kidney are shown on the left. On the right, A and B show the anatomic differences seen in subcapsular and perirenal processes. Therefore, in perirenal abscesses the abscess fluid extends outside the renal capsule, causing the capsular artery and renal fascia to deviate away from the kidney. These findings may be seen in radiologic studies. (From Meyers, M. A., Whalen, J. P., and Evans, J. A.: Am. J. Roentgenol. Rad. Ther. Nucl. Med., *121*:523, 1974. Reproduced by permission.)

kidney with little or no function in 64 per cent, calycectasis or calyceal stretching in 39 per cent, calculi in 14 per cent, and renal displacement in 4 per cent. Others have stated that intravenous urography may show a displaced renal fascia (anteriorly the fascia of Zuckerkandl and posteriorly Gerota's fascia) and renal arteriography may show displacement of the renal capsular artery away from the kidney (Meyers et al., 1974) (Fig. 14–12).

Although abdominal plain film or intrave-nous urogram may show abnormalities associated with perinephric abscess, none of these abnormalities is pathognomonic. One radiologic examination that is more specific for a perine-phric abscess is assessment of renal mobility by fluoroscopy or inspiration-expiration films. Normal kidneys that have not been operated upon should move 2 to 6 cm with respiration, but a kidney with a perinephric abscess will be fixed to surrounding tissues and will not move with respiration. In a series of 71 patients with perinephric abscesses, Salvatierra (1967) reported that only 12 patients were assessed for renal mobility and that in 10 of the 12 it was absent.

Currently, renal sonography and computerized tomography are more specific means of evaluating and localizing perinephric abscesses. Because of the fluid component of most perirenal abscesses, the perinephric collection appears as a sonolucent area, and diagnostic aspiration of this area under ultrasound guidance carries minimal morbidity (Conrad et al., 1977). Computerized tomography (CT) defines renal distortion and perirenal fluid or gas associated with perinephric abscesses in excellent anatomic detail (Wolverson et al., 1979; Mendez et al., 1979; Haaga and Weinstein, 1980; Hoddick et al., 1983). Hoddick et al. (1983), in a series of mixed renal and perirenal abscesses, concluded that CT is more sensitive than sonography for evaluation of severe renal and perirenal infections.

If a perinephric abscess is suspected and current imaging techniques are available, renal ultrasound should be performed first. Moreover, if an intravenous urogram in a patient with acute clinical pyelonephritis has abnormalities to suggest a perinephric abscess, a renal ultrasound should be performed. If the renal ultrasound does not confirm a perinephric abscess or is equivocal, and a high suspicion of abscess remains, renal CT should be performed.

Treatment. Although antimicrobial agents are useful to control sepsis and to prevent spread of infection, the primary treatment for perinephric abscess is drainage; reports of successful treatment by antimicrobial agents alone are unusual (Herlitz et al., 1981). Thorley's (1974) detailed analysis of 52 patients with perinephric abscesses supports this tenet. In this study, half the patients were admitted to medical services and the other half to surgical services; 65 per cent of those admitted to the medical service died, whereas 23 per cent of those admitted to the surgical service died. These mortality rates reflect differences in the population of patients. Those admitted to the medical services were usually sicker and had higher temperatures, more underlying diseases, and vaguer symptomatology. More importantly, none of those admitted to a medical ward had an admission diagnosis of perinephric abscess, whereas 73 per cent of those admitted to surgical wards did. Although 71 per cent of all the patients had eventual surgical treatment of their perinephric abscesses, the diagnostic delay of those patients admitted to the medical service delayed definitive treatment and consequently caused higher mortality.

Although surgical drainage, or nephrectomy if the kidney is nonfunctioning or severely infected, is the classic treatment for perinephric abscesses, renal sonography and CT make percutaneous aspiration and drainage of perirenal collections possible (Haaga and Weinstein, 1980; Elyaderani et al., 1981). Haaga and Weinstein (1980), however, consider percutaneous drainage to be contraindicated in large abscess cavities filled with thick purulent fluid.

Perinephric Abscess versus Acute Pyelonephritis. It has already been emphasized that the greatest obstacle to the treatment of perinephric abscess is the delay in diagnosis. In the series of Thorley and associates (1974) a common misdiagnosis was acute urinary tract infection. In their review, they found that two factors differentiated perinephric abscess and acute pyelonephritis: (1) Most patients wtih uncomplicated pyelonephritis were symptomatic for less than 5 days before hospitalization, whereas most with perinephric abscesses were symptomatic for longer than 5 days; and (2) no patient with an acute urinary infection remained febrile for longer than 4 days once appropriate antimicrobial agents were started. All patients with perinephric abscesses had a fever for at least 5 days, with a median of 7 days.

Patients with polycystic renal disease who undergo hemodialysis may be particularly susceptible to the progression from acute urinary infection to perinephric abscess. Of 445 patients undergoing chronic hemodialysis at the Regional Kidney Disease Program in Minneapolis, Minnesota, 5.4 per cent had polycystic kidney disease and 33.3 per cent of these developed symptomatic urinary tract infections (Sweet and Keane, 1979). Eight (62.5 per cent) developed perinephric abscesses, and three of these patients died. According to the investigators, all urinary tract infections, even those that progressed to perinephric abscesses, were promptly treated with appropriate antimicrobials, and all patients in this group became afebrile and asymptomatic when antibiotics were stopped; yet later, after varying times, all developed symptoms attributable to their perinephric abscess.

GRAM-NEGATIVE BACTEREMIA

Gram-negative bacteremia is commonly encountered by the urologist because it often follows genitourinary manipulation. Although measures to prevent or reduce bacteremia caused by genitourinary manipulation have been discussed earlier in this chapter, these measures will never eliminate all bacteremic episodes. Furthermore, the urologist deals with patients who may become bacteremic from sources unassociated with the genitourinary tract. In addition to urinary catheters, ventilatory devices and indwelling venous catheters are important sources of nosocomial infection and subsequent bacteremia. Intra-abdominal and retroperitoneal abscesses, skin, and pulmonary infections are all portals of bacteremia.

Clinical Features. The classic clinical presentation of fever and chills 1 to 2 hours after genitourinary instrumentation followed by hypotension occurs in only 30 per cent of patients with gram-negative bacteremia (McCabe and Treadwell, 1983). Others may present with nonspecific signs such as fever, hypothermia, mental status change, acidosis, tachypnea, and hyperpnea. Bacteremia may be complicated by shock, coagulation abnormalities, renal failure, and adult respiratory distress syndrome. Kreger and associates (1980b) have reported that bacteremia accompanied by shock has a 49 per cent mortality rate, as opposed to 7 per cent when unaccompanied by shock.

Metastatic infections secondary to genitourinary tract bacteremia have been described (Siroky et al., 1976). In this review of 137 patients who developed metastatic infections from bacteremia with a genitourinary source, 79 per cent had undergone prior urologic instrumentation. Fifty-nine per cent developed skeletal infections, mainly of the spine, and 29 per cent developed endocarditis, most commonly caused by *Streptococcus fecalis.*

Bacteriology. While *E. coli* is the most common organism causing gram-negative bacteremia, many nosocomial catheter-associated infections are caused by highly resistant gram-negative organisms—*Pseudomonas aeruginosa, Proteus, Providencia,* and *Serratia.* In a large series *E. coli* caused about one third of the cases, the *Klebsiella-Enterobacter-Serratia* family approximately 20 per cent, and *Pseudomonas, Proteus-Providencia,* and anaerobic species approximately 10 per cent each (Kreger et al., 1980a). Anaerobic organisms may cause bacteremia when the source is a postsurgical intra-abdominal abscess or transrectal prostatic biopsy.

Pathophysiology. Most of the clinical manifestations of bacteremia are caused by the lipid portion of the bacterial lipopolysaccharide (Wolff, 1982). This lipopolysaccharide is a lipid-carbohydrate complex that composes the cell wall of gram-negative bacteria and experimentally has been shown to activate the coagulation system and possibly initiate production of bradykinin, which causes increased vascular permeability and vasodilatation (McCabe and Treadwell, 1983). The bacteria produce fever by induction of an endogenous pyrogen from phagocytes. This pyrogen affects the anterior hypothalamus, resulting in increased heat production and reduced heat dissipation (McCabe and Treadwell, 1983).

Diagnosis and Treatment. In an evaluation of 612 patients with gram-negative bacteremia, it was reported that approximately 40 per cent of the deaths occurred within 24 hours and 60 per cent within 48 hours of the onset (Kreger et al., 1980b). The study also showed that appropriate initial antimicrobial treatment decreased the frequency of shock and improved survival rates even if shock had already developed. Use of inappropriate antimicrobial agents (drugs to which the organisms were not sensitive) did not improve the patients' morbidity or mortality. Therefore, early diagnosis and treatment with an agent to which the organism is sensitive is paramount.

Once a presumptive diagnosis of bacteremia is made, multiple blood cultures for aerobic and anaerobic organisms should be obtained. In addition, all potential sources of bacteremia must be cultured (i.e., urine, sputum, wounds). Careful attempts to identify the source of infection should be made, because the choice of appropriate antimicrobial coverage depends upon the organisms that are thought to most likely cause the infection (Table 14–6). If the urinary tract is the most likely portal of entry, an aminoglycoside (gentamicin, tobramycin, or amikacin) is usually the drug of choice, unless *Streptococcus fecalis* is suspected. If the infection is hospital-acquired, or if the patient has had multiple infections or is immunocompromised or severely ill, an aminoglycoside and anti-*Pseudomonas* penicillin (carbenicillin, ticarcillin, or piperacillin) should be used. When identification and drug sensitivities of the offending organism are known, antimicrobial therapy should be changed to use the cheapest, least toxic antibiotic with the narrowest antimicrobial coverage. Antimicrobial treatment should be continued until the patient has been afebrile for 3 to 4 days. Local infections that may have provided the focus for the bacteremia should be treated individually as appropriate.

Complications such as hypotension and renal failure should be monitored and managed with supportive measures as well outlined by McCabe and Olans (1981) (Table 14–7). Careful

TABLE 14–6. Factors Influencing Etiologic Agents in Bacteremia

Site of Origin	Precipitating Events	Most Frequent Etiologic Agent	Antibiotic(s) of Choice	Alternative
Genitourinary tract	Indwelling catheters, instrumentation	*E. coli, Klebsiella-Enterobacter-Serratia, Proteus* sp., *P. aeruginosa*	Aminoglycoside Amikacin 15 mg/kg/day Tobramycin 5 mg/kg/day Gentamicin 5 mg/kg/day	Cephalosporin
Gastrointestinal tract Bowel	Obstruction, perforation, abscesses, neoplasia, diverticuli	*Bacteroides* sp., *E. coli, Klebsiella-Enterobacter-Serratia, Salmonella*	Aminoglycoside plus clindamycin (300–600 mg every hr)	Cefoxitin (2.0 gm every 4–6 hr) Third-generation cephalosporin
Biliary tract	Cholangitis, obstruction (stones), surgical procedures	*E. coli, Klebsiella-Enterobacter-Serratia*	Aminoglycoside	Cephalosporin
Reproductive system	Abortion, instrumentation, post partum	*Bacteroides* sp., *E. coli*	Aminoglycoside plus clindamycin	Cefoxitin, third-generation cephalosporin, or chloramphenicol (50 mg/kg/day)
Vascular system	Venous cutdowns, intravenous catheters, intracardiac pacemakers, surgical procedures	*P. aeruginosa, Acinetobacter, Serratia, Enterobacter* sp.	Aminoglycoside plus carbenicillin (400–600 mg/kg/day) or ticarcillin (200–300 mg/kg/day)	Third-generation cephalosporin
Skin	Leukemia, granulocytopenia, immunosuppressive and cancer chemotherapeutic agents	*P. aeruginosa, Acinetobacter, Serratia*	Aminoglycoside and carbenicillin	Third-generation cephalosporin
Decubiti		*E. coli, Bacteroides* sp., *K. pneumoniae, Proteus* sp.	Aminoglycoside and clindamycin	Second- and third-generation cephalosporin
Respiratory tract	Tracheostomy, mechanical ventilatory assistance	*P. aeruginosa, Klebsiella-Enterobacter-Serratia, Acinetobacter, E. coli*	Aminoglycoside and carbenicillin	Third-generation cephalosporin
	Aspiration	*E. coli, Bacteroides* sp., *Klebsiella-Enterobacter-Serratia*	Aminoglycoside and penicillin (6,000,000 units daily) or clindamycin	Second- or third-generation cephalosporin

From McCabe, W. R., and Treadwell, T. L.: Monogr. Urol., *4*:Nov./Dec. 1983. Used by permission.

TABLE 14–7. MANAGEMENT OF BACTEREMIC SHOCK

1. Establishment of diagnosis
   a. Diagnosis of bacteremia
      1. Epidemiologic, clinical, and physical findings
      2. Collection of blood, urine, and other appropriate specimens for Gram stain or culture
   b. Diagnosis of etiology of shock when preceding bacteremia not recognized
      1. Hypovolemia
      2. Hemorrhage
      3. Cardiac
      4. Hypersensitivity, anaphylaxis
      5. Endocrine (adrenal insufficiency)
      6. Other (pulmonary embolism)
      7. Bacteremia
2. Appropriate antibiotic therapy
   a. Check available culture and sensitivity data
   b. Consider diagnosis, possible site of origin, nosocomiality, and possibility of anaerobes
   c. Ensure collection of appropriate cultures before administration of antibiotics
3. Volume expansion: 1000 ml of crystalloid solution over 15–20 min if congestive failure absent
4. Monitoring volume expansion: insertion of Swan-Ganz or central venous pressure (CVP) catheter
   a. Increase in wedged pulmonary artery pressure of >8 mm Hg or to levels ≥18 mm Hg suggests possible cardiac decompensation
   b. Increase in CVP of >50 mm H_2O or to level >120–140 mm H_2O with volume expansion suggests potential hazard of fluid overload
5. Continue volume expansion (15–20 ml/min) until recovery or wedged pulmonary artery pressure ≥18 mm Hg or CVP ≥120 mm H_2O
6. Vasoactive agents
7. Continued evaluation of mental status and urinary output (indwelling urethral catheter, "closed" sterile drainage system essential)
8. Ventilation: supplemental O_2 with or without intubation and assisted ventilation
9. Digitalis if congestive heart failure develops
10. Drainage of purulent accumulations; removal of foreign bodies
11. Modification of antibiotics as indicated by cultures, susceptibility tests, and renal function

From McCabe, W. R., and Treadwell, T. L.: Monogr. Urol., *4*:Nov./Dec. 1983. Used by permission.

volume expansion monitored by central venous pressure or Swan-Ganz catheter may be given as needed. If hypotension continues, vasoactive agents may be necessary to maintain adequate cardiac perfusion. Dopamine in doses of 2 to 50 μg/kg/min is commonly used. Other useful agents are listed in Table 14–8. It is still unclear whether corticosteroids are useful in the treatment of gram-negative shock.

Perhaps the most exciting development in the treatment of gram-negative bacteremia and shock involves administration of human antiserum to a mutant J5 *E. coli* lipopolysaccharide. In a randomized controlled trial in which symptomatic bacteremic patients were given either J5 antiserum or control serum close to the onset of illness, deaths were decreased from 39 per cent (42/109) in controls to 22 per cent (23/103) in those given antiserum (Ziegler et al., 1982). In patients with severe shock, death occurred in 77 per cent (30/39) of controls and 44 per cent (18/41) of the antiserum group. These investigators found that the IgM fraction of the antiserum appears to protect against the lipopolysaccharide. Although these studies are still under investigation, this adjunctive therapy may improve treatment of bacteremia.

Finally, when the patient is stable, the source of bacteremia must be sought and adequately treated. On occasion, bacteremia will continue until the focus of infection is treated; in fact, surgical treatment may be needed even though the patient is hemodynamically unstable. For instance, if the infection focus is an abscess or pyonephrosis it must be drained. Infected venous catheters need to be removed and replaced. On many occasions, however, successful treatment of the bacteremia alone also eliminates the original source of infection.

TREATMENT OF URINARY TRACT INFECTIONS

IMPORTANCE OF INITIAL STERILIZATION OF URINE

Treatment of each urinary infection must result in a sterile urine, an event that occurs within hours if the proper antimicrobial agent is used (Stamey, 1980). When therapy is continued for 10 days, it is convenient to see outpatients 1 week from the start of treatment to confirm that the urine is sterile on the seventh day. This regimen has taught us some lessons that should not be forgotten. The most important is that if the bacteriuria is suppressed to low counts, even a few hundred per ml or less, recrudescence of the bacteriuria is certain to occur; in terms of our classification, the bacteriuria remains unresolved. Thus, urine cultures obtained during therapy must not contain a single organism of the original bacterial strain, because if any number is present in the midstream voided urine during therapy there is no way to be sure that initial sterilization of the urine has occurred. Even using our technique of collecting specimens from the cystoscopy table, if the introital culture demonstrates a bacterial count several logs higher than in the midstream specimen, it is impossible to be absolutely certain that a

TABLE 14–8. Drugs Used in Management of Bacteremic Shock

Agent	Dose	Effects	Response
Dopamine	2–50 μg/kg/min	Alpha, beta₁, and "dopaminergic" effects; positive inotropic > chronotropic effects; renal and splanchnic vasodilation with doses <8 μg/kg per minute without increase in blood pressure or heart rate; vasoconstriction, reversal of renal vasodilation and ↑ in blood presure with doses per minute of ⩾10 μg/kg	↑ in blood pressure; ↑ in urine flow; improved sensorium
Isoprotenerol	1–2 μg/min	Beta₁ and beta₂, positive inotropic > chronotropic effects; vasodilation, ↑ strength and rate cardiac contractions with ↑ cardiac output and venous return	↓ CVP, ↑ cardiac output, ↑ urine output, improved sensorium; risk of tachycardia and arrhythmias
Dobutamine	2–15 μg/kg/min	Alpha and beta₁; positive inotropic effects > chronotropic effects	↑ cardiac output, ↑ urine output, improved sensorium
Norephinephrine	40–200 μg/min	Alpha and beta₁; positive inotropic effects > chronotropic effects	↑ blood pressure, ↑ cardiac output, ↑ coronary perfusion, marked peripheral vasoconstriction
Corticosteroids as single dose: Dexamethasone Methylprednisolone	6 mg/kg/min	?	Value debatable
	30 mg/kg/min	?	Value debatable

From McCabe, W. R., and Olans, R. N.: *In* Current Clinical Topics in Infectious Disease. New York, McGraw-Hill Book Co., 1981. Used by permission.

sterile bladder urine has been obtained without resorting to suprapubic aspiration of the bladder. We have repeatedly demonstrated suppression of a pretreatment bacteriuria of 10^8 bacteria per ml to a few hundred organisms on suprapubic aspiration at the height of antimicrobial therapy, only to have immediate regrowth of the infecting strain to 10^8 organisms per ml upon discontinuing treatment. For this reason, a careful clinician will demand that none of the original infecting organisms be present in the midstream urine during therapy. We have published the bacteriologic details of several patients, some with substantial focal, coarse scarring, which document an ultimate cure of their infection with nothing more than a change in antimicrobial therapy to a drug that sterilized the urine (Stamey, 1980). This principle of a sterile urine during treatment is the basis for successful antimicrobial therapy; without initial sterilization of the urine there can be no successful therapy, and, moreover, there can be no further analysis as to whether the basic problem is one of bacterial persistence or reinfection at the next recurrence.

With the duration of therapy now much shorter in symptomatic lower tract infections, and in some regimens only a single dosage, there is an even greater need to confirm a sterile urine by SPA (at least in difficult cases) since vaginal and urethral carriage is more likely to continue with ultrashort periods of therapy than with conventional treatment for 10 days. Introital carriage with the pretreatment infecting organism means that the clinician will have some of these bacteria in the voided urine; no matter how small their number, he cannot be sure he has cured the infection without suprapubic needle aspiration of the bladder. For this reason, in the assessment of clinical antibiotic trials, the definition of a "bacteriologic cure" must be scrupulously sought in the author's methodology; if cure is based on any number of the original organism per ml of urine except zero, the results should not be accepted as truly curative. Nor should we forget in clinical trials, especially those with single-dose treatment in women with symptomatic bacterial cystitis, that the spontaneous cure rate 1 month later without any therapy is 71 per cent (Mabeck, 1972).

TABLE 14–9. SERUM AND URINARY ANTIMICROBIAL LEVELS IN ADULTS

Antibiotic	Dose	Peak Serum	% Bound to Protein	T ½ Serum Peak	Mean (Active) Urine Levels*	Percentage of Dose Excreted in Urine	Percentage of Dose Active in Urine (if different)
	mg	*µg/ml*		*hr*	*µg/ml*		
Ampicillin	250 p.o. q 6 hr	3 at 2 hr	15	1	350	42	—
Carbenicillin	764 p.o. q 6 hr	11–17 at 1.5 hr	60	1.2	1000	40	—
Cephalexin	250 p.o. q 6 hr	9 at 2 hr	12	0.9	800	98	—
Colistin	75 i.m. q 12 hr	1.8 at 4 hr	≈10	2	34	75	50
Gentamicin	1 mg/kg i.m. q 8 hr (200 mg/day)	4 at 1 hr	Negligible	2	125	80	—
Kanamycin	500 i.m. q 12 hr	18 at 1 hr	Negligible	2	750	94	—
Nalidixic acid	1000 p.o. q 6 hr	34 at 2–23 hr	85	1.5	75	79	5
Nitrofurantoin	100 p.o. q 6 hr	<2		0.3	150	42	—
Penicillin-G	500 p.o. q 6 hr	1 at 1 hr	60	0.5	300	20	—
Sulfamethizole	250 p.o. q 6 hr		98	10	700	95	85
Tetracycline HCl	250 p.o. q 6 hr	2–3 at 4 hr	31	6	500	60	—
Trimethoprim/ Sulfamethoxazole	160/800 p.o. q 12 hr	1.7/32 at 2 hr	45/66	10/9	150/400	55/50	—/37
Trimethoprim	100 µ p.o. q 12 hr	1.0 at 2–4 hr	45	10	92	55	—

*These average urinary concentrations are based on the amount of biologically active drug excreted by normal kidneys at a urine flow rate of 1200 ml per 24 hours.

From Stamey, T. A.: The Pathogenesis and Treatment of Urinary Infections. Baltimore, Williams & Wilkins, 1980, p. 59. Used by permission.

SERUM VERSUS URINARY LEVELS OF ANTIMICROBIAL AGENTS

It is now generally accepted that the cure of urinary tract infections is dependent upon the antimicrobial levels achieved in the urine, not in the serum. The concentration of 13 useful antimicrobial agents in the serum and urine of healthy adults is shown in Table 14–9; observe that the urinary levels are often several hundred times greater than the serum levels. Our group at Stanford localized urinary infections to the kidneys, determined the minimal concentration (MIC) of penicillin G and nitrofurantoin required to inhibit the infecting organism, and then treated the patient with either oral penicillin G or nitrofurantoin (Stamey et al., 1965). Since neither agent is active in serum against gram-negative bacteria, the resulting cures were attributed to urinary drug levels. McCabe and Jackson (1965) in the same year treated 252 patients with "pyelonephritis"; they concluded that antimicrobial activity in the serum did not separate the cures from the failures but that inhibitory activity in the urine related directly to cure of the infection. Klastersky and coworkers (1974) serially diluted serum and urine from patients with urinary infections, inoculated their infecting organism into both fluids, and determined the bacteriostatic titers; despite using three antibiotics (gentamicin, doxycycline, and cephalexin) that have high serum concentrations, they concluded that the response of patients with urinary tract infections to therapy correlated best with the inhibitory level found in the urine.

In a major clinical effort to resolve this issue, we designed a study with a broad-spectrum antibiotic, oxytetracycline, that was widely used in the treatment of urinary tract infections (Stamey et al., 1974). Bacteriuria was diagnosed in 33 consecutive women by microscopic study of the urinary sediment; all were given 250 mg of oxytetracycline four times a day for 10 days without regard to in vitro sensitivity testing. Between the fifth and tenth days of therapy, and 1 hour after administration of an additional dose of oxytetracycline, a blood serum and urine specimen were obtained; urine and serum samples were also collected before therapy. Urine samples were cultured at regular intervals for at least 3 months in all patients. The pretreatment and "on treatment" urines were millipore-filtered and inoculated, together with their respective serums, with the original infecting organism. As seen in Table 14–10, none of the serums was inhibitory; it was urinary inhibition that correlated with antimicrobial cure of the

TABLE 14–10. ANTIBACTERIAL ACTIVITY OF SERUM AND URINE

Results	Serum Inhibitory	Urine Inhibitory
20 Cures	0/21	18/20
13 Failures	0/13	5/13

From Stamey, T. A.: The Pathogenesis and Treatment of Urinary Infections. Baltimore, Williams & Wilkins, 1980, p 58. Used by permission.

infections. Indeed, the five treatment failures in which the urine was inhibitory included the only two patients in the series with infected renal calculi (whose urines were sterilized on therapy but whose infections had recurred on the first culture after completion of treatment) and two patients whose pretreatment sensitive *E. coli* developed resistance during therapy; in these latter two instances, the "on treatment" urine was bactericidal to the pretreatment sensitive strain but noninhibitory to the resistant mutant selected during therapy.

The four studies just described constitute the main evidence that urinary levels and not serum concentrations are important in the cure of urinary infections. There are no equivalent data, to our knowledge, that support the serum position. The question of serum versus urinary levels, unfortunately, is a practical one because the policy of sensitivity-testing antibacterial agents at concentrations obtainable only in the serum prevents the physician from using drugs that are effective at the urinary level, for example, oral penicillin G for *E. coli* and *P. mirabilis,* and tetracycline for *Pseudomonas aeruginosa.* Until the United States Food and Drug Administration allows the manufacture of antimicrobial discs for urinary sensitivity testing, the practicing physician is denied an intelligent selection of these useful drugs for his patients. Fortunately, as antimicrobial sensitivity testing changes from disc diffusion testing to prepared, microdilution sensitivity trays, the clinician will have available tube dilution concentrations that accurately reflect the urinary levels as well as the serum concentrations. Those who must use FDA-controlled discs should remember that oral penicillin G at standard dosages is an excellent broad-spectrum antimicrobial agent for *E. coli* and *P. mirabilis* and that tetracycline is bactericidal to 80 per cent of the strains of *Pseudomonas aeruginosa* at the levels achieved in the urine, despite the lack of any zone of inhibition around the standard disc (based on serum levels) for these two antimicrobial agents.

BACTERIAL RESISTANCE

Table 14–1 shows that the two most common causes of unresolved bacteriuria are two different forms of bacterial resistance. Indeed, in the oxytetracycline study referred to earlier and presented in Table 14–10 (Stamey et al., 1974), 8 out of the 13 failures were due to tetracycline resistance of the *E. coli* before therapy, while 2 of the 13 patients developed resistance after having an initially sensitive pretreatment population; thus, 10 out of the 13 failures were caused by bacterial resistance. Since the clinician must first sterilize the urine if the infection is to be cured or if differentiation between bacterial persistence and reinfection is to be made, he should understand the mechanisms and implications of bacterial resistance. These have been reviewed in detail elsewhere (Stamey, 1980) but will be briefly commented upon here.

From the therapeutic view, bacterial resistance can be divided into three categories: (1) "natural" resistance, (2) selection of resistant mutants within the urinary tract during therapy, and (3) transferable ("infectious"), extrachromosomal resistance (R-factor).

Natural resistance simply refers to the absence of drug-sensitive substrate in some species of bacteria. For example, all species of *Proteus* are resistant to the polymyxin antibiotics and *Streptococcus faecalis* is always resistant to nalidixic acid.

Selection of resistant mutants within the urinary tract during therapy has a simple clinical setting. Sensitivity testing shows that the bacteriuric population is highly sensitive to a specific antimicrobial drug, but within 48 hours of therapy is replaced in the urine by an equal population of bacteria (10^5 or greater) of the original strain which is now resistant to the antimicrobial agent; sensitivity testing, however, shows that the organism remains sensitive to all antimicrobial drugs except the one used for therapy. It can be shown by elegant bacteriologic studies that the resistant organism (clone) was present *before* contact with the antimicrobial drug but only in numbers of one resistant clone per 10^5 to 10^{10} organisms, making it impossible to detect its presence clinically before therapy. How often will the urologist experience this selection of resistant clones in the course of therapy for a previously sensitive bacteriuric population? Somewhere between 5 per cent and 10 per cent of the time, which is clearly not insignificant, and a factor that must be considered in resolving bacteriuria. In personally studied series, we selected resistant mutants in 8 per cent of 25 consecutive patients treated with 250 mg of oxytetracycline four times a day, and in 7.4 per cent of 27 consecutive patients treated with 4 gm of nalidixic acid a day. The classic way to prevent selection of these resistant clones is to treat a sensitive infection with two or even three antimicrobial agents simultaneously, thereby reducing the chance of selection of a resistant mutant from 1×10^{10} to 1×10^{20} or even 1×10^{30} with three agents. Although this is necessary in the therapy of tuberculosis, in which a chronic tissue infection imposes great difficulties in exceeding the MIC of the infecting strain, it is almost never required in urinary infections, in which the opportunity to exceed the MIC by a hundred times or more occurs with many antimicrobial agents. In theory, ideal treatment for bacteriuria in reinfections of the urinary tract would include acute hydration and diuresis to reduce the total bacterial population before commencing therapy (to reduce the chance of resistant clones), and then doubling or tripling the drug dosage in the first 48 hours to exceed the MIC of the infecting organism by as much as possible despite the hydration.

Transferable, extrachromosomal drug resistance is more important to the urologist than is selection of resistant clones within the urinary tract because (1) it is much more common; (2) the transferable or "infectious" nature of R-factors produces multiply resistant strains, making therapy more difficult; and (3) R-factor resistance occurs only in the fecal flora, never within the urinary tract, which makes the latter amenable to the intelligent use of antimicrobial drugs with regard to their influence on the fecal flora. For example, transfer of R-factor resistance to nitrofurantoin is so rare that it is almost never seen; in the case of nalidixic acid, R-factor transfer has never been demonstrated. Thus, multiply resistant *E. coli* in the fecal flora that have infected the urinary tract will almost always show sensitivity to nitrofurantoin or to nalidixic acid and its analogs such as cinoxacin. Several adverse and favorable effects of specific antimicrobial agents on the fecal flora, especially in relation to transferable extrachromosomal resistance, are covered in detail in Chapter 15 in the section on prophylaxis.

DURATION OF THERAPY

For Patients with Symptomatic Acute Cystitis. Several studies have now conclusively shown that single-dose therapy is an effective way to treat the acutely symptomatic female with bacterial cystitis who has dysuria and frequency; ampicillin, amoxicillin, TMP-SMX, and sulfisoxazole have all been shown to be effective in 80 to 100 per cent of patients (Rubin et al., 1980; Buckwold et al., 1982); while earlier studies used multigram, single-dosage therapy (Bailey and Abbott, 1977; Rubin et al., 1980), the later study by Buckwold and associates (1982) demonstrated equal effectiveness with regular single-dosage TMP-SMX (160/800 mg). What these more recent studies of single-dose therapy have in common is a careful selection of symptomatic women with simple bacterial cystitis. These studies are important both because of the large population of women with recurrent acute cystitis and because the potential of treating their infections with single dosage tremendously minimizes the cost and side effects that accompany longer periods of therapy.

We should not forget Mabeck's work (1972), which showed that 71 per cent of such women achieved sterile urine with placebo therapy within 1 month of the onset of their symptoms. In this setting, it is not surprising that the addition of a single dosage of antimicrobial therapy cures 80 per cent of the infections, especially since the urine becomes sterile within hours of the first dose of antimicrobial agent. The clinician should not underestimate the considerable duration of antimicrobial inhibitory levels in the urine that follows single-dosage therapy, especially when that dosage is often in grams rather than in milligrams, or if the drug has a long half-life in the serum, such as TMP-SMX. Without doubt, many of these urines, if not most, will still be inhibitory on the third day after single-dose therapy.

We pointed out under localization of the site of urinary infections that many of these patients, despite their lower tract symptomatology, will have upper tract bacteriuria accompanying their cystitis. Several single-dose studies have attempted to distinguish between upper and lower tract bacteriuria by using the Fairley bladder-washout test (Ronald et al., 1976), the presence of radiologic abnormalities (Fairley et al., 1978), fluorescent antibody–coating (FA + or FA −) of bacteria (Fang et al., 1978; Rubin et al., 1980), or C-reactive protein (Greenberg et al., 1981). It must not be forgotten, however, that antimicrobial agents differ markedly in their pharmacologic and microbiologic activities even when chosen on the basis of sensitivity testing. If one selects an antimicrobial agent that is less potent in its rate of bacteriostatic activity (sulfonamides, for example) or its pharmacologic diffusion across epithelial membranes (ampicillin, for example), then it is absolutely certain that those patients with upper tract bacteriuria will not be cured at the same rate with single-dosage therapy as those whose bacteriuria is confined to the bladder. For one thing, among others, the transit time of the antimicrobial agent is much shorter in the upper tract than in the bladder. Indeed, if one wants to separate upper from lower tract infections on the basis of therapeutic efforts, methenamine should be the ideal drug because it can only liberate formaldehyde in bladder urine after 1 to 2 hours of stasis. In a review of the literature, one observation stands out clearly in this regard: TMP-SMX therapy, whether single dosage or a 10-day course, is extraordinarily effective *regardless* of whether tests for renal bacteriuria are positive or not. For example, in the Winnipeg study by Buckwold and associates (1982), single-dosage therapy cured 88 per cent of those patients who were FA-positive and 95 per cent of those who were FA-negative, differences that are not statistically significant. Tolkoff-Rubin and her associates (1982) cured 89 to 95 per cent of infections with single-dose TMP-SMX therapy whether the bacteria were FA-positive or FA-negative. These observations suggest, then, that methenamine (probably not single dosage) should detect all patients with renal bacteriuria and that TMP-SMX will cure both renal and bladder bacteriuria indiscriminately. It is possible, of course, that some antimicrobial agent in between these two extremes might serve to distinguish more readily between upper and lower tract bacteriuria, but is it really worth it? We think not, at least in terms of practical management of the patient (see Chapter 15).

The urologist interested in single-dose therapy should know that, at least as of 1983, the only two studies on single-dose cephalosporin therapy have not been promising (Brumfitt et al., 1970; Greenberg et al., 1981); they cured only 44 per cent and 33 per cent, respectively, of ambulatory symptomatic women.

For All Other Patients with More Complicated Infections, Especially Those with Unresolved Bacteriuria. (See Chapter 17 for the special case of true bacterial prostatitis.) Simple, symptomatic, acute bacterial cystitis, as reviewed in the foregoing section, can be treated effectively with single-dosage therapy in 80 to 100 per cent of women, depending upon the choice and dosage of antimicrobial agent. *All other bacterial infections of the urinary tract,* however, with the single exception of gonococcal urethritis, deserve at least several days of therapy. But how many? Once initial sterilization of the urine is achieved, we treat all patients when first seen—virtually regardless of how many recurrences they have had or how serious their infections— for 3 to 10 days and no longer. There are at least three reasons for this. First, it is a rare referral of a bacteriuric patient when the consulting urologist can be absolutely certain that a sterile urine was achieved at the time of previous antimicrobial efforts. Failure to culture the urine during therapy, or within a day or two of completing it, does not allow assessment of the first basic question: Has the urine ever been sterilized? In our office practice, 7 days of therapy is an especially convenient duration to answer this all-important issue. The second reason is that there are few data to indicate that full-dosage therapy for longer than 3 to 10 days offers any better cure rate. For example, Kincaid-Smith and Fairley (1969) found no difference between 2 weeks and 6 weeks of therapy while Kincaid-Smith, Friedman, and Nanra (1970) showed no difference between 1 and 2 weeks of treatment; both studies involved substantial numbers of patients with catheterization-proved infections, many of which were localized by Fairley's bladder-washout technique. Bergstrom et al. (1968) showed that in symptomatic children, both with and without reflux, there was no difference in cure rates between 10 and 60 days of sulfonamide therapy. Mabeck and Vejlsgaard (1980) treated 965 patients with UTI for 7 days; patients with fevers and loin pain were cured at the same rate as those with only dysuria and frequency, suggesting that the presence of clinical pyelonephritis is no reason to extend therapy beyond 1 week. Thus, antimicrobial therapy for longer than 3 to 10 days to cure a specific infection seems unjustified. The third reason for limiting initial therapy is the natural tendency of urinary infections, once a sterile urine is obtained, to undergo long-term remissions. This tendency in adult females (Kraft and Stamey, 1977) will be reviewed in Chapter 15. Kunin's (1970) data in children showed a 20 per cent long-term remission with each 10-day course of therapy almost regardless of the number of previous recurrences, data that were later confirmed by Govan and his colleagues at Stanford (1975).

Lastly, for those who seek evidence, in addition to that of Kincaid-Smith and Fairley (1969), Bergstrom and associates (1968), and Mabeck and Vejlsgaard (1980), that prolonged therapy is not indicated for cure of bacterial infections that involve the kidneys, recent studies using fluorescent antibody–coated bacteria (FA + or FA −) should be reassuring. Rubin and his associates (1980) cured 93 per cent of symptomatic adults who had FA + infections with 10 days of conventional therapy with TMP-SMX. Even single-dosage therapy with TMP-SMX cured 88 per cent (Buckwold et al., 1982)

and 89 per cent (Tolkoff-Rubin et al., 1982) of adult women with FA + urinary infections. In children, McCracken and colleagues (1981), using C-reactive protein (CRP) as a measure of clinical pyelonephritis, showed equivalent cures with 10 days of treatment using a cephalosporin in both CRP-positive and CRP-negative groups; 80 per cent of their CRP-positive children were febrile (≥38°C) and their E. coli strains had twice the K antigen (a marker of upper tract pathogenicity) of the CRP-negative children. Godard and associates (1980) achieved a 100 per cent cure rate of urinary tract infections in 91 female children using 3 days of full-dosage TMP-SMX; 7 children had acute pyelonephritis and 11 had asymptomatic bacteriuria. Thus, it is becoming increasingly difficult to defend the proposition that upper tract bacteriuria requires longer therapy than lower tract infections, a thesis that we have long opposed because our data at Stanford have never supported it (Stamey, 1980).

There are data on the cure rates of urinary tract infections that compare conventional 7- to 14-day antimicrobial dosage regimens with 1 day (cephalosporin—McCracken et al., 1981; TMP-SMX—Russ et al., 1980; carfecillin—Khatib, 1981), 3 days (amoxicillin—Charlton et al., 1976; TMP-SMX and penicillin G—Fair et al., 1980; TMP-SMX—Godard et al., 1980; nitrofurantoin—Lohr et al., 1981; nalidixic acid and cephalexin—Preiksaitis et al., 1981), and 4 days (doxycycline—Lockey et al., 1980) of therapy. In general, there is little difference in cure rates between any of these shorter dosage regimens and the standard 7 to 14 days of therapy. But since single-dose therapy is effective in 80 to 100 per cent of patients with simple symptomatic cystitis, and since this group of patients is so common that they usually constitute a majority of subjects entered into clinical trials, each report needs to be carefully analyzed as to the heterogeneity of the patients. What the urologist needs to know is whether these shorter regimens are equally efficacious in patients with asymptomatic bacteriuria, in those with multiply recurrent infections and renal involvement, in patients with diabetes or analgesic-abuse nephritis, in children with renal scarring and recurrent urinary infections, and in all comers with slightly reduced renal function or minimal hydronephrosis, especially with serum creatinine levels between 1.5 and 2.5 mg per dl. We *know* that 10 days of therapy has served these patients well in the past.

The information on 3 days of full-dosage therapy is especially well documented and one can make a strong argument for reducing the conventional 7 to 10 days of therapy to 3; the papers by Fair and associates (1980) in women and by Godard and associates (1980) seem especially well documented because they include both asymptomatic patients and those with clinical pyelonephritis. Three-day therapy, however, will certainly cause office inconvenience in assessing sterility of the urine on the third day, or even on the fourth day 24 hours after stopping treatment, and we will ultimately need studies with greater attention to the heterogeneity of bacteriuric patients before we adopt this regimen for all comers. By reducing 10 days of treatment to 3, however, we will soon find out whether it is acceptable or not. For example, Lacey and his colleagues (1981) have presented an interesting study of treating urinary tract infections in elderly patients in whom they compared 5 days of trimethoprim (TMP) with a 200 mg single-dose administration of TMP; the 5-day regimen was superior (94 per cent versus 67 per cent, $p < 0.01$). McCracken and associates' study (1981) was directed at comparing 1 day with 10 days of therapy with a cephalosporin. In CRP-negative children, presumably with mostly lower tract infections, the 1-day regimen was much inferior to the 10-day one ($p < 0.05$). These studies indicate that once we leave the large group of women with symptomatic bacterial cystitis, we can surely expect differences in these treatment regimens. Moreover, as we commented on TMP-SMX in the previous section on single-dose therapy, the antimicrobial agent used will continue to make a big difference in the therapeutic results. For example, Fennell and colleagues (1980) treated 85 children who had three or more urinary infections within the previous year (38 per cent of whom had abnormal radiographic studies) with 10 days of full-dosage TMP-SMX, ampicillin, or cephalexin. TMP-SMX was superior in decreasing recurrences at 2 weeks ($p < 0.01$) and 12 weeks ($p < 0.05$). Interestingly, as in many other studies (Stamey, 1980), recurrence rates were not influenced by radiologic abnormalities—another observation that makes bacterial persistence in the kidneys in the absence of stones or congenital abnormalities a very rare event given adequate antimicrobial treatment. Further evidence of remarkable differences between two drugs is the comparison of nalidixic acid and cephalexin in 3-day and 14-day trials of both FA+ and FA− infections in women (Preiksaitis et al., 1981); nalidixic acid was superior in all comparisons.

Should we not ask, then, "Is it worth distinguishing between 3-day courses of full-dosage treatment and single-dose regimens for women with acute, symptomatic bacterial cystitis, i.e., why not treat all females with urinary tract infections for 3 days as a uniform approach to therapy?" Since 3 days appears to be effective for many urinary infections more complicated than acute, symptomatic cystitis, this may be a reasonable alternative. In a general practice study by Cartwright and colleagues (1982), they noted that the mean time for dysuria and frequency to disappear in their bacteriuric patients was 4 to 5 days and that "much persuasive counseling" was needed in single-dosage therapy "if the patient was to be left without treatment for several days before their symptoms disappeared." Three days of treatment would obviate a great part of this anxiety. We wonder if the ultimate impact of single-dose therapy for acute cystitis may be in the management by the patient herself, when, at the first onset of symptoms, she self-medicates with a single tablet of appropriate drug, which should be quite effective. Moreover, if she treats early enough, the dysuria and frequency should subside earlier than 4 to 5 days.

The ultimate role of single-dose self-medication at the onset of an acute cystitis in comparison with prophylactic prevention—either with continuous or postintercourse minimal medication—as treatment strategies for recurrent symptomatic bacterial cystitis will have to be determined by further studies. In the meantime, a reasonable argument can be made for treating all ambulatory patients who present with urinary infection, symptomatic or asymptomatic, with 3 days of full-dosage therapy, making sure that none of the original infecting organisms are present in the urine between 3 and 5 days of initiating treatment. If some studies show that certain antimicrobial agents are less effective than others in achieving a sterile urine, or that they permit early and late recurrences (Preiksaitis et al., 1981; Sullivan et al., 1980), or that certain patient groups require 10 days of therapy, we will need to make allowances for these exceptions.

ANTIMICROBIAL PROPHYLAXIS FOR TRANSURETHRAL PROCEDURES

There is no question that antimicrobial prophylaxis against infective endocarditis should be given to patients with prosthetic valves or valvular heart disease who are to have genitourinary manipulation. These guidelines are published in many places (Abramowicz, 1984; Durack, 1979). For transurethral genitourinary procedures, including catheterization, catheter manipulation, cystoscopy, and urethral dilation, the regimen is as follows.

In adults—Aqueous crystalline penicillin G (2 million U) IM or IV *or* ampicillin (2.0 gm) IM or IV *plus* gentamicin (1.5 mg/kg) IM or IV *or* streptomycin (1.0 gm) IM 1 hour before the procedure; then every 8 hours for two additional doses if gentamicin and penicillin or ampicillin are used, and every 12 hours if streptomycin and penicillin or ampicillin are used.

In children—Aqueous crystalline penicillin G (30,000 U/kg) IM or IV *or* ampicillin (50 mg/kg) IM or IV *plus* gentamicin (2.0 mg/kg) IM or IV *or* streptomycin (20 mg/kg) IM with the same timing and number of doses as in adults.

For adults allergic to penicillin—Vancomycin (1.0 gm) IV infused slowly over 1 hour *plus* gentamicin (1.5 mg/kg) IM or IV given 30 minutes to 1 hour before the procedure and both drugs repeated once 8 hours later.

For children allergic to penicillin—Vancomycin (20 mg/kg) IV infused slowly over 1 hour *plus* gentamicin (2.0 mg/Kg) IM or IV with same timing and number of doses as in adults.

The issue of systemic antimicrobial prophylaxis in patients who are undergoing endoscopic procedures and who do not have cardiac valvular disorders is unsettled. The difficulty of concluding from investigative studies whether prophylaxis is indicated has been reviewed (Chodak and Plaut, 1979). In most cases these studies cannot be compared because antimicrobial agents differ, duration of catheterization differs, timing of dosing differs, and most lack control patients. To develop a rational approach to prophylaxis it must first be decided why prophylaxis is being given: to prevent infective endocarditis, to prevent bacteremia and subsequent sepsis, or to prevent postoperative urinary tract infection. Since patients with risk of infective endocarditis must receive prophylaxis, these patients will be discussed no further, but antimicrobial prophylaxis to avoid postoperative bacteremia and urinary infection will be discussed individually. If the goal is to prevent postoperative urinary infection, this probably relates more to the patient's underlying disease (e.g., bacterial prostatitis) or duration of postoperative catheterization than to the operative procedure.

Clearly, patients who have bacteriuria and undergo transurethral procedures have a high probability of becoming bacteremic. In one study, 50 per cent of the patients who had infected urine when transurethral resection of the prostate (TURP) was performed grew the same organism on blood cultures taken 2 hours later (Morris et al., 1976). In another study, of those patients with bacteriuria, 67 per cent had a positive blood culture 30 minutes after TURP started, 57 per cent became bacteremic after cystoscopy, 67 per cent became bacteremic after urethral dilation, and 17 per cent became bacteremic after urethral catheterization (Sullivan et al., 1973). In almost all of the patients who had a TURP and a positive blood culture, the bacteremia was clinically manifest by fever, hypotension, chills, or shock. From these data it can be concluded that patients who are known preoperatively to have urinary tract infections should have their urine sterilized before the procedure is started; hence in these patients preoperative antimicrobial therapy is therapeutic rather than prophylactic.

Whether or not antimicrobial prophylaxis should be given to patients with sterile urine prior to a TURP or endoscopic procedure is controversial. Morris and associates (1976) have reported that 10 per cent (10/101) of patients with initially sterile urine developed bacteremia (proven by blood culture 2 hours after TURP, even though four of these patients had been treated with prophylactic antibiotics; three of the four patients who developed gram-negative sepsis (positive blood culture and clinical signs of sepsis) had not been treated with antibiotics. In this study as in many, however, the urine was considered infected only if greater than 100,000 organisms were cultured or a repeat culture of the same organism was found; therefore, some of the patients with "initially sterile" urine may actually have been infected. In contrast, Sullivan and associates (1973) found that all patients who became bacteremic after TURP had a urinary infection at the time of their operation (Sullivan et al., 1973).

If no preoperative or postoperative antimicrobial agents are used in TURP, postoperative bacteriuria is found in 11 to 45 per cent of patients up to 1 month postoperatively (Gibbons et al., 1978; Matthew et al., 1978; Hargreave et al., 1982; Morris et al., 1976). Thus far, most prophylaxis studies have used various antimicrobials preoperatively and continued them until the catheter is removed (Gibbons et al., 1978; Nielsen et al., 1981; Lacy et al., 1971), or started them preoperatively and continued them for 5 days to 3 weeks postoperatively (Matthew et al., 1978; Gonzalez et al., 1976; Morris et al.; 1976; Falkiner et al., 1983). All but one of these studies (Gibbons et al., 1978) suggest that postoperative urinary tract infections decrease from

26 to 42 per cent to 0 to 12 per cent when various antimicrobial agents are used prophylactically (Morris et al., 1976; Hargreave et al., 1982; Nielsen et al., 1981; Lacy et al., 1971; Matthew et al., 1978). In the single study that shows no decrease (Gibbons et al., 1978), the post-TURP incidence of urinary infections in patients who received no prophylactic antibiotics is 11 per cent, which is a very low rate when compared with other studies. Furthermore, in this study catheters were routinely removed on the second postoperative day; this comparatively early catheter removal may account for the low incidence of infections in control subjects. Most of the other studies did not designate the duration of catheter drainage, but it can be inferred that it was usually longer than that cited in the Gibbons study.

From a review of these studies, several observations relating to the prevention of postoperative urinary infection may be made. First, in studies in which patients were randomized into groups that received and did not receive antibiotic prophylaxis, between 6 and 12 per cent of patients who were thought to have sterile urine were ultimately excluded because their preoperative urine was unexpectedly infected (Morris et al., 1976; Gibbons et al., 1978; Gonzalez et al., 1976; Hargreave et al., 1982). This 6 to 12 per cent incidence of infections was found in patients who had TURP after patients with catheters and those with other causes for a high probability of infection were excluded. Second, in control patients who had sterile urine 24 hours after the catheter was removed, 7 to 15 per cent were infected 1 month later (Gibbons et al., 1978; Matthew et al., 1978; Gonzalez et al., 1976). It is inferred that sterile meant fewer than 10^4 (Gibbons et al., 1978) or 10^5 (Matthew et al., 1978; Gonzalez et al., 1976) organisms cultured from urine in these studies. These data suggest either that the urine was not really sterile or that men undergoing TURP have an increased susceptibility to urinary infection in the period immediately following removal of their catheter. The latter is suggested by other studies that show indwelling catheters to be associated with increased urethral and meatal colonization (Garibaldi et al., 1980; Bultitude and Eykyn, 1973). Third, no study to date has involved prophylaxis starting only the evening before or the morning of catheter removal.

Although investigations to date do not give a definitive answer as to whether antimicrobial prophylaxis should be used in the routine healthy patient undergoing TURP, a rational approach to prophylaxis may be made. In order to approach this question, prophylaxis should be broken into two parts: (1) prophylaxis to prevent operative and perioperative bacteremia, and (2) prophylaxis to prevent postoperative urinary infection.

If it is known that the patient has a sterile preoperative urine and carries no gram-negative organisms in his urethra, probably no prophylaxis to prevent bacteremia need be given. (Sterile must mean *no* gram-negative organisms, not fewer than 10,000 or 100,000 organisms.) Unfortunately, if this is not known, or if culture results are unavailable preoperatively, 10 to 12 per cent of patients may have unsuspected bacteriuria and will have as high as a 67 per cent probability of becoming bacteremic if not treated "prophylactically." It should be assumed that any patient with an indwelling catheter is infected and must have his urine sterilized preoperatively by at least two doses of a drug that has broad coverage against gram-negative organisms (an aminoglycoside will probably achieve a sterile urine in most cases, unless multiple previous antibiotic courses have been given, or the patient has had a long hospitalization, in which case antimicrobial sensitivities will need to be obtained).

To prevent a postoperative urinary infection, which is usually a catheter-associated infection, management similar to that for removal of catheters may be followed. If the catheter is removed by 48 hours after the operation, the incidence of catheter-associated urinary infection may be so low that prophylaxis is unnecessary, as experienced by Gibbons and associates (1978), but if the catheter is left in place longer, prophylaxis may be advisable. A broad-spectrum antimicrobial agent (nitrofurantoin, cinoxacin, trimethoprim-sulfamethoxazole, tetracycline) should be started the evening before the catheter is to be removed and continued for 3 to 5 days after its removal. A urine culture should be obtained at the time the catheter is removed and on the postoperative office visit. This shorter antimicrobial therapy should minimize the creation of in-hospital resistant organisms and decrease patient cost.

Antimicrobial Prophylaxis for Transrectal Prostatic Needle Biopsy. Although perineal prostatic biopsy is common, transrectal biopsy for suspected prostatic carcinoma is popular because it is often felt to be more accurate. Infectious complications of transrectal biopsy include urinary infections, prostatitis, epididymitis, pyelonephritis, local abscess, osteomyelitis, and sepsis. It has been reported that 5 minutes after transrectal biopsy 76 per cent (16/21) of patients have bacteremia proved by blood culture (Ashby et al., 1978). Over half the organisms isolated in this study were anaerobic (mainly Bacteroides species and anaerobic streptococci). Simple cleansing enemas with povidone-iodine do not alter the infectious complications associated with the procedure, but several studies have demonstrated that appropriate antimicrobial prophylaxis may (Ashby et al., 1978; Crawford et al., 1982).

Although it is suggested that metronidazole and ampicillin or trimethoprim-sulfamethoxazole given postoperatively are satisfactory prophylaxis for transrectal biopsy, organisms resistant to both drugs were noted (Ashby et al., 1978). For this reason an aminoglycoside and metronidazole given an hour before the procedure and continued for 24 hours following the procedure might be appropriate. If oral agents need to be used, metronidazole and ampicillin or trimethoprim-sulfamethoxazole started preoperatively and continued for 48 hours postoperatively are recommended.

CATHETER-ASSOCIATED URINARY TRACT INFECTIONS

The most common site of hospital-acquired infections is the urinary tract, where approximately 40 per cent of all hospital-acquired infections occur (Stamm, 1975). The most common predisposing factor for these infections is urethral instrumentation, including catheterization. In fact, between 10 and 15 per cent of all hospitalized patients have indwelling catheters (Stamm, 1975; Fincke and Friedland, 1976).

These catheter-associated infections cause significant morbidity. Sullivan and associates (1973) reported that 8 per cent (6/75) of urethral catheterizations cause bacteremia as documented by a positive blood culture. Moreover, in one study, 20 per cent of all childhood gram-negative bacteremias were caused by urinary tract infections or prior urinary tract manipulation; similarly, 46 per cent of adult gram-negative bacteremias were from urinary infection or prior genitourinary manipulation (Dupont and Spink, 1969). Other infectious complications associated with urethral catheterization and concomitant urinary infection are acute epididymitis-orchitis, bacterial prostatitis, pyelonephritis, periurethral abscesses, and struvite bladder, and especially renal, calculi.

What constitutes bacteriuria in a catheterized patient is controversial and is discussed earlier in this chapter under diagnosis. To collect a catheter specimen, urine should be needle-aspirated from the catheter tubing using sterile technique. Cultures taken from Foley tips are useless and show less than 3 per cent correlation with subsequent and simultaneous urine cultures (Gross et al., 1974). Certainly, pyuria does not indicate bacteriuria.

When a urethral catheter is placed in a patient, the individual risks bacteremia from the manipulation and introduction of a urinary tract infection. Any patient who risks endocarditis or who has a prosthesis that might become infected should receive antimicrobial prophylaxis before catheter manipulation, as recommended earlier. The incidence of urinary infections after a single in-and-out urethral catheterization depends upon the patient's sex and general health, and on the person performing the catheterization. In their review, Stamey and Pfau (1970) found an incidence of catheterization-induced infections ranging from 1 per cent in healthy young college women to 20 per cent in hospitalized women on a medical ward.

The incidence of urinary infections in patients with indwelling catheters is directly related to the duration of catheterization. When open drainage systems are used, 95 per cent of patients (sex unspecified) became bacteriuric by 4 days (Kass and Finland, 1956). With the advent of closed drainage systems, the average daily rate of acquired bacteriuria is decreased to 4 per cent in males and 10.4 per cent in females (about half the patients received antibiotics with insertion of the catheter) (Garibaldi et al., 1974). Also with a closed system, Warren found the incidence of acquired bacteriuria to be about 5 per cent per day of catheterization (Warren et al., 1978). Others have calculated that there is only a 50 per cent cumulative probability of remaining free of infection (fewer than 10 bacteria per ml) for 4½ days after catheterization even when a closed collecting system is used (Maizels and Schaeffer, 1980).

Etiology of Catheter-Associated Infections. Catheter-associated bacteriuria may originate from three sources: (1) periurethral and perineal organisms, (2) organisms infecting the collecting bag or collecting device, and (3) bacterial infection caused by opening the closed system for irrigation, changes in tubing, or emptying the collecting bag. Kass and Schneiderman (1957) showed that 24 to 72 hours after Serratia marcescens was applied to the glans penis or vulva in 3 semicomatose patients with indwelling catheters, thousands of the organisms could be cultured from the bladder. In another study, investigators found that organisms causing catheter-associated bacteriuria could be isolated from the urethra and perineum before the bladder most of the time (Bultitude and Eykyn, 1973; Brehmer and Madsen, 1972). Maizels and Schaeffer (1980) found that bacteriuria could be attributed to the collecting bag in 45 per cent of those who became infected and to the urethra in 27 per cent.

Methods to Decrease Catheter-Associated Urinary Infections. In patients on intermittent catheterization, it has been shown by several investigators that the instillation of antibiotic solutions into the bladder just after catheterization with or without the administration of prophylactic oral antibiotics may decrease the rate of infection induced by catheterization to 0.5 to 0.6 per cent or lower (Pearman, 1971; Anderson, 1980). These methods will be discussed in greater detail in Chapter 18, Urinary Tract Infections in Spinal Cord Injury Patients. Routine use of a closed-catheter drainage system has reduced catheter-associated infections from about 90 per cent at 4 days to 30 to 40 per cent. Other means of decreasing infections have focused upon the collecting bag and urethra as sources for infection. Periodic instillations of chemicals such as hydrogen peroxide or glutaraldehyde into the collecting bag may delay the onset of bacteriuria during catheterization (Maizels and Schaeffer, 1980; Bloom and Gonick, 1969), but no devices have been completely effective in eliminating infections in the patient with the long-term indwelling catheter. Prophylactic antibiotic irrigations of closed-catheter systems have not decreased the incidence of infections and have only caused more resistant organisms (Warren et al., 1978; Dudley and Barriere, 1981). Moreover, a randomized, controlled trial of repetitive courses of cephalexin for the treatment of bacteriuria sensitive to cephalexin, in long-term catheterized patients, showed no difference in the prevalence of bacteriuria, incidence of infections, number of bacterial strains present on weekly culture, febrile days, or catheter obstructions (Warren et al., 1982). Not unexpectedly, during the study the proportion of organisms that were cephalexin-resistant increased in the cephalexin-treated group, and these organisms were resistant to many antibiotics.

Management of Catheter-Associated Urinary Infections. Whether antimicrobial prophylaxis can or should be used to prevent catheter-associated urinary infections depends upon the circumstances of the catheterization. If one-time catheterizations are followed by a single dose of an antimicrobial agent, such as nitrofurantoin 100 mg, and/or the instillation of 30 ml of neomycin/polymyxin B solution (160 mg neomycin and 300,000 units polymyxin B per liter sterile water) as Anderson (1980) used during intermittent catheterization, the incidence of infection caused by catheterization will be very low.

Patients with catheters that will be left indwelling for only a few days should be treated as patients undergoing transurethral resection of the prostate. In these patients it is reasonable to prevent the onset of infection as long as possible. Measures such as putting hydrogen peroxide into the collecting bags may be helpful. The urine should be cultured when removal of the catheter is anticipated because the urine should be sterilized when the catheter is removed. Cultures will ensure that an appropriate antibiotic is selected. Any patient who risks endocarditis must be treated with systemic antimicrobial agents when the catheter is inserted or removed.

In patients with chronic indwelling urethral catheters, no methods totally eliminate catheter-associated infections. Asymptomatic bladder bacteriuria, funguria, or pyuria should not be treated as long as the catheter remains. For catheters needing occasional irrigation, distilled water, acetic acid, or 10 per cent hemiacidrin may be used; antibiotic irrigation fluids should not be used. A patient with an elevated temperature or flank pain who has a catheter-associated infection must be treated for clinical acute pyelonephritis with the appropriate antibiotic for several days until asymptomatic. Furthermore, it is important to determine that neither the urinary tract nor the catheter drainage system is obstructive.

SHOULD PATIENTS WITH ASYMPTOMATIC BACTERIURIA BE TREATED?

The distinction between symptomatic infections and those detected on screening surveys for asymptomatic bacteriuria is considered in Chapters 15 (adults) and 16 (infants and children). There is evidence in adults (Asscher et al., 1969) and children (Savage et al., 1975; Lindberg et al., 1978) that while 80 per cent of patients with asymptomatic bacteriuria can be cured with a 7-day course of oral antimicrobial therapy, long-term cure rates are no better than placebo therapy because of reinfections in treated patients and spontaneous cures in untreated subjects.

Moreover, treatment of asymptomatic infections, which are often associated with self-agglutinating *E. coli* that have lost their O-polysaccharide surface antigens (Lindberg et al.,

1975), is frequently followed by a new *E. coli* infection with its O-surface antigens intact—antigens that are apparently responsible for acute symptoms. For this reason, unless a patient is willing to undertake long-term prophylactic regimens to prevent reinfections, a sound argument can be made against treating an asymptomatic infection just to achieve a sterile urine for a short period of time. This may especially be true for the geriatric patient with asymptomatic bacteriuria, in whom the potential side effects from unnecessary antimicrobial therapy may represent a substantial hazard.

We have, however, patients with asymptomatic bacteriuria who are convinced that they feel better generally when their urine is sterile, even though they have no specific urinary tract symptoms. About one third of patients with asymptomatic bacteriuria will develop acute symptoms within 12 months of detection if left untreated (Asscher et al., 1969; Gaymans et al., 1976). Moreover, those patients at risk for increased morbidity (see following section) from bacteriuria, such as severe diabetics, children under 4 years of age with reflux, pregnant women, and others, should not be left with asymptomatic bacteriuria.

No patient, female or male, adult or child, should be left with an asymptomatic bacteriuria caused by *Proteus* species. *Proteus* is the one infection that causes renal struvite stones if left untreated for long periods of time (see next section).

PATIENTS AT RISK OF SERIOUS MORBIDITY AND/OR RENAL SCARRING FROM RECURRENT BACTERIURIA

We have listed in Table 14–11 those patients who are at risk of either serious morbidity or renal scarring from their urinary tract infections. It is in these categories that the urologist should be particularly aggressive in resolving the urinary infection. Each will be considered briefly in this final section.

INFANTS AND CHILDREN UNDER AGE 4 YEARS WITH SEVERE REFLUX AND SYMPTOMATIC URINARY INFECTIONS

Urinary tract infection in infants and children is the subject of Chapter 16 by Professor Jan Winberg and will not be considered here. Although morbidity with chills and fever, always accompanied by bacteriuria and pyuria, can be

TABLE 14–11. SPECIAL PROBLEMS THAT PLACE PATIENTS AT RISK OF SERIOUS MORBIDITY OR RENAL SCARRING

Infants and children under age 4 years with severe reflux and UTI
Infections due to urea-splitting bacteria, which cause struvite renal stones
Congenital urinary tract anomalies that become secondarily infected
Infections in the presence of acute or chronic urinary tract obstruction
Renal papillary necrosis
Diabetes, especially with emphysematous pyelonephritis
Spinal cord injury with high pressure bladders
Pregnancy
Acute bacterial prostatitis

*Acute pyelonephritis, perirenal abscess, and gram-negative septicemia add significant morbidity and risk to any of the above conditions.

a serious and worrisome clinical presentation, most renal scarring occurs with the very earliest infections in infancy. Indeed, Dr. Winberg believes that most scarring may occur with the very first infection, rather than with later ones. The interested reader should consult his informative chapter.

INFECTIONS DUE TO UREA-SPLITTING BACTERIA THAT CAUSE STRUVITE RENAL STONES

As long as recurrent infections in adult women are caused by *E. coli*, the consequences other than symptomatic morbidity are usually not serious. Urea-splitting bacteria, however, especially the common *P. mirabilis*, cause intense alkalinization of the urine with precipitation of calcium, magnesium, ammonium, and phosphate salts and the subsequent formation of branched struvite renal stones. The bacteriologic consequences are substantial because the bacteria persist inside these struvite stones even though the urine is readily sterilized (Fig. 14–9). Indeed, struvite infection stones, together with the occasional oxalate or apatite stone that becomes secondarily infected, constitute the major cause of bacterial persistence in women in the absence of azotemia. The bacteriuria in most of these patients with struvite stones recurs almost immediately upon stopping antimicrobial therapy, usually within 5 to 7 days (Fig. 14–13).

These stones can cause serious renal damage. Figure 14–14 shows the plain film radiograph from a 52-year-old white female whose urinary tract disease was uncovered by her family doctor when he found pyuria during an examination for a febrile, flulike illness accompanied by minimal backache. She had never experienced localized flank pain; her urine cul-

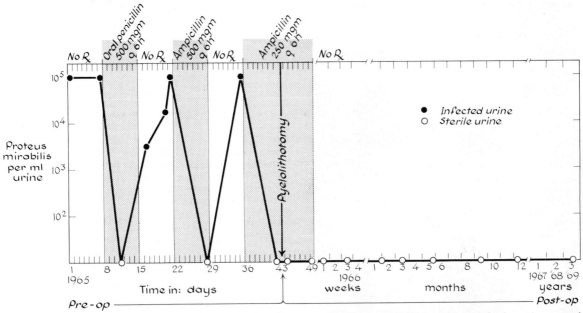

Figure 14–13. Preoperative and postoperative bacteriologic course of a 39-year-old woman with an infection stone caused by *P. mirabilis*. Note that eradication of the infection was achieved only after removal of the stone (80 per cent struvite and 20 per cent apatite) and that, in the absence of reinfection with urea-splitting bacteria, no further stones have appeared. (From Nemoy, N. J., and Stamey, T. A.: JAMA, *215*:1470, 1971. Copyright 1971, American Medical Association.)

ture grew only 10,000 *P. mirabilis* organisms per ml. Figure 14–15 represents a 20-minute intravenous urogram and Figure 14–16 a biopsy of the left kidney at the time the staghorn calculus was removed. In Figure 14–16, note the hyalinized glomeruli, the destroyed renal tubules, the inflammatory infiltrate, and the early periglomerular sclerosis. At surgery, both the left and the right renal calculi cultured large

numbers of *P. mirabilis* when the stones were crushed (Fig. 14–9). Antimicrobial agents were stopped 4 weeks after the stones were removed, and the urine has been sterile in the 3 years since surgery. The patient's creatinine has not changed from its preoperative value of 1.2 mg per dl.

All of the residual particles of struvite stones must be removed at the time of surgery

Figure 14–14. Plain film radiograph from a 52-year-old woman with bilateral struvite infection stones caused by *P. mirabilis*.

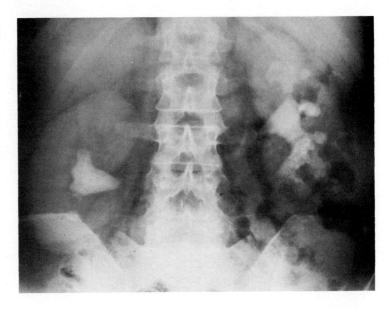

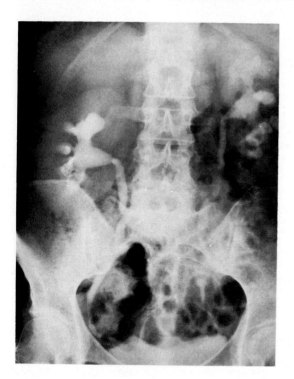

Figure 14–15. A 20-minute film from the preoperative intravenous urogram of the same patient shown in Figure 14–14. The left kidney with the staghorn calculus appears to excrete the contrast medium less well than does the right kidney. Neither ureter is obstructed below the renal pelves.

Figure 14–16. Random biopsy from the left kidney at the time of the anatrophic nephrolithotomy. The intense interstitial infiltrate with inflammatory cells, the periglomerular sclerosis, and the hyalinized glomeruli are easily seen.

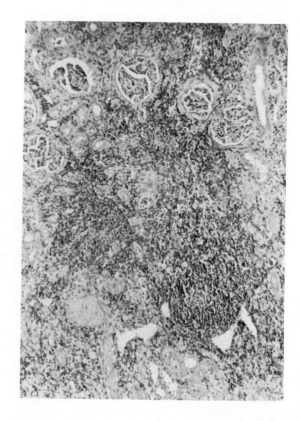

if recurrent bacteriuria from bacterial persistence in the calculus is to be prevented. Rocha and Santos (1969) have shown that soaking these stones in iodine and alcohol for 6 hours will not kill the bacteria within the interior of the stone. The importance of recognizing this fact is twofold: (1) The bacteria cannot be killed by antimicrobial therapy, even though the urine may be kept sterile for months or even years (Shortliffe et al., 1984), and (2) any fragments left behind at the time of surgical removal leave residual bacteria within the interstices of the stone; these bacteria ensure recurrence of the staghorn calculus with its attendant morbidity.

It is for this reason that we always leave a small multiholed polyethylene catheter for postoperative irrigation with Renacidin or Suby's-G solution. Using this technique, and postoperative plain film tomograms to detect residual fragments missed on the intraoperative radiographs, we published our results in 44 consecutive kidneys in 40 patients with proven struvite infection stones (Silverman and Stamey, 1983). With a mean follow-up of 7 years, there was one 4-mm stone recurrence in the left kidney (Figs. 14–14 to 14–16) in a patient whose urine had been consistently sterile for 14 months after cessation of therapy and whose calcification we believe to be around a radiolucent papilla. None of the patients had bacterial persistence postoperatively; antimicrobial agents were stopped in all within a few weeks of discharge. Among seven infections in the postoperative years, only one was *P. mirabilis,* an infection that never recurred after 10 days of treatment.

Thus, the physician should be wary of the patient with bacteriuria due to *P. mirabilis* that recurs soon after stopping antimicrobial therapy (Fig. 14–13). It is true that *P. mirabilis* is a not uncommon cause of bacteriuria (about 25 per cent of us carry this organism in our normal fecal flora), and most patients with *P. mirabilis* cystitis do not form struvite stones. But struvite stones form in those patients who have a protracted infection with *P. mirabilis,* an infection that is often asymptomatic or minimally symptomatic.

Lastly, it should be emphasized that these struvite stones, usually about 80 per cent struvite and 20 per cent apatite, often contain minimal calcium and are easily obscured on plain film radiographs of the abdomen unless the kidneys are absolutely free of overlying gas and feces. Therefore, most patients with recurrent *P. mirabilis* infection warrant plain film tomography of the kidneys. In addition, once all fragments have been surgically removed or dissolved and the patient is shown to have a sterile urine after cessation of antimicrobial therapy (the final test of successful surgery), he or she should be followed bacteriologically in case reinfection occurs with a new strain of urea-splitting bacteria, although we observed this only once in our 44 consecutive cases. This latter observation suggests some immunologic immunity to recurrent *Proteus* infections in these patients with infection renal stones.

CONGENITAL URINARY TRACT ANOMALIES THAT BECOME SECONDARILY INFECTED

Any female with a biologic susceptibility to recurrent bacteriuria (see Chapter 15) who also has a congenital anomaly can develop secondary infection of the anomaly (Table 14–2). When this occurs, her recurrent bacteriuria will be characterized by the same organism until the anomalous infected structure is surgically removed. Almost invariably after surgical resection, however, if she is followed long enough, simple reinfections with Enterobacteriaceae will appear once again. Such anomalies include nonfunctioning duplications of the renal collecting system, which accompany ectopic ureters. We reported one case in which bacteriuria due to *P. aeruginosa* had been constantly present for several years (Friedland and Stamey, 1974). Complete resection of the ureteral duplication with its ectopic ureteral orifice in the urethra cured the recurrent *P. aeruginosa* urinary infection, but the patient has experienced several simple *E. coli* infections in the 10 years since this case report.

Other anomalies include pericalyceal diverticula that lose their free communication with pelvic urine (but excrete bacteria into the urine), urachal cysts of the dome of the bladder, unilateral medullary sponge kidneys, and occasional congenital obstructions that have produced nonfunctioning kidneys into which effective urinary concentrations of antimicrobial agents cannot be delivered. Clinical examples with bacteriologic documentation of each of these congenital anomalies that can cause bacteria to persist within the urinary tract have been published (Stamey, 1980).

INFECTIONS IN THE PRESENCE OF ACUTE OR CHRONIC URINARY TRACT OBSTRUCTION

These conditions in which patients are at serious risk of renal scarring and loss of renal function are mainly iatrogenic and largely preventable. We include here those sterile calcium oxalate stones that cause acute obstruction but become secondarily infected during the course of unsuccessful efforts to remove the calculus. To be sure, women who are susceptible to reinfections of the urinary tract and who also form sterile calcium oxalate stones can develop acute obstruction in the absence of urologic intervention. The most tragic examples of chronic obstruction and bacteriuria causing serious loss of renal cortex are children with minimal reflux who develop acute ureteral obstruction following unsuccessful ureteral reimplantation. This tragedy seems even greater when we observe the normal kidneys that were present preoperatively, usually in the presence of minimal to moderate reflux, and then compare them with the scarred, shrunken kidneys of the postoperatively obstructed and infected urinary tract. We have observed the same consequences in adult males with megaloureters who had adequate to good renal function and sterile urine before they were operated upon to "improve" renal drainage; postoperatively they became obstructed and infected and eventually required dialysis and transplantation. It should not be forgotten that 15 of the 22 patients who presented to Scribner's dialysis unit with endstage renal failure (Schechter et al., 1971), in whom the primary cause was chronic pyelonephritis, had "significant obstructive or calculous disease which preceded the initial episode of urinary tract infection in each."

RENAL PAPILLARY NECROSIS

The role of infection in the development and progression of renal papillary necrosis (RPN) is controversial. Multiple predisposing conditions have been associated with the development of RPN, particularly diabetes, analgesic abuse, sickle cell hemoglobinopathy, and obstruction (Table 14–12). In the excellent review of RPN by Eknoyan and associates (1982), 67

TABLE 14–12. CONDITIONS ASSOCIATED WITH RPN

Diabetes mellitus
Pyelonephritis
Urinary tract obstruction
Analgesic abuse
Sickle cell hemoglobinopathies
Renal transplant rejection
Cirrhosis of the liver
Dehydration, hypoxia and jaundice of infants
Miscellaneous: renal vein thrombosis, cryoglobulinemia,
    renal candidiasis, contrast media injection, amyloidosis,
    calyceal arteritis, necrotizing angiitis, rapidly progressive
    glomerulonephritis, hypotensive shock, acute
    pancreatitis

From Eknoyan, G., Qunibi, W. Y., Grissom, R. T., et al.: Medicine, 61:55, 1982. Used by permission.

per cent (18/27) of the patients with RPN had an acute or chronic urinary tract infection. In only four patients (22 per cent) was pyelonephritis alone associated with RPN. In the remaining 14 patients, several of the conditions that can be associated with RPN were present in addition to the urinary infection. All four individuals with urinary tract obstruction had concomitant urinary tract infections. In nine of their RPN patients (a third), there was no evidence of infection at all. These emphasize that although any of the recognized factors in Table 14–12 may alone cause RPN, the coexistence of multiple factors, such as diabetes or obstruction and infection, increases the risk of developing RPN.

Clinically, RPN is a spectrum of disease. Patients may have an acute fulminating illness with rapid progression or may have a chronic disease that is incidentally discovered on excretory urography. Some patients may chronically pass necrotic tissue in their urine (Hernandez et al., 1975), and some may never pass papillae (Lindvall, 1978). Although the diagnosis may be made from the passage of necrotic papillae in the urine, most often it is made from the excretory urogram. The radiographs show various degrees of renal involvement with either medullary or papillary changes causing irregular sinuses or medullary cavities or classic ring shadows (Eknoyan et al., 1982; Lindvall, 1978). Retained necrotic papillae may calcify, especially in association with infection. Furthermore, this necrotic tissue may form the nidus for chronic infection. Opportunistic fungal infections have been reported (Madge and Lomvardias, 1973; Vordermark et al., 1980; Juhasz et al., 1980; Tomashefski and Abramowsky, 1981). Renal sonography may be useful to diagnose papillary necrosis (Buonocore et al., 1980; Hoffman et al., 1982).

The early diagnosis of RPN is important to improve prognosis and reduce morbidity. In addition to chronic infection, patients with analgesic abuse–associated papillary necrosis may have an increased incidence of urothelial tumors; urinary cytology examined routinely may be helpful to diagnose these tumors early (Jackson et al., 1978). In patients who have analgesic abuse–induced RPN, the disease will stabilize if the analgesic intake is stopped (Gower, 1976). Furthermore, adequate antimicrobial therapy to control infection and early recognition and treatment of ureteral obstruction caused by sloughed necrotic tissue will minimize decline in renal function. When these patients suffer from an acute ureteral obstruction due to a sloughed papilla and have a concomitant urinary infection, they are a urologic emergency. In these cases, immediate removal of the obstructing papillae by stone basket (Jameson and Heal, 1973) or acute drainage of the kidney by ureteral catheter or percutaneous nephrostomy is necessary.

DIABETES MELLITUS

Although some studies have shown that the incidence of urinary infections in young diabetic girls aged 6 to 15 years (1.6 to 2.0 per cent) (Pometta et al., 1967) and in hospitalized diabetics (Huvos and Rocha, 1959) may be no different than in nondiabetics, several more recent studies document that diabetic women have a higher incidence of infections than do nondiabetics (Vejlsgaard, 1973; Ooi and Chen, 1974; Forland et al., 1977). Two of these studies found that the incidence of infections in diabetic women ranged from 11.4 to 15.8 per cent, whereas that in matched nondiabetic women ranged from 4.5 to 4.6 per cent (Vejlsgaard, 1973; Ooi and Chen, 1974); only 2 per cent of diabetic men were found to have infections (Forland et al., 1977). These patients often have a glomerulopathy, with difficulty concentrating antimicrobial agents. In addition, they seem to be predisposed to special complications of urinary tract infections—papillary necrosis and emphysematous pyelonephritis.

Papillary Necrosis. In a review series from the United States, diabetes is the most common condition associated with papillary necrosis (Eknoyan et al., 1982). Although in diabetics urinary infection may be a primary or secondary factor in the etiology of papillary necrosis, diabetics with acute clinical pyelonephritis seem to be particularly predisposed to renal papillary necrosis (Eknoyan et al., 1982). In the study cited by Eknoyan and associates (1982), 29 of 107 diabetics (27.1 per cent) who died of acute renal infection exhibited renal papillary necrosis on gross or microscopic examination. This entity is discussed separately with other risk factors predisposing to renal loss.

Emphysematous Pyelonephritis. Emphysematous pyelonephritis is an uncommon complication of acute pyelonephritis that occurs in diabetics (although 15 per cent will have diabetes discovered only when they are found to have emphysematous pyelonephritis), with an overall mortality of 43 per cent (Freiha et al., 1979). Clinically it appears as an acute severe clinical pyelonephritis that fails to resolve during the first 2 to 3 days of treatment; its hallmark is the appearance of intraparenchymal gas. Two factors regarding the radiographic findings should be emphasized. First, emphysematous pyelonephritis must be distinguished from other entities with gas in the collecting system and around the kidney by clearly showing intraparenchymal gas. Second, reviews on emphysematous pyelonephritis emphasize that any cases reported in nondiabetic patients show no intraparenchymal gas and therefore represent conditions other than emphysematous pyelonephritis (Schultz and Klorfein, 1962; Turman and Rutherford, 1971; Spagnola, 1978; Freiha et al., 1979). The intraparenchymal gas is thought to be generated by bacterial fermentation of glucose in the necrotic infected tissue. *E. coli* is the most common etiologic organism, but any of the lactose fermenters may be involved (Freiha et al., 1979).

The diagnosis may be made from a plain abdominal radiograph, which shows mottling of the renal parenchyma with small gas bubbles extending in a radial distribution in the kidney. This is caused by gas present in the parenchymal abscesses. As the infection spreads outside the cortex the gas extends into the space between Gerota's fascia and the renal capsule, and outlines or forms thin crescents of gas around the kidney (Langston and Pfister, 1970) (Fig. 14–17). Plain film renal tomograms will establish that the gas is intraparenchymal. More recently, renal ultrasound and computerized tomography have also been used to localize the gas and extent of the infection (Conrad et al., 1979; Kim et al., 1979; Lautin et al., 1979).

Since patients with this infectious complication are usually acutely ill, rapid supportive measures should be undertaken. Patients should be started upon appropriate antimicrobial agents, and treatment of diabetes must be initiated. Obstruction of the affected kidney, if present, must be eliminated, and function of the contralateral kidney must be established, since 10 per cent of the reported cases have been bilateral (Freiha et al., 1979). Since carbon dioxide diffuses rapidly through body tissues, the observation of persistent intraparenchymal renal gas documents ineffective treatment; then surgical drainage or nephrectomy is needed (Schainuck et al., 1968). Freiha and associates (1979) have emphasized that surgical treatment must be complete extirpation because most attempts at renal sparing have been unsuccessful in retaining renal function or decreasing patient morbidity.

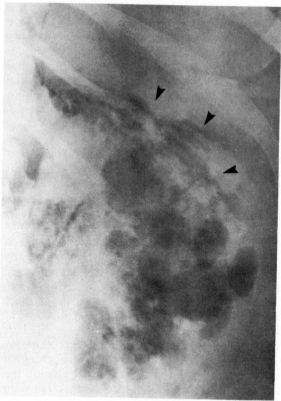

Figure 14–17. This photograph is part of an abdominal plain film taken in a female with diabetes and emphysematous pyelonephritis. The arrows mark the thin crescents of gas found around the kidney. Other areas of the kidney show small gas bubbles extending radially in the parenchyma.

SPINAL CORD INJURY WITH HIGH-PRESSURE BLADDERS

Twenty years ago, of all patients with bacteriuria, no group compared in severity and morbidity with those having spinal cord injury. Nearly all required catheterization early after their injury because of bladder spasticity or flaccidity, and significant numbers developed ureterectasis, hydronephrosis, reflux, and renal calculi. Bacteriologic and urodynamic advances in the management of these patients have vastly reduced their morbidity and mortality. In Chapter 18, Dr. Rodney Anderson discusses these special techniques and management problems that have so remarkably changed urinary tract prognosis in these patients.

PREGNANCY

The special problems that relate to bacteriuria of pregnancy, including the effects on the fetus as well as the occurrence of acute pyelonephritis, are presented in Chapter 15.

ACUTE BACTERIAL PROSTATITIS

Except in the very elderly or in immunocompromised hosts, who are highly susceptible to gram-negative bacteremia, most men with acute bacterial prostatitis mainly suffer from the serious morbidity of chills, fever, and often acute urinary retention. These patients at serious risk are discussed by Dr. Edwin Meares in Chapter 17.

PATIENTS AT RISK OF SERIOUS MORBIDITY FROM BACTERIURIA—CONCLUSION

These bacteriuric patients, then, represent those who are at substantial risk of either serious morbidity or loss of renal cortex or both. They deserve special attention and care by the urologist; they often represent true emergencies. When acute pyelonephritis, and especially perirenal abscess or gram-negative septicemia supervenes, the potential for mortality is real.

References

Abramowicz, M.: Prevention of bacterial endocarditis. Med. Lett., 26:3, 1984.

Akerlund, A. S.: Urinary antibodies to *Escherichia coli* bacteria in childhood urinary tract infections. Technical Report, University of Goteborg, Goteborg, Sweden, 1978.

Alwall, N.: Screening for urinary tract infection in nonpregnant women. Kidney Int., 8:107, 1975.

Anderson, R. U.: Prophylaxis of bacteriuria during intermittent catheterization of the acute neurogenic bladder. J. Urol., 123:364, 1980.

Anhalt, M. A., Cawood, D., and Scott, R.: Xanthogranulomatous pyelonephritis: a comprehensive review with report of 4 additional cases. J. Urol., 105:10, 1971.

Aoki, S., Imamura, S., Aoki, M., et al.: "Abacterial" and bacterial pyelonephritis. N. Engl. J. Med., 281:1375, 1969.

Ashby, E. C., Rees, M., and Dowding, C. H.: Prophylaxis against systemic infection after transrectal biopsy for suspected prostatic carcinoma. Br. Med. J., 2:1263, 1978.

Asscher, A. W., Sussman, M., Waters, W. E., et al.: The clinical significance of asymptomatic bacteriuria in the nonpregnant woman. J. Infect. Dis., 120:17, 1969.

Bailey, R. R., and Abbott, G. D.: Treatment of urinary tract infection with a single dose of amoxycillin. Nephron, 18:316, 1977.

Bailey, R. R., Little, P. J., and Rolleston, G. L.: Renal damage after acute pyelonephritis. Br. Med. J., 1:550, 1969.

Ballesteros, J. J., Faus, R., and Gironella, J.: Preoperative diagnosis of renal xanthogranulomatosis by serial urinary cytology: preliminary report. J. Urol., 124:9, 1980.

Barth, K. H., Lightman, N. I., Ridolfi, R. I., et al.: Acute pyelonephritis simulating poorly vascularized renal neoplasm, non-specificity of angiographic criteria. J. Urol., 116:650, 1976.

Bartlett, J. G., and Gorbach, S. L.: Anaerobic bacteria in suppurative infections of the male genitourinary system. J. Urol., 125:376, 1981.

Bergstrom, T., Lincoln, K., Redin, B., et al.: Studies of urinary tract infections in infancy and childhood. X. Short or long-term treatment in girls with first or second-time urinary tract infections uncomplicated by obstructive urological abnormalities. Acta Paediatr. Scand., 57:186, 1968.

Biello, D. R., Levitt, R. G., and Melson, G. L.: The roles of gallium-67 scintigraphy, ultrasonography, and computed tomography in the detection of abdominal abscesses. Semin. Nucl. Med., 9:58, 1979.

Bilges, H., Brod, J., Christ, M., et al.: Diagnosis of renal and urinary tract infection by recent techniques. Contrib. Nephrol., 16:27, 1979.

Bille, J., and Glauser, M. P.: Protection against chronic pyelonephritis in rats by suppression of acute suppuration: effect of colchicine and neutropenia. J. Infect. Dis., 146:220, 1982.

Bloom, S., and Gonick, P.: Urine sterilization in catheter drainage bottles. Invest. Urol., 6:527, 1969.

Braude, A. I.: Current concepts of pyelonephritis. Medicine, 52:257, 1973.

Brehmer, B., and Madsen, P. O.: Route and prophylaxis of ascending bladder infection in male patients with indwelling catheters. J. Urol., 108:719, 1972.

Bromberg, K., Gleich, S., and Ginsberg, M. B.: Clostridia in urinary tract infections. South Med. J., 75:1298, 1982.

Brooker, W. J., and Aufderheide, A. C.: Genitourinary tract infections due to atypical mycobacteria. J. Urol., 124:242, 1980.

Brooks, S. J. D., Lyons, J. M., and Braude, A. I.: Immunization against retrograde pyelonephritis. III. Vaccination against chronic pyelonephritis due to Escherichia coli. J. Infect. Dis., 136:633, 1977.

Brumfitt, W., Faiers, M. C., and Franklin, I. N. S.: The treatment of urinary infection by means of a single dose of cephaloxidine. Postgrad. Med. J., 46:65, 1970.

Buckwold, F. J., Ludwig, P., Godfrey, K. M., et al.: Therapy for acute cystitis in adult women: Randomized comparison of single-dose sulfisoxazole vs. trimethoprim-sulfamethoxazole. J.A.M.A., 247:1839, 1982.

Budde, E., Naumann, G., Nimmich, W., et al.: Antibody-coating of bacteria in the urine in relation to various immunologic indexes. Kidney Int., 19:65, 1981.

Bultitude, M. I., and Eykyn, S.: The relationship between the urethral flora and urinary infection in the catheterised male. Br. J. Urol., 45:678, 1973.

Buonocore, E., Vidt, D. G., and Montie, J. E.: Ultrasonography in the diagnosis of obstructive uropathy caused by papillary necrosis. Clev. Clin. Q., 47:109, 1980.

Busch, R., and Huland, H.: Correlation of symptoms and results of direct localization studies in patients with urinary tract infections. J. Urol., 132:282, 1984.

Cameron, D. D., and Azimi, F.: The value of excretory urography in the diagnosis of acute pyelonephritis. J. Urol., 112:546, 1974.

Carroll, B., Silverman, P. M., Goodwin, D. A., et al.: Ultrasonography and indium 111 white blood cell scanning for the detection of intraabdominal abscesses. Ultrasound, 140:155, 1981.

Cartwright, K. A., Stanbridge, T. N., and Cooper, J.: Comparison of once daily trimethoprim and standard co-trimoxazole in urinary infections: A clinical trial in general practice. Practitioner, 226:152, 1982.

Charlton, C. A. C., Crowther, A., Davies, J. G., et al.: Three-day and ten-day chemotherapy for urinary tract infections in general practice. Br. Med. J., 1:124, 1976.

Chodak, G. W., and Plaut, M. E.: Systemic antibiotics for prophylaxis in urologic surgery: A critical review. J. Urol., 121:695, 1979.

Coleman, B. G., Arger, P. H., Mulhern, C. B., et al.: Pyonephrosis: sonography in the diagnosis and management. Am. J. Roentgenol., 137:939, 1981.

Conrad, M. R., Bregman, R., and Kilman, W. J.: Ultrasonic recognition of parenchymal gas. Am. J. Radiol., 132:395, 1979.

Conrad, M. R., Sanders, R. C., and Mascardo, A. D.: Perinephric abscess aspiration using ultrasound guidance. Am. J. Roentgenol., 128:459, 1977.

Cotran, R. S., and Piessens, W. F.: Pathogenesis of chronic pyelonephritis. Proceedings of the 6th International Congress of Nephrology. Basel, 1976, p. 509.

Crawford, E. D., Haynes, A. L., Story, M. W., et al.: Prevention of urinary tract infection and sepsis following transrectal prostatic biopsy. J. Urol., 127:449, 1982.

Davidson, A. J., and Talner, L. B.: Urographic and angiographic abnormalities in adult-onset acute bacterial nephritis. Radiology, 106:249, 1973.

Davidson, A. J., and Talner, L. B.: Late sequelae of adult-onset acute bacterial nephritis. Radiology, 127:367, 1978.

Davies, A. G., McLachlan, M. S. F., and Asscher, A. W.: Progressive kidney damage after non-obstructive urinary tract infection. Br. Med. J., 4:406, 1972.

Dudley, M. N., and Barriere, S. L.: Antimicrobial irrigations in the prevention and treatment of catheter-related urinary tract infections. Am. J. Hosp. Pharm., 38:59, 1981.

Dupont, H. L., and Spink, W. W.: Infections due to gram-negative organisms: an analysis of 860 patients with bacteremia at the University of Minnesota Medical Center, 1958–1966. Medicine, 48:307, 1969.

Durack, D. T.: Prophylaxis of infective endocarditis. In Mandell, G. I., Douglas, R. G., and Bennett, J. E. (Eds.): Principles and Practice of Infectious Diseases. New York, John Wiley & Sons, 1979.

Eknoyan, G., Qunibi, W. Y., Grissom, R. T., et al.: Renal papillary necrosis: an update. Medicine, 61:55, 1982.

Elyaderani, M. K., Subramanian, M. P., and Burgess, J. E.: Diagnosis and percutaneous drainage of a perinephric abscess by ultrasound and fluoroscopy. J. Urol., 125:405, 1981.

Engel, G., Schaeffer, A. J., Grayhack, J. T., et al.: The role of excretory urography and cystoscopy in the evaluation and management of women with recurrent urinary tract infection. J. Urol., 123:190, 1980.

Erno, H., and Thomsen, A. C.: Immunoglobulin classes of urinary and serum antibodies in mycoplasmal pyelonephritis. Acta. Pathol. Microbiol. Scand., 88:237, 1980.

Fair, W. R., Crane, D. B., Peterson, L. J., et al.: Three-day treatment of urinary tract infections. J. Urol., 123:717, 1980.

Fair, W. R., McClennan, B. L., and Jost, R. G.: Are excretory urograms necessary in evaluating women with urinary tract infection? J. Urol., 121:313, 1979.

Fairchild, T. N., Shuman, W., and Berger, R. E.: Radiographic studies for women with recurrent urinary tract infections. J. Urol., 128:344, 1982.

Fairley, K. F., Grounds, A. D., Carson, N. E., et al.: Site of infection in acute urinary tract in general practice. Lancet, 2:615, 1971.

Fairley, K. F., Whitworth, J. A., Kincaid-Smith, P., et al.: Single-dose therapy in management of urinary tract infections. Med. J. Aust., 2:75, 1978.

Falkiner, F. R., Ma, P. T., Murphy, D. M., et al.: Antimicrobial agents for the prevention of urinary tract infection in transurethral surgery. J. Urol., 129:766, 1983.

Fang, L. S. T., Tolkoff-Rubin, N. E., and Rubin, R. H.: Efficacy of single-dose and conventional amoxicillin therapy in urinary-tract infection localized by the anti-body-coated bacteria technic. N. Engl. J. Med., *298*:413, 1978.

Favaro, S., Conventi, L., Baggio, B., et al.: Antibody-coated bacteria in the urinary sediment of rats with experimental pyelonephritis. Nephron, *21*:165, 1978.

Feldberg, M. A. M.: Bilateral adult-onset acute bacterial pyelonephritis and its late unusual sequelae. Diagn. Imaging, *51*:296, 1982.

Fennell, R. S., Luengnaruemitchai, M. Iravani, A., et al.: Urinary tract infections in children: Effect of short course antibiotic therapy on recurrence rate in children with previous infections. Clin. Pediatr., *19*:121, 1980.

Fierer, J., Talner, L., and Braude, A. I.: Bacteremia in the pathogenesis of retrograde *E. coli* pyelonephritis in the rat. Am. J. Pathol., *64*:443, 1971.

Fincke, B. G., and Friedland, G.: Prevention and management of infection in the catheterized patient. Urol. Clin. North Am., *3*:313, 1976.

Finegold, S. M.: Urinary tract infections. *In* Finegold, S. M. (Ed.): Anaerobic Bacteria in Human Disease. New York, Academic Press, 1976.

Flynn, J. T., Molland, E. A., Paris, A. M. I., et al.: The underestimated hazards of xanthogranulomatous pyelonephritis. Br. J. Urol., *51*:443, 1979.

Forland, M., Thomas, V., and Shelokov, A.: Urinary tract infections in patients with diabetes mellitus. JAMA, *238*:1924, 1977.

Forsum, U., Hjelm, E., and Jonsell, G.: Antibody-coated bacteria in the urine of children with urinary tract infections. Acta Paediatr. Scand., *65*:639, 1976.

Fowler, J. E., and Pulaski, E. T.: Excretory urography, cystography, and cystoscopy in the evaluation of women with urinary-tract infection. N. Engl. J. Med., *304*:462, 1981.

Freiha, F. S., Messing, E. M., and Gross, D. M.: Emphysematous pyelonephritis. J. Contin. Ed. Urol., *18*:9, 1979.

Friedland, G. W., and Stamey, T. A.: Recurrent urinary tract infection: With persistent Wolffian duct masquerading as duplicated urethra. Urology, *4*:315, 1974.

Funston, A. R., Fisher, K. S., van Blerk, J. P., et al.: Acute focal bacterial nephritis or renal abscess? A sonographic diagnosis. J. Urol., *54*:461, 1982.

Gadeholt, H.: Quantitative estimation of urinary sediment with special regard to sources of error. Br. Med. J., *1*:1547, 1964.

Gadeholt, H.: The cellular content in non-timed specimens of urine. Acta Med. Scand., *184*:323, 1968.

Gallagher, D. J., Montgomerie, J. Z., and North, J. D.: Acute infections of the urinary tract and the urethral syndrome in general practice. Br. Med. J., *1*:622, 1965.

Garibaldi, R. A., Burke, J. P., Britt, M. R., et al.: Meatal colonization and catheter-associated bacteriuria. N. Engl. J. Med., *303*:316, 1980.

Garibaldi, R. A., Burke, J. P., Dickman, M. L., et al.: Factors predisposing to bacteriuria during indwelling urethral catheterization. N. Engl. J. Med., *291*:215, 1974.

Gaymans, R., Haverkorn, M. J., Valkenburg, H. A., et al.: A prospective study of urinary-tract infections in a Dutch general practice. Lancet, *2*:674, 1976.

Ghosh, H.: Chronic pyelonephritis with xanthogranulomatous change. Am. J. Clin. Pathol., *25*:1043, 1955.

Gibbons, R. P., Stark, R. A., Correa, R. J., et al.: The prophylactic use-or-misuse of antibiotics in transurethral prostatectomy. J. Urol., *119*:381, 1978.

Glauser, M. P., Lyons, J. M., and Braude, A. I.: Prevention of chronic experimental pyelonephritis by suppression of acute suppuration. J. Clin. Invest., *61*:403, 1978.

Godard, C., Girardet, P., Frutiger, P., et al.: Short treat-

ment of urinary tract infections in children. Paediatrician, *9*:309, 1980.

Gonzalez, R., Wright, R., and Blackard, C. E.: Prophylactic antibiotics in transurethral prostatectomy. J. Urol., *116*:203, 1976.

Gorbach, S. L., and Bartlett, J. G.: Anaerobic infections. N. Engl. J. Med., *209*:1237, 1974.

Govan, D. E., Fair, W. R., Friedland, G. W., et al.: Management of children with urinary tract infections. The Stanford Experience. Urology, *6*:273, 1975.

Gower, P. E.: A prospective study of patients with radiological pyelonephritis, papillary necrosis and obstructive atrophy. Q. J. Med., *45*:315, 1976.

Greenberg, R. N., Sanders, C. V., Lewis, A. C., et al.: Single-dose cefaclor therapy of urinary tract infection: Evaluation of antibody-coated bacteria test and C-reactive protein assay as predictors of cure. Am. J. Med., *71*:841, 1981.

Gross, P. A., Harkavy, L. M., Barden, G. E., et al.: The fallacy of cultures of the tips of Foley catheters. Surg. Gynecol. Obstet., *139*:597, 1974.

Haaga, J. R., and Weinstein, A. J.: CT guided percutaneous aspiration and drainage of abscesses. Am. J. Roentgenol., *135*:1187, 1980.

Hampel, N., Class, R. N., and Persky, L.: Value of gallium 67 scintigraphy in the diagnosis of localized renal and perirenal inflammation. J. Urol., *124*:311, 1980.

Hanson, L. A., Ahlstedt, S., Jodal, U., et al.: The host-parasite relationship in urinary tract infections. Kidney Int., *8*:S-28, 1975.

Harding, G. K. M., Marrie, T. J., Ronald, A. R., et al.: Urinary tract localization in women. JAMA, *240*:1147, 1978.

Hargreave, T. B., Hindmarsh, J. R., Elton R., et al.: Short-term prophylaxis with cefotaxime for prostatic surgery. Br. Med. J., *284*:1008, 1982.

Harrison, R. B., and Shaffer, H. A.: The roentgenographic findings in acute pyelonephritis. J.A.M.A., *241*:1718, 1979.

Hawthorne, N. J., Kurtz, S. B., Anhalt, J. P., et al.: Accuracy of antibody-coated-bacteria test in recurrent urinary tract infections. Mayo Clin. Proc., *53*:651, 1978.

Hellerstein, S., Duggan, E., Welchert, E., et al.: Serum C-reactive protein and the site of urinary tract infections. J. Pediatr., *100*:21, 1982.

Hellerstein, S., Kennedy, E., Nussbaum, L., et al.: Localization of the site of urinary tract infections by means of antibody-coated bacteria in the urinary sediments. J. Pediatr., *92*:188, 1978.

Herlitz, H., Westberg, G., and Nilson, A. E.: A perinephric abscess in a diabetic woman: successful conservative treatment. Scand. J. Urol. Nephrol., *15*:337, 1981.

Hernandez, G. V., King, A. S., and Needle, M. A.: Nephrosis and papillary necrosis after pyelonephritis. N. Engl. J. Med., *293*:1347, 1975.

Hoddick, W., Jeffrey, R. B., Goldberg, H. I., et al.: CT and sonography of severe renal and perirenal infections. Am. J. Roentgenol., *140*:517, 1983.

Hoffer, P.: Gallium and infection. J. Nucl. Med., *21*:484, 1980.

Hoffman, J. C., Schnur, J. F., and Koenigsberg, M.: Demonstration of renal papillary necrosis by sonography. Radiology, *145*:785, 1982.

Huland, H., and Busch, R.: Chronic pyelonephritis as a cause of end stage renal disease. J. Urol., *127*:642, 1982.

Huland, H., Busch, R., and Riebel, T. H.: Renal scarring after symptomatic and asymptomatic upper urinary tract infection: A prospective study. J. Urol., *128*:682, 1982.

Huland, H., Gonnerman, D., and Clausen, C.: Bacterial

localization in patients with end stage renal disease to avoid bilateral nephrectomy before renal transplantation. J. Urol., *129*:915, 1983.

Hurwitz, S. R., Kessler W. O., Alazraki, N. P., et al.: Gallium-67 imaging to localize urinary-tract infections. Br. J. Radiol., *49*:156, 1976.

Huvos, A., and Rocha, H.: Frequency of bacteriuria in patients with diabetes mellitus. N. Engl. J. Med., *261*:1213, 1959.

Ireland, D., Tacchi, D., and Bint, A. J.: Effect of single-dose prophylactic co-trimoxazole on the incidence of gynaecological postoperative urinary tract infection. Br. J. Obstet. Gynecol., *89*:578, 1982.

Jackson, B., Kirkland, J. A., Lawrence, J. R., et al.: Urine cytology findings in analgesic nephropathy. J. Urol., *120*:145, 1978.

Jameson, R. M., and Heal, M. R.: The surgical management of acute renal papillary necrosis. Br. J. Surg., *60*:428, 1973.

Jodal, U., and Hanson, L. A.: Sequential determination of C-reactive protein in acute childhood pyelonephritis. Acta Paediatr. Scand., *65*:319, 1976.

Jodal, U., Lindberg, U., and Lincoln, K.: Level diagnosis of symptomatic urinary tract infections in childhood. Acta Paediatr. Scand., *64*:201, 1975.

Jones, S. R., Smith, J. W., and Sanford, J. P.: Localization of urinary tract infections by detection of antibody-coated bacteria in urine sediment. N. Engl. J. Med., *290*:591, 1974.

Juhasz, J., Galambos, J., and Surjan, L.: Renal actinomycosis associated with bilateral necrosing renal papillitis. Int. Urol. Nephrol., *12*:199, 1980.

Kaijser, B., and Larsson, P.: Experimental acute pyelonephritis caused by enterobacteria in animals. A review. J. Urol., *127*:786, 1982.

Kaijser, B., Hanson, L. A., Jodal, U., et al.: Frequency of *E. coli* K antigens in urinary tract infections in children. Lancet, *1*:663, 1977.

Kaijser, B., Larsson, P., and Olling, S.: Protection against ascending *Escherichia coli* pyelonephritis in rats and significance of local immunity. Infect. Immun., *20*:78, 1978.

Kallenius, G., Mollby, R., Hultberg, H., et al.: Structure of the carbohydrate part of the receptor on human uroepithelial cells for pyelonephritogenic *Escherichia coli*. Lancet, *2*:604, 1981.

Kass, E. H.: The role of asymptomatic bacteriuria in the pathogenesis of pyelonephritis. *In* Quinn, E. L., and Kass, E. H. (Eds.): Biology of Pyelonephritis. Boston, Little Brown & Co., 1960, p. 399.

Kass, E. H., and Finland, M.: Asymptomatic infections of the urinary tract. Trans. Assoc. Am. Physicians, *69*:56, 1956.

Kass, E. H., and Schneiderman, L. J.: Entry of bacteria into the urinary tracts of patients with inlying catheters. N. Engl. J. Med., *256*:556, 1957.

Kass, E. H., Silver, T. M., Konnak, J. W., et al.: The urographic findings in acute pyelonephritis: non-obstructive hydronephrosis. J. Urol., *116*:544, 1976.

Kessler, W. O., Gittes, R. F., Hurwitz, S. R., et al.: Gallium-67 scans in the diagnosis of pyelonephritis. West. J. Med., *121*:91, 1974.

Kesson, A. M., Talbott, J. M., and Gyory, A. Z.: Microscopic examination of urine. Lancet, *2*:809, 1978.

Khatib, A.: Comparative efficacy of single-and eight-day treatment of urinary tract infections with carfecillin (Uticillin). J. Int. Med. Res., *9*:186, 1981.

Kim, D. S., Woesner, M. E., Howard, T. F., et al.:

Emphysematous pyelonephritis demonstrated by computed tomography. Am. J. Radiol., *132*:287, 1979.

Kincaid-Smith, P., and Becker, G.: Reflux nephropathy and chronic atrophic pyelonephritis: a review. J. Infect. Dis., *138*:774, 1978.

Kincaid-Smith, P., and Becker, G. J.: Reflux nephropathy in the adult. *In* Hodson, J., and Kincaid-Smith, P. (Eds.): Reflux Nephropathy. New York, Masson Publishing USA, Inc. 1979, pp. 21–28.

Kincaid-Smith, P., and Bullen, M.: Bacteriuria in pregnancy. Lancet, *1*:395, 1965.

Kincaid-Smith, P., and Fairley, K. F.: Controlled trial comparing effect of two and six weeks' treatment in recurrent urinary tract infection. Br. Med. J., *2*:145, 1969.

Kincaid-Smith, P., Friedman, A., and Nanra, R. S.: Controlled trials of treatment in urinary tract infection. *In* Kincaid-Smith P., and Fairley, K. F. (Eds.): Renal Infection and Renal Scarring. Melbourne, Mercedes Publishing Co., 1970, p. 165.

King, W. W., and Cox, C. E.: Bacterial inhibition of ureteral smooth muscle contractility. I. The effect of common urinary pathogens and endotoxin in an in vitro system. J. Urol., *108*:700, 1972.

Klastersky, J., Daneau, D., Swings, G., et al.: Antibacterial activity in serum and urine as a therapeutic guide in bacterial infections. J. Infect. Dis., *129*:187, 1974.

Kohnle, W., Vanek, E., Federlin, K., et al.: Lokalisation eines Harnwegsinfektes durch Nachweis von antikörperbesetzten Bakterien im Urin. Dtsch. Med. Wochenschr., *100*:2598, 1975.

Konetschnik, F., Goldin, A. R., and Marshall, V. R.: Management of "acute renal carbuncle." Br. J. Urol., *54*:467, 1982.

Kraft, J. K., and Stamey, T. A.: The natural history of symptomatic recurrent bacteriuria in women. Medicine, *56*:55, 1977.

Kreger, B. E., Craven, D. E., Carling, P. C., et al.: Gram-negative bacteremia. III. Reassessment of etiology, epidemiology and ecology in 612 patients. Am. J. Med., *68*:332, 1980a.

Kreger, B. E., Craven, D. E., and McCabe, W. R.: Gram-negative bacteremia. IV. Re-evaluation of clinical features and treatment in 612 patients. Am. J. Med., *68*:344, 1980b.

Kuhn, J. P., and Berger, P. E.: Computed tomography of the kidney in infancy and childhood. Radiol. Clin. North Am., *19*:445, 1981.

Kunin, C. M.: The quantitative significance of bacteria visualized in the unstained urinary sediment. N. Engl. J. Med., *265*:589, 1961.

Kunin, C. M.: The natural history of recurrent bacteriuria in schoolgirls. N. Engl. J. Med., *282*:1443, 1970.

Kunz, H. H., Sieberth, H. G., Freiberg, J., et al.: Zur bedeutung der blasenpunktion fur den sicheren nachweis einer bacteriurie. Dtsch. Med Wochenschr., *100*:2252, 1975.

Lacey, R. W., Simpson, M. H. C., Lord, V. L., et al.: Comparison of single-dose trimethoprim with a five-day course for the treatment of urinary tract infections in the elderly. Age Ageing, *10*:179, 1981.

Lacy, S. S., Drach, G. W., and Cox, E.: Incidence of infection after prostatectomy and efficacy of cephaloridine prophylaxis. J. Urol., *105*:836, 1971.

Langston, C. S., and Pfister, R. C.: Renal emphysema: a case report and review of the literature. Am. J. Radiol., *110*:778, 1970.

Lark, D., O'Hanley, P., and Schoolnik, G.: Distribution of

digalactoside and dimannose receptors in human genitourinary tissue. Submitted for publication.

Lautin, E. M., Gordon, P. M., Friedman, A. C., et al.: Emphysematous pyelonephritis: optimal diagnosis and treatment. Urol. Radiol., *1*:93, 1979.

Lebowitz, R. L.: Urography in children: when should it be done? 1. Infection. Postgrad. Med. J., *64*:63, 1978.

Lewin, K. J., Fair, W. R., Steigbigel, R. T., et al.: Clinical and laboratory studies into the pathogenesis of malacoplakia. J. Clin. Pathol., *29*:354, 1976.

Lindberg, U., Claesson, I., Hanson, L. A., et al.: Asymptomatic bacteriuria in schoolgirls. VIII. Clinical course during a 3-year followup. J. Pediatr., *92*:194, 1978.

Lindberg, U., Hanson, L. A., Jodal, U., et al.: Asymptomatic bacteriuria in schoolgirls. II. Differences in *Escherichia coli* causing asymptomatic and symptomatic bacteriuria. Acta Paediatr. Scand., *64*:432, 1975.

Lindvall, N.: Radiological changes of renal papillary necrosis. Kidney Int., *13*:93, 1978.

Little, P. J., McPherson, D. R., and Wardener, H. E.: The appearance of the intravenous pyelogram during and after acute pyelonephritis. Lancet, *1*:1186, 1965.

Lockey, J. E., Williams, D. N., Raij, L., et al.: Comparison of 4 and 10 days of doxycycline treatment for urinary tract infection. J. Urol., *124*:643, 1980.

Lohr, J. A., Hayden, G. F., Kesler, R. W., et al.: Threeday therapy of lower urinary tract infections with nitrofurantoin macrocrystals: A randomized clinical trial. J. Pediatr., *99*:980, 1981.

Lomberg, L., Hanson, L. A., Jacobsson, B., et al.: Correlation of P blood group, vesicoureter reflux, and bacterial attachment in patients with recurrent pyelonephritis. N. Engl. J. Med., *308*:1189, 1983.

Lorentzen, M., and Overgaard, N. H.: Xanthogranulomatous pyelonephritis. Scand. J. Urol. Nephrol., *14*:193, 1980.

Mabeck, C. E.: Studies in urinary tract infections: I. The diagnosis of bacteriuria in women. Acta Med. Scand., *186*:35, 1969a.

Mabeck, C. E.: Studies in urinary tract infections: IV. Urinary leukocyte excretion in bacteriuria. Acta Med. Scand., *186*:193, 1969b.

Mabeck, C. E.: Treatment of uncomplicated urinary tract infection in non-pregnant women. Postgrad. Med. J., *48*:55, 1972.

Mabeck, C. E., and Vejlsgaard, R.: Treatment of urinary tract infections in general practice with sulfamethizole, trimethoprim or co-trimazine (sulphadiazine-trimethoprim). J. Antimicrob. Chemother., *6*:701, 1980.

Maderazo, E. G., Berlin, B. B., and Morhardt, C.: Treatment of malakoplakia with trimethoprim-sulfamethoxazole. Urology, *13*:70, 1979.

Madge, C. E., and Lomvardias, S.: Chronic liver disease and renal papillary necrosis with aspergillus. South Med. J., *66*:486, 1973.

Maizels, M., and Schaeffer, A. J.: Decreased incidence of bacteriuria associated with periodic instillations of hydrogen peroxide into the urethral catheter drainage bag. J. Urol., *123*:841, 1980.

Malek, R. S.: Xanthogranulomatous pyelonephritis: a great imitator. *In* Stamey, T. A. (Ed.): J. C. E. Urol. Northfield, Ill., Medical Digest, Inc. 1978, pp. 17–28.

Malek, R. S., and Elder, J. S.: Xanthogranulomatous pyelonephritis: a critical analysis of 26 cases and of the literature. J. Urol., *119*:589, 1978.

Malek, R. S., Greene, L. F., DeWeerd, J. H., et al.: Xanthogranulomatous pyelonephritis. Br. J. Urol., *44*:296, 1972.

Marple, C. D.: The frequency and character of urinary tract infections in an unselected group of women. Ann. Intern. Med., *14*:2220, 1941.

Marrie, T. J., Harding, G. K. M., and Ronald, A. R.: Anaerobic and aerobic urethral flora in healthy females. J. Clin. Microbiol., *8*:67, 1978.

Matthew, A. D., Gonzalez, R., Jeffords, D., et al.: Prevention of bacteriuria after transurethral prostatectomy with nitrofurantoin macrocrystals. J. Urol., *120*:442, 1978.

Mauro, M. A., Balfe, D. M., Stanley, R. J., et al.: Computed tomography in the diagnosis and management of the renal mass. JAMA, *248*:2894, 1982.

McAfee, J. G.: Radionuclide imaging in the assessment of primary chronic pyelonephritis. Radiology, *133*:203, 1979.

McCabe, W. R., and Jackson, G. G.: Treatment of pyelonephritis: Bacterial, drug and host factors in success or failure among 252 patients. N. Engl. J. Med., *272*:1037, 1965.

McCabe, W. R., and Olans, R. N.: Shock in gram-negative bacteremia. Predisposing factors, pathophysiology and treatment. *In* Remington, J. S., and Swartz, M. N. (Eds.): Current Clinical Topics in Infectious Diseases. New York, McGraw-Hill Book Co., 1981, pp. 121–150.

McCabe, W. R., and Treadwell, T. L.: Gram-negative bacteremia. Monogr. Urol., *4*:November/December 1983.

McCracken, G. H., Jr., Ginsburg, C. M., Namasonthi, V., et al.: Evaluation of short-term antibiotic therapy in children with uncomplicated urinary tract infections. Pediatrics, *67*:796, 1981.

McDonald, G. S. A.: Xanthogranulomatous pyelonephritis. J. Pathol., *133*:203, 1981.

McDonough, W. D., Sandler, C. M., and Benson, G. S.: Acute focal bacterial nephritis: focal pyelonephritis that may simulate renal abscess. J. Urol., *126*:670, 1981.

Mendez, G., Isikoff, M. B., and Morillo, G.: The role of computed tomography in the diagnosis of renal and perirenal abscesses. J. Urol., *122*:582, 1979.

Mendez, G., Morillo, G., Alonso, M., et al.: Gallium-67 radionuclide imaging in acute pyelonephritis. Am. J. Radiol., *134*:17, 1980.

Mendez, G., Quencer, R. M., and Miale, A.: Gallium-67 tomographic radionuclide imaging in pyelonephritis: a report of two cases. J. Urol., *120*:613, 1978.

Merimsky, E., and Feldman, C.: Perinephric abscess: report of 19 cases. Int. Surg., *66*:79, 1981.

Meyers, M. A., Whalen, J. P., and Evans, J. A.: Diagnosis of perirenal and subcapsular masses: Anatomic-radiologic correlation. Am. J. Roentgenol. Rad. Ther. Nucl. Med., *121*:523, 1974.

Miller, T., and Phillips, S.: Pyelonephritis: The relationship between infection, renal scarring, and antimicrobial therapy. Kidney Int., *19*:654, 1981.

Miller, T. E., and North, D.: The cellular kinetics of the immune response in pyelonephritis. J. Lab. Clin. Med., *78*:891, 1971.

Miller, T. E., Stewart, E., and North, J. D. K.: Immunobacteriological aspects of pyelonephritis. Contrib. Nephrol., *16*:11, 1979.

Moller, J. C., and Kristensen, I. B.: Xanthogranulomatous pyelonephritis. Acta Pathol. Microbiol. Scand., *88*:89, 1980.

Morris, M. J., Golovsky, D., Guinness, M. D. G., et al.: The value of prophylactic antibiotics in transurethral prostatic resection: a controlled trial, with observations on the origin of postoperative infection. Br. J. Urol., *48*:479, 1976.

Musher, D. M., Throsteinsson, S. B., and Airola, V. M.,

II: Quantitative urinalysis. Diagnosing urinary tract infection in men. JAMA, *236*:2069, 1976.

Neter, E.: Estimation of *Escherichia coli* antibodies in urinary tract infection: A review and perspective. Kidney Int., *8*:S-23, 1975.

Newman, C. G. H., O'Neill, P., and Parker, A.: Pyuria in infancy, and the role of suprapubic aspiration of urine in diagnosis of infection of urinary tract. Br. Med. J., *2*:277, 1967.

Nielsen, O. S., Maigaard, S., Frimodt-Moller, N., et al.: Prophylactic antibiotics in transurethral prostatectomy. J. Urol., *126*:60, 1981.

Nimmich, W., Budde, E., Naumann, G., et al.: Long-term study of humoral immune response in patients with chronic pyelonephritis. Clin. Nephrol., *6*:428, 1976.

Olsson, P. J., Black, J. R., Gaffney, E., et al.: Reversible acute renal failure secondary to acute pyelonephritis. South. Med. J., *73*:374, 1980.

Ooi, B. S., and Chen, B. T. M.: Prevalence and site of bacteriuria in diabetes mellitus. Postgrad. Med. J., *50*:497, 1974.

Parker, J., and Kunin, C.: Pyelonephritis in young women. JAMA, *224*:585, 1973.

Patel, R., Tanaka, T., Mishkin, R., et al.: Gallium-67 scan: aid to diagnosis and treatment of renal and perirenal infections. Urology, *16*:225, 1980.

Pearman, J. W.: Prevention of urinary tract infection following spinal cord injury. Paraplegia, *9*:95, 1971.

Percival, A., Brumfitt, W., and de Louvois, J.: Serum-antibody levels as an indication of clinically inapparent pyelonephritis. Lancet, *2*:1027, 1964.

Pfau, A., and Rosenmann, E.: Unilateral chronic pyelonephritis and hypertension: coincidental or causal relationship? Am. J. Med., *65*:499, 1978.

Philpot, V. B., Jr.: The bacterial flora of urine specimens from normal adults. J. Urol., *75*:562, 1956.

Pometta, D., Rees, S. B., Younger, D., et al.: Asymptomatic bacteriuria in diabetes mellitus. N. Engl. J. Med., *276*:1118, 1967.

Preiksaitis, J. K., Thompson, L., Harding, G. K. M., et al.: A comparison of the efficacy of nalidixic acid and cephalexin in bacteriuric women and their effect on fecal and periurethral carriage of Enterobacteriaceae. J. Infect. Dis., *143*:603, 1981.

Pylkkanen, J.: Antibody-coated bacteria in the urine of infants and children with their first two urinary tract infections. Acta Paediatr. Scand., *67*:275, 1978.

Ransley, P. G., and Risdon, R. A.: The pathogenesis of reflux nephropathy. Contr. Nephrol., *16*:90, 1979.

Ratner, J. J., Thomas, V. L., Sanford, B. A., et al.: Bacteria-specific antibody in the urine of patients with acute pyelonephritis and cystitis. J. Infect. Dis., *143*:404, 1981.

Ribot, S., Gal, K., Goldblat, M., et al.: The role of anaerobic bacteria in the pathogenesis of urinary tract infections. J. Urol., *126*:852, 1981.

Richet, G., and Mayaud, C.: The course of acute renal failure in pyelonephritis and other types of interstitial nephritis. Nephron, *22*:124, 1978.

Richie, J. P., Nicholson, T. C., Hunting, D., et al.: Radiographic abnormalities in acute pyelonephritis. J. Urol., *119*:832, 1978.

Roberts, J. A., Domingue, G. J., Martin, L. N., et al.: Immunology of pyelonephritis in the primate model: live versus heat-killed bacteria. Kidney Int., *19*:297, 1981.

Roberts, J. A., Roth, J. K., Domingue, G. J., et al.: Immunology of pyelonephritis in the primate model. V. Effect of superoxide dismutase. J. Urol., *128*:1394, 1982.

Rocha, H., and Santos, L. C. S.: Relapse of urinary tract infection in the presence of urinary tract calculi: The role of bacteria within the calculi. J. Med. Microbiol., *2*:372, 1969.

Ronald, A. R., Boutros, P., and Mourtada, H.: Bacteriuria localization and response to single-dose therapy in women. JAMA, *235*:1854, 1976.

Rosenfield, A., and Glickman, M.: Acute focal bacterial nephritis (acute lobar nephronia). Radiology, *132*:553, 1978.

Rubin, R. H., Fang, L. S. T., Jones, S. R., et al.: Single-dose amoxicillin therapy for urinary tract infection. JAMA, *244*:561, 1980.

Russ, G. R., Mathew, T. H., and Caon A.: Single day or single dose treatment of urinary tract infection with Co-trimoxazole. Aust. N. Z. J. Med., *10*:604, 1980.

Saiki, J., Vaziri, N. D., and Barton, C.: Perinephric and intranephric abscesses: a review of the literature. West. J. Med., *136*:95, 1982.

Salvatierra, O., Bucklew, W. B., and Morrow, J. W.: Perinephric abscess: a report of 71 cases. J. Urol., *98*:296, 1967.

Sanford, J. P., Favour, C. B., Mao, F. H., et al.: Evaluation of the "positive" urine culture. Am. J. Med., *20*:88, 1956.

Savage, D. C. L., Adler, K., Howie, G., et al.: Controlled trial of therapy in covert bacteriuria of childhood. Lancet, *1*:358, 1975.

Scarpelli, P. T., Lamanna, S., Bigioli, F., et al.: The antibody response in chronic pyelonephritis. Clin. Nephrol., *12*:7, 1979.

Schainuck, L. I., Fouty, R., and Cutler, R. E.: Emphysematous pyelonephritis, a new case and review of previous observations. Am. J. Med., *44*:134, 1968.

Schechter, H., Leonard, C. D., and Scribner, B. H.: Chronic pyelonephritis as a cause of renal failure in dialysis candidates. Analysis of 173 patients. JAMA, *216*:514, 1971.

Scherf, H., Kollermann, M. W., and Busch, R.: Nachweis antikorperbeladener bakterien im urinsediment bei kindlichen harnwegsinfektionen. Monatssch. Kinderheilk. D., *126*:23, 1978.

Schultz, E. H., and Klorfein, E. H.: Emphysematous pyelonephritis. J. Urol., *87*:762, 1962.

Sexton, C. C., Lowman, R. M., Nyongo, A. O., et al.: Malacoplakia presenting as complete unilateral ureteral obstruction. J. Urol., *128*:139, 1982.

Shimamura, T.: Mechanisms of renal tissue destruction in an experimental acute pyelonephritis. Exp. Mol. Pathol., *34*:34, 1981.

Shimizu, S., Takimoto, Y., Niimura, T., et al.: A case of prostatic malacoplakia. J. Urol., *126*:277, 1981.

Shortliffe, L. M. D., McNeal, J. E., Wehner, N., et al.: Presistent urinary infections in a young female with bilateral renal stones: Clinicopathological Conference. J. Urol., *131*:1147, 1984.

Shortliffe, L. M. D., Wehner, N., and Stamey, T. A.: Use of a solid-phase radioimmunoassay and formalin-fixed whole bacterial antigen in the detection of antigen-specific immunoglobulin in prostatic fluid. J. Clin. Invest., *67*:790, 1981a.

Shortliffe, L. M. D., Wehner, N., and Stamey, T. A.: The detection of a local prostatic immunologic response to bacterial prostatitis. J. Urol., *125*:509, 1981b.

Silver, T. M., Kass, E. M., Thornbury, J. R., et al.: The radiological spectrum of acute pyelonephritis in adults and adolescents. Radiology, *118*:65, 1976.

Silverman, D. E., and Stamey, T. A.: Management of infection stones: The Stanford Experience. Medicine, *62*:44, 1983.

Siroky, M. B., Moylan, R. A., Austen, G., et al.: Metastatic infection secondary to genitourinary tract sepsis. Am. J. Med., *61*:351, 1976.

Slotki, I. N., and Asscher, A. W.: Prevention of scarring in experimental pyelonephritis in the rat by early antibiotic therapy. Nephron, *30*:262, 1982.

Smith, J., Holmgren, J., Ahlstedt, S., et al.: Local antibody production in experimental pyelonephritis: amount, avidity, and immunoglobulin class. Infect. Immun., *10*:411, 1974.

Smith, J. W., Jones, S. R., and Kaijser, B.: Significance of antibody-coated bacteria in urinary sediment in experimental pyelonephritis. J. Infect. Dis., *135*:577, 1977.

Sotolongo, J. R., Schiff, H., and Wulfsohn, M. A.: Radiographic findings in acute segmental pyelonephritis. Urology, *19*:335, 1982.

Spagnola, A. M.: Emphysematous pyelonephritis: a report of two cases. Am. J. Med., *64*:840, 1978.

Stamey, T. A.: Editorial: A clinical classification of urinary tract infections based upon origin. South. Med. J., *68*:934, 1975.

Stamey, T. A.: Pathogenesis and Treatment of Urinary Tract Infections. Baltimore, The Williams & Wilkins Co., 1980.

Stamey, T. A., and Bragonje, J.: Resistance of nalidixic acid: A misconception due to underdosage. JAMA, *236*:1857, 1976.

Stamey, T. A., and Pfau, A.: Some functional, pathological, bacteriologic, and chemotherapeutic characteristics of unilateral pyelonephritis in man. II. Bacteriologic and chemotherapeutic characteristics. Invest. Urol., *1*:162, 1963.

Stamey, T. A., and Pfau, A.: Urinary infections—a selective review and some observations. Calif. Med., *113*:16, 1970.

Stamey, T. A., Fair, W. R., Timothy, M. M., et al.: Serum versus urinary antimicrobial concentrations in cure of urinary-tract infections. N. Engl. J. Med., *291*:1159, 1974.

Stamey, T. A., Govan, D. E., and Palmer, J. M.: The localization and treatment of urinary tract infections: The role of bactericidal urine levels as opposed to serum levels. Medicine, *44*:1, 1965.

Stamm, W. E.: Guidelines for prevention of catheter-associated urinary tract infections. Ann. Intern. Med., *82*:386, 1975.

Stamm, W. E., Counts, G. W., Running, K. R., et al.: Diagnosis of coliform infection in acutely dysuric women. N. Engl. J. Med., *307*:463, 1982.

Stanton, M. J., and Maxted, W.: Malacoplakia: a study of the literature and current concepts of pathogenesis, diagnosis and treatment, J. Urol., *125*:139, 1981.

Sullivan, M. N., Sutter, V. L., Mins, M. M., et al.: Clinical aspects of bacteremia after manipulation of the genitourinary tract. J. Infect. Dis., *127*:49, 1973.

Sullivan, T. D., Ellerstein, N. S., and Neter, E.: The effects of ampicillin and trimethoprim/sulfamethoxazole on the periurethral flora of children with urinary tract infection. Infection, *8*:339, 1980.

Sweet, R., and Keane, W. F.: Perinephric abscess in patients with polycystic kidney disease undergoing chronic hemodialysis. Nephron, *23*:237, 1979.

Teplick, J. G., Teplick, S. K., Berinson, H., et al.: Urographic and angiographic changes in acute unilateral pyelonephritis. Clin. Radiol., *30*:59, 1978.

Thiel, G., and Spühler, O.: Urinary tract infection by catheter and the so-called infectious (episomal) resistance. Schweiz. Med. Wochenschr., *95*:1155, 1965.

Thomas, E., Hillman, B. J., and Stanisic, T.: Urinary tract infection with atypical mycobacteria. J. Urol., *124*:748, 1980.

Thomas, V., Shelokov, A., and Forland, M.: Antibody-coated bacteria in the urine and the site of urinary tract infection. N. Engl. J. Med., *290*:588, 1974.

Thorley, J. D., Jones, S. R., and Sanford, J. P.: Perinephric abscess. Medicine, *53*:441, 1974.

Tolia, B. M., Iloreta, A., Freed, S. Z., et al.: Xanthogranulomatous pyelonephritis: detailed analysis of 29 cases and a brief discussion of atypical presentations. J. Urol., *126*:437, 1981.

Tolia, B. M., Newman, H. R., Fruchtman, B., et al.: Xanthogranulomatous pyelonephritis: segmental or generalized disease? J. Urol., *124*:122, 1980.

Tolkoff-Rubin, N. E., Weber, D., Fang, L. S. T., et al.: Single-dose therapy with trimethoprim-sulfamethoxazole for urinary tract infection in women. Rev. Infect. Dis., *4*:444, 1982.

Tomashefski, J. F., and Abramowsky, C. R.: Candida-associated renal papillary necrosis. Am. J. Clin. Pathol., *75*:190, 1981.

Truesdale, B. H., Rous, S. N., and Nelson, R. P.: Perinephric abscess: a review of 26 cases. J. Urol., *118*:910, 1977.

Turck, M., Goffe, B., and Petersdorf, R. G.: The urethral catheter and urinary tract infection. J. Urol., *88*:834, 1962.

Turman, A. E., and Rutherford, C.: Emphysematous pyelonephritis with perinephric gas. J. Urol., *105*:165, 1971.

VanKirk, O. C., Go, R. T., and Wedel, V. J.: Sonographic features of xanthogranulomatous pyelonephritis. Am. J. Roentgenol., *134*:1035, 1980.

Vejlsgaard, R.: Studies on urinary infections in diabetics, III. Significant bacteriuria in pregnant diabetics and in matched controls. Acta Med. Scand., *193*:337, 1973.

Vordermark, J. S., Modarelli, R. O., and Buck, A. S.: Torulopsis pyelonephritis associated with papillary necrosis: a case report. J. Urol., *123*:96, 1980.

Wadsworth, D. E., McClennan, B. L., and Stanley, R. J.: CT of the renal mass. Urol. Radiol., *48*:85, 1982.

Warren, J. W., Anthony, W. C., Hoopes, J. M., et al.: Cephalexin for susceptible bacteriuria in afebrile, long-term catheterized patients. JAMA, *248*:454, 1982.

Warren, J. W., Platt, R., Thomas, R. J., et al.: Antibiotic irrigation and catheter-associated urinary-tract infections. N. Engl. J. Med., *299*:570, 1978.

Wientzen, R. L., McCracken, G. H., Jr., Petruska, M. L., et al.: Localization and therapy of urinary tract infections of childhood. Pediatrics, *63*:467, 1979.

Winberg, J.: Personal communication. February 1983.

Winn, R. E., and Hartstein, A. I.: Anaerobic bacterial infection and xanthogranulomatous pyelonephritis. A case report. J. Urol., *128*:567, 1982.

Witten, E. M., Myers, G. H., and Utz, D. G.: Emmett's Clinical Urography. Philadelphia, W. B. Saunders Co., 1977.

Wolff, S. M.: The treatment of gram-negative bacteremia and shock. N. Engl. J. Med., *307*:1267, 1982.

Wolverson, M. K., Jagannadharao, B., Sundaram, M., et al.: CT as a primary diagnostic method in evaluating intraabdominal abscess. Am. J. Roentgenol., *133*:1089, 1979.

Ziegler, E. J., McCutchan, J. A., Fierer, J., et al.: Treatment of gram-negative bacteremia and shock with antiserum to a mutant *Escherichia coli*. N. Engl. J. Med., *307*:1225, 1982.

CHAPTER 15

Urinary Infections in Adult Women*

LINDA M. DAIRIKI SHORTLIFFE, M.D.
THOMAS A. STAMEY, M.D.

THE NATURAL HISTORY OF URINARY TRACT INFECTIONS IN WOMEN

Bacteriuria is common in women. Surveys screening for bacteriuria have shown that about 1 per cent of schoolgirls (age 5 to 14 years) (Kunin et al., 1962) have bacteriuria and that this figure increases to about 4 per cent by young adulthood and then by an additional 1 to 2 per cent per decade of age (Fig. 15–1). In addition, the older a woman is, the more likely she is to have a reinfection (Mabeck, 1972).

Whether bacteriuria is symptomatic or asymptomatic is probably not an important distinction for prognosis. Investigators who have traced patients through symptomatic and asymptomatic infections have found that many individuals who have asymptomatic infections become symptomatic at some time, and many who experience symptomatic infections then become asymptomatic with time alone. When Mabeck (1972) followed 23 untreated nonpregnant women with acute symptomatic cystitis, 21 lost their symptoms after 4 weeks but before their infection had disappeared. Conversely, when 12 pregnant women with asymptomatic untreated bacteriuria were followed, 7 of the 12 became symptomatic at some time after diagnosis (McFadyen et al., 1973). A distinction between these two groups is therefore difficult and probably not worthwhile.

Although the course of recurrent infections detected in childhood is discussed in Chapter 16, Urinary Infections in Infants and Children, the course of these infections in adult females is rarely accompanied by renal scarring and dysfunction. Little is known about the natural history of untreated bacteriuria in women because most are treated when they are diagnosed, but a few studies in which treatment with antibiotics is compared with placebo have been done. These show that 57 to 80 per cent of bacteriuric women who are untreated, or treated with placebo, clear their infections spontaneously (Guttmann, 1973; Mabeck, 1972). Mabeck (1972) found that 8 of 53 bacteriuric women placed on placebo needed to be treated with an antibiotic because of symptoms, but 32 of the remaining 45 cleared without treatment within a month, and 43 of the 45 had spontaneously cleared of bacteriuria within 5 months; only two remained persistently bacteriuric. Of those that cleared, ten became reinfected and another ten recurred with the same organism after a year; 46 per cent of the untreated women had become bacteriuric by a year later.

When women with recurrent bacteriuria are followed after treatment, about one sixth (37/219) have a very high recurrence rate (2.6 infections per year) while the remainder have only 0.32 recurrences per year (Mabeck, 1972). Similar separation was seen in a prospective study, in which only 28.6 per cent of 60 women who experienced their first symptomatic urinary tract infection had recurrent infections over the first 18 months of observation, as opposed to 82.5 per cent recurrences in 106 women who

---

*Some passages in this chapter are reproduced with permission from Stamey, T. A.: Pathogenesis and Treatment of Urinary Tract Infections. Baltimore, Williams & Wilkins Co., 1980.

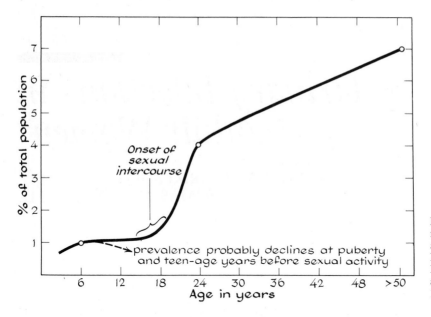

Figure 15–1. Prevalence of bacteriuria in females as a function of age. (From Stamey, T. A.: The Prevention of Recurrent Urinary Infections. New York, Science and Medicine Publishing Co., 1973. Used by permission.)

had had previous urinary infections (Harrison et al., 1974). Other investigators also have found that the probability of recurrent urinary infection increases with the number of previous infections and decreases in inverse proportion to the elapsed time between the first and second infections (Mabeck, 1972). Of these recurrent infections, 71 to 73 per cent are caused by reinfection with different organisms, rather than recurrence with the same organism (Mabeck, 1972; Guttmann, 1973).

Women with frequent recurrent infections have a rate of 0.13 to 0.22 urinary infections per month (1.6 to 2.6 infections per year) when the infections are treated with antibiotics (Guttmann, 1973; Kraft and Stamey, 1977; Mabeck, 1972). Most reinfections occurred after 2 weeks (Harrison et al., 1974) and within 5 months (Mabeck, 1972), and most occurred early in this interval (Kraft and Stamey, 1977) (Fig. 15–2). Rates of recurrence were independent of bladder dysfunction, radiologic changes of chronic pyelonephritis, and vesicoureteral reflux (Guttmann, 1973). The reinfections did not occur evenly over time. In the Stanford series, in which 23 women with frequent recurrent infections were studied with monthly urine cultures when asymptomatic and immediate cultures when symptomatic for cystitis for a mean of 3 years, 34 per cent of infections were followed by infection-free intervals of at least 6 months (average 12.8 months), and 22 of the 23 women had such an interval (Fig. 15–3); however, even these long intervals were followed by further infections (Kraft and Stamey, 1977). Similarly, Mabeck (1972) noted that some women who had frequent reinfections showed unpredictable pauses in their recurrences, further evidence to suggest that reinfections may occur in clusters.

When the Stanford data (Kraft and Stamey, 1977) on recurrent urinary infections in highly susceptible females are analyzed by examining sets of infections separated by remissions of at least 6 months, 69 per cent of the sets contain only one infection (Fig. 15–4). After this first set, the remaining sets show a 33 per cent remission rate in infections. So, a patient who has two or more infections without 6 months elapsing between any two of them, has only a 33 per cent probability of remaining free of infection for the next 6 months. Therefore, if antimicrobial prophylaxis is started after the second or any succeeding infection within a set, about a third of the women will be treated

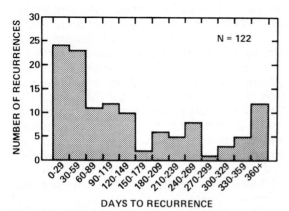

Figure 15–2. Days between recurrent urinary infections grouped by 30-day intervals. (From Kraft, J. K., and Stamey, T. A.: Medicine, *56*:55, 1977. Used by permission.)

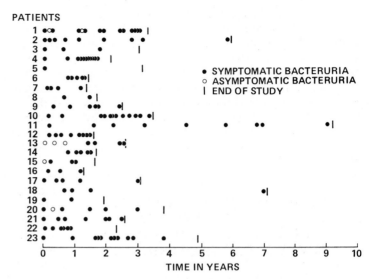

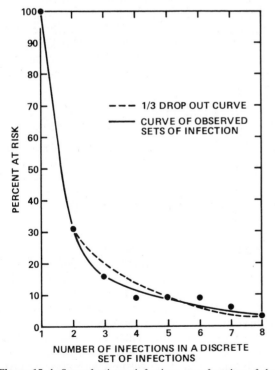

Figure 15–3. Occurrence of urinary infections in 23 women with frequent recurrent bacteriuria (From Kraft, J. K., and Stamey, T. A.: Medicine, 56:55, 1977. Used by permission.)

unnecessarily. The remaining two thirds of women still risk more infections.

Whether a patient receives no treatment at all, or short-term, long-term, or prophylactic antimicrobial treatment, the risk of recurrent

bacteriuria remains the same; treatment appears to alter only the time of recurrence. Asscher (1973) found that reinfections occurred in 17 (34 per cent) of patients treated with a 7-day course of nitrofurantoin, and 13 (29 per cent) of patients receiving placebo during a 3 to 5 year follow-up. Mabeck (1972) found that 46 per cent (20/43) of untreated patients had a recurrent infection by 12 months compared with about 40 per cent of treated patients having a recurrence. Both studies suggest that it makes little difference whether a urinary infection is cured with an antibiotic or is allowed to clear spontaneously—the ultimate risk of recurrent bacteriuria remains the same. Moreover, patients with frequent urinary infections who take prophylactic antimicrobial agents for extended periods (6 months or more) may decrease their infections during the time of prophylaxis, but the rate of infection returns to the pretreatment rate after prophylaxis is stopped (Vosti, 1975; Stamm et al., 1980). Even long interruptions in the pattern of recurrence, therefore, do not appear to alter the patient's basic susceptibility to infections.

The long-term effects of uncomplicated recurrent urinary infections are not completely known, but so far no association between recurrent infections and renal scarring, hypertension, or progressive renal azotemia has been established (Asscher et al., 1973; Freeman, 1975). Indeed, one investigator was unable to find a single case of unequivocal nonobstructive chronic pyelonephritis in 22 patients in whom chronic pyelonephritis was the cause of end-stage renal failure (Schechter et al., 1971). Similar data were reported by Huland and Busch (1982).

Figure 15–4. Sets of urinary infections as a function of the fraction of women who remain at risk of recurrent infection. After two or more infections within a set, there is a two-thirds probability of another infection during the next 6 months. A set is defined as any infection or group of infections preceded and followed by 6 months of remission. (From Kraft, J. K., and Stamey, T. A.: Medicine, 56:55, 1977. Used by permission.)

Although short-term antimicrobial treatment and prophylaxis do not seem to affect the course of recurrent urinary tract infections, pregnancy does affect this course. In these women the prevalence and rate of recurrent infection are the same, but their bacteriuria progresses to acute clinical pyelonephritis more frequently than in nonpregnant women. This variation in the natural history of recurrent infections in females is discussed in a later section.

SYMPTOMATIC INFECTIONS VERSUS THOSE INFECTIONS DETECTED ON SCREENING SURVEYS FOR BACTERIURIA

The prevalence of bacteriuria in females (Fig. 15–1) varies from less than 1 per cent in infants to 10 per cent or more in older women (Stamey, 1980). About 3 per cent to 6 per cent of sexually active women of childbearing age are bacteriuric on screening surveys; when bacteriuria is detected by screening surveys, it is conveniently called screening bacteriuria and abbreviated ScBU. Three questions need to be answered. What do we know about the urinary tracts of women with ScBU? Do they represent a separate population from those who have symptomatic infections? Is detection of their ScBU worthwhile? Answers to these questions as they relate to infants and children are discussed in Chapter 16.

ARE ADULT WOMEN WITH ScBU AT RISK OF SERIOUS RENAL DAMAGE?

In the late 1950's and early 1960's, several excellent epidemiologic studies (see Stamey, 1980 for review) were published on the 3 per cent to 6 per cent of adult women with ScBU; these studies examined such demographic parameters as age, blood pressure, concentrating ability, serologic titers, and proteinuria. Unfortunately, they never answered two critical questions: What do the kidneys look like, and what is the past history of these ScBU patients related to their bacteriuria?

Asscher and his group at Cardiff, Wales (Sussman et al., 1969; Asscher et al., 1969a; Asscher et al., 1973), answered these questions by screening 3578 asymptomatic, nonpregnant women between the ages of 20 and 65 years. Sixty-nine per cent of the 107 bacteriuric subjects (3 per cent of those screened) had had bladder irritative symptoms within a year before their bacteriuria was detected, whereas only 18 per cent of matched controls without bacteriuria had similar symptoms. These observations established that women with ScBU are not asymptomatic.

Of more importance, these investigators obtained intravenous urograms on 87 per cent of the 107 bacteriuric women and 57 per cent of 88 matched nonbacteriuric controls. One of us (TAS) had the unique opportunity to review all of these urograms in Cardiff: Every patient had a normal volume of renal cortex. Thirty-four per cent of the urograms in bacteriuric women were abnormal, but these abnormalities were minor scars, rarely involving more than a single calyx, small calculi in eight patients (four of them in the scarred kidneys), nonsurgical hydroureter and hydronephrosis, and even less important findings, such as rotation of the kidney or simple cyst. None of these patients had progressive renal cortical destruction, even though half were over 45 years of age. Moreover, when 90 per cent of the 107 bacteriuric subjects were restudied with intravenous urograms 3 to 5 years later (Asscher et al., 1973), there was no evidence that the bacteriuria had caused hypertension, azotemia, or further renal scarring. These classic studies clearly established that while women with ScBU have three times the number of abnormalities in their kidneys as matched control subjects (of the same age and parity) without bacteriuria, these abnormalities do not represent serious renal disease.

DO WOMEN WITH ScBU DIFFER FROM THOSE WITH SYMPTOMATIC BACTERIURIA?

Gaymans and his colleagues asked this question in their general practice office (Gaymans et al., 1976). They screened 95 per cent of their female patient population over the age of 14 years (1758 women); the prevalence of ScBU was 4.7 per cent, with 2.7 per cent in the age group 15 to 24 years and 9.3 per cent in women 65 years and older. Ninety per cent of the infections were caused by *E. coli*. All 1758 women were followed closely for 1 year, during which time 105 women (6 per cent) had symptomatic infections; 29 per cent of those with symptomatic infections had pre-existing ScBU. From these data, they calculated that the probability of acquiring a symptomatic infection was seven times greater in women with known ScBU than in those without (p< 0.0001).

In addition to the one third (29 per cent) with ScBU who developed symptomatic infections, another one third had only transient bacteriuria. This left only one third of Gaymans' patients who had continuous ScBU; they were older (51.2 years), had fewer upper tract symptoms, and had fewer abnormalities on intravenous urograms than those patients with ScBU who developed acute symptoms (who averaged 41 years of age).

IS DETECTION OF ScBU IN ADULT WOMEN A WORTHWHILE PUBLIC HEALTH EFFORT?

Asscher and his colleagues (1969b) emphasized that the two requirements for a useful screening procedure are that it "detects disease before irreversible damage has occurred and that the disease so detected may be effectively treated." We should add to the first requirement, of course, that the disease under study should be serious enough that detection is worthwhile. As to the second requirement, the Cardiff study showed that 80 per cent of the subjects with ScBU were cured with 7 days of oral nitrofurantoin therapy; this 80 per cent cure rate is the same as that for treating symptomatic acute infections (see Chapter 14). At follow-up a year later, however, only 55 per cent of the treated women with ScBU remained without infection, which differed little from the number of women who had spontaneous remission of their infection with placebo. Asscher and his group (1969b) concluded that successful therapy in ScBU was little different in the long run from the natural history of spontaneous remissions. Similar epidemiologic data in children is considered in Chapter 16. As will be seen, however, in the next section on urinary infections in pregnancy, screening for bacteriuria in the first trimester of pregnancy probably represents the only time that screening for bacteriuria is worthwhile.

COMMENT ON ScBU

We believe that both symptomatic and ScBU infections are integral parts of the same disease process, i.e., urinary tract infections. It is unlikely that there is any merit in separating those patients with symptomatic bacteriuria from those with ScBU.

We conclude this section with a historical note. Once the diagnosis of asymptomatic bacteriuria was placed on a firm statistical basis of $\geq 10^5$ bacteria per ml (however unsatisfactory that basis is for dealing with symptomatic infections) in 1956 (Kass, 1956), a powerful tool was placed in the hands of epidemiologic investigators for door-to-door population surveys. Indeed, there were great hopes in the late 1950's and early 1960's that the serious consequences of diseases related directly or indirectly to "pyelonephritis," such as renal failure and hypertension (Miall et al., 1962), pyelonephritis of pregnancy (Savage et al., 1967), and diabetes (Pometta et al., 1967), might be averted by early detection and treatment.

It is fair to comment in 1984 that these hopes have not been fulfilled; indeed, the work by Asscher's and Gaymans' groups have placed ScBU in its proper perspective. To that perspective, however, one must add that (1) the adult kidney (in the absence of stones, obstruction, and analgesic abuse) is astonishingly resistant to renal destruction by bacteria; (2) that hypertension, if present in patients with ScBU, is a minimal effect and the physician will do better to treat the hypertension than to treat the bacteriuria (Gallagher et al., 1965; Asscher et al., 1973); and (3) that even in progressive renal failure, bacteriuria cannot be shown to be responsible for the progression (Johnson and Smythe, 1969).

Many of us who spent much of our time seeing patients with urinary infections could not believe even in the 1960's that there was this great reservoir of silent, asymptomatic renal disease in the general population. Our suspicion was confirmed when Bill Asscher of Cardiff in 1968 allowed us to review the 143 intravenous urograms from patients and control subjects; serious renal disease, caused by bacteriuria, simply was absent in these individuals.

The failure of routine antimicrobial therapy to be much better than spontaneous cures argues against detection of ScBU by epidemiologic survey (Asscher et al., 1969b). While long-term therapy in patients with ScBU might be beneficial, patient compliance would be poor in an asymptomatic population. Moreover, the compelling observation of Gaymans and his group (1976) that the heterogeneity of the ScBU population per se requires at least 6 months of repeated cultures to intelligently separate the ScBU population into meaningful groups, is another argument against a public health approach.

All of these issues lead to the conclusion that public money is better spent in educating the physician on how to diagnose, treat, and assess the renal risk to the symptomatic patient in his office, rather than screening and treating asymptomatic populations with ScBU.

As will be seen in Chapter 16, Urinary Infections in Infancy and Childhood, the same conclusion applies to children, despite their great susceptibility to renal scarring from bacteriuria with ureteral reflux.

URINARY INFECTIONS IN PREGNANCY

Although the prevalence of bacteriuria does not change with the occurrence of pregnancy, certain anatomic and physiologic alterations associated with this state probably do change the course of bacteriuria during pregnancy. These changes may cause pregnant women to be more susceptible to pyelonephritis and may require alteration of therapy. These changes have been well summarized in several reviews (Davison and Lindheimer, 1978; Waltzer, 1981).

Anatomic and Physiologic Changes During Pregnancy

Increase in Renal Size. Renal length increases approximately 1 cm during normal pregnancy. It is thought that this does not represent true hypertrophy but is the result of increased renal vascular and interstitial volume. No histologic changes have been identified in renal biopsies (Waltzer, 1981).

Smooth Muscle Atony of the Collecting System and Bladder. The collecting system, especially the ureters, undergoes decreased peristalsis during pregnancy, and most women in their third trimester show significant ureteral dilatation (Kincaid-Smith, 1979; Davison and Lindheimer, 1978; Waltzer, 1981) (Fig. 15–5). This hydroureter has been attributed both to the muscle-relaxing effects of increased progesterone during pregnancy and to mechanical obstruction of the ureters by the enlarging uterus at the pelvic brim. Progesterone-induced smooth muscle relaxation may also cause an increased bladder capacity (Waltzer, 1981).

Bladder Changes. The enlarging uterus displaces the bladder superiorly and anteriorly. The bladder becomes hyperemic and may appear congested endoscopically (Waltzer, 1981). Estrogen stimulation probably causes bladder

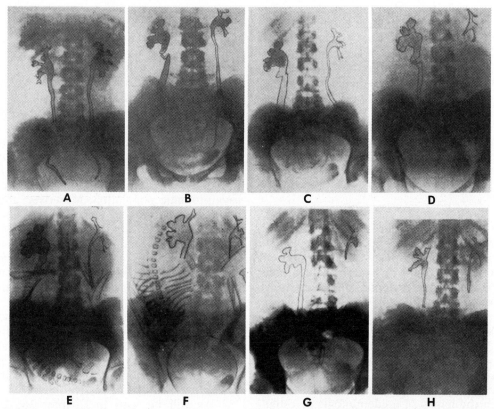

Figure 15–5. Progressive hydroureter and hydronephrosis observed on intravenous urogram during a normal pregnancy. *A,* 15 weeks; *B,* 18 weeks; *C,* 22 weeks; *D,* 26 weeks; *E,* 34 weeks; *F,* 39 weeks; *G,* 1 week post partum; *H,* 6 weeks post partum. *A* shows bilateral hydroureter and hydronephrosis as early as 15 weeks. *B* to *H* are successive urograms from one patient during a normal pregnancy. Dilation occurs mainly on the right side, and both urinary tracts are normal by 6 weeks after delivery. (From Hundley, J. M., Walton, H. J., Hibbits, J. T., Siegal, J. A., and Brack, C. P.: Am. J. Obstet. Gynecol., *30*:625, 1935.)

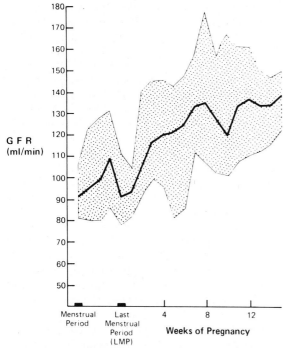

Figure 15–6. Weekly 24-hour creatinine clearance in eight women starting before conception and measured through the twelfth gestational week. The solid line represents the mean glomerular filtration rate (GFR) and the stippled area the range. (From Davison, J. M., and Lindheimer, M. D.: Clin. Obstet. Gynecol., *21*:411, 1978. Used by permission.)

hypertrophy as well as squamous changes of the urethra (Waltzer, 1981).

Augmented Renal Function. The transient increases in glomerular filtration rate and renal plasma flow during pregnancy have been well summarized by several authors and are probably secondary to the increase in cardiac output (Zacur and Mitch, 1977; Davison and Lindheimer, 1978; Kincaid-Smith, 1979; Waltzer, 1981) (Fig. 15–6). Glomerular filtration increases by 30 to 50 per cent and urinary protein excretion increases. The significance of these physiologic changes is apparent when the normal serum creatinine and urea nitrogen values for pregnant women are surveyed (Table 15–1). Values considered normal in nonpregnant women may represent renal insufficiency during pregnancy.

TABLE 15–1. Average Values for Serum Creatinine and Urea Nitrogen

	Nonpregnant Females	Pregnant Females
Serum creatine	0.7 mg/dl	0.5 mg/dl
Urea nitrogen	13.0 mg/dl	9.0 mg/dl

Data from Davison, J. M., and Lindheimer, M. D.: Clin. Obstet. Gynecol., *21*:411, 1978. Used by permission.

Davison and Lindheimer (1978) recommend that pregnant females with serum creatinine greater than 0.8 mg per dl or urea nitrogen greater than 13 mg per dl undergo further evaluation of renal function. Similarly, urinary protein in pregnancy is not considered abnormal until greater than 300 mg of protein in 24 hours is excreted.

Screening Bacteriuria in Pregnancy

The prevalence of bacteriuria found in screening pregnant females (ScBUP) is the same as that in nonpregnant females; this has been well reviewed by Stamey (1980). Beginning with a prevalence of 1.1 per cent in young schoolgirls (Kunin et al., 1962), bacteriuria appears to increase approximately 1 to 2 per cent per decade of age to attain a rate of 10 per cent by 55 to 64 years. From these data, approximately 4 to 6 per cent of females of childbearing age are bacteriuric. In Sweet's extensive review of 26 studies on the prevalence of bacteriuria in pregnant females, all of which used differing criteria to determine bacteriuria, a rate of 2.5 to 8.7 per cent is cited (Sweet, 1977). Most of the rates ranged between 4 and 7 per cent—rates no different from those found in nonpregnant females. Furthermore, of those women who had uninfected urine when first seen, fewer than 1 per cent (1/186 women) developed bacteriuria during the pregnancy in one study (McFadyen et al., 1973), and approximately 2 per cent (6/279) developed it in another (Elder et al., 1971). These are the low rates expected if the prevalence of bacteriuria in females is unaffected by pregnancy.

The site of bacteriuria in the pregnant woman probably also reflects only the situation before conception. In two studies that localized the origin of the bacteriuria, one using the Stamey ureteral catheterization technique and the other the Fairley bladder washout, upper tract infections were found in 44 and 24.5 per cent of pregnant women, respectively (Fairley et al., 1966; Heineman and Lee, 1973). In nonpregnant females with recurrent bacteriuria, Stamey has reported about a 50 per cent probability that the origin is in the upper tracts (Stamey, 1980). Using other techniques, which may reflect severity of tissue infection rather than location of infection, the results are similar; approximately 50 per cent of women with ScBUP are fluorescent antibody–positive (Fa +) (Harris et al., 1976). Fairley and associates found that the site of infection is unrelated to the likelihood that pyelonephritis will develop during pregnancy, but localization to the upper tracts may identify those women who are likely to have persistent post-partum bacteriuria (Fairley et al., 1973).

Natural History of Bacteriuria During Pregnancy

Whether treated or not, pregnant females with bacteriuria are at high risk of suffering recurrent bacteriuria. In one study that examined 148 pregnant women placed on placebo for bacteriuria, 18 per cent (27/148) developed acute pyelonephritis, 13.5 per cent (20/148) spontaneously cleared their infection, and 66 per cent (98/148) remained bacteriuric (Elder et al., 1971). When infections are cured by antibiotics, 16 and 27 per cent of the women in two studies developed a recurrent infection later in the pregnancy (Elder et al., 1971; Harris, 1979). Kincaid-Smith (1979) has shown that 6 months after delivery the rate of recurrent bacteriuria in treated women was no different from that in untreated women. Indeed, in a long-term follow-up of women who had ScBUP, 38 per cent were bacteriuric 14 years later regardless of the initial treatment (Zinner and Kass, 1971); others have reported bacteriuria to recur or persist in 20 to 30 per cent of women post partum (Sweet, 1977). Leveno and associates (1981) have shown that this risk of recurrent infection in pregnant women is independent of the duration of antimicrobial therapy and the site of infection in the urinary tract (Leveno et al., 1981). All this evidence suggests that recurrent bacteriuria in the pregnant female merely reflects a segment of the natural history of recurrent infections in females and is not a peculiarity of pregnancy.

The incidence of acute clinical pyelonephritis in pregnant women with bacteriuria is significantly increased over that in nonpregnant women. Nonpregnant women with uncomplicated urinary infections rarely develop pyelonephritis. Acute bacterial pyelonephritis is, on the other hand, frequent in pregnant women, occurring in 1 to 4 per cent of all pregnant women (Kass, 1973). In his review of 18 papers, Sweet (1977) reported that 13.5 to 65 per cent of women with ScBUP developed acute pyelonephritis during pregnancy; the average was 28 per cent. In women without ScBUP, only about 1.4 per cent developed acute pyelonephritis during pregnancy. Clearly, ScBUP increases a woman's risk of developing pyelonephritis during pregnancy.

Of the women who develop pyelonephritis during pregnancy, 60 to 75 per cent get it during the third trimester (Cunningham et al., 1973), when hydronephrosis and stasis in the urinary tract are most pronounced. Ten to 20 per cent of pregnant women who get pyelonephritis develop it again before or just after the delivery (Cunningham et al., 1973; Gilstrap et al., 1981). Moreover, a third of pregnant women who develop pyelonephritis have a documented prior history of pyelonephritis (Gilstrap et al., 1981). Treatment of ScBUP decreases the incidence of acute pyelonephritis during pregnancy from 13.5 to 65 per cent to 2.9 per cent (range of 0 to 5.3 per cent) (Sweet, 1977).

In Sweet's excellent review of bacteriuria and pyelonephritis during pregnancy (1977), he suggests that patients with a renal source of bacteriuria are more likely to have persistent post-partum bacteriuria than those with cystitis alone. In addition, those women with persistent bacteriuria may have an increased incidence of impaired creatinine clearance and urinary concentrating ability, and an increased incidence of radiographic changes compatible with chronic pyelonephritis. His review of 12 studies revealed that follow-up intravenous urograms in pregnant women with bacteriuria show an 8 to 33 per cent incidence of radiologic changes compatible with chronic pyelonephritis; the incidence of all urinary tract abnormalities in this group was 18 to 80 per cent. Zinner and Kass (1971) estimated that approximately 10 per cent of bacteriuric pregnant females have pyelographic evidence of pyelonephritis, and in their study these abnormalities were most common in women who had bacteriuria 10 to 14 years after their pregnancy. The highest incidence of radiographic changes of pyelonephritis was found in women who had their infections localized to their upper urinary tracts (Fairley et al., 1966). In this study, abbreviated intravenous urograms were performed within a few days of localization of the infection by ureteral catheterization. Thirty per cent (6) of women with upper urinary tract infections revealed radiographic renal abnormalities compatible with chronic pyelonephritis on the side to which the infection was localized, and 10 per cent (2) had nonexcretion of one kidney with infection in the contralateral one. No patient with an infection localized to the bladder showed radiographic evidence of pyelonephritis. In their evaluation of renal function, Zinner and Kass (1971) found that women who had bacteriuria during their pregnancy, and had it again 10 to 14 years later on follow-up, had significantly lower mean maximum urine osmolalities than those who were not bacteriuric on follow-up; others have found evidence of decreased creatinine clearance and concentrating ability in bacteriuric women post partum (Sweet, 1977). It is unlikely, however, that uncomplicated bacteriuria in pregnant women produces changes in kidney appearance or function different from those found in nonpregnant bacteriuric women. After following 40 bacteriuric women during pregnancy, Kincaid-Smith (1979) stated that there was no difference in renal size or function between 6 months and 4 years after delivery. Pregnancy, therefore, may provide the opportunity for bacteriuria to be discovered, but this bacteriuria probably reflects only a susceptibility to urinary infection that was present at conception. The increased likelihood that bacteriuria may progress to acute pyelonephritis during pregnancy alters the morbidity of bacteriuria for this group.

Complications Associated with Bacteriuria During Pregnancy

Prematurity and Perinatal Mortality. In the preantibiotic era, pregnant women with bacterial pyelonephritis had a high rate of infant prematurity and associated perinatal mortality (Gilstrap et al., 1981), but now acute pyelonephritis is aggressively treated with antibiotics. Whether women who have been treated for pyelonephritis or screening bacteriuria during pregnancy still deliver infants with increased prematurity and perinatal mortality is controversial. Studies designed to answer this question have not done so (Zinner, 1979). Evaluation of these studies is difficult because they define prematurity by different criteria (weight versus gestational age), define bacteriuria in different ways, fail to report statistically significant differences, and fail to mention which patients were treated. Sweet (1977) has critically reviewed these studies and concludes that the conflicting data can suggest only that pregnant women with bacteriuria have an increased incidence of prematurity. In a recent study of 487 women with acute pyelonephritis and 248 women with asymptomatic bacteriuria, Gilstrap and associates (1981) showed that ante-partum renal infections that were treated, whether symptomatic or not, did not affect pregnancy outcome. Intrapartum pyelonephritis was associated with an increased incidence of low birth weight babies, but the number of patients studied was too small for significance. In a retrospective analysis of data collected for the Col-

laborative Perinatal Project of the National Institute of Neurological and Communicative Disorders and Stroke, which analyzed over 50,000 births between 1959 and 1966, only placental growth retardation (defined as placental weight less than 40 per cent of normal) of eight prenatal disorders (amniotic fluid infection, congenital malformation, umbilical cord compression, large placental infarcts, abruptio placentae, growth-retarded placenta, Rh disease, and placenta previa) studied was significantly increased in frequency in pregnant women with pyuria and bacteriuria over that observed in normal pregnant women (Naeye, 1979). When analyzed, the higher combined perinatal mortality rate for these eight common disorders in the infected (42/1000) compared with the uninfected (21/1000) could be attributed to greater mortality from the noninfectious disorders that were accompanied by urinary infection within 15 days of delivery.

Whether clinical pyelonephritis during pregnancy causes increased risk of prematurity is still unclear, but bacteriuria in the symptomatic or asymptomatic pregnant female should be treated to avoid pyelonephritis and its possible sequelae in the mother.

Maternal Anemia. Although several studies suggest that bacteriuria untreated during pregnancy is associated with maternal anemia, not all studies support this. Some difficulties in interpreting the results of these surveys have been caused by inadequate documentation of bacteriuria. In one survey in which urine cultures were obtained by suprapubic aspiration, the data suggest that pregnant patients requiring three or more treatments for bacteriuria have lower levels of serum hemoglobin and folate than controls (McFadyen et al., 1973). In another study from England, investigators showed a statistically significant difference in the incidence of anemia between 410 bacteriuric pregnant women and 409 control pregnant women (Williams et al., 1973). In this survey, 14.6 per cent of bacteriuric women and 10 per cent of control women were anemic at the first prenatal visit. This separation increased during the third trimester (32 weeks), when 25 per cent of women treated with placebo alone had anemia, but only 16.8 of those women treated with antibiotics had anemia. Furthermore, in the 31 untreated (placebo-treated) bacteriuric women who subsequently developed pyelonephritis, the incidence of anemia was 45.2 per cent. These investigators concluded that "untreated bacteriuria increases the likelihood of developing anaemia during pregnancy and that this risk is enhanced by the development of acute pyelonephritis, even if it is treated promptly" (Williams et al., 1973).

Maternal Hypertension and Eclampsia. The data relating bacteriuria during pregnancy and hypertension and toxemia are inconclusive.

Management of Bacteriuria in Pregnancy

DIAGNOSIS OF BACTERIURIA

Since pregnant women with bacteriuria suffer such an increased risk of developing acute pyelonephritis and other complications, bacteriuria should be sought at the intial prenatal visit. The diagnosis of bacteriuria in pregnant females carries the same caveats discussed in Chapter 14 in the section on the diagnosis of bacteriuria. Even though urine specimens obtained by a nurse with the patient in the lithotomy position may be cumbersome, these special cultures might be worthwhile in the pregnant female in whom culture results are abnormal or equivocal, especially since these women are examined in the lithotomy position in any case. Suprapubic aspiration of urine will detect true bacteriuria also. Urethral catheterization, which may introduce bacteria into the bladder, should be avoided in the pregnant female, if possible. Attempts to localize the infection to upper or lower urinary tract are not thought to be helpful in the management of the bacteriuria, since recurrence rates are independent of the site of infection (Leveno et al., 1981).

If a pregnant woman has acute clinical pyelonephritis that is unresponsive to antimicrobial treatment within 48 to 72 hours, or if additional urinary tract obstruction exists, radiographic evaluation is needed. Since radiation of the fetus should be avoided, an abbreviated intravenous urogram consisting of an initial abdominal plain film, a 15-minute film, and then another film at an hour only if the collecting system was not visualized at 15 minutes is usually sufficient to determine the site and cause of obstruction, such as a stone (Waltzer, 1981). Unfortunately, renal ultrasound, which is ordinarily so useful for detecting urinary tract obstruction, is inadequate for detecting obstruction in pregnancy because normal pregnancy is accompanied by hydronephrosis. Although little is written about the use of renal nuclear scans in pregnancy, the low radiation exposure might make these studies useful for locating obstruction.

TREATMENT OF URINARY INFECTIONS IN PREGNANCY

Bacteriuria. When symptomatic or asymptomatic bacteriuria of pregnancy is diagnosed, the bacteriuria should be treated to avoid the complications already discussed. Selection of an antimicrobial agent to treat the bacteriuria must be made, however, with special considerations given to maternal and fetal toxicity. The physiologic changes of pregnancy may decrease tissue and serum drug concentrations. Maternal expanded fluid volume, distribution of drug in the fetus, increased renal blood flow, and increased glomerular filtration will decrease serum drug concentration.

Although the adverse effects of most antibiotics are the same whether or not the patient is pregnant, certain antimicrobial agents should be avoided in pregnancy (Schwarz, 1981; McGeown, 1981; Sweet, 1977; Harris, 1980; Ries and Kaye, 1974). Tetracyclines are contraindicated throughout pregnancy because they may cause acute maternal liver decompensation and fetal malformations. The chelating action of tetracycline cause hypoplasia and staining of the child's deciduous teeth. The estolate salt of erythromycin is contraindicated because it can cause cholestatic jaundice in pregnant females. Chloramphenicol, in addition to its adverse affects in adults, may accumulate to toxic concentrations in the neonate because infants may lack the ability to metabolize or excrete the drug; this toxic neonatal effect, "the gray syndrome," may cause cardiovascular collapse and high neonatal mortality. Sulfa preparations, especially long-acting forms, should be avoided during the third trimester of pregnancy because they compete for fetal billirubin binding sites on albumin and can cause neonatal hyperbilirubinemia and kernicterus. Although it is undocumented as a teratogen (Brumfitt and Pursell, 1973), most investigators feel that trimethoprim, a folic acid antagonist, should be avoided during the first trimester of pregnancy because of its potential teratogenic activity. The nitrofurantoins, a group of oxidizing drugs, can cause a hemolytic anemia in patients and fetuses with a glucose-6-phosphate dehydrogenase deficiency, a defect found in about 10 per cent of blacks in the United States, Sardinians, non-Ashkenazi Jews, Greeks, Eti-Turks, and Thais (Thompson, 1969). In these people, regeneration of glutathione, which is partially responsible for maintaining red blood cell integrity, is impaired by the enzyme deficiency, and nitrofurantoin oxidizes the hemoglobin to methemoglobin, which is further degraded. Aminoglycosides have no specific complications associated with pregnancy, but they may cause ototoxicity and nephrotoxity in both fetus and mother.

Although few data on human fetal toxicity of antimicrobial agents are available, several antimicrobial drugs that appear to be relatively safe during pregnancy have been identified (Schwarz, 1981; Harris, 1980; Sweet, 1977; Weinstein, 1979). Ideally, these drugs should achieve high urinary and low serum concentrations and affect only the bacteria. Since the penicillins and cephalosporins inhibit growth of the bacterial cell wall, and human cells have a cytoplasmic membrane without a cell wall, these drugs act specifically on the bacteria. Methenamine mandelate, when excreted in an acid urine, forms formaldehyde, which is nonspecifically bactericidal. Since the activity of this agent is dependent upon a urine pH below 5.5, this drug, although safe, has limited use. In fact, in one study in which pregnant women with bacteriuria were either placed in a control group or treated with methenamine mandelate or methenamine hippurate for the remainder of the pregnancy, only a small reduction in the incidence of pyelonephritis was noted in the treated groups. These results are poor when compared with the results of other antimicrobial agents and probably reflect the somewhat low efficacy of the methenamine. The short-acting sulfonamides can be safely used during the first two trimesters of pregnancy, since the fetus in utero handles excess unconjugated bilirubin through the placenta. Similarly, nitrofurantoin has commonly been used in pregnancy during the first two trimesters but may be contraindicated at term because it can cause a hemolytic anemia in neonates with an immature enzyme system.

Only the penicillins (penicillin, ampicillin, and synthetic penicillins) and cephalosporins, given orally or parenterally, are thought to be safe and effective during any phase of pregnancy. In this situation, oral penicillin with its extremely high urinary concentrations may be a particularly effective and inexpensive agent. Of course, as with any drugs, these drugs may still cause difficulties in women who suffer sensitivities to them. Methenamine is also probably safe during pregnancy, but it is also less efficacious than other drugs. Nitrofurantoin (in patients without glucose-6-phosphate dehydrogenase deficiencies) and the sulfonamides are generally safe during the first two trimesters. Although trimethoprim-sulfamethoxazole has been used during all phases of pregnancy without a docu-

mented increase in fetal abnormalities related to it (Brumfitt and Pursell, 1973), it probably should not be considered the drug of choice for simple infections, particularly during the first and third trimesters.

Once an appropriate antimicrobial agent is selected, the patient may be treated for 3 days (see Chapter 14, under duration of therapy); long-term treatment does not appear to reduce the risk of recurrent bacteriuria (Leveno et al., 1981). It is important to reculture the urine 1 to 2 days after treatment is completed to ensure that the urine is sterile. If it is not, the cause of bacteriuria must be determined to be lack of resolution, bacterial persistence, or reinfection. If the infection is unresolved, proper selection and administration of another drug will probably solve the problem. If the problem is bacterial persistence or rapid reinfection, then antimicrobial suppression of infection or prophylaxis throughout the remainder of the pregnancy should be considered. The antimicrobial agents and their dosage for this long-term treatment are discussed later in this chapter. When a prophylactic or suppressive agent is selected, however, the contraindications imposed by pregnancy should still be considered.

Pregnant women with acute clinical pyelonephritis should be admitted to the hospital for treatment with parenteral agents. Drugs with adequate serum and urine levels and the least potential maternal and fetal toxicity should be selected. Patients who fail to improve after 2 to 3 days of appropriate antimicrobial therapy should be evaluated for complications, such as obstruction or perinephric abscess. Since these patients suffer an increased risk of repeated pyelonephritis during their pregnancy (Gilstrap et al., 1981; Cunningham et al., 1973), they should either be monitored closely for recurrent bacteriuria or be given prophylaxis for the remainder of the pregnancy.

PREGNANCY IN WOMEN WITH RENAL INSUFFICIENCY

With current management of recurrent urinary tract infections, infections alone are no contraindication to pregnancy. In patients with renal insufficiency with or without urinary infections, Davison and Lindheimer (1978) emphasize that renal function should be carefully evaluated by both serum creatinine and creatinine clearance before a woman is counseled about conceiving or continuing a pregnancy. Although little is known about the outcome of pregnancies with varying degrees of renal insufficiency, it is known that normal pregnancy is rare if preconception serum creatinine exceeds 3 mg per dl (about 30 ml/min clearance) (Davison and Lindheimer, 1978).

One retrospective analysis of 44 pregnancies in women with pre-existing renal disease provides some helpful guidelines about the degree of renal impairment beyond which pregnancy is inadvisable (Bear, 1976). In this study, patients were divided into those with mild renal disease and serum creatinine less than 1.5 mg per dl and those with renal disease and serum creatinine greater than 1.6 mg per dl. In those with mild renal disease, 34 of 35 pregnancies resulted in normal live births, and although serum creatinine remained fixed during the pregnancy (it did not decrease as expected during a normal pregnancy), the pregnancy appeared to have no remote effect on renal function. On the other hand, pregnancy in eight patients with serum creatinine greater than 1.6 mg per dl was complicated in all cases, and the incidences of prematurity, delivery by cesarean section, hypertension, and worsening proteinuria and renal insufficiency during pregnancy were increased; four of the eight patients progressed to severe renal failure or death within 18 months. These data have caused Bear to recommend that conception is ill advised in patients with less than 50 per cent of normal renal function (serum creatinine greater than 1.7 mg/dl or less than about 50 ml/min clearance).

URETHRAL SYNDROME

The urethral syndrome is considered in detail in Chapter 24, Interstitial Cystitis and Related Syndromes. We would like, however, to present a brief overview of our approach at Stanford, which has been published elsewhere in detail (Stamey, 1980). The urethral syndrome, whether acute or chronic, usually refers to any symptoms or combination of symptoms suggestive of urinary tract infection occurring in patients considered to be uninfected. The urethral syndrome for the urologist can be divided for practical purposes into three subgroups: those patients with (1) an infectious (microbial) cause, nearly always accompanied by an inflammatory response; (2) interstitial cystitis, rarely accompanied by inflammatory cells, and (3) the "pure" urethral syndrome, which includes patients who have neither a microbial cause nor interstitial cystitis.

To exclude a microbial cause requires an awareness of two points. The first is that vaginal infection also causes dysuria and frequency in some women. Dans and Klaus (1976) found that *Neisseria gonorrhoeae, Trichomonas vaginalis, Candida albicans,* and *herpes simplex* Type 2 infections were the cause of dysuria in almost 20 per cent of their patients. To this list must be added *Chlamydia trachomatis* (Stamm et al., 1980b), which fortunately, like the other vaginal infections, also causes a purulent discharge. The second point is that either a suprapubic aspiration of the bladder urine or a carefully obtained catheterized urine (in which urethral contamination is avoided) is required to prove a sterile urine free of inflammatory cells. Many of us have repeatedly emphasized that *E. coli* and other common urinary infections may occur with few bacteria in the urine, and, as emphasized in Chapter 14, the 100,000 bacteria per ml concept has serious limitations in the symptomatic patient. Indeed, Stamm and coworkers (1982) in studying acutely dysuric women (mean age 25 years), excluding those with vaginal infections, pregnancy, diabetes, and urologic upper tract abnormalities, concluded that 100 or more bacteria per ml was diagnostic of cystitis. Moreover, suprapubic aspiration of the bladder is required to exclude anaerobic bacteria, *Ureaplasma urealyticum* (Stamey, 1980), and other potentially fastidious bacteria that require special culture conditions free of contaminants from the lower urethra and vagina for the diagnosis of cystitis.

The most practical approach for the urologist in the effort to exclude a subtle microbial cause of the urethral syndrome is to make sure that both the bladder urine obtained by needle aspiration and the urethral urine obtained by voiding are free of inflammatory cells, especially fresh polymorphonuclear leukocytes (see Chapters 6 and 14 for details). If the voided urine, especially the VB$_1$ is free of fresh leukocytes (there are always some "old" ones from the vaginal secretions that bathe the external one third of the urethra), and if the aspirated bladder urine is free of inflammatory cells, a microbial cause of the urethral syndrome is virtually excluded. With this exclusion, the urologist can then concentrate on excluding interstitial cystitis (Chapter 24); once interstitial cystitis is excluded, he is dealing with the "pure" urethral syndrome, and his troubles have just begun! We say this because many of these latter patients have an emotional basis for their discomfort and the solutions are not easy. It is in this group that urodynamic studies of the urethra may one day be useful in demonstrating neuromuscular "spasm," but this remains to be seen.

Trigonitis. It is to be hoped that the labels "trigonitis" and "urethrotrigonitis" will soon disappear from our vocabulary of ignorance. The "cobblestoned" or "granular" appearance of the trigone and floor of the vesical neck represents normal squamous epithelium in the postpubertal female. It should not be scraped off, resected, or coagulated in the false belief that "trigonitis" is present. The pathologist has encouraged the delusion by reporting biopsy material from these areas as "squamous metaplasia" rather than the normal squamous epithelium that it actually represents. Failure to recognize that vaginal inclusion epithelium covering the trigone and urethra is a normal embryologic development, plus lack of experience in cystoscopic study of normal women without bladder symptoms, is undoubtedly responsible for the cystoscopic terms "trigonitis" and "granular urethrotrigonitis." The distal third of the vagina, the urethra, and the trigone are all derived from the urogenital sinus, and thus the same squamous epithelium of the vagina usually covers the trigone and floor of the urethra (Cifuentes, 1947).

BIOLOGIC CAUSE OF RECURRENT URINARY INFECTION

If longitudinal studies are performed with frequent cultures of the vaginal vestibule and urethra in women with recurrent bacteriuria, it is clear that colonization of the vaginal and urethral mucosa precedes the occurrence of bacteriuria (Stamey, 1980; Stamey et al., 1971). Since the fecal reservoir is similar in all women, with and without urinary infections, these observations indicate that characterization of susceptibility lies in colonization of the vaginal introitus with Enterobacteriaceae from the rectal flora. Similar data in female children have confirmed these observations (Bollgren and Winberg, 1976).

Urethral colonization is determined by the vaginal bacteria. Not only are these two moist, mucosal surfaces confined anatomically by the distal labia minora, but both are derived embryologically from the urogenital sinus, they respond to the same hormones (Papanicolaou smears of the urethra show estrogen variation identical to that of vaginal epithelial cells), and several thousand of our cultures have shown their bacteriologic similarity. Thus, the urologist needs to culture only the vaginal introitus to determine urethral bacteriology (see Chapter 14).

Colonization of the Introitus with Enterobacteriaceae Precedes Bacteriuria. A representative clinical example of a 29-year-old white married female, followed through eight urinary infections over a period of 27 months, illustrates the pathogenesis of her recurrent bacteriuria.

Her first urinary infection occurred in 1963 when she was 20 years old. The next 5 years were free from infection, years that included marriage and two full-term pregnancies. The following 4 years, however, were characterized by four to five urinary infections each year. An intravenous urogram and voiding cystourethrogram were normal. Because of the unremitting pattern of her recurrences and the failure of a variety of therapeutic regimens, including urethral dilatation, she was referred to us in September 1972. Her bacteriologic course is presented in Figure 15–7A and B; cultures of the vaginal vestibule (introitus) are shown, together with the specific episodes of bacteriuria.

An intrauterine device was in place throughout the first 9 months of our observations (until 26 June 1973); a vasectomy was performed on her husband on 8 June 1973. The patient performed no vaginal douches either before or after removal of the intrauterine device.

She experienced symptoms, including urgency, frequency, and suprapubic cramping ("bladder spasms") at every infection, although on one occasion we detected bacteriuria 24 hours before the onset of her symptoms. Dysuria never occurred. Although her symptoms (especially urgency) often persisted for several days after the start of antimicrobial therapy and even in the presence of a sterile urine, she was always asymptomatic in between episodes of bacteriuria. Pyuria was usually but not invariably present, and it always cleared a few days later. She was never catheterized, or otherwise instrumented. Each infection was treated for 10 days.

As seen in Figure 15–7A, with the exception of the second 06 E. coli bacteriuria on 2 July 1973, every infection was preceded by colonization of the vaginal vestibule with the responsible pathogen. The culture immediately preceding this infection was obtained on 11 March 1973, a few hours after her gynecologist had removed an intrauterine device for prevention of pregnancy; this culture contained *Klebsiella* but no *E. coli*.

Although her first four infections showed a different organism at each succeeding bacteriuria, note that three consecutive infections were caused by 075 E. coli (Fig. 15–7A). More importantly, observe that the vaginal carriage of

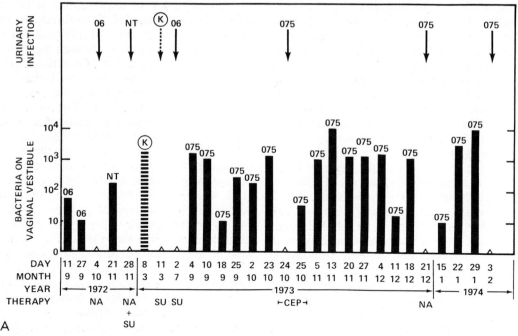

Figure 15–7. *A,* Clinical course of a 29-year-old married Caucasian woman followed through eight urinary infections in 27 months. Bacteriuric episodes are shown, together with every consecutive culture preceding the bacteriuria in which the same strain producing the infection was found on the vaginal vestibule.

Δ, without overlying bars, indicates vaginal vestibule cultures without any detectable Enterobacteriaceae. *NA* stands for nalidixic acid; *SU,* sulfonamide; and *CEP,* cephalexin. *K* refers to *Klebsiella; NT,* to nontypable *E. coli;* and numbers (06, 075), to specific serogroups of *E. coli.*

Illustration continued on opposite page

075 *E. coli* persisted at every culture between the first and second 075 bacteriuria (a period of 8 weeks) and between the second and third 075 infection (a period of 6 weeks). Anal cultures in between each 075 infection showed the same 075 *E. coli* to be the predominant strain in the feces.

The reason for pointing out these closely spaced infections with the same serogroup of *E. coli* is that not only do they clearly show the vaginal route of pathogenesis through persistence of the pathogenic strain on the vaginal mucosa, but they show equally well why the term "relapse" should not be used in defining the nature of recurrent bacteriuria. Those who use the term imply persistence within the urinary tract (kidney), while these data show persistence outside the urinary bladder. It is clear that consecutive infections with the same O-serogroup, except in the patient with infection stones or bacterial prostatitis, are actually reinfections from vaginal persistence.

During the 18 months of observation shown in Figure 15–7*A* before continuous prophylactic therapy was started on 3 February 1974, there were 66 cultures obtained when the patient was not bacteriuric. It is important to note that 22

or the 66 did not contain a single detectable colony of Enterobacteriaceae. Figure 15–7*A* shows, for simplicity, every *consecutive* culture preceding each bacteriuric episode in which the identical strain causing the bacteriuria was found on the vaginal introitus. We have pointed out repeatedly that colonization with Enterobacteriaceae is often intermittent in these susceptible patients (Stamey, 1973; Stamey and Sexton, 1975; Schaeffer and Stamey, 1977; Stamey, 1980). The longest period of time by culture that this patient's vaginal mucosa was without colonization with Enterobacteriaceae was from 1 December 1972 to 17 January 1973 (six cultures). On the other hand, her longest period of consecutive carriage of Enterobacteriaceae was from 12 March 1973 to 8 June 1973 (13 cultures).

As can be observed in Figure 15–7*A* and *B,* following the last *E. coli* 075 infection, the patient was treated for 10 days with trimethoprim-sulfamethoxazole (TMP-SMX) at full dosage of two tablets every 12 hours, and then with one-half tablet each evening at bedtime from the eleventh day for the next 6 months. Bacteriuria was absent while she was on prophylaxis and during the 4 months after she stopped taking

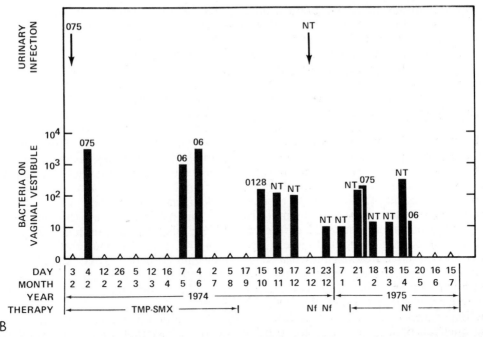

B

Figure 15–7. *Continued. B,* Same patient as shown in *A,* but illustrating the next 13 months, when continuous prophylaxis with trimethoprim-sulfamethoxazole (*TMP-SMX,* 6 months) and nitrofurantoin (*Nf,* 6 months) was used to prevent reinfections. All vaginal cultures are shown, as well as the episodes of bacteriuria.

nightly doses of TMP-SMX (Fig. 15–7*B*). Moreover, while she was on prophylaxis (February 14, 1974 to August 5, 1974), only two of nine cultures showed transient vaginal colonization with enterobacteria (*E. coli* 06). Following the bacteriuria due to nontypable (NT) *E. coli* on December 21, 1974 (which incidentally was again preceded by vaginal colonization with the same NT *E. coli*), she was treated with nitrofurantoin for 10 days (until December 31, 1974); nitrofurantoin prophylaxis, 100 mg each night, was begun after the culture of January 21, 1975. During the 6 months of nitrofurantoin prophylaxis (Fig. 15–7*B*) there were no episodes of bacteriuria, but three of six vaginal cultures showed carriage of Enterobacteriaceae, all sensitive to nitrofurantoin. The prophylactic prevention of bacteriuria is presented in the following section.

After completing 6 months of nitrofurantoin prophylaxis in July 1975, the patient was asymptomatic and free from infection until February 1976, when she became infected with a self-agglutinating *E. coli.* She responded to a short course of TMP-SMX and was well until October 1976; a nontypable *E. coli* caused the October infection. She was then well for over 1 year until December 1977 when the onset of acute lower tract symptoms caused her to self-treat herself with 5 days of TMP-SMX.

Throughout 1978, and until July 1979, she remained off all medication and was asymptomatic.

A Comparison of Introital Colonization in Women Susceptible to and Resistant to Urinary Infections. In this patient (Figure 15–7*A* and *B*) and some 50 similar to her, we have clearly shown how colonization of the vaginal vestibule precedes the occurrence of bacteriuria. The proof, however, that the basic cause of recurrent urinary infections in women lies in abnormal vaginal biologic factors depends upon the demonstration of a significant difference in enterobacterial colonization of the vaginal introitus between susceptible women and those who never have urinary infections. About 50 premenopausal women who have never had a urinary infection have volunteered for 10 consecutive, weekly cultures of the vaginal vestibule, urethra, and midstream urine. We originally compared 200 cultures from 20 control volunteers with 200 cultures from 9 women obtained in between two consecutive urinary infections (Stamey and Sexton, 1975). None of the cultures in either group was obtained during antimicrobial therapy. The difference between the two groups in colonization with any (even one) *E. coli, Proteus mirabilis, Klebsiella,* or *Pseudomonas aeruginosa* bacterium was highly significant ($p = <0.001$), meaning that the chances the two groups are similar are less than 1 in 1000. Colonization differences with *Streptococcus fecalis* were also significant ($p = 0.003$). But in addition to simple carriage per se, colonization with these fecal bacteria was shown to occur in larger numbers and to persist through consecutive cultures for longer periods in women with recurrent infections (Stamey and Sexton, 1975). It must be realized, however, that a single vaginal culture will not distinguish between the two populations. For example, 76 per cent of the 200 cultures from the normal controls never had a single detectable colony of Enterobacteriaceae, but 43 per cent of all cultures from the infection group were similarly devoid of these bacteria—just as 22 of the 66 cultures in the patient presented here (Fig. 15–7A) contained no Enterobacteriaceae. The fact that other investigators have sought to distinguish between members of the two groups by a single culture has sometimes obscured the etiologic importance of these observations.

The question of whether the 5 to 10 days of antimicrobial therapy might be causing subsequent introital colonization in women with recurrent urinary tract infections was addressed by Schaeffer and Stamey (1977). Their investigation showed no difference in colonization rates in the 30 days immediately following antimicrobial therapy and those colonization rates at later time periods, remote from potential effects of the antimicrobial agent. These studies compared 200 introital cultures in 20 control women with 198 cultures obtained from 9 women in between episodes of recurrent bacteriuria; as in the earlier study by Stamey and Sexton (1975), there is a statistically significant elevation in enterobacterial introital carriage by susceptible women over that in controls. We have reviewed elsewhere (Stamey, 1980) a number of confirmatory investigations as well as those that have failed to support these observations. In the latter group, major differences in methodology, such as the use of first voided A.M. urine cultures by the patient on dipstick agar slides, in which contaminating bacteria were assumed to come from the introital and urethral mucosa (Kunin et al., 1980), often account for the discrepancy.

These observations establish not only that bacteriuria is preceded by colonization of the vaginal introitus with the responsible organism (Fig. 15–7,A and B), but also that the biology of the vagina of women susceptible to urinary infections is different from that of normal control women who never have infections. Why are Enterobacteriaceae, *S. faecalis,* and sometimes *P. aeruginosa* more likely to colonize the mu-

cosa of the introitus and urethra in women susceptible to urinary infections? This question is the key to understanding the basic cause and prevention of recurrent bacteriuria. Between 1975 and 1978, we examined vaginal fluid in the two groups for leukocytes, estrogen indices, mucosal pH, glycogen concentrations, antibody concentrations (IgG and IgA), and bacterial agglutination titers as well as for the presence or absence of lactobacilli, *Ureaplasma urealyticum,* and *Bacteroides* species without finding significant differences; these investigations can be found in a series of ten *Studies of Introital Colonization in Women with Recurrent Infection,* published elsewhere (Stamey and Timothy, 1975a; Stamey and Kaufman, 1975; Stamey and Timothy, 1975b, Stamey and Howell, 1976; Stamey and Mihara, 1976a; Stamey and Mihara, 1976b; Fowler and Stamey, 1977; Fowler et al., 1977; Schaeffer and Stamey, 1977; Fowler and Stamey, 1978.)

In addition, we reported in 1978 (Stamey et al., 1978) that women resistant to urinary infections (who rarely colonize their vaginal introitus with fecal Enterobacteriaceae) carry specific vaginal antibody against their own fecal *E. coli,* whereas those who are susceptible have substantially less vaginal antibody directed against their colonizing strains of fecal bacteria. Although Kurdydyk and associates (1980) were unable to confirm these findings, the last chapter on the role of cervicovaginal antibody in colonization of the introitus with fecal Enterobacteriaceae, as well as the potential for vaginal immunization, is probably incomplete.

BACTERIAL ADHERENCE TO VAGINAL AND URINARY TRACT EPITHELIAL CELLS

The Role of Epithelial Cells. Because of an accumulating literature in the early 1970's on bacterial adherence to mucosal surfaces in diseases of the intestinal, respiratory, and pharyngeal tracts, and because of our frustration at Stanford over our failure to find significant differences between women susceptible to urinary infections and healthy women in the many factors that determine bacterial growth rates on mucosal surfaces in the summer of 1974 we, (Drs. Fowler and Stamey) turned our attention to a study of enterobacterial adherence to vaginal epithelial cells.

The washing human vaginal epithelial cells free of adherent organisms and then incubating them with different strains of bacteria, the investigators were able to establish the following (Fowler and Stamey, 1977): (1) Lactobacilli and *Staphylococcus epidermidis,* both normal indige-

TABLE 15–2. MEAN NUMBER OF ADHERENT BACTERIA PER CELL FOR 18 DIFFERENT
Escherichia coli O-SEROGROUPS[a]

Common Serogroups[b]		Uncommon Serogroups[c]	
O-SEROGROUPS	MEAN BACTERIA/CELL[d]	O-SEROGROUPS	MEAN BACTERIA/CELL[d]
06	49.9 ± 4.5	0128	26.1 ± 3.2
023	46.5 ± 5.3	0125	16.5 ± 1.7
050	38.9 ± 4.5	0115	11.5 ± 1.6
02	36.9 ± 3.8	0138	8.9 ± 1.5
01	25.6 ± 2.9	0135	6.1 ± 1.2
04	13.1 ± 1.5	077	3.1 ± 0.8
07	9.4 ± 0.9	0127	2.0 ± 0.4
08	6.8 ± 0.9	0111	1.0 ± 0.4
075	3.4 ± 0.5		
018	0.54 ± 0.2		
Mean = 23.1 ± 18.8[e]		Mean = 9.4 ± 8.5[e]	

P>0.1

[a]Reproduced by permission from Fowler, J. E., and Stamey, T. A., J. Urol., *117*:472, 1977.
[b]O-groups isolated from infected urine.
[c]O-groups isolated from feces.
[e]Plus or minus standard error of mean.
[e]Standard deviation.

nous organisms, avidly attached to washed epithelial cells in large numbers; (2) there was a large variation from minimal adherence (1 bacterium per epithelial cell) to substantial adherence (50 bacteria per epithelial cell) among consecutive isolates of *E. coli* that had caused urinary infections in patients (Table 15–2); and (3) most important of all, when vaginal epithelial cells were collected from 20 patients susceptible to reinfections and compared with those from 20 controls resistant to urinary infections,

the 06 *E. coli* adhered much more avidly to the epithelial cells from the susceptible women (p < 0.001) (Table 15–3).

To our knowledge, this increased adherence of pathogenic bacteria to vaginal epithelial cells is currently the only demonstrable biologic difference that can be shown in women susceptible to urinary tract infections. These studies have been confirmed in children by Källenius and Winberg (1978) and Svanborg Edén and Jodal (1979). Moreover, Schaeffer and his col-

TABLE 15–3. MEAN NUMBER OF ADHERENT *Escherichia coli* 06 PER CELL FOR PATIENTS AND CONTROLS[a]

Patient	Mean Bacteria/Cell[b]	Control	Mean Bacteria/Cell[b]
1	89.2 ± 10.3	1	50.4 ± 5.3
2	86.2 ± 9.3	2	30.3 ± 3.6
3	76.7 ± 7.1	3	28.3 ± 3.5
4	67.6 ± 7.5	4	23.8 ± 2.9
5	67.5 ± 5.7	5	23.0 ± 3.3
6	59.3 ± 7.7	6	21.2 ± 1.8
7	58.8 ± 4.4	7	20.8 ± 3.0
8	52.6 ± 5.3	8	18.8 ± 2.8
9	43.8 ± 4.5	9	18.2 ± 3.1
10	38.8 ± 3.6	10	18.2 ± 2.0
11	33.2 ± 3.9	11	18.1 ± 1.9
12	32.6 ± 4.4	12	18.0 ± 1.9
13	27.7 ± 3.2	13	15.0 ± 3.0
14	25.1 ± 2.9	14	15.0 ± 2.3
15	20.6 ± 3.3	15	14.8 ± 2.9
16	20.1 ± 2.8	16	13.5 ± 1.7
17	18.0 ± 2.6	17	12.2 ± 2.2
18	14.8 ± 1.8	18	10.6 ± 1.6
19	12.9 ± 2.4	19	8.6 ± 1.4
20	7.0 ± 1.2	20	8.1 ± 1.6
Mean = 42.6 ± 25.5[c]		Mean = 19.4 ± 9.4[c]	

P<0.001

[a]Reproduced by permission from Fowler, J. E., and Stamey, T. A., J. Urol., *117*:472, 1977.
[b]Plus or minus standard error of mean.
[c]Standard deviation.

leagues (1981) confirmed these vaginal differences in women but added the observation that the increased adherence was characteristic of the buccal epithelial cells; this important contribution emphasized that the increased receptor sites for *E. coli* on vaginal epithelial cells were not limited to the vagina, which suggests a genotypic trait for epithelial cell receptivity as a major susceptibility factor in urinary infections. In addition, Schaeffer and his associates (1982a) have recently reported that it is the adhesive ability of vaginal *E. coli* rather than anal isolates that is associated with the causation of urinary tract infections; they also reconfirmed their observation that a correlation exists between vaginal and buccal cell receptiviy to *E. coli*.

Thus, these studies individually and collectively lead to the conclusion that there is an increased epithelial cell receptivity for *E. coli* on the introtial and urethral mucosa that is characteristic of women and female children susceptible to recurrent urinary tract infections.

THE ROLE OF VIRULENCE FACTORS IN E. COLI ASSOCIATED WITH URINARY TRACT INFECTIONS

Since the intestine is the ultimate reservoir of *E. coli* for urinary infections as well as other extraintestinal infection sites, microbiologists have long been interested in the question of whether certain strains have a pathogenic advantage (uropathogenicity or nephropathogenicity) over others in causing disease. Do the *E. coli* that cause urinary tract infections colonize the vagina and urethra in a random fashion, or do only a few strains from the intestinal reservoir have some biologic advantage? For example, hemolysis of red blood cells is assumed to be a cytotoxic factor and occurs in a substantial percentage of *E. coli* stains causing urinary infections. McGeachie (1966) found hemolysis in 29 per cent of 534 strains isolated from voided urine, noting also that five common serologic O-groups (01, 04, 06, 018, and 075) accounted for 72 per cent of all the hemolytic strains he isolated. Cooke and Ewins (1975) found that hemolytic strains of *E. coli* in the periurethral flora were more likely to occur in subsequent urinary tract infections than were nonhemolytic strains in the same flora. Minshew and her associates (1978) reported that 49 per cent of their urinary tract strains caused hemolysis, in contrast to only 1 of 20 strains (5 per cent) isolated from normal enteric flora. Although the potential virulence that hemolysis imparts to some *E. coli* strains is unknown, Fried and his colleagues (1971) demonstrated that a hemolytic

E. coli (06:H31) commonly caused pyelonephritis in the kidneys of mice and rats, whereas a nonhemolytic mutant of the same *E. coli* did not.

In addition to hemolysin production, Falkow's group (Minshew et al., 1978) showed that the characteristics of colicin V production, the ability to kill allantoically inoculated 13-day-old chick embryos, and hemagglutination of human erythrocytes in the presence of D-mannose, were all more common in extraintestinal *E. coli* infections than in *E. coli* from the normal enteric flora. The ability of *E. coli* to agglutinate human erythrocytes in the presence of D-mannose was demonstrated in 59 per cent of *E. coli* from extraintestinal infections but in only 15 per cent of *E. coli* from the normal enteric flora.

Achtman and associates (Achtman et al., 1983) have identified six widespread bacterial clones among several common serotypes of *E. coli* K_1 isolates from a number of centers in Europe and the United States—implying linear descent of each clone from an ancestral cell. Using electrophoretic migration of major outer membrane proteins as their clonal markers, they proposed that O-serogroups, hemolysin, and colicin production, plasmid content, and metabolic (biochemical) properties are all independent, conserved characteristics of a limited number of clonal groups of *E. coli* K_1. It is interesting that within the K_1 isolates, none of these other properties correlated with bacterial virulence.

Bacterial Adherence as a Virulence Factor. Svanborg Edén and the Göteborg group were the first to report a correlation between bacterial adherence and the severity of urinary tract infections (Svanborg Edén et al., 1976, 1978); they showed that *E. coli* strains from children with acute pyelonephritis had high adhesive ability, whereas strains from girls with asymptomatic bacteriuria (screening bacteriuria) or normal feces had low bacterial adherence. Svanborg Edén and Hanson (1978) demonstrated that this adherence was mediated by bacterial fimbriae, or pili; these structures are nonflagellar, protein appendages that protrude from the bacterial cell surface like minute hairs. Pili can be classified by their ability to agglutinate erythrocytes of different animal species and by different sugars that are known to block the hemagglutination. This correlation between piliation and hemagglutination was first observed by Duguid and his colleagues in 1955; they also observed that hemagglutination was best demonstrated with guinea pig erythrocytes and that it was inhibited by the sugar mannose (Duguid and Gillies, 1957). Duguid (1968) reported that these mannose-sensitive pili (called Type I) were found in most strains of *E. coli* and that they represented the mechanism whereby bacteria stick to animal, plant, and fungus cells. In short, these bacterial proteinaceous "adhesins," as they are sometimes called, react with a sugar sequence on the surface of epithelial cells that is usually in the form of a glycolipid or a glycoprotein.

Källenius and Möllby (1979) were the first to recognize that the adherence of a pyelonephritic strain of *E. coli* paralleled the capacity of the strain to specifically agglutinate human rather than guinea pig erythrocytes and that this agglutination was mannose-resistant. Källenius and her associates (1980) then, by a careful examination of human erythrocyte antigens, were able to demonstrate that the terminal disaccharide of the P blood-group system, specifically the p^k glycosphingolipid (trihexosyl ceramide), was the receptor involved in the mannose-resistant hemagglutination caused by pyelonephritic strains of *E. coli*. They proposed that the critical structure was the digalactoside with the formula (α-D-Gal-p(1–4-β-D-Gal-p). Winberg's group appropriately called these p^k blood-group specific bacterial adhesins on the surface of *E. coli* "P-pili." They (Kallenius et al., 1981) examined 97 children with urinary infections and 82 healthy controls for the occurrence of *E. coli* possessing these P-pili, finding them in 91 per cent of urinary strains causing acute pyelonephritis, 19 per cent of strains causing cystitis, 14 per cent of strains causing asymptomatic bacteriuria (screening bacteriuria), but in only 7 per cent of fecal isolates from healthy controls.

While Korhonen and associates (1982) have clearly shown that the P blood group–specific bacterial adhesin on the surface of *E. coli* is located on the pilus, both mannose-resistant and mannose-sensitive adhesins can be expressed on the same *E. coli*. When large numbers of *E. coli* urinary tract strains (333) were examined for mannose-resistant and sensitive agglutination of both human and guinea pig erythrocytes (Hagberg et al., 1981), most strains with mannose-resistant hemagglutination (MRHA) of human erythrocytes simultaneously induced mannose-sensitive hemagglutination (MSHA) of guinea pig erythrocytes. Nevertheless, *E. coli* expressing MRHA attached in high numbers to human urinary tract epithelial cells, whereas those bacteria that induced only MSHA attached in low numbers and nonagglutinating strains did not attach at all.

In addition to the P blood group–specific bacterial adhesins on *E. coli* strains causing pyelonephritis, about 10 per cent of strains recognize human cells in a non-P or "X-specific" manner (Väisanen et al., 1981). Korhonen's group has identified some of these *E. coli* strains that show mannose-resistant, P blood group–independent hemagglutination of human erythrocytes as binding specifically to a 2–3 linked neuraminic acid on the erythrocyte surface (Parkkinen et al., 1983).

More recently at Stanford, Falkow's group (Low et al., 1984) have shown that the genes encoding for MRHA of human erythrocytes and for hemolysin production are closely linked on the chromosome. They have suggested that close grouping of several virulence factors might have a synergistic advantage in pathogenesis at mucosal colonization sites.

It is interesting, too, that while the association of MRHA and digalactoside P–specificity with *E. coli* causing pyelonephritis in children is "greater than any other laboratory-defined bacterial characteristic," the renal abnormalities in terms of scarring and degree of reflux are not very impressive (Väisanen et al., 1981). This observation is confirmed by the more recent report by Lomberg and associates (1983) that cases of recurrent pyelonephritis in girls with gross reflux (in whom most of the scarring historically occurs) are minimally associated with *E. coli* strains carrying P-pili. Thus, it would appear that MRHA and digalactoside P–specific pili in acute pyelonephritis are mainly of importance in nonrefluxing or minimally refluxing children.

Although these studies undoubtedly establish that bacterial adherence mediated by P-pili is a virulence factor for urinary tract infections, there are some discordant notes. For one thing, neither Fowler and Stamey (1978) nor Schaeffer and his colleagues (1982) could confirm that random rectal strains of *E. coli* that had never caused urinary tract infections in patients were any different in their capacity to adhere to squamous epithelial cells of the vaginal introitus than were bacteriuric strains isolated from the bladder. Another concern is that we have no direct in vivo measurements of adherence; all the data are based on in vitro studies of cell adherence, in which it is easy to manipulate the degree of adhesiveness with different culture conditions. Both Asscher's group (Harber et al., 1982) and ours (Stamey, 1980) have shown that bacteria taken directly from bladder urine produce very poor adherence; in our Stanford studies, standard processing of bacteria one time from urine to agar to broth increased adherence by 300 per cent.

There are some additional problems in interpreting the exciting adherence literature of the past 8 years. All of the studies, for example, by Svanborg Edén and the Göteborg group use voided epithelial cells from a female volunteer; although all their papers refer to adherence to *"uroepithelial* cells," these are, in fact, largely squamous epithelial cells (80 per cent plus) from the vagina, urethra, and trigone of the woman. It is important to recognize that we know little about attachment to transitional epithelial cells per se, which, after all, make up the bulk of the receptor sites involved in the ascent of bacteria from the bladder to the kidney. Indeed, in their initial paper on methodology, Svanborg Edén, Eriksson, and Hanson (1977) recognized that bacteria stuck much less avidly to transitional than to squamous cells. Because there have been no direct studies on bacterial adherence to transitional cells, Szabo, Shortliffe, and Stamey (1984) collected transitional cells directly from the bladder either at open surgery or by lavage with the cystoscope; only male bladders were used because of the luxuriant squamous cells present on the trigone of postpubertal females. We found that both MRHA and MSHA *E. coli* attached very well; so did *P. mirabilis,* whether the strains had caused urinary tract infection with renal stones or had resided exclusively within the rectal reservoir.

An indirect, but more complete, evaluation of epithelial receptors in the human urinary tract has been provided by David Lark, a urologist at Stanford working in the Infectious Disease Laboratory of Dr. Gary Schoolnik (Lark et al., 1984). He used an avidin-biotin peroxidase immunohistochemical method to determine both the digalactoside and the mannose receptor distribution in human biopsy material from the vagina, bladder, ureter, renal pelvis, and kidneys of patients undergoing nephroureterectomy for small-volume transitional cell carcinoma of the renal calyces. Digalactoside antibody was produced against the synthetic artificial antigen α-D-Gal-(1–4)-β-D-Gal, and mannose antibody against the α-D-Man-(1–2)-α-D-Man linkage. Tissue sections were examined under light microscopy and the brownish color reaction, indicating antibody binding to receptor, was graded as: $+++$, intense; $++$, moderate; $+$, weak; and $-$, negative. Table 15–4 shows that the digalactoside receptor is present in all genitourinary tissues examined except for the glomerulus and the loop of Henle. Of greatest interest is the increased concentration in the squamous epithelium of the vagina and the renal collecting ducts (Fig. 15–8); the intense concentration in the vaginal epithelium probably explains much of the adherence data on pathogenesis of infections at the lower urinary tract level, while the digalactoside intensity in the renal collecting ducts may partially explain the increased P-pili frequency associated with pyelonephritic *E. coli* strains. The equal distribution of the mannose receptors at all levels of the urinary tract in terms of potential ascent of *E. coli* expressing MSHA Type 1 pili may be important; there is certainly no lack of receptors to encourage adherence.

Another concern with the Göteborg studies

TABLE 15–4. Immunoperoxidase Results in Human Genitourinary Mucosa for Digalactoside and D-Mannose Receptors

Tissue	Epithelium	α-D-Gal-(1–4)-β-D-Gal Antisera	α-D-Man-(1–2)-α-D-Man Antisera
VAGINA	Squamous	$+++$	$+++$
BLADDER			
Trigone	Squamous	$+++$	$+++$
Wall	Transitional	$+$	$++$
URETER			
Distal	Transitional	$+$	$++$
Mid-	Transitional	$+$	$++$
Upper	Transitional	$+$	$++$
RENAL PELVIS	Transitional	$+$	$++$
KIDNEY			
Glomerulus		$-$	$-$
Proximal convoluted tubule		$++$	$++$
Loop of Henle		$-$	$++$
Distal convoluted tubule		$++$	$++$
Collecting unit			
Proximal		$+$	$++$
Distal		$++/+++$	$++$

Figure 15–8. Localization of α-D-gal-1-4-α-D-gal (digal) antigen on human urogenital tissue by indirect immunoperoxidase staining of Bouin's fixed sections.

A, Indirect immunoperoxidase stain with digal antibody on human vaginal tissue shows clear labeling of the squamous epithelium but also some staining of the endothelial blood vessels. × 128.

B, Indirect immunoperoxidase control shows no staining of the tissue. × 128.

C, Indirect immunoperoxidase staining on human bladder tissue shows strong labeling of the transitional epithelium with no labeling of the smooth muscle. × 400.

D, Indirect immunoperoxidase control shows absent staining of the bladder mucosa. × 400.

E, Midureter cross section shows localization of the label to the transitional epithelium. Note absence of submucosal staining. × 128.

F, Control staining on the same tissue shows total lack of stain. × 128.

G, Higher power (× 320) magnification of the renal pelvis shows the same strong mucosal localization with absent submucosal stain.

H, Control staining is absent for tissue labeling.

I, A magnification (× 320) of the renal cortical–medullary junction. Notice localization of stain to both the convoluted tubules and the collecting ducts while the interstitial tissue is unlabeled.

J, Control stain is again absent for any label.

Method: Bouin-fixed paraffin sections of human uroepithelial tissue are deparaffinized through xylol and graded alcohols. Indirect immunoperoxidase method included the primary rabbit anti-digal antibody followed by the biotinylated goat anti-rabbit IgG. After addition of the avidin-biotin-peroxidase complex (ABC), the sections were incubated with 0.05 per cent diaminobenzidine hydrochloride. For the control sections the anti-digal antibody was replaced with normal rabbit IgG. Sections were counterstained with hematoxylin. (Courtesy of David Lark, M.D.)

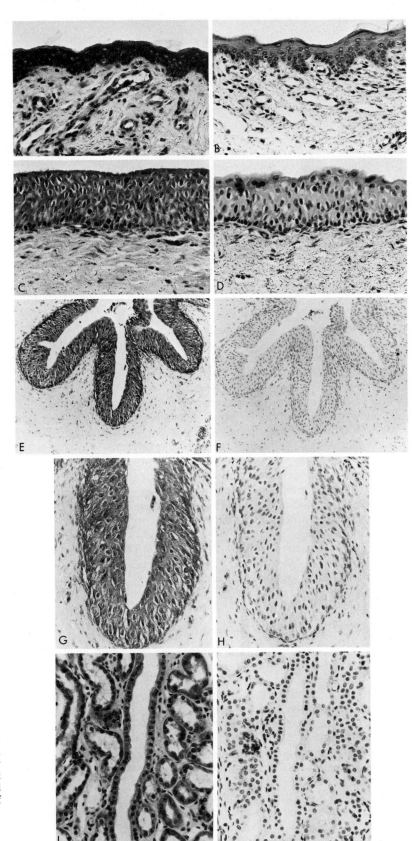

(Hagberg et al., 1981) is that the use of voided "uroepithelial" cells allows coating of the squamous epithelial cells (at least those from the vagina and urethra, which make up the majority of all cells) with Tamm-Horsfall protein, which is rich in mannose residues, binds to Type 1 pili (Orskov et al., 1980), and could lead to serious underestimation of the importance of mannose-sensitive adhesins in their attachment to squamous epithelial cells from the urethra and vagina; Ørskov and associates (1980) observed that they were unable to completely separate the mucous cells from the voided epithelial cells. Schaeffer and associates (1984) have recently re-emphasized the role of mannose-sensitive adherence of *E. coli* to vaginal cells in women with recurrent urinary infections. The observation of Ofek and his colleagues (1982) is also interesting and may be important: *E. coli* strains that were genotypically capable of producing mannose-sensitive adhesins suppressed the phenotypic expression of the adhesin during growth in human bladder urine.

Therapeutic applications of these possibilities include either vaccination with commonly shared antigens of the bacterial pili, a very complex problem at best, or bathing the urinary tract—either the bladder or the kidneys—in some way with carbohydrate analogs of the cell surface receptors so that the bacterial adhesins become bound to the analog carbohydrate rather than to the receptor on the epithelial cell surface. While this is an attractive concept, which can be readily applied in the mouse (Svanborg Edén et al., 1982) and rat (Aronson et al., 1979) models, it seems to be a cumbersome clinical maneuver when compared with the simplicity and almost total effectiveness of antimicrobial prophylaxis to prevent urinary tract infections, a subject that is covered in the next section.

OTHER HOST DEFENSE MECHANISM

There are many other host defense mechanisms, including voiding, urinary antibody, desquamation of epithelial surfaces, and antibacterial enzymes such as lysozyme and lactoferrin. In addition to these, Parsons and associates (1980) have described a surface mucin on the bladder mucosa of rabbits that they have identified as a glycosaminoglycan; its presence has not been demonstrated on the cell surface of the human bladder, nor is its relationship, if any, known to the bacteria-fixing slime (Tamm-Horsfall protein) that Ørskov and coworkers (1980) have reported in normal urine in large amounts. The mannose residues of the Tamm-

Horsfall protein are known to trap *E. coli* with Type 1 pili, an extremely ubiquitous MSHA pilus present on most *E. coli*.

PROPHYLAXIS

Prophylactic prevention of reinfections of the urinary tract is *the key* to controlling recurrent urinary tract infections. The successful management of virtually all recurrent urinary tract infections is easy if the physician understands the biology of succesful prophylaxis, recognizes the prophylactic effectiveness of four or five highly useful antimicrobial agents, and remembers the causes of bacterial persistence in the urinary tract (Table 14–2).

BIOLOGIC BASIS OF SUCCESSFUL PROPHYLAXIS: ANTIMICROBIAL EFFECT ON BOWEL AND VAGINAL BACTERIAL FLORA

The success of prophylaxis depends in large part on the effect an antimicrobial agent has on the introital and fecal reservoirs of pathogenic bacteria. Winberg and his colleagues were the first to our knowledge to emphasize that oral antimicrobial therapy causes resistant strains in the fecal flora, and subseqently resistant urinary infections (Lincoln et al., 1970; Winberg et al., 1973). The data from three studies on the effects of sulfonamide on the fecal flora are shown in Table 15–5.

The short-term therapy, 10 days or less, a resistant fecal flora is not as great a disadvantage because rapid reinfections are relatively uncommon (Kraft and Stamey, 1977). Nevertheless, the increase in resistant strains of *E. coli* as well as the proliferation of *Klebsiella, Candida albicans,* enterococci, and other pathogenic bacteria in the fecal and vaginal flora that accompanies even short-term, full dose oral administration of tetracyclines, ampicillin, sulfonamides, amoxicillin, and cephalexin in well documented (Lincoln et al., 1970; Winberg et al., 1973; Grüneberg et al., 1973; Toivanen et al., 1976; Datta et al., 1971; Hinton, 1970; Ronald et al., 1977; Sharp, 1954; Daikos et al., 1968; Preiksaitis et al., 1981). These ecologic changes may interfere with antimicrobial prophylaxis in the urinary tract and must be considered in the choice of a prophylactic agent. In long-term, low-dose tetracycline for acne vulgaris, for example, multiply drug-resistant *E. coli* were isolated from 50 per cent of the patients after 4 weeks of treatment, whereas none had been present before therapy (Möller et al., 1977). We have given healthy volunteers 10 days of ampicillin at 250

TABLE 15–5. Sulfonamide Effect on Fecal *Escherichia coli*

Drug	Per Cent Resistant					
	BEFORE	DURING	AFTER WEEK			
			1	*2*	*3*	*4*
Sulphamethoxydiazine-sulphamethoxazole (350 mg/day)[a]	1.0	77	27	11	1	0
Sulphisoxazole hospital[b] (50–200 mg/kg/day)	10	95				
Outpatient[b] (50–200 mg/kg/day)	10	66				
Sulphadimidine[c] (1/4–1.0 gm/day)		66	Continuous Prophylaxis			

[a]3 weeks of therapy (Toivanen et al., 1976)
[b]10 days of therapy (Winberg et al., 1973)
[c]Grüneberg et al., 1973
(From Stamey, T. A.: Pathogenesis and Treatment of Urinary Tract Infections. Baltimore, Williams & Wilkins Co., 1980. Used by permission.)

mg four times daily (Stamey, 1980); the effect ampicillin had in producing resistant *E. coli* in the fecal flora (17 per cent) was small indeed compared with the selecting of 83 per cent of other strains of Enterobacteriaceae that showed ampicillin resistance, a change in flora, and resistance that was always reflected on the vaginal introitus. Similar data have been reported on amoxicillin (Ronald et al., 1977). Cephalexin at 500 mg four times a day caused resistant Enterobacteriaceae in rectal swabs of 38 per cent of the patients (Preiksaitis et al., 1981).

What are the oral antimicrobial agents with minimal adverse effects on the fecal and vaginal flora? They are trimethoprim-sulfamethoxazole (TMP-SMX), nitrofurantoin, nalidixic acid (and its preferable analog, cinoxacin), cephalexin (in minimal dosage), and trimethoprim alone, as listed in Table 15–6.

Trimethoprim-Sulfamethoxazole. Näff (1971) and Knothe (1973) observed that full-dose TMP-SMX (160 mg of TMP and 800 mg of SMX twice daily) for 10 days eliminated any Enterobacteriaceae, especially *E. coli* from the feces without producing resistance; of equal importance, there was no alteration in carriage of enterococci, anaerobic lactobacteria, or the gram-negative bacteria of the Bacteroidaceae family. Overgrowth of bowel flora with either *Pseudomonas* or *Candida* was not observed.

TABLE 15–6. Oral Antimicrobial Agents Useful for Prophylactic Prevention of Reinfections of the Urinary Tract

Trimethoprim-sulfamethoxazole (TMP-SMX)
Nitrofurantoin
Nalidixic acid (preferably cinoxacin)
Cephalexin (in minimal daily dosage)
Trimethoprim

Moorhouse and Farrell (1973) reported similar findings.

We treated 28 patients at Stanford for 6 months with one-half tablet of TMP-SMX nightly (49 mg of TMP, 200 mg of SMX), screening their rectal and vaginal flora at monthly intervals for bacterial resistance (Stamey et al., 1977). Of 182 rectal cultures, only 8.8 per cent showed *E. coli* resistant to TMP-SMX and 9 of these 16 strains came from one patient. Seventy-three per cent of all rectal cultures contained no *E. coli*. Introital *E. coli* on the vagina were detected in only 8.5 per cent of all cultures, and 1 per cent showed resistant *E. coli*. No urinary tract infections occurred during TMP-SMX prophylaxis. Similar data on the fecal flora have been reported in children on long-term therapy, but the daily dose of TMP-SMX was substantially higher (Grüneberg et al., 1976).

Two patients show the remarkable effectiveness of minimal-dose, nightly prophylaxis. Both of these women were begun on prophylaxis as soon as TMP-SMX became available in the United States in 1973. The first patient was a 39-year-old, diabetic, Caucasian mother of two children who had recurrent bacteriuria, often with chills and fever, after a hysterectomy in 1971. She was referred to Stanford in April 1973, where despite antimicrobial therapy based on quantitative disc sensitivity testing, we were unable to prevent her recurrent bacteriuria between April and July 1973. An intravenous urogram showed papillary necrosis without cortical scars or calcifications. The longest interval without medication between infections was 11 days. After initial treatment, attempts to prevent further bacteriuria with nitrofurantoin prophylaxis were thwarted by nitrofurantoin-resistant *E. coli*. As can be seen in Figure 15–9, a

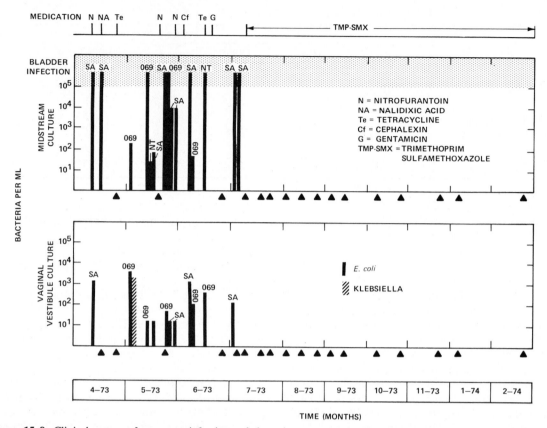

Figure 15–9. Clinical course of recurrent infections of the urinary tract in a 39-year-old diabetic woman. Quantitative cultures of the vaginal vestibule and midstream voided urine are shown with the serotypes of *E. coli*. ▲ indicates a culture in which no gram-negative bacteria were detectable in 0.1 ml of vaginal transport fluid or urine. Small colony counts of gram-positive organisms are not shown. *SA* refers to self-agglutinating *E. coli* and *NT,* to nontypable *E. coli*. (From Stamey, T. A., and Condy, M.: J. Infect. Dis., *131*:261, 1975, The University of Chicago Press, © 1975 by The Journal of Infectious Diseases.)

10-day course of TMP-SMX at full-dosage therapy was followed by one-half tablet daily at bedtime (40 mg of TMP, 200 mg of SMX). Her recurrent infections ceased, and no aerobic gram-negative bacteria could be cultured from the introital mucosa while she remained on TMP-SMX prophylaxis. We were so astonished at complete clearing of all pathogenic bacteria from the introital mucosa that we measured the concentration of TMP and SMX in her vaginal fluid. Her vaginal TMP concentrations (5 to 8.5 μg of TMP per ml) exceeded her serum levels two to three times, while SMX was undetected in the vaginal fluid. Three months after stopping TMP-SMX prophylaxis on April 8, 1974, she became reinfected with a self-agglutinating *E. coli*. In subsequent years (Stamey, 1980), 3 months has been her limit without prophylaxis before acute symptomatic reinfections occur.

Another illustrative example is a 48-year-old Caucasian mother who had her first urinary infection in 1957 and her second in 1966. She had a hysterectomy and bilateral oophorectomy in 1967 and then started taking 0.6 mg of conjugated estrogen daily. Between 1968 and 1973, symptomatic bacteriuria recurred at 4-month intervals, always with dysuria and frequency, and occasionally with fever. An intravenous urogram showed only dilation of the right upper calyx and infundibulum, without cortical scars. After we saw her in August 1973 (Fig. 15–10), she had four urinary infections in 3 months, three caused by *E. coli* 06 and one, in September, caused by *P. mirabilis*. Her vaginal introitus was colonized heavily at every culture with *E. coli* of several types, including the 06 that caused her bacteriuria as well as *P. mirabilis* and later *Klebsiella*. Three rectal cultures showed large numbers of the *E. coli* 06 and *P. mirabilis*. As can be seen in Figure 15–10, the TMP-SMX prophylaxis, started as one-half regular tablet nightly in November 1973, dramatically cleared her vaginal carriage of Enterobacteriaceae and prevented any further blad-

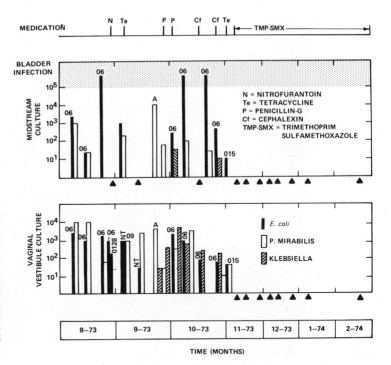

Figure 15–10. Clinical course of recurrent bacteriuria in a 48-year-old woman. Quantitative cultures of the vaginal vestibule and midstream voided urine are shown with the serotypes of *E. coli*. ▲ indicates a culture in which no gram-negative bacteria were detectable in 0.1 ml of vaginal transport fluid or urine. Small colony counts of gram-positive organisms are not shown. *NT* refers to nontypable *E. coli,* and *A,* to *Proteus mirabilis* bacteriuria, even though the colony count in the midstream urine was 10^4 per ml. The patient had been symptomatic for only a few hours, and marked pyuria accompanied infection with *P. mirabilis.* (From Stamey, T. A., and Condy, M.: J. Infect. Dis., *131*:261, 1975, The University of Chicago Press, © 1975 by The Journal of Infectious Diseases.)

der infections. Details of her follow-up after stopping prophylaxis are published elsewhere (Stamey, 1980).

Vaginal fluid measurements of TMP and SMX in these two patients and five others showed that TMP was diffusing across the non-inflamed vaginal wall, producing concentrations that exceeded serum levels (Stamey and Condy, 1975); SMX was undetectable in vaginal fluid. These observations on diffusion and concentration of TMP in vaginal fluid, and the effects of TMP-SMX in clearing of Enterobacteriaceae from the rectal flora, clearly indicate why TMP-SMX is such a powerful prophylactic agent for the prevention of reinfections in the female. These two important biologic effects occur, of course, in addition to the bactericidal levels of TMP-SMX that occur in the urine during night-time prophylaxis.

Nitrofurantoin. Most urologists recognized the efficacy of nitrofurantoin prophylaxis long before official clinical trials were performed. These studies show that once the urine is sterilized, nitrofurantoin is highly effective in preventing recurrent cystitis. Either because of its complete absorption in the upper intestinal tract or its degradation and inactivation in the intestinal tract, it produces minimal fecal resistance—about 2 per cent of fecal culures in our studies at Stanford (Stamey et al., 1977). Unlike prophylaxis with TMP-SMX, which eliminates

colonization, with nitrofurantoin colonization of the vaginal introitus with Enterobacteriaceae continues throughout therapy (36 per cent in our studies). Since the bacteria colonizing the vagina nearly always remain sensitive because of the lack of bacterial resistance in the fecal flora, prophylactic efficacy depends exclusively upon antibacterial concentrations of nitrofurantoin in the bladder urine when bacteria gain access to the bladder.

A good example of nitrofurantoin prophylaxis with cessation of susceptibility to recurrent infections is illustrated by the following patient. A 22-year-old Caucasian woman developed repeated episodes of chills, fever, and bilateral flank pain for the first 4 months of her marriage while vacationing in Europe; she required several hospitalizations. An intravenous urogram showed good renal cortex bilaterally. However, a calyceal deformity in the upper pole extended toward the capsule of the left kidney, diminutive calyces were seen below this deformed calyx, and a dilated calyx was visible in the middle of the right kidney (Fig. 15–11). The right kidney measured 12.5 cm and the left 12.1 cm, but the right mass was substantially greater than the left. The lower ureters were delicate. Her serum creatinine was 1.2 mg per dl. Although asymptomatic when she was transferred to Stanford, she was bacteriuric with an *E. coli* 050 (Fig. 15–12); ureteral catheterization studies showed

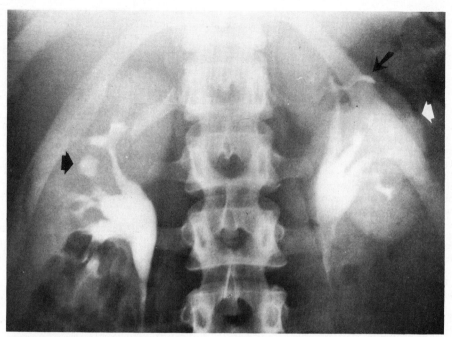

Figure 15–11. A 10-minute intravenous urogram in a 22-year-old recently married Caucasian female with a 3-month history of recurrent chills, fever, and flank pain requiring multiple hospitalizations. The blunted calix in the right kidney and the smaller, irregular left kidney with the upper calix extending to the capsule were all found to be also present on a similar urogram made 20 years earlier, at 2½ years of age.

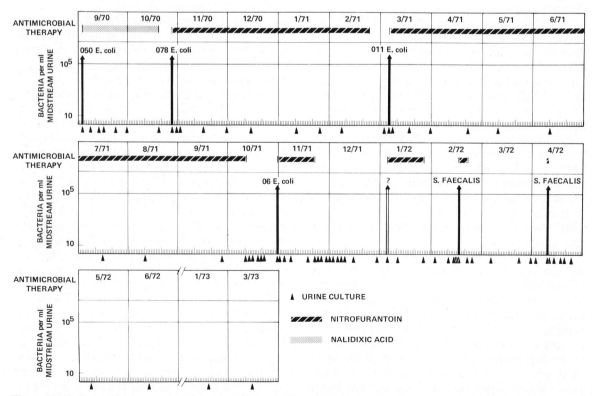

Figure 15–12. Bacteriologic course of the patient shown in Figures 15–11 and 15–13. At each reinfection after therapy was discontinued, nitrofurantoin was given for a few days at full dosage and then immediately followed by nightly prophylaxis of 100 mg. Cultures twice a year since 1973 have shown neither bacteriuria nor enterobacterial carriage on the vaginal vestibule.

TABLE 15–7. Bacterial Localization Studies in D.B., 22-Year-Old White Woman

Source[a]	Cultures	Specific Gravity[b]	Creatinine
	Escherichia coli/ml		(mg/dl)
CB	> 100,000		
WB	20		
LK$_1$	10,000	1.018	128
RK$_1$	> 10,000	1.019	126
LK$_2$	1000	1.019	116
RK$_2$	10,000	1.018	111
LK$_3$	540	1.019	118
RK$_3$	10,000	1.018	106
LK$_4$	610	1.019	
RK$_4$	8000	1.017	99

[a]CB = catheterized bladder urine; WB = washed bladder (after 2–3 liters of sterile water irrigation); LK$_1$ to LK$_4$ = serial left renal urines; RK$_1$ to RK$_4$ = serial right renal urines.

[b]Measured by refractometry.

From Stamey, T. A.: Pathogenesis and Treatment of Urinary Tract Infections. Baltimore, Williams & Wilkins Co., 1980. Used by permission.

bilateral renal bacteriuria (Table 15–7). The bladder at cystoscopy showed only that both ureteral orifices were somewhat U-shaped rather than slitlike; they were normally placed on the trigone. The patient was treated with nalidixic acid for 6 weeks (Fig. 15–12); halfway through a 6-week course of nalidixic acid, which sterilized the urine, a voiding cystourethrogram showed reflux to the kidney on the left (Fig. 15–13) and to the midureter on the right. The patient had a letter from a urologist, written 20 years before, that documented recurrent chills and fever beginning at the age of 6 weeks. When she was 2½ years old, a complete urologic evaluation, including an intravenous urogram, had been performed; the bladder appeared normal at cystoscopy, but reflux into the left ureter and kidney was demonstrated on a cystogram. This old intravenous urogram, which was obtained for review, demonstrated that the *same three abnormal calyces* were present 20 years before; these changes had been originally thought to be caused by her recent episodes of pyelonephritis following her marriage.

As can be seen in Figure 15–12, when the nalidixic acid was stopped after 6 weeks of therapy, she promptly became reinfected wih an *E. coli* 078. From that time on, each reinfection with *E. coli* that followed cessation of prophylaxis was treated with a few days of full-

Figure 15–13. A fluoroscopic spot film, showing gross reflux to the left kidney, during a voiding cystourethrogram in the same patient shown in Figure 15–11. There was also reflux to the middle of the right ureter, but not into the kidney.

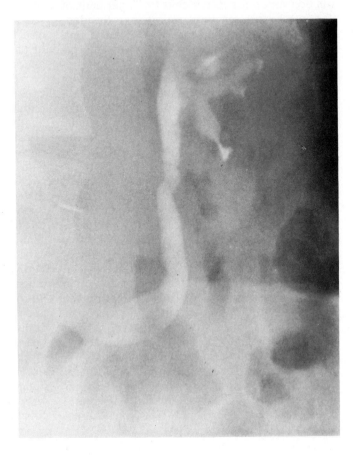

dose nitrofurantoin and followed again by nightly prophylaxis with 100-mg capsules. The *S. faecalis* infections toward the end of her recurrences were treated with very short courses. A repeat intravenous urogram in late 1972 was identical to that shown in Figure 15–11. A voiding cystourethrogram, performed with the same technique as in 1970, showed no reflux to the right ureter and only 4 cm of reflux in the terminal left ureter during voiding. The patient has been seen twice a year since 1973. One symptomatic *E. coli* infection occurred in August 1973, for which she received a few days of therapy with nitrofurantoin. Between August 1973 and the last culture taken in July 1979, she remained totally asymptomatic without antimicrobial therapy. A full-term pregnancy occurred in 1977 without complications, and bacteriuria did not occur. A second full-term pregnancy in 1980 was equally uneventful. This patient illustrates (1) the effectiveness of nitrofurantoin in long-term prophylaxis in preventing bacteriuria, and (2) the gradual loss of susceptibility to recurrent urinary infections.

The urologist should know the adverse reactions to nitrofurantoin (Holmberg et al., 1980). According to these authors, nitrofurantoin accounted for 10 per cent to 12 per cent of all adverse drug reactions reported in Sweden. The two largest groups consisted of acute pulmonary reactions (43 per cent) and allergic reactions (42 per cent). Neuropathy, blood dyscrasias, liver damage, and chronic pulmonary reactions constituted the remainder. These appeared to be acute hypersensitivity reactions, with 65 per cent to 83 per cent of the patients showing eosinophilia in their blood smears. The risk of an adverse reaction increases with age, with the greatest number occurring in patients over 50 years of age.

Cinoxacin (A Nalidixic Acid–like Drug). Nalidixic acid and its analog, cinoxacin, are useful because they produce minimal resistance among the fecal flora and serve as effective inhibitors of the transfer of R factors (Vuye, 1980); for this reason, multiply resistant *E. coli* virtually never carry resistance to nalidixic acid or cinoxacin (Stamey, 1980). The effect on the fecal flora of full-dosage nalidixic acid was qualitatively similar to TMP-SMX in that 67 per cent of 52 patients cleared all Enterobacteriaceae from their rectal cultures during oral therapy of 4 gm per day (Stamey and Mihara, 1979). Prophylactic efficacy with cinoxacin has been reported by Scheckler and associates (1982), Landes (1980), and Schaeffer and asso-

ciates (1981). The last-named investigators have also reported the effect of cinoxacin on the fecal and introital flora (Schaeffer et al., 1982b), which appears similar to that of nalidixic acid (Stamey and Mihara, 1979). An excellent review of the pharmacologic properties and therapeutic efficacy or cinoxacin in the treatment of urinary tract infections has been recently published (Sisca et al., 1983); cinoxacin has several advantages over nalidixic acid and none of the disadvantages. Although the reported prophylactic studies used 500-mg nightly dosage, a 250-mg dosage form is now available and should be equally successful in view of the high urinary concentrations achieved with cinoxacin.

Cephalexin. Fairley and his associates (1974) first reported on the prophylactic efficacy of 500 mg per day of cephalexin in preventing recurrent infections during a 6-month period of observation. Seventeen of the 22 patients remained free of infection, an impressive record because several patients had papillary necrosis, chronic pyelonephritis, and even renal calculi. Gower (1975) treated 25 women with 125 mg nightly of cephalexin for 6 to 12 months and had only one infection, while 13 of 25 women receiving a placebo had an infection. In a study of hospitalized patients with a mean age of 78 years, 125 mg per day of cephalexin was as effective as 250 mg per day in the 50 per cent of patients whose urine remained sterile (Sourander and Saarimaa, 1975).

Because of a similar favorable personal experience, and because these reports suggested minimal resistance in the fecal flora, Martinez, Kindrachuk, and Stamey (1984) studied the effect on the vaginal and rectal flora of 250 mg of cephalexin nightly for 6 months in 23 patients with reinfections of the urinary tract. Twenty-two of the 23 patients maintained a sterile urine throughout prophylaxis; a single patient developed two enterococcal urinary infections, both of which responded to nitrofurantoin. No change was detected in the rectal or vaginal carriage of Enterobacteriaceae. More importantly, not a single resistant strain of *E. coli* was detected in 154 cultures obtained at monthly intervals during cephalexin therapy. All rectal and vaginal cultures were streaked on Mueller-Hinton agar containing 32 gm per ml of cephalexin. These results are in contrast with those of Preiksaitis et al. (1981), who found rectal Enterobacteriaceae resistance in 38 per cent of patients when cephalexin was administered at a dose of 500 mg four times daily for 14 days. We conclude that cephalexin at 250 mg or less nightly is an excellent prophylactic agent because fecal resistance does not develop at this low dosage.

Trimethoprim. Kasanen and his associates in Finland (1978) studied the fecal flora in volunteers and patients who took 100 mg per day of trimethoprim for 3 weeks to 36 months; 4 of 20 patients treated for long periods developed resistant coliforms to trimethoprim (>8 μg per ml). We studied ten patients at Stanford who received 50 mg of trimethoprim once daily for a total of 63 months of prophylaxis with monthly cultures of the introitus and anal canal; only one resistant strain of *E. coli* was detected in 58 cultures. Svensson and his colleagues (1982) gave 100 mg of trimethoprim once daily for 6 months to 26 patients with recurrent urinary infections. The infection recurrence rate before prophylaxis was 26 per 100 months compared with 3.3 recurrences per 100 months during prophylaxis (p < 0.001). The postprophylactic infection rate returned to 23 recurrences per 100 months. It is important that all *E. coli* urinary infections following prophylaxis were sensitive to trimethoprim, that the number of rectal enterobacteria were markedly reduced during prophylaxis, and that although a 10 per cent incidence of trimethoprim-resistant *Enterobacter* from rectal swabs was observed less than 1 month into prophylaxis, there was no significant further accumulation of resistant bacteria. This 10 per cent incidence of trimethroprim-resistant enterobacteria is virtually the same as we found in patients receiving 40 mg of trimethoprim and 200 mg of sulfamethoxazole nightly in combination (Stamey and Condy, 1975). These studies on trimethoprim alone suggest that it should be as effective as TMP-SMX for prophylactic prevention of recurrent urinary infections. Stamm and associates (1980a) noted only one resistant strain of *E. coli* in 316 rectal, urethral, and vaginal isolates from 15 patients receiving 100 mg of trimethoprim and 15 others receiving 40 mg of TMP with 200 mg of SMX nightly for 6 months; their unbelievably low recovery of TMP-resistant *E. coli* is due to their method of sampling, which did not include streaking cultures from these colonization sites directly onto media containing trimethoprim.

These studies on TMP-SMX and trimethoprim prophylactic therapy have usually been limited to 6 months to test continuing susceptibility in patients with reinfections. Two studies (Pearson et al., 1979; Harding et al., 1982), however, continued TMP-SMX prophylaxis from 2 to 5 years without showing any increase in "breakthrough" infections or an increase in trimethoprim-resistant recurrent infections. Indeed, in the 15 patients treated for 2 years with one-half tablet of TMP-SMX thrice weekly (Harding et al., 1982), 100 of 116 cultures from the periurethral area (91 per cent) and 60 of 97 culures from the anal canal (68 per cent) showed no aerobic gram-negative bacilli at these colonization sites.

In view of all these studies that indicate minimal fecal resistance in patients who take oral TMP-SMX or trimethoprim alone, it is remarkable that Murray and associates (1982) reported TMP-resistant fecal gram-negative bacteria in 42 of 46 students who took TMP-SMX for 2 weeks in a diarrhea-preventive study in Mexico. This study would suggest that TMP-resistant strains are endemic in Mexico and should serve as a precaution to those of us who want to preserve the prophylactic efficacy of TMP-SMX in this country.

COMPARATIVE PROPHYLACTIC CLINICAL TRIALS

Several authors have compared the prophylactic efficacy of either nitrofurantoin and methenamine (Kincaid-Smith et al., 1970); methenamine mandelate, SMX, and TMP-SMX (Harding and Ronald, 1974); methenamine hippurate, nitrofurantoin, TMP, and TMP-SMX (Kasanen et al., 1974); and TMP-SMX, TMP, and nitrofurantoin (Stamm et al., 1980a). The first two and last studies included placebo-treated controls. It is clear from all these studies that any antimicrobial regimen is better than placebo therapy, that nitrofurantoin is superior to methenamine, that methenamine is better than sulfonamides, and that TMP or TMP-SMX is superior to any other regimen. For example, in the control clinical trials of Harding and Ronald (1974), there were 3.6 infections per patient year in the placebo group, 2.5 infections per patient year in the sulfamethoxazole group, 1.6 infections per patient year in the methenamine mandelate (2 gm per day) combined with ascorbic acid (2 gm per day) group, and 0.1 infection per patient year in the TMP-SMX group. It should be appreciated that in the methenamine and ascorbic acid regimen, methenamine was substantial—a dose equal to half the conventional full-dosage regimen—whereas the TMP-SMX dosage was only one eighth of the conventional daily dose (40 mg of TMP, 200 mg of SMX). In the study by Stamm and associates (1980a), the infections per patient year were comparable in the groups receiving TMP

(0.0), nitrofurantoin (0.14), and TMP-SMX (0.15), all occurring less frequently than in patients receiving placebo (2.8).

Lastly, the Winnipeg investigators (Harding et al., 1979) have also shown that thrice-weekly dosage of 40 mg of TMP and 200 mg of SMX has the same efficacy in preventing infections as described for their earlier report on nightly dosage (Harding and Ronald, 1974), which indicated an infection incidence of 0.1 per patient year of therapy.

Ronald and Harding (1981) noted that the cumulative experience with TMP 40 mg and SMX 200 mg exceeded 200 patient years, and that all studies were reporting fewer than 0.2 infections per patient year, a reduction of at least ten fold when compared with no treatment.

POSTINTERCOURSE PROPHYLAXIS

The foregoing data all relate to minimal but constant dosage with antimicrobial agents in the prevention of recurrent urinary tract infections. Constant-dosage prophylaxis has several advantages: (1) It is applicable to females of all ages, (2) it works well in sexually active women, and (3) it applies a constant, as opposed to intermittent, biologic pressure on the fecal and vaginal flora.

Postintercourse, single-dosage prophylaxis, however, is an effective way to prevent urinary tract infections in women whose recurrences are related to sexual activity. When we realized early in the 1960's that most recurrent infections were reinfections, we had women empty their bladders after sexual intercourse and take a single tablet of oral penicillin G (Stamey et al., 1965), a regimen that worked very well. Vosti (1975), using five different antimicrobial agents, documented the effectiveness of postintercourse prophylaxis in dramatically reducing the number of recurrent infections. More recently, Pfau and his colleagues in Jerusalem (Pfau et al., 1983) have shown the effectiveness of TMP-SMX, nalidixic acid, and nitrofurantoin—but not sulfonamides—in postcoital prophylaxis.

Single-tablet prophylaxis following sexual intercourse is a viable alternative in sexually active females. In those who have intercourse occasionally, it has the advantage of requiring substantially less drug than constant-dosage regimens. For those, however, who are sexually active several times per week, constant-dosage regimens are theoretically better, since they apply a constant pressure to the fecal flora rather than an intermittent one in which bacterial resistance may be encouraged. As with all antimicrobial regimens, the specific drug used for prophylaxis may make a substantial difference, depending upon its pharmacologic characteristics.

CONCLUSION

In conclusion, the urologist has in his hands the most powerful tool of his specialty—the prophylactic prevention of recurrent bacteriuria. It can save him countless hours with outpatients, dramatically reduce expenses in a medical care system overburdened with excessive cost, simplify his options in sorting out the complexities of the urethral syndrome by excluding a potential role for urinary tract infection, and lead a distressed patient to an easy, practical solution in the best tradition of our profession.

References

Achtman, M., Mercer, A., Kuseck, B., et al.: Six widespread bacterial clones among *Escherichia coli* K1 isolates. Infect. Immun., *39*:315, 1983.

Aronson, M., Medalia, O., Schori, L., et al.: Prevention of colonization of the urinary tract of mice with *Escherichia coli* by blocking of bacterial adherence with Methyl a-D-Mannopycanoside. J. Infect. Dis., *139*:329, 1979.

Asscher, A. W., Chick, S., Radford, N., et al.: Natural history of asymptomatic bacteriuria (ASB) in nonpregnant women. *In* Brumfitt, W., and Asscher, A. W.: (Eds.): Urinary Tract Infect. London, Oxford University Press, 1973, p. 51.

Asscher, A. W., Sussman, M., Waters, W. E., et al.: Asymptomatic significant bacteriuria in the non-pregnant women. II. Response to treatment and follow-up. Br. Med. J., *1*:804, 1969a.

Asscher, A. W., Sussman, M., Waters, W. E., et al.: The clinical significance of asymptomatic bacteriuria in the nonpregnant woman. J. Infect. Dis., *120*:17, 1969b.

Bear, R. A.: Pregnancy in patients with renal disease, a study of 44 cases. Obstet. Gynecol., *48*:13, 1976.

Bollgren, I., and Winberg, J.: The periurethral flora in girls highly susceptible to urinary infections. Acta Paediatr. Scand., *65*:81, 1976.

Brumfitt, W., and Pursell, R.: Trimethoprim-Sulfamethoxazole in the treatment of bacteriuria in women. J. Infect. Dis., *128*:S657, 1973.

Cifuentes, L.: Epithelium of vaginal type in the female trigone: The clinical problem of trigonitis. J. Urol., *57*:1028, 1947.

Cooke, E. M., and Ewins, S. P.: Properties of strains of *Escherichia coli* isolated from a variety of sources. J. Med. Microbiol., *8*:107, 1975.

Cunningham, F. G., Morris, G. B., and Mickal, A.: Acute pyelonephritis of pregnancy: A clinical review. Obstet. Gynecol., *42*:112, 1973.

Daikos, G. K., Kontomichalou, P., Bilalis, D., et al.: Intestinal flora ecology after oral use of antibiotics. Chemotherapy, *13*:146, 1968.

Dans, P. E., and Klaus, B.: Dysuria in women. Johns Hopkins Med. J., *138*:13, 1976.

Datta, J., Faiers, M. C., Reeves, D. S., et al.: R-factors in *Escherichia coli* in feces after oral chemotherapy in general practice. Lancet, *1*:312, 1971.

Davison, J. M., and Lindheimer, M. D.: Renal disease in pregnant women. Clin. Obstet. Gynecol., *21*:411, 1978.

Duguid, J. P.: The function of bacterial fimbriae (English translation). Arch. Immunol. Ther. Exp., *16*:173, 1968.

Duguid, J. P., and Gillies, R. R.: Fimbriae and adhesive properties in dysentery bacilli. J. Pathol. Bacteriol., *74*:397, 1957.

Duguid, J. P., Clegg, S., and Wilson, M. I.: The fimbrial and nonfimbrial hemagglutinins of *Escherichia coli.* J. Med. Microbiol., *12*:213, 1978.

Duguid, J. P., Smith, I. W., Dempster, G., et al.: Non-flagellar filamentous appendages ("fimbriae") and hemagglutinating activity in *Bacterium coli.* J. Pathol. Bacteriol., *70*:335, 1955.

Elder, H. A., Santamarina, B. A. G., Smith, S., et al.: The natural history of asymptomatic bacteriuria during pregnancy: The effect of tetracycline on the clinical course and the outcome of pregnancy. Am. J. Obstet. Gynecol., *111*:441, 1971.

Fairley, K. F., Bond, A. G., and Adey, F. D.: The site of infection in pregnancy bacteriuria. Lancet, *1*:939, 1966.

Fairley, K. F., Hubbard, M., and Whitworth, J. A.: Prophylactic long-term cephalexin in recurrent urinary infection. Med. J. Aust., *1*:318, 1974.

Fowler, J. E., Jr., and Stamey, T. A.: Studies of introital colonization in women with recurrent urinary infections. VII. The role of bacterial adherence. J. Urol., *117*:472, 1977.

Fowler, J. E., Jr., and Stamey, T. A.: Studies of introital colonization in women with recurrent urinary infections. X. Adhesive properties of *Escherichia coli* and *Proteus mirabilis:* Lack of correlation with urinary pathogenicity. J. Urol., *120*:315, 1978.

Fowler, J. E., Latta, R., and Stamey, T. A.: Studies of introital colonization in women with recurrent urinary infections. VIII. The role of bacterial interference. J. Urol., *118*:296, 1977.

Freedman, L. R.: Natural history of urinary infection in adults. Kidney Int., 8-S-96, 1975.

Fried, F. A., Vermeulen, C. W., Ginsburg, M. J., et al.: Etiology of pyelonephritis; further evidence associating the production of experimental pyelonephritis with hemolysis in *Escherichia coli.* J. Urol., *106*:351, 1971.

Gallagher, D. J. A., Montgomerie, J. Z., and North, J. D. K.: Acute infections of the urinary tract and the urethral syndrome in general practice. Br. Med. J., *1*:622, 1965.

Gaymans, R., Haverkorn, M. J., Valkenburg, H. A., et al.: A prospective study of urinary-tract infections in a Dutch general practice. Lancet, *2*:674, 1976.

Gilstrap, L. C., Leveno, K. J., Cunningham, F. G., et al.: Renal infection and pregnancy outcome. Am. J. Obstet. Gynecol., *141*:709, 1981.

Gower, P. E.: The use of small doses of cephalexin (125 mg) in the management of recurrent urinary tract infection in women. J. Antimicrob. Chemother., *1*:93, 1975.

Grüneberg, R. N., Smellie, J. M., and Leaky, A.: Changes in the antibiotic sensitivities of faecal organisms in response to treatment in children with urinary tract infection. *In* Brumfitt, W., and Asscher, A. W. (Eds.): Urinary Tract Infection. London, Oxford University Press, 1973, p. 131.

Grüneberg, R. N., Smellie, J. M., Leaky, A., et al.: Long-term low-dose cotrimoxazole in prophylaxis of childhood urinary tract infection: Bacteriological aspects. Br. Med. J., *2*:206, 1976.

Guttmann, D.: Follow-up of urinary tract infection in domicillary patients. *In* Brumfitt, W., and Asscher, A. W.

(Eds.): Urinary Tract Infection. London, Oxford University Press, 1973, p. 62.

Hagberg, L., Jodal, U., Korhonen, T. K., et al.: Adhesion, hemagglutination, and virulence of *Escherichia coli* causing urinary tract infections. Infect. Immun., *31*:564, 1981.

Harber, M. J., Chick, S., Mackenzie, R., et al.: Lack of adherence to epithelial cells by freshly isolated urinary pathogens. Lancet, *1*(8272): 586, 1982.

Harding, G. K. M., and Ronald, A. R.: A controlled study of antimicrobial prophylaxis of recurrent urinary infection in women. N. Engl. J. Med., *291*:597, 1974.

Harding, G. K. M., Buckwold, F. J., Marrie, T. J., et al.: Prophylaxis of recurrent urinary tract infection in female patients: Efficacy of low-dose thrice-weekly therapy with trimethoprim/sulfamethoxazole. JAMA, *242*:1975, 1979.

Harding, G. K. M., Ronald, A. R., Nicolle, L. E., et al.: Long-term antimicrobial prophylaxis for recurrent urinary tract infection in women. Rev. Infect. Dis., *4*:438, 1982.

Harris, R. E.: The significance of eradication of bacteriuria during pregnancy. Obstet. Gynecol., *53*:71, 1979.

Harris, R. E.: Antibiotic therapy of antepartum urinary tract infections. Int. Med. Res., *8*:40, 1980.

Harris, R. E., Thomas, V. L., and Shelokov, A.: Asymptomatic bacteriuria in pregnancy: Antibody-coated bacteria, renal function, and intrauterine growth retardation. Am. J. Obstet. Gynecol., *126*:20, 1976.

Harrison, W. O., Holmes, K. K., Belding, M. E., et al.: A prospective evaluation of recurrent urinary tract infection in women. Clin. Res., *22*:125A, 1974.

Heineman, H. S., and Lee, J. H.: Bacteriuria in pregnancy, a heterogeneous entity. Obstet. Gynecol., *41*:22, 1973.

Hinton, N. A.: The effect of oral tetracycline HCl and doxycycline on the intestinal flora. Curr. Ther. Res. Clin. Exp., *12*:341, 1970.

Holmberg, L., Boman, G., Bottiger, L. E., et al.: Adverse reactions to nitrofurantoin: Analysis of 921 reports. Am. J. Med., *69*:733, 1980.

Huland, H., and Busch, R.: Chronic pyelonephritis as a cause of end stage renal disease. J. Urol., *127*:642, 1982.

Johnson, C. W., and Smythe, C. M., Renal function in patients with chronic bacteriuria: A longitudinal study. South Med. J., *62*:81, 1969.

Källenius, G., and Möllby, R.: FEMS Microbiol. Lett., *5*:295, 1979.

Källenius, G., and Winberg, J.: Bacterial adherence to periurethral epithelial cells in girls prone to urinary-tract infection. Lancet, *2*:540, 1978.

Källenius, G., Möllby, R., Svenson, S. B., et al.: The p^k antigen as receptor for the haemagglutinin of pyelonephritic *Escherichia coli.* FEMS Microbiol. Lett., *7*:297, 1980.

Källenius, G. Möllby, R., Svenson, S. B., et al.: Occurrence of p-fimbriated *Escherichia coli* in urinary tract infections. Lancet, *2*: p. 1369, 1981.

Kasanen, A., Anttila, M., Elfving, R., et al.: Trimethoprim: Pharmacology, antimicrobial activity and clinical use in urinary tract infections. Ann. Clin. Res., *10*:1, 1978.

Kasanen, A., Kaarsalo, E., Hiltunen, R., et al.: V. Comparison of long-term, low-dosage nitrofurantoin, methenamine hippurate, trimethoprim and trimethoprim-sulfamethoxazole in the control of recurrent urinary tract infection. Ann. Clin. Res., *6*:285, 1974.

Kass, E. H.: Asymptomatic infections of the urinary tract. Trans. Assoc. Am. Physicians, *69*:56, 1956.

Kass, E. H.: The role of asymptomatic bacteriuria in the

pathogenesis of pyelonephritis. *In* Quinn, E. L., and Kass, E. H. (Eds.): Biology of Pyelonephritis. Boston, Little Brown & Co., 1960, p. 399.

Kass, E. H.: The role of unsuspected infection in the etiology of prematurity. Clin. Obstet. Gynecol., *16*:134, 1973.

Kincaid-Smith, P.: Management of renal and urinary tract disorders during pregnancy. *In* Harrison, J. H., Gittes, R. F., Perlmutter, A. D., Stamey, T. A., and Walsh, P. C. (Eds.): Campbell's Urology. Philadelphia, W. B. Saunders Co., 1979, p. 2518.

Kincaid-Smith, P., Friedman, A., and Nanra, R. S.: Controlled trials of treatment in urinary tract infection. *In* Kincaid-Smith, P., and Fairley, K. F. (Eds.): Renal Infection and Renal Scarring. Melbourne, Mercedes Publishing Co., 1970, p. 165.

Knothe, H.: The effect of a combined preparation of trimethoprim and sulphamethoxazole following short-term and long-term administration on the flora of the human gut. Chemotherapy, *18*:285, 1973.

Korhonen, T. K., Väisanen, V., Saxén, H., et al.: P-antigen–recognizing fimbriae from human uropathogenic *Escherichia coli* strains. Infect. Immun., *37*:286, 1982.

Kraft, J. K., and Stamey, T. A.: The natural history of symptomatic recurrent bacteriuria in women. Medicine, *56*:55, 1977.

Kunin, C. M., Polyak, F., and Postel, E.: Periurethral bacterial flora in women: Prolonged intermittent colonization with *Escherichia coli*. JAMA, *243*:134, 1980.

Kunin, C. M., Zacha, E., and Paquin, A. J.: Urinary-tract infections in schoolchildren. I. Prevalence of bacteriuria and associated urologic findings. N. Engl. J. Med., *26*:1287, 1962.

Kurdydyk, L. M., Kelly, K., Harding, G. K. M., et al.: Role of cervicovaginal antibody in the pathogenesis of recurrent urinary tract infection in women. Infect. Immun., *29*:76, 1980.

Landes, R. R.: Long term low dose cinoxacin therapy for the prevention of recurrent urinary tract infections. J. Urol, *123*:47, 1980.

Lark, D., O'Hanley, P., and Schoolnik, G.: Distribution of digalactoside and dimannose receptors in human genitourinary tissue. Submitted for publication.

Leveno, K. J., Harris, R. E., Gilstrap, L. C., et al.: Bladder versus renal bacteriuria during pregnancy: Recurrence after treatment. Am. J. Obstet. Gynecol., *139*:403, 1981.

Lincoln, K., Lidin-Janson, G., and Winberg, J.: Resistant urinary infections resulting from changes in the resistance pattern of fecal flora induced by antibiotics and hospital environment. Br. Med. J., *3*:305, 1970.

Lomberg, H., Hanson, L. A., Jacobsson, B., et al.: Correlation of P blood group, vesicoureteral reflux, and bacterial attachment in patients with recurrent pyelonephritis. N. Engl. J. Med., *308*:1189, 1983.

Low, D., David, V., Lark, D., et al.: Gene clusters governing the production of hemolysin and mannose-resistant hemagglutination are closely linked in *Escherichia coli* serotype 04 and 06 isolates from urinary tract infections. Infect. Immun., *43*:353, 1984.

Mabeck, C. E.: Treatment of uncomplicated urinary tract infection in non-pregnant women. Postgrad. Med., *48*:69, 1972.

Martinez, F. C., Kindrachuk, R. W., and Stamey, T. A.: Prophylactic efficacy of nightly dosage with cephalexin: Effect on the vaginal and rectal flora. Submitted for publication.

McFadyen, I. R., Eykyn, S. J., Gardner, N. H. N., et al.: Bacteriuria in pregnancy. J. Obstet. Gynaecol. Br. Commonw., *80*:385, 1973.

McGeachie, J.: Hemolysis by urinary *Escherichia coli*. Am. J. Clin. Pathol., *45*:222, 1966.

McGeown, M. G.: Treatment of urinary tract infection during pregnancy. Contrib. Nephrol., *25*:30, 1981.

Miall, W. W., Kass, E. H., Ling, J., et al.: Factors influencing arterial pressure in the general population in Jamaica. Br. Med. J., *2*:497, 1962.

Minshew, B. H., Jorgensen, J., Swanstrum, M., et al.: Some characteristics of *Escherichia coli* strains isolated from extraintestinal infections of humans. J. Infect. Dis. *137*:648, 1978.

Möller, J. K., Bak, A. L., Stenderup, A., et al.: Changing patterns of plasmid-mediated drug resistance during tetracycline therapy. Antimicrob. Agents. Chemother., *11*:388, 1977.

Moorhouse, E. C., and Farrell, W.: Effect of cotrimoxazole on faecal enterobacteria: No emergence of resistant strains. J. Med. Microbiol., *6*:249, 1973.

Murray, B. E., Rensimer, E. R., and DuPont, H. L.: Emergence of high-level trimethoprim resistance in fecal *Eschericheria coli* during oral administration of trimethoprim or trimethoprim-sulfamethoxazole. N. Engl. J. Med., *306*:130, 1982.

Naeye, R. L.: Causes of the excessive rates of perinatal mortality and prematurity in pregnancies complicated by maternal urinary-tract infections. N. Engl. J. Med., *300*:819, 1979.

Näff, H.: Über die Veränderungen der normalen Darmflora des Menschen durch Bactrim. Pathol. Microbiol., *37*:1, 1971.

Ofek, I., Goldhar, J., Eshdat, Y., et al.: The importance of mannose specific adhesins (lectins) in infections caused by *Escherichia coli*. Scand. J. Infect. Dis. (Suppl.), *33*:61, 1982.

Ørskov, I., Ørskov, F., and Birch-Andersen, A.: Comparison of *Escherichia coli* fimbrial antigen F7 with type 1 fimbriae. Infect. Immun., *27*:657, 1980.

Parkkinen, J., Finne, J., Achtman, M., et al.: *Escherichia coli* strains binding neuraminyl a2-3 galactosides. Biochem. Biophys. Res. Comm., *111*:456, 1983.

Parsons, C. L., Pollen, J. J., Anwar, H., et al.: Antibacterial activity of bladder surface mucin duplicated in the rabbit bladder by exogenous glycosaminoglycan (sodium pentosanpolysulfate). Infect. Immun., *27*:876, 1980.

Pearson, N. J., McSherry, A. M., Towner, K. J., et al.: Emergence of trimethoprim-resistant enterobacteria in patients receiving long-term cotrimoxazole for the control of intractable urinary-tract infection. Lancet, *2*:1205, 1979.

Pfau, A., Sacks, T., and Engelstein, D.: Recurrent urinary tract infections in premenopausal women: Prophylaxis based on an understanding of the pathogenesis. J. Urol., *129*:1153, 1983.

Pometta, D., Rees, S. B., Younger, D., et al.: Asymptomatic bacteriuria in diabetes mellitus. N. Engl. J. Med., *276*:1118, 1967.

Preiksaitis, J. K., Thompson, L., Harding, G. K. M., et al.: A comparison of the efficacy of nalidixic acid and cephalexin in bacteriuric women and their effect on fecal and periurethral carriage of Enterobacteriaceae. J. Infect. Dis., *143*:603, 1981.

Ries, K., and Kaye, D.: The current status of therapy in urinary tract infection in pregnancy. Clin. Perinatol., *1*:423, 1974.

Ronald, A. R., and Harding, G. K. M.: Urinary infection prophylaxis in women. Ann. Intern. Med., *94*:268, 1981.

Ronald, A. R., Jagdis, F. A., Harding, G. K., et al.: Amoxicillin therapy of acute urinary infections in adults. Antimicrob. Agents Chemother., *11*:780, 1977.

Savage, W. E., Hajj, S. N., and Kass, E. H.: Demographic and prognostic characteristics of bacteriuria in pregnancy. Medicine, *46*:385, 1967.

Schaeffer, A. J., and Stamey, T. A.: Studies of introital colonization in women with recurrent urinary infections; IX. The role of antimicrobial therapy. J. Urol., *118*:221, 1977.

Schaeffer, A. J., Chmiel, J. S., Duncan, J. L., et al.: Mannose-sensitive adherence of *Escherichia coli* to epithelial cells from women with recurrent urinary tract infections. J. Urol., *131*:906, 1984.

Schaeffer, A. J., Flynn, S., and Jones, J.: Comparison of cinoxacin and trimethoprim-sulfamethoxazole in treatment of urinary tract infections. J. Urol., *125*:825, 1981.

Schaeffer, A. J., Jones, J. M., and Dunn, J. K.: Association of *in vitro Escherichia coli* adherence to vaginal and buccal epithelial cells with susceptibility of women to recurrent urinary-tract infections. N. Engl. J. Med., *304*:1062, 1981.

Schaeffer, A. J., Jones, J. M., Falkowski, W. S., et al.: Variable adherence of uropathogenic *Escherichia coli* to epithelial cells from women with recurrent urinary tract infection. J. Urol., *128*:1227, 1982a.

Schaeffer, A. J., Jones, J. M., and Flynn, S. S.: Prophylactic efficacy of cinoxacin in recurrent urinary tract infections: Biologic effects on vaginal and fecal flora. J. Urol., *127*:1128, 1982b.

Schechter, H., Leonard, C. D., and Scribner, B. H.: Chronic pyelonephritis as a cause of renal failure in dialysis candidates. JAMA, *216*:514, 1971.

Scheckler, W. E., Burt, R. A. P., and Paulson, D. F.: Comparison of low-dose cinoxacin therapy and placebo in the prevention of recurrent urinary tract infections. J. Family Pract., *15*:901, 1982.

Schwarz, R. H.: Considerations of antibiotic therapy during pregnancy. Obstet. Gynecol., *58*:95S, 1981.

Sharp, J. L.: The growth of *Candida albicans* during antibiotic therapy. Lancet, *1*:390, 1954.

Sisca, T. S., Heel, R. C., and Romankiewicz, J. A.: Cinoxacin: A review of its pharmacological properties and therapeutic efficacy in the treatment of urinary tract infections. Drugs, *25*:544, 1983.

Sourander, L., and Saarimaa, H.: Effect of long-term treatment of urinary tract infection with a single dose in the evening. Chemotherapy, *21*:52, 1975.

Stamey, T. A.: The Prevention of Recurrent Urinary Infections. New York, Science and Medicine Publishing Co., 1973.

Stamey, T. A.: Urinary tract infections in women. *In*: Stamey, T. A.: Pathogenesis and Treatment of Urinary Tract Infections. Baltimore, Williams & Wilkins Co., 1980.

Stamey, T. A., and Condy, M.: The diffusion and concentration of trimethoprim in human vaginal fluid. J. Infect. Dis., *131*:261, 1975.

Stamey, T. A., and Howell, J. J.: Studies of introital colonization in women with recurrent urinary infections: IV. The role of local vaginal antibodies. J. Urol., *115*:413, 1976.

Stamey, T. A., and Kaufman, M. F.: Studies of introital colonization in women with recurrent urinary infections: II. A comparison of growth in normal vaginal fluid of common versus uncommon serogroups of *Escherichia coli*. J. Urol., *114*:264, 1975.

Stamey, T. A., and Mihara, G.: Studies of introital colonization in women with recurrent urinary infections: V. The inhibitory activity of normal vaginal fluid on *Proteus mirabilis* and *Pseudomonas aeruginosa*. J. Urol., *115*:416, 1976a.

Stamey, T. A., and Mihara, G.: Studies of introital colonization in women with recurrent urinary infection: VI. Analysis of segmented leukocytes on the vaginal vestibule in relation to enterobacterial colonization. J. Urol., *116*:72, 1976b.

Stamey, T. A., and Mihara, G.: The effect of nalidixic acid on faecal and vaginal carriage of Enterobacteriaceae in 54 women. *In* van der Waaij, D., and Verhoef, J. (Eds.): New Criteria for Antimicrobial Therapy: Maintenance of Digestive Tract Colonization Resistance. Proceedings of a Symposium. Amsterdam, Excerpta Medica, 1979, p. 234.

Stamey, T. A., and Sexton, C. C.: The role of vaginal colonization with Enterobacteriaceae in recurrent urinary infections. J. Urol., *113*:214, 1975.

Stamey, T. A., and Timothy, M. M.: Studies of introital colonization in women with recurrent urinary infections, I. The role of vaginal pH. J. Urol., *114*:261, 1975a.

Stamey, T. A., and Timothy, M. M.: Studies of introital colonization in women with recurrent urinary infections, III. Vaginal glycogen concentrations. J. Urol., *114*:268, 1975b.

Stamey, T. A., Condy, M., and Mihara, G.: Prophylactic efficacy of nitrofurantoin macrocrystals and trimethoprim-sulfamethoxazole in urinary infections. New Engl. J. Med. *296*:780, 1977.

Stamey, T. A., Govan, D. E., and Palmer, J. M.: The localization and treatment of urinary tract infections: The role of bactericidal urine levels as opposed to serum levels. Medicine. *44*:1, 1965.

Stamey, T. A., Timothy, M., Millar, M., et al.: Recurrent urinary infections in adult women. The role of introital enterobacteria. Calif. Med., *115*:1, 1971.

Stamey, T. A., Wehner, N., Mihara, G., et al.: The immunologic basis of recurrent bacteriuria; role of cervicovaginal antibody in enterobacterial colonization of the introital mucosa. Medicine, *57*:47, 1978.

Stamm, W. E., Counts, G. W., Running, K. R., et al.: Diagnosis of coliform infection in acutely dysuric women. N. Engl. J. Med., *307*:463, 1982.

Stamm, W. E., Counts, G. W., Wagner, K. F., et al.: Antimicrobial prophylaxis of recurrent urinary tract infections: A double-blind, placebo-contracted trial. Ann. Intern. Med., *92*:770, 1980a.

Stamm, W. E., Wagner, K. F., Amsel, R., et al.: Causes of the acute urethral syndrome in women. N. Engl. J. Med., *303*:409, 1980b.

Sussman, M., Asscher, A. W., Waters, W. E., et al.: Asymptomatic significant bacteriuria in the nonpregnant woman. I. Description of a population. Br. Med. J., *1*:799, 1969.

Svanborg Edén, C., and Hanson, L. A.: *Escherichia coli* pili as possible mediators of attachment to human urinary tract epithelial cells. Infect. Immun., *21*:229, 1978.

Svanborg Edén, C., and Jodal, U.: Attachment of *Escherichia coli* to urinary sediment epithelial cells from urinary tract infection–prone and healthy children. Infect. Immun., *26*:837, 1979.

Svanborg Edén, C., Eriksson, B., Hanson, L. A., et al.: Adhesion to normal human uroepithelial cells of *Escherichia coli* from children with various forms of urinary tract infection. J. Pediatr., *93*:398, 1978.

Svanborg Edén, C., Eriksson, B., and Hanson, L. A.:

Adhesion of *Escherichia coli* to human uroepithelial cells in vitro. Infect. Immun., *18*:767, 1977.

Svanborg Edén, C., Freter, R., Hagberg, L., et al.: Inhibition of experimental ascending urinary tract infection by an epithelial cell–surface receptor analogue. Nature, *298*:560, 1982.

Svanborg Edén, C., Hanson, L. A., Jodal, U., et al.: Variable adherence to normal human urinary tract epithelial cells of *Escherichia coli* strains associated with various forms of urinary tract infection. Lancet, *2*:490, 1976.

Svensson, R., Larsson, P., and Lincoln, K.: Low dose trimethoprim prophylaxis in long term control of chronic recurrent urinary infection. Scand. J. Infect. Dis., *14*:139, 1982.

Sweet, R. L.: Bacteriuria and pyelonephritis during pregnancy. Semin. Perinatol., *1*:25, 1977.

Szabo, R., Shortliffe, L. D., and Stamey, T. A.: Attachment of *E. coli* and *Proteus mirabilis* to uroepithelial cells. In preparation.

Thompson, R. B.: A Short Textbook of Haematology. Philadelphia, J.B. Lippincott Co., 1969.

Toivanen, A., Kasanen, A., Sundquist, H., et al.: Effect of trimethoprim on the occurrence of drug-resistant coliform bacteria in the faecal flora. Chemotherapy, *22*:97, 1976.

Väisanen, V., Tallgren, L. F., Mäkelä, P. H., et al.: Mannose-resistant haemagglutination and p antigen recognition are characteristic of *Escherichia coli* causing primary pyelonephritis. Lancet, *2*:1366, 1981.

Vosti, K. L.: Recurrent urinary tract infections: Prevention by prophylactic antibiotics after sexual intercourse. JAMA, *231*:934, 1975.

Vuye, A.: Effect of cinoxacin on the conjugal transfer of R-plasmids in *Escherichia coli*. J. Pharm. Belg., *35*:451, 1980.

Waltzer, W. C.: The urinary tract in pregnancy. J. Urol., *125*:271, 1981.

Weinstein, A. J.: Treatment of bacterial infections in pregnancy. Drugs, *17*:56, 1979.

Williams, J. D., Reeves, D. S., Brumfitt, W., et al.: The effects of bacteriuria in pregnancy on maternal health. *In* Brumfitt, W., and Asscher, A. W. (Eds.): Urinary Tract Infections. London, Oxford University Press, 1973, p. 103.

Winberg, J., Bergstrom, T., Lincoln, K., et al.: Treatment trials in urinary tract infection (UTI) with special reference to the effect of antimicrobials on the fecal and periurethral flora. Clin. Nephrol., *1*:142, 1973.

Zacur, H. A., and Mitch, W. E.: Renal disease in pregnancy. Med. Clin. North Am., *61*:89, 1977.

Zinner, S. H., and Kass, E. H.: Long-term—10 to 14 years—follow-up of bacteriuria of pregnancy. N. Engl. J. Med., *285*:820, 1971.

Zinner, S. H.: Bacteriuria and babies revised. N. Engl. J. Med., *300*:853, 1979.

CHAPTER 16

Urinary Tract Infections in Infants and Children

JAN WINBERG, M.D.

Urinary tract infection (UTI) is one of the major bacterial diseases of childhood. The risk of a newborn girl's falling ill during childhood with a symptomatic UTI is at least 3 per cent; for a boy, about 1 per cent. The incidence of asymptomatic bacteriuria (ABU) in girls of preschool and school age is approximately 1 per cent.

About half the patients with symptomatic infections (and 80 per cent of those with ABU) will develop one or several recurrent infections. Some girls of late preschool or school age will have an almost endless chain of UTI's.

Some 5 to 7 per cent of the patients with symptomatic febrile infections during the first year of life may acquire a renal scar; with later onset of the first infection this risk seems to be less. A proportion of the patients with scarring will develop renal stones, hypertension, end-stage renal disease, or complications of pregnancy. Thus, even from a qualitative point of view, UTI is a disease of major concern. These severe complications can probably be prevented by adequate care.

Adequate management usually calls for expensive microbiologic, nephrologic, and radiologic examinations and several follow-up visits after infection. The great majority of patients take antibiotics for short or long periods. UTI thus causes morbidity and inconvenience to many patients and huge costs for the family or society.

DEFINITION

UTI is the denomination for conditions that have one feature in common-presence of signif-icant amounts of bacteria in the urine. The term "UTI" is, in this chapter, used for all such conditions irrespective of the localization of the infections. There is reason to believe that several mechanisms may lead to the establishment of urinary tract infection and that, consequently, course and prognosis may differ. UTI can be classified with regard to pathogenesis, localization, and therapeutic implications.

CLASSIFICATION WITH REGARD TO PATHOGENESIS

A tentative pathogenetic classification is suggested in Table 16–1. For better understanding of the disease process, it may be valuable to split the material into such subgroups in clinical as well as in scientific work. Obstructed infections make up only a small minority of all UTI in childhood (1 to 2 per cent in girls; 5 to 10 per cent in boys) but are qualitatively important, since irreversible renal damage may occur rapidly. Gross reflux is not considered to be an obstructive complication of similar dignity as urethral valves, ureterocele, and so forth. But it is an effective means of transporting bacteria to the upper urinary tract and, when associated with intrarenal reflux, into the renal parenchyma. This probably constitutes the great impact of this common abnormality on the prognosis of UTI. Screening bacteriuria ("asymptomatic;" symptomless; covert; latent; or other terms) is revealed by examination of healthy populations, and it occurs mainly in girls. A special host-aggressor relationship in many of these patients may warrant its classification as a group in its own right, although the pathogenetic mechanism may be the same as in uncomplicated symptomatic infections.

TABLE 16–1. Classification of Urinary Tract Infection (UTI)*

Noncomplicated
Symptomatic nonobstructed, with and without slight to moderate reflux†
    Neonates
    Girls
    Boys
"Screening bacteriuria"

Complicated
With gross reflux‡
Obstructed§
Associated with a neurogenic bladder

---

*UTI is used as a common designation for conditions with significant bacteriuria.
  †Grades I–III on a IV-graded scale.
  ‡Grade IV on a IV-graded scale.
  §Valves, ureterocele, foreign bodies, stones, diverticula, and so forth.

CLASSIFICATION WITH REGARD TO THE LOCALIZATION OF THE INFECTION

Urethritis. It remains to be proven that true bacterial urethritis exists (except gonococcal).

Cystitis and Pyelonephritis. These are self-explanatory terms. Localizing measures are described on page 838.

Pyelitis. This is a term used especially in Europe to denote a febrile UTI. Bacteria reaching the renal pelvis may cause local inflammation with loin pains. It may be the forerunner of a renal invasion such as pyelonephritis. Since it is almost impossible to show that an infection involves the pelvis but not the renal tissue, there is no reason to use the term pyelitis any longer.

Chronic Pyelonephritis. This is a confusing term, since it is used in many different senses: (1) to describe certain characteristic histologic lesions of the renal parenchyma; (2) to describe focal renal parenchymal defects visible on x-ray examination and usually consisting of papillary shrinking with a defect of the corresponding part of the renal outline ("scarring"), a lesion that is often progressive; and (3) to describe a clinical condition characterized by continuous excretion of bacteria or by frequent recurrences of infection. The term chronic pyelonephritis is clearly misleading. True chronic infections of the renal parenchyma are probably rare but may occur in association with staghorn calculi and in specific infections, such as tuberculosis.

Cystourethral Syndrome (Cystourethritis; Bacterial Cystitis; Urethritis). This vague denomination is often used for patients who have the classic symptoms of "cystitis" but who are lacking significant bacteriuria. The condition is not uncommon in prepubertal girls and is often associated with uninhibited contractions of the detrusor and instability of the sphincter function. Squatting and pant-wetting are common symptoms. Pyuria, suggesting inflammation, may be present. Vulvitis and balanitis should be ruled out by inspection. The cause is unknown. Its association with UTI is complex and far from understood.

Urinary Tract Infection. In this chapter, this is used as a noncommittal term, preferred when the localization of the infection has not been determined.

CLASSIFICATION WITH REGARD TO MANAGEMENT

See Chapter 14, pages 741 to 743.

DIAGNOSTIC PROCEDURES

Demonstration of a "significant" number of bacteria in the urine is the only valid criterion for the presence of a UTI. Other commonly accepted diagnostic signs, such as pyuria, decreased concentrating capacity, elevated antibody titers, and so on, show only secondary phenomena and can therefore give only supportive evidence. Some patients with obvious infections have only small numbers of bacteria in the urine (Stamm et al., 1982; Bollgren et al., 1984). The reason for this is obscure.

Demonstration of Bacteria

Kass's (1956) definition of the limits for significant bacteriuria is statistically based. He examined whole urinary specimens (not midstream specimens) from apparently healthy adult women. The limits suggested by this study are regarded as valid for infants and children: 10,000 bacteria per ml of urine-probably contamination; 10,000 to 100,000 bacteria per ml of urine-doubtful, new culture suggested; more than 100,000 bacteria per ml of urine-probably infection. More investigations to substantiate this assumption are required. For example, the requirement of overnight incubation of bladder urine is rarely met in infants and toddlers; urgency and frequency also reduce incubation time. The prepuce and periurethral area are heavily contaminated by bacteria up to the ages of 2 to 5 years, even in healthy children (Bollgren and Winberg, 1976b), while the pubic hair seems to be a common habitat in adults. How often and to what extent these special circumstances make the urine colony count depart from Kass's values are unknown. In little boys, the overlap between normal and pathologic values seems to be especially great.

OFFICE METHODS FOR DEMONSTRATION OF BACTERIURIA

Microscopy. About 50,000 to 100,000 bacteria per ml of urine produce one rod per high-power field.

Dip Slide Culture. This is an easy and cheap method for demonstration of significant bacteriuria. The degree of accuracy is greater than that of the standard loop method routinely used for quantitative cultures (Arneil et al., 1973). It is a major advance in the diagnosis of UTI, and its use is encouraged. The set consists of a glass slide covered with blood agar on one side, and Cysteine-Lactose-Electrolyte Deficient (CLED) medium, inhibiting the growth of gram-positive organisms on the other. The slide is attached to a screw-top cap that fits into a plastic tube.* It is dipped in the urine or, even better, in the urinary stream, and the excess urine is allowed to drain off onto a scrap of paper. The slide, fitted in the plastic tube, is best incubated at 37°C, but room temperature also gives accurate results. The growth is compared with a visual scale, which gives the number of bacteria per milliliter.

A high diagnostic standard requires careful attention by the clinician in regard to (1) collection of urine, (2) transportation of urine, and (3) discontinuation of antibiotic treatment before collecting the urine for culture.

COLLECTION OF URINE

Four methods of urine collection are available: "clean catch" of midstream urine, catheterization, bladder puncture, or plastic bag collection.

*Made under the trade name of Uricult, they are marketed in this country by Metpath in New Jersey.

"Clean Catch." This should be the routine procedure, if possible using midstream urine. The preputial folds of small boys may contain large numbers of bacteria even after cleaning (Table 16–2) and must be irrigated before a culture can be taken.

Plastic Bag Collection. Reliable results can be obtained with meticulous washing of the genital region (redone if the patient has not voided within 3 hours) and detachment of the bag within 15 to 20 minutes after voiding. One should either do an immediate culture or chill the specimen to 4°C for preservation. Even with a well-trained staff, the risk of false positive results is great.

Bladder Puncture. This is mainly used for patients in the first year of life. The procedure has been described in detail (Nelson and Peters, 1965). The use of the Vacutainer System facilitates the procedure, and complications are rare. Urine obtained in this way is supposed to be sterile, but data on this point are lacking.

Indications for bladder puncture include: (1) persistent bacteriuria of doubtful significance; (2) seriously ill patients for whom rapid and accurate diagnosis is essential; (3) obstruction of bladder outflow tract or urethra; and (4) all uncircumcised boys with nonretractable prepuce if the urine contains more than 10,000 bacteria per ml of urine. It is unnecessary to confirm such a questionable culture when massive pyuria is also present.

Catheterization. This is employed if bladder puncture is not convenient, mainly for patients older than 1 year of age. The risk of infecting previously healthy patients is probably small; it may be considerable, however, in patients with a history of recurring infections (McCabe and Jackson, 1965).

TRANSPORTATION OF URINE

Bacterial multiplication starts rapidly in vitro. After 24 hours at room temperature, most urine specimens will have similar numbers of

TABLE 16–2. URINARY BACTERIA BEFORE AND AFTER PREPUTIAL IRRIGATION IN SIX NEWBORN MALES*

Day of Life	Urine Obtained Before Irrigation	First Irrigation Fluid	Second Irrigation Fluid	Urine Obtained After Irrigation
3	200,000	500,000	300	8,000
4	100,000	100,000	40,000	50
5	350,000	180,000	15,000	2,000
5	200,000	1,500,000	130,000	2,400
6	90,000	3,000,000	120,000	5,000
6	10	50,000	4,000	500

*The external genitals were cleansed with soap and water before the first urine specimen was obtained. Irrigation with two 10-ml doses of physiologic saline.

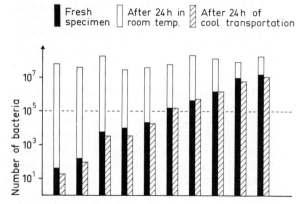

Figure 16–1. A series of urine specimens with different initial numbers of bacteria is shown. The concentration of bacteria in the same specimen after 24 hours at room temperature and after 24 hours in a cool transportation set (about +4°C) is shown. The dashed line shows the limit for significant bacteriuria. (From Kallings, L. O.: Sven. Lakartidin., *65* [Suppl. III]:30, 1968.)

bacteria irrespective of the number present at voiding (Fig. 16–1). It is mandatory that the urine be kept cold from the moment of voiding until the seeding on plates. At 0 to 4°C, the bacterial count will remain unchanged for at least 48 hours.

INFLUENCE OF ANTIBIOTICS IN THE URINE

Even at low blood levels, most antibiotics may appear in the urine in a highly concentrated, active form and can influence bacterial multiplication. Figure 16–2 shows that after administration of one 50 mg/kg dose of a short-acting sulfonamide (sulfisoxazole), the urine concentration was still sufficient to inhibit bacterial growth 48 hours later. The implication of this observation is that before culturing, therapy should be discontinued for a sufficiently long time to permit complete excretion of antibiotics. Another cause of false negative urine is perineal washing with antiseptic solutions.

Demonstration of Secondary Phenomena of Infection or Inflammation, or Both

WHITE CELL COUNT

Pyuria is only a sign of inflammation—bacterial or nonbacterial—of the genital region or urinary tract, and demonstration of it cannot replace culturing in the diagnosis of bacterial

UTI. A normal white cell count also does not exclude a UTI. In consecutive urine specimens, the number of white cells may vary between none and the number indicative of gross pyuria (Geisinger, 1931). It is more common to find a normal white cell concentration with recurrent infections than with apparent first-time infections (Fig. 16–3). Quantitative counting of urinary white cells is best done by placing the uncentrifuged urine in a counting chamber (i.e., the Fuchs-Rosenthal) (Houston, 1963).

Boys should have fewer than 10 cells per cu mm in voided specimens; girls usually also have few white cells, but counts between 50 and 100 cells per cu mm may be found without demonstrable disease. Ordinary sediment investigation is of value for demonstration of white cell casts. Presence or absence of white blood cell esterase in the urine, as demonstrated by means of paper strips (Cytur), is claimed to be a reliable index of white cell excretion. This requires confirmation.

White cell counting is helpful in three situations:

1. In making a tentative diagnosis in acutely ill patients before the results of culture are available.

2. In support of the diagnosis in patients with low-count bacteriuria due to frequency; in patients with symptoms of doubtful significance or with asymptomatic bacteriuria; and in all boys younger than 3 to 4 years old, in whom the preputial bacteria may heavily contaminate urine.

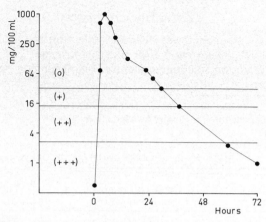

Figure 16–2. Concentration of sulfonamide in the urine (•—•) after one single dose of the short-acting sulfafurazole (Gantrisin), 50 mg/kg body weight. Common levels used for defining the degree of sensitivity are indicated: + + + equals highly sensitive, 0 equals minimal sensitivity. Even after 48 hours, biologically active sulfonamide was present in the urine. (Courtesy of Dr. K. Lincoln.)

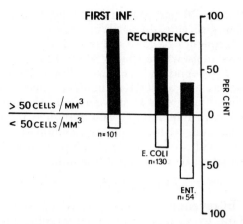

Figure 16–3. Occurrence of pyuria in girls with urinary tract infections. A count of less than 50 cells per mm³ in the uncentrifuged urine is common, especially in recurrent infection. ENT. = enterococci.

3. In suggesting renal involvement by appearance of white cell casts. Testing for proteinuria is of no help in the diagnosis of UTI. Hematuria is not uncommon.

DETERMINATION OF ANTIBODY TITER

Agglutinating and hemagglutinating antibodies to the O antigen of the infecting *Escherichia coli* can regularly be demonstrated in the serum of patients with pyelonephritis but not in those with cystitis (Percival et al., 1964; Winberg et al., 1963). The antibodies are highly specific and can be used diagnostically to verify that the isolated bacteria are the cause of the infection. This may be clinically useful as a research tool in patients with low-count bacteriuria. (See also immunology of UTI.)

RENAL FUNCTION

In acute infection of a previously healthy kidney, renal concentrating capacity is temporarily reduced. In uncomplicated infections, it improves rapidly but is not completely restored for 8 to 12 weeks (Fig. 16–4). If it does not return to normal, the possibility of obstruction of the urine flow, renal scarring, or persistent infection should be considered.

An increase in blood urea nitrogen (BUN) or serum creatinine is uncommon in uncomplicated acute pyelonephritis. If present, it suggests either obstruction with bilateral hydronephrosis or marked parenchymal reduction. During the newborn period, a BUN increase may occur even in the absence of obstruction (Bergström et al., 1967).

In scarred kidneys, all types of functional defects may be seen, including reduced ability to excrete a sodium chloride load (Aperia et al., 1971) and a lowering of the renal threshold for sodium bicarbonate reabsorption (Berg et al., 1971). The latter may be the earliest functional defect to become manifest.

Inulin and PAH clearances performed 3 to 5 days after onset of treatment for febrile infections in children have demonstrated increased values for GFR and ERPF (Berg, 1981). How-

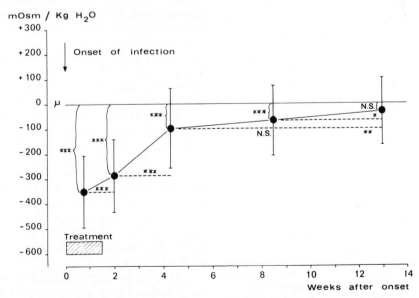

Figure 16–4. Statistical analysis of repeated concentration tests in 95 girls, selected on the basis of a rectal temperature of ⩾ 38°C, a sedimentation rate of > 20 mm/hr, and significant bacteriuria and pyuria. See text.

0 = normal mean for age (Winberg, 1959). The vertical axis gives deviation from normal mean.

*—$P < 0.05$; **—$P < 0.01$; ***—$P < 0.001$.

ever, gamma-camera studies with ^{131}I hippuran in the acute phase of untreated pyelonephritis in monkeys have shown a considerable increase in renal transit time, possibly the result of edema, and later a decrease in effective renal plasma flow (Janson and Roberts, 1978). The monkey studies may show the true effect of infection, while the clinical study may reflect the influence of early treatment on renal function.

X-ray Diagnostic Procedures

Only a few comments will be made on the place of excretion pyelograpy and micturition urethrocystography in the management of UTI. There are three main aims of these examinations:

1. To detect factors that render the kidney more susceptible to parenchymal damage, i.e., congenital or acquired obstructions of the urinary flow, calculi, gross vesicoureteral reflux, and intrarenal reflux.

2. To detect and outline renal tissue narrowing and calyceal dilatation, which may be an early sign of progressive renal scarring.

3. To check the rate of growth of the kidney, which may be a valuable aid in assessing the effect of treatment (Hodson, 1966).

Not uncommonly, urologic centers report that 25 to 50 per cent of their infected children have anatomic malformations. In general practice, the frequency of obstruction will be much

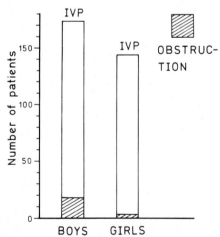

Figure 16–5. Occurrence of obstruction in 174 apparently primary infections in boys, and in 144 first or second infections in girls. Onset between birth and 16 years. Obstructions in boys: Urethral valves proven in 3 patients and suspected in 2 patients; bladder stone and diverticula in 2 patients; ureteral obstruction in 11 patients. (From Winberg, J., et al.: Acta Paediatr. Scand. [Suppl 252], 1974.)

less—5 to 10 per cent in boys and 1 to 2 per cent in girls (Fig. 16–5) (Winberg et al., 1974). The frequency of gross reflux and of scarring is discussed elsewhere (pages 848 to 854).

Ultrasound and the new radionuclide techniques as well as NMR (Chapters 7 and 8) will provide more reliable and detailed information about both function and anatomy than the traditional imaging techniques do. Gamma-camera studies with, for example, ^{131}I hippuran will be informative about ureteral function.

WHAT TO ASK THE RADIOLOGIST FOR

Intravenous Pyelography (IVP). It is important to visualize the nephrographic phase approximately 1 minute after the injection of contrast medium for evaluation of renal size and form. Symmetry in the excretion of contrast as well as the time for appearance should be noted. Morphologic changes of the parenchyma (scars, destructions, cysts) in the renal pelvices (hydronephrosis, calyceal deformities, stones) and in the ureters (obstruction, dilatation, abnormal course) should be noted. The width of the ureters should preferably be given in millimeters. Scars can be classified according to Smellie (Fig. 16–6) (Smellie et al., 1975).

Each examination should include a measurement of the kidneys. Diagrams of the normal parenchymal thickness, renal length, and area at different ages and in relation to the L1–L3 distance are available (Claësson et al., 1981 a, b, c). Area measurements are most suitable to follow the growth of the kidney, but the length measurement may be used. For demonstration of focal scarring, measurement of parenchymal thickness is superior. It should be noted that the kidney poles in little children are relatively much thicker than in older children or adults. Therefore, growth retardation in the poles is easily overlooked.

Micturition Urethrocystography (MCU). This examination should include at least one side frontal and one side projection during micturition. The frontal picture should be large enough to visualize the urethra, the bladder, and the whole of the kidneys. Morphologic changes as well as the ability of the bladder to empty and the appearance of the urethra should be noted. One film should be taken after the end of the micturition in order to evaluate the ability to empty.

If there is vesicoureteric reflux, this should be graded. There are three-, four-, and five-graded systems (Fig. 16–7). In all systems a reflux with no dilatation is probably without clinical importance. There is some disagreement

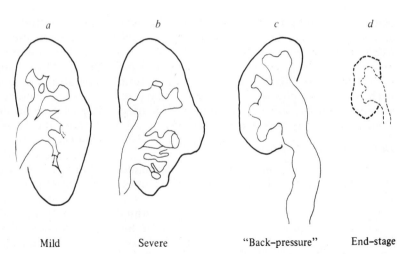

a	*b*	*c*	*d*
Mild	Severe	"Back–pressure"	End-stage

Figure 16–6. Classification of focal renal scarring according to Smellie et al. (1975). Moderate form—not more than two focal scars (a). Severe form—more than two scars; some areas with normal tissue thickness remain (b). "Back-pressure" type—in addition to a generalized deformity of the calyces (as in obstructive uropathy), the thin mantle of parenchyma shows irregular, thin areas, possibly representing scars caused by infections (c). Totally shrunken kidney with no or poor function (d). (From Smellie, J. M., et al.: Kidney Int., 8:65, 1975. Used by permission.)

as to whether vesicoureteric reflux occurs in healthy children during the first and second years of life. Gross reflux dilating the upper urinary tract is always pathologic. In such cases it should be noted whether intrarenal reflux—usually a pyelotubular backflow—is present or not.

SUGGESTED INDICATIONS FOR RADIOLOGY

Time-honored indications for IVP and MCU are given below. With increased availability of new imaging techniques—especially sonography—routines will change successively. Local equipment and experience will determine to what extent the new techniques will replace the older ones.

Apparent First Infection

1. When a mass is seen or palpated over the symphysis after micturition, indicating incomplete bladder emptying.

2. When a mass is palpated in the upper part of the abdomen, indicating hydronephrosis.

3. When blood urea nitrogen or serum creatinine is increased, or concentrating capacity is persistently lowered, or infection is associated with acidosis.

4. When blood pressure is increased.

5. When an infection fails to resolve in spite of administration of an adequate antibiotic.

6. Infants: all those with symptomatic infections.

7. Boys: all those with symptomatic infections, irrespective of age.

8. Girls: all those with febrile infections. If a first infection is associated with only lower tract symptoms and the patient is afebrile and otherwise healthy, x-ray may be unnecessary.

9. Many clinics will not have the capacity for radiologic investigation of all children with UTI. Selection of suitable patients will then be a question of the age and sex of the patient, personal experience, and how selective the material is.

Recurrent Infections

In patients with a history of recurrent infections who had not earlier been examined radiographically, an IVP and an MCU have usually been recommended. There is now reason to depart from this routine. Especially with afebrile infections, an ultrasound examination to exclude renal or ureteral dilatation, to measure renal size, and even to study the lower

Figure 16–7. Grades of reflux (no account for whether reflux is free). (From Winberg, J., et al.: *In* Kincaid-Smith, P., and Fairley, K. [Eds.]: Renal Infection and Renal Scarring. p. 293. Melbourne, Mercedes, 1971.)

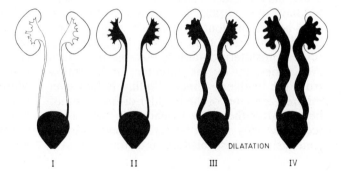

		DILATATION	
I	II	III	IV

urinary tract may be satisfactory. When ultra-sound is not available, an IVP may be sufficient. MCU is indicated only occasionally. When a girl looks healthy, grows satisfactorily and has no symptoms or signs suggesting complications such as hydronephrosis, stones, or urinary retention, she may have a fair number of infections before x-ray becomes mandatory.

Indications for Repeated IVP and MCU

Only tentative suggestions can be made. We check patients who have had febrile infections in order to monitor renal growth and calyceal appearance. Checkup is performed after about 6 months when an infection has occurred during the first year of life, and after 12 months when an infection has occurred during the second year of life. When onset has occurred later on, the checkup is performed after an interval of 2 to 3 years or more. Since preservation of renal tissue is the aim of the therapeutic efforts, we concentrate on checking the growth of the kidneys by IVU and straight films and are sparing in the use of repeated MCU in conservatively treated patients with moderate or gross reflux (Grades III and IV) (Fig. 16–7). In patients with gross reflux we are liberal with repeated IVU to see whether a progressive dilatation occurs. It is probable that IVP in many instances can be replaced by ultra-sonography. Checkup after reflux operation is discussed in Chapter 49.

Localization Studies

Localizing the site of infection is mainly a research object in studies in which it is essential to know whether an infection involves the renal parenchyma. Demonstration of persistent unilateral infection (by the Stamey technique, described later) may, however, guide elective surgery. The washout techniques, the Stamey type (Stamey et al., 1965) with ureteral catheterization, and the Fairley type (Fairley et al., 1971) using only bladder catheterization, are useful but have their pitfalls. The discharge of bacteria may be intermittent, and results may indicate bladder infection that was, in fact, renal. A reverse misinterpretation is possible if bacteria are carried up by the catheter, or by reflux, from the bladder. Another failing is that even minimal amounts of the bladder disinfectant left behind after the saline irrigation in the Fairley technique may inhibit bacterial growth and erroneously suggest bladder infection. Even if

these methods are often referred to as direct, it is questionable whether they are more so than other methods. The only truly direct one is renal biopsy, which for obvious reasons can be performed only in very selected cases.

A transitory decrease in renal concentrating capacity or an increase in serum antibody titer against the O antigen of infecting bacteria (as determined by hemagglutination or direct agglutination) is used to indicate renal involvement. While these tests seem valuable in defining groups of patients with renal infection, one must be cautious in evaluating an individual patient (Jodal et al., 1975; Lindberg et al., 1975d). A low concentrating capacity as well as a high antibody titer may have explanations other than a renal infection.

The correlation is good between concentrating capacity, antibody titer, and sedimentation rate in patients with apparent first symptomatic infection, but less good in patients with frequent recurrences or asymptomatic bacteriuria. In these instances, the infection is often caused by bacteria with a deficient cell wall. When such bacteria are used as antigen sources, measured antibody titer may be low, whereas it may be high when a laboratory strain with a more complete antigenic structure is used (Lindberg et al., 1975d). Unfortunately, it is mainly in patients with frequent recurrences or asymptomatic bacteriuria that localization studies may be needed.

Demonstration of antibody-coated bacteria in the urine has been suggested to distinguish renal from bladder infection (Thomas et al., 1974). This elegant and simple method seems less reliable in children. Determination of C-reactive protein discriminates rather well between renal and nonrenal infections in patients with symptomatic infections (Jodal et al., 1975) but not in those with asymptomatic ones (Lindberg et al., 1975d; Hellerstein et al., 1982). At present, it is difficult to say which method is most reliable. All have their drawbacks. Antibody determination involves a number of technical problems and pitfalls. Washout methods are inconvenient for the patient. Easiest to evaluate is the concentrating capacity, especially when a low value is demonstrated in two consecutive tests. Administration of DDAVP has made this test more convenient (Abyholm and Monn, 1979). Determination of C-reactive protein is easy to perform but is not reliable when most needed. The author does not think that localization studies will have much impact on management of symptomatic infection.

EPIDEMIOLOGY

SYMPTOMATIC INFECTIONS

The age and sex distribution of 596 consecutive cases of presumed first (onset) infections appearing within a defined population during a defined period of time is shown in Figure 16–8 (Winberg et al., 1974). From these data, the risk of a child's falling ill with a symptomatic UTI before the age of 11 years has been calculated to be 1.1 per cent for boys and 3.0 per cent for girls. Most infants and small children with acute symptomatic infections seem to grow out of their proneness to infections, boys usually during the second year of life, girls later on. A proportion of girls will continue to have repeated infections for many years. This explains why, even though onset infections have a peak incidence during the first year of life, girls of school age predominate among the pediatrician's patients with UTI.

SCREENING BACTERIURIA (ABU) (ASYMPTOMATIC, COVERT, LATENT, SYMPTOMLESS BACTERIURIA)*

This condition is defined here as those infections diagnosed by surveys of so-called healthy populations. The designation "asymptomatic" may not be adequate, since some of these patients feel more comfortable after eradication of bacteriuria than they did before. In apparently healthy girls between 4 and 16 years of age, the incidence is between 0.7 and 2.0 per

*Aspects other than incidence are discussed on pages 832 and 834.

cent with no definite increase with age, although a yearly acquisition rate of 0.32 per cent has been observed (Kunin et al., 1964). In males, the frequency is very low after the newborn period (Kunin et al., 1964; Meadow et al., 1969). The significance of screening bacteriuria is discussed on pages 832 and 834.

In neonates, asymptomatic bacteriuria associated with heavy pyuria may be seen in 1 to 3 per cent of males (Winberg, 1974; Lincoln and Winberg, 1964). A randomized population-based screening during the first year of life has revealed a frequency of infections of about 2.7 per cent and 0.7 per cent in males and females, respectively (Wettergren et al., 1980). The significance of both neonatal and early infantile asymptomatic bacteriuria is unknown.

BACTERIAL ETIOLOGY AND RESISTANCE PATTERN

The majority of urinary pathogens originate in the commensal flora of the bowel. The most common urinary pathogens in children are gram-negative bacteria of the family *Enterobacteriaceae*. *Escherichia coli* cause the majority of urinary tract infections, followed by *Klebsiella*, *Proteus*, and *Enterobacter*.

Among gram-positive bacteria, staphylococci and streptococci Group D (enterococci) are the most common pathogens. Out of about 150 known *E. coli* O groups, some eight to ten (01, 02, 04, 06, 07, 018, and 075) cause about two thirds of all *E. coli* urinary tract infections.

Figure 16–8. Apparently primary onset of urinary tract infection in 419 girls and 104 boys between 2 months and 16 years of age (neonates zero to 30 days old excluded). The proportion of nonfebrile infections was very small during the first year of life but increased with age. Fifty-four male and 21 female neonatal infections were not included. (From Winberg, J., et al.: Acta Paediatr. Scand. [Suppl 252], 1974.)

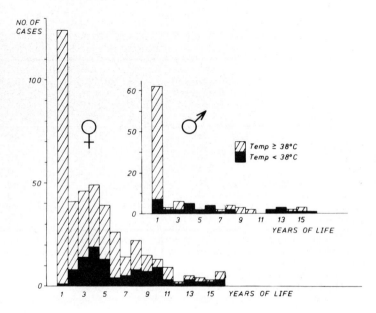

These serotypes usually also dominate in the community (Grüneberg et al., 1968). *E.coli* organisms isolated in the urine are usually of the same serotype as those dominating in the fecal flora (Grüneberg et al., 1968).

Although *E.coli* causes the majority of urinary tract infections in children, the bacterial etiology varies with the age and sex of the patient (Table 16–3) as well as with the number of previous infections. Thus, *Proteus* is a common invader in older boys, *Staphylococcus saprophyticus* is common at puberty in girls, and *Klebsiella* is seen in the newborn period. Recurrences after sulfonamide treatment are often caused by enterococci. There may, of course, be local and temporal variations of this general pattern.

Also, in patients with complications such as calculus, obstruction, or neurogenic bladder, and in children with recurrent UTI, *E.coli* is common, but the infecting strains tend to be of more uncommon species.

Staphylococci have long been considered of little significance as a cause of urinary tract infections. However, during the 1970's a particular subgroup of (coagulase-negative) staphylococci, *Staphylococcus saprophyticus*, was shown to be an important cause of urinary tract infections in young females. Also in children, pure cultures of coagulase-negative staphylococci were found in 3 per cent of patients with symptomatic UTI. The majority of infections were observed in girls from ages 11 to 16 years, and there were signs of renal involvement in several cases. The pathogenetic mechanisms of *S. saprophyticus* are not known, but these organisms have been shown to adhere well to human uroepithelium (Colleen, 1982).

The vast majority of infecting bacteria are sensitive to most commonly used antimicrobials, including sulfonamide. To these general rules, there are various exceptions. The first few months after sulfonamide therapy, a recurrence is often sulfonamide-resistant owing to an antibiotic-induced change of the intestinal flora, which subsequently determines the bacteria involved in the reinfection (see pages 856 to 858). The same occurs after ampicillin and tetracycline therapy, but not during nitrofurantoin treatment. Consequently, recurrences are rarely nitrofurantoin-resistant. The resistance pattern of the more uncommon organisms seen in patients with anatomic complications is often impossible to predict.

PATHOGENESIS AND PREDISPOSING FACTORS

INITIATION OF INFECTION

Bacteria seem to enter the urinary tract by the ascending route. It is generally assumed, but not proved that infections appearing during the newborn period are blood-borne.

Presumed ascending infection (lower plus upper) may affect 3 to 5 per cent of all girls, if those with screening bacteriuria are included. The risk of reinfection seems to increase with the number of previous infections (Fig. 16–9) and may be up to 50 times that of a previously

TABLE 16–3. ETIOLOGIC BACTERIA IN 596 APPARENT FIRST NONOBSTRUCTIVE INFECTIONS IN RELATION TO SEX AND AGE*

		Girls		Boys	
Bacteria	Neonates of Both sexes (per cent) (N = 73)	1 MO. TO 10 YRS.† (per cent) (N = 389)	10 TO 16 YRS. (per cent) (N = 30)	1 MO. TO 1 YR. (per cent) (N = 62)	1 TO 16 YRS.† (per cent) (N = 42)
E. coli	75‡	83	60	85	33
Klebsiella	11	<1	0	2	2
Proteus	0	3	0	5	33
Enterococci	3	2	0	0	2
Staphylococcus albus‖	1	<1	30	0	12§
Other bacteria	4	<1	0	3	2
Mixed	4	1	3	2	5
Unknown	1	9	7	3	10

*From Winberg, J., et al.: Acta Paediatr. Scand. [Suppl. 252], 1974.

†No difference between girls 1 mo. to 1 yr. and 1 to 10 yrs.; no difference between boys 1 to 10 yrs. and 10 to 16 yrs. except for *S. albus*.

‡Fifty-seven per cent in girls and 83 per cent in boys. X^2: p = 0.016.

§Four of the five patients were more than 11 years of age.

‖Old data. Not analyzed whether *S. epidermidis* or *S. saprophyticus*.

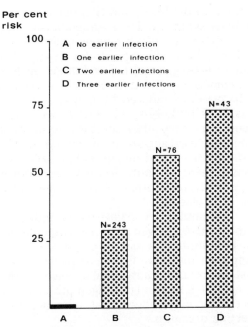

Per cent risk

Figure 16–9. Recurrence rate within 1 year of a preceding infection, related to the number of earlier infections. *(A)*, Approximate risk of a 30-day-old healthy girl having a symptomatic infection before 11 years of age. *(B)*, Observed risk in 243 girls with one earlier infection. *(C)* Observed risk in 76 patients with two earlier infections. *(D)* Observed risk in 43 patients with three earlier infections. (From Winberg, J., et al.: Acta Paediatr. Scand. [Suppl. 252], 1974.)

healthy girl (Winberg et al., 1974; Winberg et al., 1975).

The causes for the difference between *UTI-prone* and *non-UTI prone* individuals have been a matter of much speculation but are still unknown.

OBSTRUCTIVE MALFORMATION, HEMATOGENOUS VERSUS ASCENDING INFECTION, FECAL SOILING, URETHRAL LENGTH, AND "MATURATION"

The typical age and sex distribution of onset infection should help define possible pathogenetic mechanisms (see Figure 16–8). The mean number of new cases per month of life in different age periods was calculated from this population (Fig. 16–10). More than 50 males fell ill the first month of life; during the following 5 months, there were about 10 new cases per month; and in the next 6 months, there were between 1 and 2 per month. Thus, UTI in males is largely a disease of infancy. The decline in the morbidity rate for females was similar but slower.

Several possibilities must be considered to explain the slope of the curves in Figure 16–10. First, obstructive malformations cannot account for the age distribution, since patients with these were excluded. Second, the pathogenetic factors operating in the very early infections may be different from those occurring later. For example, gram-negative septicemia may explain the early peak incidence. This can, however, hardly be valid beyond the first month of life. Furthermore, asymptomatic bacteriuria, which probably is ascending rather than hematogenous, appears in between 1 and 3 per cent of newborn boys (Lincoln and Winberg, 1964; Winberg, 1974; Wettergren et al., 1980) and is not infrequent during the first 6 months of life (Wettergren et al., 1980). This suggests a decreased *local* defense at this age. Third, fecal soiling, suggested as a predisposing factor, can hardly be of decisive importance, since the rapid decrease in frequency of UTI starts during the first few months of life.

Female preponderance in UTI is usually explained with reference to the short female urethra. The successive change of the sex ratio with age demonstrated in Table 16–4 is hardly compatible with this view. It is more suggestive of a successive functional maturation of a defense mechanism or the disappearance of a predisposing factor that progresses at different speeds in the two sexes.

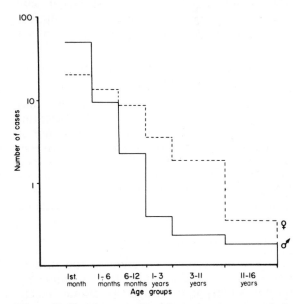

Figure 16–10. Mean number of new cases per month in different age groups in males and females; see text. (From Winberg, et al., 1974; modified by Asscher, 1980. Used by permission.)

TABLE 16–4. Sex Ratio of Onset, Nonobstructive UTI in Different Age Groups

Age	Females/Males
1 month	0.4
2 to 6 months	1.5
7 to 12 months	4.0
2 to 3 years	10.0
4 to 11 years	9.0

MEATAL STENOSIS, BLADDER NECK OBSTRUCTION, INCOMPLETE BLADDER EMPTYING, VESICOURETERAL REFLUX

So-called bladder neck obstruction and urethral meatal stenosis have often been mentioned as main causes of recurrent infections. Critical evaluation suggests that these conditions play little role, if any (Kendall and Karafin, 1972). Incomplete emptying of the urinary system (O'-Grady and Cattell, 1966; O'Grady et al., 1973) may encourage infection in some patients, especially in those with posterior urethral valves, ureterocele, bladder diverticula, neurogenic disorders (sometimes subtle), or calculus. This group is very small.

Vesicoureteral reflux has also been incriminated as a factor facilitating infection of the bladder. Evidence seems to be more against than for this hypothesis (Govan et al., 1974; Kendall and Karafin, 1972), with the possible exception of gross reflux. The role of reflux in pyelonephritis is discussed on pages 848 to 851. The micturition disturbances associated with day-wetting may in some instances predispose to UTI (Berg et al., 1977; van Gool et al., 1984).

COOLING, HYGIENE, SOCIAL CONDITIONS, AND GENETIC FACTORS

While it is well known that cooling may provoke urgency, there is so far no scientific proof that it predisposes to infection, nor is there evidence in regard to swimming, hygiene, or social condition (Stansfeld, 1966). Acute respiratory infection was reported to precede the UTI in 13 per cent of the cases. With regard to genetic factors, black girls may be more resistant to infection than white ones (Kunin, 1966).

IMMUNE RESPONSE

A gram-negative infection of the urinary tract elicits a general and a local immune response. So far, no defects in the immune mechanism have been demonstrated in patients susceptible to infections.

Immunodiffusion studies have shown that at least 20 antigens from an *E. coli* strain in addition to the O, K, and H antigens may elicit antibody synthesis. These antibodies might differ with regard to immunoglobulin class and avidity, which will explain, for example, why indirect hemagglutination and direct agglutination sometimes give different results. The antibody synthesis induced by gram-negative bacteria is of IgM, IgA, and IgG types. The last occurs especially after several infections. The commonly used agglutination methods will favor IgM antibodies and underestimate IgG. Direct measurement of antibodies will therefore give more accurate information about the distribution of Ig classes.

IgM antibodies against the O antigen may be protective, judged from experimental studies. IgG antibodies may form antigen-antibody complexes that may fixate complement and at least theoretically cause renal damage. Antibodies against K1 capsular antigen are of interest, since they may induce host tolerance to the infecting organism.

The antibodies of normal urine are of IgG and secretory IgA classes and are probably locally synthesized. Patients with repeated infections have an augmented excretion. A defect in local antibody response has so far not been explained the susceptibility to recurrent infections. Local antibodies may, however, play a role by inhibiting bacterial adhesion to epithelial surfaces and may contribute to selection of less virulent strains. See pages 839 and 840 and Table 16–5.

Determination of serum antibody response to the O antigen has been used to localize the infection. It is of limited value in the manage-

TABLE 16–5. Characteristics of *E. coli* Strains Isolated from Patients with Pyelonephritis and with ABU*

Characteristics of Urinary *E. coli*	Pyelonephritis (per cent) (N = 119)	ABU (per cent) (N = 115)
O group: 1, 2, 4, 6, 7, 16, 18, 75	80	31
Spontaneous agglutination	2	45
Serum bactericidal sensitivity		
Strains highly resistant†	69	12
Strains highly sensitive‡	4	70

*From Lindberg, U., et al.: Acta Paediatr. Scand. *64*:432, 1975.

†Less than 50 per cent of bacteria killed.

‡More than 99 per cent of bacteria killed.

ment of individual patients. Persistent high titers are sometimes seen in patients with severe renal damage. The significance of this is unknown.

The demonstration of antibody-coated bacteria in the urinary sediment is inaccurate as a sign of pyelonephritis in children. During the acute phase of pyelonephritis there is an increase of antibodies against Tamm-Horsfall protein, which is normally formed in the tubular region and excreted in the urine. The biologic significance of such a reactivity is as yet unsettled. In patients with renal scarring, the titer elevation is less (Fasth et al., 1984). There is a suppression of the cell-mediated immune response in the early phase of acute pyelonephritis (Miller et al., 1978; Ahlstedt et al., 1983). The biologic significance is unknown. The role of the inflammatory reaction in renal scarring is discussed on pages 853 and 854.

Extensive reviews of the immune response

in urinary tract infections have been published (Holmgren and Smith, 1975; Hanson et al., 1975).

PERIURETHRAL FLORA

The close proximity of the anal and urethral openings presupposes the existence of highly efficient defense mechanisms to prevent ascending infection; indeed, a first line of defense may be located in the periurethral area. As a matter of fact, dense colonization of gram-negative bacteria is only exceptionally found in this area in healthy children older than 4 or 5 years or in adult females. The mechanism by which bacteria are cleared from this area is unknown.

In contrast, in girls and adult females prone to UTI, there is often a high density of gram-negative bacteria, commonly several species at one time, even between infections. Infections are typically preceded by periurethral coloniza-

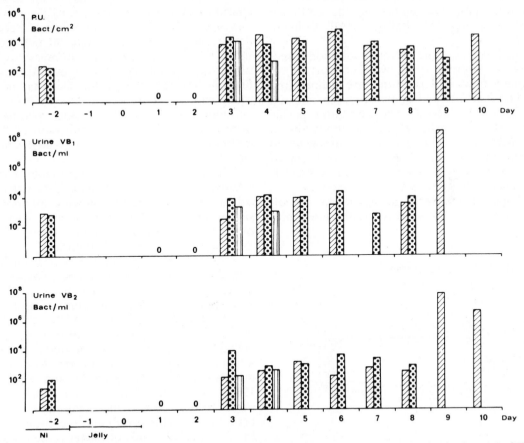

Figure 16–11. A 7-year-old girl with a history of recurrent urinary tract infection. Prophylactic nitrofurantoin (NI) was discontinued and was followed by topical application of antibiotic jelly around the urethral orifice for 2 days, after which sampling was started. The figure shows the periurethral (PU), urethral (VB1), and bladder (VB2) gram-negative flora before the appearance of UTI on day nine. Three different strains colonized the genital region, but only one invaded the bladder. This was demonstrated in four consecutive specimens. Infection was accompanied by pyuria and painful micturition. ▨ = *E. coli* O25. ▰ = *Proteus morganii*. ☐ = *E. coli* ON (not agglutinable in 68 different O-antisera) and OR (spontaneously agglutinating). (From Bollgren, I., and Winberg, J.: Acta Paediatr. Scand., 65:81, 1976.)

tion with the infecting organism (Fig. 16–11). When proneness to infection eventually disappears, as it does in many patients, the susceptibility to periurethral colonization seems to vanish as well. These observations suggest that proneness to urinary infection runs parallel to a defect of some unknown mechanism that normally clears the periurethral region of gram-negative bacteria (Stamey et al., 1971; Bollgren and Winberg 1976 a,b).

BACTERIAL ADHESION

Bacterial infections as well as physiologic colonization of mucous membranes must involve an element of interaction between the epithelial and bacterial cells; otherwise, the microorganisms would be swept away by the secretory flow of the membrane. This "adhesion" is mediated either by "unspecific" factors, such as hydrophobic or electrostatic bonds, or by specific "adhesins" (bacterial surface elements) recognizing specific receptors on the epithelial cells (Beachey, 1980; Savage, 1980; Colleen, 1982).

In *E.coli*, specific bacterial adhesion is mediated by fimbriae (pili), which consist of repeating protein molecules that are chained into hairlike structures and extend from the bacterial cell surface (Fig. 16–12). They recognize specific receptors, often carbohydrates, on the epithelial cell membrane. The ability of pathogens to adhere to mucous membranes is now recognized as a potential virulence factor. This subject is also dealt with on page 850 in Chapter 14.

"Specific" bacterial adhesion may be divided into mannose-sensitive (adhesion inhibited by mannose) and mannose-resistant (adhesion not inhibited by mannose).

Mannose-Sensitive Adhesion. This is mediated by so-called Type 1 fimbriae, which occur on most *E.coli* strains, pathogens as well as nonpathogens (Duguid and Old, 1980). They have so far not been proved to play any role in the initiation of human renal infections. Their role in lower urinary tract infections is a matter of dispute.

Mannose-Resistant Adhesion. This is a crude definition of the adhesin, telling only that adhesion is not mediated by mannose-sensitive Type 1 fimbriae. One research frontier concerns the definition and chemical characterization of specific epithelial receptors for different kinds of adhesins within the heterogeneous mannose-resistant group; another, the purification and characterization of the corresponding fimbriae.

P-Fimbriae. A disaccharide, α-D-galactose-1-4-β-D-galactose, which is part of the oligosaccharide chain of the P-blood group antigens, has been identified as the minimal receptor active element for more than 90 per cent of those *E.coli* that cause acute primary pyelonephritis in children. The in vivo importance of P-fimbriae is suggested by the fact that interference with the adhesion process by P-fimbriae antibodies or by receptor analogs modifies the infectious process. The identification of the P-fimbriae specific receptor is described in Chapter 14.

X-Fimbriae. There are a number of *E.coli* strains, usually isolated from patients with lower urinary tract infections, showing mannose-resistant adhesion, but with binding specificity other than that of P-fimbriated strains. These are provisionally named X-fimbriae.

The Host. Uroepithelial cells from infection-prone women bind *E.coli* more avidly than do cells from nonsusceptible women (Fowler and Stamey, 1977; Källenius and Winberg, 1978; Svanborg-Edén and Jodal, 1979). This holds true also for buccal cells (Schaeffer et al., 1981). Available receptors for P-fimbriated *E.coli* show a higher density in infection-prone women than in healthy controls (Svenson and Källenius, 1983). All findings may be an expression of some general "unspecific" abnormality so far unidentified. This possibility is consonant with the fact that all kinds of bacteria seem able to infect susceptible women.

CLINICAL STUDIES

E.coli expressing P-fimbriae on their surface were found in the urine of more than 90 per cent of children with a first, acute, febrile,

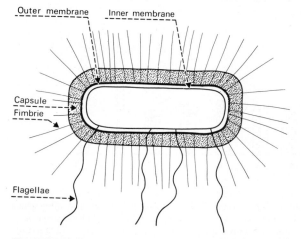

Figure 16–12. Schematic drawing of a gram-negative organism, showing the relation between fimbriae (pili) and other parts of the cell wall.

nonobstructed pyelonephritis, but were found less often in lower infections. P-fimbriae probably help the bacteria to resist the flow of urine by attaching to the uroepithelium and to the kidney cells, where the receptor active glycosphingolipids are present.

The P-fimbriated *E.coli* isolated from children with pyelonephritis also seem to dominate the periurethral and fecal flora in those children. This suggests that fecal colonization with P-fimbriated *E.coli* may be the first step in the series of events leading to overt UTI. The classic antithesis of the "special pathogenicity theory" and the "prevalence theory" of initiation of pyelonephritis may not be "either/or," but "as well as"—specially pathogenic bacteria dominate the fecal flora. Thus, factors promoting or preventing intestinal colonization may be of importance in the pathogenesis of this disease.

The finding of fecal dominance of P-fimbriated *E.coli* in infected patients may have implications for treatment. For example, persistance of P-fimbriated *E.coli* in the fecal flora may increase the risk for recurrence.

A protective effect of vaccination of monkeys with a highly purified P-fimbriae preparation suggests that immunity plays a role in the defense against infection. The very first infection in a small infant will attack a host unprotected by antifimbrial immunity and may therefore be especially dangerous. This may provide another rationale for early diagnosis and treatment of infants with pyelonephritis.

In summary, acute and recurrent UTI are complex biologic events. Recent advances in the understanding of the host-parasite interactions on a molecular level will help explain the delicate complexity of the initiation of infection and should lead to better management and prevention of renal damage. Summaries of recent advances have been published (Winberg, 1984; Svenson et al., 1984).

INITIATION OF RENAL SCARRING

This is dealt with on pages 850 to 854.

CLINICAL FEATURES

General Remarks on Symptomatology

Depending upon the clinical situation in which urinary tract infection appears, the following points merit special attention:

1. The clinical features may be influenced by age and sex of the patient, presence of anatomic disorders of the urinary tract, localization of the infection, number of earlier infections, and time interval since the last infection.

2. An infection associated with high fever is presumed to be a pyelonephritis, although the evidence for this is only indirect. Washout studies have even suggested that lower urinary tract infections might go with fever and chills (Huland et al., 1982) (see under Localization Studies). On the other hand, a renal infection may be present without any symptoms. Whether such infections will cause any renal damage is unsettled.

3. The more infections a patient has had earlier, or the closer a recurrence follows an earlier infection, the less serious the symptoms seem to be. This may be due to endotoxin tolerance (McCabe, 1963; McCabe and Anderson, 1963) or to the effect of antibodies to lipid A (Holmgren and Smith, 1975). Another explanation would be that recurrent infections are often caused by bacteria with a deficient cell wall (Lindberg et al., 1975c) and therefore probably reduced virulence (Roantree, 1971) (see page 847 and Table 16–5).

4. Such bacteria as enterococci, *Proteus, Pseudomonas,* and *Staphylococcus epidermidis* often cause fewer symptoms than does *E. coli.*

5. Increased BUN or arterial hypertension in patients older than the age of 2 months almost always indicates the existence of bilateral hydronephrosis or advanced renal parenchymal reduction.

6. Children with symptoms of frequency, urgency, burning, micturition pains, and, often, diurnal enuresis may have sterile urine or insignificant bacteriuria. The condition may or may not be associated with pyuria. Bladder-puncture studies suggest that the number of bacteria sometimes may be very small, i.e., a few thousand even in true infections (Stamm et al., 1982; Bollgren et al., 1984). Infections caused by bacteria not growing on traditional culture media may escape attention (Fairley and Birch, 1983). Renal tuberculosis should not be forgotten in countries where this disease still occurs.

7. Most commonly, children with urgency, diurnal enuresis, and other above-mentioned symptoms, but normal urinary findings, have a detrusor-sphincter overactivity or other urodynamic disturbance.

Symptomatology in Relation to Sex, Age, and Presence of Obstruction

NEONATAL INFECTIONS (1 TO 30 DAYS OLD)

It is generally thought (but by no means proven) that symptomatic neonatal urinary infections are a manifestation of a generalized septicemia. The symptoms are varied (Bergström et al., 1972) (Table 16–6). Some symptoms may precede positive urinary findings by several days. Classic symptoms of infantile urinary infections such as sluggishness, feeding difficulties, irritability, and tenderness upon touching may also be noted. A change in an initially normal weight curve may often be noted before any other symptoms and can focus early attention upon the possibility of a urinary infection.

An abnormally slow weight gain may also be noted for several weeks after successful treatment. The central nervous system symptoms in neonatal UTI (see Table 16–6) consist of generalized convulsions with loss of consciousness, marked hypotonicity or irritability, respiratory inadequacy, and absent or difficult-to-elicit primitive reflexes. Pleocytosis without demonstrable bacterial meningitis was found in one third of those who had a spinal tap. In this series, bacteremia was found in 50 per cent of those investigated; blood urea nitrogen was increased in 20 per cent. There may be marked oliguria and a temporary increase in renal size.

GIRLS AND BOYS 1 MONTH TO 3 YEARS OF AGE WITH OR WITHOUT OBSTRUCTION

A symptomatic infection of acute onset, especially if it is the first infection, usually presents with fever. Meningism, irritability, and abnormal sensitivity to touching of the skin are common symptoms, as are abdominal pains, distended abdomen, vomiting, and a certain pale or even gray color of the skin and "smelly" diapers. A few patients will have macroscopic hematuria. Otherwise, symptoms pointing to the urinary tract are usually absent.

TABLE 16–6. PROMINENT SYMPTOMS IN NEONATAL*
NONOBSTRUCTIVE UTI (N = 75)

Symptom	Per Cent
Weight loss†	76
Fever	49
Cyanosis or gray color	40
Distended abdomen	16
CNS symptoms (purulent meningitis not included)	23
Generalized convulsions	7
Purulent meningitis	8
Jaundice (conjugated bilirubin increased)	7
Other	16

*Zero to 30 days old.
†Registered for only 46 patients falling ill on days 0 to 10. Weight loss was not explained by vomiting, diarrhea, or refusal to eat.

"Failure to thrive" (feeding difficulties, sluggishness, poor gain in weight, abdominal discomfort) is a major feature of UTI during the first few years of life, according to the traditional concept. While some infections may start with such symptoms, they are more probably the typical features of long-standing infections that were overlooked during the acute febrile stage, later assuming a "low-grade" character. Diagnosis during the initial stage of febrile urinary tract infections presupposes generosity with urine cultures and sediment examinations in patients with acute febrile illness that is not readily explained by other symptoms.

OLDER GIRLS WITHOUT OBSTRUCTION

With increasing age, lower urinary tract symptoms, including enuresis, appear more frequently, as does abdominal discomfort. Pains over the loins appear during late childhood, but tenderness on palpation over the loins may be noted at a rather young age. Discrete symptoms never exclude renal involvement.

OLDER BOYS WITHOUT OBSTRUCTION

In boys over 2 years of age, generalized symptoms are few and moderate. Fever seems to occur only occasionally and is often moderate. Macro- or microscopic hematuria is common (Bergström, 1972). Micturition pains or urgency may be present. Coliform bacteria do not dominate etiologically to the same extent as in girls. *Proteus* and other atypical bacteria are relatively frequent invaders. In late-onset infection in boys, the kidneys often show focal scarring at the time of the first infection. It is probable that such patients have had early undiagnosed infections (Bergström, 1972).

INFECTIONS COMPLICATED BY OBSTRUCTION

If complicated by congenital low obstruction (urethral valves, ureterocele, prune belly syndrome, neurogenic bladder) causing bilateral hydronephrosis, infection usually starts during the first few months of life. In children with obstruction of the upper urinary tract, onset of infection may be at any age. The presenting features are the same as those of infantile infections. On physical examination, a raised bladder or a mass in the loin may be found. When an acute UTI is associated with arterial hypertension, dehydration, a high blood urea nitrogen, and electrolyte disturbances, including acidosis, this should raise the suspicion of an obstructive complication until the reverse is shown (Ericsson et al., 1955; McCrory et al., 1971). Straining at micturition, dribbling, or a poor urinary stream, often divided in portions, usually characterizes urethral obstruction; however, these symptoms may be absent even if obstruction is marked.

Screening Bacteriuria (ABU) (Asymptomatic, Covert)

GIRLS OF PRESCHOOL AND SCHOOL AGE

For definition and epidemiology see page 839.

Clinical. About one third of the patients have a past history of symptoms referable to the urinary tract. Pyuria is often absent. Reflux is seen in 20 to 35 per cent and focal renal scars in 10 to 25 per cent (Anders et al., 1974; Kunin et al., 1964; Lindberg et al., 1975b; McLachlan et al., 1975; Meadow et al., 1969). The frequency of renal scarring is the same at 4 years and at 12, indicating that the asymptomatic infection probably does not cause renal damage, at least not after the age of 4 years (McLachlan et al., 1975). Many of these patients have a small residual urine. The reason why infection is asymptomatic in some patients is not very well understood but may be due, in part, to the special characteristics of the infecting bacteria (see below).

Bacteriology. There are prominent differences between *E. coli* isolates from patients with symptomatic pyelonephritis or cystitis and those from individuals with ABU (Table 16–5). Some of the differences may be due to selection of polysaccharide-deficient mutants (Lindberg et al., 1975c; Hanson et al., 1975), which may be of low virulence (Roantree, 1971). This process may be the result of "antigenic drift," i.e., the bacteria have changed to survive the pressure from the immune response in the urinary tract. Bacteria isolated from patients with screening bacteriuria also have a low adherence capacity (Svanborg-Edén et al., 1976).

Localization. Localization of the actual infection in screening bacteriuria is difficult (Lindberg et al., 1975d; Hellerstein et al., 1982). A poor correlation was found between washout tests, concentrating capacity, C-reactive protein, antibody titers, and sedimentation rate. It is possible that the changed *E. coli* strains cannot evoke the usual inflammatory response. It is still uncertain how often the infection involves the renal parenchyma.

Therapy. A short course of antibiotics eliminates infection in more than 90 per cent of patients, but only 20 to 25 per cent remain uninfected 1 to 2 years later (Kunin et al., 1964;

Lindberg, 1975; Savage, 1975; Verrier-Jones et al., 1975). Spontaneous "cures" lasting 1 year appear in about 10 per cent (Asscher et al., 1973; Verrier-Jones et al., 1975). Recent followup studies suggest that renal function and renal growth of both scarred and unscarred kidneys are equal in medically treated as well as in untreated patients. This seems to hold true even in the presence of reflux (Verrier-Jones et al., 1982). Progress of scarring is uncommon after the age of 5 years.

Sometimes patients feel better after treatment even though they have not complained of any symptoms. On the other hand, restriction of chemotherapy may be advisable in screening bacteriuria. Thus, elimination of cell wall–deficient bacteria by therapy is sometimes followed by symptomatic recurrences (Lindberg, 1975; Asscher et al., 1969) caused by bacteria with intact cell wall emanating from the fecal reservoir (Lindberg, 1975). Restriction may also be dictated by the fact that there has been a tremendous increase in the number of side effects reported after antibiotic treatment. It would seem reasonable to limit treatment to patients with symptoms (even if slight) and with foul-smelling urine.

Course and Prognosis. ABU is often a phase in the natural history of symptomatic infections, although in some instances infections seem to begin as asymptomatic ones, as in neonates or during the first year of life (possibly also later). There is no evidence that asymptomatic bacteriuria in itself causes renal growth retardation, focal renal scarring, or renal functional impairment (McLachlan et al., 1975; Verrier-Jones et al., 1975). For example, renal scarring in patients with screening bacteriuria was observed with the same frequency at 4 years and at 12 years (McLachlan et al., 1975). A frequency of scarring of up to 25% has been reported in several studies (Meadow et al., 1969; McLachlan et al., 1975; Savage et al., 1973); the frequency has been considerably lower in other reports (Kunin et al., 1964; Lindberg et al., 1975b). This incidence is higher than the incidence of scarring in patients with symptomatic infections (Table 16–7). A reasonable interpretation is that patients with symptomatic infection have often had them diagnosed, treated, and checked, whereas many patients with screening bacteriuria represent a group whose initial symptomatic infection was not diagnosed and treated. School screening programs, including radiologic examination, seem to register events that happened long ago. If resources are restricted, it seems more urgent to screen a different group, namely infants and

TABLE 16–7. RADIOLOGIC SCARRING IN GIRLS WITH SYMPTOMATIC AND ASYMPTOMATIC BACTERIURIA

| | Per Cent with Scarring | |
	ENGLAND	SWEDEN
Symptomatic	13[a, b] (N = 281)	4.5[c, d] (N = 440)
Asymptomatic	26[e] (N = 296)	10[f] (N = 119)

[a]Referred with a history of recurrent infection.
[b]Recalculated from Smellie and Normand (1968).
[c]Followed prospectively from first symptomatic infection.
[d]From Winberg et al. (1974).
[e]From Savage et al. (1973).
[f]From Lindberg et al. (1975).

small children with fever, for urinary infections, rather than to spend money on school screening programs.

NEONATAL AND EARLY INFANTILE ASYMPTOMATIC BACTERIURIA

True, but asymptomatic, urinary excretion of bacteria may occur in 1 to 3 per cent of newborns, mainly boys (for reference, see Winberg, 1974). The significance of this finding is unknown.

Neonatal asymptomatic bacteriuria, as well as symptomatic UTI, rarely occurs before day four or five after delivery, which may explain why some studies have revealed very few, if any, neonatal infections (Edelmann et al., 1973). So far there is no clinical reason for screening healthy neonates except, possibly, premature infants (Edelmann et al., 1973).

In a population-based study of children under the age of 1 year the occurrence of asymptomatic bacteriuria has been examined by repeated cultures during the first year. At the same time, symptomatic infections occurring in the population of the same geographic area have been noted. So far, two important observations have been reported. First, an asymptomatic infection never developed into a symptomatic one. Second, patients in the group with symptomatic infections had in no instance been recorded to have had a preceding asymptomatic infection (Wettergren et al., 1980; Mårild et al., 1980).

VESICOURETERIC REFLUX (VUR) AND INTRARENAL REFLUX (IRR)—A SECOND THOUGHT

INTRODUCTION

Pioneering and comprehensive work by Hodson, Ransley and Risdon, by Smellie and

Normand, by Friedland, by Govan and associates, and by others has beyond any doubt shown that gross VUR, when associated with IRR and infections, may lead to extensive renal damage. However, the generally held view of reflux as the absolutely *dominating* factor in initiation of renal infection and renal scarring—vigorously expressed in the term "reflux nephropathy"—seems less well founded.

The reflux phenomenon and its importance are dealt with fully in Chapter 00. In this chapter, in addition to a discussion of IRR, emphasis will be on some *selected* data showing that an epidemiologic approach based on studies of patients in primary care will give a more complete picture of the overall importance of reflux. Some less often quoted studies as well as some recent data, which only partly fit prevalent opinions, will be mentioned.

Only the uncomplicated situation is considered, i.e., presence or absence of VUR in children without bladder outlet obstruction, neurogenic bladder dysfunction, true ectopia of the ureteral orifices, or prior vesicoureteral surgery, and the like.

DEVELOPMENTAL PHYSIOLOGY

Knowledge of the normal developmental physiology is a valid basis for evaluation of supposed pathologic states and their management in children. Such knowledge is unsatisfactory with regard to the vesicoureteric junction. Although the morphology and the successive prolongation of the intramural course of the ureter are well described, the developmental aspects of the valvular function, especially the competence in different ages, are but little explored.

Most studies—the majority considering children beyond the first and second years of life—so far suggest that VUR does not occur normally. There is, however, only one planned, systematic study of healthy children of different ages (Köllermann and Ludwig, 1967). This suggests a high frequency of VUR during the first year of life, with a rapid tapering thereafter (Figure 16–13) (Baker et al., 1966; Roberts, 1978). Köllermann's methodology in performing MCU has been criticized, but the results suggest at least that the morphologic maturation of the vesicoureteric junction has a functional correlate.

GENESIS OF REFLUX—GENETICS, MATURATION, OBSTRUCTION, INFECTION

A genetic predisposition seems to play a role in the onset of reflux (de Vargas et al., 1978; Jerkins and Noe, 1982). Since reflux dis-

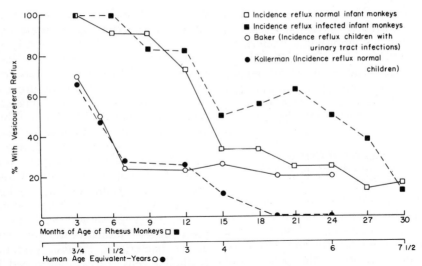

Figure 16–13. A comparison of normal infant humans and monkeys versus those with recurrent urinary tract infections. Notice that, over time, the incidence of reflux declines (thus maturation of the ureterovesical junction occurs) despite infection. (From Roberts, J. A.: South. Med. J., *71*:28, 1978. Used by permission.)

appears with growth (Smellie et al., 1975; Edwards et al., 1977), a maturation process seems to take place. It may be the rate of this functional maturation that is genetically controlled.

Obstruction is now ruled out as a major cause of VUR (for references see Gross and Lebowitz, 1981 and Ehrlich, 1982). Neither does infection seem to have any important causal role in the development of significant reflux. Although other opinions have been expressed (Kaveggia et al., 1966), the analysis of extensive material suggests "that reflux and UTI are independent variables that often coexist" (Gross and Lebowitz, 1981). This view accords with the comparison of girls with and without UTI shown in Figure 16–13. The findings in girls also correspond strikingly well to the age-adjusted frequency of VUR in monkeys.

Even if infection does not cause significant VUR—but possibly slight cases in marginally competent valves—it may interfere with the rate of maturation and lead to a delay of disappearance of reflux in both man and monkey, as suggested by the gap in reflux frequency between infected and noninfected subjects (Fig. 16–13). This would explain the often demonstrated coexistence of infection and reflux.

PYELONRENAL BACKFLOW AND RENAL DAMAGE—THE ANATOMIC VIEW

Williams (1970) was the first to suggest that in children with reflux, the difference between kidneys with and without focal scars might be a difference in local defense at the level of the papillae. This seems to have been a fruitful thought. Hodson and coworkers (1975) showed

that intrarenal reflux in the presence of severe obstruction could occur in the multipapillary kidney of the pig and cause a renal scar. Studying infants, Rolleston and associates (1975) found gross vesicoureteral reflux associated with intrarenal reflux (IRR) and infection to be predictive of future renal damage in the area with intrarenal reflux.

Ransley and Risdon (1975a, b; 1974) have explored the anatomic basis of intrarenal reflux, and found that in pigs as well as in humans, collecting ducts open at the renal papillae either with slitlike orifices or with round ones. The slitlike openings appear on the cone-shaped single papillae, while the circular ones are found in the center of the area cribrosa of the conglomerate or fused papillae. When pressure in the renal pelvis and calyces was increased in the experimental animal, the slitlike orifices tended to become occluded, while the gaping orifices of the flat or even concave area cribrosa of the compound papillae tended to remain open, and contrast was forced into the renal parenchyma. This mechanism seems very simple and would explain two things: first, why gross reflux is not invariably associated with renal damage (conglomerate papillae with gaping orifices are not always present); and second, why scarring is most common in the upper pole, followed by the lower pole, and least often in the midzone of the kidney. This distribution of scars follows the distribution of conglomerate papillae in human kidneys.

If congenital anatomic variants would be the only prerequisite for scarring, however, one would expect an equal frequency of scarring in comparable materials. This is not the case. Ten per cent were reported to have focal scars in one series of girls with asymptomatic bacteriuria (Lindberg et al., 1975b); in other series 25 per cent had them (McLachlan et al., 1975; Savage et al., 1973); and only some 5 per cent of infant girls who were followed after a symptomatic, febrile infection were affected (Winberg et al., 1974).

PYELORENAL BACKFLOW AND RENAL DAMAGE—THE FUNCTIONAL VIEW AND THE ADHERENCE CONCEPT

The way in which bacteria reach the renal tissue in patients with acute, clinical pyelonephritis long remained an enigma. Vesicoureteric reflux provided a rationale for the ascent of bacteria from the bladder to the pelvis, and intrarenal reflux for the spread into the renal parenchyma. However, among infants and children appearing in a primary care center with an acute attack of presumed clinical pyelonephritis (definition: high fever, CRP, sedimentation rate, and *E. coli* IgM antibodies; prolonged lowering of concentrating capacity as shown in Figure 16–4), only a minority had VUR demonstrable by MCU, 40 per cent in infants and 25 per cent in children (Winberg et al., 1974). In still fewer, IRR is found. Nor is progressive scarring always associated with demonstrable VUR. In a prospectively followed material from primary care, where 23 kidneys developed focal scarring, VUR with dilatation was demonstrated in only one third at the time of the first infection (Table 16–8) (Winberg et al., 1982). Similar findings have recently been reported by Winter and coworkers (1983). Furthermore, in some children with VUR the urinary tract infection (UTI) still seems to be limited to the bladder. Obviously, the mechanistic concept of pathogenesis of pyelonephritis and renal scarring—expressed in the term "reflux nephropathy" (RN)—needs an amendment and a completion.

The discrepancies between these studies and generally held views may be reconciled by some studies in the monkey suggesting a differ-

ent mechanism for pyelorenal backflow. In a series of experiments, Roberts and associates (1975, 1978, 1979, 1981, 1984) showed that some, but not all, *E. coli* strains caused ureteral paralysis and that this paralysis could be associated with an increase in ureteral perfusion pressure, flattening of a highly compliant papilla, and pyelorenal backflow. This was invariably followed by progressive renal damage. Interestingly, sonography during acute presumed pyelonephritis in infants often shows a transient dilatation of the ureter and pelvis and increased echogenicity of the renal papilla (Bollgren et al., 1984; unpublished observations).

It was later shown that a prerequisite for the effects on monkeys was the high adherence of the bacteria to monkey ureteral and renal epithelial cells, i.e., P-fimbriated (Svenson et al., 1984; Roberts et al., 1984). These experimental studies, combined with the adherence concept (page 844), might explain the obvious fact that renal infection and renal scarring are found even in the absence of gross VUR. Interestingly, the damaging effect may occur through the same final pathway as in gross VUR, i.e., pyelorenal backflow.

In this context it is also noteworthy that in the absence of gross reflux about 95 per cent of episodes of acute pyelonephritis are caused by P-fimbriated *E. coli* (highly pyelonephritogenic strains) (Källenius et al., 1982), but in the presence of gross VUR P-fimbriated *E. coli* are less common (Lomberg et al., 1983). *A cornerstone in this reasoning is the recent demonstration that inoculation of P-fimbriated E. coli into the bladder of adult nonrefluxing monkeys will result in acute and chronic pyelonephritis after a shorter or longer period of time* (Svenson et al., 1984).

In conclusion, bacterial adhesion in association with induced ureteral malfunction may lead to renal damage in the absence of VUR. See further on page 844.

STERILE REFLUX AND RENAL LESION

Hodson and coworkers have shown in the pig that sterile reflux can lead to renal scars in the areas of intrarenal reflux (Hodson et al., 1975). However, this model does require bladder neck obstruction creating a presistently increased pressure. This model will thus mimic exclusively the clinical situation of patients with obstructions or with neurogenic bladder dysfunction, as originally studied by Hutch (1952). Experimental work by Ransley and Risdon (1978), Lenaghan and associates (1972), Mendoza and Roberts (1983), and others suggests that there is no renal damage from reflux except

TABLE 16–8. DEMONSTRATION OF VUR AT THE TIME OF THE FIRST INFECTION IN 23 KIDNEYS DEVELOPING FOCAL SCARRING

Grade	Per cent
0–1	39
2	26
3	35
4	0

From Winberg, J., Bollgren, I., Källenius, G., et al.: Pediatr. Clin. North Am., *29*:801, 1982.

in association with persistently raised pressure or infection. As mentioned earlier, studies in humans show that sterile reflux does not prevent renal growth or even compensatory hypertrophy.

MANAGEMENT OF VUR—A CONSERVATIVE VIEW

Management of vesicoureteral reflux is still controversial; to quote Scott (1975), "Decisions still tend to be based on personal experience rather than applied scientific knowledge."

It is obvious that VUR, when gross and associated with IRR and infection, enhances the risk for renal scarring (Smellie et al., 1975; Rolleston et al., 1974; Filly et al., 1974; Hodson and Edwards, 1960; Smellie and Normand, 1975). Two things do not follow from this statement: (1) that VUR as shown by MCU is a prerequisite for renal infection and renal damage (see earlier), and (2) that correction of reflux improves the situation of the patient. Although operative correction of VUR has been practiced for three decades its value is still unproved. The only controlled studies, those of Elo and coworkers (1982) and the preliminary data from the Birmingham Reflux Study Group (1983), so far suggest that operation does not influence the prognosis. Uncontrolled data (Claësson et al., 1981a; Verrier-Jones et al., 1982; Smellie et al., 1981a; Govan et al., 1975) point in the same direction, i.e., that renal growth can take place even in the presence of reflux. Further data are, however, needed.

Early diagnosis, supervision of infection and renal status, and surgery in selected cases, mainly those with progressive dilation of the pelvis and minor calyces, are main points on which most people seem to agree. Table 16–9 gives some general suggestions for the management of patients with reflux. There is a great tendency for reflux to disappear spontaneously (Smellie et al., 1975). Surgery should therefore not be too readily attempted. There are excellent brief papers on vesicoureteral reflux (Girdany and Price, 1975; Lancet [leading article], 1974; Smellie and Normand, 1975; Roberts, 1984).

CONCLUSIONS

In summary, gross reflux associated with infection or with low obstruction with persistently raised pressure constitutes a major threat to the kidney. Reflux is not a prerequisite either for renal infection or for renal scarring or renal growth retardation. Strongly adhesive bacteria may reach the renal tissue in the absence of

TABLE 16–9. GENERAL SUGGESTIONS FOR MANAGEMENT OF PATIENTS WITH REFLUX UNCOMPLICATED BY OBSTRUCTION

With Susceptibility to Recurrent Infections	Without Susceptibility to Recurrent Infections
↓	↓
Long-term antibacterial prophylaxis.	Check renal concentrating power and IVP.
↓	
Repeated cultures. Check renal conc. cap. Follow renal growth ——→ with IVP. (Urethrocystography*)	If renal growth is impaired or conc. cap. persistently low, or control of infection is unsuccessful.
↓	↓
If control infection is fairly successful.	Consider operation, especially if reflux is massive, and there is
↓	progressive dilatation of
Continue conservative treatment.	upper urinary tract

*If the kidneys grow well and progressive calyceal changes do not occur, repeated urethrocystograms usually give little therapeutic guidance.

reflux demonstrable by MCU and cause renal infection and renal damage. Controlled studies have so far failed to show substantial benefit from operation of reflux uncomplicated by obstruction. The problem requires more studies.

RENAL FOCAL SCAR— "CHRONIC PYELONEPHRITIS"; "REFLUX NEPHROPATHY"

DIAGNOSTIC CRITERIA

Infections may cause renal growth retardation, focal scars, or both. Such changes may also have causes other than infection. A scar is wedge-shaped with the tip in the papilla and has a distinct demarcation from healthy renal tissue (Hepstinall, 1966). The cause of the characteristic demarcation is uncertain; distribution of intrarenal reflux and vascular or immunologic barriers have been suggested. In any case, the distribution clearly suggests the ascending nature of the infection.

Radiologic criteria have been defined by Hodson and Wilson (1965). These consist of a papillary lesion, in the most advanced cases with "clubbing," and a corresponding defect in the renal outline. It may be 24 months before a scar is visible on x-ray examination (Filly et al., 1974). Differentiation from congenital renal dysplasia may sometimes be difficult. This diagnosis should rest exclusively on strictly defined histologic criteria (Bernstein, 1968). It is striking how silently even extensive renal destruction may develop (McLachlan et al., 1975; Andersen et al., 1973).

MAIN DETERMINANTS OF RENAL SCARRING

The ultimate goal of the care of children with urinary tract infections is the prevention of progressive renal damage with its consequences, such as hypertension, complications of pregnancy, and end-stage renal disease. Prevention will become more successful if the main causes are recognized. The association of huge reflux and obstruction with scarring is well established, but there are also other determinants of renal damage following infection. These will be considered here (for review, see Winberg et al., 1982).

OBSTRUCTION

The role of obstruction, especially when associated with infection, in severe renal damage is well established and will not be dealt with here. Generous use of ultrasonography and intravenous pyelography in infants and small children with febrile infections as well as in patients with recurrent infections is recommended (see Chapter 7).

GROSS VUR AND IRR

Generous use of MCU in infants and small children with UTI will help identify this risk group so that early preventive measures can be taken (see page 856).

AGE

The growing human kidney of the young child seems to be much more vulnerable than that of the adult to both focal scarring and growth retardation. This has also been shown in the experimental animal (Asscher and Chick, 1972). Most vulnerable are kidneys of small children with gross reflux (Filly et al., 1974; Smellie et al., 1975).

Scars may already be present at the first x-ray examination. Smellie and Normand (1975) rightly pointed out that, in such instances, either the damage is congenital or the first infection, initiating the damage, went unrecognized. The latter possibility is strongly favored, since scarring and renal growth retardation (Winberg et al., 1975) are less commonly seen at the first x-ray examination in infantile infections than when the first recognized infection occurs at an older age. Table 16–10 shows that among boys with a first infection during the first year of life only 1 of 116 had a scar at the first intravenous pyelogram, whereas 6 of 116 (about 5 per cent) developed a scar later. Among those who were more than 1 year of age at the so-called first infection, focal scar was already present at the first intravenous pyelogram in one fourth. Table 16–10 indicates, first, that when infections are diagnosed during the first year and immediately treated and checked after treatment, the infection carries a rather low risk for scar formation. (The prognosis for renal growth will be dealt with on page 861.) Second, when urinary tract infection is diagnosed after the first year of life, the patient often may have had at least one earlier—probably unrecognized and untreated—infection (which causes scarring in a high percentage). As a group, girls seem to have their début infection later than boys and scars develop usually up to about age 3 to 4 years (sometimes later). The findings of McLachlan and coworkers (1975) emphasize that attempts to prevent renal damage should be directed toward very young children.

Post-mortem examinations of adults show that focal renal scars are as common in males as in females. Since urinary infections are about ten times more common in females, it has been questioned whether infections have much to do with such scars (Freedman, 1967; Kleeman and Freedman, 1960). However, a 1:1 (18/20) male to female ratio of scarring was also seen at follow-up of children with proven UTI (Winberg et al., 1974; Winberg et al., 1975). If kidneys are most vulnerable during the first year of life, this sex ratio for pyelonephritic scarring would

TABLE 16–10. Renal Scarring in Males at "First" Infection and at Follow-up

| Age at "First" UTI | N | Per Cent with Scars | |
		At "First" Infection	At Follow-up*
<1 year	116	1	5
>1 year	44	25	0

*In earlier undamaged kidneys.
From Winberg, J., Andersen, H. J., Bergström, T., et al.: Acta Paediatr. Scand. (Suppl. 252), 1974.

TABLE 16–11. Sex Distribution Among 258 Consecutive "First" Symptomatic UTI During Infancy

Age at First Infection	Male/Female Ratio	
	ABSOLUTE N	RELATIVE
0–12 months	113/145	0.8
0–6 months	102/91	1.1

From Winberg, J., Andersen, H. J., Bergström, T., et al.: Acta Paediatr. Scand. (Suppl. 252), 1974.

TABLE 16–12. Care and Prognosis in Symptomatic UTI

	Total N	Scarring	
		N	PER CENT
Adequate care at first infection	440	20	4.5
Delayed care of first infection	41	7	17

From Winberg, J., Bollgren, I., Källenius, G., et al.: Pediatr. Clin. North Am., 29:801, 1982.

be expected, since the male to female ratio for UTI among infants less than 12 months old was 0.8, and among those less than 6 months old was 1.1 (Table 16–11). Increased attention to the possibility of pyelonephritis in infants and children with unexplained fever is necessary in prevention of renal damage.

THERAPEUTIC DELAY

One important determinant of renal damage is the duration of infection before the initiation of treatment. A few days of persistent infection may be enough to cause severe renal and ureteral damage. In 41 girls in whom the first known infection was inadequately treated, the incidence of renal damage was four times as high as in 440 girls in whom diagnosis and treatment were prompt and adequate (Table 16–12).

The impact of the therapeutic delay is demonstrated in two experimental studies (Miller and Phillips, 1981; Slotki and Asscher, 1982). These investigators induced pyelonephritis in rats and delayed therapy for varying periods. With each prolongation of the interval, from 8 hours to 7 days, the renal damage became more and more severe (Table 16–13). These findings correspond very well with our clinical observations. In an analysis of causes of ureteral and renal damage, attention should be given to the duration of the first febrile infection before the start of treatment.

THE INFLAMMATORY RESPONSE

The importance of the inflammatory response for tissue damage in general has been explored during the last decade. Its relevance for initiation of parenchymal damage in renal infections has been analyzed in a series of papers (Bille and Glauser, 1982; Glauser et al., 1978). The damaging effect of the inflammatory response seems to be caused by the release of large amounts of free oxygen and hydroxyl radicals, which are highly toxic to bacteria but also to parenchymal cells. If the release of these agents exceeds the capacity of the host to metabolize them, tissue damage will occur.

The results of the studies in experimental infections can be briefly summarized as follows. In a rat experimental model, suppuration after inoculation of bacteria was maximal at 3 days. This was followed by scarring, which was extensive if the suppuration had persisted more than 3 days. Scarring became much less if suppuration was aborted through early treatment of the infection. Scarring also was slight if suppuration was aborted but infection persisted through "partial treatment" with antibiotics. Similarly and most interestingly, scarring was limited also when suppuration was aborted in the presence of an augmented number of bacteria, a situation caused by colchicine-induced depression of leukocyte migration. The *in vivo* significance of these findings has recently been shown by Rob-

TABLE 16–13. Delayed Antimicrobial Therapy versus Gross Renal Lesions

Nontreated Controls	Treated Animals	
RENAL SURFACE INVOLVED (PER CENT)	START OF THERAPY AFTER CHALLENGE	RENAL SURFACE INVOLVED (PER CENT)
	8 hours	2.5
	1 day	6
27	2 days	9
	3 days	13
	4 days	14
	7 days	21

From Miller, T., and Phillips, S.: Kidney Int., 19:654, 1981.

erts and associates (1982). Administration of superoxide dismutase—a scavenger of free radicals—prevented acute and chronic renal damage in experimental infections in monkeys.

These studies suggest that tissue damage may be caused not so much by bacteria but by the inflammatory response through O and OH free radicals liberated from leukocytes. The studies emphasize that the elapsed time between onset of infection and initiation of treatment is a critical factor in determining the extent of the renal damage. One possibility, emerging from these studies, is that renal bacteriuria not associated with pyuria may be of minor importance.

INDIVIDUAL SUSCEPTIBILITY

Some individuals are more prone to infections than others. This susceptibility is associated with an abnormal gram-negative colonization of the introitus (Stamey et al., 1971) and periurethral area (Bollgren and Winberg, 1976a), which precedes infection. Also, the anaerobic flora is abnormal (Bollgren et al., 1981). The mere presence of even abundant *E.coli* in the periurethral area is insufficient to induce infection. An additional factor in the initiation of infection must be postulated. Studies of bacterial adherence have demonstrated that uroepithelial cells from infection-prone women bind *E. coli* more avidly than do cells from nonsusceptible women (Fowler and Stamey, 1977; Källenius and Winberg, 1978). Whether such females will run a greater risk for renal damage is so far open to discussion. This is further discussed in Chapter 14 and on pages 844 and 845.

BACTERIAL VIRULENCE

A number of bacterial factors have been proposed to be associated with nephropathogenicity (Winberg et al., 1983). The ability to bind to epithelial cells by specific adhesins may be a most relevant one. The recent identification of *E.coli* adhesins (P-fimbriae) facilitating human renal infection is reviewed elsewhere.

PROPOSED HYPOTHESIS FOR INITIATION OF RENAL INFECTION

The following hypothesis for ureteral and renal infection based on the above-mentioned studies is proposed (Svenson et al., 1984). Colonization of the gut and periurethral area with P-fimbriated *E. coli* precedes ascending infection. Colonization and ascending infection are dependent on the presence of specific $Gal - \frac{1\text{-}4}{\alpha} - Gal$ receptors on the surface of the epithelial cells. Ureteral infection occurs by transport of bacteria by turbulent flow or reflux, or both. Epithelial receptors in the ureter allow local replication of bacteria. Structural damage of the ureter or endotoxin inhibition of normal autonomic neurotransmission causes ureteral hold-up of excretion and increased perfusion pressure in the ureter and renal pelvis. Pyelorenal backflow occurs at low pressure. Further bacterial attachment by P-fimbriae to tubular cells is followed by acute renal tissue inflammation. This would explain the fact that renal scarring commonly occurs without demonstrable vesicoureteral reflux. When diagnosis and treatment are immediate, damage may be avoided even when there is gross intrarenal reflux. With therapeutic delay and severe inflammatory response, renal damage will occur whether there is VUR or not.

OTHER PROPOSED FACTORS

Other factors have been suggested to induce renal damage, such as persistence of bacterial antigen; formation of immune complexes with complement fixation; cross reactions between kidney and certain *E.coli* antigens with formation of autoantibodies; a direct toxic effect of lipid A (Westenfelder et al., 1975); infection with atypical bacteria (Fairley and Birch, 1983). The possible role of such mechanisms in the pathogenesis of renal scar formation has been reviewed by Hanson and coworkers (1975) and Holmgren and Smith (1975).

DIAGNOSIS, THERAPY, AND FOLLOW-UP

GENERAL MANAGEMENT OF UTI

The goal of management is to prevent progressive renal disease. Chemotherapy and close follow-up, including radiologic and urologic exploration and, if needed, surgical treatment, are equivalent links in the management.

LOOKING FOR OBSTRUCTION—PHYSICAL AND LABORATORY EXAMINATION

The physician's first concern should be to look for evidence of obstruction of the urinary flow. One should examine thoroughly the genital organs and the abdomen, especially the suprapubic area. A raised bladder, a mass in the loin, arterial hypertension, a high BUN, or an electrolyte disturbance, including acidosis, should evoke suspicion of an obstruction (Ericsson et al., 1955). Otherwise, the main key to differentiation between obstructed and nonobstructed infections is the reaction to treatment. If the temperature has not normalized after 2 to 3 days of therapy, and if sediment has not cleared after 4 to 5 days, it is highly likely either that the bacteria are resistant to the antibiotic given or that there is an obstruction. The same is true if the renal concentrating capacity does not approach normality within 3 weeks. Such patients should have a full radiologic investigation as soon as possible.

If urethral obstruction is suspected on physical examination, the patient should have bladder drainage until an expert evaluation can be performed. If the radiologic examination confirms obstruction, the catheter should be left in place until a free urinary flow is established surgically. Direct drainage of a unilaterally obstructed pelvis may sometimes be necessary. It should be remembered that infection in itself may cause moderate dilatation of ureters and pelves (Roberts, 1975; Teague and Boyarksy, 1968), owing to muscle damage or interference with transmission of nerve impulses. When the infant is severely ill or dehydrated, or both, an intravenous drip should be set up and treatment begun at once. Appropriate parenteral antimicrobials should be given as soon as urine culture has been taken.

Follow-up. Table 16–14 gives guidelines for follow-up during and after treatment of pyelonephritis and cystitis (Winberg and Bollgren, 1980). The program might be less ambitious in girls over 5 to 6 years of age.

GENERAL POINTS ON ANTIBIOTIC THERAPY

A 10-day course of a suitable antibiotic will eradicate infection in almost 100 per cent of patients, provided bacteria are sensitive to the antibiotic (Fig. 16–14). The high rate of recurrences after a short course of antibiotic treatment was formerly interpreted as being due to recrudescence of incompletely healed infections.

TABLE 16–14. PROGRAM OF FOLLOW-UP DURING AND AFTER TREATMENT OF PYELONEPHRITIS AND CYSTITIS

Time after Onset of Treatment	Pyelonephritis (Temperature >38°C, CRP[1]-Positive)	Cystitis (Temperature <38°C, CRP-Negative)
3 days	Dipslide culture[2] WBC[3] in urine Possible IVU[4]	Dipslide culture[5] WBC
2–3 weeks	Dipslide culture[2] WBC CRP ESR Possible referral for radiologic examination[4]	Dipslide culture WBC
2 months	Dipslide culture WBC	Dipslide culture Possibly IVU[4, 5]
3–4 months	Dipslide culture WBC	Dipslide culture WBC
12 months	Dipslide culture WBC	Dipslide culture[5] WBC

Later	If possible, a checkup should
	  be performed at 24 months and
	  36 months after onset	

[1]C-reactive protein.
[2]A dipslide culture is performed and extra urine stored at 4°C for 24 hours. If the dipslide is positive, the urine is sent to a microbiologist for quantitative culture and resistance pattern.
[3]White blood cell count.
[4]See text.
[5]Can be omitted.

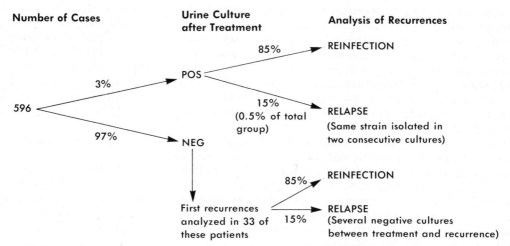

Figure 16–14. Approximate figures for immediate cure rate after treatment with sulfonamide (10 or 60 days—no difference). Only 0.5 per cent of the total group of patients had a relapse without a preceding negative culture. (From Winberg, J., et al.: Kidney Int., 8:101, 1975.)

This was the original basis for the "long-term treatment," the idea being that bacteria in the renal tissue could be eradicated only after therapy lasting weeks or months. This reason for long-term treatment is rarely, if ever, relevant, since most recurrences are reinfections; i.e., therapy for the foregoing infection has been effective, but new bacteria have invaded (Table 16–15) (Bergström et al., 1967). This is true even when recurrences appear within 2 to 3 days after discontinuation of therapy. Therefore, the current approach is to attempt eradication of infection by a short course of an antimicrobial agent, and in selected cases to follow this with a small prophylactic dose of antibiotic to prevent reinfection. Some authors prefer to put all patients on long-term prophylaxis (Normand and Smellie, 1965); others select such a regimen only for those who have repeated infections at very short intervals (Kunin, 1966; Winberg et al., 1973). Because of the high risk for renal scarring in infants and toddlers with Grade IV reflux, these patients should be given prophylaxis even before they have demonstrated susceptibility to recurrence.

Although the majority of recurrences are reinfections, a few are not. The latter are either unresolved bacteriuria or persistence of bacteria in a focus not amenable to antibiotics (see Chapter 14, page 743). A change in drug or dosage is helpful in most instances of unresolved bacteriuria, whereas surgery is the answer in most instances of persistence of bacteria.

INITIAL TREATMENT OF ACUTE INFECTIONS

Choice of antimicrobial drugs and duration of treatment should be considered in relation to the situation of the patient; whether there have been single episodes at long intervals or frequently repeated infections; whether the patient is severly dehydrated and vomiting; whether he has a neurogenic bladder or renal insufficiency; or whether the patient is a newborn. With all drugs, 10 days of therapy will eradicate infection, even in febrile pyelonephritis. Nighttime doses are not needed. Shorter courses may work as well. In afebrile infections, 5 days are probably sufficient. Some studies suggest that one single dose of a suitable drug is enough for eradication of infection (Källenius et al., 1983; Bailey, 1983). Single-dose therapy should pend further evaluation.

Single Episodes of Symptomatic Infections Separated by Long Intervals. Sulfonamide still holds its position as a good first choice in these patients, whether they have pyelonephritis or "cystitis." In vivo sulfonamide resistance has usually remained uncommon in these

TABLE 16–15. URINARY E. COLI SEROTYPES IN A GIRL
WITH 8 CONSECUTIVE INFECTIONS

Infection Number	Bacteria/ml (in millions)	E. coli Serotype
1	10	Rough:H–
2	1	O9:–
3	10	O⁻(1–146):H–
4	10	O20:H19
5	10	O20:H19
6	10	O3:H2
7	10	O73:H34
8	10	O39:H4

patients, as contrasted to those with frequently recurring infections, but local differences may exist. Cure of the infection will follow a 10-day course in almost 100 per cent of treated cases (see Figure 16–14) (Winberg et al., 1975). In addition to efficacy, solubility, frequency of side reactions, and cost should guide the choice of sulfonamide compound. Preparations with a short excretion time, such as sulfafurazole (Gantrisin) and sulfisomidine (Elkosin) have a high solubility in urine, and allergic reactions are infrequent. Sulfonamide preparations with a "long" or "half-long" excretion time do not seem to have any advantages. Even with "rapidly excreted" drugs, the antibacterial activity of urine remains high 12 to 24 hours, perhaps even 46 hours, following a single dose (see Figure 16–2) (Tschudi Madsen, 1968).

There is also some evidence that urine concentration is more essential than blood concentration in selecting treatment of UTI (Stamey et al., 1974, 1965). Considering this, it is possible that intervals between doses can be considerably prolonged. Studies to prove this are lacking, however.

In addition to sulfonamide, other suitable first-choice drugs are nitrofurantoin, amoxicillin and related penicillin substances, trimethoprim-sulfamethoxazole, trimethoprim, nalidixic acid, and third-generation cephalosporins. Indications, doses, and complications are listed in Table 16–16.

Nitrofurantoin is, in view of its limited ecologic effects (see page 859), a very suitable drug. There are, however, no controlled studies of its efficiency in treating acute febrile pyelonephritis. Gastrointestinal side effects will be few with a dosage of 3 mg/kg/24 hours. Allergic pulmonary reactions and pulmonary fibrosis have been reported with increasing frequency. These reactions seem, however, to be rare in children. Nitrofurantoin is ineffective when glomerular filtration rate is reduced to about 50 per cent of normal or less.

The previously reported rapid development of primary chromosomal resistance to nalidixic acid in a formerly sensitive bacterial population during therapy (Ronald et al., 1966) seems to occur mainly with underdosage (Stamey and Bragonje, 1976).

The combination of trimethoprim with a sulfonamide (Septrin, Bactrim, Eusaprim) has become widely used during recent years. Both compounds interfere with bacterial folate me-

TABLE 16–16. First-Choice Drugs in Management of UTI

Compound	Dosage MG/KG Body Weight/ 24 Hrs*	No. of Doses Per day	Duration of Therapy (days)	Remarks
Short-acting sulfonamide:				
Sulfafurazole	100–200	4	10	Not to be used so long as neonatal
Sulphasomidine	100	4	10	jaundice persists.
Nitrofurantoin	3	4	10	Not to be used the first month of life. Not effective when GFR is about 50 per cent of normal or less. Pulmonary side reactions reported with increasing frequency; seem so far to be rare in children. Limited ecologic side effects.
Nalidixic acid	60	3–4	10	Not to be used in newborns. Dosage at 1 to 4 months of age, 30 mg/kg/ 24 hrs. Rise in intracranial pressure described in infants and children.
Trimethoprim	6	3–4	10	Not to be used before 6 weeks of life.
Sulfamethoxazole	30			Experience with this drug limited in infants and toddlers. Diffuses into prostate and vagina.
Ampicillin	50–100	3–4	10	Neonatal infections often caused by *Klebsiella*, resistant to ampicillin.
Pivampicillin	25–50			Gastrointestinal complications very
Amoxicillin	25–50			common with ampicillin.

*First dose at waking up, the last at bedtime, one or two in between. Nighttime doses not necessary.

tabolism, but on different levels, and both have a synergistic effect in vitro.

Dosages of 5 to 7 mg/kg body weight of trimethoprim and 25 to 35 mg/kg body weight of sulfamethoxazole twice daily for 8 to 12 days are used.

Trimethoprim, unlike other antimicrobial substances, seems to concentrate by nonionic diffusion across vaginal as well as prostatic epithelium. This may play a major role in the treatment, and especially in the prevention, of certain urinary infections (Stamey and Condy, 1975; Stamey et al., 1973).

Checkup after Therapy (Table 16–14). First checkup should preferably be done after therapy has been discontinued for 2 to 3 days, and then again 2 to 3 weeks later. The next three checkups are spread out over the first year after the infection. If possible, the patients should be followed a few more years. If checkup cultures are done when urine still contains antibiotics, evaluation of the results can be difficult.

This schedule is used for all infants and small children with acute-onset, symptomatic infections. Older children with mainly lower urinary tract symptoms and no renal scarring are checked with longer intervals. Infants and small children with Grade IV reflux (see Figure 16–7) are checked each week during the first 1 to 2 months after an acute pyelonephritis. Home culture with dipslide or similar devices may be used after thorough instruction of the parents.

MANAGEMENT OF RECURRENT INFECTIONS

The cause and resistance pattern of recurrent infections are more variable than in single infections. If the patient's condition allows, therapy should be postponed until the resistance of the bacteria has been examined. If this is impracticable, a drug of a type different from that used in the preceding infection should be given. Dosage and duration of therapy are as described previously. Prophylaxis is carried through after treatment in patients with frequent reinfections. Nitrofurantoin is the drug of choice because of its insignificant effect on the gut flora (Winberg et al., 1973). Dosage is 1 mg/kg/24 hours, given as a night dose. If this does not work, the dose may be divided into one morning and one evening dose. Trimethoprim with sulfamethoxazole is a good alternative. This combination may keep the vestibular area clean (Stamey and Condy, 1975). Trimethroprim without sulfonamide has also been used as a prophylactic in a single night dose of about 2 mg/kg body weight. It is effective, but there is

some concern about increased risk for selection of resistant strains. Nalidixic acid, 20 mg/kg/24 hours, may be another alternative for prophylaxis.

With regard to duration of prophylaxis, a trial-and-error approach is suggested. Let the initial period of prophylaxis last for 2 to 4 months. If infection recurs shortly after prophylactic therapy is stopped, a new therapeutic course should be given followed by prophylaxis for half a year. After discontinuation of prophylaxis, the patient should continue to be followed with repeated cultures and so on. Some patients need prophylactic treatment for several years.

Checkup is done 2 to 3 days after each therapeutic course and at each or every second or third month during prophylaxis, depending on the susceptibility of the patient to recurrence. In patients more than 4 to 5 years old without scarring and without gross (Grade IV) reflux, the intervals between checkup examinations might be considerably prolonged. With cooperative and understanding families we see such patients once or twice a year if there are no problems. The use of dipslide (or "dip-stream") cultures (Arneil et al., 1973) facilitates checkup for both patient and doctor.

MANAGEMENT OF INFECTIONS IN PATIENTS WITH NEUROGENIC BLADDERS, SPECIFICALLY WITH MYELOMENINGOCELE—A PEDIATRICIAN'S VIEW

Therapy has three main goals: to protect the kidneys from damage, to make the patient socially continent, and to decrease the number of infections. Intermittent catheterization—clean but not sterile—has improved the situation for many of these patients (Scott and Deegan, 1982). It should be started before dilatation of the upper urinary tract has occurred. Children over 6 to 7 years of age can often learn to do it themselves. Catheterization will diminish the pressure in the upper urinary tract and in the kidneys. Infections seem to occur less frequently and to run a more benign course. During continence training, pharmacologic agents that increase bladder volume, relax the external sphincter, and stimulate detrusor contraction are often helpful.

A true obstruction of the outflow region of the bladder may complicate these cases. The patients should be cared for by the urologist and the pediatrician in cooperation. The etiology and resistance pattern of the infecting bacteria are unpredictable. In nonacute infections, therapy is best postponed until the results of culture and sensitivity tests are available. Antimicrobial therapy should be given to patients who have either urinary symptoms or a high sedimentation rate, or unspecific symptoms, such as tiredness or anorexia, that have no other obvious explanation. Antimicrobial treatment of asymptomatic infections in these patients is probably of little value. Recurrences, which usually are reinfections, are almost impossible to prevent by prophylaxis.

MANAGEMENT OF INFECTIONS IN NEWBORNS

These infections are sometimes part of a generalized septicemia. A combination of gentamicin and ampicillin is a good choice. Glomerular filtration rate is often severely reduced by infection; therefore, the serum concentration of any potentially toxic drug should be monitored. If renal infection is the only manifestation, ampicillin, 100 to 200 mg/kg body weight, may be sufficient. If response is not quick, therapy should be changed, since *Klebsiella* or *Enterobacter* is a common pathogen in this age group. When diagnosed early, neonatal *E. coli* pyelonephritis has a good prognosis (Bergström et al., 1972). Infections in this age group are often caused by *E. coli* with a K1 antigen that seems to be a virulence factor (Robbins et al., 1974). For dosage of gentamicin, see the reference by Nelson and McCracken (1972).

MANAGEMENT OF PATIENTS WITH RENAL INSUFFICIENCY AND URINARY INFECTION

The ideal qualities of an antimicrobial agent for patients with both urinary infection and renal insufficiency can be summarized as follows: (1) rapid renal excretion; (2) low toxicity, even in high serum concentrations; (3) slow metabolism in the liver; and (4) no alternative pathways of excretion. Ampicillin is a suitable drug before antibiotic sensitivity results are obtained. Sulfonamides with a short half-life are more useful than those with a long half-life. Nitrofurantoin should not be used. Gentamicin can be used, but with great caution, if the dosage is guided by assessment of serum concentration determinations. See also Asscher, 1980.

MANAGEMENT OF PATIENTS WITH SCREENING BACTERIURIA

This is dealt with on pages 847 and 848.

CHEMOTHERAPY, FECAL FLORA, AND TRANSMISSIBLE CHEMORESISTANCE (R FACTORS)

The management of UTI is seriously hampered by the increasing frequency of infections caused by organisms with R factor-mediated multiresistance. Urinary infections caused by such strains are *preceded* by the appearance of the latter in feces and in the periurethral flora (Fig. 16–15) (Winberg et al., 1973). Selective antibiotic pressure has been shown to favor intestinal colonization with resistant mutants present in the environment. This is seen with sulfonamide (Winberg et al., 1973), tetracycline (Daikos et al., 1968), ampicillin (Datta et al., 1971), and probably most other antibiotics, with one proven exception—nitrofurantoin (Winberg et al., 1973) (Fig. 16–16). The influence of environment on bacterial selection is also suggested in Figure 16–16. The difference in their effects on the physiologic bacterial reservoirs will explain the common failure of long-term prophylaxis with sulfonamide and the good protective effect of nitrofurantoin (Lippman et al., 1958; Olbing et al., 1970; Winberg et al., 1973). The influence on the periurethral flora (Winberg et al., 1973) may be especially relevant, since bacterial colonization of this area may be a predecessor to bladder infection (see Figure 16–11) (Bollgren and Winberg, 1976a; Stamey et al., 1971). Since enteric bacilli other than *E. coli* are often resistant to nitrofurantoin, this drug may be less suitable for prophylaxis in heavily contaminated hospital wards.

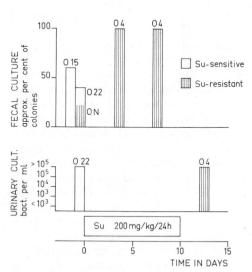

Figure 16–15. Effect of sulfonamide (Su) on the fecal flora. Treatment with sulfafurazole (Gantrisin) was in the hospital. The original, sensitive fecal strains were rapidly replaced by a resistant O4 strain because of the selective pressure. Gut sulfonamide levels amounted to 100 mg per 100 ml of feces. The recurrence at 12 days was caused by the dominating fecal *E. coli* O4. The new bacteria had an R factor–mediated resistance to sulfonamide, chloramphenicol, and ampicillin. (From Winberg, J., et al.: Clin. Nephrol., *1*:142, 1973.)

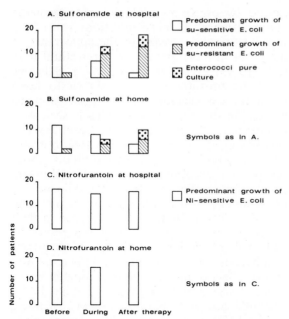

Figure 16–16. Sulfonamide *(Su)* and nitrofurantoin *(Ni)* sensitivity of the dominating fecal flora before, during, and after therapy in 74 children. (From Winberg, J., et al.: Clin. Nephrol., *1*:142, 1973.)

Recurrences following nitrofurantoin treatment are often caused by the same strain as that causing the preceding infection. Such cases were formerly evaluated as relapses of persisting renal infection, but the identicalness of organisms in two consecutive infections separated by nitrofurantoin treatment is probably better explained by reinfection from an unchanged fecal and periurethral reservoir.

In summary, the problem of resistant urinary infections should be considered in the light of the influence of therapy on the intestinal and periurethral flora. The evaluation of any drug used for treatment of UTI should be done with regard to its effect on the physiologic bacterial reservoirs. Progress will not come from the introduction of more and more potent drugs; it is more likely to come from the use of drugs with limited ecologic effects. Since resistance to nitrofurantoin, nalidixic acid (Stamey and Bragonje, 1976), and trimethoprim (Grüneberg et al., 1975) is rarely R factor-mediated, these drugs may offer some advantages for prophylaxis.

COURSE AND PROGNOSIS

These can be evaluated at different levels: the risk of recurrence, the risk of scarring and renal growth retardation, and the risk of development of hypertension or end-stage renal disease or complications of pregnancy. Some of the figures given below are from a prospective study in which the patients were diagnosed, treated, and checked at an apparent first infection (Winberg et al., 1974, 1975). If one can bring a child to puberty without renal damage, the future risk for scarring is very small, if it exists at all.

MAIN DETERMINANTS OF RENAL DAMAGE

These are dealt with on pages 852 to 854 and summarized in Table 16–17.

INFECTIONS COMPLICATED BY OBSTRUCTION

The nature of the obstruction, the success of the surgical intervention, and the time lapse between onset of infection and establishment of adequate drainage are the main factors determining the degree of permanent renal damage. Clinically, such damage—if bilateral—may manifest itself as water-losing nephropathy, generalized acidosis necessitating sodium bicarbonate replacement, uremia, or a combination of these disorders.

Repeated infections will occur in some patients even though the obstruction has been removed. In these patients, as in others with frequent recurrences, absence of symptoms or pyuria never excludes infection. Checking these patients only by history or examination of urinary sediment is inadequate. For a detailed discussion, the reader is referred to current textbooks on pediatric urology.

GIRLS WITHOUT OBSTRUCTION FALLING ILL AFTER THE NEWBORN PERIOD

Recurrence Rate. The most characteristic feature of this group of patients is their susceptibility to recurrences, which often continue to appear for many years, sometimes for decades (Lindblad and Ekengren, 1969). In such cases, it is not the infection but the inclination to acquire repeated infections that is "chronic."

TABLE 16–17. MAIN DETERMINANTS OF
RENAL DAMAGE

Anatomic obstruction
Gross VUR with IRR
Age
Therapeutic delay
Inflammatory response
Individual susceptibility
Bacterial virulence

This distinction is essential with regard to selection of therapy.

The risk of recurrence is about 30 per cent the first year after onset infection and probably somewhat less than 50 per cent for the next 5 years. An unexplained phenomenon is that reinfections tend to occur soon after the preceding infection (Fig. 16–17). The risk of recurrence seems to increase with the number of preceding infections (see Figure 16–9). This would suggest that the postulated defect of the defense mechanisms is graded.

There seems to be no obvious correlation between susceptibility to recurrence and age, localization of infection, and presence or absence of reflux. There may be a positive correlation between residual urine volume, even if small, and susceptibility to recurrence (Lindberg et al., 1975a).

From a practical point of view, it should be mentioned that in the great majority of schoolgirls with frequently recurring nonfebrile infections, scarring of a previously intact kidney will rarely, if ever, occur, and renal growth continues at a normal rate. A representative example is shown in Figure 16–18. It can be questioned whether the rigorous follow-up so often practiced in these patients is necessary.

Scarring and Renal Growth Retardation. A young girl falling ill with her first acute febrile urinary tract infection may run a risk of some 5

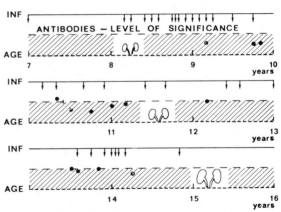

Figure 16–18. Radiographic follow-up of a girl with 33 recorded infections, which with one or two exceptions were not accompanied by fever, followed from ages 7 to 16 years. In this kind of patient renal growth is rarely influenced (see text). Infections (↑↓) and antibody titers (•) are indicated, with a dashed line at the level of significance. Within the shaded area are significant *E. coli* antibody titers.

per cent of developing a scar (Table 16–7). The risk for a boy may range from 10 to 15 per cent. These figures are for children in whom the infection is diagnosed early, treated, and checked (Winberg et al., 1974). With inadequate or delayed care, these figures may become higher (see Tables 16–12 and 16–13). In fact, scars are often already present at the first examination, especially in boys (see Table 16–10); in reports of patients not followed from their apparent first infection, the frequency of scarring is considerably greater (Lindblad and Ekengren, 1969; Smellie and Normand, 1968). A 25 per cent frequency of scarring in asymptomatic bacteriuric girls, probably representing a selection of girls with an early, unrecognized symptomatic infection, may be a measure of the approximate risk in untreated patients (Table 16–7). Scarring is often accompanied by renal growth retardation. If scarring is unilateral, there will be a compensatory hypertrophy of the undamaged kidney. Even a damaged kidney may show a remarkable catch-up growth at puberty (Fig. 16–19).

Clinically Severe Complications. It is unknown how often patients with recurrent infections will develop hypertension, uremia, distal tubular insufficiency, and obstructing stones. In the absence of obstruction, the risk of renal insufficiency and hypertension seems to be remote. Since UTI is a common disease, however, the number of patients with renal insufficiency and hypertension due to renal infections is considerable. Chantler and coworkers (1980) reported that so-called reflux nephropathy made

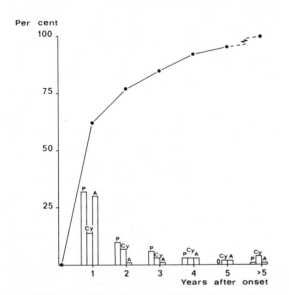

Figure 16–17. Appearance of a first recurrence after the primary infection, studied in a sample of 123 girls (aged ½ to 11 years) with at least one recurrence. Bars denote main symptom: *P*, febrile infection; *CY*, afebrile, symptomatic infection; *A*, asymptomatic infection. (From Winberg, J., et al.: Acta Paediatr. Scand. [Suppl. 252], 1974.)

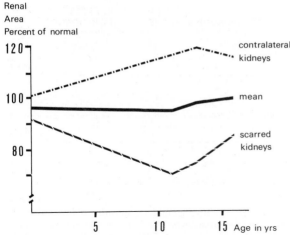

Figure 16–19. Renal parenchymal area in per cent of normal in 16 girls with unilateral scarring. The areas of the scarred and the contralateral kidneys and the mean total renal area are given as function of age. There is a catch-up growth of the scarred kidneys at puberty (Claésson et al., 1981a).

up 21 per cent of 75 children with end-stage renal disease; Holland (1979) found that among children with hypertension many had suspected focal renal damage. Complications of pregnancy, such as intrauterine fetal death, prematurity, and intrauterine growth retardation, are other possible consequences of childhood infections with renal damage.

NEONATAL INFECTIONS

Early Prognosis. These infections seem to be part of a generalized bacteremia, the course of which will determine the early prognosis.

Recurrence Rate. Early recurrences during the months following the first infection appear in about one fourth of the patients (Bergström et al., 1972). Recurrences after more than 1 year seem to be rare. This feature clearly distinguishes the infections appearing during the newborn period from those of older girls.

Scarring. The frequency of scarring following neonatal infection is unknown. In the previously mentioned study, it was seen in 2 out of 75 patients.

BOYS FALLING ILL DURING THE FIRST YEAR OF LIFE (NEONATES EXCLUDED)

Early recurrences appear as they do in girls, but infant boys, like neonates, seem to grow out of their susceptibility to infection. It is thus rare to see a recurrence more than 1 year after

the onset of infection (Winberg et al., 1975). Scarring may be more common than in girls.

OLDER BOYS (1 TO 16 YEARS OLD) WITHOUT OBSTRUCTION

There seem to be few systematic observations of UTI in boys aged 1 to 16 years. Early recurrences do occur after onset infection, as in girls; late recurrences, however, are less common. Focal renal scarring, sometimes extensive, is a common finding, even at the so-called first infection (Bergström, 1972). It is probably a consequence of earlier unrecognized infections (see Table 16–10).

GENERAL SUMMARY

Successful management of UTI requires an understanding of its pathogenesis and natural history. In patients with UTI uncomplicated by any kind of obstruction, colonization of the bowel with uropathogenic bacteria, usually *Escherichia coli*, seems to be the first step in pathogenesis. This is followed by perineal and periurethral colonization due to adherence of bacteria to urogenital epithelial cells. This adherence seems to be facilitated by a host factor, so far unknown, explaining the appearance of recurring infections by many different strains. Adherence, mediated by P-fimbriated *E. coli*, recognizing specific carbohydrate receptors on the surface of uroepithelial and renal cells, may be of particular significance for the ascent of bacteria to the kidneys, especially in children without demonstrable reflux.

The role of VUR and IRR in the pathogenesis of kidney scars may be that large numbers of nephropathogenic, mainly P-fimbriated, bacteria are carried to the renal parenchyma. It is possible that urodynamic alterations, such as ureteric paralysis, induced by P-fimbriated strains may cause IRR in the absence of VUR.

Kidney scarring following renal infection appears to be largely confined to infants and children less than 4 years of age. Scarring is a sudden phenomenon mediated by the inflammatory response, which causes a release of toxic O and OH radicals from polymorphonuclear cells. Abortion of the inflammatory response by early treatment of febrile infection may largely prevent renal scarring. The reader is referred to recent surveys and position papers (Asscher, 1980; McCurdy and Vernier, 1981; Hellerstein, 1982; Winberg et al., 1982; Bailey, 1983; Winberg, 1984; Roberts, 1983).

References

Abyholm, G., and Monn, E.: Intranasal DDAVP-test in the study of renal concentrating capacity in children with recurrent urinary tract infections. Eur. J. Pediatr., *130*:149, 1979.

Ahlstedt, S., Hagberg, M., Jodal, U., and Mårild, S.: Cell mediated immune parameters in children with pyelonephritis caused by *Escherichia coli*. Prog. Allergy, *33*:289, 1983.

Anders, D., Anders, I., and Sitzmann, F. C.: Feldstudie zur Epidemiologie inapparenter Harnweginfektionen bei Mädchen im Vorschulalter. Med. Klin., *69*:1850, 1974.

Andersen, H. J., Jacobsson, B., Larson, H., and Winberg, J.: Hypertension, asymmetric renal parenchymal defect, sterile urine and high *E. coli* antibody titre. Br. Med. J., *3*:14, 1973.

Angel, J. R., Smith, T. W., Jr., and Roberts, J. A.: The hydro-dymanics of pyelorenal reflux. J. Urol., *122*: 20, 1979.

Aperia, A., Berg, U., and Broberger, O.: Control of sodium homeostasis in children with recurrent infections and reduced glomerular filtration rates. Acta Paediatr. Scand., *60*:695, 1971.

Arneil, G. C., McAllister, T. A., and Kay, P.: Measurement of bacteriuria by plane dipslide culture. Lancet, *1*:94, 1973.

Asscher, A. W.: The Challenge Of Urinary Tract Infections. New York, Grune & Stratton, 1980.

Asscher, A. W., and Chick, S.: Increased susceptibility of the kidney to ascending *Escherichia coli* infection following unilateral nephrectomy. Br. J. Urol., *44*:202, 1972.

Asscher, A. W., McLachlan, M. S. F., Verrier-Jones, R., Meller, S., Sussman, M., and Harrison, S.: Screening for asymptomatic urinary-tract infection in schoolgirls. Lancet, *2*:1, 1973.

Asscher, A. W., Sussman, M., Waters, W. E., Evans, Joy A. S., Campbell, H., Evans, K. T., and Edmund, J.: Asymptomatic bacteriuria in the non-pregnant woman. II. Response to treatment and follow-up. Br. Med. J., *1*:804, 1969.

Bailey, R. R. (Ed.): Single Dose Therapy of Urinary Tract Infection. Sidney, Adis Health Science Press, 1983.

Baker, R., Maxted, W., Maylath, J., and Shuman, I.: Relation of age, sex, and infection to reflux: Data indicating high spontaneous cure rate in pediatric patients. J. Urol., *95*:27, 1966.

Beachey, E. H.: Bacterial Adherence. (Receptors and Recognition; series B, vol. 6). New York, Chapman and Hall, 1980.

Berg, I., Fielding, D., and Meadow, R.: Psychiatric disturbance, urgency, and bacteriuria in children with day and night wetting. Arch Dis. Child., *52*:651, 1977.

Berg, U.: Renal function in acute febrile urinary tract infection in children: Pathophysiologic aspects on the reduced concentrating capacity. Kidney Int., *30*:753, 1981.

Berg, U., Aperia, A., and Broberger, O.: Subclinical defects in renal regulation of acid base balance in children with recurrent urinary tract infections. Acta Paediatr. Scand., *60*:521, 1971.

Bergström, T.: Sex differences in childhood. Urinary tract infection. Arch. Dis. Child., *47*:227, 1972.

Bergström, T., Larson, H., Lincoln, K., and Winberg, J.: Studies of urinary tract infections in infancy and childhood. XII: Eighty consecutive patients with neonatal infection. J. Pediatr. *80*:858, 1972.

Bergström, T., Lincoln, K., Ørskov, F., Orskov, I., and Winberg J.: Studies of urinary tract infections in infancy and childhood. VIII. Reinfections vs. relapse. J. Pediatr., *71*:13, 1967.

Bernstein, J.: Developmental abnormalities of the renal parenchyma. Renal hypoplasia and dysplasia. In Sommers, S. C. (Ed.): Pathology Annual. New York, Appleton-Century-Crofts, 1968.

Billie, J., and Glauser, M. P.: Protection against chronic pyelonephritis in rats by suppression of acute suppuration: Effect of colchicine and neutropenia. J. Infect. Dis., *146*:220, 1982.

Birmingham Reflux Study Group: Prospective trial of operative versus non-operative treatment of severe vesicoureteric reflux: Two years' observation in 96 children. Br. Med. J., *287*:171, 1983.

Bollgren, I., and Winberg, J.: The periurethral aerobic flora in girls highly susceptible to urinary infections. Acta Paediatr. Scand., *65*:81, 1976a.

Bollgren, I., and Winberg, J.: The periurethral aerobic bacterial flora in healthy boys and girls. Acta Paediatr. Scand., *65*:74, 1976b.

Bollgren, I., Engstrom, C. F., Hammarlind, M., Källenius, G., Ringertz, H., and Svenson, S. B.: Low urinary counts of P-fimbriated *Escherichia coli* in presumed acute pyelonephritis. Arch Dis. Child., *59*:102, 1984.

Bollgren, I., Nord, C. E., Pettersson, L., and Winberg, J.: Periurethral anaerobic microflora in girls highly susceptible to urinary infections. J. Urol., *125*:715, 1981.

Chantler, C., Carter, J. E., Bewick, M., Counahan, R., Cameron, J. S., Ogg, C. S., Williams, D. G., and Winder, E.: 10 years' experience with regular haemodialysis and renal transplantation. Arch Dis. Child., *55*:435, 1980.

Cläesson, I., Jacobsson, B., Jodal, U., and Winberg, J.: Compensatory kidney growth in children with urinary tract infection and unilateral renal scarring: An epidemiologic study. Kidney Int., *40*:759, 1981a.

Cläesson, I., Jacobsson, B., Jodal, U., and Winberg, J.: Early detection of nephropathy in childhood urinary tract infection. Acta Radiol. [Diagn.] (Stockh.), *22*:315, 1981b.

Cläesson, I., Jacobsson, B., Olsson, T., and Ringertz, H.: Assessment of renal parenchymal thickness in normal children. Acta Radiol., *32*:305, 1981c.

Colleen, S. L. Y.: The human urethral mucosa. An experimental study with emphasis on microbial attachment. Scand. J. Urol. Nephrol., [Suppl.] 68, 1982.

Diakos, G. K., Kontomichalou, P., Bilalis, D., and Pimenidou, L.: Intestinal flora ecology after oral use of antibiotics: Terramycin, chloramphenicol, ampicillin, neomycin, paromomycin, aminodidin. Chemotherapia, *13*:146, 1968.

Datta, N., Faiers, M. C., Reeves, D. S., Brumfitt, W., Ørskov, F., and Ørskov, I.: R-factors in *Escherichia coli* in faeces after oral chemotherapy in general practice. Lancet, *1*:312, 1971.

De Vargas, A., Evans, K., Ransley, P., Rosenberg, A. R., Rothwell, D., Sherwood, T., Williams, D. I., Barratt, T. M., and Carter, C. O.: A family study of vesicoureteric reflux. J. Med. Genet., *15*:85, 1978.

Duguid, J. P., and Old, D. C.: Adhesive properties of Enterobacteriaceae. *In* Beachey, E. H. (Ed.): Bacterial Adherence. (Receptors and Recognition, series B, vol. 6). New York, Chapman and Hall, 1980, pp. 185–217.

Edelmann, C. M., Jr., Ogwo, J. E., Fine, B. P., and Martinez, A. B.: The prevalence of bacteriuria in full-term and premature newborn infants. J. Pediatr., *82*:125, 1973.

Edwards, D., Normand, I. C. S., Prescod, N., and Smellie, J. M.: Disappearance of vesicoureteric reflux during long-term prophylaxis of urinary tract infection in children. Br. Med. J., 2:285, 1977.

Ehrlich, R. M.: Vesicoureteral reflux: A surgeon's perspective. Pediatr. Clin. North Am., 29:827, 1982.

Elo, J., Tallgren, L. G., Alfthan, O., and Sarna, S.: Character of urinary tract infections and pyelonephritic renal scarring after antireflux surgery. J. Urol., 129:343, 1982.

Ericsson, N. O., Winberg, J., and Zetterström, R.: Renal function in infantile obstructive uropathy. Acta Paediatr., 44:444, 1955.

Fairley, K. F., and Birch, D. F.: Unconventional bacteria in urinary tract disease: Gardnerella vaginalis. Kidney Int., 23:862, 1983.

Fairley, K. F., Carson, N. E., Gutch, R. C., Leighton, P., Grounds, A. D., Laird, E. C., McCallum, P. H. G., Sleeman, R. L., and O'Keefe, C. M.: Site of infection in acute urinary tract infection in general practice. Lancet, 2:615, 1971.

Fasth, A., Bjure, J., Hjälmås, K., et al.: Serum autoantibodies to Tamm-Horsfall protein and their relation to renal damage and glomerular filtration rate in children with urinary tract malformations. In Hodson, C. J., Heptinstall, R. H. (Eds.): Contributions to Nephrology: Reflux Nephropathy Update. Basel, Karger, 1984. pp. 285–295.

Filly, R., Friedland, G. W., Govan, D. E., and Fair, W. R.: Development and progression of clubbing and scarring in children with recurrent urinary tract infections. Radiology, 113:145, 1974.

Fowler, J. E., Jr., and Stamey, T. S.: Studies of introital colonization in women with recurrent urinary infections: VII. The role of bacterial adherence. J. Urol., 117:472, 1977.

Freedman, L. R.: Chronic pyelonephritis at autopsy. Ann. Intern. Med., 66:697, 1967.

Geisinger, J. F.: Intermittency of pyuria at the level of the renal papillae. J. Urol., 25:649, 1931.

Girdany, B. R., and Price, S. E., Jr.: Vesicoureteral reflux and renal scarring. J. Pediatr., 86:998, 1975.

Glauser, M. P., Lyons, J. M., and Braude, A. I.: Prevention of chronic experimental pyelonephritis by suppression of acute suppuration. J Clin. Invest, 61:403, 1978.

Govan, D. E., Fair, W. R., Friedland, G. W., and Filly, R. A.: Urinary tract infections in children. Part III—Treatment of ureterovesical reflux. West. J. Med., 121:382, 1974.

Govan, D. E., Fair, W. R., Filly, R. A., and Friedland, G. W.: Management of children with urinary tract infections. The Stanford experience. Urology, 6:273, 1975.

Gross, G. W., and Lebowitz, R. L.: Infection does not cause reflux. Am. J. Roentgenol., 137:929, 1981.

Grüneberg, R. N., Leakey, A., Bendall, M. J., and Smellie, J. M.: Bowel flora in urinary tract infection: Effect of chemotherapy with special reference to cotrimoxazole. Kidney Int. 8:122, 1975.

Grüneberg, R. N., Leight, D. A., and Brumfitt, W.: Escherichia coli serotypes in urinary tract infection: studies in domiciliary, antinatal hospital practice. In O'Grady, F., and Brumfitt, W. (Eds): Urinary Tract Infections. London, Oxford University Press, 1968, p. 68.

Hanson, L. åA., Ahlstedt, S., Jodal, U., Kaijser, B., Larson, P., Lidin-Janson, G., Lincoln, K., Lindberg, U., Mattsby, I., Otling, S., Peterson, H., and Sohl, A.: The host-parasite relationship in urinary tract infections. Kidney Int. 8:28, 1975.

Hellerstein, S.: Recurrent urinary tract infections in children. Pediatr. Infect. Dis., 1:271, 1982.

Hellerstein, S., Duggan, E., Welchert, E., and Mansour, F.: Serum C-reactive protein and the site of urinary tract infections. J. Pediatr., 100:21, 1982.

Heptinstall, R. H.: Pathology of the Kidney. Boston, Little, Brown, 1966, p. 421.

Hodson; C. J.: The kidneys in urinary infection. Proc. R. Soc. Med., 59:416, 1966.

Hodson, C. J., and Edwards, D.: Chronic pyelonephritis and vesico-ureteric reflux. Clin. Radiol., 11:219, 1960.

Hodson, C. J., and Wilson, S.: Natural history of chronic pyelonephritic scarring. Br. Med. J., 2:191, 1965.

Hodson, C. J., Maling, T. M. J., McManamon, P. J., and Lewis, M. G.: The pathogenesis of reflux nephropathy (Chronic atrophic pyelonephritis). Br. J. Radiol., [Suppl.] 13, 1975.

Holland, N. H.: Reflux nephropathy and hypertension. In Hodson, J., and Kincaid-Smith, P. (Eds.): Reflux Nephropathy. New York, Masson, 1979, p. 257.

Holmgren, J., and Smith, J. W.: Immunological aspects of urinary tract infections. Progr. Allergy, 18:289, 1975.

Houston, I. B.: Pus cell and bacterial counts in the diagnosis of urinary tract infections in childhood. Arch. Dis. Child., 38:600, 1963.

Huland, H., Busch, R., and Riebel, T.: Renal scarring after symptomatic and asymptomatic upper urinary tract infection: A prospective study. J. Urol., 128:682, 1982.

Hutch, J. A.: Vesico-ureteral reflux in the paraplegic: Cause and correction. J. Urol., 68:457, 1952.

Janson, L., and Roberts, J. A.: Experimental pyelonephritis. V. Functional characteristics of pyelonephritis. Invest. Urol., 15:397, 1978.

Jerkins, G. R., and Noe, H. N.: Familial vesicoureteral reflux: A prospective study. J. Urol., 128:774, 1982.

Jodal, U., Lindberg, U., and Lincoln, K.: Level diagnosis of symptomatic urinary tract infections in childhood. Acta Paediatr. Scand., 64:201, 1975.

Källenius, G., and Winberg, J.: Bacterial adherence to periurethral epithelial cells in girls prone to urinary-tract infections. Lancet, 2:540, 1978.

Källenius, G., Kallings, L. O., and Winberg, J.: Single dose treatment of children using sulphafurazole. In Bailey, R. R. (Ed.): Single Dose Therapy of Urinary Tract Infection, Sidney, Adis Health Science Press, 1983, p. 63.

Källenius, G., Möllby, R., Svenson, S. B., Helin, I., Hultberg, H., Cedergren, B., and Winberg, J.: Occurrence of P-fimbriated Escherichia coli in urinary tract infections. Lancet, 2:1369, 1982.

Kallings, L. O.: Medicinsk behandling av urinvägsinfektioner (1). Bakteriologisk översikt. Sven. Läkartidn., 65(Suppl. III):30, 1968.

Kass, E. H.: Asymptomatic infection of the urinary tract. Trans. Assoc. Am. Physicians, 69:56, 1956.

Kaveggia, L., King, L. R., Grana, L., and Idriss, F. S.: Pyelonephritis: a cause of vesicoureteral reflux. J. Urol., 95:158, 1966.

Kendall, A. R., and Karafin, L.: Urinary tract infection in children: Fact and fantasy. J. Urol., 107:1068, 1972.

Kleeman, S. E. T., and Freedman, L. R.: The finding of chronic pyelonephritis in males and females at autopsy. N. Engl. J. Med., 263:988, 1960.

Köllermann, M. W., and Ludwig, H.: Ueber den vesicoureteralen Reflux beim normalen Kind im Säuglings- und Kleinkindalter. Z. Kinderheilk., 100:185, 1967.

Kunin, C. M.: Pattern of recurrent urinary tract infections in girls. In Symposium on Pyelonephritis. p. 1. Edinburgh, Livingstone, 1966.

Kunin, C. M., Deutscher, R., and Paquin, A.: Urinary tract infection in school children: An epidemiologic, clinical and laboratory study. Medicine, 43:91, 1964.

Leading article: VUR + IRR = CPN? Lancet, 2:1120, 1974.

Lenaghan, D., Cass, A. S., Cussen, L. J., and Stephens, F. D.: Long-term effect of vesicoureteral reflux on the upper urinary tract of dogs. J. Urol., 107:758, 1972.

Lincoln, K., and Winberg, J.: Studies of urinary tract infections in infancy and childhood. II. Quantitative estimation of bacteriuria in unselected neonates with special reference to the occurrence of asymptomatic infections. Acta Paediatr. Scand., 53:307, 1964.

Lindberg, U.: Asymptomatic bacteriuria in schoolgirls. V. The clinical course and response to treatment. Acta Paediatr. Scand., 64:718, 1975.

Lindberg, U., Bjure, J., Haugstvedt, S., and Jodal, U.: Asymptomatic bacteriuria in schoolgirls. III. Relation between residual urine volume and recurrence. Acta Paediatr. Scand., 64:437, 1975a.

Lindberg, U., Claesson, I., Hanson, L. A., and Jodal, U.: Asymptomatic bacteriuria in schoolgirls. I. Clinical and laboratory findings. Acta Paediatr. Scand., 64:425, 1975b.

Lindberg, U., Hanson, L. A., Jodal, U., Lidin-Janson, G., Lincoln, K., and Olling, S.: Asymptomatic bacteriuria in schoolgirls. II. Differences in Escherichia coli causing asymptomatic and symptomatic bacteriuria. Acta Paediatr. Scand., 64:432, 1975c.

Lindberg, U., Jodal, U., Hanson, L. A., and Kaijser, B.: Asymptomatic bacteriuria in schoolgirls. IV. Difficulties of level diagnosis and the possible relation to the character of infecting bacteria. Acta Paediatr. Scand., 64:574, 1975d.

Lindblad, B. S., and Ekengren, K.: The long term prognosis of nonobstructive urinary tract infection in infancy and childhood after the advent of sulphonamide. Acta Paediatr. Scand., 58:25, 1969.

Lippman, R. W., Wrobel, C. J., Rees, R., and Hoyt, R. A.: Theory concerning recurrence of urinary infection. J. Urol., 80:77, 1958.

Lomberg, H., Hanson, L. åA., Jacobsson, B., Jodal, U., Leffler, II., and Svanborg-Edén, C.: Correlation of P blood group, vesicoureteral reflux, and bacterial attachment in patients with recurrent pyelonephritis. N. Engl. J. Med., 308:1189, 1983.

Mackintosh, I. P., Watson, B. W., and O'Grady, F.: Theory of hydrokinetic clearance of bacteria from the urinary bladder. Invest. Urol., 12:473, 1975.

McCabe, W. R.: Endotoxin tolerance. II. Its occurrence in patients with pyelonephritis. J. Clin. Invest., 42:618, 1963.

McCabe, W. R., and Anderson, V.: Endotoxin tolerance. I. Its induction by experimental pyelonephritis. J. Clin. Invest., 42:610, 1963.

McCabe, W. R., and Jackson, G.: Treatment of pyelonephritis. Bacterial, drug and host factors in success or failure among 252 patients. N. Engl. J. Med., 272:1037, 1965.

McCrory, W. W., Shibuya, M., Leuman, E., and Krap, R.: Studies of renal function in children with chronic hydronephrosis. Pediatr. Clin. North Am., 18:445, 1971.

McCurdy, F. A., and Vernier, R. L.: Unique consequences of kidney infections in infants and children: Pathogenesis, early recognition, and prevention of scarring. Am. J. Nephrol., 1:184, 1981.

McLachlan, M. S. F., Meller, S. T., Verrier-Jones, E. R., Asscher, A. W., Fletcher, E. W. L., Mayon-White, R. T., Ledingham, J. G. G., Smith, J. C., and Johnston, H. H.: Urinary tract in schoolgirls with covert bacteriuria. Arch. Dis. Child., 50:253, 1975.

Mårild, S., Hellström, M., Jodal, U., Lidin-Janson, G., and Svanborg-Edén, C.: UTI during the first year of life in a Göteborg area 1977–79:II. Symptomatic infections. Pediatr. Res., 14:981, 1980.

Meadow, W. R., White, R. H. R., and Johnston, N. M.: Prevalence of symptomless urinary tract disease in Birmingham schoolchildren. I-Pyuria and bacteriuria. Br. Med. J., 3:81, 1969.

Mendoza, J. M., and Roberts, J. A.: Effects of sterile high pressure vesicoureteral reflux on the monkey. J. Urol., 130:602, 1983.

Miller, T., and Phillips, S.: Pyelonephritis: The relation between infection, renal scarring and antimicrobial therapy. Kidney Int. 19:654, 1981.

Miller, T. E., Scott, L., Stewart, E., and North, D.: Modification by suppressor cells and serum factors of the cell-mediated immune response in experimental pyelonephritis. J. Clin. Invest., 61:964, 1978.

Nelson, J. D., and McCracken, G. H.: The current status of gentamicin for the neonate and young infant. Am J. Dis. Child., 124:13, 1972.

Nelson, J. D., and Peters, P. C.: Suprapubic aspiration of urine in premature and term infants. Pediatrics, 36:132, 1965.

Normand, I. C. S., and Smellie, J. M.: Prolonged maintenance chemotherapy in the management of urinary infection in childhood. Br. Med. J., 1:1023, 1965.

O'Grady, F., and Cattell, W. R.: Kinetics of urinary tract infection. II. The bladder. Br. J. Urol., 38:156, 1966.

O'Grady, F., Mackintosh, I. P., Greenwood, D., and Watson, B. W.: Treatment of "bacterial cystitis" in fully automatic mechanical models simulating conditions of bacterial growth in the urinary bladder. Br. J. Exp. Pathol., 54:283, 1973.

Olbing, H., Reischauer, H. C., and Kovacs, I.: Prospektiver Vergleich von Nitrofurantoin und Sulfamethoxydiazin bei der Langzeittherapie von Kindern mit schwerer chronischrezidivierender pyelonephritis. Dtsch. Med. Wochenschr., 95:2469, 1970.

Percival, A., Brumfitt, W., and de Louvois, J.: Serum-antibody levels as an indication of clinically inapparent pyelonephritis. Lancet, 2:1027, 1964.

Ransley, P. G., and Risdon, R. A.: Renal papillae and intrarenal reflux in the pig. Lancet, 2:1114, 1974.

Ransley, P. G., and Risdon, R. A.: Renal papillary morphology in infants and young children. Urol. Res., 3:111, 1975a.

Ransley, P. G., and Risdon, R. A.: Renal papillary morphology and intrarenal reflux in the young pig. Urol. Res., 3:105, 1975b.

Ransley, P. G., and Risdon, R. A.: Reflux and renal scarring. Br. J. Radiol. (Suppl.), 14:1, 1978.

Roantree, R. J.: The relationship of lipopolysaccharide structure to bacterial virulence. In Kadis, S., Weinbaus, G., and Ajl, S. (Eds.): Microbial toxins V. Bacterial Endotoxin. New York, Academic Press, 1971 p. 1.

Robbins, J. B., McCracken, G. H., Gotschlich, E. C., Ørskov, F., Ørskov, I., and Hanson, L. A.: Escherichia coli K1 capsular polysaccharide associated with neonatal meningitis. N. Engl. J. Med., 290:1216, 1974.

Roberts, J. A.: Experimental pyelonephritis in the monkey. III. Pathophysiology of ureteral malfunction induced by bacteria. Invest. Urol., 13:117, 1975.

Roberts, J. A.: Studies of vesicoureteral reflux: A review of work in a primate model. South. Med. J., 71:28, 1978.

Roberts, J. A.: Vesicoureteral reflux in the monkey. A review. Urol. Radiol., 5:211, 1983.

Roberts, J. A., Angel, J. R., and Roth J. K., Jr.: The hydrodynamics of pyelorenal reflux: II. The effect of chronic obstructive changes on papillary shape. Invest. Urol., *18*:296, 1981.

Roberts, J. A., Roth, J. K., Jr., Domingue, G., Lewis, R. W., Kaack, B., and Baskin, G.: Immunology of pyelonephritis in the primate model: V. Effect of superoxide dismutase. J. Urol., *128*:1394, 1982.

Roberts, J. A., Kaack, B., Källenius, G., Möllby, R., Winberg, J., and Svenson, S. B.: Receptors for pyelonephritogenic *Escherichia coli* in primates. J. Urol., *131*:163, 1984.

Rolleston, G. L., Maling, T. M. J., and Hodson, C. J.: Intrarenal reflux and the scarred kidney. Arch. Dis. Child., *49*:531, 1974.

Rolleston, G. L., Shannon, F. T., and Utley, W. L.: Follow-up of vesico-ureteric reflux in the newborn. Kidney Int., *8*:59, 1975.

Ronald, A. R., Truck, M., and Petersdorf, R. G.: A critical evaluation of nalidixic acid in urinary tract infections. N. Engl. J. Med., *275*:1081, 1966.

Savage, D. C. L.: Natural history of covert bacteriuria in schoolgirls. Kidney Int., *8*:90, 1975.

Savage, D. C. L.: Adherence of normal flora to mucosal surfaces. *In* Beachey, E. H. (Ed.): Bacterial adherence. (Receptors and Recognition, series B, vol. 6). New York, Chapman and Hall, 1980, pp. 30–59.

Savage, D. C. L., Wilson, M. I., McHardy, M., Dewar, D. A. E., and Fee, W. M.: Covert bacteriuria of childhood, a clinical and epidemiological study. Arch. Dis. Child., *48*:8, 1973.

Schaeffer, A. J., Jones, J. M., and Dunn, J. K.: Association of in vitro *Escherichia coli* adherence to vaginal and buccal epithelial cells with susceptibility of women to recurrent urinary-tract infections. N. Engl. J. Med. *304*:1062, 1981.

Scott, J. E. S.: The role of surgery in the management of vesico-ureteric reflux. Kidney Int. *8*:73, 1975.

Scott, J. E. S., and Deegan, S.: Management of neuropathic urinary incontinence in children by intermittent catheterisation. Arch. Dis. Child., *57*:253, 1982.

Slotki, I. N., and Asscher, A. W.: Prevention of scarring in experimental pyelonephritis in the rat by early antibiotic therapy. Nephron, *30*:262, 1982.

Smellie, J. M., and Normand, I. C. S.: Bacteriuria, reflux and renal scarring, Arch, Dis. Child, *50*:581, 1975.

Smellie, J. M., and Normand, I. C. S.: Experience of follow-up of children with urinary tract infection. *In* O'Grady, F., and Brumfitt, W. (Eds.): Urinary Tract Infection. London, Oxford University Press, 1968, p. 123.

Smellie, J. M., Edwards, D., Hunter, N., Normand, I. C. S., and Prescod, N.: Vesico-ureteric reflux and renal scarring. Kidney Int., *8*:65, 1975.

Smellie, J. M., Edwards, D., Normand, I. C. S., and Prescod, N.: Effect of vesicoureteric reflux on renal growth in children with urinary tract infection. Arch. Dis. Child., *56*:593, 1981.

Stamey, T. A., and Bragonje, J.: Resistance to nalidixic acid: A misconception due to underdosage. JAMA *236*:1857, 1976.

Stamey, T. A., and Condy, M.: The diffusion and concentration of trimethoprim in human vaginal fluid. J. Infect. Dis., *131*:261, 1975.

Stamey, T. A., Bushby, S. R. M., and Bragonje, J.: The concentration of trimethoprim in prostatic fluid: Nonionic diffusion or active transport? J. Infect. Dis. 128 [Suppl].:686, 1973.

Stamey, T. A., Govan, D. E., and Palmer, J. M.: The localization and treatment of urinary tract infections: The role of bactericidal urine levels as opposed to serum levels. Medicine (Baltimore), *44*:1, 1965.

Stamey, T. A., Timothy, M., Millar, M., and Mihara, G.: Recurrent urinary infections in adult women. The role of introital enterobacteria. Calif. Med., *115*:1, 1971.

Stamey, T. A., Fair, W. R., Timothy, M. M., Millar, M. A., Mihara, G., and Lowery, Y. C.: Serum versus urinary antimicrobial concentrations in cure of urinary tract infections. N. Engl. J. Med. *291*:1159, 1974.

Stamm, W. E., Counts, G. W., Running, K. R., Fihn, S., Turck, M., and Holmes, K. K.: Diagnosis of coliform infection in acutely dysuric women. N. Engl. J. Med., *307*:463, 1982.

Stansfeld, J. M.: Clinical observations relating to incidence and aetiology of urinary tract infections in children. Br. Med. J., *1*:631, 1966.

Svanborg-Edén, C., Hanson, L. Å., Jodal, U., Lindberg, U., and Sohl-Åkerlung, A.: Variable adherence to normal human urinary tract epithelial cells of *Escherichia coli* strains associated with various forms of urinary tract infections. Lancet, *2*:490, 1976.

Svanborg-Edén, C., and Jodal, U.: Attachment of *Escherichia coli* to urinary sediment epithelial cells from urinary tract infection–prone and healthy children. Infect. Immun., *26*:837, 1979.

Svenson, S. B., and Källenius, G.: Density and localization of P-fimbriae specific receptors on mammalian cells: fluorescence-activated cell analysis. Infection, *11*:6, 1983.

Svenson, S. B., Källenius, G., Korhonen, T. K., Möllby, R., Roberts, J. A., Tullus, K., and Winberg, J.: Initiation of clinical pyelonephritis. The role of P-fimbriae–mediated bacterial adhesion. *In* Contributions to Nephrology: Reflux Nephropathy Update. Hodson, C. J., Heptinstall, R. H., and Winberg, J. (eds.): Basel, Karger, 1984, pp. 252–272.

Teague, W., and Boyarksy, S.: The effect of coliform bacteria upon ureteral peristalsis. Invest. Urol., *5*:423, 1968.

Thomas, V., Shelokov, A., and Forland, M.: Antibody-coated bacteria in the urine and the site of urinary tract infection. N. Engl. J. Med., *290*:588, 1974.

Tschudi Madsen, S.: Antibacterial effect of urine after single oral doses of sulphonamide. Chemotherapia, *13*:16, 1968.

van Gool, J. D., Kuijten, R. H., Donckerwolcke, R. A., Messer, A. P., and Vijverberg, M.: Bladder-sphincter dysfunction, urinary function and vesico-ureteral reflux with special reference to cognitive bladder training. *In* Hodson, C. J., Heptinstall, R. H., and Winberg, J. (Eds.): Contributions to Nephrology: Reflux Nephropathy Update. Basel, Karger, 1984, pp. 190–210.

Verrier-Jones, E. R., Meller, S. T., McLachlan, M. S. F., Sussman, M., Asscher, A. W., Mayon-White, R. T., Ledingham, J. G. G., Smith, J. C., Fletcher, E. W. L., Smith, E. H., Johnston, H. H., and Sleight, G.: Treatment of bacteriuria in schoolgirls. Kidney Int., *8*:85, 1975.

Verrier-Jones, K., Asscher, A. W., Verrier-Jones, E. R., Mattholie, K., Leach, K., and Thomson, G. M.: Glomerular filtration rate in schoolgirls with covert bacteriuria. Br. Med. J., *285*:1307, 1982.

Westenfelder, M., Galanos, C., and Madsen, P. O.: Experimental lipid A induced nephritis in the dog. Invest. Urol., *12*:337, 1975.

Wettergren, B., Fasth, A., Jacobsson, B., Jodal, U., and

Lincoln, K.: UTI during the first year of life in a Göteborg area 1977–79. I: Bacteria found at screening. Pediatr. Res., *14*:981, 1980.

Williams, D. I.: The ureter, the urologist, and the paediatrician. Proc. R. Soc. Med., *63*:595, 1970.

Winberg, J.: Determination of the renal concentration capacity in infants and children without renal disease. Acta Paediatr., *48*:318, 1959.

Winberg, J.: Screening in the newborn period. *In* Colloquium on pyelonephritis. Fourteenth International Congress on Pediatrics, 1974.

Winberg, J.: P-fimbriae, bacterial adhesion, and pyelonephritis. Arch. Dis. Child., *59*:180, 1984.

Winberg, J., and Bollgren, I.: Care of children with urinary tract infection. *In* The Management of Urinary Tract Infection, by Asscher, A. W., (Ed.): International Symposium "The Challenge of Urinary Tract Infection." Cardiff, U. K., May 14, 1980. Oxford, The Medicine Publishing Foundation, 1980.

Winberg, J., Andersen, H. J., Bergström, T., Jacobsson, B., Larson, H., and Lincoln, K.: Epidemiology of symptomatic urinary tract infection in childhood. Acta Paediatr. Scand. [Suppl. 252], 1974.

Winberg, J., Anderson, H. J., Hansen, L. A., and Lincoln, K.: Studies of urinary tract infections in infancy and childhood. Br. Med. J., *2*:524, 1963.

Winberg, J., Bergström, T., and Jacobsson, B.: Morbidity, age and sex distribution, recurrences and renal scarring in symptomatic urinary tract infection in childhood. Kidney Int., *8*:101, 1975.

Winberg, J., Bergström, T., Lidin-Janson, G., and Lincoln, K.: Treatment trials in urinary tract infection (UTI) with special reference to the effect of antimicrobials on the fecal and periurethral flora. Clin. Nephrol., *1*:142, 1973.

Winberg, J., Bollgren, I., Källenius, G., Möllby, R., and Svenson, S.: Clinical pyelonephritis and focal renal scarring. A selected review of pathogenesis, prevention, and prognosis. Pediatr. Clin. North Am., *29*:801, 1982.

Winberg, J., Bollgren, I., Källenius, G., Möllby, R., and Svenson, S.: Bacterial virulence and host defence in pathogenesis of renal infection and renal scarring. *In* Urinary Infection. Insights and Prospects, François, B., and Perrin, P. (Eds.): London, Butterworth and Co., 1983, p. 19.

Winberg, J., Larson, H., and Bergström, T.: Comparison of the natural history of urinary infection in children with and without vesico-ureteric reflux. *In* Kincaid-Smith, P., and Fairley, K. (Eds.): Renal infection and Renal Scarring. Melbourne, Mercedes, 1971, p. 293.

Winter, A. L., Hardy, B. E., Alton, D. J., Arbus, G. S., and Churchill, B. M.: Acquired renal scars in children. J. Urol., *129*:1190, 1983.

CHAPTER 17

Prostatitis and Related Disorders

EDWIN M. MEARES, JR., M.D.

INTRODUCTION

Few common ailments of the genitourinary tract confuse more patients and clinicians than do inflammations of the prostate gland. Most patients with chronic prostatitis have a poor understanding of the cause of and the outlook for their infirmity and remain generally unhappy with the results of treatment. This is unfortunate because inflammations of the prostate are common; indeed, patients with prostatitis make up a significant portion of office urologic practice.

Although many aspects of prostatic inflammations remain puzzling, some confusing issues have been resolved and new areas for study have been identified by recent investigative work. One important advance is the recognition that "prostatitis" is not one disease; rather, it occurs in several distinct forms or syndromes. These syndromes have distinctly different causes, manifestations, and sequelae. Moreover, proper clinical management and therapeutic outlooks vary considerably among these different forms. For the patient with prostatitis to truly benefit from therapy, therefore, the clinician must be specific in diagnosis and use discrimination in choosing therapeutic strategies.

TYPES OF PROSTATITIS

Currently, several distinct types of prostatitis, or prostatitis syndromes, are recognized. Since therapies and responses to treatment are different among these syndromes, the clinician must be exact in diagnosis and specific in prescribing treatment. In 1978, Drach, Fair, Meares, and Stamey proposed a new classification of common types of prostatitis syndromes: acute and chronic bacterial prostatitis, nonbacterial prostatitis, and prostatodynia.

Bacterial prostatitis is associated with bacteriuria; indeed, in cases of chronic bacterial prostatitis the pathogen persists in the prostatic secretions of untreated patients and leads to recurrent bacteriuria. In contrast, urinary tract infection rarely (if ever) occurs in patients who have nonbacterial prostatitis or prostatodynia. Patients with nonbacterial prostatitis, similar to patients with bacterial prostatitis, have excessive leukocytes and macrophages containing fat in their prostatic secretions, clearly suggesting inflammation. In contrast, patients with prostatodynia have normal prostatic expressates without signs of inflammation. Some of the similarities and differences in clinical features of the common prostatitis syndromes are shown in Table 17–1.

ETIOLOGY AND PATHOGENESIS

The causative organisms in bacterial prostatitis are similar in type and relative incidence to those responsible for urinary tract infection: Common strains of *Escherichia coli* clearly predominate. Infections caused by species of *Proteus, Klebsiella, Enterobacter, Pseudomonas, Serratia,* and other less common gram-negative organisms occur less frequently (Meares, 1980). Obligate anaerobic bacteria seldom cause prostatic infection. Most prostatic infections are caused by a single pathogen; however, infections involving two or more strains or types of bacteria occur occasionally.

TABLE 17–1. CLINICAL FEATURES OF COMMON PROSTATITIS SYNDROMES

Syndrome	History of Confirmed UTI*	Prostate Abnormal on Rectal Exam	Excessive WBCs† in EPS‡	Positive Culture of EPS‡	Common Causative Agents	Response to Antimicrobial Treatment	Impaired Urinary Flow Rate
Acute bacterial prostatitis	Yes	Yes	Yes	Yes	Coliform bacteria	Yes	Yes
Chronic bacterial prostatitis	Yes	±	Yes	Yes	Coliform bacteria	Yes	±
Nonbacterial prostatitis	No	±	Yes	No	None ? *Chlamydia* ? *Ureaplasma*	Usually no	±
Prostatodynia	No	No	No	No	None	No	Yes

*UTI = Urinary tract infection.
†WBCs = White blood cells.
‡EPS = Expressed prostatic secretions.

The role played by gram-positive bacteria in the etiology of prostatitis is controversial. Most investigators agree that enterococci cause chronic bacterial prostatitis and related recurrent enterococcal bacteriuria. However, the pathogenic role in prostatitis of other gram-positive organisms, such as coagulase-negative staphylococci, streptococci, micrococci, and diphtheroids, is questioned by many investigators. Drach reports that gram-positive bacteria are frequently localized to the prostatic secretions by culture of men with prostatitis (Drach, 1974, 1975). These normal "skin inhabitants," however, typically colonize the anterior urethra of normal men; thus, most investigators consider these organisms commensals, not pathogens (Meares, 1980). Moreover, extended studies of men who have only gram-positive bacteria (other than enterococci) on localization cultures seldom show reproducible patterns proving chronic bacterial prostatitis or a tendency for these organisms to cause urinary tract infection—a hallmark of chronic prostatitis caused by gram-negative bacteria (Meares, 1983). The recent work of several researchers suggests that gram-positive bacteria other than enterococci seldom cause significant prostatitis (Meares, 1973; Mardh and Colleen, 1975; Pfau and Sacks, 1976; Stamey, 1981; Thin and Simmons, 1983a).

The actual cause of nonacute prostatitis often is unknown. Likewise, many features of the pathogenesis of bacterial prostatitis remain uncertain. Possible routes of infection include: (1) ascending urethral infection; (2) reflux of infected urine into prostatic ducts that empty into the posterior urethra; (3) invasion by rectal bacteria, by direct extension or lymphogenous spread; and (4) hematogenous infection.

Infectious types of prostatitis sometimes are the result of sexual activity. Men develop gonococcal and nongonococcal urethritis following sexual intercourse because the urinary meatus is inoculated by vaginal organisms. It is also known that men with gonococcal prostatitis usually have histories of preceding bouts of gonococcal urethritis. Stamey (1980) finds that male sexual partners of women who have abnormal vaginal cultures due to coliforms sometimes have these same coliforms in their urethral cultures. These men generally are asymptomatic, and their urethral cultures revert to normal spontaneously. Occasionally, however, identical pathogenic bacteria are found in prostatic fluid cultures of men with chronic bacterial prostatitis and in vaginal cultures of their sexual partners, implying transmission by sexual means (Blacklock, 1974; Stamey, 1980). The frequency and importance of this mode of infection in the pathogenesis of prostatitis await documentation by additional study.

The likelihood that reflux of infected urine into prostatic ducts is important in the pathogenesis of bacterial prostatitis is enhanced by the observation that many prostatic calculi on crystallographic analysis contain constituents common to urine but foreign to prostatic secretions (Sutor and Wooley, 1974). This implies that urine must occasionally enter prostatic ducts and tissue, presumably by reflux. More direct proof of intraprostatic reflux of urine was recently observed by Kirby and associates (1982). Initially, these investigators exposed the bladder and inserted a punch suprapubic catheter into the bladder of ten male human cadavers. A carbon-particle suspension was instilled until the intravesical pressure reached 50 cm of water, and this pressure was maintained for 10 minutes. The fluid was then drained, and the bladder, prostate, and urethra were carefully removed. On section, the prostate showed macroscopic and microscopic evidence of intraductal carbon in every case. Subsequently, these investigators instilled their carbon-particle suspension via in-and-out urethral catheterization into the bladder of ten patients 2 hours prior to their undergoing transurethral prostatectomy for outflow obstruction. The patients voided prior to surgery, and at the time of surgery all visible residual carbon was washed from the bladder and urethra with irrigating fluid. The surgical specimens of seven of the ten men (70 per cent) confirmed the presence of intraductal carbon. Finally, five patients diagnosed as having nonbacterial prostatitis were selected for study. Localization specimens and cultures confirmed the absence of pathogens and greater than 20 leukocytes per high power field plus excessive macrophages in the prostatic expressates of each patient. In each patient, 400 ml of carbon suspension was instilled into the bladder through a urethral catheter, the catheter was removed, and the patient then voided spontaneously. Seventy-two hours later the prostatic expressate of each patient demonstrated an abundance of macrophages that had clearly ingested particulate carbon. These observations suggest that reflux of urine containing pathogenic bacteria into prostatic ducts and tissue is probably an important mode of prostatic infection.

Many cases of bacterial prostatitis occur as a consequence of periurethral infection associated with indwelling urethral catheterization.

METHODS OF DIAGNOSIS

GENERAL COMMENTS

The diagnosis of prostatitis is made most often by the clinician with little substantiation. The medical history and physical findings may suggest the diagnosis of a prostatitis syndrome but are not confirmatory. Acute bacterial prostatitis generally is recognized easily because its clinical manifestations are dramatic and characteristic; in contrast, the clinical features of chronic prostatitis syndromes are highly variable and inexact. Indeed, many of the signs, symptoms, and physical findings in cases of chronic bacterial prostatitis, nonbacterial prostatitis, and prostatodynia often are indistinguishable. Likewise, x-ray studies and cystourethroscopy may assist in differential diagnosis and in identifying complicating factors, but they do not confirm the diagnosis of prostatitis.

Histologic examination of prostatic tissue generally is required to diagnose unusual forms of prostatitis, such as granulomatous prostatitis.

However, since the histologic changes seen in chronic bacterial prostatitis can be produced by other conditions, they cannot be used to confirm the bacterial etiology of the inflammation. Kohnen and Drach (1979) reviewed 162 consecutive cases of surgically resected hyperplastic prostates and found an incidence of inflammation of about 98 per cent. Six distinct morphologic patterns of inflammation were observed, but no significant differences were identified among groups of cases with positive and negative evidence by culture of bacterial prostatic infection. Furthermore, in most instances the inflammatory reaction was quite focal and involved only small portions of the total gland. Thus, prostatic biopsy seems seldom indicated in the diagnosis and management of the usual case of prostatitis. Likewise, tissue culture of specimens obtained by prostatic biopsy is seldom indicated in the diagnosis of chronic bacterial prostatitis. The focal nature of the infection makes sampling errors significant. Furthermore, such tissue specimens are difficult to culture quantitatively and are easily contaminated during procurement.

EXAMINATION OF THE PROSTATIC EXPRESSATE

Microscopic examination of the expressed secretions is important in the diagnosis and classification of prostatitis but can be misleading. For example, false impressions concerning excessive leukocytes in the prostatic expressate occur in urethral disease (e.g., urethritis, strictures, condylomata, and diverticula); likewise, false impressions occur in noninfectious conditions of the prostate (e.g., uninfected prostatic calculi). The white blood cell count in prostatic fluid also rises significantly in healthy men for several hours following sexual intercourse and ejaculation (Jameson, 1967).

To localize the site of an inflammation to the urethra or prostate the clinician must always compare the microscopic appearance of the prostatic expressate with smears of the spun sediment of the first voided 10 ml of urine (urethral specimen) and the midstream urine (bladder specimen) that are obtained immediately preceding prostatic massage. What constitutes an excessive number of white blood cells (WBCs) in prostatic secretions remains controversial. Most clinicians agree that greater than 20 WBCs per high power field (HPF) is excessive; some prefer the criterion of greater than 15 WBCs per HPF; others believe that greater than 10 WBCs per HPF represents leukocytosis (Drach et al., 1978; Meares, 1980). Studies by Blacklock (1969), Anderson and Weller (1979), and Schaeffer and coworkers (1981) indicate that prostatic fluid normally contains 10 WBCs per HPF or less.

The finding of both excessive leukocytes and macrophages containing fat (oval fat bodies) is the most convincing sign of prostatic inflammation. These macrophages containing fat seldom are noticed in the prostatic secretions of healthy men, are increased about eight fold in men with nonbacterial prostatitis, and often are exceedingly prominent in the secretions of men who have bacterial prostatitis (Anderson and Weller, 1979; Meares, 1980; Stamey, 1981). Moreover, macrophages containing fat are not found in exudates arising from anterior urethritis.

EXAMINATION OF THE SEMEN

Isolated analysis or culture of the ejaculate without concomitant study of urethral and bladder specimens may be more misleading than isolated examination of the prostatic expressate. The semen not only passes through the urethra but contains fluids from several accessory glands. Cytologic examination of the semen is also complicated by the difficulty of distinguishing immature sperm from leukocytes. Mobley advocates using semen cultures to diagnose bacterial prostatitis and has based some of his clinical studies, at least in part, upon this method (Mobley, 1974, 1975, 1981). Specimens from the urethra (VB1) and bladder (VB2) must be obtained immediately before collection of the semen specimen, and all specimens must be cultured quantitatively. Comparison of the bacterial counts of the three cultures must clearly show excessive counts of bacteria in the semen; otherwise, proper interpretation of the semen culture is impossible and the diagnosis of prostatitis remains speculative. Obviously, urethral organisms of nonprostatic origin can easily contaminate the semen as it passes through the urethra during specimen procurement.

MEASUREMENT OF THE IMMUNE RESPONSE

The immune response to prostatic inflammation, especially bacterial infection, has been studied with increasing interest during the past two decades. The reader is referred to Chapter 14 for additional comments regarding the implication of immunologic markers in prostatitis.

Chodirker and Tomasi (1963) first identified and quantitatively measured immunoglobulins IgG and IgA in normal human prostatic fluid. Subsequently, Gray and coworkers (1974) used methods of immunodiffusion and immunoelectrophoresis and compared the immunoglobulin concentrations in expressed prostatic secretions of 33 healthy men with those of 48 men with prostatitis. They established normal levels of immunoglobulins IgA, IgG, and IgM with their methods and further observed that the IgA present in controls and patients seemed to be mostly secretory IgA. Among patients with "unresolved" prostatitis, they found significantly increased levels of all three immunoglobulins (especially IgA) in the prostatic secretions compared with controls. Among patients whose prostatitis was thought to have resolved, these investigators noted a return of the IgG level to normal but persistent elevation of the IgA and IgM levels at twice normal.

When studied by a method of O-specific direct bacterial agglutination, 18 of 22 men (82 per cent) with chronic *E. coli* prostatitis had elevated serum antibody titers ($\geq$1:320) against their prostatic pathogens, whereas men who had only urethritis due to *E. coli* as well as normal men had uniformly low titers ($\leq$1:160) against their urethral and fecal *E. coli*, respectively (Meares, 1977). Cure of chronic *E. coli* prostatitis results in a return to normal of elevated serum antibody titers; treatment failures result in continued elevation of antibody titers against the prostatic *E. coli* (Meares, 1978). Although this method chiefly measures IgM activity, an immunologic response in serum to prostatic pathogens in prostatitis was demonstrated.

In 1974, Thomas and associates (1974) used a direct immunofluorescence technique and observed a positive test for antibody-coated bacteria (ACB) in the urine from four of five men with prostatitis. Jones (1974) confirmed this finding and demonstrated specificity of the antibody for the infecting *E. coli* in a patient with chronic prostatitis. Various investigators subsequently studied ejaculates of patients with prostatitis and observed elevated immunoglobulin levels, especially IgA (Shah, 1976; Nishimura et al., 1977; Riedasch et al., 1978). Since semen contains fluids from several organs (not merely the prostate), and since elevated levels of IgA and positive ACB tests occur in the prostatic fluid and urine of uninfected patients with benign prostatic hyperplasia, prostatic carcinoma, bladder tumors, and bladder stones, the specificity of these observations for prostatitis is lacking (Shah, 1976; Riedasch et al., 1978).

These important early studies demonstrated elevated levels of total immunoglobulin in prostatic secretions, high levels of antigen-specific antibody in the prostatic secretions, and elevated levels of antigen-specific antibody in the serum against the prostatic pathogens in cases of chronic bacterial prostatitis.

More recently, Shortliffe and colleagues

(1981) used a solid phase radioimmunoassay and extensively studied the immune response in serum and prostatic secretions of men with acute and chronic bacterial prostatitis. They found a distinct local antibody response, mainly secretory IgA, in prostatic fluid that was independent of the serum response and that was antigen-specific for the infecting pathogen. Subsequently, Fowler and coworkers (Fowler et al., 1982; Fowler and Mariano, 1982) also used a solid phase radioimmunoassay and studied the immune response of the prostate to bacteriuria and bacterial prostatitis. Their work suggests that bacteriuria is associated with increased secretion of IgA in the prostatic fluid that is independent of prostatic infection and independent of systemic immune response. They postulate that the prostate becomes colonized routinely during episodes of urinary tract infection but that symptomatic or chronic infections are prevented by the secretion of antigen-specific IgA locally within the prostate.

Although these preliminary studies show that in bacterial prostatitis the prostate elaborates a local immune response that exceeds the response in serum, many features of this response remain uncertain. Further study and knowledge of this response may have important implications in diagnosis, clinical management, and possibly prevention of bacterial prostatitis.

DIAGNOSTIC BACTERIOLOGIC LOCALIZATION CULTURES

The simplest and most accurate way to distinguish bacterial prostatitis from nonbacterial types of prostatitis and to establish the diagnosis of chronic bacterial prostatitis is the performance of essentially simultaneous quantitative bacteriologic culture of the urethra, bladder urine, and expressed prostatic secretions. This technique was reported initially by Meares and Stamey (1968) and has served as the basis of considerable investigative work in prostatitis during the past several years. Since details regarding the collection of specimens, methods of culture, and interpretation of results are discussed in Chapter 14, additional comments will not be made here.

SECRETORY DYSFUNCTION IN PROSTATITIS

Significant alterations in the secretory products of the prostate occur in patients with prostatitis. The most profound changes are seen with documented chronic bacterial prostatitis

and are sufficiently inclusive to suggest generalized secretory dysfunction of the prostate (Table 17–2). Because the relative pH values of prostatic fluid and plasma are thought to be critically important in the nonionic diffusion of drugs across prostatic epithelium, this secretory dysfunction—especially the associated increased alkalinity of the secretions—undoubtedly affects the passage of antimicrobial agents from plasma into prostatic fluid.

That dogs and normal men secrete prostatic fluid that is slightly acidic (pH about 6.4) was suggested by Huggins and associates in 1942 and remained unquestioned for more than three decades. Indeed, Blacklock and Beavis (1974) reported that normal men have a mean prostatic fluid pH value of 6.6. In contrast, however, Anderson and Fair (1976) observed that human prostatic fluid normally is alkaline (mean pH 7.6). In 1978, Pfau and associates noted that the prostatic fluid of normal men is slightly acidic (mean pH 6.7). Subsequently, Fair and colleagues (1979) observed a mean pH value of 7.28 among 136 specimens of prostatic fluid obtained from 93 normal men and noted further a natural tendency for prostatic fluid to become increasingly alkaline with advancing age. Although these investigators disagree about the absolute pH value of normal human prostatic fluid, they uniformly agree that the prostatic fluid of men with chronic bacterial prostatitis is distinctly alkaline. Indeed, the mean pH value of prostatic fluid among their patients generally exceeded that of their controls by about ten fold.

What are the implications concerning pharmacokinetics of increased alkalinity of the prostatic secretions in patients with chronic bacterial

TABLE 17–2. ALTERATIONS IN PROSTATIC FLUID OF MEN WITH CHRONIC BACTERIAL PROSTATITIS

Increased
pH value
Ratio of LDH isoenzyme 5 to LDH isoenzyme 1*
Immunoglobuins (IgA, IgG, IgM)

Decreased
Specific gravity
Prostatic antibacterial factor (PAF)
Cation concentrations (zinc, magnesium, calcium)
Citric acid concentration
Spermine concentration
Cholesterol concentration
Enzyme concentrations (acid phosphatase, lysozyme)

*LDH = lactate dehydrogenase. Normal values are <2.
From Meares, E. M., Jr.: J. Urol., 123:141, 1980.
© The Williams & Wilkins Co., Baltimore. Used by permission.

prostatitis? One must speculate on theoretical grounds that a reversal of pH relationships between plasma and prostatic fluid, as seen in the experiments performed in dogs, must adversely alter the diffusion of antimicrobial bases and favor the diffusion of antimicrobial acids from plasma into prostatic fluid. Because the prostatic secretory dysfunction found in patients with chronic bacterial prostatitis involves multiple factors, not merely pH changes, one cannot currently predict with certainty the possible alteration in pharmacokinetics in human patients that may result from this single factor.

PROSTATIC ANTIBACTERIAL FACTOR

The prostatic fluid of dogs, rats, and normal men contains a potent antibacterial factor (PAF) that is bactericidal to most pathogens that commonly cause genitourinary tract infections. This PAF has been identified as a compound of zinc, probably a zinc salt (Fair et al., 1976). Since zinc concentrations are low and PAF activity is depressed or absent in the prostatic fluid of men who have chronic bacterial prostatitis, some clinicians believe that zinc (PAF) may serve as a natural defense against ascending genitourinary tract infection in normal men. Whether men become infected because their prostatic secretions contain inadequate levels of zinc (PAF), however, or whether zinc (PAF) is depressed as a consequence of prostatic infection remain unanswered questions. Since the prostatic fluid content of all cations, not merely zinc, is depressed in patients with chronic bacterial prostatitis, the low level of zinc observed may merely represent an effect, not an etiologic factor. Additional study is needed to resolve this important question. Depressed levels of zinc in prostatic secretion remain unaltered during therapy with oral zinc preparations (Fair et al., 1976).

PHARMACOKINETICS IN PROSTATITIS

Because clinical observations suggested that the bacteria in prostatic fluid were somehow protected from the action of antibacterial agents, various investigators employed a prostatic fistula preparation in dogs to study drug diffusion into prostatic secretions. The dogs were prepared by a standard surgical technique (Fig. 17–1), and individual antimicrobial agents

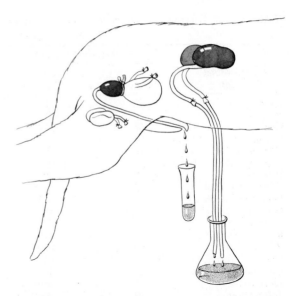

Figure 17–1. Experimental model in the dog used to study the diffusion of antibacterial agents from plasma into prostatic fluid. A ligature is placed about the bladder neck just proximal to the prostate, the ureters are ligated and cannulated above the bladder, the vasa deferens are ligated, and the foreskin is incised and sutured to the abdominal wall to expose the glans. With pilocarpine stimulation, prostatic fluid is collected directly into a flask placed under the glans penis. (From Stamey, T. A.: Pathogenesis and Treatment of Urinary Tract Infections. Baltimore, The Williams & Wilkins Co., 1980. © (1980) The Williams & Wilkins Co., Baltimore.)

were infused intravenously so that high concentrations in plasma were maintained for long periods. Prostatic secretion was then initiated and sustained by the intravenous administration of pilocarpine. Samples of plasma and prostatic fluid were collected simultaneously at appropriate intervals. In most instances the concentration of antibiotic in these samples was assayed in a large-plate, deep-well agar diffusion system or by means of paper discs.

RESULTS

The results of various diffusion studies are shown in Table 17–3. High levels of antimicrobial drugs, usually exceeding simultaneous levels in plasma, were observed only with the basic macrolides rosamicin, erythromycin, and oleandomycin and the antibacterial bases clindamycin and trimethoprim (TMP). Rosamicin, a highly lipid-soluble investigational agent, exhibits a wide range of activity in vitro against both gram-positive and gram-negative bacteria; however, the manufacturer decided recently not to market this drug because of its potential for adverse side effects. Erythromycin, oleandomycin, and clindamycin show minimal activity against the

TABLE 17–3. DIFFUSION AND PROPERTIES THAT AFFECT DIFFUSION OF CERTAIN ANTIMICROBIAL AGENTS FROM PLASMA INTO PROSTATIC FLUID IN DOGS

Antimicrobial Agent	Concentration (µg/ml)		Dissociation Characteristic	Lipid Solubility	pKa
	PLASMA	PROSTATIC FLUID			
Penicillin G	62	<0.2	Acid	No	2.7
Ampicillin	54	<0.2	Acid	No	2.5
Cephalothin	63	<0.4	Acid	No	2.5
Cephalexin	53	0.7	Amphoteric	Low	5.2, 7.3
Nitrofurantoin	15	3.2	Acid	Low	6.3
Nalidixic acid	53	<5.0	Acid	Yes	6.0
Rifampicin	17	2.0	Acid	Yes	7.9
Chloramphenicol	23	14.0	Nondissociable	Yes	. . .
Sulfamethoxazole	13	1.3	Acid	Low	6.05
Sulfisoxazole	15	0.3	Acid	Low	5.0
Polymyxin B	14	<0.5	Base	No	8–9
Kanamycin	41	2.0	Base	No	7.2
Erythromycin	16	38.0	Base	Yes	8.8
Oleandomycin	12	39.0	Base	Yes	7.6
Clindamycin	10	76.0	Base	Yes	7.6
Lincomycin	41	10.0	Base	Yes	7.6
Tetracycline	19	4.0	Amphoteric	Yes	3.3, 7.7, 9.7
Oxytetracycline	10	<2.0	Amphoteric	Low	3.3, 7.3, 9.1
Doxycycline	48	7.0	Amphoteric	Low	3.4, 7.7, 9.7
Minocycline	3.6	0.54	Amphoteric	Yes	3.4, 7.8, 9.3
Rosamicin	1.0	8.9	Base	Yes	9.1
Trimethoprim	1.2	10.0	Base	Yes	7.3

From Meares, E. M., Jr.: Rev. Infect. Dis., 4:475, 1982. Used by permission.

gram-negative bacteria that commonly cause chronic bacterial prostatitis. Chloramphenicol and lincomycin reach only medium to low levels in prostatic fluid, generally less than half the levels attained in plasma. Lincomycin shows little activity against gram-negative bacteria. Although chloramphenicol shows activity against many gram-negative bacteria in vitro, therapeutic levels are not likely to be achieved in human prostatic secretions during standard dosing; furthermore, this drug is unsuitable for long-term therapy. Most antimicrobial agents that normally are useful against the gram-negative pathogens that typically cause bacterial prostatitis reach levels that are quite low or negligible in prostatic fluid in dogs.

The explanation for these observations lies in the principles that govern the passage of drugs across biologic membranes and, in particular, the role of nonionic diffusion of weak acids and bases between membranes with different hydrogen ion concentrations. Almost all antimicrobial drugs are either weak acids or bases, and prostatic fluid in dogs is distinctly acid (pH 6.4 or less) compared with plasma (pH 7.4).

FACTORS DETERMINING DIFFUSION

The recognized factors that determine the diffusion of antimicrobial drugs from plasma across the lipid membrane of prostatic epithelium and that thus determine drug levels in prostatic fluid are shown in Figure 17–2. Except for a few water-soluble compounds of small molecular size and specific spatial configurations, only un-ionized lipid-soluble drugs that are not firmly bound to plasma proteins diffuse from the plasma across intact epithelial membranes, such as prostatic epithelium. Therefore, the pKa value of a lipid-soluble drug is of critical importance to nonionic diffusion from plasma across prostatic epithelium.

When, as in the pharmacokinetic studies performed in dogs, prostatic fluid (pH 6.4 or less) is significantly more acidic than plasma (pH about 7.4), a pH gradient complicates the diffusion of drugs from plasma into prostatic fluid. In a stable system, the uncharged (lipid-soluble) fraction of a lipid-soluble drug eventually equilibrates on each side of the membrane. In contrast, the charged fraction (non–lipid soluble) accumulates on one side. This phenomenon is called ion trapping. When plasma is more alkaline than prostatic fluid, as in the dog studies, acidic antimicrobial agents ionize to a greater extent in plasma than in prostatic fluid. The ion trapping of antimicrobial acids in such a setting, therefore, always occurs on the plasma side of the membrane, and plasma concentrations of such drugs always exceed those of the prostatic fluid. Likewise, when prostatic fluid is

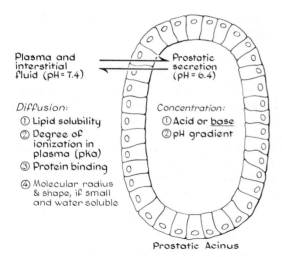

Plasma and
interstitial
fluid (pH = 7.4)

Prostatic
secretion
(pH = 6.4)

Diffusion:
① Lipid solubility
② Degree of
  ionization in
  plasma (pka)
③ Protein binding
④ Molecular radius
  & shape, if small
  and water soluble

Concentration:
① Acid or *base*
② pH gradient

Prostatic Acinus

Figure 17–2. Factors determining diffusion and concentration across biologic membranes. (From Stamey, T. A.: Pathogenesis and Treatment of Urinary Tract Infections. Baltimore, The Williams & Wilkins Co., 1980. © (1980) The Williams & Wilkins Co., Baltimore.)

more acidic than plasma, antimicrobial bases ionize to a greater extent in prostatic fluid than in plasma. Accordingly, the ion trapping of antimicrobial bases occurs on the prostatic fluid side of the membrane. Thus, their concentrations in the prostatic fluid exceed their concentrations in plasma.

Based upon a rearrangement of the Henderson-Hasselbalch equation derived by Jacobs in 1940, the theoretical partition ratios of antibiotics between acidic prostatic fluid and plasma are depicted in Figure 17–3. Note that acid antimicrobial drugs, even with favorable pKa values of 8.4 or more, can never exceed the plasma concentration of the drug. Conversely, antimicrobial drugs that are bases and that have favorably high pKa values can theoretically concentrate six fold in prostatic fluid as compared with plasma.

In 1970, Winningham and Stamey (Fig. 17–4) studied the diffusion of 17 sulfonamides from plasma into prostatic fluid in dogs. The prostatic fluid/plasma (PF/P) ratios varied from 0.02 to 0.98. A linear relation was observed between pKa value and the PF/P ratio of any given sulfonamide. The commonly used sulfonamides sulfisoxazole and sulfamethoxazole reached low levels in prostatic fluid, with PF/P ratios of 0.02 and 0.10, respectively.

The results of these diffusion studies in dogs suggest that the best therapeutic agent for curing patients with chronic bacterial prostatitis is a highly lipid-soluble antimicrobial base with minimal binding to plasma proteins and with bac-

tericidal activity against common gram-negative uropathogens.

STUDIES OF TMP IN DOGS

The development of TMP brought the hope that a genuine breakthrough in the treatment and cure of chronic bacterial prostatitis was possible. Trimethoprim, a lipid-soluble base with a favorable pKa value of 7.3 (about 50 per cent uncharged in plasma) and only moderate binding to plasma proteins (about 45 per cent bound), satisfies the theoretical requirements for accumulation in high concentration in prostatic fluid. Diffusion experiments in dogs, indeed, have shown accumulation of levels of TMP in prostatic secretions 3- to 11-fold higher than those in plasma.

The possibility of an active transport mechanism for TMP across prostatic epithelium was studied by the infusion of doses of increasing magnitude into dogs with continuously secreting prostates until the animals died from toxicity (Stamey et al., 1973). A graph of a typical experiment in one dog is shown in Figure 17–5.

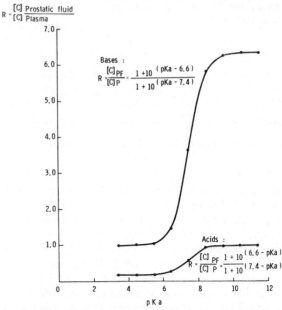

$$R = \frac{[C]\ \text{Prostatic fluid}}{[C]\ \text{Plasma}}$$

Bases :

$$R = \frac{[C]_{PF}}{[C]_P} = \frac{1 + 10^{(pKa - 6.6)}}{1 + 10^{(pKa - 7.4)}}$$

Acids :

$$R = \frac{[C]_{PF}}{[C]_P} = \frac{1 + 10^{(6.6 - pKa)}}{1 + 10^{(7.4 - pKa)}}$$

p K a

Figure 17–3. From the Henderson-Hasselbalch derivations, theoretical limits for concentration ratios are presented for acids and bases of different pK_a values. *R*, ratio of total drug in prostatic fluid to plasma; *[C]*, total concentration of each drug, charged and uncharged; *PF*, prostatic fluid; *P*, plasma; pK_a, negative logarithm of acid or base dissociation constant; 6.6 and 7.4, negative logarithms of hydrogen ion concentration in prostatic fluid and plasma. Note that *R* can only approach a ratio of 1.0 for an antimicrobial acid but can exceed 6.0 for an antimicrobial base. (From Stamey, T. A.: Pathogenesis and Treatment of Urinary Tract Infection. Baltimore, The Williams & Wilkins Co., 1980. © (1980) The Williams & Wilkins Co., Baltimore.)

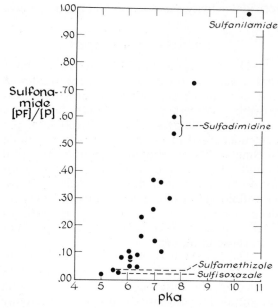

Figure 17–4. The distribution ratios, concentrations in prostatic fluid, [*PF*], divided by concentration in plasma, [*P*], of several sulfonamides are plotted against their respective pK$_a$ values. The distribution ratio of sulfanilamide approached 1.00. (From Winningham, D. G., and Stamey, T. A.: J. Urol., *104*:562, 1970. © (1970) The Williams & Wilkins Co., Baltimore.)

No evidence for the active transport of TMP into prostatic fluid was observed: Despite the progressive development of exceedingly high levels of TMP in serum, the relation of prostatic fluid/serum (PF/S) ratios remained stable.

EFFECTS OF SECRETORY DYSFUNCTION ON DRUG DIFFUSION

As mentioned previously, the secretory dysfunction associated with chronic bacterial prostatitis undoubtedly affects pharmacokinetics, especially since the prostatic secretions often become more alkaline than does plasma. The study by Stamey and associates (Fig. 17–5) of the simultaneous levels of TMP in the serum, prostatic fluid, and salivary fluid (pH 8.4) of dogs illuminates the problem created when the normal pH relation between plasma (pH 7.4) and prostatic fluid (pH 6.4) is reversed. Higher levels of TMP were attained in prostatic fluid than in the less acidic plasma. In contrast, the levels attained in salivary fluid were consistently lower than those in plasma because the salivary fluid was more alkaline. Since prostatic fluid of men with chronic bacterial prostatitis typically is more alkaline than their plasma, the diffusion of TMP into prostatic fluid of these men may

be much more limited than studies in dogs indicate.

LEVELS OF ANTIMICROBIAL DRUGS IN PROSTATIC TISSUE

Several groups of investigators have studied the prostatic tissue/serum ratios of various antimicrobial agents both in dogs and in human prostatic tissue surgically excised in the treatment of benign prostatic hyperplasia. In experiments using dogs, Nielsen and coworkers (1980) noted that levels of various penicillanic acid derivatives, including ampicillin, amoxicillin, carbenicillin, and carbenicillin indanyl sodium, in prostatic tissue significantly exceeded levels in prostatic fluid and yet were only 20 per cent to 30 per cent as high as levels in serum. More surprisingly, these investigators found a prostatic interstitial fluid/serum ratio of 0.69 for carbenicillin indanyl sodium, although this drug was not detectable in assays of prostatic tissue or prostatic fluid. Other experiments in dogs have shown that levels of minocycline and rosamicin in prostatic tissue significantly exceed their levels in serum.

Human prostatic tissue procured by means of surgical excision or by biopsy of "normal" prostates typically shows prostatic tissue/serum ratios of TMP of 2:1 to 3:1 (Meares, 1982). The concentration of TMP in prostatic tissue, therefore, exceeds that reached in serum. Hensle and

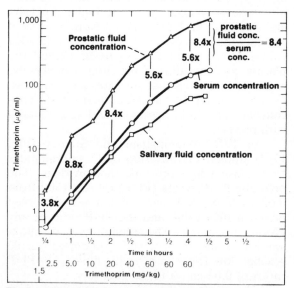

Figure 17–5. Diffusion of trimethoprim from serum into prostatic and salivary fluid in dogs. (From Stamey, T. A., Bushby, S. R. M., and Bragonje, J.: J. Infect. Dis., *128*(Suppl):686, 1973.)

associates (1977) found, similar to the finding in experiments with dogs, that tissue levels of minocycline exceeded serum levels in men undergoing prostatectomy for benign hyperplasia. Therapeutic levels of tobramycin and cephalosporins during standard dosing also have been observed in human prostatic tissue obtained by surgical excision.

The significance of these observations remains uncertain. Bacterial infections of the prostate probably involve the interstitium and stroma, not merely the ducts and acini. Whether infection of the interstitium and stroma occurs without simultaneous infection of prostatic ducts and acini, unfortunately, cannot be resolved by current diagnostic methods. Available data imply that many antimicrobial agents attain therapeutic levels in human prostatic interstitium and stroma and may effectively clear infection from those sites. However, since the pathogens in chronic bacterial prostatitis are readily recovered by culture of the prostatic secretions, it seems clear that therapeutic levels of antimicrobial drugs must be achieved within the secretions, not merely within the stroma and the interstitium. Indeed, studies performed in dogs and men uniformly show levels of TMP in prostatic tissue that greatly exceed the levels in serum. Treatment failures in bacterial prostatitis, therefore, cannot logically be equated with inadequate levels of TMP in prostatic tissue. The most reasonable explanation is the inadequate penetration of drugs into the prostatic ducts, acini, and secretions.

ACUTE BACTERIAL PROSTATITIS

CLINICAL FEATURES

Acute bacterial prostatitis is characterized by the sudden onset of moderate to high fever, chills, low back and perineal pain, urinary frequency and urgency, nocturia, dysuria, generalized malaise with accompanying arthralgia and myalgia, and varying degrees of bladder outlet obstruction. Rectal palpation usually discloses an exquisitely tender, swollen prostate gland that is partially or totally firm, irregular, and warm to the touch. The expressed prostatic secretions are packed with leukocytes and oval fat bodies and grow large numbers of the bacterial pathogen in culture. However, because bacteremia may ensue, acutely inflamed prostate glands should not be massaged unless serum

levels of an appropriate antibacterial agent have already been established. Since cystitis usually accompanies acute bacterial prostatitis, the pathogen generally may be identified by a culture of the voided bladder urine.

PATHOLOGY

Acute bacterial prostatitis results in marked inflammation of part or all of the prostate gland. Sheets of polymorphonuclear leukocytes are characteristically noted within and around the acini, along with intraductal desquamation and cellular debris. Variable tissue invasion by lymphocytes, plasma cells, and macrophages also is typical. Diffuse edema and hyperemia of the stroma are characteristic. Microabscesses may occur early in the course of the disease; large abscesses are late complications.

THERAPY

Patients who have acute bacterial prostatitis usually respond dramatically to therapy with antibacterial agents that normally diffuse poorly from plasma into prostatic fluid. Perhaps, as in acute meningitis, the intense, diffuse inflammatory reaction of the condition enhances the passage of antimicrobial agents from plasma into the prostatic ducts and acini. Patient toxicity and acute urinary retention may lead to hospitalization.

Preferred therapy in the nonallergic patient is trimethoprim-sulfamethoxazole (TMP-SMX), 160 mg TMP and 800 mg SMX, orally twice daily, until the results of the culture and sensitivity testing are known. If the pathogen is susceptible and the clinical response satisfactory, therapy is continued for 30 days to prevent chronic bacterial prostatitis. If for some reason trimethoprim-sulfamethoxazole cannot be used, initial therapy with full-dosage intravenous gentamicin plus ampicillin (3 to 5 mg/kg/day gentamicin divided into three IV doses; 2 gm ampicillin given IV every 6 hours) is recommended until the results of the sensitivity testing of the bacterial pathogen are known. If the clinical response is good, a suitable oral agent is administered instead for an additional 30 days. General supportive measures, such as adequate hydration, analgesics, antipyretics, bed rest, and stool softeners, are also employed. Urethral instrumentation should be avoided. Acute urinary retention is best managed by suprapubic needle aspiration of the bladder or placement of a punch suprapubic tube. Transurethral catheters are tolerated poorly and may create complications.

CHRONIC BACTERIAL PROSTATITIS

CLINICAL FEATURES

The clinical manifestations of chronic bacterial prostatitis are quite variable. Although chronic prostatitis may evolve from an episode of acute bacterial prostatitis, many men with chronic bacterial prostatitis have no prior history of acute prostatitis. Some men are diagnosed only because asymptomatic bacteriuria is found incidentally; however, most complain of varying degrees of irritative voiding symptoms, including dysuria, urinary urgency and frequency, nocturia, and pain perceived in various sites within the distribution of the pelvis and genitalia. Chills or fever are unusual, although postejaculatory pain and hemospermia occur occasionally. No findings on physical examination, rectal palpation of the prostate, cystoscopy, or urography are specifically diagnostic of chronic bacterial prostatitis.

The hallmark of chronic bacterial prostatitis is the occurrence of relapsing urinary tract infection caused by the same pathogen. The organism persists unaltered in prostatic fluid during therapy with most antimicrobial agents because most of these drugs accumulate poorly in prostatic secretions. The urine may be sterilized and symptoms controlled during medical therapy; however, discontinuation of drug therapy often eventually results in reinfection of the urine by the prostatic pathogen and recurrence of symptoms.

Patients with chronic bacterial prostatitis typically have prostatic expressates that on microscopic examination show excessive numbers of leukocytes and macrophages containing fat. Since "inflamed" prostatic secretions are also characteristic of nonbacterial prostatitis, however, this finding is not diagnostic of chronic bacterial prostatitis. During recent years, several biochemical and immunologic markers of bacterial infections of the prostate have evolved; however, the diagnosis is still best confirmed clinically by performance of bacteriologic cultures that localize the pathogen to the prostatic secretions (see Chapter 14). Clinical examples of the usefulness of these culture techniques in diagnosis are shown in Table 17–4.

PATHOLOGY

The histologic findings in cases of chronic bacterial prostatitis are nonspecific. In general, the inflammatory reaction is less marked and much more focal than that seen in cases of acute bacterial prostatitis. Variable infiltration by plasma cells and macrophages is prominent within and around the acini in association with focal areas of invasion by lymphocytes. Because these changes are frequently found in the prostates of patients who have no clinical or bacteriologic evidence of bacteriuria or bacterial infections, they are not diagnostic of chronic bacterial prostatitis (Kohnen and Drach, 1979).

INFECTED PROSTATIC CALCULI

Radiopaque prostatic calculi are often visible on pelvic x-ray films, and their incidence increases with advancing age of the patient. Detailed examination of surgical and autopsy specimens, however, indicates that tiny prostatic stones, often invisible on x-ray films, occur in almost every adult prostate (Fox, 1963). These stones typically are small but tend to occur in clusters. Multiple large calculi are seen most often in men who have chronic bacterial infections of the prostate. Uninfected prostatic calculi usually cause no symptoms or apparent harm; however, in men who have bacterial prostatitis, prostatic stones can become infected and serve as a source of bacterial persistence and relapsing urinary tract infection (Eykyn et al., 1974; Meares, 1974).

Ductal obstruction associated with adenomatous hyperplasia is implicated by traditional theory as the main predisposing factor in the origin of prostatic calculi. The recent examination of prostatic calculi by crystallographic analysis, however, indicates that some prostatic calculi are composed of constituents commonly found in urine but foreign to prostatic secretions—an observation suggesting that intraprostatic reflux of urine is important in the formation of certain prostatic stones. Indeed, it has been proposed to classify as "primary" or "endogenous" stones composed mainly of constituents of prostatic secretions, and to classify as "secondary" or "exogenous" stones composed mainly of constituents of urine (Sutor and Wooley, 1974; Rameriz et al., 1980).

The clinical histories of men who have chronic bacterial prostatitis with or without infected prostatic calculi are indistinguishable, except that men who have infected prostatic stones are never cured by medical therapy alone. Proof that prostatic calculi are infected requires bacteriologic culture of the washed and crushed stones; however, one generally can assume that the calculi are infected in the man who has stones and documented chronic bacterial prostatitis (Eykyn et al., 1974; Meares, 1974; Meares, 1981). Although appropriate antimicro-

TABLE 17–4. SEGMENTED CULTURES OF 15 MEN WITH CHRONIC BACTERIAL PROSTATITIS

Patient	Antibiotic	Colonies per ml				Organism
		VB1*	VB2*	EPS*	VB3*	
1	Yes	90	0	800	20	E. coli
	No	10	0	1000	20	E. coli
2	Yes	0	0	1000	0	Enterococcus
	Yes	20	0	4000	10	Enterococcus
3	Yes	50	0	165	150	E. coli
		0	0	50	20	E. aerogenes
		0	0	560	50	P. mirabilis
		0	0	140	0	P. morganii
	Yes	0	0	660	190	E. coli
		10	0	400	40	E. aerogenes
		0	0	500	20	P. mirabilis
		0	0	200	0	P. morganii
4	Yes	20	0	5000	50	Klebsiella
	Yes	50	0	100,000	1000	Klebsiella
5	No	60	0	1000	20	E. coli
	No	640	40	100,000	220	E. coli
6	Yes	0	0	5000	100	E. coli
	Yes	50	10	10,000	1500	E. coli
7	Yes	120	0	3600	370	E. coli
	No	2000	200	100,000	4000	E. coli
8	Yes	250	20	5000	330	Klebsiella
	No	0	0	50	0	Klebsiella
	No	20	0	10,000	2000	Klebsiella
9	Yes	10,000	150	100,000	10,000	E. coli
	Yes	110	0	1500	810	E. coli
10	No	2000	60	4000	250	Enterococcus
	No	600	60	4000	2000	Enterococcus
	No	260	20	7200	90	Enterococcus
	Yes	20	20	500	30	Enterococcus
11	Yes	30	0	10,000	—	E. coli
	Yes	0	0	3600	—	E. coli
12	Yes	800	20	—	5000	E. coli
	Yes	10,000	800	100,000	10,000	E. coli
13	No	0	0	10,000	600	E. coli
	Yes	0	0	7000	10	E. coli
	Yes	0	0	4000	120	E. coli
14	Yes	0	0	700	200	P. mirabilis
	Yes	30	0	1000	10	P. mirabilis
15	Yes	2500	300	20,000	10,000	Pseudomonas
	Yes	110	70	30,000	750	Pseudomonas

*VB1 = first 10 ml of urine voided (urethral culture); VB2 = midstream aliquot (bladder culture); ESP = expressed prostatic secretions from prostatic massage (prostatic culture); VB3 = first 10 ml of urine voided immediately after prostatic massage (prostatic culture).

bial therapy can usually control the symptoms and keep the urine sterile, infected prostatic calculi cannot be sterilized by medical therapy. Permanent cure of infection can be achieved, however, when all infected calculi and prostatic tissue are removed successfully by surgical means (Meares, 1981).

MEDICAL TREATMENT

Regardless of concerns and controversies about the theoretical levels of various antimicrobial agents that may be attained in human prostatic fluid, few drugs in carefully documented studies have proved successful in actually curing chronic bacterial infections of the prostate. Trimethoprim-sulfamethoxazole (TMP-SMX) currently has the best cure rates documented in reported prospective studies. Among patients who received TMP-SMX continuously for a long term (4 to 16 weeks) the rate of cure in various studies has been about 30 to 40 per cent, which significantly exceeds the cures after short-term therapy (Meares, 1980). The usual dosage is TMP-SMX, one double-strength tablet (160 mg TMP, 800 mg SMX) orally twice daily. The optimal duration of therapy has not been established with certainty. Other agents with reported usefulness in the management of chronic bacterial prostatitis include carbenicillin indanyl sodium, erythromycin, minocycline, doxycycline, and cephalexin. Studies reported from Belgium indicate remarkable success in curing bacterial prostatitis by means of direct injection of antimicrobial agents into the caudal prostate (Plomp et al., 1980; Baert et al., 1983).

Those patients who are not cured by medical therapy generally can be managed satisfactorily by continuous suppressive treatment with low-dose medication. When the organism is susceptible, TMP-SMX or nitrofurantoin is a good choice because neither is prone to produce resistant fecal bacteria and both are well suited for long-term use. The usual dosage is TMP-SMX, one single-strength tablet daily, or nitrofurantoin, 100 mg orally once or twice daily. Discontinuation of therapy, however, eventually results in recurrent symptoms and relapsing urinary tract infection.

SURGICAL TREATMENT

For those patients who have chronic bacterial prostatitis and who are not cured or adequately controlled by medical therapy, treatment by surgical means may prove necessary. Since infected calculi cannot be sterilized by means of medical therapy alone, men with chronic bacterial prostatitis and prostatic calculi often are candidates for surgical therapy. Total prostatovesiculectomy is a curative procedure but seldom is a desirable choice because of its sequelae. Provided the resectionist is successful in removing all foci of infected tissue and calculi, transurethral prostatectomy can be a curative procedure. This goal often is difficult to achieve, especially since the peripheral zones of the prostate usually contain the greatest foci of infection and stones (Blacklock, 1974).

NONBACTERIAL PROSTATITIS

CLINICAL FEATURES

Nonbacterial prostatitis (abacterial prostatitis, prostatosis), the most common prostatitis syndrome, is an inflammatory condition of unknown cause. The findings of Schaeffer and coworkers (1981) suggest that the incidence of nonbacterial prostatitis exceeds that of bacterial prostatitis by eight fold.

The symptoms are variable but include complaints such as urinary urgency and frequency, nocturia, dysuria, and pain and discomfort perceived within the pelvic, suprapubic, or genital area. Sometimes postejaculatory pain and discomfort are prominent features. Physical examination discloses no specific findings: Tender and boggy prostates are not reliable indicators of prostatitis.

Although many clinical features of chronic bacterial prostatitis and nonbacterial prostatitis are similar, one important difference bears emphasis—the patient with nonbacterial prostatitis has no positive cultures or history of documented urinary tract infection. Like patients with chronic bacterial prostatitis, however, patients with nonbacterial prostatitis have more than the normal number of leukocytes and macrophages containing fat in their prostatic expressates. Nonbacterial prostatitis appears to be either an infectious disease caused by yet unidentified pathogens or a noninfectious form of inflammation.

POSSIBLE CAUSATIVE AGENTS

Other than enterococci, gram-positive bacteria seem insignificant in the etiology of prostatitis. Yet, many clinicians still consider them pathogens in patients who otherwise would be diagnosed as having nonbacterial prostatitis. Certain gram-positive bacteria colonize the prostatic fluid merely as commensals. This possibility is suggested by a recent study performed by Fowler and Mariano (1982) in which prostatic expressates from ten uninfected controls, two bacteriuric patients, and two bacterial prostatitis patients were assayed for IgA binding to *S. epidermidis*. Despite positive cultures for *S. epidermidis* in 9 of these 14 samples, binding of IgA to *S. epidermidis* was not found in any sample. In contrast, patients with documented chronic gram-negative prostatitis showed uniform binding of IgA to the infectious pathogen.

Studies of the etiology of nonbacterial prostatitis have generally excluded causative agents such as fungi, obligate anaerobic bacteria, trichomonads, and various types of viruses.

Several investigators have found little evidence that species of *Mycoplasma* or *Ureaplasma* cause prostatitis. In 1980, however, Weidner and coworkers reported isolating *Ureaplasma urealyticum* more than twice as often from the urethra of patients with chronic prostatitis as they did from normal controls. Mean counts of these organisms in the first-voided urethral samples (VB1) differed little between the patients and controls; however, 36 of 187 patients had ureaplasma counts in their postprostatic massage specimens that exceeded the concomitant urethral counts by more than ten fold. On the basis of their bacteriologic data and the response to therapy using tetracycline, these investigators concluded that at least 16 (8.6 per cent) of the 187 patients had prostatitis caused by *U. urealyticum*. Subsequently, Brunner and associates (1983) reported finding a tenfold or greater increase in quantitative counts of *U. urealyticum* in prostatic cultures compared with urethral cultures in 82 (13.7 per cent) of 597 patients with chronic prostatitis. They concluded that these men probably had prostatitis caused by ureaplasmas, especially since 71 of the 82 patients responded favorably to therapy using tetracycline. The bacteriologic data presented in these two studies suggest that ureaplasmas occasionally are pathogens in patients who seem to have nonbacterial prostatitis. Whether ureaplasmas are true pathogens in prostatitis or merely saprophytes or contaminants awaits confirmatory study (e.g., the demonstration of an immunologic response to ureaplasmas in prostatic fluid).

The possible role of *Chlamydia trachomatis* as a causative agent in prostatitis remains controversial. Since this organism is implicated as the etiologic agent in about 40 per cent of cases of male nongonococcal urethritis and in most cases of acute epididymitis occurring in men under the age of 35, its possible role in the etiology of prostatitis seems plausible (Berger et al., 1979). Unfortunately, available data from reported studies make definitive conclusions uncertain. Bruce and associates (1981) studied early-morning urine specimens of 70 men with histories suggestive of chronic prostatitis and isolated *C. trachomatis* in 35 (50 per cent), compared with only 1 (2 per cent) of 50 normal controls. Unfortunately, the study design did not allow for localization of this organism to the prostate or for definitive conclusions regarding the etiologic role of chlamydiae in prostatitis.

Mardh and coworkers (1978) studied 53 men with nonacute prostatitis by cultural and serologic methods and concluded that *C. trachomatis* appears to play only a minor role, if any, in etiology. Indeed, *C. trachomatis* was isolated from the urethra of only 1 of 53 men and from none of 28 specimens of prostatic fluid obtained from these patients. Furthermore, an immunofluorescent test showed little or no antibody activity against chlamydiae in the serum of most, and in the prostatic fluid of even fewer, patients. Berger (1982) reported that he and his associates have been unable to isolate *C. trachomatis* from the urethra, prostatic secretions, or semen of more than 40 men with clinical and laboratory evidence of chronic nonbacterial prostatitis. Additional study of the possible etiologic role of *C. trachomatis* in cases of apparent nonbacterial prostatitis seem warranted; however, available data suggest this organism plays an unimportant role.

TREATMENT

Definitive curative therapy for patients with nonbacterial prostatitis is difficult to achieve because the underlying cause is unknown. When cultures identify no infectious agent and ureaplasmas or chlamydiae are suspected pathogens, a clinical trial using minocycline, doxycycline, or erythromycin in full dosage for 2 to 4 weeks seems reasonable. Unless symptoms improve and the inflammatory response in the prostatic secretions subsides, however, additional antimicrobial therapy is seldom warranted.

Because patients with nonbacterial prostatitis vary in their symptoms and responses to therapy, treatment strategies must be tailored individually. Once the diagnosis is established, the clinician should fully explain to the patient what is currently known about nonbacterial prostatitis. Some clinicians reassure the patient by comparing nonbacterial prostatitis with other noninfectious inflammatory conditions (e.g., arthritis): While these conditions tend to be chronic and cause intermittent symptoms, they are not infectious or contagious and do not lead to cancer or other serious diseases.

The key to successful therapy is a program tailored to relieve symptoms as well as the patient's concerns and anxieties. In general, normal sexual activity and exercise are encouraged: Dietary restrictions are advised only when patients notice that spicy foods or alcoholic beverages cause or aggravate their symptoms. Prostatic massage is used in therapy by many clinicians but has little scientific basis. Hot sitz baths effectively relieve symptoms. Irritative voiding dysfunction and discomfort may respond to anticholinergic agents (e.g., propantheline bromide, oxybutynin chloride) and anti-inflammatory agents (e.g., indomethacin, ibuprofen, naproxen). Oral zinc preparations and megavitamins have no proven efficacy in the treatment of nonbacterial prostatitis.

PROSTATODYNIA

CLINICAL FEATURES

The typical patient with prostatodynia has symptoms suggesting prostatitis but no history of documented urinary tract infection, no infectious pathogen on bacteriologic localization cultures, and no excessive numbers of inflammatory cells in his prostatic secretions. This condition is seen mainly in men aged 20 to 45 years. The predominant symptom is "pelvic" pain, not necessarily related to voiding: perineal, penile, suprapubic, scrotal, or urethral pain. Some patients complain of intermittent urinary ugency, frequency, nocturia, and dysuria; however, irritative voiding dysfunction is not a prominent complaint. Many patients are aware of variable signs of obstructive voiding dysfunction, i.e., hesitancy, a weakened stream, and even interrupted flow ("pulsating" voiding).

Typically, genitourinary examination, including palpation of the prostate gland, discloses no specific abnormality. Bacteriologic localization cultures show no infectious pathogen, and microscopy of the prostatic expressate is normal. Cystoscopy often suggests some degree of bladder neck obstruction without prostatic obstruction and mild to moderate bladder trabeculation.

NEUROLOGIC AND VIDEO-URODYNAMIC FINDINGS

Abnormal urinary flow rates typically are found in patients who have prostatitis; however, the urodynamic features of prostatodynia were not studied until recently. In 1983 the results of the prospective study of 20 consecutive men with prostatodynia who underwent complete neurologic and video-urodynamic evaluation at the Tufts–New England Medical Center were reported (Meares and Barbalias, 1983; Barbalias et al., 1983). A summary of the findings in these men is shown in Table 17–5. The most striking feature was a significant increase in maximal urethral closure pressure compared with an age- and sex-matched control group. Both peak and average urinary flow rates were typically decreased. Another prominent feature was incomplete funneling of the bladder neck during voiding with an accompanying urethral narrowing at the level of the external urethral sphincter.

POSSIBLE CAUSES

Sinaki and associates (1977) evaluated patients with a diagnosis of pyriformis syndrome, coccygodynia, levator ani spasm syndrome, proctalgia fugax, or rectal pain and believed that all patients had "tension myalgia of the pelvic floor." Subsequently, habitual contractions and spasms of the pelvic floor muscles were implicated as the primary cause of pelvic floor myalgia (Segura et al., 1979). This disorder

TABLE 17–5. CLINICAL AND VIDEO-URODYNAMIC FINDINGS IN PROSTATODYNIA

Clinical presentation: variable
Neurologic examination: normal
Pudendal neuropathy: absent ⎫
Urethral reflexes: intact   ⎬ by EMG confirmation
                                      ⎭
Type of voiding: synergistic (no dyssynergia)
Bladder capacity: often increased
Bladder contractions: voluntary (rarely involuntary) and of normal magnitude
VCUG: bladder neck obstructed or incompletely funneled
VCUG: prostatic urethra narrowed in area of EUS despite EMG silence of the EUS
Urethral pressure profile: increased maximal urethral closure pressure (at rest)
Urinary flow rate: decreased peak and average flow

EMG = electromyography; VCUG = voiding cystourethrography; EUS = external urethral sphincter.
From Meares, E. M., Jr., and Barbalias, G. A.: Semin. Urol., *1*:146, 1983. Used by permission.

often seems directly related to local painful or inflammatory conditions. Symptoms of burning or pain during voiding are atypical; instead, the predominant complaints are perineal discomfort or pain associated with sitting, running, or other activities that presumably lead to fatigue of the perineal muscles. Segura and associates believe that some men with prostatodynia actually suffer from pelvic floor tension myalgia.

Psychiatric disorders or primary emotional disturbances leading to stress have been implicated in the etiology of prostatodynia (Nilsson et al., 1975). A "chemical prostatitis" caused by intraprostatic reflux of urine may cause the symptoms in some cases of nonbacterial prostatitis and prostatodynia (Kirby et al., 1982).

The clinical and video-urodynamic findings in prostatodynia reported by Barbalias and co-workers (1983) militate against a diagnosis of pelvic floor tension myalgia. Instead, a primary abnormality involving the pelvic sympathetic nervous system is suggested, with resultant incomplete relaxation of the bladder neck and abnormal narrowing of the urethra at the level of the external urethral sphincter. Since afflicted patients appear otherwise intact neurologically, an acquired functional disorder seems plausible.

TREATMENT

Because patients with prostatodynia are not infected, antibiotics are ineffective and unwarranted in therapy. Once the diagnosis is confirmed, the goals of therapy are patient reassurance and emotional support plus measures to control symptoms.

Alpha-blocking agents are useful in treating patients with typical voiding dysfunction (Table 17–5). Clinicians vary in their choice of alpha-blocking agents and dosing schedules; however, most advise using phenoxybenzamine, 10 to 20 mg orally once or twice daily. Because phenoxybenzamine recently was implicated in mutagenicity in laboratory animals, however, many clinicians are now using an alternative alpha-blocker—prazosin, 2 to 4 mg orally once or twice daily (Meares and Barbalias, 1983). The recommended dosage and length of therapy vary according to individual drug tolerances and clinical responses. Some patients with prostatodynia improve during therapy using diazepam, 5 mg orally three times daily, with or without the concomitant use of an alpha-blocking agent. The application of techniques of biofeedback in the management of patients suffering from prostatodynia seems appealing but remains essentially untested.

OTHER TYPES OF PROSTATITIS

GONOCOCCAL PROSTATITIS

The incidence of venereal disease caused by *Neisseria gonorrhoeae* remains high throughout the world. Although the rate of isolation of *N. gonorrhoeae* from the urethras of men usually is low, among contacts of women with gonorrhea urethral infection is frequent and often symptomatic. Indeed, in one study *N. gonorrhoeae* was isolated from urethral specimens of 78 per cent of male contacts of women having gonorrhea; about half of these men were asymptomatic (Thelin et al., 1980).

That the gonococcus can infect the prostate was demonstrated in 1931 by Sargent and Irwin, who reviewed 42 cases of prostatic abscess and found that 75 per cent were caused by gonococcal infection. However, whether prostatic infection due to *N. gonorrhoeae* currently remains a significant clinical problem is uncertain. Most recent studies suggest that gonococcal prostatitis rarely occurs. Two studies, however, demonstrated positive antibody against *N. gonorrhoeae* in the prostatic fluid of patients whose cultures were negative. Danielsson and Molin (1971) used fluorescent antibody tests and detected apparent persistence of gonococci in the prostatic fluid of 40 per cent of men who were deemed cured following the usual short-term therapy on the basis of ordinary diagnostic techniques. In another study, six men had repeatedly negative cultures but positive fluorescent antibody tests against *N. gonorrhoeae* in their seminal fluid. After therapy with metacycline, five men no longer had positive antibody studies (Colleen and Mardh, 1975).

One must conclude that gonococci may invade the male accessory sex glands during acute urethral infection and that conventional therapy for gonococcal urethritis may occasionally fail to clear the gonococcus from these accessory glands. These patients may develop symptomatic prostatitis despite negative cultures for *N. gonorrhoeae*. Therefore, patients with prior histories of gonococcal urethritis who develop apparent nonbacterial prostatitis probably should receive tetracycline therapy, preferably minocycline or doxycycline, 100 mg orally twice daily for at least 2 weeks.

TUBERCULOUS PROSTATITIS

Granulomatous prostatitis due to *Mycobacterium tuberculosis* may develop as a sequela of miliary tuberculosis. The diagnosis is confirmed by recovery of the organism from prostatic fluid cultures. The reader is referred to Chapter 23 for a more detailed discussion of this topic.

PARASITIC PROSTATITIS

Prostatitic infection caused by parasites is common in certain parts of the world but uncommon in the United States. The reader is referred to Chapter 21 for a detailed discussion of this topic.

MYCOTIC PROSTATITIS

Granulomatous prostatitis caused by fungi associated with systemic mycosis (blastomycosis, coccidioidomycosis, cryptococcosis, histoplasmosis, paracoccidioidomycosis, and candidiasis) is seen occasionally in clinical practice (Schwarz, 1982). Diagnosis is usually confirmed by means of prostatic histology and cultures of prostatic fluid and tissue. Therapy is directed toward treatment of the generalized disease. The reader is referred to Chapter 22 for a more detailed discussion of fungal infections.

NONSPECIFIC GRANULOMATOUS PROSTATITIS

Nonspecific granulomatous prostatitis occurs in two forms: a noneosinophilic variety and an eosinophilic variety. Although neither variety is seen frequently in clinical practice (the eosinophilic variety is especially rare), both types are important clinically because they may be confused with prostatic carcinoma.

Noneosinophilic Variety. Noneosinophilic granulomatous prostatitis apparently represents a tissue response of the foreign body type to extravasated prostatic fluid (O'Dea et al., 1977). Acute signs and symptoms of bladder outlet obstruction associated with an enlarged, firm prostate that feels malignant characterize the clinical presentation. Fever and significant symptoms of irritative voiding dysfunction may or may not be found. Urine cultures often are sterile but may grow coliforms (mainly *E. coli*). Histologic examination of prostatic tissue obtained by biopsy or surgical excision and the exclusion by culture or other means of specific forms of infectious granulomatous prostatitis confirm the diagnosis. Some patients respond favorably to antimicrobial agents, corticosteroids, and temporary bladder drainage via a catheter; others require transurethral resection of the prostate.

Eosinophilic Variety. Particularly when associated with fibrinoid necrosis and generalized vasculitis, eosinophilic granulomatous prostatitis is a serious illness (Towfighi et al., 1972).

Because it occurs almost exclusively in patients with allergies, and especially in asthmatics, this entity also is known as allergic granuloma of the prostate. Generally, affected patients become severely ill and develop high fevers. Hemograms of the peripheral blood typically show significant eosinophilia. As the prostate gland typically becomes markedly enlarged and indurated, complete urinary retention often develops. Diagnostic confirmation requires histologic examination of prostatic tissue. Because the response to therapy using corticosteroids usually is dramatic, surgical intervention to relieve bladder outlet obstruction often is avoided. The severity of the associated generalized vasculitis and its response to therapy primarily determine the prognosis.

PROSTATIC ABSCESS

During recent years, the incidence of prostatic abscess appears to have declined and the type of infecting organism apparently has changed. In 1931, Sargent and Irwin noted that *N. gonorrhoeae* caused 75 per cent of 42 cases of prostatic abscess. Modern reports by Dajani and O'Flynn in 1968 (25 cases) and by Pai and Bhat in 1972 (24 cases) indicate that coliforms (chiefly *E. coli*) are responsible in 70 per cent of cases. Obligate anaerobic bacteria occasionally cause prostatic abscesses.

Many details concerning pathogenesis remain unclear; however, most prostatic abscesses probably are complications of acute bacterial prostatitis. Among reported cases, the youngest patient with a prostatic abscess has been a 46-day-old infant (Heyman and Lombardo, 1962); however, most have occurred in men who are in the fifth or sixth decade of life. Men who are diabetic seem especially prone to develop prostatic abscesses.

Table 17–6 indicates the signs and symptoms noted in 49 cases of prostatic abscess (25 cases reported by Dajani and O'Flynn and 24 cases reported by Pai and Bhat). That fever was found in only 41 per cent and rectal pain in only 14 per cent of the cases is surprising. Rectal examination of the prostate discloses variable findings. The gland typically is enlarged, with the affected lobe predominating, and tender to palpation. The presence of fluctuation is an important diagnostic feature; unfortunately, this finding may be missed completely or not detected until the patient has been under treatment for several days. Spontaneous rupture of

TABLE 17–6. SYMPTOMS OF PROSTATIC ABSCESS IN
49 CASES

Symptom	Number of Patients	Per Cent
Acute retention	24	49
Frequency and dysuria	24	49
Fever	20	41
Epididymo-orchitis	10	24
Rectal discomfort	7	14
Hematuria	5	10
Pus per urethram	3	6
Backache	1	2

contents of the abscess into the urethra is seen occasionally.

Once the diagnosis has been confirmed, the proper treatment consists of pathogen-specific antimicrobial therapy combined with surgical drainage. Drainage by transperineal aspiration under local anesthesia via a large-bore needle may suffice, but transurethral resection or perineal incision often is required. Proper diagnosis and therapy usually assure a good overall prognosis. Recurrent prostatic abscess is unusual.

PROSTATITIS AND INFERTILITY

During recent years, interest has grown concerning the possible relation of infections of the prostate and seminal vesicles to male subfertility and barren marriages. Despite extensive investigative study, however, controversy prevails.

A review of most studies shows that the addition of live microorganisms to normal fresh ejaculates causes decreased sperm viability (impaired motility and agglutination), but only when the inocula are massive ($>10^6$ organisms/ml) (Meares, 1980; Fowler, 1981). Since spermatozoa are not likely to be exposed to such massive concentrations of pathogens as a result of chronic prostatitis, subfertility in such cases probably does not occur on the basis of a direct effect of the pathogen on spermatozoa. Many clinicians believe, however, that the secretory dysfunction of the prostate that accompanies chronic bacterial prostatitis leads to adverse effects upon spermatozoa and resultant subfertility (Homonnai et al., 1978; Caldamone et al., 1980). Additional study seems warranted, however, to more fully examine the possible relations between infections of the prostate and seminal vesicles, secretory dysfunction of these glands, and subfertility.

SEMINAL VESICULITIS

Bacterial infections of the seminal vesicles undoubtedly occur but generally cannot be proved clinically. Whether bacterial seminal vesiculitis occurs without concomitant prostatic infection is unknown. Histopathologic studies of unselected autopsies and of autopsies performed upon men with known terminal infections of the urine suggest a low incidence of seminal vesiculitis, even when the incidence of prostatitis is high (Calams, 1955; Hyams et al., 1932). However, the incidence of seminal vesiculitis among men with clinical signs and symptoms of prostatitis apparently has not been documented well by histopathologic study.

Since "pure" vesicular fluid is virtually unobtainable for culture and analysis, the challenge of proving a case of seminal vesiculitis clinically is formidable. Semen analyses that show low volume and subnormal levels of fructose suggest secretory dysfunction of the seminal vesicles but do not confirm an infectious cause of this dysfunction. Likewise, a positive culture or abnormal cytologic examination of the ejaculate cannot be used with certainty to confirm a diagnosis of seminal vesiculitis. Seminal vesiculograms have been reported to correlate poorly with the results of surgery and histologic findings in patients with suspected seminal vesiculitis (Dunnick et al., 1982).

When a bacterial infection of the seminal vesicles is suspected, recommended therapy is the same as that for bacterial prostatitis.

References

Anderson, R. U., and Fair, W. R.: Physical and chemical determinations of prostatic secretion in benign hyperplasia, prostatitis, and adenocarcinoma. Invest. Urol., *14*:137, 1976.

Anderson, R. U., and Weller, C.: Prostatic secretion leukocyte studies in non-bacterial prostatitis (prostatosis). J. Urol., *121*:292, 1979.

Baert, L., Mattelaer, J., and deNollin, P.: Treatment of chronic bacterial prostatitis by local injection of antibiotics into prostate. Urology, *21*:370, 1983.

Barbalias, G. A., Meares, E. M., Jr., and Sant, G. R.: Prostatodynia: Clinical and urodynamic characteristics. J. Urol., *130*:514, 1983.

Berger, R. E.: Nongonococcal urethritis and related syndromes. *In* Stamey, T. A. (Ed.): 1982 Monographs in Urology. Vol. 3 (4). Princeton, N. J., Custom Publishing Services, 1982, pp. 98–125.

Berger, R. E., Alexander, E. R., Harnisch, J. P., et al.: Etiology, manifestations and therapy of acue epididymitis: Prospective study of 50 cases. J. Urol., *121*:750, 1979.

Blacklock, N. J.: Some observations on prostatitis. *In* Williams, D. C., Briggs, M. H., and Stanford, M. (Eds.):

Advances in the Study of the Prostate. London, Heinemann, 1969, pp. 37–61.

Blacklock, N. J.: Anatomical factors in prostatitis. Br. J. Urol., 46:47, 1974.

Blacklock, N. J., and Beavis, J. P.: The response of prostatic fluid pH in inflammation. Br. J. Urol., 46:537, 1974.

Bruce, A. W., Willett, W. S., Chadwick, P., et al.: The role of chlamydiae in genitourinary disease. J. Urol., 126:625, 1981.

Brunner, H., Weidner, W., and Schiefer, H-G.: Studies of the role of *Ureaplasma urealyticum* and *Mycoplasma hominis* in prostatitis. J. Infect. Dis., 147:807, 1983.

Calams, J. A.: A histopathologic search for chronic seminal vesiculitis. J. Urol., 74:638, 1955.

Caldamone, A. A., Emilson, L. B. U., Al-Juburi, A., et al.: Prostatitis: Prostatic secretory dysfunction affecting fertility. Fertil. Steril., 34:602, 1980.

Chodirker, W. B., and Tomasi, T. B.: Gamma-globulins: Quantitative relationships in human serum and nonvascular fluids. Science, 142:1080, 1963.

Colleen, S., and Mardh, P-A.: Effect of metacycline treatment of non-acute prostatitis. Scand. J. Urol. Nephrol., 9:198, 1975.

Dajani, M. D., and O'Flynn, J. D.: Prostatic abscess. Br. J. Urol., 40:736, 1968.

Danielsson, D., and Molin, L.: Demonstration of *N. gonorrhoeae* in prostatic fluid after treatment of uncomplicated gonorrheal urethritis. Acta Derm. Venereol., 51:73, 1971.

Drach, G. W.: Problems in diagnosis of bacterial prostatitis: Gram-negative, gram-positive and mixed infections. J. Urol., 111:630, 1974.

Drach, G. W.: Prostatitis: Man's hidden infection. Urol. Clin. North Am., 2:499, 1975.

Drach, G. W., Fair, W. R., Meares, E. M., Jr., and Stamey, T. A.: Classification of benign diseases associated with prostatic pain: Prostatitis or prostatodynia? J. Urol., 120:266, 1978.

Dunnick, N. R., Ford, K., Osborne, D., et al.: Seminal vesiculography: Limited value in vesiculitis. Urology, 20:454, 1982.

Eykyn, S., Bultitude, M. I., Mayo, M. E., et al.: Prostatic calculi as a source of recurrent bacteriuria in the male. Br. J. Urol., 46:527, 1974.

Fair, W. R., Couch, J., and Wehner, N.: Prostatic antibacterial factor. Identity and significance. Urology, 7:169, 1976.

Fair, W. R., Crane, D. B., Schiller, N., and Heston, W. D. W.: A re-appraisal of treatment in chronic bacterial prostatitis. J. Urol., 121:437, 1979.

Fowler, J. E., Jr.: Infections of the male reproductive tract and infertility: A selected review. J. Androl., 3:121, 1981.

Fowler, J. E., Jr., and Mariano, M.: Immunologic response of the prostate to bacteriuria and bacterial prostatitis. II. Antigen specific immunoglobulin in prostatic fluid. J. Urol., 128:165, 1982.

Fowler, J. E., Jr., Kaiser, D. L., and Mariano, M.: Immunologic response of the prostate to bacteriuria and bacterial prostatitis. I. Immunoglobulin concentrations in prostatic fluid. J. Urol., 128:158, 1982.

Fox, M.: The natural history and significance of stone formation in the prostate gland. J. Urol., 89:716, 1963.

Gray, S. P., Billings, J., and Blacklock, N. J.: Distribution of the immunoglobulins G, A and M in the prostatic fluid of patients with prostatitis. Clin. Chim. Acta, 57:163, 1974.

Hensle, T. W., Prout, G. R., Jr., and Griffin, P.: Minocycline diffusion into benign prostatic hyperplasia. J. Urol., 118:609, 1977.

Heyman, A., and Lombardo, L. J., Jr.: Metastatic prostatic abscess with report of a case in a newborn infant. J. Urol., 87:174, 1962.

Homonnai, Z. T., Matzkin, H., Fainman, N., et al.: The cation composition of the seminal plasma and prostatic fluid and its correlation to semen quality. Fertil. Steril., 29:539, 1978.

Huggins, C., Scott, W. W., and Heinen, J. H.: Chemical composition of human semen and of secretions of prostate and seminal vesicles. Am. J. Physiol., 136:467, 1942.

Hyams, J. A., Kramer, S. E., and McCarthy, J. F.: The seminal vesicles and the ejaculatory ducts: Histopathologic study. JAMA, 98:691, 1932.

Jacobs, M. H.: Some aspects of cell permeability to weak electrolytes. Symp. Quant. Biol. (Cold Spring Harbor), 8:30, 1940.

Jameson, R. M.: Sexual activity and the variations of the white cell content of the prostatic secretion. Invest. Urol., 5:297, 1967.

Jones, S. R.: Prostatitis as a cause of antibody-coated bacteria in the urine. N. Engl. J. Med., 291:365, 1974.

Kirby, R. S., Lowe, D., Bultitude, M. I., and Shuttleworth, K. E. D.: Intra-prostatic urinary reflux: An aetiological factor in abacterial prostatitis. Br. J. Urol., 54:729, 1982.

Kohnen, P. W., and Drach, G. W.: Patterns of inflammation in prostatic hyperplasia: A histologic and bacteriologic study. J. Urol., 121:755, 1979.

Mardh, P-A., and Colleen, S.: Search for uro-genital tract infections in patients with symptoms of prostatitis. Studies on aerobic and strictly anaerobic bacteria, mycoplasmas, fungi, trichomonads and viruses. Scand. J. Urol. Nephrol., 9:8, 1975.

Mardh, P-A., Ripa, K. T., Colleen, S., et al.: Role of *Chlamydia trachomatis* in non-acute prostatitis. Br. J. Vener. Dis., 54:330, 1978.

Meares, E. M., Jr.: Bacterial prostatitis versus "prostatosis": A clinical and bacteriological study. JAMA, 224:1372, 1973.

Meares, E. M., Jr.: Infection stones of the prostate gland. Laboratory diagnosis and clinical management. Urology, 4:560, 1974.

Meares, E. M., Jr.: Serum antibody titers in urethritis and chronic bacterial prostatitis. Urology, 10:305, 1977.

Meares, E. M., Jr.: Serum antibody titers in treatment with trimethoprim-sulfamethoxazole for chronic prostatitis. Urology, 11:142, 1978.

Meares, E. M., Jr.: Prostatitis syndromes: New perspectives about old woes. J. Urol., 123:141, 1980.

Meares, E. M., Jr.: Nephrology Forum: Prostatitis. Kidney Int., 20:289, 1981.

Meares, E. M., Jr.: Prostatitis: Review of pharmacokinetics and therapy. Rev. Infect. Dis., 4:475, 1982.

Meares, E. M., Jr.: Bacterial prostatitis and recurrent urinary tract infections. *In* Hoeprich, P. D. (Ed.): Infectious Diseases. 3rd ed. New York, Harper & Row, 1983, pp. 517–522.

Meares, E. M., Jr., and Barbalias, G. A.: Prostatitis: Bacterial, nonbacterial and prostatodynia. Semin. Urol., 1:146, 1983.

Meares, E. M., and Stamey, T. A.: Bacteriologic localization patterns in bacterial prostatitis and urethritis. Invest. Urol., 5:492, 1968.

Mobley, D. F.: Erythromycin plus sodium bicarbonate in chronic bacterial prostatitis. Urology, 3:60, 1974.

Mobley, D. F.: Semen cultures in the diagnosis of bacterial prostatitis. J. Urol., 114:83, 1975.

Mobley, D. F.: Bacterial prostatitis: Treatment with carbenicillin indanyl sodium. Invest. Urol., 19:31, 1981.

Nielsen, O. S., Frimodt-Moeller, N., Maigaard, S., et al.: Penicillanic acid derivatives in the canine prostate. Prostate, *1*:79, 1980.

Nilsson, I. K., Colleen, S., and Mardh, P-A.: Relationship between psychological and laboratory findings in patients with symptoms of non-acute prostatitis. *In* Danielsson, D., Juhlin, L., and Mardh, P-A. (Eds.): Genital Infections and Their Complications. Stockholm, Almquist & Wiksell International, 1975, pp. 133–144.

Nishimura, T., Mobley, D. F., and Carlton, C. E., Jr.: Immunoglobulin A in split ejaculates of patients with prostatitis. Urology, *9*:186, 1977.

O'Dea, M. J., Hunting, D. B., and Greene, L. F.: Nonspecific granulomatous prostatitis. J. Urol., *118*:58, 1977.

Pai, M. G., and Bhat, H. S.: Prostatic abscess. J. Urol., *108*:599, 1972.

Pfau, A., and Sacks, T.: Chronic bacterial prostatitis: New therapeutic aspects. Br. J. Urol., *48*:245, 1976.

Pfau, A., Perlberg, S., and Shapira, A.: The pH of the prostatic fluid in health and disease: Implications of treatment in chronic bacterial prostatitis. J. Urol., *119*:384, 1978.

Plomp, T. A., Baert, L., and Maes, R. A.: Treatment of recurrent chronic bacterial prostatitis by local injection of thiamphenicol into prostate. Urology, *15*:542, 1980.

Rameriz, C. T., Ruiz, J. A., Gomez, A. Z., et al.: A crystallographic study of prostatic calculi. J. Urol., *124*:840, 1980.

Riedasch, G., Ritz, E., Möhring, K., and Bommer, J.: Antibody coating of urinary bacteria: Relation to site of infection and invasion of uroepithelium. Clin. Nephrol., *10*:239, 1978.

Sargent, J. C., and Irwin, R.: Prostatic abscess: Clinical study of 42 cases. Am. J. Surg., *11*:334, 1931.

Schaeffer, A. J., Wendel, E. F., Dunn, J. K., and Grayhack, J. T.: Prevalence and significance of prostatic inflammation. J. Urol., *125*:215, 1981.

Schwarz, J.: Mycotic prostatitis. Urology, *19*:1, 1982.

Segura, J. W., Opitz, J. L., and Greene, L. F.: Prostatosis, prostatitis or pelvic floor tension myalgia? J. Urol., *122*:168, 1979.

Shah, N.: Diagnostic significance of levels of immunoglob-ulin A in seminal fluid of patients with prostatic disease. Urology, *8*:270, 1976.

Sharer, W. C., and Fair, W. R.: The pharmacokinetics of antibiotic diffusion in chronic bacterial prostatitis. Prostate, *3*:139, 1982.

Shortliffe, L. M. D., Wehner, N., and Stamey, T. A.: The detection of a local prostatic immunologic response to bacterial prostatitis. J. Urol., *125*:509, 1981.

Sinaki, M., Merritt, J. L., and Stillwell, G. K.: Tension myalgia of the pelvic floor. Mayo Clin. Proc., *52*:717, 1977.

Stamey, T. A.: Pathogenesis and Treatment of Urinary Tract Infections. Baltimore, Williams & Wilkins Co., 1980.

Stamey, T. A.: Prostatitis. J. R. Soc. Med., *74*:22, 1981.

Stamey, T. A., Bushby, S. R. M., and Bragonje, J.: The concentration of trimethoprim in prostatic fluid: Nonionic diffusion or active transport? J. Infect. Dis. (Suppl.), *128*:S686, 1973.

Sutor, D. J., and Wooley, S. E.: The crystalline composition of prostatic calculi. Br. J. Urol., *46*:533, 1974.

Thelin, I., Wennstrom, A-M., and Mardh, P-A.: Contact tracing in patients with genital chlamydial infection. Br. J. Vener. Dis., *56*:259, 1980.

Thin, R. N., and Simmons, P. D.: Chronic bacterial and nonbacterial prostatitis. Br. J. Urol., *55*:513, 1983a.

Thin, R. N., and Simmons, P. D.: Results of four regimens for treatment of chronic non-bacterial prostatitis. Br. J. Urol., *55*:519, 1983b.

Thomas, V., Shelokov, A., and Forland, M.: Antibody-coated bacteria in the urine and the site of urinary-tract infection. N. Engl. J. Med., *290*:588, 1974.

Towfighi, J., Sadeghee, S., Wheller, J. E., et al.: Granulomatous prostatitis with emphasis on the eosinophilic variety. Am. J. Clin. Pathol., *58*:630, 1972.

Weidner, W., Brunner, H., and Krause, W.: Quantitative culture of *Ureaplasma urealyticum* in patients with chronic prostatitis or prostatosis. J. Urol., *124*:622, 1980.

Winningham, D. G., and Stamey, T. A.: Diffusion of sulfonamides from plasma into prostatic fluid. J. Urol., *104*:559, 1970.

CHAPTER 18

Urinary Tract Infections in Spinal Cord Injury Patients

RODNEY U. ANDERSON, M.D.

ACUTE HOSPITALIZATION UROLOGIC CARE

The Intermittent Catheterization Program

The successful evolution of medical rehabilitation following spinal cord injury included new ideas about managing urinary tract infections. During World War I virtually all soldiers who had spinal cord injuries died of urosepsis, with few returning to the United States. When physicians on the front lines in World War II discovered that immediate drainage of a shocked bladder worked best, statistics improved—the mortality rate due to urosepsis declined and 50 per cent of spinal cord injury patients survived. It was during the Second World War that Sir Ludwig Guttmann, a German immigrant to England, fathered a radical but perfectly appropriate approach to the shocked neurogenic bladder; he introduced the idea of sterile intermittent catheterization of the bladder (Guttmann and Frankel, 1966). Initially only the physician, with sterile gown and gloves, was permitted to conduct this ritual for the paralyzed patient. Today most spinal cord injury centers accept intermittent catheterization (IC) as good primary management for the postinjury dysfunctional bladder. The technique probably represents the single most significant advance in urologic care of spinal cord injury.

The obvious purpose of an intermittent catheterization program is to cleanly evacuate the bladder at regular intervals, prevent bladder overdistention (greater than 500 ml), and eliminate the natural bacterial colonization that occurs with an indwelling catheter. There is no question that prevention of bacteriuria was effective under the conditions proposed by Professor Guttmann: sterile technique administered with meticulous care by the most experienced medical staff. Economic and manpower restrictions often preclude such impeccable care in most hospitals. Some compromises, including allowing the patient to do his or her own catheterization, have led to the acceptance of some bacteriuria as well as greater convenience for the patient.

Intermittent catheterization during acute hospitalization is best conducted under sterile conditions. Plastic disposable catheters of 14 or 16 French size are inexpensive, and prepackaged gloves, towels, and antiseptic add little to the cost. It is important to instruct technicians or nurses responsible for the intermittent catheterization in the delicate nature of urethral mucosa and the natural resistance offered by urinary sphincter muscles. They need to understand that one should pass a catheter into the male bladder using steady, gentle pressure, allowing fatigue of the sphincter to permit passage of the catheter into the bladder. If hematuria occurs following such a manipulation, it is most often due to superficial disruption of the urethral mucosa. A coudé tipped catheter often facilitates passage in male patients with a spastic external sphincter, patulous bulbar urethra, or benign prostatic hypertrophy. When uncontrolled sphincter spasticity is encountered, intraurethral topical anesthetics, such as lidocaine, are helpful. Consideration should also be given to routine administration of somatic muscle relaxants.

Intermittent catheterization reduces bacterial growth and prevents bladder overdistention. Rapid withdrawal of the catheter with incomplete emptying of the bladder will defeat the purpose of catheterization; therefore, the catheter should be withdrawn slowly, pausing at the level of the bladder neck to allow the last few milliliters of urine to drain out. Careful emptying down to 2 ml or less could theoretically sustain sterility in a bladder, but this is true only if bladder emptying is carried out frequently enough to abort prolonged bacterial growth (Hinman, 1977).

Frequent emptying to keep the bladder from filling beyond 500 ml is often problematic in the early days following spinal injury. This is particularly true of young, muscular individuals, in whom a pronounced fluid diuresis occurs and makes IC impractical; catheterization every 1 to 2 hours would be required to keep the bladder from overdistending. If attempts to regulate fluid intake are unsuccessful, a short-term indwelling urethral or suprapubic catheter is preferred. If indwelling catheter drainage exceeds 3 to 4 days, we prefer to place a small-diameter suprapubic catheter, easily installed via percutaneous punch.

Some rehabilitation centers prefer exclusive use of a suprapubic tube during acute care. Cook and Smith (1976) managed 43 patients with such a catheter and then removed it when the patient was ready for mobilization. They found that 40 to 50 per cent of the patients were able to maintain a sterile urine throughout the period of suprapubic drainage, an average of 38 days. Japanese workers reported on 165 cases of spinal cord injury managed initially by suprapubic cystostomy under a closed and aseptic state (Namiki, 1978). They were able to maintain sterility for a period of 30 to 48 days. The urinary drainage bag was kept free of bacteria by instilling 50 ml of 10 per cent formalin and the entire collecting system was kept closed, with the drainage duct and external urethral meatus covered with sterile gauze. The catheter was renewed approximately every week, and no bladder irrigations were performed. Seventy-seven per cent of these patients were then able to achieve a balanced bladder and void without the use of a catheter. Donovan and coworkers (1977) compared bladder rehabilitation in patients managed by IC versus manual evacuation of the bladder intermittently from a closed suprapubic catheter and found little difference in episodes of significant bacteriuria. Patients received methenamine mandelate and ascorbic acid during this time, and those managed with the suprapubic catheter achieved balanced voiding in 9 weeks as opposed to 16 weeks for the patients using intermittent catheterization.

Intermittent catheterization has proved so successful in preserving a natural state for the bladder that nonsterile conditions seem to be harmless (Lapides et al., 1976; Maynard and Diokno, 1982).* Some investigators are concerned about nonsterile techniques in the hospital environment and about poor selection of patients for prolonged intermittent catheterization (Anderson, 1980; Nanninga et al., 1982). Nanninga and his group showed that follow-up evaluations, consisting of excretory urogram, cystogram, and urinary cultures, have revealed that as many as 33 per cent of patients develop ureterectasis and hydronephrosis. Some patients develop anatomic deterioration in spite of regular intermittent catheterization and have had elevation of their serum creatinine to greater than 1.5 mg per dl. Maynard and Diokno (1982), on the other hand, reported that 28 patients on intermittent catheterization followed for 3.7 years had no evidence of hydronephrosis/hydroureter or vesicoureteral reflux. There were minor complications of cystolithiasis and nephrolithiasis and four cases of epididymitis. It is obvious from such conflicting long-term studies that patient selection is important and that those who empty the bladder on a regular basis using clean techniques do better if they have acontractile bladders. It is incumbent upon the attending physician to carefully monitor the status of the urinary tract during this mode of bladder emptying.

We may summarize recommendations for intermittent catheterization in the acute care hospital setting by suggesting that sterile technique be used on a 4- to 8-hour frequency to keep the bladder from filling beyond 500 ml and, when this is not feasible, to use a thin, polyethylene suprapubic tube, secured in a strict aseptic fashion. When the patients leave the hospital, they may then convert to clean intermittent catheterization.

---

*Nonsterile or clean intermittent catheterization implies no antiseptic preparation other than good hygiene, no sterile gloves or towels, and use of the same catheter repeatedly for about 2 weeks, rinsing it out and storing it in a dry condition.

BACTERIURIA DURING INTERMITTENT CATHETERIZATION

There is justifiable concern about the development of bacteriuria during an intermittent catheterization program, but it is difficult to define significant bacteriuria or what constitutes an infection. Clearly, many episodes of significant bacteriuria will occur and go undetected by the neurologically deprived patient. While some authors feel that any number of bacteria found on two consecutive daily catheterized urine cultures should be considered meaningful (Donovan et al., 1978), others believe that asymptomatic bacteriuria is not significant at all (Lapides et al., 1976). Urinary organisms found during IC most often represent normal skin and urethral flora, and the asymptomatic colonization by these organisms may not be harmful. The first urinary tract infection in a hospitalized patient being managed with sterile intermittent catheterization clearly represents introduction of bacteria from the distal male urethra of female introitus.

Because most urinary tract infections are asymptomatic in these patients, there are serious questions concerning prophylaxis and treatment. Although it is quite clear that mucosal alteration occurs when the bladder is colonized by bacteria (Lloyd-Davies et al., 1971), it is not generally agreed that all bacteria are harmful and that reflux or upper tract damage follows. There is not much question, however, that renal failure in spinal cord injury patients is often associated with infection (Grundy et al., 1982). Gross and Liebowitz (1981) demonstrated radiologically that infection does not cause reflux in otherwise healthy children; their data tend to refute the concept that vesicoureteral reflux is secondary to infection. Kass and associates (1981) determined that renal function is preserved in children even in the presence of persistent bacteriuria on clean intermittent catheterization. They showed that clean IC in 248 children with neurogenic bladder followed for 1 to 10 years caused no worsening of any preexisting hydronephrosis. They used low-dosage antimicrobial prophylaxis in all children with evidence of renal damage or vesicoureteral reflux, but urinary bacteria were continuously present in one third of the children. Thirty-seven per cent of those having vesicoureteral reflux suffered febrile urinary tract infections, and surgery was necessary in 60 per cent of the kidneys with Grade II reflux, or worse, resulting from these febrile urinary tract infections. No deterioration in renal function was noted in any child during follow-up of serum creatinine and blood urea nitrogen values.

Despite the questions about the seriousness of bacteriuria in spinal cord patients and the apparent harmlessness of bacteriuria in children, it seems rational to keep the urinary tract sterile, if possible. Careful watchfulness for the early establishment of bacteriuria will prevent many serious infections. Simple dipstick detection of significant levels of bacteria using a nitrite test has not been accurate enough (Lenke and Van Dorsten, 1981), and dipsticks for detection of pyuria have been advocated (Gillenwater, 1981). These chemical strips are embedded with esterase color-sensitive substances that respond to enzymes produced by polymorphonuclear leukocytes. The dipstick result compares favorably with a hemacytometer chamber count. Other than such indirect methods of detecting significant bacteria, one is left with direct sampling of the bacteria themselves. A simple dipslide culture method is convenient and inexpensive (Anderson and Hatami-Tehrani, 1979). We use dipslides as preliminary screening on a daily basis; only when the patient shows $> 10^4$ colony-forming units per ml of urine for 2 days in succession do we go to the expense of identifying the organism and performing antimicrobial sensitivities. This avoids unnecessary work-up of transient episodes of bacteriuria.

In our diligence to define urinary tract infection by quantified bacterial cultures, we neglect to seriously consider pyuria. This reliance on bacterial cultures evolved because of the clinical imprecision of quantifying pyuria under the high-power objective of the microscope. It is a poor substitute for an Addis count, leukocyte excretion rate, or careful hemacytometer count. The degree of host response to bacteriuria, in the form of pyuria, should play an important role in the evaluation and treatment of such bacterial occurrences. Our data show considerable variation in patient response to rather innocuous levels of bacteriuria (Anderson and Hsieh-Ma, 1983).

Antibody coating of bacteria (ABC) has been studied to evaluate the significance of asymptomatic bacteriuria in the setting of a neurogenic bladder. A high incidence of antibody coating of bacteria was found in patients with external condom catheters (67 per cent), ileal loop diversions (63 per cent), and suprapubic indwelling catheters (60 per cent). Newman and associates (1980) reported that about one third of patients with positive ABC tests had upper urinary tract deterioration on x-ray and concluded that the presence of ABC in the urine indicates tissue invasion with antibody response, whether the infection is renal, bladder, or prostatic. Lindan (1981), on the other hand, maintains that testing for antibody coating is a useful epidemiologic tool but is not helpful as a guide to therapy. She found no association between evidence of active tissue invasion and the ABC test but did see significant differences among the various infecting species of bacteria. *Escherichia coli, Proteus mirabilis,* and *Klebsiella* organisms made up the majority of the antibody-coated groups; typical opportunistic organisms such as *Pseudomonas, Serratia, Providencia,* and *Citrobacter* were practically never antibody coated. This was true even on retesting after periods of 6 months to 2 years of continuous carriage. Merritt and Keys (1982) compared the ABC test with the Fairley washout test in 32 patients with neurogenic bladder dysfunction and concluded that the ABC test was unreliable for localization of urinary tract infections in neurogenic bladder patients. Ureteral catheterization and urine cultures are still the definitive diagnostic method.

ANTIMICROBIAL PROPHYLAXIS DURING INTERMITTENT CATHETERIZATION

It seems only natural that patients being managed for bladder dysfunction following spinal cord injury should be prevented from colonizing the urinary tract with bacteria. The neurogenic bladder is probably more susceptible to bacterial adherence owing to structural and neurologic changes, and any urinary tract infection in the setting of a neurogenic bladder is considered a complicated infection. Lapides (1965) advocated careful avoidance of overdistention of the bladder to retain host defense mechanisms. Studies in rabbits using transmission electron microscopy, 2 months after an episode of bladder stretching, revealed intracellular separation of the cytoplasm from the plasma membrane of detrusor muscle fibers, a probable precursor of fibrosis (Lloyd-Davies and Hinman, 1971). Bacterial elimination was impaired after this overdistention as compared with control rabbits.

Inoculation occurs when the catheter carries urethral microorganisms into the bladder, numbers of which are not completely flushed out. It is logical to use prophylactic antimicrobial solutions in the bladder; solutions such as chlorhexidine digluconate and povidone-iodine have been used but are often associated with severe chemical cystitis. Bactericidal antibiotics such as kanamycin, colistin, neomycin, and polymyxin B have been used. Neomycin is a potent broad-spectrum antibiotic, but Haldorson and coworkers (1978) evaluated weekly urine cultures of patients on IC and did not find any difference in the incidence of bacteriuria between the neomycin-treated group and the control group. Rhame and Perkash (1979) reported on a series of 70 male patients managed with a combination of neomycin and polymyxin B bladder instillations and reported 52 infections over 5000 patient days. This represents one infection per 100 days of catheterization. Pearman (1979) used 50 mg of kanamycin combined with 10 mg of colistin in water instillations after catheterizations and showed markedly improved infection rates over controls—approximately 2.3 infections per 100 days' catheterization. In our rehabilitation unit we use 160 mg of neomycin and 800,000 units of polymyxin B per liter of saline, and we have found that instilling 30 ml of this solution after each catheterization is effective in reducing bacterial colonization (Anderson, 1980). This represents 1.3 infections per 100 days of catheterization.

While it is very difficult to compare prophylactic regimens using intravesical or oral antimicrobial agents, Table 18–1 lists four published series, two with controls. The major difficulty with such comparisons is variability in reporting significant levels of bacteriuria. Pearman (1979) reported any two consecutive specimens (if the patient is catheterized at least every 12 hours) showing $>10^3$ organisms or one specimen with $>10^4$ organisms to be significant. Rhame and Perkash (1979) said any specimen showing $>10^3$ was significant, and Donovan and colleagues said the appearance of the same organism in any count for 2 consecutive days was significant. The second difficulty with comparisons of antimicrobial regimens is the variability in reporting rates of infection; some are reported as infections per number of patient IC days and others as a percentage of number of catheterizations. I recommend using 2 consecutive days of growth $>10^4$ as significant bacteriuria and reporting infection rates per 100 or 1000 patient IC days; patients should then be grouped according to catheterization frequency. Organisms usually cultured from spinal cord injury patients do not often cause infections of the normal bladder: *Staphylococcus epidermidis, Candida albicans,* and other commensals. Many of these are not sensitive to antimicrobial solutions used for bladder instillations, and it was for this reason that antimicrobial therapy using oral methenamine salts was an attractive alternative. The antimicrobial action of methenamine results from its conversion to formalde-

TABLE 18–1. Effectiveness of Antimicrobial Prophylaxis During Intermittent Catheterization

Authors	Prophylaxis	No. Infections per 1000 Patient-Days' Intermittent Catheterizaton	Mean Incidence of Significant Bacteriuria per Catheterization
Donovan et al. (1978)	Methenamine mandelate	31.4 (est.)*	0.007
Pearman (1979)	Kanamycin/colistin irrigant	23 (est.)	0.008
	Controls	43 (est.)	0.014
Rhame and Perkash (1979)	Neomycin/polymyxin B irrigant	10.3	0.003 (est.)
Anderson (1980)	Oral nitrofurantoin + neosporin/polymyxin B irrigant	13	0.002
	Controls	59	0.0096

*Calculation of equivalent rates only estimated from data provided.

hyde in an acid medium. Concentration of formaldehyde in the urine is dependent upon the pH and the rate of conversion of methenamine to formaldehyde. Although this particular method of prophylaxis is often used, it is frequently misunderstood and misused, with inadequate acidification of the urine. Because the bacteria must be in contact with the formaldehyde solution for long periods of time, the drug is totally ineffective in patients with indwelling catheters. In spite of the theoretical benefits of methenamine salts in suppression or prophylaxis of urinary tract infection, there have been disappointing results (Vainrub and Musher, 1977).

It may seem excessive to administer systemic antimicrobial agents to control local and often asymptomatic bacterial colonization of the urinary bladder, but their effectiveness in reducing urinary tract bacterial colonization cannot be denied. Of all the oral antimicrobial agents used for long-term prophylaxis of urinary tract infection, nitrofurantoin leads the list of acceptable formulations. This drug has been used with great success in prevention of recurrent cystitis in an otherwise healthy female population (Stamey et al., 1977). The major objection to use of long-term antibiotic prophylaxis is natural selection of resistant organisms in the fecal flora. Nitrofurantoin does not allow such resistant mutations, presumably owing to its rapid absorption in the sterile portions of the gut. I found that 100 mg given daily during intermittent catheterization is valuable in reducing infections in IC patients (Anderson, 1980). Duffy and Smith (1982) confirmed the value of nitrofurantoin in prophylaxis during intermittent catheterization for outpatients. Nitrofurantoin is not without side effects, nor is it completely free of potentially serious unexpected reactions. Pneumonitis, peripheral neuropathy, and chronic active hepatitis have been reported (Sharp et al., 1980; Holmberg et al., 1980). Fortunately, severe adverse reactions are rare and gastrointestinal upset or skin rash constitutes the occasional unpleasant side effect, occurring less often with the macrocrystal preparation.

Trimethoprim-sulfamethoxazole (TMP-SMX) will prevent urinary tract infection in low doses; Stamey and coworkers (1977) demonstrated its ability to prevent infection at one eighth the normal dose in women with recurrent cystitis. The drug eradicates Enterobacteriaceae from the gut in 70 per cent of cases and reaches adequate inhibitory concentrations in the vaginal secretion. Merritt and associates (1982) showed significantly less bacteriuria in both bladder-retrained and IC patients using one TMP-SMX regular-strength tablet at bedtime over long periods. Selection of resistant organisms has been reported and should be watched for.

Another oral agent used successfully for long-term prophylaxis is cinoxacin, similar in molecular structure to nalidixic acid but giving higher urine concentrations and slightly wider coverage. It also tends to eliminate Enterobacteriaceae from the bowel; a 5 per cent incidence of resistent organisms has been reported. We found this preparation to be the equivalent of nitrofurantoin in preventing bacteriuria during intermittent catheterization (Anderson and Barnewolt, in preparation). It was administered as 250 mg twice daily.

Extrapolating from the results obtained from using long-term antimicrobial prophylaxis in healthy patients suffering from recurrent bladder infections, one can easily advocate their use in the spinal cord–injured. In normal women who have three infections per year, the annual cost of prophylaxis is $85.82. Treatment of three acute episodes of infection costs $392.30 (Stamm et al., 1981). With the neurogenic bladder patient susceptible to serious sequelae, such as stones, vesicoureteral reflux, bladder fibrosis, and hydronephrosis, such preventive therapy is surely appropriate.

NEUROGENIC BLADDER BALANCE AND ASSOCIATED URINARY TRACT INFECTIONS

The major objective of any urologic rehabilitation program after spinal cord injury should be to promote urinary bladder emptying with the least degree of neuromuscular disturbance, to prevent infection, to preserve renal function, and to maintain socially acceptable bladder drainage. "Bladder retraining" achieves a catheter-free status. This often means restricting large amounts of fluid intake and suppressing uninhibited detrusor contractions until the bladder may be triggered to have a contraction and empty with relaxed outlet sphincters. This is said to represent a balanced bladder. Common techniques of triggering include suprapubic tapping, tugging pubic hairs, Valsalva, and anal sphincter stretching. Bladder retraining is really a misnomer; the patient is trained to develop the ability to suppress and facilitate neurophysiologic responses. If the reflexes are not intact or significant overactivity of the detrusor exists, no amount of "training" will enable the patient to adequately empty the bladder or maintain continence. Most patients do not possess a predictable and balanced (sphincter relaxation with bladder contraction) lower urinary tract system to trigger micturition. They are left with underactive bladders with or without intact sphincter tone and voiding may occur with abdominal or manual expression, or they are left with uncontrollable reflex, contractile bladders.

Residual urine by itself does not cause urinary tract infection, but the paraplegic has a susceptible reservoir contaminated as a result of intermittent catheterization or from condom urinary drains. The goal is to achieve minimal postvoid residual volumes. Perkash (1974) reported an average intermittent catheterization duration of 78 days after acute spinal injury before a satisfactory reflex bladder was achieved. Acceptable postvoid residual volumes have been variously and arbitrarily defined as less than 100 ml or less than 25 per cent of the bladder capacity at the time of voiding. Walter

and coworkers (1977) found that bacteriuria was significantly related to residual urine; 27 per cent of patients had significant bacteriuria with greater than 100 ml postvoid volume, and 12.6 per cent had significant bacteriuria with less than 50 ml. They also showed that the duration in minutes of an uninhibited bladder contraction was inversely proportional to the frequency of bacteriuria; the patients with less sustained contractions had fewer episodes of bacteriuria, indicating the favorability of an efficient emptying mechanism. Merritt (1981) reviewed the data of 105 patients during 1190 patient weeks to determine if residual urine volumes correlated with rates of urinary tract infection and found the mean volume was 192 ml for positive culture results and 159 ml for negative results, $p < 0.01$. Progressive increase in the rate of urinary tract infection occurred between residual volumes of 100 ml and 250 ml. The rate then decreased unexpectedly for residual volumes greater than 250 ml.

URODYNAMIC MONITORING

Urodynamic assessment has permitted a redefinition of treatment goals. Frequent monitoring of neuromuscular function of the lower urinary tract after the patient develops a contractile bladder allows judicious management with pharmaceutical agents or selective surgical procedures. These studies may demonstrate sphincter dyssynergia, a common cause of poor bladder emptying in males with an upper motor neuron lesion, and help determine whether intermittent catheterization should be discontinued or reinforced with anticholinergic agents.

To detect dangerous bladder pressures and distorted neurophysiology of micturition, one should carefully measure bladder pressure during slow- or medium-rate filling with body-temperature saline. Simultaneous measurement of the external sphincter pressure reveals the coordination or discoordination of the sphincter mechanism (Karol and Anderson, 1980). Excessive bladder pressures resulting from inadequate sphincter relaxation may be lowered by using both smooth muscle neuroreceptor blocking agents (phenoxybenzamine) and somatic muscle blockers (baclofen). The studies should be repeated several days after beginning oral pharmacologic therapy to confirm the agents' effectiveness. Patients exhibiting poorly balanced contractile bladders need frequent urodynamic assessment of their micturition during the first several months after injury. Abnormal measurements of bladder function may be seen long before radiographic changes of bladder distortion or trabeculation are appreciated on x-ray with simultaneous fluoroscopy or separate cystography.

In most rehabilitation centers the tendency is to discharge the patient from the hospital without continuing intermittent catheterization if he or she is voiding. While this may be an admirable goal, each patient must be individually assessed. It is truly unacceptable if the patient returns in a few months for follow-up and x-ray reveals bladder distortion, trabeculation, and possible upper urinary tract damage in the form of reflux or hydronephrosis. These anatomic changes are preceded by detectable physiologic alterations using urodynamics or nuclear isotope methods, and such monitoring techniques are mandatory in the early months of neurogenic bladder function.

Few isolated urodynamic measurements taken by themselves reveal a bladder that is in poor balance. This is particularly true of postvoid residual urine volumes, a common measurement of bladder balance. We studied patients three different times following spinal cord injury, concentrating on those who had return of

contractile bladders and spontaneous voiding. We looked at urodynamic measurements in relation to x-ray status of a cystogram, estimating bladder trabeculation (Anderson, 1983). Table 18–2 shows the urodynamic measurements obtained in groups of male patients showing bladder trabeculation versus those with normal-appearing bladders on x-ray. Urodynamic studies could not predict that a patient would have trabeculation on x-ray, particularly if postvoid residual urine volumes were used as an indicator; postvoid residual urine volumes were actually higher in the normal-appearing bladders. Only when the measurements were considered in combination did a useful micturition index emerge (Table 18–3), and it was numerically associated with trabeculation when the group was considered as a whole, i.e., a poor micturition index was more likely to be found in a patient with bladder deterioration. This same patient group also exhibited more urinary tract infection, but it was not statistically significant. Experience from this investigation convinced us that the 4- to 9-month interval following injury most frequently reveals urodynamic changes

TABLE 18–2. Urodynamic Measurements of Subjects with Nontrabeculated and Trabeculated Bladders

Urodynamic Measurement	Interval after Injury) (Mos.)	Bladder Condition on X-Ray*	
		NORMAL (NO. PTS.)	TRABECULATED (NO. PTS.)
Bladder vol. at onset of detrusor contraction (ml)	1 to 3	356 ± 24 (32)	257 ± 57 (10)
	4 to 9	335 ± 28 (24)	207 ± 24 (23)†
	10 to 24	291 ± 42 (9)	246 ± 31 (23)
Time from detrusor contraction to flow-opening time (sec)	1 to 3	100 ± 26 (19)	172 ± 63 (14)
	4 to 9	121 ± 39 (18)	82 ± 20 (21)
	10 to 24	68 ± 21 (9)	91 ± 25 (18)
Maximum premicturition intravesical pressure (cm water)	1 to 3	70 ± 9 (28)	83 ± 9 (14)
	4 to 9	72 ± 8 (21)	128 ± 13 (21)†
	10 to 24	72 ± 13 (9)	84 ± 10 (18)
Average flow rate (ml/sec)	1 to 3	4 ± 0.6 (25)	3 ± 0.5 (14)
	4 to 9	3 ± 0.6 (17)	3 ± 0.6 (20)
	10 to 24	4 ± 0.9 (9)	3 ± 0.5 (23)
Vol. voided (ml)	1 to 3	219 ± 22 (34)	124 ± 19 (14)†
	4 to 9	171 ± 21 (17)	140 ± 22 (20)
	10 to 24	181 ± 26 (9)	131 ± 14 (18)
Postvoid residual volume (ml)	1 to 3	185 ± 22 (34)	163 ± 57 (9)
	4 to 9	186 ± 22 (34)	106 ± 19 (21)†
	10 to 24	130 ± 42 (9)	159 ± 24 (22)
Av. voiding pressure (cm water)	1 to 3	52 ± 5 (24)	60 ± 7 (14)
	4 to 9	50 ± 7 (21)	70 ± 9 (21)‡
	10 to 24	42 ± 6 (9)	50 ± 8 (18)

*Mean ± standard error.
†p < 0.01 compared with normal group in same interval after injury.
‡p < 0.05 compared with normal group in same interval after injury.
(J. Urol., 129:777, 1983. Reproduced with permission from Williams & Wilkins Co., Inc.)

TABLE 18–3. MICTURITION INDEX IN MALE SPINAL CORD INJURY PATIENTS (VOLUME VOIDED × AVERAGE FLOW RATE/AVERAGE VOIDING BLADDER PRESSURE)

Interval after Injury (Mos.)	Bladder Condition on X-Ray*	
	NORMAL (NO. PTS.)	TRABECULTED (NO. PTS.)
1 to 3	26.6 ± 7.3 (19)	5.9 ± 1.0 (14)†
4 to 9	12.8 ± 3.1 (18)	4.7 ± 1.0 (19)†
10 to 24	21.3 ± 7.2 (10)	6.9 ± 1.2 (18)†

*Mean ± standard error.
†$p < 0.05$ compared with normal group in same interval after injury.
(J. Urol., *129*:777, 1983. Reproduced with permission from Williams & Wilkins Co., Inc.)

that may require pharmacologic or surgical therapy and that bladder deterioration may occur if these conditions are left untreated.

Other forms of urinary tract monitoring are useful to detect early aberration needing attention. Lloyd and associates (1981) recommend comprehensive renal scintillation procedures after spinal cord injury for rapid diagnostic screening of the upper urinary tract. Because the preparation for an intravenous urogram is particularly cumbersome for the paraplegic or quadriplegic patient, and the incidence of undesirable side effects not insignificant, much can be said for the isotope methodology. Decreased effective renal plasma flow and obstructive patterns of excretion may be detected in patients having a normal IVP or ultrasound scan. In some instances, minor x-ray abnormalities are detected in the face of a normal isotope study, but an isotope study permits detection of subtle changes, even in a single renal unit before anatomic distortion appears. Adequate early baseline examinations permit comparison with later testing. Tempkin and associates (1983) (personal communication) studied upper urinary tract deterioration secondary to neurogenic bladder by evaluating tubular transport patterns using I-131 hippuran radionuclide renal scanning. The scans in 52 patients revealed that 85 per cent had abnormalities; radioisotope excretion delays accounted for 65 per cent of those abnormalities. These physiologic changes appeared within 1 year of injury and usually in the presence of a normal IVP. Treating the patients with anticholinergic agents (oxybutynin, 5 mg p.o.) 3 hours prior to renal scanning significantly reduced excretion delay ($p < 0.02$).

In summary, it is important to prevent urinary tract infections in spinal cord injury patients, but early and frequent urodynamic

monitoring to detect dangerously high and inefficient voiding systems is also essential for protection of the patient. When the patient is able to catheterize himself or herself, we, and most patients, prefer intermittent catheterization to wearing a urinary collecting device. We utilize anticholinergic agents to suppress bladder overactivity, which reduces the likelihood of lower tract deterioration (Fig. 18–1). If this is impossible, we strive for a low-pressure contractile system. If pharmacologic agents are ineffective, the patient should have a sphincterotomy.

LONG-TERM UROLOGIC CARE

CHRONIC INDWELLING CATHETERS

There can be no question that the urologic outcome several years after spinal cord injury and secondary neurogenic bladder depends significantly upon how carefully the patient's bladder function is balanced and how successfully urinary tract infection is avoided. Many patients, however, succumb to the convenience of an indwelling draining catheter because of frustrations with infection, poor bladder emptying (often with attendant autonomic dysreflexia), and incontinence problems. Many quadriplegics with poor detrusor function, with or without sphincter dyssynergia, cannot perform intermittent catheterization and cannot afford around-the-clock attendant care. Even a sphincterotomy may be ineffective in promoting bladder emptying, and urethral organisms reflux easily through the opened sphincters to inoculate a pool of residual urine.

Many patients do well with long-term indwelling catheters—most often in the form of suprapubic tubes—but there is no question that their complication rate is higher, that renal function is more likely to be depressed, and that squamous cell carcinoma is more common (Hackler, 1982; Kaufman et al., 1977; Barkin et al., 1983). A convincing argument for avoidance of indwelling catheters and associated hospital nosocomial urinary tract infection was presented by Platt and coworkers (1982). They showed a distinctly positive association between infection and death in patients classified as having nonfatal or ultimately fatal disease. They suggested that 14 per cent of all deaths among catheterized patients represents an excessive association with infection induced by those catheters. Their study was conducted in an older age group than most spinal cord injury patients,

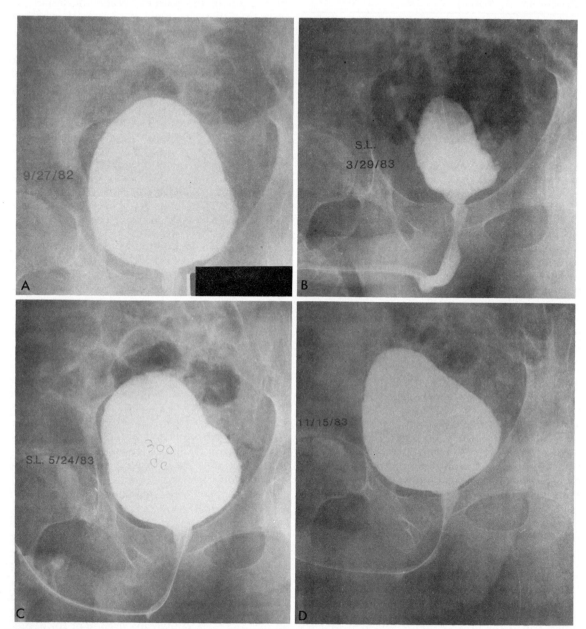

Figure 18–1. *A,* A 17-year-old male with C_7 spinal cord injury on 6-29-81 (sensory incomplete); he voids spontaneously and uses a condom urinary collecting device. Voiding cystourethrogram at 14 months post injury reveals slight bladder wall irregularity. *B,* Voiding cystourethrogram at 20 months post injury: Note severe distortion of bladder with trabeculation and right vesicoureteral reflux in spite of adequate sphincter opening. Urodynamics: External sphincter closing pressure on static profile was 140 cm water; bladder overactivity with detrusor contractions beginning at 25 ml fill (76 cm water pressure); maximum flow rate was 3 ml per second. *C,* Voiding cystourethrogram at 22 months post injury: loss of reflux and improvement of bladder distortion after treatment with oxybutynin, 5 mg t.i.d., and phenoxybenzamine, 10 mg b.i.d., for 6 weeks. Urodynamics: External sphincter closing pressure on profile was 90 cm water; maximum bladder pressure, 40 cm water at 360 ml fill; maximum flow rate was 2 ml per second. *D,* Voiding cystourethrogram at 28 months post injury shows incomplete emptying of bladder but without deterioration.

but it gives pause for thought nevertheless. Attempts to prevent infection with urethral meatal care and control of urinary drainage bag bacteria do not significantly change the morbidity of bacteriuria and cystitis (Burke et al., 1981; Maizels and Schaeffer, 1980).

Long-term urethral catheterization after spinal injury is associated with many other local complications well known to urologists (Hardy, 1968). Severe urethritis may occur with abscess formation and diverticulum development. Calculus formation in both the bladder and the upper tracts tends to accompany the indwelling catheter, but less so in patients who can maintain copious fluid intake. Acute epididymitis occurs on average in 15 per cent of males wearing urethral catheters and often follows changing of the catheter. Catheter plugging and bladder overdistention with consequent upper urinary tract infection and bacteremia are constant threats to the health of the individual.

If the need for intermittent catheterization has been overcome, males must usually wear external urinary collecting devices for their incontinence. Newer devices with self-adherent linings or double-stick soft tape wrapped around the penis facilitate comfortable wear with reasonable assurance of protection. Hirsh and associates (1979) showed that condom catheter collecting systems contribute to urinary infection, but that it depends in large part upon the management of the system. Kinking of the tube was a major reason for developing infection. Other problems besides infection interfere with the health of the male who must wear a condom catheter. Taping the condom too tightly may impede lymphatic drainage and cause edema. Cases of penile necrosis have been reported (Steinhardt and McRoberts, 1980); the sensory-deprived patient suffers insidious strangulation of the penis by the condom. Even under the best of conditions the patient must be ever alert to the possibility of skin maceration and formation of superficial ulcers. When these appear, a suprapubic catheter needs to be placed for about 2 weeks while the ulcer is treated with topical povidone-iodine or tincture of benzoin.

Urolithiasis occurs as a complication in about 6 per cent of spinal cord injury patients and is most commonly associated with infection. Many of the stones consist of struvite, a crystallization promoted by urea-splitting organisms such as *Proteus* or *Providencia* (Nikakhtar et al., 1981). Many young patients develop hypercalcemia and spill large quantities of calcium in their urine early after injury. Immobilization also leads to hypercalciuria. These patients most often have apatite (calcium-phosphate) stones, which are also susceptible to bacterial colonization and persistent bacteriuria. Upper urinary tract infection stones may require surgical removal, since antimicrobials cannot sterilize them. Occasionally, patients on intermittent catheterization may introduce a pubic hair into the bladder and create a nidus for crystallization; this may be prevented with careful catheterization and keeping the pubic hair cut short. Bladder stones manifest themselves with persistent pyuria (with or without bacteriuria), hematuria, and occasional bladder symptoms or autonomic dysreflexia. A plain-film radiograph may not reveal them, and cystoscopy is required. Most of the stones can be removed cystoscopically, using flexible tripartite grasping forceps or breaking the stone with a lithotrite and carefully washing out the fragments. An indwelling Foley catheter left in the bladder for a few days allows twice-daily instillations of 10 per cent renacidin solution, which helps to dissolve all of the remaining crystals.

One of the most frustrating clinical problems in the management of the chronic spinal cord–injured patient with a neurogenic bladder is persistent bacteriuria. The bacteriuria may be significant because it causes intermittent episodes of acute pyelonephritis, particularly if the patient has vesicoureteral reflux. Bacteriuria can be totally asymptomatic and fail to elicit low-grade pyuria. The attending physician is unsure how aggressive to be with such findings, particularly if the organism has developed resistance to all but the most potent parenteral antibiotics, such as third-generation cephalosporins or aminoglycosides. Localization of persistent bacteria may reveal infection stones in the upper collecting structures of the kidney, visible only with plain-film renal tomograms. Cystoscopic localization may exclude a prostatic reservoir of resistant bacteria. The technique includes washing the bladder thoroughly with irrigating fluid and taking a sample of this fluid for culture; it represents the maximal number of bacteria that can contaminate prostatic fluid. A prostatic massage is then performed with only a few milliliters of the irrigating fluid in the bladder. The prostatic secretion is washed into the bladder with minimal irrigating fluid and the pre- and postmassage fluids compared as to numbers of bacteria. A tenfold increase in bacterial colony counts from the postmassage specimen implicates the prostate as a source of the recurrent bacteriuria (Stamey, 1980).

It is only by a commitment to preserve the urinary tract after spinal cord injury that the attending physician can reduce the long-term morbidity and mortality associated with the neurogenic bladder. Patients must be convinced of the necessity for frequent monitoring of the urinary tract to prevent occult deterioration and its importance to a healthier and more productive life.

References

Anderson, R. U.: Prophylaxis of bacteriuria during intermittent catheterization of the acute neurogenic bladder. J. Urol., *123*:364, 1980.

Anderson, R. U.: Non-sterile intermittent catheterization with antibiotic prophylaxis in the acute spinal cord injured male patient. J. Urol., *124*:392, 1980.

Anderson, R. U.: Urodynamic patterns after acute spinal cord injury: Association with bladder trabeculation in male patients. J. Urol., *129*:777, 1983.

Anderson, R. U., and Barnewolt, B. A.: Cinoxacin vs. nitrofurantoin antimicrobial prophylaxis during intermittent catheterization after spinal cord injury. In preparation.

Anderson, R. U., and Hatami-Tehrani, G.: Monitoring for bacteriuria in spinal cord–injured patients on intermittent catheterization. Urology, *14*(3):244, 1979.

Anderson, R. U., and Hsieh-Ma, S. T.: Association of bacteriuria and pyuria during intermittent catheterization after spinal cord injury. J. Urol., *130*:299, 1983.

Barkin, M., Dolfin, D., Herschorn, S., Bharatwal, N., and Comisarow, R.: The urologic care of the spinal cord injury patient. J. Urol., *129*:334, 1983.

Burke, J. P., Garibaldi, R. A., Britt, M. R., Jacobson, J. A., and Conti, M.: Prevention of catheter-associated urinary tract infections. Am. J. Med., *70*:655, 1981.

Cook, J. B., and Smith, P. H.: Percutaneous suprapubic cystostomy after spinal cord injury. J. Urol., *48*:119, 1976.

Donovan, W. H., Kiviat, M. D., and Clowers, D. E.: Intermittent bladder emptying via urethral catheterization of suprapubic cystocath: A comparison study. Arch. Phys. Med. Rehabil., *58*:291, 1977.

Donovan, W. H., Stolov, W. C., Clowers, D. E., and Clowers, M. R.: Bacteriuria during intermittent catheterization following spinal cord injury. Arch. Phys. Med. Rehabil., *59*:351, 1978.

Duffy, L., and Smith, A. D.: Nitrofurantoin macrocrystals prevent bacteriuria in intermittent self-catheterization. Urology, *20*(1):47, 1982.

Erickson, R. P. Merritt, J. L., Opitz, J. L., and Ilstrup, D. M.: Bacteriuria during follow-up in patients with spinal cord injury: I. Rates of bacteriuria in various bladder-emptying methods. Arch. Phys. Med. Rehabil., *63*:409, 1982.

Gillenwater, J. Y.: Detection of urinary leukocytes by chemstrip-L. J. Urol., *125*:383, 1981.

Gross, G. W., and Liebowitz, R. L.: Infection does not cause reflux. Am. J. Radiol., *137*:929, 1981.

Grundy, J. D., Rainford, D. J., and Silver, J. R.: The occurrence of acute renal failure in patients with neuropathic bladders. Paraplegia, *20*:35, 1982.

Guttmann, L., and Frankel, H.: The value of intermittent catheterization in the early management of traumatic paraplegia and tetraplegia. Paraplegia, *4*:63, 1966.

Hackler, R. H.: Long-term suprapubic cystostomy drainage in spinal cord injury patients. Br. J. Urol., *54*:120, 1982.

Haldorson, A. M., Keys, T. F., Maker, M. D., and Opitz, J. L.: Nonvalue of neomycin instillation after intermittent urinary catheterization. Antimicrob. Agents Chemother., *14*:368, 1978.

Hardy, A. G.: Complications of the indwelling urethral catheter. Paraplegia, *5*:5, 1968.

Hinman, F., Jr.: Intermittent catheterization and vesical defenses. J. Urol., *117*:57, 1977.

Hirsh, D. D., Fainstein, V., and Musher, D. M.: Do condom catheter collecting systems cause urinary tract infection? JAMA, *242*:340, 1979.

Holmberg, L., Boman, G., Bottinger, L. E., Eriksson, B., Spross, R., and Wessling, A.: Adverse reactions to nitrofurantoin. Am. J. Med., *69*:733, 1980.

Kard, J. B., and Anderson, R. U.: Evaluation of synchronous water cystosphincterometry with the membrane catheter in spinal cord injury. J. Urol., *123*:907, 1980.

Kass, E. J., Koff, S. A., Diokno, A. C., and Lapides, J.: The significance of bacilluria in children on long-term intermittent catheterization. J. Urol., *126*:223, 1981.

Kaufman, J. M., Fam, B., Jacobs, S. C., Gabilondo, F., Yalla, S., Kane, J. P., and Rossier, A. B.: Bladder cancer and squamous metaplasia in spinal cord injury patients. J. Urol., *118*:967, 1977.

Lapides, J.: Role of hydrostatic pressure and distention in urinary tract infection. *In* Kass, E. H. (Ed.): Progress In Pyelonephritis. Philadelphia, F. A. Davis Co. 1965, p. 578.

Lapides, J., Diokno, A. C., Gould, F. R., and Lowe, B. S.: Further observations on self-catheterization. J. Urol., *116*:169, 1976.

Lenke, R. R., and Van Dorsten, J. P.: The efficacy of the nitrite test and microscopic urinalysis in predicting urine culture results. Am. J. Obstet. Gynecol., *140*:427, 1981.

Lindan, R.: The significance of antibody coated bacteria in neuropathic bladder urines. Paraplegia, *19*:216, 1981.

Lloyd, L. K., Dubovsky, E. V., Bueschen, A. J., Witten, D. M., Scott, J. W., Kuhlemeier, K., and Stover, S. L.: Comprehensive renal scintillation procedures in spinal cord injury: Comparison with excretory urography. J. Urol., *126*:10, 1981.

Lloyd-Davies, R. W., and Hinman, F., Jr.: Structural and functional changes leading to impaired bacterial elimination after overdistension of the rabbit bladder. Invest. Urol., *9*:136, 1971.

Maizels, M., and Schaeffer, A. J.: Decreased incidence of bacteriuria associated wtih periodic instillations of hydrogen peroxide into the urethral catheter drainage bag. J. Urol., *123*:841, 1980.

Maynard, F. M., and Diokno, A. C.: Clean intermittent catheterization for spinal cord injury patients. J. Urol., *128*:477, 1982.

Merritt, J. L.: Residual urine volume: Correlate of urinary tract infection in patients with spinal cord injury. Arch. Phys. Med. Rehabil., *62*:558, 1981.

Merritt, J. L., and Keys, T. F.: Limitations of the antibody-coated bacteria test in patients with neurogenic bladders. JAMA, *247*:1723, 1982.

Merritt, J. L., Erickson, R. P., and Opitz, J. L.: Bacteriuria during follow-up patients with spinal cord injury: II. Efficacy of antimicrobial suppressants. Arch. Phys. Med. Rehabil., *63*:413, 1982.

Namiki, T., Ito, H., and Yasuda, K.: Management of the urinary tract by suprapubic cystostomy kept under a closed and aseptic state in the acute stage of the patient with a spinal cord lesion. J. Urol., *119*:359, 1978.

Nanninga, J. B., Wu, Y., and Hamilton, B.: Long-term

intermittent catheterization in the spinal cord patient. J. Urol., *128*:760, 1982.

Newman, E., and Price, M.: Bacteriuria in patients with spinal cord lesions: Its relationship to urinary drainage appliances. Arch. Phys. Med. Rehabil., *58*:427, 1977.

Newman, E., Price, M., and Ederer, G. M.: Urinary tract infection in patients with spinal cord lesions: Antibody-coated bacteria tests as a diagnostic aid. Arch. Phys. Med. Rehabil., *61*:406, 1980.

Nikakhtar, B., Vaziri, N. D., Khonsari, F., Gordon, S., and Mirahmadi, M. D.: Urolithiasis in patients with spinal cord injury. Paraplegia, *19*:363, 1981.

Pearman, J. W.: The value of kanamycin-colistin bladder instillations in reducing bacteriuria during intermittent catheterization of patients with acute spinal cord injury. Br. J. Urol., *51*:367, 1979.

Perkash, I.: Intermittent catheterization: The urologist's point of view. J. Urol., *111*:356, 1974.

Platt, R., Polk, B. F., Murdock, B., and Rosner, B: Mortality associated with nosocomial urinary-tract infection. N. Engl. J. Med., *307*:637, 1982.

Rhame, F. S., and Perkash, I.: Urinary tract infections occurring in recent spinal cord injury patients on intermittent catheterization. J. Urol., *122*:669, 1979.

Sharp, J. R., Ishak, K. G., and Zimmerman, H. J.: Chronic active hepatitis and severe hepatic necrosis associated with nitrofurantoin. Ann. Intern. Med., *92*:14, 1980.

Stamey, T. A. (Ed.): *Pathogensis and Treatment of Urinary Infections.* Baltimore, Williams & Wilkins Co., 1980.

Stamey, T. A., Condy, W., Mihara, G.: Prophylactic efficacy of nitrofurantoin macrocrystals and trimethoprim-sulfamethoxazole in urinary infections. N. Engl. J. Med., *296*:780, 1977.

Stamm, W. E., McKevitt, M., Counts, G. W., Wagner, K. F., Turck, M., and Holmes, K. K.: Is antimicrobial prophylaxis of urinary tract infections cost effective? Ann. Intern. Med., *94*:251, 1981.

Steinhardt, G., and McRoberts, W.: Total distal penile necrosis caused by condom catheter. JAMA, *244*:11, 1980.

Stickler, D. J., Thomas, B., and Chawla, J. C.: Antiseptic and antibiotic resistance in gram-negative bacteria causing urinary tract infection in spinal cord injured patients. Paraplegia, *19*:50, 1981.

Tempkin, A. et al.: Personal communication. In preparation.

Vainrub, B., and Musher, D. M.: Lack of effect of methenamine in suppression of, or prophylaxis against, chronic urinary infection. Antimicrob. Agents Chemother., *12*:625, 1977.

Walter, S., Andersen, J. T., Hebjorn, S., and Vejlsgaard, R.: Detrusor hyperreflexia and bacteriuria. Urol. Int., *32*:117, 1977.

Yalla, S. V., Rossier, A. B., and Fam, B.: Dyssynergic vesicourethral responses during bladder rehabilitation in spinal cord injury patients: Effects of suprapubic percussion, Credé method and bethanechol chloride. J. Urol., *115*:575, 1976.

CHAPTER 19

Sexually Transmitted Diseases

RICHARD E. BERGER, M.D.

In the past decade, the incidence and variety of the known sexually transmitted diseases (STDs) have greatly increased. In addition to the five classic venereal diseases (syphilis, gonorrhea, chancroid, granuloma inguinale, and lymphogranuloma venereum), illnesses such as "idiopathic epididymitis," Reiter's syndrome, infant pneumonia, the female urethra syndrome, and acquired immunodeficiency syndrome (AIDS) have been shown to be sexually transmitted. Genital herpesvirus infection and AIDS are increasing at such a rapid rate as to cause panic in sexually active populations (Table 19–1).

The explosive increase in STDs has been accompanied by an explosion of information concerning them. The turnover in knowledge has been exceedingly rapid: What is considered accurate today may be incorrect tomorrow. The rapid changes have been due to advances in diagnostic techniques, in treatment methods, and, sometimes, even by mutations in STD organisms themselves. Changes in sexual behavior also mean STDs affect more people from a wide variety of social, economic, and ethnic backgrounds.

Thus, it is imperative that the physician treating STD make special efforts to be sure that his or her methods of diagnosis and treatment reflect the latest knowledge. Recommendations for STD treatment are periodically updated by the Centers for Disease Control (CDC). Changes that occur in the interim will need to come from a review of the current literature. The accurate diagnosis and treatment of an STD patient will allow the physician to treat not only the patient but also the sexual partner and even the couple's unborn children.

A major obstacle to the optimal treatment of STDs is, paradoxically, the inappropriate behavior of some health providers. *All* medical care personnel need to express a nonjudgmental and caring attitude toward patients with STDs. Many patients feel guilt or shame about the disease. Seeking care is often extremely difficult for them. They believe they will be singled out with a lecture on sexual ethics or that the behavior of the physician or nurse will make them feel unclean, undesirable, and unwanted as a patient. It is essential that health providers approach patients with understanding and sensitivity; otherwise, patients are very likely *not* to return for necessary treatment and their sexual partners may never be treated.

TRENDS

Sexually transmitted diseases, of course, are most common in young, sexually active people. The incidence of STD declines with age (Weström and Måardh, 1983; Bell and Hein 1984). As a result of the "baby boom" at the end of World War II, the sexually active group has been increasing in numbers. Not surprisingly, the prevalence of sexually transmitted disease has also been increasing. Since some of the most serious consequences of STDs, such as ectopic pregnancies and cervical carcinoma, may occur years after exposure to STDs, the sometimes tragic consequences of STD are also beginning to increase (Aral and Holmes, in press; Beral, 1974; Weström et al., 1981).

Rates continue to be higher in men than in women (Bell and Hein, 1984). In part, the apparently high STD rate in men may be due

TABLE 19–1. Pathogens for Which Sexual Transmission Is Important*

Agent	Disease or Syndrome
BACTERIA	
Neisseria gonorrhoeae	Urethritis, epididymitis, proctitis, cervicitis, endometritis, salpingitis, perihepatitis, bartholinitis, pharyngitis, conjunctivitis, prepubertal vaginitis, ?prostatitis, accessory gland infection, amniotic infection syndrome, disseminated gonococcal infection, chorioamnionitis, premature rupture of membranes, premature delivery
Chlamydia trachomatis	Urethritis, epididymitis, proctitis, cervicitis, endometritis, salpingitis, perihepatitis, bartholinitis, prepubertal vaginitis, otitis media in infants, ?chorioamnionitis, ?premature rupture of membranes, ?premature delivery, inclusion conjunctivitis, nasopharyngitis, infant pneumonia, trachoma, lymphogranuloma venereum
Mycoplasma hominis	Postpartum fever, ?salpingitis
Ureaplasma urealyticum	Nongonococcal urethritis, ?chorioamnionitis, ?premature delivery, infant pneumonia
Treponema pallidum	Syphilis
Gardnerella vaginalis	*Gardnerella*-associated ("nonspecific") vaginosis, neonatal sepsis
Haemophilus ducreyi	Chancroid
Calymmatobacterium granulomatis	Donovanosis (granuloma inguinale)
Shigella sp.	Enterocolitis
Campylobacter sp.	Enteritis, proctocolitis
Streptococcus agalactiae	Neonatal sepsis and meningitis
VIRUSES	
Herpes simplex virus	Initial and recurrent genital herpes, aseptic meningitis, neonatal herpes, cervical dysplasia and carcinoma, ?carcinoma in situ of the vulva
Hepatitis B virus	Acute hepatitis B, chronic active hepatitis, persistent (unresolved) hepatitis, polyarteritis nodosa, chronic membranous glomerulonephritis, ?mixed cryoglobulinemia, ?polymyalgia rheumatica, hepatocellular carcinoma
Hepatitis A virus	Acute hepatitis A
Cytomegalovirus	Heterophil-negative infectious mononucleosis, congenital infection, gross birth defects and infant mortality, neonatal brain damage, ?cervicitis, protean manifestations in the immunosuppressed host
Genital papilloma virus	Condyloma acuminatum, laryngeal papilloma, ?cervical dysplasia and carcinoma
Molluscum contagiosum	Genital molluscum contagiosum
PROTOZOA	
Trichomonas vaginalis	Vaginitis
Entamoeba histolytica	Enteritis, liver abscess
Giardia lamblia	Enteritis
FUNGI	
Candida albicans	Vulvovaginitis, balanitis
METAZOA	
Phthirius pubis	Pubic lice infestation
Sarcoptes scabiei	Scabies
Enterobius vermicularis	Proctitis

*From Holmes, K. K., et al.: Urol. Clin. North Am., *11*:3, 1984.

to the fact that symptoms and signs in men may be more obvious, with men more often seeking medical care. Also, men may have more sexual partners than women (Weström et al., 1981; Sorensen, 1972; Hunt, 1974). Certain STDs (syphilis, hepatitis, and gonorrhea) occur much more frequently in homosexual men than heterosexual men (Bell and Hein, 1984; Crawford et al., 1977; William, 1981).

Sexually transmitted diseases are becoming more frequent in women. Women's sexual behavior may be becoming like men's: More women are having intercourse at an earlier age, and the number of sexual partners a women is likely to have is increasing. This change in behavior has led to a proportional increase in STDs in women, along with an increase in the serious consequences often associated with

STDs: pelvic inflammatory disease (PID), infertility, ectopic pregnancy, and so forth (Bell and Hein, 1984).

Socioeconomic factors affect the prevalence and types of STDs. Persons of lowest socioeconomic status have the highest morbidity rates (Pedersen and Bonin, 1971). In the United States, Orientals have the lowest reported incidence of STDs; blacks have the highest, and whites occupy the middle category (Pedersen and Bonin, 1971; Weström et al., 1981).

Certain types of STDs apparently affect some groups more than others. Strains of gonorrhea that cause systemic disease are more common in blacks than whites (Knapp et al., 1978; Crawford et al., 1977). Genital herpes infection is more common in whites than in blacks (Corey, in press). Urban populations have higher rates of STDs than rural residents. In 1979, the 63 largest cities in the United States reported 53 per cent of the cases of gonorrhea and 65 per cent of the cases of syphilis, but only 27 per cent of the total population lived in those cities (U.S. Department of Health and Human Services CDC Statistics, 1981).

CONTACT TRACING

Examination and treatment of the sexual partners of the patients with STDs are essential to prevent re-infection, to prevent complications in sexual partners, and to limit spread of the disease in the community. *Sexual partners (especially in cases infected with syphilis,* Neisseria gonorrhoeae *or* Chlamydia trachomatis*) should be treated on the basis of contact. If partners are treated only if they become symptomatic, as many as 50 per cent of cases will remain untreated* (Johnson, 1979). *Furthermore, if cultures of partners are done and if the partner is treated only if the culture is positive, patients will be lost to follow-up, may possibly re-infect their partners, and may have increased risk of possible serious consequences of their infections.* Since approximately 60 per cent of patients who have one STD will have at least one other, examination of the patients and their partners for other STD and treatment of that disease are highly recommended (Wentworth et al., 1973).

URETHRITIS

Gonococcal Urethritis in Men

Gonococcal urethritis (GU) is associated with the gram-negative diplococcus, *N. gonor-*

rhoeae. The incubation period for GU varies from 3 to 10 days, but exceptions are very common. For example, some strains of gonococci will produce symptoms in a period as short as 12 hours. Others may take as long as 3 months to manifest themselves (Harrison, 1984).

EPIDEMIOLOGY

Most cases of gonococcal urethritis are acquired during intercourse. For a man, the risk of acquiring gonorrhea during a single episode of intercourse with an infected partner is approximately 17 per cent (Greenberg, 1979). This risk increases as the number of sexual contacts with an infected partner increases. Not only can the gonococcus be transmitted by direct vaginal exposure, but there is increasing evidence that infection may be transmitted through oral sex with a partner whose pharynx is infected. There have been cases of gonorrhea that have been acquired from infected secretions without vaginal penetration.

SYMPTOMS AND SIGNS

Classically, gonococcal urethritis produces urethral discharge and burning on urination. The discharge is usually profuse and purulent, but it may be scant or even absent. *Gonococcal urethritis may be asymptomatic in 40 to 60 per cent of the contacts of partners with known gonorrhea* (Crawford et al., 1937; John and Donald, 1978; Portnoy et al., 1974). *Without treatment, even symptomatic gonorrhea will improve. However, the host may remain a carrier and be potentially infective* (McCutchan, 1981).

PREVENTION

Gonorrhea may be prevented by the regular use of condoms, postcontact antibiotics, and intravaginal application of antiseptics and antibiotics. Although condoms can prevent urethrally acquired gonorrhea, most men do not use this protection (Hooper et al., 1978).

Unfortunately, the indiscriminate use of prophylactic antibiotics can result in the development of resistant strains of gonococci (Harrison, 1979). The impact of intravaginal bacteriostatic agents is currently unknown (Cates et al., 1982). Researchers are working to develop immunization against *N. gonorrhoeae* (Marx, 1980), but immune vaccines are not yet available.

DIAGNOSIS

Laboratory procedures are essential for the accurate diagnosis of gonorrhea. *Because gonococcal infections occur in areas that have extensive normal bacterial noncontaminated flora such as the urethra, it is extremely important to collect noncontaminated specimens.* Urethral specimens must be obtained from within the urethra and *not* simply from a drop of discharge. Collect specimens with a calcium alginate (Calgiswab, Inolex) urethrogenital swab; wait at least 1 hour (preferably 4 hours) after the patient has urinated before swabbing. Swabs need to be inserted 2 to 4 cm into the urethra and rotated gently. Cotton swabs should be avoided because of a bacteriocidal effect (Kellogg et al., 1976). If there is a history of oral-genital contact, also collect pharyngeal swabs. In homosexual men and all women, obtain rectal swabs. Directly inoculate swabs on the culture medium. The same swab may be used for Gram staining. If this is not possible, collect two specimens. The swab should be rolled onto the slide as white blood cells may be disrupted if roughly rubbed. The slide then can be heat-fixed and air-dried and examined immediately. Trained laboratory personnel who regularly read Gram stains can make the diagnosis of gonorrhea with approximately a 99 per cent specificity and 95 per cent sensitivity (Granato et al., 1981).

Because the gonococcus is an extremely friable organism, the preferred method of diagnosis is to plate the urethral swab onto the culture medium directly. Transport media should be used to take specimens to the laboratory when direct plating of specimens cannot

be done (James-Holmquest, et al., 1973). Although there are a number of serologic and fluorescent antibody tests available for diagnosis, the high sensitivity and specificity of the Gram stain make these tests unnecessary in most instances (Harrison, 1984).

The rapid increase in the resistance of gonorrhea to the commonly used antibiotics means that cultures for N. gonorrhoeae *are now an absolute necessity.* The emergence of penicillin- and tetracycline-resistant strains of gonococci has made it mandatory to perform cultures on patients from geographic areas where resistant organisms are prevalent. The modified Thayer-Martin and New York City media (Thayer, 1966; Granato et al., 1981; Riccardi and Felman, 1979) are the most effective. Details of the culturing of gonococci obtained from the American Society of Microbiology (Kellogg et al., 1976).

TREATMENT

Gonococcal urethritis was initially treated by instillation of antiseptic agents into the urethra (Kampmeier, 1983). In the mid-1930's, sulfa drugs were used successfully. However, resistance quickly developed (Campbell, 1944; Dees and Colston, 1937). During the 1940's, gonococcal urethritis was treated successfully with penicillin. Since then, the amount of penicillin needed to treat gonorrhea has steadily

TABLE 19–2. TREATMENT OF GONOCOCCAL URETHRITIS IN MEN*

Treatment	Advantages	Disadvantages
Tetracycline, 500 mg orally q.i.d. for 7 days, or doxycycline, 100 mg orally b.i.d. for 7 days	1. Effective against coexisting chlamydial infections	1. Compliance required 2. May encourage tetracycline resistance 3. Ineffective against anorectal infections
Amoxicillin, 3.0 gm or ampicillin 3.5 gm, with 1 gm probenecid orally	1. Single dose	1. Ineffective against coexisting chlamydial infections 2. Ineffective against anorectal and pharyngeal infections
Aqueous procaine penicillin G: 4.8 million units i.m. with 1.0 gm of probenecid	1. Single dose	1. Injection 2. Possible procaine reaction 3. Possible anaphylaxic 4. Ineffective against coexisting chlamydial infections
Amoxicillin, 3.0 gm orally, or ampicillin, 3.5 gm with 1 gm probenecid orally, *plus* tetracycline, 500 mg orally q.i.d. for 7 days, or doxycycline, 100 mg p.o. b.i.d. for 7 days	1. Adequate single-dose treatment for gonorrhea 2. Effective against chlamydial infections	1. Efficacy and side effects not evaluated

*Modified from Berger, R. E.: Semin. Urol., *1*:138, 1983.

increased (Harrison et al., 1978). In 1976, the gonococcus acquired a plasmid for penicillinase production, making some strains *totally* resistant to penicillin (John and Donald, 1978). Since 1972, the CDC has issued recommendations for the treatment of gonorrhea. The summary of the current CDC recommendations for treatment of gonorrhea with their advantages and disadvantages is listed in Table 19–2. Penicillin, ampicillin, and amoxicillin regimens are all extremely effective in eradicating urethritis in individuals with penicillin-sensitive organisms. However, the current *recommended* treatment for gonococcal urethritis includes a tetracycline or a tetracycline derivative, because about 30 per cent of men with gonococcal urethritis also will be infected with *C. trachomatis*. Although *N. gonorrhoeae* is usually sensitive to penicillin, *C. trachomatis* is not sensitive to penicillin. Both *C. trachomatis* and *N. gonorrhoeae* are usually sensitive to tetracycline. If rectal or pharyngeal gonorrhea is present, however, penicillin is still the drug of choice. Spectinomycin, cefoxitin, cefotaxime, and trimethoprim-sulfamethoxazole are recommended for patients with penicillinase-producing *N. gonorrhoeae* (PPNG) (Table 19–3).

It is extremely important that all patients treated for gonorrhea have adequate follow-up. Three to 7 days after therapy, repeat all cultures and examine the patient. Rectal cultures in women and pharyngeal and rectal cultures in homosexual men must be repeated. If symptoms of urethritis persist, the patient could still be infected or could have developed postgonococcal urethritis. All patients who still have gonococci in their urethral secretions should be treated—immediately—for PPNG. Test the antibiotic sensitivities of the organism. If the organism was susceptible to the original medication, the patient's persistent illness is most likely due to re-infection.

Nongonococcal Urethritis in Men

The incidence of nongonococcal urethritis (NGU) has increased faster than any other sexually transmitted disease except, perhaps, Herpes simplex II (Aral and Holmes, 1984) (Fig. 19–1). The morbidity of clinical infections and complications of NGU may be equal to and perhaps greater than that of gonococcal disease (Table 19–4). However, since NGU infections are not reported to health authorities, the sexual partners of infected patients often are not examined or treated. Therefore, the incidence of NGU and its associated infections will probably continue to increase.

Young men are prime candidates for contracting NGU. Nongonococcal urethritis more often affects men of higher socioeconomic status than does gonococcal urethritis (Wiesner, 1977). Urethritis in homosexual men is less likely to be nongonococcal and more likely to be gonococcal.

ETIOLOGY

Nongonococcal urethritis is a syndrome with several causes and not an etiologic diagnosis (Table 19–5). *The most important and potentially dangerous pathogen involved in NGU is* C. trachomatis. *C. trachomatis* can be blamed for 30 to 50 per cent of NGU cases (Alani et al, 1977; Bowie et al., 1977, 1980; Segura et al., 1977; Wong et al., 1977; Paavonen et al., 1977; Terho et al., 1978b; Csango et al., 1978; Ripa et al., 1978; Perroud and Miedzybrodzka, 1978; Bowie et al., 1978; Swartz et al., 1978; Lassus et al., 1979; Coufalik et al., 1979; Taylor-Robinson and McCormack, 1979).

Bowie et al. (1977) have summarized evidence in favor of *C. trachomatis* in the etiology of NGU:

1. Chlamydia can be isolated from the urethra of 25 to 60 per cent of men who have

TABLE 19–3. Antibiotics Effective Against PPNG

Spectinomycin	2 gm intramuscularly (single dose)
Cefoxitin	2 gm intramuscularly, plus 1 gm of probenecid by mouth
Cefotaxime	1 gm intramuscularly
The following regimens are effective but have not been approved by the FDA:	
Cefaclor	500 mg orally four times daily for 5 days
Sulfamethoxazole/trimethoprim	Nine single-strength tablets in a single daily dose for 3 days total therapy

*Modified from Harrison, W. O.: Urol. Clin. North Am., *11*:45, 1984.
Abbreviations: PPNG = Penicillinase-producing *Neisseria gonorrhoeae;* FDA = Food and Drug Administration.

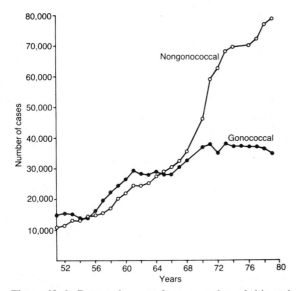

Figure 19–1. Reported cases of gonococcal urethritis and nongonococcal urethritis in men in clinics in England and Wales, 1951–1979. (From Aral, S. O., and Holmes, K. K.: *In* Holmes, K. K., et al. (Eds.): Sexually Transmitted Diseases. New York, McGraw-Hill Book Company, In press. Used by permission.)

TABLE 19–4. DISEASES ASSOCIATED WITH THE SEXUAL TRANSMISSION OF NEISSERIA GONORRHOEAE AND CHLAMYDIA TRACHOMATIS*

N. gonorrhoeae	C. trachomatis
Urethritis	Urethritis
Cervicitis	Cervicitis
Salpingitis	Salpingitis
Bartholinitis	Bartholinitis
Perihepatitis	Perihepatitis
Arthritis	Reiter's syndrome
Urethral syndrome	Urethral syndrome
Proctitis	Proctitis
Conjunctivitis	Conjunctivitis
Endocarditis	Endocarditis
Asymptomatic	Pneumonia
	Otitis media
	Asymptomatic

*From Berger, R. E.: *In* Stamey, T. A.: Monographs in Urology, Burroughs Wellcome, 1982.

NGU (Alani et al., 1977; Bowie et al., 1977*c*, 1980; Segura et al., 1977; Wong et al., 1977; Paavonen, 1978; Terho, 1978; Csango, 1978; Ripa et al., 1978; Perroud and Miedzybrodzka, 1978; Swartz et al., 1978; Lassus et al., 1979; Coufalik et al., 1979; Taylor-Robinson and McCormack, 1979). Conversion and the formation of IgM antibodies against *C. trachomatis* can be demonstrated in men with NGU with positive urethral cultures for *C. trachomatis*.

2. Up to 80 per cent of sexual contacts in men with *C. trachomatis* also will have *C. trachomatis* (Linder, 1911; Holmes et al., 1975; Richmond and Sparling, 1976).

3. Differential responses to therapy can be demonstrated in chlamydia-positive and chlamydia-negative cases (Bowie et al., 1976; Coufalik et al., 1979; Handsfield et al., 1975).

4. Postgonococcal urethritis develops in men who contract gonococcal and chlamydial infection simultaneously (Alani et al., 1977; Segura et al., 1977; Richmond et al., 1972; Oriel et al., 1975; Vaughn-Jackson et al., 1977; Terho, 1978*a*; Bowie et al., 1978) and who are treated with penicillin to which chlamydia is not sensitive.

Chlamydia trachomatis can be recovered from the urethra in 25 to 60 per cent of heterosexual men with NGU, in 4 to 35 per cent of men with gonorrhea, and in 0 to 7 per cent of men seen in STD clinics without symptoms of urethritis (Schachter, 1978). Although asymptomatic infection seems to be infrequent in men seen in STD clinics, asymptomatic infection occurs in 50 per cent of the contacts of women with chlamydia cervical infections (Thelin et al., 1980).

TABLE 19–5. ETIOLOGY OF SEXUALLY TRANSMITTED NONGONOCOCCAL URETHRITIS (NGU)*

	Acute†	Persistent‡	Recurrent§
Chlamydia trachomatis	30–50%	0%	0–5%
Ureaplasma urealyticum	30–40%	40–50%	10–20%
Neither	20–30%	50–60%	70–80%
Trichomonas vaginalis	1–2%	5–10%	1–2%
Herpes simplex virus	1–2%	5–10%	0%
Yeasts	Rare	Rare	Rare
Gardnerella vaginalis	Rare	Rare	Rare
Staphylococcus saprophyticus	Rare	?Never	?Never
Corynebacterium genitalium	Rare	?Never	?Never
Others	?	?	?

*From Bowie, W. R.: Urol. Clin. North Am., *11*:55, 1984.
†Acute NGU = Less than 1 month's duration, without prior treatment for that episode.
‡Persistent NGU = Persists unchanged or only minimally improved at the end of 1 week of tetracycline.
§Recurrent NGU = Recurs within 6 weeks of starting treatment, without intercourse with a new or untreated partner.

From 20 to 50 per cent of men with NGU may have infections with *Ureaplasma urealyticum*. Information on the pathogenic role of *U. urealyticum* in the etiology of NGU has been difficult to interpret because genital colonization with this organism is directly proportional to the patient's number of previous sexual partners. With three to five partners, specimens from 40 per cent of men and 70 per cent of women will contain ureaplasma (Taylor-Robinson and McCormack, 1980).

Evidence for the role of *U. urealyticum* in NGU has come from several sources. When men with relatively few sexual partners and no history of urethritis are examined, the rate of isolation of *U. urealyticum* is significantly higher in those men with negative chlamydia cultures than in those with positive cultures (Bowie et al., 1977c). Treatment studies have also shown a pathogenic role for chlamydia. Bowie et al. (1976) found that men with *C. trachomatis*–negative, *U. urealyticum*–positive urethritis responded poorly to sulfonamides but well to aminocyclotol, to which *U. urealyticum* but not *C. trachomatis* is sensitive. It has also been shown that NGU persists in a group of chlamydia-negative patients with NGU who have persistence of ureaplasma (Root et al., 1980; Stimson et al., 1981; Swartz et al., 1978). Furthermore, endourethral inoculation of ureaplasma in nonhuman primates has produced colonization of urethritis (Taylor-Robinson and McCormack, 1980). Of the 14 serotypes of *U. urealyticum,* some may be more pathogenic than others. So far, there is no convincing evidence that *U. urealyticum* harms women or the children to whom they give birth.

In 20 to 30 per cent of cases of men with acute urethritis, the cause cannot be determined. Although these men may show improvement or even be cured with antibiotics, the cause of their urethral inflammation cannot be definitely determined (Bowie et al., 1981). Herpes simplex virus (Holmes et al., 1975), cytomegalovirus, *Trichomonas vaginalis,* and other organisms have not been convincingly shown to be associated with the majority of these cases (Bowie et al., 1977; Swartz et al., 1978).

There is no evidence that drinking caffeinated beverages or alcohol may cause urethritis, nor has it been shown that stripping the urethra will cause urethritis.

DIAGNOSIS

The usual incubation period for nongonococcal urethritis is 1 to 5 weeks. Longer incubation periods often occur. The usual symptoms include dysuria and urethral discharge. Diagnosis of NGU requires demonstration of urethritis and exclusion of infection with *N. gonorrhoeae.* Urethral discharge is often scant; however, it may be thick and purulent. Discharge may not be present and the patient may complain only of urethral itch (Jacobs and Kraus, 1975). Asymptomatic infection is common, especially among contacts of women with known cervical chlamydia infection.

The man suspected of having urethritis ideally should be examined after 4 hours of urinary continence so that discharge may be reliably demonstrated (Fig. 19–2). On Gram stain urethral swab, more than four polymorphonuclear leukocytes per field in five 1000-power oil immersion fields correlate with urethritis. Alternatively, the presence of 15 or more polymorphonuclear leukocytes in five random 400-power fields of the spun sediment of the first-void urine correlates with urethritis (Bowie, 1978; Swartz et al., 1978). *When urethritis is suspected but urethral inflammation cannot be detected, the patient should be examined in the early morning before voiding.* Simmons (1978) found that of 200 men with genitourinary symptoms without urethritis on initial examination, 108 had urethritis diagnosed when examined in the early morning.

Cultures for the detection of *C. trachomatis* should be employed when available. Because *C. trachomatis* is an intracellular parasite of columnar epithelium (Fig. 19–3), the appropriate specimen for culture is an endourethral swab rather than urethral exudate or urine. The specimen must be taken carefully from 2 to 4 mm inside the urethra and placed in special transport media. It then may be frozen to $-70°$ C and stored, or kept at $4°$ C and delivered to the laboratory, where it should be inoculated promptly. Preliminary culture results are available 2 to 3 days after inoculation. Although many physicians believe that cultures are unnecessary, *C. trachomatis* is a dangerous pathogen, and culture results may serve both as guide to therapy and as proof of cure.

TREATMENT

Since NGU is a syndrome that can be caused by many different organisms that respond differently to treatment, results of therapy are inconsistent. The current recommendations from the Centers for Disease Control are based on chlamydia infection and are given in Table 19–6.

The cause of the urethritis appears to be

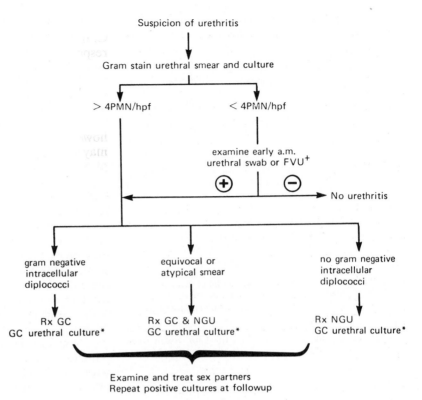

Figure 19–2. Flow chart for the management of urethritis.

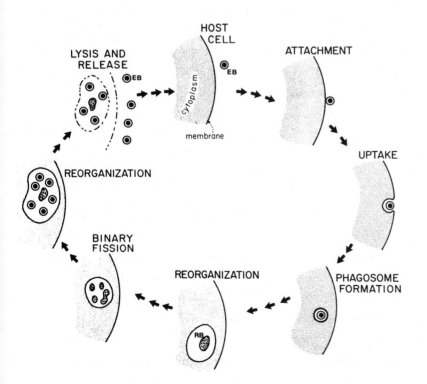

Figure 19–3. Life cycle of *Chlamydia trachomatis*. (From Krieger, J. N., Urol. Clin. North Am., *11*:15, 1984.)

TABLE 19–6. MANAGEMENT OF NONGONOCOCCAL
URETHRITIS (NGU)*

A. Investigation
 1. Careful physical examination
 2. Demonstrate a polymorphonuclear leukocyte
    response—Gram stain or first voided urine
    sediment
 3. Exclude *Neisseria gonorrhoeae* infection—Gram
    stain ± culture
 4. Reassess in the morning prior to voiding if
    necessary

B. Initial Management of NGU if Diagnosed
 1. Seven days of treatment with tetracycline 500 mg
    q.i.d., or minocycline or doxycycline, 100 mg
    twice daily or erythromycin 500 mg q.i.d. for 7
    days
 2. Treat partner(s) appropriately

C. Management of Persistent or Recurrent NGU
 1. Question about compliance and re-exposure
 2. Examine carefully for less usual causes of uethritis
 3. Demonstrate urethritis
 4. Treat any specific cause that can be elucidated
 5. If a specific etiology is not found or *Ureaplasma
    urealyticum* is present, treat with erythromycin
    base 500 mg q.i.d. for 14 days

*Modified from Bowie, W. R.: Urol. Clin. North Am.,
11:55, 1984.

the best indicator of response to therapy. Men
with *C. trachomatis* respond the best and men
with neither *C. trachomatis* nor *U. urealyticum*
respond the worst to therapy (Bowie et al.,
1981).

*In the absence of culture, NGU should be
assumed to be caused by* C. trachomatis. *C.
trachomatis* can be isolated from 30 to 60 per
cent of female partners of men with NGU (Alani
et al., 1977; Paavonen et al., 1978; Terho,
1978*b*; Lassus et al., 1979; Holmes et al., 1975;
Oriel et al., 1975). Therefore, as part of the
management of urethritis, every attempt should
be made to treat the patient's sexual partner
promptly. In general, the same regimen used to
treat the male should be used to treat the
female.

RECURRENCE

Recurrent or persistent NGU may be due
to:

1. Re-infection with the initial organism
(usually from re-exposure to the same sexual
partner who has not been treated).

2. Persistence of the original organism due
to antibiotic resistance.

3. Idiopathic failure, usually in cases where
chlamydia or ureaplasma are not found.

Recurrence that is due to re-infection often
can be prevented if the sexual partner is treated
concurrently. Exposure to a different infected
partner is difficult to prevent. When both male

and female partners are treated concurrently
with a tetracycline regimen, *C. trachomatis* is
almost never isolated at the time of recurrence.
Since C. trachomatis *causes major morbidity
whereas the other organisms involved in NGU
cause minimal morbidity, every effort should be
made to eradicate and confirm the eradication of*
C. trachomatis. Cultures are most helpful in this
respect.

Recurrence caused by resistance to tetracycline therapy is almost never due to *C. trachomatis*. However, *U. urealyticum* can be isolated in 20 to 30 per cent of men at the time of
recurrence (Bowie et al., 1981). *Chlamydia trachomatis* usually is not resistant to tetracycline;
however, tetracycline-resistant *U. urealyticum*
may be one cause of persistent urethritis (Root
et al., 1980; Stimson et al., 1981). To eradicate
the infection, treat patients with erythromycin
for 1 to 2 weeks. Treatment of sexual partners
with erythromycin also may be indicated (Table
19–6).

Not surprisingly, the urologist often sees
patients with urethral discharge or symptoms
who have had multiple courses of antibiotics
effective against both *C. trachomatis* and *U.
urealyticum*. *It is imperative that urethritis and
urethral inflammation be properly diagnosed in
these patients*. Sometimes patients can express a
small amount of mucoid material from the urethra; however, this does not contain inflammatory cells, and therefore the patient cannot be
considered to have true urethritis. If the patient
does continue to have a discharge, cultures for
T. vaginalis should be performed and smears
examined for fungi with 10 per cent potassium
hydroxide. Examination of the sexual partner
may be of help in determining the etiology,
especially with *T. vaginalis* infection. If no pathogens are detected, urethroscopy and cystoscopy should be performed to detect possible
intraurethral lesions.

COMPLICATIONS IN MEN

In most cases, chlamydia-negative urethritis
does not cause severe complications in men.
Some cases of salpingitis and resulting infertility
in females are related to neither gonococcal nor
chlamydia infection; however, it is not known
whether nonchlamydial urethritis in men can
lead to transmission and complications in their
female partners.

It is essential that male patients with chlamydia-negative urethritis be given correct information and emotional reassurance. Many men
are ridden with guilt at the thought of spreading
a sexually transmitted disease. In general, the

physician can tell the patient that chlamydia-negative recurrent urethritis is a nuisance, but usually is of no serious consequence to the patient's health, or that of his wife, girl friend, or children.

Urethritis in Women

Sexually transmitted diseases are a frequent cause of the urethral syndrome in women. Although women, unlike men, usually do *not* have a urethral discharge, *N. gonorrhoeae* and *C. trachomatis* may be common pathogens in the female urethra. These organisms have been isolated from the urethra of 10 per cent of women in venereal disease clinics (Wallin et al., 1981). Dysuria occurs in approximately 20 per cent of women with chlamydial or gonococcal infections attending venereal disease clinic (Paavonen, 1979; Wong et al., in press). When these women present in other settings, the physician may erroneously diagnose bladder infection. Urinalysis may often show pyuria, but culture for routine urinary pathogens will be sterile. Curran et al. in 1975 found gonorrhea in 30 per cent of the women who presented to the emergency room with symptoms of urinary tract infection. Of 13 patients with insignificant growth on their routine urine cultures, eight were actually infected with *N. gonorrhoeae*. Of 32 women with the urethral syndrome, pyuria, and sterile bladder urine, 11 were found to have chlamydia infection (Stomm et al., 1980). Since

women with urinary symptoms caused by *C. trachomatis* or *N. gonorrhoeae* potentially may suffer more serious consequences from their infection than those with coliform bladder infection, it is essential that the physician accurately diagnose and appropriately treat patients with the urethral syndrome (Fig. 19–4).

Other STDs may cause urinary symptoms. Women with *primary genital herpes infection* will often have dysuria (Corey et al., 1983). Vaginitis is also a common cause of dysuria. Diagnosis is made by pelvic examination and examination of the vaginal secretions (Komaroff et al., 1978; Wallin et al., 1981). Stamm et al. (1980, 1984) have seen ureaplasmas in quantities of greater than 10^3 organisms per milliliter from six of ten (60 per cent) women with acute urethral syndrome of unknown etiology and pyuria, but in only nine of 26 (35 per cent) women with acute urethral syndrome without pyuria. The significance of ureaplasma in the etiology of the urethral syndrome requires further study.

EPIDIDYMITIS

Acute epididymitis is a clinical syndrome resulting from acute inflammation, pain, and swelling of the epididymis. It should not be confused with *chronic* epididymitis, which involves chronic pain in the epididymis and testicle, usually without swelling.

Acute epididymitis has been a major cause

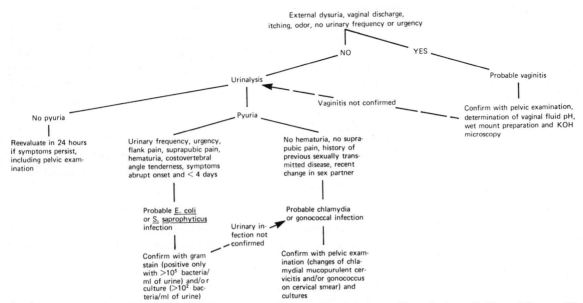

Figure 19–4. Flow chart for the management of dysuria and frequency in women. (From Latham, R. H., and Stamm, W. E.: Urol. Clin. North Am., *11*:95, 1984. Used by permission.)

of loss of work. In the military, it is a major cause of hospital admissions to urology wards (Hanley, 1966; Shapiro and Breschi, 1973; Sufrin, 1980). Complications from acute epididymitis include abscess formation, testicular infarction, and development of chronic pain and infertility (Gartman, 1961; Bietz, 1959; Pelouse, 1941).

ETIOLOGY

Until recently, most of the cases of epididymitis in young men were considered to be "idiopathic." Physicians thought that inflammation resulted from *sterile* urine being forced down the vas deferens while the patient strained against a closed external urethral sphincter. Graves and Engle in 1950 developed a dog model that tended to confirm this theory. However, in military studies, fewer than 10 per cent of patients with epididymitis had a history of straining (Mittemeyer et al., 1966). In a series of civilian patients, only two of 50 patients had a history of straining, and both of these patients were concurrently infected with *C. trachomatis* (Berger et al., 1979). Although the reflux of sterile urine down the vas deferens may occur when men with normal urinary tracts strain, such reflux probably would not cause pyuria and urethritis seen in the vast majority of these young men.

Epididymitis caused by sexually transmitted organisms occurs mainly in sexually active males under the age of 35 (Olier, 1981; Berger et al., 1979). The majority of cases of epididymitis in children and older men, on the other hand, are due to the common urinary pathogens.

Epididymitis is usually caused by spread of infection from the urethra or bladder. The most common etiology of epididymitis in any particular group appears to be the most common cause of genitourinary infection in that group. Although epididymitis is uncommon in children, the most common cause of epididymitis is the coliform organisms that cause bacteriuria. In men under the age of 35, bacteriuria is uncommon while urethritis from *N. gonorrhoeae* and *C. trachomatis* is common. The most common cause of epididymitis in young men is therefore due to the organisms that cause urethritis (Berger, 1978; Berger et al., 1979). Approximately two thirds of men under age 35 with noncoliform, nongonococcal epididymitis have *C. trachomatis* as the etiology. In men over age 35, sexually transmitted urethritis is uncommon. Bacteriuria secondary to acquired obstructive urinary disease, however, is relatively common. The most common cause of epididymitis in older men is the organisms that cause bacteriuria (Berger, 1978; Berger et al., 1979).

A small group of men in all age groups may have epididymitis that is due to systemic disease such as tuberculosis, Cryptococcus, Brucella, and other organisms that cause systemic infections (Gottesman, 1974; Kazzaz and Salmo, 1974; Mitchell and Huins, 1974; Thomas et al., 1981; William et al., 1979).

Recently, a truly noninfectious cause of epididymitis has been described secondary to treatment with the antiarrhythmic drug amiodarone (Gasparich et al., in press). This disease did not respond to antibiotic therapy, was not associated with ureteral or urinary inflammation, involved only the head of the epididymis, and responded favorably to a decrease in the dosage of amiodarone.

DIAGNOSIS

In acute epididymitis, the inflammation and swelling usually begin in the tail of the epididymis and may spread to involve the rest of the epididymis and testicular substance. The spermatic cord is usually tender and swollen. Although men with epididymitis resulting from urethritis that causes sexually transmitted organisms always have a history of sexual exposure, exposure can be 30 days prior to onset. Watson (1979) found that half of the men with gonococcal epididymitis did not have a urethral discharge. If the patient is examined immediately after obtaining a urinalysis, urethritis and urethral discharge may be missed because white cells and bacteria have been washed out of the urethra during urination (Fig. 19–5).

The microbial etiology of epididymitis can usually be determined easily by examination of a Gram-stained urethral smear for urethritis, and Gram stain of midstream urine specimen for gram-negative bacteriuria. The presence of intracellular gram-negative diplococci on the smear will correlate with the presence of *N. gonorrhoeae*. The presence of only white cells on urethral smear will indicate the presence of NGU. *Chlamydia trachomatis* will be isolated in approximately two thirds of these patients (Berger et al., 1979).

DIFFERENTIAL DIAGNOSIS FROM TORSION

It is imperative for the physician to make the differential diagnosis between epididymitis and torsion promptly. Delay in accurate diagnosis of torsion can result in the patient losing a testicle. Mistakes are also made in men ages 18 to 35, in whom both epididymitis and torsion are common.

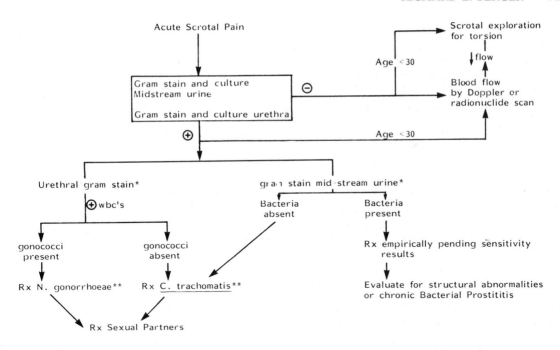

Figure 19–5. Flow chart for the management of acute epididymitis. (From Berger, R. E.: *In* Stamey, T. A. (Ed.): Monogr. Urol., *3*:99, 1982. Used by permission.)

The presence of urethritis probably indicates that the patient has an epididymitis and not a torsion.

Physical examination in early epididymitis shows swelling limited to the tail of the epididymis. However, 15 per cent of cases of early torsion also have swelling only in the epididymis (Delvillar et al., 1972).

Radionuclide scanning of the scrotum is probably the most accurate method of diagnosis; however, it may be not readily available (Abu-Sleiman et al., 1979). Doppler ultrasound of the scrotum may be of use if the operator is experienced. In order to press the Doppler probe firmly against the testicle, perform a spermatic cord block with 1 per cent xylocaine. In men with epididymitis, the arterial pulse of the ipsilateral testicle should be louder than the pulse in the contralateral testicle. The pulse in the ipsilateral testicle will be softer or absent than the contralateral testicle in men with torsion. If a pulse is heard in the ipsilateral testicle, the testicular artery should be compressed at the external inguinal ring. If the pulse disappears, it is truly coming from the testicle and probably a torsion has not occurred. If the pulse remains,

the impulse may be coming from inflamed scrotal vessels and torsion may still be present (Pederson, 1975). In case of any doubt, it is always safer to perform scrotal exploration promptly.

TREATMENT

The recommended treatment for acute epididymitis is presented in Table 19–7. Treatment is directed at the specific etiologic organism. Since gonococcal urethritis is associated with concomitant *C. trachomatis* infection in approximately 30 to 50 per cent of cases, tetracycline is the drug of choice in men with *N. gonorrhoeae* or *C. trachomatis* infection. Tell the patient to rest in bed; provide pain medication, and make sure patient relaxes with his scrotum elevated on a towel. Elevation will improve lymphatic drainage. Treat all patients with antibiotics. Injection of the spermatic cord with a local anesthetic and oral nonsteroidal anti-inflammatory drugs may be of symptomatic benefit (Costas and Van Blerk, 1973; Lapides et al., 1964; Moore et al., 1971; Smith, 1971). In a controlled trial, Moore et al. (1971) found prednisone to be of no value as an adjunct to antibiotic therapy

TABLE 19–7. TREATMENT OF ACUTE EPIDIDYMO-ORCHITIS*

A. Epididymo-orchitis secondary to bacteriuria
  1. Urine culture and sensitivity
  2. Prompt administration of broad-spectrum antimicrobial (e.g., tobramycin and/or cephalosporin)
  3. Bed rest and scrotal evaluation
  4. Strongly consider hospitalization
  5. Evaluate for underlying urinary tract disease

B. Epididymo-orchitis secondary to sexually transmitted urethritis
  1. Gram stain of urethral smear
  2. Administer:
    a. Tetracycline, 500 mg orally q.i.d. for at least 10 days, or
    b. Doxycycline, 100 mg orally b.i.d. for at least 10 days, or alternatively
    c. Amoxicillin, 500 mg orally q.i.d. for at least 10 days (gonococcal epididymitis)
    d. Erythromycin, 500 mg orally q.i.d. for at least 10 days (nongonococcal epididymitis)
  3. Bed rest and scrotal elevation
  4. Examine and treat sexual partners

*Adapted from Berger, R. E.: Semin. Urol., *1*:143, 1983.

in the treatment of epididymitis. Men with epididymitis due to urethritis-causing organisms seldom have structural urinary tract pathology. Younger boys and older men who have epididymitis secondary to bacteriuria often have structural urologic abnormalities. Men and boys with bacteriuria should undergo radiographic and cystoscopic evaluation for structural urinary abnormalities.

PELVIC INFLAMMATORY DISEASE

Pelvic inflammatory disease is one of the most severe consequences of STDs in women. It has been linked to infection with *N. gonorrhoeae, C. trachomatis,* anaerobic bacteria, and possibly mycoplasmas. Since at least three of these four groups of organisms are sexually transmitted, it is essential that the urologist be aware of the serious sequelae of the transmission of the organisms. Untreated male contacts with urethral gonorrhea and/or chlamydia are a major source of infection for both initial and recurrent episodes of PID.

More than 80 per cent of the male sexual partners of women with gonococcal PID will have gonococcal urethritis. These men are often asymptomatic. Identification and treatment of infected male contacts should decrease the rate of recurrent PID in their partners.

CONSEQUENCES

Pelvic inflammatory disease is very common. The cost of caring for acute infection and its sequelae is over $1 billion per year (Curran, 1980).

Infertility. Pelvic inflammatory disease can lead to serious and permanent consequences, including infertility: Following a single episode of PID, 12 per cent of patients will be sterile; after two episodes, 35 per cent will be sterile; and after three attacks, 75 per cent will be sterile (Weström, 1975). Of women who have had one episode of salpingitis, 25 per cent will develop another (Falk, 1965). The damage caused by the first occurrence may make the patient more susceptible to further problems. In virtually all cases, PID-caused infertility is due to tubal occlusion.

Infertility increases in direct proportion to the severity of the pelvic infection. *Infertility is more likely to occur in patients with non-gonococcal rather than gonococcal PID* (Weström, 1975). Weström (1975) estimated that of every 29 females born in 1950, one is sterile because of tubal occlusion by the age of 30.

Ectopic Pregnancy. The most common cause of ectopic pregnancy is fallopian tube damage caused by PID. *Approximately half of all women with ectopic pregnancy have had previous PID* (Weström, 1980). Indeed, the risk of ectopic pregnancy in women who have PID is seven to ten times greater than in women who never have had this infection (Weström, 1975 and 1980). The increasing rate of PID is one factor in the doubling of the number of ectopic pregnancies in the United States in the last 10 years (Fig. 19–6).

Pain. Chronic abdominal pain is a sequela of PID in approximately 15 per cent of women who have salpingitis. This pain is probably related to pelvic adhesions around the tubes and ovaries.

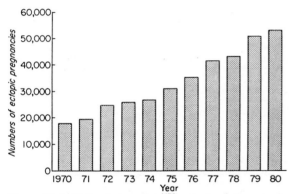

Figure 19–6. Estimated number of ectopic pregnancies in the United States, 1970–1980: Hospital Discharge Survey. (From Aral, S. O., and Holmes, K. K.: *In* Holmes, K. K. et al. (Eds.): Sexually Transmitted Diseases, New York, McGraw-Hill Book Co. In press. Used by permission.)

ETIOLOGY

From 10 to 70 per cent of women who acquire *N. gonorrhoeae* cervical infection develop PID (Table 19–8). Bacterial virulence may explain why some women develop PID and others do not (Draper et al., 1980). The presence of bacteriocidal antibodies may protect against the development of PID (Måardh et al., 1977 and 1981; Gjonnaess et al., 1982).

Chlamydia trachomatis is also a major cause of PID (Table 19–9). The number of cases that are due to *C. trachomatis* may be greater than the number due to *N. gonorrhoeae* (Måardh et al., 1981, Gjonnaess et al., 1982). *Chlamydia has been isolated from 20 to 50 per cent of women with PID* (Måardh et al., 1977 and 1981; Gjonnaess et al., 1982; Sweet et al., 1979; Paavonen, 1980). Women with *C. trachomatis* infection may have milder symptoms than women with *N. gonorrhoeae,* but tubal damage is just as severe (Svensson et al., 1980).

Serology tests have implicated mycoplasms in the etiology of PID. Increases in IgG anti-bodies to *Mycoplasma hominis* are identified in 20 per cent of patients with PID (Eschenbach et al., 1975). Significant elevations to IgM have also been seen. Rises in antibody titers to *U. urealyticum* also are seen in approximately 20 per cent of patients with PID (Henry-Suchet et al., 1980).

Various anaerobic and aerobic bacteria have been isolated in 30 to 60 per cent of women with nongonococcal salpingitis, and in 20 to 50 per cent in women with acute gonococcal salpingitis. Anaerobes seem to be more common in women who have infection associated with intrauterine devices (IUDs) (Eschenbach et al., 1975; Eschenbach, 1984).

DIAGNOSIS

The diagnosis of PID can be difficult. A wide spectrum of symptoms varies from very mild to very severe. A history of abdominal pain is not definitive because *half of the women with salpingitis severe enough to cause tubal occlusion do not have pain severe enough to make them seek medical attention* (Eschenbach, 1984). These women may present with urethritis and mild lower abdominal pain. The physician may misdiagnose cystitis because of the pyuria seen on urinalysis.

By examination, unilateral salpingitis occurs in less than 10 per cent of cases (Falk et al., 1965). *Grossly abnormal cervical discharge is found in half the patients.* Fever may or may not be present. Only 45 per cent of patients with confirmed salpingitis have a high white blood cell count or an erythrocyte sedimentation rate elevated about 15 mm/hr (Jacobson and Weström, 1969).

Gram stain of cervical secretions, despite the fact that it is often negative, can be of great help in diagnosis. Gram stain is positive for gonorrhea in only 67 per cent of women who have *N. gonorrhoeae* recovered from the cervix. However, if typical gram-negative diplococci are

TABLE 19–8. RECOVERY OF ORGANISMS FROM THE ABDOMEN OF WOMEN WITH CERVICAL *Neisseria gonorrhoeae* AND ACUTE PELVIC INFLAMMATORY DISEASE*

Author	No. of Patients	GC Isolated	GC Only	GC and Aerobe and/or Anaerobe	Aerobe and/or Anaerobe	Chlamydia or Mycoplasma	% Sterile
Eschenbach et al., 1975	21	33%	28%	5%	24%	10%	32%
Monif et al., 1976	28	39%	18%	21%	22%	N.D.	39%
Sweet et al., 1979	13	61%	31%	31%	31%	0	8%

*From Eschenbach, D.: Urol. Clin. North Am., *11*:65, 1984.
Abbreviations: N.D. = Not done; GC = gonococcus.

TABLE 19–9. FREQUENCY OF *Chlamydia trachomatis* RECOVERY AND ANTIBODY FROM WOMEN WITH ACUTE PELVIC INFLAMMATORY DISEASE*

Author	No. of Patients	Cervical Chlamydia	Abdominal Chlamydia	Significant Antibody Change
Sweet et al., 1979	39	5%	0	23%
Eschenbach et al., 1975	100	20%	2%	10%
Paavonen, 1980	228	30%	N.D.	19%
Måardh, Ripa, et al., 1977	53	36%	30%	N.D.
Måardh, Lind, et al., 1981	60	38%	N.D.	37%
Henry-Suchet, et al., 1980	56	46%	12%	46%

*From Eschenbach, D.: Urol. Clin. North Am., *11*:65, 1984.
Abbreviation: N.D. = Not done.

found in leukocytes on a cervical smear, it is certain that the patient has gonococcal salpingitis. If five or more polymorphonuclear leukocytes are seen per high power field (hpf), the patient has cervicitis. This condition may be caused by *N. gonorrhoeae* or *C. trachomatis*, both of which can cause salpingitis (Paavonen et al., 1982).

TREATMENT

A summary of the treatment for salpingitis is given in Table 19–10. At the present time, it is probably best to admit all patients to the hospital so that they can be treated with intravenous antibiotics.

TABLE 19–10. GUIDELINES FOR THE TREATMENT OF ACUTE PELVIC INFLAMMATORY DISEASE*

Antibiotic	Dose	Duration (Days)
HOSPITALIZED PATIENTS		
Regimen A		
Hospital regimen		
Doxycycline	100 mg IV Q 12 h	≥4
Cefoxitin	2 gm IV Q 6 h	≥4
Discharge regimen		
Doxycycline	100 mg p.o. b.i.d.	Total 10–14 days
Regimen B		
Hospital regimen		
Clindamycin	600 mg IV Q 6 h	≥4
Tobramycin or gentamicin	2 mg/kg loading then 1.5 mg/kg IV Q 8 h	≥5
Discharge Regimen		
Clindamycin	450 mg p.o. q.i.d.	Total 10–14 days
Regimen C		
Hospital regimen		
Doxycycline	100 mg IV Q 12 h	≥4
Metronidazole	1 gm IV Q 12 h	≥4
Discharge Regimen		
Doxycycline	100 mg p.o. b.i.d.	Total 10–14 days
NONHOSPITALIZED PATIENTS		
Loading dose *(choice of one)* with 1.0 gm probenecid		
Cefoxitin	2.0 gm I.M.	
Amoxicillin	3.0 gm p.o.	
Ampicillin	3.5 gm p.o.	
Aqueous procaine penicillin G	4.8 MV I.M.	
Followed with *(choice of one)*		
Doxycycline	100 mg p.o. Q 6 h	10–14 days
Tetracycline	500 mg p.o. Q 6 h	10–14 days

*Modified from Centers for Disease Control: Sexually Transmitted Disease: Treatment Guidelines 1982. M.M.W.R. (Suppl), *31*:43S, 1982.

VAGINITIS

Vaginitis is often considered the province of the gynecologist; however, many patients will go to a urologist because their symptoms mimic those of a bladder infection. The urologist plays an important role in the proper identification and treatment of these conditions. In women with lower urinary tract complaints, vaginitis must be differentiated from infections with coliform bacteria, *N. gonorrhoeae,* and *C. trachomatis.* Treatment of vaginitis can be based on specific etiologic diagnosis derived from the examination of vaginal secretions (Table 19–11). In a normal female, the vaginal discharge is clear, white or gray, and nonhomogeneous. The pH of the vaginal fluid is less than 4.5. Microscopical epithelial cells with distinct borders are present. Leukocytes are rare. If 10 per cent potassium hydroxide (KOH) is added to the secretion, amines are not released and there is no "fishy" odor.

Trichomonas Vaginitis

Trichomonas vaginalis is a pear-shaped protozoon with three to five flagella projecting from its base and an undulating membrane that runs lengthwise along the parasite. Although accounting for less than 2 per cent of the etiology of NGU in men (Holmes et al., 1975), *T. vaginalis* is highly pathogenic for the human vagina. Women with vaginal trichomonas almost always show an inflammatory reaction manifested by a neutrophil response (Whittington, 1957) and are usually symptomatic.

DIAGNOSIS

The diagnosis of trichomonas vaginitis is made from history and physical examination. The most common symptoms include vaginal itching, dysuria, and discharge. A few women will present with dysuria and frequency, suggesting bladder involvement. The pH of the vaginal fluid is greater than 4.5. On a saline-wet mount, leukocytes and motile trichomonads are seen. An addition of 10 per cent KOH to the vaginal secretion may liberate a fishy odor owing to amines. The saline-wet preparation will detect approximately 70 per cent of infections (Fouts and Kraus, 1980). The most sensitive method for detecting trichomonas is culture.

TREATMENT

Metronidazole is the only available systemic trichomonicide in the United States (Table 19–12). It may be given in a single 2-gm dose or as a 250-mg dose three times a day for 7 days. The efficacy of these two regimens is roughly equal. The single-dose regimen uses considerably less total metronizazole and is more reliable. Patients should avoid drinking alcohol. In women who fail the first treatment, a repeat of the same dosage will eradicate the organism in about 85 per cent of cases. Persistent infection may be caused by drug resistance. If possible, susceptibility studies should be performed prior to retreatment (Lossick, 1982). Considerably higher doses of metronidazole may be necessary to eradicate resistant strains.

Since the major cause of vaginal trichomoniasis relapse is re-infection, the sexual partners of women with trichomonas also should be treated. In the male, the wet mount preparation

TABLE 19–11. DIAGNOSIS OF VAGINITIS*

	Discharge Appearance	pH Discharge	Amine Odor on Adding 10% Potassium Hydroxide	Microscopy
Normal	Clear to gray, nonhomogeneous	<4.5	No	Rare PMNs† epithelial cells with distinct borders
Trichomonas	Gray, possibly frothy	≥4.5	Yes	Many PMNs,† *trichomonas*
Yeast	White adherent plaques	<4.5	No	Many PMNs,† yeasts, and pseudomycelia with 100%
Nonspecific vaginitis	White-gray	≥4.5	Yes	Rare PMNs, "clue cells"

*From Berger, R. E.: In Stamey, T. A.: Monographs in Urology. Burroughs-Wellcome, 1982.
†Leukocytes may also be present in vaginal fluids as a result of *Chlamydia trachomatis* or *Neisseria gonorrhoeae.*
Abbreviations: PMN = Polymorphonuclear neutrophil leukocyte; KOH = potassium hydroxide.

TABLE 19–12. TREATMENT OF VAGINITIS

Trichomonas vaginitis:
Metronidazole* 250 mg orally 3 times daily for 7 days
or
Metronidazole* 2 gm orally, single dose
or
Clotrimazole† 100 mg intravaginally daily for 7 days

Candida vaginitis:
Miconazole 100 mg intravaginally daily for 7 days
Clotrimazole 100 mg intravaginally daily for 7 days
Nystatin 10,000 units intravaginally b.i.d. for 14 days

Nonspecific vaginitis:
Metronidazole* 500 mg orally twice daily for 7 days
Ampicillin 500 mg orally four times daily for 7 days

*Contraindicated in pregnancy.
†50% cure rate

of urethral secretions is very insensitive and treatment must be initiated on the basis of exposure unless cultures are available. Trichomonas can be identified in 13 to 80 per cent of male sex partners of infected women. In men, spontaneous resolution is common. It has been suggested (Krieger and Rein, 1982) that the zinc levels in the general secretions of males may protect them against most strains of *Trichomonas vaginalis*.

Candidal Vaginitis

ETIOLOGY AND DIAGNOSIS

Candida species are common inhabitants of the mouth, vagina, and large intestines of healthy individuals (Drake and Maiback, 1973). There is a poor correlation between the isolation of Candida and the presence of clinical vaginitis. Clinical disease occurs most often in diabetics, pregnant women, and patients on antibiotic therapy, especially tetracycline compounds. Candidal organisms are frequently shared by sexual partners; however, it is unlikely that candidal vaginitis is a sexually transmitted disease. The frequent colonization of the gastrointestinal tract makes autoinoculation a possible source of re-infection (Eddie, 1968; Thin et al., 1979).

The most prominent clinical feature of Candidal vaginitis is an intense itching. On examination, there are white adherent plaques on the vaginal wall. Discharge is often minimal. On a 10 per cent KOH preparation, leukocytes, yeast, and pseudomycelia are seen. The pH of the vaginal fluid is less than 4.5. The sensitivity of KOH preparation is dependent upon adequate sampling and ranges from 38 to 84 per cent

(Eddie, 1968; Miles et al., 1977). Culture may be needed for diagnosis in some cases.

TREATMENT

Because of the high incidence of asymptomatic colonization, treatment for Candida is given only to women with clinical disease. Nystatin, the mainstay of treatment, is given in vaginal tablets of 10,000 units twice daily for 14 days. Other treatments include myconazole, 100 mg intravaginally daily for 7 days, and clotrimazole, 100 mg intravaginally for 7 days. Routine treatment of the male sexual partner is not necessary.

Nonspecific Vaginitis

ETIOLOGY

Nonspecific vaginitis is usually associated with *Gardnerella vaginalis* infections (Holmes et al., 1981; McCormack et al., 1977). This organism was previously known as *Hemophilus vaginalis*, or *Corynebacterium vaginale*. However, this organism may be found in as many as 68 per cent of all women without evidence of vaginal disease (Totten et al., 1982). *Gardnerella vaginalis* has even been identified in virginal women and prepubertal girls. Almost all women with nonspecific vaginitis have the organism in their vaginal secretions (Holmes et al., 1981).

Recent evidence has suggested that anaerobes play an essential part in the development of nonspecific vaginitis. Increased numbers of gram-positive and gram-negative anaerobic bacteria have been found in women with nonspecific vaginitis (Spiegel et al., 1980). *Gardnerella vaginalis* does *not* produce volatile amines that cause the characteristic odor associated with this syndrome (Chen et al., 1979). Anaerobes, however, can produce these substances. There is also a high ratio of succinate to lactate in the vaginal secretions of women with nonspecific vaginitis probably as a result of anaerobic metabolism (Malouf et al., 1981). On microscopy, characteristic "clue cells" are seen (Fig. 19–7).

DIAGNOSIS

Concomitant cervical infection with *C. trachomatis* or *N. gonorrhoeae* is not uncommon in women with vaginitis. If many leukocytes and no Candida or trichomonas are visible, cervical infection with these organisms should be suspected.

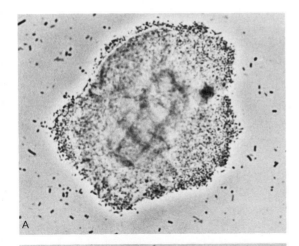

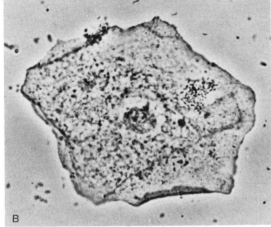

Figure 19–7. *A,* "Clue cell" seen in patient with "nonspecific vaginitis." *B,* Normal vaginal epithelial cell. (From Vontver and Eschenbach, 1981.)

TREATMENT

Metronidazole at dosages of 500 mg twice a day for 7 days is uniformly effective in treatment (Malouf et al., 1981; Spiegel et al., 1980). Because of the potential oncogenic potential of metronidazole, some authors use ampicillin for initial treatment and reserve metronidazole for treatment failures. In vitro activity of sulfonamides is very poor, but the high local levels achieved with intravaginal therapy may occasionally be effective. Most investigators discount the efficacy of sulfonamides in this disease (Jones et al., 1982). As a result of the high prevalence of *G. vaginalis* in asymptomatic individuals, treatment of this organism without clinical disease is not indicated. Furthermore, there is probably no indication for concomitant treatment of the sexual partners.

GENITAL ULCERS

The diagnosis of acute genital ulcers presents a perplexing problem. The initial clinical impressions of even the most experienced specialist of sexually transmitted disease may be wrong 40 per cent of the time (Chapel et al., 1977). *In only three instances is the presentation of the ulcer pathognomonic:*

1. A fixed drug-eruption is always triggered by the ingestion of one particular medication.

2. A group of vesicles on an erythematous base which does not follow a neural distribution is pathognomic for herpes simplex infection.

3. A genital ulcer that develops acutely during sexual activity is diagnostic of trauma (Kraus, 1984) (Table 19–13).

If the clinical picture does not fit any of these pathognomonic presentations, the physician must include premalignant processes, such as erythroplasia of Queyrat; malignant processes, such as squamous cell carcinoma; and nonmalignant processes, such as syphilis, chancroid, genital herpes, lymphogranuloma venereum, granuloma inguinale, fixed drug eruptions, and traumatic ulcers in the differential diagnosis. Although the symptoms of each of these diseases do differ, the natural variability, influence of secondary infection, and possible coexistence of more than one disease entity make the differential diagnosis extremely difficult. The quest for the proper diagnosis and treatment, therefore, needs to be based largely on laboratory examination. A flow diagram illustrating the evaluation and management of a patient with acute ulcers is presented in Fig. 19–8. The test most valuable for malignant lesions is biopsy; for genital herpes it is viral culture; for syphilis it is dark-field examination and serologic tests; for chancroid it is selective me-

TABLE 19–13. CLINICAL PRESENTATIONS USEFUL IN GENITAL ULCER DIFFERENTIAL DIAGNOSIS*

Presentation	Diagnosis
Grouped vesicles†	Genital herpes
Onset during sexual activity†	Traumatic ulcer
Recurrences associated with the same systemic medicine†	Fixed drug reaction
Deep ulcer with undermined border	Chancroid
Firm, rolled, elevated ulcer border	Granuloma inguinale
Painless, firm, indurated ulcer	Syphilis

*From Kraus, S. J.: Urol. Clin. North Am., *11*:155, 1984.
†Pathognomonic.

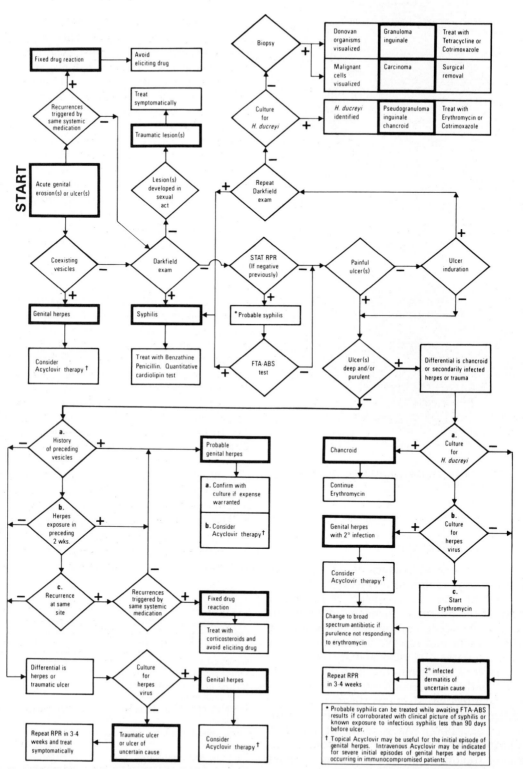

Figure 19–8. Evaluation and management of acute genital ulcers and erosions in sexually active patients. (From Kraus, S. J.: Urol. Clin. North Am., *11*:155, 1984.)

TABLE 19–14. Laboratory Aids in the Diagnosis of Acute Genital Ulcers*

Diagnosis	Preferred Test†	Ancillary Tests
Genital herpes	Viral culture	Tzanck smear Fluorescent antibody smear
Syphilis	Darkfield examination	Serologic tests (RPR, VDRL, FTS-ABS, MHA-TP)
Chancroid	Selective medium culture	
Granuloma inguinale	Crush preparation	Histology
Lymphogranuloma venereum	Serologic test (LGV complement fixation or *C. trachomatis*‡ microimmunofluorescence)	*C. trachomatis* culture
Traumatic ulcer	None	
Fixed drug reaction	None	

*From Kraus, S. J.: Urol. Clin. North Am., *11*:155, 1984.
†Based on sensitivity, specificity, and availability.
‡*Chlamydia trachomatis.*
Abbreviations: RPR = Rapid plasma reagin test; VDRL = Venereal Disease Research Laboratory test, FTS-ABS = fluorescent treponemal antibody absoption test; LGV = lymphogranuloma venereum test; MHA-TP = microhemagglutination test.

dium culture for *Hemophilus ducreyi;* for granuloma inguinale, a crush preparation for the cytologic or histologic identification of *Calymmatobacterium granulomatis* is necessary; and for lymphogranuloma venereum, a serologic test and chlamydia culture are required (Table 19–14).

Since the treatment for each of these diseases differs significantly (Table 19–15), a correct differential diagnosis is essential.

GENITAL HERPES INFECTIONS

Genital herpes simplex virus (HSV) is a disease of great concern to physicians and patients. The increasing incidence of the infection in men and women (Fig. 19–9), the risk of transmission to sexual partners, the high morbidity and even mortality of infant infections, the association with cervical cancer, and the absence of curative therapy have made it imperative that all physicians be able to diagnose, counsel, and treat the patient with genital herpes (Nahmias, 1973*a, b*).

Herpes simplex virus is a double-stranded DNA virus that may cause persistent or latent infections. Two antigenic types may be distinguished (Nahmias and Roizman, 1973*b*). Types I and II may be distinguished by DNA restriction enzyme analysis or monoclonal antibodies directed against glycoproteins (Balachandran et al., 1982; Goldstein et al., 1983; Peterson et al., 1983; Richman et al., 1982).

The majority of patients with genital herpes infection have Type II virus. However, Type I

TABLE 19–15. Antimicrobial Therapy for Infectious Genital Ulcers*

Infectious Process	Drug of Choice	Alternative Drug
Chancroid	Erythromycin, 500 mg 4 times a day for 10 days	Sulfamethoxazole-trimethoprim 1 double-strength tablet b.i.d. × 10 days
Genital herpes	5% acyclovir ointment 6 times a day for 7 days (initial episode)†	
Granuloma inguinale	Tetracycline 500 mg 4 times a day until healed	Sulfamethoxazone-trimethoprim 1 double-strength b.i.d. until healed
Lymphogranuloma venereum	Tetracycline, 500 mg 4 times a day for 2 weeks	Erythromycin 500 mg p.o. q.i.d. × 2 weeks
Syphilis (primary)	Benzathine penicillin G, 2,400,000 units intramuscularly	Tetracycline 500 mg p.o. q.i.d. × 15 days

*From Kraus, S. J.: Urol. Clin. North Am., *11*:155, 1984.
†Does not prevent recurrence of herpes.

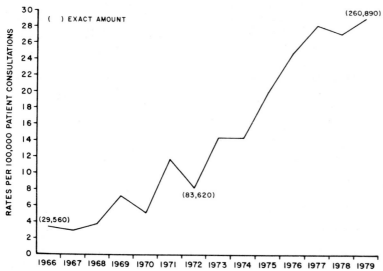

Figure 19–9. Estimated rates of patient consultations for genital herpes seen by physicians in private practice in the United States, 1966–1979. (From Centers for Disease Control: Genital herpes infection—United States, 1966–1979. M.M.W.R., *31*:137, 1982.)

*Data Source: IMS America, NDTI.

herpes, which is commonly associated with oral infections, has been reported in 10 to 25 per cent of cases (Corey et al., 1983*a*; Reeves et al., 1981). Herpes simplex virus is seen in 5 per cent of STD clinic visits. In college students, HSV infections are ten times more common than gonorrhea or syphilis (Scriba, 1978).

Although the risk of transmission from a single exposure is unknown, genital herpes infection may be transmitted by either genital or oral-genital contact. Although it is not inevitable if one infected partner has genital herpes for the other to acquire it, partners are at risk even when the infection is asymptomatic. The risk of transmission, however, is lower when couples avoid sexual contact during clinical recurrences (Mertz et al. 1981 and 1983*b*).

CLINICAL COURSE

The signs and symptoms from first-episode genital herpes are much more severe than those from recurrent disease. HSV Types I and II produce primary genital infections of equal severity. First-episode disease is also much more severe in persons without prior HSV oral infection (primary first-episode disease) than is first-episode genital herpes in persons with prior HSV oral infection (nonprimary first-episode disease). The symptoms and signs of first-episode and recurrent genital herpes are presented in Table 19–16. Dysuria is present in 44 per cent of men and 83 per cent of women. Herpes simplex virus can be isolated from the urethras of most of these patients, suggesting a true

urethritis. The virus may cause NGU in men and urethral syndrome in women in the absence of external lesions (Corey et al., 1983). The clinical illness of primary genital herpes tends to be more severe in women (Table 19–17). Recurrent genital herpes is usually milder. HSV Type II causes 99 per cent of recurrent genital herpes. The cases of recurrence with HSV Type I primary infections are fewer than for primary HSV Type II infections (Corey et al., 1983*a*; Reeves et al., 1981). In contrast to primary herpes, which is often bilateral, recurrent disease is often unilateral. Local symptoms are milder, and systemic symptoms are unusual. Urethral isolation can be obtained in fewer than 2 per cent of men (Corey et al., 1983). Extragenital skin lesions, usually from autoinoculation, are found in 10 per cent of men and 26 per cent of women with primary genital herpes (Corey et al., 1983).

Neurologic complications are also common in patients with primary infections. Thirteen to 36 per cent of patients develop mild meningitis with spinal fluid leukocytosis (Brenton, 1980). One per cent of patients with primary genital herpes develop severe sacral or autonomic nervous system dysfunction (Caplan et al., 1977; Corey et al., 1983; Goldmeier et al., 1975; Goldmeier, 1979; Jacobs et al., 1980, Oates and Greenhouse, 1978; Riehle and Williams, 1979), resulting in urinary retention. Patients may complain of constipation, weakness, impotence, and sensory loss. Cystometrics may reveal a hypotonic curve with decreased sensation. Catheter-

TABLE 19–16. Virus Type, Signs, and Symptoms in Patients with Genital Herpes Seen at the University of Washington*

	First Episode Genital Herpes		Recurrent Genital Herpes
	Primary	Nonprimary	
Number of patients	209	77	362
Percent female	68%	57%	40%
Percent with HSV-2	90%	99%	99%
Mean duration viral shedding (days)	11.3	6.8	4.1
Per cent shedding virus from cervix	87%	65%	12%
Mean number of lesions at onset	16.3	9.5	6.4
Mean lesions area (mm²) at onset	525	158	59
Per cent with bilateral lesions	84%	45%	11%
Per cent forming new lesions	75%	45%	37%
Mean duration lesions (days)	19.0	15.5	10.0
Per cent with tender lymphadenopathy	80%	–	26%
Mean duration local pain (days)	11.9	8.7	4.7
Per cent with systemic symptoms	62%	16%	8%

*Abstracted from Corey, L., et al.: *98, 958*, 1983; adapted from Mertz, G. J., and Corey, L.: Urol. Clin. North Am., *11*:103, 1984.

ization for a period of weeks may be necessary before bladder function returns. On the other hand, some patients may be unable to urinate because of local pain. These latter patients may be managed by voiding into a tub of warm water (Mertz and Corey, 1984). Herpes simplex virus encephalitis has a mortality of 70 per cent and is usually associated with HSV Type I (Craig and Nahmias, 1973).

In homosexual men, HSV is the second most common cause of proctitis after gonorrhea (Goldmeier et al., 1975; Goldmeier, 1979; Goodell et al., 1983).

DIAGNOSIS

Vesicles grouped on an erythematous base that do not follow a neural distribution are essentially pathogenic for genital herpes. Confirmation of the diagnosis and the diagnoses of outpatient cases are based on laboratory meth-

TABLE 19–17. Signs and Symptoms in Patients with Primary and Recurrent Genital Herpes*

	Primary Genital HSV-2		Recurrent Genital Herpes	
	Males	Females	Males	Females
Number	63	126	218	144
Mean duration viral shedding (days)	10.5	11.8	4.2	3.9
Mean duration of all lesions (days)	16.5‡	19.7	10.6	9.3
Per cent forming new lesions	76%	74%	43%†	29%
Mean number of lesions at onset	15.7	15.4	7.5	4.8
Mean lesions area at onset (mm²)	427	550	63	54
Per cent with HSV isolated from urethra	28%†	82%	NA	NA
Per cent with dysuria	44%†	83%	9%	27%
Per cent with urethral/vaginal discharge	27%†	85%	4%	45%
Mean duration of lymphadenopathy (days)	8.6‡	15.4	9.2	6.9
Per cent with systemic symptoms (fever, malaise, etc.)	39%†	68%	5%†	13%
Per cent with headache, photophobia, and nuchal rigidity	13%†	36%	NA	NA
Per cent with local pain	95%	99%	67%†	88%
Median duration of local pain (days)	10.9	12.2	3.9‡	5.9

*Abstracted from Corey L., et al.: Ann. Intern. Med., *98*:958, 1983; adapted from Mertz, G. J., and Corey, L.: Urol. Clin. North Am., *11*:103, 1984.
†P<0.05 by Chi-square for males versus females.
†P<0.05 by Student's *t*-test for males versus females.

ods. Papanicolaou (Pap) smears of lesions will demonstrate intranuclear inclusions in 50 to 60 per cent of culture-positive cases (Brown et al., 1979; Goldstein et al., 1983; Corey and Holmes, 1983). Immunofluorescent techniques will reveal 70 per cent of culture-positive cases (Moseley et al., 1981).

Virus isolation by culture is the most sensitive of techniques for diagnosing herpes virus infections. Results can be available in 5 days (Goldstein et al., 1983). Serum antibody to HSV infections can be measured by a number of methods (Ashley and Corey, 1981; Balachandran et al., 1982; Cappel et al., 1980). No test presently available is completely reliable in differentiating Type I from Type II infection (McClung et al., 1976; Rawls et al., 1970). Serologic tests are now useful only to document a history of past infection.

TREATMENT

At the time of this writing, acyclovir is the only drug that has shown efficacy in the treatment of genital herpes. Topical, intravenous, and oral forms are effective for first-episode genital herpes. Oral acyclovir has been shown effective therapeutically and prophylactically in recurrent genital herpes infections. While other forms of therapy may be harmless, patients should be discouraged from using potentially harmful, as well as ineffective, forms of therapy, such as bacille Calmette Guérin (BCG), smallpox vaccination, or photodynamic inactivation (Felbee et al., 1973; Kern and Schiff, 1959; Miller, 1979; Myers et al., 1975). Levamisole, topical adenine arabinoside (aRA-A), IDU, idoxuridine (IDU), IDU plus dimethylsulfoxide (DMSO), ether, and betadine have all been shown to be ineffective in the treatment of primary genital herpes. Interferon, arilone, isoprinosine, 2-deoxy-D-glucose (2-DG) lysine, laser therapy, and phosphonoformate require further testing (Bierman, 1978; Bierman et al., 1981; Blough and Giuntoli, 1979; Jones et al., 1976; Kern et al., 1982; Milman et al., 1978; Pavin et al., 1978; Scheibel and Jessen, 1979).

Acyclovir acts on viral thymidine kinase as a guanine analog. It is selectively phosphorylated in the virus and acts as an inhibitor of viral DNA polymerase and also acts as a chain terminator (Ashley and Corey, 1981).

The oral acyclovir (200 mg orally five times per day for 5 to 10 days) and intravenous acyclovir (5 mg/kg every 8 hours for 5 days) appear more effective than topical therapy (5 per cent acyclovir in polyethlene glycol) in the treatment of primary genital herpes. Oral acyclovir offers considerable economic advantage over intravenous therapy (Mertz et al., 1982; Nilson et al., 1982; Corey et al., 1983b; Mindel et al., 1982; Wallin et al., 1981). In any form, acyclovir decreases the duration of viral shedding, time to crusting of lesions, time to healing of lesions, and duration of pain and itching in primary genital herpes. Only the oral and intravenous forms decrease dysuria, vaginal discharge, systemic symptoms, and the development of new lesions.

In the treatment of recurrent herpes, topical acyclovir has shown little effect (Corey et al., 1982b; Reichman et al., 1983; Spruance et al., 1982). However, oral acyclovir has been shown to significantly decrease the duration of viral shedding and time to crusting of recurrent lesions. Oral acyclovir did not significantly decrease the duration of local pain or itching (Reichman et al., in press). To have maximal effect, it must be given during the prodrome. Routine use may not be warranted, since symptoms are not affected and viral shedding is only shortened by 1 to 2 days.

Prophylactic oral acyclovir (200 mg orally two to five times per day) may sufficiently decrease recurrence (Douglas et al., 1983). More information on the long-term side effects and efficacy are needed before this form of therapy can be recommended.

As with treatments for other STDs, resistance to acyclovir has already occurred (Burns et al., 1982; Caplan et al., 1977; Crumpacker et al., 1982). Use of acyclovir outside its prescribed indications should be discouraged.

GENITAL WARTS

All wart viruses belong to the papilloma species, which are DNA-containing viruses (Dunn and Ogilvie, 1968; Oriel and Almeida, 1970; Oriel, 1971). Papilloma virus infection stimulates rapid cell division and duplication of virus particles. Patients transmit the disease when released viral particles from lesions come in contact with another person (Coggin and zur Hausen, 1979). A relationship between genital warts and cervical carcinoma is now receiving significant research attention (Syrjanen, 1981). It is possible that this "minor" venereal disease may cause significant health problems.

Although warts have a typical appearance, they can be confused with condolomata lata of syphilis, molluscum contagiosum, granuloma inguinale, benign neoplasms, and carcinoma.

Typically, warts are found near mucous membranes on stratified squamous epithelium of skin. They often are found at the urinary meatus, fossa navicularis of the urethra, anus, cervix, vagina, and vulva. They also may occur on the penis, scrotum, labia majora, and perianal area.

If a patient has external warts near an orifice, examine the patient internally. About half of the patients with perianal warts also have warts in the anal canal. Furthermore, 10 per cent of women with warts on the vulva will have warts on the cervix (Carr and Williams, 1977; Meisels and Fortin, 1976; Oriel, 1971; Pollack et al., 1978; Powell, 1978). Cervical warts may be misdiagnosed as cervical dysplasia. Men with meatal warts should undergo urethroscopy if the warts are recurrent or if there is persistent bloody discharge; both of these signs indicate urethral warts.

The CDC has provided site-specific treatment recommendations for warts (Table 19–18). Approximately two thirds of these sexual partners will develop genital warts (Barrett et al., 1954; Oriel, 1971 and 1983). Since patients with warts often have concurrent STD, examine patients and their partners for this possibility.

MOLLUSCUM CONTAGIOSUM

Molluscum contagiosum is a dermatologic disease that has a sexual mode of transmission (Brown et al., 1981; Lynch and Minkin, 1968). It is caused by a DNA-containing pox virus that replicates in the cytoplasm of infected cells. The incubation period is usually from 2 to 7 weeks, but can vary from as little as 1 week to as long as 6 months.

The lesions are smooth, pink or pearly-colored, and dome-shaped. A small dimple impression on the top is the outstanding diagnostic feature. Often, milky-white material can be expressed from the lesion (Felman and Nikitas, 1983). Often, the lesions are asymptomatic. Confirmation of the diagnosis can be made by characteristic molluscum body (Reed and Parkinson, 1977) on biopsy.

The lesions of molluscum contagiosum usually spontaneously regress in 2 to 3 months (Brown et al., 1981). Treatment, however, can prevent transmission. Treatment can be with cryotherapy, podophyllyn, phenol- or sulfa nitrate, and curettage. Examine patients for other STDs.

TABLE 19–18. Site-Specific Treatment of Genital Warts

Site	Treatment
External genital and perianal	*Primary* 10–25% podophyllin in compound tincture of benzoin weekly for 4 weeks *Secondary* Cryotherapy, electrosurgery, surgical removal
Vaginal and cervical	*Primary* Cryotherapy, electrosurgery, surgical removal *Secondary* 10–25% podophyllin in compound tincture benzoin (Be absolutely sure area is dry before removing speculum).
Meatal	*Primary* 10–25% podophyllin in compound tincture benzoin weekly for 4 weeks *Secondary* Cryotherapy, electrosurgery, and surgical removal
Urethral	*Primary* 5% S-Fluoruracil or thiotepa (podophyllin should not be used)
Anorectal	*Primary* 10–25% podophyllin in compound tincture benzoin (avoid exposure to normal mucosa) *Secondary* Cryotherapy, electrosurgery, surgical removal
Oral warts	*Primary* Cryotherapy, electrosurgery, and sugical removal

INFANT AND MATERNAL SEXUALLY TRANSMITTED DISEASES

Although seldom treated by the urologist, prenatal and infant sexually transmitted diseases are one of the reasons (along with PID) that it is so important to accurately diagnose and treat the more minor manifestations of the STD pathogens in adults.

During pregnancy, husbands may have sexual partners other than their wives (Asal and Holmes, 1984). As a result, there is an increased risk of sexually transmitted infection in pregnant women. Such infections can cause serious damage to the mother or the fetus.

Gonorrhea in the pregnant mother may result in chorioamnionitis and postpartum endometritis, low birth weight, and premature delivery (Monif, 1978; Rabin et al., 1983; Bejar et al., 1981). Chlamydia infection has been associated with endometritis (Martin et al., 1982; Wagner et al., 1980; Westrom and Mardh, 1982). Furthermore, both *M. hominis* and *U. urealyticum* have been associated with chorioamnionitis, postpartum endometritis, and spontaneous abortion (Harwick et al., 1970; Rabin et al., 1983; Wallace et al., 1978) (Table 19–19).

Ophthalmia neonatorum is the most common consequence of maternal gonococcal infection. The risk of ocular infection to infants of mothers with gonorrhea is approximately 25 per cent (Chacko et al., 1982; Hammerschlag et al., 1980; Rothenberg, 1979). Rare neonatal consequences of gonorrhea include sepsis, meningitis, and arthritis.

The rate of chlamydia infection in pregnant mothers varies from 8 to 12 per cent (Alexander and Harrison, 1983). The infant may contract infection-causing inclusion conjunctivitis or chlamydia pneumonia from an infected mother during birth. Twenty to 40 per cent of infants born to chlamydia-positive mothers become chlamydia carriers, and 5 to 15 per cent develop pneumonia (Harrison et al., 1978). *C. trachomatis* is now one of the leading causes of infant pneumonia.

Infants are almost certain to become infected with syphilis if the birth mother is so infected. Fortunately, syphilis is relatively rare. Prevention requires serologic screening of mothers both early and late in pregnancy. Always treat the sexual partners of the infected patients.

Herpes virus Type II also may be transmitted to the infant during birth. Although neonatal herpes is rare, it can be devastating. Systemic herpes infection can cause death in as many as eight out of ten infants (Nahmias and Visentine, 1983). Herpes virus is transmitted to the infant only when it is actively secreted by the mother at the time of delivery. In a primary infection, the risk of transmission is 70 per cent. If the mother has recurrent herpes, the chance of transmission is less than 10 per cent (Nahmias and Visentine 1983). Prevention of these infections requires that the physician exercise extreme care in diagnosing the infection. Currently, women excreting the virus up to 6 weeks before delivery are advised to have cesarean sections.

Other pathogenic agents, such as cytomegalovirus and streptococcus, that can be transmitted sexually also may be related to severe prenatal problems. A summary of the more common STDs in infants is presented in Table 19–20.

HEPATITIS AND ENTERIC INFECTIONS

In the past, viral hepatitis and enteric infections were not viewed as STDs. Now, however, many of these infections are known to be sexually transmitted in some cases (Table 19–21). Hepatitis A and B may be transmitted by sexual contact and through other close physical contact. Enteric infections, such as amebiasis, giardiasis, shigellosis, campylobacteriosis, and enteric viruses may be transmitted directly by the oral-fecal route.

Most of these sexually transmitted enteric infections occur in homosexual men. Fecal contact is made in two ways: through anal-receptive intercourse, and by anilingus. Both of these sexual practices are common among homosexuals, but are much less frequent among heterosexuals. Approximately 10 per cent of the population may be homosexual or bisexual (Kinsey et al., 1948). In at least one study, 31 per cent of the men who were homosexual also had sexual contact with women (Judson et al., 1980). Enteric diseases contracted by homosexual contact may also be transmitted to female partners. Approximately one third of hepatitis B cases may be attributable to homosexual contacts; 25 per cent are acquired by heterosexual contact. Thirty to 80 per cent of homosexual men test seropositive for hepatitis B (Judson, 1981). Female partners of men with hepatitis B are also at risk; in one study, 20 to 27 per cent developed hepatitis 3 to 12 months following exposure (Judson, 1981). For treatment information, check the articles listed at the end of this chapter.

Hepatitis A is also spread by sexual contact (Christenson et al., 1982; Corey and Holmes, 1980). Hepatitis A is more prevalent in homosexual men than heterosexual men. In heterosexuals, the incidence of seropositivity is directly proportional to the number of sexual partners (Christenson et al., 1982; Corey and Holmes, 1980; McFarlane et al., 1981).

At this time, there is little evidence that non-A, non-B hepatitis, which accounts for 70 per cent of post-transfusion hepatitis, has a sexual mode of transmission (Robinson, 1982).

Proctitis is another syndrome found in homosexual men. This syndrome may be caused

TABLE 19–19. MATERNAL AND FETAL RISKS OF SEXUALLY TRANSMITTED ORGANISMS*

Organism	Maternal Infection Rate (%)	Predominant Type of Transmission	Maternal Effects	Fetal Effects	Postpartum Effects	Treatment	Prevention
Neisseria gonorrhoeae	1–5	Perinatal	Urethritis, cervicitis, salpingitis, disseminated, gonococal infection, ?infertility, ?ectopic pregnancy	Chorioamnionitis, premature birth, low birth weight	Endometritis	Penicillin or ampicillin (?with erythromycin for concurrent chlamydial infection	Screening, culture, first prenatal visit and late in third trimester
Chlamydia trachomatis	2–25 (usually 8–12)	Perinatal	Cervicitis, salpingitis, perihepatitis, ?infertility, ?ectopic pregnancy	Chorioamnionitis, premature birth, low birth weight	Endometritis	Erythromycin	Screening, culture
Mycoplasma hominis	20–50	Perinatal	?	Placentitis, spontaneous abortion	Endometritis	?	?
Ureaplasma urealyticum	50–75	Perinatal	?	Placentitis, chorioamnionitis, premature birth, low birth weight	–		
Group B streptococcus	15–35	Perinatal	Sepsis (rare)	Septic abortion, premature birth, low birth weight	Endometritis, sepsis	None for carrier state	Penicillin prophylaxis infant
Syphilis	<0.01	Transplacental	Range of manifestations of adult syphilis	Spontaneous abortion, stillbirth, premature birth, low birth weight	–	Penicillin	Serologic screening in pregnancy, first trimester: for high-risk groups, third trimester also
Herpes virus infections Herpes simplex virus (HSV)	1–5	Perinatal	Range of manifestations	Spontaneous abortion (rare)	–	None	Screening cultures, cesarean section
Cytomegalovirus (CMV)	1–12	Perinatal	None	Spontaneous abortion, congenital disease	–	None	None

*From Alexander, E. R.: Urol. Clin. North Am., *11*:131, 1984.

TABLE 19–20. NEONATAL RISKS OF SEXUALLY TRANSMITTED ORGANISMS*

Organism	Maternal Infection Rate	Infant Effects	Transmission Risk from In-Fected Mother	Prevention	Treatment of Neonate
Neisseria gonorrhoeae	1–5	Conjunctivitis, sepsis, meningitis	4–30% Rare	Screening culture mother late pregnancy	Penicillin
Chlamydia trachomatis	2–25 (usually 8–12)	Conjunctivitis, pneumonia, bronchiolitis, otitis media	25–50%	Erythromycin or tetracycline ocular prophylaxis	Erythromycin
Mycoplasma hominis	20–50	Sepsis	Rare	—	—
Ureaplasma urealyticum	50–75	Pneumonia			
Group B steptococcus	15–35	Sepsis, meningitis, pneumonia, arthritis, osteomyelitis, cellulitis	70% infection, 1% disease	Penicillin, neonatal prophylaxis	Penicillin, ampicillin with aminoglycoside
Syphilis	0.01	Prematurity, stillbirth, neonatal death, congenital syphilis	50% 50%	Serologic screening in early and late pregnancy	Penicillin
Herpes Virus Infections Herpes simplex virus (HSV)	1–5	Disseminated, central nervous system, localized	5% recurrent at delivery, 50% primary at delivery	Culture screening in pregnancy, cesarean section	Vidarabine, acyclovir
Cytomegalovirus (CMV)	1–12	Disseminated (rare), congenital (0.5–2%), acquired (40–60%)		None	None

*From Alexander, E. R.: Urol. Clin. North Am., *11*:131, 1984.

TABLE 19–21. SEXUALLY TRANSMITTED AGENTS THAT CAUSE INFECTIONS OF THE LIVER, INTESTINES, AND ANORECTUM

Target Organ	Infectious Agents
Liver	Hepatitis B virus
	Hepatitis A virus
	Hepatitis non-A, non-B Agent(s)
Intestines	*Giardia lamblia*
	Entamoeba histolytica
	Cryptosporidium species
	Shigella species
	Campylobacter fetus
	Strongyloides species
Anorectum	*Neisseria gonorrhoeae*
	Chlamydia trachomatis
	Treponema pallidum
	Herpes simplex virus
	Human papilloma virus

*From Judson, F. N.: Urol. Clin. North Am., *11*:177, 1984.

TABLE 19–22. IMMUNE ABNORMALITIES IN ACQUIRED IMMUNODEFICIENCY SYNDROME (AIDS)*

In vivo:
  Cutaneous anergy
  Impaired antibody production to neoantigens

In vitro:
  Cell-mediated
    Lymphopenia (total, T-cells)
    Helper T-lymphocytes ($\downarrow$ No. and %) (OKT4, Leu-3)
    Suppressor/cytotoxic T-lymphocytes (variable No., $\uparrow$ %) (OKT8, Leu-2)
    Helper:suppressor ratio $\downarrow$ (H.S., OKT4:OKT8, Leu-3:Leu-2)
    Lymphocyte blastogenesis $\downarrow$ to mitogens and antigens
    Natural killer cell activity $\downarrow$

  Humoral
    Spontaneous Ig production $\uparrow$
    Induced IG production $\downarrow$
    Lymphocyte blastogenesis $\downarrow$ to B-cell mitogens

*From Collier, A. C., and Handsfield, H. H.: Urol. Clin. North Am., *11*:187, 1984.

by *N. gonorrhoeae, C. trachomatis,* or Herpes simplex virus. Culture is the best method of diagnosis (Klein et al., 1977; Deheragoda, 1977; Quinn et al., 1981*a,b;* Klotz et al., 1983).

ACQUIRED IMMUNODEFICIENCY SYNDROME

The acquired immunodeficiency syndrome (AIDS) is defined by the occurrence of a disease that is predictive of a deficit in cell-mediated immunity occurring in a person with no known cause for diminished resistance to that disease (Collier and Handsfield, 1984) (Table 19–22). The infections predictive of and associated with the AIDS syndrome are listed in Table 19–23. In addition, AIDS is often associated with Kaposi's sarcoma. The incidence of AIDS has increased dramatically since the syndrome was first reported in 1978. From 1978 to 1983, 2259 cases were reported (Centers for Disease Control, 1983).

Several groups run a particularly high risk of contracting AIDS (Table 19–24): The majority of AIDS patients are homosexual men (Darrow et al., 1983, Detels et al., 1983; Juffe et al., 1983; Marmor et al., 1982); intravenous drug abusers (17 per cent) (Masur et al., 1982; Small et al., 1983); Haitian immigrants (5 per cent) (Pitchenik et al., 1983; Leonidas and Hyppolite, 1983; Barry et al., 1983); and hemophiliacs (less than 4 per cent). Median age is 36 years. The majority of AIDS victims have come

from several large metropolitan centers such as New York, San Francisco, and Los Angeles.

The etiology of AIDS is unknown. Immunologic paralysis from repeat exposure to STD (Sonnabend et al., 1983), immunosuppression, continuous exposure to semen products (Anderson and Tarter, 1982; Hurtenbach and Shearer, 1982; Witkin and Sonnabend, 1983), and transmissible microbiologic agents may cause AIDS. Evidence supporting a transmissible agent includes:

1. Clusters of cases.

2. The occurrence of immunodeficiency in infants born to infected mothers (Rubinstein et al., 1983; Oleske et al., 1983).

3. The occurrence in nonpromiscuous sexual partners of AIDS patients (Harris, 1983).

4. The occurrence of AIDS in low-risk adults and neonates receiving transfusions (Ammann et al., 1983).

TABLE 19–23. COMMON OPPORTUNISTIC INFECTIOUS AGENTS ASSOCIATED WITH ACQUIRED IMMUNODEFICIENCY SYNDROME (AIDS)*

Fungi: *Candida* sp., *Cryptococcus neoformans, Aspergillus* sp., *Histoplasma capsulatum*

Bacteria: *Mycobacterium avium–intracellulare, Mycobacterium tuberculosis, Nocardia* sp.

Viruses: Cytomegalovirus, Epstein-Barr virus, Herpes simplex virus, Varicella-zoster virus

Protozoa: *Pneumocystis carinii, Toxoplasma gondii, Cryptosporidium* sp.

*Modified from Collier, A. C., and Handsfield, H. H.: Urol. Clin. North Am., *11*:187, 1984.

TABLE 19–24. POPULATIONS AT RISK FOR ACQUIRED IMMUNODEFICIENCY SYNDROME (AIDS)*

Category†	Per Cent of Reported Cases
Homosexual or bisexual men	71.4
Intravenous drug users	16.9
Haitian immigrants	5.3
Hemophiliacs	0.7
Other/none	2.7
Unknown/incomplete information	3.0

*Modified from Collier, A. C., and Handsfield, H. H.: Urol. Clin. North Am., *11*:187, 1984.

†Hierarchical categories; persons with multiple characteristics are listed in the highest appropriate category only.

Several agents, including cytomegalovirus, Epstein-Barr virus, human leukemia virus, and other related retroviruses have been implicated (Mangi et al., 1974; Rinaldo et al., 1980; Rogers et al., 1983, Blattner et al., 1983). It is hoped that work in progress will lead to the cure of this deadly syndrome.

References

Trends and Contact Tracing

Amsel, R., Totten, P. A., Spiegel, C. A., et al.: Nonspecific vaginitis: Diagnostic criteria and microbial and epidemiological associations. Am. J. Med., *74*:14, 1983.

Aral, S. O., and Holmes, K.K.: Epidemiology of sexually transmitted diseases. *In* Holmes, K. K., Måardh, P-A., Sparling, P. F., et al. (Eds.): Sexually Transmitted Diseases. New York, McGraw-Hill Book Co., 1984.

Armstrong, B., and Holman, D.: Increasing mortality from cancer of the cervix in young Australian women. Med. J. Aust., *1*:460, 1981.

Baird, P. J.: Serologic evidence for the association of papillomavirus and cervical neoplasia. Lancet, *2*:17, 1983.

Bell, T. A. and Hein, K.: Adolescents and sexually transmitted diseases. *In* Holmes, K. K., Måardh, P-A., Sparling, P. E., et al. (Eds.): Sexually Transmitted Diseases. New York, McGraw-Hill Book Co., 1984.

Beral, V.: Cancer of the cervix: A sexually transmitted infection? Lancet, *1*:1037, 1974.

Brunham, R. C., Kuo, C-C., Stevens, C. E., et al.: Treatment of concomitant *Neisseria gonorrhoeae* and *Chlamydia trachomatis* infections in women: Comparison of trimethoprim-sulfamethoxazole with ampicillin-probenecid. Rev. Infect. Dis., *4*:491, 1982.

Centers for Disease Control: Acquired immunodeficiency syndrome (AIDS) Update—United States. MMWR, *32*:309, 1983.

Centers for Disease Control: Annual summary 1981. Reported morbidity and mortality in the United States. MMWR, *30*:38, 43, 82, 1982.

Centers for Disease Control: Condyloma acuminatum—United States, 1966–1981. MMWR, *32*:306, 1983.

Centers for Disease Control: Follow-up on penicillaminase-producing *Neisseria gonorrhoeae*—worldwide. MMWR, *26*:153, 1977.

Centers for Disease Control: Genital herpes infection—United States, 1966–1979. MMWR, *31*:137, 1982.

Centers for Disease Control: Hepatitis surveillance, report number 46, U.S. Department of Health and Human Services, March 1981, pp 20–25.

Centers for Disease Control: Penicillaminase-producing *Neisseria gonorrhoeae*—Los Angeles. MMWR, *72*:181, 1983.

Centers for Disease Control: Penicilin-resistant gonorrhea—North Carolina. MMWR, *32*:273, 1983.

Centers for Disease Control: Sexually transmitted diseases: Treatment guidelines 1982. MMWR, *31*(Suppl):355, 1982; Rev. Infect. Dis., *4*:5729, 1982.

Corey, L.: General herpes. *In* Holmes, K. K., Måardh, P-A., Sparling, P. F., et al. (Eds.): Sexually Transmitted Diseases. New York, McGraw-Hill Book Co., 1984.

Corey, L., Reeves, W. C., and Holmes, K. K.: Cellular immune response in genital herpes simplex virus infection. N. Engl. J. Med., *299*:986, 1978.

Crawford, G., Knapp, J. S. Hale, J., et al.: Asymptomatic gonorrhea in men: Caused by gonococci with unique nutritional requirements. Science, *196*:1352, 1977.

Creasman, W. T., and Parker, R. T.: Management of early cervical neoplasia. Clin. Obstet. Gynecol., *18*:233, 1975.

Falk, H. C.: Interpretation of the pathogenesis of pelvic infection as determined by cornual resection. Am. J. Obstet. Gynecol., *52*:66, 1946.

Fichtner, R. R., Aral, S. O., Blount, J. H., et al.: Syphilis in the United States: 1967–1979. Sex. Transm. Dis., *10*:77, 1983.

Fraser, J. J., Rettig, P. J., and Kaplan, D. W.: Prevalence of cervical *Chlamydia trachomatis* and *Neisseria gonorrhoeae* infections in female adolescents. Pediatrics, *71*:333, 1983.

Graham, S., Rawls, W., Swanson, M., et al.: Sex partners and herpes simplex virus type 2 in the epidemiology of cancer of the cervix. Am. J. Epidemiol., *115*:729, 19082.

Harris, R. W. C., Brinton, L. A., Cowdell, R. H., et al.: Characteristics of women with dysplasia or carcinoma *in situ* of the cervix uteri. Br. J. Cancer, *42*:359, 1980.

Holmes, K. K., Bell, T. A., and Berger, R. E.: Epidemiology of sexually transmitted diseases. Urol. Clin. North Am., *11*:3, 1984.

Holmes, K. K., and Handsfield, F. H.: Sexually transmitted diseases. *In* Petersdorf, R. G., Adams, R. D., Braunwald, E., et al. (Eds.): Harrison's Principles of Internal Medicine. New York, McGraw-Hill Book Co., 1983.

Hunt, M.: Sexual Behavior in the Seventies. Chicago, Playboy Press, 1974, pp. 150–152.

Jick, H., Hannan, M. T., Stergachis, A., et al.: Vaginal spermicides and gonorrhea. JAMA, *248*:1619, 1982.

Johnson, R. E.: Epidemiologic and prophylactic treatment of gonorrhea: A decision analysis review. Sex. Transm. Dis., *6*:159, 1979.

Jones, R. B., Ardery, B. B., Hui, S. L., et al.: Correlation between serum antichlamydial antibodies and tubal factor as a cause of infertility. Fertil. Steril., *38*:553, 1982.

Judson, F. N.: Epidemiology and control of nongonococcal urethritis and genital chlamydial infections: A review. Sex. Transm. Dis., *8*(Suppl):117, 1981.

Judson, F. N., Penley, K. A., Robinson, M. E., et al.: Comparative prevalence rates of sexually transmitted diseases in heterosexual and homosexual men. Am. J. Epidemiol., *112*:836, 1980.

Kinghorn, G. R., and Waugh, M. A.: Oral contraceptive

use and prevalence of infection with *Chlamydia trachomatis* in women. Br. J. Vener. Dis., *57*:187, 1981.

Knapp, J. S., Thornsberry, C., Schoolnik, G. K., et al.: Phenotypic and epidemiolgic correlates of auxotype in *Neisseria gonorrhoeae*. J. Infect. Dis., *138*:160, 1978.

Mirrett, S., Reller, L. B., and Knapp, J. S.: *Neisseria gonorrhoeae* strains inhibited by vancomycin in selective media and correlation with auxotype. J. Clin. Microbiol., *14*:94, 1981.

Moore, D. E., Foy, H. M., Daling, J. R., et al.: Increased frequency of serum antibodies to *Chlamydia trachomatis* in infertility due to distal tubal disease. Lancet, *2*:574, 1982.

Mosher, W. D.: Infertility trends among U.S. couples: 1965–1976. Fam. Plann. Perspect., *14*:22, 1982.

National Center for Health Statistics: Births, Marriages, Divorces, and Deaths for March 1982. Monthly Vital Statistics Report 31:No. 3, June 21, 1982.

Pedersen, A. H. B., and Bonin, P.: Screening females for asymptomatic gonorrhea infection. Northwest. Med., *70*:255, 1971.

Perine, P. L., Morton, R. S., Piot, P., et al.: Epidemiology and treatment of penicillinase-producing *Neisseria gonorrhoeae*. Sex. Transm. Dis., *6*(Suppl):152, 1979.

Phillips, L., Potterat, J. J., Rothenberg, R. B., et al.: Focused interviewing in gonorrhea control. Am. J. Publ. Health, *70*:705, 1980.

Pollack, E. S., and Horn, J. W.: Trends in cancer incidence and mortality in the United States, 1969–1976. J. Natl. Cancer Inst., *64*:1091, 1980.

Poretz, D. M.: The private practice of infectious disease. J. Infect. Dis., *147*:417, 1983.

Rubin, G. L., Ory, H. W., and Layde, P. M.: Oral contraceptives and pelvic inflammatory disease. Am. J. Obstet. Gynecol., *144*:630, 1982.

Schmerin, M. J., Jones, T. C., and Klein, H.: Giardiasis: Association with homosexuality. Ann. Intern. Med., *88*:801, 1978.

Scott, R. M., Snitbhan, R., Bancroft, W. H., et al.: Experimental transmission of hepatitis B virus by semen and saliva. J. Infect. Dis., *142*:67, 1980.

Senanayake, P., and Kramer, D.: Contraception and the etiology of pelvic inflammatory disease: New perspectives. Am. J. Obstet. Gynecol., *138*(Part 2):852, 1980.

Sorensen, R. C.: Adolescent Sexuality in Contemporary America. New York, World Publishing Co., 1972. p. 122.

Stamm, W. E., Wagner, K. F., Amsel, R., et al.: Causes of the acute urethral syndrome in women. N. Engl. J. Med., *303*:409, 1980.

St. John, R. K., Blount, J., and Jones, O.: Pelvic inflammatory disease in the United States: Incidence and trends in private practice. Sex. Transm. Dis., *8*:56, 1981.

St. John, R. K., Jones, O. G., Blount, J. H., et al.: Pelvic inflammatory disease in the United States: Epidemiology and trends among hospitalized women. Sex. Transm. Dis., *8*:62, 1981.

Thayer, J. D., and Martin, J. E.: A selective medium for the cultivation of *N. gonorrhoeae* and *N. meningitidis*. Public Health Rep., *79*:49, 1964.

U.S. Bureau of the Census: Current Population Reports. Series P-25, No. 917, Preliminary estimates of the population in the United States, by age, sex and race: 1970 to 1981. Washington, D.C., U.S. Govt. Print. Office, 1982.

U.S. Department of Health and Human Services, Public Health Services, Centers for Disease Control: STD Fact Sheet, Edition 35.

Wentworth, B. B., Bonin, P., Holmes, K. K., et al.: Isolation of viruses, bacteria and other organisms from venereal disease clinic patients: Methodology and problems associated with multiple isolations. Health Lab. Sci., *10*:75, 1973.

Weström, L., Bengtsson, L. P. H., and Måardh, P-A.: Incidence, trends, and risks of ectopic pregnancy in a population of women. Br. Med. J., *282*:15, 1981.

Weström, L., and Måardh, P-A.: Pelvic inflammatory disease: epidemiology, clinical manifestations, and sequelae. *In* Holmes, K. K., and Måardh, P-A. (Eds.): International Perspectives on Neglected Sexually Transmitted Diseases: Impact on Venereology, Infertility, and Maternal and Infant Health. New York, McGraw-Hill Book Co., 1983.

William, D. C.: Hepatitis and other sexually transmitted diseases in gay men and lesbians. Sex. Transm. Dis., *8*(Suppl):330, 1981.

William, D. C.: Sexually transmitted disease in gay men: An insider's view. Sex. Transm. Dis., *6*:278, 1979.

Windall, J. J., Hall, M. M., Washington, J. A., et al.: Inhibitory effects of vancomycin on *Neisseria gonorrhoeae* in Thayer-Martin medium. J. Infect. Dis., *142*:775, 1980.

Zelnik, M., and Kantner, J. F.: Sexual activity, contraceptive use and pregnancy among metropolitan teenagers: 1971–1979. Fam. Plann. Perspect. *12*:230, 1980.

Gonococcal Urethritis in Men

Aral, S. O., and Holmes, K. K.: Epidemiology of sexually transmitted diseases. *In* Holmes, K. K., Måardh, P-A., Sparling, P. F., et al. (Eds.): Sexually Transmitted Diseases. New York, McGraw-Hill Book Co., 1984.

Ashford, W. A., Golash, R. G., and Hemming, V. G.: Penicillaminase-producing *Neisseria gonorrhoeae*. Lancet, *2*:657, 1976.

Austin, T. W., Brooks, G. F., Bethel, M., et al.: Trimethoprim-sulfamethoxazole in the treatment of gonococcal urethritis. J. Infect. Dis. *128*:S666, 1973.

Babione, R. W., Hedgecock, L. E., and Ray, J. P.: Navy experience with oral use of penicillin as a prophylaxis. U.S. Armed Forces J., *3*:973, 1952.

Basaca-Sevilla, V., Riel, R. S., Sevilla, J. S., et al.: The prevalence of *Neisseria gonorrhoeae* and penicillinase-producing *N. gonorrhoeae* in the Philippines. Phil. J. Microbiol. Infect. Dis., *9*:45, 1980.

Berg, S. W., and Harrison, W. O.: Spectinomycin as primary treatment of gonorrhea in areas of high prevalence of penicillinase-producing *Neisseria gonorrhoeae*. Sex. Transm. Dis., *8*:38, 1981.

Berg, S. W., Kilpatrick, M. E., Harrison, W. O., et al.: Cefoxitin as single-dose treatment for urethritis caused by penicillinase-producing *Neisseria gonorrhoeae*. N. Engl. J. Med., *301*:509, 1979.

Berger, R. E.: Urethritis and epididymitis. Semin. Med., *1*:38, 1983.

Brooks, G. F., Gotschlich, E. C., Holmes, K. K., et al.: Immunobiology of *Neisseria gonorrhoeae*. Washington, D. C., American Society for Microbiology, 1978.

Brown, S. T., Thompson, S. E., Biddle, J. W., et al.: Treatment of uncomplicated gonococcal infection with trimethoprim-sulfamethoxazole. Sex. Transm. Dis., *9*:9, 1982.

Campbell, D. J.: Gonorrhea in North Africa and the central Mediterranean. Br. Med. J., *2*:44, 1944.

Cates, W., Jr., Weisner, P. J., and Curran, J. W.: Sex and spermicides: Preventing unintended pregnancy and infection. JAMA, *148*:1636, 1982.

Centers for Disease Control: Global distribution of penicillinase-producing *Neisseria gonorrhoeae* (PPNG). MMWR, *31*:1, 1982.

Centers for Disease Control: Penicillaminase-producing *Neisseria gonorrhoeae*—Los Angeles. MMWR, *32*:181, 1983.

Centers for Disease Control: Pencillin-resistant gonorrhea—North Carolina. MMWR, *32*:273, 1983.

Centers for Disease Control: Sexually transmitted disease: Statistical letter. U.S. Dept. Health Human Services.

Centers for Disease Control: Sexually transmitted disease: Treatment guidelines 1982. MMWR, *31*(Suppl):35S, 1982.

Centers for Disease Control: Spectinomycin-resistant penicillinase-producing *Neisseria gonorrhoeae*—worldwide. MMWR, *31*:632, 1982.

Crawford, G., Knapp, J. S., Hale, J., et al.: Asymptomatic gonorrhea in men. Science, *196*:1352, 1937.

Dees, J. E., and Colston, J. A. C.: The use of sulfonilamide in gonococcic infections: A preliminary report. JAMA, *108*:1855, 1937.

Elmros, T., and Larrsen, P. A.: Survival of gonococci outside the body. Br. Med. J., *2*:403, 1972.

Engelbrecht, H. E., Movson, I. J., and Van den Bulcke, C.: Urethral stricture in males. S. Afr. J. Radiol., *5*:28, 1967.

Frazier, J. J., Miller, J., and Pickering, L. K.: Orbital cellulitis due to *Neisseria gonorrhoeae* in an enucleated socket. Arch. Ophthalmol., *97*:2345, 1979.

Gilbaugh, J. H., and Fuchs, P. C.: The gonococcus and the toilet seat. N. Engl. J. Med., *301*:91, 1979.

Granato, P. A., Schneible-Smith, C., and Weiner, L. B.: Use of New York City medium for improved recovery of *N. gonorrhoeae* from clinical specimens. J. Clin. Microbiol., *13*:963, 1981.

Greenberg, S. H.: Male reproductive tract sequelae of gonococcal and nongonococcal urethritis. Arch. Androl., *3*:317, 1979.

Halverson, C. W., Keys, T. F., and Clarke, E. J., Jr.: *In vitro* susceptibility of *Neisseria gonorrhoeae* to different antibiotics. Milit. Med., *134*:1427, 1969.

Handsfield, H. H., Lipman, T. O., Harnisch, J. P., et al.: Asymptomatic gonorrhea in men. N. Engl. J. Med., *290*:117, 1974.

Handsfield, H. M., Murphy, V. L., and Holmes, K. K.: Dose-ranging study of ceftriaxone for uncomplicated gonorrhea in men. Antimicrob. Agents Chemother. *290*:839, 1981.

Harrison, W. O.: Cefaclor in the treatment of uncomplicated gonococcal urethritis. Postgrad. Med. J., *55*:85, 1979.

Harrison, W. O.: Gonococcal urethritis. Urol. Clin. North Am., *11*:45, 1984.

Harrison, W. O., Hooper, R. R., Kilpatrick, M. E., et al: Penicillin-resistant gonorrhea: Alternative therapy. *In* Seigenthaler, W., and Luthy, R. (Eds.): Current Chemotherapy. Washington, D.C., American Society for Microbiology, *1*:194–195, 1978.

Harrison, W. O., Hooper, R. R., Wiesner, P. J., et al.: A trial of minocycline given after exposure to prevent gonorrhea. N. Engl. J. Med., *300*:1074, 1979.

Harrison, W. O., Hooper, R. R., Wiesner, P. J., et al.: Prevention of gonorrhea: Evaluation of prophylactic antibiotics. Proc. 13th Intersci. Conf. Antimicrob. Agents Chemother., abstract 64, Washington, D.C., American Society for Microbiology, 1973.

Holmes, K. K., Counts, G. W., and Beaty, H. N.: Disseminated gonococcal infection. Ann. Intern. Med., *74*:979, 1971.

Holmes, K. K., Wiesner, P. J., and Pederson, A. H. B.: The gonococcal arthritis dermatitis syndrome. Ann. Intern. Med., *75*:470, 1971.

Hooper, R. R., Wiesner, P. J., Harrison, W. O., et al.:

Cohort study of venereal diseases: 1. Risk of transmission from infected women to men. Am. J. Epidemiol., *107*:235, 1978.

James-Holmquist, A. N., Wende, R. D., Mudd, R. L., et al.: Comparison of atmospheric conditions for culture of clinical specimens of *Neisseria gonorrhoeae*. Appl. Microbiol., *26*:466, 1973.

John, J., and Donald, W. H.: Asymptomatic urethral gonorrhea in men. Br. J. Vener. Dis., *54*:322, 1978.

Judson, F. N.: Gonococcal urethritis—Diagnosis and treatment. Arch. Androl., *3*:329, 1979.

Kampmeier, R. H.: Introduction of sulfonamide therapy for gonorrhea. Sex. Transm. Dis., *10*:81, 1983.

Katsman, L.: Gonorrheal abscess of the penis. Vestn. Dermatol. Venerol., *5*:64, 1980.

Kellogg, D. S., Holmes, K. K., and Hill, G. A.: Cumitech 4: Laboratory diagnosis of gonorrhea. Washington, D. C., American Society for Microbiology, 1976.

Kleibl, K.: Primary gonococcal abscess on the raphe perinei. Czech. Dermatol., *54*:9, 1979.

Kvale, P. A., Keys, T. F., Johnson, D. W., et al.: Single oral dose ampicillin-probenecid treatment of gonorrhea in the male. JAMA, *215*:1449, 1971.

Lancaster, D. J., Berg, S. W., Harrison, W. O., et al.: Treatment of penicillin-resistant gonorrhea with cefotaxime. Drug Ther. (Spec. Suppl.), 87, Oct. 1981.

Marx, J. L.: Vaccinating with bacterial pili. Science, *209*:1103, 1980.

McCutchan, J. A.: Gonorrhea and nongonococcal urethritis. *In* Braude, A. I. (Ed.): Medical Microbiology and Infectious Disease. Philadelphia, W. B. Saunders Co., 1981.

McCutchan, J. A., Adler, M. W., and Berrie, J. R. H.: Penicillinase-producing *Neisseria gonorrhoeae* in Great Britain, 1977–1981. Br. Med. J., *285*:337, 1982.

Miller, M. A., Millikin, P., Griffin, P. S., et al.: *Neisseria meningitidis* urethritis: A case report. JAMA, *242*:1656, 1979.

Moore, G., Pittard, W. B., III, Mosca, N., et al.: gonorrhea detection by urine sediment culture. JAMA, *224*:1499, 1973.

Morton, R. S.: The gonococcus. *In* Gonorrhea. London, W. B. Saunders Co., 1977, pp. 25–61.

Neisser, A.: Zbl. Med. Wiss., *17*:497, 1879.

Phillips, I.: Beta-lactamase-producing, penicillin-resistant gonococcus. Lancet, *2*:656, 1976.

Portnoy, J., Mendelson, J., Clecner, B., et al.: Asymptomatic gonorrhea in the male. Can. Med. Assoc. J., *110*:169, 1974.

Riccardi, N. B., and Felman, Y. M.: Laboratory diagnosis in the problem of suspected gonococcal infection. JAMA, *242*:2703, 1979.

Rothenberg, R., and Judson, F. N.: The clinical diagnosis of urethral discharge. Sex. Transm. Dis., *10*:24, 1983.

Soendjojo, A.: Gonococcal urethritis due to fellatio. Sex. Transm. Dis., *10*:41, 1983.

Sparling, P. F.: Treatment of gonorrhea: What effect will antibiotic resistance have in the future? Sex. Transm. Dis., *6*:120, 1979.

Thayer, J. D., and Martin, J. E.: Improved medium selective for cultivation of *Neisseria gonorrhoeae* and *Neisseria meningitidis*. Public Health Rep., *81*:559, 1966.

van Klingeren, B., van Wijngaarden, L. J., Dessens-Kroon, M., et al.: Penicillinase-producing gonococci in the Netherlands in 1981. J. Antimicrob. Chemother., *11*:15, 1983.

Watson, R. A.: Gonorrhea and acute epididymitis. Milit. Med., *144*:784, 1979.

Willcox, R. R.: Amoxycillin in the treatment of gonorrhea. Br. J. Vener. Dis., *48*:504, 1972.

Nongonococcal Urethritis in Men

Alani, M. D., Darougar, S., Burns, D. C., et al.: Isolation of *Chlamydia trachomatis* from the male urethra. Br. J. Vener. Dis., *53*:1977.

Aral, S. O., and Holmes, K. K.: Epidemiology of sexually transmitted diseases. *In* Holmes, K. K., Måardh, P-A., Sparling, P. F., et al. (Eds.): Sexually Transmitted Diseases. New York, McGraw-Hill, 1984.

Berger, R. E., Alexander, E. R., Harnisch, J. P., et al.: Etiology, manifestations and therapy of acute epididymitis: Prospective study of 50 cases. J. Urol., *121*:750, 1979.

Berger, R. E.: Nongonococcal urethritis and related syndromes. *In* Stamey, T.A. (Ed.): Monographs in Urology. Burroughs Wellcome, 1982.

Bowie, W. R.: Comparison of Gram stain and first voided urine sediment in the diagnosis of urethritis. Sex. Transm. Dis., *5*:39, 1978.

Bowie, W. R.: Nongonococcal urethritis. Urol. Clin. North Am., *11*:55, 1984.

Bowie, W. R.: Treatment of chlamydial infections. *In* Måardh, P-A., et al. (Eds.): Chlamydial Infections. Amsterdam, Elsevier Biomedical Press, 1982, pp. 231–244.

Bowie, W. R., Alexander, E. R., Floyd, J. F., et al.: Differential response of chlamydial and ureaplasma-associated urethritis to sulfafurazole (sulfisoxazole) and aminocyclitols. Lancet, *2*:1276, 1976.

Bowie, W. R., Alexander, E. R., and Holmes, K. K.: Etiologies of postgonococcal urethritis in homosexual and heterosexual men: Roles of *Chlamydia trachomatis* in *Ureaplasma urealyticum*. Sex. Transm. Dis., *5*:151, 1978*a*.

Bowie, W. R., Alexander, E. R., Stimson, J. B., et al.: Therapy for nongonococcal urethritis: Double-blind randomized comparison of two doses and two durations of minocycline. Ann. Intern. Med., *95*:306, 1981.

Bowie, W. R., Floyd, J. F., Stimson, J. B., et al.: Double-blind comparison of two doses and two durations of minocycline therapy for nongonococcal urethritis. *In* Siegenthaler, W., and Luthy, R. (Eds.): Current Chemotherapy: Proceedings of the 10th International Congress of Chemotherapy. Zurich Sept. 18–23, 1977*a*. Washington, D.C., American Society for Microbiology, 1978*b*.

Bowie, W. R., Pollock, H. M., Forsyth, P. S., et al.: Bacteriology of the urethra in normal men and men with nongonococcal urethritis. J. Clin. Microbiol., *6*:482, 1977*b*.

Bowie, W. B., Wang, S. P., Alexander, E. R., et al.: Etiology of nongonococcal urethritis: Evidence for *C. trachomatis* and *U. urealyticum*. J. Clin. Invest., *59*:735, 1977*c*.

Bowie, W. R., Yu, J. S., Fawcett, A., et al.: Tetracycline in nongonococcal urethritis. Comparison of 2 g and 1 g daily for 7 days. Br. J. Vener. Dis., *56*:332, 1980.

Bureau of the Census. U.S. Department of Commerce: Current population reports: Population estimates and projections. Projections of the number of households and families, 1979–1995. Series P25, No. 805, 1979.

Centers for Disease Control: Sexually transmitted disease: Treatment guidelines 1982. MMWR, *31*:33S, 1982.

Coufalik, E. D., Taylor-Robinson, D., and Csonka, G. W.: Treatment of nongonococcal urethritis with rifampicin as a means of defining the role of *Ureaplasma urealyticum*. Br. J. Vener. Dis., *55*:36, 1979.

Csango, P. A.: *Chlamydia trachomatis* from men with nongonococcal urethritis: Simplified procedure for cultivation and isolation in replicating McCoy cell culture. Acta Pathol. Microbiol. Scand. (B), *86*:257, 1978.

Ford, D. K., da Roza, D. M., and Schulzer, M.: The specificity of synovial mononuclear cell responses to microbiological antigens in Reiter's syndrome. J. Rheumatol., *9*:561, 1982.

Handsfield, H. H., Alexander, E. R., Wang, S. P., et al.: Differences in the therapeutic response of chlamydia-positive and chlamydia-negative forms of nongonococcal urethritis. J. Am. Vener. Dis. Assoc., *2*:5–9, 1975.

Harrison, W. O., Hooper, R. R., Wiesner, P. J., et al.: A trial of minocycline given after exposure to prevent gonorrhea. N. Engl. J. Med., *300*:1074, 1979.

Holmes, K. K., Handsfield, H. H., Wang, S.P., et al.: Etiology of nongonococcal urethritis. N. Engl. J. Med., *292*:1199, 1975.

Jocobs, N. F., and Kraus, S. J.: Gonococcal and nongonococcal urethritis in men. Clinical and laboratory differentiation. Ann. Intern,. Med., *82*:7, 1975.

Keat, A. C., Maini, R. N., Nkwazi, G. C., et al.: Role of *Chlamydia trachomatis* and HLA-B27 in sexually acquired reactive arthritis. Br. Med. J., *1*:605, 1978.

Lassus, A., Paavonen, J., Kousa, M., et al.: Erythromycin and lymecycline treatment in Chlamydia-positive and Chlamydia-negative nongonococcal urethritis—A partner-controlled study. Acta Derm. Venereol., *59*:278, 1979.

Linder, K.: Gonoblennurrhoe, Finsehlussblennorrhoe, und trachoma. Albrecht von Graefes. Arch. Klin. Exp. Opthalmol., *78*:345, 1911.

McCabe, M. E., Fiumara, N. J., and McCormack, W. M.: Effect of three regimens for the treatment of gonorrhea on the incidence of postgonococcal urethritis. Presented at the First Sexually Transmitted Diseases World Congress, San Juan, Puerto Rico, November 15–21, 1981, abstract no. 130.

Martin, D. H., Pollack, S., Kuo, C-C., et al.: Urethral chlamydial infection in men with Reiter's syndrome. *In* Måardh, P-A., et al. (Eds.): Chlamydial Infections. Amsterdam, Elsevier Biomedical Press, 1982.

Meares, E. M., Jr., and Stamey, T. A.: Bacteriologic localization patterns in bacterial prostatitis and urethritis. Invest. Urol., *5*:492, 1968.

Oriel, J. D., Reeve, P., Thomas, B. J., et al.: Infection with Chlamydia group A in men with urethritis due to *Neisseria gonorrhoeae*. J. Infect. Dis., *131*:376, 1975.

Oriel, J.D., Reeve, P., Wright, J. T., et al.: Chlamydia infection of the male urethra. Br. J. Vener. Dis., *52*:46, 1976.

Paavonen, J., Kousa, M., Saikku, P., et al.: Examination of men with nongonococcal urethritis and their sexual partners for *Chlamydia trachomatis* and *Ureaplasma urealyticum*. Sex. Transm. Dis., *5*:93, 1978.

Perroud, H. M., and Miedzybrodzka, K.: Chlamydial infection of the urethra in men. Br. J. Vener. Dis., *54*:45, 1978.

Podgore, J. K., Holmes, K. K., and Alexander, E. R.: Asymptomatic urethral infections due to *Chlamydia trachomatis* in male U.S. military personnel. J. Infect. Dis., *146*:828, 1982.

Richmond, S. J., Hilton, A. L., and Clark, S. K. R.: Chlamydial infection: Role of chlamydia subgroup A in nongonococcal and postgonococcal urethritis. Br. J. Vener. Dis., *48*:437, 1972.

Richmond, S. J., and Sparling, P. F.: Genital chlamydial infections. Am. J. Epidemiol., *103*:428, 1976.

Ripa, K. T., Måardh, P-A., and Thelin, I.: *Chlamydia trachomatis* urethritis in men attending a venereal disease clinic: A culture and therapeutic study. Acta Derm. Venereol., *58*:175, 1978.

Root, T. E., Edwards, L. D., and Spengler, P. J.: Nongonococcal urethritis: A survey of clinical and laboratory features. Sex. Transm. Dis., *7*:59, 1980.

Schachter, J.: Chlamydial infections. N. Engl. J. Med., *298*:423, 490, 540, 1978.

Schachter, J., Hanna, I., Hill, E. C., et al.: Are chlamydia infections the most prevalent venereal disease? JAMA. *231*:1252, 1975.

Segura, J. W., Smith, T. F., Weed, L. A., et al.: Chlamydia and nonspecific urethritis. J. Urol., *117*:720, 1977.

Shepard, M. C., and Lunceford, C. D.: Serological typing of *Ureaplasma urealyticum* isolates from urethritis patients by an agar growth inhibition method. J. Clin. Microbiol., *8*:566, 1978.

Simmons, P. D.: Evaluation of the early morning smear investigation. Br. J. Vener. Dis., *54*:128, 1978.

Stimson, J. B., Hale, J., Bowie, W. R., and Holmes, K. K.: Tetracycline resistant *Ureaplasma urealyticum*: A cause of persistent urethritis. Ann. Intern. Med., *94*:192, 1981.

Swartz, S. L., Kraus, S. J., Herrmann, K. L., et al.: Diagnosis and etiology of nongonococcal urethritis. J. Infect. Dis., *138*:445, 1978.

Taylor-Robinson, D., Evans, R. T., Coufalik, E. D., et al.: *Ureaplasma urealyticum* and *Mycoplasma hominis* in chlamydial and non-chlamydial nongonococcal urethritis. Br. J. Vener. Dis., *55*:30, 1979.

Taylor-Robinson, D., and McCormack, W. M.: The genital mycoplasmas. N. Engl. J. Med., *302*:1003, 1980.

Terho, P.: *Chlamydia trachomatis* in gonococcal and postgonococcal urethritis. Br. J. Vener. Dis., *54*:326, 1978*a*.

Terho, P.: *Chlamydia trachomatis* in nonspecific urethritis. Br. J. Vener. Dis., *5*:93, 1978*b*.

Thelin, I., Wennstrom, A-M., and Måardh, P-A.: Contact tracing in patients with genital chlamydial infection. Br. J. Vener. Dis., *56*:259, 1980.

Vaughan-Jackson, J. D., Dunlop, E. M. C., Daroughar, S., et al.: Urethritis due to *Chlamydia trachomatis*. Br. J. Vener. Dis., *53*:180, 1977.

Wiesner, P. J.: Selected aspects of the epidemiology of nongonococcal urethritis. *In* Hobson, D., and Holmes, K. K. (Eds.): Nongonococcal Urethritis and Related Oculogenital Infections. Washington, D.C., The American Society for Microbiology, 1977.

Wong, J. L., Hines, P. A., Brasher, M. D., et al.: The etiology of nongonococcal urethritis in men attending a venereal disease clinic. Sex. Transm. Dis., *4*:4, 1977.

Urethritis in Women

Bailey, R. R.: Significance of coagulase-negative staphylococci in urine. J. Infect. Dis., *127*:179, 1973.

Brooks, D., and Maudar, A.: Pathogenesis of the urethral syndrome in women and its diagnosis in general practice. Lancet, *2*:893, 1972.

Brumfitt, W., Hamilton-Miller, J. M. T., Ludlam, H., et al.: Lactobacilli do not cause frequency and dysuria syndrome. Lancet, *2*:393, 1972.

Corey, L., Adams, H. G., Brown, Z. A., et al.: Genital herpes simplex virus infections: Clinical manifestations, course, and complications. Ann. Intern. Med., *98*:958, 1983.

Counts, G. C., Stamm, W. E., McKevitt, M., et al.: Treatment of cystitis in women with a single dose of trimethoprim-sulfamethoxazole. Rev. Infect. Dis., *4*:484, 1982.

Curran, J. W., Rendtorff, R. C., Chandler, R. W., et al.: Female gonorrhea: Its relation to abnormal uterine bleeding, urinary tract symptoms, and cervicitis. Obstet. Gynecol., *45*:195, 1975.

Dove, G. A., Bailey, A. J., Gower, P. E., et al.: Diagnosis of urinary tract infection in general practice. Lancet, *2*:1281, 1972.

Drabu, Y. J., and Sanderson, P. J.: Urine culture in urethral syndrome. Lancet, *1*:37, 1980.

Engel, G. Schaeffer, A. J., Grayhack, J. T., et al.: The role of excretory urography and cystoscopy in the evaluation and management of women with recurrent urinary tract infection. J. Urol., *123*:1909, 1980.

Fair, W. R., McClennan, B. L., and Jost, R. G.: Are excretory urograms necessary in evaluating women with urinary tract infection? J. Urol., *121*:313, 1979.

Fowler, J. E., and Pulaski, E. T.: Excretory urography, cystography, and cystoscopy in the evaluation of women with urinary-tract infection. N. Engl. J. Med., *304*:462, 1981.

Gallagher, D. J. A., Montgomerie, J. Z., and North, J. D. K.: Acute infections of the urinary tract and the urethral syndrome in general practice. Br. Med. J., *1*:622, 1965.

Gargan, R. A., Brumfitt, W., and Hamilton-Miller, J. M. T.: Do anaerobes cause urinary infections? Lancet, *1*:37, 1980.

Greenberg, R. N., Rein, M. F., Sander, C. V., et al.: Urethral syndrome in women. JAMA, *245*:1106, 1981.

Handsfield, H. H.: Gonorrhea and nongonococcal urethritis: Recent advances. Med. Clin. North Am. *62*:925, 1978.

Hovelius, B., Måardh, P-A., and Bygren, P.: Urinary tract infections caused by *Staphylococcus saprophyticus*: Recurrences and complications. J. Urol., *122*:645, 1979.

Jordon, P. A., Iravani, A., Richard, G. A., et al.: Urinary tact infection caused by *Staphylococcus saprophyticus*. J. Infect. Dis., *142*:510, 1980.

Kass, E. H.: Asymptomatic infections of the urinary tract. Trans. Assoc. Am. Physicians, *69*:56, 1956.

Kindall, L., and Nickels, T. T.: Allergy of the pelvic urinary tract in the female: A preliminary report. J. Urol., *61*:222, 1949.

Komaroff, A. L., Pass, T. M., McCue, J. D., et al.: Management strategies for urinary and vaginal infections. Arch. Intern. Med., *138*:1069, 1978.

Kraft, J. K., and Stamey, T. A.: The natural history of symptomatic recurrent bacteriuria in women. Medicine, *56*:55, 1977.

Latham, R. H., and Stamm, W. E.: Urethral syndrome in women. Urol. Clin. North Am., *11*:95, 1984.

McLean, P., and Emmett, J. L.: Internal urethrotomy in women for recurrent infection and chronic urethritis. J. Urol., *101*:724, 1969.

Mond, N. C., Percival, A., Williams, J. D., et al.: Presentation, diagnosis, and treatment of urinary tract infections in general practice. Lancet, *1*:514, 1965.

Paavonen, J.: *Chlamydia trachomatis*–induced urethritis in female partners of men with nongonococcal urethritis. Sex. Transm. Dis., *6*:69, 1979.

Sellin, M., Cooke, D. I., Gillespie, W. A., et al.: Micrococcal urinary tract infections in young women. Lancet, *2*:570, 1975.

Smith, D. R.: Stress reaction linked to urinary frequency. Med. World News. July 20, 1962.

Stamm, W. E., Counts, G. W., Running, K. R., et al.: Diagnosis of coliform infection in acutely dysuric women. N. Engl. J. Med., *307*:463, 1982.

Stamm, W. E., Running, K., Hale, J., et al.: Etiologic role of *Mycoplasma hominis* and *Ureaplasma urealyticum* in women with the acute urethral syndrome. Sex. Transm. Dis. (Suppl.), *10*:271, 1983.

Stamm, W. E., Wagner, K. F., Amsel, R., et al.: Causes of the acute urethral syndrome in women. N. Engl. J. Med., *303*:409, 1980.

Steensberg, J., Bartels, E. D., Bay-Nielson, H., et al.:

Epidemiology of urinary tract diseases in general practice. Br. Med. J., 4:390, 1969.

Tapsall, J. W., Taylor, P. C., Bell, S. M., et al.: Relevance of "significant bacteriuria" to aetiology and diagnosis of urinary tract infection. Lancet, 2:637, 1975.

Wallin, J. E., Thompson, S. E., Zaidi, A., et al.: Urethritis in women attending an STD clinic. Br. J. Vener. Dis., 57:50, 1981.

Wong, E. S., Fennel, C., and Stamm, W. E.: Urinary tract infections among women attending a sexually transmitted disease clinic. Sex. Transm. Dis., 11:18, 1984.

Epididymitis

Abu-Sleiman, R., Ho, J. E., and Gregory, J. G.: Scrotal scanning. Present value and limits of interpretation. Urology, 13:326, 1979.

Amar, A. A.: Trichomonas vaginalis epididymitis. JAMA, 200:417, 1917.

Barker, K., and Roper, R. P.: Torsion of the testis. Br. J. Urol., 36:35, 1964.

Beck, A. D., and Taylor, D. E.: Post-prostatectomy epididymitis: A bacteriological and clinical survey. J. Urol., 104:143, 1970.

Berger, R. E.: Acute epididymitis. Sex. Transm. Dis., 8:286, 1981.

Berger, R. E.: Nongonococcal urethritis and related syndromes. In Stamey, T. E. (Ed.): Monographs in Urology. Burroughs-Welcome, 1982.

Berger, R. E., Alexander, E. R., Harnish, J. P., et al.: Etiology, manifestations and therapy of acute epididymitis: Prospective study of 50 cases. J. Urol., 121:750, 1979.

Berger, R. E., Alexander, E. R., Monda, G. D., et al.: *Chlamydia trachomatis* as a cause of acute "idiopathic" epididymitis. N. Engl. J. Med., 298:301, 1978.

Berger, R. E., Holmes, K. K., Mayo, M.E., et al.: The clinical uses of epididymal aspiration cultures in the management of selected patients with acute epididymitis. J. Urol., 124:60, 1980.

Bietz, O.: Fertilitatsuntersuchungen bei der unspezifichen Epididymitis. Hautarzt, 10:134, 1959.

Bormel, P.: Current concepts of the etiology and treatment of epididymitis. Med. Bull. U.S. Army, Europe, 20:332, 1963.

Bowie, W. R.: Urethritis in men. In The Diagnosis and Treatment of Sexually Transmitted Diseases. Boston, John Wright PSG Inc., 1983.

Bruce, A. W., Chadwick, P., Willet, W. S., et al.: The role of chlamydiae in genitourinary disease. J. Urol., 126:625, 1981.

Bullock, K. N., and Hunt, J. M.: The intravenous urogram in acute epididymo-orchitis. Br. J. Urol., 53:47, 1981.

Costas S., and Van Blerk, P. J. P.: Incision of the external inguinal ring in acute epididymitis. Br. J. Urol., 45:555, 1973.

David, W. H., and Scardino, P. L.: Meningitis presenting as epididymitis. South. Med. J., 65:936, 1972.

Delvillar, R. G., Ireland, G. W., and Cass, A. S.: Early exploration in acute testicular conditions. J. Urol., 108:887, 1972.

Doolittle, K. H., Smith, J. P., and Saylor, M. L.: Epididymitis in the prepubertal boy. J. Urol., 96:364, 1966.

Drach, G. W.: Sexuality and prostatitis: A hypothesis. J. Am. Vener. Dis. Assoc., 3:87, 1976.

Drach, G. W.: Trimethoprim-sulfamethoxazole therapy of chronic bacterial prostatitis. J. Urol., 11:637, 1974.

Drummond, A. C.: Trichomonas infection of the prostate gland. Am. J. Surg., 31:98, 1936.

Eykyn, S., Bulitude, M. I., Mayo, M. E., Lloyd-Davies,

R. W., et al.: Prostatic calculi as a source of recurrent bacteruria in the male. Br. J. Urol., 46:527, 1974.

Fisher, I., and Morton, R. S.: Epididymitis due to *Trichomonas vaginalis*. Br. J. Vener. Dis., 45:252, 1969.

Furness, G., Kamat, M. K., Kaminski, Z., et al.: The relationship of epididymitis to gonorrhea. Invest. Urol., 11:312, 1974.

Furness, G., Kamat, M. K., Kaminski, Z., et al.: Epididymitis after the luminal spread of NSU corynebacteria and gram-negative bacteria from the fossa navicularis. Invest. Urol., 11:486, 1974.

Gartman, E.: Epididymitis: A reappraisal. Am. J. Surg., 101:756, 1961.

Gasparich, J. P., Mason, J. T., Greene, H. L., Berger, R. E. and Krieger, S. N.: Amiodarone-associated epididymitis: Drug-related epididymitis in the absence of infection. J. Urol. In press.

Gierup, J., Hedenberg, C., and Osterman, A.: Acute nonspecific epididymitis in boys. Scand. J. Urol. Nephrol., 9:5, 1975.

Gislason, T., Noronha, R. F. X., and Gregory, J. F.: Acute epididymitis in boys: A 5-year retrospective study. J. Urol., 124:533, 1980.

Gottesman, J. E.: Coccidioidomycosis of prostate and epididymitis with urethrocutaneous fistula. Urology, 4:711, 1974.

Graham, J. B., and Grayhack, T. T.: Epididymitis following unilateral vasectomy and prostatic surgery. J. Urol., 87:582, 1962.

Graves, R. S., and Engel, W. J.: Experimental production of epididymitis with sterile urine: Clinical implications. J. Urol., 64:601, 1950.

Hanley, H. G.: Nonspecific epididymitis. Br. J. Surg., 53:875, 1966.

Holder, L. E., Martin, J. R., Holmes, E. R., et al.: Testicular radionuclide angiography and static imaging: anatomy, scintigraphic interpretation, and clinical indications. Radiology, 125:739, 1977.

Johannisson, G., Lowhagen, G-B., and Nilsson, S.: *Chlamydia trachomatis* and urethritis in men. Scand. J. Infect. Dis. (Suppl.), 32:87, 1981.

Kamat, M. H., Del Gaizo, A., and Seebode, J. J.: Epididymitis: Response to different modalities of treatment. J. Med. Soc. N.J., 67:227, 1970.

Kazzaz, B. A., and Salmo, N. A.: Epididymitis due to *Schistosoma haematobium* infection. Trop. Geogr. Med., 26:333, 1974.

Kessler, D., Berger, R. E., and Holmes, K. K.: Epididymitis in heterosexual and homosexual men. Presented at the 5th Meeting of International Society of STD Research, Seattle, August 1983.

Kohler, P. F.: An inquiry into the etiology of acute epididymitis. J. Urol., 87:918, 1962.

Krieger, J. N.: Urologic aspects of trichomoniasis. Invest. Urol., 18:411, 1981.

Kristensen, J. K., and Scheibel, J. H.: Acute epididymitis. Ugeskr. Laeger., 143:3550, 1981.

Lapides, J., Harwig, K. R., Anderson, E. C., et al.: Oxyphenbutazone therapy for mumps orchitis and acute epididymitis and osteitis pubis. J. Urol., 98:526, 1964.

Lommel, C.: Beitrage zur Kenntnis der Antiperistaltik das Vas Deferens. Ztschr. Urol. Chir., 3:214, 1914.

Måardh, P-A., Colleen, S., and Sylwan, J.: Inhibiting effect on the formation of chlamydial inclusions in McCoy cells by seminal fluid and some of its constituents. Invest. Urol., 17:510, 1980.

McClellan, D. S., Cottrell, T. L. C., and Lloyd, F. A.: Effect of varidase on acute nonspecific epididymitis. J. Urol., 8:633, 1960.

McDonald, J. H., and Heckel, N. J.: Acute pneumococcal epididymitis. Ill. Med. J., *95*:304, 1949.

Medlar, E. M., Spain, D. M., and Holiday, R. W.: Postmortem compared with clinical diagnosis of genitourinary tuberculosis in adult males. J. Urol., *61*:1078, 1949.

Megali, M., Garsel, E., and Lattimer, J. K.: Reflux of urine into ejaculatory ducts as a cause of recurring epididymitis in children. J. Urol., *108*:978, 1972.

Mitchell, C. J., and Huins, T. J.: Acute brucellosis presenting as epididymo-orchitis (letter). Br. Med. J., *2*:557, 1974.

Mittemeyer, B. T., Lennox, K. W., and Borski, A. A.: Epididymitis: A review of 610 cases. J. Urol., *85*:370, 1966.

Møller, B. R., and Mårdh, P-A.: Experimental epididymitis and urethritis in Grivet monkeys provoked by *Chlamydia trachomatis*. Fertil. Steril., *34*:275, 1980.

Moore, C. A., Lockett, B. L., Lennox, K. W., et al.: Prednisone in the treatment of acute epididymitis: A cooperative study. J. Urol., *106*:578, 1971.

Nickel, W. R., and Plumb, R. T.: Other infections and inflammations of the external genitalia. *In* Harrison, J. H., Gittes, R. F., and Perlmutter, A. D. (Eds.): Campbell's Urology. 4th ed. Philadelphia, W. B. Saunders Co., 1978, p. 640.

Nilsson, T., and Fischer, A.: Acute epididymitis: Investigation, etiology, and treatment with doxycycline. Curr. Ther. Res., *65*:732, 1979.

Nilsson, S., Obuant, K., and Persson, P. S.: Changes in the testes parenchyma caused by acute nonspecific epididymitis. Fertil Steril., *19*:748, 1968.

Oates, J. K.: Sexually transmitted disease. *In* Blandy, J. F. (Ed.): Urology. Oxford, Blackwell Scientific Publications, 1976.

Olier, C.: Diagnosis of acute chlamydial epididymitis. Prog. Reprod. Biol., *8*:161, 1981.

Pedersen, J. F., Holm, H. H., and Hald, T.: Torsion of the testes diagnosed by ultrasound. J. Urol., *113*:66, 1975.

Pelouze, P. S.: Epididymitis. *In* Gonorrhea in the Male and Female. Philadelphia, W. B. Saunders Co., 1941.

Perri, A. J., Slachta, G. A., Feldman, A. E., et al.: The Doppler stethoscope and the diagnosis of the acute scrotum. J. Urol., *116*:98, 1976.

Quinto, O.: Swelling of scrotum in infants and children and nonspecific epididymitis. Acta Chir. Scand., *110*:417, 1956.

Reisman, D. D.: Epididymitis owing to ectopic ejaculatory duct: A case report. J. Urol., *117*:540, 1977.

Rosenbloom, D.: Chronic prostatitis: A psychosexual approach. Cal. Med., *82*:454, 1954.

Ross, C. J., Gow, J. G., and St. Hill, C. A.: Tuberculosis epididymitis: A review of 170 patients. Br. J. Surg., *48*:663, 1961.

Schachter, J.: Chlamydia infection. N. Engl. J. Med., *298*:490, 540, 1978.

Scheibel, J. H., Anderson, J. T., Brandenhoff, P., et al.: Chlamydia trachomatis in acute epididymitis. Scand. J. Urol. Nephrol., *17*:47, 1983.

Schmidt, S., and Hinman, F.: The effect of vasectomy upon the incidence of epididymitis after prostatectomy: An analysis of 810 operations. J. Urol., *63*:872, 1950.

Shapiro, S.A., and Breschi, C. C.: Acute epididymitis in Vietnam: Review of 52 cases. Milit. Med., *138*:643, 1973.

Smith, D. R.: Treatment of epididymitis by infiltration of the spermatic cord with procaine HCl. J. Urol., *46*:74, 1971.

Sufrin, G.: Acute epididymitis. Sex. Transm. Dis., *8*:132, 1980.

Svend-Hansen, H., Nielsen, P., and Pedersen, N.: The value of routine intravenous urography in acute epididymitis. Int. J. Urol. Nephrol., *9*:245, 1977.

Thomas, D., Simpson, K., Ostojic, H., et al.: Bacteremic epididymo-orchitis due to *H. influenzae* type B. J. Urol., *126*:832, 1981.

Tozzo, P. J.: Semen analysis in unilateral epididymitis. N.Y. State J. Med., *1*:2769, 1968.

Watson, R. A.: Gonorrhea and acute epididymitis. Milit. Med., *144*:785, 1979.

William, D. C., Felman, Y. M., and Corsaro, M. C.: *Neisseria meningitidis*: Probable pathogen in two related cases of urethritis, epididymitis, and acute pelvic inflammatory disease. JAMA, *242*:1653, 1979.

Williams, C. B., Litvak, A. S., and McRoberts, W. J.: Epididymitis in infancy. J. Urol., *125*:125, 1979.

Wolin, L. H.: On the etiology of epididymitis. J. Urol., *105*:531, 1971.

Pelvic Inflammatory Disease

Barlett, J, G., Onderdonk, A. B., Drude, E., et al.: Quantitative bacteriology of the vaginal flora. J. Infect. Dis., *136*:271, 1977.

Buchanan, T. M., Eschenbach, D. A., Knapp, J. S., et al.: Gonococcal salpingitis is less likely to recur with *Neisseria gonorrhoeae* of the same principal outer membrane protein (POMP) antigenic type. Am. J. Obstet. Gynecol., *138*:978, 1980.

Centers for Disease Control: Sexually transmitted disease: Treatment guidelines 1982. MMWR (Suppl.), *31*:43S, 1982.

Chaparro, M. V., Ghosh, S., Nashed, A., et al.: Laparoscopy for the confirmation and prognostic evaluation of pelvic inflammatory disease. Int. J. Gynecol. Obstet., *15*:307, 1978.

Curran, J. W.: Economic consequences of pelvic inflammatory disease in the United States, Am. J. Obstet. Gynecol., *138*:848, 1980.

Draper, D. L., James, J. F., Brooks, G. F., et al.: Comparison of virulence markers of peritoneal and fallopian tube isolates with endocervical *N. gonorrhoeae* isolates from women with acute salpingitis. Infect. Immun., *27*:882, 1980.

Eschenbach, D.: Acute pelvic inflammatory disease. Urol. Clin. North Am., *11*:65, 1984.

Eschenbach, D. A.: Acute pelvic inflammatory disease. Presented at the 13th Interscience Conference on Antimicrobial Agents and Chemotherapy, Washington D.C., Sept. 19–21, 1973.

Eschenbach, D. A.: Epidemiology and diagnosis of acute pelvic inflammatory disease. Obstet. Gynecol., *55*:142S, 1980.

Eschenbach, D. A., Buchanan, T. M., Pollock, H. M., et al.: Polymicrobial etiology of acute pelvic inflammatory disease. N. Engl. J. Med., *293*:166, 1975.

Eschenbach, D. A., Harnisch, J. P., and Holmes, K. K.: Pathogenesis of acute pelvic inflammatory disease: Role of contraception and other risk factors. Am. J. Obstet. Gynecol., *128*:838, 1977.

Eschenbach, D. A., and Holmes, K. K.: The etiology of acute pelvic inflammatory disease. Sex. Transm. Dis., *6*:224, 1979.

Falk, V.: Treatment of acute non-tuberculous salpingitis with antibiotics alone and in combination with glucocorticoids. Acta Obstet. Gynecol. Scand., *44* (Suppl. 6):3, 1965.

Falk, V., and Krook, G.: Do results of culture for gonococci vary with sampling phase of menstrual cycle? Acta Derm. Venereol., 47:190, 1967.

Flesh, G., Weiner, J. M., Cortlett, R. C., et al.: The intrauterine contraceptive device and acute salpingitis. Am. J. Obstet. Gynecol., 135:402, 1979.

Forslin, L., Falk, V., and Danielsson, D.: Changes in the incidence of acute gonococcal and nongonococcal salpingitis. Br. J. Vener. Dis., 54:247, 1978.

Gerzof, S. G., Robbins, A. H., Johnson, W. C., et al.: Percutaneous catheter drainage of abdominal abscesses: A five year experience. N. Engl. J. Med., 305:653, 1981.

Gjonnaess, H., Dolaken, K., Ånestad, G., et al.: Pelvic inflammatory disease: Etiologic studies with emphasis on chlamydial infection. Obstet. Gynecol., 59:550, 1982.

Hagar, W. D., Douglas, B., Majmudar, B., et al.: Pelvic colonization with Actinomyces in women using intrauterine contraceptive devices. Am. J. Obstet. Gynecol., 135:680, 1979.

Henry-Suchet, J., Catalan, F., Loffredo, V., et al.: Microbiology of specimens obtained by laparoscopy from controls and from patients with pelvic inflammatory disease or infertility with tubal obstruction: Chlamydia trachomatis and Ureaplasma urealyticum. Am. J. Obstet. Gynecol., 138:1022, 1980.

Holmes, K. K., Eschenbach, D. A., and Knapp, J. S.: Salpingitis: Overview of etiology and epidemiology. Am. J. Obstet. Gynecol., 138:893, 1980.

Holtz, F.: Klinishe studien über die nicht tuberkulose salpingoophoritis. Acta Obstet. Gynecol. (Suppl.), 10:5, 1930.

Jacobson, L., and Westroöm, L.: Objectionalized diagnosis of acute pelvic inflammatory disease. Am. J. Obstet. Gynecol., 105:1088, 1969.

Jones, R. B., Ardery, B. R., Hui, S. C., et al.: Correlation between serum antichlamydial antibodies and tubal factor as a cause of infertility. Fertil. Steril., 38:553, 1982.

Kasper, D. L., Eschenbach, D. A., Hayes, M. E., et al.: Quantitative determination of the serum antibody response to the capsular polysaccharide of Bacterioides fragilis subspecies fragilis in women with pelvic inflammatory disease. J. Infect. Dis., 138:74, 1978.

Lee, N. D., Rubin, G. L., Ory, H. W., et al.: Type of intrauterine device and the risk of pelvic inflammatory disease. Obstet. Gynecol., 62:1, 1983.

Måardh, P-A.: An overview of infectious agents of salpingitis, their biology and recent advances in methods of detection. Am. J. Obstet. Gynecol., 138:933, 1980.

Måardh, P-A., Lind, I, Svensson, L., et al.: Antibodies to Chlamydia trachomatis, Mycoplasma hominis and Neisseria gonorrhoeae in sera from patients with acute salpingitis. Br. J. Vener. Dis., 57:125, 1981.

Måardh, P-A., Ripa, T., Svensson, L., et al.: Role of Chlamydia trachomatis infection in acute salpingitis. N. Engl. J. Med., 296:1377, 1977.

Måardh, P-A., and Weström, L.: Tubal and cervical cultures in acute salpingitis with special reference to Mycoplasma hominis and T-strain mycoplasmas. Br. J. Vener. Dis., 46:179, 1970.

McGee, Z. A., Melly, M. A., Gregg, C. R., et al.: Virulence factors of gonococci: Studies using human fallopian tube organ culture. Immunobiology of N. gonorrhoeae. In Brooks, G. F., Gotschlich, E. L., Holmes, K. K., et al. (Eds.): Washington, DC, American Society for Microbiology, 1978, p. 258.

Mishell, D. R., and Moyer, D. E.: Association of pelvic inflammatory disease with the intrauterine device. Clin. Obstet. Gynecol., 12:179, 1969.

Møller, B. R., Freundt, E. A., Block, F. T., et al.: Experimental infection of the genital tract of female Grivet monkeys by Mycoplasma hominis. Infect. Immun., 20:258, 1979.

Møller, B. R., and Måardh, P-A.: Experimental salpingitis in Grivet monkeys by Chlamydia trachomatis. Acta Pathol. Microbiol. Scand. 88:107, 1980.

Monif, G. R. G., Welkos, S. L., Baer, H., et al.: Cul-de-sac isolates from patients with endometritis-salpingitis-peritonitis and gonococcal endocervicitis. Am. J. Obstet. Gynecol., 126:158, 1976.

Moore, D. E., Spadoni, L., Foy, H-M., et al.: Increased frequency of serum antibodies to Chlamydia trachomatis in infertility due to tubal disease. Lancet, 2:514, 1982.

Paavonen, J.: Chlamydia trachomatis in acute salpingitis. Am. J. Obstet. Gynecol., 138:957, 1980.

Paavonen, J., Brunham, R. C., Kiviat, N., et al.: Cervicitis: Etiologic, clinical and histopathologic findings. In Måardh, P-A., Holmes, K. K., Oriel, J. D., et al. (Eds.): Chlamydial Infection. New York, Elsevier Biomedical Press, 1982.

Paavonen, J., Brunham, R. C., Kiviat, N., et al.: Clinical and histologic evidence of endometritis among women with cervicitis. In Måardh, P-A., Holmes, K. K., Oriel, J. D., et al. (Eds.): Chlamydial Infection. New York. Elsevier Biomedical Press, 1982.

Randtorff, R. C., Curran, J. W., Chandler, R. W., et al.: Economic consequences of gonorrhea in women. Am. J. Vener. Dis. Assoc., 1:40, 1974.

Ripa, K. T., Møller, B. R., Måardh, P-A., et al.: Experimental acute salpingitis in Grivet monkeys provoked by Chlamydia trachomatis. Acta Pathol. Microbiol. Scand. [B], 87:65, 1979.

Senanayake, P., and Kramer, D. G.: Contraception and the etiology of pelvic inflammatory disease: New perspectives. Am. J. Obstet. Gynecol., 138:852, 1980.

Sparks, R. A., Purrier, B. G. A., Watt, P. J., et al.: The bacteriology of the cervical canal in relation to the use of an intrauterine contraceptive device. In Insler, V., and Bettendorf, G. (Eds.): The Uterine Cervix in Reproduction. Stuttgart, Thieme, 1977.

Spiegel, C. A., Amsel, R., Eschenbach, D. A., et al.: Anaerobic bacteria in nonspecific vaginitis. N. Engl. J. Med., 303:601, 1980.

St. John, R. K., Blount, J., and Jones, O. G.: Pelvic inflammatory diseases in the United States: Incidence and trends in private practice. Sex. Transm. Dis., 8:56, 1981.

St. John, R. K., Jones, O. G., Blount, J. H., et al.: Pelvic inflammatory disease in the United States. Epidemiology and trends among hospitalized women. Sex. Transm. Dis., 8:62, 1981.

Svensson, L.: Chlamydial Salpingitis. Doctoral Dissertation, Lund University, 1983.

Svensson, L., Weström, L., Ripa, K. T., et al.: Differences in some clinical and laboratory parameters in acute salpingitis related to culture and serologic finding. Am. J. Obstet. Gynecol., 138:1017, 1980.

Sweet, R. L., Mill, J., Hadley, K. W., et al.: Use of laparoscopy to determine the microbiologic etiology of acute salpingitis. Am. J. Obstet. Gynecol., 134:68, 1979.

Taylor, K. S. W., Wassen, J. F., deGraaff, C., et al.: Accuracy of grey-scale ultrasound diagnosis of abdominal and pelvic abscesses in 220 patients. Lancet, 1:83, 1978.

Thompson, S., Holcomb, G., Cheng, S., et al.: Antibiotic therapy of outpatient pelvic inflammatory disease. Presented at 20th Interscience Conference on Antimicrobial Agents and Chemotherapy. New Orleans, Sept. 22-24, 1980.

Weström, L.: Effect of acute pelvic inflammatory disease on fertility. Am. J. Obstet. Gynecol., 121:707, 1975.

Weström, L.: Incidence, prevalence, and trends of acute pelvic inflammatory disease and its consequences in industrialized countries. Am. J. Obstet. Gynecol., 138:880, 1980.

Weström, L., Bengtsson, L. P., and Måardh, P-A.: The risk of pelvic inflammatory disease in women using intrauterine contraceptive devices as compared to non-users. Lancet, 2:221, 1976.

Weström, L., Iosif, S., Svensson, L., et al.: Infertility after acute salpingitis: Results of treatment with different antibiotics. Curr. Ther. Res., 26:752, 1979.

Weström, L., and Måardh, P-A.: Epidemiology, etiology and prognosis of acute salpingitis: A study of 1457 laparoscopically verified cases in nongonococcal urethritis and related disease. In Hobson, D., and Holmes, K. K. (Eds.): Nongonococcal Urethritis and Related Diseases. Washington, D. C., American Society for Microbiology, 1977.

Zucherman, H., Kahane, A., and Carmel, S.: Antibacterial activity of human cervical mucus. Gynecol. Invest., 6:265, 1975.

Vaginitis

Austin, T. W., Smith, E. A., Darwish, R., et al.: Metronidazole in a single dose for the treatment of trichomoniasis: Failure of a 1 g single dose. Br. J. Vener. Dis., 58:121, 1982.

Balsdon, M. J., Rosedale, N., Blatchford, N. R., et al.: The systemic treatment of recurrent vaginal candidosis: An evaluation of oral ketoconazole therapy. Curr. Ther. Res., 31:511, 1982.

Berger, R. E.: Nongonococcal urethritis and selected syndromes. In Stamey, T. E. (Ed.): Monographs in Urology. Burroughs-Wellcome, 1982.

Borten, M., and Friedman, E. A: Duration of colposcopic changes associated with trichomonas vaginitis. Obstet. Gynecol., 51:111, 1978.

Bramley, M., and Kinghorn, G.: Do oral contraceptives inhibit Trichomonas vaginalis? Sex. Transm. Dis., 6:261, 1979.

Caison, S. G., Dawson, S. G., Hilton, E. T., et al.: Comparison of culture and microscopy in the diagnosis of Gardnerella vaginalis infection. J. Clin. Pathol., 35:550, 1982.

Chen, K. C. S., Forsyth, P. S., Buchanan, T. M., et al.: Amine content of vaginal fluid from untreated and treated patients with nonspecific vaginitis. J. Clin. Invest., 63:828, 1979.

Criswell, B. S., Ladwig, L. L., Gardner, H. L., et al.: Haemophilus vaginalis vaginitis by inoculation from culture. Obstet. Gynecol., 33:195, 1969.

Diamond, L. S.: The establishment of various trichomonads of animals and man in axenic cultures. J. Parasitol., 43:488, 1957.

Drake, T. E., and Maibach, H. I.: Candida and candidiasis. Postgrad. Med., 53:83, 120, 1973.

Eddie, D. A. S.: Laboratory diagnosis of vaginal infections caused by Trichomonas and Candida species. J. Med. Microbiol., 1:153, 1968.

Elegbe, I. A., and Botu, M.: A preliminary study on dressing patterns and incidence of candidiasis. Am. J. Public Health, 72:176, 1982.

Elegbe, I. A., and Elegbe, I.: Quantitative relationships of Candida albicans infections and dressing patterns in Nigerian women. Am. J. Public Health, 73:450, 1983.

Feinberg, J. G., and Whittington, M. J.: A culture medium for Trichomonas vaginalis Donne and species of Candida. J. Clin. Pathol., 10:327, 1957.

Fouts, A. C., and Kraus, S. J.: Trichomonas vaginalis: Reevaluation of its clinical presentation and laboratory diagnosis. J. Infect. Dis. 141:137, 1980.

Francioli, P., Shio, H., Roberts, R. B., et al.: Phagocytosis and killing of Neisseria gonorrhoeae by Trichomonas vaginalis. J. Infect. Dis. 147:87, 1983.

Gabriel, G., and Thin, R. N. T.: Clotrimazole and econazole in the treatment of candidosis. Br. J. Vener. Dis., 59:56, 1983.

Gardner, H. L.: Infectious vulvovaginitis. In Monif, G. R. F. (Ed.): Infectious Diseases in Obstetrics and Gynecology. New York, Harper & Row, 1982.

Gardner, H. L., and Dukes, C. D.: Haemophilus vaginalis vaginitis: A newly defined specific infection classified "non-specific vaginitis." Am. J. Obstet. Gynecol., 69:962, 1955.

Goldberg, R. L., and Washington, J. A.: Comparison of isolation of Haemophilus vaginalis (Corynebacterium vaginale) from peptone-starch-dextrose agar and Columbia colistin-nalidixic acid agar. J. Clin. Microbiol., 4:245, 1976.

Handsfield, H. H.: Sexually transmitted diseases. Hosp. Pract., 17:99, 1982.

Harris, J. R. W.: Introduction, epidemiology and social aspects of candidiasis. In Morton, R. S., and Harris, J. R. W. (Eds.): Recent Advances in Sexually Transmitted Diseases. Edinburgh, Churchill Livingstone, 1975.

Hasenclever, H. F., and Mitchell, W. O.: Antigenic studies of Candida: Observation of two antigenic groups in Candida albicans. J. Bacteriol., 82:570, 1961.

Heath, J. P.: Behavior and pathogenicity of Trichomonas vaginalis in epithelial cell cultures. Br. J. Vener. Dis., 57:106, 1981.

Holmes, K. K., Handsfield, H. H., Wang, S. P., et al.: Etiology of nongonococcal urethritis. N. Engl. J. Med., 292:1199, 1975.

Holmes, K. K., Speigel, C., Amsel, R., et al.: Nonspecific vaginosis. Scand. J. Infect. Dis. (Suppl.), 26:110, 1981.

Hurley, R.: Candidal vaginitis. Proc. R. Soc. Med. (Suppl. 4), 70:1, 1977.

Jones, B. M., Kinghorn, G. R., and Geary, I.: In vitro susceptibility of Gardnerella vaginalis and Bacteroides organisms associated with nonspecific vaginitis to sulfonamide preparations. Antimicrob. Agents Chemother., 21:870, 1982.

Kinghorn, G. R., Jones, B. M., Chowdhury, F. H., et al.: Balanoposthitis associated with Gardnerella vaginalis infection in men. Br. J. Vener. Dis., 58:127, 1982.

Kozinn, P. J., Taschdjian, C. L., and Wiener, H.: Incidence and pathogenesis of neonatal candidiasis. Pediatrics, 21:421, 1958.

Krieger, J. N., and Rein, M. F.: Zinc sensitivity of Trichomonas vaginalis: In vitro studies and clinical implications. J. Infect. Dis., 146:341, 1982.

Kuberski, T.: Trichomonas vaginalis associated with nongonococcal urethritis and prostatitis. Sex. Transm. Dis. 7:135, 1980.

Kudelko, N.: Allergy in chronic monilial vaginitis. Ann. Allergy, 29:266, 1971.

Kupferberg, A. B., Johnson, G., and Sprince, H.: Nutritional requirements of Trichomonas vaginalis. Proc. Soc. Expert. Biol. Med. 67:304, 1948.

Lanceley, F., and McEntegart, M. G.: Trichomonas vaginalis in the male: The experimental infection of a few volunteers. Lancet, 1:668, 1953.

Leopold, S.: Heretofore undescribed organism isolated from

the genitourinary system. U.S. Armed Forces Med., 4:263, 1953.

Levin, S., Zaidel, L., and Bernstein, D.: Intrauterine infection of fetal brain by Candida. Am. J. Obstet. Gynecol., 130:597, 1978.

Levine, B. B., Siraganian, R. R., and Schenkeim, I.: Allergy to human seminal plasma. N. Engl. J. Med., 290:916, 1974.

Lossick, J. G.: Single dose metronidazole treatment for vaginal trichomoniasis. Obstet. Gynecol., 56:508, 1978.

Lossick, J. G.: Treatment of Trichomonas vaginalis infections. J. Infect. Dis. (Suppl.), 4:801, 1982.

Malouf, M., Fortier, M., Morin, G., et al.: Treatment of Haemophilus vaginalis vaginitis. Obstet. Gynecol., 57:711, 1981.

McCormack, W. M., Hayes, C. H., Rosenec, B., et al.: Vaginal colonization with Corynebacterium vaginale. J. Infect. Dis., 136:740, 1977.

McGuire, L. S., Guzinski, G. M., and Holmes, K. K.: Psychosexual functioning in symptomatic women with and without signs of vaginitis. Am. J. Obstet. Gynecol., 137:600, 1980.

McLennon, M. T., Smith, J. M., and McLennon, C. E.: Diagnosis of vaginal mycosis and trichomoniasis: Reliability of cytologic smear, wet smear and culture. Obstet. Gynecol., 40:231, 1972.

Mead, P. B., Gibson, M., Schentag, J. J., et al.: Possible alteration of metronidazole metabolism by phenobarbital (letter). N. Engl. J. Med., 306:1490, 1982.

Miles, M. R., Olsen, L., and Rogers, A.: Recurrent vaginal candidiasis: Importance of an intestinal reservoir. J.A.M.A., 238:1836, 1977.

Milne, J. D., and Warnock, D. W.: Effect of simultaneous oral and vaginal treatment on the rate of cure and relapse in vaginal candidosis. Br. J. Vener. Dis., 55:362, 1979.

Milson, I., and Forssman, L.: Treatment of vaginal candidosis with a single 500 mg clotrimazole pessary. Br. J. Vener. Dis. 58:124, 1982.

Nielson, M. H., and Nielson, R.: Electron microscopy of Trichomonas vaginalis: Interaction with vaginal epithelium in human trichomoniasis. Acta Pathol. Microbiol. Scand., 83:305, 1975.

Oriel, J. D., Partridge, B. M., Denny, M. J., et al.: Genital yeast infections. Br. Med. J., 4:761, 1972.

Palacios, H. J.: Hypersensitivity as a cause of dermatologic and vaginal moniliasis resistant to topical therapy. Ann. Allergy, 37:110, 1976.

Panja, S. K.: Treatment of trichomoniasis with metronidazole rectal suppositories. Br. J. Vener. Dis., 58:257, 1982.

Pheifer, T. A., Forsyth, P. S., Durfee, M. A., et al.: Nonspecific vaginitis: Role of Haemophilus vaginalis and treatment with metronidazole. N. Engl. J. Med., 298:1427, 1978.

Piot, P., VanDyck, E., Totten, P., et al.: Biotyping of Gardnerella vaginalis (abstract). In Programs and abstracts of the 82nd annual meeting. American Society for Microbiology, Washington, DC, 1982.

Polonelli, L., Archibusacci, C., Sestito, M., et al.: Killer system: A simple method for differentiating Candida albicans strains. J. Clin. Microbiol., 17:774, 1983.

Soliman, M. A., Ackers, J. P., and Catterall, R. D.: Isoenzyme characterization of Trichomonas vaginalis. Br. J. Vener. Dis., 58:250, 1982.

Spiegel, C. A., Amsel, R., Eschenbach, D., et al.: Anaerobic bacteria in nonspecific vaginitis. N. Engl. J. Med., 303:601, 1980.

Spiegel, C. A., Eschenbach, D. A., Amsel, R. A., et al.: Identification of curved motile anaerobic bacteria associated with bacterial (nonspecific) vaginosis (ab-

stract). In Programs and abstracts of the 82nd annual meeting, American Society for Microbiology, Washington, D.C., 1982.

Swartz, S. L., Kraus, S. J., Hermann, K. L., et al.: Diagnosis and etiology of nongonococcal urethritis. J. Infect. Dis., 138:445, 1978.

Thin, R. N., Rendell, P., and Wadsworth, J.: How often are gonorrhea and genital yeast sexually transmitted? Br. J. Vener. Dis., 55:278, 1979.

Totten, P. A., Amsel, R., Hale, J, et al.: Selective differential human blood bilayer media for isolation of Gardnerella (Haemophilus) vaginalis. J. Clin. Microbiol., 15:141, 1982.

Warnock, D. W., Speller, D. C. E., Day, J. K., et al.: Resistogram method for differentiation of strains of Candida albicans. J. Appl. Microbiol., 46:571, 1979.

Weston, T. E. T., and Nicol, C. S.: Natural history of trichomonal infections in males. Br. J. Vener. Dis., 33:80, 1963.

Whittington, M. J.: Epidemiology of infections with Trichomonas vaginalis in light of improved diagnostic methods. Br. J. Vener. Dis., 33:80, 1957.

Wiesner, P. J., Jones, O. E., and Blount, J. H.: World trends in sexually transmitted diseases: The situation in the United States. In Catterall, R.D., and Nicol, C. S. (Eds.): Sexually Transmitted Diseases. New York, Academic Press, 1976.

Genital Ulcers

Brown, S. T., Jaffe, H. J. W., Zaidi, A., et al.: Sensitivity and specificity of diagnostic tests for genital infection and Herpesvirus hominis. Sex. Transm. Dis., 6:10, 1979.

Centers for Disease Control: Sexually transmitted disease: Treatment guidelines 1982. Rev. Infect. Dis., 4:5729, 1982.

Chapel, T. A., Brown, W. J., Jeffries, C., et al.: How reliable is the morphological diagnosis of penile ulcerations? Sex. Transm. Dis., 4:150, 1977.

Hammond, G. W., Lian, C. J., Wilt, J. C., et al.: Comparison of specimen collection and laboratory techniques for isolation of Haemophilus ducreyi. J. Clin. Microbiol., 7:39, 1978.

Hart, G.: Chancroid donovanosis lymphogranuloma venereum. DHEW (Centers for Disease Control) Publication No. 75-8302.

Kraus, S. J.: Evaluation and management of acute genital ulcers on sexually active patients. Urol. Clin. North Am., 11:155, 1984.

Kraus, S. J., Kaufman, H. W., Albritton, W. L., et al.: Chancroid therapy: A review of cases confirmed by culture. Rev. Infect. Dis., 4:S848, 1982.

Kraus, S. J., Werman, B. S., Biddle, J. W., et al.: Pseudogranuloma inguinale caused by Haemophilus ducreyi, Arch. Dermatol., 118:494, 1982.

Sottnek, F. O., Biddle, J. W., Kraus, S. J., et al.: Isolation and identification of Haemophilus ducreyi in a clinical study. J. Clin. Microbiol., 12:170, 1980.

Genital Herpes Infections

Adam, E., Kaufman, R. H., Mirkovic, R. R., et al.: Persistence of virus shedding in asymptomatic women after recovery from herpes genitalis. Obstet. Gynecol., 54:171, 1979.

Adams, H. G., Benson, E. A., Alexander, E. R., et al.: Genital herpetic infection in men and women: Clinical course and effect of topical application of adenine arabinoside. J. Infect. Dis., 133:A151, 1976.

Ashley, R. L., and Corey, L.: Analysis of the humoral immune response to HSV in primary genital herpes patients (abstract). International Symposium on Medical Virology. Anaheim, California, Oct. 1981.

Aston, D. L., Cohen, A., and Spindler, M. A.: Herpesvirus hominis infection in patients with myeloproliferative and lymphoproliferative disorders. Br. Med. J., 4:462, 1972.

Balachandran, N., Frame, B., Chernesky, M., et al.: Identification and typing of herpes simplex viruses with monoclonal antibodies. J Clin. Microbiol., 16:205, 1982.

Baringer, J. R.: Recovery of herpes simplex virus from human sacral ganglions. N. Engl. J. Med., 291:828, 1974.

Becker, W. B., Kipps, and McKenzie, D.: Disseminated herpes simplex virus infection: Its pathogenesis based on virological and pathological studies in 33 cases. Am. J. Dis. Child., 115:1, 1968.

Bierman, S. M.: Double-blind crossover study of levamisole as immunoprophylaxis for recurrent herpes progenitalis. Cutis, 21:352, 1978.

Bierman, S. M., Kirkpatrick, W., and Fernandez, H.: Clinical efficacy of ribavirin in the treatment of genital herpes simplex virus infection. Chemotherapy, 27:139, 1981.

Blough, H. A., and Giuntoli, R. L.: Successful treatment of human genital herpes infections with 2-deoxy-D-glucose. J.A.M.A., 241:2798, 1979.

Bolognese, R. J., Corson, S. L., Fuccillo, D. A., et al.: Herpesvirus hominis type II infections in asymptomatic pregnant women. Obstet. Gynecol., 48:507, 1976.

Brenton, D. W.: Hypoglycorrhachia in herpes simplex type 2 meningitis. Arch. Neurol., 37:317, 1980.

Brooks, S. L., Rowe, N. H., Drach, J. C., et al.: Prevalence of herpes simplex virus in a professional population. J. Am. Dent. Assoc., 102:31, 1981.

Brown, S. T., Jaffee, H. W., Zaidi, A., et al.: Sensitivity and specificity of diagnostic tests for genital infection with herpesvirus hominis. Sex. Transm. Dis., 6:10, 1979.

Buchman, T. G., Roizman, B., Adams, G., et al.: Restriction endonuclease fingerprinting of herpes simplex virus DNA: A novel epidemiological tool applied to a nosocomial outbreak. J. Infect. Dis. 138:488, 1978.

Buchman, T. G., Roizman, B., and Nahmias, A. J.: Demonstration of exogenous genital reinfection with herpes simplex virus type 2 by restriction endonuclease fingerprinting of viral DNA. J. Infect. Dis., 140:295, 1977.

Burnett, J. W., and Katz, S. L.: A study of the use of 5-iodo-2'-deoxyuridine in cutaneous herpes simplex. J. Invest. Dermatol., 40:7, 1962.

Burns, W. H., Saral, R., Santos, G. W., et al.: Isolation and characterization of resistant herpes simplex virus after acyclovir therapy. Lancet, 1:421, 1982.

Caplan, L. R., Kleman, F. J., and Berg, S.: Urinary retention probably secondary to herpes genitalis. N. Engl. J. Med., 297:920, 1977.

Cappel, R., De Cuyper, F., Berg, S., et al.: Efficacy of a nucleic acid free herpetic subunit vaccine. Arch. Virol., 65:15, 1980.

Centers for Disease Control: Adverse reactions to smallpox vaccinations—1978. MMWR, 28:265, 1979.

Centers for Disease Control: Genital herpes infection, United States, 1966–1979. MMWR, 31:137, 1982.

Centifanto, Y. M., Drylie, D. M., Deardourff, S. L., et al.: Herpesvirus type 2 in the male genitourinary tract. Science, 178:318, 1972.

Chang, T., and Fiumara, N.: Treatment with levamisole of recurrent herpes genitalis. Antimicrob. Chemother., 13:809, 1978.

Coen, D. M., and Schaffer, P. A.: Two distinct loci confer resistance to acycloguanosine in herpes simplex virus type 1. Proc. Natl. Acad. Sci. USA, 77:2265, 1980.

Corey, L., Adams, H. G., Brown, Z. A., et al.: Genital herpes simplex virus infection: Clinical manifestations, course and complications. Ann. Intern. Med., 98:958, 1983a.

Corey, L., Benedetti, J., Critchlow, C., et al.: Double-blind controlled trial of topical acyclovir in genital herpes simplex virus infections: The Seattle experience. Am. J. Med., 73:326, 1981a.

Corey, L., Fife, K. H., Benedetti, J. K., et al.: Intravenous acyclovir for the treatment of primary genital herpes. Ann. Intern. Med., 98:914, 1983b.

Corey, L., and Holmes, K. K.: Genital herpes simplex virus infection: Current concepts in diagnosis, therapy and prevention. Ann. Intern. Med., 98:973, 1983.

Corey, L., Nahmias, M. E., Guinan, M. E., et al.: A trial of topical acyclovir in genital herpes simplex virus infections. N. Engl. J. Med., 306:1313, 1982b.

Corey, L., Reeves, W. C., Chiang, W. T., et al.: Ineffectiveness of topical ether for the treatment of genital herpes simplex virus infection. N. Engl. J. Med., 299:237, 1978.

Craig, C. P., and Nahmias, A.: Different patterns of neurologic involvement with herpes simplex virus types 1 and 2: Isolation of herpes simplex virus from the buffy coat of two adults with meningitis. J. Infect. Dis., 127:365, 1973.

Crumpacker, C. S., Schnipper, L. E., Marlowe, S. L., et al.: Resistance to antiviral drugs of herpes simplex virus isolated from a patient treated with acyclovir. N. Engl. J. Med., 306:343, 1982.

Crumpacker, C. S., Schnipper, L. E., Zaia, J. A., et al.: Growth inhibition by acycloguanosine of herpesvirus isolated from human infections. Antimicrob. Agents Chemother., 15:642, 1979.

Davidson-Parker, J. D.: A double-blind trial of idoxuridine in recurrent genital herpes. J. Antimicrob. Chemother., 3(Suppl.):131, 1977.

Deardourff, S. L., Deture, F. A., Drylie, D. M., et al.: Association between herpes hominis type 2 and the male genitourinary tract. J. Urol. 112:126, 1974.

Deture, F. A., Drylie, D. M., Kaufman, H. E., et al.: Herpesvirus type 2 isolation from seminal vesicle and testes. Urology, 7:541, 1976.

Deture, F. A., Drylie, D. M., Kaufman, H. E., et al.: Herpes virus type: Efficacy and long-term follow-up. Presented at the 23rd Interscience Conference on Antimicrobial Agents and Chemotherapy. Las Vegas, Nevada, Oct. 24, 1983.

Duenas, A., Adam, E., Melnick, J. L., et al.: Herpesvirus type 2 in a prostitute population. Am. J. Epidemiol., 95:583, 1972.

Eberle, R., and Courtney, R. J.: Assay of type-specific and type-common antibodies to herpes simplex virus types 1 and 2 in human sera. Infect. Immun., 31:1062, 1981.

Elion, G. B., Furman, P. A., Fyfe, J. A., et al.: Selectivity of action of an antiherpetic agent, 9-(2-hydroxyethoxymethyl) guanine. Proc. Natl. Acad. Sci. USA, 74:5716, 1977.

Felber, T. D., Smith, E. B., Knox, J. M., et al.: Photodynamic inactivation of herpes simplex. JAMA, 223:289, 1973.

Field, H. J., and Darby, G.: Pathogenicity in mice of strains of herpes simplex virus which are resistant to acyclovir in vitro and in vivo. Antimicrob. Agents Chemother., 17:209, 1980.

Friedrich, E. G., Jr., and Masukawa, T.: Effect of providone-iodine on herpes genitalis. Obstet. Gynecol., *45*:337, 1975.

Goldmeier, D.: Herpetic proctitis and sacral radiculomyelopathy in homosexual men. Br. Med. J., *2*:549, 1979.

Goldmeier, D., Bateman, J. R. M., and Rodin, P.: Urinary retention and intestinal obstruction associated with anorectal herpes simplex virus infection. Br. Med. J., *1*:425, 1975.

Goldstein, L. C., Corey, L., McDougall, J., et al.: Monoclonal antibodies to herpes simplex viruses: Use in antigenic typing and rapid diagnosis. J. Infect. Dis. *147*:829, 1983.

Goodell, S. E., Quinn, T. C., Mkrtichian, E. E., et al.: Herpes simplex proctitis in homosexual men: Clinical, sigmoidoscopic, and histopathological findings. N. Engl. J. Med., *308*:868, 1983.

Grauballe, P. C., and Vestergaard, B. F.: ELISA for herpes simplex virus type 2 antibodies (letter). Lancet, *2*:1038, 1977.

Guinan, M. E., MacCalman, J., Kern, E. R., et al.: Topical ether and herpes simplex labialis. JAMA, *243*:1059, 1980.

Hatherley, L. I., Hayes, K, and Jack, I.: Herpes virus in an obstetric hospital: II. Asymptomatic virus excretion in staff members. Med. J. Aust., *2*:273, 1980.

Hevron, J. E.: Herpes simplex virus meningitis. Obstet. Gynecol., *49*:622, 1977.

Hilletman, M. R., Larson, V. M., Lehman, E. D., et al.: Subunit herpes simplex 2 vaccine. *In* Nahmias, A. J., Dowdle, W. R., and Schwinazi, R. F. (Eds.): The Human Herpesviruses. New York, Elsevier, 1981.

Ishiguro, T., Ozaki, Y, Matsunami, M., et al.: Clinical and virological features of herpes genitalis in Japanese women. Acta Obstet. Gynecol. Scand., *61*:173, 1982.

Jacobs, S. C., Hebert, L. A., Piering, W. F., et al.: Acute motor paralytic bladder in renal transplant patients with anogenital herpes infection. J. Urol. *123*:426, 1980.

Jacome, D. E., and Yanez, G. F.: Herpes genitalis and neurogenic bladder and bowel. J. Urol., *124*:752, 1980.

Jones, B. R., Coster, D. J., Falcon, M. G., et al.: Topical therapy of ulcerative herpetic keratitis with human interferon. Lancet, *2*:128, 1976.

Jose, D. G., and Minty, C. C. J.: Levamisole in patients with recurrent herpes infection. Med. J. Aust., *2*:390, 1980.

Josey, W., Nahmias, A., and Naib, Z.: The epidemiology of type 2 (genital) herpes simplex virus infection. Obstet. Gynecol. Surv., *27*:295, 1972.

Josey, W., Nahmias, A., Naib., Z. M., et al.: Genital herpes simplex infection in the female. Am. J. Obstet. Gynecol., *96*:493, 1966.

Kalinyak, J. E., Fleagle, G., and Docherty, J. J.: Incidence and distribution of herpes simplex virus types 1 and 2 from genital lesions in college women. J. Med. Virol., *1*:275, 1977.

Kern, A. B., and Schiff, B. L.: Smallpox vaccinations in the management of recurrent herpes simplex: A controlled evaluation. J. Invet. Dermatol., *33*:99, 1959.

Kern, E. R., Glasgow, L. A., Klein, R. J., et al.: Failure of 2-deoxy-D-glucose in treatment of experimental cutaneous and genital herpes simplex virus (HSV) infections. J. Infect. Dis., *146*:159, 1982.

Kern, E. R., Glasgow, L. A., Overall, J. C., et al.: Treatment of experimental herpesivrus infections with phosphonoformate and some comparison with phosphonacetate. Antimicrob. Agents Chemother., *14*:817, 1978.

Kitces, E. N., et al.: Herpes simplex virus vaccine: Protec-

tion from stomatitis, ganglionitis, encephalitis and latency. IARC Sci. Publ., *24* (part 2):1027, 1978.

Klastersky, J., Cappel, R., Snoeck, J. M., et al.: Ascending myelitis in association with herpes simplex virus. N. Engl. J. Med., *287*:182, 1972.

Klein, P. J., Friedman-Kien, A. E., and DeStefano, E.: Latent herpes simplex virus infections in sensory ganglia of hairless mice prevented by acycloguanosine. Antimicrob. Agents Chemother., *15*:723, 1979.

Klein, R. J., Friedman-Kien, A. E., and Yellin, P. B.: Orofacial herpes simplex virus infection in hairless mice: Latent virus in trigeminal ganglia after topical antiviral treatment. Infect Immun., *20*:130, 1978.

Knox, S. R., Corey, L., Blough, H. A., et al.: Historical findings in subjects from a high socioeconomic group who have genital infections with herpes simplex virus. Sex Transm. Dis., *9*:15, 1982.

Korsager, B., Spencer, E. S., Mordhorst, C., et al.: Herpesvirus hominis infections in renal transplant recipients. Scand. J. Infect. Dis., *7*:11, 1975.

Linnemann, C. C., Jr., Buchman, T. G., Light, I. J., et al.: Transmission of herpes simplex virus type 1 in a nursery for the newborn: Identification of viral isolates by DNA "fingerprinting." Lancet, *1*:964, 1978.

Linnemann, C. C., First, M. R., Alvira, M. M., et al.: Herpesvirus hominis type 2 meningoencephalitis following renal transplantation. Am. J. Med., *61*:703, 1976.

Lonsdale, D. M.: A rapid technique for distinguishing herpes simplex virus type 1 from type 2 by restriction enzyme technology. Lancet, *1*:849, 1979.

MacCallum, F. O., and Juel-Jensen, B. E.: Treatment of herpes simplex virus skin infection with IDU in dimethylsulfoxide: Results of double-blind controlled trial. Br. Med. J., *2*:805, 1966.

McClung, H., Seth, P., and Rawls, W. E.: Relative concentration in human sera of antibodies to cross reacting and specific antigens of HSV types 1 and 2. Am. J. Epidemiol., *104*:192, 1976.

Mertz, G., and Corey, L.: Genital herpes simplex virus interacts in adults. Urol. Clin. North Am., *11*:103, 1984.

Mertz, G. J., Jourden, P., Peterman, G., et al.: Herpes simplex virus type-2 glycoprotein subunit vaccine: Tolerance and immunogenicity. Am. Fed. Clin. Res., Western Section. Carmel, California, Feb. 1983*a*.

Mertz, G. J., Jourden, J., Remington, M., et al.: Risk of transmission of genital herpes. Presented at the 5th International Meeting, International Society for STD Research, Seattle, Aug. 1–3, 1983*b*.

Mertz, G. J., Jourden, J., Winter, C., et al.: Sexual transmission of initial genital herpes (HSV): Implications for prevention. (Abstract 622) 21st Interscience Conference on Antimicrobial Agents and Chemotherapy (ICAAC). Chicago, 1981.

Mertz, G. J., Reichman, R., Dolin, R., et al.: Double-blind placebo controlled trial of oral acyclovir for first-episode genital herpes. Presented at the 22nd Interscience Conference on Antimicrobial Agents and Chemotherapy (ICAAC). Miami Beach, Oct. 1982.

Meyers, J. D., Flournoy, N., and Thomas, E. D.: Infection with herpes simplex virus and cell-mediated immunity after marrow transplant. J. Infect. Dis., *142*:338, 1980.

Miller, J. B.: Treatment of active herpes virus infections with influenza virus vaccine. Ann. Allergy, *43*:295, 1979.

Milman, N., Scheible, J., and Jessen, O.: Failure of lysine treatment in recurrent herpes simplex labialis. Lancet, *2*:942, 1978.

Mindel, A., Adler, M. W., Sutherland, S., et al.: Intravenous acyclovir treatment for primary genital herpes. Lancet, *1*:697, 1982.

Mintz, L.: Recurrent herpes simplex infections at a smallpox vaccination site. JAMA, *247*:2704, 1982.

Mitchell, C. D., Bean, B., Gentry, S. R., et al.: Acyclovir therapy for mucocutaneous herpes simplex infections in immunocompromised patients. Lancet, *1*:1389, 1981.

Morriseau, M. A., Phillips, C. A., and Leadbetter, G. W., Jr.: Viral prostatitis. J. Urol., *103*:767, 1970.

Morrison, R. E., Miller, M. H., Lyon, L. W., et al.: Adult meningoencephalitis caused by herpesvirus hominis type 2. Am. J. Med., *56*:540, 1974.

Moseley, R., Corey, L., Winter, C., et al.: Comparison of the indirect immunoperoxidase and direct immunofluorescence techniques with viral isolation for the diagnosis of genital herpes simplex virus infection. J. Clin. Microbiol., *13*:913, 1981.

Muller, S. A., Herrmann, E. C., Jr., and Winkelmann, R. K.: Herpes simplex infections in hematologic malignancies. Am. J. Med., *52*:102, 1972.

Myers, M. D., Oxman, M. N., Clark, J. E., et al.: Failure of neutral-red photodynamic inactivation in recurrent herpes simplex virus infections. N Engl. J. Med., *293*:945, 1975.

Nahmias, A. J., Josey, W. E., Naib, Z. M., et al.: Antibodies to herpesvirus hominis types 1 and 2 in humans. Am. J. Epidemiol., *91*:539, 1970.

Nahmias, A. J., Naib, Z. M., and Josey, W. E.: Prospective studies of the association of genital herpes simplex virus infection and cervical anaplasia. Cancer Res., *33*:1491, 1973*a*.

Nahmias, A. J., and Roizman, D.: Infection with herpes simplex virus 1 and 2. N Engl. J. Med., *29*:667, 719, 781, 1973*b*.

Nilsen, A. E., Aasen, T., Halsos, A. M., et al.: Efficacy of oral acyclovir in the treatment of initial and recurrent genital herpes. Lancet, *2*:571, 1982.

Oates, J. K., and Greenhouse, P. R.: Retention of urine in anogenital herpetic infection. Lancet, *1*:691, 1978.

Pazin, G. J., Armstrong, J. A., Lam, M. T., et al.: Prevention of reactivated herpes simplex infection by human leukocyte interferon after operation on the trigeminal root. N. Engl. J. Med., *301*:225, 1979.

Peterson, E. P., Schmidt, O. W., Goldstein, L. C., et al.: Typing of clinical HSV isolates using mouse monoclonal antibodies to HSV-1 and HSV-2: Comparison with type-specific rabbit antisera and restriction endonuclease analysis of viral DNA. J. Clin. Microbiol., *17*:92, 1983.

Price, R. W., Walz, M. A., Wohlenberg, C., et al.: Latent infection of sensory ganglia with herpes simplex virus: Efficacy of immunization. Science, *188*:938, 1975.

Quinn, T. C., Corey, L., Chaffee, R. G., et al.: The etiology of anorectal infections in homosexual men. Am. J. Med., *71*:395, 1981.

Rattray, M. D., Corey, L., Reeves, W. C., et al.: Recurrent genital herpes among women: Symptomatic versus asymptomatic viral shedding. Br. J. Vener. Dis., *54*:262, 1978.

Rawls, W. E., Gardner, H. L., Flanders, R. W., et al.: Genital herpes in two social groups. Am. J. Obstet. Gynecol., *110*:682, 1971.

Rawls, W. E., Iwamoto, K., Adam, E., et al.: Measurement of antibodies to herpesvirus types 1 and 2 in human sera. J. Immunol., *104*:599, 1970.

Reeves, W. C., Corey, L., Adams, H. G., et al.: Risk of recurrence after first episodes of genital herpes: Relation to HSV type and antibody response. N. Engl. J. Med., *305*:315, 1981.

Reichman, R. C., Badger, G. J., Guinan, M. E., et al.: Topically administered acyclovir in the treatment of recurrent genital herpes simplex genitalis: A controlled trial. J. Infect. Dis., *147*:336, 1983.

Reichman, R. C., Badger, G. J., Mertz, G. J., et al.: Treatment of recurrent genital herpes infections with oral acyclovir: A controlled trial. JAMA (in press).

Richman, D. D., Cleveland, P. H., and Oxman, M. N.: A rapid enzyme immunofiltration technique using monoclonal antibodies to serotype herpes simplex virus. J. Med. Virol., *9*:299, 1982.

Riehle, R. A., and Williams, J. J.: Transient neuropathic bladder following herpes simplex genitalis. J. Urol., *122*:283, 1979.

Russell, A. S., Brisson, E., and Grace, M.: A double-blind, controlled trial of levamisole in the treatment of recurrent herpes labialis. J. Infect. Dis., *137*:597, 1978.

Saral, R., Burns, W. H., Laskin, O. L., et al.: Acyclovir prophylaxis of herpes simplex virus infections: A randomized double-blind controlled trial in bone marrow transplant recipients. N. Engl. J. Med., *305*:63, 1981.

Scheibel, M., and Jessen, O.: Lysine prophylaxis in recurrent herpes simplex labialis: A double-blind controlled cross over study. Acta Derm. Venereol. (Stockh.), *60*:85, 1979.

Schnipper, L. E., and Crumpacker, C. S.: Resistance of herpes simplex virus to acycloguanosine: Role of viral thymidine kinase and DNA polymerase loci. Proc. Natl. Acad. Sci. USA, *77*:2270, 1980.

Scriba, M.: Protection of guinea pigs against primary and recurrent genital herpes infections by immunization with live heterologous or homologous herpes simplex virus: Implications for herpes virus vaccine. Med. Microbiol. Immunol., *166*:63, 1978.

Silvestri, D. L., Corey, L., and Holmes, K. K.: Ineffectiveness of topical idoxuridine in dimethylsulfoxide for therapy of genital herpes. JAMA, *248*:953, 1982.

Skinner, G. R. B., Woodman, C. B. J., Hartley, C. E., et al.: Preparation and immunogeneity of vaccine Ac NFU1$_1$(S;$^-$) MRC towards the prevention of herpes genitalis. Br. J. Vener. Dis., *58*:381, 1982.

Skoldenberg, B., Jeansson, S., and Wolontis, S.: Herpes simplex virus 2 and acute aseptic meningitis. Scand. J. Infect. Dis., *2*:227, 1975.

Spruance, S. L., Crumpacker, C. S., Schnipper, L. E., et al.: Topical 10% acyclovir (ACV) in polyethylene glycol (PEG) for herpes simplex labialis: Results of treatment begun in the prodrome and erythema stages. Presented at the 22nd Interscience Conference on Antimicrobial Agents and Chemotherapy (ICAAC). Miami Beach, Oct. 1982.

St. Geme, J. W., Prince, J. G., Burke, B. A., et al.: Impaired cellular resistance to herpes simplex virus in Wiskott-Aldrich syndrome. N. Engl. J. Med., *273*:229, 1965.

Stamm, W. E., Wagner, K. F., Amsel, R., et al.: Causes of the acute urethral syndrome in women. N. Engl. J. Med., *303*:409, 1980.

Stone, W. J., Scowden, E. B., Spannuth, C. I., et al.: Atypical herpesvirus hominis type 2 infection in uremic patients receiving immunosuppressive therapy. Am. J. Med., *63*:511, 1977.

Straus, S. E., Smith, H. A., Brickman, C., et al.: Acyclovir for mucocutaneous herpes simplex virus infection in immunosuppressed patients. Ann. Intern. Med., *96*:270, 1982.

Sumaya, C. V., Marx, J., and Ullis, K.: Genital infections with herpes simplex virus in a university student population. Sex. Transm. Dis., *7*:16, 1980.

Sutton, A. L., Smithwick, E. M., Seligman, S. J., et al.:

Fatal disseminated herpesvirus hominis type 2 infection in an adult with associated thymic dysplasia. Am. J. Med., 56:545, 1974.

Vontver, L. A., Reeves, W. C., Rattray, M., et al.: Clinical course and diagnosis of genital herpes simplex virus infection and evaluation of topical surfactant therapy. Am. J. Obstet. Gynecol., 133:548, 1979.

Wade, J. C., Newton, B., McLaren, C., et al.: Intravenous acyclovir to treat mucocutaneous herpes simplex virus infection after marrow transplantation. Ann. Intern. Med., 96:265, 1982.

Wallin, J., Lernestedt, J-O., Lycke, E., et al.: Therapeutic efficacy of trisodium phosphonoformate in treatment of recurrent herpes labialis. In Nahmias, A. J., Dowdle, W. R., and Schwinazi, R. F. (Eds.): The Human Herpesviruses. New York, Elsevier, 1981.

Wentworth, B. B., Bonin, P., Holmes, K. K., et al.: Isolation of viruses, bacteria and other organisms from venereal disease clinic patients: Methodology and problems associated with multiple isolations. Health Lab. Sci., 10:75, 1973.

Wheeler, C. E., Jr., and Abele, D. C.: Eczema herpeticum, primary and recurrent. Arch. Dermatol., 93:162, 1966.

Whitley, R. J.: Topical acyclovir in mucocutaneous herpes simplex virus infections of immunocompromised hosts. Am. J. Med. (in press).

Genital Warts

Barrett, T. J., Silbar, J. D., and McGinley, J. P.: Genital warts—a venereal disease. J.A.M.A., 154:333, 1954.

Carr, G., and William, D. C.: Anal warts in a population of gay men in New York City. Sex. Transm. Dis., 4:56, 1977.

Centers for Disease Control: Sexually transmitted disease: Treatment guidelines 1982. MMWR, 31:335, 1982.

Coggin, J., and zur Hausen, H.: Papillomaviruses and cancer. Cancer, 39:545, 1979.

Dunn, A. E., and Ogilvie, M. M.: Intranuclear virus particles in human genital wart tissue: Observations on the ultrastructure of the epidermal layer. J. Ultrastruct. Res., 22:282, 1968.

Friedrich, E. G., Wilkinson, E. J., and Fu, Y. S.: Carcinoma in situ of the vulva: A continuing challenge. Am. J. Obstet. Gynecol., 136:830, 1980.

Ghosh, A. K.: Cryosurgery of genital warts in cases in which podophyllin treatment failed or was contraindicated. Br. J. Vener. Dis., 53:49, 1977.

Hahn, G. A.: Carbon dioxide laser surgery in the treatment of condyloma. Am. J. Obstet. Gynecol., 141:1000, 1981.

Malison, M. D., Morris, R., and Jones, L. W.: Autogenous vaccine therapy for condyloma acuminatum. Br. J. Vener. Dis., 58:62, 1982.

Malison, M. D., and Salkin, D.: Attempted BCG immunotherapy for condylomata acuminata. Br. J. Vener. Dis., 57:148, 1981.

Margolis, S.: Therapy for condyloma acuminatum: A review. Rev. Infect. Dis., 4:5829, 1982.

Margolis, S.: Genital warts and molluscum contagiosum. Urol. Clin. North Am., 11:163, 1984.

Meisels, A., and Fortin, R.: Condylomatous lesions of the cervix and vagina: I. Cytological patterns. Acta Cytol., 20:505, 1976.

Meisels, A., Fortin, R., and Roy, M.: Condylomatous lesions of the cervix and vagina: II. Cytologic, colposcopic and histopathologic study. Acta Cytol., 21:379, 1977.

Morton, R. S.: The Other STD's: A Synopsis. Washington, D.C., DHHS Publication, 40–45, 1979.

Oriel, J. D., and Almeida, J. D.: Demonstration of virus particles in human genital warts. Br. J. Vener. Dis., 37:37, 1970.

Oriel, J. D.: Condylomata acuminata as a sexually transmitted disease. Dermatol. Clin., 1:93, 1983.

Oriel, J. D.: Genital warts. Sex. Transm. Dis., 8:326, 1981.

Oriel, J. D.: Natural history of genital warts. Br. J. Vener. Dis., 47:1, 1971.

Pollack, H. M., de Benedictis, T. J., Marmar, J. L., et al.: Urethrographic manifestations of venereal warts (condylomata acuminata). Radiology, 126:643, 1978.

Powell, L. L.: Condyloma acuminatum: Recent advances in development, carcinogenesis and treatment. Clin. Obstet. Gynecol., 21:1061, 1978.

Quality Assurance Guidelines for STD clinics—1982. Washington, D.C., DHHS Publication No. 00–4066, 1982.

Syrjanen, K. J.: Current views on the condylomatous lesions of the uterine cervix and their possible relationship to cervical squamous cell carcinoma. Obstet. Gynecol. Surg., 35:685, 1981.

von Krogh, G.: The beneficial effect of 1 per cent 5-fluorouracil in 7 per cent ethanol on therapeutically refractory condylomas in the preputial cavity. Sex. Transm. Dis., 5:137, 1978.

von Krogh, G.: Penile condylomata acuminata: An experimental model for evaluation of topical self-treatment with 0.5 per cent–1 per cent ethanolic preparations of podophyllotoxin for three days. Sex. Transm. Dis., 8:179, 1981.

Molluscum Contagiosum

Brown, S. T., and Weinberger, J.: Molluscum contagiosum: Sexually transmitted disease in 17 cases. J. Am. Vener. Dis. Assoc., 1:35, 1974.

Brown, S. T., Nalley, J. F., and Kraus, S. J.: Molluscum contagiosum. Sex. Transm. Dis., 8:227, 1981.

Centers for Disease Control: Sexually transmitted diseases: Treatment guidelines 1982. MMWR, 31:335, 1982.

Felman, Y. M., and Nikitas, J. A.: Genital molluscum contagiosum. Cutis, 26:28, 1980.

Felman, Y. M., and Nikitas, J. A.: Sexually transmitted molluscum contagiosum. Dermatol. Clin. 1:103, 1983.

Lynch, P. J., and Minkin, W.: Molluscum contagiosum of the adult: Probable venereal transmission. Arch. Dermatol., 98:141, 1968.

McFadden, G., Pace, W. E., Purses, J., et al.: Biogenesis of poxviruses: Transitory expression of molluscum contagiosum early functions. Virology, 94:297, 1979.

Margolis, S.: Genital warts and molluscum contagiosum. Urol. Clin. North Am., 11:163, 1984.

Morton, R. S.: The other STD's: A synopsis. Washington, D.C., DHHS Publication, 40–45, 1979.

Pirie, G. D., Bishop, P. M., Burke, D. C., et al.: Some properties of purified molluscum contagiosum virus. J. Gen. Virol., 13:311, 1971.

Quality Assurance Guidelines for STD Clinics, 1982. Washington, D.C., DHHS Publication No. 00–4066, 1982.

Reed, R. J., and Parkinson, R. P.: The histogenesis of molluscum contagiosum. Am. J. Surg. Pathol., 1:161, 1977.

Infant and Maternal Sexually Transmitted Diseases

Alford, C. A., Stagno, S., Pass, R. F., et al.: Epidemiology of cytomegalovirus. In Nahmias, A. J., Dowdle, W. R., and Schwinazi, R. F. (Eds): The Human Herpesviruses. New York, Elsevier, 1981.

Alexander, E. R.: Maternal and infant sexually transmitted diseases. Urol. Clin. North Am., 11:131, 1984.

Alexander, E. R., and Harrison, H. R.: Role of *Chlamydia trachomatis* in perinatal infection. Rev. Infect. Dis., 5:713, 1983.

Alexander, E. R., Harrison, H. R., Lewis, M., et al.: Strategies for prevention of infant chlamydial disease. *In* Måardh P-A., et al. (Eds.): Chlamydial Infections, Vol. 2. Fernstrom Foundation Series. Amsterdam, Elsevier, 1982.

Amstey, M. S., and Stedman, K. T.: Asymptomatic gonorrhea in pregnancy. J. Am. Vener. Dis. Assoc., 3:14, 1976.

Aral, S. O., and Holmes, K. K.: Epidemiology of Sexually Transmitted Disease. *In* Holmes, K. K., Måardh, P-A, Sparling, P. F., et al. (Eds.): Sexually Transmitted Diseases. New York, McGraw-Hill Book Co., 1984.

Baker, C.: Prevention of neonatal Group B streptococcal disease. Pediatr. Infect. Dis., 2:1, 1983.

Baker, C. F., Goroff, D. R., Alpert, S., et al.: Vaginal infection with Group B streptococcus. J. Infect. Dis., 136:137, 1977.

Bejar, R., Curbelo, V., Davis, C., et al.: Premature labor: II. Bacterial sources of phospholipase. Obstet. Gynecol., 57:479, 1981.

Centers for Disease Control: Syphilis trends: U.S. 1982. MMWR, 31-355, 1982.

Chacko, M. R., Phillips, S., and Jacobson, M. S.: Screening for pharyngeal gonorrhea in the urban teenager. Pediatrics, 70:620, 1982.

Dworsky, M. E., and Stagno, S.: Newer agents causing pneumonitis in early infancy. Pediatr. Infect. Dis. 1:188, 1982.

Franciosi, R. A., Knostman, J. D., and Zimmerman, R. A.: Group B streptococcal neonatal and infant infection. J. Pediatr., 82:707, 1973.

Gold, E., and Nankervis, G. A.: Cytomegalovirus. *In* Evans, A. S. (Ed.): Viral Infections of Humans: Epidemiology and Control. New York, Plenum, 1976.

Hammerschlag, M. R., Chandler, J. W., Alexander, E. R., et al.: Erythromycin ointment for ocular prophylaxis of neonatal chlamydial infection. JAMA, 244:2291, 1980.

Harrison, H. R., Alexander, E. R., Weinstein, L., et al.: Cervical *Chlamydia trachomatis* and mycoplasma infections in pregnancy. JAMA, 2501721, 1983.

Harrison, H. R., English, M. G., Lee, C. K., et al.: *Chlamydia trachomatis* infant pneumonitis: Comparison with matched controls and other infant pneumonitis. N. Engl. J. Med., 298:702, 1978.

Harwick, H. J., Purcell, R. H., Iuppa, J. B., et al.: *Mycoplasma hominis* and abortion. J. Infect. Dis., 121:260, 1970.

Holmes, K. K., Counts, C. W., and Beatty, H. N.: Disseminated gonococcal infection. Ann. Intern. Med., 74:979, 1971.

Ingall, D., and Nevins, L.: Syphilis. *In* Remington, J. S., and Klein, O. J. (Eds.): Infectious Disease of the Fetus and Newborn Infant. 2nd ed. Philadelphia, W. B. Saunders Co., 1983.

Jordan, M. C., Rousseau, W. E., Noble, G. R., et al.: Association of cervical cytomegalovirus with venereal disease. N. Engl. J. Med., 288:932, 1973.

Kass, E. H., and McCormack, W. M.: Genital mycoplasmas as a cause of excess premature delivery. Trans. Assoc. Am. Physicians, 94:261, 1981.

Lang, D. J., and Kummer, J. F.: Cytomegalovirus in semen: Observations in selected populations. J. Infect. Dis., 132:472, 1975.

Martin, D. H., Koutsky, L., Eschenbach, D. A., et al.: Prematurity and perinatal mortality in pregnancies complicated by maternal *Chlamydia trachomatis* infection. JAMA, 247:1585, 1982.

McCormack, W. M.: Colonization with genital mycoplasmas in women. Am. J. Epidemiol., 97:240, 1973.

Monif, G. R. G.: Gonorrhea and pregnancy. Perinatal Care, 2:12, 1978.

Morenstein, G. B., Todd, W. A., Brown, G., et al.: Group B hemolytic streptococcus: Randomized controlled treatment study at term. Obstet. Gynecol., 55:315, 1980.

Nahmias, A. J., and Visentine, A. M.: Herpes simplex. *In* Remington, J. S., and Klein, O. J. (Eds.): Infectious Disease of the Fetus and Newborn Infant. 2nd ed. Philadelphia, W. B. Saunders Co., 1983.

Rabin, G. L., Peterson, H. B., Darfnean, S. F., et al.: Ectopic pregnancy in the United States, 1970 through 1978. JAMA, 249:1725, 1983.

Rathbun, K. C.: Congenital syphilis: A proposal for improved surveillance, diagnosis and treatment. Sex. Transm. Dis., 10:102, 1983.

Rathbun, K. C.: Congenital syphilis. Sex. Transm. Dis., 10:93, 1983.

Regan, J. A., Chao, S., and James, L. S.: Premature rupture of membranes, preterm delivery and Group B streptococcal colonization of mothers. Am. J. Obstet. Gynecol., 141:186, 1981.

Rothenberg, R.: Ophthalmia neonatorum due to *Neisseria gonorrheae*. Sex. Transm. Dis., 6:187, 1979.

Siegel, J. D., McCracken, G. H., Threlkeid, N., et al.: Single dose penicillin prophylaxis against neonatal Group B streptococcal infections: A controlled trial in 18,738 newborn infants. N. Engl. J. Med., 303:769, 1980.

Taylor-Robinson, D., and McCormack, W. M.: The genital mycoplasmas. N. Engl. J. Med., 302:1003, 1063, 1980.

Wagner, G. P., Martin, D. H., Koutsky, L., et al.: Puerperal infectious morbidity: Relationship to route of delivery and to antepartum *Chlamydia trachomatis* infection. Am. J. Obstet. Gynecol., 138:1028, 1980.

Wallace, R. J., Jr., Alpert, S., Brown, K., et al.: Isolation of *Mycoplasma hominis* from blood cultures in patients with post partum fever. Obstet. Gynecol., 51:181, 1978.

Wallin, F., and Forgsren, A.: Group B streptococci in venereal disease clinic patients. Br. J. Vener. Dis., 51:401, 1975.

Weström, L., and Måardh, P-A.: Genital chlamydial infections in the female. *In* Måardh, P-A., et al. (Eds.): Chlamydial Infections, Vol. 2. Fernstrom Foundation Series, Amsterdam, Elsevier, 1982.

Whittley, R. J., Nahmias, A. J., Soong, S. J., et al.: Vidarabine therapy of neonatal herpes simplex virus infection. Pediatrics, 66:495, 1980.

Whittley, R. J., Nahmias, A. J., Visentine, A. M., et al.: Natural history of herpes simplex virus infection of mother and newborn. Pediatrics, 66:489, 1980.

Yow, M. D., Mason, E. O., Leeds, L. J., et al.: Ampicillin prevents intrapartum transmission of Group B streptococcus. JAMA, 241:1245, 1979.

Hepatitis and Enteric Infections

Anders, B. J., Lauer, B. A., Paisley, J. W., et al.: Double-blind placebo controlled trial of erythromycin for treatment of campylobacter enteritis. Lancet, 1:131, 1982.

Bader, M., Pedersen, A. H. B., Williams, R., et al.: Venereal transmission of shigellosis in Seattle–King County. Sex. Transm. Dis., 4:89, 1977.

Bancroft, W. H., Snitbhan, R., Scott, R. M., et al.: Transmission of hepatitis B virus to gibbons by exposure to human saliva containing hepatitis B surface antigen. J. Infect. Dis., *135*:79, 1977.

Blacklow, N. R., and Cukor, G.: Viral gastroenteritis. N. Engl. J. Med., *304*:397, 1981.

Blazer, M. J., and Reller, L. B.: Campylobacter enteritis. N. Engl. J. Med., *305*:1444, 1981.

Blazer, M. J., Wells, J. G., Feldman, R. A., et al.: Campylobacter enteritis in the United States: A multicenter study. Ann. Intern. Med., *98*:360, 1983.

Centers for Disease Control: Cryptosporidiosis: Assessment of chemotherapy in males with acquired immune deficiency syndrome (AIDS). MMWR, *31*:589, 1982a.

Centers for Disease Control: Immune globulins for protection against viral hepatitis. MMWR, *30*:423, 1981.

Centers for Disease Control: Inactivated hepatitis B vaccine: Recommendations of the Immunization Practices Advisory Committee. Ann. Intern. Med., *97*:379, 1982b.

Centers for Disease Control: Sexually transmitted disease: Treatment guidelines 1982. MMWR, *31* (Suppl.):335, 1982c.

Christenson, B., Bröstrom, C. H., Bottiger, M., et al.: An epidemic outbreak of hepatitis A among homosexual men in Stockholm. Am. J. Epidemiol., *116*:599, 1982.

Corey, L., and Holmes, K. K.: Sexual transmission of hepatitis A in homosexual men: Incidence and mechanism. N. Engl. J. Med., *302*:435, 1980.

Deheragoda, P.: Diagnosis of rectal gonorrhea by blind anorectal swabs compared with direct vision swabs taken via a proctoscope. Br. J. Vener. Dis., *53*:311, 1977.

Dritz, S. K., Ainsworth, T. E., Back, A., et al.: Patterns of sexually transmitted diseases in a city. Lancet, *2*:3, 1977.

Drugs for parasitic infections. Med. Lett. Drugs Ther., *24*:5, 1982.

Garcia, L. S., Bruckner, D. A., Brewer, T. L., et al.: Techniques for the recovery and identification of *Cryptosporidium* oocysts from stool specimens. J. Clin. Microbiol., *18*:185, 1983.

Gilman, R. H., Spira, W., Rabbani, H., et al.: Single-dose ampicillin therapy for severe shigellosis in Bangladesh. J. Infect. Dis., *143*:164, 1981.

Goldmeier, D.: Proctitis and herpes simplex virus in homosexual men. Br. J. Vener. Dis., *56*:111, 1980.

Goodell, S. E., Quinn, T. C., Mkrtichian, E., et al.: Herpex simplex virus proctitis in homosexual men. N. Engl. J. Med., *308*:868, 1983.

Hurwitz, A. L., and Owen, R. L.: Venereal transmission of intestinal parasites. West. J. Med., *128*:89, 1978.

Judson, F. N.: Epidemiology of sexually transmitted hepatitis B infections in heterosexuals: A review. Sex. Transm. Dis., *8*(Suppl.):336, 1981.

Judson, F. N.: Sexually transmitted viral hepatitis and enteric pathogens. Urol. Clin. North Am. *11*:177, 1984.

Judson, F. N., Penley, K. A., Robinson, M. E., et al.: Comparative prevalence rates of sexually transmitted diseases in heterosexual and homosexual men. Am. J. Epidemiol., *112*:836, 1980.

Kean, B. H., William, D. C., and Luminais, S. K.: Epidemic of amoebiasis and giardiasis in a biased population. Br. J. Vener. Dis., *55*:375, 1979.

Kinsey, A. L., Pomeroy, W. B., and Martin, C. E.: Sexual Behavior in the Human Male. Philadelphia, W. B. Saunders Co., 1948.

Klein, E. J., Fisher, L. S., Chow, A. W., et al.: Anorectal gonococcal infection. Ann. Intern. Med., *86*:340, 1977.

Klotz, S. A., Drutz, D. J., Tam, M. R., et al.: Hemorrhagic proctitis due to lymphogranuloma venereum serogroup L₂. N. Engl. J. Med., *308*:1563, 1983.

Mao, J. S., Yu, P. H., Ding, Z. S., et al.: Patterns of shedding of hepatitis A virus in feces and of antibody responses in patients with naturally acquired type A hepatitis. J. Infect. Dis., *142*:654, 1980.

McFarlane, E. S., Embil, J. A., Manuel, F. R., et al.: Antibodies to hepatitis A antigen in relation to number of lifetime sexual partners in patients attending a STD clinic. Br. J. Vener. Dis. *57*:58, 1981.

McMillan, A., Sommerville, R. G., and McKie, P. M. K.: Chlamydial infection in homosexual men. Br. J. Vener. Dis., *57*:47, 1981.

Meyers, J. D., Kuhoric, H. A. and Holmes, K. K.: *Giardia lamblia* infection in homosexual men. Br. J. Vener. Dis., *53*:54, 1977.

Oriel, J. D.: Anal warts and anal coitus. Br. J. Vener. Dis., *47*:373, 1971.

Oriel, J. D.: Genital warts. Sex. Transm. Dis., *8*:326, 1981.

Pickering, L. K., DuPont, H. L., and Androlarte, J.: Single-dose tetracycline for shigellosis in adults. JAMA, *239*:853, 1978.

Phillips, S. C., Mildvan, D., William, D. C., et al.: Sexual transmission of enteric protozoa and helminths in a venereal disease clinic population. N. Engl. J. Med., *305*:603, 1981.

Quinn, T. C., Corey, L., Chatter, R. G., et al.: Campylobacter proctitis in a homosexual man. Ann. Intern. Med., *93*:458, 1980.

Quinn, T. C., Corey, L., Chatter, R. G., et al.: The etiology of anorectal infections in homosexual men. Am. J. Med., *71*:395, 1981a.

Quinn, T. C., Goodell, S. E., Mkrtichian, E., et al.: *Chlamydia trachomatis* proctitis. N. Engl. J. Med., *305*:195, 1981b.

Reiner, N. E., Judson, F. N., Bond, W. M., et al.: Detection of asymptomatic rectal mucosal lesions and hepatitis B surface antigen at sites of sexual contact in homosexual men with persistent hepatitis B virus infection: Evidence for de facto parenteral transmission. Ann. Intern. Med., *96*:170, 1982.

Robinson, D. A.: Infective dose of *Campylobacter jejuni* in milk. Br. Med. J., *282*:1584, 1981.

Robinson, W. S.: The enigma of non-A, non-B hepatitis. J. Infect. Dis., *145*:387, 1982.

Sargeaunt, P. G., Oates, J. K., Maclennan, I., et al.: *Entamoeba histolytica* in male homosexuals. Br. J. Vener. Dis., *59*:193, 1983.

Schmerin, M. J., Gelston, A., and Jones, T. C.: Amebiasis. An increasing problem among homosexuals in New York City. JAMA, *238*:1386, 1977.

Schmerin, M. J., Jones, T. L., and Klein, H.: Giardiasis: Association with homosexuality. An. Intern. Med., *88*:801, 1978.

Schreeder, M. T., Thompson, S. E., Hadler, S. C., et al.: Hepatitis B in homosexual men. Prevalence of infection and factors related to its transmission. J. Infect. Dis., *146*:7, 1982.

Tzipori, S.: Cryptosporidiosis in animals and humans. Microbiol. Rev., *47*:84, 1983.

Waugh, M. A.: Anorectal Herpesvirus hominis infection in men. J. Am. Vener. Dis. Assoc., *3*:68, 1976.

William, D. C., Shookhoff, H. B., Felman, Y. M., et al.: High rates of enteric protozoal infections in selected men attending a venereal disease clinic. Sex. Transm. Dis. *5*:155, 1978.

Acquired Immunodeficiency Syndrome

Ammann, A., Cowan, M. J., Wara, D. W., et al.: Acquired immunodeficiency in an infant: Possible transmission by means of blood products. Lancet, *1*:956, 1983.

Anderson, D. J., and Tarter, T. H.: Immunosuppressive effects of mouse seminal plasma components in vivo and in vitro. J. Immunol., *128*:535, 1982.

Barré-Sinoussi, F. B., Chermann, J. C., Rey, F., et al.: Isolation of a T-lymphotropic retrovirus from a patient at risk for acquired immune deficiency syndrome (AIDS). Science, *220*:868, 1983.

Barry, M., Stansfield, S. K., and Bia, F. J.: Haiti and the Hospital Albert Schweitzer, Ann. Intern. Med., *98*:1018, 1983.

Blatter, W. A., Blayney, D. W., Robert-Guroff, M., et al.: Epidemiology of human T-cell leukemia/lymphoma virus. J. Infect. Dis., *147*:406, 1983.

Blattner, W. A., Takatsuki, K., and Gallo, R. C.: Human T-cell leukemia-lymphoma virus and adult T-cell leukemia. JAMA, *250*:1074, 1983.

Brynes, R. K., Chan, W. C., Spira, T. J., et al.: Value of lymph node biopsy in unexplained lymphadenopathy in homosexual men. JAMA, *250*:1313, 1983.

Bygbjerg, I. C.: AIDS in a Danish surgeon (Zaire, 1976). Lancet, *1*:925, 1983.

Centers for Disease Control: Acquired immune deficiency syndrome (AIDS): Precautions for clinical and laboratory staffs. MMWR, *31*:577, 1982a.

Centers for Disease Control: A cluster of Kaposi's sarcoma and *Pneumocystis carinii* pneumonia among homosexual male residents of Los Angeles and Orange Counties, California. MMWR, *31*:305, 1982b.

Centers for Disease Control: Cryptosporidiosis: Assessment of chemotherapy of males with acquired imune deficiency syndrome (AIDS). MMWR, *31*:589, 1982c.

Centers for Disease Control: Diffuse, undifferentiated non-Hodgkin's lymphoma among homosexual males—United States. MMWR, *31*:277, 1982d.

Centers for Disease Control: An evaluation of the acquired immunodeficiency syndrome (AIDS) reported in health care personnel—United States. MMWR, *32*:358, 1983a.

Centers for Disease Control: Human T-cell leukemia virus infection in patients with acquired immune deficiency syndrome: Preliminary observations. MMWR, *32*:233, 1983b.

Centers for Disease Control: Kaposi's sarcoma and *Pneumocystis* pneumonia among homosexual men—New York City and California. MMWR, *30*:305, 1981a.

Centers for Disease Control: *Pneumocystis* pneumonia—Los Angeles. MMWR, *30*:250, 1981b.

Centers for Disease Control: Prevention of acquired immune deficiency syndrome (AIDS): Report of interagency recommendations. MMWR, *32*:101, 1983c.

Centers for Disease Control: The safety of hepatitis B virus vaccine. MMWR, *32*:134, 1983d.

Centers for Disease Control: Sexually transmitted disease: Statistical letter, calendar year 1981. Atlanta, Georgia, U.S. Department of Health and Human Services, 1983e.

Centers for Disease Control: Update: Acquired immunodeficiency syndrome (AIDS)—United States. MMWR, *31*:507, 1982e; *32*:465, 1983f.

Centers for Disease Control: Task force on Kaposi's sarcoma and opportunistic infections. N. Engl. J. Med., *306*:248, 1982f.

Clumeck, N., Mascart-Lemone, F., de Maubeuge, J., et al.: Acquired immune deficiency syndrome in black Africans. Lancet, *1*:642, 1983.

Collier, A. C., and Handsfield, H. H.: Acquired immune deficiency syndrome. Urol. Clin. North. Am., *11*:187, 1984.

Conte, J. E., Hadley, W. K., Sande, M., et al.: Infection-control guidelines for patients with the acquired immunodeficiency syndrome (AIDS). N. Engl. J. Med., *309*:740, 1983.

Current, W. L., Reese, N. C., Ernst, J. V., et al.: Human cryptosporidiosis in immunocompetent and immunodeficient persons. N. Engl. J. Med., *308*:1252, 1983.

Darrow, W., Jaffe, H. W., and Curran, J. W.: Passive anal intercourse as a risk factor for AIDS in homosexual men. Lancet, *2*:160, 1983.

Desforges, J.: AIDS and preventative treatment in hemophilia. N. Engl. J. Med., *308*:94, 1983.

deShazo, R. D., Andes, W. A., Nordberg, J., et al.: An immunologic evaluation of hemophiliac patients and their wives. Ann. Intern. Med., *99*:159, 1983.

Detels, R., Fahey, J. L., Schwartz, K., et al.: Relation between sexual practices and T-cell subsets in homosexually active men. Lancet, *1*:609, 1983.

Drew, W. L., Conant, M. A., Miner, R. C., et al.: Cytomegalovirus and Kaposi's sarcoma in young homosexual men. Lancet, *1*:125, 1982.

Dzik, W., and Neckers, L.: Lymphocyte subpopulations altered during blood storage. N. Engl. J. Med., *309*:435, 1983.

Essex, M., McLane, M. F., Lee, T. H., et al.: Antibodies to cell membrane antigens associated with human T-cell leukemia virus in patients with AIDS. Science, *220*:859, 1983.

Ewing, E. P., Spira, T. J., Chandler, F. W., et al.: Unusual cytoplasmic body in lymphoid cells of homosexual men with unexplained lymphadenopathy. N. Engl. J. Med., *308*:819, 1983.

Fernandez, R., Mouradian, J., Metroka, C., and Davis, J.: The prognostic value of histopathology in persistent generalized lymphadenopathy in homosexual men. N. Engl. J. Med., *309*:185, 1983.

Friedman-Kien, A., Laubenstein, L. J., Rubinstein, P., et al.: Disseminated Kaposi's sarcoma in homosexual men. Ann. Intern. Med., *90*:693, 1982.

Gallo, R. C., Sarin, P. S., Gelmann, E. P., et al.: Isolation of human T-cell leukemia virus in acquired immune deficiency syndrome. Science, *220*:865, 1983.

Gerstoft, J., Malchow-Møller, A., Bygbjerg, I., et al.: Severe acquired immunodeficiency in European homosexual men. Br. Med. J., *285*:17, 1982.

Giraldo, G., Beth, E., Kourilsky, F. M., et al.: Antibody patterns to herpes viruses in Kaposi's sarcoma: Serological association of European Kaposi's sarcoma with cytomegalovirus. Int. J. Cancer, *15*:839, 1975.

Goldsmith, J. C., Moseley, P. L., Monick, M., et al.: T-lymphocyte subpopulation abnormalities in apparently healthy patients with hemophilia. Ann. Intern. Med., *98*:294, 1983.

Gottlieb, M. S., Groopman, J. E., Weinstein, W. M., et al.: The acquired immunodeficiency syndrome. Ann. Intern. Med., *99*:208, 1983.

Gottlieb, M., Schroff, R., Schanker, H. M., et al.: *Pneumocystis carinii* pneumonia and mucosal candidiasis in previously healthy homosexual men. N. Engl. J. Med., *305*:1425, 1981.

Greene, J. B., Sidhu, G. S., Lewin, S., et al.: *Mycobacterium avium–intracellulare*: A cause of disseminated life-threatening infection in homosexuals and drug abusers. Ann. Intern. Med., *97*:539, 1982.

Harris, C., Small, C. B., Klein, R. S., et al.: Immunodeficiency in female sexual partners of men with the acquired immunodeficiency syndrome. N. Engl. J. Med., *308*:1181, 1983.

Harwood, A. R., Osoba, D., Hofstader, S. L., et al.: Kaposi's sarcoma in recipients of renal transplants. Am. J. Med., *67*:759, 1979.

Hersey, P., Bradley, M., Hasic, E., et al.: Immunologic effects of solarium exposure. Lancet, *1*:545, 1983.

Hughes, W.: *Pneumocystis carinii* pneumonia. N. Engl. J. Med., *297*:1381, 1977.

Hughes, W. T., Kuhn, S., Chaudhary, S., et al.: Successful chemoprophylaxis for *Pneumocystis carinii* pneumonitis. N. Engl. J. Med., *297*:1419, 1977.

Hurtenbach, U., and Shearer, G. M.: Germ cell–induced immune suppression in mice. J. Exp. Med., *155*:1719, 1982.

Hymes, K., Cheung, T., Greene, J., et al.: Kaposi's sarcoma in homosexual men—a report of eight cases. Lancet, *2*:598, 1981.

Jaffe, H. W., Choi, K., Thomas, P. A., et al.: National case-control study of Kaposi's sarcoma and *Pneumocystis carinii* pneumonia in homosexual men, Part I: Epidemiologic results. Ann. Intern. Med., *99*:145, 1983.

Judson, F. N.: Fear of AIDS and gonorrhea rates in homosexual men. Lancet, *2*:159, 1983.

Kornfeld, H., Stouwe, R. A. V., Lange, M., et al.: T-lymphocyte subpopulations in homosexual men. N. Engl. J. Med., *307*:729, 1982.

Krown, S. E., Real, F. X., Cunningham-Rundles, S., et al.: Preliminary observations on the effect of recombinant leukocyte A interferon in homosexual men with Kaposi's sarcoma. N. Engl. J. Med., *308*:1071, 1983.

Lane, H. C., Masur, H., Edgar, L. C., et al.: Abnormalities of B-cell activation and immunoregulation in patients with the acquired immunodeficiency syndrome. N. Engl. J. Med., *309*:453, 1983.

Leonidas, J. R., and Hyppolite, N.: Haiti and the acquired immunodeficiency syndrome. Ann. Intern. Med., *98*:1020, 1983.

Levy, J. A., and Ziegler, J. L.: Acquired immunodeficiency syndrome is an opportunistic infection and Kaposi's sarcoma results from secondary stimulation. Lancet, *2*:78, 1983.

Liautaud, B., Laroche, C., Duvivier, J., et al.: Le sarcome de Kaposi (maladie de Kaposi) est-il fréquent en Haiti? Presented at the 18th Congrès des Médecins Francophones de l'Hêmisphère Américain, Port au Prince, Haiti, April 12–16, 1982.

Ma, P., and Soave, R.: Three-step stool examination for cryptosporidiosis in 10 homosexual men with protracted watery diarrhea. J. Infect. Dis. *147*:824, 1983.

Mangi, R. J., Niederman, J. C., Kelleher, J. E., et al.: Depression of cell-mediated immunity during acute infectious mononucleosis. N. Engl. J. Med., *291*:1149, 1974.

Marmor, M., Friedman-Kien, A. E., Laubenstein, L., et al.: Risk factors for Kaposi's sarcoma in homosexual men. Lancet, *1*:1083, 1982.

Masur, H., Michelis, M. A., Greene, J. B., et al.: An outbreak of community-acquired *Pneumocystis carinii* pneumonia. N. Engl. J. Med., *305*:1431, 1981.

Masur, H., Michelis, M. A., Wormser, G. P., et al.: Opportunistic infection in previously healthy women. Ann. Intern. Med., *97*:533, 1982.

Mathur, U., Enlow, R. W., Spigland, I., et al.: Generalized lymphadenopathy: A prodrome of Kaposi's sarcoma in male homosexuals (abstract 853). Presented at the Interscience Conference on Antimicrobial Agents and Chemotherapy, Miami Beach, October 4–6, 1982.

Meuwissen, J. H., Tauber, I., Leeuwenberg, A. D., et al.: Parasitologic and serologic observations of infection with Pneumocystis in humans. J. Infect. Dis., *136*:43, 1977.

Miller, J. R., Barrett, R. E., Britton, C. B., et al.: Progressive multifocal leukoencephalopathy in a male homosexual with T-cell immune deficiency. N. Engl. J. Med., *307*:1436, 1982.

Miller, L. G., Goldstein, G., Murphy, M., and Gins, L. C.: Reversible alterations in immunoregulatory T-cells in smoking. Chest, *82*:526, 1982.

Miyoshi, I., Kobayashi, M., Yoshimoto, S., et al.: ATLV in a Japanese patient wih AIDS. Lancet, *2*:27, 1983.

Morris, L., Distenfeld, A., Amorosi, E., et al.: Autoimmune thrombocytopenic purpura in homosexual men. Ann. Intern. Med., *96*:714, 1982.

Moss, A. R., Bacchetti, P., Gorman, M., et al.: AIDS in the "gay" areas of San Francisco. Lancet, *1*:923, 1983.

Oleske, J., Minnefor, A., Cooper, R., et al.: Immune deficiency syndrome in children. JAMA, *249*:2345, 1983.

Pifer, L. L., Hughes, W. T., Stagno, S., and Woods, D.: *Pneumocystis carinii* infection: Evidence for high prevalence in normal and immuosuppressed children. Pediatrics, *61*:35, 1978.

Pitchenik, A., Fischl, M. A., Dickinson, G. M., et al.: Opportunistic infections and Kaposi's sarcoma among Haitians: Evidence of a new acquired immunodeficiency state. Ann. Intern. Med., *98*:277, 1983.

Pitchenik, A., Fischl, M. A., and Spira, T. J.: Acquired immune deficiency syndrome in low-risk patients. JAMA, *250*:1310, 1983.

Reiner, N. E., Judson, F. N., Bond, W. W., et al.: Asymptomatic rectal mucosal lesions and hepatitis B surface antigen at sites of sexual contact in homosexual men with persistent hepatitis B virus infection. Ann. Intern. Med., *96*:170, 1982.

Rinaldo, C. R., Carney, W. P., Richter, B. S., et al.: Mechanisms of immunosuppression in cytomegaloviral mononucleosis. J. Infect. Dis., *141*:488, 1980.

Ritchie, A. W. S., Oswald, I., Micklem, H. S., et al.: Circadian variation of lymphocyte subpopulations: A study with monoclonal antibodies. Br. Med. J., *286*:1773, 1983.

Rogers, M. F., Morens, D. M., Stewart, J. A., et al.: National case-control study of Kaposi's sarcoma and *Pneumocystis carinii* pneumonia in homosexual men, Part 2: Laboratory results. Ann. Intern. Med., *99*:151, 1983.

Rubinstein, A., Sicklick, M., Gupta, A., et al.: Acquired immunodeficiency with reversed T4/T8 ratios in infants born to promiscuous and drug-addicted mothers. JAMA, *249*:2350, 1983.

Siegal, F. P., Lopez, C., Hammer, G., et al.: Severe acquired immunodeficiency in male homosexuals, manifested by chronic perianal ulcerative herpes simplex lesions. N. Engl. J. Med., *305*:1439, 1981.

Small, C. B., Klein, R. S., Friedland, G. H., et al.: Community-acquired opportunistic infections and defective cellular immunity in heterosexual drug abusers and homosexual men. Am. J. Med., *74*:433, 1983.

Snider, W. D., Simpson, D. M., Aronyk, K. E., and Nielsen, S. L.: Primary lymphoma of the nervous system associated with acquired immune-deficiency syndrome. N. Engl. J. Med., *308*:45, 1983.

Sonnabend, J., Witkin, S. S., and Purtilo, D. T.: Acquired immunodeficiency syndrome, opportunistic infections, and malignancies in male homosexuals. JAMA, *249*:2370, 1983.

Sterry, W., Marmor, M., Konrads, A., et al.: Kaposi's sarcoma, aplastic pancytopenia, and multiple infections in a homosexual (Cologne, 1976). Lancet, *1*:924, 1983.

Stevens, C. E.: No increased incidence of AIDS in recipients of hepatitis B vaccine. N. Engl. J. Med., *308*:1163, 1983.

Taylor, J. F., Templeton, A. C., Vogel, C. L., et al.: Kaposi's sarcoma in Uganda: A clinicopathological study. Int. J. Cancer, *8*:125, 1971.

Trainin, Z., Wernicke, D., Ungar-Waron, H., and Essex, M: Suppression of the humoral antibody response in natural retrovirus infections. Science, *220*:858, 1983.

Vandepitte, J., Verwilghen, R., and Zachee, P; AIDS and cryptococcosis (Zaire, 1977). Lancet, *1*:925, 1983.

Venet, A., Dennewald, G., Sandron, D., et al.: Bronchoal-veolar lavage in acquired immunodeficiency syndrome. Lancet, *2*:53, 1983.

Vieira, J., Frank, E., Spira, T. J., and Landesman, S. H.: Acquired immune deficiency in Haitians. N. Engl. J. Med., *308*:125, 1983.

Waltzer, P. D., Perl, D. P., Krogstad, D. J., et al.: *Pneumocystis carinii* pneumonia in the United States. Ann. Intern. Med., *80*:83, 1974.

Witkin, S. S., and Sonnabend, J.: Immune response to spermatozoa in homosexual men. Fertil. Steril., *38*:337, 1983.

Visible Lesions of the Male Genitalia

WALTER R. NICKEL, M.D.,
ROBERT T. PLUMB, M.D.

Within the past ten years we have welcomed the statement that, due to vaccination, smallpox had been eradicated on a worldwide basis. Today there is a prevailing policy of health departments and practitioners to treat all suspicious genital lesions with broad-spectrum antibiotics when first seen. This tends to eliminate the need for diagnostic laboratory procedures. Often the patient is well toward recovery before even a preliminary report is available. Therefore, some of the discussion of syphilis, chancroid, lymphogranuloma venerum, and granuloma inguinale, as with smallpox, may seem to be a historical review. Except for herpes simplex and the growing tragic outlook for victims of acquired immunodeficiency syndrome (AIDS) sexually transmitted diseases have been "low key" for the past 40 years.

SYPHILIS

Chancre

In a discussion of the inflammatory lesions of the male genital tract, it seems correct to begin with syphilis. The syphilitic chancre (hard chancre), which in the past has been more commonly the province of the urologist than it is at present, is merely the pale foreshadowing of many more seriously generalized tissue reactions. Syphilis has been called the great imitator. It is caused by the penetration of the *Treponema pallidum,* the specific spirochete isolated first by Schaudinn in 1905. It gains entrance through the intact or abraded skin or mucous membrane. The penis is the usual site of primary involvement in the male. The sites of predilection on the penis are the glans and prepuce, but other sites, such as the meatus, areas within the urethra, and the surface of the shaft, are not uncommon.

The chancre begins as a hyperemic or erythematous spot, usually in a single localized area. In a day or two, desquamation occurs with surrounding induration, forming either a hard papule or a more characteristic ulcerated lesion (Fig. 19–10), usually within a week. The firm, rubbery hardness of the ulcer is due to the vascular sclerosis (endarteritis), with pronounced lymphocytic, plasma cell, and epithelioid cell infiltration. Typically, the lesion is a painless, rather clean, shallow ulcer with rolled indurated borders. Usually solitary, it persists in a rather quiescent fashion, slowly and spontaneously involuting as the secondary stage develops (Figs. 19–11 and 19–12) or until treated, whereupon it heals without scarring. Often the primary chancre develops a unilateral painless satellite of discrete, rubbery lymph nodes, which in doubtful cases may yield by needle aspiration the spirochete for dark-field examination. Treat-

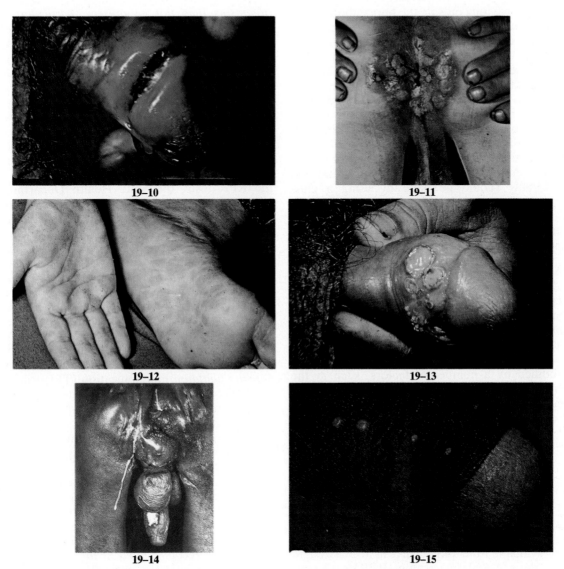

Figure 19–10. Primary syphilis, hard chancre.

Figure 19–11. Condylomata lata of secondary syphilis. (Courtesy of the Department of Dermatology, University of Southern California.)

Figure 19–12. Secondary syphilis on the palms and soles.

Figure 19–13. Chancroid multiple lesions due to autoinoculation.

Figure 19–14. Lymphogranuloma venereum, late advanced stage with scarring, producing sinus tracts of the buttocks and perineal body. (Courtesy of the Department of Dermatology, University of Southern California.)

Figure 19–15. Granuloma inguinale of the frenulum of the penis with typical velvety granulations. (Courtesy of the Department of Dermatology, University of Southern California.)

ment in this early stage is usually accompanied by a febrile reaction (Herxheimer reaction).

Treponema pallidum is a delicate parasite that multiplies by transverse fission. Since it does not live long outside the human body, slide identification is feasible only with fresh material. Using a dark-field condenser, the experienced observer can easily distinguish the organism from other treponemas by its size, morphology, and movements. It is a tightly wound, spiral organism, undulating slowly forward and backward on its own axis, so that it is easily kept in the microscopic field. It bends only in the middle, and it is usually much smaller than other spirochetal denizens of the area. Proper collection of material to be studied is important and preferably should be done by using a glass pipette. The ulcer should be cleaned and serum alone should be expressed from it, for pus and red cells interfere considerably with the examination.

The average interval from infectious exposure to appearance of the chancre is 10 to 30 days. Much longer incubation periods have been reported, but these are open to question. The time of development of positive serologic reactions ranges from 3 weeks to 3 months after inoculation.

The severity of infection appears to be modified by a number of factors, such as the amount of the inoculum, the degree of racial immunity, and a certain natural immunity. Infection is systemic from the outset.

Diagnosis

In the diagnosis and differential diagnosis of chancre, emphasis should be placed upon the value of the dark-field microscope. In smaller communities in which dark-field examination is not available, the physician can use a reagin test, the rapid plasma reagin (RPR) card test, which can be performed in most laboratories. As a screening test this is replacing the VDRL (Venereal Disease Research Laboratories) test and is generally equivalent to it; statements about the VDRL test apply equally to the RPR test.

The Bulletin of the Department of Health, Education and Welfare (HEW) (1976) contains the following comments on the diagnosis of primary syphilis: *The diagnosis of primary syphilis is definite if* T. pallidum *is demonstrated by dark-field microscopy or by fluorescent antibody (FTA) techniques. (Commensal spirochetes of the oropharynx may be mistaken for* T. pallidum;

therefore caution must be used in interpreting specimens from this site.)

Failure to demonstrate T. pallidum *cannot exclude the possibility of syphilis, since sufficient organisms may not be present, particularly if topical or systemic antimicrobials are being used.*

Repeated examinations daily for 3 days with no intervening local or systemic treatment, or aspiration of enlarged regional lymph nodes may be necessary to demonstrate the organism in some patients.

If positive, the RPR and VDRL tests indicate past or present infection and, following the titer, can indicate the body's response. In questionable cases, but usually only after at least two negative results from either the VDRL or the RPR tests, the State Health Department laboratories will perform more specific tests. The quickest and least expensive, the fluorescent treponema antibody-absorption (FTA-ABS) test, is also the most specific and sensitive test available and gives positive results in almost every patient with syphilis regardless of whether adequate, inadequate, or no treatment has been given. An occasional biological false-positive (BFP) test result for syphilis has been reported, but these are rare, and this test remains the most sensitive one currently available. Performance of the expensive and more difficult *Treponema pallidum* immobilization (TPI) test has been phased out and replaced by the microhemagglutination test (MHA-TP), which can be automated and quantitated.

The HEW Bulletin (1976) comments on the serologic diagnosis of primary syphilis as follows: *A reagin test for syphilis, such as the VDRL or RPR, should be obtained at the patient's initial visit. Patients with typical lesions and a reactive reagin test should be treated for primary syphilis even if direct examination for spirochetes is negative. Treponemal serologic tests are not recommended in the presence of a non-reactive reagin test, regardless of the nature of the lesion. If the initial reagin test is non-reactive, repeat reagin tests should be performed one week, one month, and three months later. Non-reactive reagin tests over three months exclude syphilis as a cause of such lesions.*

Secondary Syphilis

Secondary syphilitic lesions may be present anywhere on the body and the genitalia. The skin involvement is highly variable, but is usually bilaterally symmetrical and consists of macular papular or papulosquamous eruptions. In moist areas or mucous surfaces, these eruptions are apt to be eroded (mucous patches), especially on the glans penis or scrotum or in the perianal region. These lesions develop into elevated flat papules or plaques (condylomata lata) (Fig. 19–11) in these same areas. These are the most infectious lesions of syphilis and are teeming with spirochetes. At this stage, syphilitic lesions are usually obvious elsewhere on the skin, appearing first on the palms and soles (Fig. 19–12).

The lesions from which syphilitic chancres must be differentiated include chancroid, granuloma inguinale, lymphogranuloma venereum, balanitides of varying etiology, carcinoma, scabies, psoriasis, lichen planus, leukoplakia, erythroplasia, herpes simplex, and a host of other entities.

The ulcers of *chancroids* have a short incubation period (2 to 5 days) and are dirty, ragged, and painful (Fig. 19–13). They spread by apposition (autoinoculation) and tend to produce early inguinal adenitis with much periadenitis, matting, and suppuration. The adenopathic lesions of syphilis are nonmatting, discrete, and freely movable, with no tendency to suppurate unless secondarily infected. Differentiation may be made by microscopic identification of the spirochete or Ducrey's bacillus. Both infections may be present in the same lesion. *Granuloma inguinale* is a superficial affliction of the skin with red, velvety granulations rolling toward the periphery in a serpiginous outline. Buboes are uncommon. Tissue biopsy demonstrates the Donovan bodies. The penile lesion of lymphogranuloma inguinale is usually so insignificant and evanescent that it escapes notice in the majority of cases. In cases of inguinal adenitis without penile lesions, *lymphogranuloma venereum* (see later discussion) or bacterial infection must be considered. A negative serologic reaction for syphilis provides further supportive evidence that the adenitis arises from some other cause.

Balanitides of varying causes will be found devoid of spirochetes and replete with the causative bacteria. Carcinoma of the penis has so often been treated as a venereal infection that biopsy and tissue examination should be made an integral part of the investigation of the majority of indurated or ulcerative genital lesions of more than 2 weeks' duration. Scabies, lichen planus, herpes simplex, and psoriasis are usually typical clinically, but serologic tests should be routine. Tertiary gummatous lesions of the genitalia would indeed be a rarity.

The treatment of syphilis today is not usually in the province of the urologist. For those using this text as a reference in rural or isolated areas, however, the following recommended treatment, which has not altered appreciably for several years, is included, especially since there may be other concomitant infections.

Treatment

The following schedule is based on that published by the Public Health Service Centers for Disease Control (1982):

Patients with early syphilis (primary, secondary, or latent syphilis of less than 1 year's duration) should receive the following:

Benzathine penicillin G, 2.4 million units total by intramuscular injection at a single session. Benzathine penicillin G is the drug of choice, because it provides effective treatment in a single visit.

Patients who are allergic to penicillin should receive one of the following:

1. Tetracycline hydrochloride,* 500 mg four times a day by mouth for 15 days.

2. Erythromycin (stearate, ethylsuccinate, or base), 500 mg four times a day by mouth for 15 days.

These antibiotics appear to be effective but have been evaluated less extensively than penicillin.

CHANCROID

Chancroid, or soft chancre (Fig. 19–13), has been known since ancient times. Prior to identification of its etiologic agent, it was often confused with the chancre of syphilis. The coexistence of syphilis and chancroid has been so common that chancroid has often been described as the masker of syphilis. It is much more universally prevalent than syphilis. In the United States chancroid so far has remained a rare disease. A notable increase in incidence occurs in wartime in all overseas troops, especially those in the tropics (Gaisin and Heaton, 1975).

Chancroid is a predominantly local and regional disease of rather superficial nature; untoward late systemic morbidity has never been ascribed to it. The causative agent is the *Hemophilus ducreyi,* a gram-negative, short,

---

*Food and some dairy products interfere with absorption. Oral forms of tetracycline should be given 1 hour before or 2 hours after meals.

plump rod occurring predominantly in parallel chains (like a school of fish or railroad tracks). This disease is contracted by contact with abraded skin or mucous membrane, usually during coitus, and thereafter is fostered by poor genital hygiene and general unsanitary habits. Further lesions may develop in adjacent areas by autoinoculation.

In the male the initial sites of predilection are the parafrenular areas and the coronal sulcus. The incubation period is relatively short, reported by some as 1 to 2 days and usually no longer than a week. Sexual relations with prostitutes has accounted for a significant factor in the etiology of infection; in addition, prostitutes may be asymptomatic carriers (Gaisin and Heaton, 1975).

By means of inoculation studies utilizing the bubo fluid from inguinal chancroidal abscesses, Willcox (1950) had frequent opportunities to observe the step-by-step development of the local lesion. According to his studies, the lesion appears first as an erythematous area, which blends into a small papule within 24 hours and is followed by a distinctly inflamed button at 48 hours, a pustule at 96 hours, and rapid subsequent ulceration. The ulcer may be linear, serpiginous, or circumferential, and its borders are not indurated. The sore may penetrate deeply; its base may be granular or membranous and is frequently covered with a purulent exudate. The ulcer is painful and bleeds easily. If uncomplicated, it will heal within 2 or 3 weeks simply by cleansing, with soft cicatrization closing in from the periphery. The pathologic picture, which is not specific, is one of lymphocytic infiltration that may undermine the superficial borders of the ulcer for some distance.

The varying types of lesions that have been described result primarily from the secondary infection, which may develop in the unattended ulceration and is furthered by the presence of a redundant prepuce, which causes the retention of infected secretions. Thus, simple ulcerative and inflammatory soft chancres have been delineated. The mixed lesions are frequently the cause of clinical confusion, owing to the concurrence of syphilitic and chancroidal characteristics.

The secondary manifestations of chancroid may be classified as local, regional, and systemic. *Phimosis* due to inflammatory edema is frequent and propagates increased destruction by the infection. Severe paraphimosis may result if unwise manipulation of the prepuce succeeds in retracting it past the corona. *Phagedenic chancroid* used to occur more commonly in the past. At present, earlier treatment has prevented the deep-seated infections that could destroy the glans penis partially or completely and formerly resulted occasionally in gangrene with scarring and urethral stricture.

Inguinal lymphatic involvement develops in most cases and may vary from mild adenitis and periadenitis to bilateral abscesses; unilateral involvement, however, is more common. The matted periadenitis distinguishes the chancroidal lesion from the syphilitic, for there is matting of the nodes together with attachment to the skin that is rarely seen in syphilis. The enlarged nodes are tender and will persist either to resolution or fluctuation within 1 or 2 weeks. Prolonged chronic adenitis with lymphatic blockage must be ascribed more readily to concomitant lymphogranuloma venereum. A systemic phase usually is dependent upon the extent of inguinal infection and consists of fever, malaise, and occasionally anemia.

Diagnosis

Despite the suggestive clinical features of chancroid—the soft, painful, dirty, frequently malodorous ("smell the diagnosis"), multi-designed lesions (Fig. 19–13) with the typical matted adenopathy and buboes—reiteration of the fundamental tenet in the diagnosis of penile lesions is necessary: *The organism must be demonstrated when possible.* Academically, cultural characteristics of autoinoculation and absolute identification of the bacillus are desirable. But for all practical purposes in an antibiotic age, treatment in the physician's office and in health departments is most often completed before an absolute diagnosis is made. Differential distinction between chancroid, syphilis, lymphogranuloma venereum, and granuloma inguinale may be suspected by the shorter incubation period of chancroid, the multiplicity of lesions, the type of ulceration, the spreading by adjacent inoculation, and the character of the adenitis.

Herpes progenitalis and nonspecific ulcerations are usually of little import in the differential diagnosis. They may be ruled out by inspection and subsequent smear.

Erosive balanitis and gangrenous balanitis demand the protection of a long prepuce, and the adenopathy seen therein is usually not tender. Difficulty may be encountered in garnering Ducrey's bacillus from the ulcers; Levin (1941) estimated that only 20 to 60 per cent of cases may be diagnosed by smear. On the other hand, other workers have been able to isolate the organism with methyl green–pyronine, Giemsa, and Gram stains in almost 90 per cent of the cases. The use of human blood as a culture medium for the *Hemophilus ducreyi* organisms is necessary for definitive identification (Breen, 1967). Autoinoculation and heteroinoculation techniques (Willcox, 1950), though cumbersome, will usually permit demonstration of the organism.

Treatment

Prior to the advent of antibiotic agents, the treatment of chancroid involved attempts at prophylaxis, in which soap and water and calomel ointment rubs were utilized immediately after suspicious exposure. Subsequent to the appearance of the lesion, simple cleanliness allowed the tissues to combat the infection in a great many cases. Antibiotic creams such as Chloromycetin and erythromycin have been found to be not only prophylactic but therapeutic as well (Deacon, 1956).

A dorsal slit to relieve balanoposthitis or to perform circumcision is contraindicated during the active stage of the infection because of the risk of spread along the incision. Similarly, when necessary, aspiration is preferable to incision of large inguinal abscesses to prevent chronic discharging sinuses.

The introduction of the sulfonamides has tremendously reduced the frequency of complications incident to chancroidal infection. Sulfonamides, while they may have theoretical superiority because they do not mask the syphilitic infection, are in practice definitely inferior to tetracycline. Each of the antibiotics in small doses is capable of postponing the appearance of the syphilitic chancre for as long as several months, thus necessitating careful and prolonged follow-up study for not only clinical but also serological signs of syphilis. For this reason, adequate syphilitic treatment should be instituted in all cases of chancroid at the outset.

The Centers for Disease Control (1982) recommend initial treatment with erythromycin 500 mg orally four times a day for a minimum of 10 days, or with trimethoprim/sulfamethoxazole (160 mg/800 mg) orally twice a day for at least 10 days. The patient must be carefully observed for evidence of sufonamide toxicity, granulocytopenia, renal changes, and cutaneous sensitization. A large fluid intake and alkalinization are helpful in the reduction of renal toxicity.

Penicillin has been found to be of no value in the treatment of chancroid. Whatever effect it may have is upon secondary coccal invaders or the fusospirochetal organisms that can produce the destructive phagedenic stage of the disease. Under these circumstances penicillin may be used, but a broad-spectrum antibiotic is preferable. The majority of the antibiotics have been investigated both experimentally (Willcox, 1963) and clinically, and the tetracyclines, chloramphenicol, and the more recently introduced antibiotics all appear to be prophylactic against heteroinoculative bubo material. These drugs have achieved prompt remission of the disease in doses of 2 to 4 gm daily for 10 to 15 days. (Prophylaxis for syphilis requires the larger dose.) Probably the best cure rate is achieved with combined treatment (Kerber, 1969) utilizing sulfonamide drugs and tetracycline.

LYMPHOGRANULOMA VENEREUM

Lymphogranuloma venereum is a venereal disease that has received increasing attention as a result of studies concerning the high incidence of previous infection or latency (as evidenced by extensive utilization of the complement fixation and Frei skin tests), and as a result of the demonstration by electron microscopic studies (Schachter et al., 1970) of the specific causative organism, *Chlamydia trachomatis*. Specific identification in any individual case is accomplished by using the patient's blood serum for microimmunofluorescence (micro IF) tests (Wang and Grayston, 1974).

These organisms, formerly classified as a large virus in the psittacosis–lymphogranuloma venereum group, have been reclassified separately as *Chlamydia* (formerly, *Bedsonia*) because of their more rickettsial-like morphologic and biochemical characteristics. The more important of the characteristics, according to Moulder (1966), include the relatively large size, obligate intracellular method of reproduction, structure, metabolism, and DNA and RNA content.

The genus *Chlamydia* includes two species. *Chlamydia trachomatis* includes strains that cause such specific diseases as lymphogranuloma venereum, trachoma, inclusion conjunctivitis, and a very common form of nongonococcal urethritis. The other species, *Chlamydia psittaci*, causes psittacosis and ornithosis.

Although lymphogranuloma venereum begins on the genitals, it soon becomes systemic. Clinical manifestations, however, occur essentially in three forms: (1) glandular form; (2) an anorectal form (Fig. 19–14); and (3) occasionally, a persistent genital form. Each may be associated with a wide variety of systemic symptoms (Abrams, 1968). As is true of the majority of such diseases, lymphogranuloma is encountered more often in people in the lower economic and cultural strata, in tropical and semitropical climates, and in large metropolitan areas (Becker, 1976).

Lymphogranuloma is acquired primarily during coitus. Descriptions of the incubation period have ranged from 2 days to 3 weeks, the discrepancy undoubtedly being due to the frequent evanescence of the primary lesion and the inaccuracy of the history of exposure.

Initially, an erosion, papule, or vesicle appears commonly on or near the coronal sulcus, but it may appear anywhere upon the penis. It tends to heal quickly subsequent to its painless, nonindurated, and frequently unnoticed existence. Occasionally, a mildly febrile systemic reaction is present. Within 1 to 4 weeks or perhaps longer the inguinal nodes begin to show involvement. Unilateral adenitis is more common; periadenitis with matting or fusing of the nodes and fixation to the skin is followed by subsequent suppuration. Unless treated or unless spontaneous subsidence occurs, sinus tracts are formed as outlets for the purulent exudate. Extension to the deep pelvic nodes, especially in women, and to the perirectal lymphatics has been frequently reported, and proctitis with subsequent rectal strictures has been ascribed to this mode of spread. The dominance of rectal involvement (Fig. 19–14) is perhaps more satisfactorily explained by the attraction of the rectal columnar epithelium for the lymphogranuloma organism, a factor that is reminiscent of the preference of the psittacosis organism for the respiratory columnar epithelium. On this basis, involvement of the rectum may be more correctly assumed to occur by surface spread from the genitals (Goldgreber, 1957).

The third clinical type of lymphogranuloma is that which smolders in the penile tissues and is accompanied by subacute chronic involvement in the groin. This results eventually in severe stenosis of the lymphatic channels of the penis and scrotum with subsequent development of elephantiasis.

After resolution of the acute lymphatic stage of the disease, the condition becomes chronic, and evidence of activity may be difficult to detect; however, secondary invaders, coupled with the organism in a more latent form, continue to proliferate in the rectal strictures, and other granulomatous reactions derive from this chronic mixed type of infection.

Diagnosis

The diagnosis and differential diagnosis of lymphogranuloma venereum may be difficult. After the identification of various closely related chlamydia types, which caused in particular a common type of nongonococcal urethritis (NGU), we made an inquiry of the Centers for Disease Control of the Public Health Service. We specifically asked to know the effect of chlamydia associated with NGU on the Frei test. The reply (from Stephen J. Kraus, Clinical Research Investigator, VD Control Division) stated, "The Frei test is no longer available in the United States and it was phased out before *C. trichomatis* was found to be an etiology of NGU. For these reasons, the influence of *C. trichomatis* on the Frei test is unknown." The complement fixation reaction also might not be as specific for lymphogranuloma as previously believed.

The present microimmunofluorescent serologic approach (Wang and Grayston, 1974), now a research tool, seems to offer the best specificity in the differential diagnosis of lymphogranuloma venereum and even other closely related venereal diseases caused by the *Chlamydia* species, especially NGU. Tissue culture and egg yolk tests are also research tools used in making this diagnosis. Biopsy to rule out carcinoma of the rectum is required (Rainey, 1954).

The type of primary lesion, the presence of discrete nonsuppurative adenitis, and the finding of the *T. pallidum* organism in the dark-field examination confirms the diagnosis of a lesion as syphilitic. The dirty, autoinoculable lesions of chancroid with their short incubation period and the concomitance of buboes, both replete with Ducrey's bacilli on smear, will distinguish the soft chancre. Absence of Donovan bodies in the granulation tissue of lymphogranuloma on biopsy will rule out granuloma inguinale.

Treatment

Treatment with tetracycline, 500 mg four times a day taken 1 hour before meals without milk, continued for 2 to 3 weeks should produce a clinical response. If this response is not obvious, alternative drugs—erythromycin 500 mg four times a day orally, doxycycline 100 mg twice a day orally, or sulfamethoxazole or other sulfonamides in equivalent dose, 1 gm twice a day orally—should be used at least 2 weeks, or concomitant use of drugs should be considered. Steroids have been used in the scarring types of lymphogranuloma such as rectal stricture or stenosis. Adequate aggressive therapy in the bubo stage will probably lessen any later sequelae.

Therapeutic response can be measured by following the lymphogranuloma complement fixation test titer, and changes here will indicate the need for repeating the treatment.

The bubo should not be incised, but they can be drained with a large needle, which is inserted into the fluctuant abscess through uninvolved skin adjacent to it. This tends to prevent slow-healing sinus tracts.

Adequate medical management should precede any consideration of surgical intervention to correct chronic lymphedema or fibrous changes involving the penis, scrotum, and thighs. The Kondoleon and Torek principles have been applied (Weinstein and Roberts, 1950) with some success in combination with plastic reconstructive operations.

GRANULOMA INGUINALE

Granuloma inguinale is included here more because of its predilection for the genitals than because of actual knowledge about its mode of transmission. Considered for many years to be a tropical disease, it appears to be a disappearing disease and is now rarely seen. Although Donovan first identified the encapsulated bacillus that bears his name, *Calymmatobacterium (Donovania) granulomatis*, and postulated its etiologic capacity in the granulation reactions typical of the disease, it remained for Greenblatt et al. (1939) and Anderson et al. (1945) to demonstrate, through embryonic yolk sac cultivation experiments, the undoubted relationship of the organisms to the entity. Packer and Goldberg (1950), in commenting upon the enigma of the transmissibility of the disease, noted that even though injection of bacteria-free suspensions of Donovan bodies into a donor permits their growth and multiplication, the role of the Donovan body in the production of the lesion may not necessarily be primary. From the fact that the mate of a person with clinically proven granuloma inguinale may remain free of the disease despite prolonged cohabitation, it must be assumed that the contagious aspects of the problem are little understood. Goldberg (1966) affords us the interesting postulation that not only is the relationship of the Donovan body to the Enterobacteriaceae group suggested by serologic similarities but that experimental assessments of growth requirements for the organism may strengthen the prediction that both active and dormant strains depend for their perpetuation upon an enteric pool. The inconsistencies of the contagious aspects of the disease could possibly be related to these findings. It is the incipiency of the primary lesions in the genital tract, along with the fact that direct inoculation of a donor produces the disease at the site of inoculation (Dienst et al., 1950), that accounts for the inclusion of granuloma inguinale in the group of coitally acquired diseases.

The Donovan body is a gram-negative, encapsulated, nonmotile, usually intracellular bacillus that appears to be intimately related to the Friedlander *Klebsiella pneumoniae* branch of the Escherichieae group, based on the demonstration of a common hapten in the capsule of each. It is almost entirely confined to the black population, to the extent that inferences as to inherent susceptibility have been made.

After an indeterminate incubation period the initial lesion appears as a nodule on the penis or groin or in the perineal area; it soon ruptures to unfold bright red, velvety granulation tissue of insignificant depth (Fig. 19–15). Daughter lesions may develop and coalesce; the primary one may simply spread circumferentially or progress in any direction. Involvement of the inguinal nodes is not common early in this disease. Secondary infection, frequently fusospirochetal, almost invariably supervenes to transform the lesion into a fetid accumulation of exuberant granulations, in the crevices of which purulent matter lurks consistently. Exquisite pruritus is fairly constant in the early stages. The lesions gradually roll onward, almost like waves, to involve at times amazing amounts of the body surface. Superficial and profound cicatricial healing occurs as the disease progresses. Erosive changes may occur on the penis that can produce extensive destruction, and, with scar tissue proliferation, bizarre deformities.

Anyone who has ever seen the disease in its chronic extensive form can realize the magnitude of the disturbance that may occur. There are even now a few cases of these exceptionally destructive lesions (Fitz et al., 1975) or of granuloma *en cuirasse*, wherein the body from the knees to the chest is a solid wall of chronically infected cicatrization, which causes almost complete invalidism.

Before the antibiotic era, the untreated disease progressed chronically until either the secondary infection was no longer controllable or death from other causes supervened. Symptomatology was related to the effects of the concomitant infection rather than to the granulations themselves, except when urethral encroachment produced signs of obstruction. In cases of extensive genitoinguinal scarring, lymphatic stasis may be so severe that it produces genital elephantiasis.

Diagnosis

The diagnosis of granuloma inguinale can be suspected from the expanding velvety granulations and later from the typical chronic scarring manifestations. Material from clean subsurface areas obtained by scraping or by biopsy using touch-smear techniques is subjected to Wright's stain. The Donovan bodies may be seen in encapsulated bacillary or occasionally coccoid forms; they take a deep blue stain with a surrounding pink capsule and are ensconced in large mononuclear cells. Careful scrutiny will always reveal the organisms if present.

In the differential diagnosis, tuberculosis can be ruled out by the more rapid and deeply destructive elements that are encountered with the acid-fast organisms; demonstration of typical histologic caseation and the tubercle bacilli either by smear or animal inoculation may be resorted to if doubt exists. Primary and secondary syphilis are seldom other than concomitant offenders, and here the dark-field examination can demonstrate that the moist, fragile, elevated, easily distinguishable condylomata teem with spirochetes; primary chancres do not show the tendency toward peripheral progression or the sloping everted edges that are characteristic of granuloma inguinale. The dark-field and serologic tests will prove diagnostic. Gumma may necessitate histologic study prior to differentiation. Carcinoma can easily mimic granuloma inguinale in its chronicity and its exuberance, but the depth of ulceration, persistent localization of the primary lesion, and biopsy will reveal a true neoplasm. Recent delineation of reactivity of sera from patients with carcinoma of the penis when tested with *Donovania* antigen reinforces a relationship that has often been suspected (Goldberg, 1966). Biopsy is mandated in any chronic genital lesion so that carcinoma may be ruled out. The typical dirty, rapidly developing and spreading ulcers of chancroid will not be confused readily with granuloma inguinale if they are secondarily infected; in such cases aspiration and identification of the proper organisms will confirm the diagnosis. Lymphogranuloma venereum will be confused with granuloma inguinale only in its initial and late elephantiasic stages. The usual evanescence of the lymphgranulomatous primary lesion will indicate its proper category. Biopsy and differentiation of causative organisms can corroborate the impressions garnered clinically.

It is when the investigation for the Donovan body is relatively infrequent that the diagnosis has been missed. Clinics in which there is a routine battery of tests for all the common genital lesions will seldom fail to make the proper diagnosis.

Treatment

Because of the unsatisfactory results of older treatment of this condition with Fuadin, tartar emetic, Podophyllin, and surgery, antibiotics were a real bonanza in the treatment of this chronic disease.

When streptomycin and later tetracycline were introduced, the curative powers of these drugs in a disease of such chronicity were hardly believable, but as report followed report in substantiation of complete cure, it was believed that total eradication of the disease, regardless of stage, could be achieved. The initial success obtained with streptomycin, wherein only 10 per cent of the patients relapsed after one course of treatment (Novy, 1950), has been augmented during the past two decades by reports on the efficacy of the majority of the antibiotics, with the notable exception of penicillin. As in so many instances, organism resistance to streptomycin has occurred, and in view of the wide choice of effective medications available at the present time, it is now seldom employed.

The conclusion of Dienst et al (1950), Pariser et al. (1950), Kornblith (1950), and others that response to medication bears no relationship to the duration of the disease, sex, or previous therapy has been firmly established. An apparently important factor in determining the length of therapy is the extent of the lesion. The treatment of choice today is tetracycline or erythromycin, 4 gm daily for 2 weeks. Robinson's (1951) experience that relapses usually occur within the first 6 months after therapy has been amply documented. His criteria for immediate retreatment—i.e., perpetuation of revocable Donovan bodies within a few days of completion of treatment or upon recrudescence in healed lesions—continue to be valid. It is gratifying to note the efficacy of so many therapeutic entities, since fairly extensive followups have demonstrated that few, if any, patients fail to respond to treatment with the same or different agents. Surgical measures are still applicable in some patients who require plastic reconstruction; such surgery can be approached in conjunction with utilization of antibiotics with every probability of success. The masking effect of antibiotics upon the lesions of syphilis should be reiterated, and careful serologic follow-up study is advised. Toxic reactions to antibiotics have been well publicized and represent an acknowledged hazard. Peripheral blood studies must be secured periodically to avoid granulocytic depression during prolonged or recurrent treatment schedules.

References

Abrams, A. J.: Lymphogranuloma venereum. J.A.M.A., *205*:199, 1968.

Anderson, K., Demonbreum, W. A., and Goodpasture, E. W.: An etiologic consideration of *Donovania granulomatis* cultivated from granuloma inguinale in embryonic yolk. J. Exp. Med., *81*:25, 1945.

Barrow, J.: Granuloma inguinale in a Jamaican and his wife. Br. J. Vener. Dis., *34*:34, 1958.

Becker, L. E.: Review: Lymphogranuloma venereum. Int. J. Dermatol., *15*:26, 1976.

Breen, J. L.: The venereal diseases. J. Am. Health Assoc., *15*:26, 1967.

Butts, D. C. A.: Granuloma inguinale. A preliminary report on certain microscopic observations. Am. J. Syph., *21*:544, 1937.

Butts, D. C. A., and Olansky, S.: Observations on the cause and transmission of granuloma inguinale. Arch. Derm. Syph., *54*:524, 1946.

Centers for Disease Control Morbidity and Mortality Weekly Report: Sexually transmitted diseases treatment guidelines 1982. MMWR, *31*:25, 1982.

Coutts, W. E.: Genitourinary lesions in lymphogranuloma venereum. J. Urol., *49*:595, 1943.

Deacon, W. E., Olansky, S., Albritton, D. C., et al.: Experimental chancroid prophylaxis and treatment. Antibiot. Med., *2*:143, 1956.

Dienst, R. B., Chen, C. H., and Greenblatt, R. B.: Granuloma inguinale. Urol. Cutan. Rev., *53*:537, 1949.

Dienst, R. B., Chen, C. H., and Greenblatt, R. B.: Experimental transfer of chemoresistant granuloma inguinale. Am. J. Syph., *34*:289, 1950.

Fitz, G. S., Hubler, W. R., Jr., Dodson, R. F., and Randolph, A.: Mutilating granuloma inguinale. Arch. Dermatol., *111*:1464, 1975.

Gaisin, A., and Heaton, C. L.: Chancroid: Alias the soft chancre. Int. J. Dermatol., *14*:188-197, 1975.

Goldberg, J.: Studies on granuloma inguinale. Br. J. Vener. Dis., *42*:205, 1966.

Goldgreber, M. B.: Specific disease simulating non-specific ulcerative colitis. Ann. Intern. Med., *47*:939, 1957.

Greenblatt, R. B.: Granuloma inguinale, lymphogranuloma venereum. *In* Current Therapy, 1960. pp. 398-399. Philadelphia, W. B. Saunders Co., 1960.

Greenblatt, R. B., Dienst, R. B., Pund, E. R., and Torpin, R.: Experimental and clinical granuloma inguinale. J.A.M.A., *113*:1109, 1939.

Jannach, J. R.: Granuloma inguinale of the epididymis. Br. J. Vener. Dis., *34*:31, 1958.

Kerber, R. E.: Treatment of chancroid. Arch. Dermatol., *100*:604, 1969.

Kornblith, B. A.: Lymphogranuloma venereum and granuloma inguinale. J. Insur. Med., *5*:30, 1949-50.

Levin, E. A.: The diagnosis of chancroid. Urol. Cutan. Rev., *45*:587, 1941.

Marmell, M.: Granuloma inguinale: Treatment with methacycline. N.Y. J. Med., *64*:804, 1964.

Moulder, J. W.: The relation of the psittacosis group (chlamydiae) to bacteria and viruses. Ann. Rev. Microbiol., *20*:107, 1966.

Novy, F. G., Jr.: The newer antibiotics in dermatology. Calif. Med., *72*:201, 1950.

Packer, H., and Goldberg, J.: Complement fixation studies in granuloma inguinale. Am. J. Trop. Med., *30*:387, 1950.

Pariser, H., Goldberg, S. Z., and Mitchell, G. H.: Streptomycin in the treatment of granuloma inguinale. Arch. Dermatol. Syph., *62*:261, 1950.

Rainey, R.: The association of lymphopathia inguinale and cancer. Surgery, *35*:221, 1954.

Robinson, H. M., Jr.: The treatment of granuloma inguinale, lymphogranuloma venereum, chancroid and gonorrhea. Arch. Dermatol. Syph., *64*:284, 1951.

Schachter, J., Dawson, C. R., Balas, S., and Jones, P.: Evaluation of methods for detecting acute TRIC agent infections. Am. J. Ophthalmol., *70*:381, 1970.

United States Department of Health, Education and Welfare. Centers for Disease Control: Bulletin, No. 980376. Atlanta, Center for Disease Control, 1976.

Wang, S., and Grayston, J. T.: Human serology in *Chlamydia trachomatis* infection with microimmunofluorescence. J. Infect. Dis., *130*:388, 1974.

Willcox, R. R.: Effectiveness of antichancroidal drugs tested by autoinoculation of bubo fluid. Am. J. Syph., *34*:378, 1950.

Willcox, R. R.: The treatment of chancroid. Br. J. Clin. Pract., *17*:455, 1963.

CHAPTER 20

Cutaneous Diseases of External Genitalia

WALTER R. NICKEL, M.D.
ROBERT T. PLUMB, M.D.

Cutaneous lesions of the genitalia are uncommon, often intriguing, and challenging to diagnose. Even though they are visible they may be overlooked. Training programs in urology are not apt to stress recognition of them, and clinical practitioners are usually concerned with the medical and surgical management of more serious and life-threatening illnesses.

In the life span of a physician's practice some of these lesions of the external genitalia might never, or only rarely, be encountered. The more common of these cutaneous diseases are presented here, some in pictorial form. Mere identification of some of these diseases, when no treatment is indicated or when there is no satisfactory treatment even in the most expert hands, is often enough to reassure the patient.

Biopsy of these accessible lesions is often helpful or necessary. Microscopic interpretation should be entrusted only to a physician specializing in dermatopathology.

VIRAL DISEASES (See also Chapter 19)

This expanding group, except for herpes zoster, is discussed in Chapter 19, Sexually Transmitted Disease. Herpes zoster, for any practical purpose, has never been considered a transmissible disease.

These segmentally distributed grouped vesicles of the male penis (Fig. 20–1) are only part of the usually systemic symptoms associated with herpes zoster. There is usually a day or two of antecedent severe pain before skin le-

sions appear; sometimes some other surgically oriented disease is diagnosed from the history.

As with herpes simplex, there has been no specific treatment. There have been proponents of treatment with antibiotics, gamma globulin, or parenteral steroids, but it is especially important to control pain in the early stage of this disease. The possibility that herpes zoster may be the premonitory sign of underlying disease in an apparently well person must never be overlooked.

There may be real promise of a more specific therapy from reports (Serota et al., 1982; Peterslund et al., 1981) of cases in which acyclovir was given intravenously. The reports include immunosuppressed and nonimmunosuppressed patients. The beneficial results of treatment were very encouraging.

INFLAMMATIONS AND INFECTIONS

Erythemas

Erythema Multiforme. This disease can present on the penis or scrotum as bullae that resolve to form multicolored (red to brown), annular, iris-like lesions. Confirmatory similar lesions are found elsewhere on the skin of the elbows, knees, palms, and oral or anal regions. A severe debilitating form (Stevens-Johnson syndrome) with extensive erosive involvement of every body orifice (Fig. 20–2) is accompanied by systemic symptoms of fever and general prostration. The cause, especially in recurrent cases, is often unknown. Known precipitating factors are viral infections (herpes simplex), vaccinations, drugs of any type, other acute or chronic infections, and rheumatoid states.

Treatment of this self-limited condition should be directed toward removing the cause, when known. In the majority of cases, however, local treatment with steroid creams and short-term use of oral or parenteral steroids is the treatment of choice. In the rarer severe debilitating type (Stevens-Johnson syndrome), hospitalization may be necessary.

Dermatitis Herpetiformis. The cause of dermatitis herpetiformis is unknown, and urologically the presence of large bullae of the genitalia is considered for interest only. It is dramatic to see these large blistering lesions arising on a noninflammatory base (Fig. 20–3). Such patients, when encountered, are referred to a dermatologist.

About the only condition that could present with these large bullae is pemphigus vulgaris. A distinctly different, more recently described bullous disease that has been confused with pemphigus and dermatitis herpetiformis is bullous pemphigoid. This is seen in a predominantly older population and is a much more benign condition. Both pemphigus and bullous pemphigoid usually respond to systemic steroids.

Bullous diseases can be so confusing clinically that often the accurate diagnosis rests with immunofluorescent studies of an active lesion.

Urticaria (Angioneurotic Edema, Hives)

Urticaria is characterized by a marked, sudden appearance of erythema and coincident edema of the skin, often the foreskin or shaft of the penis, associated with extreme pruritus. There is usually similar urticarial involvement elsewhere. There is a multiplicity of possible causes, including food, vaccines, and drugs, and of these, penicillin is a common offender.

Treatment consists of avoiding the specific agent, if known, but again, usually prompt relief can be obtained from oral antihistamine drugs combined with short-term use of oral or parenteral steroids. Local applications are of little value in this disease, which sometimes has extensive skin involvement.

Dermatitis Medicamentosa (Fixed Drug Eruption)

In rare instances a person given the same drug a second or third time will develop a localized, fixed tissue allergy (Fig. 20–4). With each subsequent administration of the drug a definite, angry-appearing, red to purple area of the skin will develop at the same site within 24 to 36 hours. With cessation of the drug the whole process will disappear in 2 to 6 days. This fixed drug eruption is common on the glans penis, and the most commonly incriminated drugs are those of the sulfa, phenolphthalein, tetracycline, and barbital groups. Once seen the eruption is easily recognized. Generalized drug eruptions can involve the genitalia coincidentally as macular erythema or hemorrhagic manifestations. In adults the serious and dramatic disease toxic epidermal necrolysis is one of the most striking examples of drug-related diseases.

Papulosquamous Lesions

Seborrheic Dermatitis and Intertrigo. General use of the term "intertrigo" seems to be declining. This is probably because placing it under the designation seborrheic dermatitis (Fig. 20–5), which also sometimes involves predictable areas of the body such as the scalp, chest, back, axillae, umbilicus, and groin, represents a more accurate diagnostic concept. The cause in either case is unknown, and there is no general agreement on the possible relationship to bacterial infection.

The disease begins as erythematous scaling papules that become larger scaling plaques involving the glans penis, shaft, scrotum, and groin as well as areas such as those listed above. They may assume an annular configuration similar to that found in psoriasis, pityriasis rosea, Reiter's disease, or even lichen planus, from which they must be differentiated.

Treatment of an isolated plaque of seborrheic dermatitis of the glans penis can be a real challenge, especially in a fastidious male. The local use of any of the steroid creams is the first choice of therapy; however, in refractory cases, an addition of 2 per cent Ichthyol, 5 per cent sodium sulfacetamide, or 3 per cent Vioform may be helpful. Because of the difficult differential diagnosis involved, the refractory type has been referred to as seborriasis.

Psoriasis. Psoriasis begins as a small erythematous papule. These papules enlarge or coalesce to form typical red, elevated, scaling, psoriatic plaques. Probably owing to the moistness of the genital region, the plaques of psoriasis (Fig. 20–6) are usually much redder in the groin and on the shaft and glans penis than elsewhere on the body. In these moist areas the characteristic silver scale is apt to be absent. The presence of typical psoriatic plaques on the scalp, knees, elbows, and sacral region, often with nail involvement, confirms the diagnosis.

Psoriasis in the genital region is notoriously

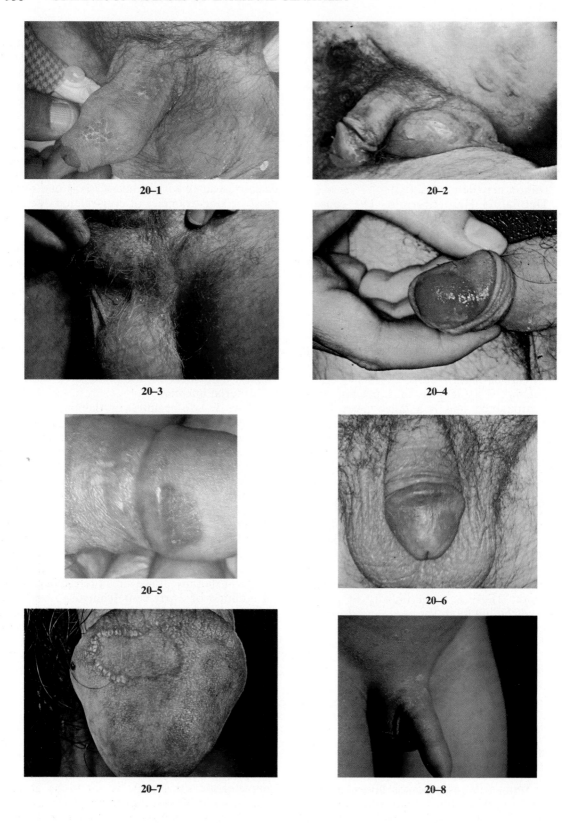

20–1

20–2

20–3

20–4

20–5

20–6

20–7

20–8

refractory to treatment. Systemic steroids in this very chronic and recurrent condition are rarely indicated. No really effective and safe systemic treatment has been evolved. Local steroids, alone or in combination with water-soluble tar (Balnetar, liquor carbonis detergens) in a 5 to 10 per cent concentration, are still valuable. Sun exposure (ultraviolet light) to the point of tanning the exposed parts, with or without local treatment, is often effective even on covered areas of the body. The spa treatment of bathing and sunshine offers the best overall results in this disease, the cause of which is still unknown.

Lichen Planus. Lichen planus (Fig. 20–7) has no known cause. Most suddenly developing and extensive cases are associated with tension, worry, anxiety, and personal intimate psychosomatic stresses. Typical lesions on the glans penis, shaft, or scrotum begin as tiny, flat-topped papules. As they develop they often form an annular configuration. When fully developed they have a lacelike, retiform, silvery appearance that might be mistaken for leukoplakia of the glans. Similar lesions found elsewhere on the body, especially on the wrists and buccal mucosa, are confirmatory. This disease is self-limiting but is predictably recurrent.

Treatment with antimalarial drugs has been of value, but the systemic use of steroids orally or parenterally usually clears the disorder in 2 to 8 weeks. Local steroid creams are effective, especially when used with an occlusive plastic cover at night.

Pityriasis Rosea. Pityriasis rosea (Fig. 20–8) is another disease with an unknown cause; it occurs more often in the 10- to 40-year-old age group. Rarely are two cases seen in the same family at the same time. The lesions are characteristically ovoid, slightly reddened, and elevated and have peripheral scaling. The lesions may occur on the shaft of the penis coincidentally along with typical lesions on other parts of the body that may show a segmental distribution. The occurrence in the groin of the oval, scaling, heraldic plaque (mother spot) is most often diagnosed as ringworm. In diagnosis, the use of 10 per cent potassium hydroxide digestion in examination of the scales, as described later under Candidiasis, is helpful, especially if potassium hydroxide examination is negative. The diagnosis is confirmed by finding other typical lesions on the body.

Treatment of pityriasis should be undertaken with the knowledge that this is a self-limited disease that clears in 4 to 8 weeks without complication. Antihistamines are helpful for the usual mild itching. Local treatment with sunshine or ultraviolet light and the twice-daily use of a mild keralytic lotion will materially shorten the course of the disease. The simplest such lotion contains 5 per cent salicylic acid, 5 per cent liquor carbonis detergens, and 10 per cent glycerine in a 70 per cent alcoholic solution.

Contact Eczema or Contact Dermatitis (Dermatitis Venenata). Contact dermatitis of the genitalia usually involves both the penis and the scrotum. Local agents (Fig. 20–9) such as blue ointment, ammoniated mercury, local anesthetics, local antiseptics, plants (particularly poison oak or poison ivy), and materials used in new unwashed underwear are some of the more common contacts. In the sensitive person there is an acute onset, sometimes with massive edema (Fig. 20–10), sufficient to cause angulation of the penis (especially in plant dermatitis). This acute appearance, followed in a few days by dull red, scaling, swollen skin and continuing itching, is a common occurrence, especially if the cause is not removed. There may be a lack of other evidence of contact dermatitis in acute cases, especially in hunters. These people carefully wash vigorously after a day in the forest to

---

Figure 20–1. Herpes zoster of the shaft and foreskin.

Figure 20–2. Severe type of erythema multiforme, Stevens-Johnson type. Every body orifice is involved.

Figure 20–3. Bullous lesions of penis and scrotum in dermatitis herpetiformis.

Figure 20–4. Dermatitis medicamentosa (fixed drug eruption).

Figure 20–5. Seborrheic dermatitis of the glans.

Figure 20–6. Psoriasis of the male genitalia.

Figure 20–7. Lichen planus of the glans with typical annular configuration. (Courtesy of the United States Naval Hospital, San Diego, California.)

Figure 20–8. Pityriasis rosea involving the male genitalia.

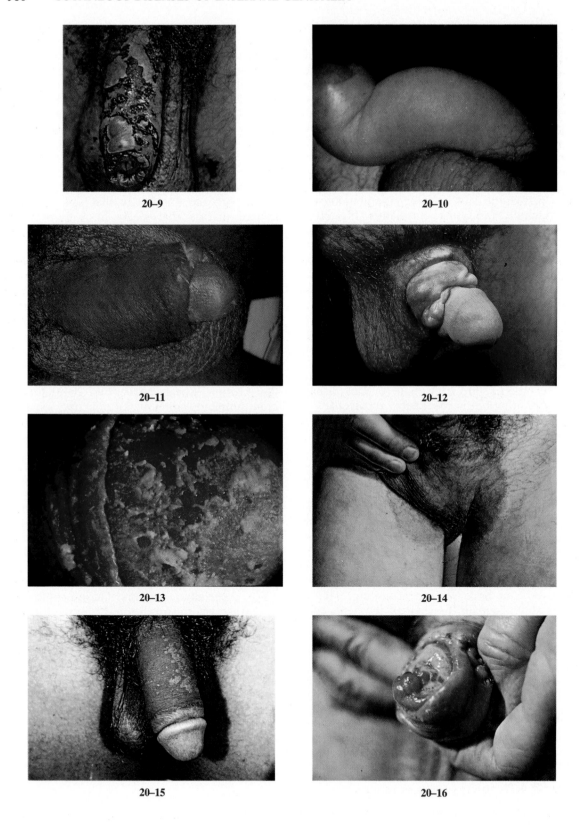

20–9

20–10

20–11

20–12

20–13

20–14

20–15

20–16

prevent dermatitis from plants but forget to wash the genitalia, which had been contaminated at the time of urination earlier in the day.

Treatment of this condition is elimination of the contactant when possible, and use of local steroid creams or lotions as well as oral antihistamines. In more severe cases a short course of oral or parenteral steroids is beneficial.

Psychosomatic Dermatoses

Localized Neurodermatitis (Lichen Simplex Chronicus). Localized neurodermatitis, lichen simplex chronicus (Fig. 20–11), is discussed here because the appearance of chronic contact dermatitis and chronic localized neurodermatitis of the genitalia is similar. Both of these conditions result finally in a chronic, dull red, scaling, edematous dermatitis that involves both penis and scrotum most commonly, but often only the scrotum. If the patient has good insight he will realize that fear, tension, anxiety, sexual frustrations, or even some erotic satisfaction from scratching is the cause of a continuing problem. Neurodermatitis may be present for years in spite of every therapeutic approach.

Treatment requires a frank discussion with the patient of the probable underlying stress factors so that he can realize what he contributes to the problem. In general, the treatment is otherwise the same as that for chronic contact dermatitis. In this condition tranquilizing drugs are of value.

Factitial Conditions. Every large clinic or medical school has at least one or two famous cases of self-inflicted, genitally oriented skin or skin-related conditions. The most common of these are instances of the application of constricting bands around the penis as a means of self-mutilation. Others involve local trauma caused by the insertion of a foreign material, usually paraffin or some oily material (Fig. 20–12), into the shaft of the penis, producing a foreign-body granulomatous reaction. This results in a large stony-hard, unchanging configuration of the penis. Surgery is required for this condition when recognized, and microscopic examination will reveal the "Swiss cheese" appearance of the tissue caused by puddling of different-sized fat globules in these granulomatous masses.

Fungus and Fungus-Mimicking Diseases

These diseases, which have heterogeneous causes, are grouped together because they are commonly confused, owing to their often clinically similar manifestations.

Erythrasma. Erythrasma, a fairly uncommon disease, is initially almost always mistaken clinically for a fungus infection. It is a bacterial infection, however, caused by *Corynebacterium minutissimum*. It occurs in the axillae and especially in the groin as a marginated, pinkish brown, slightly scaling dermatitis. Potassium hydroxide examination is negative for fungi because this is a gram-positive organism susceptible to many oral and local antibiotics. Examination with a Wood's light in a totally dark room will reveal the typical coral-red fluorescence in the involved area of skin.

Treatment with oral erythromycin (1 gm daily for 10 days) and the local use of erythromycin cream will result in complete clearing.

Candidiasis (Moniliasis). Candidiasis is caused by a yeast of the genus *Candida (Monilia),* of which the most common species is *Candida albicans.* This infection is more common in the uncircumcised male. It presents as an angry red pruritic balanitis covered with whitish, curdlike flecks (Fig. 20–13) of material composed of solid masses of strands of the yeast organisms. Placing these curdlike masses on a

---

Figure 20–9. Acute contact dermatitis from potassium permanganate wet compresses.

Figure 20–10. Acute contact dermatitis of the penis and foreskin with intense edema, producing "angulation."

Figure 20–11. Lichen simplex chronicus of the penis and scrotum.

Figure 20–12. Factitial lesion of lipogranuloma.

Figure 20–13. Candidiasis (moniliasis) of the glans. Note the curdlike appearance.

Figure 20–14. Tinea cruris with marginated sharp borders.

Figure 20–15. Tinea versicolor of the penile shaft.

Figure 20–16. Granuloma of the glans, showing foreign body response microscopically. Condition cleared with biopsy and exteriorization.

glass slide, adding a drop of 10 per cent potassium hydroxide, coverslipping, and then digesting with heat (do not boil) will provide a thin film in which yeast or fungal elements can be seen by direct examination. In potassium hydroxide examination the light source on the microscope must be reduced by closing the substage condenser almost completely in order to visualize these translucent organisms.

Candidal involvement in the groin in both males and females, particularly after ingestion of oral antibiotics (especially in pregnant women, diabetics, or women on the "pill"), is suggested by scattered satellite lesions beyond the main area of dermatitis. These present as fine vesiculopustules, some of which have already ruptured, and are also positive for *Candida* with potassium hydroxide examination. In diagnosis the use of cultures in areas where candida are normally found is not too valuable. If the problem is recurrent, the sexual partner should be examined to confirm a "Ping-Pong" type of reinfection, especially in the uncircumcised male.

TREATMENT. Nystatin (Mycostatin) 3 per cent concentration carried as a cream, ointment, or lotion used either alone or mixed with steroids or antibacterial preparations (Mycolog) has been standard and usually effective treatment. Recently, other preparations considered more effective against fungi and candida (monilia) have been developed: clotrimazole (Lotrimin, Mycelex), miconazole (Monistat, Miconizol), econazole (Spectazole).

Griseofulvin is of no value against candida. Ketoconazole (Nizoral) orally is highly effective against candida. If ketoconazole is used more than 3 weeks the blood, and particularly the liver, must be carefully monitored.

Tinea Cruris. This fungus infection (Fig. 20–14) is very common in males, usually in the groin, but is less common on the scrotum and penis. For unknown reasons this infection is more rare in females. The usual offending fungus in tinea of the groin is the *Epidermophyton* or *Trichophyton* group. These superficial mycoses characteristically present as clinically marginated, scaling, pruritic dermatitis. Scrapings of scale from the margin, when digested with 10 per cent potassium hydroxide (for method, see under Candidiasis), reveal hyphal elements that are usually broader and straighter and have a sharper angulation (branching) than candida and do not show the yeast bodies of candida. The problem of treating this disease has almost been solved by the use of oral griseofulvin and local antifungal remedies.

Local treatment using one-quarter strength Whitfield's ointment is still effective, but undecylenic acid preparations, tolnaftate, and the imidazol derivatives, Lotrimin, Micatin, and Halotex seem to be effective also. With more efective oral and local treatment, the use of cultures for routine identification has decreased.

TREATMENT. Locally, almost any of the old treatments are effective in varying degrees—Desenex ointment, Whitfield's ointment, and others. To these the newer clotrimazole (Lotrimin and Mycelex), haloprogen (Halotex), miconazole (Monistat), econazole (Spectazole), and tolnaftate (Tinactin) should be added. Systemic use of griseofulvin or ketoconazole (Nizoral) is often combined with the above for 3- to 4-week periods. Prolonged use of either of these two drugs requires laboratory monitoring to include liver function studies.

Tinea Versicolor. This very superficial fungus infection (Fig. 20–15) is caused by *Pityrosporon orbiculare (Malassezia furfur)*. Initially, the skin lesions have a droplet or guttate appearance, which is followed by coalescence to form lesions of variable size, most often on the chest, back, and arms. Extensions to the abdomen, thighs, genitalia, scrotum, and shaft of the penis are observed. Scrapings examined with 10 per cent potassium hydroxide reveal the stubbled cigar-like organisms and numerous clumps of spores ("spaghetti and meatballs").

TREATMENT. At present, with any treatment, this disease tends to be recurrent. Locally, selenium sulfide (Selsun) or sodium thiosulfate (Tinver), clotrimazole (Lotrimin and Mycelex), miconazole (Monistat), and econazole (Spectazole) are prescribed most often.

Ketoconazole systemically seems to be very effective and offers promise. Whether the disease will recur with its use is still debated. If this drug is used for more than 2 or 3 weeks the patient's blood must be monitored to include liver function studies. Griseofulvin is of no value.

Granulomas

Nonspecific Granulomas. Nonspecific superficial granulomas (Fig. 20–16) have been observed on the glans penis. Clinically they present as small, inflammatory, firm nodules with an eroded surface. Biopsy, which is usually curative, reveals a superficial granulomatous reaction. It is not known whether the lesions are generated from glandular or cystic causes or from *Mycobacterium balnei*. Those on the scrotum are most often keratin granulomas arising from manipulation of a small cyst.

Tuberculosis. See Chapter 23.

Lichen Nitidus. The cause of lichen nitidus (Fig. 20–17), an uncommon and bizarre skin condition, is unknown. Characteristically it appears as tiny pinhead-sized, flat papules studded on the shaft of the penis; there may be a few or many. Microscopically there is a nest of epithelioid cells in the space between two expanded rete pegs just beneath the epidermis. The lesions are asymptomatic and of no consequence; one need only reassure the patient of their banal transient nature.

Hidradenitis Suppurativa. The cause of hidradenitis suppurativa (Fig. 20–18) is unknown. It is generally believed that this scarring chronic condition results from some type of inflammation involving the apocrine sweat glands. They have been referred to as *secondary sex glands* or as scent glands that occur only in certain areas of the body. The genitalia are rich in apocrine glands as are the scalp, axillae, breast, umbilicus, and the groin and scrotal areas. Early in the disease these lesions yield almost no pus and painfully form and reform, producing cordlike or ropelike scarring. They do not heal completely but form chronic draining sinuses wherever the apocrine glands exist. This condition can be so disabling that extensive plastic surgery may be necessary as a last resort to exteriorize and remove the lesions; skin grafts in the areas of the groin and scrotum may even be required. The extent of the problem and the heroic approach to it have been moderated by the concomitant use of steroids and antibiotics.

INFECTIONS AND INFLAMMATIONS

Balanitis and Balanoposthitis

By definition these diseases from any cause can be traced in almost every case to the presence of a foreskin, which may be redundant and phimotic, thereby predisposing to infections. This preputial cloak harbors beneath it normally desquamating epithelial cells, glandular secretions, and *Mycobacterium smegmatis,* and provides an inviting, warm, moist culture medium for any incidental organisms that may be present. It is obvious, therefore, that personal daily hygiene will prevent most instances of simple balanitis and balanoposthitis. From a strictly medical standpoint all adult, sexually active males would profit from circumcision if it has not already been done.

One must be alert to the real possibility that balanitis and balanoposthitis can be harbingers of other, more serious diseases and therefore cannot be dismissed as simple local unhygienic inflammations, especially if they become chronic or persistent. In Table 20–1 some common and uncommon diseases are listed along with methods for their diagnosis.

In many instances of unresponsive vulvovaginitis it is found that the sexual partner is perpetuating the disease by means of a chronic, seemingly nonspecific, and relatively mild balanoposthitis that is due to a variety of organisms and underlying pathologic processes (Catterall, 1966).

TABLE 20–1. Common Causes of Balanoposthitis and Means of Differentiation

Disease	Investigation
Amoebiasis	Direct microscopic examination
Balanitides (organic and traumatic)	Bacteriology; history; course
Balanitis circumscripta plasmacellularis	Histology
Candidiasis	Potassium hydroxide examination
Drug eruptions	History; course
Eczematous eruptions	History; response to treatment
Erythroplasia of Queyrat	Histology
Extramammary Paget's disease	Histology
Exudative discoid and lichenoid chronic dermatoses	History; other lesions; course
Granuloma inguinale	Bacteriology
Kaposi's sarcoma	Histology; other lesions
Keratoderma blennorrhagica	Histology; course
Leukoplakia	Histology
Lichen planus	Other lesions; histology
Lichen sclerosis et atrophicus	Histology; other lesions
Lymphogranuloma venereum	Virology; immunology
Neurodermatitis	Course; response to treatment
Pemphigus	Histology; other lesions; course
Precancerous lesions	Histology
Psoriasis	Other lesions; histology
Scabies	Potassium hydroxide
Squamous cell carcinoma	Histology

Erosive and Gangrenous Balanitis

In an era of antibiotics, any balanitis due to a mixed type of microbial infection that progressed to a gangrenous stage would be uncommon. The etiologic organisms, the short and borrelia-like spirochete and the stubby, fusiform, curved vibrio, inhabit the mouth and often the smegma of normal males. It is suspected that salivary contact by fellatio occurs, and the organisms, alighting upon an already unclean and irritated area, may then produce infection. The incubation period varies from 3 days to 1 week. The first signs of involvement may be small red erosions on the glans or undersurface of the prepuce, with concomitant development of much preputial exudation; the purulent discharge may be accompanied by phimosis. If the disease is unchecked, confluent ulcerations will develop along with considerable edema of the penis. The gangrenous phase appears after much induration, reddening, and swelling of the prepuce, which turns black; the gangrene may be accompanied by necrosis of the glans and portions of the shaft. In certain instances the entire penis has been destroyed within a comparatively short time. In the advanced stages, the inguinal nodes reflect the severity of the inflammatory reaction, becoming large but not tender. Constitutional symptoms of infection are common.

The diagnosis may be assumed from the rapid and destructive course of the disease, but the organisms are plentiful in smears and cultures made from the lesions, and identification of the symbiotic organisms is comparatively easy. The spirochete is longer and coarser than *Treponema pallidum,* and its morphology and movement are entirely different. Since mixed infections may occur, darkfield examination must be made, and smears must be inspected for Ducrey's bacillus. The primary lesions of syphilis are hardly ever as exudative, dirty, or rapidly spreading. There is no undermining of the erosive and gangrenous ulcers as there is in chancroid, and the adenitis never matches the chancroidal adenitic involvement in extent or fluctuant course.

Since anaerobic conditions are necessary for growth of the offending organisms, simple exposure to air and local cleansing has in the past been effective. Formerly this treatment, used with peroxide powder and arsphenamine and, in severe cases, a dorsal slit, was the extent of therapy. With the advent of penicillin and other systemic and local antibiotics, the treatment is specific and effective; however, even now a dorsal slit procedure is sometimes necessary.

Balanitis Circumscripta Plasmacellularis (Zoon, 1952)

This disorder is essentially diagnosed by microscopic examination. It occurs on the glans penis and has the same clinical appearance as erythroplasia of Queyrat. The lesions of balanitis circumscripta plasmacellularis (Fig. 20–19) sometimes appear shiny red and smooth rather than red, velvety, and granular as in typical cases of erythroplasia of Queyrat. This clinical similarity has given rise to the designation of the benign form of erythroplasia of Queyrat. Microscopically, the primary change in erythroplasia of Queyrat is the atypical epithelial alterations.

By definition the microscopic changes in balanitis circumscripta plasmacellularis occur in the dermis, where the inflammatory infiltrate is composed largely of plasma cells. The epithelium is thinned and does not actively participate. Predictably, plasma cells in greater numbers are found in any inflamed genital location.

PARASITES

Scabies

Scabies (Fig. 20–20) is caused by the itch mite, *Sarcoptes scabiei,* and is usually contracted from the bed partner. The disease can be transmitted by sleeping alone in the same bed or in a sleeping bag recently used by an infected person. Children who indulge in close contact games transmit it among themselves. Infected hospital personnel sometimes transmit the disease to the patients. The profound itching of scabies usually begins after the person goes to bed and becomes warm, at which time the mites become active. Itching is so intense that the victims sometimes almost mutilate the skin, producing linear excoriations and ecchymotic marks. On the male genitalia typical lesions are represented by inflammatory papules or nodules with some swelling of the soft tissue from scratching. These are obvious on the glans, shaft, and scrotum and are often crusted. They can be secondarily infected and may be mistaken for some more formidable disease.

Genital lesions in scabies are particularly diagnostic in the fastidiously clean person who washes his hands frequently, and, as a result, scabies lesions are not so apt to be formed on the wrists, fingers, and webs of the fingers.

Demonstration of the scabetic mite is usually possible if a thin sliver of skin from a papule is removed with a razor blade, placed on a glass slide, and digested with heat and 10 per cent potassium hydroxide. If the actual mite is not demonstrated, the eggs are easily identified and are diagnostic.

Formerly, sulfur in different combinations of ointments was the treatment of choice. At present the use of Kwell lotion is favored because it is effective, clean to use, and odorless. Instructions to the patients include: Bathe before beginning treatment; apply the lotion to all parts of the skin from the neck down twice a day for 2 days; bathe after completing treatment and then change bed linens and clothing, and wash or dry clean linens and clothing that have been worn. This is very effective treatment, but in some cases the inflammatory papules on penis and scrotum are slow to resolve even though all parasites are dead.

Pediculosis Pubis (Phthiriasis, Crab Lice)

Infections with the crab louse (Figs. 20–21 and 20–22) should be suspected whenever there is itching in the hairy portions of the pubis, thighs, and scrotum. The presence of nits attached to the hair shafts near the skin surface or the presence of the embedded louse at the orifice of the hair shaft is diagnostic. These lice are easily seen with the naked eye and resemble an airplane, owing to the extended claws clamped on a hair. The axillae and eyelashes are sometimes involved.

Here again, Kwell applied as a shampoo once for 5 minutes to all hair-bearing areas and then repeated 1 week later will completely eradicate the disease (avoid contact with eyes). This is also effective treatment against the unhatched nits; the presence of empty shells still attached to hair shafts after several weeks does not mean active disease. Microscopic examination following this treatment will reveal that the unhatched crab louse has been destroyed.

VASCULAR LESIONS

Angiokeratoma, Fordyce Type

Angiokeratomas of the Fordyce type (Fig. 20–23) are found on the scrotum and penile shaft and sometimes perimeatally. These are of unknown cause and do not appear until adult life. They do not tend to disappear, and no treatment is indicated. Recognition of this Fordyce type is important because those of the Fabry type imply further trouble. The angiokeratomas are dark blue or reddish. They may bleed when traumatized or may mimic melanoma if they become thrombosed. Microscopi-

cally, the abundant blood vessels forming these lesions are intimately related to the keratin layer of the skin, hence the name angiokeratoma. Very often there will be microscopic evidence of an organizing thrombus in one of these superficial vessels.

As stated, no treatment is necessary for these nonthreatening lesions except for cosmetic reasons or repeated bleeding. In such a case, simple electrosurgical desiccation is sufficient.

Lymphangiokeratoma

Lymphangiokeratomas (Figs. 20–24 and 20–25) exist in the same location as angiokeratomas and present with the appearance of a small, translucent glass bead (frog-spawn appearance). This is a congenital lesion and appears at an earlier age. It may be associated with more extensive underlying lymphangioma.

Angiokeratoma, Fabry Type (Angiokeratoma Corporis Diffusum Universale, Glucolipid Lipidosis) (Fig. 20–26)

This is a serious, hereditary, sex-linked disorder in which there is deposition of a specific glucolipid throughout the organs and vessels of the body. It is thought to result from some enzymatic defect. The angiokeratomatous lesions that begin to appear at puberty are clinically identical with those of the Fordyce type in appearance and location, but the similarity ceases there. In the Fabry type of angiokeratoma, the vascular lesions continue to proliferate on the buttocks, abdomen, umbilical region, elbows, fingers, lips, and oral mucous membranes.

Deposition of the glucolipid is found in the walls of blood vessels as vacuolated spaces in examination of skin biopsy material. Symptoms of continued evidence of the disease are found in the eye, kidneys, nervous system, and heart. Males with this disease die before 50 years of age.

Varices (Varicose Veins)

Varicose veins (Fig. 20–27) of the male genitalia are usually related to varicosities found elsewhere. Often a history of varicose veins as a family trait or the presence of pressure on the veins elsewhere explains their presence.

The veins become a problem only when they become large, thereby adding a sense of increased weight to the scrotum; surgical treatment may be indicated in this case. In a mild case a suspensory may be adequate to remove symptoms. The complication of hemorrhage or

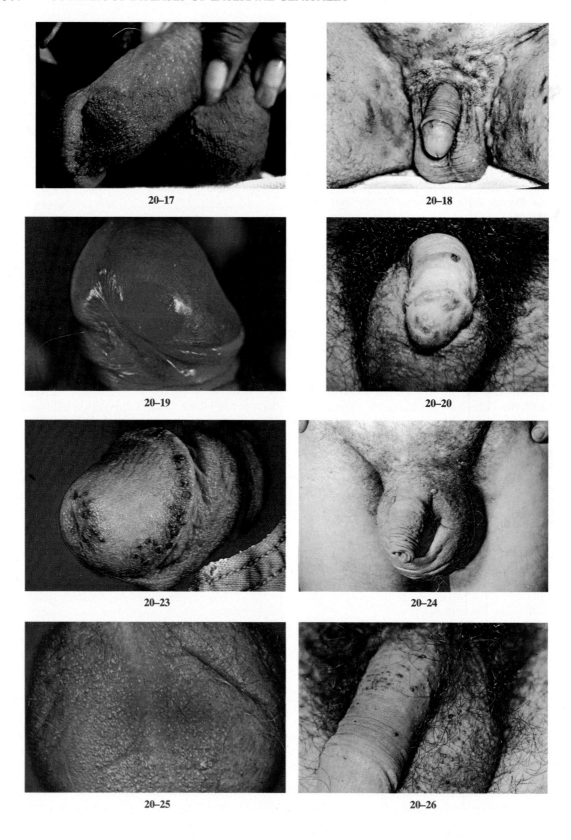

20–17

20–18

20–19

20–20

20–23

20–24

20–25

20–26

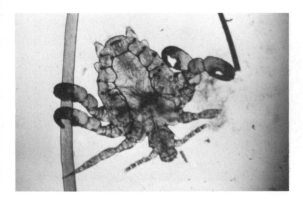

Figure 20–21. Crab louse.

thrombosis should be approached by proper surgical intervention.

Hemangioma

This is most often a congenital lesion. In such patients a strawberry or cavernous hemangioma (Fig. 20–28) persists into adult life rather than undergoing spontaneous involution as usual. Hemangiomas may occur anywhere on the genitalia and in the authors' experience are more common in female infants.

In most cases hemangiomas are no longer treated because the vast majority undergo spontaneous involution. Cryotherapy, sclerosing solutions, and surgical procedures may on rare occasions be used. Radiation, formerly used with good effect, is now in disfavor.

Pyogenic Granuloma (Proudflesh)

An excessive proliferation of new blood vessels in a localized area, referred to as pyogenic granuloma, arises sometimes spontaneously but most often following slight injury, abrasion, or a minor surgical procedure. The

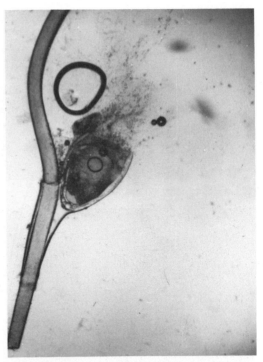

Figure 20–22. Nit of crab louse on pubic hair.

increased moisture of the scrotal area is especially favorable to this proliferation.

Complete local destruction by surgery or by electrosurgical procedures is adequate treatment; care must be taken that the underlying vascular component in the dermis is included in the procedure.

Sclerosing Lymphangitis

In a description (Nickel and Plumb, 1962) of this condition as a nonvenereal sclerosing lymphangitis (Fig. 20–29), it was noted that several of our early patients were physicians.

Figure 20–17. Typical tiny flat papules of the penile shaft in lichen nitidus.

Figure 20–18. Hidradenitis suppurativa of the male genitalia and groin. (Courtesy of the University of California, Los Angeles, California.)

Figure 20–19. Balanitis circumscripta plasmacellularis (Zoon) (benign erythroplasia).

Figure 20–20. Scabies of the penis.

Figure 20–23. Perimeatal and coronal angiodermatoma (Fordyce type). (Courtesy of Dr. William Carson.)

Figure 20–24. Lymphangioma of the genitalia, scrotal enlargement.

Figure 20–25. Lymphangioma of the scrotum showing "frog spawn" appearance of surface lymphangiokeratomas.

Figure 20–26. Angiokeratoma corporis diffusum (Fabry's disease). The penis and scrotum are involved before more serious manifestations develop.

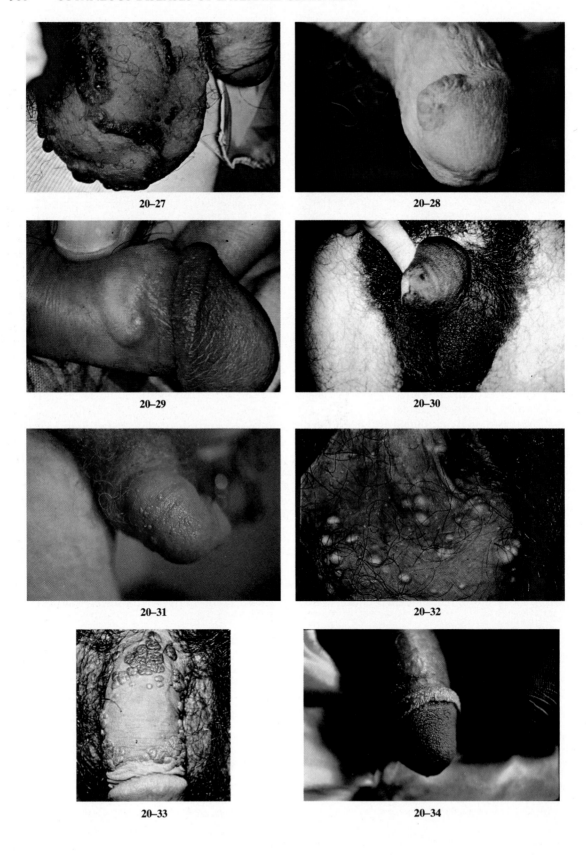

20–27

20–28

20–29

20–30

20–31

20–32

20–33

20–34

These lesions present as translucent, rather firm masses with a wormlike configuration that may encircle 70 per cent of the penis. Typically they appear on the shaft behind the corona, but we have observed sclerotic, pencil-like lesions on the dorsal penis extending onto the pubis. Microscopically there is a marked thickening of the wall of the involved lymph vessel.

The cause of this condition is unknown. It is self-limited, and therefore reassurance of the patient is all that is necessary.

Traumatic Hematoma

This can be dramatic clinically (Fig. 20–30) without too much disability and usually resorbs without intervention.

Lymphedema and Lymphostasis

Following hemipelvectomy a massive lymph stasis developed in the penis, which assumed an angular configuration. Vesicles filled with lymph developed on the skin. These ruptured easily and clear lymph continued to drain. The picture (Fig. 20–31) was taken from the posterior view to more adequately show the lymph vesicles in the angulated configuration of the markedly swollen penis.

BENIGN NEW GROWTHS

Cysts

Epithelial inclusion cysts (Fig. 20–32), often multiple, are fairly common on the scrotum. When these are incised they are found to be filled with a whitish, cheesy material that proves microscopically to be keratin. Extensive excision of the multiple lesions is usually unnecessary because simple incision and expression of the contents will result in eradication.

Clinically identical lesions, again usually multiple, when subjected to biopsy and microscopic examination, may be found to be instances of localized calcinosis of the skin. These lesions show no residue of any previous cyst or hemorrhage or any other explanation for what appears to be a primary instance of calcinosis cutis.

Seborrheic Keratoses (Seborrheic Verruca)

These acquired warty growths usually occur as flattened gray to brown pigmented lesions (Fig. 20–33) on the shaft of the penis or in the groin or pubic region. They lack the predilection for moist areas noted in condyloma acuminatum. They may assume a linear configuration and may be a kind of wart related to other viral warts.

Treatment by electrosurgical destruction is most satisfactory for these usually multiple lesions. Cryocautery using liquid nitrogen is also used, producing necrosis and sloughing of the lesions.

Pearly Penile Papules, Hirsutoid Papillomas of the Corona

Pearly-appearing papules (Johnson and Baxter, 1964) (Fig. 20–34), which are scattered in a crownlike excrescence from the corona of the penis, are usually most developed in young adults. Their bizarre appearance is of interest, but no therapy is indicated. Microscopically they are angiofibromas.

Nevi and Melanomas

Ordinary pigmented nevi are rare on the genitalia compared with other portions of the body. Because the glans penis and foreskin are quasi-mucous membranes it is the authors' opinion that pigmented moles in this area should be

---

Figure 20–27. Varices of the scrotum.

Figure 20–28. Hemangioma of the adult male glans.

Figure 20–29. Sclerosing (nonvenereal) lymphangitis. Note the wormlike configuration from the sclerotic vessel.

Figure 20–30. Traumatic hemorrhage in the penis and scrotum.

Figure 20–31. Massive stasis edema of penis forming lymph vesicles, following hemipelvectomy.

Figure 20–32. Epithelial inclusion cysts of the scrotum.

Figure 20–33. Seborrheic verruca type lesion found in dry areas.

Figure 20–34. Pearly penile papules; hirsutoid papillomas of penis.

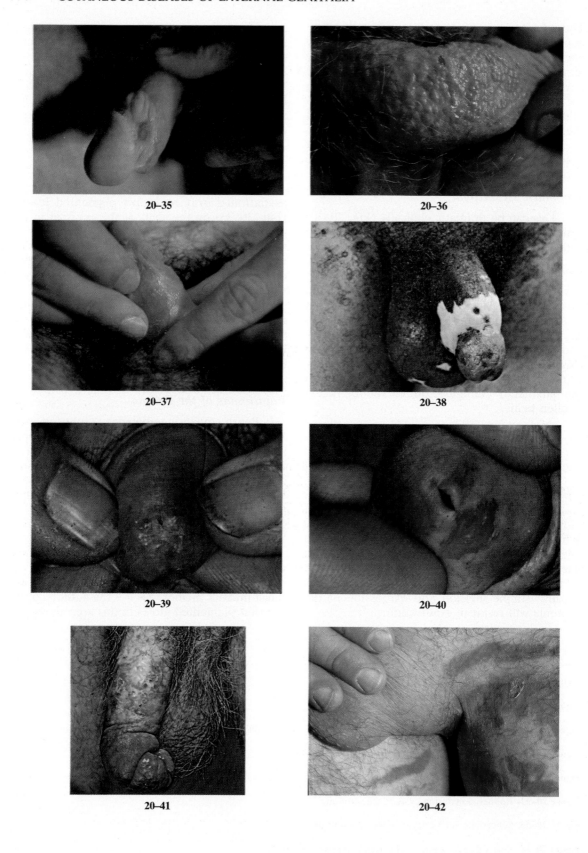

20–35

20–36

20–37

20–38

20–39

20–40

20–41

20–42

removed. The nevus pictured here, which appeared in a young male, was microscopically reported as a "junction nevus" (Fig. 20–35). Malignant melanomas in this area are likewise rare.

Syringomas

The nodular or warty-appearing lesions are more common on the face (eyelids), neck, and axillae. They appear usually at puberty and tend to be familial. They are asymptomatic, and again they present only a cosmetic problem. This is one instance in which a biopsy is the only way to make an accurate diagnosis (Fig. 20–36). Microscopically there are collections of ductal structures presenting as small cysts, some of which have a comma-like tail.

Sebaceous Gland Hyperplasia

Aberrant sebaceous glands are very common on the mucosal surface of the mouth, especially the labial and buccal mucosa (Fordyce disease). They are acquired lesions that can appear as clustered whitish papules on the quasimucosal surfaces of the penis (Fig. 20–37). They are "cosmetic," and patients need only reassurance.

ATROPHIC AND OTHER PIGMENTARY DISORDERS

Vitiligo

The cause of vitiligo (Fig. 20–38) is unknown. It appears spontaneously in all age groups and results in total and usually permanent progressive pigmentary loss. In the white leukodermic areas the melanocytes have ceased to function. Loss of pigment without atrophy may first appear in the perimeatal region, but it is only part of a more generalized pigment loss.

The condition is asymptomatic and cosmetic only. Until the advent of methoxsalen and its derivatives no treatment was offered. Results even with this drug have been disappointing. Psoralen drugs depend upon their photosensitive effect to produce quicker erythema and, ideally, repigmentation. They must be used daily with sun exposure for months if they are to have any beneficial effect.

Lichen Sclerosus et Atrophicus and Balanitis Xerotica Obliterans

Considering the microscopic picture alone, balanitis xerotica obliterans and lichen sclerosus et atrophicus, whether in male or female, are the same disease. There is one notable difference, however, because on rare occasions in men the atrophic sclerotic process produces meatal stenosis (Fig. 20–39), which requires meatotomy.

The cause of this disease is unknown; it is often part of the same disease process elsewhere on the body. The foreskin is often involved in these atrophic sclerotic changes, which result in phimosis. The involved skin shows an expanding area of white pigment loss. This is accompanied by extreme atrophy of the skin and poor cohesion of the epidermis to the underlying sclerotic homogeneous connective tissue, which accounts for the ecchymotic, hemorrhagic changes (Fig. 20–40) of the glans that accompany even mild trauma. In the male this disease is not considered precancerous.

All treatments are disappointing. Local steroids have been used, with debatable results. Administration of vitamin E locally and orally likewise has not been dramatically beneficial.

Figure 20–35. Pigmented nevus, junctional type, in young male.

Figure 20–36. Syringomas. These warty-appearing lesions require biopsy for diagnosis.

Figure 20–37. Aberrant sebaceous glands behind corona of penis. (Courtesy of Dr. Judith Adler.)

Figure 20–38. Vitiligo of the glans.

Figure 20–39. Meatal stenosis in balanitis xerotica obliterans.

Figure 20–40. Hemorrhage in this atrophic skin of balanitis xerotica obliterans.

Figure 20–41. Radiation dermatitis of the penis following treatment of Peyronie's disease. (Courtesy of the United States Naval Hospital, San Diego, California.)

Figure 20–42. Acute phase of striae cutis distensae from steroid creams.

Meatotomy in meatal stenosis may be a surgical emergency if neglected.

Radiation Dermatitis

This atrophic and sclerotic condition (Fig. 20–41) can occur after radiation treatment for Peyronie's disease. Such treatment for this disease is being phased out.

Atrophies

Striae Cutis Distensae. These discolored areas in the groin appear suddenly in some persons using steroid preparations locally. The acute lesions (Fig. 20–42) appear red—almost hemorrhagic—and slowly assume an atrophic white appearance when the medication is stopped.

GANGRENE

Primary idiopathic spontaneous fulminating gangrene of the penis, in contradistinction to the gangrenous conditions that may involve the penis secondarily or as the terminal picture of many infectious and other pathologic processes, is a distinct entity. Commonly associated with gangrene of the scrotum, it was first described by Fournier. The loosely contrived cellular structure of the penis and the scrotum in particular are essential factors that allow the sequence of events to occur. Debility predisposes to its onset. It is fortunately not often seen, for the mortality rate has been estimated to be 17 to 27 per cent. The organisms responsible for the majority of cases are the hemolytic streptococcus and staphylococcus, but *Escherichia coli*, diphtheroids, and *Bacillus fragilis* have also been incriminated. Histologically the presence of thrombosed vessels at the periphery of the lesions has led to the postulation that the characteristic distribution and rapid progress are due to vascular thrombotic episodes and deprivation of blood supply to the tissues (Thomas, 1956).

A scratch or unobserved abrasion may be the portal of entry, and the characteristic features are soon fulfilled. The onset is sudden in a previously healthy individual, and progression of the gangrenous state is rapid (Tan, 1964). The disease may be confined to the penis with only erythema noticeable on the adjacent scrotum. Usually within 24 hours of the onset of redness and swelling of the penis, an exudative, moist desquamation begins. Crepitation in the pitting surface may be noticed prior to the occurrence of gangrene, which spreads rapidly to involve the entire penis. Spontaneously a line of demarcation appears, and within the confines of the gangrenous area sloughing gradually occurs down to the primary fascial planes. The corpora and testicles are not involved. The process may at times be seen to envelop the entire pubic region. In a few days the necrosis sloughs away, and hemorrhage may occur in the uninvolved base. Granulation tissue soon covers the area, and healing proceeds. Systemic symptoms may be severe throughout the course of the disease, chills, fever, and pain being common. Complete regeneration of tissue occurs within 4 to 6 weeks.

Diagnosis is self-evident from the history, clinical appearance, and fulminating course of the process, but the organisms responsible must be isolated so that the appropriate chemotherapeutic and antibiotic agents may be utilized, in conjunction with local and general supportive measures. Early and extensive débridement of devitalized tissue has materially shortened the duration of the disease and is employed as soon as the progress of the cellulitis has been halted by the antibiotics. Irrigations with antiseptic solutions, the use of streptococcal and gasgangrene antisera, and blood transfusions, which were the sole methods of therapy in the past, may be employed subsequent to initial control with one of the antibiotics. Recent authors have advised the use of hyperbaric oxygen (HBO) at 3 atmospheres one to two times daily.

Secondary gangrene occurs in the penis infrequently; diabetes and arteriosclerosis may be productive of it. Somewhat more commonly, the venereal disease, cavernositis, the balanitides, and local abscesses secondary to the periurethral results of stricture and infection may all, if untreated, occasion the development of gangrene. The therapeutic rationale is dependent upon control of the primary disease, but extensive surgical repair or amputation may be required.

Gangrene of the Scrotum

This condition occurs following a wide variety of inciting conditions (Fig. 20–43). Gangrenous necrosis of the scrotal skin and wall is relatively common after urinary extravasations. It may also occur in the presence of other underlying urinary tract diseases, such as paraphimosis, penile erosions, inguinal adenitis, prostatoseminal vesiculitis, and epididymitis. The connection between the underlying disease and the relatively sudden and generalized gangrenous process is not always obvious. It is

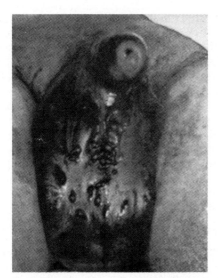

Figure 20–43. Streptococcus scrotal gangrene.

grene was first clinically described in 1885 by Fournier, and since that time it has been given such terms as "Fournier's gangrene," "streptococcus gangrene," "scrotal gangrene," "spontaneous fulminating gangrene," "essential gangrene," and "idiopathic gangrene." It usually occurs in middle or later life, but 26 cases have been described in children. In 1945 Mair, in analyzing 240 cases of reported gangrene in the scrotum to that date, found that 125 were of the "spontaneous" type. The onset is dramatically sudden, having been described as "explosive," even occurring in the middle of the night and awakening the patient. An otherwise healthy individual may be suddenly seized with pain in the scrotum, following which edema and swelling soon appear. The scrotum becomes tense, painful, reddened, warm, glossy, and, as mortification develops, moist. The gangrene is usually limited at the demarcation of the scrotum but has been known to spread under Colles' and Scarpa's fasciae to the abdomen and even to the axilla. It is usually accompanied by chills, fever, nausea, vomiting, and prostration. It must be differentiated from erysipelas, which usually begins in a limited area and spreads with a perceptible red, raised margin at the periphery. In the latter, the constitutional symptoms are paramount in comparison with the local symptoms. With careful examination, it should not be difficult to differentiate this acute process from acute epididymitis, acute orchitis, hydrocele, or torsion of the testis.

This spontaneous, relatively rare, and inexplicable gangrene is thought to result from an infection. The redundancy of the scrotal tissues is believed to favor the occurrence of such gangrene. It is thought that ingress of the organisms into the wall of the scrotum can occur by one of several mechanisms. Organisms might enter the skin through minute abrasions, possibly by trauma from the fingernails. Embolic bacteria from remote sites in the body have been considered, even though this condition occurs without any history or antecedent genitourinary-tract or general disease. A logical causative factor in many cases could be minute and unrecognizable periurethral phlegmons, through which bacteria progress from the urethra into the scrotal tissue without abscess formation or extravasation of urine. Urethral strictures and perirectal abscess are known causes.

In the majority of reported instances there is emphysema of the tissue, and actual gas is often encountered upon surgical incision. From a clinical standpoint, it is significant that those cases that have crepitation usually show more

known to occur after mechanical, chemical, or thermal injuries to the scrotum. Atrophic disturbances, diabetes, alcoholism, and general debility have led to extensive scrotal gangrene. Embolism of the internal hypogastric arteries from an aneurysm of the aorta has resulted in scrotal gangrene. A case has been reported by Meleney due to *Entamoeba histolytica*.

A peculiar form of scrotal gangrene has been observed in the last two decades in association with the rickettsial disease Rocky Mountain spotted fever, which has become prevalent in this country. Gangrene in these cases is due to proliferation of endothelial cells in the walls of the blood vessels, with necrosis of the smooth musculature. This leads to thrombosis, and in severe cases dependent parts of the body, such as the scrotum, become gangrenous. Secondary infection may accelerate the gangrenous process.

Before the era of antibiotics, scrotal gangrene was not a rarity. Randall observed 147 cases at the Philadelphia General Hospital in a period of 16 years. In many of these cases the gangrene also involved the penis. In these modern times, most patients seek medical attention soon after urinary extravasation or the beginning of a periurethral phlegmon, at which time administered antibiotics are usually successful in aborting the development of such extensive gangrenous processes.

A remarkable form of "spontaneous gangrene" involving the scrotum occurs in which there is no evidence of pre-existing disease either in the genitourinary tract or elsewhere (Fig. 20–43). This relatively sudden scrotal gan-

constitutional symptoms, such as high fever and evidence of toxemia. The bacteriology in this remarkable disease is incomplete, but anaerobic streptococci, either alone or with other organisms, have been reported in 28 to 44 cases studied (Mair, 1945). A wide variety of other organisms, including hemolytic streptococci, *Proteus,* and especially the gas-forming anaerobes, have also been encountered. It is well known that anaerobes normally inhabit the male urethra, and it is believed by some observers that the primary infective agents are the anaerobic bacilli that are usually overgrown by streptococci in cultures from this area.

Treatment. Treatment of gangrene of the scrotum is two fold. The first stage is recognition and treatment of any underlying etiologic disease process of the urinary tract when it exists. In urinary extravasation immediate diversion of the urinary stream may be necessary. The second objective is directed toward the probable bacteria involved. In this respect, the early recognition of the pregangrenous state and the institution of proper antibiotic therapy is extremely important. Combined broad-spectrum antibiotics are advised, on the assumption that it is likely to be a mixed infection. Prompt surgical drainage and débridement of the tense, swollen scrotal tissue in either the pregangrenous or the gangrenous state relieves tension and drains the edema. Multiple scrotal incisions with the insertion of drains, followed by irrigations of the tissue with 1:5000 potassium permanganate solution or zinc peroxide, frequently is of value. Zinc peroxide is more efficacious than hydrogen peroxide because it liberates oxygen more slowly. Recently, the use of HBO has been recommended for 90 minutes at 3 atmospheres of pressure.

NONVENEREAL INFECTIONS OF THE SCROTUM

The scrotum is subject to infections by all pyogenic and specific organisms as well as to many diseases indigenous to tropical areas. In general, infections of the scrotum are not dissimilar to infections of skin and subcutaneous tissues elsewhere in the body, but some differences are manifest because of the nature of the scrotal wall. The scrotal skin is in the form of transverse rugae, which tend to render the skin folds inaccessible to air, especially when the dartos is contracted, and this may interfere with resistance to bacteria. The scrotum is situated in a well-protected area, unfavorable for proper ventilation, and, with numerous sweat glands, it is prone to become moist. Bacteria from the rectum and urethra are prevalent on the surface, but there is evidently a local tissue resistance to the organisms so commonly found in this area. Contact with adjacent mesial surfaces of the thighs is often a deterrent to healing processes. The especially loose, fat-free, and contractile scrotal wall reacts to infection with considerable edema. The resulting tenseness leads to excoriation and interference with vascularity, both of which may lower the resistance to infections. In spite of these factors, the scrotum heals readily after most infections and after surgery.

Abscess of the Scrotal Wall

Primary abscesses of the scrotal wall are not uncommon. These occur from infections of the hair follicles or sweat glands or through abrasions of the skin. They behave as localized abscesses or furuncles elsewhere and are treated similarly, i.e., with warm wet compresses and incision and drainage. Antibiotics may be used. Even though such localized abscesses are painful and disabling, they usually are not as serious as abscesses of the scrotal wall secondary to extension of periurethral phlegmons, anorectal abscesses, or suppurative lesions of the epididymis or testis. Scrotal wall abscesses usually become apparent several days after instrumentation of an infected urethra. The skin becomes red and edematous with an area of fluctuation. Incision and drainage may lead to formation of a urinary fistula. Cultures of the pus usually reveal organisms of the coccal and coliform group.

Abscess not infrequently develops after vasectomy from infection at the proximal end of the divided vas. Tuberculosis and rare specific infections may also cause scrotal wall suppuration. Infecting organisms can metastasize to the scrotum from a distant focus, as in a reported case due to *Corynebacterium diphtheria.*

Treatment. Incision and drainage of the abscess are essential. Large portions of the scrotal skin may become necrotic. Débridement may be necessary. The scrotal skin regenerates rapidly; however, on occasion, with an extensive abscess or poor healing, hernia testis may occur (Fig. 20–44). The use of broad-spectrum antibiotics or specific drug therapy, when indicated, may help keep the process localized.

Infected Fistulae

Before the era of antibiotics, infected fistulae were not an uncommon occurrence in the practice of urology. Most patients have multiple sinuses, which are the end result of periurethral

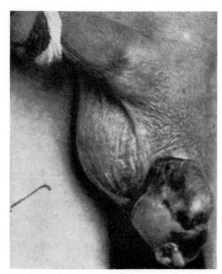

Figure 20–44. Hernia testis secondary to scrotal abscess in a young adult.

abscesses developing around the bulbous urethra. They often occur spontaneously in association with a urethral stricture, after trauma, or after the passage of sounds for dilatations. Urinary fistulae often heal temporarily but usually reopen with episodes of abscess formation. In such fistulae there is considerable granulation and infected scar tissue extending from the external fistulous opening to the urethra. Treatment is not only excision of the tract but also excision of the fistulous opening in the urethra. A single fistula can often be cured with wide exposure of the tract and removal of scar tissue down to the urethra, followed by closure of the urethral opening. In multiple fistulae with more extensive involvement of the urethra, a wide excision of the urethral wall and periurethral inflammatory tissue may be necessary. This often leads to an extensive urethral defect, so that various reconstructive operations are required. It may be necessary to close the urethral defect with whole or split-thickness skin grafts. If the urethra is not adequately repaired and considerable scar tissue forms during healing, stricture and periurethral inflammation are likely to recur with re-formation of abscesses and the reappearance of fistulae.

Scrotal fistulae were at one time common after tuberculosis of the epididymis in which caseous areas gradually extended to the surface, but tuberculous fistulae are now relatively uncommon. Untreated tertiary syphilis with gumma of the testis not uncommonly erodes through the scrotal walls in a manner similar to that in caseous tuberculosis. A case of actinomycosis of the scrotal wall was reported by Anderson and Jenkins (1938). This patient had chronic recurring anal fistulae for a number of years. He was seen after a long interval, during which time fistulae had appeared on the side of the scrotum. The wall was thickened, indurated, and painless and had typical chronically infected, draining sinuses. Microscopic section from the margins of fistulae revealed colonies of *Actinomyces*. Fistulae have also been described following a number of tropical parasitic diseases (see Chapter 21).

Scrotal Erysipelas

Scrotal erysipelas is a diffuse streptococcal infection of the scrotal skin and subcutaneous tissue occurring as a result of surgical incisions, wounds, scrotal abscesses, and fistulae. It is seen especially in debilitated and senile individuals. This type of cellulitis may also result from retrograde lymphatic infection into the scrotum from acute inguinal adenitis due to malignancy, chancroid infection, and other conditions. Erysipelas in the lower abdomen or adjacent skin areas may progress into the scrotum. This infection of the scrotum may be so intense as to become gangrenous (see earlier section on gangrene). It usually develops from a single area with a definite margin and gradually involves the entire scrotum. The soft, loose tissues of the scrotum become markedly swollen, tense, smooth, and warm. Blebs may form on the surface. The infecting organism is usually a streptococcus and a number of antibiotics are effective. The scrotum should always be elevated to enhance the circulation and reduce edema. Local applications of heat and, especially, wet solutions, as described in most textbooks, are not helpful and are not indicated.

ORCHITIS

Acute infection involving solely the testis is a relatively rare occurrence in clinical urology. The rich blood and lymphatic supply of the testicle gives it a high threshold of resistance so that metastatic infection occurs rarely. There are three pathways whereby orchitis may develop: metastatic via the blood, via lymph vessels, and ascending through the vas deferens and epididymis to the testicle. Almost every known infectious process has at times metastasized to the testicle as a primary infection, but in the majority of instances the orchitis is secondary to an extension of inflammations existing in the epididymis so that the process is usually an epididymo-orchitis. Orchitis, in general, may be divided into the following categories: pyogenic, viral, spirochetal, traumatic, chemical, mycotic, parasitic, and idiopathic, in which organisms and a primary focus of infection cannot be demonstrated.

Nonspecific Orchitis

Any pyogenic bacterium causing a septicemia may, on occasion, result in pyogenic orchitis. The usual etiologic agents are *Escherichia coli, Klebsiella pneumoniae,* streptococcus, staphylococcus, and *Pseudomonas aeruginosa,* as well as other organisms. In this form of orchitis the testicle is tense, swollen, and bluish, with many punctate hemorrhages on the surface. Multiple foci of necrosis are found, accompanied by considerable edema and interstitial infiltration of polymorphonuclear cells. The seminiferous epithelium is evidently easily damaged as a result of the ischemia. The process may progress to suppuration involving the whole testis, in which event an abscess of the testicle results. The most common cause of suppurative orchitis and abscess formation is epididymitis, complicating urinary tract infection, prostatectomy, catheterization, or instrumental procedures.

Acute pyogenic orchitis with or without abscess formation is usually ushered in with high fever and sudden pain in the involved testicle. The pain radiates to the inguinal canal and is usually accompanied by nausea and vomiting. The involved testis is swollen, tense, sometimes exquisitely tender, and at times fluctuant. There is usually an acute associated hydrocele that becomes a pyocele if the abscess ruptures. The scrotal skin may show some redness and edema. It is frequently difficult clinically to distinguish between acute orchitis, acute epididymitis, and epididymo-orchitis unless the epididymis can be palpated. In children, orchitis may be confused with torsion of the spermatic cord and strangulated hernia, especially if a congenital hydrocele of cryptorchidism is present. Delineation of the scrotal contents may be difficult even after aspiration of the fluid from the tunica vaginalis.

Treatment

Treatment of orchitis is essentially medical, including specific treatment of the underlying disease process. The patient is maintained with bed rest and adequate elevation of the scrotum. Hot or cold compresses are used only for symptomatic relief. The extent of the involvement depends upon the intensity of the inflammatory process and the virulence of the infecting organism. Aspiration of the symptomatic hydrocele may give considerable relief. Abscess of the testis is extremely rare and usually requires orchiectomy. Incision and drainage only result in sloughing and gradual extrusion of the parenchyma. Chemotherapeutic or antibiotic treatment is indicated according to the nature of the specific etiologic agent. With almost routine use of drugs early in all infectious processes in medicine today, there is less suppurative epididymitis and subsequent orchitis. Under the influence of drugs an infected epididymis is now safely removed, allowing the secondary inflammatory process in the testis to subside. Secondary atrophy and sterility from fibrosis and destruction of the tubules and ductal system frequently occur in orchitis of any form.

Traumatic Orchitis

This condition is considered by most urologists to be the result of an infectious process resulting from a lowered resistance of the injured tissues to bacteria. Enlargement of the testis (also spermatic cord and epididymis) may follow trauma, vas ligation, or surgical manipulation, without a history of preliminary disease or inflammation. Histologic studies in some cases reveal a nonspecific granulomatous reaction evidently due to proteins from extravasated sperm following an obstruction or traumatic procedures. The tissue reaction includes giant cells and resembles that of tuberculosis. It is probable that granulomatous orchitis in the past has sometimes been confused with tuberculous infection. Chemical substances, such as iodine, thallium, lead, carbon disulfide, and alcohol, have been alleged to cause destruction of the seminiferous tubules.

In all cases of direct or indirect trauma resulting in a lump in the testis, it must be remembered that a *minor trauma may first call the attention of the patient to a malignant testicular tumor.*

Specific Orchitis

Acute orchitis also may occur in rare instances during such systemic diseases as diphtheria, typhus fever, glanders, influenza, undulant fever, leprosy, dengue fever, typhoid fever, syphilis, paratyphoid fever, varicella, variola, mumps, scarlet fever, tuberculosis, amebiasis, schistosomiasis, sporotrichosis, actinomycosis, rickettsial diseases, malaria, filariasis (see later section on funiculitis), infectious mononucleosis, bilharziasis, and, on extremely rare occasions, in many other unusual diseases. Orchitis may occur as a complication of localized foci of infection elsewhere in the body, such as sinusitis, tonsillitis, furunculosis, osteomyelitis, endocarditis, acute rheumatic fever, acute articular fever, cellulitis, and gout. In some cases the testicular necrosis associated with the above diseases does not show demonstrable organisms in the testis and the pathologic process may be a result of the action of bacterial toxins on the testicle. Epidemics of obscure orchitis, usually epididymo-orchitis, have occurred in Malta and elsewhere, with as many as 60 cases having been seen during a single epidemic. The clinical picture is one of prodromal fever associated with mild constitutional symptoms without evidence of urinary-tract infection. Urologists have observed sporadic cases of epididymo-orchitis of a similar nature. Two such obscure cases included a boy of 8 years and a young man of 21 years of age. These cases of orchitis were not due to mumps. In the first case, orchitis recurred after an interval of several months, and in the second case, mumps orchitis was known to have existed 5 years previously on the opposite testis. Both cases were refractory to antibiotics.

Mumps Orchitis. Orchitis in mumps, because of its frequency, merits special consideration. Mumps is a highly incapacitating but self-limited viral disease complicated by orchitis in approximately 18 per cent of cases. It is exceedingly rare before puberty. Onset of the orchitis is usually 4 to 6 days after the appearance of parotitis, but it may occur without parotid involvement. A small epidemic of mumps orchitis has been observed without parotitis. In about 70 per cent of cases the orchitis is unilateral, with some degree of atrophy of the involved testis in 50 per cent of cases. Inclusion of the epididymis in this process is not rare. Sterility is infrequently a sequela of unilateral mumps. Baumrucker (1946) found only seven cases of sterility in 95 patients with testicular atrophy after mumps orchitis.

The signs and symptoms are essentially those of other interstitial types of orchitis. Nausea, vomiting, and chills may be present in severe cases. Testicular swelling is a prominent feature, although it is not remarkable in the first 48 hours. Mumps orchitis usually subsides in 7 to 10 days.

Treatment of mumps orchitis is medical and surgical. Bed rest, scrotal support, and either hot or cold applications are advised, although the value of these procedures is unsubstantiated. Considerable enthusiasm has been registered in recent years for the use of gamma globulin, diethylstilbestrol, and convalescent serum from individuals who have had mumps within a period of 3 to 4 months. Pooled plasma may result in temperature reduction within 24 hours in an occasional instance, but it is doubtful that it alters the general course of established orchitis. There is some evidence that it may reduce the incidence of orchitis by 65 to 75 per cent. Gamma globulin, given after the onset of parotitis, has been reported to reduce the incidence of orchitis. Early reports of the effectiveness of diethylstilbestrol in reducing the incidence of orchitis and favorably affecting the course of the disease have not been substantiated by more extensive studies. It is possible, however, that diethylstilbestrol in adequate doses (3 to 5 mg or more a day) may diminish the degree of pain, swelling, and fever. There is little evidence that there is any effect on the subsequent degree of testicular atrophy.

The preventive and therapeutic values of ACTH, cortisone, and prednisone have been extensively studied. Although there is a difference of opinion, it is probably safe to state that these drugs, prophylactically administered, perhaps lower the incidence of orchitis occurring in a series of adult mumps parotitis. The statistical advantage is probably offset by the inherent undesirable effects of the hormones. From the point of view of therapy of established mumps orchitis, Smith and Bishir (1958) reported some reduction only of pain with massive doses of cortisone, the local findings and clinical course of the disease being otherwise essentially unaltered; they stated that the incidence of complicating infections in these patients does not render the treatment worthwhile. Mongan (1959) reported no statistical advantage in the use of prednisone over placebos (thiamine) or no treatment in a series of 30 military personnel.

Surgical treatment of severe mumps orchitis has consisted of tapping the hydrocele to reduce the pressure in the tunica. Simple needle aspiration of the testicle is of no value. Many urologists advocate an "H" type of incision into the tunica albuginea after exposing the testicle to release intratesticular tension. Follow-up reports are too few in number to be of value in appraisal of this procedure, but there is evidence that, if it is done within the first 2 days of acute swelling, it results not only in relief of symptoms but also in a marked reduction of subsequent atrophy. The difficulty is in deciding which cases will respond favorably to radical therapy. The majority of patients begin to show improvement during the period when this type of therapy would be valuable. It should be reserved for those severe cases in which it appears that there is going to be considerable persistent swelling of the testicle.

INFECTIONS OF THE SPERMATIC CORD

Inflammation of the spermatic cord may primarily involve either the vas or one of the other major structures of the cord (vessels, lymphatics, and connective tissue). In many instances all or a combination of these structures are involved. Acute, subacute, and chronic inflammations may be encountered without evidence of disease elsewhere in the genital tract, but the vast majority of infections of the spermatic cord occur as a complication of prostatitis, seminal vesiculitis, and especially infections of the epididymis and testicle. The infectious process reaches the cord from these organs either through the lumen of the vas or by way of the lymphatics, although in rare instances funiculitis is a metastatic process from disease elsewhere in the body.

The most common infectious process today in the spermatic cord is vasitis after trauma or operative procedures to the prostate and posterior urethra. Most funicular infections are due to the ordinary pyogenic organisms. Several categories of acute inflammation of the spermatic cord constitute clinical entities worthy of recording.

Deferentitis

Inflammation restricted to the vas deferens, as a segmental infection unassociated with infections elsewhere in the genital tract, is rare but has been reported on a number of occasions. Usually there develops a variably tender, indurated, fibrous, and nodular enlargement of the vas from the epididymis to the inguinal area. Surgical exploration and removal of chronic segmental lesions in certain cases have revealed tuberculosis. Some segmental lesions have been known to appear with gonococcal urethritis and to disappear with treatment and improvement in the latter. *Granulomas* of the spermatic cord and testis have been recognized following

trauma and vas ligation. They occur as a painful mass in the cord resulting from the extravasation or penetration of sperm into the tissues, around which a histologic reaction containing giant cells develops. *Vasitis nodosa* has been described by Benjamin (1943) as a peculiar beading and nodularity involving the vas deferens just above the epididymis. These tiny, firm nodules on the wall of the vas show epithelium-lined spaces. They are probably the result of a previously unrecognized vasitis of unknown origin.

Funiculitis

This generally refers to inflammations of the tissues of the cord except the vas deferens. It should be stressed that most acute inflammations, especially tuberculosis, *Chlamydia,* and pyogenic infections associated with epididymitis, frequently involve all tissues of the cord and especially the lymphatics. Funiculitis may be acute, subacute, or chronic, and there are several well-known varieties.

Endemic funiculitis is an entity that has been known since the eighteenth century and on occasion has been epidemic. This acute inflammation occurs as a cellulitis of the cord. It may be associated with fever and symptoms of general toxemia; however, in other instances the symptoms are extremely mild. There is slight thickening and induration of the cord, which may progress to several inches in diameter and in which abscess formation and necrosis occur. In subacute and chronic cases the cord contains fibrous nodules. The pathologic findings are striking, consisting of thrombosis of the veins in the pampiniform plexus, sometimes with pus formation. The testicle, epididymis, and other tissues of the cord where infections ordinarily occur are usually normal. The vas in these cases, as a rule, cannot be palpated because it is obscured by the general enlargement of the entire spermatic cord. The etiology is entirely unknown, but from incomplete bacteriologic studies the cause is thought to be a streptococcus. This type of funiculitis occurs sporadically in temperate climates. We have observed one case in which there was a fusiform tender enlargement of the entire spermatic cord without epididymitis, prostatitis, or infection in the urinary tract or elsewhere. In our case, administration of modern antibiotics resulted in immediate resolution, and no insight as to the etiology was gained.

Lymphogranuloma venereum funiculitis has been encountered on a few occasions. It is usually a retrograde lymphatic involvement of the cord, apparently from infection of the deep iliac nodes by this virus. In the largest number of instances, the vas along with the other structures of the cord is involved. There is also a peculiar and characteristic involvement of the veins and arteries of the cord, which are evidently secondarily infected by passage of the virus through the wall during the primary lymphangitis.

Syphilitic funiculitis is a rare disease, there being only seven confirmed cases up to 1920. It occurs 4 to 9 years after the primary lesions and is characterized by irregular masses in the spermatic cord, which have the firm and elastic consistency of gummae. There is not anything pathognomonic about this condition, and the diagnosis can only be suspected with the finding of syphilis elsewhere in the body and the rapid disappearance of the tumors after the application of specific antiluetic therapy.

References

Abeshouse, B. S.: Torsion of the spermatic cord. Urol. Cutan. Rev., *40*:699, 1936.

Ablin, R. J., and Curtis, W. W.: Condyloma acuminata: Treatment by autogenous vaccine. Ill. Med. J., *147*:343, 1975.

Abrams, A. J.: Lymphogranuloma venereum. JAMA, *205*:199, 1968.

Anderson, C. W., and Jenkins, R. H.: Actinomycosis of the scrotum. N. Engl. J. Med., *219*:953, 1938.

Anderson, K., Demonbreum, W. A., and Goodpasture, E. W.: An etiologic consideration of Donovania granulomatis cultivated from granuloma inguinale in embryonic yolk. J. Exp. Med., *81*:25, 1945.

Armstrong, J. A., and Reed, S. E.: Nature and origin of initial bodies in lymphogranuloma venereum. Nature, *201*:371, 1964.

Baker, W. J., and Ragins, A. B.: Actinomycosis of the testicle. J. Urol., *56*:547, 1946.

Baumrucker, G. O.: Incidence of testicular pathology. Bull. U.S. Army Med. Dept., *5*:312, 1946.

Becker, L. E.: Review: Lymphogranuloma venereum. Int. J. Dermatol., *15*:26, 1976.

Benjamin, J. A., Robertson, T. D., and Cheetam, J. G.: Vasitis nodosa: A new clinical entity simulating tuberculosis of the vas deferens. J. Urol., *49*:575, 1943.

Blau, S., and Hyman, A. B.: Erythroplasia of Queyrat. Acta Derm. Vener., *35*:44, 1955.

Bofverstedt, B.: Condylomata acuminata. Acta Derm. Vener., *47*:376, 1967.

Breen, J. L.: The venereal diseases. J. Am. Health Assoc., *15*:26, 1967.

Brown, F. R.: Testicular pain. Lancet, *1*:994, 1949.

Brown, P. B.: Erythroplasia of Queyrat. Br. J. Plast. Surg., *19*:378, 1966.

Bruns, T. N. C., Lauvetz, R. J., Kerr, E. S., and Ross, G., Jr.: Buschke-Lowenstein giant condyloma acuminata: Pitfalls in management. Urology, *5*:773, 1975.

Buckley, T. L.: Brucellosis of the male genitalia. Calif. West. Med., *48*:175, 1938.

Burhans, R. A.: Treatment of orchitis of mumps. J. Urol., *54*:547, 1945.

Butts, D. C. A.: Granuloma inguinale. A preliminary report on certain microscopic observations. Am. J. Syph., *21*:544, 1937.

Butts, D. C. A., and Olansky, S.: Observations on the cause and transmission of granuloma inguinale. Arch. Derm. Syph., *54*:524, 1946.

Callomon, F.: Metastische Hodenerkrankungen bei akuten Infektionskrankheiten, ihr Vorkommen und ihre Erkennung. Derm. Z., *67*:193, 1933.

Campbell, R. R.: Streptococcal scrotal and penile gangrene. Surg. Gynecol. Obstet., *34*:780, 1922.

Candel, S.: Immune serum globulin (gamma globulin) in prophylaxis of orchitis. Mil. Surgeon, *99*:199, 1946.

Candel, S., Wheelock, M. C., and Grimaldi, G. J.: Mumps orchitis with discussion of plasma prophylaxis. U.S. Navy Med. Bull., *45*:97, 1945.

Catterall, R. D.: Candida albicans and the contraceptive pill. Lancet, *2*:803, 1966.

Cawley, E. P., and Grekin, R. H.: Parafavus restricted to the scrotum. Arch. Derm. Syph., *60*:435, 1949.

Chaudhury, D. S.: A case report of gangrenous balanitis in leprosy. Leprosy Rev., *37*:225, 1966.

Ch'i An-Sheng: Further observations on tuberculosis of the penis. Chinese Med. J., *82*:328, 1963.

Cooke, R. A., and Rodrique, R. B.: Amebic balanitis. Med. J. Aust., *1*:114, 1964.

Corbett, M. B., Sidell, C. M., and Zimmerman, M.: Idoxuridine in the treatment of cutaneous herpes simplex. JAMA, *196*:441, 1966.

Coutts, W. E.: Genitourinary lesions in lymphogranuloma venereum. J. Urol., *49*:595, 1943.

Cronqvist, S.: Spermatic invasion of the epididymis. Acta Pathol. Microbiol. Scand., *26*:786, 1949.

Curtis, A. C., and Cawley, E. P.: Histoplasmosis of the penis. J. Urol., *57*:781, 1947.

Cusumano, C. L., and Monie, R. G.: A word of caution concerning photodynamic inactivation therapy for herpes hominus infections. Obstet. Gynecol., *45*:335, 1975.

Dawson, D. F.: Giant condyloma and verrucous carcinoma of genital area. Arch. Pathol., *79*:225, 1965.

Deacon, W. E.: VDRL chancroid studies TV. Experimental chancroid prophylaxis and treatment. Antibiot. Med., *2*:143, 1956.

Dienst, R. B., Chen, C. H., and Greenblatt, R. B.: Granuloma inguinale. Urol. Cutan. Rev., *53*:537, 1949.

Dienst, R. B., Chen, C. H., and Greenblatt, R. B.: Experimental transfer of chemoresistant granuloma inguinale. Am. J. Syph., *34*:189, 1950.

Donovan, C.: Malaria. Indian Med. Gaz., *40*:411, 1905.

Dretter, S. P., and Klein, L. A.: The eradication of intraurethral condyloma acuminata with 5 percent 5-fluorouracil cream. J. Urol., *113*:195, 1975.

Epstein, E.: Regional Dermatologic Diagnosis. Philadelphia, Lea & Febiger, 1950.

Ewell, G. H.: Traumatic epididymo-orchitis. JAMA, *113*:1105, 1939.

Fitz, G. S., Hubler, W. R., Jr., Dodson, R. F., and Randolph, A.: Mutilating granuloma inguinale. Arch. Dermatol., *111*:1464, 1975.

Fournier, J. A.: Étude clinique de la gangrene foudroyante de la verge. Semaine Med., *4*:69, 1884.

Frankland, A. W.: Deficiency scrotal dermatitis in P.O.W.'s in the Far East. Br. Med. J., *1*:1023, 1948.

Friedman, N. B., and Garske, G. L.: Inflammatory reactions involving spermatic granuloma and granulomatous orchitis. J. Urol., *62*:363, 1949.

Friedman, S.: Queyrat's erythroplasia with carcinomatous invasion: Report of an unusual case. J. Urol., *69*:813, 1953.

Gaisin, A., and Heaton, C. L.: Chancroid: Alias the soft chancre. Int. J. Dermatol., *14*:188, 1975.

Gall, E. A.: The histopathology of acute mumps orchitis. Am. J. Pathol., *23*:637, 1947.

Garrow, I., and Werne, J.: Metastatic epididymitis. Urol. Cutan. Rev., *51*:3, 1947.

Gartman, E.: Intraurethral condyloma. J. Urol., *75*:717, 1956.

Gellis, S. S., McGuiness, A. C., and Peters, M.: Study on prevention of mumps orchitis by gamma globulin. Am. J. Med. Sci., *210*:661, 1945.

Gibson, T. E.: Idiopathic gangrene of scrotum. J. Urol., *23*:125, 1930.

Goldberg, J.: Studies on granuloma inguinale. Br. J. Vener. Dis., *42*:205, 1966.

Goldgreber, M. B.: Specific disease simulating non-specific ulcerative colitis. Ann. Intern. Med., *47*:939, 1957.

Govan, D. E., and Perkash, I.: Urethral catheterization. Invest. Urol., *5*:394, 1968.

Graves, R. S., and Engel, W. J.: Experimental production of epididymitis with sterile urine; clinical implications. J. Urol., *64*:601, 1950.

Greenbaum, S. S.: Scrotum: Dermatologic lesions. *In* Piersal, G. W., and Bortz, E. L. (Eds.): The Cyclopedia of Medicine, Surgery, and Specialties. Philadelphia, F. A. Davis, 1940.

Greenblatt, R. B.: Granuloma inguinale, lymphogranuloma venereum. *In* Current Therapy, 1960. Philadelphia, W. B. Saunders Co., 1960, pp. 398–399.

Greenblatt, R. B., Dienst, R. B., Pund, E. R., and Torpin, R.: Experimental and clinical granuloma inguinale. JAMA, *113*:1109, 1939.

Harvard, B. M.: Acute monilial balanitis. J. Urol., *85*:374, 1961.

Haury, B., Rodeheaver, G., Stevenson, T., et al.: Streptococcal cellulitis of the scrotum and penis with secondary skin gangrene. Surg. Gynecol. Obstet., *141*:35, 1975.

Herman, L., and Klauder, J. V.: Studies of the prenatal transmission of syphilis. I. Syphilis of the testicle. Am. J. Med. Sci., *159*:705, 1920.

Hinman, F.: Principles and Practice of Urology. Philadelphia, W. B. Saunders Co., 1935.

Hinman, F., and Johnson, C. M.: The differential diagnosis of acute fat necrosis in the scrotum. J. Urol., *41*:726, 1939.

Hoyne, A. L., Diamond, J. H., and Christian, J. R.: Diethylstilbestrol in treatment of mumps orchitis. JAMA, *140*:663, 1949.

Iannuzzi, G.: Le Epididimiti e Orchiti Specifiche e Aspecifiche. Roma, 1942.

Isaac, A. G.: Orchitis and epididymitis due to undulant fever. J. Urol., *40*:201, 1938.

Jannach, J. R.: Granuloma inguinale of the epididymis. Br. J. Vener. Dis., *34*:31, 1958.

Jansen, T. G., Dillaha, C. J., and Honeycutt, W. M: Bowenoid conditions of the skin. South. Med. J., *60*:185, 1967.

Johnson, B. L., and Baxter, D. L.: Pearly penile papules. Arch. Dermatol., *90*:166, 1964.

Jones, R. B., Hirschmann, J. V., Brown, G. S., and Tremann, J. A.: Fournier's syndrome: Necrotizing subcutaneous infection of the male genitalia. J. Urol., *122*:279, 1979.

Kass, E. H., and Sossen, H. S.: Prevention of infection of urinary tract in presence of indwelling catheters. JAMA, *169*:1181, 1959.

Kaufman, J. J., and Silver, B. B.: Tuberculous ulcer of the penis. J. Urol., *72*:226, 1954.

Kerber, R. E.: Treatment of chancroid. Arch. Dermatol., *100*:604, 1969.

Kornblith, B. A.: Lymphogranuloma venereum and granuloma inguinale. J. Insur. Med., *5*:30, 1949–50.

Lamb, R. C., and Juler, G. L.: Fournier's gangrene of the scrotum. Arch. Surg., *118*:38, 1983.

Levin, E. A.: The diagnosis of chancroid. Urol. Cutan. Rev., *45*:587, 1941.

Lisser, H., and Hinman, F.: Syphilis of the epididymis without involvement of the testicle. Am. J. Syph., *2*:465, 1918.

Lynn, J. M., and Nesbit, R. M.: Influence of vasectomy upon the incidence of epididymitis following transurethral prostatectomy. J. Urol., *59*:72, 1948.

Machacek, G. F., and Weakley, D. R.: Giant condylomata. Arch. Dermatol., *80*:82, 1960.

Mackay-Dick, J.: Infective mononucleosis. J. R. Army Med. Corps, *82*:279, 1944.

Mair, G. B.: Idiopathic gangrene of scrotum. Lancet, *1*:464, 1945.

Marmell, M.: Granuloma inguinale: Treatment with methacycline. N.Y. J. Med., *64*:804, 1964.

Marmell, M.: Donovanosis of the anus in the male: An epidemiological consideration. Br. J. Vener. Dis., *34*:213, 1958.

Marmell, M.: Oleandomycin in the treatment of Donovanosis. Antibiot. Med. Clin. Ther., *3*:263, 1956.

Mathe, C. P.: Suppurative orchitis; its diagnosis and treatment. J. Urol., *34*:324, 1935.

McCord, C. P., and Minister, D. K.: Lead orchitis. JAMA, *82*:1104, 1924.

McDaniel, W. E.: Four venereal diseases. J. Ky. Med. Assoc., *62*:281, 1964.

McDonald, D. F., Hulet, W. H., and Cowan, J. W.: Scrotal gangrene treated with oxygen under high pressure. J. Urol., *113*:364, 1975.

McDonald, J. H., and Heckel, N. J.: Acute pneumococcal epididymitis. Ill. Med. J., *95*:304, 1949.

McGavin, D.: Thrombosis of pampiniform plexus. Lancet, *2*:368, 1935.

McLachlan, A. E. W.: Syphilitic epididymitis. Br. J. Vener. Dis., *14*:134, 1938.

Merricks, J. W., and Cottrell, T. L.: Erythroplasia of Queyrat. J. Urol., *69*:807, 1953.

Michelson, H. E.: Syphilis of the epididymis. JAMA, *73*:1431, 1919.

Mongan, E. S.: The treatment of mumps orchitis with prednisone. Am. J. Med. Sci., *237*:749, 1959.

Moulder, J. W.: The relation of the psittacosis group (chlamydiae) to bacteria and viruses. Ann. Rev. Microbiol., *20*:107, 1966.

Neumann, H.: Neurodermatitis circumscripta venenosa scroti. Zentralbl. Haut Geschlechtskr., *62*:617, 1939.

Nickel, W. R., and Plumb, R. T.: Nonvenereal sclerosing lymphangitis. Arch. Dermatol., *86*:761, 1962.

Nixon, N., and Lewis, D. B.: Mumps orchitis; surgical treatment. J. Urol., *56*:554, 1946.

Norton, R. J.: Use of diethylstilbestrol in orchitis due to mumps. JAMA, *143*:172, 1950.

Novy, F. G., Jr.: The newer antibiotics in dermatology. Calif. Med., *72*:201, 1950.

O'Connor, F. M.: Erythema multiforme exudativum. Arch. Dermatol., *77*:532, 1958.

Oeconomos, N.: Deferentitis considered as a clinical entity. Urol. Cutan. Rev., *52*:388, 1948.

Packer, H., and Goldberg, J.: Complement fixation studies in granuloma inguinale. Am. J. Trop. Med., *30*:387, 1950.

Pariser, H., Goldberg, S. Z., and Mitchell, G. H.: Streptomycin in the treatment of granuloma inguinale. Arch. Dermatol. Syph., *62*:261, 1950.

Peterslund, N. A., Ipsen, J., Schonheyder, H., Seyer-Hansen, K., Esmann, V., and Juhl, H.: Acyclovir in herpes zoster. Lancet, *2*:827, 1981.

Pinck, B. D.: Surgical treatment of mumps orchitis. Urol. Cutan. Rev., *51*:257, 1947.

Pinkus, H., and Gould, S. E.: Extramammary Paget's disease and intraepidermal carcinoma. Arch. Dermatol. Syph., *39*:479, 1939.

Poynter, J., and Levy, J.: Balanitis xerotica obliterans. Br. J. Urol., *39*:420, 1967.

Queyrat, R.: Erythroplasie du gland. Bull. Soc. Franc. Dermatol. Syph., *22*:378, 1911.

Rainey, R.: The association of lymphopathia inguinale and cancer. Surgery, *35*:221, 1954.

Rambar, A. C.: Use of convalescent serum in the treatment and prophylaxis of orchitis. Am. J. Dis. Child., *71*:1, 1946.

Robinson, H. M., Jr.: The treatment of granuloma inguinale, lymphogranuloma venereum, chancroid and gonorrhea. Arch. Dermatol. Syph., *64*:284, 1951.

Rolnick, H. C.: Syphilis of the epididymis. J. Urol., *12*:147, 1924.

Ronchese, F.: Calcification and ossification of steatomas of the scrotum. Arch. Dermatol. Syph., *49*:12, 1944; with correction, *49*:304, 1944.

Rondall, A.: Idiopathic gangrene of scrotum. J. Urol., *4*:219, 1920.

Rosenberg, W.: Abscess of the testicle. J. Urol., *34*:44, 1935.

Roshan, P. D.: Autopsy studies in syphilis. J. Vener. Dis. Inform., *27*:293, 1946.

Rowe, R. J.: Evaluation of chloromycetin as an adjunct to the surgical management of lymphogranuloma venereum and segmental ulcerative colitis. Am. J. Surg., *81*:42, 1951.

Rudolph, R., Soloway, M., DePalma, R. G., et al.: Fournier's syndrome: Synergistic gangrene of the scrotum. Am. J. Surg., *129*:591, 1975.

Schachter, J., Dawson, C. R., Balas, S., and Jones, P.: Evaluation of methods for detecting acute TRIC agent infections. Am. J. Ophthalmol., *70*:381, 1970.

Schmidt, S. S., and Hinman, F.: The effect of vasectomy upon the incidence of epididymitis after prostatectomy. J. Urol., *63*:872, 1950.

Semon, H. C. G.: An Atlas of the Commoner Diseases. Baltimore, The Williams & Wilkins Co., 1947.

Serota, F. T., Starr, S. E., Bryan, C. K., Koch, P. A., Plotkin, S. A., and August, C. S.: Acyclovir treatment of herpes zoster infections: Use in children undergoing bone marrow transplantation. JAMA, *247*:2132, 1982.

Serri, F.: Le orchioepidimiti da pneumobacillo di Friedlander. G. Ital. Dermatol. Sif., *87*:291, 1946.

Slotkin, G. E.: Industrial epididymitis and epididymo-orchitis. N.Y. State J. Med., *39*:1096, 1939.

Smith, I. M., and Bishir, J. W.: Treatment of mumps orchitis with ACTH and cortisone. N. Engl. J. Med., *258*:120, 1958.

Smith, R. G.: Plasma treatment of mumps orchitis. U.S. Navy Med. Bull., *44*:159, 1945.

Sobel, N.: Chancroid. *In* Current Therapy, 1960. Philadelphia, W. B. Saunders Co., 1960, p. 395.

Steinberg, J., and Straus, R.: Sperm invasion of the epididymis. J. Urol., *57*:498, 1947.

Stengel, A., Jr.: Mumps orchitis. Am. J. Med. Sci., *191*:340, 1936.

Stokes, J. H.: Modern Clinical Syphilology. Philadelphia, W. B. Saunders Co., 1946.

Stokes, J. H., Besancon, J. H., and Schoch, A. G.: Infectious recurrence and mucocutaneous relapse in syphilis. JAMA, *96*:344, 1931.

Sutton, R. L., and Sutton, R. L., Jr.: Handbook of Diseases of the Skin. St. Louis, C. V. Mosby Co., 1949.

Tan, R.: Fournier's gangrene of the scrotum and penis. J. Urol., *92*:508, 1964.

Thomas, J. F.: Fournier's gangrene. J. Urol., *75*:719, 1956.

Thompson, L.: Syphilis of the genital organs of the male and the urinary organs. Am. J. Syph., *4*:706, 1920.

Trasoff, A., and Goodman, D. H.: Rheumatic orchitis associated with rheumatic pericarditis and effusion. Med. Ann. D. C., *13*:149, 1944.

Tunbridge, R. E., and Gavey, C. J.: Epidemic epididymo-orchitis in Malta. Lancet, *1*:775, 1946.

United States Department of Health, Education and Welfare. Center for Disease Control: Bulletin, No. 980376. Atlanta, Center for Disease Control, 1976.

Variot, G.: Nigritie congénitale du scrotum et hyperpigmentation des petites livres chez des enfants nouveau-nés. Bull. Mém. Soc. Anthrop. (Paris) 6s, *1*:76, 1910.

Veenema, R. J., and Lattimer, J. K.: Genital tuberculosis in the male. J. Urol., *78*:65, 1957.

Wang, S., and Grayston, J. T.: Human serology in *Chlamydia trachomatis* infection with microimmunofluorescence. J. Infect. Dis., *130*:388, 1974.

Wang, S., and Grayston, J. T.: Immunologic relationship between genital TRIC, lymphogranuloma venereum and related organisms in a new microtitre indirect immunofluorescence test. Am. J. Ophthalmol., *70*:367, 1970.

Weber, F. P.: A note on supposed "calcinosis" of the scrotum. Br. J. Dermatol. Syph., *48*:312, 1936.

Weinstein, M., and Roberts, M.: Elephantiasis and the Kondolean operation. Am. J. Surg., *79*:327, 1950.

Wershub, L. P.: Urology and Industry. Springfield, Ill., Charles C Thomas, 1956.

Wesselhoeft, C., and Vose, S. N.: Surgical treatment of severe orchitis in mumps. N. Engl. J. Med., *227*:277, 1942.

Wesson, M. B.: "Traumatic orchitis": A misnomer. JAMA, *91*:1857, 1923.

Weyrauch, H. M., and Gass, H.: Urogenital complications of dengue fever. J. Urol., *55*:90, 1946.

Wilensky, A. O., and Samuels, S. S.: Acute deferentitis and funiculitis. Ann. Surg., *78*:785, 1923.

Wilhelmi, O. J.: Use of corticosteroids in urologic practice. J. Urol., *82*:375, 1959.

Willcox, R. R.: Effectiveness of antichancroidal drugs tested by auto inoculation of bubo fluid. Am. J. Syph., *34*:378, 1950.

Willcox, R. R.: The treatment of chancroid. Br. J. Clin. Pract., *17*:455, 1963.

Zak, V. I.: Actinomycosis of the penis. Urologia Moskva, *23*:65, 1958.

Zoon, J. J.: Balanoposthite chronique circonscrite benigue à plasmocytes. Dermatologica, *105*:1, 1952.

CHAPTER 21

Parasitic Diseases of the Genitourinary System*

FRANZ VON LICHTENBERG, M.D.
JAY STAUFFER LEHMAN, M.D.†

Parasitic disease is a major health problem today, especially in developing countries, but the human urogenital tract is regularly affected by only a few species of parasites. Three will be discussed in some detail.

Schistosoma haematobium, a digenetic blood fluke, can cause life-threatening uropathy; filarial roundworms of the genera *Wuchereria* and *Brugia* can give rise to funiculoepididymitis, hydrocele, genital elephantiasis, or chyluria; and *Trichomonas vaginalis,* a protozoan flagellate, can cause troublesome, but rarely severe, urogenital symptoms. Sexually transmitted protozoal enteric diseases, especially among male homosexuals, have recently come into the limelight of professional and public attention and will also be discussed briefly. Genitourinary involvement due to other parasites is either subordinate to systemic manifestations, or rare; only brief descriptions of these entities will be given here. Finally, proteinuria or—more rarely—renal failure may complicate endemic malaria, schistosomiasis, and, probably, other parasitic infections; our present understanding of these associations will be outlined.‡

In the aggregate, millions of people have parasitic infections of the genitourinary tract; accurate prevalence figures for urinary schistosomiasis and for filariasis are available for only a few well-studied census populations; as many as 40 to 60 per cent of adult women seen in gynecologic practices are said to harbor trichomonads. In each instance, however, the number of symptomatic infections is substantially lower than the total number. One must therefore clearly distinguish between *parasitic infection* and *parasitic disease,* which constitutes a variable fraction of total prevalence, depending on intensity of infection and other complex pathogenic factors.

At a time when many endemic infections are beginning to come under better control, schistosomiasis and filariasis continue to increase. Irrigational agriculture tends to spread vector snail populations, and human crowding in tropical cities favors mosquito-host contact. At the same time, modern population mobility and jet travel are bringing "tropical diseases" to the doorsteps of physicians who lack familiarity with their management.

The single most important requirement for recognition of parasitic infections is still *awareness,* based on knowledge of parasitic life cycles, pathology, and geographic distribution, which must be retained beyond the time of brief medical school exposure. There must also be *careful history taking,* including the question of "unde venis?" ("Where have you been?"), and there must be knowledgeable and competent *parasitologic laboratory back-up,* currently available in only a few health centers.

Management of parasitic diseases tran-

*The authors wish to acknowledge support for their research and in the preparation of this manuscript by NIH–NIAID Grant R-22-AI-02631-25, and Grant 280-0160 of the Edna McConnell Clark Foundation, N.Y.

†Dr. Jay Stauffer Lehman died in 1979, but his contributions to this chapter have since required only minor revision. To honor Dr. Lehman's substantial legacy to American Tropical Medicine and to preserve the memory of this outstanding young physician and epidemiologist, his authorship is being continued.

‡Disseminated toxoplasmosis in renal transplant patients undergoing immunosuppressive therapy is discussed separately in Section XV, Chapter 66.

scends urogenital manifestations and must be addressed to the whole patient. Decisions on when and how to use parasiticidal drugs require a thorough understanding of the patient's pathologic condition and up-to-date knowledge of the best available drugs for the different parasites. Such information is often difficult to obtain from standard texts, and consultation is advisable for physicians with limited experience in such matters.

Assistance can be obtained from key faculty of university- or government-sponsored health centers that maintain tropical disease training programs, including, in the continental United States, the Centers for Disease Control in Atlanta, which maintain both a laboratory consulting service and a drug repository for parasitic diseases, with liaison to the various state laboratories.*

URINARY SCHISTOSOMIASIS

First recognized by Egyptian physicians of the XIIth Dynasty (1900 B.C.), schistosomiasis haematobia has been a scourge of the great agricultural civilizations of the Middle East for millennia, and it is still today a major cause of disease and death in these fertile river valleys. It is also endemic throughout most of Africa, and through Southwest Asia as far as Iran, posing a risk for visitors to any of the regions named.

Infection is acquired by exposure to water that harbors the infected bulinid snail host. In endemic foci, it usually first manifests itself in children or adolescents by apparently inconsequential hematuria, followed by an asymptomatic period that may persist indefinitely or may be followed by obstructive uropathy, with or without bacterial superinfection, leading to renal failure and death. A wide spectrum of other pathologic and clinical manifestations can occur, and there is an apparent correlation with the occurrence of urothelial cancer. Clinical management and prognosis depend to a considerable extent on the intensity of infection and on the stage of the pathologic condition; an understanding of the natural history of the disease is therefore essential.

Biology and Life Cycle

The life cycle of digenetic trematodes consists of a sexual reproductive phase, namely egg laying, which is carried out by long-lived adult worms in the blood vessels of the definitive mammalian host, and an asexual phase represented by sporocyst development inside the specific snail intermediate host. The results of sexual multiplication, the miracidia, and of asexual multiplication, the cercariae, must each migrate through fresh water in order to complete the cycle by penetrating the snail or the mammalian skin, respectively (Fig. 21–1).

The normal habitat of the adult *Schistosoma haematobium* comprises postcapillary vesical and pelvic venules of man (other mammals are only sporadically infected); these vessels are largely tributaries of the caval system but are connected to the portal venous system via collaterals. The worms measure about 1.5 cm in length, the male being lanceolate with a central fold ("gynecophorous canal") that grasps the slender, rounded female in permanent copula. Although worm pairs are attached to the endothelium by their acetabula and are in intimate contact with the vessel in which they nest, no clotting or inflammation occurs around them while they produce and lay between 200 and 500 eggs per day; thus, during its estimated median life span of 5 to 10 years (Warren et al., 1974), even a single worm pair will spawn several million eggs. According to experimental data, about one fifth of the eggs are excreted via the urine or feces, while the rest are deposited in situ (i.e., the urogenital and pelvic organs) or are swept to the lung, liver, and other widespread sites via the blood stream (Cheever and Anderson, 1971). Local egg deposition by *S. haematobium* is clustered (several eggs at one time), so that a few worms, strategically placed, can produce significant lesions.

S. haematobium eggs measure about 80 by 150 nm, are ovoid, tannish in color, thin-shelled, and terminally spined (Fig. 21–2); unlike the laterally spined *Schistosoma mansoni* eggs, they are not acid-fast upon appropriate staining. The only other schistosome that is pathogenic for humans and has similar terminally spined eggs, *Schistosoma intercalatum,* is rarely seen ouside limited foci in the Republic of Zaire; thus, the finding of terminally spined eggs in urine or urinary organ tissue is, for practical purposes, pathognomonic of *S. haematobium* infection.

Egg maturation begins in utero from a single oocyte stage, and it continues after posture for several days until the miracidium forms. Mature miracidia remain viable within eggs for less than 3 weeks (probably only about 12 days); if not extruded into water within that period, they die and the eggs become "dark," i.e., degenerate. In active infection, all egg stages from immature to degenerate are therefore

---

*Centers for Disease Control, Bureau of Epidemiology, Parasitic Disease Branch, Atlanta, Georgia.

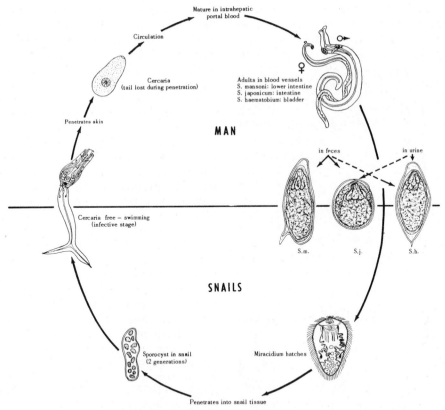

Figure 21–1. The life cycle of a schistosome. (From U.S. Department of Health and Human Services, Public Health Service Publications, U.S. Government Printing Office, Washington, D.C.)

seen, while in cured or inactive infection only degenerate (dark) eggs appear in the tissues or excreta. Eggs frequently become calcified in *S. haematobium* infection; after decalcification, most of these eggs are seen to contain dead but morphologically preserved miracidia.

Upon deposition into fresh water, eggs swell osmotically, and miracidia break the shell and emerge as autonomous, short-lived, ciliated larvae that engage in active swimming and host-seeking. Guided by phototropism and by snail trace materials (Chernin, 1974), they encounter snails of one or another local *Bulinus* species (e.g., *B. truncatus* in Egypt, *B. globosus* in subsaharan Africa), penetrate them, migrate through their tissue, and transform into successive generations of mother-and-daughter sporocysts, from which cercariae are eventually produced. This enormous, asexual multiplication from a single miracidium to up to 10^5 cercariae compensates for the attrition suffered during the aquatic part of the life cycle.

Cercariae continue to be shed by infected snails for several days or weeks. They consist of a body (ca. 175 μm), i.e., an undifferentiated, but genotypically male or female miniature worm, and a forked muscular tail (ca. 220 μm) that propels the body through water by energetic, vibratory movements. The cercariae penetrate the unbroken mammalian corneal skin layer, at which time the tail drops off. If penetration is not accomplished within a few hours after shedding, cercariae become lethargic and die.

Upon successful penetration of a susceptible host, the cercarial body undergoes a sudden and radical adaptation to the new, isotonic environment—with attendant mortality of up to two thirds of all penetrating organisms—and, after a variable resting stop in the dermis (Fig. 21–3), the new schistosomulum begins its migratory and maturation process, which in the case of *S. haematobium* may require as long as 80 to 110 days.

Migration routes are not completely known, but they include blood and lymph vessels, and possibly tissue spaces as well. Concentrations of schistosomula occur in the lung at 4 to 7 days, and in the liver from about the second week onward as growth of the worms accelerates. Finally, homing, pairing, and nesting of adults are completed, and oviposition begins,

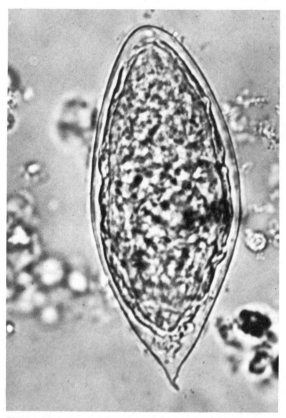

Figure 21–2. Egg of *Schistosoma haematobium*, as seen in urinary sediment. × 800. (Courtesy of Dr. Steven Pan, Harvard School of Public Health.)

hesitantly at first, but soon followed by a steep ascent to the maximal egg-laying level, which is thereafter maintained in somewhat irregular fashion, until the ultimate decline and death of the worms.

In overview, the delicately balanced life cycle just described would seem to depend on so many fortuitous conjunctions that it could easily be disturbed, but like other prodigies of nature it has proved remarkably hardy and has resisted many human attempts to interrupt it.

Distribution and Epidemiology

Transmission of *S. haematobium* occurs throughout the African continent, including the islands of Madagascar and Mauritius. In Southwest Asia, it is found in Southern Yemen, Yemen, Saudi Arabia, Israel, Lebanon, Syria, Turkey, Iraq, and Iran. There is also a small focus in the Indian state of Maharashtra, the easternmost location known. Outside these zones, all diagnosed cases have been imported (Wright, 1973).

Within the vast endemic regions, preva-

lence and infection intensity vary widely, as does the public health importance of the disease. Typically, these are highest in regions in which irrigational agriculture is long established, such as the Nile Valley and Delta. In most countries, transmission of *S. haematobium* is fairly widespread; where it coexists with *S. mansoni,* the former is usually more extensive and the latter more focal. In Israel, foci are now few and highly circumscribed, and in Cyprus the last few foci have apparently been eradicated. Conversely, countries in which transmission is actually or predictably on the increase are quite numerous, especially around large water projects in the Sudan, and around the Aswan Dam and Lake Volta (Vander Schalie, 1974). Regional strains of *S. haematobium* are thought to vary in "virulence" because of differences in the vector snail species or because of unknown factors involving the parasite, but this matter will require further definition.

In endemic settings, first exposure occurs most frequently in children of preschool or school age, and it is followed by repeated additional exposures. In those communities in which exposure is primarily a matter of swimming and bathing, or of clothes-washing in rivers or lakes, infection may decrease in adults; on the other hand, fishermen, boatyard workers, and others with occupational water contact may continue to be exposed (Gilles et al., 1965). The distribution among the sexes also seems to depend on exposure patterns that, in many communities, are biased toward the male. Little is known about the relationship between exposure patterns and acquired resistance in man. In some heavily exposed human groups, such as the canal-cleaners of the Sudan, remarkably little overt disease has been noted, and recent cohort studies of infected children suggest that infection levels may stabilize at a time when repeat exposures are still continuing (Bradley and McCullough, 1973). In fact, the case for acquired human immunity is probably better documented for *S. haematobium* than for other schistosome species.

In both clinical and autopsy studies, the prevalence of infection and its intensity, as measured by egg excretion or by tissue egg load, have been found to be related. Tissue egg load, in turn, is related to the pathologic condition. Autopsy studies in Nigeria and in Egypt (Smith et al., 1974, 1975; Edington et al., 1970a and b) have shown that severe uropathy is uncommon in populations with frequency of infection at autopsy of less than 30 per cent but it increases significantly when this threshold is exceeded.

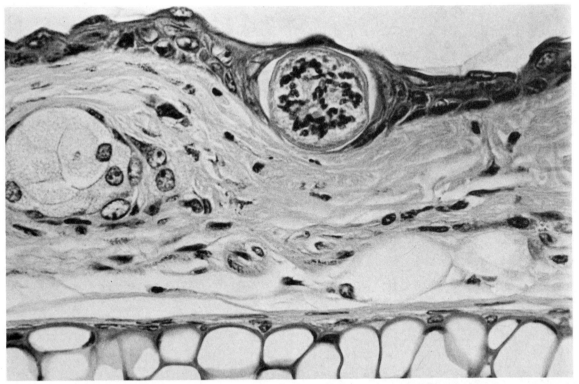

Figure 21–3. Schistosomulum traversing the epidermis of the mouse ear. × 800.

Pathology and Pathogenesis

Although cercarial penetration and migration elicit cellular responses and immunologic reactions, these are rarely severe enough to cause clinical symptoms (see later). Most clinical disease is related to egg deposition.

The basic tissue response to schistosome eggs is the formation of granulomas ("pseudotubercles") around them, i.e., an accumulation of macrophages, lymphoid cells, and eosinophils that is elicited by antigens released from the egg (Fig. 21–4) and is modulated by the cell-mediated immunity of the host or by an interplay between cellular and humoral factors (Warren, 1973a). Experimentally, individual schistosome granulomas have been shown to enlarge and plateau at 8 days in the sensitized host, concomitant with egg maturation, and slowly to involute within 4 to 6 months (von Lichtenberg, 1973, 1962). (See Figs. 21–5 and 21–6.) In patent human infections, all stages of this process are simultaneously present. In addition, the early pathologic effects of *S. haematobium* infection, known principally from primate studies (Sadun et al., 1970), have a diffuse inflammatory component seen in the sites of active egg laying when large numbers of eggs are amassed.

Grossly, the early schistosomal bladder shows sessile, polypoid mucosal patches, covered by partly eroded, hyperemic mucosa,

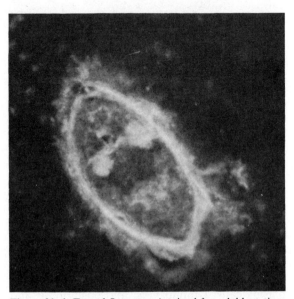

Figure 21–4. Egg of *S. mansoni* stained for soluble antigen by the direct immunofluorescent technique. Note positivity of apical glands and around eggshell in the granuloma center.

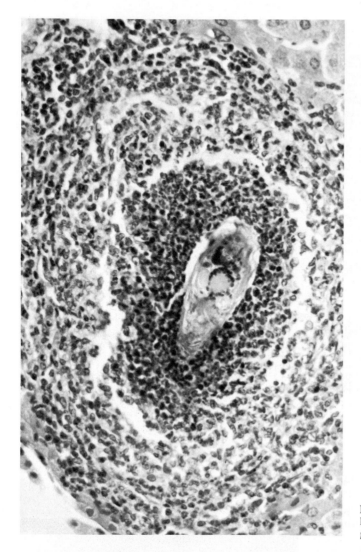

Figure 21–5. Early schistosome granuloma in the liver, showing mature miracidium and numerous granulocytes. × 420.

sharply delimited and composed of edematous granulation tissue (Figs. 21–7 and 21–8). Underlying the polypoid patch one finds scattered granulomas and nesting adult worm pairs. There is, as well, a scattering of eggs and smaller lesions in the flat portions of the bladder mucosa. Ureteral patches tend to be concentric, and the lumen may show narrowing or fusiform dilatation at their level. Similar lesions may appear in the rectum.

Histologically, in the early lesions, numerous eggs may be seen permeating the mucosa and submucosa. Scattered granulomas are large and abscess-like, with numerous eosinophils; the granulation tissue between them is rich in plasma cells, lymphocytes, and eosinophils and is markedly edematous. Polypoid patches are clinically observed mainly in children through their early teens, largely by pyelogram, in which they appear as bulky rounded rarefactions, and most often are midline or symmetric on the posterior wall of the bladder. More rarely, similar lesions are seen in association with the advanced pathologic state that predominates in adult bladders. Polypoid patches almost certainly undergo spontaneous reversion in some patients and have been found to undergo rapid involution or disappearance following antischistosomal therapy (Lucas et al., 1966).

During the chronic active stage of infection—usually the second or third decade of life—schistosomal bladders show "sandy patches," i.e., relatively flat, granular, tannish mucosal lesions of variable depth (as determined by the amount of egg deposition), often less sharply defined than the early exudative lesions just described (Figs. 21–9 and 21–10). Whether sandy patches evolve out of polypoid patches,

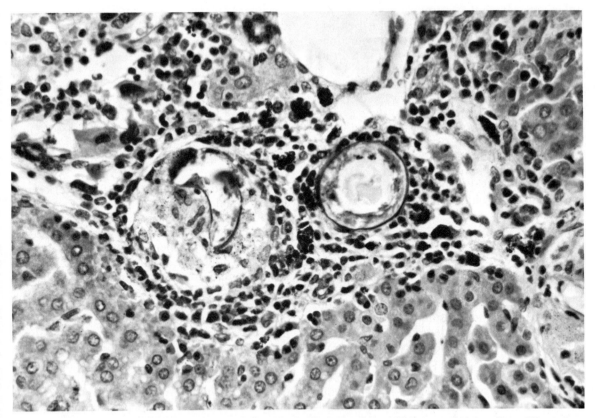

Figure 21–6. Late *S. haematobium* granuloma in the liver, showing calcified egg and giant cell. × 420.

or arise de novo, or both, has not been settled. Sandy patch distribution in the bladder ranges from a single locus to nearly total bladder involvement; in the latter case, it may be more difficult to define endoscopically or by autopsy gross examination but can be sensed as a slightly gritty or "sandy" feel to the touch. Hyperemia and erosion are less prominent and more focal in these lesions than at the earlier stages, but deep, linear ulcers may form in patches that have become thickly encrusted and stiff. What is termed a calcified bladder is, essentially, a thick, circumferential, coalescent sandy patch that may be a few millimeters to over 1 cm deep, and it contains sufficient numbers of calcified eggs to appear as a shell-like radiopaque edge on x-ray films of the bladder, or as a cloudy veil on frontal projection. A variant of the sandy patch is the fibrous patch, in which scar tissue accumulates, thus hiding the sandy elements and substituting tough, keloid-like tissue. Sandy or fibrous patches around the ureteral orifices can produce variable distortion, such as narrowing or incompetence, or a golf-ball hole appearance; much more rarely, the urethral infundibulum, or the urethra itself, is stiffened or narrowed, but trigonal retraction

and deformity, as reported in early texts, are not seen in schistosomiasis unless there is associated bacterial cystitis (see later). Similarly, ureteral stenosis directly attributable to encroachment by sandy or fibrous patches is less common than is ureteral dilatation.

Microscopically, while oviposition persists, groups of intact, viable eggs may be seen mixed with calcific egg deposits, and eggs continue to be excreted in relatively substantial proportions into the urine. Responses to viable eggs vary; in the most active sites, numerous plasma cells and eosinophils continue to be present. The bulk of sandy patches, however, is made up of masses of calcified eggs, packed closely together within a delicate fibrous matrix infiltrated by sparse lymphocytes. These deposits largely occupy the submucosal layer; lesser numbers of eggs are scattered throughout the muscular and outer layers of the bladder. As activity of infection declines, inflammatory reaction also tends to subside; eosinophils and plasma cells disappear, and lymphoid cell infiltrates become less prominent. By the time the cell reaction disappears, worm pairs can no longer be found, and all the eggs have become calcified or nonviable.

Urothelial changes accompany all stages of

infection. Mucosal hyperplasia takes the form of Brunn's nests, with thickening of the surface layer; squamous metaplasia is very common, though substantial keratinization is not. Epithelial dysplasia is variable, but it can be quite severe, with atypical syncytial cells showing dense hyperchromatic convoluted nuclei, which are also noted in urinary sediments and cytologic smears. In Egyptian cases, cyst formation (cystitis cystica), sometimes with calcification of the epithelial cyst contents (cystitis cystica calcinosa), is not uncommon. Glandular metaplasia also occurs, with the epithelium exhibiting mucus-producing goblet cells so as to resemble colonic mucosa.

The relationship of these lesions to schistosome infection or to associated bacterial cystitis, or to both, is often difficult to judge, but bladders showing extensive lymph follicle formation (cystitis lymphofollicularis) are usually associated with *Salmonella* superinfection, rather than with schistosomal infection alone.

Parasite-bacteria interaction may also be of importance in aggravating obstructive uropathy and in potentiating kidney damage. It is clear from autopsy statistical analysis that obstructive uropathy can result from schistosomal involvement alone, in the absence of any other etiologic factor; in fact, there is a direct correlation between the intensity of infection, as judged by tissue egg load, and the frequency of obstructive uropathy (Edington et al., 1970a). However, it has also been shown that schistosomal obstructive uropathy predisposes to both vesical and renal bacterial infection, similar to but perhaps even more commonly than obstructive uropathy due to other causes.

While schistosomal obstructive uropathy tends to be bilateral, it is frequently asymmetric, and there is extreme variation in the distribution of affected ureteral segments (Figs. 21–11 and 21–12). In autopsy statistics, severe ureteral involvement and especially high involvement tend to correlate with high infection intensity. However, even at low intensity a strategically placed single obstructive ureteral patch can have severe consequences. This event has been observed both in human patients and in experimental primates, and it is a reminder that low-level infections cannot be disregarded.

In the ureter, several types of lesions have been observed, related to stage and infection intensity. A common type of cylindrical hydroureter affects predominantly the lower ureteral segments, with widening and sinuosity of the distal portion (Figs. 21–9 and 21–10). Although the lower ureter usually has more *S.*

haematobium eggs, it is difficult to account for cylindrical ureterectasis, especially in the mildly infected patient. It has been suggested that this may be caused by interference with peristaltic function or by reflux rather than by true anatomic obstruction. Cylindrical dilatation in early infection is reversible by treatment, and a large proportion of obstructive uropathy reported in post-mortem studies is due to relatively innocuous, minimal ureteral dilatation, which often appears to have been asymptomatic and nonprogressive.

Segmental obstruction of the ureter by mural or ostial schistosomal patches (Figs. 21–11 and 21–12) is potentially more serious. This "stenotic" lesion more frequently causes severe hydroureter, hydronephrotic atrophy, and cessation of function of the homolateral kidney; clinical and autopsy data suggest its occurrence at a relatively early age, especially when stenotic involvement is bilateral.

Schistosomal infection in the endemic population is often additive to, and interrelated with, other pathologic background urinary tract conditions, such as lower and upper urinary tract bacterial infections, obstruction due to prostatism, or urinary stone formation. Pyelonephritis and other forms of parenchymal kidney disease are relatively frequent overall in Egypt and in other African countries, but only pyelonephritis (and not glomerulonephritis or arterionephrosclerosis) is more frequent and severe in association with schistosomiasis haematobia (Smith et al., 1974; Edington et al., 1970a).

The relationship between urinary schistosomiasis and bladder cancer has been a subject of unending debate over several decades. Although reliable statistics are lacking, bladder cancer is more frequent, occurs at an earlier age, and is more often of the squamous variety in Egypt and in some other endemic areas than in industrialized countries. Skeptics point out that bladder cancer frequency is also greater in some nonendemic African environments, but most researchers favor the hypothesis that schistosome infection might act as a cocarcinogen (Cheever, 1978). We have already mentioned the frequency of hyperplasia/metaplasia/dysplasia of the urothelium seen both in the presence and in the absence of true neoplasm. What has not been elucidated is the fate of these lesions with or without treatment of the underlying infection. Prospective studies would be difficult to carry out, given the insidious manner in which bladder cancer tends to arise in the patient with schistosomiasis. Not only are symptoms such as

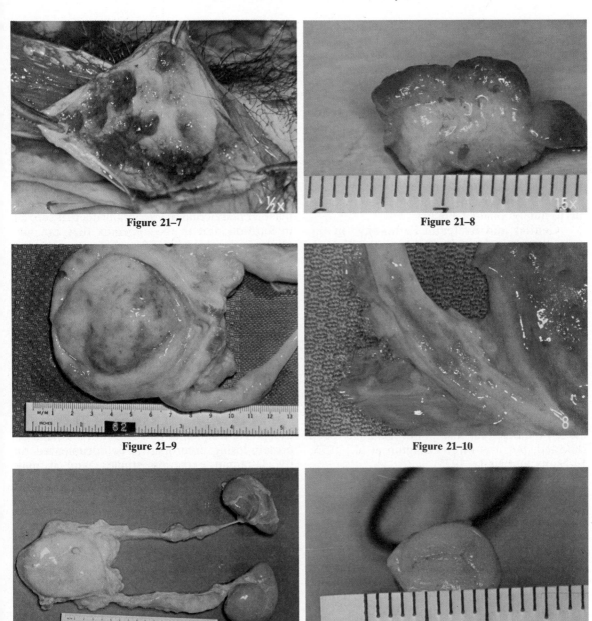

Figure 21–7. Polypoid *S. haematobium* patches in the chimpanzee bladder 7 months after infection. (See text.)

Figure 21–8. Cross section of bladder wall at the site of a polypoid patch, illustrating edema, hyperemia, and superficial mucosal erosion.

Figure 21–9. Sandy patches in the chimpanzee bladder, 17½ months after infection. Note dilation of lower ureters.

Figure 21–10. Sandy patches in the lower ureter (close-up).

Figure 21–11. Bilateral hydroureter in a chimpanzee 7 months after infection with *S. haematobium,* showing fusiform dilations and narrowings; note ureteral asymmetry.

Figure 21–12. Cross section through a ureteral patch shows encroachment on muscle layer and compression of lumen.

hematuria present prior to and after cancer development, but x-ray images and even cytopathologic findings may well be equivocal until a neoplasm has reached an advanced stage.

Transitional cell tumors resembling Grade I human bladder carcinomas have been reported in the capuchin monkey *Cebus apella* experimentally infected with *S. haematobium,* and in a few other primate species (Kuntz et al., 1972). In these experiments, urothelial dysplasia seemed to be linked with relatively high bladder egg loads. None of these putative tumors has as yet shown invasiveness or metastasis comparable to human bladder tumors.

Genital and Systemic Pathology. In the male, the *seminal vesicles* are regularly affected; indeed, schistosome eggs or blood, or both, may appear in the ejaculate before they appear in the urine. Although significant inflammatory and fibrous lesions of this organ are common, clinical evidence of male infertility due to schistosomiasis is rare. Prostatic involvement is generally moderate, and it does not seem to cause urethral obstruction, although the verumontanum is not uncommonly involved. Eggs are occasionally found in the cord, epididymis, and testis, where they may cause nodularity or induration, but little else. Schistosomal involvement of the scrotal and penile skin has been reported, but it is rare (Edington et al., 1975; El-Mofty and Nada, 1975).

Egg deposition can occur anywhere in the female genital tract. Occasionally, granulomatous involvement of the uterine cervix gives rise to complaints similar to those of chronic cervicitis, as well as to a suspicious granular or polypoid appearance at culdoscopy. Other localizations are minor, including the ovaries and fallopian tubes. Ovarian egg deposition and granulomas have been found proximal to normal graafian follicles, and when infertility is found in patients with schistosomiasis, other causes must first be ruled out (Williams, 1967).

At term in pregnancy, schistosome eggs have been found in the placenta and amniotic fluid (Sutherland et al., 1965) but documented reports of eggs in aborti or stillborn fetuses are not extant. Experimentally, a degree of unresponsiveness to injected schistosome eggs that appears to be transitory has been noted in the offspring of infected female mice (Hang et al., 1974; Lewert and Mandlowitz, 1969); how this tolerance or specific suppression is transmitted is not yet understood, but the relative absence of clinically acute schistosomiasis in children living in endemic areas has often been commented upon.

Scattered eggs have been found everywhere along the digestive tract, but the rectosigmoid and appendix are the sites most commonly affected. The stools may become positive for eggs before the urine, but, on the whole, rectal involvement is more erratic than that of the urinary tract, and quantitative stool egg excretion does not correlate well with infection intensity. Both the lower colon and the appendix can be the site of bilharziomas, i.e., of tumor-like granulomatous and fibrous masses, which may appear elastic and lobulated to the touch and may contain numerous eggs, though fewer in number than could account for the total fibrotic mass. Bilharziomas are generally deep or serosal in location, but in the appendix they can virtually replace the organ and encroach on its lumen. The reasons for the more frequent appendicular involvement by *S. haematobium* compared with that by *S. mansoni* are not clear, nor is the relationship of these infections to acute appendicular symptoms when they occur (Edington et al., 1975; El-Mofty and Nada, 1975).

Schistosomal colonic polyposis, in which the mucosa is studded with broadly or narrowly stalked granulomatous masses covered by inflamed mucosa, has been reported almost exclusively from Egypt. This lesion can give rise to dysentery, to anemia due to blood loss, and to protein-losing enteropathy, as documented by [^{51}Cr]albumin excretion studies, and it may therefore seriously impair the patient's health (Lehman et al., 1958). Polyposis is more closely associated with severe *S. mansoni* infection but is also known to arise in *S. haematobium* or combined infections.

Depending on the intensity of *S. haematobium* infection, greater or lesser numbers of eggs or granulomas, or both, are invariably found in the liver and lung at autopsy. However, in contrast to *S. mansoni* infection, liver fibrosis and pulmonary arteritis are rarely, if ever, seen in *S. haematobium* infections. Indeed, egg loads that would be associated with severe pathologic effects in the case of *S. mansoni* seem to cause only minimal architectural damage in the liver and lung in *S. haematobium* infections (Sadun et al., 1970).

Ectopic Lesions. Scattered schistosome eggs have been found by systematic tissue digest at autopsy in most human organs and tissues not already mentioned (Alves, 1958; Gelfand, 1950). Such localizations are often erratic in distribution but somewhat related to overall infection intensity. The kidney and pancreas are frequently positive for eggs, but these focal lesions lack clinical expression. This is also true when the central nervous system is the target of sporadic eggs; however, massed ectopic egg deposition may occur, especially at the level of the spinal cord, and may give rise to severe neurologic symptoms (Bird, 1967; Wakefield et al., 1962). (See later.)

Clinical Manifestations

Persons living in an endemic area rarely give a history suggestive of cercarial penetration or swimmer's itch. Noninfected persons entering such an area and becoming infected later in life may report such an event. Likewise, acute schistosomiasis is rarely encountered among endemic populations, whereas a noninfected traveler upon first, presumably heavy, exposure, may develop a protean syndrome of fever, lymphadenopathy, splenomegaly, eosinophilia, urticaria, and other manifestations of a serum sickness-like disease (Hiatt et al., 1979; Warren, 1973a; Diaz Rivera et al., 1956). Acute schistosomiasis generally occurs 3 to 9 weeks after infection, roughly coincident with the initiation of egg laying, but it may precede the appearance of eggs in the urine. Clinically, acute schistosomiasis is much more fulminant in *Schistosoma japonicum* infection and is rarely life-threatening in *Schistosoma haematobium* infection. The acute disease is self-limiting, and the infection enters a patent and active period in which eggs are deposited in tissues, traverse the bladder mucosa, and are excreted in the urine.

The signs and symptoms of the active phase of *S. haematobium* infection are classically those of hematuria and dysuria. Hematuria is described as terminal and, on occasion, gives rise to blood loss anemia. In general, however, patients are not greatly inconvenienced by their symptoms at this stage of the disease. In some highly endemic areas, nearly all the young people at some time or another suffer complaints of dysuria and hematuria, and this becomes absorbed into a background of minor complaints; indeed, in some communities hematuria in males is regarded as a normal sign of puberty.

During the active stage of infection, polypoid patches (see Pathology and Pathogenesis, preceding) may reach extremely large size and become frank, pedunculated polyps. If this occurs near the bladder outlet, they may temporarily or completely obstruct bladder emptying, causing combinations of urinary retention and incontinence. Occasionally a single large polypoid patch at the ureterovesical junction obstructs urine flow partially or completely. Therefore, hydroureter and hydronephrosis are frequently seen at this early stage of infection. Nevertheless, other than colicky flank pain,

there is often little to indicate that early obstructive uropathy is developing (Lehman et al., 1973).

After some time, measured in years, the active phase of infection enters a more quiescent period, in which egg deposition and excretion continue but symptoms are less noticeable. It should be stressed, however, that although clinical disease is not as immediately apparent, silent obstructive uropathy is occurring during this phase as polypoid patches are replaced by sandy patches and fibrosis, and the bladder and ureters undergo what is probably largely irreversible damage (see Pathology and Pathogenesis, preceding). Because of the slow, insidious nature of these effects, hydroureter and hydronephrosis may reach enormous proportions without intervening symptoms. In areas in which severe uropathy is highly prevalent, it is not uncommon in radiographs to encounter nonfunctioning kidneys, presumably secondary to urinary schistosomiasis, in patients who are apparently well.

In patients who develop bladder ulceration, particularly in the area of the trigone, pain may be intense and is often referred to the glans penis or to the perineal region. Bladder ulcer is frequently associated with superimposed bacterial infection.

As patients enter the inactive phase of infection (in which viable eggs are no longer detected in urine or tissues), obstructive uropathy may continue and worsen because of fibrosis and stenosis of the bladder and ureter and also because of the lack of tonicity and a peristalsis of the ureter. Calcification and fibrosis in the bladder wall produce, in some patients, a small, contracted bladder with little functional capacity (as small as 50 ml). Incontinence results. Urinary tract stone formation occurs, either in the bladder or in the ureter, particularly in endemic areas such as Egypt, which fall in the "stone belt" (Ghorab, 1962). At this late stage the majority of clinical manifestations continue to be associated with complications of the disease, such as bladder ulcer, stone formation, and obstructive uropathy rather than with the infection itself.

Bacterial Urinary Tract Infections in Urinary Schistosomiasis. The more readily explicable infections are those due to coliform organisms, such as *E. coli,* or to *Klebsiella* and *Pseudomonas,* which are presumably secondary to instrumentation of the urinary tract, by either cystoscope or catheter (Lehman et al., 1973). Such iatrogenic infections are frequently encountered in hospitalized patients. Another type of infection, which as yet is poorly understood, involves chronic infection of the urinary tract by *Salmonella* species, including *Salmonella typhi* and *S. paratyphi.* Urinary tract carriage of *Salmonella* is very frequently associated with intermittent bacteremia; the etiologic basis of this situation has yet to be determined, but there is a definite association between schistosomiasis and chronic *Salmonella* infections and some indication that the *Salmonella* organisms may, in fact, be residing on or in the worms themselves (Young et al., 1973). Patients with schistosomiasis and concomitant chronic salmonellosis may be seriously ill, suffering from profound weakness, usually with intermittent fever and refractory anemia. The spleen is enlarged. Nephrotic syndrome, perhaps due to an immune-complex mechanism, has been reported as a complication (Highashi et al., 1975). Significantly, these complications often respond to antischistosomal drug treatment alone or in combination with antibiotics.

Physiologic Alterations Secondary to Urinary Schistosomiasis. The basic physiologic alterations noted in urinary schistosomiasis are due to obstructive uropathy. In this sense, urinary schistosomiasis is not different from other forms of obstructive uropathy, and the reader is referred to Section III, The Pathophysiology of Urinary Obstruction (Chapters 9 and 10). Clinically, the first test of renal function to be altered is maximal urine concentration. Findings in the 18-hour concentration test become abnormal early in schistosomal hydronephrosis, and until obstructive uropathy reaches a very severe degree, these are the only routine renal function test findings that are clearly affected. Superimposed urinary tract infection similarly reduces urine concentration, and when both urinary tract obstruction and bacterial infection are present, the effects upon urinary concentrating mechanisms may be additive (Lehman et al., 1971). The extreme of this situation is frank polyuria and a diabetes insipidus–like syndrome. Only very late in the course of obstructive uropathy due to schistosomiasis is the glomerular filtration rate affected. Some patients with remarkably obstructed urinary tracts and severe bilateral hydronephrosis maintain their creatinine clearance adequately. This, however, may be a very precarious situation, and the superimposition of a urinary tract or systemic bacterial infection can initiate rapid deterioration of renal function, leading to uremia and possibly death (Lehman et al., 1970). It should be emphasized that there are to date no good clinical or epidemiologic studies that indicate the frequency with which renal failure complicates severe obstructive urinary schistosomiasis.

Ectopic Manifestations. The colonic polyposis syndrome has already been mentioned under Pathology and Pathogenesis. Spinal cord involvement—depending on whether schistosome egg deposition involves the nerve roots or the leptomeninges, or extends throughout the neural structures of the cord—gives rise to different neurologic syndromes of radiculitis, simulated spinal cord tumor, or transverse myelitis (the most severe).

An important clinical feature of this localization of the infection is that it can appear suddenly, in the absence of other clinical manifestations of schistosomiasis, when infection is mild or latent and eggs in the stools or urine are detected only with difficulty or not at all (Bird, 1967; Wakefield, 1962).

Diagnosis is of extreme urgency, since motor deficit often progresses at a rapid rate and may result in permanent paraplegia unless the condition is recognized and treated. A good clinical history is essential, including report of exposure to schistosome-infected waters; eosinophils in significant numbers are found in the spinal fluid in half or more of the patients. The circumoval precipitin antibody is found in the spinal fluid of patients with central nervous system involvement by a schistosomiasis (Yogore et al., 1975). Negative findings in urine or stool examination do not rule out this diagnosis!

Present standards of treatment favor early laminectomy for relieving local edema and cord compression, and for obtaining a diagnostic tissue sample. Antischistosomal treatment can be instituted simultaneously or earlier, but its effect on the outcome depends on the stage of pathologic condition already present. Some cases of the disease have responded to drug treatment alone, while in others the patients have sustained permanent deficits despite treatment. Massed schistosome lesions in the brain are exceptional in schistosomiasis haematobia, but some have been reported in Oriental schistosomiasis.

Diagnosis

Diagnostic techniques in urinary schistosomiasis can be divided into two general categories. The first deals with tests and techniques aimed at diagnosing infection and intensity of infection by *Schistosoma haematobium,* and the second deals with the diagnosis of the consequences and sequelae of the infection.

Diagnosis of Infection. The detection of terminally spined eggs of *S. haematobium* in a urinary sediment is diagnostic of infection with the parasite. In moderate to heavy infections, eggs will almost always be present in a routine urinary sediment, and the diagnosis is hence easy. In lighter infections, routine urinalysis will not always reveal the presence of eggs, and the sedimentation or filtration, or both, of larger volumes of urine, up to and including 24-hour collections, will be necessary. Since egg excretion follows a diurnal periodicity, with maximal egg excretion occurring between the hours of 10 A.M. and 2 P.M., a midday sample of urine has the greatest likelihood of containing eggs. The eggs of *S. haematobium* are easily counted by filtering a known aliquot of urine through filter paper and staining the eggs with triketohydrindene hydrate (Ninhydrin) under controlled conditions of heat and humidity. The purple-stained eggs are then counted under low magnification, and the number of eggs occurring per volume of urine or per 24 hours is calculated (Bell, 1963). An alternative method, suitable for epidemiologic studies, is nuclepore filtration (Peters et al., 1976) or nylon mesh filtration (Mott, 1983). Screening of infected young people in an endemic setting can be conveniently accomplished with a dipstick method for detecting blood in the urine (Pugh et al., 1980). Day-to-day egg excretion for individuals varies considerably, but, in general, it tends to remain high for high-volume egg excretors, and low for low-volume egg excretors. Quantification of the numbers of eggs in a given sample of urine and, in particular, of a 24-hour sample of urine, has come to be a method for estimating the intensity of infection with *S. haematobium*. Of course, such an assessment assumes that there is a correlation between the number of eggs appearing in the urine and the worm burden. In general terms, the assessment of infection intensity by quantification of urine egg excretion has proved to be of value in epidemiologic studies of the impact of the infection upon groups of people.

Pathologic studies suggest that egg excretion in the urine is in part a function of the stage of schistosomiasis. In early, active infection, e.g., in schoolchildren, 24-hour urinary egg counts correlate relatively well with tissue egg loads. This phase ends sometime during the second or third decade of life and, thereafter, the proportions of eggs shed from the progressively more inactive lesions decrease. As a result, in older, less active or inactive infection, severe tissue involvement can be accompanied by minimal egg excretion, to the point at which a single examination may miss detection of an infected individual with up to 10^6 eggs per gram of urinary tract tissue. As a further consequence, epidemiologic studies based on the detection of eggs in the urine may ignore many inactive cases; radiographic findings are really better indices of severity than are urinary egg counts in the older age groups (Lehman et al., 1973).

Eggs may often be seen in tissue obtained by rectal or bladder mucosal biopsy. In the absence of eggs from multiple urine specimens, rectal biopsy should be attempted prior to bladder biopsy, as the chances of finding characteristic eggs are nearly as good by the former method. A squash preparation of the biopsy material between glass slides is preferable to routine pathologic section and staining, and it often permits a judgment about whether viable eggs are present, signifying active infection.

Immunologic methods, such as skin testing and serologic techniques, have been advanced as diagnostic tools in schistosomiasis. The most widely used tests at present are the fluorescent antibody, bentonite and latex flocculation, complement fixation, and circumoval precipitin tests (Kagan, 1974). In a recent WHO-sponsored collaborative serodiagnostic study, tests performed with egg-derived antigenic fractions, especially the ELISA method, have shown high sensitivity-specificity for detecting *S. mansoni* infection. *S. haematobium* egg antigens are not widely available, however, and the detection of eggs therefore remains the diagnostic cornerstone in that infection (Mott and Dixon, 1982). It must also be remembered that although a positive immunologic test may tell with reasonable specificity that a person has had prior exposure to schistosome infection, it in no way indicates the present status of the infection. Skin tests and serologic tests may remain positive in the absence of eggs or living worms. Therefore, immunologic testing is probably of value only as an epidemiologic tool to indicate changing trends in large populations.

Diagnosis of Sequelae and Complications of Urinary Schistosomiasis. Radiography is by far the most important diagnostic tool in the evaluation of the patient with urinary schistosomiasis. Important alterations of the urinary tract due to schistosomiasis are not subtle and may be interpreted with relative ease by an aware physician. A plain x-ray film of the abdomen may reveal calcification within the urinary tract or in other organs. The classic presentation of a calcified bladder, which at times appears like a fetal head resting in the pelvis, is pathognomonic of chronic urinary schistosomiasis (Fig. 21–13). The seminal vesicles, prostate, posterior urethra, distal ureters, and, rarely, the colon may also be calcified.

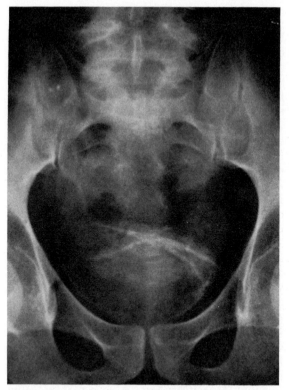

Figure 21–13. Plain x-ray film, showing bladder calcification in a patient with *Schistosoma haematobium* infection.

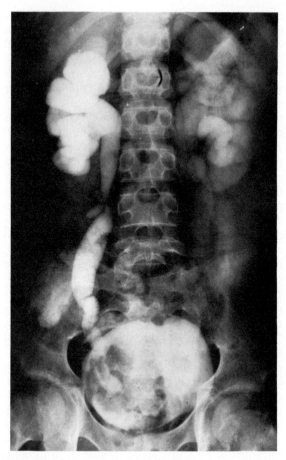

Figure 21–14. Intravenous urogram in a 15-year-old Egyptian boy with *Schistosoma haematobium* infection. Note the massive space-occupying lesion in the bladder and similar lesions in the right lower ureter.

Intravenous urography (von Lichtenberg and Swick, 1929) is indicated in every patient with *S. haematobium* infection, although in endemic areas it is obviously not feasible or even possible to attempt this. However, the evaluation of an individual patient should include a standard urogram, including delayed films as necessary. Readily observable lesions include hydroureter, hydronephrosis, ureteral stenosis, and bladder and ureteral filling defects (polypoid lesions). (See Figs. 21–14 to 21–16.) In the presence of severe obstructive uropathy, delayed films are frequently needed to visualize greatly distended ureters and kidneys. If visualization is not obtained, an infusion urogram can be done on a subsequent day. Postvoiding films may give some indication of bladder retention due to bladder neck obstruction. The use of the cystourethrogram will indicate the presence of vesicoureteric reflux.

Cystoscopy has in the past been widely used as a diagnostic tool in urinary schistosomiasis. Many lesions are visually characteristic, and biopsy may be performed at the same time. However, in our opinion and that of other writers, instrumentation of the urinary tract for diagnostic purposes has been overemployed in

schistosomiasis and may, in fact, account for many of the serious and resistant urinary tract infections that are increasingly seen in patients hospitalized for treatment of advanced urinary schistosomiasis. Particularly in Egypt, where instrumentation is frequently performed, chronic urinary tract infections with organisms such as *Klebsiella* and *Pseudomonas* are being encountered with increasing frequency.

As an adjunct to urography, renography by radioisotopic techniques has been used in several institutions, particularly for evaluating responses to treatment, but this must be considered an experimental rather than a diagnostic tool.

Treatment

Medical Management. Recent progress in developing safe and effective antischistosomal drugs has simplified both the decision to treat schistosome infection and the form of the treat-

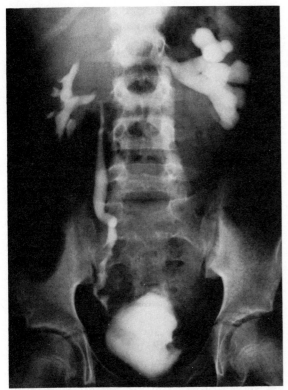

Figure 21–15. Intravenous urogram in another Egyptian boy, showing scalloping of the bladder and right lower ureter by schistosomal polypoid lesions.

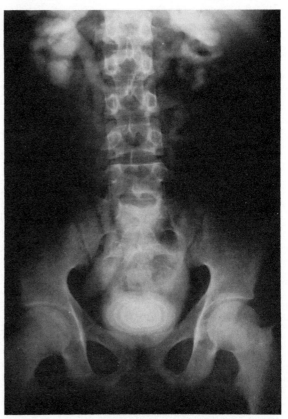

Figure 21–16. Intravenous pyelogram at 2½ hours in a 23-year-old Egyptian farmer who was shedding numerous viable eggs of *S. haematobium* in the urine. Note hydronephrosis, poor excretory function, and unusual, large, laminated bladder calculus. (Courtesy of Dr. Stuart Young, NAMRU III, Cairo.)

ment itself. There is now no valid reason to withhold medical treatment from persons with either light or advanced infections, as long as the indications and safeguards prescribed for the various drugs are observed. Treatment should not be given, however, without first defining the parasitologic status and disease condition of the person to be treated or without a follow-up to determine response, detect residual pathology that might require surgical correction, and teach the (endemic) patient how to avoid re-exposure (Davis, 1982).

Of the three species of schistosomes pathogenic for humans, *Schistosoma haematobium* is the most amenable to treatment. It responds well to metrifonate (Bilharcil), to hycanthone mesylate (Etrenol), to praziquantel (Biltricide), to niridazole (Ambilhar), and to Oltipraz (Cook, 1982; Davis, 1982). There is no longer any need to use the antimonial compounds, tartar emetic or stibophen (Fuadin), which were formerly the mainstay of therapy despite their relative toxicity. Oxaminiquine (Vansil), while highly effective against *S. mansoni*, is ineffective against other schistosome species. The aim of treatment is a reduction in worm burden, if not total parasitologic cure. In fact, in endemic areas, there may be rationale for leaving an individual with a few remaining worms, if concomitant immunity plays a major role in immunity to reinfection. Ideally, schistosomicidal treatment should begin at the earliest possible stage of patent infection, since the reversibility of lesions declines at progressively later stages (von Lichtenberg, 1975). Treatment at a prepatent stage is rarely achieved, even though findings in serologic tests may already have become positive, but both experimental and clinical data suggest that treatment during acute schistosomiasis (as seen in visitors to endemic areas) and in children during the early chronic active stage can prevent the irreversible pathologic effects. Conversely, before late infection is treated, it must be established whether the infection is active. If only dark eggs lacking miracidia with intact organelles or flame cell movement are found, treatment may not be indicated.

METRIFONATE. This organophosphate compound is now the drug of first choice for treatment of *Schistosoma haematobium* infection in its endemic setting. When given by mouth, in the form of 100 mg tablets, it is slowly metabolized to the anticholinesterase compound dichlorvos, known as an insecticide. Its presumed mode of action is to block the worm's cholinesterase, thereby paralyzing it. At the same time, it lowers the patient's own plasma cholinesterase and erythrocyte cholinesterase levels, but these return to normal without clinical manifestations of toxicity. Only rarely have nausea, vomiting, and bronchospasm been reported as side effects. The recommended dose is 7.5 to 10 mg per kg, given in three oral doses at intervals of 14 days. Cure rates have generally been in the 70 to 80 per cent range, and no major adverse reactions have been observed among the thousands of individuals treated. No contraindications are known. Relapses are uncommon. There seems to be no obstacle to extending treatment to four or more doses, if advisable. Should overdose occur and cholinergic symptoms arise, atropine can be administered. Metrifonate has been used in large-scale antischistosoma chemotherapy in several control projects. It seems to be a safe and effective drug for *S. haematobium* infection but not for *S. mansoni* or for *S. japonicum*. Its sole disadvantage is the need for multiple successive doses, which limits it applicability among people living in poorly accessible or dispersed places or under nomadic conditions.

PRAZIQUANTEL. This heterocyclic pyrazinoisoquinolin compound is effective against all three major human schistosomes as well as against numerous other trematodes and platyhelminths. It is more expensive than metrifonate but is effective against *S. haematobium* in a single oral dose. It is currently in the process of being licensed for general use by the FDA and is likely to become the antischistosomal drug of choice in the near future, especially in the developed countries.

Praziquantel appears to interfere with the ion transport mechanism of the schistosome tegument, resulting in rapid fluxes of Ca^+ and Na^+ into the worms and sudden contraction of the parasite's musculature. Cure rates for *S. haematobium* infection have ranged from 83 per cent to 100 per cent; animal toxicity studies have shown tolerance for well over 20 times therapeutic levels of the drug, and mutagenicity testing in various systems has been essentially negative. In human trials the drug has been remarkably free of toxic side effects, and complaints have been limited to epigastric pain, abdominal discomfort, nausea, anorexia, diarrhea, dizziness, headache, and occasionally pruritus or urticariform drug eruptions and fever. Mostly, these symptoms have been mild and have lasted for less than 24 hours. Some may have been related to the death of worms. Forty mg per kg given in a single oral dose is the recommended procedure for *S. haematobium*. Higher or multiple doses are required for *S. mansoni* or *S. japonicum*. Praziquantel is available in tablets of 600 mg for oral administration.

OTHER SCHISTOSOMICIDAL DRUGS. Hycanthone and niridazole, while highly effective against both *S. haematobium* and *S. mansoni*, are now considered less desirable for therapy, since both have shown mutagenic activity in vitro and carcinogenicity in mice and hamsters. Prior to the advent of less hazardous drugs, niridazole had shown particularly excellent curative effect in *S. haematobium*-infected children; hycanthone was widely used against *S. mansoni* in children and adults. Two other experimental drugs, Oltipraz and Amoscanate, are currently in advanced stages of experimental trial but are not generally available. Oltipraz has shown promise in use against *S. mansoni* and *S. haematobium* and Amoscanate against all three major human schistosomes, but toxicity and side effects of these two compounds still remain to be fully evaluated. Amoscanate administered together with a broad-spectrum antibiotic has not caused jaundice or other side effects that had been noted in earlier trials. It has been particularly effective against *S. japonicum*.

Until licensed by the FDA, praziquantel is available in the United States on an investigational basis from Miles Pharmaceuticals, 400 Morgan Lane, West Haven, Connecticut 06516. Outside the United States it is distributed by Bayer A.G., Wupperthal, Federal Republic of Germany. Metrifonate is available through the Parasitic Disease Division, Center for Infectious Diseases, Center for Disease Control, Atlanta, Georgia 30333. That division can also be consulted for guidance in the use of antischistosomal drugs and other antiparasitic compounds. For a more detailed discussion of the current status of pharmacology and therapy, consult Davis (1982).

Finally, it is quite clear that low-level schistosome infections are well tolerated by many persons and in the majority of cases will not produce symptomatic chronic disease or lead to silent obstructive uropathy. However, because of the possibility that a single space-occupying lesion in the ureter may obstruct urine flow partially or completely, and because of the hazard of ectopic lesions, continued evaluation of patients with active *S. haematobium* infection is advised. If drug treatment has been given, follow-up urinary tract examinations should be performed at 3 months to assess cure or reduction in egg excretion. Retreatment may be advisable in selected circumstances.

Surgical Management. A wide variety of surgical procedures have been employed in the treatment of various complications of urinary schistosomiasis. In general terms these are reserved for complications that have not responded to adequate medical treatment within a reasonable time of follow-up. Strictures of the ureter have been thought generally amenable to surgical intervention, and, depending upon the extent and location of the stricture, procedures involving excision or dilatation have been used. When the ureterovesical junction is involved, a variety of plastic operations for attempting to reconstruct a functional valve have been developed. Most of these procedures are variants of the Leadbetter-Politano operation (Leadbetter and Leadbetter, 1961). When a ureter is hopelessly obstructed, nephrostomy is performed as a last resort, particularly in the face of superimposed bacterial infection.

Lesions of the bladder also necessitate various types of surgical intervention. Chronic deep bladder ulcers generally require partial cystectomy. Obstructing polypoid lesions that are resistant to antischistosomal therapy may need to be resected either in an open or a closed procedure. Bladder neck obstruction may be treated by dilatation or excision of the trigonal plate. The chronically contracted bladder has been managed variously by vesical denervation, urinary shunting, and overdistention under anesthesia. Cancer of the bladder in association with urinary schistosomiasis is generally of the squamous cell type and diagnosed late. Surgical treatment frequently involves a radical anterior pelvic exenteration, if possible.

Prognosis

Considering the tens of millions of people affected with *S. haematobium,* many of whom have mild infections, the prognosis is generally good (Warren, 1973b). Many individuals with schistosomiasis have annoying symptoms but do not develop significant urinary tract lesions. There are, however, no good population-related data on morbidity and mortality due to this infection and its sequelae. There is reasonable evidence to support the hypothesis that the impact of schistosomiasis on a community is determined by the overall intensity of infection and the risk of reinfection. Similarly, the long-term prognosis for an individual will depend on his worm burden, the degree and location of the individual lesion secondary to egg deposition, and the stage of the pathologic lesions.

The prognosis for persons with demonstrable urinary tract lesions has improved with the advent of newer and better antischistosomal drugs. In children, the active stage of the infection and the polypoid-type lesion associated with this stage are readily treatable. Polypoid lesions and obstructive uropathy secondary to them have been shown in many instances to resolve rapidly following antischistosomal treatment.

Visitors to endemic foci (missionaries, tourists, and so forth) will most often present after a single exposure, in a relatively early stage of schistosome infection that is generally responsive to therapy, even when the egg count is relatively high. A more unfortunate variant of this type of presentation, and an avoidable one, is the incompletely cured and followed-up case of early infection, the patient now returning with recurrent symptoms.

For patients with later, more chronic stages of schistosomiasis, in which obstructive uropathy is more often associated with sandy patches and fibrosis, the prognosis is less clear. Some individuals seem to tolerate remarkably advanced obstructive uropathy with little, if any, deterioration in renal function. Bacterial superinfection of the urinary tract is clearly a bad prognostic event, and such infections should be treated as vigorously as possible. The older patient with severe bilateral obstructive uropathy and a small, contracted bladder who has a hospital-acquired bacterial urinary tract infection resistant to most antibiotics has a generally poor prognosis. The patient with bladder cancer in association with schistosomiasis also has a very poor prognosis.

It must be remembered that in all developing countries in which schistosomiasis is highly prevalent other important endemic disease states present similar and continuous threats to the health and survival of indigenous populations.

Prevention and Control

Individuals who avoid contact with water inhabited by snails infected with *S. haematobium* will effectively prevent contracting this infection. Travelers in endemic areas should be advised of the hazard of infected streams, rivers, ponds, and lakes, and should avoid bathing in or otherwise entering such water. If contaminated water is inadvertently contacted, brisk rubbing of the skin following exposure, dry or with alcohol, may prevent cercarial penetration. Boiling of water effectively kills cercariae. At present, there is no prophylactic drug available.

Measures to control the transmission of infection have utilized several basic approaches, including (1) destruction of the snail host; (2) elimination of urine and fecal contamination of water; and (3) reduction of contact with infected water. Obviously, in many endemic areas, measures such as these may be expensive, unfeasible, or poorly tolerated by the local population. Worldwide there has been little success in the control of schistosomiasis; in many areas prevalence is actually increasing. Mass therapy, by drugs, has been looked to for effective control, and currently the major control campaigns instituted by the governments of Brazil, Egypt, and the People's Republic of China all include drug treatment as part of their plan. Favorable short-term results have been reported from each of these campaigns, but their long-term effects may not become known for some time. Research toward a vaccine is in a stage of exploration, and it is uncertain whether a safe and effective vaccine for human use can be developed (WHO, 1974).

GENITAL FILARIASIS

The most widespread lymphatic filarial parasite is *Wuchereria bancrofti*, which has periodic nocturnal, periodic diurnal, and subperiodic variants (the last limited to the Pacific area). *W. bancrofti* is a human parasite without known animal reservoirs; not so, organisms belonging to the genus *Brugia*, limited to the Far East, of which three species are currently recognized: *B. malayi*, *B. pahangi*, and the "Timor filaria." *Brugia* can infect primates and domestic animals spontaneously and has been transmitted to laboratory hosts. Nonlymphatic filarial parasites (*Loa, Dipetalonema, Dirofilaria* spp.) only exceptionally cause urogenital manifestations, but *Onchocerca volvulus*, the agent of African river blindness, is known to cause hanging groin and scrotal elephantiasis and will be described separately.

All lymphatic filarial species are transmitted by mosquitoes; their clinical manifestations are similar and begin after a relatively long prepatent period. Acute hypersensitivity or febrile reactions may occur, often including transitory genital edema or hydrocele; major attacks result in funiculoepididymitis or orchitis. Filarial attacks may repeat themselves at irregular and often lengthy intervals, eventually resulting in chyluria or in permanent deformity from elephantiasis or hydrocele. Microfilaremia is regularly detected only during established infection, but not in the initial or late stages, and a variety of amicrofilaremic ("occult") filarial syndromes occur. Episodic or relentlessly progressive filariasis tends to be associated with considerable patient anxiety and discomfort and is frequently incapacitating, the more so since only limited therapeutic recourses are available. In its socially stigmatizing aspect it is comparable to leprosy as one of the great plagues of the tropics. At the same time, minor and stationary filarial manifestations, especially hydrocele, tend to be ignored, and their public health importance is often underestimated. Current prospects for control of filarial transmission remain dim in most endemic areas.

Biology and Life Cycle

The lymphatic filariae are elongated nematodes (up to 100 mm by 0.3 mm for the female *W. bancrofti*) and are viviparous. The cycle proceeds directly from man to mosquito and back through a regular sequence of larval moults. The most common urban vector of *W. bancrofti* is the ubiquitous *Culex pipiens fatigans*, but filariae have adapted to a wide variety of *Culex, Anopheles, Aedes*, and *Mansonella* mosquitoes under differing ecologic settings.

Female mosquitoes suck up microfilariae (first-stage larvae) with their blood meals; larvae rapidly mature and moult, becoming infective in their third stage, when they move to the salivary glands. During the next mosquito bite, infective larvae are discharged onto the puncture wound inflicted by the stylet, together with a droplet of saliva, and thus traverse the epidermis. They cannot enter unbroken skin but are able to cross the normal conjunctiva or buccal mucosa (Sullivan and Chernin, 1976; Ah et al., 1974*b*); aquatic transmission from dead mosquitoes to man (as originally postulated by P. Manson) is therefore a potential alternate pathway, but this is surely a rare event.

Little is known as yet about the prepatent period of filariasis (which was experimentally shown to range from 53 to 131 days for *Brugia* and is probably longer for *Wuchereria*), except that the host lung vessels are entered via the blood stream within minutes. The last two larval moults occur in the lymphatics of the definitive host at or near the final nesting sites of the adult male and female worm, and these moults have been shown to coincide with bouts of local inflammatory activity, and with early, episodic clinical symptoms; similar bouts occur during early mating. Better knowledge of the dynamics of filarial transmission is needed to understand reasons for the regional differences in infection intensity and in localization of lesions. Many variables will have to be sorted out before we can explain certain peculiarities, such as the frequent involvement of the upper extremities and breast in some endemic areas (especially the South Pacific), or the comparative rarity of elephantiasis in relation to hydrocele in others (especially Puerto Rico). Little is known about the effect of host immunity resulting from repeated infection, if any; both partial resistance to reinfection and partial enhancement have been recently demonstrated in different experimental systems and with different filarial organisms (Ah et al., 1974a; Klei et al., 1974).

Adult filarial worms prefer to live in the larger lymphatic vessels and trunks of man, more rarely in distended lymphatic capillaries or in the lymph node sinuses, and still more rarely in serous cavities. Those occasional worms that enter blood vessels are swept into the pulmonary artery, where they die, giving rise to focal arteritis and pulmonary infarction similar to those caused by human infection with the dog heartworm, *Dirofilaria immitis* (Beaver and Cran, 1974). Much of the mature female *Wuchereria* body cavity is occupied by her paired uterus containing all stages of embryos from eggs to mature microfilariae (see Fig. 21–18). Discharge of microfilariae into the blood seems to be regulated by a feedback system that tends to maintain a reasonably constant individual level of microfilaremia, variable from host to host. There is, however, no constant relationship between worm number and microfilaremia level. In fact, microfilaremia is found in only an estimated 30 to 40 per cent of all cases of infection.

Transfer experiments have established the longevity of microfilariae as on the order of several months. Thus, microfilarial periodicity is not the result of periodic release from the worm uterus, but of a release from parenchymal capillary beds (lung, spleen, and so forth) to the peripheral circulation. A variety of drugs and anesthetics can quickly and temporarily affect this distribution. Despite long and careful research efforts, the regulatory mechanisms that produce the circadian rhythms of microfilaremia remain unknown; however, it is abundantly clear that the timing of maximal microfilaremia in each endemic focus corresponds rather well to the time of maximal biting frequency of the mosquito vector.

Distribution and Epidemiology

Few tropical countries can boast that they are free of *Wuchereria* transmission, except for tropical parts of the continental United States and of Australia. However, prevalence of infection varies greatly when microfilarial surveys are compared, from sporadic in Puerto Rico to nearly 50 per cent in parts of southern India. Neither percentage reflects the total prevalence of infection, and the latter one probably indicates a near-holoendemic condition. In most endemic foci, both microfilaremia and filarial pathologic effects show greater frequencies in males, particularly as regards urogenital manifestations.

Within each endemic country, bancroftian filariasis tends to concentrate in the coastal lowlands and plains and to be less frequent and severe in mountainous terrain. Many of the flatter and smaller archipelagos of the South Pacific are holoendemic, including the area east of the International Date Line, where subperiodic filariasis is common. Removal of the patient from an endemic area to a temperate or cold environment is reputed to influence favorably the clinical course of filarial edema, but adequate records of this phenomenon are not available.

In contrast to that of *Wuchereria*, *Brugia* distribution is relatively focal and is limited to rural populations of tropical Southeast Asia, extending from the western coast of India to New Guinea, the Philippines, and Japan. Both day- and night-biting mosquitoes are involved in transmission, and a variety of circadian patterns of microfilaremia has been reported in different endemic foci (Sasa and Tanaka, 1972). Given the finding of spontaneously infected jungle mammals and primates, it appears likely that animal reservoirs may play a role in transmission to humans, especially in sites such as New Guinea.

Two patterns have been observed in the age distribution of microfilaremia: In some populations, there is a linear increase well into the fourth decade, and subsequently microfilaremia continues at a high plateau; in fact, microfilaremia has been followed for as long as 14 years in some patients. In other foci there is a fall in prevalence beginning in the patients' twenties or thirties, with only sporadic microfilaremia in older age groups. The second pattern is more common, particularly where transmission is moderate or low. (Often, the fall in microfilaremia seems to coincide with the onset of permanent pathologic effects in members of the same population.)

As already indicated, a large proportion of those infected with filariae are asymptomatic and may remain so permanently, as shown by autopsy studies in which small numbers of worms, live and dead, have been detected in patients of mature ages, without history of any complaints attributable to filariasis (Galindo et al., 1962). Most of these minimal infections are probably urban and may well represent the bulk of endemic infections, the symptomatic cases representing the "tip of the iceberg." The severest pathologic conditions are found in stable, rural agricultural or fishing communities in which filarial transmission has been continuous for many years. It can therefore be assumed that repetitive, prolonged exposure is necessary for lesions such as elephantiasis or lymph scrotum to arise.

Pathology and Pathogenesis

From the epidemiologic findings mentioned earlier, as well as from animal experiments, it is evident that host reactions to microfilariae are distinct from those to adult worms. Experimentally, microfilaria-vaccinated hosts can be made amicrofilaremic, although adult worms develop normally and their uteri contain microfilariae (Wong et al., 1969). Longitudinal studies of experimental *Brugia* infection in cats have shown circulating eosinophils to rise at or near the time when microfilaremia begins a rapid decrease (Denham et al., 1972).

Human occult filariasis (see later) is characterized by circulating eosinophilia and dense eosinophilic infiltration of the affected lymph nodes or lung, accompanied by granulomas around damaged or dead microfilariae that show stellate hyaline surface precipitates (M-K bodies*). This resembles the Splendore-Hoeppli phenomenon seen in schistosomiasis and in cutaneous phycomycosis, which is thought to represent antigen-antibody precipitates (Williams et al., 1969; Danaraj et al., 1966; Lie, 1962). Granulomatous reactions to microfilariae also occur without M-K precipitates and can be seen in the spleen at autopsy in human patients (Fig. 21–17), as well as in filaria-infected baboons (Orihel and Moore, 1975). Perhaps these various phenomena represent a spectrum of host reactivity against microfilarial antigens that can range from delayed to reaginic hypersensitivity,

---

*Meyers-Kouvenaar bodies.

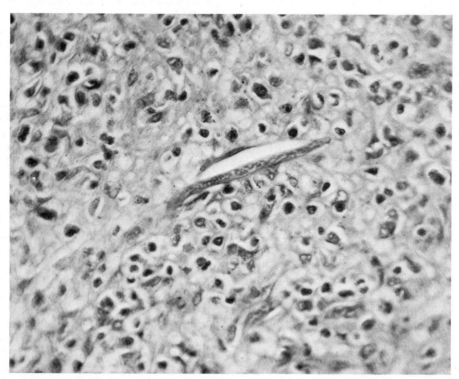

Figure 21–17. Microfilaria of *W. bancrofti* in splenic granuloma found at autopsy. Most of the surrounding cells are macrophages and eosinophils. × 380.

the central problem being the absence of host reactivity to microfilariae in so many chronically infected individuals. Recent studies have shown that microfilarial antigens can elicit T-suppressor cells, which inhibit the production of specific antimicrofilarial antibodies by B-lymphocytes in microfilaremic individuals and in experimental animal models (Piessens, 1982).

The most significant—and the majority of the urogenital—pathologic effects of lymphatic filariasis are elicited by the *adult worms*. The course of filariasis can be subdivided into, first, the prepatent period; second, early established infection; and third, late infection. Further variation results from localization of the lesions, and from presence or absence of complications.

The Prepatent Period. This is known principally from experimental *Brugia* infection in the cat, dog, and jird, but a few tissue specimens were obtained from military patients in a comparable stage of infection during World War II (Wartman, 1947). Characteristically, these lesions are relatively diffuse in relation to the number and size of the developing worms and are felt by many to represent reactions to exoantigens, rather than to somatic antigens of live or dead worms; this would also best explain the timing and episodic nature of this pathologic condition.

When worms can be found histologically, the lymph vessels in which they are coiled appear dilated or varicose ("lymphangiectasis") but only mildly inflamed, with a few eosinophils and lymphocytes nearby. There is nevertheless considerable edema, vasodilatation, and inflammatory infiltration of the surrounding tissues, or of the lymphatic drainage sites, including hydrocele (von Lichtenberg, 1957). Lymph nodes show enlargement by lymphoreticular proliferation as well as eosinophilia, but whether lymph node involvement contributes to the edematous condition is not clear. In a detailed study of *Brugia*-infected dogs, tags of moulted tegument and rounded structures suggesting filarial eggs were found in the infiltrate (Schacher and Sahyoun, 1967). In human cases, adult worms only occasionally have been identified in biopsy material, but the type of inflammation in the tissues and lymph nodes was felt to be distinctive. The lesions of prepatent filariasis usually remit spontaneously or after treatment and appear to be largely reversible.

Early Established Infection. In contrast to lesions of prepatent filariasis, those of established infection do not totally remit, but either persist actively or result in significant scarring and lymphatic obstruction. Lesions may appear in the worm nesting areas (funiculoepididymitis, orchitis, filarial lymphangitis, filarial abscess) or in their lymphatic distribution (hydrocele, lymphadenitis, genital edema, and so forth), or both. Often (but not always) when tissue is surgically excised, dying or dead adult filariae are detected in the specimen, and many believe this finding to be related to the severity of the filarial attack. The pathologic lesions vary from a mild, nodular inflammation sometimes simulating neoplasm to extensive exudation simulating acute bacterial disease (Figs. 21–18 and 21–19). In both instances, the lymphatics on which the reaction is centered become obliterated, usually far beyond the site occupied by the dying worm itself (von Lichtenberg, 1957). Histologically, nodular lesions show chronic granulomatous inflammation around cuticular fragments or entire segments of a necrotic nematode, surrounded by giant cells and macrophages; similar, but smaller, granulomas can occur in the draining lymph nodes, and in the absence of parasite fragments, they may be misdiagnosed as tubercles. Often, the granulomatous process is segmental in that adjacent worm portions appear intact, or calcified, with only mild foreign body reaction (Fig. 21–20). Tissue eosinophilia is a useful diagnostic hint, but this varies and may be absent. The surrounding tissues and the more distant lymphatic territories show edema and chronic inflammatory infiltrate dominated by lymphoid cells. These frequently aggregate around vessels, or in the wall of the lymphatic itself, where they sometimes protrude in the form of an inflammatory polyp (polypoid lymphangitis). When inflammation is more violent, lymph—or fibrin thrombi or red cell extravasation—is frequently seen in association with the inflammatory process (Fig. 21–19). Sometimes, adjacent veins are also heavily inflamed, and may thrombose (von Lichtenberg, 1957). The most acute, exudative filarial lesions, especially when subcutaneous in location, may grossly resemble a boil, become fluctuant, and on incision yield a rich, whitish purulent exudate that surrounds a dying worm and is subsequently proved to be bacteriologically sterile (O'Connor and Hulse, 1935). Histologically these filarial abscesses contain variable mixtures of neutrophils and eosinophils. The inflammatory process often ascends in a cordlike fashion along a lymph vessel, with exudate found even at remote levels and aggregates of granulocytes seen in regional lymph nodes. The pathogenesis of the most violent filarial attacks is, as yet, poorly understood. In the opinion of many, they are set off by an

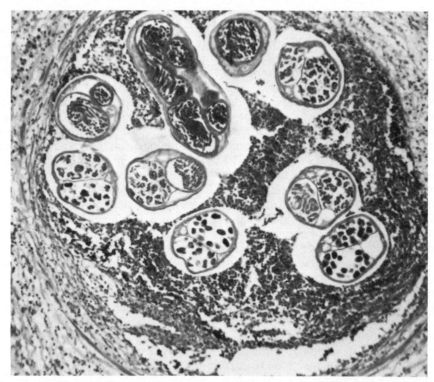

Figure 21–18. Intact, adult *W. bancrofti* female in acutely inflamed lymph vessel of epididymis. Note developmental stages of microfilariae in worm uterus. × 100.

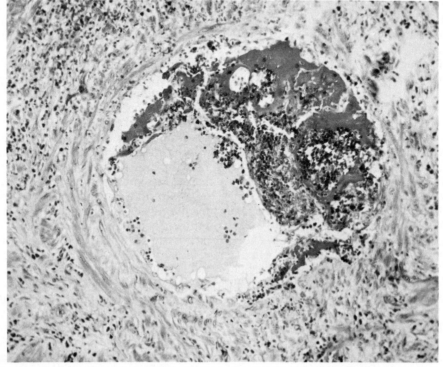

Figure 21–19. Inflamed lymph vessel of cord distant from site of adult filarial worm, showing diffuse inflammation and thrombosis with fibrin and red cells. × 100.

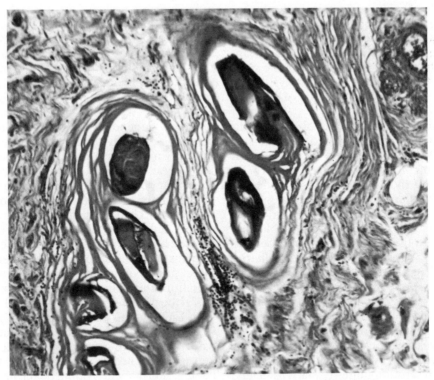

Figure 21–20. Coiled, calcified adult filaria with concentric fibrosis and minimal lymphoid infiltrate found in epididymis of a patient with hydrocele. × 200.

Arthus reaction that depends on the interaction of filarial somatic antigens from dying worms with host antibody and damages the endothelia of blood and lymphatic vessels. Delayed hypersensitivity has also been implicated, especially in granulomatous reactions to the more slowly dying worms.

Eventually, filarial inflammatory episodes—whether clinical or subclinical—abate, leaving in their wake obliterated lymphatics surrounded by poorly organized granulation and scar tissue. The nodules surrounding dead worms subsequently shrink; if inflammation has been mild and worms have undergone calcification, such scars may be only a few millimeters in size and difficult to detect except by tissue-clearing methods (Galindo et al., 1962). (See Fig. 21–20.) Conversely, after severe attacks, inflammation may continue smoldering and result in a palpable mass, or in a cordlike induration of the affected zone. The pathologic conditions arising from lymph vessel obstruction vary according to the location as described later; their common feature is the accumulation of edema or of hydrocele fluid rich in protein, and in cholesterol, in association with a predominantly lymphocytic infiltrate.

Late Infection. Neither the pathology nor the pathophysiology of filarial lymphatic obstruction has been fully clarified, but it is clear from lymphangiographic studies that obliteration of lymphatic vessels is initially bypassed by collateral formation; in due course, these collaterals themselves become partly obstructed and, at some point in time, become insufficient for adequate lymph drainage. A factor that would tend to enhance lymphatic obstruction is the observed localization of adult filariae at progressively more distal points during successive reinfections. Thus, when cats' legs are first exposed to *Brugia*, the initial worms tend to localize in the popliteal trunk; subsequent worms will most often lodge in lymphatics below that level, choking off collaterals (Ewert, 1971). On late lymphangiograms, lymphedematous tissues show rich networks of intercommunicating lymph vessel branches extending into superficial dermal layers that are, however, poorly connected to the central drainage points from the inguinofemoral and iliac trunks upward (Kanetkar et al., 1966; Cohen et al., 1961). There is as yet no consensus on whether filariasis results in dilatation of normally present lymphaticovenous fistulae.

The role of phlebosclerosis and phlebothrombosis in developing lymphedema remains unclear but is probably important over a period of time. These vessels often show significant pathologic effects, and—particularly in the spermatic cord—their anatomic pathways make them highly susceptible to stasis or chronic obstruction.

A relationship of lymphatic obstruction to filarial infection intensity had long been surmised and has now been proved in experimental *Brugia* infection of dogs and cats (Ewert, 1971). It has also been shown that filariasis alone can produce lymphedema in heavy infections but that swelling and inflammation occur more prominently and more extensively if the blocked extremity is exposed to virulent streptococcal superinfection as soon as the first adult filarial worms have matured (Bosworth and Ewert, 1975). Nevertheless, the respective roles of filariae and of bacterial and fungal organisms remain a subject of continuing controversy. There is no evidence of a bacterial role in chyluria. Filarial hydrocele is only rarely found to be superinfected by bacteria, but elephantiasis or lymph scrotum quite regularly is. Thus, exposure to bacteria probably plays an important role, and by the time lymphedema has become established in an extremity, it would be difficult to avoid, especially in subjects who are farmers or laborers.

Another subject not yet fully clarified is the topography of worms in Bancroft's filariasis and its relationship to delayed pathologic effects. Very little is known about the favored sites in female patients, but serial autopsy studies of male patients indicate that the tail of the epididymis and the lower spermatic cord are among the most constant worm localization sites and are often the only ones found in mild infections (Galindo et al., 1962). Correspondingly, funiculoepididymitis is the most frequent direct manifestation of filariasis in the male, and hydrocele the most frequent indirect one.

Assuming that superinfection results in a saturation of the preferred habitat and therefore in the spread of adult filariae to increasingly distant sites, occupancy of the inguinal or femoral lymphatic trunks might bring about edema of the scrotum or lower extremities; higher filarial localizations at the level of the kidney hilus would bring about lymph varix, which—by rupture into a renal calyx—would cause chyluria. In keeping with this hypothesis, all the manifestations named, other than epididymitis and hydrocele, are more frequent in areas of high filarial transmission and in heavily infected

individuals; however, direct proof is unavailable, and locating filariae during human autopsies is notoriously difficult. Thus far no filariae have been found in the cisterna chyli or thoracic duct.

The results of permanent lymphatic obstruction can be seen in purest form in chyluria, in which protein- and lipid-rich lymph fluid escapes directly into urine, rendering it cloudy or milky, depending on the size of the leak. In hydrocele, similar fluid is stored in the scrotal cavity, varying from clear, slightly viscid material (Fig. 21–21) to a frankly milky or even cheesy appearance. Long-term storage of this fluid is irritating to the tunica and results in thickening, chronic lymphoplasmocytic inflammatory infiltration, and sometimes calcification (Figs. 21–22 and 21–23). Once these secondary changes take place, the scrotal contents become increasingly vulnerable to trauma and further irritation; this may result in minor bleeding and in further calcium and cholesterol deposition (von Lichtenberg and Medina, 1957).

The edema of filarial elephantiasis is, likewise, of the high-protein, high-cholesterol type and in this respect differs from hydrostatic edema. Permanent lymphedema in the subcutaneous tissue and dermis is regularly accompanied by lymphoid cell infiltrates, often centering around dilated superficial lymphatics that

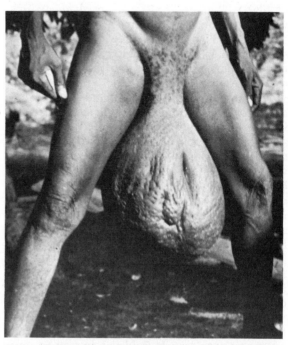

Figure 21–21. Huge hydrocele and scrotal elephantiasis. (Courtesy of Dr. B. H. Kean. Reproduced from Zaiman, H.: A Pictorial Presentation of Parasites.)

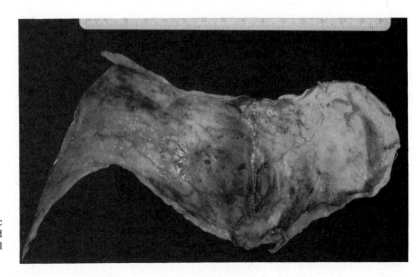

Figure 21–22. Excised hydrocele sac with marked fibrous thickening and focal calcification, plus recent focal hemorrhages.

may show polypoid lymphangitis or lymph thrombi. Such vessels can sometimes be visualized directly or by dye injection in locations where the overlying dermis is thin, especially the scrotum. There may also be perivascular infiltration and thickening of blood vessels as this process continues. In due course, fibroblastic and epithelial proliferation follow. Plump fibroblasts deposit additional ground substance and eventually build up a thick, dense layer of collagen. The epidermis becomes thickened, with focal condylomatous or papillomatous proliferations and with hyperkeratosis, and it acquires the pachydermal appearance from which elephantiasis derives its name (Fig. 21–24). The

underlying dermis is at first boggy but eventually becomes tough. There seems to be no limit to the connective tissue and epidermal growth, and grotesque enlargement of the penis, scrotum, or extremity can be the end result. At that stage, bacterial or fungal superinfection is extremely common and may result in recurrent lymphangitis, erysipelas, chronic festering ulcer, or persisting fungal crusting, thus aggravating the vicious cycle already established.

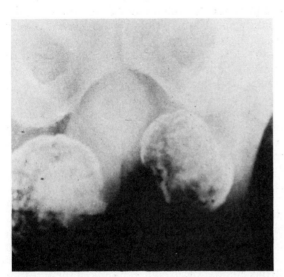

Figure 21–23. Bilateral intrascrotal calcifications in a filariasis patient. (Courtesy of Dr. B. H. Kean. Reproduced from Zaiman, H.: A Pictorial Presentation of Parasites.)

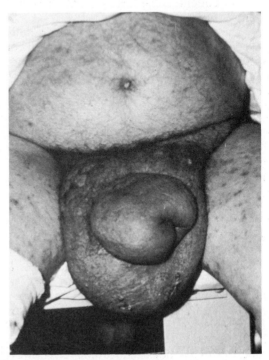

Figure 21–24. Elephantiasis of the penis and scrotum. (Courtesy of Dr. M. Wittner. Reproduced from Zaiman, H.: A Pictorial Presentation of Parasites.)

Clinical Manifestations

Prepatent Filariasis. Clinically, the earliest tissue changes of filariasis often coincide with fever or general symptoms; with swelling, reddening, or itching; or with formation of a small hydrocele in the affected region, sometimes visible only by transillumination. Episodic fever may recur ("fiebre de la costa"), as may the local symptoms, but as a rule these abate and are followed by clinical remission. Medical treatment (see later) is highly effective at this stage.

Funiculoepididymitis. Most symptomatic cases of filarial funiculoepididymitis are seen in patients prior to their fourth decade of life. The course of the attack may be single, with remission, or repetitive and progressive. Although the lower, intrascrotal portions of the cord are preferred, the high, intra-abdominal portions also can be involved. Besides local pain, which often radiates to the testis or mimics the pain of ureteral colic, there can be systemic symptoms, such as fever, chills, and anorexia; there is often marked psychologic alarm and anxiety.

Tissue swelling may be cordlike or lumpy to the touch, and in some instances may mimic the findings of an intrascrotal tumor or torsion of the cord. There may be accompanying hydrocele or soft tissue edema. Peripheral leukocytosis is frequent, sometimes with marked eosinophilia.

The picture may be further complicated by varicocele or thrombosis of the spermatic cord, which adds to the local pathologic lesion and to the pain and discomfort. In a number of documented instances, there has been bacterial superinfection of an acutely inflamed filarial cord, resulting in exquisite pain, high fever, septic thrombophlebitis, and pyemia or endocarditis. This alarming, and sometimes lethal, complication is, fortunately, rare. A nonfilarial form of thrombophlebitis of the cord has also been reported from India (Castellani, 1931).

Little is known of the outcome of the funicular filarial attack if properly diagnosed and left without surgical treatment, except that relatively mild cases have involuted spontaneously, with or without later recurrence. Because it is frequently impossible to rule out a more malignant condition, in many cases an operation is ultimately performed, at which time the homolateral testis is not infrequently sacrificed. Firm standards with regard to surgical indications have not been formulated; however, consideration should be given to the fact that filarial involvement is frequently bilateral, and contralateral funiculitis, although rarely reported, is a definite menace. In addition, even in severe funiculitis, the spermatic cord—unlike that in ascending bacterial infection—is usually intact and patent, and sterility due to filarial involvement must be a rare event.

The present authors are of the opinion that a rational therapeutic approach to filarial funiculoepididymitis requires a thorough work-up of the patient; evaluation of the etiologic basis, whether filarial or bacterial, or both; appropriate antibiotic treatment for the latter, if present; and conservative surgical correction of the former by decompression or excision of filarial nodules, preserving the testis and cord whenever possible. When funiculoepididymitis is recurrent, painful, and deforming, or is complicated by blood vessel involvement, more radical surgery is probably still justified. New approaches are obviously needed, including funicular lymphangiography or functional studies of the lymph flow, or both.

Orchitis. This complication is rarely seen in pure form and shares many of the features described under Funiculoepididymitis (see preceding section), which it may accompany. Its main importance derives from its capacity to simulate a rapidly developing malignant tumor of the testis.

Hydrocele. Differentiation of filarial from idiopathic hydrocele is often difficult on either clinical or laboratory grounds, but there are some features that may permit an inferential judgment; even though microfilariae or adult worms are rarely detected in the hydrocele fluid, the presence of a milky or sediment-rich hydrocele fluid constitutes an immediate clue, as does the presence of nodules along the cord or in the epididymis. With respect to the tunica, a very thick, fibrous covering should also arouse suspicion, especially if there are cholesterol or calcium deposits. Indeed, calcification of the tunica is so rare in idiopathic hydrocele that its presence is strongly suggestive of an infectious etiologic basis, especially of filariasis. Excision of the hydrocele sac, if possible intact, is the treatment of choice; an alternative method is inversion with partial excision (Jachowski et al., 1962). Small hydroceles that do not grow substantially can of course be ignored.

Scrotal and Penile Elephantiasis, Lymph Scrotum. Mild scrotal edema is not unusual either during the early phase of infection or in conjunction with established hydrocele. Penile edema is a more unusual event, and the monstrous elephantiasic enlargements of the scrotum or penis often depicted in textbooks of tropical medicine occur largely in populations that have no access to modern medical care, such as in tribesmen in remote jungle regions. Occasionally, however, such record-sized penile or scrotal lesions come under the care of a urologist—one such case was seen in Japan (Sato et al., 1974)—and enter the literature of urologic oddities. In leg elephantiasis the differential diagnosis between filaria and other etiologic possibilities (as in elephantiasis nostras) may be difficult, but genital elephantiasis is only rarely due to other factors, such as malignancy, lymph node surgery, or radiation. The only treatment currently available is excision and plastic reconstruction by full-thickness skin grafting (Jantet et al., 1961); unless associated bacterial infection is present, surgical healing is often quite satisfactory, despite a tendency for lymph weeping during and after surgery. Data on the frequency of recurrence are not available, but it must be regarded as a distinct danger in the long run, since the pathophysiologic condition underlying elephantiasis has really not been corrected.

Lymph scrotum is an extreme case of scrotal edema, in which blistering and weeping of lymph occur spontaneously; this condition is practically pathognomonic of severe filarial infection and is uncommon, except in certain geographic foci. Obviously, lymph scrotum can become a difficult problem, since the moist intercrural area is easily superinfected by bacteria or fungi, this resulting in festering skin ulcers or systemic sepsis, or both. This condition is difficult to treat medically, but excision can sometimes be effective.

Chyluria. This complication has been found in patients with or without microfilaremia, usually young adults, and is probably an earlier event in the natural history of filariasis than is genital elephantiasis. Until recently, the eruption of a lymphatic varix into the urinary collecting system had been a mere postulate, but this has now been directly demonstrated by lymphangiography. Lymph fistulae were found to be relatively distal, near the renal calyces (Tani and Akisada, 1970), and the thoracic duct was neither involved nor deformed. In some patients, two or more fistulae could be found. This could best be explained by lymphatic blockage with proximal dilatation, probably elicited by dying worms.

Chyluria may initially alarm the patient, but usually not for long, and thus, over a period of time, it can result in a relatively large-scale protein loss. In some patients, albumin synthesis may not generate sufficient colloid to keep them from becoming hypoproteinemic. In most, however, chyluria is intermittent, and protein loss is much less than is commonly found in protein-losing enteropathy; it may, in fact, correct itself spontaneously and responds rather promptly to bed rest, as well as to the use of abdominal binders that raise the intra-abdominal pressure sufficiently to stop the leak of low-pressure lymphatic fluid (Ahrens, 1970). Moreover, retrograde lymphangiography, a diagnostic procedure, appears to have a sclerosing effect on lymphatic fistulae and has been found to close them with curative effect in 48 per cent of patients so treated, and to ameliorate additional patients (Gandhi, 1976). This fortunate circumstance has made it unnecessary in most cases to attempt surgical correction, which is, at best, a difficult endeavor because the varix is often hard to find and to eliminate at the time of surgery. Radical procedures, such as nephrectomy, must be regarded as a form of surgical overkill.

Diagnosis

As in urinary schistosomiasis, a distinction should be made between diagnosis of infection and diagnosis of disease states resulting from infection.

Diagnosis of Infection. The detection of *Brugia* or *Wuchereria* microfilariae in peripheral blood is diagnostic. Proper identification is based on the presence or absence of sheathing and on the number and position of nuclei in the caudal end (Hunter et al., 1976; Taylor, 1960). Samples must be taken at times when maximal microfilaremia is known to occur, e.g., midnight in the case of nocturnal periodic *W. bancrofti*. Peripheral blood smears are best examined after lysing of red cells and staining with Giemsa or Leishman's stain. Various concentration methods are used to detect microfilariae, including filtration of volumes of hemolyzed blood. Microfilariae should also be searched for in chylous urine or hydrocele fluid. Immunologic tests exist, including complement fixation and skin tests. These are group-specific and useful only in suggesting a filarial etiologic basis for lymphedematous states. Histologic identification of adult worms in surgical or autopsy material is, of course, important, but routine biopsy is not advised, as worms are often few and difficult to find, and removal of enlarged lymph nodes may further prejudice lymph drainage. It should be noted that blood eosinophilia, while suggestive, is not invariably present.

Recognition of Amicrofilaremic Filariasis. Amicrofilaremic disease occurs in four different settings: (1) in early symptomatic cases, especially nonresidents exposed for the first time (military personnel, tourists); (2) in the late stages of filariasis, whether symptomatic or asymptomatic; (3) after treatment with diethylcarbamazine; and (4) as a distinctive syndrome (Danaraj et al., 1966; Lie, 1962). The latter syndrome, variously named occult filariasis, eosinophilic lung, or Meyers-Kouvenaar syndrome, is characterized by marked, sustained peripheral eosinophilia only temporarily affected by corticosteroids but responsive to antifilarial drugs; absence of classic filarial lesions such as lymphedema or funiculoepididymitis; presence of lymphadenopathy that can be marked enough to simulate lymphoma; and striking pulmonary infiltrates, often associated with allergic manifestations, especially asthma. The frequency of this syndrome varies markedly between endemic foci and is particularly predominant in Singapore and in southern India. It has been shown that the basophils and mast cells of tropical eosinophilia patients discharge histamine more vigorously when stimulated with microfilarial antigen than do cells of normal persons or of filaria-infected persons without the hypereosinophilic syndrome (Ottesen et al., 1979).

Diagnosis of Filarial Disease States. Careful history taking and physical examination are important in suggesting a filarial cause of lymphedema. It is noteworthy that all of the late filarial lesions have nonfilarial counterparts. This is possibly true even of chyluria, since it has never been proved that all endemic cases in the Far East are actually infected by filariae. Tuberculosis, schistosomiasis haematobia, and gonorrhea may produce funiculoepididymitis. Nonfilarial elephantiasis can be elicited by malignancies, by surgery, or by x-irradiation, or their combinations, and there exist idiopathic, infectious, and hereditary forms of lymphedema (such as elephantiasis nostras), some of them found in tropical areas where filarial transmission is absent. In the case of hydrocele, if one includes all minor intrascrotal collections, this is, of course, much more frequent than generally realized in tropical and nontropical populations. Idiopathic hydrocele with or without varicocele or hernia, or both, is indeed a frequent malady of older men. It can be shown, however, that in areas of filarial transmission hydrocele occurs at an earlier median age and is significantly increased in overall frequency (Jachowski et al., 1962).

Lymphangiography may help distinguish filariasis from other causes of lymphatic obstruction, especially from those conditions in which lymph vessels are reduced in their number and competence (Jantet et al., 1961). Also, calcified worms may rarely be demonstrable on plain x-ray film and may be of diagnostic help. Serodi-agnosis of filariasis, though obviously a desirable goal, has been hampered by cross reactions between antigens of different filarial species and other parasitic helminths. Through the use of modern techniques, such as monoclonal antibodies, antigen specificity should be improvable, perhaps to the point of future clinical applicability.

Treatment

Medical Management. In the treatment of lymphatic filariasis two objectives must be kept in mind: (1) elimination of the adult parasite in order to stop further progression of disease; and (2) abolition of microfilaremia in order to interrupt vector-borne transmission of the infection, a matter of public health concern. Unfortunately, there is as yet no wholly satisfactory drug regime for achieving *both* of these objectives; indeed, there is considerable discussion regarding the primacy of each of these aims and about the correct therapeutic route for achieving them. Most workers, however, agree that persons with patent microfilaremia should be treated.

The established antifilarial drug is diethylcarbamazine (DEC) (Hetrazan, Banocide), which promptly abolishes microfilaremia for at least several weeks. The evidence that DEC kills adult filariae as well is, at best, equivocal, but long-term low-dose treatment with this drug is reported to reduce the frequency of elephantiasis in comparison with untreated control subjects (Partono et al., 1981). In advanced filariasis, DEC has little effect on established pathology. Moreover, it is known to cause allergic "Mazotti reactions" in patients treated for *Onchocerca volvulus* infection and similar, though usually milder, allergic side effects in patients infected by *Wuchereria* or *Brugia* sp. Therefore, in patients with very high microfilarial counts, DEC should be started at low dosage (3 mg per kg body weight per day) and increased gradually in order to avoid severe symptoms. The recommended schedule otherwise is 6 mg per kg per day for a total course of 72 mg per kg in *W. bancrofti* infection versus 4 mg per kg per day for a total of 60 mg per kg in *B. malayi* disease. There is some variation of opinion regarding optimal scheduling and dose, and, in any case, the schedule should be adjusted to the patient's reaction to the drug. Headache, fever, nausea, vomiting, and allergic manifestations, as well as local pain and swelling over lymph nodes and along lymphatics, occur. Generalized and allergic symptoms usually respond to antihistamines.

New and experimental drugs currently under development include the benzimidazole compounds mebendazole and flubendazole, already in wide use as broad-spectrum antihelmintics, which have recently been used in onchocercal infection with promising clinical results. Allergic reactions and other side effects were fewer with these drugs than after the usual DEC treatment; however, experience with these drugs in lymphatic filariasis is still very limited. In any case, many authorities now concur that an effective anti–adult filarial drug is the desideratum and, when available, will eventually replace DEC. Until that time, the reader is best advised to turn to an experienced tropical medicine consultant or to the Parasitic Disease Section of the Center for Disease Control, Atlanta, Georgia, which maintains a repository of antifilarial drugs and can furnish detailed information about their use. Hints for the nonsurgical therapy of chyluria are given on page 1009.

Foot and skin care is of obvious importance in the management of lymphedema. Superimposed bacterial infections, particularly those with streptococci, should be treated vigorously.

Surgical Management. Genital elephantiasis is often amenable to surgical intervention, and a variety of procedures have been devised to remove edematous tissue and to reconstruct the scrotum or vulva. For local management, the reader is referred to the preceding sections dealing with specific complications.

Prognosis

Acute Filariasis in the Recently Infected Patient. The experience in the World War II Pacific theater has shown that early filariasis can produce considerable physical and psychologic discomfort. The migratory nature of the tissue swellings, the sometimes marked itchiness, the localization in the genital area, plus the uncertain prognosis frequently combined to threaten the patient's self-confidence, particularly if he was familiar with the chronic deformities of filariasis seen in endemic populations. However, long-term follow-up has revealed that only a small proportion of incidentally infected patients developed either hydrocele or elephantiasis years after they were first found infected. Treatment during the early stage of disease can reliably eliminate the infection, and if elephantiasis has not developed, it is unlikely to follow.

Late Chronic Stages. The prognosis of elephantiasis in patients receiving medical treatment is not known, although it is unusual for marked progression to continue. In some treated patients, elephantiasis will continue to progress, whereas in other patients a slow improvement has been noted.

Prevention and Control

Diethylcarbamazine has been used as a prophylactic drug, given in a small monthly dose. Major control methods include the use of residual insecticides, such as DDT, and the reduction of mosquito-breeding sites.

UROGENITAL TRICHOMONIASIS

Trichomonas vaginalis is a flagellate protozoan; it most frequently colonizes the vagina and cervix of postpubertal women and the anterior urethra of the male sexual partners. Chronic infections are largely asymptomatic, or attended by minimal itching and burning. New infection, or its spread to the female urethra or the posterior male urethra or prostate is more likely to give rise to detectable pathologic lesions and to clinical complaints. Although the penis, vulva, and other contiguous sites are occasionally invaded, disseminated infection is unknown in man; thus, the parasite is considered a near-commensal, or a weak pathogen, and most of its clinical importance derives from its simulation of more serious venereal and nonvenereal urogenital infections.

Biology and Life Cycle

The trichomonads and their nearest relatives, the ameboflagellates, include many nonpathogenic species, as well as animal parasites. *T. vaginalis* is the only known trichomonad that is pathogenic for humans and is known in only a single form: a 15- to 18-μm cell body shaped like a turnip or spinning top, with a single nucleus and three to four anterior flagella. Under high magnification, the undulating membrane, axostyle, and posterior flagellum become visible (Fig. 21–25). In a fresh preparation, trichomonads appear as relatively refringent objects smaller than host cells, and moving with a random sort of flitting motion, faster than that of granulocytes. The organisms multiply by binary fission, and no intermediary or animal hosts are known, although some strains of trichomonads are pathogenic when transmitted to baby mice and to female rabbits. *T. vaginalis* has now been cultured axenically in special media, and its strain characteristics and cell biology are being studied by sophisticated biotechnology. Thus far, however, success has been limited in

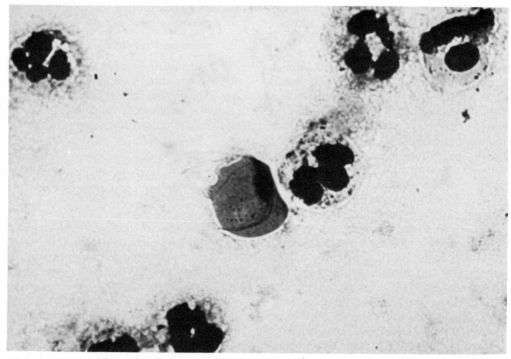

Figure 21–25. Trichomonas vaginalis, as seen in Giemsa-stained smear of urethral exudate. Note axostyle and flagella. × 1000. (Courtesy of Dr. Steven Pan, Harvard School of Public Health.)

understanding the basis for strain differences in pathogenicity (Honigberg, 1978).

Distribution and Epidemiology

Little is known about the frequency of asymptomatic infection, except that it is rare in prepubertal girls but common in sexually active women. Neonatal infection has also been reported (Farouk et al., 1974), alone or associated with candidiasis of the vestibulum vaginae. This age distribution has been attributed to the change in pH and bacterial environment of the vagina concomitant with the estrous cycle. In selected groups of gynecologic patients, frequencies of 40 to 60 per cent infection have been reported (Baumeister and Hollinger, 1941), but only one in seven such women has complaints attributable to trichomoniasis. Transmission is largely by sexual intercourse, most frequently heterosexual. By implication, examination of the index patient's sexual partners is warranted. However, unlike the case in syphilis, acquisition of the parasite under unhygienic bathroom conditions has been sufficiently documented so as to be a plausible source (Burgen, 1963). Little is known about the natural history of untreated trichomoniasis in the male, except that organisms tend to become scanty or to disappear in time in some individuals, while persisting in others, especially those with urethral stenosis of other causes. It also should be noted that the parasite is relatively resistant to cold temperature, but not to acid pH below 4.

Pathology and Pathogenesis

Relatively little is known about the feeding (by cytostome) and metabolism of trichomonads, and the mechanism that converts a commensal into a pathogen is therefore poorly understood. It has, however, been shown that *T. vaginalis* is capable of activating complement (Gillin and Sher, 1981). Mouse inocula suggest that strain variation exists with regard to pathogenicity, as is also true in the case of *Histomonas meleagridis*, the turkey parasite (Honigberg, 1970). An activation mechanism similar to that of *Entamoeba histolytica* has also been postulated, based on the transmission of a "virulence factor" from bacteria to the protozoan organism (Honigberg, 1978; Wittner and Rosenbaum, 1970). A relatively rich bacterial flora is indeed present in the *Trichomonas* habitat and is subject to population changes. As in amebiasis, broad-spectrum antibiotics have been found somewhat useful in suppressing pathologic effects and infection from trichomonads, but far less than specific therapy (see later).

Conversely, it is reasonable to believe that part of the pathology seen in symptomatic trichomoniasis may be the effect of bacterial superinfection, especially in cases showing relatively severe inflammation. Part of the host response to trichomonads is immunologically determined, since it has been observed that males show more violent urethritis upon reinfection than during the initial episode, even though it was treated. Further study of this subject is obviously needed, and it is unfortunate that the scientific community has almost ignored this interesting organism.

Regardless of localization site, pathologic lesions, when present, are largely exudative, with reddening of the mucosa, occasional edema, and variably showing reddish spots, small blisters, or granules. In the uterine cervix, this is described as "strawberry mucosa." Such lesions may be accompanied by marked tenderness and burning sensation, especially when touched or manipulated. The exudate is described as predominantly lymphoplasmocytic but may include polymorphonuclear leukocytes or eosinophils, especially if there is focal erosion or ulceration (which occurs rarely, and in such cases the role of bacteria is difficult to assess). The exudate as seen grossly on the mucosa or expressed from the urethra is usually creamy white or yellowish and frothy. Trichomonal pathology in the prostate or seminal vesicles has not been adequately investigated.

As far as available, histopathologic studies of other infected sites (mainly the uterine cervix) have shown chronic active inflammation, with or without mucosal erosion and without specific histologic features (Frost, 1974).

Clinical Manifestations

According to localization site, there can be trichomonal vaginitis, female or male urethritis, cystitis, prostatovesiculitis, and very rarely vulvar or preputial lesions. Combinations do, of course, occur. Since the pH of the childhood vagina does not permit trichomonal growth, the patients are typically adults, of sexually active ages.

The most common symptoms are itching, burning, tenderness, and discharge from either the vagina or the urethra, especially before or during micturition, sometimes with increased frequency of voiding. The discharge is typically described as scanty and frothy, often most noticeable in the morning, prior to first urination. Redness and irritation of the urethral meatus is frequently a main complaint. A common mode of presentation to the physician is worry about gonorrhea. Another common complaint is

chronic vaginitis or mild dyspareunia, or both, in female patients. In prostatovesiculitis or cystitis, there may in addition be mild pollakiuria and dull perineal or pelvic pain or discomfort. On rectal examination, the prostate and vesicles may feel enlarged and boggy or may be tender, but the more dramatic symptoms of bacterial genitourinary infection are lacking. It is important to be aware of the possible coincidence of trichomonal infection in patients whose genitourinary complaints are due to another cause. This is particularly important with respect to cervical carcinoma. Although hematuria due to trichomonads has been reported (Sanjurjo, 1970a), this is probably unusual and invites a fuller examination of possible causes. There have also been reports of renal trichomoniasis (Manwell, 1934), penile skin ulcers (Sowmini et al., 1972; Soubigou et al., 1938), and other lesions, but these are certainly unusual manifestations, if indeed due solely to the parasites.

Diagnosis

In cases in which acute symptoms appear, there are usually plenty of organisms, and the diagnosis is easily confirmed by examination of the fresh exudate diluted in a drop of warm physiologic saline and viewed under a middle-power microscope. Exudate from the vagina or urethral meatus, or vesicoprostatic fluid obtained by massage, may be used. The refringence and motility of the organisms are characteristic, and—if desired—their morphologic detail can be checked on air-dried, alcohol-fixed smears, stained with a Giemsa or Papanicolaou variant. An early-morning urethral specimen is especially useful if parasites are scanty. If these procedures fail, a sediment of a few milliliters of urine should be examined in the same manner. Urethral scrapings with a sterile platinum loop may sometimes be necessary. The last resort is culture, carried out in an experienced parasitologic laboratory.

Not infrequently, trichomonads are first detected in a Papanicolaou smear at the time of cytologic studies performed for other reasons in females, and, more rarely, in cervical or vaginal biopsy material, where they may actually be relatively difficult to recognize because of shrinkage and admixture with host exudate cells (Fig. 21–26). When detected in conjunction with cervical epithelial dysplasia, there may be some debate about the significance of that association, but the consensus is that, unlike the case of herpes simplex virus II or of the human papilloma viruses, this can be discounted (Bechtold and Reicher, 1952).

Very recently, an ELISA test for detecting

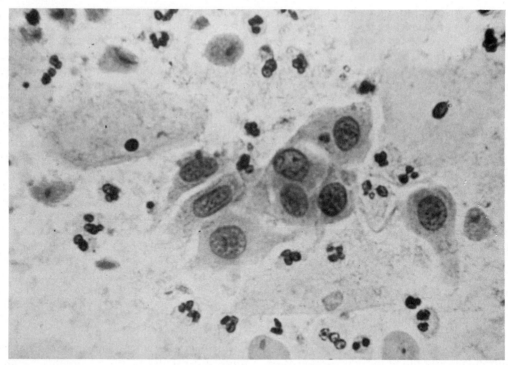

Figure 21–26. *T. vaginalis* in Papanicolaou smear from cervix, showing epithelial dysplasia. × 800. (From Reagan, J. W., and Patten, S. F., Jr.: Cytology of the Female Reproductive Tract. Chicago, American Society of Clinical Pathologists, 1967.)

antitrichomonas antibody has been developed. If its sensitivity/specificity proves satisfactory, this should become a useful tool for population screening. Serodiagnosis is unlikely, however, to replace the direct demonstration of *Trichomonas* in the clinical diagnosis of individual patients.

Treatment

Metronidazole (Flagyl) has revolutionized treatment, and oral drug administration has generally replaced repetitive topical maneuvers such as have been commonly used in the past (Sanjurjo, 1970a). Although metronidazole was shown to be mutagenic for bacterial tester strains and although there have been reports of carcinogenicity resulting from high-dose administration to rodents, no convincing evidence has yet come forth that therapeutic use of metronidazole results in long-term toxic effects to humans, such as fetal abnormalities or increased incidence of malignant tumors (Roe, 1982). To the contrary, since the efficacy of metronidazole against anaerobic bacterial pathogens became better recognized, it has now been administered to ever larger numbers of patients, sometimes with lifesaving effects yet still without evidence that it might have caused them irreparable

harm. Thus, metronidazole exemplifies the difficulties of predicting long-term toxicity for man from the animal studies currently used for that purpose. It is still the consensus, however, that use of metronidazole should be avoided in pregnant women. The status of other 5-nitroimidazole derivatives (tinidazole, ornidazole, nimorazole, and so forth) is currently under investigation.

A small number of *T. vaginalis* strains have shown resistance to repeated courses of metronidazole treatment, although these organisms show normal susceptibility to the drug under anaerobic conditions in vitro (Müller, 1982). The biochemical basis of that resistance is related to aerobic metabolism but is not fully understood. Unfortunately, resistance should be similar for alternate 5-nitroimidazole–derived drugs serving as potential substitutes. If such a resistant strain of *T. vaginalis* is encountered, efforts should be made to isolate the strain for research purposes and appropriate consultation should be obtained.

Metronidazole is changed to a toxic derivative by reduction of its nitro group and is then quickly converted to inactive compounds to be excreted. Nitroreduction is effected by the redox system of anaerobic organisms and is responsible for the drug's specificity. The drug's ultimate targets are the microbial DNA, RNA, and proteins. Administration is oral.

For vaginitis, metronidazole is given in three daily doses of 250 mg each (a total daily dosage of 750 mg) for 10 days. Additionally, one 500-mg vaginal suppository daily for 10 days will improve cure rates.

For symptomatic trichomoniasis in males, and for asymptomatic trichomoniasis in males and females, the oral regime given above will generally also be effective. Indications for treatment of asymptomatic infection have not been worked out, but in a sexually active individual it would seem reasonable to treat. Both male and female partners should be treated simultaneously to interrupt a cycle of reinfection.

Undesirable drug effects have been reported: dryness of the mouth, unpleasant taste, diarrhea, and penile burning. More serious is a possible central nervous system effect common to the nitrofurans, manifested by depression, insomnia, hallucinations, dizziness, and headache. Urticaria and temporary leukopenia may occur. As far as is known at present, all these manifestations are promptly reversed upon discontinuance of the drug. Patients should be cautioned to avoid alcoholic beverages during the course of treatment, as metronidazole may cause a disulfiram (Antabuse) type of reaction.

Prevention

Treatment of contacts is of obvious importance, as is personal hygiene. Sexual abstinence during the treatment period should be encouraged for a variety of reasons, including the possible mutagenic effect of the drug. Otherwise, a condom should be used during intercourse.

OTHER PARASITIC DISEASES OF THE GENITOURINARY TRACT

Grouped in this section are parasitic infections that are relatively rare, or in which urogenital manifestations are usually overshadowed by other disease processes. These include the two other human schistosomes, *S. mansoni* and *S. japonicum*, the filarial worm *Onchocerca*, the intestinal helminth *Oxyurus*, the larval tapeworm of hydatid disease, and *Entamoeba histolytica*, with all of its protean manifestations. The remainder of parasites in this group can be considered chance findings or medical curiosities.

SCHISTOSOMIASIS MANSONI AND JAPONICA

Although bladder and pelvic organ deposition of *S. mansoni* eggs is regularly demonstrated by autopsy digest, it is rarely substantial; in the Egyptian focus, the *S. mansoni* egg load was found to be approximately 100 times less than that of *S. haematobium* when eggs of both species were present (Smith et al., 1974). Little is known about genitourinary involvement by *S. japonicum*. Clinically, "ectopic urogenital lesions" of schistosomiasis mansoni and japonica behave much like the stray pelvic lesions described in *S. haematobium* infection, i.e., they can manifest themselves as chronic cervicitis, as asymptomatic intrascrotal lumps, or—rarely—even as subcutaneous granulomas of the penile or perineal skin. Eggs may also reach the kidney and urinary passages and may be shed in the urine, or in the ejaculate, usually in small numbers. The main significance of such findings is to direct attention to more substantial schistosomal lesions of the gastrointestinal tract, liver, and pulmonary vasculature or of the central nervous system.

ONCHOCERCIASIS

Onchocerca volvulus is the agent of African river blindness and of severe, debilitating, chronic dermatitis. Onchocerciasis is common throughout tropical Africa, and endemic foci also exist in Central and South America, with some regional variation in the clinical picture. This filaria differs sharply from *Brugia* and *Wuchereria* in that (1) it is transmitted by black flies of the *Simulium* species; (2) its adult worms inhabit the subcutaneous tissue and are large enough to cause palpable fibrous nodules, in which they are encapsulated; and (3) microfilariae are diffusely distributed throughout the dermis, also appearing in the anterior eye chamber but not in the peripheral blood. Diagnosis and estimation of infection intensity are made by microscopic examination of skin scrapings.

The late stages of onchocercal infection, when blindness and atrophic dermatitis are usually the principal manifestations, produce hanging groin and scrotal elephantiasis. A few hanging groins have been successfully excised by surgery with good primary wound closure. Excised surgical specimens have shown atrophy and fibrosis of the inguinal lymph nodes with subcutaneous edema and fibrosis superimposed on the usual onchocercal dermatitis (Connor et al., 1970); the pathogenesis of these lesions has not been clarified, except that they have been shown to occur in areas where *Wuchereria* or

Brugia infection are not endemic and cannot therefore be attributed to filariae other than *Onchocerca* (Connor et al., 1970).

Most patients with onchocercal hanging groin are from endemic areas of rural Africa, where prevention of infection is today of high priority if the agricultural food supply of those zones is to be ensured and further developed. An excellent World Health Organization monograph on onchocerciasis is available (Buck, 1974). Therapy has been a difficult problem. Recently, encouraging results have been reported with mebendazole and with Ivermectin (Aziz, 1982).

PELVIC OXYURIASIS

The common intestinal pinworm, *Oxyuris (Enterobius) vermicularis,* which is ubiquitous worldwide, will occasionally migrate from its nocturnal swarming site, the anus, into the vagina and upward, reaching the peritoneal cavity via the uterus and fallopian tube. In that unnatural habitat, worm movement and egg laying will continue for some time before the worms die. This can be accompanied by active inflammation involving the pelvic peritoneum, with pain, fever, simulated acute appendicitis, or other bizarre manifestations that are seldom attributed to their true cause. At a later stage, dead worms and eggs become enclosed by granulomas and adhesions, which are sometimes detected years later as an incidental surgical finding. Because these granulomas grossly resemble miliary tubercles, they may cause confusion until eggs in these foci have been correctly identified (Symmers, 1950). Although oxyuris eggs differ from those of schistosomes in size, shape, and absence of spine, they do occasionally show Hoeppli phenomena. It is unusual to find *Ascaris* eggs in the same pelvic location without severe peritonitis or perforation (Waller and Othersen, 1971). Thus, the correct parasitologic diagnosis is of obvious importance, the more so since treatment of pelvic oxyuriasis—if still indicated—is simply effected with pyrvinium pamoate or other systemic anthelmintics.

HYDATID DISEASE

There is virtually no part of the human anatomy in which hydatid cysts have not appeared, but renal hydatids constitute a small proportion (about 2 per cent) relative to the principal sites, the liver and lung (Musacchio and Mitchell, 1966; Borrell and Barnes, 1933). The hydatid is the larval form of *Taenia echin-*

ococcus (Echinococcus granulosus), whose definitive host is the dog and whose intermediary host is the sheep. The major endemic sites of hydatidosis are superimposable with areas of sheep-raising, such as Australia, Argentina, Greece, Spain, the Middle East, and so forth. In many of these areas progress has been made in preventing transmission, but previously infected patients will carry their cysts for most of their remaining lifetimes. In addition, there are feral life cycles that may explain the sporadic occurrence of human cases in sites in which sheep are absent; echinococcal cysts of other species are found in Alaska, Siberia, and parts of Europe *(E. multilocularis)* (Rausch, 1967) and in Central America *(E. vogeli)* (D'Alessandro et al., 1979). In each instance, the cysts are acquired by man, the accidental host, through unwitting ingestion of tapeworm eggs excreted in the feces of dogs or of alternate feral hosts.

In the kidney, or in other urogenital sites, most of the evolution of pathologic lesions is dominated by the slow, concentric growth of the hydatid cyst over a number of years. Hydatid cysts can be asymptomatic or give rise to pressure symptoms and dull flank pain, depending upon the location and size. While viable and growing, the cyst wall is a thick, laminated polysaccharide parasite membrane on which the parasite's germinal epithelium is anchored (Fig. 21–27). The cyst is enveloped by a host fibrous shell with mild inflammatory reaction. Epithelial sprouts are formed inwardly, giving rise to scolices and daughter cysts that repeat the patterns found in the mother cyst; each scolex contains a small tapeworm head recognizable by its crown of hooklets (Fig. 21–27). Water-clear cystic fluid of high protein and antigen content bathes the germinal structures. The cysts can reach up to 20 cm in diameter, but they usually rupture at some earlier point (Fig. 21–28).

Rupture can occur as a slow leak resulting in the involution of the cyst, which fills with debris, cholesterol, and "hydatid sand" composed of dead and/or viable scolices, daughter cysts, and hooklets and which eventually calcifies; or rupture may be dramatic, attended by systemic anaphylactoid symptoms or by spillage of cystic products into the peritoneum or the blood stream. New metastatic cysts may thus arise in other organs. Rupture into the renal pelvis gives rise to acute flank pain followed by voiding of scolices or daughter cysts, with or without hematuria and/or obstruction of urinary passages (Musacchio and Mitchell, 1966; Borrell and Barnes, 1933). This unusual complication is diagnosed by locating the scolices or single

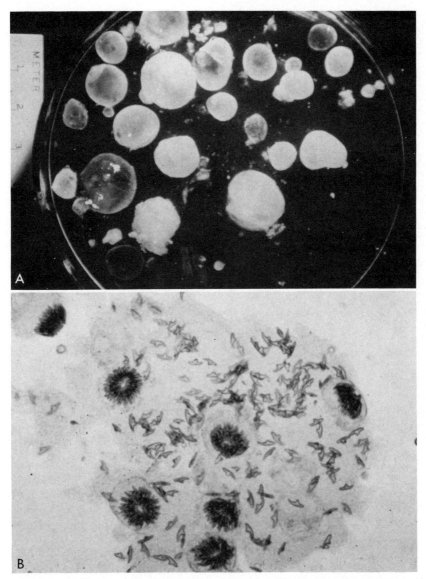

Figure 21–27. *A,* Hydatid daughter cysts and hydatid sand. *B, E. granulosus* scolices and hooklets seen by microscopic examination of hydatid sand. (Reproduced from Zaiman, H.: A Pictorial Presentation of Parasites.)

hooklets in the urinary sediment, for which darkfield observation may be useful. The hooklets are refringent and small, measuring about 5 μm, and must be searched for carefully. More frequent than this sudden clinical presentation is a chronic dull flank or lower back discomfort due to cystic pressure, rarely with microscopic hematuria. The cysts, being focal, seldom affect renal function. The diagnosis can be made by radiographs or CAT scans, which show the spherical cyst, its relatively thick wall, a fluid content, and often some calcification of the cystic wall. When the x-ray appearance is not fully characteristic, the Casoni skin test with hydatid fluid antigen has proved useful, and complement fixation and hemagglutination inhibition tests are also available (through state laboratories or the Center for Disease Control in Atlanta). In most cases the diagnosis, *once suspected,* presents little difficulty. Treatment, if warranted, is by surgical excision. This is definitely an elective procedure, except in the case of those few hydatid cysts that have become superinfected by bacteria and thus constitute

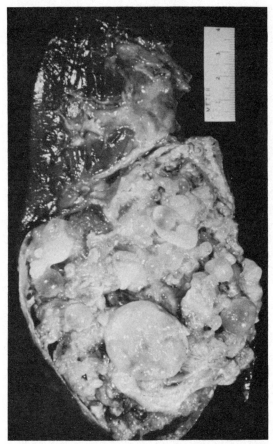

Figure 21–28. Echinococcosis of the human kidney.

the nidus of a chronic, difficult-to-eradicate urinary infection. Allergic manifestations of hydatid disease may require corticosteroids.

AMEBIASIS

In invasive infections by *Entamoeba histolytica,* the kidney is the fifth most common site of abscess localization (Brandt and Perez Tamayo, 1970). The abscess is, however, almost invariably accompanied by other invasive lesions, particularly by liver abscesses. The right kidney is more frequently involved, and the pathologic lesion is similar to that seen in the liver; hematuria may be a prominent manifestation, especially if the growing abscess induces renal vein thrombosis. The outcome of this condition, whether or not diagnosed during life, is frequently lethal, and medical therapy (metronidazole, emetine, or chloroquine) must be promptly instituted. Surgery, if necessary, should be performed only after drug therapy has taken hold; otherwise, disastrous spread of amebic infection is likely to occur (Grigsby, 1969).

Amebic ulceration of the perineum—e.g., anal skin, scrotum, and penis—can occur in continuity with rectal ulcers or by fecal contamination of abraded skin. These lesions, although rare, are extremely destructive and can permanently damage or scar the affected area (Engman and Meleney, 1931). Clinical awareness is important, since such lesions often resemble bacterial or fusospirillar ulcers, but their burrowing margins, necrotic, discolored surface, and indolence should furnish a clue eventually leading to microscopic identification of amebae in freshly collected necrotic exudate, or on iron hematoxylin–stained permanent smears. These procedures are preferable to biopsy diagnosis. The patient groups most likely to present such lesions are children in endemic areas where there is poor hygiene and a scarce water supply. Most of them have had past or present dysenteric symptoms as well. Amebiasis of the urethra and bladder has been described but is usually part of devastating invasive amebiasis with other systemic manifestations for which the patient has sought medical help. Good reviews on the pathology (Brandt and Perez Tamayo, 1970), surgery (Grigsby, 1969), and medical management of amebiasis (Barrett-Connor, 1972; Powell, 1969) are available.

SEXUALLY TRANSMITTED PROTOZOAL ENTERIC INFECTIONS

Sporadic instances of amebic ulcer of the penis have long been known to occur among individuals practicing anal intercourse. These shaggy, undermining ulcers can be confused with other venereal and nonvenereal skin infections unless fresh scrapings are examined for *Entamoeba histolytica* trophozoites. In some instances such lesions have been surgically excised after proving resistant to empirical antibiotics and have been diagnosed only after histopathologic study. Occasionally, the elementary bodies of *Chlamydia trachomatis,* found in its various venereal lesions, have been mistaken for protozoal parasites.

Transmission of enteric pathogens by variant sexual practices such as cunnilingus or anal eroticism has become an increasingly prevalent problem in medical practice. The protozoa *Entamoeba histolytica, Giardia lamblia,* and *Cryptosporidium* sp. as well as bacterial and viral pathogens are known causes of the "gay bowel syndrome," an entity most familiar to physicians in metropolitan venereal disease clinics (Owen, 1980). Stool examination for cysts or trophozoites of these organisms is useful in homosexual or bisexual patients whose sexual preferences expose them to this hazard regardless of whether they currently show symptoms or not. A large proportion of treatable *Giardia* and amebic infections are clinically silent yet constitute a potential source of transmission. Thus, the rule of contacting the partners of infected index cases, if feasible, applies here as it does in other venereal infections (Owen, 1980). The clinical and pathologic manifestations of venereally transmitted amebiasis or giardiasis, when they occur, are the same as in the general population. With regard to cryptosporidiasis, its endemicity and morbidity are still unknown, as this infection has only recently been recognized in humans. The infection is detected either by histopathologic study of small bowel biopsy material or by a flotation method for stool extracts that is not yet widely used. Rarely, homosexual patients with the acquired immune deficiency syndrome (AIDS) have experienced chronic intestinal malabsorption and even lethal infection by this agent (Weinstein et al., 1982).

STRAY PARASITES OF UROGENITAL ORGANS

Many nematode species that have migratory larvae, or can produce ectopic lesions, have been sporadically detected in urogenital organs or urine; among these are *Strongyloides stercoralis* (in strongyloides hyperinfection) (Whitehill and Miller, 1944), *Toxocara canis* (visceral larva migrans) (Dent et al., 1965), and *Armillifer armillatus* (a primitive pentastomid acquired from reptiles, seen chiefly in Africa and in Southeast Asia) (Hopps, 1971; Lindner, 1965; Cannon, 1942). Rare organisms that have at one time or another been reported in human urine are flies and insect larvae (Sanjurjo, 1970*b*), and even fish—*Vandelia cirrhosa*, or Candiru, a small Amazonian catfish (Lins, 1945).

EFFECT OF PARASITIC INFECTIONS ON THE KIDNEY

As laboratory and pathology services have become more available in tropical countries, it has been noted that the frequencies of proteinuria and of nephrosis-nephritis are greater in several geographically dispersed tropical areas than is commonly reported from temperate, industrialized countries. Children and young adults seem to be particularly affected. Populations with greater propensity to renal parenchymal damage generally also present a large diversity of endemic infectious and parasitic diseases, including malaria, schistosomiasis, salmonellosis, leprosy, filariasis, hepatitis, and streptococcal infection. Thus, it is often difficult in individual cases or population groups to relate proteinuria or renal disease to any single etiologic factor. It is nevertheless important to be aware of nephropathy as a prominent health hazard in the tropics and when possible to perform appropriate screening on individuals belonging to high-risk groups, even if they are symptom-free.

Some of the etiologic factors of tropical nephropathies have recently been better defined. The long-suspected relationship between malaria and the nephrotic syndrome has been directly, as well as experimentally, confirmed by the demonstration of malarial antigen and specific antibody globulin in the glomerular basement membrane of nephrotic children infected with *P. malariae* and in macaque and *Aotus* monkeys with primate malarias (Voller et al., 1973; Ward and Conran, 1969). This nephropathy is not unique to quartan malaria but is more frequently associated with *P. malariae*, possibly because of the long and frequently subclinical course of that infection. Glomerular damage in malarial nephrosis appears to involve both the classic and the alternate complement pathway. The course of malarial nephrosis is often chronic and progressive and is relatively unresponsive to corticosteroid treatment. Affected patients have hyperglobulinemia and show distinctive serum protein clearance patterns (Soothill and Hendrickse, 1967). Eradication of quartan malaria in an endemic focus substantially decreases the number of cases of childhood nephrosis (Gilles and Hendrickse, 1963).

A suspected relationship between proteinuria, nephropathy, and schistosomiasis mansoni has also been partially confirmed. On population survey, significantly higher urinary protein excretion was found in schistosome-infected than in noninfected individuals in a malaria-free zone of Brazil, even though few of the surveyed individuals had any of the severe manifestations of schistosomiasis (Lehman et al., 1975). Mesangial glomerular proliferation with focal membranous change is the most frequent finding at autopsy in patients with *S. mansoni* infections and is significantly increased in those with hepatosplenic disease, i.e., with pipestem liver fibrosis resulting from severe infection (Andrade et al., 1971). These changes (Fig. 21–29) have also been experimentally reproduced in chimpanzees (Cavallo et al., 1974) and, in somewhat

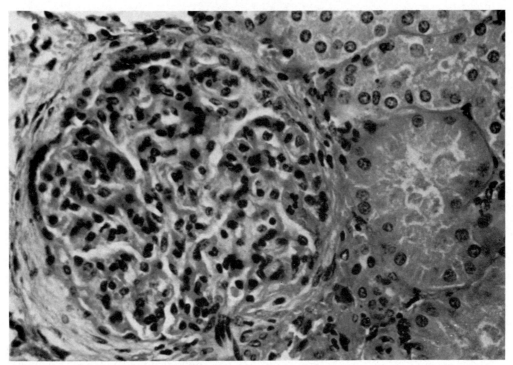

Figure 21–29. Glomerulus of experimental primate with schistosomal nephropathy. Note mesangial and capsular proliferation and neutrophils in glomerular loops. × 420.

lesser form, in other experimental animals (Hillyer and Lewert, 1974). The pathogenesis of this unique, and relatively benign, nephropathy, which ends in renal failure in relatively few patients, remains uncertain and is currently a subject of active investigation. It is known that circulating antigen of schistosome gut origin (von Lichtenberg et al., 1974) (Fig. 21–30) is detectable in severe experimental and in human *S. mansoni* infection. Several observers have noted deposition of immunoglobulins and complement fractions in the mesangium and to a lesser extent in the glomerular loops of human and experimental specimens studied by immunofluorescence (de Brito et al., 1971). In a few clinical specimens and, more consistently, in experimental animals, schistosome antigens have also been demonstrated in these lesions (Moriearty and de Brito, 1977).

Similar findings are beginning to emerge from studies of patients with lepromatous leprosy, and in this case the finding of specific immune complexes in the glomeruli has also recently been claimed. The antigen in this case appears to be a protein-linked polysaccharide, which has also been found in the arteriolar lesions of erythema nodosum leprosum rather than the well-known waxlike mycobacterial

phospholipids. In filariasis, evidence of nephropathy is thus far only experimental, involving renal antigen-antibody complexes and electronmicrographic abnormalities in *Dirofilaria*-infected dogs and in *Brugia*-infected hamsters (Klei et al., 1974). Whether nephritis occurs in chronic human lymphatic filariasis is not yet known. It should also be noted that in leprosy and in filariasis, renal amyloidosis is a known complication of human and of experimental infection, respectively.

In trypanosomiasis, experimental evidence is somewhat ahead of clinical studies. In acute Rhodesian sleeping sickness, the cause of renal failure appears to be diffuse intravascular coagulation rather than nephritis, and the chronic Gambian form has not yet been studied nephrologically. However, nephritic kidney changes have been reported in cattle infected with *Trypanosoma congolense,* and recently marked proliferative nephritis was seen in macaques experimentally infected with *T. rhodesiense,* within a few weeks of the onset of infection. This renal lesion also involves both the classic and the alternate complement pathway (Nagle et al., 1974).

In conclusion, it appears that in tropical countries endemic parasitic infections are added

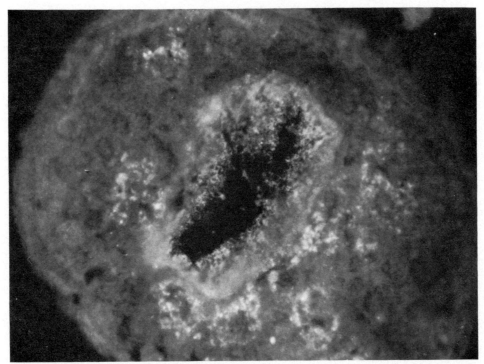

Figure 21–30. Cross section of female *S. mansoni,* stained for "circulating antigen" by the indirect immunofluorescent method. Esophagus and its lumen show positive staining. Approximately × 400.

to other causes of nephropathy that exist in temperate zones, and a variety of disease entities are probably now lumped together under the label "tropical mesangiocapillary glomerulonephritis." More research is urgently needed, especially since better knowledge of parasite-related nephropathies may enlarge our general understanding of the pathogenesis of renal diseases, and their prevention.

References

Ah, H. S., McCall, J. W., and Thompson, P. E.: Vaccination against experimental *Brugia pahangi* infection in dogs. *In* Proceedings of the Third International Congress on Parasitology, Munich, Germany, Vol. 3, pp. 1236–1237, 1974a.

Ah, H. S., Klei, T. R., McCall, J. W., and Thompson, P. E.: *Brugia pahangi* infections in Mongolian jirds and dogs following the ocular inoculation of infective larvae. J. Parasitol., *60*:643, 1974b.

Ahrens, E. H., Jr.: Clinical research on patients with chyluria. Jpn. J. Trop. Med., *11*:53, 1970.

Alves, W.: The distribution of schistosoma eggs in human tissues. Bull. W. H. O., *18*:1092, 1958.

Andrade, Z. S., Andrade, S. G., and Sadigursky, M.: Renal changes in patients with hepatosplenic schistosomiasis. Am. J. Trop. Med. Hyg., *20*:77, 1971.

Aziz, M. A.: Efficacy and tolerance of Ivermectin in human onchocerciasis. Lancet, *2*:171, 1982.

Barrett-Connor, L.: Chemoprophylaxis of amebiasis and trypanosomiasis. Ann. Intern. Med., *77*:797, 1972.

Baumeister, C., and Hollinger, N.: *Trichomonas* infection of the male genitourinary tract. Arch. Surg., *43*:433, 1941.

Beaver, P. C., and Cran, I. R.: *Wuchereria*-like filaria in an artery, associated with pulmonary infarction. Am. J. Trop. Med. Hyg., *23*:869, 1974.

Bechtold, E., and Reicher, N. B.: The relationship of *Trichomonas* infestations to false diagnoses of squamous carcinoma of the cervix. Cancer, *5*:422, 1952.

Bell, D. R.: A new method for counting *Schistosoma mansoni* eggs in faeces: With special reference to therapeutic trials. Bull. W. H. O., *29*:525, 1963.

Bird, A. V.: Spinal cord complications of bilharziasis. S. Afr. Med. J., *39*:158, 1967.

Borrell, J. H., and Barnes, J. M.: Renal manifestations of hydatid diseases. N.Y. State J. Med., *33*:1390, 1933.

Bosworth, W., and Ewert, A.: The effect of streptococcus on the persistence of *Brugia malayi* and the production of elephantiasis in cats. Int. J. Parasitol., *5*:583, 1975.

Bradley, D. J., and McCullough, F. S.: Egg output stability and the epidemiology of *Schistosoma haematobium.* II. An analysis of the epidemiology of endemic *S. haematobium.* Trns. R. Soc. Trop. Med. Hyg., *67*:491, 1973.

Brandt, H., and Perez Tamayo, R.: Pathology of human amebiasis. Hum. Pathol., *1*:351, 1970.

Buck, A. A. (Ed.): Onchocerciasis: Symptomatology, pathology, diagnosis. Geneva, World Health Organization, 1974.

Burgen, J. A.: *Trichomonas vaginalis* infection from splashing in water closets. Br. J. Vener. Dis., *39*:248, 1963.

Cannon, D. A.: Linguatulid infestation of man. Ann. Trop. Med. Parasitol., *36*:160, 1942.

Castellani, A.: Endemic funiculitis, brief general account. J. Trop. Med., *34*:373, 1931.

Cavallo, T., Galvanek, E. G., Ward, P. A., and von Lichtenberg, F.: The nephropathy of experimental hepatosplenic schistosomiasis. Am. J. Pathol., 76:433, 1974.

Cheever, A. W.: Schistosomiasis and neoplasia (Editorial). J. Natl. Cancer Inst., 61:13, 1978.

Cheever, A. W., and Anderson, L. A.: Rate of destruction of *Schistosoma mansoni* eggs in the tissues of mice. Am. J. Trop. Med. Hyg., 20:62, 1971.

Chernin, E.: Some host-finding attributes of *Schistosoma mansoni* miracidia. Am. J. Trop. Med. Hyg., 23:320, 1974.

Cohen, L. B., Nelson, G., Wood, A. M., Manson-Bahr, P. E. C., and Bowen, R.: Lymphangiography in filarial lymphedema and elephantiasis. Am. J. Trop. Med. Hyg., 10:843, 1961.

Connor, D. H., Morrison, N. E., Kerdel-Vegas, F., Berkoff, H. A., Johnson, F., Tunnicliffe, R., Failing, F. L., Hale, L. N., Lindquist, K., et al.: Oncocerciasis: Oncocercal dermatitis, lymphadenitis and elephantiasis in the Ubangi territory. Hum. Pathol., 1:553, 1970.

Cook, I. A.: Treatment. *In* Nash, T. E. (Moderator): Schistosome infection in humans: Perspectives and recent findings. Ann. Intern. Med., 97:740, 1982.

D'Alessandro, R. L.: *Echinococcus vogeli* in man with a review of polycystic disease in Colombia and neighboring countries. Am. J. Trop. Med. Hyg., 28:303, 1979.

Danaraj, T. J., Pacheco, W., Shanmugaratnam, K., and Beaver, P. C.: The etiology and pathology of eosinophilic lung (tropical eosinophilia). Am. J. Trop. Med. Hyg., 19:181, 1966.

Davis, A.: Management of the patient with schistosomiasis. *In* Jordan, P., and Webbe, G. (Eds.): Schistosomiasis, Epidemiology, Treatment and Control. pp. 184–226. London, William Heinemann Medical Books, 1982.

de Brito, T., Gunji, J., Camargo, M. E., Ceravolo, A., and da Silva, L. C.: Glomerular lesions in experimental infection of *Schistosoma mansoni* in *Cebus apella* monkeys. Bull. W. H. O., 45:419, 1971.

Denham, D. A., Ponnudurai, T., Nelson, G. S., Frances, G., and Rogers, R.: Studies with *Brugia pahangi:* I. Parasitological observations on primary infections of cats *(Felis catus)*. Int. J. Parasitol., 2:239, 1972.

Dent. J. H., Nichols, R. L., Beaver, P. C., Carrera, G. M., and Staggers, R. J.: Visceral larva migrans; with a case report. Am. J. Pathol., 32:777, 1965.

de Serres, F. J., Guest Editor: Workshop on long-term toxicity of antischistosomal drugs. J. Toxicol. Environ. Health, 1(2):173, 1975.

Diaz Rivera, R. S., Ramos Morales, F., Koppisch, E., Garcia Palmieri, M. R., Cintron Rivera, A. A., Marchand, E. J., and Torregrosa, M. V.: Acute Manson's schistosomiasis. Am. J. Med., 21:918, 1956.

Edington, G. M., Nwabuebo, I., and Junaid, T. A.: The pathology of schistosomiasis in Ibadan, Nigeria, with special reference to the appendix, brain, pancreas and genital organs. Trans. R. Soc. Trop. Med. Hyg., 69:153, 1975.

Edington, G. M., von Lichtenberg, F., Nwabuebo, I., Taylor, J. R., and Smith, J. H.: Pathologic effects of schistosomiasis in Ibadan, Western State of Nigeria. I. Incidence and intensity of infection; distribution and severity of lesions. Am. J. Trop. Med. Hyg., 19:982, 1970a.

Edington, G. M., von Lichtenberg, F., Nwabuebo, I., Taylor, J. R., and Smith, J. H.: Pathogenesis of lesions of the bladder and ureters. Am. J. Trop. Med. Hyg., 20:244, 1970b.

El-Mofty, A. M., and Nada, M.: Cutaneous schistosomiasis. Egypt. J. Bilharz., 2:23, 1975.

Engman, M. F., and Meleney, H. E.: Amebiasis cutis. Arch. Dermatol. Syph., 24:1, 1931.

Ewert, A.: Distribution of developing and mature *Brugia malayi* in cats at various times after a single inoculation. J. Parasitol., 74:1039, 1971.

Farouk, L., Al-Salihi, Curran, J. P. and Wang, J. S.: Neonatal *Trichomonas vaginalis:* Report of 3 cases and review of the literature. Pediatrics, 53:196, 1974.

Frost, J. K.: Protozoa. *In* Novak, E. R., and Woodruff, J. D. (Eds.): Novak's Gynecologic and Obstetric Pathology. 7th ed., pp. 679–680. Philadelphia, W. B. Saunders Co., 1974.

Galindo, L., von Lichtenberg, F., and Baldizon, C.: Bancroftian filariasis in Puerto Rico: Infection pattern and tissue lesions. Am. J. Trop. Med. Hyg., 11:739, 1962.

Gandhi, G. M.: Role of lymphangiography in management of filarial chyluria. Lymphology, 9:11, 1976.

Gelfand, M.: Schistosomiasis in south central Africa, a clinicopathological study. Cape Town, Juta, 1950.

Ghorab, M. M. A.: Ureteritis calcinosa—A complication of bilharzial ureteritis and its relation to primary ureteric stone formation. Br. J. Urol., 34:33, 1962.

Gilles, H. M. and Hendrickse, R. G.: Nephrosis in Nigerian children: Role of *Plasmodium malariae;* effect of antimalarial treatment. Br. Med. J., 2:27, 1963.

Gilles, H. M., Lucas, A., Linder, R., Cockshot, S. G., et al.: *Schistosoma haematobium* infection in Nigeria. III. Infection in boatyard workers at Epe. Ann. Trop. Med. Parasitol., 59:451, 1965.

Gillin, F. D., and Sher, A.: Activation of the alternate complement pathway by *Trichomonas vaginalis*. Infect. Immun., 34:268, 1981.

Grigsby, W. P.: Surgical treatment of amebiasis. Surg. Gynecol. Obstet., 128:609, 1969.

Hang, L. M., Boros, D. L., and Warren, K. S.: Induction of immunologic hyporesponsiveness to granulomatous hypersensitivity in *Schistosoma mansoni* infection. J. Infect. Dis., 130:515, 1974.

Hiatt, R. A., Sotomayor, Z. R., Sanchez, G., Zombrana, M., and Knight, W. B.: Factors in the pathogenesis of acute schistosomiasis mansoni. J. Infect. Dis., 139:659, 1979.

Higashi, G. I., Farid, Z., Bassily, S., and Miner, W. F.: Nephrotic syndrome in schistosomiasis mansoni complicated by chronic salmonellosis. Am. J. Trop. Med. Hyg., 24:713, 1975.

Hillyer, G. V., and Lewert, R. M.: Studies on renal pathology in hamsters infected with *Schistosoma mansoni* and *Schistosoma japonicum*. Am. J. Trop. Med. Hyg., 23:404, 1974.

Honigberg, B. M.: Trichomonads. *In* Jackson, G. J., Herman, R., and Singer, I. (Eds.): Immunity to Parasitic Animals. Vol. 2, pp. 469–550. New York, Appleton-Century Crofts, 1970.

Honigberg, B. M.: Trichomonads of importance in human medicine. *In* Kreier, J. P. (Ed.): Parasitic Protozoa. Vol. 2, pp. 469–550. New York, Academic Press, 1978.

Hopps, H. C.: Pentastomiasis. *In* Marcial-Rojas, R. (Ed.): Pathology of Protozoal and Helminthic Diseases. pp. 970–989. Baltimore, The Williams & Wilkins Co., 1971.

Hunter, G. W., Swartzwelder, J. C., and Clyde, D. F.: Morphology of the Filarioidea. *In* Hunter, G. W., Swartzwelder, J. C., and Clyde, D. F.: Tropical Medicine. 5th ed., pp. 492–494. Philadelphia, W. B. Saunders Co., 1976.

W.H.O.: Immunology of schistosomiasis. Memorandum of a meeting of investigators held in Nairobi, December 11–17, 1974.

Is Flagyl dangerous? Med. Lett. Drugs Ther., *17*(13):53 (June 20), 1975.

Jachowski, L. A., Gonzalez-Flores, B., and von Lichtenberg, F.: Filarial etiology of tropical hydroceles in Puerto Rico. Am. J. Trop. Med. Hyg., *11*:220, 1962.

Jantet, G. H., Taylor, G. W., and Kinmonth, J. B.: Operations for primary lymphedema of the lower limbs: Results after 1–9 years. J. Cardiovasc. Surg. (Torino), *2*:27, 1961.

Kagan, I. G.: Current status of serologic testing for parasitic disease. Hosp. Pract., *9*:157, 1974.

Kanetkar, A. V., Deshmukh, S. M., Pradham, R. S., Kelhar, M. D., and Sen, P. K.: Lymphangiographic patterns in filarial oedema of lower limbs. Clin. Radiol., *17*:258, 1966.

Klei, T. R., Crowell, W. A., and Thompson, P. E.: Ultrastructural glomerular changes associated with filariasis. Am. J. Trop. Med. Hyg., *23*:608, 1974.

Klei, T. R., McCall, J. W., Malone, J. B., and Thompson, P. E.: Superinfections of *Brugia pahangi* in the Mongolian jird. Proc. Third Int. Cong. Parasitol., Munich, Germany, *2*:617, 1974.

Kuntz, R. E., Cheever, A. W., and Myers, B. J.: Proliferative epithelial lesions of the urinary bladder of nonhuman primates infected with *Schistosoma haematobium*. J. Natl. Cancer Inst., *48*:223, 1972.

Leadbetter, G. W., Jr., and Leadbetter, W. F.: Ureteral re-implantation and bladder neck reconstruction. JAMA *175*:349, 1961.

Lehman, J. S., Jr., Farid, Z., and Bassily, S.: Mortality in urinary schistosomiasis. Lancet, *2*:822, 1970.

Lehman, J. S., Jr., Farid, Z., Bassily, S., and Kent, D. C.: Hydronephrosis, bacteriuria, and maximal urine concentration in urinary schistosomiasis. Ann. Intern. Med., *75*:49, 1971.

Lehman, J. S., Jr., Farid, Z., Smith, J. H., Bassily, S., and El-Masry, N. A.: Urinary schistosomiasis in Egypt: Clinical, radiological, bacteriological and parasitological correlations. Trans. R. Soc. Trop. Med. Hyg., *67*:384, 1973.

Lehman, J. S., Mott, K. E., de Souza, C. A. M., Leboriero, O., and Muniz, T. M.: The association of schistosomiasis mansoni and proteinuria in an endemic area. A preliminary report. Am. J. Trop. Med. Hyg., *24*:616, 1975.

Lehman, J. S., Farid, Z., Bassily, S., Kent, D., Haxton, J., and Wahab, M.: Intestinal protein loss in schistosomal polyposis of the colon. Gastroenterology, *59*:433, 1958.

Lewert, R. M., and Mandlowitz, S.: Schistosomiasis: Prenatal induction of tolerance to antigens. Nature, *224*:1029, 1969.

Lie, K. J.: Occult filariasis: Its relationship with tropical pulmonary eosinophilia. Am. J. Trop. Med. Hyg., *11*:646, 1962.

Lindner, R. R.: Retrospective x-ray survey for *Porocephalus*. J. Trop. Med. Hyg., *68*:155, 1965.

Lins, E. E.: The solution of incrustations in the urinary bladder by a new method. J. Urol., *53*:702, 1945.

Lucas, A. O., Adeniyi-Jones, C.C., Cockshot, W. P., and Gilles, H. M.: Radiological changes after medical treatment of vesical schistosomiasis. Lancet, *1*:631, 1966.

Mahmoud, A. A., and Warren, K. S.: Anti-inflammatory effects of tartar emetic and niridazole: Suppression of schistosome egg granuloma. J. Immunol., *112*:222, 1974.

Manwell, E. J.: Urinary symptoms in relation to *Trichomonas vaginalis* infestation. N. Engl. J. Med., *211*:567, 1934.

Moran, C. J., Ryder, G., Turk, J. L., and Waters, M. F. R.: Evidence for circulating immune complexes in lepromatous leprosy. Lancet, *2*:572, 1972.

Moriearty, P. L., and Brito, E.: Elution of renal anti-schistosome antibodies in human schistosomiasis mansoni. Am. J. Trop. Med. Hyg., *26*:717, 1977.

Mott, K. E.: Unpublished observations, 1983.

Mott, K. E., and Dixon, H.: Collaborative study of antigens for immunodiagnosis of schistosomiasis. Bull. W.H.O., *60*:729, 1982.

Müller, M.: Mode of action of metronidizole on anaerobic organisms. *In* Finegold, S. M. (Ed.): First United States Metronidazole Conference (Tarpon Springs, Florida, Feb. 19–20, 1982). New York, BMI Biomedical Information Corporation, 1982, pp. 67–82.

Musacchio, F., and Mitchell, N.: Primary renal echinococcosis: A case report. Am. J. Trop. Med. Hyg., *15*:168, 1966.

Nagle, R. B., Ward, P. A., Lindsley, H. B., Sadun, E. M., Johnson, A. J., Berkaw, R. E., and Hildebrandt, P. H.: Experimental infections with African trypanosomes. VI. Glomerulonephritis involving the alternate pathway of complement activation. Am. J. Trop. Med. Hyg., *23*:15, 1974.

O'Connor, F. W., and Hulse, C. R.: Studies in filariasis. I. In Puerto Rico. Puerto Rico J. Public Health Trop. Med., *11*:167, 1935.

Orihel, T. C., and Moore, P. J.: *Loa loa:* Experimental infection in two species of African primates. Am. J. Trop. Med. Hyg., *24*:606, 1975.

Ottesen, E. A., Neva, F. A., Paranjare, R. S., Tripathy, S. P., Thirnvengadm, K. V., and Beaven, M. A.: Specific allergic sensitization to filarial antigens in tropical eosinophilia syndrome. Lancet, *1*:1158, 1979.

Owen, R. L.: Sexually transmitted enteric disease. *In* Remington, J. S., and Swartz, M. N. (Eds.): Current Clinical Topics in Infectious Diseases. New York, McGraw-Hill Book Co., 1980, pp. 1–29.

Partono, F., Purnomo, Oemijati, S., and Soewarta, A.: The long-term effects of repeated diethylcarbamazine administration with special reference to microfilaremia and elephantiasis. Acta Trop., *38*:217, 1981.

Peters, P. A., Warren, K. S., and Mahmoud, A. A. F.: Rapid, accurate quantification of schistosome eggs via nuclepore filters. J. Parasitol., *62*:154, 1976.

Piessens, W. F.: Immunology of lymphatic filariasis and onchocerciasis. *In* Cohen, S., and Warren, K. S.: Immunology of Parasitic Disease. 2nd ed., pp. 622–653. Oxford, Blackwell Scientific Publications, 1982.

Powell, S. J.: Drug therapy of amoebiasis. Bull. W.H.O., *40*:953, 1969.

Pugh, R. N. H., Bell, D. R., and Gittes, H. M.: Malumfasi endemic diseases research project XV. The potential medical importance of bilharzia in northern Nigeria: A suggested rapid, cheap and effective solution for control of *Schistosoma haematobium* infection. Ann. Trop. Med. Parasitol., *74*:597, 1980.

Rausch, R. L.: On the occurrence and distribution of *Echinococcus* sp. (Cestoda, Taeniidae) and characteristics of their development in the intermediate host. Am. J. Parasitol., *42*:19, 1967.

Roe, F.: The safety of metronidazole: A few clouds but no rain. *In* Finegold, S. M. (Ed.): First United States Metronidazole Conference (Tarpon Springs, Florida, Feb. 19–20, 1982). New York, BMI Biomedical Information Corporation, 1982, pp. 113–124.

Sadun, E. H., von Lichtenberg, F., Cheever, A. W., Erickson, D. G., and Hickman, R. L.: Experimental infection with *Schistosoma haematobium* in chimpanzees. Parasitologic, clinical, serologic and pathological observations. Am. J. Trop. Med. Hyg., *19*:427, 1970.

Sanjurjo, L. A.: Trichomoniasis. *In* Campbell, M. F., and Harrison, J. H. (Eds.): Campbell's Urology. 3rd ed., p. 503. Philadelphia, W. B. Saunders Co., 1970*a*.

Sanjurjo, L. A.: Strongylosis. *In* Campbell, M. F., and Harrison, J. H. (Eds.): Campbell's Urology. 3rd ed., pp. 508–509. Philadelphia, W. B. Saunders Co., 1970*b*.

Sasa, M., and Tanaka, H.: A new method for statistical analysis of the microfilarial periodicity survey data. (Abstr. 35.) *In* Joint Conference on Parasitic Diseases. pp. 104–106. Japan-U.S. Cooperative Medical Science Program, Hiroshima, July 18–20, 1972.

Sato, H., Otsuji, Y., Maeda, T., Irie, Y., Nakashima, A., Imamura, K., and Fukuoka, Y.: A case of huge penile and scrotal elephantiasis. (Abstr. F 12.) *In* Joint Conference on Parasitic Diseases. Japan-U.S. Cooperative Medical Science Program, Unzen, Nagasaki, Aug. 17–19, 1974.

Schacher, J. F., and Sahyoun, P. F.: A chronological study of the histopathology of filarial disease in cats and dogs caused by *Brugia pahangi*. Trans. R. Soc. Trop. Med. Hyg., *61*:234, 1967.

Smith, J. H., Elwi, A., Kamel, I. A., and von Lichtenberg, F.: A quantitative analysis of urinary schistosomiasis in Egypt. I. Pathology and pathogenesis. Am. J. Trop. Med. Hyg., *23*:1054, 1974.

Smith, J. H., Elwi, A., Kamel, I. A., and von Lichtenberg, F.: A quantitative analysis of urinary schistosomiasis in Egypt. II. Evolution and epidemiology. Am. J. Trop. Med. Hyg., *24*:806, 1975.

Soothill, J. F., and Hendrickse, R. G.: Some immunological studies of the nephrotic syndrome of Nigerian children. Lancet, *2*:629, 1967.

Soubigou, M. M., Dulisquet, and Gaudin: Ulcerous balanitis due to *Trichomonas vaginalis*. Bull. Soc. Pathol. Exot., *31*:52, 1938.

Sowmini, C. N., Vijayalakshmi, K., Chellamuthia, C., and Sundaram, S. M.: Infections of the median raphe of the penis. Report of 3 cases. Br. J. Vener. Dis., *49*:469, 1972.

Sullivan, J. J., and Chernin, E.: Oral transmission of *Brugia pahangi* and *Dipetalonema viteae* to adult and neonatal jirds. Int. J. Parasitol., *6*:75, 1976.

Sutherland, J. C., Berry, A., Hynd, M., and Proctor, N. S. F.: Placental bilharziasis. Report of a case. S. Afr. J. Obstet. Gynaecol., *3*:76, 1965.

Symmers, W. St. C.: Pathology of oxyuriasis. A.M.A. Arch. Pathol., *50*:475, 1950.

Tani, S., and Akisada, M.: Lymphographical findings of the lymphaticopelvic fistulization in filarial chyluria. Jpn. J. Trop. Med., *11*:55, 1970.

Taylor, A. E. R.: Studies on the microfilaria of *Loa loa*, *Wuchereria bancrofti*, *Brugia malayi*, *Dirofilaria immitis*, *Dirofilaria repens* and *Dirofilaria aethiops*. J. Helminthol., *34*:13, 1960.

Vander Schalie, H.: Aswan Dam revisited. Environment, *16*:18, 1974.

Voller, A., Davies, D. R., and Hutt, M. S. R.: Quartan malarial infections in *Aotus trivirgatus,* with special reference to renal pathology. Br. J. Exp. Pathol., *54*:457, 1973.

von Lichtenberg, A., and Swick, M.: Klinische Prüfung des Uroselectans. Klin. Wochenschr., *8*:2089 (Nov. 5), 1929.

von Lichtenberg, F.: Schistosomiasis as a world-wide problem: Pathology. J. Toxicol. Environ. Health, *1*:175, 1975.

von Lichtenberg, F.: Comparative histopathology of schistosome granulomas in the hamster. Am. J. Pathol. *72*:149, 1973.

von Lichtenberg, F.: Host response to eggs of *Schistosoma mansoni*. I. Granuloma formation in the unsensitized laboratory mouse. Am. J. Pathol. *41*:711, 1962.

von Lichtenberg F.: The early phase of endemic Bancroftian filariasis in the male. Pathological study. J. Mt. Sinai Hosp., *24*:983, 1957.

von Lichtenberg, F., and Medina, R.: Bancroftian filariasis in the etiology of funiculoepididymitis, periorchitis hydrocele in Puerto Rico (statistical study of surgical and autopsy material over a 13-year period). Am. J. Trop. Med. Hyg., *6*:739, 1957.

von Lichtenberg, F., Bawden, M. P., and Shealey, S. H.: Origin of circulating antigen from the schistosome gut. An immunofluorescent study. Am. J. Trop. Med. Hyg., *23*:1088, 1974.

Wakefield, G. S., Carroll, J. D., and Speed, D. E.: Schistosomiasis of the spinal cord. Brain, *85*:535, 1962.

Waller, C. E., and Othersen, H. B., Jr.: Ascariasis: Surgical complications in children. Am. J. Surg., *120*:50, 1971.

Ward, P. A., and Conran, P. B.: Immunopathology of renal complications in simian malaria and human quartan malaria. Milit. Med., *134*:1228, 1969.

Warren, K. S.: The pathology of schistosome infections. Helminthol. Abstr., *42*:592, 1973*a*.

Warren, K. S.: Regulation of the prevalence and intensity of schistosomiasis in man. Immunology or ecology? J. Infect. Dis., *127*:595, 1973*b*.

Warren, K. S., Mahmoud, A. A. F., Cummings, P., Murphy, D. J., and Houser, H. B.: Schistosomiasis mansoni in Yemeni in California. Duration of infection, presence of disease, therapeutic management. Am. J. Trop. Med. Hyg., *23*:903, 1974.

Wartman, W. B.: Filariasis in American Armed Forces in World War II. Medicine, *26*:333, 1947.

Weinstein, L., Edelstein, S. M., Madara, J. L., Falchuk, K. R., McManus, B. M., and Trier, J. S.: Intestinal cryptosporidiosis complicated by disseminated CMV infection. Gastroenterology, *81*:584, 1981.

Whitehill, R., and Miller, H. M: Infestations of the genitourinary tract by *Strongyloides stercoralis*. A case report. Bull. Johns Hopkins Hosp., *75*:169, 1944.

Williams, A. O.: Pathology of schistosomiasis of the uterine cervix due to *S. haematobium*. Am. J. Obstet. Gynecol., *98*:784, 1967.

Williams, A. O., von Lichtenberg, F., Smith, J. H., and Martinson, F. D.: Ultrastructure of phycomycosis and associated Splendore-Hoeppli phenomenon. Arch. Pathol., *87*:459, 1969.

Wittner, M., and Rosenbaum, R. M.: Role of bacteria in modifying virulence of *Entamoeba histolytica*: Studies of amebae from axenic cultures. Am. J. Trop. Med. Hyg., *19*:755, 1970.

Wong, M. M., Fredericks, H. J., and Ramachandran, C. P.: Studies on immunization against *Brugia malayi* infection in the rhesus monkey. Bull. W.H.O., *40*:493, 1969.

Wright, W. H.: Geographical distribution of schistosomes and their intermediate hosts. *In* Ansari, N. (Ed.): Epidemiology and Control of Schistosomiasis (Bilharziasis), pp. 32–249. Basel, S. Karger, 1973.

Yogore, M. G., Jr., Lewert, R. M., and Reyes, V. A.: Cerebral schistosomiasis japonica in the Philippines: Immunoprecipitins in the cerebrospinal fluid. Paper presented to American Society of Tropical Medicine and Hygiene, Fiftieth Annual Meeting, New Orleans, La., Nov. 11, 1975.

Young, S. W., Higashi, G. I., and Kamel, R.: Interaction of Salmonellae and schistosomiasis in host-parasite relations. Trans. R. Soc. Trop. Med. Hyg., *67*:797, 1973.

CHAPTER 22

Fungal Infections of the Urinary Tract

JAN SCHÖNEBECK

INTRODUCTION

Bacteriuria and its various facets are well known to every urologist and are rarely a diagnostic or therapeutic problem. The threshold for significant bacteriuria is established; we know the implication of asymptomatic bacteriuria and that the fear of chronic bacterial pyelonephritis felt in the 1960's was exaggerated.

The implication of funguria is less well known and not so extensively studied. Many physicians seem to be rather hesitant about what to do when faced with a funguric patient. However, our present knowledge undoubtedly allows some guidelines to be drawn. It is evident that there are many similarities between bacteriuria and funguria—but there are also important differences.

Animal experiments have shown that many fungi have the ability to attack the urinary tract. Renal metastases in a systemic fungal infection are common; in disseminated candidiasis the frequency is about 90 per cent (Lehner, 1964), in cryptococcosis about 50 per cent (Salyer and Salyer, 1973), and in aspergillosis 19 per cent (Young et al., 1970). Many different yeast species may be found on culture of the urine in hospitalized patients (Ahern et al., 1966). However, clinical experience tells us that important fungal infections of the urinary tract in man are almost exclusively limited to *Candida albicans*. This chapter is thus mainly confined to different aspects of urinary tract infection caused by this organism. Some cases of *Torulopsis glabrata* infection, a few of *Aspergillus* and *Penicillium* species, and occasional cases of sporotrichosis, phycomycosis, and infection by some other rare

fungi have been published. They are briefly discussed at the end of this chapter.

Actinomyces occasionally infects the kidneys, 11 cases being reported by Cumming and Nelson in 1929. It is—in spite of its name—no longer classified as a fungus and is therefore not discussed here.

Candida albicans is a yeast fungus that in man normally lives as a saprophyte in the oral cavity, in the vagina, in the intestinal canal, but mainly in the colon, where it exists with, and is suppressed by, the normal bacterial flora. It usually occurs in the unicellular form (Fig. 22–1). Characteristic of *Candida* species is their ability to form (pseudo)hyphae (Fig. 22–2). Both forms may be found in urinary tract infections, but invasive candidiasis is nearly always in the pseudomycelial form.

EXPERIMENTAL CANDIDIASIS OF THE URINARY TRACT

Some knowledge of experimental data greatly facilitates the understanding of the clinical picture of real *Candida* infection.

In 1960 and 1963 Louria and coworkers showed that if *Candida albicans* is injected intravenously in mice, the kidney is the only organ in which progressive infection occurs in surviving animals. This is probably because yeast fungi enter the tubules, where they seem to be protected from the inflammatory reaction. From the tubules they may reinvade the renal parenchyma. The kidney is thus the organ most severely affected in generalized candidiasis.

Hurley and Winner (1963) confirmed these findings. By injecting a smaller amount of candida organisms and observing the animals for

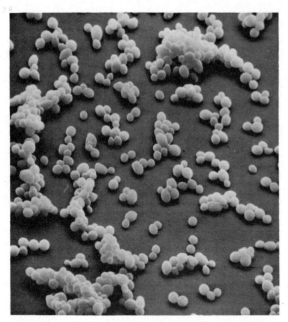

Figure 22–1. *Candida albicans* (yeast form). Scanning electron microscopy × 1200. (From Schönebeck, J.: Scand. J. Urol. Nephrol. Suppl. 11, 1972.)

some weeks they found that the *acute* renal infection with disseminated candida abscesses in the kidney cortex was followed by a *chronic* stage. Early in this chronic stage the cortical infections subsided but fungal mycelium was seen in the tubules, the kidney pelves, and the ureters. After 3 weeks the kidney pelves were

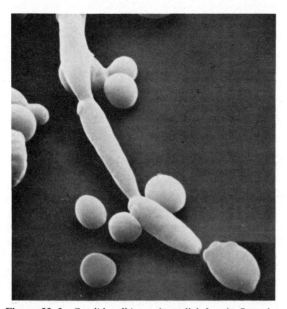

Figure 22–2. *Candida albicans* (mycelial form). Scanning electron microscopy × 6000. (From Schönebeck, J.: Scand. J. Urol. Nephrol. Suppl. 11, 1972.)

dilated and their lumens occupied by proliferating, intermingling mycelium-fungus balls. Finally, the hydronephrosis progressed and the kidney parenchyma was converted to a thin atrophic ring in which no fungi could be demonstrated.

CANDIDA RESERVOIR AND ROUTES OF SPREAD

The *Candida* reservoir in the patient's own intestinal tract is—as with bacterial infections—the source of infection in most cases of urinary tract candidiasis. The routes of spread appear to be via the lymphatics and blood stream (hematogenous infection) or from the anus via the urethra and urinary bladder to the kidneys (ascending infection). The hematogenous route has been conclusively proved by a fairly heroic autoexperiment by Krause and associates (1969). A healthy volunteer ingested 80 gm (10^{12} cells) of *Candida albicans*. Positive blood and urine cultures were obtained after some hours. The amount ingested may seem large, but following antibiotic therapy the number of *Candida* cells per ml of feces may rise to 10^9 (Cohn, 1957). The first step of the ascending route (from the anus via the urethra to the bladder) has never been proved but, as in the case of bacterial infection, seems probable. If *Candida albicans* is injected into the urinary bladder of rabbits it can be demonstrated in the kidneys in 32 per cent of cases (Parkash et al., 1970). Cultures taken from the renal pelvis at autopsy of a case of candida cystitis (death from heart attack) and of two patients in whom an ileal conduit had been created and who died a few days postoperatively were positive for *Candida albicans* (Schönebeck, 1972; Schönebeck et al., 1972). Although hematogenous spread cannot be excluded, these cases as well as some other examples of patients who died following uretersigmoidostomy and were found to have candida infection of the kidneys (Lehner, 1964; Crosby, 1967) indicate that candida cells may ascend via the ureters. It should be noted that after such operations the ureteral orifices often reflux, which facilitates fungal ascent to the kidneys.

Occasionally the source of infection may be fairly unusual. McLeish and coworkers (1977) described two patients receiving kidney homografts from a donor whose urine culture yielded *Candida albicans* greater than 10^5 per ml. When the recipients were treated with large doses of cortisone, they developed candida infections, one of them passing a fungus ball in the urine.

Candiduria was described in the late nineteenth century, and occasional cases of candida infection of the urinary tract were published during the first half of the twentieth century. Serious infections due to candida previously affected mainly patients with grave, often incurable, underlying diseases. In such cases the infection was a terminal event and the lack of effective therapy made little difference in the overall prognosis. The present situation is different. Candida infections, systemic or of the urinary tract, now occur in patients who have undergone kidney transplantation or other major surgical procedures and in those treated with antibiotics, steroids, and cytotoxic agents. Many of these patients would have a good prognosis if the fungus infection could be eliminated. Furthermore, therapeutic options have improved dramatically during the last few decades. It is therefore important that the canduric patient is correctly evaluated and treated.

FACTORS FAVORING THE DEVELOPMENT OF CANDIDURIA

In the route of spread from the gut to the kidneys, many factors may promote candiduria. The importance of an increase of the *Candida* flora of the intestine was shown by the oral ingestion experiment of Krause and coworkers (1969). The most common way, however, to increase this flora is the administration of antibiotics. This can even lead to fecal cultures that yield a pure culture of *Candida*. Antibiotic treatment is a recognized cause of candiduria (Bergmann and Lipsky, 1964; Schönebeck, 1972; Hamory and Wenzel, 1978).

The administration of cortisone (Louria et al., 1963) or of cytostatic agents (Folb and Trounce, 1970) as well as radiation therapy (Hurley, 1966) also favors the development of candiduria, probably by weakening cellular defense mechanisms.

Local conditions in the urinary tract are also important. After invading the kidneys, the candida organisms penetrate to the kidney tubules, where they seem to be protected from the body's defense mechanisms. The optimal pH for candida growth is 5.1 to 6.4 (Johnson, 1954). Thus, the normal acidity of the urine is another candida-promoting factor.

Glucosuria favors candida growth at glucose concentrations exceeding 1.5 gm per liter (Johnson, 1954), which means that diabetes, especially if it is poorly controlled, is another promoting factor. Alloxan-induced diabetes renders mice more susceptible to progressive renal infection when *Candida albicans* cells are administered intravenously (Andriole and Hasenclever, 1962). Foreign bodies (indwelling catheters) are commonly associated with funguria (Schönebeck, 1972); rarely, stones of the urinary tract (Hodgin, 1969) and impairment of the fungicidal properties of prostatic secretion may be of importance (Gip and Molin, 1970).

In making a statistical analysis of factors predisposing to candiduria, Klimek and associates (1979) found the most significant factors in their patients to be central venous catheters, drains (other than Foley catheters), broad-spectrum antibiotics, and cortisone.

Urine Sampling Technique. In diagnosing urinary tract candidiasis it is most important that the urine samples be properly collected. Thus, when yeastlike fungi are found in the urine sediment or on urine culture, the finding should always be checked by culture or an adequately collected urine sample. In women, the urine is easily contaminated with the vaginal or fecal flora; therefore, only catheterized or aspirated samples give reliable results. In men, samples collected by the clean voided midstream technique are usually satisfactory (Schönebeck and Ånséhn, 1972). Fungi readily grow on ordinary agar plates. However, if a fungus infection is suspected, the bacteriologist should always be told, as culture on Sabouraud agar plates is preferable.

Significant Candiduria. It has been suggested that in candiduria—as in bacteriuria—the number of organisms per volume of urine could be of help in deciding whether the candiduria is of significance, that is, whether or not it is a sign of invasive infection. The threshold of significance has been variously put at 10^3 organisms per ml (Perry, 1964), 10^4 per ml (Goldberg et al., 1979), and 10^5 per ml (Freis, 1971). Wise and coworkers (1976) have, however, proved that the infection may be life-threatening when urinary counts are as low as 15,000 organisms per ml, which is in accordance with my own experience (Schönebeck, 1972). On the other hand, quite large numbers of candida may occasionally be present in the urine, apparently without being of any clinical importance (Haley, 1965; Schönebeck and Ånséhn, 1972). This may be the case in patients with indwelling catheters (Wise et al., 1976) and in patients with a freshly created ileal conduit or cecocystoplasty (Schönebeck and Ånséhn, 1972). The important point in evaluating candiduria is not its magnitude but its relationship to the total clinical picture. If the patient's general condition is good, there need be no hurry to interfere even if the colony count of candida in the urine is "significant." If a funguric patient falls seriously ill, treatment should be instituted immediately, whether the candiduria is "significant" or not.

As pointed out by Lehner (1964), candiduria may precede candidemia in systemic candidiasis and thus be a warning signal.

CLINICAL PICTURES

The presentation of urinary tract candidiasis may be variable, but a useful outline is presented in Table 22–1.

Asymptomatic candiduria is always pathologic, as fungi are never found in the urine of normal, healthy persons (Schönebeck and Ånséhn, 1972). In following 40 such patients, Schönebeck (1972) found that the asymptomatic candiduria usually disappeared spontaneously when predisposing factors (indwelling catheters, antibiotic therapy, and diabetes) were discontinued or treated. However, it could be present for years and it was possible for such patients to undergo major surgical procedures and to be treated with broad-spectrum antibiotics without the candiduria turning to manifest infection. If, on the other hand, the patient's general condition deteriorated, symptomatic infection could become evident. This occurred in four patients: one with cardiac infarct, one with untreated pernicious anemia, and two with postoperative hydronephrosis following resection of the urinary bladder. Asymptomatic candiduria can give rise to complications in spite of the patient's

being in excellent general condition; this was observed in a man with a kidney transplant in which the fungi aggregated to form bezoars obstructing the ureter, causing anuria (Schönebeck et al., 1970).

After the creation of an ileal conduit or cecocystoplasty, asymptomatic candiduria is a normal finding and may be massive (Schönebeck and Ånséhn, 1972). Even in these cases it usually disappears spontaneously in some months.

Asymptomatic candiduria is most often a harmless condition. It usually disappears spontaneously when predisposing factors are dealt with, but it may continue for years. Under certain conditions, however, it may turn into symptomatic infection, or give rise to bezoar formation or both.

Candida Septicemia and Pyelonephritis. Candida pyelonephritis occurs in two main forms: (1) multiple abscess formation primarily in the renal cortex; and (2) diffuse fungal infiltration of the tips of the papillae or infiltration along the collecting tubules, sometimes leading to papillary necrosis. These forms often occur together, and the first probably precedes the second. Both may be accompanied by bezoar formation. In candida septicemia, multiple abscesses—mainly localized to the renal cortex—are a secondary phenomenon. Clinical experience (Louria et al., 1962; Lehner, 1964) and experimental studies on animals (Louria et al., 1960; Hurley and Winner, 1963) have shown that the kidney is the principal target organ in generalized candidiasis. Multiple abscesses, however, may be present in the absence of septicemia (Taylor and Rundle, 1952; Cowan et al., 1962) and are often probably an expression of primary disease of the urinary tract.

The symptoms of candida pyelonephritis are variable. The patient is usually seriously ill, with high fever, progressive uremia, and flank pain. The onset may be fairly acute, with sudden anuria due to obstruction of the tubules (Fig. 22–3) or sometimes—when combined with bezoar formation—of the renal pelves or the ureters. A clinical picture that has been claimed to be pathognomonic of renal candidiasis is that of progressive uremia in combination with marked variation in urine volume (Taylor and Rundle, 1952). This sign has also been described by Tannenberg (1923) and by Schönebeck and Winblad (1971). Progressive uremia may dominate the clinical picture (Gillam and Wadelton, 1958).

Three cases have been described in which the candida infection has extended beyond the kidney parenchyma, thus forming a perinephric

TABLE 22–1. Presentation of Urinary Tract Candidiasis

Asymptomatic Candiduria	⟶ Spontaneous disappearance
	⟶ Urinary tract candidiasis with symptoms

Manifest Candidiasis of the Urinary Tract	
Classic picture of infection (with or without bezoar formation)	Septicemia
	Pyelonephritis
	Cystitis
	Progressive renal failure
Bezoar formation (without symptoms of infection)	Anuria
	Ureteral colic

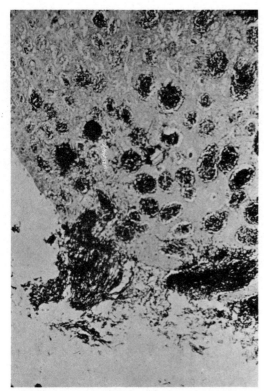

Figure 22–3. Section of necrotic tip of renal papilla with clusters of fungi adjacent to the papilla and filling the distal distended part of the collecting tubules. Magnification × 12. (From Schönebeck, J., and Winblad, B.: Scand. J. Urol. Neprhol. 5:281, 1971.)

abscess (Tennant et al., 1968; Cromie and Buck, 1978; Noe and Tonkin, 1982).

Candida Cystitis. Cystitis due to yeastlike fungi was described at the end of the last century; diabetics with funguria showed fermentation of the sugar in the urine (Senator, 1891), producing pneumaturia and sometimes markedly decreasing the sugar content of the urine. Pneumaturia in fungal cystitis has also been described by Gibberd and Williams (1962). In one patient the pneumaturia was so severe that micturition sounded like the passing of flatus (Müllern-Aspegren, 1921). Pneumaturia is by no means pathognomonic of fungus infection, as it can also be due to an *E. coli* infection or to a vesicointestinal fistula. Urinary frequency and, occasionally, hematuria are nowadays the most common symptoms; pneumaturia being rare since diabetes is usually well treated. At cystoscopy the bladder epithelium may be diffusely reddened and sometimes covered by white, often confluent patches. Olanescu and coworkers (1956) described a cystoscopic appearance that *they* considered pathognomonic of candida cystitis: numerous reddened papules

about the size of a grain of rice surrounded by a paler margin in the epithelium of the bladder. Apart from these areas the bladder was not especially inflamed. Cystitis is often associated with bezoar formation.

Bezoar Formation. One of the main differences between bacterial and fungal infections is the formation of bezoars. Some fungi—e.g., *Candida* species—grow long and threadlike, forming pseudomycelia (Fig. 22–2). These threads intermingle into small clusters that aggregate to form bezoars (Figs. 22–4 and 22–5). Their size is usually that of a grain of wheat, but they may be large enough to fill the urinary bladder. Schönebeck (1972) reviewed 24 cases from the literature and presented 5 of his own cases. Since then, 15 to 20 additional cases have been described. Urinary tract bezoars may form in the renal pelvis or in the urinary bladder. They occur at all ages, and both sexes are about equally affected. Bezoars can form in the seriously ill patient with candida pyelonephritis or in the asymptomatic patient with candiduria. As a rule, predisposing factors are present (e.g., diabetes, antibiotics, a kidney transplant) but bezoar formation has also been reported in a previously healthy patient (Beland and Piette, 1973).

The clinical picture is variable. It can be one of progressive uremia with variable urine output or acute anuria caused by obstruction of the collecting tubules, of the renal pelvis (Fig. 22–3), or of the ureters. If the bezoar obstructs

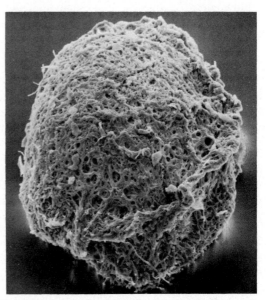

Figure 22–4. *Candida albicans* bezoar grown in a test tube. Scanning electron microscopy × 240. (From Schönebeck, J.: Scand. J. Urol. Nephrol. Suppl. 11, 1972.)

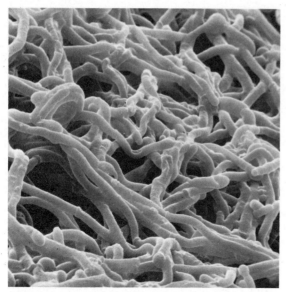

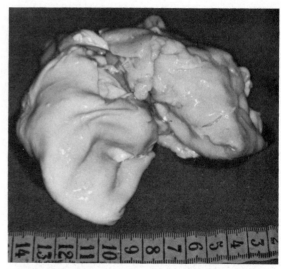

Figure 22–6. Large bladder bezoar after suprapubic removal.

Figure 22–5. Same as Figure 22–4. Magnification × 2400. The bezoar consists of intermingling pseudomycelial threads. (From Schönebeck, J.: Scand. J. Urol. Nephrol. Suppl. 11, 1972.)

the ureter, the patient may experience pain resembling renal colic or, if a solitary kidney is present, may become anuric. If the ball is located in the urinary bladder the patient usually experiences frequency and urgency. Bladder bezoars may grow as large as 10 cm in diameter; they can be seen radiographically as large, laminated, partly radiodense spheres in the bladder region (Margolin, 1971; Harold et al., 1977). Small bezoars passing spontaneously may be the only symptom of bezoar formation in the urinary bladder (Bartkowiak, 1964). The large ones may require a suprapubic cystotomy for removal (Chisholm and Hutch, 1961).

The small bezoars usually consist entirely of intermingled mycelia, but this is not always the case with the large bladder bezoars. Histopathologic examination of multiple sections from such a bezoar (Fig. 22–6) from a 48-year-old diabetic man with pneumaturia and intractable cystitis showed the mass to consist mainly of structureless, amorphous material with few scattered clusters of fungi in the yeast—as well as in the mycelial—form (Schönebeck, 1984). The radiographic appearance was quite typical (Fig. 22–7). At cystoscopy the bezoar looked like a grayish-white, rounded but somewhat irregular mass (Fig. 22–8) (Schönebeck, 1984).

Diagnosis of *Candida* infection of the urinary tract is based on the clinical picture and repeated culture of correctly sampled urine and blood.

An IVP and, if necessary, a retrograde urogram should be obtained. Serologic detection of antibodies (precipitins or agglutinins) is limited by false positive and false negative findings, but a rising titer may be helpful in chronic patients or in patients with a kidney transplant. A glance through the microscope at a urine sediment—nowadays an investigation unfortunately often replaced by various tape tests—can in some minutes make the diagnosis. The fungi may be found in the yeast and/or the mycelial

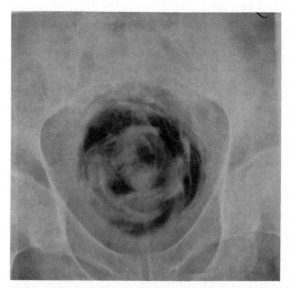

Figure 22–7. X-ray appearance of large bladder bezoar in the bladder of a 48-year-old diabetic man.

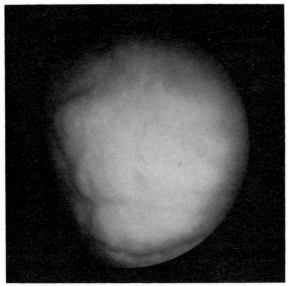

Figure 22–8. Cystoscopic appearance of large bladder bezoar. (From Schönebeck, J.: Atlas of Cystoscopy. Copenhagen, Schulz Medical Information, 1984.)

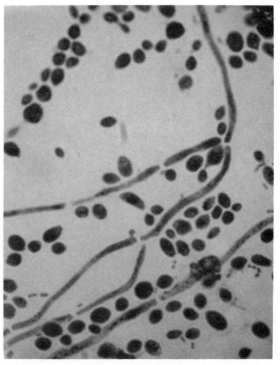

Figure 22–9. *Candida albicans* (yeast and mycelial forms) in urine sediment. Magnification × 400.

phase (Fig. 22–9) and also engulfed by polymorphonuclear leukocytes (Fig. 22–10).

Treatment. Faced with a funguric patient, the clinician must realize that the most important point is not the magnitude of the funguria but its relationship to the total clinical picture. A very useful systematic approach to the evaluation and treatment of candiduria (Fig. 22–11) has been suggested by Janosko and McRoberts (1979).

The seriously ill or potentially seriously ill patient with candiduria should be treated with intravenous amphotericin B and/or 5-fluorocytosine perorally. An IVP should be performed as soon as possible; if it is normal, medical therapy should be continued. If bezoars are

Figure 22–10. *Candida albicans* (yeast form) in urine sediment and engulfed by a polymorphonuclear leukocyte. The yeasts are the translucent oval bodies in the middle and right upper part of the cell.

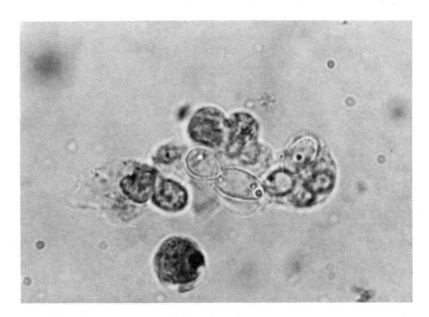

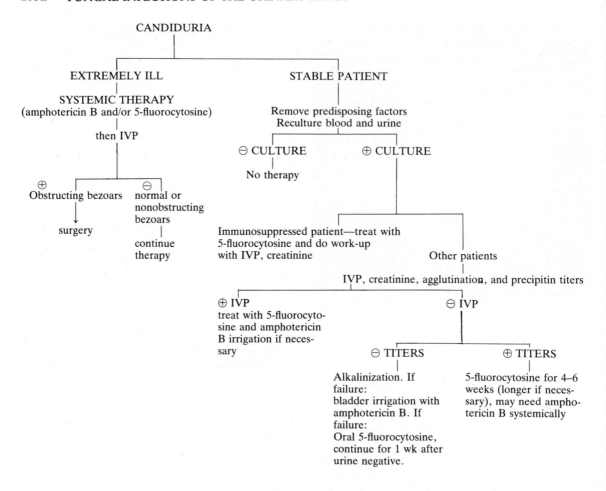

Figure 22–11. A systematic approach to the evaluation and treatment of candiduria. (Modified from Janosko, E. D., and McRoberts, J. W.: South. Med. J., 72:1578, 1979.)

present, surgery may be necessary, especially if the bezoars are obstructing the renal pelvis or ureter.

If the patient is clinically stable, an effort to allow spontaneous clearance of the funguria should be made. As a first step, catheters and intravenous lines should be removed—or replaced if this is not possible. Antibiotics, immunosuppressive agents, and cortisone should, if possible, be discontinued and the urine recultured in the ensuing days. Quite often the candiduria will disappear (Schönebeck, 1972).

If candiduria persists, the immunosuppressed patient should be treated. Before therapy is begun, all patients should be evaluated with a serum creatinine and sometimes a creatinine clearance and an IVP to determine involvement of the upper urinary tract. Blood samples should be cultured; *Candida* precipitin and agglutinin titers may be useful if serial blood samples are available. Umenai and Ishida (1977) found that positive titers often indicate deep

tissue invasion, but others have not found this measure to be so useful. If the IVP shows evidence of pyelonephritis, papillary necrosis, or bezoar formation, alkalinization of the urine and 5-fluorocytosine perorally should be started. If this treatment fails, amphotericin B can be substituted for 5-fluorocytosine. Obstructing bezoars are treated surgically. If the IVP is normal, simple alkalinization of the urine may suffice to eradicate the fungus (Schönebeck, 1972) or bladder irrigation with amphotericin B can be tried. This has been proved to be an efficient and harmless therapy (Cuétara et al., 1972; O'Connel and Hardner, 1973; Wise et al., 1982). If it fails, 5-fluorocytosine perorally could be tried.

DRUGS. When systemic therapy is indicated, two drugs are currently recommended: amphotericin B and 5-fluorocytosine. Available is also ketoconazole, although its efficacy in urinary tract infection is not yet fully established.

Amphotericin B binds to cell membrane

sterols, resulting in increased permeability of the membrane and ultimately to cell death. It is not absorbed from the intestinal tract and has to be given parenterally or as a local instillation. After intravenous injection, very little appears in the bile or urine. The main advantage of this drug is its effectiveness against many different fungi that rarely develop resistant strains. The main disadvantage with the drug is its high renal toxicity; a reduction in glomerular filtration rate of about 40 per cent may be anticipated. However, renal function generally returns to normal or near-normal after therapy. If one is not acquainted with the use of amphotericin B, the instructions should be carefully studied before treatment is started. In emergency cases it is given as an intravenous infusion, 0.3 mg per kg body weight in 500 to 1000 ml 5 per cent dextrose in water, the full 24 hours' dosage in 6 to 8 hours. The dose is increased to 0.6 mg per kg on the second and subsequent days (Cohen, 1982). In candida cystitis, irrigation with 1000 ml of water (not saline) containing 50 μg per ml has proved very useful. It does not seem to be absorbed from the bladder and no side effects have been observed (Wise et al., 1982). Irrigation via nephrostomy or ureteral catheters (Blum, 1966; Sales and Mundy, 1973) may also be effective in candida infections localized to the kidneys.

5-Fluorocytosine is a synthetic pyrimidine derivative that interferes with the fungal nucleic acids and disrupts the production of proteins. It is not taken up by mammalian cells. Although toxic effects (elevated transaminases, gastrointestinal symptoms, leukopenia, and a few cases of agranulocytosis) have been described, they are not common. This and the fact that it is readily absorbed from the intestinal tract are the main advantages of this drug. Major drawbacks are its narrow spectrum (mainly candida infections and cryptococcosis) and the selection of resistant strains. Primary resistance to the drug in *Candida albicans* is less than 10 per cent but in other *Candida* strains it is more common, slightly less than 30 per cent (Schönebeck and Ånséhn, 1973). Approximately 90 per cent of the compound is absorbed orally, and about 90 per cent is excreted unchanged in the urine. It is dialyzable; the serum concentration is hardly detectable after hemodialysis. The therapeutic serum level is between 25 and 100 μg per ml. Subtherapeutic levels increase the chance of selecting resistant strains, while greater than therapeutic levels increase the incidence of toxic side effects (Normark and Schönebeck, 1972). The dose is easily adjusted based on creatinine

TABLE 22–2. 5-FLUOROCYTOSINE THERAPY IN RENAL FAILURE

Normal renal function	Recommended dose 50 mg/kg body weight weight every 6 hours
Renal insufficiency	
Creatinine clearance	
25–40 ml/min	50 mg/kg body weight every 12 hours
12.5–25 ml/min	50 mg/kg body weight every 24 hours
12.5 ml/min	A single dose of 50 mg/kg body weight followed by regular control of 5-FC concentration in serum

From Schönebeck, J., et al.: Chemotherapy, *18*:321, 1973.

clearance (Table 22–2); renal insufficiency is no contraindication to use the drug.

Ketoconazole is a synthetic imidazole and is effective orally. It has few side effects and a broad spectrum of activity. The urine is cleared of candida in only about half of the patients with funguria (Graybill, 1983), which is explained by the fact that very little of the drug appears in the urine. Although some excellent therapeutic results have been reached, failures are common (Graybill, 1983). The place of the drug in fungal infections of the urinary tract has not yet been settled.

Other Candida Species in Urinary Tract Infection. Although *Candida albicans* is by far the most common fungal organism to infect the urinary tract, other *Candida* species, *C. parapsilosis, C. krusei, C. guilliermondi, C. tropicalis,* and *C. stellatoidea,* may also cause infection (Price et al., 1967; Sales and Mundy, 1973; O'Connel and Hardner, 1973; Kraatz et al., 1977; Grüneberg and Leakey, 1976). The clinical picture and prognosis are similar to those in *Candida albicans* infection, although primary resistance to 5-fluorocytosine is more common in other *Candida species* (about 28 per cent) than in *Candida albicans* (about 7 per cent) (Schönebeck and Ånséhn, 1973).

OTHER FUNGI THAT CAUSE URINARY TRACT INFECTION

Torulopsis Glabrata. The genus *Torulopsis* belongs to the same group as the genus *Candida. Torulopsis glabrata* occurs as spherical or oval yeastlike cells somewhat smaller than *Candida.* It does not form pseudohyphae; torulopsis infections are therefore not associated with the formation of bezoars. The organism is usually saprophytic and may be cultured from the urine of asymptomatic patients (Schönebeck and Ånséhn, 1972), but it may also give rise to symptomatic and sometimes serious urinary tract infection. Kauffman and Tan (1974) published 11 cases, 7 of which had been previously reported. Ten were women. The average age was 62 years, and the youngest patient was 35. Nine were diabetics, five had been treated with antibiotics, and five had urinary tract obstruction, which, if unrelieved, made eradication of the infection possible. Four patients died. Ladehoff and Bach (1974) reported a generalized *Torulopsis glabrata* infection in a 60-year-old diabetic woman. The primary site of infection was the urinary tract.

DIAGNOSIS. The clinical picture is indistinguishable from bacterial pyelonephritis with subsequent bacteremia; the diagnosis depends on culturing the fungus from urine samples. Blood cultures should also be obtained. An IVP and urethrocystoscopy should be done to exclude urinary tract obstruction.

TREATMENT. Although primary resistance to 5-fluorocytosine is less than 10 per cent (Marks et al., 1971; Schönebeck, 1972), this drug was a failure in four of five cases, owing to the emergence of resistant strains. Amphotericin B was used systemically or instilled locally in the urinary tract in three patients without eradication of the organism. Two patients were cured, one after alkalinization of the urine and one after local instillation of Mycostatin. The clinical experience is evidently too small to allow any conclusions as to therapy, but the following seems reasonable: Urinary tract obstruction must be rapidly relieved, the urine alkalinized, and, as resistance to 5-fluorocytosine develops rapidly, amphotericin B is preferred despite its greater toxicity. Clinically important resistance to this drug probably does not develop either in *Torulopsis glabrata* or in *Candida* species.

Aspergillosis. The kidneys are involved in about 10 per cent of the cases of disseminated aspergillosis (Young et al., 1970). Only four cases have been described in which the kidney was the only organ affected. Two of these patients were otherwise completely healthy. One had a bezoar of the renal pelvis (Comings et al., 1962) and the other an abscess of the right kidney (Mende and Sawicka, 1964). The third patient was a narcotic addict who passed a fungus ball through the urethra. He also had positive sputum cultures but no clinical signs of aspergillosis except for renal involvement (Melchior et al., 1972). The last patient was a 22-year-old man with diabetes treated with cortisone because of episcleritis. He repeatedly passed fungus balls; surgical removal of those fungus balls from the right renal pelvis was necessary. He was the only patient in whom both kidneys were involved (Warshawsky et al., 1975). In two cases *Aspergillus fumigatus* was isolated and in another *Aspergillus flavus*. In the last patient the species was not stated. Therapy in these cases has been mainly operative, the involved kidney being removed in the first two cases. Amphotericin B should be given systemically and, in suitable cases, may be instilled via nephrostomy tubes.

Cryptococcosis. In cryptococcosis the CNS is the main target organ. The kidneys are involved in about 50 per cent of the cases with dissemination (Salyer and Salyer, 1973). The renal lesions are most often focal and are not associated with severe functional impairment; they are therefore of minor interest. However, Randall and coworkers (1968) described four cases in which hematuria, pyuria, and azotemia preceded the symptoms of meningitis. Autopsy or biopsy of these cases showed papillary necrosis associated with cryptococci. Cryptococci may also be found in the prostate, sometimes causing symptoms of prostatism; biopsy can be misinterpreted as granulomatous prostatitis or prostatic carcinoma (Voyles and Beck, 1946; Tillotson and Lerner, 1965). It is, however, evident that these cases are exceptional and that cryptococcosis is in general of minor importance in urinary tract pathology. Treatment should consist of 5-fluorocytosine or amphotericin B or both. Both drugs given simultaneously is probably the best therapy.

Penicillosis. Salisbury (1868) mentioned that he had found *Penicillium* species in urinary tract diseases. Since then only two cases have been described. The first one was a 61-year-old female with chronic cystitis and bladder bezoars. Following suprapubic removal of multiple masses, subsequently proved to be *Penicillium glaucum,* her symptoms resolved (Chute 1911). The second patient was a 65-year-old man complaining of right-sided lumbar pain. He spontaneously passed pink material, which, on microscopic examination, consisted of mycelia, and on culture proved to be *Penicillium citrinum.* The fungus was localized to the right kidney. No therapy was given. The patient was followed for several years without evidence of deterioration (Gilliam and Vest, 1951).

Sporotrichosis. Only one case of renal

sporotrichosis has been described (Rochard et al., 1909). A 29-year-old woman had a nephrectomy because of pyelonephritis and a palpable mass. Cultures of the pus from the kidney grew *Sporotrichum Schenk de Beurmann*.

Phycomycosis. Two cases of isolated renal phycomycosis have been described. The first patient (Prout and Goddard, 1960) survived after nephrectomy and amphotericin B treatment. The second (Langston et al., 1973) died in spite of amphotericin B therapy. In this second case, both kidneys were affected with large necrotic areas confined to the medullary regions, primarily involving the papillae.

South American Blastomycosis. Silveira and colleagues (1976) described a case of South American blastomycosis of the ureter. However, this was part of a generalized infection, as was the case for two similar reports published in 1956 by Silva and in 1973 by Billis and Silveira.

Transplanted Fungal Infection. Twenty per cent of patients have funguria following kidney transplant (Schönebeck, 1972), and fungal infections are a well-known problem in these patients. Perhaps less well known is the fact that fungal infections may be transferred with a transplanted kidney. One such case of histoplasmosis (MacLean et al., 1965), one of cryptococcosis (Ooi et al., 1971), and two of candidiasis (McLeish et al., 1977) have been published.

References

Ahearn, D. G., Jannach, J. R., and Roth, F. J.: Speciation and densities of yeasts in human urine specimens. Sabouraudia, 5:110, 1966.

Andriole, V. T., and Hasenclever, H. F.: Factors influencing experimental candidiasis in mice I. Alloxan diabetes. Yale J. Biol. Med., 35:96, 1962.

Bartkowiak, Z.: The phenomenon of yeast globules in course of candidiasis of the urinary tract. Sci. Lett. Poznan, 13:47, 1964.

Beland, G., and Piette, Y.: Urinary tract candidiasis: Report of a case with bilateral ureteral obstruction. Can. Med. Assoc. J., 108:472, 1973.

Bergmann, M., and Lipsky, H.: Über die Pilzbeziedlung des Urogenitaltraktus. Med. Klin., 59:732, 1964.

Billis, A., and Silveira, E.: Blastomicose sul-americana do ureter. Rev. Assoc. Med. Bras., 19:463, 1973.

Blum, J. A.: Acute monilial pyohydronephrosis: Report of a case successfully treated with amphotericin B continuous renal pelvis irrigation. J. Urol., 96:614, 1966.

Chisholm, E. R., and Hutch, J. A.: Fungus ball *(Candida albicans)* formation in the bladder. J. Urol., 86:559, 1961.

Chute, A. L.: An infection of the bladder with *Penicillium glaucum*. Boston Med. Surg. J., 144:420, 1911.

Cohen, J.: Antifungal chemotherapy. Lancet, 1:532, 1982.

Cohn, I., Jr.: Yeast growth during pre-operative preparation of the colon with antibiotics. Monogr. Ther., 2:43, 1957.

Comings, D. E., Turbow, B. A., Callahan, D. H., and Waldstein, S. S.: Obstructing aspergillus cast of the renal pevis. Arch. Intern. Med., 110:255, 1962.

Cowan, D., Dillon, J., Talbot, B., and Bridge, R.: Renal moniliasis: A case report and discussion. J. Urol., 88:594, 1962.

Cromie, W. J., and Buck, B. E.: Pan-nephric candidal abscess. Urology, 11:187, 1978.

Crosby, D. L.: Fatal candidiasis following colonic sterilisation with neomycin and bacitracin. Br. J. Urol., 39:479, 1967.

Cuétara, M. D., Mallo, N., and Dalet, F.: Amphotericin lavage in the treatment of candidial cystitis. Br. J. Urol., 44:475, 1972.

Cumming, R. E., and Nelson, R. J.: Actinomycosis of the urinary tract. Surg. Gynecol. Obstet., 3:352, 1929.

Folb, P. I., and Trounce, J. R.: Immunological aspects of *Candida* infection complicating steroid and immunosuppressive drug therapy. Lancet, 1:112, 1970.

Freis, A.: Das auftreten systemischer Candidamykosen im zusammenhang mit grundkrankheit und vorbehandlung. Arzneim. Forsch., 21:320, 1971.

Gibberd, F. B., and Williams, E. R.: Pneumaturia due to *Candida albicans*. Br. Med. J., 2:300, 1962.

Gillam, J. F., and Wadelton, D. H.: A case of renal moniliasis. Br. Med. J., 1:985, 1958.

Gilliam, J. S., Jr., and Vest, S. A.: Penicillium infection of the urinary tract. J. Urol., 65:484, 1951.

Gip, L., and Molin, L.: On the inhibitory activity of human prostatic fluid on *Candida albicans*. Mykosen, 13:61, 1970.

Goldberg, P. K., Kozinn, P. J., and Wise, G. J.: Incidence and significance of candiduria. JAMA, 241:582, 1979.

Graybill, J. R.: Potential and problems with ketoconazole. *In* Proceedings of a Symposium on New Developments in Therapy for Mycoses. Am. J. Med., 74:86, 1983.

Grüneberg, R. N., and Leakey, A.: Treatment of candidal urinary tract infection with nitrofuratel. Br. Med. J., 2:908, 1976.

Haley, L. D.: Yeast infections of the lower urinary tract. 1. In vitro studies of the tissue phase of *Candida albicans*. Sabouraudia, 4:98, 1965.

Hamory, B. H., and Wenzel, R. P.: Hospital-associated candiduria: Predisposing factors and review of the literature. J. Urol., 120:444, 1978.

Harold, D. L., Koff, S. A., and Kass, E. J.: *Candida albicans* "fungus ball" in bladder. Urology, 9:662, 1977.

Hodgin, U. G.: Cystitis due to *Candida pseudotropicalis*. Rocky Mount. Med. J., 66:30, 1969.

Hurley, R.: Pathogenicity of the genus *Candida*. *In* Winner, H., and Hurley, R. (Eds.): Symposium on Candida Infections. London, Livingstone, 1966, pp. 12–25.

Hurley, R., and Winner, H. I.: Experimental moniliasis in the mouse. Br. J. Pathol. Bacteriol., 86:75, 1963.

Janosko, E. D., and McRoberts, J. W.: Evaluation and treatment of urinary candidiasis. South. Med. J., 72:1578, 1979.

Johnson, S. A.: *Candida (Monilia) albicans*. Arch. Derm. Syph., 70:49, 1954.

Kauffman, C. A., and Tan, J. S.: Torulopsis glabrata renal infection. Am. J. Med., 57:217, 1974.

Klimek, J. J., Sayers, R., Kelmas, B. W., and Quintiliani, R.: Statistical analysis of factors predisposing to candiduria. Conn. Med., 43:364, 1979.

Kraatz, G., Bernhardt, H., and Ranft, R.: Pilzbesiedlung der ableitenden harnwege bei chronischer pyelonephritis. Zschr. Urol., 70:1, 1977.

Krause, W., Matheis, H., and Wulf, K.: Fungaemia and funguria after oral administration of *Candida albicans*. Lancet, 1:598, 1969.

Ladehoff, P., and Bach, A.: Sepsis med *Torulopsis glabrata* formenlig udgående fra nyrefocus. Ugeskr. Laeger, *136*:2031, 1974.

Langston, C., Roberts, D. A., Porter, G. A., and Bennett, W. M.: Renal phycomycosis. J. Urol., *109*:941, 1973.

Lehner, T.: Systemic candidiasis and renal involvement. Lancet, *1*:1414, 1964.

Louria, D. B., Brayton, R. G., and Finkel, G.: Studies on the pathogenesis of experimental *Candida albicans* infections in mice. Sabouraudia, *2*:271, 1963.

Louria, D. B., Fallon, N., and Browne, H. G.: The influence of cortisone on experimental fungus infections in mice. J. Clin. Invest. *39*:1435, 1960.

Louria, D. B., Stiff, D. P., and Bennett, B.: Disseminated moniliasis in the adult. Medicine, *41*:307, 1962.

MacLean, L. D., Dossetor, J. B., Gault, M. H., Oliver, J. A., Inglis, F. G., and MacKinnon, K. J.: Renal homotransplantation using cadaver donors. Arch. Surg., *91*:288, 1965.

Margolin, H.: Fungus infections of the urinary tract. Semin. Roentgenol., *6*:323, 1971.

Marks, M., Steer, P., and Eickhoff, T.: In vitro sensitivity of *Torulopsis glabrata* to amphotericin B, 5-fluorocytosine and clotrimazole (Bay 5097). Appl. Microbiol., *22*:93, 1971.

McLeish, K. R., McMurray, S. D., Smith, E. J., and Filo, R. S.: The transmission of *Candida albicans* by cadaveric allografts. J. Urol., *118*:513, 1977.

Melchior, J., Mebust, W. K., and Valk, W. L.: Ureteral colic from a fungus ball: Unusual presentation of systemic aspergillosis. J. Urol., *108*:698, 1972.

Mende, R., and Sawicka, A.: Aspergillosis of the kidney. Case Report. Pol. Tyg. Lek., *19*:308, 1964.

Müllern-Aspegren, U.: Uréthrite et cystite à saccharomyces avec "prematurie." Acta Derm. Venereol., *2*:126, 1921.

Noe, H. N., and Tonkin, I. L.: Renal candidiasis in the neonate. J. Urol., *127*:517, 1982.

Normark, S., and Schönebeck, J.: In vitro studies of 5-fluorocytosine resistance in *Candida albicans* and *Torulopsis glabrata*. Antimicrob. Agents Chemother., *3*:114, 1972.

O'Connel, C. J., and Hardner, G. J.: Thrush of urinary bladder due to *Candida guilliermondii*. N.Y. State J. Med., *73*:1685, 1973.

Olanescu, C., Streja, M., and Zaharia, Z.: Infectious funguiques de l'appareil urinaire. J. Urol. Med. Chir., *2*:771, 1956.

Ooi, B. S., Chen, T. B., Lim, C. H., Khoo, O. T., and Chan, K. T.: Survival of a patient transplanted with a kidney infected with *Cryptococcus neoformans*. Transplantation, *11*:428, 1971.

Parkash, C., Chugh, T. D., Gupta, S. P., and Thanik, K. D.: Candida infection of the urinary tract—an experimental study. J. Assoc. Physicians India, *18*:497, 1970.

Perry, J.: Opportunistic fungal infections of the urinary tract. Texas State J. Med., *60*:146, 1964.

Price, W. E., Webb, E. A., and Smith, B. A.: Urinary tract candidiasis treated with amphotericin. Br. J. Urol., *98*:523, 1967.

Prout, G. R., and Goddard, A. R.: Renal mucormycosis. N. Engl. J. Med., *263*:1246, 1960.

Randall, R. E., Jr., Stacy, W. K., Toone, E. C., Prout, G. R., Jr., Madge, G. E., Shadomy, H. J., Shadomy, S., and Utaz, J. P.: Cryptococcal pyelonephritis. N. Engl. J. Med., *279*:60, 1968.

Rochard, Rubens, Duval, and Bodoleo: Pyelonéphrite sporotrichose. Gazette des Hospiteau Paris, 1147, 1909.

Sales, J. L., and Mundy, H. B.: Renal candidiasis: Diagnosis and management. Can. J. Surg., *16*:139, 1973.

Salisbury, J. H.: On the parasitic forms developed in parent epithelial cells of the urinary and genital organs and their secretions. Am. J. Med. Sci., *55*:371, 1868.

Salyer, W. R., and Salyer, D. C.: Involvement of the kidney and prostate in cryptococcosis. J. Urol., *109*:695, 1973.

Schönebeck, J.: Asymptomatic candiduria. Scand. J. Urol. Nephrol., *6*:136, 1972.

Schönebeck, J.: Atlas of Cystoscopy. Copenhagen, Schultz Medical Information, 1984.

Schönebeck, J.: Studies on Candida infection of the urinary tract and on the antimycotic drug 5-fluorocytosine. Scand. J. Urol. Nephrol. (Suppl. 11), 1972.

Schönebeck, J., Andersson, L., Lingårdh, G., and Winblad, B.: Ureteric obstruction caused by yeast-like fungi. Scand. J. Urol. Nephrol., *4*:171, 1970.

Schönebeck, J., and Anséhn, S.: The occurrence of yeast-like fungi in the urine under normal conditions and in various types of urinary tract pathology. Scand. J. Urol. Nephrol., *6*:123, 1972.

Schönebeck, J., and Ånséhn, S.: 5-fluorocytosine resistance in *Candida* species and *Torulopsis glabrata*. Sabouraudia, *11*:10, 1973.

Schönebeck, J., and Winblad, B.: Primary renal Candida infection. Scand. J. Urol. Nephrol., *4*:171, 1971.

Schönebeck, J., Winblad, B., and Ånséhn, S.: Renal candidosis complicating caeco-cystoplasty. Scand. J. Urol. Nephrol., *6*:129, 1972.

Senator, H.: Ueber pneumaturie im allgemeinen und bei diabetes mellitus insbesondre. Internat. Beitr. Wissenschaftl. Med. Berlin. Bb III, p. 317, 1891.

Seneca, H., Longo, F., and Peer, P.: Candida pyelonephritis and candiduria: The clinical significance of *Candida albicans* in the urine. J. Urol., *100*:266, 1968.

Silva, W. B.: Registro de um caso de blastomicose sulamericana generalizada con comprometimento cardiaco. An. Fac. Med. Univ. Recife, *16*:235, 1956.

Silveira, E., Billis, A., Trevisan, M., and Veira, R.: South American blastomycosis of the ureter. Am. J. Trop. Med. Hyg., *25*:530, 1976.

Tannenberg, J.: Doppelseitige soorerkrankung des nierenbeckens bei einem diabetiker. Zeitschr. Urol., *17*:82, 1923.

Taylor, H., and Rundle, J.: Acute moniliasis of the urinary tract. Lancet, *1*:1236, 1952.

Tennant, F. S., Remmers, A. R., Jr., and Perry, J. E.: Primary renal candidiasis. Arch. Intern. Med., *122*:435, 1968.

Tillotson, J. R., and Lerner, A. M.: Prostatism in an eighteen-year-old boy due to infection with *Cryptococcus neoformans*. N. Engl. J. Med., *273*:1150, 1965.

Umenai, T., and Ishida, N.: The significance of candiduria. Tohoku J. Exp. Med., *122*:59, 1977.

Voyles, G. Q., and Beck, E. M.: Systemic infection due to *Torula histolytica* (cryptococcus hominis). Arch. Intern. Med., *77*:504, 1946.

Warshawsky, A. B., Keiller, D., and Gites, R. F.: Bilateral renal aspergillosis. J. Urol., *113*:8, 1975.

Wise, G. J., Goldberg, P., and Kozinn, P. J.: Genitourinary candidiasis: Diagnosis and treatment. J. Urol., *116*:778, 1976.

Wise, G. J., Kozinn, P. J., and Goldberg, P.: Amphotericin B as a urologic irrigant in the management of noninvasive candiduria. J. Urol., *128*:82, 1982.

Young, R. C., Bennett, J. E., Vogel, C. L., Carbone, P. P., and DeVita, V. T.: Aspergillosis. The spectrum of the disease in 98 patients. Medicine, *49*:147, 1970.

CHAPTER 23

Genitourinary Tuberculosis

JAMES G. GOW, M.D.

INTRODUCTION AND HISTORICAL REVIEW

Over the last two decades there has been a profound, if gradual, change in the manner in which genitourinary tuberculosis is approached. It is a change that mirrors the approach taken by many disciplines in medicine. The ideology of optimism has given way to the idealogy of concern, as the feeling that the future will always be better than the past has not been realized; yet is it not very rare for any future that is to span 20 years to be predictable? When it is considered that tuberculosis precedes recorded history, the results obtained in the treatment of all manifestations of the disease have been one of the outstanding achievements of the generation.

The disease known as consumption was observed in humans as long as 7000 years ago (Myers, 1952). The remains of ancient skeletons have shown the characteristic changes of tuberculosis, indicating that the disease affected man about 4000 B.C., and it was known to be a common disease in Egypt in about 1000 B.C. (Morse et al., 1964). In 375 B.C., Hippocrates described phthisis, a lingering disease that becomes worse in winter, results in emaciation, and causes diarrhea in its terminal phase (Jenkins and Wolinsky, 1965). Galen in 180 A.D. had considerable interest in consumption, and his methods of treatment were followed for the next 1500 years. In 1696, Richard Wiseman wrote that "scrofula or the Kings-Evil was a difficult problem that confronted physicians and surgeons daily."

During the 1700's in Europe, tuberculosis infections reached epidemic proportions, and nearly one quarter of the deaths in England at that time were due to consumption (Colby, 1954; Flick, 1925). The infectious nature of the disease was established by Villemin, who showed in experiments carried out between 1865 and 1868 that tuberculosis could be transferred from man or cattle to rabbits. In 1879, Cohnheim presented his elimination theory. According to his hypothesis, tubercle bacilli in the blood were eliminated in the urine, so that the bacilli were supposedly lodged in a focus somewhere in the urinary tract. On March 24th, 1882, Robert Koch announced that he had discovered the cause of tuberculosis, and 3 weeks later he published his first article, describing the pathogenesis of the disease and outlining Koch's postulates, which have since become the basis of studies in all infectious diseases. He had observed the organism in all cases of the disease, he had grown the organism outside the body, and he had reproduced the disease in a susceptible host.

In 1885, Nocard isolated the avian form of the tubercle bacillus, and in 1889 Theobald Smith described the bovine variety. The acid-fast nature of the bacillus was discovered by Ehrlich in 1882. Thirty years after Cohnheim's hypothesis, Ekehorn (1908) proposed his direct hematogenous theory, which suggested that the bacilli were transported like emboli to the renal capillaries, where they lodged and formed a tuberculous focus. According to this theory, the remainder of the kidney and the rest of the urinary tract were secondarily infected via the urine. This theory was accepted and formed the basis of the belief that tuberculosis could be treated by nephrectomy.

The pathogenesis of renal tuberculosis remained obscure until Medlar (1926) published his classic studies on 30 patients who had died from pulmonary tuberculosis, none of whom had any clinical evidence of genitourinary disease. He reviewed 100,000 serial sections from the kidneys of these patients. Microscopic lesions were found in these kidneys, nearly all in the cortex and nearly all bilateral. It was Medlar (1949) who suggested that these lesions should be termed "metastatic" rather than "secondary," as it was clear that the kidneys had become infected through the blood stream, and that the term "secondary" should be used to describe the pathologic changes.

The next milestone was reached in 1955, when Coulaud succeeded in inducing primary tuberculous lesions in the renal cortex of rabbits; 2 years later, Wildbolz (1937) used the term "genitourinary tuberculosis," emphasizing that renal and epididymal tuberculosis were not separate diseases but local manifestations of the same blood-borne infection.

The last and greatest historical event was the discovery of the antituberculous drugs, starting with streptomycin in 1943, followed by para-aminosalicylic acid in 1946, isoniazid in 1952, and rifampicin in 1966.

INCIDENCE

The incidence of new cases of tuberculosis is a good index of the progress of the disease. Although, it does not reflect all the humans suffering or the number of cases that require treatment, it reveals the trend of the problem and gives some idea of the effect of the control measures. To be of value, any statistics must include a high proportion of all new cases, which can be detected only in countries with an efficient organization. Therefore, there will always be differences between reports from developed and developing countries—in the latter the incidence is many times higher, a trend that has quickened since the advent of chemotherapy. Moreover, in developed countries all forms of tuberculosis have tended to infect the older age groups, whereas in many developing countries the disease has continued to affect adolescents and young adults. The World Health Organization has estimated that throughout the world there are 10 million new cases of all forms of tuberculosis, mostly in the Third World countries. In developed countries the annual decline is about 12 per cent, whereas in developing countries the decline hardly has been noticed (W.H.O., 1981). In the United States, 13 per 100,000 population are affected (U.S. Department of Health, 1980, 1982). Table 23–1 shows the reduction in the notification of pulmonary and genitourinary tuberculosis in the 5 years from 1975 to 1979 in Great Britain.

Whereas the incidence of pulmonary tuberculosis has continued to decline in the United Kingdom in the last two decades, that of nonpulmonary tuberculosis, apart from genitourinary tuberculosis, has remained static. Worldwide, the genitourinary disease accounts for only 14 per cent of the nonpulmonary manifestations, and only 20 per cent are from the white population (Lane, 1982).

The consistently steady decline of the genitourinary manifestation is almost certainly due to the effective chemotherapeutic treatment of the primary pulmonary focus. Nevertheless, new cases are always being seen, and urologists must be aware of the possible diagnosis. According to the foregoing figures, the incidence in the United States and United Kingdom is about 13 per 100,000 population, but in some Third World countries the incidence can be as high as 400 per 100,000 inhabitants (Lowell, 1976), a daunting prospect when it is realized that one case of sputum-positive tuberculosis can affect as many as 30 other people, some of whom will undoubtedly develop the renal manifestation. The disease will therefore remain a serious problem while so many cases remain undiagnosed and untreated. It is also significant for the urologist that whereas in the Western world only between 8 and 10 per cent of patients with pulmonary tuberculosis develop renal tuberculosis, as many as 15 to 20 per cent in the underdeveloped countries are found with *Mycobacterium tuberculosis* in the urine (Freedman, 1979). A lot more is known today about the incidence and treatment of tuberculosis, but until the identification of infected cases becomes more effective, the ultimate goal of complete eradication will remain in the far distance.

EPIDEMIOLOGY

There is now general agreement that the annual tuberculous infection rate is the best single indicator for evaluating the tuberculous problem and its trend in developed and devel-

TABLE 23–1. REDUCTION IN THE NOTIFICATION OF PULMONARY AND GENITOURINARY TUBERCULOSIS IN THE UNITED KINGDOM, 1975–1979

	Pulmonary Tuberculosis	Genitourinary Tuberculosis
1975	9900	995
1976	8951	753
1977	6510	641
1978	6314	559
1979	6453	435

oping countries and that it is an index expressing the importance of tuberculosis within the community (Styblo, 1980).

In developed countries, there is reliable evidence that (1) the tuberculous incidence has been falling since the turn of the century; (2) under present conditions, irrespective of any treatment, it is diminishing at the rate of 5 per cent per annum; and (3) this decrease in infection rate is exponential (Sutherland, 1976).

This means that under present conditions of human resistance and environment, the tubercle bacillus eventually will be eradicated (provided that the present balance against it is maintained), although eradication might take many years.

The situation changes if the impact of modern chemotherapy is added to the natural regression rate. Although it is difficult to estimate the impact of chemotherapy on the overall tuberculous situation, a conservative estimate is that case-finding and treatment accelerated the decrease in the incidence by about 7.8 per cent annually. This percentage, when added to the 5 per cent annual natural decrease, results in a total fall in the risk of infection by more than 12 per cent per annum, which will lead to a complete eradication before the end of the century.

In developing countries, the situation is very different. In Lesotho and Uganda (W.H.O., 1969) and in Algeria and Tunis, Sutherland and coworkers (1971) showed that there was very little downward trend over a period of 10 years. The risk of infection remained at about 2.6 per cent, so that there will be a gradually increasing number of infected cases. The disease will therefore remain a major problem, as there will be no tendency for self-elimination. It is estimated that, accepting an annual risk of infection of 3 per cent, 26 per cent of the population will be infected at the age of 10 years and 45 per cent at the age of 20 years.

It is a salutary exercise to estimate what would happen if, in such countries, the annual infection rate were made to decrease by 5 per cent. If that were to happen, there would be a reduction of the risk of infection from 3 per cent in 1980 to 0.7 per cent in 2010, and an increase in the proportion of unaffected population from 55 per cent to 68 per cent (Styblo, 1980).

The two basic methods for planning efficient tuberculous control are (1) bacillus Calmette-Guérin (BCG) inoculation, and (2) case-finding and treatment. In developed countries the time may not be far distant when mass BCG vaccination will be no longer necessary and then be discontinued, as the economic consideration

and complications outweigh any possible benefits, especially as case-finding and treatment have reached such a high degree of efficiency and the few additional cases that may occur can be treated by the highly effective short-course regimens available.

In developing countries, BCG immunization must play a major part in the control of the disease if it can be effectively organized, and for it to be efficient it must be carried out soon after birth.

Case-finding remains the major weakness of any antituberculous program, and it is calculated that only one third of smear-positive cases are diagnosed (Farga, 1972) and that any improvement is going to be difficult in the foreseeable future for reasons of population dispersal, poor transport, inadequate medical facilities, insufficient laboratories, and poor socioeconomic conditions. It is vital, however, for the eventual control of the disease that this problem be tackled energetically, because, as said previously, one smear-positive patient can infect up to 30 other persons. In the developing world the necessary services are still totally inadequate and economic facilities are just as much a problem as medical resources.

With modern short-course chemotherapy, the results are bound to be successful, and an improvement in the identification of smear-positive cases from 30 per cent to 50 per cent will make a considerable impact on the overall worldwide tuberculosis problem. Using the present effective drugs the rate at which patients can be rendered almost noninfectious is quite dramatic, because the organisms in the sputum of most patients with pulmonary disease are reduced about a thousandfold in 2 to 3 weeks. In those with renal tuberculosis it is almost impossible to isolate *M. tuberculosis* from the urine after 2 weeks, so that at the end of this time they can be considered noninfectious. "Find, isolate, treat, and educate" should be the slogan that motivates all workers who are tackling the problem of tuberculosis in the developing countries.

IMMUNOLOGY

The Immune Response. The development of any infectious disease depends upon the reaction between the invasive properties of the pathogen and the immune response of the host. The immunologic response associated with an invading pathogen consists of recognition, responses, and reaction (Grange, 1980). The immune system consists of two main classes of lymphocytes, the T cells and the B cells. The T cells do not produce antibodies but synthesize lymphokines, which make macrophages more aggressive to invading parasites. The B cells, however, develop into plasma cells, which very rapidly produce antibodies. Both these classes of cells are complementary and are essential for the rapid elimination of bacteria. It is the magnitude of the cell-mediated response that determines the progress of the disease in man. However, these two factors vary in importance between different bacteria; in the case of the *M. tuberculosis* it is the cell-mediated response that is most important, and it is doubtful whether the production of antibodies plays any major part in host defense.

Bacille Calmette-Guérin (BCG). At a time when effective antibiotic therapy for tuberculosis is taken for granted, it is salutary to remember that the discovery of prophylactic measures against many infecitons (a more logical approach) antedated the discovery of powerful drugs by about 200 years. Early attempts to induce immunity against tuberculosis with tuberculin and various vaccines failed; it was not until Calmette and Guérin (1925) discovered the method of attenuating the virulence of the *M. tuberculosis* by repeated subculture, eventually obtaining a permanently avirulent strain that they called BCG, that any success was achieved. This vaccine, which has been given since its discovery in 1925, has a low but definite complication rate.

The degree of protection is very variable, from 80 per cent in United Kingdom urban schoolchildren and North American Indians to nil in Georgia (U.S.A.) schoolchildren and Southern Indian general population (Ten Dam et al., 1976).

It has been suggested that BCG acts not by preventing infection but by limiting the multiplication and spread of the *M. tuberculosis*. Stanford and associates (1981) proposed that two different acquired mechanisms of cell-mediated response to mycobacteria exist, one of which confers good host protection and the other of which does not. Early contact with environmental mycobacteria primes the host to respond in one of these two ways, which of the two being determined by the species of *Mycobacterium* to which the host is first exposed. Once primed, the pattern of response is established for life and subsequent BCG vaccination will merely boost the established response. When the initial mycobacteria are those that prime the host with the less effective of the two mechanisms, the BCG will confer little or no benefit. This hypothesis helps to explain the geographic variations of the efficacy of BCG.

Despite the variation of the response, the procedure is safe and inexpensive. It is recommended at the present time that every effort be made to pursue the school vaccination program so that all tuberculin-negative children at the age of 11 or 12 years in developed countries should be inoculated with BCG. In developing countries, the vaccine should be given as soon as possible after birth, since otherwise many will be dead by the age of 13 years (Ten Dam and Hitze, 1980).

Today, however, the use of BCG still remains controversial. In the first place, protection lasts for only 15 years. Second, there will be a proportion of subjects in any age group who will have been infected, and BCG cannot affect this number. Third, there is a change of complications—lymphadenitis, lupus vulgaris, and BCG–itis. Fourth, it cannot influence the incidence of infected cases. Because of these inconsistencies, some Western countries have already stopped mass BCG vaccination, taking the view that possible complications outweigh any possible benefits. However, despite these reasons, this view is considered unwise, because epidemics of tuberculosis do occur and are not merely diseases of immigrants, chronic bronchitics, and alcoholics. The most recent epidemic was reported by Hill and Stevenson (1983), who published the details of an epidemic of 41 new tuberculous patients, only 7 of whom had been vaccinated with BCG.

MYCOBACTERIUM

In morphology the *Mycobacterium* varies considerably from short cells to long filaments, which can under certain conditions show branching. It is 2.4 μm long and 0.2 to 0.5 μm wide. The mycobacterium cell has a thick wall separated from the cell membrane by a translucent zone. The organisms have no true capsule or flagella, are nonmotile, and are pathogenic.

The cell wall itself is a complex structure composed of four layers. The innermost layer consists of murein (peptidoglycan), as in other bacteria, while the outer three layers are composed of ropelike complexes of peptides, polysaccharides, and lipids, set in a homogeneous matrix. The lipids account for between 40 and 50 per cent of the weight of the bacterium.

M. tuberculosis is the most virulent and infective of all mycobacteria, although the precise nature of this high virulence remains unknown (Barksdale and Kim, 1977). The cytoplasm of the mycobacterium does not differ essentially from that of other bacteria. *M. tuberculosis* is strictly aerobic and can multiply in air alveoli, whereas the *M. bovis* is partially anaerobic, a property that is used to help differentiate between the two. For example, the *M. tuberculosis* will grow on the surface of an egg-enriched medium, while the *M. bovis* is usually seen a few millimeters below the surface. It grows only within a restricted range of temperature, the optimum being 35° C, and on culture the first colonies are seen after 3 to 4 weeks. The *M. bovis* is a much more important organism in underdeveloped countries because there is no pasteurization of milk.

The mycobacteria differ from other organisms in that they show quite different responses to antibiotic treatment. There are certain factors that may explain some of the differences. In the first place, mycobacteria are extremely slow-growing. *E. coli* and other common pathogens have a doubling time of about 20 minutes, whereas *M. tuberculosis* divides only once every 20 to 24 hours. Most antibiotics work only when the metabolic machinery is functioning, which means that the organisms are susceptible only when they are dividing; as long as they are not dividing, the metabolism does not get blocked by the antibiotic and they survive in its presence. The second factor that distinguishes the tuberculous infection from, say, the *E. coli* infection, is that there is effective cooperation between the antibiotic and the phagocytes in the latter case. Organisms such as *E. coli,* whose division may have been slowed or stopped, can be phagocytized. Once inside the cell, the oxidative and lysosomal enzymes usually kill the phagocytized organism. This is not so in the case of *M. tuberculosis,* as that organism is quite resistant to the various intracellular killing mechanisms, certainly early in the infection before cellular immunity is fully developed. Therefore, the *M. tuberculosis,* once it has been phagocytized, can survive and even travel around in the phagocytic cell. It is also interesting that despite the lack of any significant humoral antibody response, phagocytes manage to ingest *M. tuberculosis,* possibly owing to the affinity between the waxy coat and the cell membrane lipids.

It is probably true that the concentration of antibiotics is substantially lower inside phagocytes, and also the intracellular pH may not favor some antibacterials, as most are effective only at a particular pH. It is this population of *M. tuberculosis* that is susceptible to pyrazinamide, which enters phagocytes and which is at its most active at a pH o 5.5 (see further on).

Next, there is another factor that is peculiar to the mycobacterium, namely, a proportion of the organisms are able to become dormant and lie in tissues for a long time, even a lifetime, without dividing and are thus not susceptible to any antibiotic action.

Finally, there is the well-known fact that *M. tuberculosis* is much more prone than most bacteria to develop resistance, especially when antibiotics are given singly.

Nontuberculous mycobacteria. In the early 1950's, when it had become routine practice to culture *M. tuberculosis,* it was soon realized that other mycobacteria were important pathogens for man, and a new concept about mycobacterial infection was reached. These organisms became known as nontuberculous mycobacteria (Wolinsky, 1979).

The organisms are classified into two groups, human pathogens and human nonpathogens (Table 23–2). They produce lesions similar to those of *M. tuberculosis* but usually of lower virulence.

Nontuberculous mycobacteria rarely cause pathogenic changes in the genitourinary system. Only five cases of renal disease have been reported since 1956, two due to *M. kansasii* (Woods et al., 1956) and three to *M. avium-intracellulare* (Pergament et al., 1974). Three cases of epididymitis have been recorded, all

TABLE 23–2. CLASSIFICATION OF MYCOBACTERIA

Human Pathogens	Human Nonpathogens
Mammalian tubercle bacilli (tuberculous complex) M. tuberculosis M. bovis (including BCG strain) M. africanum	Slowly growing M. gordonae M. gastri M. terrae complex M. flavescens
M. leprae	Rapidly growing M. smegmatis M. vaccae M. parafortuitum complex
Slowly growing potential pathogens M. avium-intracellulare M. scrofulaceum M. kansasii M. ulcerans M. marinum M. xenopi M. szulgai M. simiae	
Rapidly growing potential pathogen M. fortuitum complex	

due to *M. xenopi* (Hepper et al., 1971). One case of granulomatous prostatitis due to a combination of *M. kansasii* and *M. fortuitum* has also been reported (Lee et al., 1977).

The principles of treatment are the same as those for *M. tuberculosis* disease, using intensive multidrug regimens. However, as the nontuberculous mycobacteria are often resistant to one or more of the first-line drugs, it is important to obtain an early, complete spectrum of drug sensitivities. Even so, treatment poses problems. There are many documented cases in which nontuberculous mycobacteria have been found in the urine, none of which have caused any disease. Nevertheless, if sensitive organisms are found, it is prudent to give a 3- or 4-month intensive course of chemotherapy.

PATHOGENESIS

In assessing the progress of any tuberculous infection, it is important to differentiate between people who have had no prior exposure to *M. tuberculosis* and those who have previously been infected. The former manifestation is called a primary focus or primary disease, and in this type of infection the mycobacterium lodges within the macrophage. At this stage, the macrophages have no capacity for controlling the disease. The organisms therefore multiply, but only at a slow rate, because of their inherent capacity; hence, the condition resulting from the infection may require several weeks to become manifest. When the *M. tuberculosis* organisms have multiplied sufficiently, an inflammatory reaction occurs. In spite of this reaction there is still little resistance to the multiplication of the bacteria, and rapid spread therefore occurs, first by way of the lymphatics and then through the blood stream. Within about 4 weeks, however, the rate of multiplication decreases and the dissemination ceases. At this stage, two immunologic manifestations occur. First, the individual shows evidence of delayed hypersensitivity, and second, the macrophages acquire the ability to inhibit the multiplication of virulent *M. tuberculosis*. This type of immunity is known as acquired cellular immunity.

PRIMARY AND SECONDARY TUBERCULOSIS

The difference between primary and secondary, or reactivation, tuberculosis depends on the multiplication and spread of the infection, i.e., before the development of delayed hypersensitivity. Although the term "reactivation" is used for chronic tuberculosis, in some cases it is likely that dormant bacilli, through changed circumstances, have begun to multiply and produce recurrence of the disease. Among these changed circumstances are debilitating disease, trauma, corticosteriod administration, immunosuppressive therapy, diabetes, and anemia.

It must be realized that genitourinary tuberculosis is caused by metastatic spread of organisms through the blood stream. It therefore produces the appearance of secondary tuberculosis, which can occur either by reactivation of old infection or by reinfection from an active case.

The initial lesion is characterized by destruction due to the inflammatory reaction caused by retained hypersensitivity. The disease is very slow to progress, and if it does, it extends as necrosis of adjacent tissue develops, which is, again, caused by hypersensitive inflammation. Necrosis is the outstanding feature of renal tuberculosis. Consequently, the destruction caused makes control of the disease more difficult. However, as the antituberculous drugs enter cavities, there is no delay in the response to treatment.

PATHOLOGY

TUBERCULOSIS OF THE KIDNEY

Renal tuberculosis is a secondary manifestation of the disease and is caused by a blood-borne metastatic organism, as there is already a hypersensitive reaction produced by the previous primary infection in the lungs. This infection may have happened many years previously. It is contracted by inhaling droplets of exhaled infected bronchial secretions. However, most of these metastatic lesions heal, as the bacteremia is not intense.

Once a person has been infected, he may harbor live *M. tuberculosis* organisms for the rest of his life. These can become reactivated if the appropriate circumstances occur.

When the organisms reach the kidney, they settle in the blood vessels, usually those close to the glomeruli, and cause microscopic foci that have the classic features of secondary tuberculosis. Polymorphonuclear leukocytes disappear early from the lesion. Macrophages appear, and a low-grade inflammatory reaction continues. Next, granulomas form. These consist of a central Langhans' giant cell surrounded by lymphocytes and fibroblasts. Because the person will have developed some immunity, the microscopic appearances are those of a more chronic lesion. Lymphocyte infiltration increases; macrophages appear in large numbers, many being transformed to epithelioid cells and others mediating the destruction of the phagocytized bacilli. The further course of the infection will depend on the infecting dose, the virulence of the organism, and the resistance of the host. If the bacterial multiplication is checked, tubercles are replaced by fibrous tissue, but if they continue to multiply they form further tubercles that coalesce with a central area of caseous necrosis. The factor that determines virulence in strains of *M. tuberculosis* is not known.

The healing process starts by the formation of reticula around the lesions. This eventually matures into fibrous tissue. Later, calcium salts are deposited, producing the classic calcified lesion, which is clearly visible on urography.

In the kidney these lesions slough into parts of the collecting system, and produce tuberculous bacilluria. They may go on increasing in size until they reach a papilla, which is invaded and destroyed. With further progress a calyx is ulcerated, causing the typical ulcerocavernous lesion. The cavities usually are not large, and it is rare at the present time to see extensive cavitative destruction of renal tissue. If the defense mechanisms of the body are powerful enough to control the infection, fibrous tissue reaction occurs. This causes strictures in the calyceal stem or at the pelviureteric junction. As a result, chronic abscesses form in the parenchymatous tissue, which are always larger than the urographic appearances suggest. Once a calyceal stem becomes stenosed, it is extremely rare for communication to be restored. Very occasionally, one moiety of a duplex kidney is involved. In every case in the author's experience the disease has remained confined to the moiety originally infected, and if surgery is required, it is never necessary to remove the whole kidney.

Renal Calcification. Calcification is becoming a growing hazard in renal tuberculosis. Its incidence is slowly increasing so that its presence is assuming more and more importance in the management of renal tuberculosis (Antonio and Gow, 1975).

From the early 1950's to 1964, 24 per cent of patients had calcification somewhere in the renal tract (Gow, 1965), whereas in a survey taken between 1975 and 1980, 53 per cent of patients show some form of renal calcification. Marszalak and Dhai (1982) reported only 20 per

cent of their series of 95 patients seen between 1977 and 1980, however. The etiology remains obscure, as there is no evidence to support a different pathogeneses for tuberculous calcification and for discrete renal calculi. Occasionally, precipitating factors that are known to be associated with calculous disease are found, e.g., recumbency, high calcium intake, recurrent urinary infection, obstructive uropathy, and hypercalciuria, but there is no common denominator. It is not without significance that 28 per cent of all large areas of calcification that were excised had viable *M. tuberculosis* in the calcified matrix (Wong, 1980).

In the management of this complication, the aim should be to retain as much functioning renal tissue as possible. Small lesions can be kept under review on an annual basis and can continue to be managed conservatively, provided that there is no increase in size. This review should continue for 10 years or more, as the writer has seen a sudden increase in size that required surgical intervention. Nevertheless, most small calcified lesions will remain unchanged for more than 20 years. Larger areas of calcification (Fig. 23–1) should be excised, and nonfunctioning kidneys with extensive calcification (Fig. 23–2) should be removed. Calcification or calculi occuring after chemotherapeutic treatment has been completed should be managed in the same way as any other uncomplicated calcification of the renal tract.

Hypertension and Renal Tuberculosis. Many renal diseases have been associated with hypertension ever since Goldblatt and coworkers (1934) showed that obstruction of the renal artery of one kidney produced this disease. All the associated renal diseases have one common factor, i.e., the reduction in the blood supply to part or the whole of the kidney, and, as this is a universal pathologic change in renal tuberculosis, it might be thought that the two conditions would be associated much more commonly than they are. In 1940, Nesbit reported the first case of hypertension associated with renal tuberculosis, cured by nephrectomy (Nesbit and Ratliff, 1940). This was followed in 1956 by the account of a study by Smith. Since then there have been many studies of different groups of patients with genitourinary tuberculosis. Braasch (1940) reported a double incidence in patients with severe renal tuberculosis when compared with the incidence of all patients with hypertension. These figures were confirmed by Flechner (Flechner and Gow, 1980). Hsiung and coworkers (1965) reported that of 30 patients treated by nephrectomy, 25 were greatly improved, but the long-

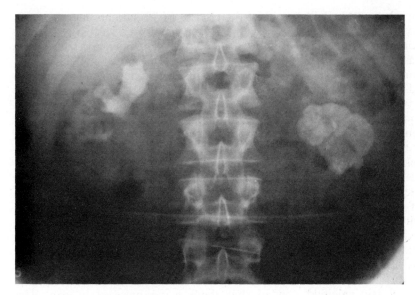

Figure 23–1. Moderate calcification in a tuberculous kidney.

term follow-up studies were inadequate. Schwartz and Lattimer (1967), however, reported that only 1 hypertensive patient out of 20 showed any improvement in blood pressure.

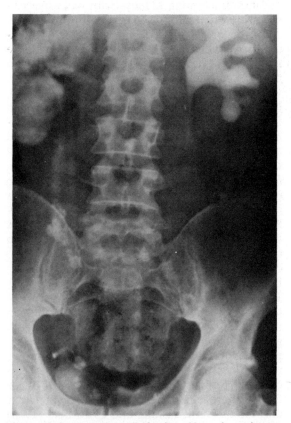

Figure 23–2. Extensive calcification. Note the quiescent disease in the right kidney and the calcification in the seminal vesicles.

In the series quoted by Flechner and Gow (1980), 64.7 per cent with unilateral nonfunctioning or poorly functioning kidneys had a fall in blood pressure after nephrectomy. These figures are consistent with those of Marks and Pontasse (1973) and Hsiung and associates (1965), so that it is apparent that two thirds of patients with extensive unilateral tuberculous nephropathy will achieve a substantial fall in blood pressure following nephrectomy. The results in this special group are far better than the 25 per cent that is generally accepted as the standard for hypertensive patients with other unilateral nephropathies. To what degree the extent of the disease is responsible can be predicted by the selective measurement of renal vein renin in unilateral tuberculous kidneys. This may be an important investigation before proceeding to nephrectomy in the doubtful case, as there are many patients with genitourinary tuberculosis who have hypertension that is not related to the tuberculous disease. These patients should have medical treatment for the hypertension, combined with antituberculous chemotherapy.

TUBERCULOSIS OF THE URETER

Tuberculous ureteritis is always an extension of the disease in the kidney. Its effects are very variable. The site most commonly affected is the ureterovesical junction, and this infection may progress to stricture formation.

The stricture may be long or short, and can cause extensive hydronephrosis. Occasionally, the disease is manifested by a stricture at the pelviureteric junction. This is always secondary to extensive disease of the kidney and, if not recognized early, can rapidly cause complete destruction. Only rarely is the disease seen in the middle third. Very occasionally, the whole of the ureter is involved. In these cases the kidney shows extensive disease, is often nonfunctioning, and is calcified (Fig. 23–3). Nephroureterectomy is the only possible treatment.

TUBERCULOSIS OF THE BLADDER

Bladder lesions are always secondary to renal tuberculosis. The earliest forms of infection invariably start around one or another ureteric orifice, which becomes red, inflamed, and edematous (Fig. 23–4). As the area of mild inflammation progresses, bullous granulations appear and these may completely obscure the ureteric orifice (Fig. 23–5); if a retrograde pyelogram is required, endoscopic resection of these granulations has to be carried out so that the ureteric orifice can be identified.

Tuberculous ulcers may be present but are rare and are a late finding. They are irregular in outline and superficial, with a central inflamed area usually surrounded by raised granulations. Initially, they are in close proximity to the ureteric orifices, but as the disease progresses they can appear in any part of the bladder (Fig. 23–6). Patchy cystitis with granulations on the fundus or the base is a late development. If the disease progresses, the inflammation spreads deep into the muscle, which eventually is replaced by fibrous tissue. This starts around the ureteric orifice, which contracts and can either produce a stricture or become withdrawn, rigid, and dilated, assuming the classic golf-hole appearance (Fig. 23–7). These ureters are usually rigid in the lower third and invariably give rise to ureteric reflux. With modern chemotherapy this is now a rare occurrence. Healed mucosal lesions have a stellate appearance, caused by bands of fibrous tissue that meet at a central point, usually the site of the initial area of severe infection (Fig. 23–8).

Occasionally, the whole of the bladder is covered by angry, inflamed, velvety granulations with ulceration, and once this stage has been reached it is very unlikely that, even with modern chemotherapy, there will be sufficient recovery of the bladder to ensure an adequate capacity (Fig. 23–9).

Tubercles are very infrequent, but if they are seen they are always close to the ureteric orifices. If isolated tubercles are visible away from the ureteric orifices, which appear normal on inspection and give a clear efflux, it must be assumed that they are not caused by the *M. tuberculosis* and are almost certainly malignant, making biopsy essential.

In very extensive disease involving the ureter, bladder, and seminal vesicles, fistulae into the rectum are rare complications (Patoir et al., 1969).

TUBERCULOSIS OF THE TESTIS

Tuberculosis of the testis is nearly always secondary to infection of the epididymis, which in most cases is blood-borne because of the extensive blood supply of the epididymis, particularly the globus minor (Macmillan, 1954).

A very rare presentation is a tuberculous orchitis with no epididymal involvement. It is impossible to differentiate such a swelling from a tumor, and early exploration is therefore required.

Eleven per cent of cases have a renal lesion at autopsy, which confirms the evidence of a direct hematogenous infection of these organs (Riehle and Jayavaman, 1982).

TUBERCULOUS EPIDIDYMITIS

Although for many years the route of infection of the epididymis remained a source of controversy, it is now accepted that all the tuberculous foci in the epididymis are the result of metastatic spread of organisms via the blood stream. The disease usually starts in the globus minor because of its greater blood supply compared with other parts of the epididymis (Macmillan, 1954). Retrovasal migration of organisms may occur in acute epididymitis after prostatectomy, but abnormalities in the posterior urethra and extensive destructive lesions in tuberculous prostatitis are rarely seen. Furthermore, in a series of prostatic biopsies carried out by the author in 20 patients with proven tuberculous epididymitis, only 1 showed evidence of tuberculous infection, signifying that disease, if present in the remainder, could not have been extensive. Although this evidence is not conclusive, because it is acknowledged that only small pieces of prostate were examined, it suggests that if the disease had been substantial enough to produce a tuberculous epididymitis, more than 1 out of 20 would have been diseased. Furthermore, tuberculous epididymitis may be associated with renal disease, but this is by no means universal, the renal focus is often microscopic and therefore excretes a small number of tubercle bacilli. Because of this, the chances of any organisms' migrating up the vas deferens must be remote. If this were the common route of infection, tuberculous epididymitis would be expected to be a common concomitant to severe tuberculous cystitis when *M. tuberculosis* organisms are constantly present in the urine, whereas this, in fact, is rare.

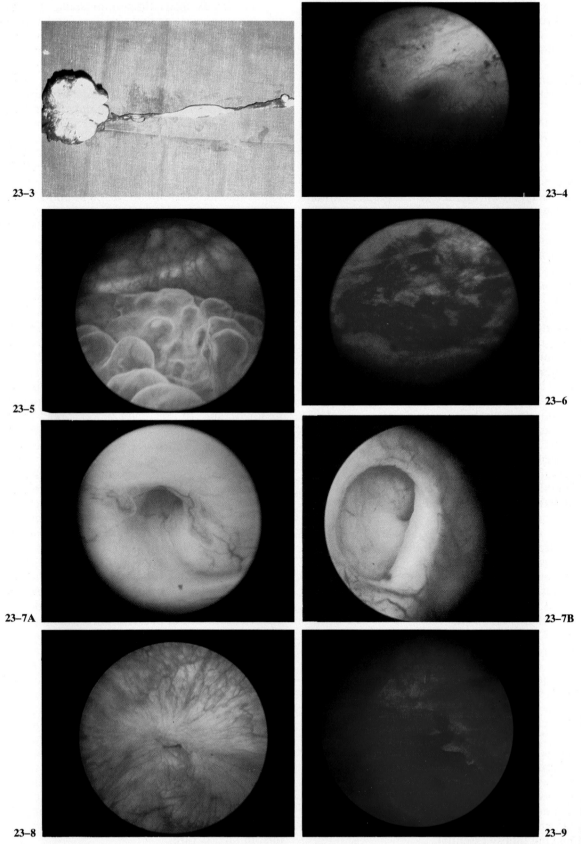

Figures 23–3 to 23–9. *See legends on opposite page.*

Lastly, the tuberculous epididymitis may be the first and only presenting symptom of genitourinary tuberculosis, as an intravenous urogram shows a normal ureter and upper urinary tract and *M. tuberculosis* cannot be isolated from the urine. The diagnosis is made by culturing *M, tuberculosis* from a discharging sinus or after epididymectomy.

As with other forms of tuberculosis, epididymitis is showing a decreasing incidence in the Western world, but is still endemic in many Third World regions. The disease usually develops in young, sexually active males, and in 70 per cent of patients there is a previous history of tuberculosis.

The usual presentation is a painful, inflamed scrotal swelling. The globus minor alone is affected in 40 per cent of cases. In extensive disease, there may be generalized epididymal induration with beading of the palpable vas and even involvement of the testis.

In earlier series (Ross et al., 1961), lesions were noted to be bilateral in 34 per cent of cases, but this is now an unusual presentation.

It should be remembered that external injury causing severe tissue damage may reactivate a dormant tuberculous focus that was previously unidentified, so that it produces a focus of the disease (Kretschmer, 1928). The presentation of tuberculous epididymitis and a history of trauma with a previous history of tuberculosis may have medicolegal importance. The writer has seen two cases of tuberculous epididymitis occurring after scrotal trauma, one 32 years and the other 35 years after tuberculosis of the spine had been treated in infancy.

The management of tuberculous epididymitis may pose problems when *M. tuberculosis bacteria* are not isolated from the urine. In the acute phase the inflammatory reaction involves the testis, so that it is difficult to differentiate the lesion from an acute epididymo-orchitis.

Occasionally, a discharging sinus may be found posteriorly. If there is no sinus and the *M. tuberculosis* organisms are absent from the urine, the disease should be observed while an appropriate antibiotic, such as co-trimoxazole, is taken. If there is no improvement after 2 to 3 weeks, antituberculous chemotherapy should be started. If after a further 3 weeks the lesion becomes nodular, firm, and painless, the testis should be explored without delay, as two cases of seminoma presenting in conjunction with tuberculosis have been reported (Gow, 1957, 1963).

Tuberculosis of the tunica vaginalis with no disease in the epididymis or testis may rarely present with the finding of multiple nodules on palpation (Kato, 1970).

MALE GENITAL TRACT

Tuberculous Prostatitis. Tuberculosis of the prostate is rare, and in many cases the diagnosis is made by the pathologist or is found incidentally after a transurethral resection. Very rarely, in acute fulminating cases, the disease spreads rapidly and cavitation may lead to a perineal sinus (Sporer and Auerback, 1978).

The route of infection is invariably the hematogenous spread of organisms in the same way as in the kidney. There is no evidence that infection is caused by continuous contact with urine from a kidney with active disease. Advanced lesions that destroy tissue may cause a reduction in the volume of semen, a sign that may help in diagnosis (Lattimer and Weschler, 1978).

On palpation, the gland is nodular, is hardly ever tender, and is rarely enlarged. Soft areas are extremely uncommon.

THE TRANSMISSION OF GENITAL TUBERCULOSIS. The transmission of genital tuberculosis from husband to wife is very rare. Lattimer and coworkers (1954) could find only eight reports

---

Figure 23–3. Extensive tuberculosis of the kidney and ureter with calcification and stricture formation.

Figure 23–4. Acutely inflamed ureteric orifice.

Figure 23–5. Tuberculous bullous granulations.

Figure 23–6. Acute tuberculous ulcer.

Figure 23–7. *A,* Tuberculous golf-hole ureter. *B,* Tuberculous golf-hole ureter, severely withdrawn.

Figure 23–8. Healed tuberculous lesion.

Figure 23–9. Acute tuberculous cystitis with ulceration.

in the literature. This is surprising, since many men with genital tuberculosis have *M. tuberculosis* in the semen. Recently, a study was made (Sutherland et al., 1982) when the husbands of 229 women with proven tuberculosis of the genital tract were examined. Sixteen had a past history of various types of tuberculosis. Urologic examination was performed on 128 husbands, and active genitourinary tuberculosis was found in 3.9 per cent. As in these cases, the diagnosis of the husband's disease may be made only after the lesion has appeared in the wife. The lesions respond rapidly to chemotherapy.

Although this form of the disease is unlikely to be seen in the Western world, it could appear in the underdeveloped countries, and a painful swollen inguinal gland in the female that is proven to be tuberculous should alert the clinician to the possible diagnosis of genital tuberculosis in the male partner.

Tuberculosis of the Penis. Tuberculosis of the penis is a very rare manifestation of the disease. Up to 1971 only 139 cases had been reported in the literature (Lal et al., 1971). Many years ago it was not uncommonly seen as a complication of ritual circumcision, when it was the usual practice for the operators, many of whom had open pulmonary tuberculosis, to suck the circumcised penis (Lewis, 1946). At the present time, tuberculosis of the penis always occurs in adults and is primary or secondary, depending on the presence or absence of coincidental pulmonary tuberculosis.

Primary tuberculosis occurs with coital contact from disease already present in the female genital tract or from contamination from infected clothing (Narayana et al., 1976; Agarwalla et al., 1980). In rare incidences the penile lesion may be caused by reinoculation from the male partner through an infected ejaculate. Secondary penile tuberculosis occurs as a secondary manifestation from active pulmonary tuberculosis.

In all cases the lesion presents as a superficial ulcer of the glans, which clinically is indistinguishable from malignant disease, although it can also progress to cause a tubercular cavernositis with involvement of the urethra (Veukataramaiah et al., 1982). The diagnosis is confirmed by biopsy. All lesions rapidly respond to antituberculous chemotherapy.

Tuberculosis of the Urethra. Tuberculosis of the urethra is very rare. Symes and Blandy (1973) quoted only 16 cases previously reported in the literature. It is caused by the spread from another focus in the genital tract; its rarity is difficult to understand, in view of the almost constant exposure of the urethra to infected urine. The presentation can be either acute or chronic. In the acute phase there is a urethral discharge with involvement of the epididymis, prostate, and other parts of the renal tract, so the diagnosis is not difficult because organisms will always be isolated. The initial treatment is intensive chemotherapy.

In the chronic condition the diagnosis is more difficult, as the disease presents as urethral obstruction. The disease may be quiescent, but there will invariably be a history of tuberculosis, even though it may have occurred many years previously. The management of this type of stricture is the same as for any other urethral stricture, but a course of antituberculous treatment should be given to cover the surgery to guard against the reactivation of a latent focus, which might be present in the dense fibrous tissue. Internal urethrotomy has yet to be evaluated, but it should have some place in the initial management of chronic tuberculous urethral strictures.

CLINICAL FEATURES

TUBERCULOSIS IN THE WESTERN WORLD

As the patient will usually present with rather vague urinary tract symptoms, a careful history is important. This may not be easy, since the memory for details is often confused and the length of illness uncertain. Furthermore, urologists are at a disadvantage in that they rarely see more than one or two cases a year, so that the diagnosis does not readily come to mind. Once the disease has been considered, a family history is important, not only for close members of the family but also for any other probable contacts. A history of previous tuberculosis in the patient may also be significant, as he may have had some form of the disease many years previously. When the diagnosis is made, all members of the family, including grandchildren, as well as frequent visitors and contacts should be examined. It must be stressed that urologists should always be aware of the diagnosis in a patient presenting with vague, longstanding urinary symptoms for which there is no obvious cause. When the patient is told of the diagnosis, he immediately realizes that he has not been well for some time.

TUBERCULOSIS IN IMMIGRANTS

The incidence of tuberculosis is much higher in immigrants than in the native population. In Great Britain the notification rate of nonpulmonary tuberculosis has been 70 to 80 times higher in immigrants from India than in the native white population (Innes, 1981). This is probably due to a more virulent strain of *M. tuberculosis* and the lower host resistance. It has been shown that the longer an immigrant lives in Great Britain before he develops the disease, the more apt the disease is to be like the pattern of the country of his adoption (Davies, 1980). Tuberculosis in immigrants is much more a disease of the young, but only 4 per cent is genitourinary (Davies, 1980).

TUBERCULOSIS IN THE DEVELOPING COUNTRIES

Tuberculosis in the developing countries is a much more acute disease and largely affects the younger age group and children. Because of poor socioeconomic conditions and lack of control, the disease is prevalent and the risk of infection serious. The genitourinary manifestation is becoming more widespread; in a recent survey in India, 20 per cent of patients with pulmonary disease also had genitourinary lesions, many of which required surgical treatment.

SYMPTOMS AND SIGNS

The symptoms and signs of genitourinary tuberculosis vary in both intensity and duration. The age and sex incidence had remained unchanged over many years, males predominating over females in the ratio of 2 to 1. Most patients were in the age group 20 to 40 years, but during the last few years, as in the pulmonary disease, there has been a notable increase in the numbers between the ages of 45 and 55 and over 70 years.

The patient usually complains of increasing painless frequency of micturition, at first during the night but later by both day and night, that has not responded to the usual antibiotic treatment. Urgency is uncommon, unless there is extensive bladder involvement. The urine is normally sterile and usually contains more than 20 pus cells per high-power field. However, in the author's series, 20 per cent of patients did not have any abnormal pus cells in the urine. A superimposed infection is found in 20 per cent of cases, 90 per cent of which are due to *E. coli*. The symptoms are commonly intermittent and have been present for some time before the patient seeks medical advice. However, he is invariably vague as to the precise time the symptoms actually started.

Hematuria, which is almost without exception total and intermittent, is present in only 10 per cent of cases but microscopic hematuria should not be ignored. Renal and suprapubic pain is a rare presenting symptom and usually means extensive involvement of the kidney and the bladder. Suprapubic pain is always accompanied by severe frequency. Ureteric colic is uncommon and occurs only when either a small flake of calcification or a clot passes down the ureter.

Hemospermia was noted in only 4 cases in the writer's series and is a rare presenting symptom (Gow, 1976). However, Yu and coworkers (1977) reported an 11 per cent incidence in 65 tuberculosis patients reviewed over a period of 10 years. All these patients had other clinical evidence of genitourinary tuberculosis. Tuberculosis should always be excluded in patients who are seen with repeated attacks of hemospermia as the only presenting symptom, even though there is no other evidence of genitourinary tuberculosis.

Recurrent cystitis is also a warning sign, and an *E. coli* infection that responds to antibiotics but recurs repeatedly should alert the urologist, because in these cases tuberculosis must be excluded. If the disease is not confirmed and the symptoms persist or recur, investigation should be carried out repeatedly, as *M. tuberculosis* is notoriously difficult to isolate from the urine when there are only small lesions.

The only first presenting symptom in a few patients is a painful testicular swelling. It is often difficult to differentiate between tuberculosis and nonspecific epididymo-orchitis in the absence of any radiologic changes and a cutaneous sinus, so early-morning specimens of urine should be examined.

Rarely, the diagnosis is an incidental finding and is made following the transurethral resection of the prostate, when the pathologist reports foci of tuberculosis. There may or may not be evidence of disease elsewhere in the urinary tract, but all these patients require the full course of antituberculous chemotherapy.

The classic triad of lassitude, loss of weight, and anorexia is never seen in the early stages of the disease.

Lastly, it is important to emphasize that the presenting symptoms may be minimal and that this in no way reflects the true nature of the disease, since even with very few symptoms the disease can be advanced and of long standing.

TUBERCULOSIS IN CHILDREN

Genitourinary tuberculosis has always been one of the most uncommon manifestations of the disease in children. There are two possible reasons. First, the incidence of renal complication is small in relation to the number of children with primary infection. Second, the symptoms of renal tuberculosis do not appear for some years after the primary infection, and this period varies from 3 to more than 10 years (Ustvedt, 1947). In view of this, it is very unlikely that the disease will be seen until the age of 10 years or more.

The clinical presentation varies. Some children will have other forms of tuberculous lesions, others will present with frequency of micturition and occasional hematuria, and another group will present with painful swelling of the epididymis. In children, pyuria is almost a constant finding and red cells are frequently found, but the culture for nonspecific organisms is invariably sterile.

The treatment is the same course of chemotherapy as is given to adults, with a reduced dose, according to the age of the child.

INVESTIGATIONS

TUBERCULIN TEST

The tuberculin test is carried out by intradermal injection of a protein-purified derivative of tuberculin. When it is injected, an inflammatory reaction develops at the site and reaches a maximum between 48 and 72 hours. This reaction consists of a central indurated zone surrounded by an area of inflammation; it is assessed by measuring the diameter of the indurated area. The response is cell-mediated through the T-lymphocyte mediator. The problem is to interpret the results accurately, as any expression of sensitivity is an individual peculiarity, which depends on the person's ability to respond to the local concentration of the injection at that particular time. Such a response may also be modified by malignancy, deficiency states such as iron or vitamin C deficiencies, steroids, irradiation, and liver diseases. However, an indurated area over 10 mm in diameter is considered a positive reaction. Positive tests must also be interpreted with caution, as nonspecific reactions do occur, probably owing either to mycobacteria other than *M. tuberculosis* or to a previous injection with BCG. Positive reactions are considered to be an indication that the person has been infected, provided that he has not been vaccinated with BCG, but cannot be regarded as an indication of active tuberculous disease or that the symptoms are caused by tuberculosis. *M. tuberculosis* infection is far more common than tuberculous disease.

Nevertheless, areas of 5 mm or less suggest little or no mycobacterial activity because of the high degree of acquired immunity, whereas reactions greater than 15 mm in diameter indicate a high degree of hypersensitivity, which probably reflects active disease (Youmans, 1975).

A positive test is of more help when it is known that a previous test was negative, since in that case the infection may be recent and is likely to produce a lesion that requires treatment.

URINE EXAMINATION

The urine is examined for red cells and pus cells, and its pH and concentration are noted. It is also cultured for nonspecific organisms that are tested for antibiotic sensitivities. Secondary bacterial infection is not common with tuberculosis and is found in only about 20 per cent of cases. The usual organism is *E. coli*. At least three, but preferably five, consecutive early-morning specimens of urine should be cultured, each onto two slopes; a plain Löwenstein-Jensen to isolate *M. tuberculosis,* BCG, and the occasional nontuberculous mycobacteria; and a pyruvic egg medium containing penicillin to catch the *M. bovis*.

Improvements in technique have allowed laboratories to dispense with routine guinea-pig inoculations; in a series of 200 urinary specimens 14 out of 41 specimens of urine were positive on culture when the animal inoculations were negative, whereas only 1 specimen was positive on animal inoculation when the culture was negative. The important technical advances appear to be the use of sulfuric acid to control contamination and also the variety of media (Marks, 1972). There is now very little place for animal inoculation in isolating the mycobacterium.

Each specimen of urine should be inoculated as soon as possible after collection, since the longer the urine remains in contact with organisms the less likely it is that the mycobacterium will grow (Bjornesjo, 1956). Infections will be missed if specimens are collected and then pooled for culture studies.

Sensitivity tests should always be carried out when the cultures are positive, in order that the most effective course of chemotherapy can be started. Sensitivity tests should be performed on streptomycin, isoniazid, pyrazinamide, ethambutol, and rifampicin. It is very unusual to find an organism that is resistant to these antibiotics. Most secondary infections will be controlled by a combination of streptomycin and rifampicin, and therefore no other specific treatment need be started unless the organisms are still present 2 weeks after commencement of the antituberculous course.

BLOOD

A full blood count erythrosedimentation rate (ESR), and urea and electrolyte values should be carried out in every case. In addition, if calcification is present, a complete biochemical assessment of calcium metabolism is performed. If the ESR is elevated, it should be measured at monthly intervals, as it gives some indication of response to treatment.

RADIOGRAPHY

Plain X-Ray. Straight x-ray of the urinary tract is important, as it may show calcification in the renal areas and in the lower genitourinary tract. Tuberculous ureteric calcification is not common unless there is extensive renal calcification. Nevertheless, it must be distinguished from that seen in bilharziasis. In the former, all calcification is intraluminal and appears as a cast of the ureter, which is thickened and not dilated (Hartman et al., 1977). In schistosomiasis the calcification is mural, and the ureter is generally dilated and tortuous.

Calcification rarely occurs in the bladder wall and seminal vesicles. A calcified psoas abscess can simulate renal calcification, and an intravenous urogram should be carried out if there is any doubt of the diagnosis.

Plain x-ray of the chest and spine is also carried out to exclude any evidence of old or active pulmonary or spinal disease.

Intravenous Urography. The introduction of the high-dose intravenous urogram has been a big advance in the investigation of renal tract pathology and has made retrograde pyelography a largely unnecessary, or a very infrequent, investigation in genitourinary tuberculosis. Tomography may be combined with an intravenous urogram if more precise information is required. In addition, image-intensified endoscopy allows dynamic study of the diseased ureter, particularly at the pelviureteric junction. This functional information relating to ureteral peristalsis is an established part of the investigation of ureteric pathology, as it gives an indication of the extent of the disease, the peristaltic activity, the amount of fibrosis that is present, and the length of a stricture, particularly at the ureterovesical junction.

The renal lesion may appear as a distortion of a calyx (Fig. 23–10), as a calyx that is fibrosed and completely occluded (the lost calyx [Sherwood, 1980], Fig. 23–11), as multiple small calyceal deformities (Fig. 23–12), or as severe calyceal and parenchymal destruction (Fig. 23–13).

Calcification may be present. It is always associated with a calyceal lesion and can be minimal or extensive. Occasionally, one (Fig. 23–14) or, very rarely, both (Fig. 23–15) moieties of a duplex kidney are involved.

A nonfunctioning or extensively diseased kidney indicates irreversible tuberculous disease. Tuberculous ureteritis is manifested by dilatation above a ureterovesical stricture or, if the disease is more advanced, by a rigid fibrotic ureter with multiple strictures.

The cystographic phase of the intravenous urogram can give valuable information about

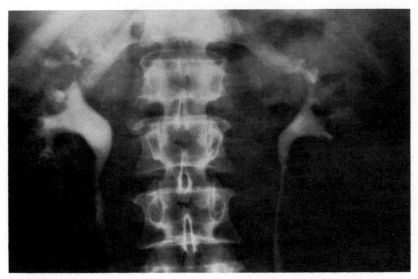

Figure 23–10. Distortion of the right upper pole calyx, with the typical stellate appearance.

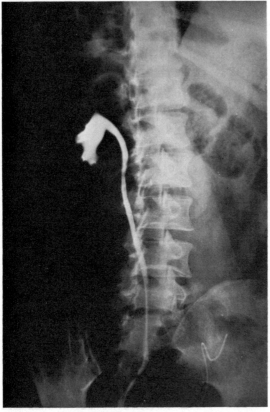

Figure 23–11. Occluded calyx.

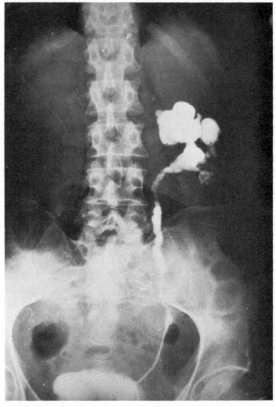

Figure 23–13. Severe calyceal and parenchymal destruction.

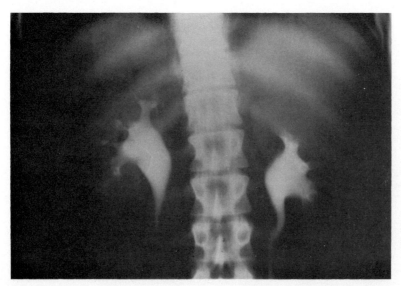

Figure 23–12. Multiple calyceal deformities.

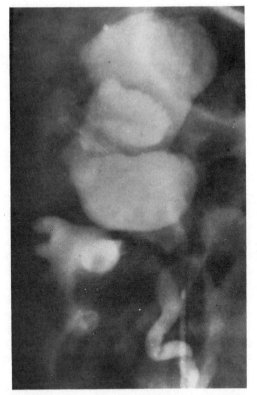

Figure 23–14. Involvement of one moiety of duplex kidney.

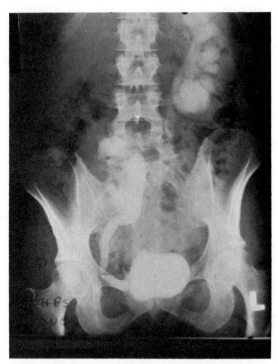

Figure 23–16. Contracted irregular bladder, with diseased left and right kidney, the right being ectopic. Note stricture at the lower end of the right ureter.

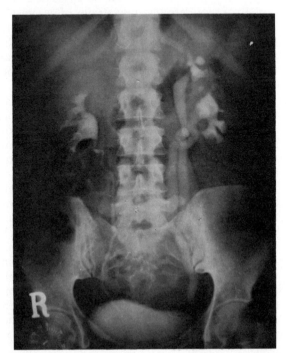

Figure 23–15. Involvement of both moieties of duplex kidney. Note also the stricture at the lower end of the ureter.

the condition of the bladder, which may be small and contracted (the thimble bladder [Fig. 23–16]); or irregular, with filling defects and bladder asymmetry.

Retrograde Pyelography. As said previously, retrograde pyelography is now a rare investigation. There are two indications for its use. The first is a stricture at the lower end of the ureter, where it is necessary to try to delineate (a) the length of the stricture, and (b) the amount of obstruction and dilatation above the stricture. The examination is performed under direct vision, using an image intensifier. The contrast agent should be introduced through a bulb-ended catheter, Braasch or Chevassu, the tip of which is inserted into the ureteric orifice. As in intravenous urography, it is important to combine a dynamic study with the examination, so that ureteric function can be assessed.

The second indication is ureteric catheterization, which may be required to obtain urine samples for culture from each kidney when it is not certain from which side the organisms are coming. In such cases a No. 7 French catheter is passed into the renal pelvis. To increase the output of urine, 40 mg of furosemide is given half an hour before the cystoscopy or, alternatively, 20 gm of mannitol is infused intravenously during the examination.

Percutaneous Antegrade Pyelography. This investigation is becoming more important as an alternative to retrograde ureterography in the case of a large kidney. It is particularly useful in visualizing a nonfunctioning.kidney or in determining the condition of all excretory pathways above an obstruction. It can also be used to aspirate the contents of the renal pelvis so that they can be sent for diagnostic examination. This technique can be used as well for aspirating the contents of tuberculous cavities, which can be sent for estimation of the quantity of drugs that has penetrated the walls. Sometimes chemotherapeutic agents can be inoculated into the cavity.

Arteriography. This invasive radiologic investigation is of limited value and should never be considered as a method of routine evaluation in a patient with genitourinary tuberculosis. Occasionally, it may be used for assessing the amount of renal parenchymal damage or for delineating arterial circulation when partial nephrectomy is being planned. It will also mark the precise area of destruction of a kidney, which is often more extensive than would be suggested by intravenous urography. It has one important application when there is a possibility of coincidental renal tumor with tuberculosis. The writer has now seen five such cases.

Radioisotope Investigation. Renal scanning affords information of functional renal tissue and parenchymal abnormalities. It gives details regarding the extent of the disease. However, renal tuberculosis is well seen on intravenous urography, and it is doubtful whether radioisotope investigation would add anything to this investigation. It may be useful, however, in assessing the response to treatment and the eventual optimal renal function.

Cystoscopy. Endoscopy has little importance in making the diagnosis of genitourinary tuberculosis. It has some place, however, in assessing the extent of the disease or the response to chemotherapy.

It must always be carried out under general anaesthesia with a muscle relaxant to reduce the risk of hemorrhage. The phase of bladder filling should be performed under direct vision.

Bladder Biopsy. Bladder biopsy is contraindicated in the presence of acute tuberculous cystitis or even when there are areas of inflammation, either in the bladder or close to the ureteric orifice, that are suspicious of tuberculosis. The writer has never seen a case in which a biopsy was positive for tuberculosis when the urine has been sterile. Biopsy is acceptable only in cases in which tubercles, or an ulcer some distance from a normal ureteric orifice, are present because, when such lesions are seen, a diagnosis of carcinoma must be excluded.

MANAGEMENT

Western World. No longer is it necessary to treat patients in the hospital, except in special circumstances, such as when the disease is extensive, the symptoms severe, and the home environment totally inadequate for the care of the patient. In Third World countries, however, it is usually essential to admit the patients to ensure that the drugs are taken consistently. Patients are seen weekly as outpatients, liver function assessment is carried out, and the urine is inspected to note the color, which will be brown if the rifampicin is being taken regularly. If surgery is required, it is scheduled as a planned procedure and the patient is admitted 6 weeks after the start of the intensive course of treatment.

The urologist should supervise the chemotherapy and not abdicate his responsibilities by allowing the drug regimens to be dictated by colleagues in other medical disciplines. Certainly, any problems should be discussed, especially if there are resistant strains of organism, but the urologist should always be responsible for the overall management of the patient. Otherwise, irreversible severe damage to the renal tract may occur, and kidneys may even be destroyed.

The aim should be to treat the active disease, to make the patient noninfectious as soon as possible, to preserve the maximal amount of renal tissue, and to provide every member of the community with the best available treatment.

Developing Countries. The situation in these areas is very different. Living conditions are poor, tuberculous infection is everywhere, malnutrition is common, and other diseases such as malaria, gastroenteritis, and worm infestation are indigenous, so that the resistance to an infection with *M. tuberculosis* is low. Although pulmonary tuberculosis is the most common type, genitourinary tuberculosis is being seen more and more in an acute form, so that the physician should always be aware of this diagnosis.

Management of the disease will depend on the resources and facilities of the region involved, but hospital admission for surgical treatment will be necessary for a high proportion of patients with genitourinary tuberculosis.

Antituberculous Drugs

Antituberculous drugs are divided into three groups: primary agents, secondary agents, and minor agents (Table 23–3).

PRIMARY AGENTS

Isoniazid. Isoniazid (isonicotinic acid hydrazide) was discovered in 1952. It is highly active against *M. tuberculosis*, inhibiting most strains in a concentration of 0.05 to 0.2 μg per ml. The precise action is unknown. It has been postulated that it interferes with the biosynthesis of nucleic acids (Wimpenny, 1967). It also inhibits the synthesis of mycolic acids in *M. tuberculosis* by affecting the enzyme mycolase synthetase, which is unique to *Mycobacterium*. The inhibiting concentration against this enzyme is low and is comparable to the M.I.C. (minimum inhibitory concentration) of the drug against *M. tuberculosis* (Kucers, 1979).

Some unchanged isoniazid is excreted by the kidneys, but most of it is in the inactive form of acetyl-isoniazid. Nevertheless, 70 per cent of all administered isoniazid is excreted by the kidneys (Mitchell et al., 1976). It is widely distributed in the body, and body tissue levels similar to serum levels are obtained. It readily penetrates caseous material and does enter macrophages (Bennett et al., 1977). There is no cross resistance with rifampicin.

Rifampicin. Rifampicin is one of a group of antibiotics that is isolated from *Streptomyces mediterranei*. It is highly active against *M. tuberculosis,* and its MIC is 0.20 μg per ml. Rifampicin acts by inhibiting bacterial RNA synthesis, as it interferes with DNA-directed RNA polymerase of sensitive bacteria (Hartmann et al., 1967).

Rifampicin is lipid-soluble and so enters macrophages. It is excreted in the urine; with a 600-mg oral dose, peak concentrations of 100 μg per ml are reached in the urine after 8 hours, and a lethal concentration is detectable for 36 hours (Kunin et al., 1969).

Streptomycin. Streptomycin was isolated from *Streptomyces griseus* in 1944. It belongs to a group of antibiotics known as the aminoglycosides. The usual MIC for *M. tuberculosis* is 8 μg per ml. Like other aminoglycosides, it interferes with bacterial protein synthesis by its ability to bind to a particular protein or proteins of the 30 S unit of bacterial ribosomes, so that faulty proteins are produced (Luzzatto et al., 1968). It penetrates the walls of tuberculous abscesses in lethal concentrations even in caseous material (Fellander et al., 1952). It also rapidly diffuses into body tissues and is excreted by glomerular filtration. High concentrations are obtained in the urine, 200 to 400 μg per ml after a 1-gm intramuscular injection, and for a period of 24 hours after injection the MIC of 8 μg per ml is retained.

Pyrazinamide. Pyrazinamide, a derivative of nicotinamide, was synthesized in 1952 and was shown to possess some activity against *M. tuberculosis*, especially in an acid medium. Its usual MIC is 20 μg per ml, but this is found only if the drug is tested in an acid medium with a pH of 5.5. The precise mechanism of action of pyrazinamide is unknown. Its metabolized pyrozinoic acid may be involved in the activity of pyrazinamide and its activity is enhanced in an environment with a pH of less than 5.5. It is excreted in the urine and urine concentration reaches a peak in 2 hours and then falls exponentially for 48 hours. Its half-life is 9 hours (Elland, 1969), but the lethal concentration is retained in the urine after a single dose of 1 g for a period of up to 36 hours.

SECONDARY AGENTS

Ethambutol. Ethambutol was discovered in 1961 and was found to have a high degree of antituberculous activity. Minimum inhibitory concentrations are between 1 and 2 μg per ml and rarely are higher than 5 μg per ml.

Ethambutol is active against *M. tuberculosis* strains resistant to isoniazid and other commonly used antituberculous drugs. It is well

TABLE 23–3. CLASSIFICATION OF ANTITUBERCULOUS DRUGS

Classification	Agent	Activity
Primary agents	Rifampicin Isoniazid Pyrazinamide Streptomycin	Bacteriocidal
Secondary agents	Ethambutol Ethionamide Cycloserine Viomycin	Bacteriostatic
Minor agents	Kanamycin Thiocetazone	Bacteriostatic

absorbed after oral administration, with a normal dose of 25 mg per kg of body weight. The peak serum level of about 5 μg per ml is reached in approximately 4 hours. About 80 per cent is excreted in the urine as active unchanged drug, and this excretion occurs within 24 hours of administration. High concentrations of active drug are obtained in the urine.

MODE OF ACTION. Ethambutol appears to enter the cells of *M. tuberculosis*. Its precise mechanism is not known, but it is probable that it inhibits *mycobacteria* synthesis. It exerts its maximal inhibitory effect against *mycobacteria* at a neutral pH. The other secondary and minor agents, kanamycin and thiocetazone, are now very rarely used.

Chemotherapy

For the last three decades it was considered almost a heresy to suggest that treatment should be less than 18 to 24 months, as the results had been so good—achieving almost the 100 per cent success in some centers that were able to impose exemplary control on the patients. To think of anything less was to invite relapses and the emergence of resistant strains of the organism.

During this time, though, discerning physicians, who realized the difficulties of long courses of treatment both to the patient and to the supervising staff, were attempting shorter regimens, but all failed. However, with the discovery in 1966 of rifampicin, a drug as potent against *M. tuberculosis* as isoniazid, the scene changed. Shorter courses of treatment became much more likely to succeed and to be a distinct possibility for routine treatment, as two powerful fully bacteriocidal drugs had become available.

Since the early 1970's, considerable research into short-course treatment has been conducted. All of this is in the pulmonary disease, but nevertheless it is equally relevant to the genitourinary manifestation.

To appreciate the reasoning for adopting short-course treatment it is necessary to understand the mechanisms of drug action and to study the thousands of patients who have been treated by various combinations during the last 10 years.

Mechanism of Drug Action. The mechanisms of short-course chemotherapy have been based largely on the experimental work on mice at the Pasteur Institute, the work of Professor Mitchison's Unit, and a large number of cooperative clinical trials in many countries. Each of these trials was designed to compare the effectiveness of short-course regimens and, in addition, to assess the contribution of individual drugs (Fox, 1980).

Grosset (1978) summarized the mouse experiments.

1. Pyrazinamide and rifampicin are very potent sterilizing drugs in experimentally infected mice.

2. The most important sterilizing combinations are isoniazid plus pyrazinamide and isoniazid plus rifampicin.

3. Adding streptomycin or ethambutol makes little or no contribution to the sterilizing capacity of the two foregoing combinations.

Following experimental and clinical work, Mitchison (1980) suggested that there were four bacterial populations (Fig. 23–17). The first is a population of rapidly dividing bacilli, which are killed by all the bacteriocidal drugs. The second is the intermittent metabolizers, which metabolize for periods of little more than a few hours. These are killed by rifampicin, because of the speed with which its bacteriocidal action starts, whereas they would not be affected by other drugs, especially isoniazid, as there is a lag period of 1 day before the drug begins to exert its bacteriocidal effect (Dickinson and Mitchison, 1981). The third group are those in the acid environment of macrophages. These are destroyed by pyrazinamide, whose activity is greatly enhanced in an acid medium. The last group are the completely dormant organisms, which are not affected by any of the antituberculous drugs and are not likely to cause any disease.

As a result of this hypothesis, various drug combinations have been studied, and it was shown that combinations with isoniazid have the highest bacterial activity (Jindani et al., 1980). Isoniazid is therefore the key bacteriocidal drug, with rifampicin and pyrazinamide having definitive sterilizing roles on special populations.

The re-emergence of pyrazinamide as a vital drug is particularly gratifying since in the 1950's it was relegated to the second line because of its toxicity, which was due to the administration of unnecessarily high doses. It is a drug that has little value in preventing drug resistance but that is an essential part of sterilizing regimens.

Streptomycin is often added to make a quadruple combination, especially for the initial 2 months of intensive therapy. It is uncertain whether or not it is necessary, especially in drug-sensitive infection. However, it should still be

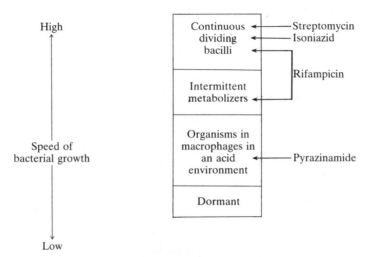

Figure 23–17. Different bacterial populations within the lesions in man. (Modified from Mitchison, D. A.: J. R. Coll. Physicians, *14*:91, 1980.)

used in severe cases until more definitive evidence is available.

Choice of Drug Regimens for Drug-Sensitive Infections. The British Thoracic Association (1980) showed unequivocally that for regimens that did not contain pyrazinamide there was a definite superiority for the 9-month over the 6-month duration. There is now, however, abundant evidence that there are many effective 6-month regimens, all of which have in common the initial use of rifampicin, isoniazid, and pyrazinamide. Combining trials in East Africa, Singapore, and the Second British Association Study, 422 patients have been treated for 6 months and only 4 (1 per cent) have relapsed bacteriologically (Fox, 1981). All these patients received daily streptomycin, isoniazid, rifampicin, and pyrazinamide for the first 2 months, followed either by isoniazid, rifampicin, and pyrazinamide, or by isoniazid and rifampicin for an additional 4 months. A further trial in Hong Kong (Hong Kong/B.M.R.C., 1981) showed that streptomycin, isoniazid, rifampicin, and pyrazinamide given three times a week for 6 months was just as effective, as there was only 1 per cent bacteriologic relapse.

Effectiveness of Regimens Shorter than 6 Months. There is now growing evidence that regimens shorter than 6 months may be equally effective. Mehrotra (1981) showed that only 1 per cent of patients treated with streptomycin, isoniazid, rifampicin, and pyrazinamide daily for 3 months, followed by rifampicin and isoniazid daily for 6 weeks, relapsed bacteriologically. This may have wide implications for Third World countries.

Regimens for Smear-Negative but Cul-ture-Positive Disease. This group is particularly important for patients suffering genitourinary manifestations, as the majority are in this category. The results of two studies in Hong Kong (Girling, 1981; Chen, 1981) are significant. It was quite definite that neither 2- nor 3-month courses were adequate; it is also doubtful whether 4 months would be sufficient, although patients given streptomycin, isoniazid, rifampicin, and pyrazinamide three times a week for 4 months did not show any relapses up to 8 months after cessation of treatment. Nevertheless, a longer period of review is necessary before a definite opinion can be given. Six months of treatment with the same four drugs given three times a week did not produce any bacteriologic relapses.

From these studies the evidence is that, for the treatment for pulmonary tuberculosis, rifampicin, isoniazid, and pyrazinamide with or without streptomycin are the drugs of choice for the initial intensive treatment period, followed by rifampicin and isoniazid either continuously three times a week or twice a week, with the whole course to last 6 months. There is no place for ethambutol or other bacteriostatic drugs in the initial treatment of sensitive organisms.

In Third World countries this ideal may have to be relaxed and a lower success rate accepted. Supervision and attendance are more difficult, cost is a major factor, social and cultural traditions play an important part, and more patients are likely to abscond. Despite the cost, rifampicin should be included in all regimens, as the length of the course can be kept to a minimum; even if the patients do fail to keep appointments, there is a greater chance of successful treatment, and a consequent reduction of the rate of infection.

How do the Results of these Extensive Investigations Affect the Genitourinary Manifestations? There are certain aspects of the genitourinary disease that make it likely to respond better to short-course chemotherapy. In the first place, there are far fewer organisms in renal than in pulmonary disease, and these are discharged into the urine intermittently. Second, there are high concentrations of isoniazid, rifampicin, pyrazinamide, and streptomycin in the urine. Third, isoniazid and rifampicin pass freely into renal cavities in high concentration. Lastly, all the drugs reach an adequate concentration in kidney, ureters, bladder, and prostate. The two recommended alternative regimens for genitourinary tuberculosis are shown in Figure 23–18.

As has been stated, the value of streptomycin in the initial phase is still undecided; it is suggested, however, that it be given for cases of extensive disease with severe symptoms, as it has such a high concentration in the urine. The continuation phase is given three times a week for 2 months, but future evidence may confirm that it is just as successful when given twice a week. The course should finish after 4 months, as all but 1 per cent or less will be cured. The writer has had only one relapse in 140 patients treated with short-course regimens.

Pyrazinamide 25 mg/kg body wt./day maximum dose 2 gm daily	
Isoniazid 300 mg daily	600 mg 3 times a week
Rifampicin 450 mg daily	900 mg 3 times a week
2 months	2 months

Streptomycin 1 gm daily	
Isoniazid 300 mg daily	
Rifampicin 450 mg daily	Isoniazid 600 mg 3 times a week
Pyrazinamide 25 mg/kg body wt./day maximum dose 2 gm daily	Rifampicin 900 mg 3 times a week
2 months	2 months

Figure 23–18. Alternative regimens for treatment of genitourinary tuberculosis.

It is far better to treat the very rare relapse when it occurs than to needlessly treat all the others, because recurrent organisms almost invariably remain sensitive to the four first-line drugs.

The only exceptions to this regime of treatment are, first, patients who are undergoing renal transplantation when there is a previous history of any form of tuberculosis. These patients should receive rifampicin, 900 mg, and isoniazid, 600 mg, three times a week for 1 year or longer, as with the immunosuppressive drugs there is always the danger of reactivation of dormant bacilli. The second exception is patients who are receiving hemodialysis for end-stage renal tuberculosis. In these patients, rifampicin and isoniazid can be given in the normal dose, as they are largely metabolized in the liver and the part that remains unchanged is removed by the dialysate on the days of dialysis. The drugs should be given immediately after the dialysis is finished. Streptomycin is removed by dialysis, but because of its ototoxicity it is recommended that daily blood concentration should be estimated to ensure that the peak serum levels do not rise above 20 μg per ml.

There are very few published data on patients undergoing dialysis who are also receiving pyrazinamide therapy. However, as this drug is largely metabolized in the liver, it should not be withdrawn from routine chemotherapy regimens, provided the liver function tests are carefully monitored.

Use of Steroids. Another approach to shortening the duration of chemotherapy was suggested by Tripathy (1978). He attempted to reduce the host resistance by means of steroids, so that the bacilli would become more vulnerable to the action of the antituberculous drugs. However, after a 6-week course of prednisolone there was no evidence that the steroids influenced the sterilizing activity of regimens that included isoniazid, rifampicin, and pyrazinamide. Steroids, however, may be useful in cases of acute tuberculous cystitis. At least 20 mg t.d.s. of prednisolone given with the four antituberculous drugs for 4 weeks helps to alleviate the severe bladder symptoms and allows an earlier appraisal of the subsequent management. This high dose of prednisolone is required, as rifampicin reduces the effectiveness and bioavailability of prednisolone. McAllister and co-workers (1983) showed that when rifampicin is given with prednisolone, the amount of drug available to the tissues was reduced by 66 per cent.

TOXICITY

ANTITUBERCULOUS DRUGS

Antituberculous drugs do not often cause serious problems, but when they do, it is usually in the first few weeks of treatment. As soon as toxic reactions occur, however, they must be rapidly and efficiently managed; otherwise, there is the risk that the patient's treatment may be jeopardized and recovery prolonged.

The two main reactions are hypersensitivity to the antituberculous drugs and jaundice.

Hypersensitivity. Although all the antituberculous drugs can produce hypersensitivity reactions, streptomycin, rifampicin, thiocetazone, and para-aminosalicylic acid are most commonly involved. As the latter two are rarely used, the first two are the only ones of any significance.

The clinical manifestations are a macular rash, which is irritable and accompanied by pyrexia. More general reactions may occur, including periorbital swellings, conjunctivitis, aching limbs, generalized lymphadenopathy, and even, very rarely, Stevens-Johnson syndrome (British Medical Research Council, 1973).

MANAGEMENT. The minor reactions can be treated by antihistamines and do not require alteration in the course of treatment. If the reaction is severe, all the drugs should be stopped until the symptoms have subsided. Once the patient has recovered, the management should be (1) identification of the drug responsible for the reaction, and (2) resumption of adequate chemotherapy as soon as possible.

To identify the drug, each should be challenged in turn, first using the drugs that are least likely to cause reactions, so that effective treatment can be continued. The challenging doses are outlined in Table 23–4 (Girling, 1982).

TABLE 23–4. CHALLENGE DOSES FOR DETECTING HYPERSENSITIVITY TO ANTITUBERCULOUS DRUGS

	Challenging Dose	
Drug	DAY 1	DAY 2
Isoniazid	50 mg	300 mg
Rifampicin	75 mg	300 mg
Pyrazinamide	250 mg	1000 mg
Ethionamide	125 mg	375 mg
Cycloserine	125 mg	250 mg
Ethambutol	100 mg	500 mg
Streptomycin	125 mg	500 mg

Adapted from Girling, D. J.: Drugs, *23*:56, 1982.

Desensitization can be carried out rapidly using a dose equal to or less than the first challenging dose, if necessary under steroid cover, but it should always be performed under the shield of three antituberculous drugs to which the patient is not hypersensitive.

Hepatotoxicity. It is important to appreciate that transient increases in liver enzyme concentrations occur during the early weeks of treatment with any antituberculous drugs and that they are not significant, since they soon return to normal (Baron, 1974). They must be distinguished, however, from clinical hepatitis, which occurs in less than 1 per cent of patients.

Combinations of antituberculous drugs, especially those including pyrazinamide, were at first considered potentially toxic and were more likely to produce jaundice because all the drugs were metabolized in the liver. Furthermore, pyrazinamide had gained a reputation for being hepatotoxic because when it was first used it was given in very high doses, and it is known that hepatitis is dose-related (McLeod et al., 1959). When it is used in combinations in dosage of less than 35 mg per kg of body weight daily, no unacceptable hepatotoxicity has been experienced. This evidence is based on the treatment of thousands of patients in many countries (Fox, 1978).

MANAGEMENT. When jaundice and associated symptoms occur, all drugs should be stopped. If the jaundice is due to the drugs, recovery is usually rapid, and when it is complete, treatment with the same regimen can usually be restarted. However, liver function should be carefully monitored until the course is finished, and it may be wise to recommence treatment initially three times a week for 3 or 4 weeks.

Other Reactions. Other reactions to the drugs may occur infrequently. Isoniazid may cause urticarial rash and neurologic disturbances, which can be controlled by pyridoxine, 20 mg daily; it is a wise precaution to give this drug if the daily dose of isoniazid exceeds 900 mg.

Rifampicin can give rise to gastrointestinal disturbances, to thrombocytopenic purpura and the "flu syndrome," and, very rarely, to acute renal failure.

Pyrazinamide can cause nausea, anorexia, and arthralgia. Streptomycin is ototoxic, which is reversible if the drug is withdrawn immediately upon appearance of symptoms.

Ethambutol can cause retrobulbar neuritis and should be stopped if ocular changes occur.

This reaction is always dose-related, so this drug must be carefully regulated. All these symptoms disappear when the drug is immediately discontinued.

Rifampicin and the Contraceptive Pill. Rifampicin can cause the failure of oral contraceptive steroid therapy owing to changes in the kinetics of the estrogen component, which causes a rapid breakdown so that the levels fall below the concentration required for contraception. It may also cause disturbing menstrual disorders. Reimers and associates (1974) reported five pregnancies in 88 women on oral contraception who were being treated for tuberculosis with rifampicin. In this same group of 88, 68 had some menstrual changes. Efforts have been made to overcome this reaction with rifampicin by increasing the dose of estrogens, but the results have been too unpredictable owing to the individual variation of patients' responses. Some responses show a fivefold shorter half-life, whereas others may be only 1.5 to 2. It is suggested that female patients in the childbearing years adopt some other form of contraception when being treated with rifampicin, especially as the treatment is relatively short-term and the metabolism of estrogens returns to normal within 3 to 4 weeks after the drug has been stopped.

Antituberculous Drugs in Pregnancy. The diagnosis of tuberculosis of any form in a young woman is always a cause for anxiety, especially when pregnancy and the possible adverse effects of drugs are considered. If possible, young women should be advised against pregnancy until the treatment is completed, but if the patient is already pregnant when the diagnosis is made, the risks to the patient against those to the fetus must be assessed. Unless there is severe renal failure, in which case pregnancy should be terminated, the pregnancy is allowed to continue, as most reported anomalies have been caused by much higher doses than are used in humans. Rifampicin in the series of Snider and coworkers (1980) produced a higher incidence of limb defects, but this has not been confirmed. Moreover, there is very little evidence of any increased risk of toxemia or neonatal mortality in women with a history of renal tuberculosis, provided that renal function and blood pressure are normal. Because it is difficult to assess the toxicity of one drug when the treatment is a combination of three or more agents, it is advisable to give rifampicin three times a week rather than every day during the first 3 months of the pregnancy, and to add pyridoxine, 20 mg daily, to the regimen as long as isoniazid is being taken.

Antituberculous Drugs in the Nursing Mother. Rifampicin is present in milk but is not known to do any harm. There are also significant amounts of isoniazid in milk, with a consequent theoretical risk of neurotoxicity, so both mother and baby should be given pyridoxine. Very little ethambutol is found in milk, making the risks of ocular toxicity negligible.

Antituberculous Drugs in Renal Failure. Streptomycin is excreted almost totally unchanged in the urine; in oliguric patients its half-life is increased from the normal 2 to 3 hours to between 60 and 70 hours. Isoniazid is metabolized mostly in the liver, less than 25 per cent being excreted unchanged in the urine; in oliguria its half-life is hardly altered, remaining between 2 and 5 hours.

Rifampicin is also largely metabolized in the liver, only 30 per cent of the drug being excreted in the urine, so that in oliguria its half-life stays at between 2 and 5 hours.

Pyrazinamide has a half-life of 6 hours and is largely metabolized in the liver. Only 4 per cent is excreted unchanged in the urine, so that only in very severe renal failure will its dose need to be reduced (Stollmeyer et al., 1968).

Ethambutol, like streptomycin, is excreted in the urine, 80 per cent being unchanged. Because of its dose-related toxicity, it should be avoided in all cases of renal failure, as in oliguria its half-life is increased from 2 to 4 hours to more than 15 hours.

The creatinine clearance (ml/min) is the most accurate way to judge the best dose regimen in the presence of renal failure (Bennett et al., 1977). Table 23–5 shows the recommended doses in the presence of various degrees of renal insufficiency (Blythe, 1979). It should be the rule that streptomycin and ethambutol are not used in the presence of tuberculous renal failure.

Topical Drugs. Topical agents have only a minor role in the management of genitourinary tuberculosis at the present time. In severe cystitis a combination of 5 per cent rifampicin and 1 per cent isoniazid made up in normal saline can be used for slowly irrigating the bladder. Ten ml of 1 per cent lidocaine should be added to every 100 ml of the solution, as it helps to relieve the severe bladder symptoms. If, however, bladder fibrosis is already under way, it can have no lasting effect. The same solution can be used to irrigate the pelvis of a kidney after the repair of an obstruction at the pelviureteric junction and can be instilled into a closed renal abscess after the contents have been aspirated. A cream of the same combined concentration can be used as a dressing for discharging tuberculous sinuses.

TABLE 23–5. RECOMMENDED DOSES IN THE PRESENCE OF VARIOUS DEGREES OF RENAL IINSUFFICIENCY

		Frequency of Administration			
		CREATINE CLEARANCE (ML/MIN)			
Drug	**Dose**	> 100 ML/MIN	80–50 ML/MIN	50–10 ML/MIN	< 10 ML/MIN
Streptomycin	1 gm	1 × 24 hrs	1 × 48 hrs	1 × 72 hrs	1 × 96 hrs
Isoniazid	300 mg	1 × 24 hrs	1 × 24 hrs	1 × 36–48 hrs	1 × 60–72 hrs
Rifampicin	450 mg	1 × 24 hrs	1 × 24 hrs	1 × 24 hrs	1 × 48 hrs
Pyrazinamide	25 mg/kilo body wt	1 × 24 hrs	1 × 24 hrs	1 × 24 hrs	1 × 48 hrs
Ethambutol	25 mg/kilo body wt	1 × 24 hrs	1 × 24 hrs	1 × 48 hrs	1 × 72 hrs

SURGERY

Surgical treatment has undergone many changes in the last 30 years. Figure 23–19 shows the surgical treatment carried out in the author's unit from 1947 to 1981. During the last 4 years there has been a steady increase, which coincides with the introduction of short-course chemotherapeutic treatment. Surgery continues to be an essential part of the modern philosophy of the management of genitourinary tuberculosis, and about 80 per cent of patients now require some operative procedure (Fig. 23–19).

EXCISION OF DISEASED TISSUE

Nephrectomy. The indications for nephrectomy are (1) a nonfunctioning kidney with or without calcification, (2) extensive disease involving the whole kidney together with hypertension and pelviureteric obstruction, and (3) coexisting renal carcinoma. This is a rare occurrence, but if suspected, arteriograms should always be carried out.

The management of nonfunctioning or severely diseased tuberculous kidneys has been controversial and has varied from nephrectomy to conservative treatment with long-term chemotherapy. Bloom and associates (1970) and

Horne and Tulloch (1975) advocated conservative treatment, stating the adequate chemotherapy could control the tuberculous disease. Kerr and coworkers (1969, 1970), however, recommended the removal of diseased organs, and Wong and Lan (1980) reported that 89.3 per cent of all nonfunctioning kidneys had been destroyed and required nephrectomy. In only 3 out of 28 cases was reconstruction possible.

It can still be argued that modern effective chemotherapy will kill all organisms. However, there is no proof that this is so, and in any case it is never possible to salvage nonfunctioning kidneys. With short-course chemotherapy, it is therefore advisable to remove a large focus and allow the drugs to destroy the residual mycobacteria, but it is also a sound surgical practice to excise a nonfunctioning and potentially dangerous organ. Short-course chemotherapy has altered the whole philosophy of the surgical management of extensive disease of the genitourinary tract, but it is now most important that these lesions be explored, either to try to restore function or, more likely, to remove irreparable disease.

Flechner and Gow (1980) reviewed 300 cases of genitourinary tuberculosis. There were 73 patients with nonfunctioning or poorly func-

Figure 23–19. The changing pattern of surgery.

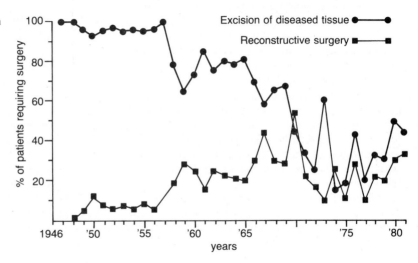

tioning kidneys. Three of the four patients who did not have a nephrectomy developed complications, flank sinuses, abscesses, and hypertension. Osterhage and coworkers (1980) investigated the activity of *M. tuberculosis* after efficient chemotherapy on the basis of histologic preparations after nephrectomy. Despite sterilization of the urine, 50 per cent of the patients showed active tuberculosis. No cultures of the diseased tissue were taken, so an opinion based on histologic evidence may be suspect. Nevertheless, it is further evidence to support nephrectomy in extensive renal disease in patients undergoing short-course regimens.

Ureterectomy. Nephroureterectomy is rarely indicated. As much of the ureter as possible that can be removed through the nephrectomy incision should be carried out and the lower end transfixed and ligated.

The writer has been required to go back on only one occasion in over 400 nephrectomies for removal of the ureter, and that was a patient in whom a stone had formed. This is a rare complication and not an indication for ureterectomy.

Partial Nephrectomy. This procedure is becoming less and less common and is very rarely required, since with modern chemotherapy the response of a local lesion in the kidney is rapid and complete. There are only two indications: (1) the localized lesion containing calcification that has failed to respond after 6 weeks of intensive chemotherapy, and (2) an area of calcification that is slowly increasing in size and is threatening to gradually destroy the whole kidney. Partial nephrectomy can never be justified in the absence of calcification.

There are only a very few points in the technique that need special emphasis. Cooling is not required. If possible, only the artery to the area that is being resected should be ligated. The capsule should be stripped from the renal cortex so that it can be used for strengthening the suture line in the final closure of the defect. All the vessels in the renal cortex and medulla are carefully and conscientiously ligated independently after localization by frequently releasing the clamp that is controlling the appropriate vessel. The calyces are closed by a continuous catgut or Dexon suture. The perirenal fat is carefully dissected off the kidney and retained so that it can be stitched over the suture line. The wound should be drained for a few days.

Cavernotomy. Cavernotomy has hardly any place in the modern management of genitourinary tuberculosis, since with modern x-ray techniques the contents of an abscess can be aspirated under the control of the image intensifier. This is a very satisfactory method of treatment and largely obviates surgery. It also allows the instillation of antituberculous drugs into the cavity as well as the aspiration of its contents, which can be cultured for viable organisms and from which the quantity of antituberculous drugs can be estimated. If there is extensive calcification in the wall, a careful control must be exercised; otherwise, there may be a slow but insidious extension that will ultimately destroy the kidney. Once this process starts, a partial nephrectomy should be carried out.

Epididymectomy. The incidence of tuberculous epididymitis is declining, but epididymectomy is still required. The main indication is a caseating abscess that is not responding to chemotherapy. Another indication is a firm swelling that has slowly increased in size despite antibiotics and antituberculous chemotherapy.

Involvement of the testis is uncommon, and orchiectomy is required in only 5 per cent of cases. Ligation of the contralateral vas is never needed; the writer has seen a number of patients who have fathered children following unilateral epididymectomy for tuberculosis. The only serious complication is testicular atrophy, which occurs in 6 per cent of patients. It is always confined to the severe cases, in which, because of the inflammation surrounding the cord, there is extreme difficulty in dissecting the globus major from the vascular pedicle. Epididymectomy should be performed through a scrotal incision. The globus minor is dissected first, followed by the body of the epididymis, and finally the globus major. The vas is then isolated and brought out in the groin through a separate stab incision to prevent the formation of a subcutaneous abscess.

RECONSTRUCTIVE SURGERY

Stricture of the Ureter. The most common site at which tuberculous stricture is found is the ureterovesical junction. It may, however, also occur at the pelviureteric junction and, rarely, in the middle third of the ureter. Very occasionally, it may involve the entire ureter, causing complete stenosis, fibrosis, and even calcification. If the whole ureter is involved, there is invariably extensive disease in the kidney, so reconstructive surgery in this type of stricture is impossible.

Pelviureteric Strictures. Strictures at this level are very uncommon; the writer has seen only eight such cases in his entire experience of the disease. The explanation is that by the time the patient presents for treatment, a combination of an acute tuberculous infection with an obstruction at the pelviureteric junction will have destroyed the greater part of the kidney.

The urologist fortunate enough to be confronted with genitourinary tuberculosis accompanied by kidney disease in which the kidney is functioning but in which there is pelviureteric obstruction should be prepared to relieve the obstruction at the earliest possible moment, even within 2 to 3 weeks after the start of chemotherapy. If the operation can be delayed for 5 to 6 weeks, however, the results will be better. The immediate progress should be monitored by an intravenous urogram, which is taken weekly, and if there is significant deterioration, immediate surgery should be carried out.

Both the Anderson-Hynes and the Culp techniques give satisfactory results. The anastomosis is made over a Silastic stent, which is left in situ for 3 weeks. Pyelostomy is an essential part of the technique, since it not only allows free drainage but also permits instillation of a combination of 5 per cent isoniazid and 1 per cent rifampicin, once daily. The pyelostomy tube is clamped off the day after the Silastic stent is removed and is withdrawn once it is established that urine is draining satisfactorily. With this technique and modern chemotherapy, the chances of a secondary nephrectomy are very small. A pyelostomy can be performed even in the presence of inflammation. However, if the inflammation is severe at the time of surgery, it is advisable to leave the stent in for 5 to 6 weeks and carry out instillation with antituberculous drugs for a similar period. Very rarely, an intrapelvic stricture involving all the major calyces is present (Fig. 23–20). A reconstruction should be attempted by dissecting out the sinus using the Gil-Vernet technique and restoring the pelvis by bivalving the ureter and forming an anastomosis with the upper and lower dilated calyces.

Strictures of the Middle Third of the Ureter. Strictures at this level are very rare indeed. Should they occur, the best method of treatment is by the Davis intubation ureterostomy technique (Davis et al., 1948; Smart, 1961). This is contingent on the integrity of some part of the urothelium; if this condition is met, the ureter will regenerate around an indwelling tube over a linear incision. The Silastic stent should be left in for at least 6 weeks and can be brought out either through the skin or through the urethra. A double-J stent is an

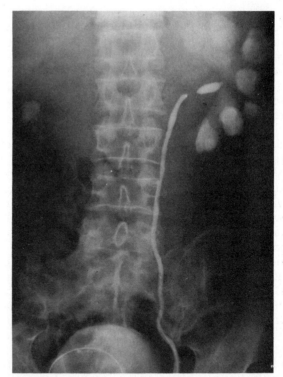

Figure 23–20. Multiple intrapelvic strictures with calyceal dilatation.

admirable piece of equipment for this operation. Recurrent stricture, however, is always likely to be a complication; all patients should therefore be followed up most carefully and intravenous urogram carried out at 3-month intervals for at least 12 months, to guard against this serious complication.

Strictures of the Lower End of the Ureter. Strictures of the lower end of the ureter occur in approximately 9 per cent of patients. These can be managed medically or by dilatation or surgery.

MEDICAL MANAGEMENT. When obstruction at the lower end of the ureter is present at the start of chemotherapy, it requires careful observation. It is not, however, necessary to put the patient on corticosteroids immediately, as a number of these strictures will be due to edema, which will respond to chemotherapy. A satisfactory regime is to start the patient on normal chemotherapy and to perform an intravenous urogram, with one radiographic view at 25 minutes, taking a 17-inch by 14-inch picture at weekly intervals, and noting progress. If there is deterioration or no improvement after 3 weeks, corticosteroids, 20 mg t.d.s. should be given, together with the other chemotherapy. This is a large dose of steroids, but as previously pointed out, rifampicin doubles the excretion of cortisone, and therefore a much larger dose is needed to achieve the desired effect. The same management is continued with the weekly intravenous urogram; if there is deterioration or no improvement after a 6-week period, surgical reimplantation is carried out, if an initial attempt at dilatation has failed.

URETERIC DILATATION. Endoscopic dilatation has been referred to by many authors, but few large series of patients have been reviewed. Murphy and coworkers (1982) reported the results of the management of 97 strictures seen in 92 patients over a period of 25 years. Dilatation was successful in 51 ureters (64 per cent), and failed to relieve the strictures in 29. Dilatation failed in 17 ureters owing to technical difficulties. The dilatation is performed under general anesthesia by passing either a No. 8 French Braasch catheter or two No. 5 French ureteric catheters up the affected side. The dilatation is repeated every 2 weeks initially, and later every 1 to 2 months, until the upper renal tract is stabilized. In Murphy's series, the mean number of dilatations per patient was four. In view of the high failure rates and the number of general anesthetics required, it is unlikely that this technique will be adopted except in special cases.

SURGICAL MANAGEMENT. Most ureteric strictures are less than 2 inches in length (Fig. 23–21) and commence in the intermural part of the bladder. The area of fibrosis is localized and, unless a large part of the ureter is involved, is confined to the intermural part or an area just proximal to it. Above the fibrotic area there is often a dilated segment, and unless the stricture has been present for a considerable time, the muscle will improve after the obstruction has been relieved and the recommencement of normal peristalsis will occur. These ureters should be reimplanted into the bladder. A reflux-preventing technique is to be employed whenever possible, and, for success to be guaranteed, a submucous tunnel of at least 5 cm is necessary.

An accurate assessment of the length of the stricture and the function of the ureter is obtained by retrograde ureterogram, using a bulb catheter and watching the peristaltic function of the ureter on an image intensifier. Cystoscopy is essential to study the bladder so that an area free from infection is chosen for the reimplantation whenever it is necessary.

The tuberculous infection is nearly always localized to the area around the infected ureteric orifice, so that there should be no difficulty in reanastomosing the ureter into an intact bladder.

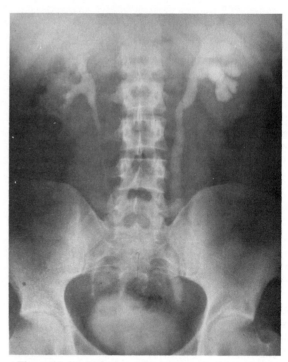

Figure 23–21. Stricture at the lower end of the ureter.

If the stricture is longer than 2 inches, however, a direct reimplantation cannot be achieved. In these cases, either a psoas hitch (Turner-Warwick, 1965) or a Boari flap procedure (Gow, 1968) may be necessary. Both give equally satisfactory results, provided that a reflux-preventing technique is used in the same way as for direct reimplantation. Using the latter technique, strictures as long as 14 to 15 cm can be excised and the remaining ureter reimplanted. If the Boari procedure is selected, it is helpful to distend the bladder by running in 200 to 250 ml of saline. In this way the bladder flap can be accurately delineated and planned. It should be remembered that a larger area of the bladder than would seem necessary will be required, as there is always considerable contraction of the flap when the bladder is decompressed. The bladder and bladder flap are closed in two layers, and indwelling catheter drainage is maintained for 8 to 10 days. Some urologists advocate using a stent through the anastomosis to the renal pelvis and out through the urethra. This is not considered necessary, and the writer has experienced few complications without this addition to the technique.

Two-layer closure is important, the first being continuous interlocking suture. Before final closure, the bladder is again distended with fluid so that any leaks can be identified and closed. The bladder flap and ureter are then sutured to the psoas muscle to avoid any kinking at the level of the ureterovesical flap. The wound is closed with drainage down to the anastomosis, which is removed after 4 to 5 days.

Ureteroureterostomy. This technique can be used when an extensive stricture involves one or both ureters. After the ureteroureterostomy, either the longer of the two ureters can be anastomosed into the bladder or a Boari flap can be fashioned using a reflux-preventing technique. With modern chemotherapy the risks are negligible.

AUGMENTATION CYSTOPLASTY

The urinary bladder, besides being a contractile organ for expelling urine, is also a reservoir. Therefore, in determining the appropriate treatment there are two aspects to be considered. The main symptoms that warrant consideration of an augmentation cystoplasty are an intolerable frequency both day and night, together with pain, urgency, and hematuria. An intravenous urogram will reveal a small, contracted, hypertonic bladder, which normally empties completely. The appearance on cystoscopy is a diffuse velvet inflammation with a capacity of less than 100 ml. A superimposed secondary infection is invariably present in the initial stages. The word "augmentation" must be emphasized. The procedure is not a cystectomy, which should be reserved for carcinoma, interstitial cystitis, or total chemical or physical destruction of the bladder, but a method of increasing the bladder capacity while retaining as much of the bladder as possible. This is important if voiding is to be satisfactory, as the mural pressure of the cecum or colon is only, on average, 16 cm of water, which is insufficient force to empty the bladder. Hence, if very little bladder remains, voiding will depend entirely on abdominal pressure (Dounis et al., 1979; Gleason et al., 1972).

Many patients will show deterioration of renal function, caused by either reflux or obstruction. The writer agrees with Kuss (Kuss et al., 1970) that renal failure is no contraindication to surgery, and that patients with a creatinine clearance of more than 15 ml per minute should be accepted for augmentation cystoplasty. Indeed, there are many examples of patients with poor renal function who show a marked improvement after this procedure, and the writer knows of no case in which the renal function has deteriorated after surgery. Enuresis, incontinence, and psychiatric disturbances

are a contraindication to this procedure, and in these cases, if surgery is necessary, a urinary diversion is the only treatment.

The ileum was the first part of the bowel to be used, but the loop method employed suffered from loop stagnation and a narrowing of the anastomosis. Even the patch ileocystoplasty advocated by Tasker (1953) failed to overcome all the problems. The colon was the next part of the gastrointestinal tract to be tried, and even though there was significant ureteric reflux, it still continues to give satisfactory results (Duff et al., 1970). Its advantages are a longer colonic mesentery, safer ureteral surgery, and complete extraperitoneal vesicocolic anastomosis. However, it is essential to investigate the colon by a barium enema prior to surgery to exclude the presence of diverticular disease.

In 1965, Gil-Vernet advocated the use of the cecum together with the terminal ileum. The technique using the caecum has certain advantages. Mucus discharge, infection, and residual urine are less, and if the urine has to be diverted, reimplantation into the ileum is a safe and reliable procedure, provided that an antireflux procedure, as suggested by Leadbetter (1951), is adopted. As the ileocecal valve is competent in 80 per cent of patients, the intussusception technique advocated by Hendren (1980) is not recommended. Splitting of the cecum also has disadvantages, since it then becomes a patch, which reduces the voiding power of the cecal implant. Whatever arguments are proposed in favor of either a colocystoplasty or a cecocystoplasty, there is no doubt that both are satisfactory methods and that the choice of the segment of bowel has not influenced the long-term results (Smith et al., 1977). The main advantage of the cecum is in reimplantation of the ureters, since then the ileum can be used and reflux can more easily be prevented. In addition, there is no fashioning of the bowel, it is easily rotated, it is isoperistaltic, and there is no absorption of solutes (Dounis et al., 1980).

All patients should have at least 4 weeks of extensive chemotherapy before surgery. Urethral flow rates are also an essential part of the preoperative preparation. A reduced flow rate in the female is treated by bladder neck dilatation, with incisions at the 3 and 9 o'clock positions, using the Otis urethrotome. In the male, either a transurethral resection or a bladder neck incision is carried out. Both these procedures should be performed 3 weeks before the augmentation. There is a fine line between retention and incontinence, and precise accuracy is difficult to achieve, so that the resection has to be carefully performed and may have to be repeated. It is better to repeat the procedure once, or even twice, rather than to have an incontinent patient.

The YV-plasty suggested by Chan (Chan et al., 1980), is not recommended, as it increases the risk of incontinence.

Certain aspects of the technique are worth emphasizing. A good bowel preparation is important: A combination of oral neomycin, 1 gm t.d.s., and metronidazole, 200 mg t.d.s., for 48 hours before surgery, with a retention enema of 500 ml of 5 per cent povidone-iodine, following a colonic washout has given excellent results.

If a ureteroileal anastomosis is indicated, it should be performed before the vesicocolic anastomosis; otherwise, the technical difficulties may be insuperable. As little of the bladder as possible should be resected. Inflammation of the bladder is no contraindication to surgery, but a two-layer closure and the routine use of the omentum wrapped round the anastomosis reduce the complications. Gentamicin, 160 mg IV is given just before the bowel is resected.

Lower urinary tract infection is occasionally seen as a postoperative complication. It is often symptomless and difficult to eradicate, so that low-dose antibiotics continuously for 6 months or longer may be required.

Occasionally, patients present with a long-standing urinary diversion and wonder whether the normal anatomy can be restored. It may be possible, but a careful study of the defunctioned bladder must be carried out to ensure that the disease is quiescent, that there is no bladder outlet obstruction, and that there is adequate detrusor activity. For this purpose, a full urodynamic screening is necessary.

The gastrocystoplasty as advocated by Leong (1978) is a recent technique that requires further evaluation and a prolonged follow-up before it can be considered as an alternative to the proven existing methods.

URINARY DIVERSION IN TUBERCULOSIS

Although in previous years, urinary diversion was an accepted method of treatment in a few isolated cases, now it is rarely necessary. There are only three indications for permanent urinary diversion: (1) a history of psychiatric disturbance or obvious subnormal intelligence, (2) enuresis, and (3) intolerable diurnal symptoms with incontinence that has not responded to chemotherapy or bladder dilatation. Ileal or colonic conduits are both satisfactory methods.

Ureterosigmoid anastomosis is not recommended, as in this type of case incontinence often rapidly occurs. However, if it is considered, before the procedure is carried out, the patient's control of fluid in the rectum should be determined. For this, 250 ml of normal saline is run into the rectum, and the patient is asked to retain the fluid while ambulant for as long as possible. Unless there is complete control for more than 2 hours, ureterosigmoid anastomosis is contraindicated.

References

Agarwalla, B., Mohanty, G. P., Sahu, L. K., and Rath, R. C.: Tuberculosis of the penis—report of two cases. J. Urol., *124*:927, 1980.

Antonio, D., and Gow, J. G.: Renal calcification in genitourinary tuberculosis—a clinical study. Int. Urol. Nephrol., *7*:289, 1975.

Barksdale, L., and Kim, K. S.: Mycobacterium. Bacteriol. Rev., *41*:217, 1977.

Baron, O. N., and Bell, J. L.: Serum enzyme changes in patients receiving anti-tuberculous therapy with rifampicin or p-aminosalicylic acid plus isoniazid and streptomycin. Tubercle, *55*:115, 1974.

Bennett, W. M., Singer, I., Golper, T., Ferg, P., and Coggins, C. J.: Guidelines for drug therapy in renal failure. Ann. Intern. Med., *86*:754, 1977.

Bjornesjo, K. B.: Tuberculostatic factor in normal human urine. Am. Rev. Tub. Pulm. Dis., *73*:967, 1956.

Bloom, S., Wechsler, H., and Lattimer, J. K.: Results of a long-term study of non-functioning tuberculous kidney. J. Urol., *104*:760, 1970.

Blythe, W. B.: The management of intercurrent medical and surgical problems in the patient with chronic renal failure. *In* Earley, L. E., and Gottschalk, C. W. (Eds.): Strauss and Welt's Diseases of the Kidney. 3rd ed. Boston, Little, Brown & Co., 1979, p. 523.

Braasch, W. F., Walters, W., and Hammer, H. J.: Hypertension and the surgical kidney. JAMA, *115*:1837, 1940.

British Medical Research Council: Co-operative controlled trial of standard regimen of streptomycin, P.A.S. and isoniazid and three alternative regimens of chemotherapy in Britain. Tubercle, *54*:99, 1973.

British Thoracic Association: Short course therapy in pulmonary tuberculosis. Lancet, *1*:1182, 1980.

Calmette, A., and Guérin, C.: Essai de prémunition par le B.C.G. contra l'infection tuberculeuse de l'homme et des animaux. Presse Med. (Paris), *33*:825, 1925.

Chan, S. L., Ankerman, G. J., Wright, J. E., and McLoughlin, M. G.: Caecocystoplasty in the surgical management of the small contracted bladder. J. Urol., *124*(3):338, 1980.

Chen, W.: Hong Kong Chest Services/British Medical Research Council controlled trial of four three-times weekly regimens and a daily regimen all given for six months for pulmonary tuberculosis. 12th International Congress of Chemotherapy, Florence, 1981.

Cohnheim, J.: Die Tuberkulose von Standpunkte der Infectionskchre. Leipzig, 1879.

Colby, F. H.: Tuberculous infections and inflammations of the urinary tract. *In* Campbell, M. (Ed.): Textbook of Urology, Vol. 1, p. 525. Philadelphia, W.B. Saunders Co., 1954.

Coulaud, M. D.: Étude éxperimentale de la tuberculose renale du lapin. J. Urol. (Paris), *39*:572, 1935.

Davies, P. D. O.: Tuberculosis epidemiology and treatment. Hosp. Update, August 1980, p. 777.

Davis, D. M., Strong, G. H., and Drake, W. M.: Intubated ureterostomy. Experimental work and clinical results. J. Urol., 59:851, 1948.

Dickinson, J. M., and Mitchison, D. A.: Experimental models to explain the high sterilising activity of rifampicin in the chemotherapy of tuberculosis. Am. Rev. Respir. Dis., 123:367, 1981.

Dounis, A., and Gow, J. G.: Bladder augmentation—a long term review. Br. J. Urol., 51:264, 1979.

Dounis, A., Abel, B. J., and Gow, J. G.: Caecocystoplasty for bladder augmentation. J. Urol., 123(2):164, 1980.

Duff, F. A., O'Grady, J. F., and Kelly, D. J.: Colocystoplasty. Br. J. Urol., 42:704, 1970.

Ekehorn, G.: Die Ausbreitumgswerse der Nieren tuberkulose in der tuberkulosen Niere. Folia Urol., 2:412, 1908.

Elland, G. A.: Absorption metabolism and excretion of pyrazinamide in man. Tubercle, 50:144, 1969.

Farga, V.: The avenues of the Union (Editorial). Bull. Int. Union Tuberc., 47:49, 1972.

Fellander, M., Hiertoun, T., and Wallmark, G.: Studies on the concentration of streptomycin in the treatment of bone and joint tuberculosis. Acta Tuberc. Scand., 27:176, 1952.

Flechner, S. M., and Gow, J. G.: Role of nephrectomy in the treatment of non-functioning or very poorly functioning unilateral tuberculous kidney. J. Urol., 123(6):822, 1980.

Flick, L. F.: Development of Our Knowledge of Tuberculosis. Lancaster, Pa., Wickersham Printing Co., 1925.

Fox, W.: The current status of short course chemotherapy. Bull. Int. Union Tuberc., 53:268, 1978.

Fox, W.: Short course chemotherapy for tuberculosis. In Flenley, D. C. (Ed.): Recent Advances in Respiratory Medicine. 2nd ed. Edinburg, Churchill Livingstone, 1980, p. 183.

Fox, W.: Whether short course chemotherapy. Br. J. Dis. Chest, 75:331, 1981.

Freedman, L. R.: In Earley, L. E., and Gottschalk, C. W. (Eds.): Strauss and Welt's Diseases of the Kidney. Boston, Little, Brown & Co., 1979, p. 859.

Gil-Vernet, J. M., Jr.: The ileocolic segment in urological surgery. J. Urol., 94:418, 1965.

Girling, D. J.: Hong Kong Chest Service/Tuberculous Research Centre, Madras/British Medical Research Council Study of three-month and two-month regimens for smear-negative pulmonary tuberculosis. 12th International Congress of Chemotherapy, Florence, 1981.

Girling, D. J.: Adverse effects of anti-tuberculous drugs. Drugs, 23:56, 1982.

Gleason, M. D., Gittes, R. F., Bottaccini, M. R., and Byrne, J. C.: Energy balance of voiding after caecal cystoplasty. J. Urol., 108:259, 1972.

Goldblatt, H., Lynch, J., Hanzal, R. F., and Summerville, W. W.: Studies on experimental hypertension. J. Exp. Med., 59:347, 1934.

Gow, J. G.: Carcinoma of the epididymis. Urologia, 24:594, 1957.

Gow, J. G.: Seminoma of the epididymis. Urologia, 30:589, 1963.

Gow, J. G.: Renal calcification in genito-urinary tuberculosis. Br. J. Surg., 52:283, 1965.

Gow, J. G.: The results of the reimplantation of the ureter by the Boari technique. Proc. R. Soc. Med., 61:128, 1968.

Gow, J. G.: Genito-urinary tuberculosis. In Blandy, J. P. (Ed.): Urology. Oxford, Blackwell Scientific Publications, 1976.

Grange, J. M.: Mycobacterial Disease. 1st ed. London, Arnold, 1980, p. 32.

Grosset, J.: The sterilising value of rifampicin and pyrazinamide in experimental short-course chemotherapy. Tubercle, 59:287, 1978.

Hartman, G. W., Segura, J. W., and Hattery, R. R.: In Witten, D. M., Myers, G. H., and Utz, D. C. (eds.): Emmett's Clinical Urography. 4th ed. Philadelphia, W. B. Saunders Co., 1977, pp. 898–921.

Hartmann, G., Honikel, K. O., Knüsel, F., and Nüesch, J.: The specific inhibition of the D.N.A.-directed R.N.A. Synthesis by rifampicin. Biochim. Biophys. Acta, 145:843, 1967.

Hendren, W. H.: Re-operative ureteral reimplantation. Management of the difficult case. J. Pediatr. Surg., 15:770, 1980.

Hepper, N. C. G., Karlson, A. G., Leary, F. J., and Soule, E. H.: Genito-urinary infection due to Mycobacterium kansasii. Mayo Clin. Proc., 46:387, 1971.

Hill, J. D., and Stevenson, D. K.: Tuberculosis in unvaccinated children, adolescents and young adults: a city epidemic. Br. Med. J., 286:1471, 1983.

Hong Kong Chest Service/British Medical Research Council.: Controlled trial of four thrice-weekly regimens and a daily regimen all given for six months for pulmonary tuberculosis. Lancet, 1:171, 1981.

Horne, N. W., and Tulloch, W. S.: Conservative management of renal tuberculosis. Br. J. Urol., 47:481, 1975.

Hsiung, J. C., Miao, T. C., and Che'n, C. C.: An investigation into hypertension due to renal tuberculosis. Chin. Med. J., 84:327, 1965.

Innes, J. A.: Non-respiratory tuberculosis. J. R. Coll. Physicians Lond., 15(40):227, 1981.

Jenkins, D. E., and Wolinsky, E.: In Baum, G. R. (Ed.).: Textbook of Pulmonary Diseases. Boston, Little, Brown & Co., 1965, p. 257.

Jindani, A., Aber, V. R., Edwards, E. A., and Mitchison, D. A.: The early bacteriocidal activity of drugs in patients with pulmonary tuberculosis. Am. Rev. Respir. Dis., 121:939, 1980.

Kato, T.: A case of tuberculosis of the tunica vaginalis propria testis associated with hydrocoele. Acta Urol. Jpn., 16:597, 1970.

Kerr, W. K., Gale, G. L., and Peterson, K. S. S.: Reconstructive surgery for genito-urinary tuberculosis. J. Urol., 101:254, 1969.

Kerr, W. K., Gale, G. L., Struthers, N. W., Peterson, K. S. S., Couthard, H. S., Greatrex, G. E., Gross, J., Wigle, W. D., and Ashley, M. J.: Prognosis in reconstructive surgery for urinary tuberculosis. Br. J. Urol., 42:672, 1970.

Koch R.: Die atilogie der Tuberkulose. Berl. Klin. Wochenschr., 15:221, 1882.

Kretschmer, H. L.: Tuberculosis of the epididymis. Surg. Gynecol. Obstet., 47:652, 1928.

Kucers, A., and Bennett, N. McK.: The Rise of Antibiotics. London, William Heinemann Medical Books, 1979, p. 805.

Kunin, G. M., Brandt, D., and Wood, H.: Bacteriolologic structures of rifampicin, a new semi-synthetic antibiotic. J. Infect. Dis., 119:132, 1969.

Kuss, R., Bilker, M., Camey, M., Chatelain, C., and Lassan, J. P.: Indications and early and late results of intestinocystoplasty. A review of 185 cases. J. Urol., 103:53, 1970.

Lal, M. M., Sekhon, G. S., and Dhall, J. C.: Tuberculosis of the penis. J. Ind. Med. Assoc., 56:316, 1971.

Lane, D. J.: Extrapulmonary tuberculosis. Med. Int., 1(21):983, 1982.

Lattimer, J. K., Colmore, H. P., Sanger, G., Robertson,

H., and McLellan, F. C.: Transmission of genital tuberculosis from husband to wife via the semen. Am. Rev. Tub., *69*:618, 1954.

Lattimer, J. K., and Wechsler, M.: Genito-urinary tuberculosis. In Harrison, J. H., et al. (Eds.): Campbell's Urology. 4th ed. Vol. 1., Ch. 15. Philadelphia, W. B. Saunders Co., 1978.

Leadbetter, W. F.: Consideration of problems incident to performance of uretero-enterostomy: report of a technique. J. Urol., *65*:818, 1951.

Lee, L. W., Burgler, L. W., Price, E. B., and Cassidy, E.: Granulomatous prostatitis. Association with isolation of *Mycobacterium fortuitum*. JAMA, *237*:2408, 1977.

Leong, C. H.: Use of the stomach for bladder replacement and urinary diversion. Ann. R. Coll. Surg. Engl., *60*:283, 1978.

Lewis, E. L.: Tuberculosis of the penis. A report of 5 new cases and a complete review of the literature. J. Urol., *56*:737, 1946.

Lowell, A. N.: Tuberculosis in the World. Washington, D.C., U.S. Department of Health, Education and Welfare, P.H.S. Center for Disease Control. Publication No. CDC76-8317, 1976.

Luzzatto, L., Apirian, D., and Schlessinger, D.: Mechanism of action of streptomycin in *E. coli;* interruption of the ribosome cycle at the initiation of protein synthesis. Proc. Natl. Acad. Sci. U.S.A., *60*:873, 1968.

Marks, J.: Ending the routine guinea pig test. Tubercle, *53*:31, 1972.

Marks, L. S., and Pontasse, E. F.: Hypertension from renal tuberculosis. Operative cure predicted by renal vein renin. J. Urol., *109*:149, 1973.

Marszalak, W. W., and Dhai, A.: Genito-urinary tuberculosis. S. Afr. Med. J., *62*(6):158, 1982.

McAllister, W. A. C., Thompson, P. J., Al-Habet, S. M., and Rogers, H. J.: Rifampicin reduces effectiveness and bioavailability of prednisolone. Br. Med. J., *286*:923, 1983.

MacLeod, M. N., Hay, D., and Stewart, S. M.: The use of pyrazinamide plus isoniazid in the treatment of pulmonary tuberculosis. Tubercle, *40*:14, 1959.

Macmillan, E. W.: Blood supply of the epididymis in man. Br. J. Urol., *26*:954, 1954.

Medlar, E. M.: Cases of renal infection in pulmonary tuberculosis. Evidence of healed tuberculous lesions. Am. J. Pathol., *2*:401, 1926.

Medlar, E. M., Spain, D. M., and Holliday, R. W.: Postmortem compared with clinical diagnosis of genito-urinary tuberculosis in adult males. J Urol., *61*:1078, 1949.

Mehrotra, M. L., Gautam, K. D., and Chaube, C. K.: Shortest possible acceptable effective ambulatory chemotherapy in pulmonary tuberculosis. Preliminary report. Am. Rev. Respir. Dis., *124*(3):239, 1981.

Mitchell, J. R., Zimmerman, H. J., Ishak, K. G., Thorgeirsson, W. P., Timbrell, J. A., Snodgrass, W. R., and Nelson, S. D.: Isoniazid, clinical spectrum, pathology and probable pathogenesis. Ann. Intern. Med., *84*:181, 1976.

Mitchison, D. A.: Treatment of tuberculosis. J. R. Coll. Physicians Lond., *14*:91, 1980.

Morse, D., Brothwell, D. R., and Ucko, P. J.: Tuberculosis in ancient Egypt. Am. Rev. Respir. Dis., *90*:524, 1964.

Murphy, D. M., Fallon, B., Lane, V., and O'Flynn, J. D.: Tuberculous stricture of ureter. Urology, *20*(4):382, 1982.

Myers, J. A.: Chemotherapy in tuberculosis (Editorial). Dis. Chest, *22*:598, 1952.

Narayana, A. S., Kelly, D. G., and Duff, F. A.: Tuberculosis of the penis. Br. J. Urol., *48*(4):274, 1976.

Nesbit, R. M., and Ratliff, R. K.: Hypertension associated with unilateral nephropathy. J. Urol., *43*:427, 1940.

Osterhage, H. R., Fischer, V., and Hanbensak, K.: Positive histological tuberculous findings, despite stable sterility of the urine on culture. Eur. Urol., *6*(2):116, 1980.

Patoir, G., Spy, E., and Cordier, R.: Trois cas de fistules vésico ou urethro-rectales tuberculeuses. J. Urol. Nephrol., *75*:210, 1969.

Pergament, M., Gonzales, R., and Fraley, E. E.: Atypical mycobacteriosis of the urinary tract—a case report of extensive disease caused by the Battey bacillus. JAMA, *229*:816, 1974.

Reimers, D., Nocke-Finck, L., and Breuer, H.: Rifampicin and "Pill" do not go well together. JAMA, *227*:608, 1974.

Riehle, R. A., and Jayavaman, K.: Tuberculosis of the testis. Urology, *20*(1):43, 1982.

Ross, J. C., Gow, J. G., and St. Hill, C. A.: Tuberculous epididymitis. Br. J. Urol., *48*:663, 1961.

Schwartz, D. T., and Lattimer, J. K.: Incidence of arterial hypertension in 540 patients with renal tuberculosis. J. Urol., *98*:651, 1967.

Sherwood, T.: Uroradiology. Oxford, Blackwell Scientific Publications, 1980.

Smart, R. W.: An evaluation of intubation ureterotomy, with a description of surgical technique. J. Urol., *85*(4):512, 1961.

Smith, H. W.: Unilateral nephrectomy in hypertensive disease. J. Urol., *76*:685, 1956.

Smith, R. B., Van Cangh, P., Skinner, D. G., Kaufman, J. J., and Goodwin, W. E.: Augmentation enterocystoplasty—a critical reveiw. J. Urol., *118*:35, 1977.

Snider, D. E., Jr., Layde, P. M., Johnson, M. W., and Lyle, H. A.: Treatment of tuberculosis during pregnancy. Am. Rev. Respir. Dis., *122*:65, 1980.

Sporer, A., and Auerback, M. D.: Tuberculosis of the prostate. Urology, *11*(4):362, 1978.

Standford, J., Shield, M., and Rook, G.: How environmental mycobacteria may predetermine the protective efficacy of B.C.G. Tubercle, *62*:55, 1981.

Stollmeyer, K. D., Bean, R. E., and Kubica, G. P.: The absorption and excretion of pyrazinamide. Am. Rev. Respir. Dis., *98*:70, 1968.

Styblo, K.: Recent advances in epidemiological research in tuberculosis. Adv. Tuberc. Res., *20*:1, 1980.

Sutherland, A. M., Glen, E. S., and MacFarlane, J. R.: Transmission of genito-urinary tuberculosis. Health Bull. *40*:2, 1982.

Sutherland, I.: Recent studies in the epidemiology of tuberculosis based on the risk of being infected by the tubercle bacillus. Adv. Tuberc. Res., *19*:1, 1976.

Sutherland, I., Styblo, K., Sampalik, M., and Bleiker, M. A.: Annual risk of tuberculous infection in 4 countries, derived from the results of tuberculosis surveys in 1948–52. Bull. Int. Union Tuberc., *47*:123, 1971.

Symes, J. M., and Blandy, J. P.: Tuberculosis of the male urethra. Br. J. Urol., *45*:432, 1973.

Tasker, J. H.: Ileocystoplasty: a new technique. Experimental study with the report of a case. Br. J. Urol., *25*:349, 1953.

Ten Dam, H., and Hitze, K.: Does B.C.G. vaccination protect the newborn and young infants? Bull. W.H.O., *58*:37, 1980.

Ten Dam, H., Tounan, K., Hitze, K., and Guld, J.: Present knowledge of immunisation against tuberculosis. Bull. W.H.O., *54*:255, 1976.

Tripathy, R. C.: Tuberculous Chemotherapy Centre, Madras. Madras study of short course chemotherapy in pulmonary tuberculosis. Proceedings of the XXIVth World Conference of the International Union Against Tuberculosis. Brussels, 5–9, Sept., 1978.

Turner-Warwick, R. T.: The psoas hitch procedure. Institute of Urology film, London, 1965.

U.S. Department of Health and Human Services: Annual Summary. Morbid. Mortal. Weekly Rep. 80, 1980.

U.S. Department of Health and Human Services: Morbid. Mortal. Weekly Rep. *31*:123, 1982.

Ustvedt, H. J.: The relation between renal tuberculosis and primary infection. Tubercle, *28*:22, 1947.

Veukataramaiah, N. R., Van Raalte, J. A., and Dutla, S. N.: Tuberculous ulcer of the penis. Postgrad. Med. J., *58*:59, 1982.

Wildbolz, H.: Ueber Urogenital Tuberkulose Schweiz. Med. Wochenschr., *67*:1125, 1937.

Wimpenny, J. W. T.: Effect of isoniazid on biosynthesis on *Mycobacterium tuberculosis* var. *bovis* B.C.G. J. Gen. Microbiol., *47*:379, 1967.

Wiseman, R.: A treatise of the Kings-Evill. Eight Chirurgical Treatises. 3rd ed. London, Tooke and Meredith, 1696.

Wolinsky, E.: Non-tuberculous mycobacteria and associated diseases. Am. Rev. Respir. Dis., *119*:107, 1979.

Wong, S. H., and Lan, W. Y.: The surgical management of non-functioning tuberculous kidneys. J. Urol., *124*(2):187, 1980.

Woods, L. E., Butler, V. B., and Pollak, A.: Human infection with the yellow acid fast bacillus. A report of fifteen additional cases. Am. Rev. Tuberc., *73*:917, 1946.

World Health Organization: The W.H.O.-assisted tuberculosis control programme in Lesotho. Epidemiological findings and an evaluation of two different case finding programmes. Nairobi, W.H.O., 1969.

World Health Organization: Magnitude of the tuberculosis problem of the world. Wkly. Epidemiol. Rec., *50*:393, 1981.

Youmans, G. P., Paterson, P. Y., and Sommers, H. M.: The Biological and Clinical Basis of Infectious Diseases. Philadelphia, W. B. Saunders Co., 1975, p. 347.

Yu, H. H. Y., Wong, K. K., Lim, T. K., and Leong, C. H.: Clinical Study of haemospermia. Urology, *10*(6):562, 1977.

CHAPTER 24

Interstitial Cystitis and Related Syndromes

EDWARD M. MESSING, M.D.

Interstitial Cystitis

The evaluation and management of a patient with interstitial cystitis present a diagnostic and therapeutic challenge even to the highly skilled urologist. This syndrome is defined by the triad of chronic, unexplained irritative voiding symptoms; sterile, cytologically negative urine; and characteristic cystoscopic findings. Although few urologic disorders have identical clinical features, documentation of all three must be made before a diagnosis of interstitial cystitis can be established.

HISTORY OF TERMINOLOGY

Interstitial cystitis was probably first recognized by Nitze in 1907. He found inflammation of the vesical submucosa in patients with suprapubic pain whose bladder mucosa appeared to crack during maximal distention at cystoscopy. He called this entity cystitis parenchymatosa. Subsequently, Knorr (1908) and Hunner (1914) identified the same disease, the latter popularizing it as a "rare type of bladder ulcer." Hunner distinguished this entity from those previously reported by Mercier (1836), Tait (1870), Skene (1887), and Fenwick (1896), who referred to infectious ulcers as interstitial cystitis. Since 1914, other names for this disease have included "elusive ulcer" (Howard, 1944; Hunner, 1920), paracystitis (Geraghty, 1917), punctate ulcer (Reed, 1919), circumscribed panmural ulcerative cystitis (Keene, 1920), submucous ulcer (Bumpus, 1921) linear ulcer (Herbst, 1920), panmural fibrosis (Crenshaw, 1934), sub-

mucous cystitis (Donahue, 1929), panmural cystitis (Bowers and Lattimer, 1957), submucous fibrosis (Frontz, 1928), cystitis lymphopathia (Powell, 1949), cystitis infiltranscircumscripta (Peterson and Hager, 1929), and bladder fissure (Herbst et al., 1937), but it is most commonly referred to as Hunner's ulcer (Kretschmer, 1922). The widespread acceptance of this term is unfortunate, however, since ulcers, whose original description has been attributed to the optical deficiencies of primitive cystoscopes (Walsh, 1978), are rarely present (Messing and Stamey, 1978; Walsh, 1978). This misrepresentation has prevented many endoscopists from diagnosing this disease.

EPIDEMIOLOGY

Interstitial cystitis most often occurs in middle-aged women (Herbst et al., 1937; Hunner, 1914; Smith and Dehner, 1972; Higgins, 1941; Winsbury-White, 1933; Oravisto et al., 1970; Kinder and Smith, 1958; Warres, 1961; Messing and Stamey, 1978; Oravisto, 1975). It is from 6 to 11 times more common in females than in males (Walsh, 1978; O'Conor, 1955; Oravisto, 1975; Messing and Stamey, 1978). The condition has been reported in children (Geist and Antolak, 1970; Chenowith and Claywater, 1960; McDonald et al., 1953) and the elderly (Guerrier et al. 1965; Oravisto, 1975; Messing and Stamey, 1978). Owing to medical and technologic advances over the past 60 years, as well as differences in diagnostic criteria, it is difficult to estimate its actual incidence from the literature. Reported frequencies, which range from 0.07 per cent (Bowers and Lattimer, 1957) to 0.15 per cent (Kretschmer, 1922) of all urologic hospital admissions, and 0.25 per cent to 0.5 per cent (von Garrelts, 1966) of new urology outpatients, are probably low. In the Helsinki area it occurs in at least 1.8 per 10,000 females (Oravisto, 1975). Geographic and racial differences have not been reliably evaluated.

Symptoms are usually present for 3 to 5 years (Oravisto, 1975) before the correct diagnosis is established. Typically, there is rapid initial progression of symptoms, which soon stabilize. Subsequent major deterioration is unusual even without treatment (Oravisto, 1975).

ETIOLOGY

The etiology of interstitial cystitis is unknown, and it is possible that a variety of factors result in its development. Infectious, lymphovascular, neurogenic, endocrinologic, psychoneurotic, and inflammatory (including autoimmune) mechanisms have been implicated primarily by epidemiologic and anecdotal clinical observations. The roles of defective bladder protective layers and irritative substances in the urine are unsubstantiated. Investigations have been hampered by the disease's relative rarity, nonuniform diagnostic criteria, and lack of a naturally occurring or experimentally induced animal model.

A variety of other disorders have been reported to occur in association with interstitial cystitis. These include collagen diseases (e.g., lupus erythematosus [Gordon et al., 1973]); rheumatoid arthritis (Oravisto et al., 1970; Silk, 1970) and polyarteritis (Oravisto et al., 1970); autoimmune diseases (e.g., thyroiditis [Silk, 1970]); pelvic (Bowers and Lattimer, 1957; Hunner, 1920), gastrointestinal (Bowers and Lattimer, 1957), and pharyngeal (Hunner, 1918a; Meisser and Bumpus, 1921) infections; and allergic conditions (Hand, 1949; Higgins, 1941; Oravisto et al., 1970; Messing and Stamey, 1978; Rosin et al., 1979). With the possible exception of allergy, none has occurred with sufficient regularity to imply a causal relationship.

Infection. Aware of differences between this disease and the condition previously described by Fenwick (1896) and Skene (1887), Hunner proposed that interstitial cystitis resulted from chronic bacterial infection of the bladder wall secondary to hematogenous dissemination (Hunner, 1915; 1918a). Subse-

quently, others (Meisser and Bumpus, 1921; Winsbury-White, 1933; Coutts and Vargas-Zalazar, 1945; Ellenberg, 1942; Stamm et al., 1980) also suggested a role for infection of the bladder lumen or wall by a variety of microorganisms. However, the inability of antibiotic therapy to relieve symptoms (Keene, 1925; Franksson, 1957; Messing and Stamey, 1978) and studies using sophisticated culturing and histologic methods (including electron microscopy) (Hanash and Pool, 1970; Collan et al., 1976) have conclusively demonstrated that no known infectious organism (with the possible exceptions of proviral forms or slow-growing viruses) in the urine or bladder is responsible for this disease.

Obstruction of Vascular and Lymphatic Channels. Based upon the finding of submucosal edema and fibrosis in interstitial cystitis (see further on), its relative frequency in middle-aged females, and clinical anecdotes that temporally relate onset or exacerbation of symptoms to pelvic infections or surgery, chronic lymphatic obstruction (Powell, 1945; Coutts and Vargas-Zalazar, 1945) and vascular insufficiency (Engel, 1939) have been proposed as etiologic factors. These mechanisms have been supported neither by experimental models (Powell, 1945; Herbst et al., 1937) nor by clinical reports of symptomatic improvement by operations such as cystocystoplasty (Turner-Warwick and Handley-Ashken, 1967) and cystolysis (Worth and Turner-Warwick, 1973; Leach and Raz, 1983; Freiha et al., 1980), which interfere with vesical lymphatic drainage and blood flow.

Neurogenic. Prompted by the prominence of pain and early reports of focal inflammation in and around intramural and perivesical nerve bundles (Hand, 1949; Smith, 1952; Franksson and Bohm, 1957), Hand proposed in 1949 that local perineuritis may be responsible for this condition. Meirowsky (1969) later demonstrated that submucosal edema, fibrosis, and mononuclear cell infiltration of the bladder without gross ulceration can be induced in monkeys by providing chronic irritative stimuli to sacral nerve roots. Based on these encouraging findings, a variety of denervating operations, including presacral neurectomy (Milner and Garlick, 1959; Pearl and Strauss, 1938; Whitfield et al., 1957; Franksson and Bohm, 1957), sacral neurectomy (Meirowsky, 1969), cystolysis (Worth and Turner-Warwick, 1973; Freiha et al., 1980; Leach and Raz, 1983), and transvaginal trigonal nerve disruption (Ingelman-Sundberg, 1959), were advocated for severely symptomatic patients. Unfortunately, the results of all of these procedures are unpredictable, and follow-up cystoscopy demonstrating true resolution in those individuals whose symptoms improved is lacking. Since sensory denervation of the bladder often increases bladder capacity (Milner and Garlick, 1959; Pearl and Strauss, 1938; Whitfield et al., 1957) and eliminates pain, follow-up cystoscopy is necessary to support a neurogenic etiology. Further discrediting such a hypothesis is the failure of several authors to confirm the histologic observations that prompted Hand's original proposal (Skoluda et al., 1974; Messing and Stamey, 1978; Collan et al., 1976).

Endocrinology. The development or exacerbation of interstitial cystitis after oophorectomy (Powell, 1944); its relative rarity in males, children, and elderly women (Oravisto, 1975); and anecdotal reports of remissions or exacerbations during pregnancy or administration of birth control pills all suggest that the sex hormonal milieu may influence the course of this disease and play a role in its etiology (Powell, 1944, 1949). However, no experimental or clinical trial has supported this contention and symptomatic responses to hormonal changes are completely unpredictable. Furthermore, because of lack of rigid diagnostic criteria and follow-up cystoscopy, those successes attributed to hormonal therapy may have occurred for other diseases (e.g., endometriosis [Warres, 1962]), that can symptomatically resemble interstitial cystitis.

Psychoneurosis. For over 50 years, urologists have been impressed that particular personality traits are common to many patients with interstitial cystitis (Hunner, 1930; Bowers et al., 1958; Walsh, 1978; Worth and Turner-Warwick, 1973). However, we are unaware of any systematic study of this factor. Because of the severity of symptoms, the length of time they have been endured before a correct diagnosis has been made, the unpredictable response to any but the most drastic treatment, and the insinuations of frustrated physicians, any evaluation of underlying neuroses would be confounded. Furthermore, we are unaware of therapeutic triumphs attributed to psychotherapy that have been confirmed by follow-up cystoscopic evaluation. Therefore, until evidence to the contrary is provided, we suggest that neurotic traits are more a response to this chronic debilitating condition than its cause.

Inflammation. Fister (1938) first pointed out similarities between interstitial cystitis and systemic lupus erythematosus (SLE), and since that time this disease has anecdotally been associated with other connective tissue (Oravisto et al., 1970; Silk, 1970; Young, 1935; Shipton, 1965) or autoimmune (Silk, 1970) disorders.

Epidemiologic similarities between interstitial cystitis and collagen diseases such as SLE; failure to demonstrate a common infectious, endocrinologic, anatomic, neurogenic, or neoplastic etiology; presence of nonspecific chronic inflammation and edema (see further on); occasional association with allergic disorders; and initially enthusiastic therapeutic trials with a variety of steroidal (Hoyt, 1952; Guerrier et al., 1965; Weaver and Tyler, 1950) and nonsteroidal (Guerrier et al., 1965; Walsh, 1978) anti-inflammatory agents have all been offered as supportive evidence. Experimentally, the most suggestive data center on a weakly positive fluorescent antinuclear antibody (FANA) test reported by Jokinen and coworkers (1972a, b) in a majority of patients with interstitial cystitis, deposits of various immunoglobulins in the mucosa and submucosa of interstitial cystitis bladders reported by Gordon and associates (1973), and the presence of antibladder antibodies in the serum of patients with interstitial cystitis found by Silk (1970), Gordon and coworkers (1973), and Grossman (1982) (against the human bladder cancer cell line T-24). For the reasons that follow, however, each of these lines of evidence must be seriously questioned.

Jokinen and colleagues (1972a) originally reported that 85 per cent of their patients had positive FANA tests in > 1:10 dilution (a very low titer, and not diagnostic of SLE); a percentage that has been reduced to 53 per cent in subsequent publications (Oravisto, 1980). Despite similarities in diagnostic criteria, we have been unable to confirm these findings (Messing and Stamey, 1978), and because of a false negative rate of at least 47 per cent, this test cannot be recommended for diagnostic purposes.

Gordon and coworkers (1973) demonstrated the presence of IgA, IgM, and IgG in the submucosa and muscle layers of the bladder in five of eight patients with interstitial cystitis. However, they also found that an even higher percentage of patients with other bladder diseases had similar immunoglobulin deposition. Normal controls were not evaluated. Jokinen and colleagues (1972b) detected no immunoglobulins in the bladder basement membrane of patients with interstitial cystitis after adsorbing fluorescein-labeled antihuman immunoglobulin with acetone-treated rat liver particles to make sure that this reagent was reacting specifically with human antibodies. Only if the adsorbent contained human immunoglobulin–like molecules could the discrepancy between the findings of Jokinen and Gordon and their coworkers be explained. We have also been unable to confirm the observations of Gordon and associates (Messing and Stamey, 1978).

Employing indirect immunofluorescence, Silk (1970) and Gordon and coworkers (1973) found circulating antibladder antibodies in the sera of 9 of 20 and 5 of 5 interstitial cystitis patients, respectively. However, after appropriately adsorbing sera from similar patients with rodent and human nonbladder target tissues to remove nonspecific antibodies, Jokinen and colleagues (1972b) were not able to confirm the findings of either Silk or Gordon and coworkers, who had not performed similar adsorptions. Grossman (1982) reported that adsorbed sera from 9 of 16 interstitial cystitis patients still reacted with a human transitional cell carcinoma cell line, T-24. However, such sera also reacted even more vigorously with melanoma and renal cell carcinoma cell line targets, and criteria used to diagnose interstitial cystitis were not rigid.

Further challenging the concept of an immune pathogenesis are clinical observations including the independent histologic studies of Skoluda and associates (1974), Collan and coworkers (1976), and Messing and Stamey (1978), who found far less inflammation than had previously been described in this disease (Smith and Dehner, 1972). Moreover, in those case reports of patients with severe SLE who developed a bladder syndrome symptomatically and cystoscopically identical to interstitial cystitis, marked vasculitis has always been seen on bladder biopsy (de la Serna and Alarcon-Segovia, 1981; Boye et al., 1979; Weisman et al., 1981), a finding notably absent from the typical interstitial cystitis bladder (see later). The highly variable response to immunosuppressants and anti-inflammatory agents (see further on) also fails to support an inflammatory mechanism. Finally, the immediate and permanent relief of all symptoms upon urinary diversion without bladder removal (Messing and Stamey, 1978) and recurrence of interstitial cystitis–like lesions in intestinal segments of patients who have undergone intestinal cystoplasties (McGuire et al., 1973; Messing and Stamey, 1978) would not be expected if inflammation directed against bladder tissue were responsible for the disease. These observations remain unexplained whether one postulates antibladder immunity (Gordon et al., 1973; Silk, 1970) or antitissue immunity with the bladder as a target organ (Oravisto, 1980).

An alternative hypothesis implicates the bladder as a shock organ for systemic allergic responses (Zondek and Bromberg, 1947). Evidence for this theory is based on two observations: (1) the increased incidence of known allergies in interstitial cystitis patients (14 to 30 per cent) (Hand, 1949; Messing and Stamey, 1978), and (2) the reported abundance of mast cells in deeper layers of the interstitial cystitis bladder. We will discuss the etiologic significance of the latter findings in the section on pathology.

Deficiencies in Bladder Lining. The glycosaminoglycans (GAG) layer on the luminal surface of the bladder's transitional epithelium may have a protective function (Parsons et al., 1980). Deficiencies in this layer may provide intraluminal agents (e.g., microorganisms, carcinogens, crystals) unusual access to the bladder wall, causing some forms of bacterial cystitis (Hanno et al., 1978), tumors (Kaufman et al., 1980), or stones (Gill et al., 1982). Parsons and colleagues (1983) have suggested that similar GAG layer deficiencies may allow normally excluded, and as yet unspecified, components of urine to reach the deeper layers of the bladder, resulting in chronic irritation as well as the symptoms, cystoscopic findings, and histologic appearance characteristic of interstitial cystitis. To support this hypothesis, they have treated patients with an oral heparin analog, sodium pentosanpolysulfate (SP-54), and have reported gratifying symptomatic relief in over 80 per cent (Parsons et al., 1983). While the details of this study will be discussed later, GAG layer deficiencies have not been demonstrated in bladder biopsies from any patient with interstitial cystitis using immunohistologic or electron microscopic techniques (Collan et al., 1976). In addition, few patients whose symptoms improved with SP-54 have undergone either follow-up cystoscopy or repeat biopsy (to demonstrate regeneration of the GAG layer). Thus, while this therapy may represent an important clinical advance (see later), the GAG layer's role in interstitial cystitis is purely speculative.

"Toxic" Substances in the Urine. A corollary to Parsons' hypothesis that defects in protective mechanisms allow substances normally present in urine to gain access to and irritate the deeper layers of the bladder wall is the suggestion that patients with interstitial cystitis may excrete abnormal amounts or types of irritants (Messing and Stamey, 1977). The bladder, because of its reservoir function, would be particularly susceptible to the effects of such agents. That substances in the urine can penetrate an intact bladder mucosa into the deeper layers has been demonstrated in rodents for several chemicals, including tryptophan and its metabolites, glycine, glucose (Morris and Bryan, 1966), and epidermal growth factor (> 5,000 MW) (Messing et al., 1984). Other agents that may be implicated include normally excreted vasoactive amines (e.g., bradykinin) and angiogenic factors (Chodak et al., 1981). To our knowledge, investigations in these directions have not been pursued.

CLINICAL PRESENTATION

History and Physical Examination. The symptoms of interstitial cystitis—intense frequency, urgency, nocturia, and suprapubic or pelvic pain that is somewhat diminished by voiding (Messing and Stamey, 1978; Hand, 1949)—are familiar to all urologists. Less than one third of patients experience burning upon urination (Messing and Stamey, 1978), which is more typical of infectious cystitis, urethritis, and tumors. Dyspareunia is not uncommon but is very hard to evaluate in patients who are experiencing such florid pelvic symptoms. Incontinence is uncommon and generally of the urgency type (Leach and Raz, 1983). Patients often will be told they have other urologic diseases, including urinary infections and prostatitis (Messing and Stamey, 1978), without objective evidence to support such diagnoses. They also may have allergies (Hand, 1949; Messing and Stamey, 1978; Rosin et al., 1979), but only rarely have pelvic, gastrointestinal, and autoimmune diseases. Even those with positive FANAs almost never have a history of collagen diseases (Jokinen et al., 1972a; Messing and Stamey, 1978). Physical examination (including pelvic and neurologic examinations) is usually normal (Messing and Stamey, 1978), although increased anterior vaginal tenderness (Lapides, 1975) may be elicited.

Laboratory Tests. Urinalysis and culture and cytologic examination of the urine remain the most important laboratory investigations. Urinalysis is usually normal, with less than 10 per cent of patients having more than five red blood cells per high power field, and no more than 30 per cent having more than five white cells per high power field (and only one third of these having more than ten white cells per high power field [Messing and Stamey, 1978]). Cultures are invariably sterile, since the diagnosis of interstitial cystitis cannot be made in the face of bacterial, fungal, mycobacterial, chlamydial, parasitic, mycoplasmal, gonococcal, or other infections. In patients with recurrent or persistent bacteriuria, sterilization of the urine must

be accomplished and maintained for protracted periods before a diagnosis of interstitial cystitis is possible. Since carcinoma in situ can present with identical symptoms and cystoscopic findings, urinary or bladder lavage specimens must not contain atypical cells on cytologic examination (Utz and Zincke, 1974; Smith and Badenoch, 1965; Walsh, 1978; Messing and Stamey, 1978). The role of prostatic massage in diagnosing this condition appears to be limited to ruling out other causes of irritative voiding symptoms, and we are unaware of abnormal prostatic secretions occurring in men with interstitial cystitis. We no longer routinely test for FANA, since it appears to be of little diagnostic value or demonstrated utility as a marker of disease progression, remission, or response to treatment in those individuals with a positive test (Jokinen et al., 1972a, b).

Radiologic Studies. With the exception of ruling out other disorders, radiographic studies such as intravenous urography and voiding and static cystography are of no value in diagnosing interstitial cystitis. They should be performed if indicated by findings on urinalysis, physical examination, or history and as a baseline measurement prior to the institution of various therapeutic modalities (particularly open surgery). In our experience, most patients have undergone these studies prior to referral.

Cystoscopy. Since there are no other objective findings, the diagnosis of interstitial cystitis requires cystoscopy. With the possible exception of infectious (particularly tuberculous or fungal), toxic (e.g., cyclophosphamide, formalin), and radiation cystitises, and neoplasms (particularly carcinoma in situ), we are unaware of other diseases with a cystoscopic picture similar to the one described by Hand (1949), Walsh (1978), and ourselves (Messing and Stamey, 1978). It is critical to recognize, however, that two cystoscopic findings often associated with interstitial cystitis, a reduced bladder capacity and a Hunner's (or for that matter, any) ulcer are frequently not found (Hand, 1949; Oravisto and Alfthan, 1976; Walsh, 1978; Messing and Stamey, 1978). The herald lesions of this disease are "glomerulations" (Walsh, 1978): pinpoint petechial hemorrhages that develop throughout the bladder after hydrodistention under 70 cm of water pressure (Table 24–1). Anesthesia is usually required to allow sufficient distention of the bladder for the petechiae to be detected (Table 24–2) (Messing and Stamey, 1978; Kastrup et al., 1983).

We have divided our patients into two categories based upon bladder capacity under

TABLE 24–1. Cystoscopic Evaluation

Evaluation Data	Early (N = 28)	Classic (N = 24)
Bladder capacity >450 cc	27	1
With anesthesia <450 cc	1	23
Bloody drainage of fluid (last 50 to 100 cc)		
Yes	25	23
No	1	0
Not described	2	1
Hunner's ulcer		
Yes	0	15
No	28	9
Fissures, linear scars		
Yes	0	23
No	26	0
Not described	2	1
Glomerulations		
Many	20	17
Few	8	6
Not described	0	1
"Splotchy" hemorrhages		
Many	7	20
Few	15	4
Not described	6	0
Trabeculations		
Many	2	3
Few	3	6
None	16	2
Not described	7	13
Other abnormalities		
Yes	1	4
No	27	18
Not described	0	2

From Messing, E. M., and Stamey, T. A.: Urology, *12*:381, 1978. Used by permission.

anesthesia. These groups roughly correspond to the stages of Hand (1949) and Oravisto and Alfthan (1976). During the first distention in a patient with over 400-ml capacity, the bladder looks normal or has only faint trabeculations. After capacity is reached, the terminal portion of the drained irrigating fluid is blood-tinged. Upon redistention, glomerulations appear, often in unequal distribution, throughout the bladder (Walsh, 1978; Messing and Stamey, 1978). During the initial passage of the cystoscope, and at the time of the first emptying, the endoscopist must take care to avoid traumatizing the wall of the bladder. A diagnosis of interstitial cystitis cannot be made if the only areas of hemorrhage result from the collapsed bladder hitting the cystoscope's tip. In those individuals whose capacity is below 400 ml, the initial distention usually reveals scars and fissures that crack and ooze blood as capacity is reached. Again, the terminal portion of the evacuated irrigating fluid is bloody, and upon redistention, glomerulations appear often in the same distribution and density as occur in patients with large-capacity interstitial cystitis. We have made an extensive effort to quantitate these findings, but observe that with the possible exception of bladder capacity (Messing and Stamey, 1978; Hand, 1949), severity of symptoms rarely correlates with degree of endoscopic pathology.

TABLE 24–2. Cystoscopy With and Without Anesthesia in Patients With Early or Classic Interstitial Cystitis

	Interstitial Cystitis			
	Early (N = 9)		Classic (N = 7)	
	Anesthesia			
Evaluation	With	Without	With	Without
Bladder capacity	9	2	1	0
> 450 cc	0	7	6	7
< 450 cc				
Bloody fluid (last 50 to 100 cc	9	2	6	1
Yes	0	7	0	5
No	0	0	1	1
Not described				
Hunner's ulcer	0	0	6	2
Yes	9	9	1	5
No				
Fissure, scar	0	0	7	4
Yes	9	9	0	3
No				
Glomerulation	9	1	7	0
Yes	0	7	0	7
No	0	1	0	0
Not described				
"Splotchy" hemorrhages	9	3	7	4
Yes	0	6	0	3
No				

Reprinted with permission from the article "Interstital Cystitis, Early Diagnosis, Pathology, and Treatment". From Messing, E. M., and Stamey, T. A.: Urology, *12*:381, 1978. Used by permission.

We have performed cystoscopy on many patients under anesthesia who had intrinsically normal bladders (Messing and Stamey, 1978) (those women undergoing endoscopic suspension of the vesical neck for stress urinary incontinence [Stamey, 1973]) or various forms of vesical pathology and are convinced that findings typical of interstitial cystitis are rarely present in other individuals. Although patients with both large and small bladders (under anesthesia) appear to have the same disease, we are unaware (both in our experience and from the literature) of individuals who have converted from one type of cystoscopic appearance to the other (spontaneously or with therapy) (Oravisto, 1975).

Histopathology. Despite numerous attempts at histopathologic description (Bumpus, 1921; Collan et al., 1976; Smith, 1952; Simmons, 1961; Smith and Dehner, 1972; Jacobo et al., 1974, Skoluda et al., 1974; Messing and Stamey, 1978), the diagnosis of interstitial cystitis remains entirely based on clinical and cystoscopic criteria. Lack of uniformity in reports can be attributed to several factors, including marked variation in patient selection and lack of appropriate normal and pathologic controls. Biopsies are also of dubious clinical value because they are often of inadequate depth (Messing and Stamey, 1978) and necessary stains are not performed.

Of the recent studies on this subject, the one by Smith and Dehner (1972) is the most influential. However, these authors selected material from cases in the Armed Forces Institute of Pathology files that fit "historical criteria of a chronic edematous pan-cystitis with mast cell infiltration and a poor therapeutic response" rather than studying pathologic specimens from all patients with clinical histories and cystoscopic findings typical of interstitial cystitis. Furthermore, over 80 per cent of their patients who had urine cultured had infected urine at the time of biopsy, a situation not typical of interstitial cystitis. Finally, these authors did not examine any control specimens. In two more recent publications by a different group (Larsen et al., 1982; Kastrup et al., 1983) the diagnosis of interstitial cystitis was based primarily on symptomatology rather than upon cystoscopic findings. At least one quarter of their patients lacked the development of glomerulations after bladder distention and would have been eliminated (using the criteria outlined in this chapter) from other reports (Oravisto and Alfthan, 1976; Messing and Stamey, 1978). Larsen and colleagues (1982) studied biopsies from an ill-defined group of poorly matched patients (pathologic controls) and used no normal controls. Kastrup and coworkers (1983) provided sex- and age-matched pathologic controls but failed to define their underlying disease, leading the reader to conclude that more than one third of their controls may have had interstitial cystitis. Such deficiencies are not unique to these two studies. For example, in our own report we included age- and sex-matched normal controls but studied a highly heterogeneous population of pathologic controls with a limited number of subjects in each group (Messing and Stamey, 1978). The absence of controls has also detracted from the value of studies by Hand (1949), Hunner (1914), Walsh (1978), and Collan and coworkers (1976).

Histologic abnormalities are found in all areas of the bladder that contain any endoscopic evidence of disease and do not reflect the degree of cystoscopic pathology noted in the particular biopsy site (Hand, 1949). Thus, it makes little difference in what region biopsy is done as long as it has some endoscopic evidence of interstitial cystitis. The classic description of a chronic, transmural pancystitis with marked involvement of deeper layers with inflammation and fibrosis (Hand, 1949; Smith and Dehner, 1972) has been expanded to include a broader picture of a normal mucosa, edema and vasodilation of the lamina propria, and only occasional inflammation or fibrosis in the muscularis (Messing and Stamey, 1978; Collan et al., 1976; Skoluda et al., 1974). Walsh (1978) reported an eosinophil infiltrate in the submucosa and muscularis, but this has not been seen by others (Messing and Stamey, 1978; Collan et al., 1976; Kastrup et al., 1983; Smith and Dehner, 1972). Similarly, perineural inflammation has been reported (Smith and Dehner, 1972; Hand, 1949; Smith, 1952; Kinder and Smith, 1958) without confirmation by other researchers (Messing and Stamey, 1978; Collan et al., 1976; Kastrup et al., 1983). Thus, even the concept of a nonspecific chronic inflammatory infiltrate through all layers of the bladder, previously considered typical of this disease, has not been substantiated.

Using similar criteria for patient selection, a number of investigators (Collan et al., 1976; Skoluda et al., 1974; Messing and Stamey, 1978) concluded that under routine hematoxylin and eosin examination with light microscopy, the single abnormality invariably found was submucosal edema and vasodilation. Thus, H & E examination reveals no pathognomonic findings and does not suggest etiology.

Several groups have reported that an abundance of mast cells appears to reside in the deeper layers of the bladder (Simmons and Bunce, 1958; Bohne et al., 1962; Silk, 1970; Smith and Dehner, 1972; Collan et al., 1976; DeJuana and Everett, 1977; Larsen et al., 1982; Kastrup et al., 1983). Since, under appropriate immunologic or mechanical stimulation, these cells are known to release granules containing vasoactive amines that cause smooth muscle contraction and neural stimulation (Riley and West, 1953; Fisher, 1960), this finding may be of etiologic, mechanistic, and therapeutic importance. Special stains that interact with heparin (toluidine blue, Giemsa) (Lillie, 1965; Pearse, 1968) or enzymes (Leder, 1964; Pearse, 1968) contained within the granules must be performed for their identification. In addition, deep biopsies are essential, since if an increased number of mast cells exists, it occurs only in the muscularis (Messing and Stamey, 1978; Kastrup et al., 1983). Since mast cells are found in normal bladders (Messing and Stamey, 1978), suitable controls are required to demonstrate their abundance in interstitial cystitis. Employing highly quantitative methodology, Larsen (1982) and Kastrup (1983) and their coworkers found a statistically significant increase in the number of mast cells in the muscular layers of bladders with interstitial cystitis. Using somewhat less rigid quantification, we did not find such a difference (Messing and Stamey, 1978). Variations in subject and control populations may explain this discrepancy. Interestingly, a statistically significant increase in the amount of histamine in the bladders of interstitial cystitis patients could not be shown by Kastrup and associates (1983), thus rendering the observation of mast cell abundance of uncertain significance.

A particularly intriguing finding by Larsen and coworkers (1982) was that, of 11 patients with symptoms characteristic of interstitial cystitis but without typical cystoscopic findings, 7 had an increased number of mast cells in the muscularis. Further follow-up of these patients is awaited, since if they subsequently develop appropriate cystoscopic abnormalities, mast cells may be implicated in the etiology or may serve as an important marker of interstitial cystitis.

While these findings are of interest, they are of negligible value to the urologist trying to make a diagnosis. Even if the appropriate special stains are performed and muscle is included in the biopsy, impractically rigid scoring criteria, which count the number of mast cells in the muscularis per mm^2 of tissue, must be adhered

to in order to attain the 12 per cent false negative and a 5 per cent false positive rates reported by Kastrup and colleagues (1983). Moreover, false positive and false negative rates triple if an error of one or two is made in the average number of mast cells counted. Thus, to make these observations applicable to the routine clinical situation, a pathologist who is relatively unfamiliar with the deeper layers of the bladder* and with special mast cell stains must count mast cells accurately in a precisely measured area of tissue.

Other Tests. The majority of interstitial cystitis patients are women, and symptoms sometimes fluctuate with menstrual and menopausal events and may be mimicked by conditions such as endometriosis. For these reasons, many patients referred to us have previously been subjected to extensive gynecologic evaluations, including pelvic ultrasound, CAT scan, laparoscopy, and even laparotomy. Although undoubtedly indicated in some patients, these studies clearly do not assist in the diagnosis of interstitial cystitis.

Similarly, we have found urodynamic studies to be irrelevant unless physical findings, the presence of marked incontinence, or the absence of pain as a prominent clinical feature indicate a need for their performance. Unanesthetized interstitial cystitis patients almost always have such reduced bladder capacity and pelvic discomfort that artifactual information is obtained. This leads to misdiagnoses and delays the institution of effective therapy. We are convinced, however, that urodynamic studies should be performed prior to most of the open surgical procedures to be discussed in the next section.

TREATMENT

General Principles. Interstitial cystitis is an uncommon disease of uncertain etiology that can be promptly and accurately diagnosed—but rarely is. Responsibility for this delay must be shared by nonurologic physicians to whom patients present and urologists who lack awareness of the simple means required to establish a diagnosis. However, even the knowledgeable urologist may procrastinate in his evaluation because he knows that interstitial cystitis neither

---

*Even academic pathologists with an abiding professional interest in the subject cannot agree more than 50 per cent of the time if an infiltrating transitional cell carcinoma of the bladder invades the muscularis (Gilchrist, 1983).

is a threat to health nor, with the exception of total urinary diversion, does it have any certain or simple treatment. Guidelines for its management include awareness and acceptance by both physician and patient that (1) the disease offers little actual risk to health and life; (2) it is almost never a manifestation of an underlying disease that does present such a risk; (3) symptoms rarely progress and occasionally abate spontaneously (Oravisto, 1975); (4) delaying therapy does not render the patient less likely to respond when treatment is given or more likely to have worsening of symptoms, bladder capacity, or cystoscopic appearance; and (5) using available modalities, symptoms may be made tolerable but rarely will be totally and permanently eliminated.

While such explanations do little for a physician's sense of effectiveness, they are greatly appreciated by patients who have been offered numerous diagnoses and unsuccessful remedies and whose motives and emotional stability have been questioned by frustrated physicians, by relatives and friends, and by themselves. In addition, such candor reassures patients who may fear that they harbor a life-threatening disease, and it is of great help in planning and administering effective treatment. This approach can be employed only by the urologist who has established the diagnosis using the criteria outlined.

Traditional therapy for interstitial cystitis has been clinically and scientifically unsatisfactory. Many regimens have been heralded in preliminary reports, only to be abandoned within several years (a fate sure to befall some discussed below). Therapeutic modalities have included systemic and topical medications as well as endoscopic and open surgery. Open surgical procedures have been designed to reduce bladder sensation, increase bladder capacity, or prevent urine from contacting the bladder. Some examples of each follow, including some of primarily historical interest.

A. Medical therapy
  1. Systemic medication
    a. Removal of allergenic foods plus intramuscular injection of adrenalin (Duke, 1922).
    b. Intravenous injection of Mercurochrome (Eisenstadt and McDougall, 1931); gold sodium thiosulfate with bismuth intramuscularly (Fister, 1938); intramuscular injections of emetine hydrochloride (Henline, 1941); emetine chloride (Kreutzman, 1941); and ACTH (Weaver and Tyler, 1950).
    c. Oral administration of estrogen (Powell, 1944); potassium iodide (Hand, 1949); α-tocopherol (Van Dusen and Mustain, 1951); banthine (Riskind and Zide, 1952); and potassium para-amino benzoate (McCrea, 1960).
    d. Oral administration of steroidal (cortisone [Hoyt, 1952], prednisolone [Guerrier et al., 1965]) and nonsteroidal (oxyphenbutazone [Guerrier et al., 1965] and benzydamine [Walsh, 1978]) anti-inflammatory agents.
    e. Administration of antihistamines (Pyribenzamine [Simmons and Bunce, 1958] and cimetidine) or mast cell–stabilizing factors such as heparin (Weaver et al., 1963).
    f. Oral administration of sodium pentosanpolysulfate (SP-54) (Parsons et al., 1983).
  2. Local treatment
    a. Catheter drainage (Keyes, 1922).
    b. Bladder distention by tidal irrigations (Longacre, 1936); condom (Bohne and Fetz, 1954); balloon catheter (Kearns, 1932); delayed micturition (Ormond, 1937); or hydraulic distention (Bumpus, 1930).
    c. Intravesical instillation of bichloride of mercury (Hunner, 1914); gomenol oil (Hunner, 1914); boric acid (Hunner, 1914); Thompson fluid (Hunner, 1914); silver iodide (Keene, 1920); Argyrol (Stevens, 1923); Mercurochrome (Keene, 1925); triphenylmethane (Davis, 1941); Amniotin oil (Eiknev, 1941); cajuput oil (Baker and Callahan, 1959); iodophor (Warres, 1962); histamine and hyaluronidase (Powell, 1949); dimethyl sulfoxide (DMSO) (Stewart et al., 1967; Fowler, 1981; Ek et al., 1978); silver nitrate (Dodson, 1926; Pool and Rives, 1944; Hanash and Poole, 1970); or Clorpactin WCS-90 (Wishard et al., 1957; O'Conor, 1955; Murnaghan et al., 1969; Messing and Stamey, 1978).
    d. Transcutaneous electrical nerve stimulation (Fall et al., 1980).
B. Surgical procedures
  1. Endoscopic
    a. Urethral and ureteral dilation (Hunner, 1920).
    b. Local injections directly into and around ulcers with absolute alcohol (Alexander and Christi, 1936); ad-

renalin and procaine (Rose, 1951); Hydrocortone hyaluronidase (Shulte and Reynolds, 1956), and hydrocortisone (Weaver et al., 1963).

c. Prolonged bladder distention with the Helmstein balloon (Walsh, 1978), including use with bladder rupture (Higson et al., 1978).

d. Endoscopic resection (Greenberg et al., 1974), or fulguration (Barnes, 1947; Kreutzmann, 1922).

2. Open surgical procedures

a. Open resection (Hunner, 1914; Geraghty, 1917; Reed, 1919; Herbst, 1920) and fulguration (Furniss, 1917; Kretschmer, 1920) of ulcers.

b. Reduce bladder sensation

(1) Neurosurgical procedures, including resection of presacral nerves (Learmonth, 1931; Quinby, 1931); presacral neurectomy and sacral ganglionectomy (Pearl and Strauss, 1938); anterolateral cordotomy (Nesbit, 1947); and differential sacral neurectomy (Moulder and Meirowsky, 1956).

(2) Bladder denervations via transvaginal approach (Ingelman-Sundberg, 1959); cystocystoplasty (Turner-Warwick and Handley Ashken, 1967; Worth and Turner-Warwick, 1973); and cystolysis (Worth and Turner-Warwick, 1973; Freiha and Stamey, 1980; Leach and Raz, 1983).

c. Bladder augmentation, including ileo- (Ferris, 1955), sigmoidal, and cecocystoplasties (von Garrelts, 1966), without and with supertrigonal cystectomy (McGuire et al., 1973; Badenoch, 1971).

d. Urinary diversion with or without cystectomy, including ureterosigmoidostomy (Lower and Schlumberger, 1939) and ileal loop (Badenoch, 1971).

This plethora of treatments implies that each one is only partially effective and that most clinicians fail to confirm preliminary enthusiastic reports. Only those measures that remain in vogue will be discussed in the following sections.

Treatment During Diagnostic Cystoscopy. Since the diagnosis of interstitial cystitis requires hydraulic distention during the cystoscopic examination under anesthesia, it should be remembered that this procedure alone has been known to be of therapeutic value for over 50 years (Bumpus, 1930). Although degree of distention and criteria to determine responsiveness vary, approximately 30 per cent of patients are afforded considerable, if temporary, relief by this treatment. To be considered efficacious, all proposed therapies must therefore improve upon this standard.

Kerr (1971) and Greenberg and coworkers (1974) have independently advocated transurethral fulguration and resection of visible ulcers at diagnosis but have indicated that recurrences are frequent. Both studies claimed considerable improvement after such treatment but failed to cite criteria for this conclusion. We have observed minimal success with this modality (Messing and Stamey, 1978), and it is clearly useless in individuals with no ulcers.

Systemic Agents. Systemic treatment with steroidal and nonsteroidal anti-inflammatory agents and with immunosuppressants has been suggested once hydraulic distention is performed and interstitial cystitis diagnosed conclusively. Corticosteroids have been found to be effective by Badenoch (1971) in 70 per cent of patients; however, recurrence rates, duration of remissions, and complications of therapy are not discussed. This series is the largest and most optimistic, but we agree with Walsh (1978) that "the response to steroids is totally unpredictable and . . . in cases in which there is a response the dose needed is considerable" (Walsh, 1978; Messing and Stamey, 1978).

Azathioprine and, to a lesser degree, chloroquine and/or oxychloroquine with aspirin were found by Oravisto and Alfthan (1976) to relieve pain in 50 to 60 per cent of patients but were far less effective for reducing urinary frequency. A starting dose of 150 mg of azathioprine was given daily and was tapered to 50 to 100 mg per day after subjective improvement occurred (usually within 2 weeks). Therapy was well tolerated but histologic or cystoscopic follow-up in apparent successes was not discussed. We are unaware of reports confirming these findings and have no experience with the use of these agents for interstitial cystitis.

Benzydamine (1-benzo-3-[3-(dimethylamino)propoxy]-1 H-indazole) is an anti-inflammatory analgesic, which was reported by Walsh in 1978 to eliminate pain in 73 per cent of his patients. As with azathioprine, frequency was not markedly relieved and cystoscopic appearance rarely changed. This drug is not available in this country, but we found it of no value in two patients who obtained it from abroad.

Anti-H-1 histamines, such as Pyribenzamine, or systemic or local heparin instillations

(Simmons, 1961; Weaver et al., 1963) have been employed because of reports of excess mast cells in the interstitial cystitis bladder. The results of these treatments have not been encouraging (DeJuana and Everett, 1977).

Parsons and associates (1983) presented a series in which 83.5 per cent of patients experienced subjective clinical improvement after oral ingestion of the heparin analog sodium pentosanpolysulfate (SP-54). Symptomatic relief required continued treatment and rarely occurred before 3 months. No patient experienced complications from long-term administration of this medication. The rationale for its use is to supplement the GAG layer, which these investigators suggest is deficient in interstitial cystitis. However, there is no evidence to support this contention (in interstitial cystitis or any other human disease) or that this medication could reverse such a deficiency if it did exist. Furthermore, criteria for inclusion of patients and evaluation of therapeutic responses are scant in this report. SP-54 is still unavailable for general use, but follow-up of the initial series by Parsons and coworkers with independent confirmation is eagerly awaited.

Local Instillations

DIMETHYL SULFOXIDE (DMSO). Since the initial report by Stewart and colleagues in 1967, several subsequent reports by this group (Stewart et al., 1972; Shirley et al., 1978) and others (Ek et al., 1978; Fowler, 1981) have confirmed moderate efficacy with minimal toxicity (transient elevation of serum lactate dehydrogenase) for DMSO. Owing to its strict adherence to diagnostic criteria, Fowler's study is probably the most pertinent. He found complete symptomatic relief in 15 per cent of patients and mild improvement in another 65 per cent, which was usually sustained for at least 4 months. Continuous therapy was required. Improvements were strictly subjective, with little measurable change in bladder capacity noted. Although far more limited than that of most of the reported series, our experience with DMSO has been much less favorable. However, this remedy has achieved widespread popularity in this country and abroad, in large part because of its relative benignity and ease of administration (it requires neither anesthesia nor inpatient care). All authors have followed the protocol outlined by Shirley and coworkers (1978).

CLORPACTIN WCS-90. While initial successes independently reported by Wishard and associates (1957) and OConor (1955) using 0.2 per cent Clorpactin WCS-90 instillations were not widely accepted, the report by Murnaghan

and colleagues (1969) has been confirmed by our group (Messing and Stamey, 1978). Seventy-two per cent of patients in our series experienced dramatic and sustained improvement following several intravesical instillations of a 0.4 per cent solution of Clorpactin WCS-90. As many as six instillations (the first two given at 4-week intervals and the last four given weekly or every other week) constituted a course of therapy. Hydraulic distention was not performed with each instillation, and thus therapeutic response could not be attributed to the effects of repeat hydraulic distentions. Each treatment required full anesthesia. With the exception of severe irritative symptoms for a day or two (often requiring narcotic analgesics and anticholinergics), instillations were well tolerated (Messing and Stamey, 1978) if vesicoureteral reflux was not present (Messing and Freiha, 1979). These observations continue to hold true, and we have noted that at least one third of patients achieve nearly total long-lasting relief after only one or two instillations. We therefore routinely instill Clorpactin at the time of initial cystoscopic examination under anesthesia (see further on). However, owing to the inconvenience, discomfort, expense, and risks (primarily of multiple anesthetics), we take great effort to involve patients in the decision to proceed with repeated treatments.

SILVER NITRATE. Silver nitrate in combination with bladder fulguration can improve symptoms temporarily in approximately 50 per cent of patients (Pool and Rives, 1944; DeJuana and Everett, 1977; Hand, 1949; Burford and Burford, 1958). However, diagnostic and response criteria are obscure in most studies claiming such benefit. In the technique outlined by Pool and Rives (1944), hospitalization is required for each instillation and patients with vesicoureteral reflux are to be excluded from treatment.

Open Surgery. While the list of surgical procedures proposed for treating interstitial cystitis is substantial, it is generally believed that such therapy should be reserved for patients who fail conservative management with several established modalities. We also feel that prior to any open surgical procedure for this disease, urodynamic evaluation (unnecessary for urinary diversion) and radiographic studies should be obtained to provide baseline information for objective postoperative evaluation.

BLADDER DENERVATION. Pain relief has been reported following neurosurgical procedures, including presacral neurectomy, bilateral cordotomy, and selected sacral neurectomies and rhizotomies. However, these procedures are suboptimal because localized denervation can be accomplished by operations that approach these nerves at an end-organ level, thus avoiding side effects inherent with more proximal nerve sectioning (where selectivity can less accurately be achieved). Although essentially of historical interest, these operations should be kept in mind if intractable pain persists and patients are not candidates for total urinary diversion.

LOCALIZED DENERVATION. Turner-Warwick and Handley-Ashken in 1967 described a localized bladder denervation operation for interstitial cystitis—cystocystoplasty. This procedure consisted of a supertrigonal transection of the bladder, transection of the inferior vesical pedicles and nerves, and reanastomosis of the fundus of the bladder to the trigone. To avoid devascularization, care was taken not to interfere with the superior vesical pedicles or the peritoneal attachments of the bladder. While an impressive case report was presented in this and a subsequent publication, no data were provided to document a "generally satisfactory experience" with this procedure (Worth and Turner-Warwick, 1973). The second paper described a new operation, cystolysis, in which bladder denervation was achieved by blunt dissection and transection of the superior vesical and the ascending branches of the inferior vesical neurovascular pedicles with careful preservation of the ureteric sheath. The anterior bladder wall was attached to the posterior rectus muscle to prevent the bladder from falling into the pelvis. Distal and posterior dissection was not mentioned. Although periods of follow-up were variable and in many cases brief, the authors claimed total relief of pain in all individuals and considerable improvement in voiding frequency in 9 of 11. Worth and Turner-Warwick emphasized that preoperative bladder capacity under anesthesia must be normal to realize a favorable result. Worth (1980) published a long-term follow-up, and while statistics were not provided, results were not as favorable as initially reported. However, the author concluded that "good symptomatic improvement" occurred in "the majority of" correctly selected patients. More recently, Freiha and Stamey (1980) and Leach and Raz (1983) performed modifications of this operation on patients refractory to "medical management," with improvement noted in 5 of 5 patients from the former series and 14 of 15 patients in the latter. In both series, however, follow-up was brief and few patients experienced total elimination of symptoms. Urodynamic data presented by both groups demonstrate that postoperative urinary retention can occur, which requires intermittent catheterization on a long-term or permanent basis. The limited anecdotal experience reported by Walsh (1978) of complications should remind the occasional performer of this operation that it is still experimental and not without risk. As with most treatments, in no series have follow-up cystoscopies been reported in patients considered to be surgical successes.

Although others may disagree (Walsh, 1982, personal communication to T. A. Stamey), we believe that individuals with truly intractable symptoms (particularly pain) and normal bladder capacity under anesthesia should be offered cystolysis. However, candidates must understand that relief is not guaranteed and that intermittent catheterization may be necessary.

AUGMENTATION CYSTOPLASTY. Cystolysis or cystocystoplasty will not effectively reduce urinary frequency in those individuals who have small-capacity bladders (under anesthesia). For such patients, intestinal cystoplasty has been recommended (Worth and Turner-Warwick, 1973). As several groups have pointed out, supertrigonal cystectomy is essential in order to prevent symptomatic and cystoscopic recurrences (Worth and Turner-Warwick, 1973; McGuire et al., 1973; Messing and Stamey, 1978).

This differs from operations described for contracted bladders from other causes (e.g., tuberculous cystitis), in which considerably more bladder is retained to further maximize capacity without allowing the intestinal segment to function as a diverticulum. We generally prefer performing cecocystoplasties. Persistent mucousuria and difficulties in bladder emptying (particularly in males) may necessitate prolonged intermittent catheterization and must be discussed with patients prior to surgery. Prior to patient selection, it is important to determine that there is no endoscopic evidence of interstitial cystitis on the trigone. Preoperative cystoscopy demonstrated considerable involvement of the trigone in the two individuals we have seen who have had symptomatic and endoscopic recurrences after intestinal cystoplasties. Since this operation is associated with considerable morbidity, we do not recommend it for patients with trigonal involvement under the rationale that little is lost and total urinary diversion can always eventually be performed. Our limited personal experience is not as favorable as that reported by Worth and Turner-Warwick (1973) and nearly parallels that of Smith and coworkers (1977), in which approximately two thirds of patients experienced excellent or total relief (Freiha et al., 1980). We currently recommend this operation for individuals with small-capacity bladders whose trigones are free of endoscopic evidence of interstitial cystitis.

URINARY DIVERSION. For the patient who has failed all other forms of therapy, total urinary diversion can essentially guarantee immediate and permanent cure (Messing and Stamey, 1978; Freiha et al., 1980). Cystectomy is not necessary to achieve this relief, and it is our experience that even patients who have not had their bladders removed awaken from surgery aware that their pain is entirely gone. We perform a cystectomy at the time of diversion in qualified older patients, since we have cared for three individuals (Messing and Stamey, 1978; Messing and Freiha, 1979) who have required subsequent cystectomy for pyovesica or the development of carcinoma in the defunctionalized bladder. In younger patients we have been more reluctant to remove the bladder owing to the (albeit unlikely) possibility that a medical remedy for this disease may be forthcoming. In defense of this policy, to our knowledge the only case in which a patient has not experienced total symptomatic relief with urinary diversion without cystectomy was reported by Wishard and coworkers (1957). In this instance culture data were not obtained, so we cannot determine whether persistence of interstitial cystitis or an infectious process made the delayed cystectomy necessary.

GUIDELINES FOR DIAGNOSIS AND MANAGEMENT

Diagnostic Evaluation. Regardless of age or sex, individuals with symptoms of interstitial cystitis, and at times those with just severe frequency and urgency (Messing and Stamey, 1978) who have sterile, microscopically clear urine, warrant cystoscopy under anesthesia to diagnose (or rule out) interstitial cystitis. Patients with pyuria should have appropriate cultures (including those for *Chlamydia* [Stamm et al., 1980], mycobacteria, fungi, *N. gonorrhoeae* and *Ureaplasma*) to document sterility of the urinary tract prior to endoscopy. If the history is suggestive (e.g., sexual promiscuity or urethritis in consorts) or if cultures are difficult to obtain, a therapeutic trial with an antibiotic for *Chlamydia* or *Ureaplasma* (e.g., tetracycline, doxycycline, or erythromycin [Stamm et al., 1981]) is not unreasonable. Extensive gynecologic evaluation and trials of hormonal therapy

are not needed unless physical examination or history indicates the presence of pelvic masses, endometriosis, or other conditions that may symptomatically resemble interstitial cystitis.

Once the urologist is satisfied that the patient has neither an infectious nor a neoplastic process, and unless the history indicates a need for other studies (e.g., urodynamics for severe incontinence), we recommend cystoscopy under anesthesia. We obtain urinary cytology prior to cystoscopy, not because the result would influence our decision to perform this procedure, but because our examination and biopsy regimen would be entirely different if we suspected carcinoma in situ, which in our experience and that of others (Utz and Zincke, 1974; Smith and Badenoch, 1965) may be indistinguishable endoscopically from interstitial cystitis. Cystoscopy without full anesthesia is not undertaken, since it is usually unsatisfactory for diagnosing interstitial cystitis (Messing and Stamey, 1978; Hand, 1949; Kastrup et al., 1983) and patients find the procedure intolerable.

When the diagnosis has been established, we recommend that biopsies be performed to eliminate serious conditions that endoscopically and symptomatically may be mistaken for interstitial cystitis, such as carcinoma in situ or eosinophilic and toxic cystitises. If diffuse involvement of the bladder wall is encountered, a single biopsy from a representative area will suffice. However, individual biopsies must be done on particularly suspicious areas or a focal area of malignancy may be overlooked. Since the primary need for the biopsy is to rule out other more serious diseases and not to diagnose interstitial cystitis (see earlier), we believe that the cold-cup technique, which minimizes mucosal destruction, should be employed. Unless discrete ulcers are seen, we have not found it beneficial to fulgurate any areas but biopsy sites.

After biopsy and fulguration are completed, and if our findings are consistent with a diagnosis of interstitial cystitis, we instill one liter of a 0.4 per cent solution of Clorpactin WCS-90 under 15 to 20 cm of water pressure (Messing and Stamey, 1978). This is done without performing cystography unless we infer from the configuration or position of the ureteral orifices that vesicoureteral reflux may be present. We have noted no serious complication from the instillation of this agent at the time of bladder biopsy (Messing and Stamey, 1978), although treatment is withheld if bladder perforation is suspected. Because we question the role of biopsy in diagnosing interstitial cystitis, we do not wait for histopathologic confirmation of our clinical and endoscopic impression before giving Clorpactin. However, we do not instill it in individuals with irritative voiding symptoms who lack the cystoscopic features of interstitial cystitis, since we have not found this treatment helpful in these patients.

Thus, at the time of the diagnostic examination under anesthesia, we not only perform hydrodistention but administer the first Clorpactin instillation. Once the diagnosis is established, we counsel the patient on what is known about this condition, stressing the following positive features: (1) the likelihood that no further progression or deterioration will occur; (2) that interstitial cystitis does not pose a risk to health or life; (3) that at least 10 per cent of patients experience lasting spontaneous remissions (Oravisto, 1975); and (4) that with the combination of a single hydraulic distention (under 70 cm of water pressure) and one Clorpactin WCS-90 instillation, over 25 per cent of patients receive the only treatment necessary (Messing and Stamey, 1978). Patients usually find this information, as well as the confirmation that an organic disease is responsible for their symptoms, reassuring.

If symptoms have not been satisfactorily relieved in 1 month, a second Clorpactin instillation is recommended (Messing and Stamey, 1978). Although in our 1978 series hydrodistention was not performed on any but the initial instillation in order to distinguish therapeutic effects, we see no reason to avoid combining these. If symptoms at this stage are not very severe, we encourage patients to refrain from further Clorpactin treatments unless exacerbations occur. For those individuals whose symptoms have not been sufficiently relieved by the first two Clorpactin instillations to warrant expectant management, and who, because of logistic, financial, medical, or discomfort reasons are reluctant to undergo several additional weekly instillations of Clorpactin, we suggest a series of DMSO treatments as described by Stewart and coworkers (1967). It is possible that we have observed fewer successes with this agent than other authors have because we do not treat patients with minimal symptoms or those with favorable responses to one or two Clorpactin instillations.

None of our patients who failed the second Clorpactin instillation have responded to standard systemic medications (e.g., anti-inflammatory agents, antihistamines, anticholinergics, tranquilizers, β-adrenergics, and analgesics, alone or in combination). However, over 50 per cent have been dramatically helped by repeated Clorpactin instillations. Alternative modalities that are still experimental include trials with sodium pentosanpolysulfate (which currently can be given only by Dr. Parsons; see earlier) or an oral inhibitor of mast cell degranulation, ketotifen (Greenwood, 1982) (obtained through contact with Dr. Robert Burns of Sandoz Laboratories), on the presumption that increased mast cell activity may be responsible for some of the symptoms in this disease.

Occasionally, patients fail to improve despite undergoing full courses of Clorpactin instillations and are not satisfied in knowing that their symptoms are unlikely to worsen. Carefully advising them of complications such as prolonged urinary retention, and without guaranteeing cure, we recommend cystolysis if they have a large-capacity bladder, and cecocystoplasty with supertrigonal cystectomy if they have a small-capacity bladder without endoscopic evidence of interstitial cystitis involving the trigone. Urinary diversion is reserved for patients who have failed these operations or who have small-capacity bladders with trigonal involvement.

Following these approaches, interstitial cystitis can be promptly and definitively diagnosed and usually managed effectively.

References

Alexander, J. C., and Christi, A. B.: Submucous injection of alcohol for relief of pain in Hunner ulcer. Urol. Cut. Rev., 40:793, 1936.

Badenoch, A. W.: Chronic interstitial cystitis. Br. Med. J., 43:718, 1971.

Baker, W. J., and Callahan, D. H.: Interstitial cystitis. J. Urol., 81:112, 1959.

Barnes, R. W.: Treatment of interstitial cystitis. Calif. Med., 66:347, 1947.

Bohne, A. W., and Fetz, R. J.: Interstitial cystitis: an adjunct in its treatment. Arch. Surg., 69:831, 1954.

Bohne, A. W., Hodson, J. M., Rebuck, J. W., and Reinhard, R. E.: An abnormal leukocyte response in interstitial cystitis. J. Urol., 88:387, 1962.

Bowers, J. E., and Lattimer, J. K.: Interstitial cystitis. Int. Abst. Surg., 105:313, 1957.

Bowers, J. E., Schwarz, B. E., and Leon, M. J.: Masochism and interstitial cystitis: a case report. Psychosomat. Med., 20:296, 1958.

Boye, E., Morse, M., Huttner, I., et al.: Immune complex–mediated interstitial cystitis as a major manifestation of systemic lupus erythematosus. Clin. Immunol. Immunopathol., 13:67, 1979.

Bumpus, H. C.: Submucous ulcer of the bladder in the male. J. Urol., 5:249, 1921.

Bumpus, H. C.: Interstitial cystitis; its treatment by overdistension of the bladder. Med. Clin. North Am., 13:1495, 1930.

Burford, E. H., and Burford, C. E.: Hunner ulcer of the bladder: a report of 187 cases. J. Urol., 79:952, 1958.

Chenowith, C. V., and Claywater, E. W.: Interstitial cystitis in children. J. Urol., 83:150, 1960.

Chodak, G. W., Scheiner, C. J., and Zetter, B. R.: Urine from patients with transitional cell carcinoma stimulates migration of capillary endothelial cells. N. Engl. J. Med., *305*:869, 1981.

Collan, Y., Alfthan, O., Kivilaakso, E., and Oravisto, K. J.: Electronic microscopic and histological findings in urinary bladder epithelium in interstitial cystitis. Eur. Urol., *2*:242, 1976.

Coutts, W. E., and Vargas-Zalazar, R.: Chronic interstitial cystitis and lymphogranuloma venereum. Urol. Cut. Rev., *49*:166, 1945.

Crenshaw, J. L.: Late results of pan-mural fibrosis of the bladder. Trans. Am. Assoc. Genitourin. Surg., *27*:109, 1934.

Davis, E.: Aniline dyes in treatment of Hunner ulcer. J. Urol., *46*:899, 1941.

DeJuana, C. P., and Everett, J. C.: Interstitial cystitis. Urology, *10*:325, 1977.

de la Serna, A. R., and Alarcon-Segovia, D.: Chronic interstitial cystitis as an initial major manifestation of systemic lupus erythematosus. J. Rheum., *8*:808, 1981.

Dodson, A. I.: Hunner's ulcer of the bladder: report of 10 cases. Virginia Med. Month. *53*:305, 1926.

Donahue, P. S.: Submucous cystitis. J. Urol., *29*:465, 1929.

Duke, W.: Elusive ulcer of the bladder (Discussion). Surg. Gynecol. Obstet., *35*:759, 1922.

Eiknev, W. C.: Interstitial cystitis. Urol. Cut. Rev., *45*:385, 1941.

Eisenstadt, J. S., and McDougall, T. G.: Rupture of the bladder through Hunner ulcer. Am. J. Surg., *14*:477, 1931.

Ek, A., Engberg, A., Frodin, L., and Jonsson, G.: The use of dimethyl-sulfate (DMSO) in the treatment of interstitial cystitis. Scand. J. Urol. Nephrol., *12*:129, 1978.

Ellenberg, J.: Fibrotic bladder due to G. C. infection. J. Mt. Sinai Hosp. (New York), *9*:876, 1942.

Engel, W. J.: Interstitial cystitis. Cleve. Clin. Q., *6*:307, 1939.

Fall, M., Carlsson, C., and Erlandson, B.: Electrical stimulation in interstitial cystitis. J. Urol., *123*:1920, 1980.

Fenwick, E. H.: The clinical significance of the simple solitary ulcer of the urinary bladder. Br. Med. J., *1*:1133, 1896.

Ferris, D. O.: An operation to increase the capacity of a contracted urinary bladder. Proc. Mayo Clin., *30*:305, 1955.

Fisher, E. R.: Tissue mast cells. JAMA, *173*:121, 1960.

Fister, G. M.: Similarity of interstitial cystitis to lupus erythematosus. J. Urol., *40*:37, 1938.

Fowler, J. E.: Prospective study of intravesical dimethyl sulfoxide in treatment of suspected early interstitial cystitis. Urology, *18*:21, 1981.

Franksson, C.: Interstitial cystitis: a clinical study of 59 cases. Acta Chir. Scand., *113*:51, 1957.

Franksson, C., and Bohm, E.: Interstitial cystitis and sacral rhizotomy. Acta Chir. Scand., *113*:63, 1957.

Freiha, F. S., and Stamey, T. A.: Cystolysis: a procedure for the selective denervation of the bladder. J. Urol., *123*:360, 1980.

Freiha, F. S., Faysal, M. H., and Stamey, T. A.: The surgical treatment of intractable interstitial cystitis. J. Urol., *123*:632, 1980.

Frontz, W. A.: Observations on the pathology, clinical diagnosis and treatment of submucous fibrosis (localized cystitis). South. Med. J., *21*:899, 1928.

Furniss, H. D.: Fulguration of Hunner ulcers. Am. J. Obstet., *24*:655, 1917.

Geist, R. W., and Antolak, S. J.: Interstitial cystitis in children. J. Urol., *104*:922, 1970.

Geraghty, J. T.: Infections of the bladder with special reference to localized resistant areas of cystitis. Surg. Gynecol. Obstet., *24*:655, 1917.

Gilchrist, K.: Personal communication, 1983.

Gill, W. G., Jones, K. W., and Ruggiero, K. J.: Protective effects of heparin and other sulfated glycosaminoglycans on crystal adhesion to injured urothelium. J. Urol., *127*:152, 1982.

Gordon, H. L., Rossen, R. D., Hersh, E. M., and Yiuin, J. J.: Immunologic aspects of interstitial cystitis. J. Urol., *109*:228, 1973.

Greenberg, E., Barnes, R., Stewart, S. and Furnish, T.: Transurethral resection of Hunner's ulcer. J. Urol., *111*:764, 1974.

Greenwood, C.: The pharmacology of ketotifen. Chest, *82* (Suppl.):45S, 1982.

Grossman, H. B.: Antibodies to a bladder cancer tumor–associated antigen in patient with interstitial cystitis. Surg. Forum (68th Ann. Clinical Congress Am. Coll. Surg.), *33*:657, 1982.

Guerrier, H. P., Roberts, J., and Slade, N.: Anti-inflammatory agents in the management of interstitial cystitis. Br. J. Urol., *37*:88, 1965.

Hanash, K. A., and Pool, T. L.: Interstitial and hemorrhagic cystitis: viral, bacterial and fungal studies. J. Urol., *104*:705, 1970.

Hand, J. R.: Interstitial cystitis. J. Urol., *61*:291, 1949.

Hanno, P. M., Parsons, C. L., Shrom, S. H., et al.: The protective effect of heparin on experimental bladder infection. J. Surg. Res., *25*:324, 1978.

Henline, R. B.: Comments to paper: Kreutzmann, H. A. R.: The treatment of Hunner's ulcer with deep X-ray therapy. J. Urol., *46*:907, 1941.

Herbst, R. H.: Ulcer of the bladder. Surg. Clin. Chicago, *4*:867, 1920.

Herbst, R. H., Baumrucker, G. O., and German, K. L.: Elusive ulcer (Hunner) of the bladder with an experimental study of the etiology. Am. J. Surg., *38*:152, 1937.

Higgins, C. C.: Hunner ulcer of the bladder. Ann. Intern. Med., *15*:708, 1941.

Higson, R. H., Smith, J. C., and Whelan, P.: Bladder rupture: an acceptable complication of distension therapy? Br. J. Urol., *50*:529, 1978.

Howard, T. L.: My personal opinions on interstitial cystitis. J. Urol., *51*:526, 1944.

Hoyt, H.: Cortisone in urologic conditions with report of a trial in interstitial cystitis. J. Urol., *66*:526, 1952.

Hunner, G. L.: A rare type of bladder ulcer in women: report of cases. Trans. South. Surg. Gynecol. Assoc., *27*:257, 1914.

Hunner, G. L.: A rare type of bladder ulcer in women: report of cases. Boston Med. Soc. J., *172*:660, 1915.

Hunner, G. L.: Elusive ulcer of the bladder. Am. J. Obstet., *78*:374, 1918a.

Hunner, G. L.: A rare type of bladder ulcer. JAMA, *70*:203, 1918b.

Hunner, G. L.: Intractable bladder symptoms due to urethritis. J. Urol., *4*:503, 1920.

Hunner, G. L.: Neurosis of the bladder. J. Urol., *24*:567, 1930.

Ingelman-Sundberg, A.: Partial denervation of the bladder. A new operation for the treatment of urge incontinence and similar conditions in women. Acta Obstet. Gynecol. Scand., *38*:487, 1959.

Jacobo, E., Stamler, F. W., and Culp, D. A.: Interstitial cystitis followed by total cystectomy. Urology, *3*:481, 1974.

Jokinen, E. J., Alfthan, O. S., and Oravisto, K. J.: Antitissue antibodies in interstitial cystitis. Clin. Exp. Immunol., *11*:333, 1972a.

Jokinen, E. J., Lassus, A., Salo, O. P., and Alfthan, O. S.: Discoid lupus erythematosus and interstitial cystitis. The presence of bound immunoglobulins in the bladder mucosa. Ann. Clin. Res., *4*:23, 1972b.

Kastrup, J., Hald, T., Larsen, S., and Nielson, V. G.: Histamine content and mast cell count of the detrusor muscle in patients with interstitial cystitis and other types of chronic cystitis. Br. J. Urol., *55*:495, 1983.

Kaufman, J. E., Stauffer, C., Schmidt, J. D., and Parsons, C. L.: The effect of tryptophan metabolites on the anti-adherence nature of the bladder surface sulfonated glycosaminoglycan. Presented at Annual Meeting, American Urological Association, San Francisco, May 18–22, 1980.

Kearns, W. M.: A new method to bring about dilatation of the contracted bladder. Urol. Cut. Rev., *36*:184, 1932.

Keene, F. B.: Circumscribed panmural ulcerative cystitis. Ann Surg., *71*:479, 1920.

Keene, F. B.: Elusive ulcer of the bladder. Am. J. Obstet., *10*:380, 1925.

Kerr, W. S., Jr.: Interstitial cystitis: treatment by transurethral resection. J. Urol., *105*:664, 1971.

Keyes, E. L.: Character and treatment of bladder ulcers. J. Urol., *8*:167, 1922.

Kinder, C. H., and Smith, R. D.: Hunner's ulcer. Br. J. Urol., *30*:338, 1958.

Knorr, R.: Die Cystoskopie und Urethroskopie beim Weibe. Berlin, Urban und Schwarzenberg, 1908, p. 211.

Kretschmer, H. L.: Elusive ulcer of the bladder. Trans. Am. Assoc. Genitourin. Surg., *15*:417, 1922.

Kretschmer, H. L.: Elusive ulcer of the bladder: 44 cases. JAMA, *86*:739, 1926.

Kreutzmann, H.: The treatment of Hunner's ulcer of the bladder by fulguration. Calif. Med., *20*:128, 1922.

Kreutzmann, H.: The treatment of Hunner's ulcer with deep X-ray therapy. J. Urol., *46*:907, 1941.

Lapides, J. Observations on interstitial cystitis. Urology, *5*:610, 1975.

Larsen, S., Thompson, S. A., Hald, T., et al.: Mast cells in interstitial cystitis. Br. J. Urol., *54*:283, 1982.

Leach, G. E., and Raz, S.: Interstitial cystitis. *In* Raz, S. (Ed.): Female Urology. Philadelphia, W. B. Saunders Co., 1983, pp. 351–356.

Learmonth, J. R.: Neurosurgery in disease of the urinary bladder. J. Urol., *26*:13, 1931.

Leder, L. D.: Über die selektive fermentcytochemische Darstellung von neutrophilen myeloschen Zellum und Gewebsmastzellen in Paraffinschitt. Klin. Wochenschr. *42*:553, 1964.

Lillie, R. D.: Histopathologic Technic and Practical Histochemistry. 3rd ed. New York, McGraw-Hill Book Co., 1965, pp. 159–165.

Longacre, J. J.: The treatment of contracted bladder with controlled tidal irrigation. J. Urol., *36*:25, 1936.

Lower, W. E., and Schlumberger, F. C.: Bilateral simultaneous ureterosigmoidostomy for chronic interstitial cystitis. Cleve. Clin. Q., *6*:181, 1939.

McCrea, L. E.: Interstitial cystitis. J. Urol., *84*:311, 1960.

McDonald, H. P., Upchurch, W., and Sturdivant, C. E.: Interstitial cystitis in children. J. Urol., *70*:890, 1953.

McGuire, E. J., Lytton, B., and Corog, J. L.: Interstitial cystitis following colocystoplasty. Urology, *2*:28, 1973.

Meirowsky, A. M.: The management of chronic interstitial cystitis by differential sacral neurectomy. J. Neurosurg., *30*:604, 1969.

Meisser, J. G., and Bumpus, H. C.: Focal infections in relation to submucous ulcer of the bladder and to cystitis. J. Urol., *6*:285, 1921.

Mercier, L. A.: Mémoire sur certaines perforatuns spontanées de la vessie non décrites jusqu'à ce jour. Gaz. Med. Paris, *4*:257, 1836.

Messing, E. M., and Freiha, F. S.: Complication of Clorpactin WCS-90 therapy for interstitial cystitis. Urology, *13*:389, 1979.

Messing, E. M., and Stamey, T. A.: Interstitial cystitis: a review of 62 cases and report of a myoactive substance isolated from the overdistended bladder. Presented at Annual Meeting, Western Section American Urological Association, San Francisco, March 1977.

Messing, E. M., and Stamey, T. A.: Interstitial cystitis: early diagnosis, pathology, and treatment. Urology, *12*:381, 1978.

Messing, E. M., Reznikoff, C. A., and Erturk, F.: Epidermal growth factor and normal urothelium. Presented at 4th Annual National Bladder Cancer Project Workshop, Sarasota, Fla., January 4–7, 1984.

Milner, W. A., and Garlick, W. B.: Selective sacral neurectomy in interstitial cystitis with a minimum eighteen month follow-up. S. Afr. Med. J., *33*:116, 1959.

Morris, C. R., and Bryan, G. T.: Absorption of ^{14}C-labeled tryptophan and its metabolites, glycine and glucose, by the urinary bladder of the mouse. Invest. Urol., *3*:577, 1966.

Moulder, M. K., and Meirowsky, A. M.: Management of Hunner's ulcer by differential sacral neurectomy. J. Urol., *75*:261, 1956.

Murnaghan, G. F., Saalfeld, J., and Farnsworth, R. H.: Interstitial cystitis treatment with Clorpactin WCS-90. Br. J. Urol., *42*:744, 1969.

Nesbit, R. M.: Anterolateral cordotomy for refractory interstitial cystitis with intolerable pain. J. Urol., *57*:741, 1947.

Nitze, M.: Lehrbuch der cystoskopie: ihre Technik und klinische Bedeutung. Berlin, J. E. Bergman, 1907, pp. 205–210.

O'Conor, V. J.: Clorpactin WCS-90 in interstitial cystitis. Q. Bull. Northwest Med. Sch., *29*:392, 1955.

Oravisto, K. J.: Epidemiology of interstitial cystitis. Ann. Chir. Gynaecol. Fenn., *64*:75, 1975.

Oravisto, K. J., and Alfthan, O. S.: Treatment of interstitial cystitis with immunosupression and chloroquine derivatives. Eur. Urol., *2*:82, 1976.

Oravisto, K. J., Alfthan, O. S., and Jokinen, E. J.: Interstitial cystitis, clinical and immunologic findings. Scand. J. Urol. Nephrol., *4*:37, 1970.

Oravisto, K. J.: Interstitial cystitis as an autoimmune disease. A review. Eur. Urol., *6*:10, 1980.

Ormond, J. K.: Interstitial cystitis. J. Urol., *33*:376, 1937.

Parsons, C. L., Schmidt, J. D., and Pollen, J. Y.: Successful treatment of interstitial cystitis with sodium pentosanpolysulfate. J. Urol., *130*:51, 1983.

Parsons, C. L., Stauffer, C., and Schmidt, J. D.: Bladder-surface glycosaminoglycans: an efficient mechanism of environmental adaption. Science, *208*:605, 1980.

Pearl, F., and Strauss, B.: Presacral neurectomy and sacral ganglionectomy. J. Urol., *39*:645, 1939.

Pearse, A. G. E.: Histochemistry. 3rd ed., Boston, Little, Brown & Co., 1968, pp. 330–341, 775–776.

Peterson, H., and Hager, B. H.: Interstitial cystitis: report of cases. Calif. West. Med., *31*:262, 1929.

Pool, T. L., and Rives, H. F.: Interstitial cystitis. J. Urol., *51*:520, 1944.

Powell, T. O.: Studies on lymphatics of female urinary bladder. Surg. Gynecol. Obstet., *78*:605, 1944.

Powell, T. O.: Studies on the etiology of Hunner ulcer. J. Urol., *53*:823, 1945.

Powell, T. O.: Treatment of Hunner ulcer. Urol. Cut. Rev., *53*:397, 1949.

Quinby, W. C.: Resection of the presacral nerve in the

painful bladder of interstitial cystitis. Trans. Am. Assoc. Genitourin. Surg., *24*:335, 1931.

Reed, C. A.: Irritable bladder in women. JAMA, *72*:332, 1919.

Riley, J. F., and West, G. B.: The presence of histamine in tissue mast cells. J. Physiol., *120*:528, 1953.

Riskind, L. A., and Zide, H. A.: Banthine in urologic disorders. J. Urol., *68*:636, 1952.

Rose, D. K.: Infiltration treatment of Hunner ulcer. J. Urol., *65*:1021, 1951.

Rosin, R. D., Griffiths, T., Sofras, F., et al.: Interstitial cystitis. Br. J. Urol., *51*:524, 1979.

Shipton, E. A.: Hunner's ulcer (chronic interstitial cystitis), a manifestation of collagen disease. Br. J. Urol., *37*:443, 1965.

Shirley, S. W., Stewart, B. H., and Mirelman, S.: Dimethyl sulfoxide in treatment of inflammatory genitourinary disorders. Urology, *11*:215, 1978.

Shulte, T. L., and Reynolds, L. R.: Transurethral intramural injection of hydrocortone hyaluronidase for Hunner's ulcers. J. Urol., *75*:63, 1956.

Silk, M.: Bladder antibodies in interstitial cystitis. J. Urol., *103*:307, 1970.

Simmons, J. L.: Interstitial cystitis: an explanation for the beneficial effect of an antihistamine. J. Urol., *85*:149, 1961.

Simmons, J. L., and Bunce, P. L.: On the use of antihistamine in the treatment of interstitial cystitis. Am. Surg. *24*:664, 1958.

Skene, A. J.: Diseases of the Bladder and Urethra in Women. New York, William Wood and Co., 1887.

Skoluda, D., Wegner, K., and Lemmel, E. M.: Critical notes on immune pathogenesis of interstitial cystitis. Urologe [A], *13*:15, 1974.

Smith, B. H., and Dehner, L. P.: Chronic ulcerating cystitis (Hunner's ulcer). A study of 28 cases. Arch. Pathol., *93*:76, 1972.

Smith, G. G.: Interstitial cystitis. J. Urol., *67*:903, 1952.

Smith, J. C., and Badenoch, A. W.: Carcinoma of the bladder simulating chronic cystitis. Br. J. Urol., *37*:93, 1965.

Smith, R. B., Van Cangh, P., Skinner, D. G., et al.: Augmentation enterocystoplasty: a critical review. J. Urol., *118*:35, 1977.

Stamey, T. A.: Endoscopic suspension of the vesical neck for urinary incontinence. Surg. Gynecol. Obstet., *136*:547, 1973.

Stamm, W. E., Running, K., McKevitt, M., et al.: Treatment of the acute urethral syndrome. N. Engl. J. Med., *304*:956, 1981.

Stamm, W. E., Wagner, K. F., Amsel, R., et al.: Causes of the acute urethral syndrome in women. N. Engl. J. Med., *303*:409, 1980.

Stevens, A. R.: Panmural cystitis: Unusual case. Trans. Am. Assoc. Genitourin. Surg., *16*:225, 1923.

Stewart, B. H., Branson, A. C., Hewitt, C. B., et al.: The treatment of patients with interstitial cystitis with special reference to intravesical DMSO. J. Urol., *107*:377, 1972.

Stewart, B. H., Persky, L., and Kiser, W. S.: The use of dimethyl sulfoxide (DMSO) in the treatment of interstitial cystitis. J. Urol., *98*:671, 1967.

Tait, L.: On the cure of the chronic perforating ulcer of the bladder by the formation of an artificial vesicovaginal fistula. Lancet, *54*:738, 1870.

Turner-Warwick, R., and Handley-Ashken, M.: The functional results of partial, subtotal and total cystoplasty with special reference to ureterocystoplasty, selective sphincterotomy and cystocystoplasty. Br. J. Urol., *39*:3, 1967.

Utz, D. C., and Zincke, H.: The masquerade of bladder cancer in situ as interstitial cystitis. J. Urol., *111*:160, 1974.

Van Dusen, R. E., and Mustain, R.: Alpha-tocopherol in treatment of interstitial cystitis. J. Urol., *65*:1033, 1951.

von Garrelts, B.: Interstitial cystitis: thirteen patients treated operatively with intestinal bladder substitutes. Acta Chir. Scand., *132*:436, 1966.

Walsh, A.: Interstitial cystitis. *In* Harrison, J. H., Gittes, R. F., Perlmutter, A. D., Stamey, T. A., and Walsh, P. C. (Eds.): Campbell's Urology. 4th ed. Philadelphia, W. B. Saunders Co. 1978, pp. 693–707.

Walsh, A.: Personal communication to T. A. Stamey, 1982.

Warres, H. L.: The role of hyperemia in the treatment of chronic interstitial cystitis. J. Urol., *86*:57, 1961.

Warres, H. L.: Interstitial cystitis. J. Urol., *87*:542, 1962.

Weaver, R. G., and Tyler, F. H.: The use of ACTH in interstitial cystitis. Proc. Second Clin. ACTH Conf., Philadelphia, Blakiston, 1950.

Weaver, R. G., Dougherty, T. F., and Natoli, C.: Recent concepts of interstitial cystitis. J. Urol., *89*:377, 1963.

Weisman, M. H., McDonald, E. C., and Wilson, C. B.: Studies of the pathogenesis of interstitial cystitis, obstructive uropathy, and intestinal malabsorption in a patient with systemic lupus erythematosus. Am. J. Med., *70*:875, 1981.

Whitfield, R. D., Myers, P. W., Milner, W. A., and Campbell, E.: Selective sacral neurectomy for Hunner's ulcer with neurohistologic observations. Surg. Forum, *7*:567, 1957.

Winsbury-White, H.: Spread of infection from cervix to urinary tract. Br. J. Urol., *5*:249, 1933.

Wishard, W. N., Nourse, N. H., and Mertz, J. H.: Use of Clorpactin-WCS-90 for relief of symptoms due to interstitial cystitis. J. Urol., *77*:420, 1957.

Worth, P. H. L.: The treatment of interstitial cystitis by cystolysis with observations on cystoplasty. A review after 7 years. Br. J. Urol., *52*:232, 1980.

Worth, P. H. L., and Turner-Warwick, R.: The treatment of interstitial cystitis by cystolysis with observations on cystoplasty. Br. J. Urol., *45*:65, 1973.

Young, J. E.: Hunner ulcer of the bladder. Cleve. Clin. Q., *2*:51, 1935.

Zondek, B., and Bromberg, Y. M.: Endocrine allergy: clinical reactions of allergy to endogenous hormones and their treatment. J. Obstet. Gynaecol. Brit. Emp., *54*:1, 1947.

Urethral Syndrome

DEFINITION

The urethral syndrome is an entity in which patients suffer from frequency, urgency, dysuria, and, at times, suprapubic and back pain and urinary hesitancy, in the absence of objective urologic findings. While it is usually termed the female urethral syndrome, there is no reason to believe that a similar condition does not occur in males (e.g., prostatodynia) or in children of either sex. Despite this consideration, we will limit our discussion to the symptom complex found in adult women.

"LACK OF OBJECTIVE FINDINGS"

Since the symptoms outlined are indistinguishable from those caused by urinary infections, tumors, stones, interstitial cystitis, and many other entities, it is important to rule out these conditions before diagnosing the urethral syndrome. To avoid confusion, therefore, it is assumed that women with the urethral syndrome have absolutely negative urinalyses on initial (VB_1) and midstream (VB_2) collections; sterile urine and urethral swab cultures (for *Trichomonas*, mycobacteria, fungi, *Chlamydia, Ureaplasma, N. gonorrhoeae*, and bacterial pathogens); cytologically normal urinary and bladder lavage specimens; and no cystoscopic findings typical of bladder or urethral malignancies, condylomata, diverticula, or chronic cystitises, such as interstitial or eosinophilic cystitis. In addition, patients will not be included who have objective findings of neurologic disorders (e.g., multiple sclerosis) or collagen diseases (e.g., systemic lupus erythematosus), or who have a history of severe pelvic, vaginal, or lower abdominal trauma, radiation therapy, exposure to toxins, or recurrent episodes of bacteriuria or other infections. Pelvic examination (with the possible exception of mild anterior distal vaginal tenderness), gynecologic history, and, if performed, radiologic studies of the urinary tract, including intravenous urography and cystourethrography, must reveal no abnormalities that could explain the symptoms. Although these exclusions may seem excessively broad, entities with such objective findings would normally be diagnosed during standard (primarily outpatient) evaluations and are discussed elsewhere in the text.

EPIDEMIOLOGY

Epidemiologic data similar to those for interstitial cystitis are not available for the urethral syndrome, in large part because of inconsistencies in the criteria used to define it. Most authors (Mabry et al., 1981; Smith, 1979; Carson et al., 1979; Kaplan et al., 1980) believe that the urethral syndrome occurs more commonly in women during the reproductive years, but it is also seen in children (Kaplan et al., 1980) and the elderly. Variations in racial and geographic incidence have not been reported.

ETIOLOGY

Popular hypotheses as to the causes of the urethral syndrome implicate obstructive (urethral stenosis or glandular enlargement along the urethra), infectious, neurogenic, and psychogenic mechanisms. Other factors, such as hormonal imbalances (Zondek and Bromberg, 1947), reactions to ingested or environmental chemicals (Bell, 1975), and allergic conditions (Gilmore and Vane, 1971) have been proposed with little supporting evidence and are not widely accepted.

Urethral Obstruction. The proposition that symptoms are caused by a stenotic urethra and are thus surgically treatable has had many advocates (Roberts and Smith, 1968; Farrar et al., 1973; O'Donnell, 1978; Splatt and Weedon, 1977; Davis, 1955; Richardson, 1969). Each has claimed excellent results for procedures that dilate, resect, mobilize, incise, or widen the urethra. Unfortunately, diagnostic criteria are poorly documented in each report. Moreover, these procedures involve some risk for incontinence and are of uncertain, and usually temporary, efficacy (Mabry et al., 1981; Schmidt and Tanagho, 1981). Most important, no objective evidence supports an anatomically obstructive etiology. Histologic studies purporting to show increased fibrosis in tissues surrounding the distal urethra are nonquantitative, poorly controlled, and because of failure to account for sampling errors, not compelling (Splatt and Weedon, 1977, 1981). In addition, only 1 of 63 women with the urethral syndrome seen at Duke University was found to have a stenotic urethra when urethral calibration was performed (Mabry et al., 1981). Thus, while obstructive phenomena may play a role in the unusual case, they cannot be implicated as a common cause of the urethral syndrome.

Infection. The role of infection in the urethral syndrome has been investigated by many authors (Bruce et al., 1973; Gallagher, 1965; Cox et al., 1968; Stamm et al., 1980; Maskell et al., 1979; Smith, 1979; Panja, 1983). Most proponents of an infectious etiology base their arguments upon two observations that explain why infections are not detected by routine clinical microbiologic laboratory culturing and reporting practices: (1) Patients with true urinary infections often have less than 10^5 bacterial pathogens per ml of urine (Smith, 1979); and (2) fastidious organisms often colonize the urinary tract (Bruce et al., 1973; Smith, 1979; Stamm et al., 1980; Maskell et al., 1979), which require special collection, culturing, and incubation techniques for detection and identification. However, the vast majority of women with lower urinary tract symptoms and colonization with such organisms have pyuria (more than 5 white cells per high power field) in their VB_1 and VB_2 collections (Stamm et al., 1980; Stamm, 1983; Maskell et al., 1979; Panja, 1983) and thus do not lack the objective findings necessary to diagnose the urethral syndrome. Maskell and coworkers (1979) are alone in reporting that as many as one third of female patients with lower urinary tract colonization with fastidious organisms considered responsible for irritable voiding symptoms lacked pyuria. However, considering the abundance of reports associating pyuria with infection, this probably occurs rarely.

An additional reason for believing the urethral syndrome has an infectious (or inflammatory) etiology is the finding of urethritis or pseudomembranous trigonitis on cystoscopic examination (Smith, 1979; Parkes and Boreham, 1980). However, such observations may be artifactual in that urethroscopy in the female is rarely performed without prior urethral traumatization. This is caused by placement of local anesthetic (which effects severe vasodilation), calibration, and blind passage of the cystoscope sheath over an obturator into the bladder, with urethroscopy being performed only when the scope is withdrawn. In addition, cobblestoning and erythema of the urethra and trigone with an occasional exudate (Smith, 1979; Splatt and Weedon, 1981) are in large part under hormonal influence (Fair et al., 1970). This parallels cyclic menstrual fluctuations, details of which are rarely obtained in the typical urologic interview. Furthermore, since these findings are present neither in all individuals having the urethral syndrome (Carson et al., 1980) nor in all with true bacterial cystitis, their significance is obscure. As might be anticipated, attempts to obliterate these lesions by endoscopic techniques, including instillations, urethral suppositories, fulgurations, cryosurgery, and urethral dilations (Mabry et al., 1981; Splatt and Weedon, 1977; Parkes and Boreham, 1980), do not consistently relieve symptoms. Finally, followup endoscopy to document their disappearance in patients who do improve has not been reported. When not artifactual, these endoscopic findings remain of interest. However, they hardly support the concept of an inflammatory or infectious etiology.

Neurogenic. Three groups in this country have reported that symptoms in the urethral syndrome were due to spasm of the external urethral sphincter (Raz and Smith, 1976; Schmidt and Tanagho, 1981; Kaplan et al., 1980). Evidence consisted of a staccato or prolonged flow phase during uroflowimetry (Kaplan et al., 1980) and increased external sphincter tone detected on urethral pressure profilimetry (Raz and Smith, 1976; Schmidt and Tanagho, 1981) or by transcutaneous electrodes (Kaplan et al., 1980). Each group suggested that multiple factors may be responsible for these observations, including a functional etiology in many patients. Gratifying responses to therapy with diazepam (Kaplan et al., 1980; Raz and Smith, 1976) or electrical stimulation in a biofeedback setting (Schmidt and Tanagho, 1981) do little to support a neurogenic as opposed to a psychogenic etiology. Moreover, invasive studies (e.g, cystometrometry and urethral pressure profilimetry) on a sensitive urethra further traumatized by instrumentation produce biasing artifacts. Kaplan and associates (1980) tried to evaluate patients noninvasively by performing uroflow studies and recording transcutaneous electromyographic (EMG) potentials. However, to avoid instrumentation, they had to resort to a technology (transcutaneous EMG) that is of limited utility in adults and that examines activity of the entire pelvic floor rather than specifically that of the external urethral sphincter (Kaplan et al., 1980). In summary, these studies present a urodynamic picture that can be produced voluntarily in the neurologically intact individual and thus provide meager evidence to support an underlying neurogenic etiology.

Psychogenic Etiology. In addition to urodynamic data that may implicate a psychogenic etiology (Kaplan et al., 1980; Schmidt and Tanagho, 1981), Carson and coworkers (1979, 1980) found specific psychologic pathology in the majority of patients to whom they administered the Minnesota Multiphasic Personality Inventory (MMPI). Most patients scored consistently higher on the hypochondriasis, hysteria, and schizophrenia scales than a group of age- and sex-matched, historical, "medical patient" controls. The MMPI configuration most commonly seen was "conversion-V" which is found in patients who manifest "psychophysiological reactions to deal with tension and anxiety" (Carson et al., 1980). The authors suggested that psychogenic causes may be etiologically important, since 13 out of the 15 patients referred for subsequent psychiatric counseling achieved total resolution of their symptoms following such therapy. While it may be difficult to diagnose psychopathology in a patient who has taken the MMPI in the absence of a psychiatric interview, these findings corroborate the clinical observations of others (Mabry et al., 1981; Zufall, 1978). Thus, if the condition is strictly defined as occurring in women in the absence of pyuria (and with sterile urine and negative urine cytology), evidence for an anatomic, infectious, inflammatory, or neurogenic cause of the urethral syndrome is weak. Conversely, external sphincter spasm of possible psychogenic origin may well be implicated.

DIAGNOSIS

Patients with the urethral syndrome are first seen by primary care physicians or gynecologists. Thus, by the time urologic evaluation is sought, gynecologic conditions that can cause irritable voiding symptoms have usually been eliminated. In the initial urologic evaluation, pelvic and neurologic examinations should be repeated, and microscopic examination of the urinary sediment and urine culture is essential. Although patients are often told that they have recurrent urinary infections, these episodes are usually poorly documented (Mabry et al., 1981). Between 55 per cent (Panja, 1983) and 70 per cent (Stamm, 1983) of such patients will have

---

*See the discussion by Stamm (1983) for the merits of examining a drop of unspun urine on a hemocytometer rather than looking at spun urinary sediment, in order to quantitate pyuria.

pyuria.* With extensive culturing for typical urinary pathogens (instructing laboratories to identify organisms with colony counts of less than 10^5 per ml) and more fastidious organisms, a diagnosis other than the urethral syndrome can be established.

Radiographic Studies. The yield of radiologic evaluation, including intravenous urography and cystourethrography, has been reviewed by several authors (Carson et al., 1980; Mabry et al., 1981; Zufall, 1978), who have concluded that these studies are rarely justified in patients with the urethral syndrome. However, individuals with lower ureteral stones or urethral diverticula not suspected by history, physical examination, laboratory tests, or cystoscopy may require x-ray studies for diagnosis. Thus, while radiographic evaluation of the urinary tract is almost always normal in the urethral syndrome, it may be warranted to rule out other uncommon causes for similar symptoms. Intravenous urography with a postvoid film will usually suffice. Radiologic evaluation is mandatory in the presence of an abnormal urinalysis (particularly hematuria).

Urodynamic Studies. Unless incontinence is a major component of the symptom complex (usually urge incontinence), or physical examination or history clearly demonstrates a neurologic deficit, urodynamic studies merely confirm the fact that these patients have a painful urethra. Uroflowimetry (Schmidt and Tanagho, 1981; Kaplan et al., 1980) is potentially the most diagnostic of such tests.

Cystoscopy. Since the observation of urethral and trigonal erythema immediately after instrumentation is not diagnostic of the urethral syndrome (see earlier) (Carson et al., 1980), the purpose of cystoscopy is to rule out other diseases with similar symptomatology. Because interstitial cystitis is likely to be the source of lower tract irritative symptoms in the presence of sterile, cytologically unremarkable urine and normal urinalysis, we believe cystoscopy should be performed under full anesthesia (Messing and Stamey, 1978). Urethral (Splatt and Weedon, 1977) or bladder biopsies appear to be of negligible value in the absence of objective endoscopic or cytologic findings and are indicated only as considered appropriate to rule out other diseases.

Psychiatric Testing. We do not routinely obtain a psychiatric evaluation unless we infer that symptoms are related to emotionally charged events. Similarly, since it is not known how many individuals with objective causes of lower urinary tract symptoms score the conversion-V pattern on MMPI testing that many urethral syndrome patients do (Carson et al., 1979, 1980), we do not routinely perform this study either. Clearly, if the MMPI is obtained, it must be backed up with sophisticated interpretation and a psychiatric interview.

TREATMENT

Patients with the urethral syndrome can be divided into two groups: those with pyuria (greater than 5 cells per high power field or greater than 10 white blood cells per ml) (Stamm, 1983), and those without pyuria. In the presence of pyuria, care must be taken in culturing the urine to make sure that an infection with less than 10^5 gram-negative rods per ml is not occurring. If such is found, appropriate antibiotic therapy should be initiated. If urine specimens cultured by traditional aerobic incubation techniques are sterile, urine and urethral swab specimens should be cultured for anaerobic organisms, gonococci, *Chlamydia,* and *Ureaplasma.* Pending results of such cultures, patients may be started on a trial of doxycycline (Stamm et al., 1981). If symptoms are not improved and pyuria not relieved, we switch to erythromycin, which has been found to be successful against most of the anaerobes that can be responsible for this disease (Maskell et al., 1979) as well as *Chlamydia* and *Ureaplasma.* If symptoms are still not relieved or if pyuria persists, a more detailed work-up for sterile pyuria must be undertaken, which eliminates such causes as mycobacterial infection, stones, or tumors.

Infections are far less likely in the absence of true pyuria in the VB$_1$ or VB$_2$ (Stamm et al., 1980; Panja, 1983; Stamm, 1983). For women with documented histories of prior recurrent urinary infections, we initiate a course of long-term, low-dose, antimicrobial prophylaxis (e.g., trimethoprim-sulfamethoxazole or nitrofurantoin). This is done because patients with recurrent bacteriuria occasionally experience irritable voiding symptoms when their urine is uninfected (Kraft and Stamey, 1977), and then develop documented bacteria within several months (Kraft and Stamey, 1977; Gallagher et al., 1965). If symptoms are not relieved or if women without pyuria have no documented history of bacteriuria, we perform special cultures only after interstitial cystitis is ruled out. Erythromycin is the first agent we try pending culture results, owing to the finding of Maskell and coworkers (1979) that 33% of patients who did

not have pyuria were still symptomatically infected with anaerobes sensitive to this antibiotic.

The woman without pyuria or other objective findings whose symptoms persist despite a trial with erythromycin presents a great diagnostic and therapeutic challenge. The list of treatments for such patients has been exhaustively reviewed by others (Smith, 1979; Mabry et al., 1981; Zufall, 1978; Carson et al., 1980) and includes: endoscopic (Roberts and Smith, 1968; Davis, 1955; Farrar et al., 1973) and open surgical procedures (O'Donnell, 1978; Richardson, 1969) designed to eliminate urethral stenosis; fulguration, scarification, resection, or cryosurgical procedures (Carson et al., 1980; Mabry et al., 1981; Parkes and Boreham, 1980), which obliterate cystoscopically apparent urethritis or trigonitis; bladder instillations with a variety of anti-inflammatory or cauterizing agents, including DMSO (Shirley and Stewart, 1978) and silver nitrate (Carson et al., 1980); systemic therapy with anticholinergics, α-adrenergic blockers (Raz and Smith, 1976), and skeletal muscle relaxants (Kaplan et al., 1980), which are believed to control the underlying urodynamic abnormalities described with this entity; electrical stimulation and biofeedback (Schmidt and Tanagho, 1981) to correct psychogenic causes; and psychotherapy (Carson et al., 1979, 1980). While numerous other treatments have also been proposed, they are currently less popular.

Reported results were variable for each modality, nonrigid criteria were used to determine diagnosis and therapeutic response, and duration of follow-up was very brief or not mentioned. Nonetheless, 30 to 67 per cent of patients undergoing surgical treatment experienced improvement in a large retrospective study performed by Carson and associates (1980) and a prospective series by Mabry and colleagues (1981). In a personal retrospective series, Zufall (1978) found almost identical results but, in addition, reported similar efficacy for antibiotics and anticholinergics. The most impressive finding of these studies was that the best results (85 per cent in Carson et al., 1980 and 100 per cent in Zufall, 1978) occurred in patients managed by observation only. While these women probably had milder symptoms than did those undergoing specific therapy, high rates of spontaneous remission must be considered in evaluating results of any treatment.

Perhaps the most appealing approach is that of Kaplan and coworkers (1980) and Schmidt and Tanagho (1981), who employed skeletal muscle relaxants or electrostimulation combined with biofeedback techniques (women were shown their uroflow studies and EMGs). They noted dramatic improvement in almost all patients. Such findings are consistent with those of Carson and associates (1980) for urethral syndrome patients referred for psychiatric therapy (87 per cent improvement). Although in the report of Carson and associates (1980), patients had manifestations of psychiatric illness in addition to urinary symptoms, the overall results for "mind over bladder" therapy should be kept in mind by urologists who recommend more invasive treatments.

A recent observation by Larsen and co-workers (1982) may also influence management of this syndrome. These investigators found that over 25 per cent of patients who were believed to have interstitial cystitis, based upon symptomatology and preoperative evaluation (see earlier), lacked that disorder's typical cystoscopic findings under anesthesia. Two thirds of such patients were found to have an elevated number of mast cells in the muscularis on bladder biopsy. It is possible that such individuals should be considered to have the urethral syndrome and could be helped by oral agents that stabilize mast cells, such as ketotifen (Greenwood, 1982). This medication has properties similar to those of cromolyn sodium but is excreted in much higher concentrations in the urine. Reports of follow-up cystoscopy on these individuals to determine whether they develop interstitial cystitis will be of great interest.

Similarities between the urethral syndrome and interstitial cystitis are superficial, the findings of Larsen and associates (1982) notwithstanding. The former condition occurs in many patients, whereas the latter occurs in few. Furthermore, interstitial cystitis can be definitively diagnosed by demonstrating typical cystoscopic findings when symptomatic patients are examined under anesthesia in the presence of totally sterile and cytologically normal urine (Messing and Stamey, 1978). Those patients with irritable voiding who lack these findings, and who have no evidence of pyuria, infection, or any other pathology (see earlier) that could explain their symptoms, can be considered to have the urethral syndrome. Diagnostic evaluation should be limited to those tests that rule out serious underlying conditions and pursued only as symptoms dictate. Treatment should be oriented toward a conservative approach, since this is usually as effective as surgery, far less expensive, and less subject to risk (Schmidt and Tanagho, 1981; Raz and Smith, 1976).

References

Bell, I. R.: The kinin system theory of mechanism for food and chemical sensitivities. Presented at the Ninth Advanced Seminar in Clinical Ecology, Toronto, November 8, 1975.

Bruce, A. W., Chadwick, P., Hassen, A., and VanCott, G. F.: Recurrent urethritis in women. Can. Med. Assoc. J., 108:973, 1973.

Carson, C. C., Osborne, D., and Segura, J. W.: Psychologic characteristics of patients with female urethral syndrome. J. Clin. Psychol., 35:312, 1979.

Carson, C. C., Segura, J. W., and Osborne, D. M.: Evaluation and treatment of the female urethral syndrome. J. Urol., 124:609, 1980.

Cox, C. E., Lacy, S. S., and Hinman, F., Jr.: The urethra and its relationship to urinary tract infection. II. The urethral flora of the female with recurrent urinary infection. J. Urol., 99:632, 1968.

Davis, D. M.: Vesical orifice obstruction in women and its treatment by transurethral resection. J. Urol., 73:112, 1955.

Fair, W. R., Timothy, M. M., Miller, M. A., and Stamey, T. A.: Bacteriologic and hormonal observations of the urethra and vaginal vestibule in normal, premenopausal women. J Urol., 104:426, 1970.

Farrar, D. J., Green, N. A., and Handley-Ashken, M.: An evaluation of Otis urethrotomy in female patients with recurrent urinary tract infections. Br. J. Urol., 45:610, 1973.

Gallagher, D. J., Mongomerie, J. Z., and North, J. D.: Acute infections of the urinary tract and the urethral syndrome in general practice. Br. Med. J., 1:622, 1965.

Gilmore, N. J., and Vane, J. R.: Hormones released into the circulation when the urinary bladder of the anesthetized dog is distended. Clin. Sci., 41:69, 1971.

Greenwood, C.: The pharmacology of ketotifen. Chest, 82 (Suppl.):455, 1982.

Kaplan, W. E., Firlit, C. F., and Schoenberg, H. W.: The female urethral syndrome: external sphincter spasm as etiology. J. Urol. 124:48, 1980.

Kraft, J. K., and Stamey, T. A.: The natural history of symptomatic recurrent bacteriuria in women. Medicine, 56:55, 1977.

Larsen, S., Thompson, S. A., Hald, T., et al.: Mast cells in interstitial cystitis. Br. J. Med., 54:283, 1982.

Mabry, E. W., Carson, C. C.,and Older, R. A.: Evaluation of women with chronic voiding discomfort. Urology, 18:244, 1981.

Maskell, R., Pead, L., and Allen, J.: The puzzle of "urethral syndrome": a possible answer. Lancet, 1:1058, 1979.

Messing, E. M., and Stamey, T. A.: Interstitial cystitis: early diagnosis, pathology and treatment. Urology, 12:381, 1978.

O'Donnell, R. P.: Cystourethritis (letter). Urology, 12:236, 1978.

Panja, S. K.: Urethral syndrome in women attending a clinic for sexually transmitted diseases. Br. J. Vener. Dis., 59:179, 1983.

Parkes, A. C., and Boreham, P.: Cryosurgery for the urethral syndrome: preliminary communication. J. R. Soc. Med., 73:428, 1980.

Raz, S., and Smith, R. B.: External sphincter spasticity syndrome in female patients. J. Urol. 115:443, 1976.

Richardson, F. H.: External urethroplasty in women: technique and clinical evaluation. J. Urol., 101:719, 1969.

Roberts, M., and Smith, P.: Non-malignant obstruction of the female urethra. Br. J. Urol., 40:694, 1968.

Schmidt, R. A., and Tanagho, E. A.: Urethral syndrome or urinary tract infection? Urology, *18*:424, 1981.

Shirley, S. W., Stewart, B. H., and Mirelman, S.: Dimethyl sulfoxide in treatment of inflammatory genitourinary disorders. Urology, *11*:215, 1978.

Smith, P. J.: The management of the urethral syndrome. Br. J. Hosp. Med., *22*:578, 1979.

Splatt, A. J., and Weedon, D.: The urethral syndrome: experience with the Richardson urethroplasty. Br. J. Urol., *49*:173, 1977.

Splatt, A. J., and Weedon, D.: The urethral syndrome: morphological studies. Br. J. Urol., *53*:263, 1981.

Stamm, W. E.: Measurement of pyuria and its relation to bacteriuria. (Symposium on Body Fluids and Infectious Diseases). Am. J. Med., *75*:53, 1983.

Stamm, W. E., Running, K., McKevitt, M., et al.: Treatment of the acute urethral syndrome. N. Engl. J. Med., *304*:956, 1981.

Stamm, W. E., Wagner, K. F., Amsel, R., et al.: Causes of the acute urethral syndrome in women. N. Engl. J. Med., *303*:409, 1980.

Zondek, B., and Bromberg, Y. M.: Endocrine allergy: clinical reactions of allergy to endogenous hormones and their treatment. J. Obstet. Gynaecol. Brit. Emp., *54*:1, 1947.

Zufall, R.: Ineffectiveness of treatment of urethral syndrome in women. Urology. *12*:337, 1978.

URINARY LITHIASIS

CHAPTER 25

Urinary Lithiasis

GEORGE W. DRACH, M.D.

INTRODUCTION

Urologists have been defined forever as surgeons because of their methods of dealing with urinary lithiasis. Anthropologic history provides evidence that urinary calculi existed as long as 7000 years ago and perhaps more. The "specialty" of urologic surgery was even recognized by Hippocrates, who, in his famous oath for the physician, stated, "I will not cut, even for the stone, but leave such procedures to the practitioners of the craft" (Clendening, 1942). The recognition of different varieties of urinary calculi also resulted in more varieties of medical treatment, most of which failed. During the last decade, however, many major advances have greatly improved our understanding of the causes of stone disease. Although not all calculi can be cured, patients who develop one of the five major types of urinary calculi now have at least a 50 per cent chance of cure or control with medical therapy alone. Surgery continues to be important as one aspect of treatment of urinary calculi, but it is now only one step in the total therapeutic plan for patients with urinary lithiasis.

Literature referred to in this chapter was reviewed through July 1983. A few important works published after this date have been included. Considerable selection has been exercised by the author in choosing the literature for the references for this chapter. Most references are from English language journals. Selected journals in languages other than English may have extensive reports regarding urinary lithiasis, but only concepts summarized adequately in English abstracts are given here. References to all topics covered are included alphabetically in the bibliography. Certain reviews have been selected and listed separately as a rapid introduction to research, patient evaluation, or treatment of urinary lithiasis. Finally, several research symposia in urinary lithiasis have been conducted within the past decade. These have resulted in authoritative volumes with valuable information about worldwide research on urinary lithiasis. Most are available as soft- or hard-bound books. A separate list of proceedings of these research symposia has also been included.

This chapter will attempt to summarize the facts and theories necessary for the understanding and care of patients with urinary calculi. A brief historical review is followed by epidemiologic factors in the incidence of urolithiasis, such as heredity, age, sex, geography, environment, and occupation or economic level. Next, aspects of etiology will be discussed in general terms with reference to both clinical and laboratory research. There is much literature on urinary lithiasis that describes crystallization processes in urine. It is the author's opinion that an understanding of these processes is critical to our future understanding of urinary stone disease. Therefore, we will review in depth the principles of crystallization in biologic systems as they pertain to urinary systems.

Thereafter, we will pursue some specific aspects of diagnosis of urinary calculi and discuss the necessary clinical, radiologic, and laboratory studies. An attempt will be made to survey the problem of renal damage caused by stones in a discussion of the pathophysiology of obstruction due to urinary calculi, nephrocalcinosis, and urinary tract epithelial changes related to urinary lithiasis. Having progressed through the etiologic and diagnostic aspects of urinary lithiasis, we will next classify the individual patient with regard to the type of stone and degree of activity of his disease. Based upon this classification, we will discuss specific treatments available for specific types of stone disease.

Finally, we will discuss some practical aspects of management of stones that have passed out of the kidneys or formed in other specific anatomic locations. This includes stones of the ureter, bladder, prostate, and urethra. We will also summarize some recent observations on stone disease in children.

Urinary lithiasis represents a realm of sharing between the urologist and his medical colleagues. In some instances, medical specialists with training in endocrinologic diseases perform nonsurgical evaluation and treatment of urinary stone disease. In many instances, however, this is not possible or feasible. Decisions about evaluation and treatment of patients with urinary lithiasis often rest with the urologist. Urologists must therefore understand all aspects of the etiology, diagnosis, and surgical and nonsurgical treatment of urinary lithiasis.

HISTORY

Ancient man was undoubtedly afflicted with stone just as man is now. Riches (1968) refers to a stone that was found in the pelvis (presumably bladder) of an Egyptian skeleton estimated to be over 7000 years old. Perhaps because of the admonition of Hippocrates, surgical treatment of bladder calculi was for centuries traditionally left to numbers of wandering lithotomists. By the 17th and 18th centuries many of these men had become famous. Wangensteen et al. (1969) refer to some of the more famous lithotomists of that time. They included Colot, Fr. Jaques, Rau, Fr. Come, and others. Soon, however, surgeons trained in anatomy and other aspects of medical practice recognized that traveling lithotomists were not as adept at their calling as might be desired. Many of these well-trained individuals, whom Wangensteen et al. classified as "professionals," began to take an interest in urinary lithiasis. Most of their interest centered upon improvement of techniques for removal of bladder calculi. As an example, Dupuytren, who is famous in many areas of medicine and surgery, developed a new type of perineal instrument for removal of bladder calculi (Drach, 1974a). Celsius, Franco, and Cheselden were other great contributors to the development of improved lithotomy techniques. Civiale and Bigelow, although separated in time by half a century, were instrumental in the development of practical lithotrity and litholopaxy techniques that are still used. Sir Henry Thompson became famous for his interest in medical therapy of bladder stone and suggested the possibility of treatment of bladder stone by dissolution (Thompson, 1873, cited by Thorwald, 1956). Only after this period of improvement in surgery did a significant amount of attention turn to medical treatment of urolithiasis, although naturopaths had tried unsuccessfully to treat "disease of the stone" for centuries. Galen, for example, treated stone disease with wine and honey, parsley and caraway seed; and Howship recommended administration of alkalis or acids to arrest calculi, as did Sir Astley Cooper (cited by Wesson, 1935).

As Europeans moved to America, they brought with them their predisposition to form bladder calculi. Wangensteen et al. (1969) summarized several reviews of lithotomy practice in America during the years 1810 to 1853. Vogel (1970) noted that in America, urinary calculous disease was isolated predominantly to immigrant Europeans. For instance, he reviews the statement that "savages were unacquainted with a great many diseases that afflict the Europeans, such as the gout, dropsy, gravel." Citing another reference, he notes that North Carolina Indians were "never troubled by scurvy, dropsy, or stone." In 1559, an Inca reporter (cited by Vogel) stated that he thought that corn was the factor that prevented occurrence of urinary calculi in native American Indians. Many Indian herbal treatments were adapted to the treatment of urinary calculus or gravel by the Americans. Thus, Vogel mentions the use of haw or hawthorne tree, persimmon, sarsaparilla, and decoctions of multiple other leaves and twigs as remedies for stone.

In contrast, Beck and Mulvaney (1966) reported two urinary calculi associated with the bony remains of two Indians buried in Fulton County, Illinois and Marion County, Indiana. Both stones were predominantly carbonate apatite, although one contained a small amount of struvite. Dating of these archeologic sites placed one inhabitant at 1500 B.C. and the other at 1500 A.D. Since, as we shall see, pure apatitic calculi usually accompany metabolic disease, it seems possible that these calculi were caused by such a disease and that, indeed, idiopathic urinary stone disease rarely afflicted native American Indians. Some authors (notably Prien, 1971, and Joly, 1931) have used this observed capability of transference of European urinary stone disease to the New World to challenge the theory (to be presented later in this chapter) that geographic distribution of urinary calculi has any importance whatsoever.

Whether or not stone disease of early centuries was governed more by heredity or by environment, there is no doubt that bladder calculi were an endemic part of life prior to the twentieth century (Ellis, 1969; Ostergaard, 1973). King (1971) and Prien (1971) noted the historical trend away from bladder calculi toward upper urinary tract calculi whenever a country becomes more industrialized and diet becomes more nutritious. When agrarian and primitive pursuits remain the primary way of life for a population, the incidence of bladder stone disease continues to be high, as it is in Thailand (Lonsdale, 1968b; Suvachittanont et al., 1973). By the early 1900's, observers of urinary stone disease had already begun to notice an increased occurrence of renal and ureteral calculi and a decreased occurrence of bladder calculi in Europe, the British Isles, and America. This change seemed to parallel increased industrialization.

By 1950, investigators began to report some significant physiologic observations that were associated with the production of urinary calculi. These included the importance of diet, especially in association with uric acid bladder calculi (Gutman and Yu, 1968). Hypercalciuria was clearly defined as one factor contributing to the formation of calcium calculi (Flocks, 1939), and hypercalciuria due to hyperparathyroidism was identified and separated from idiopathic hypercalciuria (Albright and Reifenstein, 1948; Flocks, 1940). The importance of nucleation of stones in the kidney was studied intensively by Randall (1937), who described his famous "Randall's plaques." Urinary crystals and colloid were described, and the "crystalloid" and "colloid" composition of all stones was determined (Wesson, 1935). The effects of infection on stone formation were noted to be different from the effects of excessive excretion of crystalloids in the absence of infection. Much groundwork was laid for the worldwide resurgence of research into the etiology and prophylaxis of urolithiasis that followed World War II. The remainder of this chapter is concerned mostly with the immense amount of information about urinary stone disease gained since 1950.

The history of stone disease implies that many diverse factors might be involved in its causation: heredity, environment, age, sex, urinary infection, the presence of metabolic diseases, and dietary excesses or deficiencies. Review of epidemiologic aspects of urinary calculi begins our survey of urolithiasis.

EPIDEMIOLOGIC ASPECTS OF UROLITHIASIS

Andersen (1973) presents an interesting multifaceted theory of epidemiology of urinary calculi. He notes that the incidence of upper tract urinary calculi varies greatly with age, anatomic site, and geographic distribution and that there are unexplained increases during different periods of history. He feels therefore that there are at least two separate epidemiologic factors involved in the genesis of urinary calculi. The first of these may be considered intrinsic. Intrinsic factors are related to the inherited biochemical or anatomic makeup of the individual. For example, African Bantu natives and the related North American Negro tend to have very few urinary calculi (Modlin, 1967; Pantanowitz et al., 1973). A subcategory of this racial or ethnic factor includes any familial tendency toward generation of calculi. Familial inheritance of calcium stone disease has been reported by Resnick et al. (1968) and McGeown (1960) and reviewed by Finlayson (1974). No true sex-linked inheritance of urinary lithiasis has been defined, but Transbol and Frydendal (1973) have reported that male relatives of patients with hypercalciuric stone disease were more often affected than female relatives. Intrinsic factors of urolithiasis, then, include ethnic, racial, and familial background and any inherited physiologic or anatomic predisposition to urinary calculi. Most of these factors will be discussed further in the sections on specific types of calculi, although the effects of heredity, age, and sex on incidence of calculi will be discussed in this section.

Superimposed upon these apparent intrinsic factors are those that Andersen (1973) terms extrinsic. Another term for these might be "environmental factors." These include climate, water available for drinking, dietary patterns of populations and of households of people with urinary calculi, the presence or absence of trace elements in foodstuffs and drinking water, and different occupations. Some of these extrinsic factors seem to be definitely related to the occurrence of urinary calculi, but first let us review several intrinsic factors.

Intrinsic Factors

HEREDITY

Underlying all epidemiologic concepts of causation of urinary calculi is the role of heredity. Numerous authors have noted that urinary calculi are relatively rare in the North American Indian, the Negroes of Africa and America, and the native-born Israeli. It would appear that resistance to urinary stone disease has been part of the natural selection of individuals for persistence of their race in areas that have relatively hot climates. Conversely, the incidence of stone disease is known to be highest in some of the colder temperate areas of the world populated primarily by Eurasians and Caucasians. Although the incidence of bladder stones seems to be related primarily to dietary habits and malnutrition in underdeveloped and primitive countries, dietary improvement over the years has probably resulted only in a change of the site of occurrence of urinary calculi from bladder to kidney (Sutor, 1972). In other words, the hereditary capability of forming stones persists while the anatomic site of presentation has changed.

Interest in the familial incidence of urinary calculi in relation to heredity is not new. We find evidence of studies of this nature by Gram (1932) and Goldstein (1951), and more recently, genetic studies have been performed by Resnick et al. (1968) and McGeown (1960). These authors conclude that urolithiasis requires a polygenic defect (more than one gene is involved). In addition, genetic predisposition to urinary lithiasis has partial penetrance, so that the severity of stone disease may differ from generation to generation even though the individual has the gene defects necessary for urinary lithiasis.

White et al. (1969) caution against accepting familial or hereditary theories of stone formation too readily, however. They studied stone formers and their spouses and similar pairs of non–stone formers. They noted that urinary calcium excretion was significantly higher in spouses of stone formers than in control persons of the same sex in non–stone forming households. Hence, household diet as well as familial tendencies must be considered in theories of etiology of urinary lithiasis.

Renal tubular acidosis is one hereditary disease that has certainly been associated with frequent episodes of urinary lithiasis. Nephrolithiasis and nephrocalcinosis have been reported to occur in almost 73 per cent of patients with this disease (Dretler et al., 1969; Marquardt, 1973). Incomplete renal tubular acidosis also appears to be transmitted as a hereditary trait that results in urinary lithiasis. Cystinuria is a prime example of familial transmission of a type of urinary lithiasis that is definitely hereditary. Cystinuria is known to be expressed when two recessive genes for cystinuria are present; that is, it is a homozygous recessive disease (Crawhall and Watts, 1968). The genetic defect is that of excessive excretion of cystine, ornithine, lysine, and arginine (mnemonic: COLA). Only cystine becomes insoluble in urine. Inter-

estingly, some patients with cystinuria do not develop urinary calculi (King, 1967, 1971). It therefore appears that at least two gene defects (again polygenic) are required to predispose some cystinurics toward formation of cystine urinary calculi. Hence, only stone-forming cystinurics carry the additional gene defect that causes them to form urinary calculi of cystine.

AGE AND SEX

Figure 25–1 shows the typical age and sex distributions of incidence of urinary calculi in a group of 119 patients (Drach, unpublished observations). Note that the peak age incidence of urinary calculi occurs in the third to fifth decades. About three males are afflicted for every female. These observations are generally confirmed by most individuals who have studied age and sex incidence of urinary calculi (Blacklock, 1969; Fetter and Zimskind, 1961; Inada et al., 1958). Several authors have pointed out that the maximum incidence of urinary lithiasis appears to occur in the 30- to 50-year age group (Bailey et al., 1974; Burkland and Rosenberg, 1955; Fetter and Zimskind, 1961; Frank et al., 1959; Prince and Scardino, 1960). But when does urolithiasis begin? If we ask the patients depicted in Figure 25–1 their age at the onset of their disease, we obtain the results shown in Figure 25–2. Note that the majority of patients report onset of disease in the second decade of life, with decreasing onset through the third, fourth, and fifth decades. If we combine this fact with the apparent observation in Figure 25–1 that the maximum incidence of disease occurs in the fifth decade, we recognize that urinary

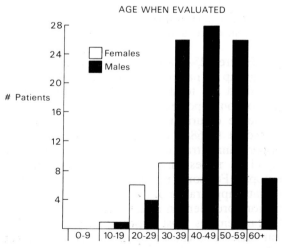

Figure 25–1. Age and sex distribution for 119 patients who were evaluated completely for their recurrent renal lithiasis. A male to female ratio of 3:1 is evident. Compare with Figure 25–2.

TRIGGER OR LIMIT CONCEPT OF CALCULUS FORMATION

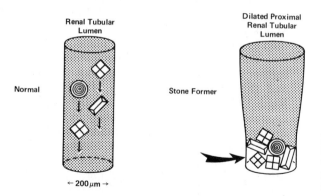

Figure 25–9. "Triggering" of urolithiasis may occur when many crystals or spherules aggregate to occlude a urinary tubule (arrow), or a single crystal may become lodged in the tubule and then grow larger as urine in the metastable zone of saturation flows by.

faces. It is likely that both processes are important in the creation of urinary calculi.

EPITAXY

One other aspect of crystallization that has received considerable attention is epitaxy (Hench, 1972; Lonsdale, 1968a,b; Seifert, 1967). If a crystal has a pattern or organization of ions that is regular and predictable, this structure is called a lattice. This surface lattice may resemble very closely that of a second but different type of crystal. Depending upon the closeness of resemblance, the second type of crystal may actually be able to grow upon the surface of the first. For example, let us suppose

that urine is supersaturated for a period of time with uric acid. For some reason, such as dehydration combined with the intake of a meal containing a large amount of purine, the concentration of uric acid goes up markedly. The formation product for uric acid is exceeded, and a number of uric acid crystals form by the "free nucleation" process. When these nuclei form, they "pull" uric acid out of solution, and the concentration of free uric acid in the urine decreases. Let us suppose that the amount of decrease is sufficient to keep the growth of uric acid nuclei to a relatively low rate. Our patient, however, who is still dehydrated, eats a large dish of rhubarb pie for dessert and quenches his

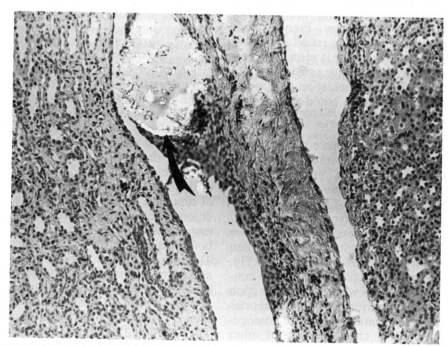

Figure 25–10. Randall's plaque (arrow): Subepithelial collection of calcified material has acquired additional calcium oxalate crystals and has begun to erupt through the epithelium. (100 ×, partly crossed polars.)

Hodgkinson and Nordin, 1971; Lonsdale, 1968*a*,*b*; Mullin, 1972; Thomas, 1974; Walton, 1965, 1967; Williams, 1974*a*,*b*).

CRYSTAL NUCLEATION

Nucleation of crystals occurs when active ions and molecules in a solution no longer flow randomly in a completely dissociated fashion but cluster together closely enough to form the earliest crystal structure that will not dissolve. This structure has the form of a lattice that is characteristic of that crystal. If this process occurs spontaneously in a pure solution (such as sodium plus chloride in distilled deionized water), the process is called homogeneous nucleation. But pure solutions are difficult to create. Dust particles, glass chips, and other contaminants may enter the solution and serve as nuclei. The analogy is that of a chemical catalyst: Other particles that start nucleation "catalyze" the process. This type of secondary nucleation is probably most likely to occur in urine and is referred to as heterogeneous nucleation. No matter what type of nucleation occurs, it requires energy to "push" the crystal nucleus together (Uhlmann and Chalmers, 1965). The energy required for nucleation is higher than that required for simple crystal growth, and is provided when the amount of supersaturation is high enough (metastable region) to cause nucleation. According to Walton (1965), the physical factors that tend to control nucleation are those of interfacial energy, the temperature, and the frequency of collision. Frequency of collision increases as supersaturation increases, and therefore, enough energy is ultimately created to allow nucleation. Once satisfactory energy has been achieved, nucleation may occur in one of several fashions as noted above.

CRYSTAL GROWTH

Once nucleation has occurred in the complex solution known as urine, certain nuclei may continue to grow if the urine remains supersaturated. Not only will such nuclei continue to grow in the zone above the formation product (the zone that permits spontaneous nucleation), they will continue to grow even if the saturation of urine falls into the metastable zone between solubility product and formation product (Fig. 25–8). The concept of increasing the urine concentration to the level where the formation product is exceeded is critical to certain theories of urinary stone formation in which homogeneous nucleation is a critical event. In other theories, however, saturation is required only to the range of metastable supersaturation; it is

postulated that adequate heterogeneous nuclei are already created by biologic processes in the kidney (Carr, 1969; Drach and Boyce, 1972; Malek and Boyce, 1973; Randall, 1937). Stones then grow on these preformed nuclei.

These two concepts of nucleation may be further separated into the free particle theory and the fixed particle theory (Finlayson and Reid, 1978). In free particle nucleation, multiple crystals are formed simultaneously in the upper urinary system when the formation product of a substance is exceeded. One concept of free particle nucleation also allows for the fact that urine probably contains multiple, previously formed microliths in the kidney papillae that are subsequently excreted and may then serve as nuclei for other ions. To conform to this theory, however, these particles must float freely in urine and must serve as nuclei for further growth or aggregation of crystals. In the theory of fixed particle nucleation, it is suggested that because of excessive concentration of certain ions in certain areas of kidney, precipitation of crystals or spherules may occur in the renal papillae either within the tubular lumina or beneath the surface of the papillae (Drach and Boyce, 1972; Finlayson and Reid, 1978; Hautmann et al., 1980; Malek and Boyce, 1973; Randall, 1937; Resnick et al., 1978; Resnick and Boyce, 1978; Vermeulen and Lyon, 1968) (Figs. 25–9 and 25–10). These particles remain "fixed" and serve as nuclei for further growth.

CRYSTAL AGGREGATION

Another concept is necessary to promote our understanding of the probable genesis of urinary calculi. This concept is that of aggregation. If multiple nuclei and crystals are formed spontaneously and float freely, these nuclei become active kinetically and bounce about in the urine. If they remain small, free, and independent within the solution, they will then pass through the urinary tract within a given amount of time and will be voided. Under certain conditions, however, these nuclei can grow and may come close enough to each other to be bound together by various chemical forces. Therefore, nuclei or larger growing crystals may aggregate to form larger crystal masses. Should these become large enough to become lodged in a given position in the urinary tract they may then continue to grow by one of two processes. They may add additional crystals to their surfaces by the process of aggregation, or they may grow by adding new crystal mass to their sur-

TRIGGER OR LIMIT CONCEPT OF CALCULUS FORMATION

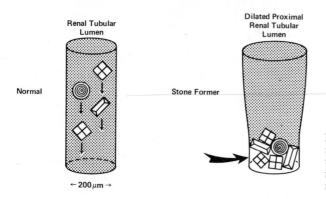

Figure 25–9. "Triggering" of urolithiasis may occur when many crystals or spherules aggregate to occlude a urinary tubule (arrow), or a single crystal may become lodged in the tubule and then grow larger as urine in the metastable zone of saturation flows by.

faces. It is likely that both processes are important in the creation of urinary calculi.

EPITAXY

One other aspect of crystallization that has received considerable attention is epitaxy (Hench, 1972; Lonsdale, 1968a,b; Seifert, 1967). If a crystal has a pattern or organization of ions that is regular and predictable, this structure is called a lattice. This surface lattice may resemble very closely that of a second but different type of crystal. Depending upon the closeness of resemblance, the second type of crystal may actually be able to grow upon the surface of the first. For example, let us suppose

that urine is supersaturated for a period of time with uric acid. For some reason, such as dehydration combined with the intake of a meal containing a large amount of purine, the concentration of uric acid goes up markedly. The formation product for uric acid is exceeded, and a number of uric acid crystals form by the "free nucleation" process. When these nuclei form, they "pull" uric acid out of solution, and the concentration of free uric acid in the urine decreases. Let us suppose that the amount of decrease is sufficient to keep the growth of uric acid nuclei to a relatively low rate. Our patient, however, who is still dehydrated, eats a large dish of rhubarb pie for dessert and quenches his

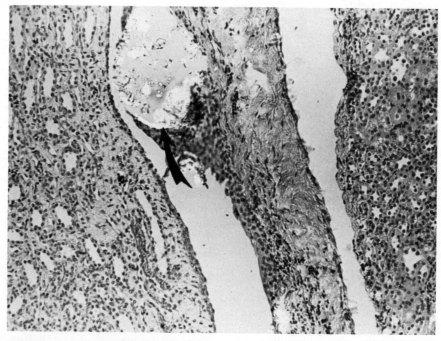

Figure 25–10. Randall's plaque (arrow): Subepithelial collection of calcified material has acquired additional calcium oxalate crystals and has begun to erupt through the epithelium. (100 ×, partly crossed polars.)

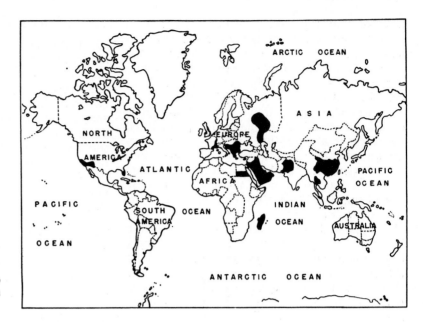

Figure 25–3. World stone map showing selected areas with high incidence of urolithiasis.

occurrence of idiopathic urinary lithiasis. Low-incidence areas include Central and South America, most of Africa, and those areas of Australia populated by native aborigines. Many of the areas with a low incidence of stone disease have warm climates and large populations of native inhabitants. One wonders again whether the processes of natural selection have previously eliminated those individuals with genetic tendencies toward development of urinary lithiasis.

In addition to different incidences for all urinary calculi combined, there are differences in types of urinary stone disease in different areas of the world. Lonsdale (1968a and b), and Sutor and Wooley (1970b, 1971, 1974) have reported extensive geographic surveys of types of urinary calculi. They have noted, for example, that stones from Great Britain, Scotland, and the Sudan are similar and are composed primarily of mixed calcium oxalate and calcium phosphate. In other areas of the world, most upper urinary tract calculi are composed mainly of magnesium ammonium phosphate (struvite). Sutor et al. (1974a) note that many oxalate but few struvite calculi were found in stone collec-

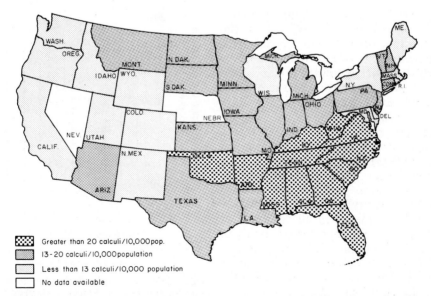

Greater than 20 calculi/10,000 pop.

13 - 20 calculi/10,000 population

Less than 13 calculi/10,000 population

No data available

Figure 25–4. Geographic distribution of urinary lithiasis in the United States in 1974, based on a hospital discharge survey. (From Sierakowski, R., Finlayson, B., and Landes, R.: Urol. Res., 1:157, 1978. Used by permission.)

tions of the Royal Navy. Hence, it seems to confirm that struvite stones are associated primarily with upper urinary tract infection in the female. Sexual differences in the type and incidence of stones affect the geographic and occupational distribution of urolithiasis.

A number of children's stones from underdeveloped areas such as Thailand were analyzed by Sutor et al. (1974b). They stated that approximately 89 per cent of these stones contained ammonium acid urate or calcium oxalate or both. Examination of the nuclei of these calculi suggested that ammonium urate was the primary component. In their series, uric acid also appeared to be more common in adult lower urinary tract stones than in upper urinary tract stones. Hence, in geographic areas where the incidence of bladder stone disease exceeds that of upper tract calculi, uric acid, urate, and perhaps calcium oxalate calculi should predominate.

Upper urinary tract calculi composed of uric acid tend to be more common in certain geographic areas. Representative areas include Czechoslovakia and Israel (Herbstein et al., 1974), and possibly Chicago (Gutman and Yu, 1968). Conversely, Hazarika et al. (1974) report that upper urinary tract calculi analyzed in India contained mostly calcium oxalate or calcium phosphate. Uric acid or ammonium urate calculi were rarely encountered. Pantanowitz et al. (1973) reported that calcium oxalate and phosphate were found in 53 per cent of 256 South African stones analyzed by them. Most of the remaining stones in this series contained "triple phosphates."

In summary, geography has some influence on the incidence of urinary calculi and on the types of calculi that occur within a given area. However, the capability of individuals to transport the intrinsic tendency toward urinary stone formation from area to area makes it likely that the major tendencies contributing to urinary lithiasis are inherent in the individual. The effects of geography represent one aspect of environment superimposed upon the intrinsic factors. Andersen (1973) further stated in his stone formation hypothesis (presented previously) that, given an intrinsic predisposition toward urinary lithiasis, "dietary structure provides the baseline of stone incidence in all countries or regions." He points out that certain types of geography tend to establish dietary patterns. Geography has an effect in terms of temperature and humidity, which also seem to influence the incidence of human urinary calculi.

CLIMATIC AND SEASONAL FACTORS

It is difficult to find direct evidence for the influence of climate on the occurrence of urinary lithiasis. Several authors, however, have attempted to show a relationship between higher environmental temperature and increased seasonal incidence of urinary stone disease. For example, Prince et al. (1956) related their observations on seasonal variation in incidence of urinary calculi to high summer temperatures in the southeastern United States. Figure 25–5 is derived from data presented in their article. Peak incidence of lithiasis occurred in July, August, and September, which are also the months with the highest average temperatures. The relative humidity in their area ranged between 70 and 80 per cent throughout the year and therefore did not appear to be related to the peak incidence of urinary stone disease. Prince and Scardino (1960) followed this study with a prospective analysis of 922 occurrences of ureteral stone. Once again, the peak incidence occurred in July, August, and September. In examining their later report, one notes that the highest incidence of urinary calculi appears to occur 1 to 2 months following the achievement of the maximum mean annual temperature in their area.

An interesting contrast to these studies by Prince and Scardino is found in the communication by Bateson (1973). He reports incidence

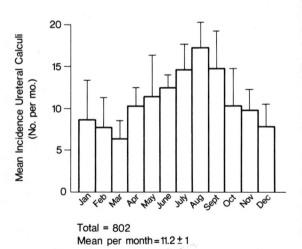

Seasonal Incidence of Ureteral Calculi*
(Southeastern U.S.A.)

Total = 802
Mean per month = 11.2 ± 1

*Derived from data in Prince et al. 1956 by using only years 1949-1954

Figure 25–5. Greatest incidence of ureteral stones occurs in summer months June through September.

Monthly Incidence of Free (Ureteral) Urinary Calculi*
(Perth, Western Australia)

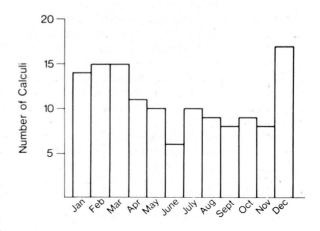

Figure 25–6. Compare with Figure 25–5. Greatest incidence of ureteral stones occurs in the months of December through March during the Australian summer.

*Derived from data in Bateson, 1973

of upper urinary tract calculi in the area surrounding Perth in Western Australia. Figure 25–6 shows the incidence of calculi per month in 188 of his patients. The peak incidence of urinary calculi occurs in December through March. This coincides with the peak maximum summer temperatures in that geographic area. A comparison of Figures 25–5 and 25–6 indicates that in both areas increased mean environmental temperatures seem to be related to an increased incidence of urinary calculi. Summer in Perth, Western Australia, usually includes the months of December through March, while summer in Savannah, Georgia, includes May through September. Mean temperatures in Perth for the summer months are near 83.2° F, while mean temperatures in summer in Savannah are about 79.2° F. Bateson states that the dry climate contributes to the formation of stones; in contrast, the relative humidity for the area near Savannah is near 75 per cent.

Rivera (1973) studied the seasonal incidence of urinary calculi in the area surrounding San Juan, Puerto Rico. Maximum incidence of urolithiasis in this northern hemisphere region occurred in July through October in most years. Highest average monthly temperatures in the area occurred in the months of August and September. During the study some unusual seasonal changes occurred, including unusual coolness during periods when relatively high temperatures would be expected. There was a decrease in the number of calculi during these unexpected cool periods. Rivera concluded that urinary calculi follow a recurrent annual cycle

with increased occurrence during the hot months. Peak incidence immediately followed periods of higher temperature, increased humidity, increased precipitation, and slower winds. Al-dabbagh and Fahadi (1977) drew similar conclusions. In contrast, Elliott (1975) concluded from a 10-year study of seasonal variations in urolithiasis that peak stone incidence occurred during periods of above average temperature and *below* average rainfall. In view of the conflicting data accumulated from dry regions, it appears that mean temperature remains the most critical factor.

Parry and Lister (1975) present an alternative viewpoint that implicates increased exposure to sunlight as a cause of increased urinary calcium excretion. This may lead to increased incidence of urolithiasis. But Blacklock (1969) reported a higher incidence of urinary calculi in below-decks naval personnel who worked in a hot environment (cooks, boiler stokers) than in above-decks personnel who supposedly receive more sunlight. The sunlight theory requires much more prospective study to prove its value.

Elevated environmental temperature seems to be definitely related to increased risk of stone disease in populations capable of forming stones. High temperatures increase perspiration, which may result in increased concentration of urine. This hyperconcentration could contribute to stone formation in many ways. For example, if the individual has, as noted previously, an inborn tendency toward formation of calculi, dehydration would result in decreased urine volume and increased urinary

concentration of these molecules as well as excessive urinary acidity (Toor et al., 1964). These two changes promote crystallization of the respective molecules. Hallson and Rose (1977) have shown increased crystalluria in stone-formers during summer months. In persons with a tendency to form calcium calculi, urinary concentrations of calcium oxalate and phosphate would increase until large crystals could form, possibly aggregrating into stones. Patients with a tendency toward formation of uric acid or cystine calculi would have an additional risk because acid urine holds much less uric acid or cystine in solution. One admonition to stone formers as derived from these studies, then, might be to "keep cool."

WATER INTAKE AND URINARY LITHIASIS

Two factors involved in the relationship between water intake and urolithiasis are the volume of water ingested as opposed to that lost by perspiration, and the mineral or trace element content of the water supply of the region. One of the prevailing assumptions in the literature of urolithiasis is that increased water intake and increased urinary output decrease the incidence of urinary calculi in those patients who are predisposed to the disease. One can find multiple references to the validity of this statement. In their survey of urolithiasis in the United States, Burkland and Rosenberg (1955) questioned urologists about their opinions of methods of preventing recurrence of urinary stone disease. "Forcing water" received the highest total number of positive responses (along with elimination of infection and elimination of urinary obstruction). In addition, authorities who discuss the treatment of urinary calculi stipulate that encouraging increased water intake is critical to success. We find this opinion reaffirmed in reviews by Drach, (1976a), Smith and Boyce (1969), Finlayson (1974), and Thomas (1975). Finlayson points out the theoretical criticism that urine dilution by increased water intake may actually increase ion activity coefficients of the elements in urine. Ion collisions would increase and might contribute to increased formation of crystals. (These points will be discussed further in the section on crystallography.) But water diuresis does reduce the average time of residence of free crystal particles in urine and also dilutes absolutely the components of urine that may crystallize. Finlayson concludes that the dilutional effects of water diuresis probably outweigh the changes in ion activity and therefore do help to prevent stone formation. For example, in pa-

tients who form urinary calculi of calcium oxalate, Finlayson (1974) demonstrated that increased urine flow causes a reduction in urine oxalate concentration. However, to be significantly effective, a urine output of more than 3600 milliliters per day would be theoretically necessary. Few patients are able to ingest enough water to create such a high urinary output unless they are re-educated to increase water drinking.

Environment, family education, heredity, and other factors are associated with various habits of ingestion of fluids, especially water. Lonsdale (1968b) pointed out that habitual low levels of water intake may have been related to the high incidence of uric acid stones of British adults in earlier times. A revealing series of studies of water drinking habits was reported by Frank et al. (1959, 1966). They first investigated very thoroughly the epidemiologic aspects of occurrence of urinary lithiasis in native and immigrant groups populating Israeli communities. They noted that the areas of highest incidence of urolithiasis were the warmer desert regions as opposed to the cooler mountainous areas. Within these desert areas the incidence of calculi formation was highest among immigrants from Europe, lower in individuals from East and North Africa, and lowest in the native-born population of Israel. Overall incidence of calculi rose markedly after age 18. The authors selected one factor as the most important in increasing risk of stone disease—namely, low urinary output in an area of high environmental temperatures. They also felt that low urinary output was secondary to the transfer of home-country drinking habits to Israel by the immigrants. In this group, water intake remained low in spite of climatic changes. To further test this hypothesis, they selected one village and attempted to increase the consumption of water by the population by emphasizing that water drinking would decrease the incidence of urinary calculi. In a second village no attempt was made to increase water drinking or to educate the people about calculous disease, but observations on water drinking and on incidence of stone disease were continued. Without giving any further explanations to the second village, the authors conducted surveys of average daily urinary output in both villages. Their educational program on water drinking appeared to be effective. Between 1962 and 1965 there was a consistent difference in the average urinary output of individuals in the two villages. Those in the "educated" village produced an average of 200 to 300 ml more urine per day than those in

the control village. (The authors reported an interesting incidental observation. In the control village there was little difference between the average summer urinary output [1041 ml per day] and the average winter output [1060 ml per day].) The posteducation incidence of urinary calculi was 0.07 per cent in the village with high urinary output and 1.80 per cent in the village with low urinary output, a highly significant difference. This well-performed study implies that low daily urinary volume is a very important factor in the causation of urolithiasis. In support of Frank et al. (1959), Blacklock (1969) reported that by increasing urinary output from approximately 800 to 1200 ml per day, incidence of urinary calculi in sailors decreased by 86 per cent. Those who treat urinary lithiasis with medications need to remember these reports of the effectiveness of increased urinary output alone.

Although volume of water drinking and subsequent urinary output play a part in causing urolithiasis, other investigators have suggested that the mineral content of water may contribute to causation of stone disease. Data are conflicting, however (Churchill et al., 1980; Shuster et al., 1982). Some say that excessive water hardness (usually calcium sulfate) contributes to calculi (Rose and Westbury, 1975), while others say that excessive softness (as when sodium carbonate is predominant) causes increased incidence of stone disease (Evans et al., in press; Sierakowski et al., 1978; Juuti and Heironen, 1980). Additionally, the presence or absence of certain trace elements in water has been implicated in the formation of urinary calculi. For example, zinc is an inhibitor of calcium crystallization (Elliot and Eusebio, 1967), and low urinary levels of zinc could therefore increase a tendency toward stone formation. Yet Yendt and Cohanim (1973) reported improvement in their stone-forming patients after treatment with thiazides. Urinary zinc concentrations in most of these patients also fell. Proof that water hardness or softness or trace element content is critical to stone formation will require a well-constructed prospective study similar to that conducted on water drinking by Frank et al. (1959, 1966).

DIET

There can be little doubt that dietary intake of various foods and fluids that result in increased urinary excretion of substances that produce stones has a significant effect on the incidence of urinary calculi. Ingestion of excessive amounts of purines (uric acid) (Hodgkinson, 1976), oxalates (Thomas, 1975), calcium, phosphate, and other elements often results in excessive excretion of these components in urine. Effects of diet in relation to specific types of urinary calculi will be reviewed in a later section of this chapter.

One must be very cautious about assuming that the dietary patterns of an individual are the same as those of the community in which he lives. Lonsdale (1968b) points out that stone-forming patients may have exceptional dietary patterns because of previous habits, or because they cannot assimilate the normal diet. Peculiar dietary excesses may also occur, such as use of large amounts of Worcestershire sauce with its high oxalate content (Finlayson, personal communication; Holmes, 1971), vegetarian diet in childhood urolithiasis, or habitual excessive ingestion of milk products in the form of ice cream. Not only the diet but also its source may be important. Identical vegetables grown in different parts of Thailand contain amounts of oxalate that differ by 50 per cent or more (Suvachittanont et al., 1973). Practical problems associated with analysis of total diet for a large group of people make dietary studies highly suspect. In addition, the diet most important is that of the individual stone-forming patient; a careful dietary history is critical to the evaluation of every stone former.

OCCUPATION

Lonsdale indicated (1968b) that urinary calculi are much more likely to be found in individuals who have sedentary occupations. Blacklock (1969) reported that the incidence of urinary calculi was higher in administrative and sedentary personnel of the Royal Navy than in the manual worker. The highest rates of incidence were found in cooks and engine room personnel, and, as discussed previously, these were probably associated with work conditions that included a hot environment. The rate of stone formation was lowest in the "active" group of Royal Marines. Mates (1969) performed an extensive survey of regional differences in occurrence of stone disease in Czechoslovakia. He reported that of all epidemiologic factors studied, the occupation of the individual was of greatest importance. The lowest incidence of stone disease in his country was found in agricultural and border populations. The highest incidence was found in industrial areas, and within these it was especially high among those with sedentary occupations and among Civil Service employees. (Mates then described an interesting method for prevention of stone

disease based on his epidemiologic study: "A large consumption of beer and butter is associated with minimal stone disease.") Andersen (1973) emphasized that the relationship between diet and heredity is the major determinant for urolithiasis but that occupation is also important. He postulates that the economic level of living (related to occupation) and the diet predicated by this level are as likely to be involved in the genesis of upper urinary tract calculi as they have been in the genesis of primary or endemic stones of the bladder. Sutor et al. (1974a) correlated occupation with incidence of urinary calculi in 856 patients. Professional and managerial classes had a much higher than expected incidence of calculi, while skilled and partly skilled workers had the expected frequency. Unskilled laborers had a slightly lower than expected incidence, and manual workers had a much lower than expected frequency of urinary calculi. Occupation also tends to determine exposure to other factors such as high environmental temperature, which may then increase a tendency toward formation of urinary calculi.

Robertson and colleagues performed extensive studies of the relationship between occupation, social class, and risk of stone formation (Robertson et al., 1979b; Robertson et al., 1979a and b). They confirmed that the risk of formation of calcium urinary calculi was increased in the most affluent countries, regions, societies, or individuals. These persons have more disposable income to spend on animal protein, which leads to increased urinary concentrations of calcium, oxalate, and uric acid (Robertson et al., 1979a and b). In fact, they have gone so far as to suggest the alternative to high-protein (rich man's) diets in their paper, "Should recurrent calcium oxalate stone-formers become vegetarians?" (Robertson et al., 1979c). Hence, it becomes difficult to assess whether occupation itself is a primary factor in stone disease or whether it merely establishes other aspects of environment such as diet, heat exposure, and water drinking; alterations in these latter factors may then be the real instigators of urolithiasis.

In summary, this review of the epidemiology of urinary lithiasis leads us to conclude that the following factors all appear to play some part in the genesis of urinary calculi: heredity, age, sex, geographic location, environmental temperature, water intake, diet, social class, and occupation of the individual. Given the fact that for urolithiasis to occur, the individual must have the capability of forming urinary calculi, we will now discuss the physical and chemical factors that play a part in the formation of urinary calculi.

PRESENT THEORETICAL BASIS OF ETIOLOGY OF URINARY LITHIASIS

Modern concepts of etiology of urinary calculous disease may be separated conveniently into four major theories (Table 25–1): (1) the supersaturation/crystallization theory; (2) the matrix nucleation theory; (3) the inhibitor absence theory; and (4) epitaxy (Coe et al., 1980; Elliot, 1973b; Finlayson, 1974, 1978; Malek and Boyce, 1973; Pak, 1983; Resnick and Boyce, 1978; Scott, 1975; Vermeulen and Lyon, 1968; Williams, 1974a). Robertson et al. (1976) developed a combined theory of saturation of urine with crystallizable agents versus inhibition by certain proteins. In 1981 they presented an extended combined theory, in which the major factors contributing to, for example, calcium crystallization, were evaluated by discriminant analysis (Robertson and Peacock, 1983). They showed that risk of calcium oxalate crystallization was related to six factors (in the order of importance): Calcium oxalate crystallization increased as urinary concentrations of oxalate, uric acid, pH, and calcium increased, it decreased as urinary concentrations of protein inhibitors and total volume increased.

To understand the present theories of the causation of stone disease it is necessary first to explain some of the basic processes involved in crystallization in biologic systems. We will also discuss some aspects of renal anatomy that are critical to the application of these crystallization processes to urinary lithiasis. Finally, we will examine urinary excretion patterns of some substances that are critical in the formation of specific types of calculi. Specific discussions of each type of calculus will follow this general introduction to etiology.

Processes of Crystallization

As Finlayson (1974) emphasized, it is impossible to discuss present-day concepts of stone

TABLE 25–1. MODERN THEORIES OF ETIOLOGY OF CALCIUM STONE DISEASE

Supersaturation/crystallization
Matrix initiation
Inhibitor lack
Epitaxy
Combinations of above

disease without becoming acquainted with the vocabulary of biologic crystallization. Therefore, we will introduce at this point some descriptions and examples of crystallization processes so that our use of these words in discussing diagnosis and treatment of urolithiasis will make sense. Terms to be reviewed include saturation and the saturation concentration; supersaturation; solubility product; formation product or formation saturation; metastable region of supersaturation; crystal nucleation; crystal growth; crystal aggregation; epitaxy; and zeta potential.

SATURATION

If increasing amounts of substances capable of crystallizing are added to pure water at a given pH and temperature, eventually a high enough concentration is reached for crystals to form. When crystals begin to form, we say that the solution has become saturated with the substance. There is a specific limit to the amount of solids or solute that can be held in solution. When this amount is exceeded, crystals must form. Crystallization of a single substance such as cystine or uric acid will occur when enough of the substance is added to water at given pH and temperature to saturate the solution. When two or more substances are combined to form the crystal, as is the case with table salt (sodium chloride) or calcium oxalate, the level of saturation is governed by the product of the concentrations of the two (or more) substances. The point at which saturation is reached and crystallization begins is referred to as the solubility product (SP). It is defined as the product of the molar concentrations of the two substances at the point at which saturation is reached.

Note that pH and temperature are always specified for any crystallization process. Alteration in either factor may greatly alter the amount of substance or solute that may be held in solution. Perhaps the best known illustration of the effects of temperature on solubility is the increased solubility of sugar in hot water. For all practical purposes, there need be no concern about temperature in our discussion of urolithiasis because it must occur at body temperature, near 37° C. One must be cautious in analyzing the results of some in vitro studies of stone crystallization, however, because many such studies are performed at room temperature rather than at body temperature (Finlayson, 1974). Since urine varies widely in pH, this factor must be considered in any explanation of urolithiasis, as we shall see.

Saturation and solubility product are easy to define in water, but urine is a much more complex solution. In urine, when the concentration of a substance reaches the point at which saturation would occur in water, crystallization does not occur as expected. Urine has the ability to hold more solute in solution than does pure water. Although all elements and molecules in urine are suspended in water, the mixture of many electrically active ions in urine causes interactions that change the solubility of their elements. Such a solution is called polyionic, and the definition of saturation or solubility product of a given substance in this type of solution becomes very complex and difficult. In addition, many organic chemical molecules such as urea, uric acid, citrate, and the complex mucoproteins of urine all mutually affect the solubility of other substances. For example, citrate is known to combine with calcium to form a soluble complex. It therefore prevents some calcium from combining with oxalate or phosphate and becoming crystalline. As a corollary to this statement, Finlayson (1974), Elliot (1973a), Welshman and McGeown (1975), Nicar et al. (1983), Menon and Mahle (1983), and Schwille et al. (1982) have reported that deficiency in urinary citrate is one of many factors found in the urine of stone formers.

Electrical attraction or repulsion of ions in biologic solutions is also involved in the stone-forming crystallization process. Rollins and Finlayson (1973) studied electrical fields of urine-like solutions and the effects of various additives on the electrical attraction of urinary substances. This type of biologic electrical activity is called zeta potential (Gardner, 1969).

In an attempt to simplify the study of urinary stone disease, many investigators have tried to eliminate urinary components that they believe do not contribute to or detract from a tendency to form urinary calculi. The most elemental of these solutions requires, for calcium oxalate crystals, the presence of calcium, oxalate, sodium, and chloride ions (Finlayson and Roth, 1973). But even this simple solution does not adequately explain all the ionic activity present in urine, nor does it explain other ionic effects on stone formation. A further discussion of ionic activity and its relationship to urolithiasis is beyond the scope of this chapter. The interested reader is referred to the works of Finlayson (1978), Robertson et al. (1968 and 1972a), Nordin et al. (1979), and Isaacson (1968) for further information. It is, however, important to stress that the presence of such a large number of ionically active substances does change the solubility of any given element or substance in urine.

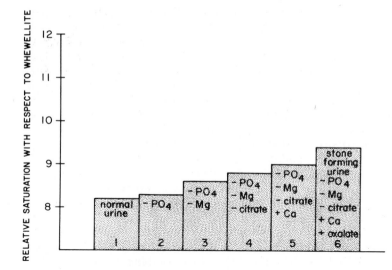

Figure 25-7. Effect of certain urinary components on degree of saturation of urine with whewellite (calcium oxalate monohydrate). Removal of some (PO_4, magnesium, citrate) or addition of others (calcium, oxalate) results in increased saturation and increased risk of precipitation of stone crystals. (Used with permission of Birdwell Finlayson, M.D.)

SUPERSATURATION

The most significant and beneficial effect of these ionic and protein-elemental interactions is to increase the solubility of various substances that otherwise might crystallize in the concentrations present in urine (Fig. 25–7). Hence, if a given amount of calcium and oxalate that would crystallize when placed in a solution of water at given pH and temperature is placed in urine, it will be held in solution. If the amount of calcium and oxalate is increased progressively in the same volume of urine at constant pH and temperature, the calcium and oxalate will stay in solution even though the solubility product has been exceeded. In doing this, we are actually creating supersaturation. This zone of supersaturation is called the metastable region and is illustrated in Figure 25–8. The amount of substance in urine can be increased to a point at which urine will no longer hold it in solution. Then spontaneous nucleation of the crystals begins. The area of supersaturation between the solubility product and spontaneous urinary crystallization is the *metastable region* for a given substance.

The point at which spontaneous nucleation of crystals occurs is known as the formation product (FP) for urine. This means that although urine contains multiple and complex solubilizing factors for that particular crystal, the amount of substance in urine may eventually become so great that it is capable of crystallizing in spite of the solubilizers and inhibitors that are present (Breslau and Pak, 1980; Dyer and Nordin, 1967; Finlayson, 1974; Fleisch, 1965;

PROCESSES OF CRYSTALLIZATION RELATED TO STONE FORMATION

Figure 25-8. Concepts of crystallization in urine summarized. See text for full discussion of various zones.

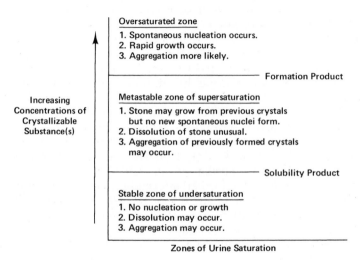

sistence of their race in areas that have relatively hot climates. Conversely, the incidence of stone disease is known to be highest in some of the colder temperate areas of the world populated primarily by Eurasians and Caucasians. Although the incidence of bladder stones seems to be related primarily to dietary habits and malnutrition in underdeveloped and primitive countries, dietary improvement over the years has probably resulted only in a change of the site of occurrence of urinary calculi from bladder to kidney (Sutor, 1972). In other words, the hereditary capability of forming stones persists while the anatomic site of presentation has changed.

Interest in the familial incidence of urinary calculi in relation to heredity is not new. We find evidence of studies of this nature by Gram (1932) and Goldstein (1951), and more recently, genetic studies have been performed by Resnick et al. (1968) and McGeown (1960). These authors conclude that urolithiasis requires a polygenic defect (more than one gene is involved). In addition, genetic predisposition to urinary lithiasis has partial penetrance, so that the severity of stone disease may differ from generation to generation even though the individual has the gene defects necessary for urinary lithiasis.

White et al. (1969) caution against accepting familial or hereditary theories of stone formation too readily, however. They studied stone formers and their spouses and similar pairs of non–stone formers. They noted that urinary calcium excretion was significantly higher in spouses of stone formers than in control persons of the same sex in non–stone forming households. Hence, household diet as well as familial tendencies must be considered in theories of etiology of urinary lithiasis.

Renal tubular acidosis is one hereditary disease that has certainly been associated with frequent episodes of urinary lithiasis. Nephrolithiasis and nephrocalcinosis have been reported to occur in almost 73 per cent of patients with this disease (Dretler et al., 1969; Marquardt, 1973). Incomplete renal tubular acidosis also appears to be transmitted as a hereditary trait that results in urinary lithiasis. Cystinuria is a prime example of familial transmission of a type of urinary lithiasis that is definitely hereditary. Cystinuria is known to be expressed when two recessive genes for cystinuria are present; that is, it is a homozygous recessive disease (Crawhall and Watts, 1968). The genetic defect is that of excessive excretion of cystine, ornithine, lysine, and arginine (mnemonic: COLA). Only cystine becomes insoluble in urine. Inter-

estingly, some patients with cystinuria do not develop urinary calculi (King, 1967, 1971). It therefore appears that at least two gene defects (again polygenic) are required to predispose some cystinurics toward formation of cystine urinary calculi. Hence, only stone-forming cystinurics carry the additional gene defect that causes them to form urinary calculi of cystine.

AGE AND SEX

Figure 25–1 shows the typical age and sex distributions of incidence of urinary calculi in a group of 119 patients (Drach, unpublished observations). Note that the peak age incidence of urinary calculi occurs in the third to fifth decades. About three males are afflicted for every female. These observations are generally confirmed by most individuals who have studied age and sex incidence of urinary calculi (Blacklock, 1969; Fetter and Zimskind, 1961; Inada et al., 1958). Several authors have pointed out that the maximum incidence of urinary lithiasis appears to occur in the 30- to 50-year age group (Bailey et al., 1974; Burkland and Rosenberg, 1955; Fetter and Zimskind, 1961; Frank et al., 1959; Prince and Scardino, 1960). But when does urolithiasis begin? If we ask the patients depicted in Figure 25–1 their age at the onset of their disease, we obtain the results shown in Figure 25–2. Note that the majority of patients report onset of disease in the second decade of life, with decreasing onset through the third, fourth, and fifth decades. If we combine this fact with the apparent observation in Figure 25–1 that the maximum incidence of disease occurs in the fifth decade, we recognize that urinary

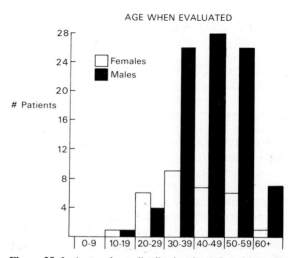

Figure 25–1. Age and sex distribution for 119 patients who were evaluated completely for their recurrent renal lithiasis. A male to female ratio of 3:1 is evident. Compare with Figure 25–2.

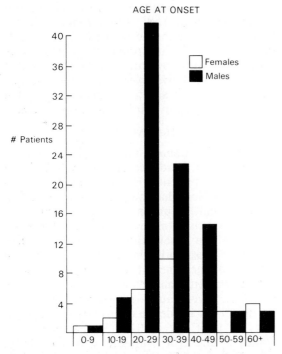

Figure 25–2. Age and sex distribution of 119 patients at the time of first episode of proven renal lithiasis. Only 6 per cent of males had onset after age 50, but 25 per cent of females had onset after age 50. As noted in the text, this later onset of some stone disease in females was correlated with renal infection or metabolic diseases, especially hyperparathyroidism.

calculous disease has a tendency to persist over long periods of an individual's life. Blacklock (1969), in a long-term study of individuals in the military services, found that the chance of having one or more recurrences of urinary calculous disease during a period of many years was 67 per cent for the male patient with idiopathic urinary lithiasis. Coe (1977) reports peak risk of recurrence of calculi at 1½ and 8 years.

Figures 25–1 and 25–2 also show that in this group of patients females constitute about one third the total number. This is the same proportion reported in most other studies of incidence of urinary calculi by sex. However, Lonsdale (1968b) observed that incidence of upper urinary tract calcification is approximately equal in males and females at the time of autopsy. For some reason, therefore, the symptomatic appearance of urinary calculous disease is more prevalent in males. Add to this the fact that in females most upper urinary tract calculous disease is caused by chronic urinary tract infection or metabolic defects such as cystinuria or hyperparathyroidism, and we recognize that most upper urinary tract lithiasis throughout the

world is accounted for by recurrent idiopathic calcific or uric calculi in males.

Several authors have commented upon the apparently equal tendency toward urinary lithiasis in males and females during childhood (Malek and Kelalis, 1975; Prince and Scardino, 1960). This observation, coupled with reports that increased serum testosterone levels resulted in increased endogenous oxalate production by the liver (Liao and Richardson, 1972), led Finlayson (1974) to postulate that lower serum testosterone levels may contribute to some of the protection women (and children) enjoy against oxalate stone disease. Welshman and McGeown (1975) have demonstrated increased urinary citrate concentrations in the urine of females, and they postulate that this may aid in protecting females from calcium urolithiasis.

Extrinsic Factors

GEOGRAPHY

Given the fact that heredity, age, and sex must have important effects on the incidence of urinary lithiasis, numerous other studies also attempt to relate high or low incidence to the geographic distribution of this disease. Figure 25–3 is a world stone map that shows areas of relative high incidence of urinary calculi. There is a noticeable increase in urinary calculi in mountainous or tropical areas. Boyce et al. (1956) performed an extensive study of the incidence of calculous disease in the United States. Their results are put into more modern terms by Sierakowski et al. (Fig. 25–4). A similar survey of the United States had been conducted earlier by Burkland and Rosenberg (1955) and had shown essentially the same results. Whereas Boyce and colleagues tended to emphasize reports of stone disease on the East Coast, Burkland and Rosenberg emphasized disease in the western United States. Results shown in Fig. 25–4 summarize the entire United States. All groups agreed that the areas of highest incidence of urolithiasis in the United States are the northwest, the southeast, and the arid southwest. Finlayson (1974) reviewed several worldwide geographic surveys and stated that the United States is relatively high in the incidence of urinary calculous disease for its population. Other high-incidence areas are the British Isles, Scandinavia, the Mediterranean countries, northern India and Pakistan, northern Australia, Central Europe, portions of the Malayan peninsula, and China. In certain other areas of the world there is a relatively low

thirst with four glasses of very strong iced tea. The pie and tea contain large amounts of oxalate. Because of the warm weather, he also eats a large dish of ice cream, thereby supplying a sufficient amount of dietary calcium. A large amount of calcium and oxalate then reaches the urine, and the formation product for calcium oxalate is exceeded. In such a case, one would expect a certain number of crystals of calcium oxalate to form, and this may happen. Since multiple nuclei of uric acid are already present in the urine, however, calcium oxalate may actually grow more easily upon the previously formed uric acid crystals. Calcium oxalate and uric acid do have crystal lattices that are similar enough to permit this process of epitaxy, or the deposit of one type of crystal upon the surface of another. In fact, it is not unusual to find that urinary calculi have a nucleus of uric acid and a surface covering of calcium oxalate. The degree to which epitaxy may be important in the formation of a particular crystal depends upon the relationship between the amount of supersaturation for that crystal and that for the crystal that forms on its surface by epitaxy. In the hypothetical case presented above, supersaturation with calcium oxalate was very great, and therefore the slight mismatch between the lattices of uric acid and calcium oxalate could be overcome by the high degree of supersaturation and the high driving force toward precipitation of calcium oxalate. In some situations the degree of mismatch between the surface lattices of two crystals is so great that epitaxy is not likely to occur. It is for this reason that cystine crystals rarely deposit upon the surface of a previously formed nucleus of uric acid or calcium oxalate. The mismatch in surface lattices is too great.

Epitaxy requires oriented overgrowth of one crystal on the surface of another. Because of this requirement, physicians have the opportunity to modify crystal surfaces to prohibit epitactic overgrowth and to interfere with stone formation and growth. In some concepts of inhibition of stone formation this theory is used as the basis of attempts to poison growing surfaces of crystals. At the present time, however, no known method of interfering with stone growth includes epitaxy or inhibition of epitaxy as its primary mechanism of action (Finlayson, 1974; Lonsdale, 1968a).

Relationship Between Time Allowed for Crystal Growth and Size of Passages

One final aspect of our review of crystallization processes must be considered before we proceed to a discussion of the application of these principles to urinary lithiasis. In a simple water solution the growth of a crystal occurs over a period of time. For a given crystal, this growth may be estimated by measuring the increase in size or weight per unit of time. In a static solution such as that in a test tube in a laboratory, this is a relatively simple procedure. One can take a portion of the mixture, weigh and count the crystals in this portion, and estimate the total mass of crystals present in the container. The crystals will continue to grow as long as additional solutes are added to the solution to promote supersaturation. If solutes are not added, however, the growth will continue only until the level of crystallizable solute in the supernatant has dropped below the solubility product. At this point, we say that supersaturation has been relieved, and growth ceases.

But normal urine is not a static solution. It flows continuously, and new solutes are continuously excreted. Therefore, crystals may form best at the point of greatest supersaturation of urine, usually the renal papillae (Fig. 25–9) (Vermeulen and Lyon, 1968; Hautmann et al., 1980; Jordan et al., 1978). As soon as these crystals form, they can flow within 3 to 5 minutes into the renal pelvis, down the ureter, and into the bladder, where they remain for a period of approximately 3 to 6 hours. Transit time of urine from the normal kidney to the normal bladder is estimated to be from 5 to 10 minutes.

The lumen of the nephron is smallest at the level of the collecting duct, where its diameter is 50 to 200 micrometers. Anatomically, this portion occurs in the renal papilla (Finlayson, 1974). If the crystal does not have time to grow large enough to obstruct any renal tubule, it then passes into the ureter, where the minimum diameter that can cause obstruction within 10 minutes is approximately 2 millimeters. (This statement is a clinical observation based on the fact that the majority of urinary calculi that cause symptoms are greater than 2 millimeters in diameter (Lehtonen, 1973; Sutor and Wooley, 1975; and many others.) After the crystal has reached the bladder, it may still grow and may achieve a size that exceeds 6 millimeters in diameter; such a crystal could still be voided through the urethra without difficulty.

To summarize this theory, urinary crystals form in the small lumen of the renal tubule and progress through the renal pelvis to the ureter, into the bladder, and out the urethra. Even if crystals grow as they progress through the urinary tract, they are able to pass because the conduits become progressively larger toward the outside.

For a urolith to achieve adequate size to create symptoms we must suppose that within the brief period of time in transit from kidney to bladder the supersaturation of urine is so great that the crystal will grow very rapidly into a structure that can pass no farther through the system. To try to avoid this problem, the urinary tract is anatomically constructed like an inverted cone. The diameters are smallest in the renal tubule and become progressively larger in the ureter, the bladder, and the urethra. Teleologically, it's a good system that allows passage of any possible small particles. But if a particular crystal becomes stuck, growth can continue for long periods of time whenever urinary supersaturation or aggregation of new crystals occurs. Hence, if somehow the crystal mass becomes lodged in the renal papilla or tubule it is no longer able to move through the system (Figs. 25–9 and 25–10). It resides at that point and continues to grow in supersaturated urine. Intermittent layered growth of stones has been reviewed by Lonsdale (1968a). If the crystal breaks off or breaks away from the renal papilla when it is smaller than the size required to obstruct the ureter, it will pass through the system without causing symptoms. But if it attains a diameter of greater than approximately 2 millimeters, it may pass into the ureter and create urinary obstruction. Then it becomes a symptomatic urinary calculus.

What about bladder calculi? A calculus of 2 to 3 millimeters may pass through the ureter and into the bladder with relatively few symptoms. But let us suppose it enters a bladder in which there is obstruction of the urinary outlet. (This occurs especially often in males; bladder calculi are extremely rare in females.) If, because of prostatic obstruction or a narrow bladder neck, the stone cannot enter the urethra but remains in the base of the bladder or in a diverticulum, it can then continue to grow whenever the urine is supersaturated with the substances that created the stone. Such stones may achieve enormous size, the largest reported weighing over 1 kilogram (Becher et al., 1978).

Inhibitors of Crystallization

Perhaps no aspect of urinary calculous disease has generated so much interest and confusion as urinary inhibitors of crystallization. Elliot (1983) studied calcium oxalate solubility in urine and pointed out that the solubility of calcium oxalate in urine is not greatly different in stone patients from that in normal persons. For example, he reports that the calcium oxalate solubility products in active stone formers and normal individuals were not significantly different. On the other hand, Robertson and Peacock (1972) have shown that calcium stone formers tend to excrete considerably more oxalate and calcium than do normal persons. But they also showed moderate overlap in the degree of saturation between normal and stone-forming groups. Recall also that many cystinurics do not form calculi. Therefore, in spite of the fact that these people have an excessive amount of cystine in their urine, for some reason they do not develop the processes of crystallization associated with urinary calculi. How can we explain the fact that some individuals with supersaturated urine seem to be capable of holding more crystallizable urinary substances in solution? The answer given by many investigators is a relative lack of crystallization inhibitors in the urine of stone formers.

Inhibitors may be classified as predominantly organic or inorganic. Of the inhibitors within the organic group perhaps the most famous is the peptide inhibitor first described by Howard et al. (1967) and studied extensively by Robertson et al. (1969) and Smith et al. (1969). This low molecular weight peptide enables the urine to hold in solution considerably greater amounts of calcium than is possible when it is absent. These investigators have indicated that stone formers have a significant lack of this inhibitor in their urine. The major criticism of this particular inhibitor is the fact that the test substrate used is rachitic rat cartilage. Although the inhibitor studied may be effective in prohibiting calcification of rat cartilage, rat cartilage is as yet unreported as a component of human urinary calculi. Later, Barker et al. (1974), working in the laboratory of Howard, published findings indicating that most inhibition that they found in urine could be accounted for by the polyelectrolyte interactivity of the multiple ions of urine. More recently, higher molecular weight glycoproteins have been shown to inhibit calcium oxalate crystallization (Drach et al., 1983; White et al., 1983). Much more investigation in this area of stone disease is needed.

Other organic inhibitors may be present. Matrix (to be defined later) may have the ability to inhibit the formation of urinary calculi (Gill, personal communication). Yet Boyce and his colleagues continue to indicate that particular structures of matrix may be important in enhancing the formation of urinary calculi. For example, an enhancing substance known as substance A in matrix was described by Boyce (Boyce, 1967, 1968, 1969; King, 1967, 1971). Attempts to confirm the presence of this substance A in the matrix of urinary calculi led to conflicting results (Bichler et al., 1976). Foye et al. (1976), however, described a significant difference between the composition of uromucoids in normal people and that in stone-forming persons. The uromucoid of stone formers contains more sulfhydryl groups (-SH) than does normal uromucoid. This increase in -SH is believed to explain the fact that the uromucoid of stone formers binds more calcium than does normal uromucoid. Hence, normal uromucoid may not be inhibitory, but, in contrast to uromucoid from stone formers, it does not promote stones by excessive calcium binding. It remains conceivable that particular types of matrix may be more active in coating the surface of crystals that form in urine. This may be particularly true when crystals reach a certain size. Matrix coating may inhibit stone formation by producing surface (zeta potential) charges that prevent further deposition of crystal or that inhibit aggregation. The individual coated crystals may then repel rather than aggregate (Riddick, 1968; Rollins and Finlayson, 1973). As a related example, Schmidt-Nielsen (1964) has published fascinating observations on the excretion of "gelatinous" urine by desert mammals. In this very concentrated urine, the crystals of oxalate that are excreted are uniformly coated by mucous substances that are similar to human matrix substance. Large crystals and stones do not occur.

Other organic substances undoubtedly have some importance in the inhibitory processes of urine. Amino acids, specifically alanine, may be important in improving the solubility of calcium substances in some types of urinary lithiasis (Chow et al., 1973; Elliot and Eusebio, 1967). On the other hand, in humans, the contribution of these substances to the solubilization of stones seems minimal (Finlayson, 1974).

Urinary citrate, as shown previously, appears to have some part in the solubilization of calcium, oxalate, and phosphate in urine (Fig. 25–7). Certainly, citrate is found to be decreased in patients who form urinary calculi that contain calcium (Elliot, 1973a; Finlayson, 1974; King, 1967, 1971; Miller et al., 1958; Welshman and McGeown, 1976; Williams, 1974a, b). Urea increases the solubility of some components of urine, especially uric acid (Porter, 1966), but it does not seem to influence calcium precipitation (Finlayson et al., 1972).

INORGANIC INHIBITORS OF CRYSTALLIZATION

Most inhibitors of crystallization that have been reported are related to inorganic elements that affect the calcium phosphate or calcium oxalate systems. Foremost among these are phosphates, especially pyrophosphate (Fleisch and Bisaz, 1964). Investigations leading to the elucidation of the effects of the –P–O–P–(pyrophosphate) structure were summarized by Fleisch (1965). Most subsequent reviews of inorganic inhibitors include pyrophosphate as one major component (Drach et al., 1983). In fact, Thomas (1975) feels that one of the major effects of oral administration of large doses of orthophosphate is the increased urinary excretion of pyrophosphate. Conversely, oral administration of pyrophosphate does not result in an increase in renal excretion of pyrophosphate. Therefore, no medications containing pyrophosphate have been devised for treatment of urinary lithiasis. The action of phosphate as a crystal poison of calcification has been known for many years. Simkiss (1964) reviewed the multiple effects that phosphates may have upon calcifying biologic systems and found that orthophosphates themselves do not appear to have a direct effect upon urinary stone formation of the calcigerous type. In fact, administration of orthophosphates to patients who have a tendency toward phosphate stone (whether magnesium phosphate or calcium phosphate) can actually increase the rate of stone formation.

When it is excreted into urine in significant amounts, magnesium, a divalent cation, tends to increase the solubility of calcium, phosphate, and perhaps oxalate (Moore and Gowland, 1975). A high calcium/magnesium ratio has been implicated as one of the causes of calcigerous renal calculi (King, 1967; Oreopoulos et al., 1975). Prien and Gershoff (1974) and Melnick et al. (1971) have used this observation to justify administration of magnesium to many patients who chronically form calcigerous urinary calculi. They have reported a satisfactory decrease in tendency toward calcium stone formation after therapy. This approach will be discussed further in a later section.

As mentioned previously, some authors have implicated trace metals in inhibition of urinary stone formation, especially stones of the calcigerous type. Zinc seems to be the most frequently mentioned of these substances (Elliot and Eusebio, 1967; Elliot and Ribeino; 1973).

In Figure 25–7, adapted from Finlayson (1974), the cumulative effects of some organic or inorganic inhibitors on the solubilization of urinary calcium are shown. The effects of these multiple components are roughly additive, and therefore each contributes partly to the solubilization of calcium. For this reason, it is likely that calcium stone formers have deficiencies in not one but several of the inhibitors that should be present in urine (Drach, 1976b). This may be why patients who form stones are often found to have low levels of urinary citrate as well as magnesium and other inhibiting elements. Should they also have a burst of supersaturation of urine with calcium and oxalate at the same time, it is likely that stone formation would begin and would proceed rapidly.

MATRIX

Noncrystalline protein-like matrix of urinary calculi was first described by Anton von Heyde in 1684 (cited by King, 1967). The exact influence of matrix upon formation and crystallization of urinary calculi has been hotly debated for years. Boyce and his colleagues have pursued the role of matrix in stone formation since their earliest report in 1954 (Boyce, 1969). Extensive investigations have characterized matrix as a derivative of several of the mucoproteins of urine. Matrix content of a given stone varies, but most solid urinary calculi have a matrix content of about 3 per cent by weight (Boyce and King, 1959). On the other hand, matrix calculi, composed of an average of 65 per cent of matrix by weight, may occur, especially in association with urinary infection (Allen and Spence, 1966; Mall et al., 1975). Finally, the matrix content of some calculi may be very small; uric acid calculi, for example, may have a matrix content of less than 2 per cent.

Chemical analysis of stone matrix reveals it to be about 65 per cent protein, 10 per cent hexose, 3 to 5 per cent hexosamine, and 10 per cent bound water (Boyce, 1968). Uromucoid, the major mucoid component of urine, is very similar in composition to matrix, except that it also contains about 3.5 per cent sialic acid, whereas matrix has none. Malek and Boyce (1973) have postulated that this distinctive lack of sialic acid may be due to cleavage of the acid from uromucoid molecules by the renal enzyme sialidase. This results in creation of a matrix laid down upon minerals, such as calcium, which may be the first step in stone formation.

Whether matrix truly initiates stone formation or plays a part in causation of stone disease continues to be uncertain. Vermeulen and coworkers (Finlayson et al., 1961; Vermeulen and Lyon, 1968) have in several investigations indicated that matrix may be only an adventitious coprecipitate with the crystals that form stones. Sutor and O'Flynn (1973) demonstrated that matrix crept into a previously crystallized mass placed by a patient in her bladder. However, as Finlayson (1974) concludes, simple coprecipitation cannot explain all the interactions observed between stone crystals and ma-

trix. For example, polymerization of matrix must occur in order to form the matrix stone, and Watanabe (1972) feels that matrix functions to bridge stone crystals together. Matrix must originate in the renal tubules, probably in the proximal tubule (Herrman, 1963; Keutel, 1965; Malek and Boyce, 1973). Malek and Boyce demonstrated that kidneys of patients with idiopathic calcium lithiasis show a large number of intranephronic calculi in the renal tubules. These microliths are laminated structures of matrix and crystals that mimic the structures of larger stones. Such microliths were not found in kidneys of patients who formed struvite, uric acid, or cystine stones. Therefore, matrix-related growth or aggregation of these small intranephronic stones may be one primary event in the causation of calcigerous lithiasis.

Boyce et al. (1962) described one component that is immunologically unique to stone matrix and is different from any of the other mucoids of urine. This "substance A" was found on the matrix of all calcigerous stones, in the kidneys of patients who had stone disease, and in the urine of calcium stone-forming patients. It could also be found in the urine of patients who had other reasons for renal inflammation such as infection, infarction, or cancer (Boyce, 1969; Keutel and King, 1964). Moore and Gowland (1975) conducted extensive studies into immunologically distinct reactants of stone matrix and uromucoids of urine. They were not able to find a single distinct protein such as protein A but instead found three or four antigens unique to stones. They detected these "stone-specific antigens" in the urine of 85 per cent of stone formers but in no normal individuals. The exact relationship between these antigens, matrix A, and stone formation remains unclear. In addition, Bichler et al. (1976) have challenged the observations that total uromucoid excretion is elevated in active stone formers. They found no significant difference in uromucoid excretion rates between 49 normal persons and 79 stone formers. As noted previously, the uromucoid of stone formers does bind more calcium than that of normal persons (Foye et al., 1976). Matrix undoubtedly plays some role in stone formation. Whether it is active or passive, qualitative or quantitative, enhancing or inhibitory remains to be seen.

MODERN THEORIES OF ETIOLOGY OF URINARY LITHIASIS

After the previous discussion of processes of crystallization, inhibitors, and matrix we can progress to theories of the etiology of urinary stone formation (Table 25–1).

SUPERSATURATION/CRYSTALLIZATION

Uric acid and cystine calculi form whenever urine with a tendency to remain at an acid pH becomes oversaturated with uric acid or cystine. Stone growth or dissolution is directly and linearly related to these two factors, as will be described further in the sections covering these specific types of calculi. Magnesium ammonium phosphate (struvite) calculi form whenever the product of the concentration of these ions exceeds the saturation product and when the urine remains alkaline for long periods of time. Therefore, three of the five major types of urinary calculi can be explained primarily by our first theory of stone formation—supersaturation of urine with a substance that can crystallize in urine at a given pH.

INHIBITOR LACK

Unfortunately, we find that supersaturation alone does not completely explain even these three types of calculi, and certainly not calcium phosphate or calcium oxalate stone formation. Many normal persons have urinary supersaturation with the substances mentioned previously. They will form crystals, but the crystals remain small and are passed easily. So we must resort to the effects of some types of inhibitors that prevent or at least limit crystal growth and aggregation in normal urine. Neither the supersaturation theory nor the inhibitor theory can stand alone. It seems necessary to combine both to have a cogent theory of stone formation. Robertson and colleagues (1976) have produced such a theory for calcium oxalate urinary lithiasis; their studies show that for calcium oxalate calculi, an index of supersaturation versus inhibition can be determined for an individual, and that stone formers have higher indices—that is, stone formers show greater supersaturation and less inhibition of crystallization and stone formation.

MATRIX INITIATION

Where does the matrix fit in? Matrix, as mentioned previously, may inhibit crystal growth, interfere with crystal aggregation, and even enhance stone growth. At the present time the uromucoid of normal persons is thought to be a beneficial inhibitor of crystallization and stone formation, whereas the matrix of stone formers represents uromucoid with some qualitative defect that alters its ability to inhibit crystallization or even causes it to promote stone formation (Finlayson, 1974).

INTRANEPHRONIC AND FIXED NUCLEATION

Some investigators of urinary stone disease still criticize the supersaturation/crystallization/inhibition/matrix theories because they encompass only those events that occur in urine. These workers state that the major process that ultimately leads to stone formation is aggregation of small crystals formed previously in the kidney. Some investigators believe that the initial nucleation and growth of nuclei and crystals begin in the renal (intranephronic) tissue, while others believe that the process begins freely in renal tubular urine. Hence, nucleation, growth, inhibitors, matrix, and aggregation are all believed to be important in stone formation by one group or another. All may be important.

To summarize, we have discussed multiple theories of causation of urinary stones, whether formed of cystine, calcium, uric acid, or other crystallizable elements. The proponents of the intranephronic theory of urinary stone disease believe that disease begins within the renal tubular cell. Excretion of multiple calcified nuclei from these cells into the urine allows growth of crystals in the previously supersaturated urine. In such a theory there is no need for a free nucleation phase. The ability to study such submicroscopic nuclei has been limited, however, and their importance in the genesis of stone disease is not yet understood. Intranephronic calculosis is probably most important in calcium stone disease.

EXTRANEPHRONIC AND FREE PARTICLE NUCLEATION

Proponents of the extranephronic theory of urinary stone formation believe that it all happens in urine; their arguments can be separated into three major divisions. There are those who believe that urinary supersaturation with a given element results in spontaneous crystallization of that element. Since we now know that crystal growth in urinary solutions does not proceed rapidly enough to postulate formation of a single large mass that obstructs the ureter or bladder (Finlayson and Dubois, 1973; Miller et al., 1977), concepts of aggregation or agglomeration of spontaneously nucleated crystals must be prepared to explain formation of a larger mass. We know also that inhibitors of multiple organic or inorganic types exist in urine. It is theorized that these crystal inhibitors affect the surfaces of crystals and prevent them from aggregating or from growing larger. Some investigators feel that one of these inhibitors may be uromucoid itself. When uromucoid is deficient or different in its composition from normal uromucoid, perhaps inhibition no longer occurs. Hence, one possibility in the matrix theory of stone formation is the fact that uromucoid normally acts as an inhibitor (Drach et al., 1982). Patients with stone disease may lack some significant component of uromucoid or produce additional components that decrease its inhibiting action.

One of the major problems in the study of urinary lithiasis has been the difficulty of measuring the kinetics of crystallization in nucleation and growth of urinary calculi. At what point and how rapidly does nucleation occur? How fast does the crystal grow? Does aggregation occur or not? The approaches of Robertson et al. (1973, 1976), Gill et al. (1974), and Miller et al. (1977) offer possibilities for thorough study of these aspects of urinary crystallization. The methodology used by Miller et al. was first used by Finlayson (1972), who used a constant crystallizer with a volume of 2500 ml to approximate the continuously flowing kidney/urine system. This process was modified to create a constant crystallizer with a volume of 110 ml, which more closely approximates the components of the urinary system.

FINAL THEORY

Whether nucleation, growth, or aggregation is the most important component in formation of urinary calculi is not yet known. One can surmise, however, from the massive amount of investigation that has been conducted, that basic crystallization processes are critical to the formation of urinary calculi. For this reason, we must now define those aspects of renal function that allow supersaturation of urine and thereby formation of urinary calculi. This final theory of urolithiasis is an attempt to combine all the elements discussed previously.

First, renal function must be adequate for the excretion of excess amounts of crystallizable substances. In some instances, excess excretion is the result of some particular defect of renal tubular function (e.g., cystinuria). Second, the kidney must be able to adjust its pH excretion to conform to that required to crystallize the substance. The net result of these two requirements is the ability of the kidney to excrete an excessive amount of a given substance at a pH that allows precipitation of that substance. Third, the urine must have a complete or relative absence of a number of inhibitors of crystallization of the crystallizable components (Fig. 25–7). It seems unlikely at the present time that a single inhibitor is responsible for solubilizing all urinary substances. One element that definitely has a part in this process, however, is

uromucoid. Whether or not uromucoid is normally intended to be an inhibitor of crystallization or aggregation and whether it is deficient or defective in some stone formers is uncertain.

Fourth, one concept that is often forgotten is that the crystal mass must reside in the urinary system for a time sufficient to allow growth or aggregation of the crystal mass to a size large enough to obstruct the urinary passage through which it is proceeding. Trapping of nuclei in the kidney provides time for growth. Hence, stasis may have an important part in the genesis of urinary calculi if it holds the crystal mass in a particular position long enough to allow significant growth. This relationship with time is probably the reason that, as mentioned previously, the urinary system is built like an inverted cone in which the diameters are smallest in the renal tubules, larger in the ureter, and greatest in the urethra.

These observations on urinary stone disease form the basis of our understanding and treatment of almost all human urinary stone diseases. In the next section, we will assume that a patient has whatever defect is necessary, has formed a symptomatic calculus, and requires initial diagnosis and treatment of his or her acute urinary lithiasis. We will then discuss aspects of continued evaluation and treatment for specific types of stone disease.

INITIAL DIAGNOSIS AND THERAPY OF URINARY LITHIASIS

General Observations

A urinary calculus usually announces its presence with an acute episode of renal or ureteral colic. Bladder colic differs from ureteral colic and will be discussed separately in the section on bladder calculus. Uroliths create problems in patients only when they become trapped in some segment of the urinary tract. In general, this segment is one of five portions of the upper urinary tract. First, stones may become impacted in a calyx of the upper urinary tract. Individual calyces may therefore become distended and painful and create hematuria. An alternative form of this process is the occurrence of stone in a calyceal diverticulum, which is usually a congenital abnormality (Middleton and Pfister, 1974) (Fig. 25–11). The second area in which a calculus may become impacted is the ureteropelvic junction. It is here that the rela-

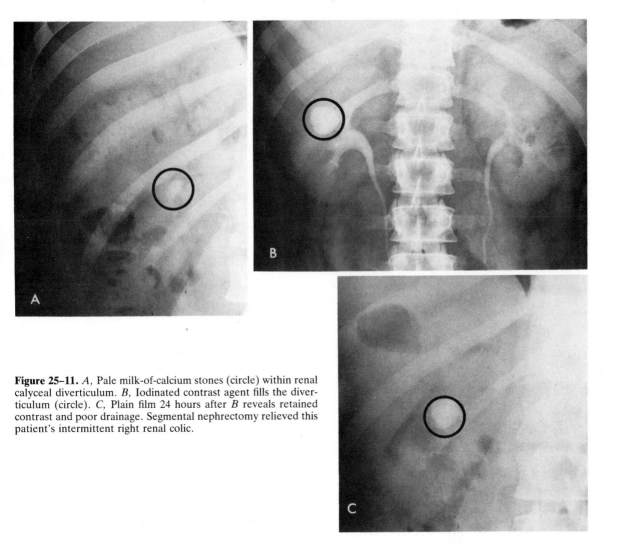

Figure 25–11. *A*, Pale milk-of-calcium stones (circle) within renal calyceal diverticulum. *B*, Iodinated contrast agent fills the diverticulum (circle). *C*, Plain film 24 hours after *B* reveals retained contrast and poor drainage. Segmental nephrectomy relieved this patient's intermittent right renal colic.

tively large diameter of the renal pelvis (1 cm) abruptly decreases to that of the ureter (2 to 3 mm). A third area of impaction is at or near the pelvic brim, where the ureter begins to arch over the iliac vessels posteriorly into the true pelvis. The fourth area, especially in females, is the area of the posterior pelvis, where the ureter is crossed anteriorly by pelvic blood vessels and the broad ligament. Finally, the most constricted area through which the urinary calculus must pass is the ureterovesical junction (Fig. 25–12).

Several authors have studied the approximate sizes of calculi that appear to be capable of passing through these constricted areas (see previous discussion). In general, it is believed that all urinary calculi with a maximum diameter of up to 4 to 5 milliliters are capable of passing through the ureter. Although some 90 per cent of such calculi may pass spontaneously, it is always extremely difficult to predict correctly the 10 per cent that do not pass (Fig. 25–34).

RENAL COLIC

Renal colic is a symptom complex that is characteristic for the presence of upper urinary tract calculi. A typical episode occurs during the night or early morning hours, is abrupt in onset, and usually affects a patient who is sedentary or at rest. It is the partially obstructing, continuously moving calculus that appears to create

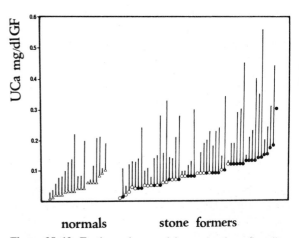

Figure 25–13. Fasting urinary calcium excretions (baseline values) and post–oral calcium load values (vertical bars) of normal and stone-forming persons, ranked in ascending order. (0 = normocalciuric; ● = hypercalciuric patients). (From Lien, J., and Keane, P.: J. Urol., *129*:401, 1983. Used by permission.)

the greatest amount of colic. The extreme crescendo of pain begins in the area of the flank, courses laterally around the abdomen, and generally radiates to the area of the groin and testicle in the male, or to the labia majora and round ligament in the female. It has been surmised that this radiation of pain is related to the blood supply of the cord and testicular or ovarian vessels by the testicular or ovarian artery, which has its origin from the aorta very near the renal artery. Autonomic nerve fibers that serve both kidney and testicle or ovary become involved in the transmission of pain sensations to the spinal cord and brain. Recent research suggests that prostaglandins are involved in genesis of pain of renal and ureteral colic (Wahlberg, 1983). As the stone moves to the midureter, pain generally tends to radiate to the lateral flank and abdominal area. With impaction of the stone in a particular area of the ureter for a period of time, local inflammatory changes occur, and the most painful area then may actually be located around the area of impaction of the calculus. If the stone eventually moves toward the bladder, severe renal colic may once again occur. When ureteral stones are near the bladder, patients often develop the urinary symptom of urgency.

Since the autonomic nervous system transmits visceral pain, confusion about the source of the pain is not uncommon and is related to the diffuse spreading of strong stimuli to other areas of similar anatomic innervation. The celiac ganglion serves both kidneys and stomach, so nausea and vomiting are commonly associated

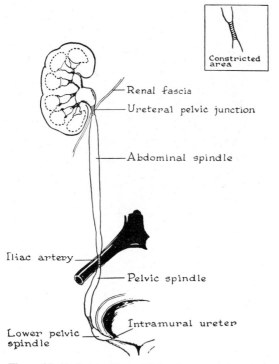

Figure 25–12. Points of constriction in a normal ureter.

with renal colic. In addition, ileus or other intestinal stasis associated with local irritation is not infrequent. Similarity of these symptoms to those of the gastrointestinal tract causes urinary lithiasis and colic to be confused with a number of abdominal diseases. Among these are gastroenteritis, acute appendicitis, colitis, and salpingitis.

PHYSICAL SIGNS

Physical signs of urinary calculous disease are characteristic. The first of these is the fact that the patient almost always has "moving irritation." That is, individuals with urinary lithiasis rarely can find comfort in any given position. They sit, stand, pace, recline, and move continuously in an attempt to shake off whatever it is that is creating their discomfort. Fever is rarely present unless urinary infection occurs along with the calculus. Pulse rate may be elevated by virtue of pain and agitation, and blood pressure is sometimes above normal in a patient in whom it has previously been normal. Grunting respirations are not uncommon, especially at the peak of colic, and may be similar to those of an individual who has respiratory distress.

Examination of the chest is necessary and should reveal a normal chest. Examination of the abdomen in general reveals moderate deep tenderness on palpation over the location of the calculus. In addition, the kidney may show moderate to marked tenderness, especially upon palpation or upon fist percussion over the posterior flank.

URINALYSIS

Urinalysis in most patients with urinary lithiasis reveals the presence of microscopic or gross hematuria. Some patients do not demonstrate hematuria, especially if the calculus has created complete obstruction. In some instances of urinary calculus without pain, hematuria may be the only presenting complaint, or it may be discovered incidentally on routine physical examination. Although such painless hematuria may be due to other causes, silent urinary calculus remains one of the diseases that must be ruled out. Moderate pyuria may occur even in patients with uninfected urinary lithiasis. When significant numbers of pus cells are present in the urine, however, a thorough search for infection should be made. This is particularly true of females, in whom urinary infection is likely to be the most common cause of urinary lithiasis. Urinalysis sometimes reveals an additional finding that may be helpful in diagnosing

the type of calculus present. On occasion, patients who are in an active phase of urinary lithiasis will have in their urine crystals of the same type that are creating the calculus. Therefore, the observation of cystine, uric acid, or calcium oxalate crystals in the urine may be an indication of the type of calculus ultimately found.

Radiographic examination of the urinary tract is the next step in the evaluation of the patient with suspected urinary lithiasis. In fact, it forms the cornerstone of the initial evaluation of the patient and establishes, in general, the presence of calculous disease and its severity.

Radiographic Examination for Urinary Lithiasis

PLAIN ABDOMINAL FILMS

In the initial evaluation the first routine radiographs ordered are plain KUB (kidney-ureter-bladder) radiographs. A representative film is illustrated in Figure 25–14. Plain films of the abdomen often show densities that are not clearly stones but may represent other calcified densities such as pelvic phleboliths. It is then

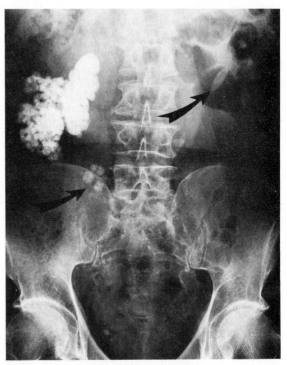

Figure 25–14. Multiple right renal, right ureteral (arrow), and left renal (arrow) calculi appear on this plain abdominal film. Patient also had an obstructing left lower ureteral matrix calculus that is not visible.

helpful to obtain additional plain films in the right posterior oblique, left posterior oblique, or lateral position. In most patients, the position and outline of the kidneys can be seen on the plain film. The position of the ureter is characteristically parallel to the lateral processes of the lumbar spine. It then crosses over the pelvic brim and turns somewhat laterally into the true pelvis (Figs. 25–12 and 25–14). Therefore, the observation of a radiodense calculus in the area of the kidney or along the course of the ureter, along with typical signs of colic and hematuria, may be sufficient for diagnosis of urinary stone.

RADIODENSITY OF CALCULI

Radiodensity of calculi is more variable than we are led to believe. It is widely known that calculi that contain calcium, such as calcium oxalate and calcium phosphate calculi, are radiodense (Boyce et al., 1956; Emmett and Witten, 1971; Lalli, 1974). Roth and Finlayson (1973), through some unique radiographic techniques, have shown that calcium phosphate (apatite) stones are the most radiopaque and have a density like that of bone. Calcium oxalate calculi are almost as opaque. Magnesium ammonium phosphate (struvite) calculi are somewhat less radiopaque than calcium calculi. Cystine calculi must be considered partly radiodense. Roth and Finlayson estimate that cystine stones are approximately 0.45 times as radiopaque as calcium oxalate calculi. In addition, they note that cystine calculi are at least 40 times more opaque than uric acid stones. Figure 25–15 compares calcium, magnesium, cystine, and uric acid calculi in a single radiograph. In addition, Figures 25–14 through 25–18 and Figure 25–20 show the relative radiodensities of stones on plain abdominal films of patients with bladder or upper tract calculi.

The degree of radiodensity is one factor in visualization of the calculus on the plain film, but the structure and configuration of the calculus also contribute. For example, calcium oxalate calculi must be at least 2 mm thick to appear on most radiographs. If the calculus measures 1 × 2 mm in size, it can be seen only when the x-rays course through it parallel to the greatest diameter. For this reason, stones will sometimes disappear in one plane of the radiograph and reappear in another. For cystine calculi, a degree of thickness approximating 3 to 4 mm is necessary for the stone to be visualized at all. Calculi of ammonium acid urate have slight radiodensity, but even large calculi of uric acid have no radiodensity at all in comparison to surrounding soft tissues.

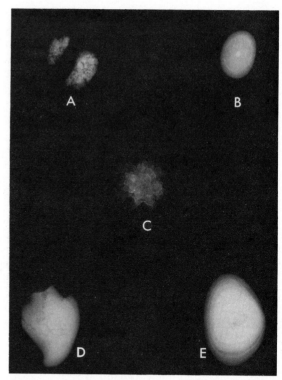

Figure 25–15. Radiodensities in air (to improve contrast) of five human calculi. *A,* Calcium oxalate. *B,* Calcium phosphate. *C,* Uric acid. *D,* Cystine. *E,* Magnesium ammonium phosphate. Note that only the uric acid calculus is truly radiolucent.

Therefore, only calculi of relatively pure uric acid or of matrix (Fig. 25–16) can be considered truly radiolucent. It is these calculi that create the greatest diagnostic problem based upon plain abdominal films. For differentiation of these calculi, radiographic studies employing some type of contrast media are necessary. The most common type of study performed in a patient with suspected stones who is not allergic to renal contrast media is the intravenous urogram. Basic techniques for this study are covered elsewhere in this text and will not be reviewed here. Only those aspects of intravenous urography of special importance to urinary lithiasis will be discussed.

INTRAVENOUS UROGRAM

Aside from the observation of a radiodense calculus somewhere in the path of the urinary tract, the first indication of the presence of urolithiasis is delay in the appearance of the contrast medium in the nephrogram following injection of contrast. This implies obstruction by calculus. As Lalli (1974) points out, observation of such a delay indicates that the usual 5-, 10-, and 20-minute pyelographic films are

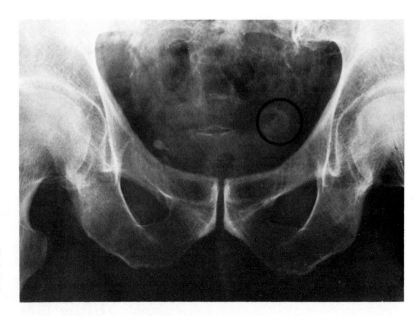

Figure 25-16. Matrix calculus of left lower ureter outlined faintly by iodinated contrast (circle). This type of calculus must also be considered radiolucent.

not likely to be useful in defining the location and presence of the calculus. Therefore, it is better to extend the period of observation and obtain films at perhaps 20, 30, and 60 minutes. In this way, the patient avoids the unnecessary inconvenience of reclining on the radiographic table for an excessive period of time and benefits from the decreased amount of radiation exposure. Delayed films may be obtained several hours or even one day following the injection of contrast material (Fig. 25-17). Should there be difficulty in visualization after one dose of contrast, reinjection of contrast agent may be useful. If there is still no visualization, retrograde pyelography may be indicated.

Recently, there has been an increase in the use of infusion pyelography for detection of all types of urologic disorders. Lalli (1974) has observed that brisk diuresis may be created by performance of intravenous pyelography or urography. Occasional reports of spontaneous rupture of the renal pelvis or ureter due to obstructing calculus have appeared in the literature, but the author is impressed with the increased numbers of reports of spontaneous urinary extravasation following the use of infusion pyelography (Amin and Howerton, 1974; Aubert, 1973; Borkowski and Czapliczki, 1974; Munster and Hunter, 1968; Quencer and Foster, 1972; Reece and Hackler, 1974; Silver et al., 1973; Van Regemorter and Hardy, 1973; Wart et al., 1973). Although extensive comparative information is not yet available, it may be just as useful and safer to perform single or repeated bolus injections of iodinated contrast material as necessary. On the other hand, Claypool and

colleagues (1975) have indicated that the infusion technique is more likely to give a definitive diagnosis more rapidly than bolus injection methods. Combinations of contrast studies with computerized tomographic scanning can be very specific in defining stone location and type.

RENAL ANGIOGRAPHY

Renal angiography may be useful in further definition of stone disease in selected patients. Figure 25-18 illustrates such a patient. This figure reveals an extremely large calculus that resembles a calcium oxalate stone in its density and configuration. Intravenous urography revealed malrotation of the kidney or possible horseshoe kidney. The patient was acutely ill, and it was felt that emergency surgery might be necessary. Multiple renal arteries and abnormal anatomy were suspected. Renal angiography revealed a single major artery to this kidney. An extended anterior pyelolithotomy was selected as the preferred method of surgery.

RADIOISOTOPE METHODS

Radioisotope renography and scanning have contributed to diagnosis of obstruction and location of calculus in a number of patients, particularly those who are otherwise sensitive to contrast material. Use of these techniques is demonstrated in Figure 25-19. In this patient, who was markedly sensitive to intravenous contrast agent, not only the location of the calculus but also the degree of urinary obstruction was clearly defined. The patient ultimately passed a small calculus spontaneously.

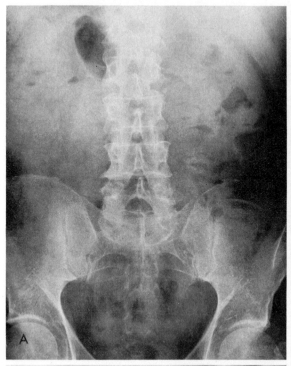

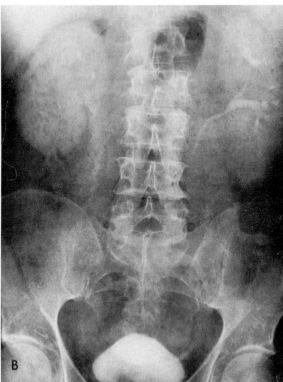

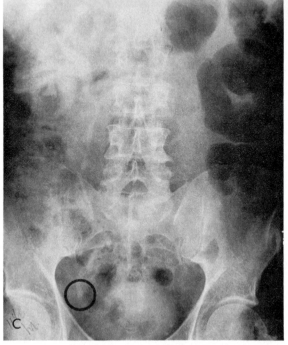

Figure 25–17. Value of delayed radiographs. *A*, KUB radiograph of patient with acute right renal colic and hematuria. No obvious calculus. *B*, Radiograph 20 minutes after infusion of iodinated contrast. Prolonged right nephrogram and poor right ureteral filling. *C*, Radiograph 11½ hours after infusion. Mild right hydroureteronephrosis down to a small lucent filling defect (circle). Patient subsequently passed a 3-mm uric acid calculus.

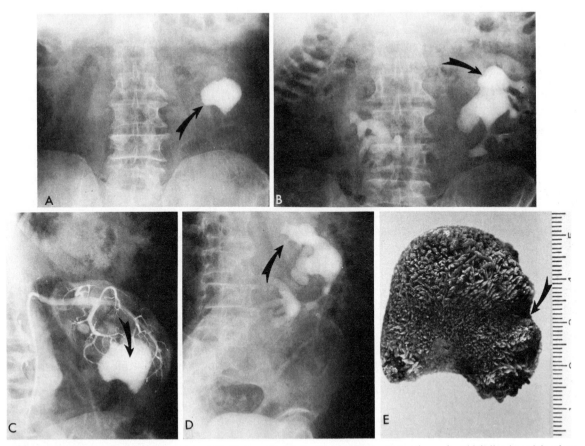

Figure 25–18. Value of angiography. *A* and *B*, Plain radiograph reveals large calculus (arrow), which lies in pelvis of an apparent horseshoe kidney. *C*, Renal angiography demonstrates malrotation without horseshoe formation and reveals excellent location for extended pyelolithotomy (arrow) and pyeloplasty. *D*, Postoperative intravenous urogram reveals improved upper pole drainage. *E*, Large calculus of pure calcium oxalate was removed intact. Notches on border (arrow) occurred adjacent to renal papillae.

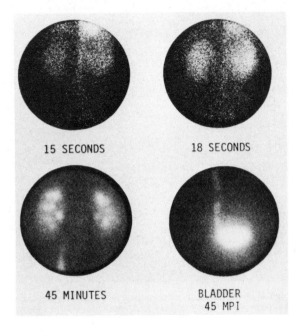

Figure 25–19. Radioisotopic renal scans may be helpful in detecting an obstructing calculus. Ureteral fullness near the bladder at 45 minutes in this very ill patient who was allergic to intravenous iodinated contrast material led to consideration of a right ureteral calculus.

In other instances, when radiographic or radioisotope methods are not successful, *retrograde pyelography* is necessary. This may also be true in cases of relatively radiolucent calculi that are difficult to locate by intravenous pyelography. Such a patient is illustrated in Figure 25–20. In this instance, the calculi turned out to be two small cystine calculi, which could be seen only with difficulty on plain films and were not clearly defined by intravenous urography.

ULTRASOUND SCANNING

Ultrasound scanning of the kidney, ureter, and bladder is useful. We have found it helpful in defining some relatively large urinary calculi in our patients. Figure 25–21 illustrates the ultrasound appearance of relatively large calculi filling the lower portion of the kidney. The ultrasound scan also showed that there was significant renal substance present and indicated that the kidney was relatively hydronephrotic. This led to the decision to remove the calculus surgically to preserve renal function.

The progressive evaluation of symptomatology, physical examination, urinalysis, and radiographic evaluation generally constitute the preliminary examination of a patient with urinary calculous disease. After a urolith is diagnosed, a decision is required about the degree of seriousness of the disease process. The primary decision is whether to apply surgical therapy or wait. The author has reviewed some of these surgical indications previously (Drach, 1974*b*). Surgical removal of stone is necessary when there is evidence of significant obstruction, progressive renal deterioration, refractory pyelonephritis, or unremitting pain. Stone obstruction of an infected kidney requires emergency surgery.

Early Management and Treatment

The majority of patients with urinary lithiasis require prompt therapy for pain relief. Most patients gain relief from the intramuscular injection of 50 to 100 mg of meperidine or 10 to 15 mg of morphine, depending on body size and severity of pain. Liberal use of narcotics to treat the pain of urolithiasis has resulted in some patients who fake symptoms. Most are drug addicts who are attempting to get illicit drugs.

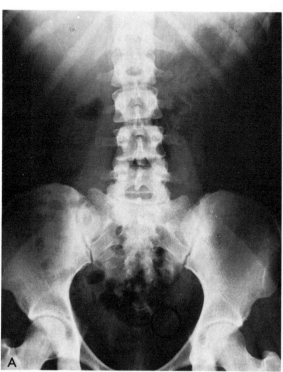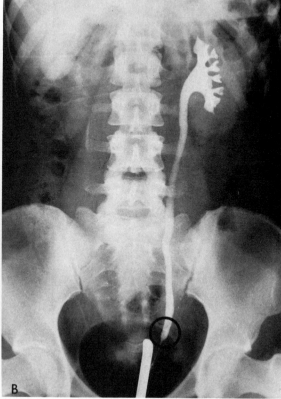

Figure 25–20. Retrograde pyelography (*A* and *B*) confirmed presence of two ureteral cystine calculi (circles) obstructing the left ureter. Sepsis was present, and stones were removed by manipulation.

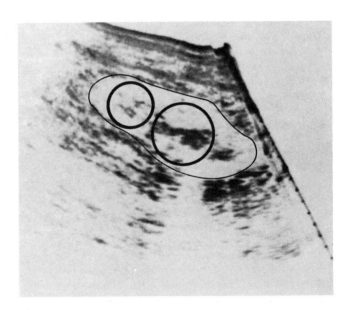

Figure 25–21. Ultrasound left renal scan, posterior view, of patient with duplicated left kidney. Upper portion (small circle) reveals normal small pelvocalyceal echoes. Lower portion is enlarged (outline) and contains dense dark echoes consistent with renal calculus (large circle).

Drug addicts most frequently relate a story that sounds too much like a textbook. In addition, they are almost always "allergic" to intravenous contrast media and indicate that their previous stones are known to be radiolucent uric acid or matrix and therefore cannot be seen on plain radiographs. The absence of uric acid crystals or infection in the urine of such patients helps increase suspicion of drug dependency. The presence of hematuria in a patient who claims stone disease should not be taken as an absolute indication of the presence of this disease. In the author's experience, drug addicts have successfully added blood to their urine by incising the lateral edges of their fingers or biting the inner edges of their cheeks and spitting into the urinary specimen, or even going so far as to insert a pin into the urethral meatus inside the glans penis. On the other hand, once certain evidence of urinary calculus has been established, real patients are extremely thankful for whatever pain relief can be obtained.

Hospitalization may be necessary for those individuals who have so much gastrointestinal upset that they cannot retain food or fluids. In addition, they may become exhausted by the loss of sleep and other discomforts created by stone disease. Other patients may not be able to take or retain oral pain medication and may require narcotic injections at frequent enough intervals to require hospitalization.

It is an almost universal adage in urology that fluids must be forced upon the stone patient, whether given intravenously or orally. Studies on urodynamics indicate that an increase in diuresis generally decreases the rate of ureteral peristalsis. If so, one wonders whether forced water drinking serves to propel the stone through the urinary system or to decrease peristalsis and thereby inhibit urinary colic.

Some authors have advised the use of antispasmodic or anti-inflammatory agents in the treatment of urinary calculous disease (Peters and Eckstein, 1975). In particular, aminophylline or indomethicin (Buck et al., 1983; Flannigan et al., 1983) therapy has been advised. The author has attempted to use these drugs on several occasions with variable results. A long-term, carefully controlled study of these medications is necessary before they are accepted.

Most patients with urinary calculous disease do not require surgery or hospitalization and can be followed as outpatients. Since urinary calculi are often less than 4 to 5 mm in size and the great majority of these will pass spontaneously, such patients need only pain relief and instructions about recovery of the calculus. It should be emphasized to the patient that it is critical to recover any calculus or gravel that is passed. One of several commercially available funnel-like straining devices can be provided. In the author's experience, however, the simplest way for the patient to observe passage of a urinary calculus is to urinate into a clear glass jar. The density of the calculus causes it to fall to the bottom, and since most calculi are larger than 1 mm the patient can recognize and recover it. Stone analysis is performed on any calculus that is recovered, whether by the patient, at surgery, or by any other method. Stone analysis provides information about stone composition and allows us to plan future therapy for the majority of patients with urinary calculous disease.

One other aspect of stone disease must be covered at this point. How long does one wait for passage of a calculus in a patient with partial or complete obstruction of the urinary tract before one becomes concerned about significant damage to renal function? Conversely, does urinary obstruction due to calculus have any significant effect upon the kidney?

Pathophysiology of Urinary Obstruction Associated with Lithiasis

One may divide the pathophysiologic effects of stone on the kidney and ureter into two categories: first, functional results of partial or complete obstruction; and second, results of local irritation by stone. To these two categories must be added associated effects of any infection, which will alter the effects of obstruction and local irritation.

RENAL FUNCTION CHANGES

Renal or ureteral obstruction, partial or complete, produces a progressive decrease in excretory functions of the kidneys, according to studies performed in dogs. Little similar information on humans is available. After obstruction, a rapid redistribution of renal blood flow from medullary to cortical nephrons occurs; this results in decreased glomerular filtration rate (GFR) and renal plasma flow (RPF), reflecting a decrease in both glomerular and tubular function (Lackner and Barton, 1970). Finkle and Smith (1970) and Vaughan et al. (1971) observed similar decreases in function and agreed that these decreases resulted from decreased renal blood flow. Stecker and Gillenwater (1971) observed a significant concentration defect and reduced urinary acid excretion following partial ureteral obstruction lasting up to 16 weeks in dogs. Moody et al. (1975) divided renal response to ureteral occlusion into three phases: at 0 to 1½ hours, ipsilateral renal blood flow and ureteral pressures both rose; at 1½ to 5 hours, renal blood flow fell while ureteral pressures continued to rise; and at 5 to 18 hours, renal blood flow and ureteral pressures both fell. Vaughan et al. (1970) showed further that contralateral renal blood flow increased as function and renal blood flow of the obstructed kidney decreased.

Obstruction results not only in decreased renal function but also in fairly rapid changes in ureteral peristaltic function. Gee and Kiviat (1975) observed hypertrophy of rabbit ureteral musculature after only 3 days of obstruction. If obstruction continued for 2 weeks, connective tissue deposits (scar) occurred between muscle bundles, and such changes were "marked" at 8 weeks. Rose et al. (1975) observed effects of chronic ureteral obstruction in 24 dogs. They concluded that chronic ureteral obstruction resulted in decreased peristalsis and decreased pressure generation. They noted that the presence of urinary infection in addition "totally impaired" ureteral function. Perhaps this is why fewer stones in patients with infection pass spontaneously (Westbury, 1974). Such infection must, of course, involve the obstructed kidney. Pyonephrosis and pyelonephritis with stone create destructive renal changes, as described in another chapter. Obstruction by stone worsens these changes. Stone obstruction also inhibits the cure of pyelonephritis because decreased renal function results in decreased excretion of antibiotics and inhibits drainage of infected urine. Relief of obstruction after up to 8 weeks results in a rapid increase in ipsilateral renal blood flow and partial reversal of functional defects (Vaughan et al., 1970, 1971). Finkle et al. (1970) proposed that measurement of tubular clearance of water (T_CH_2O) following mannitol diuresis may be useful in assessing the amount of renal tubular function remaining after relief of chronic obstruction. They feel that the major effects of obstruction are on the tubules (Finkle and Smith, 1970). Stecker and Gillenwater (1971) state, however, that the glomerular-tubular balance is maintained in the obstructed kidney, and relief of obstruction results in improvement of both glomerular filtration rate and renal plasma flow.

Of practical interest to the urologic surgeon is the answer to the question of how long to wait before operating for stone. If infection exists behind the obstruction, the answer is clear: Operate as quickly as possible. If no infection exists and pain or discomfort is minimal, one must judge each case individually. With complete obstruction, it appears that renal deterioration (at least in dogs) begins within 18 to 24 hours. Within 5 days and certainly by 2 weeks some irreversible renal functional loss has occurred. After 16 weeks of obstruction, only "slight recovery" can be expected (Stecker and Gillenwater, 1971). Partial obstruction modifies the above figures but may still result in some irreversible functional damage. Schweitzer (1973) studied chronic partial obstruction in animals and concluded that renal damage occurs early. He suggested that surgical intervention of some kind may well be necessary earlier than is usually practiced if renal damage is to be avoided completely.

PATHOLOGIC CHANGES

Local changes created by stone include histopathologic evidence of inflammation and anatomic evidence of distortion. Locally there may be desquamation of epithelium, ulceration of the tissue contiguous to the calculi, and fibrosis. When a large stone occupies a thickened pelvis, interstitial fibrosis and leukocytic and round-cell infiltration are evident microscopically. Additional changes are influenced by the extent of obstruction of the outflow of urine from the renal pelvis.

Generally, the obstruction produced by the calculus at the outlet of the kidney is incomplete and promotes the formation of intrarenal hydronephrosis. As the calculus enlarges, it will assume the configuration of the renal pelvis, and the urine usually courses around it into the ureter. This adaptability, along with the fibrosis and hypertrophy of the walls of the pelvis, explains the relative infrequency of pelvic dilatation (Hinman, 1979). Hydronephrosis is evidenced by blunting of the calyces and later by various degrees of dilatation of the individual calyces. Atrophy and destruction of renal parenchyma follow, and, as this process progresses, the dilated calyces may stretch almost to the renal capsule.

Infection is sometimes superimposed, and various lesions such as calculous pyelonephritis, calculous pyohydronephrosis, and perinephritis may develop. With the introduction of infection, multiple stones may form; renal function is rapidly impaired, and the renal parenchyma is destroyed.

CALCULOUS PYELONEPHRITIS

Calculous pyelonephritis may become the most prominent lesion. The gross appearance of the kidney is influenced by the extent and virulence of the infection. With severe infection the renal pelvis is thickened, and miliary abscesses may develop in the swollen vascularized cortex of the kidney. With further ravages of infection, the cortex becomes thin, the infundibula of the calyces become obstructed, and localized areas of pyonephrosis are discernible as the calyces become dilated. The kidney becomes adherent to adjacent tissue surfaces. When infection is chronic, the kidney is small and pale because of the fibrous tissue reaction.

Microscopically, the wall of the renal pelvis is thickened, the mucous membrane is edema-

tous, and desquamation of the epithelium and ulceration may occur. The tubules are filled with inflammatory debris and blood cells. Many of the tubules may be destroyed as the renal cortex is thinned out. Interstitial fibrosis, round-cell infiltration, and localized areas of polymorphonuclear leukocytes occur.

Calculous pyohydronephrosis may develop when infection is superimposed on a kidney that is the site of calculous hydronephrosis. Three types of this pyohydronephrosis are recognized: atrophic, giant, and intermediate.

The atrophic kidney is very small and densely adherent to the adjacent perinephric fat. Most of the renal parenchyma is destroyed, leaving a shell of tissue attached to the pelvis. On microscopic study, little normal tissue is visible; interstitial fibrosis and round-cell infiltration are evident.

The giant hydronephrotic kidney consists of a large multilocular sac that may fill the entire flank. The surface is irregular, owing to the variable size of the tremendously dilated calyces. Multiple stones or a solitary calculus may be present in the pelvis. Again, microscopic examination shows little normal renal parenchyma. The walls of the calyces are fibrotic, perhaps thickened, and in many instances the large dilated calyces are separated by fibrous tissue septa. The perirenal fat is thickened and is especially adherent in the region of the renal pelvis.

The intermediate pyohydronephrotic kidney varies in appearance according to the degree of disease. The kidney is not as large as that of the giant type. The surface is nodular, and the elevated areas are fluctuant because of the dilated calyces and the thinning of the cortex. The capsule is thickened and adherent. Microscopically, more recognizable parenchyma, including glomeruli and tubular structures, is present; the calyceal walls are thin and are separated from the renal capsule by fibrous tissue. In other areas, round-cell and leukocytic infiltration occurs. The perinephric fat is thickened.

NEPHROCALCINOSIS

Nephrocalcinosis is the term applied to small diffuse calcifications distributed throughout the renal parenchyma. These calcifications usually occur in the renal papillae (Fig. 25–22).

REPLACEMENT LIPOMATOSIS (XANTHOGRANULOMATOUS PYELONEPHRITIS)

A kidney damaged by calculi may be the site of replacement lipomatosis. Roth and Davidson (1938) reviewed a series of 70 previously

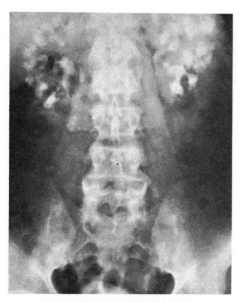

Figure 25-22. Nephrocalcinosis.

TABLE 25-2. METHODS OF STONE ANALYSIS
Chemical
Qualitative "spot" tests*
Quantitative analysis
Chromatographic and autoanalyzer methods
Optical
Binocular dissection microscopy with petrographic
(polarization) microscopy*
Instrumental
Radiographic crystallography*
Infrared spectroscopy
Thermoanalytic
Scanning electron microscopy
Transmission electron microscopy

*Commonly used methods

reported cases and added 37 new cases. They concluded that neither calculi nor inflammation was specific or necessary for the development of replacement lipomatosis. Of 33 cases reviewed by Kutzmann (1931), the coexistence of calculi and pyelonephritis was reported in 26. *Proteus mirabilis* is most often the causative agent (Goodman et al., 1979; Malek and Elder, 1978). Destruction of renal parenchyma appears to be a prerequisite for replacement lipomatosis; the fatty masses replace the destroyed tissue. Computerized tomographic scanning and ultrasonography have greatly improved the noninvasive diagnosis of this condition (Subramanyam et al., 1982).

SQUAMOUS CELL CARCINOMA

A striking relationship between renal calculi and squamous cell carcinoma of the renal pelvis has been observed. Gilbert and McMillan (1934) presented a collective review of 55 cases of squamous cell carcinoma of the renal pelvis. In 1939, Higgins reviewed 59 cases and added 5 others, 3 of which were complicated by renal calculi. In a later collective review, Gahagan and Reed (1949) reported that calculi occurred in 48 of 106 cases of squamous cell carcinoma of the renal pelvis.

Analysis of Uroliths

Following acute treatment, stone recovery is of paramount importance. In their review of incidence of urinary calculi, Burkland and Ro-

senberg (1955) asked urologists their opinion about the importance of stone analysis. The replies indicated that many urologists did not believe that analysis of calculi was important in planning the treatment course for the patient. It is to be hoped that modern attitudes have changed. Most therapy for stone disease is now based on analysis of calculi.

Based on information presented previously in this chapter, it is obvious that an individual who forms calculi will usually produce more than one during the course of his life. To prevent formation of future calculi, we must know the calculus type usually formed by that patient. Smith (1974a) has indicated that stone analysis is extremely important in planning therapy. Of the group of patients that he placed in the "indeterminate activity" category, fully one third (37 per cent) developed a new calculus within the year following evaluation. One would suspect, therefore, that the incidence of repeat urinary calculus is significantly high. Estimates vary from 8 to 80 per cent.

Westbury (1974) indicated that the degree to which a stone former is able to reproduce the pattern of chemical composition of the initial calculus depends to a large extent upon the sterility of the urine. He states that "excluding the presence of urinary infection for each patient liable to urolithiasis there is an inherent set of factors which seem to determine the composition of all of the stones formed by that patient." As Westbury points out, it is only the advent of urinary infection that results in change of composition of calculi in many patients. It is also important to determine whether the patient's infection was present prior to (and therefore caused) stone formation, or whether it was the result of catheterization, cystoscopy, or other manipulations necessary for treatment of the original stone. In the latter case, the patient develops a superimposed urinary infection that

TABLE 25–3. Spot Tests to Determine Presence of Common Crystalloids in Urinary Calculi*

Chemical	Method	Finding
1. Uric acid	Powdered stone; 1 drop 20% sodium carbonate; 2 drops uric acid reagent	Prompt deep blue color (pale blue is negative)
2. Phosphate	Powdered stone†; 4–5 drops ammonium molybdate (3.5 gm in 75 ml water and 25 ml concentrated nitric acid)	Distinct yellow precipitate (may be warmed)
3. Oxalate	(a) Powdered stone; 2–3 drops 10% HCl; if no effervescence, cool and add pinch of manganese dioxide; do not mix	Tiny bubbles of gas explosively released from bottom of test tube
	(b) Char small fragment of spatula and add 2 drops 10% HCl‡	Foaming effervescence
4. Carbonate	Relatively large sample of powdered stone; 8–10 drops 10% HCl (save for 5, 6, 7a)	Foaming effervescence
5. Calcium	Acid extract§; 2–3 drops 20% NaOH	Fine white precipitate or film from oxalate stones; dense precipitate from phosphate stone
6. Magnesium	Acid extract; 2–3 drops of 20% NaOH; 2–3 drops "M" (p-nitrobenzene-azoresorcinol, 1 mg in 100 ml normal NaOH)	Reddish-purple reagent slowly becomes defintely blue (precipitate forms)
7. Ammonium	(a) Acid extract; 2–3 drops of 20% NaOH; 2–3 drops Nessler's solution	Yellowish-orange precipitate
	(b) Powdered stone; 2–3 drops Nessler's solution	Yellowish-organge precipitate
8. Cystine	(a) Powdered stone; 1 drop NH_4OH; 1 drop 5% NaCN (wait 5 minutes); 2–3 drops 5% sodium nitroprusside	Beet red color; on standing may fade to orange red
	(b) Char over flame‡	Hydrogen sulfide odor

*From Winer, J. H.: JAMA, *169*:1715, 1959.

†Performed on microslide, it is easier to see precipitate. (Other tests are best performed on artist's spot plate on which several calculi can be analyzed simultaneously.)

‡Simple alternate methods require heat to char stone fragment in platinum spatula. Technical errors can be avoided by washing surface and taking samples by scraping various layers and nucleus with knife.

§With use of medicine dropper, tip plugged with wisp of cotton, acid extract from no. 4 is taken up, cotton is removed, and filtrate is divided for nos. 5, 6, and 7.

---

alters the type of stone even though the original stone disease was of the noninfected type.

METHODS

Many types of analysis of urinary calculi have been proposed (Table 25–2). The most common and most practical type for the clinical laboratory is chemical analysis. Table 25–3 describes chemical spot test techniques for analysis of urinary calculi. Hammerstein (1896) probably initiated most of the chemical analytical procedures performed up to the present time. Numerous authors have since pointed out that there are limitations to the use of qualitative chemical methodology for testing urinary calculi (Hazarika et al., 1974b; Hodgkinson et al., 1969; Laskowski, 1965; Murphy and Pyrah, 1962).

Schneider et al. (1973) compared chemical, x-ray defraction, infrared spectroscopy, and thermoanalytical procedures in analysis of urinary calculi. They found all of these methods accurate in detecting the components of urinary calculi. However, they felt that the chemical

methods were best for practical use in the hospital laboratory; there was only a 2 per cent error in detection of components of calculi by this method. Domanski (1937) has questioned the usefulness of chemical analysis. He pointed out, for example, that although it was possible by chemical reaction to liberate ammonium from pure uric acid stones, ammonium was not really a significant component of uric calculi. Carbonates also were often released from calculi in which they were not really present. This occurred because the chemical test for carbonates was not accurate in the presence of oxalate.

Prien and Frondel (1947) pointed out clearly the difficulty of accurate identification and analysis of the components of urinary calculi by chemical techniques alone. They emphasized the greater accuracy of optical crystallography and x-ray crystallography. Therefore, the great majority of precise analyses of urinary calculi recently have been performed by petrographic or crystallographic methods. Foremost among these has been petrographic microscopy. Prien and Frondel (1947), Prien and Prien (1968), and Prien (1963, 1974) have continuously updated their observations on petrographic analysis of urinary calculi. Sutor and colleagues (Sutor, 1968; Sutor and Scheidt, 1968) subsequently evaluated methods of crystallographic stone analysis that utilized x-ray and optical crystallography. She points out, for example, that the x-ray defraction technique allows some minor components of mixed urinary calculi to go undetected. As much as 20 to 30 per cent of the lesser component may go undetected unless certain corrective factors are applied. These factors are discussed in her evaluation (Sutor, 1968).

Many chemical and instrumental techniques of analysis such as x-ray crystallography are criticized because in preparation for such analysis the calculus is usually ground up in a mortar and pestle. The nucleus and various layers of growth are thereby mixed. On the other hand, proponents of chemical analysis criticize optical crystallography because the observer selects only small portions of the stone for analysis. If the stone is not fractured or cut, only surface analysis is performed. Elliot (1973a) therefore recommended the use of optical crystallographic examination combined with initial careful dissection of the stone under a binocular stereoscopic microscope. In this way separate layers and segments of the stone may be analyzed. In calcium oxalate calculi, he found that calcium oxalate monohydrate (whewellite) composed the nucleus or initiating crystal of two thirds of all stones. The majority of surface deposits were composed of calcium oxalate dihydrate (weddellite). These observations were confirmed by Bastian and Gebhardt (1974), who reported that whewellite was five times more frequent in the nucleus than weddellite. They also described nuclei of pure apatite overgrown with various forms of calcium oxalate or even uric acid (epitaxy). In addition, occasional nuclei of struvite, whitlockite (tricalcium-phosphate), or cystine were found. Microanalysis revealed that the nuclei were composed of many small clumps of crystallites. They concluded that the initiation of stone disease was a process of aggregation, as we have discussed previously. None of these observations would have been possible if the stones had been pulverized for chemical analysis.

Laskowski (1965) has attempted to combine the most beneficial methods of optical crystallography with chemical analysis to give a definitive analysis of the calculus. He utilized the technique described by Elliot (1973a) for initial microdissection of the calculus, with subsequent petrographic examination under the polarizing microscope. He then performed spot microchemical tests to confirm the presence or absence of particular ions. Using his methods, one can determine very precisely the composition of almost all urinary calculi without expensive instruments. Additional comments on the importance of analysis have been made by Berman (1975), Catalina and Cifuentes (1970), Finlayson (1974), Herring (1962), Lagergren (1955), Lonsdale (1968b), and Lonsdale and Sutor (1972). Sutor and Wooley (1969) have gone so far as to analyze calculi dating back to medieval times in London. Sutor et al. (1974b) have summarized the results of their extensive geographic survey of urinary calculi (see previous section on geography).

Infrared spectroscopic analysis of urinary calculi has been reported by Hazarika and Rao (1974), Kister et al. (1974), and Takasaki (1971, 1975b), and thin-section transmission electron microscopic analysis of calculi has been reported by Meyer et al. (1971). Their analyses of uric acid, oxalate, and phosphate stones reveal that the material is very finely divided and highly aggregated. The review of Cifuentes et al. (1973) has several chapters that describe additional methods of analysis of urinary calculi.

For the practicing urologist, the most useful methods are chemical analysis and petrographic microscopy through the polarizing microscope. Because it is relatively easy to instruct laboratory personnel in these techniques, almost no small hospital laboratory or large clinic should be without the methodology and ability to analyze urinary calculi (Fig. 25–23). As noted previously, Laskowski (1965) presents an excellent combined method for evaluation of urinary calculi. Similar methodology is presented in *Laboratory Microscopy* by Freeman and Beeler (1974). For those individuals who do not have these references available, summaries of the chemical methods and of optical crystallography are provided in this chapter (Tables 25–3 and 25–4).

INCIDENCE OF TYPES OF URINARY LITHIASIS

Table 25–5 summarizes the observations of a number of investigators on reported incidence of urinary calculi as analyzed by various methods. Several interesting points emerge. As noted in the section on geography, there are some specific geographic areas with relative malnutrition and primitive development where bladder calculi of uric acid may predominate. But in most of the world today the most common type of calculus is mixed calcium oxalate and calcium

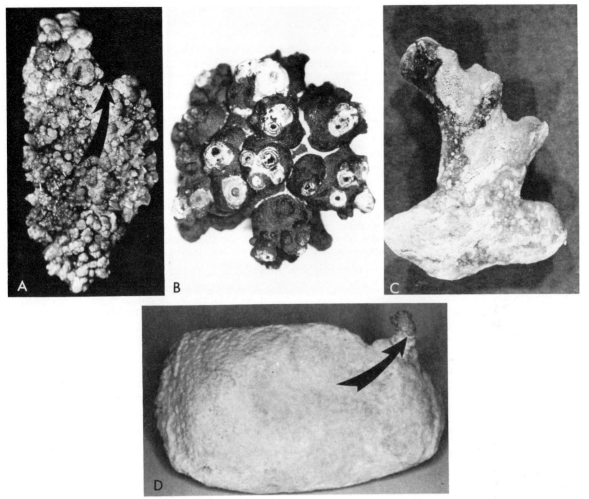

Figure 25–23. Examples of urinary calculi. *A,* Calcium oxalate monohydrate (whewellite). Actual size 5 × 8 mm. Arrow indicates indentation of point of attachment of stone to papilla. This is sometimes called a "mulberry stone." *B,* Uric acid calculus. Actual size 2.3 cm. Sometimes called a "jack stone." *C,* Staghorn calculus of magnesium ammonium phosphate (struvite). Actual size 4.5 × 7 cm. *D,* Bladder calculus of magnesium ammonium phosphate (struvite), which has formed on a piece of nonabsorbable suture (arrow). Patients who produced stones in *C* and *D* both had chronic urinary infection caused by *Proteus mirabilis.*

phosphate. Again, the relative proportion of uric acid calculi stays approximately the same the world over. Also, we see roughly the same proportions of cystine calculi. It seems, then, that throughout the world approximately the same percentage of population is afflicted with a given type of urinary lithiasis.

Also, although we have discussed several methods of analysis of urinary calculus components, they all tend to lead us to the same result—namely, definition of five basic types of urinary calculus. Only minor differences occur. For example, Herring (1962) reported calcium oxalate calculi collectively in his review and did not further separate them into those that were pure and those that were mixed calcium oxalate

and calcium phosphate calculi. Herring used crystallographic methods, and as Sutor has discussed in her reviews (Sutor, 1968; Sutor and Scheidt, 1968), there are limitations in x-ray crystallography for complete analysis of calculus components. As noted above, there is a possibility of missing one component if it represents 30 per cent or less of the total proportion of the calculus. Hence, Herring's approach to analysis may have resulted in some error in the quantitative analysis of urinary calculi.

Mixed urinary calculi, as can be seen from Table 25–5, are very common. Hodgkinson and Marshall (1975) performed extensive quantitative chemical analyses of pure and mixed urinary calculi. They showed clearly that calculi of

TABLE 25–4. DETERMINATION OF CRYSTALLINE COMPOSITION OF URINARY CALCULI BY OPTICAL CRYSTALLOGRAPHY USING SPECIFIC GRAVITY OILS*†

Using 1.550 oil, crossed polars, and ¼ wave (red) filter, Becke line method:
  A. If both indices of crystal are greater than 1.550, stone could be uric acid, cystine, tricalcium phosphate, calcium oxalate monohydrate, urates. Go to Group A, below.
  B. If both indices of crystal are less than 1.550, stone could be calcium oxalate dihydrate, magnesium ammonium phosphate, calcium hydrogen phosphate. Go to group B, below.
  C. If crystal has one index greater than and one index less than 1.550, stone could be calcium oxalate monohydrate, carbonate apatite, urates, hydroxyl apatite, calcium hydrogen phosphate. Go to Group C, below.

If under group A, use 1.750 oil
  1. If crystal has one index greater and one index less than 1.750, stone is *uric acid*.
  2. If crystal has both indices greater than 1.750, or one index greater and one equal to 1.750, stone is *urates*.
  3. If crystal has both indices less than 1.750, stone could be cystine, calcium oxalate monohydrate, or tricalcium phosphate.
    If under group 3, use 1.574 oil
    a. If both indices of crystal are greater than 1.574, stone could be cystine, or tricalcium phosphate.
    b. If one index is greater and one less than, or if both indices are less than 1.574, stone is *calcium oxalate monohydrate*.

If under group a, use 1.650 oil
  I. If both indices are less than 1.650, stone is *tricalcium phosphate*.
  II. If one index is greater than and one less than 1.650, stone is *cystine*.
If under group B, use 1.538 oil
  1. If both indices are less than 1.538, stone is *magnesium ammonium phosphate*.
  2. If both indices are greater than 1.538, stone is *calcium hydrogen phosphate*.
  3. If one index is greater than and one less than 1.538, stone is *calcium oxalate dihydrate*.
If under group C, use 1.700 oil
  1. If one index is greater than and one less than 1.700, or if both indices are greater than 1.700, stone is *urates*.
  2. If both indices are less than 1.700, stone could be calcium oxalate monohydrate, carbonate apatite, hydroxyl apatite, or calcium hydrogen phosphate.
    If under group 2, use 1.504 and 1.640 oils
    a. If one index of crystal is less than 1.504, stone is *calcium oxalate monohydrate*.
    b. If one index of crystal is greater than 1.640, stone is *calcium oxalate monohydrate*.
    c. If no crystals have an index greater than 1.640 or less than 1.504, stone could be carbonate apatite, hydroxyl apatite, or calcium hydrogen phosphate.
      If under group c, use 10% HCl
      I. If effervescence occurs, stone is *carbonate apatite*.
      II. If no effervescence occurs, stone is *hydroxyl apatite*.

*Method of Urology Research Laboratory, University of Arizona.
†References:
  Prien, E. L., and Frondel, C.: J. Urol. *57*:949, 1947.
  Wahlstrom, E. E.: Optical Crystallography. New York, John Wiley & Sons, Inc., 1965.

TABLE 25–5. SOME COMPARATIVE INCIDENCES OF FORMS OF URINARY LITHIASIS (PER CENT OF STONES ANALYZED)

Form of Lithiasis	USA*	USA†	Israel‡	Japan§	Great Britain¶
Pure calcium oxalate	33		14	17.4	39.4
Mixed calcium oxalate and phosphate	34	73	64	50.8	20.2
Pure calcium phosphate	6	8		3.2	13.2
Magnesium ammonium phosphate (struvite)	15	9	12	17.4	15.4
Uric acid	8	7.63	9	4.4	8
Cystine	3	0.88	2	1.0	2.8
Artifacts and other	1	1.5		5.8	1.0

*Prien, E. L., Sr., and Gershoff, S. F.: J. Urol., *112*:509, 1974.
†Herring, L. C.: J. Urol., *88*:545, 1982.
‡Herbstein, F. H., Kleeberg, J., Shalitin, Y., et al.: Isr. J. Med. Sci., *10*:1493, 1974.
§Takasaki, E.: Calc. Tiss. Res., *7*:232, 1971.
¶Westbury, E. J.: Br. J. Urol., *46*:215, 1974.

mixed composition (which includes calcium oxalate, magnesium ammonium phosphate, and calcium phosphate) are prevalent in their Leeds population. The major component in the largest number of their calculi was calcium oxalate. They noted a decrease in the proportion of calcium phosphate and magnesium ammonium phosphate in their calculi between the years 1965 and 1974. More recently, therefore, the calculi in the population of Leeds are likely to be composed of larger proportions of calcium oxalate. Urinary infection tends to increase the percentage of phosphate in a urinary calculus. So too does the presence of metabolic diseases such as hyperparathyroidism, renal tubular acidosis, and medullary sponge kidney. All four of these disease states result in a more alkaline urine. It is this alkalinity that is believed to contribute to the deposition of phosphate in calculi. Hodgkinson and Marshall presume that improved diagnosis and treatment of these conditions have contributed to the decreased proportions of phosphates in urinary calculi. One other interesting comment is made by Hodgkinson and Marshall. The observed number of bladder stones has remained constant at about 20 per year during the entire period of observation noted in their report. Hence, they conclude that the incidence of bladder stone disease has reached a basal level for their particular population.

Knowledge of the percentage composition of a urinary calculus contributes to the ability to predict the most probable cause of that calculus. Therefore, it is critical that the laboratory be capable of providing accurate quantitative analysis of the calculus by suitable methods. Only then can the urologist and his colleagues formulate a therapeutic plan that will be useful in preventing future stone disease in that patient.

EVALUATION AND TREATMENT OF SPECIFIC TYPES OF MEDICALLY ACTIVE UROLITHIASIS

Fortunately, renal calculous disease that creates stones of pure calcium phosphate, magnesium ammonium phosphate, uric acid, and cystine, which account for 30 per cent of all patients with urinary lithiasis, usually results from conditions that are relatively easy to diagnose and for which we have good therapeutic measures. These therapeutic measures include diet, fluid therapy, drug treatment, and surgery.

Similar but somewhat less effective therapy exists for the remaining 70 per cent of patients (those with calcium stones). In this section, we will discuss all aspects of treatment except surgery. Surgery for urinary lithiasis is discussed under surgery of specific areas of the urinary tract in other sections of this textbook.

General Aspects of Diagnosis and Treatment

A stone episode may be one of a series of recurrent stones in a given patient, or it may be the initial incident. Nevertheless, the therapeutic steps are essentially the same. The first step is to provide emergent, acute therapy, which has been discussed earlier. In addition, categorization of stone-formation activity is made. The main reason for this categorization is to decide whether surgical intervention is necessary. The sizes of calculi that are likely to pass spontaneously have been discussed in the sections on incidence and on ureteral stones. We should remember, however, that even very small calculi may become totally impacted in the ureter, causing obstruction and resultant damage to the kidney. Results of obstruction associated with urinary calculi have been discussed in the section on pathophysiology. In addition, if urinary infection is present, there will be deterioration of kidney function related to the infectious process.

One way or another, it is imperative to recover the stone. Stone analysis is performed, and the type of calculus is then known. At the present time, mixed calcium oxalate/calcium phosphate calculi are extremely common. In the great majority of these stones, however, the largest component is calcium oxalate as the crystallizing agent. The forms of calcium oxalate that precipitate may be monohydrate (whewellite) or dihydrate (weddellite) or both. It is possible that at some future time different causes for the crystallization of these two types of oxalate stone may be found, but at present we know of no difference in the crystallization process other than the degree of hydration of the crystal (Berenyi et al., 1972). Therefore, both types of oxalate calculi are treated by the same methods.

One point must be re-emphasized. If a stone is associated with a urinary tract infection, the physician must decide whether the infection is the primary cause of the stone (as it is in most patients with struvite calculi) or if the infection is secondary to urinary manipulation or instrumentation for treatment of stone disease in the

TABLE 25–6. MAJOR URINARY ABNORMALITIES ASSOCIATED WITH SUPERSATURATION AND STONE

Type of Stone Former	pH*	Component
Cystine	Acid	Cystine excess
Uric acid	Acid	Relative uric acid excess
Calcium phosphate	Alkaline	Relative calcium excess
Calcium oxalate		
Idiopathic	†	Calcium and oxalate excess
Hyperoxaluric	†	Oxalate excess
Renal tubular acidosis	Alkaline	Perhaps calcium and phosphate excess
Magnesium ammonium phosphate (infected)	Very alkaline	Relative magnesium, ammonium, and phosphate excess

*Urinary pH that persists and promotes precipitation.
†Calcium oxalate precipitation occurs throughout pH range of normal urine.

past. In the former case, therapy is directed toward eradication of infection and removal of the stone. Prevention of future calculi is then dependent upon the continued elimination of urinary infection and maintenance of acidity of the urine. In the latter case, both infection and stone must usually be eliminated by surgery, but the prophylactic plan must allow for control of both infection and the primary urinary stone-forming process. The term "infection stones" refers only to those calculi that are caused primarily by the splitting of urea by bacteria in the urine, with subsequent elevation of urinary pH and formation of struvite crystals. Stones that are not *caused* by infection are considered to be different from stones of infection and are not treated in the same way. This point cannot be emphasized too strongly.

Sections of this chapter dealing with specific types of calculus should be reviewed thoroughly before initiating therapy. Table 25–6 summarizes the basic defects that contribute to supersaturation and presumably to stone formation in patients. Let us now review separately the evaluation and treatment of the stone-forming patient, based on stone analysis.

Uric Acid Lithiasis

SPECIAL ASPECTS OF ETIOLOGY

Early in his development, man suffered one significant genetic mutation as he branched off from other anthropoids. This mutation resulted in the disappearance of the enzyme uricase from human organs, especially the liver. As Gutman and Yu (1968) and Yu (1981) point out, this mutation left man without the ability to convert uric acid by-products of purine metabolism into the substance allantoin, which is freely water-soluble when excreted by the kidneys.

Most animals filter uric acid through the glomerulus and rapidly reabsorb it through renal tubular cells. It recirculates through blood to the liver, where the enzyme uricase transforms it to allantoin. Allantoin then returns to the circulation and is easily excreted by the kidneys. Only the Dalmatian coach hound, of all mammals, has a risk of uric acid urinary lithiasis equal to that of man, but it has a different enzymatic defect. The end result is that man has levels of uric acid in his system that are ten times greater than those of other mammals (Fanelli, 1977; Watts, 1976; Yu, 1981).

Man not only produces excessive, relatively water-insoluble uric acid, he also excretes urine that is predominantly acid because of the acid end products of metabolism. When uric acid enters human urine it exists in two forms. One is free uric acid. The other is the urate salt, which forms a complex mostly with sodium. Sodium urate is approximately 20 times more soluble in water than free uric acid. As Seegmiller (1973) notes: "The limited solubility of uric acid in acidic aqueous solution is obviously the most fundamental property responsible for its formation of renal calculi."

As noted in Figure 25–24, the pK_a of uric acid is 5.75. At that point, half of the uric ions exist as free uric acid and the other half are associated with other ions as the urate salt. Persistent excretion of urine below pH 5.75 contributes to increased concentration of the relatively insoluble uric acid. Peters and Van Slyke (1968) have calculated that urinary saturation with uric acid is achieved with 60 mg per liter at pH 5.0 and 37°C, but urine at pH 6.0 can contain 220 mg per liter (Fig. 25–25). The average male excretes approximately 400 mg of uric acid per day in a volume of slightly over a liter; therefore, urine is often supersaturated with uric acid. Fortunately, this uric acid is usually kept in solution through variations in urinary pH and through interaction with other molecules in the urine, probably mucoid mole-

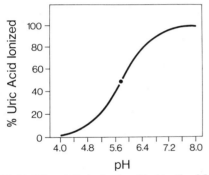

Figure 25–24. Dissociation of uric acid. At pK$_a$ of 5.75 one-half of uric acid is ionized as urate salts and is therefore soluble. As pH increases, more becomes ionized and soluble. (From Gutman, A. B., and Yu, T. F.: Am. J. Med., *45*:756, 1968.)

Excretion of Metabolic Acid into Urine

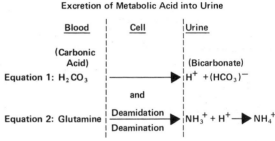

Figure 25–26. Simplified illustration of excretion of metabolic acid end-products by urine. Free acid (equation 1) arrives at the kidney via blood as carbonic acid, traverses the renal cell, and enters the urine in ionized form. In urine, free acid is measured as pH by meters or paper strips. Some acid is bound in the form of glutamine (equation 2), which is enzymatically cleaved within the renal cell to produce ammonia (NH_3^+), which diffuses rapidly into the urine. Here the ammonia quickly combines with another H^+ to become ammonium (NH_4^+). Ammonium remains in the urine. Amounts contributed to acid excretion by ammonium are measured by determining the titratable acidity of urine. If little H^+ is excreted as ammonium (an alkaline ion), the urine maintains an acid pH.

cules (Porter, 1966; Seegmiller, 1973; Sperling et al., 1965; Yu and Gutman, 1973) and urea.

Patients who persistently form uric acid stones often have prolonged periods of acidity in their urine. Normal individuals have variation in pH of urine that results, especially in daytime hours, in postprandial alkaline tides that take the pH well above 6.5. Urine in normal individuals also varies remarkably throughout the day in its content of acid or ammonium. Both represent acid excretion. Excretion of acid by the kidney may be summarized by two equations (Fig. 25–26). At any given time, depending upon the amount of acid presented to the kidney, the relative amounts of hydrogen ion or ammonium that are excreted may increase or decrease. In general, the processes of oxidation in the body result in the production of excess acidity, and therefore most urine excreted by the average human contains more free acid. For this reason the mean urinary pH of the average individual is approximately 1 full pH unit lower than blood, or pH 6.4. Marked changes in urine pH can also result from ingestion of foods containing acid or alkaline, environmental changes, and the presence or absence of other diseases such as respiratory illness, cardiac disease, and so on. These diseases may result in a combination of reduced daily urinary volume and acid urine. Patients with uric acid lithiasis have a tendency to maintain a urine pH of below 6.0, and often the pH is fixed in the range of 5.0 (Cifuentes et al., 1973; Gutman and Yu, 1968; Rapaport et al., 1967; Thomas, 1975; Williams, 1974a; Yu and Gutman, 1973; Yu, 1981). Yu and Gutman postulate that the most likely explanation for persistent low urinary pH in these patients is a disturbance in the renal regulation of ammonium. Most such patients show a partial deficiency in renal production of ammonium. Less ammonium then becomes available for urine buffering. In Figure 25–26, note that ammonium is produced from glutamine by enzymatic reactions in the renal tubular cell. It is excreted by diffusion through cell walls as NH_3. When it enters the renal tubular lumen, it quickly combines with a free ion of hydrogen, forming the NH_4^+ ion. The net result is buffering of urine to a more alkaline pH. Therefore, the acid load originally presented to the urine is converted to an alkaline load. In this way the titratable acidity (free H^+ ion) actually decreases, and the urine becomes less acid. If ammonium is not excreted, urine remains more acid.

In summary, three factors must be involved in the creation of uric acid urolithiasis. First,

Amount of Uric Acid or Urate Suspended in Urine at Different pH (mgm/liter)

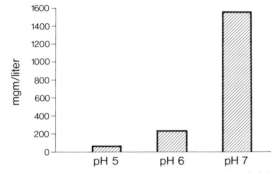

Figure 25–25. Amounts of uric acid or urate suspended by and soluble in 1 liter of urine at three different pH levels. By comparison with Figure 25–24, note that the maximum solubility of uric acid is achieved near pH 7.

there must be a relative hyperuricosuria or chronic oversaturation of urine with uric acid. Second, such patients usually have a tendency toward excretion of excessively acid urine. Finally, patients with uric acid urolithiasis often excrete a reduced volume of urine. Such patients may be chronically dehydrated by medication or by occupations in a hot environment, or they may live in a hot climate (Atsmon et al., 1963; Toor et al., 1964).

Awareness of these three factors immediately suggests three forms of therapy. First, an increase in daily fluid intake will increase urine output and dilute urinary uric acid. Second, an attempt should be made to alkalize the urine. Third, excessive uric acid excretion should be decreased. Methods for performing this last alteration vary. As with many other elements in the urine, urinary uric acid arises from two sources, endogenous production within the tissues of the body and diet. The relative contribution of these two sources to urinary uric acid varies in each individual. Zollner and Griebsch (1973) observed no difference in intestinal purine absorption in normal and hyperuricemic persons. Hyperuricemic persons, however, did demonstrate below-normal renal clearances of uric acid at any given level of plasma uric acid. These authors also noted that, in spite of their observations on intestinal absorption, dietary limitation of purine intake (the precursor of most uric acid) did decrease serum and urinary uric acid levels. Similar results were obtained after administration of allopurinol. Seegmiller (1973) reports that only one fourth of patients with hyperuricemic gout excrete excess uric acid when on a purine-free diet. Therefore, only one fourth of patients with this type of hyperuricemia can be producing excessive purine endogenously. In contrast, three fourths of these individuals probably acquire excess urinary uric acid from their diet. Controversy about this point exists, however. Cifuentes and colleagues (1973) do not believe that diet is important in control of uric acid lithiasis, but May and Schindler (1973), reporting multiple observations in their patients, indicated that dietary control is important. The author believes that both diet and endogenous production are important in the control of uric acid lithiasis.

CLASSIFICATION OF URIC ACID LITHIASIS

By definition, if patients form uric acid calculi their urine must be supersaturated with uric acid. They therefore have hyperuricosuria. Because of the great variation in solubility of uric acid with variation in urinary pH, it is not possible to establish a precise definition of exactly how much uric acid per day can be considered excessive without taking into consideration total urinary volume and urinary pH (See Figs. 25–24 and 25–25).

The upper limit of normal concentration for serum uric acid is reported by most laboratories to be between 6.5 and 7.0 mg per dl for men and about 5.5 mg per dl for women (Gutman and Yu, 1968). Based on serum levels, most authors tend to classify patients with uric acid lithiasis into two broad groups, those with hyperuricemia and those with normal serum uric acid concentration. Gutman and Yu further subdivide uric acid nephrolithiasis into four major categories.

Their first category is termed idiopathic uric acid lithiasis. These individuals do not have hyperuricemia, and the amount of urinary excretion of uric acid per day is within normal ranges. The major physiologic abnormality in these patients is a consistently low urine pH. If urine pH is measured throughout the day, an alkaline tide does not appear as is normal. Patients with chronic diarrheal states, those with ileostomy, and those who take medications to acidify urine may be included in this category (Williams, 1974a).

Their second category includes uric acid nephrolithiasis associated with hyperuricemia such as the Lesch-Nyhan syndrome. This latter disease is of interest because such patients have a definable deficiency in an enzyme, hypoxanthine-guanine phosphoribosyltransferase. DeVries and Sperling (1973) have also reported a mutation of a similar enzyme system in a family with a tendency toward gout. Therefore, there is increasing belief that hyperuricemia with uric acid urolithiasis represents an inborn error of metabolism. In an additional group of patients in this category there is myeloproliferative or other neoplastic disease with increased endogenous production of uric acid.

A third category consists of patients who develop uric acid lithiasis because of excessive loss of water to the environment. This may be due to excessive perspiration or to gastrointestinal losses such as that associated with ileitis, colitis, and similar conditions.

The final category includes patients who develop uric acid lithiasis because of ingestion of uricosuric drugs or overindulgence in foods high in purine and proteins (organ meats, sardines). Such drugs include salicylates, thiazides, and others.

Note that of the foregoing categories only one involves hyperuricemia. The other three involve only excessive urinary excretion of uric acid (hyperuricosuria) enhanced by consistent low volume and pH.

EVALUATION OF PATIENTS

From the foregoing it can be seen that evaluation of such patients requires measurement of serum and urinary acid levels, assessment of responses of urinary uric acid to ingestion of dietary purines, and observation of daily urinary pH conducted by measuring and recording the pH of every voiding with Nitrazine pH paper. If the patient also has evidence of hyperuricemia, evaluation should include a brief survey to rule out myeloproliferative or neoplastic disease.

Special diagnostic aspects of uric acid lithiasis include recognition that this is the *only* solid urinary calculus that is radiolucent. In addition, uric acid lithiasis may be associated with urinary obstruction through showers of small crystals rather than with a single large crystalline structure. For this reason, microscopic examination of the urine can be helpful both in diagnosing uric acid urolithiasis and in determining success of therapy. Patients under medical control should not have evidence of uric acid crystals in their urine at any time.

THERAPY

With the exception of some physicians who feel that diet has no part in the treatment of individuals with uric acid lithiasis, most investigators agree on the regimen that should be used to treat such patients. The initial and immediate therapy involves instruction of the patient and testing to guarantee that he is getting enough fluids to ensure urinary output in excess of 1500 ml per day or even 2000 ml per day. In hot climates this may require intake of enormous quantities of fluid. Increased urinary output also results in some increase in urinary pH owing to diuretic effects of water. Since endogenous uric acid production continues at a basal rate in all individuals, it is best to advise the patient to consume a diet that limits protein intake to less than 90 grams per day (see Appendix A). This amount is enough to maintain body protein balance.

If patients have the renal defect that produces consistently acid urine, they should be given medications to alkalize the urine to a level between pH 6.5 and 7.0. In treatment of uric acid stones it is not necessary to alkalize the urine above pH 7.0. In fact, excessive alkalization may be detrimental, since such patients may then begin to form stones that precipitate in alkaline solution, such as apatite or struvite. Patients should be instructed to test their urine

with Nitrazine or other suitable pH paper in order to maintain pH in the proper range. Uric acid calculi can easily be dissolved by nonsurgical therapy if the urine pH and uric acid are kept within the undersaturated range and if the patient has no other problem that makes surgery necessary.

Medications that may be used for alkalization therapy include sodium bicarbonate, 650 mg or more every 6 to 8 hours, or comparable amounts of liquid preparations of balanced citrate in dosages of about 15 ml three times or four times daily (Drach, 1976a; Thomas, 1975). Freed (1975) suggested alkalization of urine with a regimen that combines use of sodium bicarbonate, 1 gm three times a day, with administration of acetazolamide, 250 mg once a day. Problems of hypertension and cardiovascular and renal problems due to sodium or potassium overload are thereby avoided. Patients rarely cooperate with long-term administration of alkali, so careful monitoring is essential. Long-term alkalization may not be necessary for control of most patients with uric acid stones. Dietary protein limitation and increased urinary output may suffice. Urinary alkalization seems advisable during periods when attempts at stone dissolution are under way.

If the patient has hyperuricemia, it is advisable that he be given allopurinol, 300 to 600 mg per day. This medication may be given as a single tablet or in divided doses. Allopurinol was originally developed for the treatment of gout and of hyperuricemia associated with malignant disease (Rundles et al., 1966). Occasional side effects may occur, including rash and activation of acute arthritis associated with primary gout. According to Gutman and Yu (1968), this activation of arthritis often occurs in spite of colchicine prophylaxis in doses of up to 1 mg per day or more. Other patients develop diarrhea or abdominal cramps. The incidence of these side effects ranges from 5 to 6 per cent (Gutman and Yu, 1968; Rundles et al., 1966; Thomas, 1975). To review, therapy of uric acid lithiasis requires increasing urinary volume, limiting dietary purines and protein, possibly alkalizing urine, and perhaps administering allopurinol.

Cystine Urinary Lithiasis

SPECIAL ASPECTS OF ETIOLOGY

Cystinuria is an inherited defect in renal tubular reabsorption of four amino acids, cystine, ornithine, lysine, and arginine. Smith (1974b) has suggested use of the mnemonic

COLA to remember these four amino acids. Cystinuria is inherited as an autosomal recessive trait. However, some individuals who are heterozygous for the disease do show evidence of excretion of excessive cystine and the other three dibasic amino acids in their urine. Some authors further divide this heterozygous form of cystinuria into separate forms. When it is completely recessive (Type I), there is no amino aciduria. Incompletely recessive forms (Types II and III) show increased urinary excretion of cystine in the range of 150 to 300 mg in 24 hours. These patients usually do not form calculi.

The amino acid transport defects exist both in the renal tubular cells and in the intestinal mucosa. Although patients with this disease sometimes have small stature, presumably due to excessive urinary loss of lysine, the only clinical symptom of importance is the occurrence of urinary calculi. The incidence of clinically evident cystinuria is believed to be approximately 1 per 20,000 (Smith, 1974b). Methionine is the probable dietary precursor of cystine (Crawhall and Watts, 1968), and normal individuals in general excrete less than 100 mg of cystine in their urine per day. Since approximately 300 to 400 mg of cystine per liter of urine is soluble within the pH range of 4.5 to 7.0 (Fig. 25–27), a normal individual rarely if ever exceeds the solubility product for cystine. In contrast, patients with homozygous cystinuria usually excrete amounts of cystine in excess of 600 mg per day. The upper limit of solubility of cystine per gram of creatinine appears to be 180 mg. Cystine, like uric acid, is much less soluble in acid than in alkaline urine. It differs from uric acid in that its improved solubility becomes apparent only at pH levels above 7.2. Elevation of the pH to 7.8 almost doubles the solubility of cystine (Fig. 25–27) (Dent and Senior, 1955).

EVALUATION

Urinary stones of cystine should be suspected in the initial evaluation of individuals with family histories of stone disease, in recurrent disease in those under 30 years of age (Pavanello et al., 1981), and in individuals who have radiographic evidence of slightly dense, laminated, "ground-glass" calculi (Fig. 25–20). Cystine stones should always be diagnosed whenever the characteristic hexagonal crystals are seen in urine. One screening test for cystinuria utilizing cyanide nitroprusside can detect concentrations of cystine in excess of approximately 75 mg/gm creatinine (Smith, 1974b). False positive reactions due to medication and

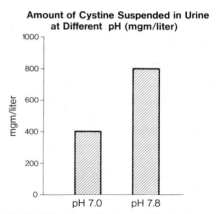

Amount of Cystine Suspended in Urine at Different pH (mgm/liter)

Figure 25–27. Elevation of urinary pH also improves the solubility of cystine. In contrast to uric acid (Fig. 25–25), urine pH increasing from 7.0 to over 7.8 doubles the solubility of cystine. Therapy is therefore directed at attempting to keep the urinary pH near 8.

positive tests in non–stone forming heterozygous cystinurics may produce confusing results. A confirmatory quantitative determination of total urinary cystine must be performed by chromatographic methods if the screening test is positive. Knowledge of the total urinary cystine concentration also determines the amount of therapy necessary to prevent stone formation.

THERAPY

One of the most helpful ways to devise therapy for cystinuria is to measure the total daily cystine excretion in urine. Most cystinurics who excrete 300 to 800 mg per day can be controlled by urinary dilution and alkalization similar to that given for uric acid lithiasis. Cystine solubility in urine increases two to three times at pH above 7.5, so every attempt should be made to keep urinary pH above this level. Sodium bicarbonate, 12.6 gm or more per 24 hours, in equally divided doses or 100 ml of balanced citrate solution per day in divided doses should provide adequate alkalization.

Fluid intake should continue around the clock and should ensure urinary output of 3 to 4 *liters* per day. Patients should drink two large glasses of water every 2 hours while awake and once during the night to force this amount of urine. If increased urinary output doesn't awaken them to urinate, they must set a separate alarm clock to awaken them during sleep.

Dietary restriction of methionine is theoretically sound but results in a very unpalatable diet that most patients cannot tolerate, and the resulting reduction in cystine excretion is small. Patients should not, however, overload their diet with methionine-containing proteins. Dietary methionine restriction may be used as a last resort in patients who cannot be controlled by other methods of treatment (see Appendix B).

It is seldom necessary to add D-penicillamine to the treatment plan for these patients. However, D-penicillamine therapy may speed attempts to dissolve cystine calculi. D-penicillamine, up to 1.5 gm per day in divided doses, usually reduces pure urinary cystine excretion to below 400 mg per day. After administration of D-penicillamine, most urinary cystine combines with D-penicillamine to form cystine-s-penicillamine, which is soluble in urine. Effectiveness of D-penicillamine can be assessed by testing a 24-hour urinary specimen for free cystine with nitroprusside and for penicillamine disulfide with 3 per cent FeCl (Lotz et al., 1965). Unfortunately, many patients develop allergic or idiosyncratic reactions to penicillamine, including arthralgia, rash, nephrotic syndrome, or other manifestations. These complications plus high cost limit the use of D-penicillamine.

Several authors have now reported the use of alpha-mercaptopropionylglycine (MPG) to treat patients with cystinuria and stones (Johansen et al., 1980; Koide et al., 1982; Pak, 1982). Once again, urinary cystine solubility and excretion are enhanced by formation of thiol disulfide compounds in a manner similar to D-penicillamine. In one report on the treatment of 35 patients (Koide et al., 1982), the daily dosages ranged from 600 to 1800 mg per day for stone dissolution and 300 to 1500 mg per day for prophylaxis. Complete or significant dissolution occurred in 7 of 21 patients treated for this purpose. Side effects occurred in 16 patients, but most patients were able to be adapted to the drug when reintroduced to it gradually. Hence, it seems that this compound may be better tolerated than the present D-penicillamine. It is to be hoped that MPG will soon be available in all countries. In summary, therapy for cystine stones includes greatly increased urinary volume, vigorous alkalization of urine, occasionally D-penicillamine, and rarely dietary restriction of methionine.

Stones of Urinary Infection

SPECIAL ASPECTS OF ETIOLOGY

Calculi composed of magnesium ammonium calcium phosphate or "struvite" stones and those few due to carbonate-apatite are the subject of this portion of our discussion. It has already been noted that uric acid and cystine calculi are produced by simple physicochemical processes that occur with acidic urinary pH and associated hyperexcretion; the urine is therefore supersaturated with one or the other insoluble molecule. Magnesium ammonium phosphate stones are caused by a similar but reverse situation due to urinary pH. Clark and Nordin (1969) indicate in their introduction to a renal stone research symposium that "this type of stone (struvite) is also probably due to simple precipitation from supersaturated solution." Barnhouse (1968) and Griffith and Musher (1973) have probably advanced our knowledge about the physical chemistry of production of struvite calculi as much as any investigators. Our understanding of this disease has been a progressive deepening of awareness that stones of infection are always associated with urea-splitting bacteria and subsequent elevation of urinary pH due to increased bacterial ammonium production (Fig. 25–28).

Griffith (1979) reviewed and confirmed observations of previous investigators that the basic abnormality in the formation of struvite calculi is maintenance of a urinary pH of greater than 7.2 (Barnhouse, 1968; Elliot et al., 1959; Nemoy and Stamey, 1971; Priestley and Osterberg, 1936). The situation, as noted earlier, is opposite to that characteristic of uric acid and cystine calculi. In the case of magnesium ammonium phosphate ($MgNH_4PO_4 \cdot 6H_2O$), urine is undersaturated at the normal mean physiologic pH of approximately 5.85 (Elliot et al., 1959). The presence of bacteria in the urine of the type that can split urea provides the conditions necessary for precipitation of magnesium ammonium phosphate (Fig. 25–29). Remember also that many of these calculi have small quantities of calcium phosphate mixed in their lattice (Hodgkinson and Marshall, 1975).

Struvite calculi account for the great majority of staghorn calculi encountered in urologic practice in most countries. They can grow to immense size and indeed achieve the appearance of a true staghorn, as shown in Figures 25–23C and 25–30. Nemoy and Stamey (1971), Thompson and Stamey (1973), and Jennis et al. (1970) have reviewed previous studies and con-

Bacterial Urease

$$NH_2CO\,NH_2\,(UREA) + H_2O \longrightarrow 2NH_3 + H_2CO_3$$

$$2NH_3 + H_2O \longrightarrow NH_4 + OH$$

Figure 25–28. Production of ammonium by the action of bacterial urease on urea to form NH_3, which quickly becomes NH_4. Because of the excess of NH_4, the urine remains alkaline even if renal excretion of acid is normal.

MAGNESIUM AMMONIUM PHOSPHATE (STRUVITE)
CALCULI: MECHANISMS OF FORMATION AND DISSOLUTION

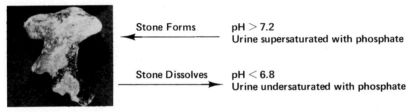

Stone Forms   pH > 7.2
⟵―――――――――   Urine supersaturated with phosphate

Stone Dissolves   pH < 6.8
―――――――――⟶   Urine undersaturated with phosphate

Figure 25–29. Factors in formation of magnesium ammonium phosphate (struvite) calculi related to persistent alkaline urine.

firmed the fact that struvite and other urinary calculi not only are caused by action of bacteria on urine but also contain numerous infective bacteria within their structures. These authors have also shown that the penetration of antibiotics into these stones is inadequate for cure, so the presence of an infected urinary calculus acts as a source for continued urinary infection. As long as infected urinary stones exist anywhere in the urinary tract it is unlikely that the urinary system can be sterilized by antibiotics or other methods.

Recurrence of struvite urinary calculi following surgical removal is usually due to retention of small fragments of stone within the kidney or to failure to eradicate urinary infection completely. Boyce and Elkins (1974) reviewed their series of 100 consecutive surgical procedures to remove staghorn calculi. They report stone recurrence in 17.7 per cent of their patients. They strongly emphasize that complete removal of every visible fragment of calculus is necessary during the operative procedure. Thereafter, patients must be observed carefully to keep the urinary tract totally free of infection *forever*. Hence, maintenance of a sterile urine is a very large part of any postsurgical plan for removal of infected staghorn urinary calculi (Drach, 1974*b*).

The reported incidence of stone recurrence following such operations varies. Sutherland (1954) reports a very high recurrence rate. Nemoy and Stamey (1971) have observed retained calculi in 4 out of 11 operations, an incidence of 36 per cent. Blaivas et al. (1975) reported the need for treatment of postoperative recurrent stones in ten patients, although the proportion of this to the total number of stone operations they performed is not presented. Incidence of postoperative recurrence seems to depend greatly upon uncertain factors and ranges between 20 and 70 per cent. Hence,

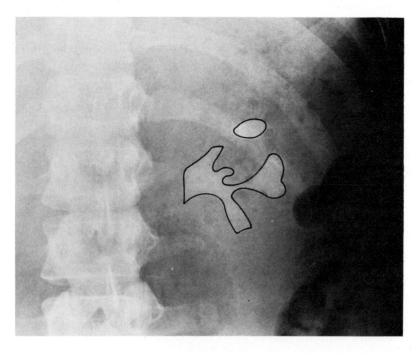

Figure 25–30. Struvite calculi (outline) may be relatively radiolucent and may be confused with cystine calculi. This calculus proved to be composed of pure struvite.

improved methods for continued postoperative treatment and control of such patients are obviously needed.

Two other urologic conditions appear to contribute to infection and to the tendency to form magnesium ammonium phosphate calculi. The first is the presence of a foreign body in the urinary tract, and the second is neurogenic bladder associated with trauma, stroke, and similar conditions. Such patients often carry residual urine and frequently require urinary catheter drainage; subsequently, they acquire urinary infection. The presence of a catheter or any other foreign body nucleus in the urinary tract (Fig. 25–23D) creates a situation that often results in magnesium ammonium phosphate calculi. In patients with neurogenic bladder it is difficult to ascertain whether it is the catheter or other foreign body that actually initiates the infection stone or whether it is the infection itself. Both factors are probably important.

As an example, Griffith and Musher (1973) in their series of struvite stone experiments used the foreign body method of Vermeulen and colleagues (1964, 1968) to create magnesium ammonium phosphate calculi on zinc discs placed in the bladders of rats that were infected with *Proteus* species. Hence, one cannot separate the effects of infection from those of foreign body in their reports. Dalton et al. (1975) reviewed the literature regarding formation of struvite calculi on foreign body nuclei. They point out that formation of foreign body calculi not associated with infection could be prevented by massive diuresis, which for man would require approximately 15 liters of output per day. However, when infection is present even massive diuresis is of no help. They listed over 30 separate agents that have acted as foreign body nuclei for urinary calculi. Among the most common are sutures (Fig. 25–23D), and their investigation was concerned particularly with suture material. They stated that nearly all types of suture material currently in use (including chromic catgut) have been demonstrated to support stone formation, and thus the "prevention of suture exposure to the urinary stream seems prudent."

In patients with neurogenic bladder, it has been supposed that recumbency and abnormalities of calcium and magnesium balance in urine contribute to stone disease. But there are investigations indicating that stone formation in such patients is not likely to be caused by excessive excretion of calcium, secondary hyperparathyroidism, or other metabolic effects (Burr, 1972; Burr and Walsh, 1974; Claus-Walker et al.,

1973; Jennis et al., 1970). The most likely cause is urinary infection, which leads to persistent alkaline urine pH that then results in urine supersaturation with magnesium ammonium phosphate. The formation product for struvite may be exceeded, and spontaneous nuclei of stones can form. If a catheter is also present, it represents the nucleus, and only the solubility product need be exceeded for struvite stone growth to occur. As shown in our simple chemical equation in Figure 25–28, an environment of constant elevation of urinary pH of over 7.2 is thereby achieved, at the concentrations of magnesium, ammonium, and phosphate in the urine of infected individuals at a body temperature of 37°C. No more is needed for growth of struvite crystals.

Classification of Infected Urinary Calculi. Infection as the cause of magnesium ammonium phosphate urinary calculi must be differentiated from infection that is the result of treatment of previous calculi of different composition. Cox (1974) has made this differentiation in his analysis of a series of patients who had urinary tract infection associated with renal lithiasis (Table 25–7). The table clearly separates those patients with infection that caused stones from those who have stones and then acquire infection. A decision about whether infection occurred following treatment of a particular type of urinary calculus other than struvite is important in planning the therapy of the patient. Westbury (1974) has pointed out that individuals who have had urinary calculi of a particular type are highly likely to have similar calculi caused by the same pathologic deficit. After infection, the subsequent composition of future calculi is not as clearly predictable. Therefore, admixtures of larger amounts of calcium phosphate and magnesium ammonium phosphate (struvite) become more common in analysis of subsequent stones in infected patients (Hodgkinson and Marshall, 1975; Westbury, 1974).

EVALUATION OF PATIENTS

Individuals with chronic urinary infection should always be considered to have a higher risk of formation of urinary calculi than individuals without infection. For this reason, occasional radiographic evaluation of the urinary tract is advisable in patients with chronic urinary infection. The majority of patients with clinical stone disease and infection present with evidence of a clinical syndrome that is a combination of pain due to urinary obstruction from calculus and pain and fever related to acute urinary tract infection. They often have or have

TABLE 25–7. BACTERIOLOGIC DATA ON PATIENTS WITH RENAL LITHIASIS,
NORTH CAROLINA BAPTIST HOSPITAL, 1968–1970*

	Group 1†	Group 2	Group 3	Group 4
Number of patients in group	200	70	100	35
Per cent of patients infected	37	8	35	83
Infecting bacteria (no. of patients)				
E. coli	40(54%)	4	13(37%)	4(13%)
Klebsiella	5	0	1	0
Enterobacteriaceae	3	0	2	2
P. mirabilis	7	0	10	10
Indole-positive Proteus‡	3	0	3	3
Pseudomonas	5	0	3	7
Staphylococcus	2	1	1	1
Enterococcus	4	1	1	1
Other or mixed	5	0	1	2

*From Cox, C. E.: Urol. Clin. North Am., *1*:279, 1974.
†Patient groups:
    Group 1. Two hundred urologic patients without urolithiasis.
    Group 2. Seventy urologic patients with urolithiasis without prior instrumentation.
    Group 3. One hundred patients with urolithiasis with prior instrumentation.
    Group 4. Thirty-five patients with staghorn calculi. All but three had had previous instrumentation.
‡*Proteus morganii, P. vulgaris,* and *P. rettgeri*

had indwelling urinary catheters. Foreign bodies must be suspected if there has been penetrating injury or abdominal surgery. Urinary infection must be documented by culture and identification of causative organisms. Drug sensitivities for proper treatment of these organisms should be determined by accepted techniques.

THERAPY

In all patients with infected stones, the basis of therapy is either eradication or complete suppression of urinary tract infection. The majority of urea-splitting organisms are of the *Proteus* species. On the other hand, organisms such as *Pseudomonas, Klebsiella,* staphylococci (especially *S. epidermidis*), and even *Mycoplasma* are capable of producing bacterial urease (Friedlander and Braude, 1974; Griffith et al., 1976). *E. coli* apparently does not produce urease (Griffith, 1979). Therapy should be directed toward long-term treatment with antibiotics specific for the infecting organism. Treatment of these chronically infected patients continues for months or years, not just weeks. Once again, stimulation of copious urinary output by ingestion of large amounts of fluids decreases urinary concentrations of magnesium, ammonium, and phosphate and helps relieve supersaturation of urine with these ions. Restriction of dietary phosphate and a decrease in intestinal absorption of phosphate by administration of aluminum hydroxide gels (which bind intestinal phosphate) (Marshall and Green,

1952) may be necessary to decrease urinary phosphate supersaturation (Appendix D). Certainly, patients who have urinary infection and who are prone to struvite stone formation should not be given medications that contain magnesium or phosphate.

Whenever possible, foreign bodies should be removed. Newer techniques of management of neurogenic bladder by bladder training, intermittent catheterization, urinary diversion, or use of prosthetic valves (see Chapter 11) allow many patients who formerly would have required catheter drainage to be free of catheters. If catheters must be used, the author has found that twice-daily irrigations with only 20 to 50 ml of solutions of 0.25 per cent or 0.5 per cent acetic acid greatly reduce struvite encrustation and calculi. Teflon coating of latex catheters and use of pure silicone catheters or tubes also decrease rapidity of struvite encrustation. No material compatible with the body exists that will *never* allow stone encrustation.

As noted by Nemoy and Stamey (1971), one cannot expect to clear the urinary tract of infection as long as stones are present. For this reason, many patients with infected urinary calculi require surgical removal of such calculi. Aspects of surgical approaches to the treatment of stone disease are covered elsewhere in this text. One aspect of medical treatment that has again achieved great importance is the dissolution of calculi by irrigation techniques. Acidic solutions proposed by Suby et al. (1942) and

Suby and Albright (1943) have been used for many years. Mulvaney (1960) and later Mulvaney and Henning (1962) reported on the use of hemiacidrin for dissolution of urinary calculi of struvite. Nemoy and Stamey (1971), Blaivas et al. (1975), and Jacobs and Gittes (1976) reviewed the development of hemiacidrin irrigation and the problems associated with it. For many years, reports in the literature indicated that this agent was extremely toxic and may have caused death. However, these authors state that in reviewing the literature they felt that the great majority of patients who had toxicity with this irrigation technique were actually afflicted with severe urinary infection and sepsis. All groups therefore now strongly recommend that the irrigation-dissolution technique be used only in patients in whom the urinary tract infection is completely under control. Hypermagnesemia must also be watched for (Cato and Tulloch, 1974).

Albright et al. (1948) observed that citric acid solutions would disintegrate predominantly calcium (apatite) stones not only because of the acid pH of the solutions but also because of the formation of a calcium and citrate ion complex. Subsequent to the introduction of the "buffered" citrate solution by Albright, solutions G and M were developed by Suby. Solution G contains citric acid monohydrate, 32.5 gm; anhydrous magnesium oxide, 3.84 gm; anhydrous sodium carbonate, 4.37 gm; and distilled water, 1000 ml. The pH of this solution is 3.95. Solution M is less acid (pH 4.6) than solution G and is made by adding 32.5 gm of citric acid monohydrate, 3.84 gm of anhydrous magnesium oxide, and 8.84 gm of anhydrous sodium carbonate to 1000 ml of distilled water. These solutions have not always been effective in dissolving phosphate calculi. Mulvaney (1960), as noted, reported his experience with a new solvent designed especially for struvite and apatite calculi. This solution was called hemiacidrin (Renacidin). He stated that calcium phosphate, magnesium ammonium phosphate, and magnesium phosphate stones were soluble, but the solvent appeared to have little effect on calcium oxalate and uric acid calculi. Startling beneficial results have been reported in some instances using these and other solutions to attack the renal calculi directly through irrigation of the renal pelvis and calyces by means of ureteral catheters. These irrigations have sometimes been carried out for weeks, but the occasional morbidity associated with the procedure has prevented its wide acceptance.

The technique for management of irrigation in suitable patients is thoroughly outlined in the article by Nemoy and Stamey (1971) and in Stamey's recent text (1982). It is necessary at this point to emphasize that the package insert for hemiacidrin (10 per cent Renacidin) contains this warning: "It is contraindicated for therapy or preventive therapy above the ureteral-vesical junction; therefore it is contraindicated for ureteral catheters, or pyelostomy tubes or renal lavage for dissolving calculi." For this reason, the composition of Suby's G and M solutions has also been given. Those individuals who do not wish to accept the responsibility for use of Renacidin in the kidney may prefer to irrigate with one of Suby's solutions.

Whichever solution is used, the technique remains essentially the same as that described by Nemoy and Stamey. These authors state first that it is absolutely necessary that no irrigation be attempted until the urine is completely sterile. If surgery has been performed, a nephrostomy tube is left in place postoperatively. On the other hand, if the patient is in poor clinical condition and surgery is contraindicated, a large double-lumen Tiemann ureteral catheter (5 to 7 French) may be inserted through the bladder into the renal pelvis. With either method, the renal pelvis is first irrigated with a sterile saline solution at a rate of 120 ml/hour for 24 to 48 hours beginning on the fourth or fifth postoperative day. The height of irrigation is adjusted to the lowest level necessary to maintain flow rate at 120 ml/hour. If there is leakage around the surgical drain or through the incision, irrigation is stopped until additional healing occurs. The patient is observed carefully for development of fever or any flank discomfort. Occurrence of either of these conditions necessitates immediate cessation of irrigation.

If after 48 hours the patient's condition remains satisfactory and there is no infection, no leakage, and no fever or flank discomfort, irrigation with an appropriate irrigating solution is begun. Flow rate is continued at 120 ml/hour through the irrigating tube or catheter. Nemoy and Stamey (1971) and Jacobs and Gittes (1976) explained that their patients are instructed to stop the irrigation themselves if there is evidence of flank pain at any time. The progress of irrigation is followed by obtaining x-ray tomographs of the calculi at intervals. Irrigation is continued for 24 to 48 hours after the last radiographically visible fragments have disappeared. In some instances the rate of irrigation may be reduced to prevent irritation of the kidney or bladder, or sterile saline solutions may be alternated with irrigating solutions.

These authors emphasize that the presence of infected urine, fever, or persistent flank pain is an absolute contraindication to continued irrigation.

Treatment of urinary tract infection, maintenance of high fluid intake and output, and possible irrigation of calculi to dissolve them provide only partial answers to medical treatment of infection stones. Some new approaches have been reported but are still in the experimental phase. Griffith and colleagues (1973, 1975, 1976a, 1979) have reported upon the use of acetohydroxamic acid to inhibit action of bacterial urease. This drug treatment results in decreased urinary pH, and about 60 per cent of patients show subsequent inhibition of the formation of struvite calculi and occasional dissolution of calculi that may be present. According to these authors, this medication is well tolerated by humans. The usual dosage is 750 mg per day in divided doses. Andersen (1975) has reported upon a similar urease inhibitor, benurestat. When such drugs become more widely available, they may result in dissolution of many calculi without need for surgery.

It must be re-emphasized at this point that the presence of obstruction by calculus in association with urinary infection constitutes an absolute indication for surgical relief of obstruction. Whether this is accomplished by insertion of ureteral catheter, nephrostomy, or open surgery for removal of obstructing calculus depends upon the urologist's assessment of the patient's condition. Excretion of antibiotics by the obstructed kidney is severely limited, and therefore one cannot expect antibiotics to be effective in controlling the renal damage and sepsis associated with urinary infection complicated by obstruction due to stone.

Calcium Urinary Lithiasis

SPECIAL ASPECTS OF ETIOLOGY

Table 25–5 indicates that calcium urinary calculi are the most common calculi worldwide. As noted in the introduction to this chapter, the incidence of bladder calculi has decreased following progressive improvement in nutrition and the industrial advancement of many of the primitive societies of the world. The result has been a continuously increasing incidence of upper urinary tract calculi composed predominantly of calcium oxalate or of calcium oxalate and calcium phosphate. Hodgkinson et al. (1975) commented upon the relative decrease over the past centuries in the amount of phosphate found in mixed calculi; the proportion of the calcium oxalate calculi is indeed increasing continuously.

The three stones discussed previously (uric acid, cystine, and struvite) all form in accordance with simple chemical laws of precipitation in urine. In some cases, the presence of certain urine components increases the solubility of these substances above their solubility product; nevertheless, if the concentration of their molecules rises above the respective formation product at a given pH and temperature of 37°C, precipitation of crystals occurs. When a large number of these molecules precipitate to form crystals, then by aggregation or other processes mentioned previously, an object large enough to obstruct urinary passages—i.e., a stone—results.

For many years, there has been controversy about whether calcium urinary lithiasis obeys the same physical rules. Laboratory studies reveal that calcium oxalate and calcium phosphate urinary crystals do form spontaneously when the formation product for these molecules in urine is exceeded. Any preformed crystals or nuclei will continue to grow as long as urinary supersaturation with calcium and phosphate or oxalate exists. Hence, in the laboratory, calcium crystals do precipitate as expected.

Note that for calcium oxalate and calcium phosphate calculi it is the *product* of the two ions that predicts propensity to crystallize. Marshall and Robertson (1976) have produced a nomogram that predicts crystallization when only the calcium and oxalate concentrations of urine are known. Hence, if the formation product for calcium phosphate is 35, the ratio of calcium to phosphate of either 1 to 35 or 35 to 1 may allow crystallization. In reality, such ratios allow inefficient crystallization and rarely occur in humans. Better crystallization occurs with ratios in the midrange, such as 7 to 5 (Oreopoulos et al., 1975), which are found in human urine.

In an attempt to sort out the interrelationship of various theories and also to place them in perspective with regard to certain diseases that are associated with calcium calculi, we will review first those observations associated only with hypercalciuria. This will include a discussion of absorptive hypercalciuria and renal leak hypercalciuria. We will then proceed to a discussion of those diseases that result in both hypercalcemia and hypercalciuria, such as hyperparathyroidism and others that may be confused with hyperparathyroidism or idiopathic renal hypercalciuria. Then we will discuss those states associated with excessive excretion of urinary oxalate or hyperoxaluria. Absolute hyperoxaluria will be illustrated by primary hyperoxaluria, the congenital disease in which individuals excrete enormous amounts of oxalate in the urine because of enzymatic defects in the kidneys and other body tissues. We will then move on to review so-called idiopathic and acquired hyperoxaluria, the relative hyperoxalurias sometimes noted in patients who form recurrent oxalate urinary calculi. Apatite urinary calculi (calcium phosphate) will be discussed in the context of hypercalciuria. Once we have reviewed the etiology of the various types of calcium urinary lithiasis, we will attempt to classify these patients in order to design appropriate therapy for them.

CALCIUM AND THE KIDNEY

Normal serum calcium in humans averages 9.6 mg/dl. Of this, approximately 45 per cent is free ionic calcium, and 55 per cent is protein-bound, mostly to albumin. It is for this reason that measurement of total serum calcium also requires a knowledge of serum protein concentrations. Measurement of serum ionized calcium is complex and does not seem to improve prediction of the amount of ionized calcium as derived from a nomogram of total serum calcium and serum protein (Figure 25–31). Only free ionic serum calcium is filtered by the glomerulus. If effective renal blood flow is estimated at 600 ml/min, then about 47 grams of calcium

are filtered daily, or about 32.4 mg/min, Since normal persons rarely excrete more than 200 mg/day, it is obvious that normal renal reabsorption of calcium is excellent. In addition to conserving body calcium, this process also serves to produce a urine that is usually undersaturated with calcium. There is, however, a tubular maximum for reabsorption of calcium. When this is exceeded by an increased serum calcium load presented to the kidney, as in intestinal hyperabsorption or hyperparathyroidism, excessive renal calcium loss results (Copp, 1969; Kleeman et al., 1958). Hypercalciuria results (Henneman et al., 1958; Pak et al., 1974).

HYPERCALCIURIA AND CALCIUM URINARY LITHIASIS

In general, investigators of urinary lithiasis have indicated that substantial numbers of patients with idiopathic calcium stone disease excrete excessive amounts of calcium in their urine during any 24-hour period. Flocks (1939) described this first. For many years, most observations of hypercalciuria were based on analysis of 24-hour urine collections. Perhaps the most difficult thing to reconcile with these observations is that the critical factor necessary for precipitation of calcium phosphate or calcium oxalate in urine is the instantaneous concentration of the two elements in urine, not the 24-hour concentration (Marshall and Robertson, 1976). It is quite possible for the patient to exceed the formation product for these ions in urine in an interval of only 15 to 30 minutes. At that point rapid crystallization can occur, and, if it is associated with aggregation, trapping in the urinary system, or growth of previously formed nuclei, stone formation may begin and growth can continue even when supersaturation decreases to a relatively low level (although it must be greater than the solubility product). Hence, many classic studies that report hypercalciuria of 24-hour urinary specimens are now questioned. Is it possible to ascertain instantaneous hypercalciuria in stone formers unless one follows them around 24 hours a day and analyzes every urinary specimen? Chambers and Dormandy (1969) have proposed just such an analysis, but most laboratories find it impractical. How can we resolve this dilemma?

DETECTION OF HYPERCALCIURIA

The variability of supersaturation of urine with calcium oxalate or calcium phosphate throughout the day has led to the development of numerous tests that attempt to detect hypercalciuria and thereby to estimate quickly the

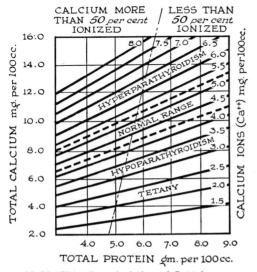

Figure 25–31. Chart for calculation of Ca++ ion concentration from total protein and total calcium of serum or plasma. (From McLean, F. C., and Hastings, A. B.: Am. J. Med. Sci., *189*:602, 1935.)

TABLE 25–8. WHEN IS THE PATIENT HYPERCALCIURIC?

Author(s)	Patient's Diet	Definition	
		MALES	FEMALES
Coe, 1975	Not listed	>300 mg/day	>250 mg/day
Drach, 1975	400 mg calcium	>100 mg/daytime (12 hours)	
Pak, 1974	400 mg calcium	>200 mg/day	>200 mg/day
Smith, 1974	1 gm calcium	>275 mg/day	>250 mg/day
Williams, 1974	Not listed	>300 mg/day	>250 mg/day
Nordin, 1972	"When urinary excretion is excessive for dietary intake"		
Chambers and Dormandy, 1969	"If urine osmolality is over 530 milliosmols, any value >22 mg/dl"		
Finlayson, 1974	Whenever urine is "supersaturated with calcium" and another ion with which it may precipitate		
Thomas, 1975	Analysis of 24-hr calcium excretion is "not clinically useful"		
Broadus, 1978	1000 mg calcium >4 mg/kg/day, either sex		

tendency of an individual to form stones. Some modifications, for example, test specimens from 2 or 4 or 12 hours of urine collection only (Drach, 1976b; Pak et al., 1975). Previously, excretion rates per 24-hour day were routine, but Finlayson (1974), Robertson et al., (1976), Pak et al. (1974), and King (1967, 1971) have pointed out that excretion of urinary calcium by stone formers varies so greatly that 24-hour specimens produce less information because of averaging. Various methods have been suggested to overcome these objections. Pak et al. (1975) proposed a brief test for absorptive hypercalciuria that utilizes only a 2-hour fasting and 4-hour postprandial urinary specimen. Chambers and Dormandy (1969), as noted previously, have proposed use of a 20-hour "urinary series" in which every urinary specimen passed is analyzed for calcium, phosphorus, oxalate, and other ionic constituents. Drach (1976b) proposed two 12-hour periods of urinary collection that correspond to a nighttime fasting period (9:00 P.M. to 9:00 A.M.) with generally low urinary calcium, and a daytime period (9:00 A.M. to 9:00 P.M.), which reveals the effects of diet on excretions. Broadus et al. (1978) have proposed that a 24-hour urinary collection while the patient is ingesting 1000 mg/day calcium will reveal absorptive hypercalciuria if calcium excretion is more than 4 mg/kg/day. Pak (1982) combines several 24-hour urinary collections

and an oral calcium loading test in categorizing his patients. Each method has its limitations and is not foolproof. Investigators continue to look for *the* test that will predict that significant hypercalciuria exists in the patient who has a tendency toward calcium lithiasis (Table 25-8).

Most clinicians must continue to rely upon analysis of 12- or 24-hour urine specimens to predict whether hypercalciuria exists. Table 25–8 lists some levels above which patients are said to be hypercalciuric. Note that there is considerable disagreement about the level of urinary calcium that must be exceeded for hypercalciuria to exist. Our problem is one of definition: We are really attempting to detect urinary supersaturation with calcium rather than only hypercalciuria. If one patient excretes 300 mg of calcium per day but his urine is not supersaturated at this level, perhaps this is not hypercalciuria for him. Perhaps "hypercalciuria" exists only when elevated urinary calcium results in urinary supersaturation and renal calcium deposition or stone formation. Hence, in the future it is more likely that we will test for calcium supersaturation, as Pak and Chu (1973) have done.

If hypercalciuria is detected, it is useful to place the patient in the proper category of causation of hypercalciuria. Four major causes exist (Table 25–9). The first is absorptive hypercalciuria, which is the result of excessive

TABLE 25–9. HYPERCALCIURIAS OF UROLITHIASIS

Term	Presumed Cause
Intestinal hyperabsorption	Excessive intestinal absorption of calcium
Renal leak	Failure of kidney to reabsorb tubular calcium
Bone resorption	Excessive calcium mobilized from bone
Carbohydrate load	Form of renal leak

TABLE 25–10. General Aspects of Separation of Hypercalciurias

Type of Hypercalciuria	Serum Calcium	Urine Cyclic AMP	Serum PTH	Fasting Urine Calcium	Bone Density	Intestinal Absorption
Primary hyperparathyroidism (bone-resorptive)	↑	↑	↑	↑	Low	↑
Renal stones, absorptive	Nl*	Nl or low	Nl or low	Nl	Nl	↑
Renal stones, "renal leak"	Nl	↑	↑	↑	?	Nl
Renal stone, normocalciuric	Nl	Nl	Nl	Nl	Nl	Nl

*Nl = Normal.

intestinal absorption of calcium presented to the gut (Pak et al., 1974). Pak (1982) now subdivides this group into Type I (hypercalciuric on a low-calcium diet) and Type II (hypercalciuric on a normal calcium diet). He also defines a Type III patient: hypercalciuria associated with hypophosphatemia. The second cause is renal leak hypercalciuria, which results when renal tubules fail to reabsorb calcium normally, thereby losing or leaking calcium into urine (Coe and Davalach, 1974). Third is the hypercalciuria of hyperparathyroidism, which occurs because excessive parathyroid hormone produces excessive resorption of bone. Intestinal calcium absorption may also be increased. The calcium load presented to the kidneys becomes too great to be efficiently reabsorbed, and excessive urinary calcium results. Fourth, many other metabolic diseases result in hypercalciuria. Most of those associated with calcium stone disease are discussed later in this chapter. The differentiation of any type of hypercalciuria depends first upon the exclusion of metabolic diseases or hyperparathyroidism. Then, separation of absorptive hypercalciuria or renal leak hypercalciurias can be performed using the methods described by Pak (1982), Coe and Davalach (1974), or Broadus et al. (1978). A summary derived from their observations is presented in Tables 25–10 and 25–11. An additional dietary test may be necessary to detect certain

individuals who excrete excessive urinary calcium after excessive carbohydrate intake. These patients develop a brief hypercalciuria after a high-carbohydrate meal, such as six donuts (Lemann et al., 1969; Thom et al., 1978). The mechanism is unclear, but some data suggest that the carbohydrate ingestion triggers a decreased renal reabsorption of calcium and hence a "renal leak" hypercalciuria in some oxalate stone formers and their susceptible relatives (Gittes et al.; 1967).

Coe et al. (1982) and Lien and Keane (1983) question whether one can distinguish between different forms of hypercalciuria such as "absorptive" or "renal leak." Both groups have concluded from studies of 27 and 52 patients, respectively, that the two defects may in reality be extremes of a continuum of behavior. As Coe hypothesizes: "A uniform elevation of intestinal calcium absorption and a variable defect of renal calcium reabsorption could explain our results far better than the hypothesis of distinct absorptive and renal forms of hypercalciuria."

Finlayson (1974) and Pak (1982) have covered hypercalciurias extensively in their reviews.

HYPERPARATHYROIDISM

Hyperparathyroidism produces a combination of all previously described absorptive renal and bony calcium defects. There is hyperab-

TABLE 25–11. Oral Calcium Load Method for Defining Hypercalciurias Excluding Carbohydrate-Induced Hypercalciurias*

Classification	Serum Calcium	Fasting Urine Calcium (mg/mg Cr)	Post-Calcium Load Urine (mg/mg Cr)	Fasting cAMP (Urine) (μm/gm Cr)	Lost-Load cAMP (Urine) (μm/gm Cr)
Absorptive hypercalciuria	Normal	<0.11	>0.2	<5.52	<3.4
Renal leak hypercalciuria	Normal	>0.11	<0.2	>6.86	<5.0
Hyperparathyroidism	High (>10.3)	>0.11	>0.2	$\overline{\times}6.55$ ±2.26	>4.60
Normocalciuric nephrolithiasis	Normal	<0.11	<0.2	$\overline{\times}3.42$ ±0.96	$\overline{\times}2.82$ ±0.84
Normal control	Normal	<0.11	<0.2	<6.86	$\overline{\times}3.00$

*Modified from Pak, C. Y., Ohata, M., Lawrence, E. C., et al.: J. Clin. Invest., *54*:387, 1974.

sorption of calcium through the gut with increased reabsorption of bone and an increased renal loss of calcium due to hypercalcemia in spite of increased reabsorption (Kleeman et al., 1958). The most significant diagnostic difference other than elevated serum calcium to separate patients with hyperparathyroidism from those with absorptive hypercalciuria or renal leak hypercalciuria is a moderate increase in parathyroid hormone levels.

Hyperparathyroidism causes significant numbers of urinary calculi, and removal of the parathyroid glands eliminates the tendency toward urinary calculi in the majority of patients with this affliction (Harrison and Rose, 1973). However, older concepts of hyperparathyroidism now must include consideration of a number of new factors that relate to calcium homeostasis and stone formation. These include the precise control of serum calcium by parathyroid hormone, thyrocalcitonin, vitamin D, and the renal hormone 1,25-dihydroxycholecalciferol (1,25 DHCC) (Fig. 25–32). In addition, the importance of cyclic 3':5'-adenosine monophosphate (AMP) as the intrarenal messenger for parathyroid hormone has been established (Chase and Aurbach, 1967), and urinary cAMP determinations may aid diagnosis of hyperparathyroidism (Murad and Pak, 1972; Stewart and Broadus, 1981).

Serum calcium concentration is regulated by a labile reservoir of calcium at the surface of the bone, which responds to increased or decreased parathyroid hormone (PTH) concentration. Parathyroid hormone is a relatively small polypeptide with a molecular weight of 9000 and is produced by the parathyroid gland. Purified PTH has both bone calcium mobilizing and renal phosphaturic actions, and the effects of the hormone both on bone and on kidneys probably are mediated through the formation of cyclic AMP at the cell membrane. Through a combination of mobilization of calcium from the bone, increased renal tubular resorption of calcium, and increased intestinal absorption of calcium, increased serum PTH increases serum calcium concentration. The hormone may have minor direct effects on the gastrointestinal tract, but it may result in increased intestinal calcium absorption by causing renal synthesis and release of 1,25 DHCC (Fig. 25–32).

Physiologic studies have indicated that the secretion of PTH by the parathyroid glands is controlled directly by the serum calcium level, with an increase in hormone concentration when serum calcium is decreased and vice versa. Studies of the role of the phosphate ion in controlling PTH secretion indicate that the effect of phosphate is secondary to any effects produced on the serum concentration of calcium. Hence,

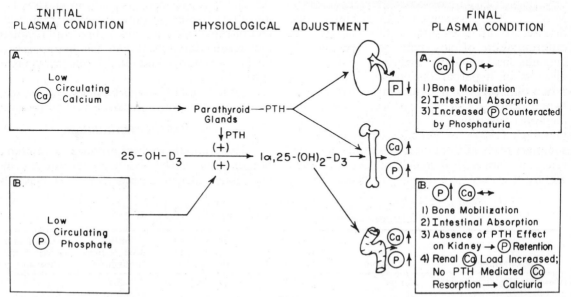

Figure 25–32. One model for homeostatic control of calcium and phosphate through the integrated functions of parathyroid hormone (PTH) and 1,25 dihydroxyvitamin D_3 (1,25 D_3, referred to in text as 1,25 DHCC). When either plasma calcium (A) or phosphate (B) is depleted, the kidneys are stimulated to convert circulating 25-hydroxyvitamin D_3 to 1,25 D_3. For calcium, this reaction is mediated by PTH, but for phosphate no intermediary has been found. Combined results of PTH and 1,25 D_3 activities are shown for kidney, bone, and gut. The resulting adjustments in plasma for low calcium are shown in box *A*, and those for low phosphate are shown in box *B*. (From Haussler, M. R., et al.: Clin. Endocrinol., 5:151A, 1976.)

hyperphosphatemia stimulates the parathyroid glands only indirectly by inducing hypocalcemia, a mechanism that is probably involved in stimulating the parathyroid gland in chronic renal failure. The parathyroid glands store only small amounts of hormone; hence, they show a high rate of protein synthesis when stimulated by hypocalcemia.

Copp et al. (1962) demonstrated a hormone that they thought originated in the parathyroid gland. This hormone, which they called calcitonin, decreased blood calcium content. It was later shown that the calcium-lowering hormone came from the thyroid gland, and the name was changed to thyrocalcitonin (TCT). Parafollicular cells adjacent to the thyroid follicles produce TCT. This hormone appears to act directly on bone to inhibit calcium mobilization, an action that is antagonistic to but not dependent on the presence of PTH. Thyrocalcitonin appears to play only a minor role in calcium homeostasis in man and may be secreted only at times of severe hypercalcemia. It functions independently of PTH (Gittes et al., 1967). It may, however, be useful as a therapeutic agent in treating Paget's disease.

Parathyroid hormone, TCT, and cAMP revolutionized our concepts of calcium metabolism and hyperparathyroidism, but the role of the kidney in the function of these hormones and messengers was believed to be secondary until it was discovered that the kidney was the major source of the active form of vitamin D_3, a substance called 1,25-dihydroxycholecalciferol (1,25 DHCC). The final activation of its immediate precursor in blood, 25-hydroxycholecalciferol, results in "active" vitamin D_3, or 1,25 DHCC, by attachment of a hydroxl at position 25 in the kidney. This vitamin acts primarily on the intestinal mucosa to promote calcium and phosphorus absorption by gut. It does not require PTH to be active on intestinal mucosal cells, but it does require PTH to promote production by renal cells (DeLuca, 1976). Figure 25–32 shows the interrelationship of all these concepts.

In a given individual, the concentration of serum calcium is the most precisely controlled biologic component of the serum that has been studied to date (Copp, 1969; Drach and King, 1970; Harris, 1970). To maintain this serum calcium level, the body has three mechanisms—gut absorption of calcium, bone deposition and resorption of calcium, and renal and fecal excretion of calcium. Laboratory determination of serum calcium used to be imprecise, but precision has improved over the years and, therefore,

normal limits in serum have been defined (Harris, 1970). At the present time, most hospital laboratories define the range as 9.0 mg/dl to 10.5 mg/dl. In one Mayo Clinic series (Keating, 1961), male patients in an older age group were found to have hyperparathyroidism even with serum calcium levels as low as 10.1 to 10.2 mg/dl. They noted a small regression of serum calcium with age in males, so the normal serum calcium level at age 20 can be at an upper limit of 10.2 mg/dl, while at the age of 80 the upper limit of normal is 10.0 mg/dl. In females, there is a slight increase in normal serum calcium levels with age. In this group, the upper limit of serum calcium at age 20 is 10.0 mg/dl, but the upper limits climbed slowly to 10.1 mg/dl at age 80. Putting these two observations together, it is likely that the upper limit of normal serum calcium levels for most humans is at or below 10.2 mg/dl. The author is well aware that this upper limit is much lower than that published by many laboratories. However, with improvements in analysis of serum calcium it is likely that this level will continue to be shown to be an absolute upper limit for most humans.

Another concept that must be considered with regard to hyperparathyroidism is the *degree* of control that the parathyroid gland manifests over serum calcium. We are aware of the inverse control relationship between parathyroid hormone and serum calcium. We also know that this is modified somewhat by thyrocalcitonin (although not much in humans) and by 1,25-vitamin D_3. In general, elevation of serum calcium in normal humans results in suppression of and decreased excretion of parathyroid hormone. This, in turn, results in adjustment of serum calcium to a lower level. Abnormally low levels of serum calcium lead to excretion of more parathyroid hormone, with the resultant tendency to increase serum calcium to normal. The half-life of serum parathyroid hormone is believed to be about 20 minutes, which provides a quick reaction to changes in serum calcium.

Patients with hyperparathyroidism usually manifest abnormal control of serum calcium (Drach and King, 1970). Both the absolute level of serum calcium and the day-to-day control of serum calcium can be abnormal. Therefore, a stone-forming patient with hyperparathyroidism may have brief episodes of hypercalcemia interspersed with periods during which he is normocalcemic. As noted previously, the ability to increase serum calcium above the normal level temporarily increases the calcium load to the kidneys and may result in hypercalciuria and stone formation. For this reason, the author and others have proposed that it is possible that urinary calculous disease due to "idiopathic" hypercalciuria may actually be an intermittent and intermediate form of hyperparathyroidism that is midway between normal and overt hyperparathyroidism. This hypothesis has not been proved.

One of the answers to the problem of hyperparathyroidism was thought to be the measurement of serum immunoreactive parathyroid hormone. Unfortunately, this test has not been fully accurate. Great variations in measurement of parathyroid hormone by different laboratories led to confusion. No suitable standard method or standard value exists, so no comparisons can be made between laboratories. On the other hand, careful control of dietary calcium intake along with observation of the fasting serum calcium level with simultaneous measurement of serum parathyroid hormone has resulted in the designation of some normal zones for both elements. The elevation of serum calcium or parathyroid hormone, or both, strongly hints at hyperparathyroidism. The work of Arnaud (1973) and his colleagues (Arnaud and Strewler, 1981) has been critical in defining these relationships.

Based on the foregoing observations of the effects of PTH on serum or urinary components, a number of confirmatory tests have been devised for the diagnosis of hyperparathyroidism. The first and most important of these is multiple observation of serum calcium levels, sometimes over a prolonged period of time. On occasion, patients with urinary calculous disease have serum calcium concentrations that are clearly elevated and abnormal only intermittently. The concomitant presence of urinary calculous disease of calcium type (or on rare occasions, magnesium ammonium phosphate type) and *any* elevated serum calcium level is a compelling reason to suspect hyperparathyroidism. The author recalls one patient in whom a total of 53 serum calcium determinations were made over a period of 5 years. It was only at the end of this period that overt hyperparathyroidism with hypercalcemia became evident. The patient underwent exploratory surgery, and a large parathyroid adenoma was removed. Stone formation ceased immediately. The patient has not had another urinary calculus in 3 years, whereas she was passing an average of one calculus every 2 months prior to surgery. This case is presented only to emphasize the fact that prolonged observations of serum calcium may be necessary to discover this disease (Johansson et al., 1975).

If elevated or upper normal levels of serum calcium are found, simultaneous determination of serum parathyroid hormone should be performed. If both serum calcium and serum parathyroid hormone are elevated in the absence of other diseases that may cause these abnormalities, the presumptive diagnosis of hyperparathyroidism may be made (Waterhouse and Heinig, 1976, Arnaud and Strewler, 1981). The treatment for this disease remains surgical, and a surgical consultant should be contacted.

Many adjunctive tests have been proposed for diagnosis of hyperparathyroidism. Among these are the phosphate reabsorption test (Reynolds et al., 1960; Schrott et al., 1972), the steroid suppression test (Strott and Nugent, 1968), measurement of urinary cyclic AMP (Murad and Pak, 1972), and many others. Many of these have been reviewed (Keating, 1961; Schrott et al., 1972; Smith, 1974; Strott and Nugent, 1968). The author agrees with other reviewers that the false positive and false negative percentage of error (25 per cent) in all of these tests makes them of borderline usefulness as absolute diagnostic indicators of parathyroid disease (Lafferty, 1981). If elevated serum calcium and elevated serum parathyroid hormone are present, and one or more other indicators of the disease, such as urinary calculi or peptic ulcer, are also evident, surgical exploration for parathyroid lesion should be advised. One must be very careful to exclude other diseases that may cause hypercalcemia, however (Table 25–12). The final diagnosis of hyperparathyroidism is still made by surgical exploration and demonstration of parathyroid adenoma or hyperplasia.

Renal lesions resulting from hyperparathyroidism and nephrocalcinosis have been defined. Histologic examination reveals marked deposition of calcium, excreted calcium bodies, and other debris in the renal tubules of patients who have hyperparathyroidism. There appear to be two aspects to the renal disease process. The first is a direct interference with the physiologic function of the kidney cells. If hypercalcemia caused by excess parathyroid hormone is re-

TABLE 25–12. SOME DISEASES THAT MAY BE ASSOCIATED WITH HYPERCALCEMIA AND HYPERCALCIURIA

Hyperparathyroidism	Metastatic malignant
Vitamin D intoxication	neoplasms
Idiopathic infantile	Leukemia
hypercalcemia	Lymphoma
Sarcoidosis	Milk-alkali syndrome
Multiple myeloma	Myxedema
Hyperthyroidism	Adrenal insufficiency

lieved, this functional aspect of hyperparathyroidism can be reversed (Drach and Boyce, 1972). However, there are secondary mechanical and anatomic aspects of cell death and deposition of calcium in the kidney that persist for long periods of time following relief of hyperparathyroidism. Therefore, nephrocalcinosis of this disease may persist for a long time after treatment. In spite of this, the formation and production of new urinary calculi cease in most patients following removal of parathyroid adenoma or hyperplasia (Harrison and Rose, 1973; Stubbs and Myers, 1973).

HYPERCALCEMIC CRISIS

Acute parathyroid intoxication (parathyroid crisis) may necessitate emergency therapy for hypercalcemia if the patient is to be saved. Parathyroid crisis usually occurs when the serum calcium content approaches a level of 17 mg/dl or higher. It is characterized by a rapid pulse, progressive lethargy, nausea, vomiting, abdominal discomfort, and azotemia. When the serum calcium reaches 20 mg/dl, respiratory distress, renal failure, and coma develop, and the patient may then die of cardiac arrest.

Definitive treatment of parathyroid crisis requires parathyroidectomy. Serum calcium content may also be temporarily decreased by the intravenous administration of inorganic phosphates or sulfates. The mechanism by which inorganic phosphates lower the serum calcium level is not known, but it is not related to increased excretion of calcium in the urine. Inorganic phosphate may also be given orally, depending upon how rapid an effect is needed. The usual daily dose of inorganic phosphate ranges from 1 to 3 gm. In patients with renal failure, small doses should be used to prevent hypotension and secondary acute tubular necrosis.

Intravenous administration of isotonic sodium sulfate solution (containing 38.9 gm sodium sulfate decahydrate in water) will produce an increase in the urinary excretion of calcium. This increased calcium excretion may be due to an increased glomerular filtration rate produced by rehydration and the effect of sodium ion on calcium resorption in the proximal renal tubules or a complex effect of the nonresorbable sulfate anion on the renal tubule. Sodium sulfate produces a more rapid decrease in serum calcium content than does the administration of inorganic phosphates; sodium chloride produces a similar effect but to a lesser degree.

Other drugs that reverse hypercalcemia are furosemide, ethacrynic acid, corticosteroids, mithramycin, calcitonin, and estrogens. One of the most rapid ways to effect reversal is hemodialysis. Paterson (1974) has reviewed all the foregoing methods and still recommends intravenous phosphates as the drug of first choice.

OTHER DISEASES THAT MAY CAUSE HYPERCALCEMIA AND HYPERCALCIURIA

There are a number of diseases that increase the serum concentration and urinary excretion of calcium and may be confused with hyperparathyroidism or idiopathic hypercalciuria (Table 25–12). Although the investigation of these diseases is beyond the realm of most urologists, one should be aware of their existence. Included in this group are idiopathic infantile hypercalcemia (Williams, 1974a), sarcoidosis (Ellman and Parfitt, 1960), multiple myeloma (Sherwood et al., 1967), hyperthyroidism (Williams, 1974a), leukemia (Sherwood et al., 1967), lymphoma (Sherwood et al., 1967), and milk-alkali syndrome (Smith, 1974a). The diseases that are most important to and most likely to be seen by the urologist are vitamin D intoxication, immobilization syndrome, and renal tubular acidosis. Williams (1974a) confirms that, aside from idiopathic hypercalciuria and hyperparathyroidism, the diseases most commonly associated with calcium urolithiasis are renal tubular acidosis and vitamin D intoxication, but he also includes hyperthyroidism. We will now briefly discuss a few of these more common diseases.

Vitamin D Intoxication. Excessive amounts of vitamin D (more than 100,000 units per day for many months) ingested or injected will cause hypercalcemia and hypercalciuria. When administration of vitamin D is stopped, serum and urinary calcium levels return to normal slowly because large amounts of the vitamin are stored in fat. Stone formation also ceases.

Immobilization Syndrome. Abrupt total immobilization due to casts, traction, or quadriplegia may lead to marked loss of calcium from bone with resultant hypercalciuria. Space travel also causes immobilization syndrome. Treatment involves exercises when possible, avoidance of excessive calcium in the diet, forcing of fluids to provide urine output in excess of 2000 ml per day, and perhaps administration of oral orthophosphate if no urinary infection exists (Thomas, 1974). Stones associated with urinary infections should be treated as infection stones.

Renal Tubular Acidosis. In 1936, Butler, Wilson, and Farber described a clinical syndrome characterized by persistent dehydration, hyperchloremia, hypokalemia, metabolic acidosis, and nephrocalcinosis. This was the first clinical report of the syndrome now called distal renal tubular acidosis (it has a variety of other names such as hyperchloremic acidosis, Butler-Albright syndrome, idiopathic acidosis, Lightwood's syndrome, and tubular insufficiency without glomerular insufficiency).

Renal tubular acidosis results in an inability to excrete acid urine; the fasting urinary pH always exceeds 5.5. There are two forms of the disease. *Proximal* (Type I) renal tubular acidosis results from a defect in carbonic anhydrase of the proximal tubule. These patients do not form renal calculi. *Distal* (Type II) renal tubular acidosis probably results from decreased hydrogen ion secretion in the distal renal tubule, with impairment of the conservation of fixed base. An acid load test (Dretler et al., 1969) reveals that these patients do not excrete metabolic acids normally. Distal tubular secretion of potassium increases in an attempt to offset the deficiency of hydrogen ion secretion, but this adjustment does not compensate completely, and increased amounts of calcium and sodium are also excreted in the urine. Hydrogen ions are retained, while sodium, potassium, and calcium are lost. One consequence is hypercalciuria. With the continued loss of sodium in the urine the serum sodium concentration is depressed, stimulating the osmoregulatory system to suppress the release of antidiuretic hormone. This produces water diuresis in an attempt to maintain iso-osmolarity of the body fluids. Consequent to the increased loss of fluids, there is a contraction of extracellular fluid and intravascular volume. As this contraction reaches a critical level, the volume control system is brought into action to maintain extracellular fluid volume. Contraction of plasma volume is also a potent stimulus of aldosterone. Increased aldosterone increases sodium and chloride resorption by the kidney in almost equal amounts, resulting in a relative hyperchloremia. This defect, coupled with hydrogen ion retention, results in metabolic acidosis.

The characteristic serum biochemical abnormalities resulting from all this are a reduced serum carbon dioxide combining power, decreased PCO_2 and serum pH, hyperchloremia, and hypokalemia. The serum calcium and phosphorus levels are normal, but the urine is alkaline in the presence of hypercalciuria. These factors predispose to formation of calculi, usually of calcium phosphate (Dretler et al., 1969).

Some patients have an incomplete form of renal tubular acidosis in which metabolic acidosis is not present and some acid in an acid load test can be excreted. Yet these patients do not acidify the urine below pH 5.5 when not challenged by excessive metabolic acid. Most also have hypercalciuria (Marquardt, 1973; Sommerkamp and Schwerk, 1973; Young and Martin, 1972) and some have hyperuricemia (Fellstrom et al., 1983).

Bone lesions of renal tubular acidosis are osteomalacic—there is a failure to calcify already formed osteoid matrix. Pseudofracture lines (described by Milkman, 1934) are not true fractures but localized linear areas of decreased bone formation bounded on either side by areas of hyperostosis that suggest linear fractures.

Correction of metabolic acidosis and restoration of fixed base occurs following administration of a balanced sodium citrate solution that may also contain potassium. Stone formation ceases with such therapy, although nephrocalcinosis may persist. The objectives of medical treatment are to relieve acidosis, to reduce hyperchloremia and hypercalciuria, and to improve renal reabsorption of calcium. For maintenance therapy, "Shohl's solution" may be used in divided doses. This liquid medication consists of 98 gm of sodium citrate, 140 gm of citric acid, and 1000 ml of water. When edema is present and sodium is to be avoided, or if potassium replacement is necessary, potassium citrate may be used in this prescription instead of sodium citrate. Albright's solution can be used as a substitute: It consists of 75 gm of sodium citrate, 25 gm of potassium citrate, 140 gm of citric acid, and 1000 ml of water. This solution is particularly effective when hypokalemia is present. Average dosages are 15 ml three or four times daily. When renal insufficiency is present, the patient must be closely observed for potassium intoxication and development of metabolic alkalosis. Because of the inherent inability of the kidneys to excrete acids, including chloride radicals, dietary salt should be restricted.

Claus-Walker et al. (1973) have shown that one of the significant differences between patients with calcium urinary lithiasis and normal persons is a deficiency of potassium excretion in the urine. Patients with renal tubular acidosis, on the other hand, have excessive excretion of potassium in their urine in exchange for the hydrogen that is retained in their system owing to the defect of the disease. Hence, urinary potassium does not seem to have any direct relationship to formation of calcium urinary calculi.

CALCIUM UROLITHIASIS ASSOCIATED WITH HYPEROXALURIA

We have seen that in many conditions the amount of urinary calcium may be elevated, and this increase may be associated with urinary calculi. The most common type of stone disease, however, is calcium oxalate urolithiasis. For this reason, a number of investigators emphasize the effect of increased oxalate rather than calcium on the precipitation of calcium oxalate in urine (Elliot, 1983; Hautmann et al., 1980; Menon and Mahle, 1983; Valyasevi and Dhanamitta, 1974; Yanagawa et al., 1983). Robertson and his coworkers (1969, 1972a, b, 1973, 1974, 1976, 1978) have produced increasingly strong evidence indicating that the amount of urinary oxalate at any given time is roughly ten times more important in determining the precipitation of calcium oxalate than the quantity of either calcium or phosphate in urine. Their most recent report indicates that one can actually separate stone formers from normal persons by utilizing a biaxial comparison of the saturation of urine with calcium oxalate versus the presence of "inhibitor." These observations combine the supersaturation/crystallization and inhibitor theories. Gill et al. (1974) used radioisotopic methods to measure the saturation of urine with calcium oxalate and to predict the propensity for growth of preformed calcium oxalate nuclei. Finally, Miller et al. (1977) have devised a system that measures directly the nucleation rate, growth rate, and total crystal mass of calcium oxalate crystals produced by urine specimens. Each of these methods provides some information that is useful in predicting calcium oxalate stone disease, but all are still in the stage of research development and have not been proved valuable in clinical practice. Therefore, we are left with the process of determining amounts of calcium, oxalate, phosphate, magnesium, sodium, and chloride in urine in order to predict, by calculation, the saturation of urine with calcium oxalate or phosphate. Finlayson et al. (1973) measured only these components of urine and published a system of computer calculations that permit a fairly accurate estimation of the degree of calcium oxalate saturation of urine.

One major factor that has been detrimental to the study of the effects of oxalate on urolithiasis has been the difficulty of analysis of oxalate, whether in serum or in urine. Methods for determination of oxalate in biologic systems may be roughly divided into three types. The first method is quantitation of oxalate by enzymatic reduction with oxalase and measurement of the carbon dioxide liberated by the reaction (Elliot et al., 1970). The margin of error in this method is about 5 per cent. The second method is an analysis performed by chromatographic titration (Hodgkinson, 1970). The analysis method is somewhat more accurate but still does not give completely reproducible results, especially for determination of serum oxalate. Finally, radioisotopic dilution methods have also been devised. However, analysis of duplicate samples of serum oxalate from the same specimen using two different types of oxalate analysis does not give similar values. The amounts of oxalate in urine, however, are so much higher than those in serum that the present enzymatic and chromatographic or radioisotopic dilution techniques give values that are useful in clinical practice.

Urinary oxalate has two major sources of origin in the human. The first is endogenous production by means of enzymatic cleavage of glyoxalate to form oxalic acid and glycine. The second source is absorption of excess oxalate via the gut from foods and liquids (Table 25–13). In serum, oxalate is found in very low amounts. Once excreted, urinary oxalic acid rapidly forms a complex with the multiple cationic salts and ions available and becomes oxalate salt. Oxalate is soluble when combined with most components of urine such as magnesium. Only when it forms a complex with calcium in high concentrations does it become insoluble. Then crystalline precipitation of calcium oxalate occurs. As noted previously, this spontaneous precipitation occurs whenever the product of concentrations of calcium and oxalate exceeds the *formation* product (Marshall and

TABLE 25–13. SOME LIQUIDS AND FOODS THAT CONTAIN LARGER AMOUNTS OF OXALATE*

Liquids	
MODERATE AMOUNTS	
Apple juice	
Beer	
Coffee	
Cola	
Instant tea	
HIGH AMOUNTS	
Cocoa	
Cranberry juice	
Grape juice	
Grapefruit juice	
Fresh tea	
Foods	
Asparagus	Almonds
Beets	Cashew nuts
Cactus fruits	Concord grapes
Greens	Cranberries
Plums	Currants
Raspberries	
Rhubarb	
Spinach	

*Modified from Thomas, W. C., Jr.: Urol. Clin. North Am., *1*:261, 1974; see also Appendix C.

Robertson, 1976). Calcium oxalate crystals may also grow on preformed nuclei whenever the *solubility* product is exceeded.

The importance of oxalate in the process cannot be denied. The upper limit of normal urinary excretion of oxalate for man is approximately 35 mg/day. The upper limit of urinary excretion of calcium ranges between 200 and 300 mg/day, according to most investigators (Table 25–8). An increase of one tenth in oxalate (to a level of 38.5 mg/day) equals an increase of ten times one-tenth in urinary calcium (from 200 to 400 mg/day). The presence of 400 mg of calcium and 38.5 mg of oxalate in a 24-hour urine specimen with a volume of approximately 1.5 liters would almost guarantee precipitation of calcium oxalate.

It is here that there is a peculiar difference between stone formers and normal persons. It is not unheard of for a normal human on occasion to excrete 45 mg of oxalate and 300 mg of calcium per day. Indeed, these individuals will produce multiple small crystals of oxalate. However, the size of these crystals is limited to approximately 7 to 12 microns. Once the larger size is approached, additional small crystals are formed, but larger crystals do not grow or form by aggregation. It is only when the system goes awry that urinary calculi form. As noted previously, calculus formation is presumably related to the formation of larger crystals, aggregates of crystals, and crystal masses that obstruct or occlude some portion of the urinary tract. Whether or not we accept the theory that excessive amounts of oxalate lead to calculi, we know that some conditions of hyperoxaluria result in calculi. We will review those processes of excessive oxalate excretion and calculi formation by examining first the disease condition known as primary hyperoxaluria.

Hyperoxaluria. Primary hyperoxaluria is a congenital illness characterized by the endogenous formation of excessive amounts of oxalate in tissues without any associated pyridoxine deficiency. This rare congenital defect can be further separated into two types. Type I hyperoxaluria is labeled glycolic aciduria and is due to a deficiency of soluble 2-oxoglutarate: glyoxylate carboligase. Type II is called L-glyceric aciduria but results in similar findings of excessive urinary oxalate excretion. The enzymatic deficiency is D-glyceric dehydrogenase. Patients with primary hyperoxaluria and urinary stone disease develop evidence of the disease early in life, often in childhood. They have extensive nephrocalcinosis and renal failure, and most die prior to the age of 30. The use of oral phosphates to treat this abnormality will be discussed later, but no drug currently known alters the enzymatic defect. Treatment is usually not successful (Hall et al., 1960; Hockaday et al., 1967; Watts, 1973).

Acquired hyperoxaluria is a relatively new condition recognized to be associated with enteric diseases. Patients with regional ileitis, colitis, and, more recently, postoperative intestinal bypass have been demonstrated to excrete excessive amounts of oxalate in the urine (Dickstein and Frame, 1973; Fikri and Casella, 1975; Smith and Hofman, 1974). It appears that rapid intestinal transit, shortness of bowel, and lack of bacterial activity in the bowel contribute to excessive absorption of oxalate products. The turnover of oxalate in the serum of these patients is extremely rapid, and increased amounts of oxalate are excreted by the kidneys. Because the effects of urinary oxalate on crystallization are ten times greater than the effects of calcium (according to the theory presented previously) and because a calcium to oxalate ratio of even 1 to 35 could result in stones, these patients are extremely prone to develop urinary calculi even though their calcium excretion levels may not be excessively high. If we add the fact that they are chronically dehydrated by diarrhea and also tend to have relatively acid urine, it is not surprising that they form calculi easily. There have also been reports that postoperative patients who have undergone a Bricker (ileal loop) procedure develop this type of calculous disease (Dretler, 1973; Koff, 1975; Ratiazzi et al., 1975; Singer et al., 1973).

Idiopathic Hyperoxaluria. Up to this point we have concentrated upon calculi associated with hyperoxaluria for which a cause may be demonstrated. We now must consider those individuals who have "idiopathic" hyperoxaluria. As mentioned previously, the presence of oxalate in urine depends upon endogenous production and oral intake. For each individual there seems to be a basal level of production of oxalate that is characteristic of his or her system. On a regular diet without excessive ingested oxalate, most individuals do not have increased urinary oxalate concentrations (Drach, 1976*b*; Robertson and Peacock, 1972). However, if they eat or drink foods containing high amounts of oxalate, some patients will have a rapid increase in urinary oxalate excretion. Examples of such high oxalate foods are given in Table 25–13. Ingestion of soluble oxalates in particular increases urinary excretion of oxalates in many patients.

Another possibly important aspect of oxalate metabolism is the fact that serum oxalate levels are related directly to the testosterone concentration in blood. This is the probable reason that excretion of oxalate by females is on the average considerably less than that by males (Finlayson, 1974; Thomas, 1975). Welshman and McGeown (1975), however, believe that the major urinary difference between males and females is a deficiency in citrate excretion by the former. In addition, in a study of 64 stone-forming patients, the author was unable to find any correlation between serum testosterone levels and urinary oxalate excretion (Drach, unpublished observations). Based upon these facts, it is obvious that the best possible modification of oxalate excretion by a "normal" or stone-forming individual with idiopathic disease is achieved mostly by limitation of oral oxalate intake. At the present time there is no known way to interfere with endogenous production of oxalate. Succinimide has been proposed (Hodgkinson et al., 1975), but these authors surveyed the effects of this drug in animals and found relatively little response. They continue to recommend limitation of dietary intake for control of oxalate excretion.

In calcigerous lithiasis, we are therefore faced with multiple possible causes. Excessive urinary calcium or oxalate or deficient inhibitors such as phosphate or magnesium may trigger stone disease unpredictably. Hence, stone disease occurs intermittently. When is a patient actively forming stones?

ATTEMPTS TO ESTIMATE ACTIVITY OF CALCIUM STONE DISEASE

An additional complexity in the study of calcium stone disease revolves around the fact that stones may be initiated and formed entirely of either calcium oxalate or calcium phosphate or, more commonly, of mixtures of the two components. Which component is critical in initiating the formation of stones? Several investigators have attempted to clarify this problem. Pak (1973) and his colleagues proposed that supersaturation of urine with calcium and phosphate with precipitation of brushite was the nucleus for formation of calcium stones. They not only substantiated this theory by in vitro testing in their own laboratories but also indicated that stone analyses often showed that the nidus of a calculus was indeed calcium phosphate even though the surface growth was calcium oxalate (Elliot, 1973a; Prien, 1974). The form of phosphate that is present is apatite, however, not brushite, and not all stones have phosphate nuclei.

Other investigators have approached the problem of stone activity differently. As mentioned previously, Robertson and colleagues (1976) have proposed a method of evaluation in which the ionic activity products of urinary calcium, phosphorus, and oxalate are compared with the total amount of crystal inhibition present. When the ion product of these substances increases enough or the inhibition factors decrease enough, crystallization and presumably urinary stone formation occur. Gill et al. (1974) have proposed a method of estimation of stone-forming activity in which a radioisotopic dilution procedure is used to measure the degree of supersaturation of calcium and oxalate in urine. When urine supersaturation of these individuals reaches a critical point, therapy could be initiated. Sarig and her colleagues (1982) have, for example, devised a diagnostic index (D.I.) derived from rapidity of calcium oxalate precipitation in urines. Stone formers could be separated from normal persons with an error rate of 13.5 per cent, with the inverse error rate being 19.2 per cent. Marshall and Barry (1973) observed that saturation of urine with calcium oxalate exists in patients with pure oxalate stones, but saturation with calcium phosphate and calcium oxalate exists in patients with mixed calculi. Hence, it may ultimately be necessary to measure urine saturation with both components to correctly predict calcium stone formation activity. Breslau and Pak (1980) have described methods for such estimation using their activity product ratio (APR) to predict saturation of urine with calcium oxalate or phosphate. They also estimate a formation product ratio (FPR) that gives an upper border for the limit of metastability (see Fig. 25–8) of urine, or the point at which spontaneous nucleation of crystals will occur. This limit is found to be lower in stone formers than in normal persons and implies that afflicted patients have less crystallization inhibitor in their urines.

All of these investigations attempt to approach the problem of nucleation, growth, and aggregation of urinary calculi and try to define those individuals who are actively forming calcium stones. A tendency toward calcium urolithiasis persists for such a long period that it is necessary to know, if possible, when patients are at a high risk of stone formation. At that time, they can be treated with medication, whereas taking medication for 10 years to avoid the production of one calculus is not satisfactory to most patients. Although all the methods listed are still in the early stages of development, we will soon be able to predict when stone formers are "active." Therapy can then be initiated or increased. Until then, we must simply use clinical judgment and treat those patients who have recurrent symptomatic calcium stone disease.

CLASSIFICATION OF PATIENTS WITH CALCIUM UROLITHIASIS

Therapy of calcigerous urinary calculi is based primarily on the identification of any primary factors that may cause the disease. Therefore, patients are first categorized according to the presence of any other metabolic disease that may be contributing to their problem. Patients with hyperparathyroidism are treated by exploration and parathyroidectomy. Therapy for renal tubular acidosis consists of reversal of the acidosis and correction of potassium imbalance, including administration of bicarbonate and/or citrate solutions of sufficient quantity to bring serum pH back to normal. Patients who develop calculi in association with other metabolic diseases (Table 25–12) should have those diseases treated first. Stone formation usually ceases, and any residual stones can be treated subsequently. If none of the foregoing diseases is present, we must look for the defect likely to be associated with "idiopathic" calcium urinary calculi (Table 25–10).

EVALUATION OF PATIENTS WITH CALCIUM UROLITHIASIS

The minimum basic evaluation of any patient with calcium urolithiasis is presented in Table 25–14. Performance of the studies indicated will rule out the overt presence of most of the diseases mentioned in Table 25–12 and in previous portions of this section. Utilizing these studies, patients with hyperparathyroidism, renal tubular acidosis, hyperoxaluria, hyperthyroidism, vitamin D intoxication, sarcoidosis, and hypercalciuria related to a hypercorticoid state (which may be drug-induced) can often be identified. In some instances, however, certain metabolic diseases may be barely perceptible, as in "normocalcemic hyperparathyroidism" or "incomplete renal tubular acidosis." Such patients have usually been initially classified as having "idiopathic hypercalciuria." If stone formation continues in spite of therapy, a complete metabolic evaluation by a team specializing in the study of calcium stone formation is usually advisable.

If, however, a preliminary survey results in no obvious diagnosis of severe metabolic disease, patients are usually placed in the classification of "idiopathic hypercalciuria" or "acquired hyperoxaluria." As we shall see,

TABLE 25–14. MINIMUM LABORATORY EVALUATION OF THE PATIENT WITH METABOLICALLY ACTIVE* CALCIUM UROLITHIASIS

Serum	Urine†
Creatinine	Creatinine
Sodium	Sodium
Potassium	Chloride
Carbon dioxide	Calcium
Chloride	Phosphorus
Calcium (fasting)‡	Magnesium
Phosphorus	Uric acid
Uric acid	Oxalate
Magnesium	Osmolality (fasting)
Total protein	Culture
Albumin	Fasting pH ($\times 3$)
Osmolality (fasting)	
Thyroid function tests	
Serum pH	

*Metabolically active—defined by Smith (1947a) as formation of more than one stone per year.

†See text: The author prefers to divide urinary collections into 12-hour overnight (9:00 P.M. to 9:00 A.M.) and daytime (9:00 A.M. to 9:00 P.M.) periods.

‡Serum parathyroid hormone is determined if any serum calcium exceeds 10 mg/dl.

treatment of these conditions is similar, and precise evaluation and classification beyond this point is at present not productive. Some hints may be gained from evaluation, however.

Figure 25–7 illustrates the cumulative effects on calcium solubility in urine of certain organic and inorganic inhibitors. The author (Drach, 1976b) and others have studied urinary constituents in stone formers and have shown that "idiopathic" stone formers tend to have one or more urinary excesses or deficiencies that may promote calcium stone formation. These include absorptive or renal leak hypercalciuria (Pak et al., 1974, 1975), hyperoxaluria due to dietary excess or acquired from intestinal disease (Smith, 1974a; Thomas, 1974), urinary magnesium lack (Oreopoulos et al., 1975; Drach 1976b), and excessive uric acid (Coe and Raisen, 1973; Coe and Davalach, 1974). In general, patients are placed on some type of therapy directed at alleviating the most obvious deficiency found in urine. As noted previously, Robertson et al. (1979b) have combined six of these urinary risk factors in urine into one "risk factor index," which seems to correlate well with incidence of recurrent stone formation.

THERAPY OF IDIOPATHIC CALCIUM UROLITHIASIS

There exists, then, a very large group of individuals known as idiopathic calcium oxalate/phosphate stone formers with some small urinary abnormality. Therapeutic advice to these

TABLE 25–15. Drug Treatment for Calcium Stone disease

Drug	Postulated Effect on Urine	Average Adult Dosage	Contraindications	Side Effects
Neutral phosphate	Increases solubility of calcium	250 to 500 mg 4 times a day	Urinary infection or poor renal function	Diarrhea
Magnesium oxide	Increases urinary magnesium; decreases urinary calcium	150 mg 4 times a day	Urinary infection or poor renal function	Diarrhea
Hydrochlorthiazide	Same as above	50 mg 2 times a day	Hypokalemia, other diuretics	Hypokalemia
Allopurinol	Inhibits epitaxy	300 mg/day	Previous sensitivity	Activates gout

patients has been extensive and variable over the years, but several general treatment factors are apparently valid. Once again, the maintenance of a large fluid intake and high urinary output and avoidance of dehydration are critical preventive measures. Whenever the urinary concentration of calcium oxalate and phosphate can be decreased by increased water drinking, the risk of stone formation decreases (Finlayson, 1974). Some patients, however, because of their lifestyle or because they have excessive absorption or excretion of calcium, oxalate, or phosphate, are unable to increase water drinking. These patients should definitely be advised to avoid excessive amounts of calcium and oxalate in their diet. The amount of phosphate in the diet does not seem to be critical, and excess dietary phosphate may actually bind gut calcium. A typical low-calcium, low-oxalate diet is included in Appendix C. Carbohydrate-induced hypercalciuria can be remedied by avoiding excessive dietary carbohydrate and drinking fluids when eating carbohydrates. Interestingly, low-calcium, low-oxalate diets tend also to be low-carbohydrate diets.

In addition to the therapeutic cornerstones of increased fluid intake and dietary restriction, some medications may be useful in the treatment of calcigerous urinary calculi. These drugs and their uses are summarized in Table 25–15.

There is continuous controversy about whether commonly used oral neutral phosphates or oral thiazides (Thomas, 1975; Yendt and Cohanim, 1973; Pak, 1982) constitute better therapy for calcium urolithiasis. Table 25–16 attempts to summarize the pros and cons of these medications.

When thiazides are used as therapy for calcium urinary calculi, the therapeutic response is usually based on decreased urinary calcium excretion; hence, these drugs are especially useful in hypercalciuric patients. This effect requires decreased vascular volume. It has been noted that increased dietary salt intake and increased vascular volume negate the hypocalciuric effects of thiazides (Griffith, personal communication). It is therefore advisable for patients who receive thiazide treatment to restrict dietary salt intake to that necessary for cooking.

Physicians sometimes wonder what medication should be used initially in treating stone patients. Table 25–17 summarizes a method used by the author that will at least imply possible defects in the patient's urine or serum (Drach, 1976b). As noted previously, one usually prescribes a drug that is designed to correct the most obvious urinary defect and is not otherwise contraindicated for that patient. Several experimental drugs in addition to these have

TABLE 25–16. Oral Neutral Phosphates Versus Thiazides

Phosphates		Thiazides	
BENEFITS	PROBLEMS	BENEFITS	PROBLEMS
Urine calcium decreases	Diarrhea	Dosage once or twice daily	Hypokalemia
Urinary crystals decrease	Risk of infection Urine oxalate increases	No diarrhea No apparent risk if infection occurs	Hyperuricemia
	Large tablets	Urine calcium decreases	"Weakness"
	Frequent gastritis		

TABLE 25–17. Hints at Selection of Patients for Anticalcium Stone Therapy

Serum or Urinary Defect Found	Therapy Likely to Succeed
Hypercalcemia and hypercalciuria with elevated PTH	Surgical removal of abnormal parathyroid glands
Hypercalcemia, hypervitaminosis D	Stop excessive vitamin D
Hypercalciuria, immobilization	Exercises, large fluid output, low-calcium diet
Hypercalciuria, hyperthyroidism	Treat hyperthyroidism
Hypercalciuria, hyperabsorption	Neutral phosphates
Hypercalciuria, renal leak	Thiazides
Relative hypercalciuria, magnesium deficit $\left(\dfrac{MG \times 100}{Ca}\right) \leq 33$	Magnesium oxide
Hyperuricemia and hyperuricosuria with calcium urolithiasis	Allopurinol
Intestinal hyperabsorption, hyperoxaluria	High-calcium, very low oxalate diet plus (perhaps) cholestyramine

been proposed, especially in Europe. Cellulose phosphate has been used clinically in Europe and in the United States (Pak et al., 1974). Its mode of action is similar to that of neutral phosphate tablets. That is, gut calcium is bound by phosphate and not absorbed. However, cellulose phosphate avoids the sodium or potassium overload that is sometimes associated with neutral phosphate tablets (Pak, 1982). One potential problem associated with any oral phosphate is that urinary oxalate excretion is apparently increased by the use of these drugs (Elliot et al., 1970). Diphosphonates have also been proposed to prevent calcium urinary stones. Reports of the use of these substances are early, and their efficacy has not yet been proved (Ohata and Pak, 1974). Several potentially serious complications, especially osteomalacia, have been reported. Hence, we are left with a limited number of drugs that appear to affect calcium urolithiasis beneficially. In most pa-

tients, however, the use of the drugs listed in Table 25–15 has been effective in reducing long-term incidence of urinary stone disease. Roughly 70 to 90 per cent of patients so treated may expect cessation of new stone formation (Coe, 1977; Pak, 1982).

Investigators of stone disease are still looking for the perfect treatment for this condition. Perhaps the most frustrating aspect of stone disease is its intermittent activity (Table 25–18) and the fact that patients who are treated may decide that they are cured after several years and stop treatment, only to discover that their disease returns after medication and dietary treatment cease. Also, the overall incidence of calcium stone disease is increasing. More attention to specific etiologic factors, prediction of "activity of stone disease," and development of specific therapeutic measures are necessary before calcium urolithiasis disease can be brought under control.

TABLE 25–18. Estimation of Stone Disease Activity* and Need for Treatment

Condition	Symptoms and Signs	Recommend
Surgically active	Renal colic Obstruction Infection Intractable pain	Urologic consultation for possible surgical removal
Metabolically active	Formation of new stone within the past year Growth of known stone within the past year Documented passage of stone or gravel within the past year	Preventive measures† plus specific drugs (Table 25–15)
Metabolically and surgically inactive	None of the above for 1 year	Preventive measures† only; observation
Indeterminate	Uncertain activity or period of observation less than 1 year	Preventive measures† only; observation

*After Smith, L. H.: Urol. Clin. North Am., *1*:241. 1974*a*.
†Refers to increased daily urinary volume and appropriate diet. See text.

Rare Forms of Urinary Lithiasis

MATRIX CALCULI

Matrix calculi are found predominantly in individuals with infections due to urease-producing organisms. *Proteus* species are especially likely to be associated with matrix calculi. Boyce has defined matrix calculi as those stones composed of coagulated mucoids with very little crystalline component. Several clinical reports of these stones have appeared (Allen and Spence, 1966; Mall et al., 1975). They are radiolucent and may be confused with uric acid calculi. However, their association with alkaline urinary tract infection usually assists in making a presumptive diagnosis, because uric acid calculi are usually formed in acid-sterile urines. In most instances, surgical manipulation is required for their removal, since they are not dissolvable by any means yet known.

HEREDITARY XANTHINURIA

Hereditary xanthinuria results in the production of xanthine calculi. This rare calculus is also radiolucent and may be confused with a uric acid calculus. Radiographic crystallographic analysis of the stone is usually necessary to confirm this type of calculus. Quantitative urinary chromatography for xanthine reveals the presence of excessive excretion of this substance. No effective therapy exists (Dent and Philpot, 1954; Frayha et al., 1973; Pearlman, 1950). Occasionally, patients who are given allopurinol for treatment of uric acid urolithiasis or gout will begin to form xanthine calculi (Seegmiller, 1968) because allopurinol blocks conversion of xanthine to uric acid. The most specific therapy for xanthine stone appears to be increased urinary volume.

SILICATE CALCULI

Silicate urinary calculi occur in domestic animals with some degree of frequency (Joekes et al., 1973), but they are extremely rare in humans. Patients who have chronically taken large doses of silicate-containing antacids have developed small silicate calculi (Joekes et al., 1973). Once again, stone analysis is necessary to ascertain this type of calculus. Treatment is directed at alteration of antacid therapy.

TRIAMTERENE CALCULI

Triamterene is often used singly or in combination with hydrochlorothiazide in the treatment of hypertension. This latter combination tends to avoid potassium depletion, which may result from oral hydrochlorothiazide alone. Un-

fortunately, however, some few patients (0.4 per cent of 50,000 calculi) may incorporate triamterene into stones or have stones composed almost entirely of triamterene. It seems, therefore, that triamterene should be used with great caution in stone formers (Ettinger et al., 1980; Werness et al., 1982).

2,8 HYDROXYADENINE CALCULI

These very rare, radiolucent calculi occur in the presence of deficient adenine phosphoribosyl transferase, an inherited metabolic defect. Homozygous and heterozygous genotypes have both produced this condition. Treatment should be by low-purine diet and oral allopurinol administration (Witten et al., 1983).

SPURIOUS CALCULI

Spurious or fake urinary calculi are not at all unusual. Most stone analysis laboratories report that approximately 1 to 2 per cent of all calculi submitted are produced outside the human body. Sutor and O'Flynn (1973) reported one patient who inserted boiler scale into her bladder in order to mimic the production of urinary calculi. In this case it was observed that although matrix was not present when boiler scale was formed on the boiler, it did infiltrate the entire substance of the calculus after it had been placed in the bladder. The author was acquainted with a patient whose wife stated that she had extracted urinary calculi from his urethra. The patient was convinced that he had calculi. It was only after confrontation with the fact that the calculi were composed of standard creekbed stones that the wife admitted that she had palmed the calculi, placed them in the urethra, and subsequently expelled them under the eyes of her husband.

The emergency rooms of North America's hospitals are occasionally visited by individuals who fake urinary calculous disease (usually due to "uric acid stones") for secondary gain to obtain drugs (Sharon and Diamond, 1974). The standard story of these individuals is that they know they have stone disease, uric acid stone disease, and they are allergic to intravenous urogram dye. A high degree of suspicion is in order when an individual from out of town arrives with this story, has a severe degree of pain, and dramatizes this pain to an excessive degree. Several patients have developed a true "Münchausen syndrome" and have traveled the United States with their supposed stone disease (Atkinson and Earll, 1974). However, it is better to give an addict meperidine than to withhold it from a true sufferer of ureteral colic.

URINARY LITHIASIS OF CHILDREN

Prior to this century, the major incidence of urinary lithiasis was bladder stones of children. As nations have increased their productivity and moved into the industrial age, average income and therefore food quality have improved. These events have resulted in the gradual disappearance of endemic bladder stone disease from previously afflicted populations, so that such stones are now found mostly in North Africa, the Middle and Near East, Burma, Thailand and Indonesia (VanReen, 1981).

Most pediatric bladder calculi in the endemic areas are composed of acid urate (Brockis et al., 1981) or calcium oxalate, or mixtures thereof. Urine pH in such children is nearly always acidic (Aurora et al., 1970) in the absence of infection. In the presence of infection, struvite becomes more common, but infections seem to be an unusual complication of the uninstrumented child with bladder stone. Perhaps the occurrence of such stones can be traced to the common practice in endemic areas of feeding infants human breast milk and cereal foods, such as polished rice or millet. Human breast milk, in contrast to cow's milk, is very low in phosphorus, as is polished rice (Andersen, 1962; Thalut et al., 1976). Such low-phosphate diets result in high peaks of urinary ammonia excretion (Brockis et al., 1981). Perhaps also important, Valyasevi and Dhanamitta (1974) showed that ingestion of vegetable oxalate contributed to the high degree of crystalluria often seen in these children. They then fed the children oral neutral orthophosphate and stated that such supplementation "practically eliminated (calcium oxalate) crystalluria and crystal clumping."

Urologic disease such as obstruction and reflux may coexist with bladder stone of nutritional etiology, and Taneja et al. (1970) have recommended that such children undergo a complete urologic study: voiding cystourethrograms, intravenous urography, and endoscopic examination. They base these recommendations on the occurrence of obstructive lesions in 38.5 per cent and reflux in 41 per cent of 52 afflicted children who were studied completely.

If we exclude endemic bladder calculi of children in developing countries, we observe that the majority of urinary stones of children affect the upper tracts, just as in adults. The subject of childhood urolithiasis in industrialized countries has been ably reviewed by a number of authors (Malek and Kelalis, 1975; Paulson, 1972, 1974; Mitchell, 1981; Borgmann and Nagel, 1982; O'Regan et al., 1982; Noe et al., 1983; Steele et al., 1983).

It appears from the aforementioned reviews that the incidence of stones in patients under 15 or 16 years of age is about 7 per cent of all patients seen for stones (Borgmann and Nagel, 1982). The male:female ratio is 1:1, which differs from the 3:1 or 4:1 ratio seen in adults. Two major types of stones occur: lower or upper tract stones associated with infection and neurogenic bladder or urologic anomaly, and "idiopathic" stones. Some 20 to 30 per cent of children with stones present with *painless* hematuria, so that exclusion of stone disease becomes one of the most important aspects of differential diagnosis of painless hematuria of children.

Stapleton et al. (1982) have studied 21 children who had uncomplicated calcium urolithiasis. They demonstrated that significant hypercalciuria did occur in stone-forming children. It is necessary to set different limits and standards of calcium excretion for children, e.g., renal hypercalciuria if fasting UCa/UCr exceeded 0.21 and absorptive hypercalciuria if post–calcium load UCa/UCr exceeded 0.31. Perhaps this is the reason that many previous authors did not find hypercalciuria in their studies of pediatric urolithiasis. Noe, who was a participant in the aforementioned study, subsequently reported (Noe et al., 1983) that 91 per cent of 47 pediatric urinary stone patients had "factors causing or predisposing to stone disease." Of these, 53 per cent had metabolic causes; 19 per cent, urologic anomalies; 15 per cent, infectious cause; and 4 per cent, immobilization syndrome, with the remaining 9 per cent unexplained.

Children with urolithiasis may have classic metabolic diseases such as hyperparathyroidism, renal tubular acidosis, cystinuria (Pavanello et al., 1981), primary hyperoxaluria, or diseases that produce an excessive excretion of uric acid, such as Lesch-Nyhan syndrome or leukemia. Any metabolic evaluation should include screening for these defects.

Adolescents are not spared. Rambar and MacKenzie (1978) studied 31 adolescents who had stones. In 13 per cent the stones were related to inborn errors of metabolism, such as cystinuria or primary oxalosis. Three of their patients developed stones in their transplanted kidneys. Twenty-two (71 per cent) required some type of surgical procedure to relieve stone obstruction or related problems. Other authors (Borgmann and Nagel, 1982; Noe et al., 1983) report the need for surgical intervention in 70 to 94 per cent of pediatric urolithiasis patients. Interestingly, once the surgical correction has been performed, the recurrence rate for stones in the pediatric age group seems to be lower than that for adults, or at least "no greater" than for adults (Steele et al., 1983).

Diagnosis of urinary calculous disease in children is similar to that in adults: pain (although 20 to 30 per cent presented with painless hematuria as noted earlier), hematuria, and radiologic evidence of calculi. One significant radiologic difference has been reported by Breatnach and Smith (1983). In a group of 50 children who had intravenous urography for calculi, "increased nephrographic density was never seen" and "the adult intravenous urogram pattern of acute ureteric obstruction was not seen." Since, however, 80 per cent of these children had associated urinary infection, generalized ureteral dilation and calyectasis were quite common and may have masked the typical radiologic signs of stone obstruction. The occurrence of lucent calculi (uric acid and, to some degree, cystine) requires urography. It has been reported to approach 10 per cent of childhood calculi (Rambar and MacKenzie, 1978; Steele et al., 1983), but the more common incidence figure for radiolucent calculi in children approximates 3 to 4 per cent (Borgmann and Nagel, 1982).

Some physicians tend to avoid intravenous urography in younger children because of excessive radiation exposure. Certainly, genitalia and gonads should be shielded whenever possible. Higher degrees of radiation can be avoided by the performance of a tailored urogram as proposed by Lalli (1974). Only those radiographs necessary to make a proper diagnosis are taken. This technique requires the attention and presence of a perceptive urologist or radiologist.

Treatment of patients in the pediatric age group is similar to that for adults and, as noted earlier, often includes initial surgical removal of stone(s) and correction of any urinary defects. Most of the authors referred to previously agree that thorough metabolic evaluation of children is warranted to discover the cause of their urolithiasis. Thereafter, appropriate therapy can be assigned. The usual admonitions to increase fluid intake and output seem universally accepted. Cystinuria, primary hyperoxaluria, hyperuricosuria, and rarer forms of stone disease respond to the specific therapies noted previously. Hypercalciuria has been treated by dietary limitation of calcium and oxalate with or without neutral orthophosphates (Noe et al., 1983). These investigators have also treated renal leak hypercalciuria with thiazides (2 mg/kg/day), but use of thiazides in children has been questioned by Steele et al. (1983).

CONSIDERATIONS REGARDING SPECIFIC LOCATIONS OF CALCULI

Renal Calculi

Calculi too large to pass spontaneously range in size from 1 cm to the large staghorn stones that occupy the renal pelvis and calyces. Surgical removal is usually necessary. Occasionally, in a patient in poor general health, an asymptomatic staghorn calculus may be discovered during the course of a general health examination. In such a patient, if the function of the sound kidney is adequate, a conservative policy of observation may be advisable but only if it is clearly understood that if sepsis, pain, or evidence of decreased function should appear, operation may be required (Libertino et al., 1971). However, the presence in the kidney of calculi too large to pass spontaneously is a potential hazard. Even with our newest chemotherapeutic agents, eradication of infection is not possible until infected calculi have been removed. Individual consideration of each case is necessary, and the urologist's clinical judgment may be taxed to the utmost in some instances to determine whether to pursue a policy of watchful waiting or to advocate immediate surgical intervention.

Bilateral renal calculi present additional problems. In most instances, infection is present. Occasionally, even with multiple calculi, the urine is sterile. Surgical intervention is not always advisable in patients with bilateral stones. Aged persons with bilateral renal calculi may live fairly comfortably and eventually succumb to other disease. In such patients, operation would be a hazardous procedure. In a young patient with the same type of bilateral lithiasis, surgical intervention may be advisable in the hope of preserving renal function and eliminating infection in the urinary tract.

It is important to reiterate that individualization of each patient's problems is essential in planning surgical and other treatment for renal lithiasis. Factors in one patient may require treatment different from that which would be instituted if such complications were not present. As a general rule, it is well to lean toward conservatism and preservation of renal function in regard to surgical treatment.

Types of Operation. See Chapter 62.

Ureteral Calculi—Some Specific Considerations

AGE

Stone in the ureter is essentially a disease of middle life; it is rare in childhood and unusual in old age. In a series of 857 patients (Higgins, 1939), 69 per cent of ureteral calculi occurred in patients aged 20 to 50 years. (The age range of the entire series of patients spanned 20 to 72 years.) Age incidence was similar in the series reported by Bumpus and Thompson (1925), Scholl (1936) and Furlow and Bucchiere (1976) and also noted in Figure 25–1.

SEX

Ureteral calculi occur much more often in men than in women. Jeanbrau (Joly, 1931) reported the ratio as 61 per cent in men and 39 per cent in women; Bumpus and Scholl reported 68 per cent in men and 32 per cent in women; and Ravich observed 69.8 per cent in men and 30.2 per cent in women. In the Cleveland Clinic (Higgins, 1939) series of 857 patients, 79 per cent were men and 21 per cent were women. These authors' figures also agree with those noted in Figure 25–1.

SITE OF ORIGIN

It is now generally believed that ureteral calculi originate in the kidney and then pass into the ureter. Their cause is thus the same as that of renal lithiasis. Calculi that develop primarily in the ureter are rare. Perhaps this is because the smooth mucosal lining of the ureter is constantly bathed with urine, and accumulations of crystals are promptly washed into the bladder. Available reports indicate that in those rare instances in which ureteral stones are primary, they have been formed in association with ureteroceles, neoplasms, ureters with blind endings, ectopic ureters, sacculations, or dilated segments of the ureter proximal to a stricture.

SITE OF IMPACTION

Certain anatomic characteristics determine where a stone may become impacted as it moves down the ureter. The points of relative constriction discussed earlier in this section (Fig. 25–12) occur at or just below the ureteropelvic junction; where the ureter crosses the iliac vessels; at the base of the broad ligament in women and at the area of the vas deferens in men; where the ureter enters the external muscular coat of the bladder; and at the vesical orifice. Two points of angulation also are present: at

the place where the ureter crosses the iliac vessels and enters the true pelvis, and at the point where it enters the bladder. These normal anatomic variations probably explain the frequency with which calculi become impacted in certain portions of the ureter more often than in others.

In Higgins' series (1939) of 251 consecutive cases, the calculus was at the ureteropelvic junction or in the upper third of the ureter in 39 patients, in the lumbar portion or middle third in 23, in the pelvic portion in 155, and in the intramural portion in 34. Thus, 61.7 per cent of calculi were in the pelvic ureter when first seen; if the stones in the intramural portion are added, 75.3 per cent of stones were in the lower third of the ureter. In a second series of 350 consecutive cases (Higgins, 1939), the corresponding figure is 77 per cent. Geraghty and Hinman (1915) reported a combined incidence of 73.4 per cent of stones in the pelvic and intramural portions of the ureter; Joly (1931) stated that half the number of stones impacted in the ureter were found in the pelvic portion, and, if those in the intramural portion are included, the figure was approximately 70 per cent. It is evident that the majority of impacted ureteral stones will be found in the pelvic portion of the ureter, a statement confirmed in recent reviews by the author (Drach, 1978, 1983)(Fig. 25–33).

SIZE, WEIGHT, AND SHAPE

The size of the ureteral calculus is of considerable importance clinically, but of equal importance is the caliber of the ureter below the stone. Calculi range in size from a few millimeters to 10 centimeters in length and width.

Numerous authors have tried to relate the

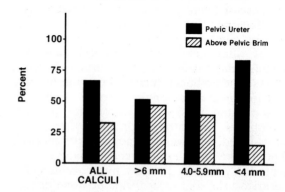

Figure 25–33. Distribution of ureteral calculi by size at time of presentation (253 patients). (From Drach, G. W.: Urol. Clin. North Am., *10*:709, 1983. Data adapted from Carstensen and Hansen: Acta Chir. Scand. (Suppl.), *433*:66, 1973.)

possibility of spontaneous passage of ureteral calculi to the size of the calculus. To become impacted, calculi usually must have one diameter in excess of 2 mm. If the smaller diameter is less than 4 mm, spontaneous stone passage is likely (Prince and Scardino, 1960; Sandergard, 1956; Drach, 1983). Stones that weigh more than 0.1 gm, have a small diameter of more than 1 cm, or are associated with urinary infection are not as likely to pass spontaneously (Sutor and Wooley, 1975) (Fig. 25–34). Some ureteral calculi become very large. Heath (1922) removed a calculus 2.5 by 15 cm that weighed 65.8 gm. Tennant (1924) removed a ureteral stone that weighed 66 gm, and Joly (1931) cites one case reported by Federoff in which the calculus weighed 52 gm. Despite occasional reports of such giant stones, ureteral calculi are rarely more than 2 cm in length. Their shape often varies according to the length of time the stone has been in the ureter. A calculus recently expelled from the kidney is usually round or ovoid. After stones have resided in the ureter for some time, the longitudinal diameter becomes greater than the transverse.

If it is inside a very dilated ureter, the stone may remain round, move freely in the ureter, and act as a ball-valve. Multiple calculi may also remain round or ovoid in a dilated ureter. They may become faceted as they rub beside one another in undilated ureters, in which free movement is not possible. Greatly elongated calculi in the pelvic portion of the ureter may even assume the curvature of this segment.

In the great majority of patients, a single stone develops. In his series of 350 cases of ureteral calculi seen at the Cleveland Clinic, Higgins (1939) noted the presence of multiple ureteral stones in only 7 and bilateral ureteral calculi in 6 patients. Braasch and Moore (1915) observed multiple stones in 17 patients in a series of 278 cases of ureteral stones.

LATERALITY

Ureteral calculi are equally frequent on the left and right sides, although in certain patients stone formation seems to be limited to one side. Kretschmer (1942), in a review of 500 cases, stated that 45.8 per cent of calculi were on the right side and 51.8 per cent occurred on the left. Bumpus and Thompson (1925) and Scholl (1936) reported that ureteral calculi were observed with equal frequency on the two sides; in Higgins' series, 47 per cent were present in the right ureter and 53 per cent in the left.

COMPOSITION

Since ureteral calculi originate in the kidney, they are the same chemical types as renal stones. Small calculi of calcium oxalate occur most frequently. Uric acid, cystine, and struvite stones occur less commonly but can be more difficult to define because of their decreased radiodensity. If infection supervenes, layers of struvite may be formed over previously deposited substances such as uric acid. Unusual radiographic appearances of stones with "hollow" centers result.

PATHOLOGIC CHANGES CAUSED BY URETERAL CALCULI

Impaction of calculi in the ureter produces various pathologic changes influenced by the extent and duration of obstruction and the presence or absence of infection (see earlier section on pathophysiology of obstruction). When a small calculus passes through the ureter readily or with moderate delay, no lasting pathologic changes are discernible and the caliber of the ureter soon returns to normal. When obstruction is incomplete and no infection exists, the duration of blockage is then of greatest importance, as noted earlier in this chapter.

Periureteritis and ureteritis may be pronounced in the area around the calculus. Calculi may rarely ulcerate through the ureter. At the site of impaction the ureter is usually fixed to the adjacent fat and contiguous structures by inflammatory changes. In early stages, the extent of dilatation of the ureter above the calculus may be pronounced and tortuosity develops. In later stages, the ureter is thickened by fibrous-

Figure 25–34. Combined data from two studies provide an estimate of percentages of stones first seen in the pelvic ureter and their likelihood of retention *for 1 year.* (From Drach, G. W.: Urol. Clin. North Am., *10*:709, 1983.)

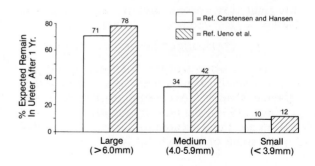

tissue infiltration. Microscopically, round-cell infiltration and fibrosis are observed. When infection is present, stricture formation is more prevalent below the calculus than if infection is absent. The degree of ureteral inflammation is also increased by infection, which also decreases ureteral peristalsis and may therefore contribute to greater dilatation of the ureter proximal to the calculus (Rose et al., 1975).

When infection is absent, various degrees of hydronephrosis may ensue. When infection supervenes, rapid destruction of renal parenchyma occurs also. The appearance of the kidney may vary from that of chronic pyelonephritis to a huge pyonephrotic sac. The changes depend upon the extent of retrograde pressure on the kidney and the virulence of the infecting organism.

SYMPTOMS

A calculus passing down the ureter may cause symptoms of colic, as previously described (see section on initial diagnosis and therapy). The patient may experience a single attack of colic followed by the expulsion of the stone, or he may have several episodes as the calculus traverses the course of the ureter more slowly. The first pain is usually severe and occurs in the flank in the region of the costovertebral angle. Later, pain is sometimes felt in the region of the umbilicus and may follow the course of the ureter through the posterior abdomen, or it may be referred to the genitalia. As the stone nears the bladder, the patient may experience frequency, urgency, and strangury. Dysuria and tenesmus may be pronounced. The pain of renal colic may sometimes be referred to the perineum, bladder, penis, or testicles. Stone impaction in the ureter may also cause atypical symptoms. Unusual referral of ureteral colic pain to the thigh, hip, or knee has been reported. In Higgins' series (1939), only 56 per cent of patients gave a fairly typical history of an attack of colic with subsequent intermittent pain or discomfort. On other occasions, the pain of colic may become relatively steady and fixed, although it is often aggravated by exertion. On the right side, chronic ureteral stone pain may falsely suggest cholecystitis or appendicitis.

ROENTGENOGRAPHIC OBSERVATIONS

The structures of the bony pelvis may obscure a small calculus that casts a faint radiographic shadow. According to Peterson and Holmes (1937), the most frequently overlooked calculi are those located in a small area medial to the spine of the ischium just above a transverse line joining the lowest part of the ischial spines. In 100 cases Peterson and Holmes found that 96 per cent of calculi were diagnosed by roentgenographic study and only 4 per cent were "invisible." The roentgenogram usually reveals a single shadow, but in some instances evidence of multiple stones may be seen. In general, the shadow cast by a stone that has been in the ureter for some time is elongated and fusiform, with the long axis parallel to the course of the ureter.

When the procedure is not contraindicated by some other condition, an excretory urogram should be obtained after initial plain films are made. The status of both kidneys is determined and the degree of hydronephrosis and intensity of obstruction of the kidney, as evidenced by the rate of elimination of the contrast medium on the involved side, is interpreted. The degree of dilatation of the ureter above the calculus is noted. Failure to visualize the contrast medium when obstruction is complete does not signify that the kidney is destroyed and functionless. Excellent renal function may return after obstruction is relieved, especially when the obstruction has occurred recently. In many instances, enough information results from the excretory urogram to allow decisions to be made about immediate management of the patient. Dourmashkin (1945) stated that routine retrograde pyelography should be avoided in cases of calculous ureteral obstruction that present no diagnostic problem and may be diagnosed by other means. Of a series of 1550 cases of ureteral calculi, retrograde pyelography was resorted to in only 118 cases, chiefly in patients with uric acid calculi or in those in whom the stone was not recognized immediately for various reasons. These observations remain true nearly 40 years later.

Nichols and Lower (1933) stressed the value of plain stereoscopic films in determining the relative anteroposterior position of all calcareous deposits along the course of the ureter. Such films are also important in excluding areas of increased density due to the pelvic bones, enterolithiasis, or phleboliths and dense areas on the external surface of the body. Introduction of an opaque catheter into the ureter is frequently a valuable procedure. After the catheter passes beyond the obstruction, anteroposterior and oblique exposures may be made with the catheter in place, or two exposures may be made on the same film with the tube shifted according to the Kretschmer stereoscopic technique. This will demonstrate the relation of the stone to the lumen of the ureter. If, however, the ureter is dilated, the calculus may be a considerable distance from the catheter and still be in the ureter.

It may be difficult to differentiate shadows cast by ureteral stones from those made by intestinal contents, mesenteric glands, phleboliths, atheromatous plaques, or lesions on the skin. Intestinal contents rarely cause confusion if the patient is properly prepared before roentgenographic study. Mesenteric glands move with changes in position and usually do not have a uniform density. Phleboliths in pelvic veins may be confused with ureteral stones. Phleboliths usually are round and cast dense shadows lateral to the course of the normal ureter. Their centers are often radiolucent.

Failure to see an obstruction or nonvisualization of a calculus on the initial film does not always exclude the possibility that a small stone is present in the ureter. The stone may be too small to obstruct the passage of the catheter or it may have been dislodged by the introduction of the catheter. If the stone can be bypassed with a ureteral catheter, renal function tests, bacteriologic cultures of urine, or retrograde pyelograms may be performed. In other instances, if the ureteral catheter fails to pass the obstruction, the stereoscopic roentgenogram may at least show the tip of the catheter in contact with the stone.

FACTORS THAT INFLUENCE CHOICE OF TREATMENT

Few urologic problems require weighing of so many factors as does treatment of an obstructing calculus in the ureter (Anderson, 1974; Drach, 1978, 1983; Furlow and Bucchiere, 1976). The questions that arise in each case include whether operation should be performed for immediate relief of the obstruction; whether stone manipulation should be done; or whether a period of watchful waiting should be undertaken. The most significant factors to be considered in making decisions about proper management of each case are discussed in the following paragraphs.

The economic status and occupation of the patient will influence the type of treatment to be carried out. A sudden attack of recurrent ureteral colic in a person who works with machinery, an engineer, or a pilot may endanger his own life and the lives of those around him or dependent upon him. A laborer who has a stone passing slowly down the upper ureter (with arrest of its progress from time to time occasioning severe attacks of colic) may frequently be restored more rapidly to his gainful occupation with no greater financial burden when the calculus is removed by means of a simple muscle-splitting incision.

Duration of symptoms is another important factor. The patient who has had repeated episodes of severe colic deserves relief. When the symptoms and obstruction are of long duration, further delay in treatment may lead to irreparable renal damage. Should one wait 2 days or 2 weeks for spontaneous passage of a stone? In one series of 350 cases of ureteral calculi, 54.1 per cent of the stones that passed spontaneously did so within 16 days after the patient was first examined (Higgins, 1939).

The size of the calculus also influences the clinical course and the choice of treatment. As noted previously, the larger the calculus (over 4 mm), the less likely it is that it will pass spontaneously (Carstensen and Hansen, 1973). These authors also report that over 90 per cent of these small calculi will pass within 3 months.

Status of renal function is a prime consideration in making decisions about treatment for ureteral stones. When the excretory urogram reveals slight hydronephrosis or dilatation of the ureter above the calculus, it signifies that the urine is flowing around the stone and that the stone is causing little obstruction. If repeat roentgenograms reveal little or no progress in the descent of the calculus and no obstruction, one may wait for spontaneous passage, but any progressive obstruction must be relieved. Cessation of pain does not always mean that obstruction has been relieved but may really signify onset of complete obstruction.

Any preferred method of treatment for ureteral calculi should have as its prime objective the preservation of function of the kidney on the affected side. Clinical evidence of renal damage, which is confirmed by intravenous urograms indicating complete ureteral obstruction, or a progressively enlarging hydronephrosis signifies that conservative treatment is unwarranted, and surgical intervention should be instituted promptly.

The degree of impaction is also significant in deciding upon the course of treatment. A stone that remains in the same position week after week probably will not pass spontaneously. According to Joly (1931), if the stone has not moved downward within a period of a month or 6 weeks, watchful waiting should be abandoned, and other methods of treatment should be instituted. The status of the opposite kidney must always be kept in mind. In patients with a solitary kidney, any continuing obstruction is grave and demands relief.

The age and general condition of the patient may influence the procedure to be advocated. Elderly, debilitated patients may not tolerate instrumentation well. Severe febrile reactions may result. In children, because of technical difficulties in passing cystoscopes of adequate size, lack of complete cooperation, and the necessity for repeated administration of anesthetics, open surgery is frequently the procedure of choice.

In the presence of an obstructing calculus, infection is indicated by hyperpyrexia and leukocytosis. Prompt surgical intervention with establishment of free drainage is a lifesaving measure and may prevent the development of gram-negative bacteremia. To prepare such a patient for operation, some surgeons first insert an indwelling ureteral catheter, which provides temporary drainage and is of inestimable value in halting a septic course. In elderly men, associated disease such as prostatic hypertrophy may make manipulative procedures technically difficult. In such cases, open stone removal or at least nephrostomy drainage may be the preferred procedure.

In general, a small ureteral stone accompanied by infrequent attacks of colic but not associated with infection or progressive hydronephrosis may be observed in the hope that the stone will pass spontaneously. Progression of the calculus is noted, and the status of the kidney is periodically assured by means of roentgenograms. If impaction occurs, active measures must be taken. Various drugs such as neostigmine and the antispasmodics (e.g., atropine) have been used to facilitate the passage of the calculus. Aminophylline, Tandearil, and other agents have also been suggested (Holmlund, 1974; Lehtonen, 1973), but there are no clear reports of drug effectiveness in promoting stone passage (Peters and Eckstein, 1975; Rutishauser, 1971). Hence, the results of drug treatment are inconsistent and vary considerably among different urologists.

MANIPULATION

Braasch and Moore (1915) list eight contraindications for manipulative treatment of ureteral calculi: (1) when the caliber of the stone exceeds 2 cm; (2) when there is considerable periureteritis; (3) when the kidney is either hydronephrotic or pyohydronephrotic; (4) when the stone is known to have been present for a long time; (5) when several unsuccessful attempts have already been made to remove it; (6) when cystoscopy is poorly tolerated; (7) when congenital anomalies of the genital organs

are present; and (8) when a severe febrile reaction or acute pyelonephritis follows the first manipulative procedure.

Opinions about mechanical stone removers vary. Most urologists agree with Coppridge (1940), who stated that their use should be restricted to stones in the lower third of the ureter. When the ureter is completely obstructed at any level, one or more catheters should be passed, if possible, to establish drainage from the kidney. These are usually withdrawn after 12 to 24 hours.

Various mechanical devices have been recommended for stone manipulation, and the large number of instruments available today for the removal of ureteral stones indicates that no one instrument or method is suitable in all instances. Likewise, serious complications may result from the use of such instruments. Perforation of the ureter, ureteral avulsion, stricture, and stone basket incarceration may occur (Drach, 1978).

Currently, the best procedure for management of small stones in the upper and middle thirds of the ureter in the absence of infection or significant obstruction is one of watchful waiting. If the calculus is 1 cm or less in diameter and is moving spontaneously down the ureter, manipulative treatment should be delayed until the stone is in the pelvic region. Then, if manipulation is advisable, catheter or basket extractors are employed. If the stone is in the upper or middle portion of the ureter and is producing complete obstruction as shown by intravenous urography, surgical intervention is advocated. If the stone is in the intramural segment and does not pass spontaneously, a ureteral meatotomy may be performed, and the stone may be removed with an extractor. One must remember that such meatotomies may result in reflux or stricture. When manipulative procedures are not feasible for reasons previously mentioned, and spontaneous expulsion cannot occur, surgical intervention is advisable.

RECURRENCE

The results of operations for ureteral stone are usually satisfactory. An instance has been reported of a recurrence of primary stone in the ureter, perhaps associated with deposition of phosphates on a suture that had been passed into the lumen of the ureter during its closure after ureterolithotomy (Dalton et al., 1975), but most recurrent ureteral calculi originate in the kidney and lodge again in various portions of the ureter.

The important features, then, in the management of patients with ureteral calculi are prompt diagnosis, early removal of the calculus, whether spontaneously, by manipulative procedures, or by open operation, followed by adequate postoperative evaluation and possibly prophylactic or specific therapy. These measures are usually followed by gratifying results.

SURGICAL TREATMENT

See Chapter 68.

Vesical Calculi

As mentioned in the introduction, in certain parts of the world the incidence of vesical calculi is high, while in other areas there has been a steady and pronounced decrease in incidence of stones in the bladder since the nineteenth century, when vesical calculi were unusually prevalent. This decrease has been attributed to dietary and nutritional progress.

Age. As an etiologic factor in calculi of the bladder, age incidence varies in different parts of the world. According to Joly (1931), in England and France during the nineteenth century, calculous disease was largely limited to children; now it is a disease of adult life (Hodgkinson and Marshall, 1975). The decrease in vesical calculi in childhood is probably due to improvement in diet and nutrition. In some areas of the world, such as Thailand and Indonesia, bladder calculi continue to occur in children.

Sex. Vesical calculus is predominantly a disease of the male sex in all races and nationalities. In a review of calculous disease of the bladder in the Canton Hospital, Thompson (1921) stated that only 2 per cent of cases occurred in women. In the United States the increased frequency of vesical calculi in men occurs in men over 50. Vesical calculi appear to be definitely associated with obstruction of the bladder neck due to bladder neck contracture, prostatic enlargement, stricture of the urethra, or diverticulum of the bladder.

Hence, in men, factors that give rise to retention of urine, such as stricture of the urethra, prostatic hypertrophy, diverticulum of the bladder, cystoceles, and neurogenic bladder, are associated with the formation of vesical calculi. Urinary infection especially promotes formation of struvite stones in these patients. Other bladder stones are formed on foreign bodies, such as sutures or catheters, or on objects introduced into the bladder via the urethra by the patient (Dalton et al., 1975) (Fig. 25–35).

Composition. The composition of the calculus in the bladder is influenced by the pH and degree of saturation of the urine. In the United States, calcium oxalate is the most common constituent of calculi. In Europe, uric acid and urate stones are most prevalent. The bladder is more often infected than the kidney, and therefore the incidence of struvite calculi due to bladder infection is higher than that of struvite calculi in the kidney.

Usually a single stone is observed in the bladder, but in the presence of retained urine, multiple stones—2 or 3 to 100 or more—may be present in 25 to 30 per cent of cases (Fig. 25–36). It has also been noted that when there is diverticulum of the bladder, multiple stones are formed more frequently. Multiple stones may become faceted, and the size of the stones varies tremendously; they may be extremely small or they may weigh more than 1000 gm. Randall (1937) described a calculus weighing 1816 gm. The longitudinal circumference was

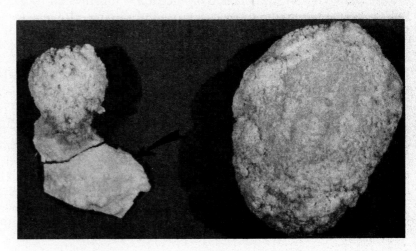

Figure 25–35. Bladder calculi of struvite removed from a patient who had had an indwelling Foley balloon retention catheter for 5 months. Catheter had been removed 3 months previously. Arrow points to thin curved portion of calculus, which fits the curvature of a catheter balloon.

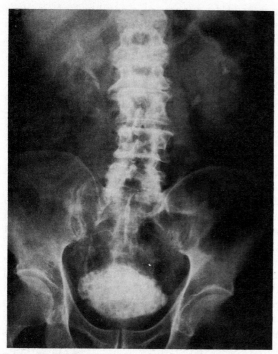

Figure 25–36. This patient with frequency, urgency, and microhematuria had a "normal" plain abdominal radiograph. Intravenous pyelogram revealed hundreds of small uric acid bladder calculi.

48 cm and the transverse circumference was 40 cm. The bulk of the calculus was composed of calcium phosphate.

Pathologic Changes. In the absence of infection, a smooth stone may be present in the bladder for some time without causing inflammatory changes in the bladder wall. Generally, the calculus produces sufficient mechanical irritation to cause chronic inflammatory changes. The earliest cystoscopic change is usually increased vascularity, which is followed by development of areas of congestion and reddening of the mucosa. With the introduction of infection, bullous edema, pronounced congestion, and ulceration appear.

When the calculus obstructs the urethral orifice, signs of back pressure are evident in the form of coarse trabeculation, with cellules and diverticulum formation. Pus may be noted on the floor of the bladder and on the stone. The bladder wall is thickened, and fibrous tissue reaction occurs in the muscular layer. In cases of long duration, pericystitis may occur, with adherence of the bladder to the adjacent fat in the pelvis; rarely, perforation of the bladder may occur.

Symptoms. In some patients, especially those with prostatic enlargement and residual urine, there may be no symptoms referable to the bladder calculus or calculi. In such patients, the complaints are predominantly those of prostatic obstruction, and the calculi are found during the course of urologic examination.

Typical symptoms of vesical stone are voiding pain and hematuria. The discomfort may be dull, aching, or sharp lower abdominal pain, which is aggravated by exercise and sudden movement. Severe pain usually occurs near the end of micturition. Pain is also produced by the movement of the calculus as it strikes the base of the bladder. Relief may be afforded by assuming a recumbent position. Terminal hematuria may occur.

In boys, the pain may be referred to the tip of the penis (along the course of the second and third sacral nerves) or to the scrotum; in boys or girls the pain may be referred to the perineum via the third and fourth sacral nerves. On occasion, referred pain may lodge in the back, the hip, or even the heel or sole of the foot.

Besides pain, there may be an interruption of the urinary stream from impaction of the stone in the internal urethral orifice. Frequency and dysuria are then usually present. Frequency of urination is enhanced by activity, and urgency is present in from 40 to 50 per cent of patients, while interruption of the stream occurs in about 30 to 40 per cent of patients. In the presence of infection, the usual symptoms of cystitis are superimposed; nocturia occurs, urgency is increased, and terminal pain is pronounced. Priapism and nocturnal enuresis may occur in children.

DIAGNOSIS OF VESICAL CALCULUS

History. Although a presumptive diagnosis may be tentatively made from a history of pain aggravated by exercise, interruption of the urinary stream, and terminal hematuria, these symptoms are not pathognomonic of this disease, for they may be produced by other lesions in the bladder.

Physical Examination. Physical examination is rarely of value in establishing a diagnosis, but instances have been cited in which a large stone was palpable on rectal, vaginal, or abdominal examination. Sensing the bladder stone by feeling it "clink" on a urethral sound is an age-old technique of detecting bladder stone.

Laboratory Findings. Albumin, erythrocytes, and leukocytes are usually found in the urine, but these are also commonly found with other lesions of the urinary tract. If infection has occurred, bacteria are often seen in the stained sediment or detected in urinary cultures.

Roentgenographic Study. Often no evidence of vesical calculi is seen in plain roentgenograms because of the presence of uric acid in many of the calculi and also because of overlying prostatic tissue (Fig. 25–36). It has been stated that more than 50 per cent of bladder stones are not discernible on roentgenograms. Nichols and Lower (1933) reported that cystoscopic examination was the surest method for detecting vesical calculi, whereas roentgenography was the most reliable procedure for detecting calculi in a bladder diverticulum.

Stones in the bladder, as seen on the roentgenogram, are often ovoid, with the long axis occupying a transverse position. These shadows must be differentiated from phleboliths, masses in the intestines, and calcified lymph nodes.

The most accurate and certain means of diagnosis is cystoscopic examination, as the absence of a shadow on the roentgenogram does not preclude the presence of a vesical calculus.

TREATMENT

Since obstructive lesions and infection seem to play a role in the formation and enlargement of vesical calculi, their eradication will minimize the occurrence of stone. Obstruction must be relieved, bladder stasis corrected, and foreign bodies removed whenever possible.

Owing to drug sensitivity studies, many infections of the bladder that in the past were classified as drug-resistant may now be eradicated. Relief of obstruction and eradication of bladder infection are valuable prophylactic procedures in prevention of further episodes of bladder calculi.

While satisfactory results have been reported from the use of Suby's G or M solutions, treatment with these agents is protracted and is now rarely employed. Renacidin may be used to dissolve phosphate calculi and may prove beneficial in irrigating indwelling suprapubic or urethral catheters to prevent formation of calculus. It has produced little bladder irritability when used in a 10 per cent solution. Daily irrigations with 0.25 per cent or 0.5 per cent acetic acid solution also serve as beneficial prophylaxis against recurrent struvite calculi when catheters must be left indwelling. Conversely, uric acid calculi may be dissolved by irrigation with alkaline solutions.

Two surgical methods of treatment are available—litholapaxy and suprapubic lithotomy. The choice of operation is influenced by the age and physical condition of the patient, the size and hardness of the calculus, and the presence or absence of coexisting pathologic lesions involving the urethra, the bladder neck, or the bladder itself.

Calculi of the Prostate and Seminal Vesicles

CLASSIFICATION

True prostatic calculi are those that develop in the tissues or acini of the gland and are not to be confused with so-called false calculi that may be urinary calculi lodged in a dilated prostatic urethra or in a pouch of the urethra. Similarly, a calculus present in an abscess cavity that communicates with the urethra should not be considered a true prostatic calculus.

ETIOLOGY

True prostatic calculi are formed by the deposition of calcareous material on corpora amylacea. Corpora amylacea are small round or ovoid bodies present in the alveoli of the prostate gland. They are rare in boys but frequent in men. Corpora amylacea have a laminated structure composed of lecithin and a nitrogenous substance of an albuminous nature, which is apparently formed around desquamated epithelial cells. Inorganic salts (calcium phosphate and calcium carbonate) impregnate the corpora amylacea, converting them into calculi. Sutor and Wooley (1974b) observed that some prostatic calculi probably arise from precipitation of salts found in normal prostatic fluid, that is, calcium and magnesium phosphates; other authors have held that the corpora amylacea may serve only as nuclei. Infection also contributes to formation of some prostatic calculi.

INCIDENCE

The frequency of prostatic calculi is not known, since in many instances they are noted incidentally during a routine roentgenographic survey. Joly (1931) observed 34 cases of prostatic calculi in a series of 636 cases of urinary calculi, an incidence of 5.3 per cent. Stones in the seminal vesicles are an extremely rare condition. White (1928) reported one case (not confirmed by vesiculotomy); the patient was 48 years old. White found only one other case reported in the literature.

Prostatic calculi are rarely observed in boys and are infrequent in men less than 40 years of age. The majority occur in men aged 50 to 65 years. Calculi in the seminal vesicles also occur more frequently in elderly men.

PHYSICAL CHARACTERISTICS

Prostatic calculi vary in number from a single one to several hundred. Generally, they are multiple and range in size from 1 mm to 3 or 4 cm in diameter. They are brownish gray and round or ovoid. Small stones are usually smooth, but large and multiple calculi occupying a single cavity may be definitely faceted. They are usually firm in consistency but can be readily crushed.

Calculi in the seminal vesicles may be single or multiple and are brown. The nucleus is composed of epithelial cells and a mucoid substance that is covered with lime salts. The stones are smooth and hard and range in size from 1 to 2 mm to 1 cm in diameter.

COMPOSITION

Generally, stones in the prostate are composed of calcium phosphates. Huggins and Bear (1944) observed that the organic components, which compose about 20 per cent of the calculus, include proteins (8 per cent), cholesterol (from 3.7 to 10.6 per cent), and citrate (from 0.17 to 2.9 per cent). True prostatic calculi are composed solely of calcium phosphate trihydrate (whitlockite) and carbonate (Sutor and Wooley, 1974b). Whenever such nuclei or nuclei of urinary stones become trapped in prostatic ducts, they are exposed to the urine and may therefore have the same composition as urinary calculi. The amount of carbonate is somewhat less than that in bone; otherwise, chemical and roentgenographic analyses show a close similarity between the inorganic constituents of prostatic calculi and bone salts. Huggins and Bear also stated that corpora amylacea may occasionally be seen in the anterior segment of the prostate, but corpora amylacea occur mostly in the posterior segment, where most true calculi of the prostate are found.

PATHOLOGIC CHANGES

In the presence of minute calculi, the only pathologic change in the prostate may be chronic inflammation with areas of round cell infiltration. The acini may be filled with debris and desquamated epithelial cells, and the acini themselves may or may not be dilated.

When large calculi are present, the ducts and acini may be dilated, and the surrounding cavities may vary in size and shape. Their epithelial lining is absent, and round cell infiltration and fibrosis are observed between the acini.

Occasionally, in the presence of a large calculus, little normal prostatic tissue is identifiable. Calculi are found either in the mouths of the ducts or deep in the gland. They are not usually observed in the adenomatous element of the gland but are adherent to the surface of a surgically removed adenoma. This explains the finding of calculi adjacent to the plane of nucleation of the adenoma at the time of suprapubic prostatectomy. When there has been infection or suppuration of long standing, periprostatitis may occur along with possible abscess formation and eventual rupture into the urethra. When there is a calculus in the seminal vesicle, chronic inflammatory changes with fibrosis are usually present, and the duct may be completely blocked.

SYMPTOMS

There are no symptoms pathognomonic of calculous disease of the prostate gland, and in many cases there may be no suspicion of its presence. Symptoms, when present, may be due to prostatic hypertrophy, stricture of the urethra, or chronic prostatitis. Prostatic calculi contain and harbor bacteria, just as infected renal calculi do (Eykyn et al., 1974). In some instances, small prostatic calculi may be brought in by the patient after he has passed them spontaneously with the urine. This patient may complain of dull aching pain in the lower back, perineum, or penis. Difficulty in voiding, lack of force of the stream, and dribbling will occur if there is concomitant urethral stricture or prostatic hypertrophy. Sometimes urethral discharge exists because of chronic prostatitis.

Hematuria is not usually observed, but terminal urinary bleeding may be present. Abscess formation due to calculi is uncommon but may occur. A patient with prostatic abscess has severe deep pain in the perineum and rectum that is aggravated by defecation. Temperature is elevated, and general constitutional symptoms may be pronounced. The prostate gland is exquisitely tender to palpation. If cystitis is present, dysuria, nocturia, and frequency of micturition occur. A stone in the seminal vesicle may be silent and produce no symptoms. In the cases reported, hematospermia, painful erections, and perineal discomfort at the time of ejaculation have occurred (Drach, 1975).

PHYSICAL DIAGNOSIS OF PROSTATIC CALCULI

The diagnosis is established by rectal palpation of the prostate gland, urethroscopic examination, and roentgenographic study (Fig.

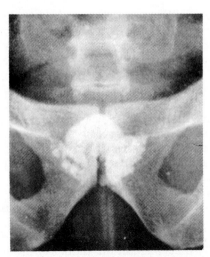

Figure 25–37. Prostatic calculi.

25–37). On rectal examination, the prostate gland may be enlarged, or there may be no findings that suggest calculi. Prostatic enlargement occurs in about 70 per cent of cases. The prostate is firm and movable, and the borders are well defined. When the calculi are large, crepitation may be elicited in 18 to 20 per cent of cases; crepitation is usually most evident near the base of the gland. The consistency of the gland and its contour will vary. It may be smooth or nodular, firm or hard. In the presence of large calculi, localized areas of stony hardness are noted. In 18 to 22 per cent of cases, nodules are palpable, while the remaining tissue is of normal consistency. These nodules may be confused with prostatic carcinoma.

When a calculus is present in a seminal vesicle, the prostate is usually of normal consistency, while the involved vesicle is stony hard and fixed. Crepitation is elicited if multiple calculi are present.

Prostatic calculi, as noted earlier, may be wrongly interpreted upon physical examination as carcinoma. The prostate gland with carcinomatous involvement is usually fixed, but in the presence of calculi it usually is movable. In carcinoma of the prostate, the gland is stony hard, and extension toward the seminal vesicle is often demonstrable. Crepitation is absent in cases of carcinoma, and usually the tissue between any multiple nodules is not of normal consistency. Determination of acid-phosphatase concentration, needle biopsy of the prostate, and roentgenographic study may separate prostatic carcinoma from prostatic calculi.

Calculi in the prostate gland must also be differentiated from tuberculosis, which is more frequently observed in young than in old patients. One or both vesicles may be involved, and tuberculosis of the epididymis may be present.

Panendoscopic examination may reveal only the presence of prostatic enlargement in patients with prostatic calculi. Occasionally a grating is felt upon passing the urethroscope. Rectal palpation of the prostate with the instrument in the urethra may confirm crepitation. A small calculus sometimes protrudes into and obstructs the urethra.

Roentgenographic study usually confirms diagnosis of prostatic calculi (Fig. 25–37). Three characteristic types of shadows may be observed. Diffuse shadows may be generally distributed throughout the gland, since such calculi are extremely small and occupy much of the gland. In other, more frequently observed types, there are so-called horseshoe or ring arrangements. In the ring type, the shadows surround a clear central portion formed by the urethra. In the horseshoe type, the stones are present on both sides of the gland but are absent anterior to the urethra, as evidenced by the clear space that is the opening of the horseshoe. In other instances, a large solitary calculus is observed, or the prostate gland appears to be completely replaced by calculus formation.

A diagnosis of stone in the seminal vesicle is made by rectal palpation, which demonstrates a hard, tender, smooth nodule in the vesicle. Large calculi may be revealed by roentgenographic study, which shows mottled shadows in the region of the vesicle.

TREATMENT

In so-called cases of silent asymptomatic prostatic calculi, no treatment is indicated. Three methods of treatment are available when surgical relief is necessary.

In recent years enthusiasm has been expressed for the transurethral removal of prostatic stones. This procedure may produce temporary relief, but it does not guarantee removal of all calculi, and recurrent stone formation may ensue. It may be utilized in young patients to avoid impairment of sexual activity or in the aged patient who is a poor surgical risk. Suprapubic removal may be advocated in the presence of a large stone or stones or when there is significant prostatic hypertrophy. Perineal prostatotomy may be indicated for the removal of some deep stones in the prostate. In the presence of multiple calculi, total perineal prostatectomy and bilateral seminal vesiculectomy will usually afford a cure.

RECURRENCE

Recurrence of prostatic calculi may follow prostatotomy. New stones can form in the remaining cavities of the gland. False recurrences—that is, stones overlooked at the time of operation—may be observed. Therefore, after operation, roentgenograms should be obtained before the patient is dismissed from the hospital. True or new calculus formation may also occur after transurethral resection. Complete elimination of signs follows total retropubic or perineal prostatectomy.

Urethral Calculi

IN THE MALE

The majority of urethral calculi in the male consist of stones expelled from the bladder into the urethra. Their progress through the urethral canal may be arrested with final impaction in the urethral canal. Rarely, a calculus may form primarily in the urethra when stricture is present, or it may form in a pouch or diverticulum that opens into the urethra.

Incidence. Among natives in the Oriental countries, urethral calculi are common in children because stones of the bladder are also frequent.

Position and Composition. A stone's progress through the normal urethra may be arrested in the prostatic urethra, the bulb, the anterior portion of the perineal urethra, the fossa navicularis, or the external meatus. It may also become impacted at the site of a urethral stricture. Englisch (1904), in a review of 361 cases, observed that in 41.2 per cent the stones were in the posterior urethra; in 18.8 per cent they were in the bulb; in 28.4 per cent they were in the scrotal and penile portions; and in 11.3 per cent they were in the fossa navicularis.

Calculi that migrate to the urethra obviously have the same constituents as bladder or upper urinary tract calculi, because they originate in either the bladder or the kidney. If there is associated infection, a primary urethral calculus is composed of struvite. Usually only a single stone is encountered.

Symptoms. While urinating, the patient with a urethral calculus may experience a sudden stoppage and be therefore unable to empty the bladder. Dribbling also occurs. Pain occasioned by the stone in the urethra may be rather severe and may radiate to the head of the penis. When the calculus is lodged in the posterior urethra, the pain is referred to the perineum or the rectum. When the calculus is lodged in the anterior urethra, the pain may be localized at the site of impaction, and the patient will be aware of a palpable mass. With increased efforts to void, the calculus may be expelled. Complete obstruction requires temporary catheterization or, if that is not possible, immediate removal of the stone.

A stone may be present in a diverticulum of the urethra for an extended period without producing symptoms. A urethral discharge may be observed, the result of infection in the diverticulum. The patient may be aware of a lump that has gradually increased in size and hardness on the undersurface of the penis. This lump may at times become exquisitely tender. There is usually no change in the caliber of the stream of urine and no dribbling.

Diagnosis. Diagnosis may be established by palpation of the penis or the perineum. Rectal palpation may disclose the presence of a calculus in the posterior urethra. The tentative diagnosis may be confirmed by panendoscopic examination or roentgenography (Fig. 25–38). Likewise, a grating may be felt upon attempts to pass a sound.

Treatment. Treatment is influenced by the size, shape, and position of the calculus and by the status of the urethra. At times, a stone in the anterior urethra may be grasped and removed with forceps; pressure is exerted simultaneously on the urethra proximal to the stone so that it is not forced into the bladder. A small stone may sometimes be gently massaged or milked outward, so that it can be expelled. Removal of a stone via the urethroscope may be advisable. When a stricture obstructs passage

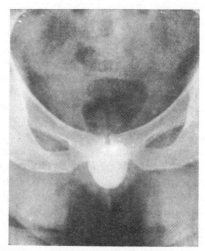

Figure 25–38. Calculus in a diverticulum of the urethra (female).

of the stone, a preliminary internal urethrotomy may be performed. When a large stone has been impacted for some time in the urethra, an external urethrotomy may be required. A calculus lodged in the fossa navicularis can be removed by meatotomy.

A calculus recently impacted in the posterior urethra frequently may be pushed back into the bladder and then crushed. When the stone is large and definitely fixed, it may be removed by the perineal or suprapubic route, depending upon the personal preference of the surgeon. A urethrovesical calculus is best removed by the suprapubic route. External urethrotomy of the penile urethra should be avoided, if possible, because of the danger of fistula formation.

When the calculus occupies a urethral diverticulum, diverticulectomy should also be performed. In past years, recurrence was frequently reported, and many of the stones re-formed in the diverticulum. At present, correction of urethral strictures, diverticulectomy, and adequate therapy to eradicate the infection are followed by extremely satisfactory end results.

IN THE FEMALE

The occurrence of urethral calculi in women is infrequent in comparison with that in men. This may be attributed to two factors—the short urethra in women that permits passage of any calculus and the infrequency of vesical calculi in women. Calculi in the female urethra are usually associated with a urethral diverticulum or a urethrocele (Fig. 25–38).

The urethral diverticulum is a pouch formed by dilatation of a portion of the urethrovaginal septum, and it communicates with the urethral canal. The opening of the pouch into the urethra may be wide or narrow and tubular. If the mouth of the diverticulum is wide, it is doubtful that calculus formation can occur, for stone formation in a diverticulum is usually due to urinary stasis and stagnation with infection, which allows the precipitation of urinary salts. Theoretically, therefore, the presence of a calculus in a diverticulum would presuppose a narrow opening between the urethra and the diverticulum.

Symptoms and Diagnosis. The symptoms of urethral diverticulum, with or without calculus, are those of infection of the lower urinary tract, including frequency, dysuria, nocturia, pyuria, and, in rare instances, hematuria. Pain during coitus is a prominent symptom. Occasional discharge of pus may occur; this gives the patient only temporary relief. Vaginal examination discloses a hard mass in the anterior vaginal wall.

Treatment. The treatment of a urethrocele or diverticulum containing a calculus is surgical, with excision of the sac containing the calculus. The surgical technique varies according to the personal preference of the operating surgeon.

Preputial Calculi

In regard to pathogenesis, there are three types of preputial calculi. First are calculi arising from inspissated smegma that becomes impregnated with lime salts; these are soft in consistency, brown, and single or multiple. The second type is calculi that form in stagnant urine retained in the sac because of phimosis. These may be multiple or single, round or faceted, and are composed of magnesium ammonium phosphate or calcium phosphate. Third are calculi that have been expelled from the bladder into the urethra and have gained entrance into the preputial sac via the urethral meatus or by ulceration through the fossa navicularis. Most of these are grayish and are usually composed of phosphates.

Preputial calculi usually form when phimosis is present; in this country these calculi are rare. Thompson (1921) reported 116 cases from the Canton Hospital. The condition is rarely observed in childhood; it is primarily a disease of adult life. There may be no symptoms referable to the calculus, although the patient may be aware of the presence of a lump for a considerable period. The usual symptoms are those of balanoposthitis. A discharge from the small opening in the foreskin, edema, and, in the late stages, ulceration may be present. Carcinoma may also coexist when the calculus has been present for a long time.

The diagnosis is established by palpation of the stone.

When an acute infection is present, a dorsal slit should be performed to establish drainage. The ultimate treatment consists of circumcision.

ROLE OF SURGERY IN THE TREATMENT OF URINARY CALCULI

Most of this chapter has been concerned with the etiology, diagnosis, and nonsurgical therapy of urinary calculi. It may be anticipated, however, that approximately 50 per cent or more of patients with urinary calculous disease will at some time or other require treatment by surgical means. For this reason, development of a surgical plan for many patients is critical. It must include all aspects of the medical treatment of urinary calculi, including possible preoperative antibiotic therapy, adjustment of fluid intake, correction of dietary and metabolic abnormalities, and complete elimination of all obstructing calculi from the kidneys, ureters, and bladder so that postoperative preventive medical therapy may be effective. If even small stone nuclei are left within the kidney, it is possible for new crystals to grow upon the surface of the retained nucleus and to re-create stone disease. Only by total prevention of stone formation in the patient can one achieve the goals of combined surgical and medical therapy and prevent further complications.

FUTURE OUTLOOK FOR HUMAN UROLITHIASIS

It is clear that there have been major advances in our understanding of the etiology, diagnosis, and treatment of urinary calculous disease of all types. The cause of stone disease due to cystinuria, hyperuricosuria, or infection has been defined as simple physicochemical excesses of particular elements in the urine at a given pH and temperature of 37°C. It now appears that calcium oxalate and calcium phosphate urinary lithiasis may also be based on relatively simple physicochemical processes of supersaturation of urine with these substances. But whether calcium oxalate and/or calcium phosphate supersaturation is the sole initiating event is at present difficult to determine. Because these crystals often form in the urine of normal individuals, it is not likely that the simple precipitation of either element is the one causative factor in calcium stone disease. It seems much more likely that patients with calcium stone disease lack some limiting factor or inhibitor that prohibits the growth and aggregation of "normal" crystals before they grow too large to be passed from the urinary tract. Matrix may be important in this process as either a normal inhibitor or an abnormal initiator of stone growth.

There is still much to be done in discovery of new treatments for stone disease. Many of our present drug treatments are used empirically, and their mechanisms of action in improving urinary lithiasis are not known. Many drugs succeed despite paradoxical effects on urine components. For example, oral phosphate treatment of calcium oxalate urinary lithiasis reduces the concentration of urinary calcium, but it simultaneously increases the concentration of urinary oxalate and phosphate, which should enhance calcium oxalate or phosphate precipitation. May we presume that there is a greater degree of decrease in calcium than of increase in oxalate or phosphate? If so, how can we measure these differences? The publications by Robertson and colleagues (1976, 1983) may give us a means to do this, and the work of Pak and colleagues (1974, 1982) in defining precipitation of brushite as a possible factor in the initiation of urolithiasis may lead to the answers to some of these questions.

Whatever the mode of medical treatment ultimately instituted, the major problem of urinary stone disease is the fact that the patient discovers it himself. When he arrives at the physician's office he already *has* stone disease. In many instances, he is already beyond the point of medical therapy, and surgical intervention is required. The real advances in treatment of stone disease will come when we can survey prospectively at reasonable cost all high-risk individuals and ascertain early in life the defects that may predispose them to urinary calculous disease. Perhaps approaches such as the diagnostic index of Sarig et al. (1982) will help us in the prospective detection of risk of urinary lithiasis. Based upon this information, a plan of lifetime prophylaxis can be designed so that the significant morbidity and mortality of urinary lithiasis will not become a problem for them (Scott, 1975).

References

Admirand, W. H., Earnest, D. L., and Williams, H. E.: Hyperoxaluria and bowel disease. Trans. Assoc. Am. Physicians, *84*:307, 1971.

Albright, F., and Reifenstein, E. C., Jr.: Parathyroid Glands and Metabolic Bone Disease. Baltimore, The Williams & Wilkins Co., 1948.

Albright, F., Suby, H., and Sulkowitch, H. W.: *In* Parathyroid Glands and Metabolic Bone Disease. Baltimore, The Williams & Wilkins Co., 1948.

Al-Dabbagh, T. G., and Fahadi, K.: Seasonal variations in the incidence of ureteric colic. Br. J. Urol., *49*:269, 1977.

Alken, C. E., May, P., and Braun, J. S.: Analysis of treatment results in uric acid lithiasis with and without hyperuricemia. Adv. Exp. Med. Biol., *41*:535, 1974.

Allen, T. D., and Spence, H. M.: Matrix stone. J. Urol., *95*:284, 1966.

Amar, A. D.: Bladder filling maneuver for visualization of calculus in lower ureter. JAMA, *219*:621, 1972.

Amin, H. A.: Urethral calculi. Br. J. Urol., *45*:192, 1973.

Amin, M., and Howerton, L. W.: Spontaneous rupture of the ureter. South. Med. J., *67*:1498, 1974.

Andersen, D. A.: Benurestat, a urease inhibitor for the therapy of infected urolithiasis. Invest. Urol., *12*:381, 1975.

Andersen, D. A.: Environmental factors in the etiology of urolithiasis in urinary calculi. *In* Rapado, A., and Hodgkinson, A. (Eds.) New York, S. Karger, 1973.

Andersen, D. A.: Historical and geographical differences in the pattern of incidence of urinary stones considered in relation to possible aetiological factors. *In* Hodgkinson, A., and Nordin, B. E. C. (Eds.): Renal Stone Research Symposium, p. 7. London, J. & A. Churchill Ltd., 1969.

Andersen, D. A.: The nutritional significance of primary bladder stone. Br. J. Urol., *34*:160, 1962.

Anderson, E. E.: The management of ureteral calculi. Urol. Clin. North Am., *1*:357, 1974.

Anderson, E. E., Rundles, R. W., Silberman, H. R., et al.: Allopurinol control of hyperuricosuria; a new concept in the prevention of uric acid stones. J. Urol., *97*:344, 1967.

Andren-Sandberg, A.: Permanent impairment of renal function demonstrated by renographic follow-up in ureterolithiasis. Scand. J. Urol. Nephrol., *17*:81, 1983.

Arnaud, C. D.: Parathyroid hormone: Coming of age in clinical medicine. Am. J. Med., *55*:577, 1973.

Arnaud, C. D., and Strewler, G. J.: Primary hyperparathyroidism. Semin. Nephrol., *1*:376, 1981.

Atkinson, R. L., Jr., and Earll, J. M.: Munchausen syndrome with renal stones. JAMA, *230*:89, 1974.

Atsmon, A., De Vries, A., and Frank, M.: Uric Acid Lithiasis. Amsterdam, Elsevier Publishing Co., 1963.

Aubert, J.: Calculous anuria and spontaneous rupture of the kidney pelvis. Importance of intravenous urography in the anuric patient. Acta Urol. Belg., *41*:396, 1973.

Aurora, A. L., Teneia, O. P., and Gupta, D. N.: Bladder stone disease of childhood. II. A clinico-pathological study. Acta Paediatr. Scand., *59*:385, 1970.

Auvray, P.: Ureterocele and lithiasis. Acta Urol. Belg., *40*:720, 1972.

Ayvazian, J. H.: Xanthinuria and hemochromatosis. N. Engl. J. Med., *270*:18, 1964.

Bach, D., Hesse, A., and Vahlensieck, W.: Citric acid excretion in stone-formers and healthy controls on normal and standard diet. Urologe [A], *19*:220, 1980.

Baggio, B., Gambaro, G., Ossi, E., Favaro, S., and Borsatti, A.: Uncreased urinary excretion of renal enzymes in idiopathic calcium oxalate nephrolithiasis. J. Urol., *129*:1161, 1983.

Bailey, R. R., Dann, E., Greenslade, N. F., et al.: Urinary stones: A prospective study of 350 patients. N.Z. Med. J., *79*:961, 1974.

Baker, R., and Connelly, J. P.: Bilateral and recurrent renal calculi: Evidence indicating renal collagen abnormality and results of salicylate therapy. JAMA, *160*:1106, 1956.

Barker, L. M., Pallante, S. L., Eisenberg, H., et al.: Simple synthetic and natural urines have equivalent anticalcifying properties. Invest. Urol., *12*:79, 1974.

Barnhouse, D. H.: In vitro formation of precipitates in sterile and infected urines. Invest. Urol., *5*:342, 1968.

Bastian, H. P., and Gebhardt, M.: The varying composition of the nucleus and peripheral layers of urinary calculi. Urol. Res., *2*:91, 1974.

Bateson, E. M.: Renal tract calculi and climate. Med. J. Aust., *2*:111, 1973.

Becher, R. M., Bhupendra, M. T., and Newman, H. R.: Giant vesical calculus. JAMA, *239*:2272, 1978.

Beck, C. W., and Mulvaney, W. P.: Apatitic urinary calculi from early American Indians. JAMA, *195*:168, 1966.

Bennett, A. H., and Colodny, A. H.: Urinary tract calculi in children. J. Urol, 109:318, 1973.

Berenyi, M.: Models for the formation of uric acid and urate stones. Int. Urol. Nephrol., *4*:199, 1972.

Berenyi, M., Frang, D., and Legrady, J.: Theoretical and clinical importance of the differentiation between the two types of calcium oxalate hydrate. Int. Urol. Nephrol., *4*:341, 1972.

Berlin, T., Bjorkhem, I., Collste, L., Holmberg, I., and Wijkstrom, H.: Relation between hypercalciuria and vitamin D3–status in patients with urolithiasis. Scand. J. Urol. Nephrol., *16*:269, 1982.

Berman, L. B.: Renal geology. JAMA, *231*:865, 1975.

Berson, S. A., and Yalow, R. S.: Parathyroid hormone in plasma in adenomatous hyperparathyroidism, uremia and bronchiogenic carcinoma. Science, *154*:907, 1966.

Bichler, K. H., et al.: Uromucoid excretion of normal individuals and stone formers. Br. J. Urol., *47*:733, 1976.

Blacklock, N. J.: The pattern of urolithiasis in the Royal Navy. *In* Hodgkinson, A., and Nordin, B. E. C. (Eds.): Renal Stone Research Symposium, p. 33. London, J. & A. Churchill, Ltd., 1969.

Blacklock, N. J., and Macleod, M. A.: Calcium-47 absorption in urolithiasis. Br. J. Urol., *46*:377, 1947a.

Blacklock, N. J., and Macleod, M. A.: The effect of cellulose phosphate on intestinal absorption and urinary excretion of calcium. Some experience in its use in the treatment of calcium stone formation. Br. J. Urol., *46*:385, 1974b.

Blaivas, J. G., Pais, V. M., and Spellman, R. M.: Chemolysis of residual stone fragments after extensive surgery for staghorn calculi. Urology, *6*:680, 1975.

Bone, H. G., Zerwekh, J. E., Britton, F., and Pak, C. Y. C.: Treatment of calcium urolithiasis with diphosphonate: Efficacy and hazards. J. Urol., *121*:568, 1979.

Boquist, L., Lindqvist, B., Osterberg, Y., et al.: Primary oxalosis. Am. J. Med., *54*:673, 1973.

Borden, T. A.: Methylene blue and experimental stone disease in the rat. Invest. Urol., *4*:161, 1966.

Borgmann, V., and Nagel, R.: Urolithiasis in childhood—a study of 181 cases. Urol. Int., *37*: 198, 1982.

Borkowski, A., and Czapliczki, M.: Nontraumatic extravasation from the ureter. Int. Urol. Nephrol., *5*:271, 1974.

Bourke, E., and Costello, J.: The clinical importance of oxalic acid. Ir. Med. J., *68*:93, 1975.

Boyce, W. H.: Some observations on the ultrastructure of idiopathic human renal calculi. *In* Finlayson, B., Hench, L. L., and Smith, L. G. (Eds.): Urolithiasis: Physical Aspects, p. 97. Washington, D.C., National Academy of Sciences, 1972.

Boyce, W. H.: Organic matrix of native human urinary concretions. *In* Hodgkinson, A., and Nordin, B. E. C. (Eds.): Renal Stone Research Symposium, p. 93. London, J. & A. Churchill, Ltd., 1969.

Boyce, W. H.: Organic matrix of human urinary concretions. Am. J. Med., *45*:673, 1968.

Boyce, W. H.: The renal tubule in the genesis of renal calculi. *In* Proceedings of the Third International Congress of Nephrology, Washington, D.C., 1966. Vol. 2, p. 354. New York, S. Karger, 1967.

Boyce, W. H., and Elkins, I. B.: Reconstructive renal surgery following anatrophic nephrolithotomy: Follow-up of 100 consecutive cases. J. Urol., *111*:307, 1974.

Boyce, W. H., and Garvey, F. K.: The amount and nature of the organic matrix in urinary calculi: A review. J. Urol., *76*:213, 1956.

Boyce, W. H., and King, J. S., Jr.: Crystal-matrix interrelations in calculi. J. Urol., *81*:351, 1959.

Boyce, W. H., Garvey, F. K., and Strawcutter, H. E.: Incidence of urinary calculi among patients in general hospitals, 1948–1952. JAMA, *161*:1437, 1956.

Boyce, W. H., King, J. S., and Fielden, M. L.: Total nondialysable solids (TNDS) of human urine. XIII. Immunological detection of a component peculiar to renal calculous matrix and to urine of calculous patients. J. Clin. Invest., *41*:1180, 1962.

Boyce, W. H., McKenny, W. M., Long, T. T., et al.: Oral administration of methylene blue to patients with renal calculi. J. Urol., *97*:783, 1967.

Braasch, W. F., and Moore, A. B.: Stones in the ureter. JAMA, *65*:123, 1915.

Breatnach, E., and Smith, S. E. W.: The radiology of renal stones in children. Clin. Radiol., *34*:59, 1983.

Breslau, N. A., and Pak, C. Y. C.: Urinary saturation, heterogeneous nucleation, and crystallization inhibitors in nephrolithiasis. *In* Coe, F. L., Brenner, B. M., and Stein, J. H. (Eds.): Nephrolithiasis. New York, Churchill-Livingstone, 1980.

Brickman, A. M., Ellison, A. F., Kliger, A. S., Lang, R., and Broadus, A. E.: Low urine volume in stone formers. Ann. Intern. Med., *93*:644, 1980.

Brickman, A. S., Massry, S. G., and Coburn, J. W.: Changes in serum and urinary calcium during treatment with hydrochlorothiazide: Studies on mechanisms. J. Clin. Invest., *51*:945, 1972.

Broadus, A. E., and Thier, S. O.: Metabolic basis of renal-stone disease. N. Engl. J. Med., *300*:839, 1979.

Broadus, A. E., Dominguez, M., and Barrter, F. C.: Pathophysiologic studies in idiopathic hypercalciuria: use of an oral calcium tolerance test to characterize distinctive hypercalciuric subgroups. J. Clin. Endocrinol. Metab., *47*:751, 1978.

Brockis, J. G., Bowyer, R. C., McCulloch, R. K., Taylor, T. A., Wisniewski, Z. S., et al.: Pathophysiology of endemic bladder stones. In press.

Brueziere, J., Gueriot, J. C., and Begue, P.: Idiopathic renal lithiasis in infants. Report of 40 cases. J. Urol. Nephrol. (Paris), *80*:589, 1974.

Buck, A. C., Lote, C. J., and Sampson, W. F.: The influence of renal prostaglandins on urinary calcium excretion on idiopathic urolithiasis. J. Urol., *129*:421, 1983.

Bumpus, H. C., Jr., and Thompson, G. J.: Ureteral stones. Surg. Clin. North Am., *5*:812, 1925.

Bunts, R. C.: Management of urological complications in 1000 paraplegics. J. Urol., *79*:733, 1958.

Burch, P. R. J., and Dawson, J. B.: Aetiological implications of the sex and age distribution of renal lithiasis. *In* Hodgkinson, A., and Nordin, B. E. C. (Eds.): Renal Stone Research Symposium, p. 71. London, J. & A. Churchill, Ltd., 1969.

Burkland, C. E., and Rosenberg, M.: Survey of urolithiasis in the United States. J. Urol., *73*:198, 1955.

Burr, R. C.: Urinary calcium, magnesium, crystals and stones in paraplegia. Paraplegia, *10*:56, 1972.

Burr, R. C., and Walsh, J. J.: Urinary calcium and kidney stones in paraplegia. Report of an attempted prospective study. Paraplegia, *12*:38, 1974.

Busby, D. E.: Urinary calculus. Space Life Sci., *1*:279, 1968.

Butler, A. M., Wilson, J. L., and Farber, S. J.: Dehydration and acidosis with calcification at renal tubules. J. Pediatr., *8*:489, 1936.

Butt, A. J.: Historical survey of etiologic factors in renal lithiasis. *In* Etiologic Factors in Renal Lithiasis, p. 6. Springfield, Ill., Charles C Thomas, 1956.

Care, A. D., Duncan, T., and Webster, D.: Thyrocalcitonin and its role in calcium homeostasis. J. Endocrinol., *37*:115, 1967.

Carlson, K. P., Bates, H. N., and Boyce, W. H.: Death due to parathyroid crisis. J. Urol., *84*:219, 1960.

Carr, R. J.: Aetiology of renal calculi: Micro-radiographic studies. *In* Hodgkinson, A., and Nordin, B. E. C. (Eds.): Renal Stone Research Symposium, p. 123. London, J. & A. Churchill, Ltd., 1969.

Cartstensen, H. E., and Hansen, T. S.: Stones in the ureter. Acta Chir. Scand. (Suppl.), *433*:66, 1973.

Catalina, R., and Cifuentes, L.: Calcium oxalate: Crystallographic analysis in solid aggregate in urinary sediment. Science, *169*:183, 1970.

Cato, A. R., and Tulloch, A. G. S.: Hypermagnesemia in a uremic patient during renal pelvic irrigation with prenacidin. J. Urol., *111*:313, 1974.

Cattolica, E. V., and Hinman, F.: Spontaneous passage of large calculi from true and false ureteroceles. Urol. Int., *28*:65, 1973.

Caulfield, J. B., and Schrag, P. E.: Electron microscopic study of renal calcification. Am. J. Pathol., *44*:365, 1964.

Chabal, J., Goudot, E. E., and Odoulami, H.: Urinary lithiasis in African children in Senegal (45 cases). Bull. Soc. Med. Afr. Noire Lang. Fr., *17*:195, 1972.

Chakmakjian, Z. H., and Bethune, J. E.: Sodium sulfate treatment of hypercalcemia. N. Engl. J. Med., *275*:862, 1966.

Chambers, E. L., Jr., Gordon, G. S., Goldman, L., et al.: Tests for hyperparathyroidism; tubular reabsorption of phosphate, phosphate deprivation, and calcium infusion. J. Clin. Endocrinol., *16*:1507, 1956.

Chambers, R. M., and Dormandy, T. L.: Hypercalciuria—relative and absolute. *In* Hodgkinson, A., and Nordin, B. E. C. (Eds.): Renal Stone Research Symposium, p. 233. London, J. & A. Churchill, Ltd., 1969.

Chase, L. R., and Aurbach, G. D.: Parathyroid function and renal excretion of 3′,5′-adenylic acid. Proc. Natl. Acad. Sci., *58*:518, 1967.

Chertow, B. S., Baylink, D. J., Wergedal, J. E., et al.: Decrease in serum immunoreactive parathyroid hormone in rats and in parathyroid hormone secretion in vitro by 1, 25-dihydroxycholecalciferol. J. Clin. Invest., *56*:668, 1975.

Chow, F. H., Hamar, D. W., Udall, R. H., et al.: Urinary calculi matrices and urine polyelectrolytes. Proc. Soc. Exp. Biol. Med., *144*:912, 1973.

Chulkaratana, S., Van Reen, R., and Valyasevi, A.: Studies of bladder stone disease in Thailand. XV. Factors affecting the solubility of calcium oxalate. Invest. Urol., *9*:246, 1971.

Churchill, D. N., Maloney, C. M., Bear, J., Bryant, D. G., Fodor, G., and Gault, M. H.: Urolithiasis—a study of drinking water hardness and genetic factors. J. Chron. Dis., *33*:727, 1980.

Cifuentes, L., Rapado, A., Abehsera, A., et al.: Uric acid lithiasis and gout. *In* Urinary Calculi. International Symposium on Renal Stone Research, p. 115. Basel, S. Karger, 1973.

Clark, P. B., and Nordin, B. E. C.: The problem of the calcium stone. *In* Hodgkinson, A., and Nordin, B. E. C. (Eds.): Renal Stone Research Symposium, p. 1. London, J. & A. Churchill, Ltd., 1969.

Claus-Walker, J., Campos, R. J., Carter, R. E., et al.: Electrolytes in urinary calculi and urine of patients with spinal cord injuries. Arch. Phys. Med. Rehabil., *54*:109, 1973.

Claypool, H. R., Lind, T. A., Haber, K., and Freundlich, I.: Comparison of drip infusion and bolus techniques in excretory urography as a routine examination. Ariz. Med., 1975.

Clendening, L.: Sourcebook of Medical History, p. 14. New York, Dover Publications, Inc., 1942.

Coe, F. L.: Calcium–uric acid nephrolithiasis. Arch. Intern. Med., *138*:1090, 1978.

Coe, F. L.: Treated and untreated recurrent calcium nephrolithiasis in patients with idiopathic hypercalciuria, hyperuricosuria, or no metabolic disorder. Ann. Intern. Med., *87*:404, 1977.

Coe, F. L.: The performance of a computer system for metabolic assessment of patients with nephrolithiasis. Comput. Biomed. Res., *7*:40, 1974.

Coe, F. L., and Davalach, A. G.: Hypercalciuria and hyperuricosuria in patients with calcium nephrolithiasis. N. Engl. J. Med., *291*:1344, 1974.

Coe, F. L., and Raisen, L.: Allopurinol treatment of uric acid disorders in calcium stone formers. Lancet, *1*:129, 1973.

Coe, F. L., Keck, J., and Norton, E. R.: The natural history of calcium urolithiasis. JAMA, *238*:1519, 1977.

Coe, F. L., Margolis, H. C., Deutsch, L. H., and Strauss, A. L.: Urinary macromolecular crystal growth inhibitors in calcium nephrolithiasis. Min. Electrolyte Metab., *3*:268, 1980.

Cohanim, M., and Yendt, E. R.: The effects of thiazides on serum and urinary zinc in patients with renal calculi. Johns Hopkins Med. J., *136*:137, 1975.

Cook, D. A.: Treatment of renal stones: Cellulose phosphate or magnesium. N. Engl. J. Med., *291*:1034, 1974.

Copp, D. H.: Endocrine control of calcium homeostasis. J. Endocrinol., *43*:137, 1969.

Copp, D. H., McPherson, G. D., and McIntosh, H. W.: Renal excretion of calcium in man; estimation of Tm-Ca. Metabolism, *9*:680, 1960.

Copp, D. H., Cameron, E. C., Cheney, B. A., Davidson, A. G., and Henze, K. G.: Evidence for calcitonin—a new hormone from the parathyroid that lowers blood calcium. Endocrinology, *70*:638, 1962.

Coppridge, W. M.: Clinical management of ureteral stones. South. Med. J., *33*:18, 1940.

Cox, C. E.: Symposium on renal lithiasis. Urinary tract infection and renal lithiasis. Urol. Clin. North Am., *1*:279, 1974.

Crawford, J. E., Cremty, E. P., and Alexander, A. E.: The effect of natural and synthetic polyelectrolytes on the crystallization of calcium oxalate. Aust. J. Chem., *21*:1967, 1968.

Crawhall, J. C., and Watts, R. W. E.: Cystinuria. Am. J. Med., *45*:736, 1968.

Crawhall, J. C., Scowen, E. F., and Watts, R. W. E.: Effect of penicillamine on cystinuria. Br. Med. J., *1*:588, 1963.

Dalton, D. L., Hughes, J., and Glenn, J. F.: Foreign bodies and urinary stone. Urology, *6*:1, 1975.

DeLuca, H. F.: Vitamin D endocrinology. Ann. Intern. Med., *85*:367, 1976.

Dempsey, E. F., Forbes, A. P., Melick, R. A., et al.: Urinary oxalate excretion. Metabolism, *9*:52, 1960.

Dent, C. E., and Philpot, G. R.: Xanthinuria: Inborn error (or deviation) of metabolism. Lancet, *1*:182, 1954.

Dent, C. E., and Senior, B.: Studies on the treatment of cystinuria. Br. J. Urol., *27*:317, 1955.

Dent, C. E., and Sutor, D. J.: Presence or absence of inhibitor of calcium oxalate crystal growth in urine of normals and of stone formers. Lancet, *2*:775, 1971.

Deren, J. J., Porusk, J. G., Levitt, M. G., et al.: Nephrolithiasis as a complication of ulcerative colitis and regional enteritis. Ann. Intern. Med., *56*:843, 1962.

DeVries, A., and Sperling, O.: Familial gouty malignant uric acid lithiasis due to mutant phosphoribosylpyrophosphate synthetase. Urologe [A], *12*:153, 1973.

Dhanamitta, S., Valyasevi, A., and VanReen, R.: Studies of bladder stone disease in Thailand. XI. Effect of 4-hydroxy-L-proline and orthophosphate supplementations on crystalluria. Am. J. Clin. Nutr., *23*:372, 1970.

Dickstein, S. S., and Frame, B.: Urinary tract calculi after intestinal shunt operations for the treatment of obesity. Surg. Gynecol. Obstet., *136*:257, 1973.

Domanski, T. J.: Renal calculi: A new method of qualitative analysis. J. Urol., *37*:399, 1937.

Dourmashkin, R. L.: Cystoscopic treatment of stones in the ureter with special reference to large calculi based on a study of 1550 cases. J. Urol., *54*:245, 1945.

Drach, G. W.: Stone manipulation: Modern usage and occasional mishaps. Urology, *12*:286, 1978.

Drach, G. W.: Transurethral ureteral stone manipulation. Urol. Clin. North Am., *10*:709, 1983.

Drach, G. W.: Urolithiasis. *In* Conn, H. F. (Ed.): Current Therapy, p. 552. Philadelphia, W. B. Saunders Co., 1976a.

Drach, G. W.: Contribution to therapeutic decisions of ratios, absolute values and other measures of calcium, magnesium, urate or oxalate balance in stone formers. J. Urol., *116*:339, 1976b.

Drach, G. W.: Prostatitis: Man's hidden infection. Urol. Clin. North Am., *2*:499, 1975.

Drach, G. W.: Baron Dupuytren, lithotomist (1777–1835). Invest. Urol., *11*:424, 1974a.

Drach, G. W.: Symposium on renal lithiasis. Perioperative aspects of renal stone surgery. Urol. Clin. North Am., *1*:299, 1974b.

Drach, G. W., and Boyce, W. H.: Nephrocalcinosis as a source for renal stone nuclei. Observations on human and squirrel monkeys and on hyperparathyroidism in the squirrel monkey. J. Urol., *197*:897, 1972.

Drach, G. W., and King, J. S.: Estimating aberrant homeostasis: Variance in serum calcium as an aid in diagnosis of hyperparathyroidism. Clin. Chem., *16*:792, 1970.

Drach, G. W., Kraljevich, Z., and Randolph, A.: Effects of high molecular weight urinary molecules on crystallization of calcium oxalate dihydrate. J. Urol., *127*:805, 1982.

Drach, G. W., Robertson, W. G., Scurr, D. S., and Randolph, A. D.: Pyrophosphate inhibition of calcium oxalate dihydrate crystallization in simulated urine: continuous flow studies. World J. Urol., *1*:146, 1983.

Drach, G. W., Smith, M. J. V., and Boyce, W. H.: Medical therapy of renal calculi. J. Urol., *104*:635, 1970.

Dretler, S. P.: The pathogenesis of urinary tract calculi occurring after ileal conduit diversion. I. Clinical study. II. Conduit study. III. Prevention. J. Urol., *109*:204, 1973.

Dretler, S. P., Coggins, C. H., McIver, M. A., and Their, S. O.: The physiologic approach to renal tubular acidosis. J. Urol., *102*:665, 1969.

DuPreez, H. M., and Cremin, B. J.: Urinary calculi in childhood. A clinical and radiological study. S. Afr. Med. J., *47*:1025, 1973.

Dyer, R., and Nordin, B. E. C.: Urinary crystals and their relation to stone formation. Nature, *215*:751, 1967.

Dzhavad-Zade, M. D., and Mamedova, Y. A.: Primary hyperoxaluria in the etiology of urolithiasis and pyelonephritis in children. Pediatria, *62*:9, 1973.

Ehrig, U., Harrison, J. E., and Wilson, D. R.: Effect of long-term thiazide therapy on intestinal calcium absorption in patients with recurrent renal calculi. Metabolism, *23*:139, 1974.

Eisman, J. A., et al.: 1,25-Dihydroxyvitamin D in biological fluids: A simplified and sensitive assay. Science, *193*:1021, 1976.

Elder, T. D., and Wyngaarden, J. B.: The biosynthesis and turnover of oxalate in normal and hyperoxaluric subjects. J. Clin. Invest., *39*:1337, 1960.

Elliot, J. S.: Calcium oxalate urinary calculi: Clinical and chemical aspects. Medicine, *62*:36, 1983.

Elliot, J. S.: Structure and composition of urinary calculi. J. Urol., *109*:82, 1973a.

Elliot, J. S.: *In* Cifuentes, L., Rapado, A., and Hodgkinson, A. (Eds.): Urinary Calculi. International Symposium on Renal Stone Research, p. 24. Basel, S. Karger, 1973*b*.

Elliot, J. S., and Eusebio, E.: Calcium oxalate solubility: The effects of trace metals. J. Invest. Urol., *9*:428, 1967.

Elliot, J. S., and Ribeiro, M. E.: The urinary excretion of trace metals in patients with calcium oxalate urinary stone. Invest. Urol., *10*:253, 1973.

Elliot, J. S., Ribeiro, M. E., and Eusebio, E.: The effect of oral phosphate upon the urinary excretion of oxalic acid. Invest. Urol., 7:528, 1970.

Elliot, J. S., Sharp, R. D., and Lewis, L.: The solubility of struvite in urine. J. Urol., *81*:366, 1959.

Elliott, J. P., Jr.: A stone season. A ten-year retrospective study of 768 surgical stone cases with respect to seasonal variation. J. Urol., *114*:574, 1975.

Ellis, H.: A History of Bladder Stone. Oxford, Blackwell, 1969.

Ellman, P., and Parfitt, A. M.: The resemblance between sarcoidosis with hypercalcemia and hyperparathyroidism. Br. Med. J., *2*:108, 1960.

Emmerson, B. T.: Pathogenesis and management of uric acid calculi. Br. J. Urol., *44*:729, 1972.

Emmett, J. L., and Witten, D. M.: Calculous disease of the genitourinary tract. *In* Clinical Urography, p. 607. Philadelphia, W. B. Saunders Co., 1971.

Englisch, J.: Über eigelagerte und eingesachte Steine der Harnröhre. Arch. Klin. Chir., *72*:487, 1904.

Ettinger, A., Oldroyd, N. O., and Sorgel, F.: Triamterene urolithiasis. JAMA, *244*:2443, 1980.

Evans, J., Sierakowski, R., Hemp, G., et al.: The correlation between the incidence of urolithiasis and local water quality in the United States. (in press).

Eykyn, S., et al.: Prostatic calculi as a source of recurrent bacteriuria in the male. Br. J. Urol., *46*:527, 1974.

Fanelli, G. M.: Urate excretion. Annu. Rev. Med., *28*:349, 1977.

Farmer, R. G., Mir-Madjlessi, S. H., and Kiser, W. S.: Urinary excretion of oxalate, calcium, magnesium, and uric acid in inflammatory bowel disease. Cleve. Clin. Q., *41*:109, 1974.

Farmer, R. G., Mir-Madjlessi, S. H., and Kiser, W. S.: Proceedings: Urinary excretion of oxalate, calcium, magnesium, and uric acid in inflammatory bowel disease and relationship to urolithiasis. Gut, *14*:828, 1973.

Fellstrom, B., Backman, U., Danielson, B. G., Johansson, G., Ljunghall, S., and Wilkstrom, B.: Uricemia and urinary acidification in renal calcium stone disease. J. Urol., *129*:256, 1983.

Fetter, T. L., and Zimskind, P. D.: Statistical analysis of patients with ureteral calculi. JAMA, *186*:21, 1961.

Fikri, E., and Casella, R. R.: Hyperoxaluria and urinary tract calculi after jejunoileal bypass. Am. J. Surg., *129*:334, 1975.

Finkle, A. L., and Smith, D. R.: Parameters of renal functional capacity in reversible hydroureteronephrosis in dogs. V. Effects of 7 to 10 days of ureteral constriction on RBF-Kr, C-In, Tc-H₂O, C-PAH, osmolality, and sodium reabsorption. Invest. Urol., *8*:299, 1970.

Finkle, A. L., Karg, S. J., and Smith, D. R.: Parameters of renal functional capacity in reversible hydroureteronephrosis in dogs. VI. Response to mannitol challenge by the chronically obstructed canine kidney and its clinical implication. J. Urol., *104*:368, 1970.

Finlayson, B.: Physicochemical aspects of urolithiasis. Kidney Int., *13*:344, 1978.

Finlayson, B.: The treatment of urinary stone disease. Aust. N.Z.J. Surg., *50*:13, 1980.

Finlayson, B.: Perspectives in hypertension and nephrology. (in press).

Finlayson, B.: Symposium on renal lithiasis. Renal lithiasis in review. Urol. Clin. North Am., *1*:181, 1974.

Finlayson, B.: The concept of a continuous crystallizer. Invest. Urol., *9*:258, 1972.

Finlayson, B., Reid, F., The expectation of free and fixed particles in urinary stone disease. Invest. Urol. 15:442, 1978.

Finlayson, B., Roth, R., and Dubois, L.: Perturbation of calcium ion activity by urea. Invest. Urol., *10*:138, 1972.

Finlayson, B., and Dubois, L.: Kinetics of calcium oxalate deposition in vitro. Invest. Urol., *10*:429, 1973.

Finlayson, B., and Miller, G. H.: Observations on the kinetics of experimental foreign body lithiasis. J. Urol., *104*:169, 1970.

Finlayson, B., and Roth, R. A.: Appraisal of calcium oxalate solubility in sodium chloride and sodium-calcium chloride solutions. Urology, *1*:142, 1973.

Finlayson, B., and Smith, A.: Spectrophotometry of the stability constant of CaC₂O₄ based on competition between murexide and oxalate for Ca². J. Chem. Eng. Data. (in press).

Finlayson, B., Roth, R. A., and Dubois, L.: Calcium oxalate solubility. *In* Cifuentes, L., Rapado, A., and Hodgkinson, A. (Eds.): Urinary Calculi. International Symposium on Renal Stone Research, p. 1. Basel, S. Karger, 1973.

Finlayson, B., Smith, A., and Dubois, L.: The stability constants of magnesium oxalate complexes. Invest. Urol., *13*:20, 1975.

Finlayson, B., Vermeulen, W., and Stewart, R. J.: Stone matrix and mucoprotein from urine. J. Urol., *86*:355, 1961.

Flannigan, G. M., Clifford, R. P. C., Carver, R. A., Yule, A. G., Madden, N. P., and Towler, J. M.: Indomethacin—an alternative to pethidine in ureteric colic. Br. J. Urol., *55*:6, 1983.

Fleisch, H.: Some new concepts on the pathogenesis and the treatment of urolithiasis. Urol. Int., *19*:372, 1965.

Fleisch, H., and Bisaz, S.: The inhibitory effect of pyrophosphate on calcium oxalate precipitation and its relation to urolithiasis. Experientia, *20*:276, 1964.

Flocks, R. H.: Prophylaxis and medical management of calcium urolithiasis: The role of the quantity and precipitability of the urinary calcium. J. Urol., *44*:183, 1940.

Flocks, R. H.: Calcium and phosphorus excretion in the urine of patients with renal or ureteral calculi. JAMA, *113*:1466, 1939.

Forsman, P. J., and Jenkins, M. E.: Primary hyperparathyroidism in childhood presenting as renal stones. Nebr. Med. J., *57*:87, 1972.

Foye, W. O., et al.: Degree of sulfation in mucopolysaccharide sulfates in normal and stone forming urines. Invest. Urol., *14*:33, 1976.

Frank, M., and DeVries, A.: Prevention of urolithiasis. Arch. Environ. Health, *13*:625, 1966.

Frank, M., DeVries, A., Atsmon, A., et al.: Epidemiological investigation of urolithiasis in Israel. J. Urol., *81*:497, 1959.

Fraser, D., Russell, R. G. G., Pohler, C., et al.: The influence of disodium ethane-1-hydroxyl-1, 1-diphosphonate (EHDP) on the development of experimentally induced urinary stones in rats. Clin. Sci., *42*:197, 1972.

Frayha, R. A., Salti, I. S., Abuhaidar, G. I., et al.: Hereditary xanthinuria and xanthine urolithiasis: An additional three cases. J. Urol., *109*:871, 1973.

Freed, S. Z.: The alternating use of an alkalizing salt and

aceta-zolamide in the management of cystine and uric acid stones. J. Urol., *113*:96, 1975.

Freeman, J. A., and Beeler, M. F.: Laboratory Medicine—Clinical Microscopy, p. 97. Philadelphia, Lea & Febiger, 1974.

Friedlander, A. M., and Braude, A. I.: Production of bladder stones by human T mycoplasmas. Nature, *247*:67, 1974.

Friedman, J., and Raisz, L. G.: Thyrocalcitonin: Inhibitor of bone resorption in tissue culture. Science, *150*:1465, 1965.

Furlow, W. L., and Bucchiere, J. J.: The surgical fate of ureteral calculi: review of Mayo Clinic experience. J. Urol., *116*:559, 1976.

Gahagan, H. O., and Reed, W. K.: Squamous cell carcinoma of the renal pelvis; review of the literature. J. Urol., *62*:139, 1949.

Gardner, B.: Studies of the zeta potential of cells and a silica particle in varying concentrations of albumin, calcium, sodium, plasma and bile. J. Lab. Clin. Med., *73*:202, 1969.

Garrett, R. A., and Holland, J. M.: Milk-of-calcium in caliceal diverticulum. J. Urol., *109*:927, 1973.

Garten, V. A., and Head, R. B.: Nucleation in salt solutions. J. Chem. Soc., *69*:514, 1973.

Gaston, E. A., and Ferrucci, J.: Calculus formation in urethral diverticulum in woman; report of a case. N. Engl. J. Med., *221*:379, 1939.

Gee, W. F., and Kiviat, M. D.: Ureteral response to partial obstruction. Smooth muscle hyperplasia and connective tissue proliferation. Invest. Urol., *12*:309, 1975.

Gentile, A.: True prostatic calculus. J. Urol., *57*:746, 1947.

Geraghty, J. T., and Hinman, F.: Ureteral calculus; special means of diagnosis and newer methods of intravesical treatment. Surg. Gynecol. Obstet., *20*:515, 1915.

Ghazali, S., Barratt, T. M., and Williams, D. I.: Childhood urolithiasis in Britain. Arch. Dis. Child., *48*:291, 1973.

Ghosh, B. N., Mathur, S. C., and Bhat, H. S.: Primary hyperparathyroidism in renal calculi. Int. Surg., *58*:625, 1973.

Gibbs, D. A., and Watts, R. W. E.: The identification of the enzymes that catalyse the oxidation of glyoxylate to oxalate in the 100,000 g supernatant fraction of human hyperoxaluric and control liver and heart tissue. Clin. Sci., *44*:227, 1973.

Gilbert, J. B., and McMillan, S. F.: Cancer of the kidney; squamous cell carcinoma of renal pelvis with special reference to etiology. Ann. Surg., *100*:429, 1934.

Gill, W. B., and Vermeulen, C. W.: Oxamide crystalluria and urolithiasis. Rat and in vitro observations. Invest. Urol., *1*:339, 1964.

Gill, W. B., and Vermeulen, C. W.: Causation of stones by two co-acting agents—Diamox and operative insult on the urinary tract. J. Urol., *88*:103, 1962.

Gill, W. B., Jones, K. W., and Ruggiero, K. J.: Protective effects of heparin and other sulfated glycosaminoglycans on crystal adhesion to injured urothelium. J. Urol., *127*:152, 1982.

Gill, W. B., Silvert, M. A., and Roma, M. J.: Supersaturation levels and crystallization rates of calcium oxalate from urines of normal humans and stone formers determined by a 14C-oxalate technique. Invest. Urol., *12*:203, 1974.

Gittes, R. F., Wells, S. A., and Irvin, G. L., III: New role for the parathyroid glands in calcium homeostasis. J. Urol., *97*:1082, 1967.

Glazenburg, J.: The effect of hydrochlorothiazide on the renal excretion of oxalic acid and on the formation of oxalate stones in the urinary tract. Arch. Chirurg. Neirlandicum, *23*:216, 1971.

Glenn, J. F.: Bladder stones. From lithotrity to ultrasound. Urol. Clin. North Am., *1*:375, 1974.

Goldsmith, R. S., and Ceccarelli, F. E.: Diagnosis of occult hyperparathyroidism by a new rapid calcium infusion test. J. Urol., *89*:487, 1963.

Goldsmith, R. S., and Ingbar, H. S.: Inorganic phosphate treatment of hypercalcemia of diverse etiologies. N. Engl. J. Med., *274*:1, 1966.

Goldstein, A. E.: Familial urological diseases. Am. Surg., *17*:221, 1951.

Goodman, M., Curry, T., and Russell, T.: Xanthogranulomatous pyelonephritis: a local disease with systemic manifestations. Medicine, *58*:171, 1979.

Gram, H. C.: Heredity of oxalic urinary calculi. Acta Med. Scand., *78*:268, 1932.

Grant, A. M. S., Baker, L. R. I., and Neuberger, A.: Urinary Tamm-Horsfall glycoprotein in certain kidney diseases and its content in renal calculi. Clin. Sci., *44*:377, 1973.

Gregory, J. G., Starkloff, E. B., Miyai, K., et al.: Urologic complications of ileal bypass operation for morbid obesity. J. Urol., *113*:521, 1975.

Griffith, D. P.: Urease stones. Urol. Res., *7*:215, 1979.

Griffith, D. P., and Musher, D. M.: Acetohydroxamic acid: Potential use in urinary infection caused by urea-splitting bacteria. Urology, *5*:299, 1975.

Griffith, D. P., and Musher, D. M.: Prevention of infected urinary stones by urease inhibition. Invest. Urol., *11*:228, 1973.

Griffith, D. P., Bragin, S., and Musher, D. M.: Dissolution of struvite urinary stones. Experimental studies in vitro. Invest. Urol., *13*:351, 1976*a*.

Griffith, D. P., Musher, D. M., and Campbell, J. W.: Inhibition of bacterial urease. Invest. Urol., *11*:234, 1973.

Griffith, D. P., Musher, D. M., and Itin, C.: Urease: The primary cause of infection-induced urinary stones. Invest. Urol., *13*:346, 1976*b*.

Grove, W. J., Vermeulen, C. W., Goetz, R., et al.: Experimental urolithiasis. II. The influence of urine volume upon calculi experimentally produced upon foreign bodies. J. Urol., *64*:549, 1950.

Gutman, A. B., and Yu, T. F.: Uric acid nephrolithiasis. Am. J. Med., *45*:756, 1968.

Hages, B. H., and Magath, T. B.: The etiology of incrusted cystitis with alkaline urine. JAMA, *85*:1352, 1925.

Hagler, L., and Herman, R. H.: Oxalate metabolism. Am. J. Clin. Nutr., *26*:758, 1973.

Hall, E. G., Scowen, E. F., and Watts, R. W.: Clinical manifestations of primary hyperoxaluria. Arch. Dis. Child., *35*:108, 1960.

Hallson, P. C., and Rose, G. A.: Seasonal variations in urinary crystals. Br. J. Urol., *49*:227, 1977.

Hammerstein, G.: On calcium and its solubility in presence of inorganic salts with special reference to occurrence of crystalluria. Comp. Renal Trans. Lab. Carlsberg, *17*:83, 1929.

Hammersten, O.: Lehrbuch der Physiologischen Chemie, p. 837. Wiesbaden, J. F. Bergmann, 1896.

Harris, E. K.: Distinguishing physiologic variation from analytic variation. J. Chron. Dis., *23*:469, 1970.

Harrison, A. R., and Rose, G. A.: Medullary sponge kidney. Urol. Res., *7*:197, 1979.

Harrison, A. R., and Rose, G. A.: The late results of parathyroidectomy in patients with calculus or nephrocalcinosis. *In* Cifuentes, L., Rapado, A., and Hodgkinson, A. (Eds.): Urinary Calculi. International Symposium on Renal Stone Research, p. 354. Basel, S. Karger, 1973.

Hartung, R.: The significance of uric acid in calcium oxalate nephrolithiasis. Munch. Med. Wochenschr., *117*:387, 1975.

Haussler, M. R., Baylink, D. J., Hughes, M. R., et al.: The assay of 1,25-dihydro-oxyvitamin D₃: Physiologic and pathologic modulation of circulating hormone levels. Clin. Endocrinol., *5*:151A, 1976.

Hautmann, R., Lehmann, A., and Komor, S.: Calcium and oxalate concentrations in human renal tissue: the key to the pathogenesis of stone formation. J. Urol., *123*:317, 1980.

Hazarika, E. Z., and Rao, B. N.: Spectrochemical analysis of urinary tract calculi. Indian J. Med. Res., *62*:776, 1974.

Hazarika, E. Z., Balakrishna, and Rao, B. N.: Upper urinary tract calculi: Analysed by x-ray diffraction and chemical methods. Indian J. Med. Res., *62*:443, 1974*a*.

Hazarika, E. Z., Rao, B. N., Kapur, B. M., et al.: Lower urinary tract calculi analysed by x-ray diffraction and chemical methods. Indian J. Med. Res., *62*:893, 1974*b*.

Heath, P. M.: Large ureteral calculus. Br. J. Surg., *10*:153, 1922.

Hedstrand, H., and Ljunghall, S.: Glucose tolerance in idiopathic calcium-stone formation. Lancet, *1*:1251, 1975.

Hench, L. L.: Factors in protein-mineral epitaxis. *In* Finlayson, B., et al. (Eds.): Urolithiasis: Physical Aspects, p. 203. Washington, D.C., National Academy of Sciences, 1972.

Henneman, P. H., Benedict, P. H., Forbes, A. P., et al.: Idiopathic hypercalciuria. N. Engl. J. Med., *259*:802, 1958.

Herbstein, F. H., Kleeberg, J., Shalitin, Y., et al.: Chemical and x-ray diffraction analysis of urinary stones in Israel. Isr. J. Med. Sci., *10*:1493, 1974.

Herring, L. C.: Observations of 10,000 urinary calculi. J. Urol., *88*:545, 1962.

Herrman, G.: Nachweis der Beldung von Harnmucoid mit Hilfe der Immuno-Fluorescenz. Verh. Dtsch. Ges. Inn. Med., *69*:178, 1963.

Higgins, C. C.: Factors in recurrence of renal calculi. JAMA, *113*:1460, 1939.

Higgins, C. C., and Roen, P. R.: Report of a case of calculus-containing urethral diverticulum in a woman. J. Urol., *49*:715, 1943.

Hinman, F.: Directional growth of renal calculi. J. Urol., *121*: 700, 1979.

Hioco, D.: Idiopathic hypercalciuria and normocalcemic hyperparathyroidism. Rev. Rhum. Mal. Osteoartic., *40*:651, 1973.

Hockaday, T. D. R., Clayton, J. E., Frederick, E. W., et al.: Primary hyperoxaluria. Medicine, *43*:315, 1967.

Hodgkinson, A.: Uric acid disorders in patients with calcium stones. Br. J. Urol., *48*:1, 1976.

Hodgkinson, A.: Relations between oxalic acid, calcium, magnesium and creatinine excretion in normal men and male patients with calcium oxalate kidney stones. Clin. Sci. Mol. Med., *46*:357, 1974.

Hodgkinson, A.: Determination of oxalic acid in biological material. Clin. Chem., *16*:547, 1970.

Hodgkinson, A., and Marshall, R. W.: Changes in the composition of urinary tract stones. Invest. Urol., *13*:131, 1975.

Hodgkinson, A., and Nordin, B. E. C.: Physical chemistry of calcium stone formation. Biochem. J., *122*:5P, 1971.

Hodgkinson, A., and Wilkinson, R.: Plasma oxalate concentration and renal excretion of oxalate in man. Clin. Sci. Mol. Med., *46*:61, 1974.

Hodgkinson, A., Bissett, P., and Tye, J.: Effect of succinimide and other drugs on oxalate excretion by rats. Urol. Int., *30*:465, 1975.

Hodgkinson, A., Marshall, R. W., and Cochran, M.: Diurnal variations in calcium phosphate and calcium oxalate activity products in normal and stone-forming urines. Isr. J. Med. Sci., *7*:1230, 1971.

Hodgkinson, A., Peacock, M., and Nochalson, M.: Quantitative analysis of calcium containing urinary calculi. Invest. Urol., *6*:549, 1969.

Holmes, G.: Worcestershire sauce and the kidneys. Br. Med. J., *3*:252, 1971.

Holmlund, D.: Tanderil in the treatment of ureteral stone disease. Helv. Chir. Acta, *41*:333, 1974.

Holzbach, R. T., and Pak, C. Y.: Metastable supersaturation. Physico-chemical studies provide new insights into formation of renal and biliary tract stones. Am. J. Med., *56*:141, 1974.

Horton, W. A., and Calli, L. J., Jr.: Multiple endocrine adenomatosis presenting as Zollinger-Ellison syndrome, nonbeta islet cell adenoma, parathyroid adenoma, renal calculi, bronchial carcinoid, insulinoma, hepatic hamartoma, etc. Birth Defects, *7*:275, 1971.

Howard, J. E., Thomas, W. C., Barker, L. M., et al.: The recognition and isolation from urine and serum of a peptide inhibitor to calcification. Johns Hopkins Med. J., *120*:119, 1967.

Huggins, C., and Bear, R. S.: Course of prostatic ducts and anatomy; chemical and x-ray diffraction analysis of prostatic calculi. J. Urol., *51*:37, 1944.

Inada, T., Miyazaki, S., Omori, T., et al.: Statistical study on urolithiasis in Japan. Urol. Int., *1*:150, 1958.

Isaacson, L. C.: Urinary ionic strength, osmolality and specific conductivity. Invest. Urol., *5*:406, 1968.

Iur'eva, E. A., Kazanskaia, I. V., Korovina, N. A., et al.: Clinical biochemical and genetic analysis of nephrolithiasis in children. Vopr. Okhr. Materin. Det., *19*:32, 1974.

Jacobs, S. C., and Gittes, R. F.: Dissolution of residual renal calculi with hemiacidrin. J. Urol., *115*:2, 1976.

Jennis, F., Larson, J. N., Neale, F. C., et al.: Staghorn calculi of the kidney: Clinical bacteriological and biochemical features. Br. J. Urol., *42*:511, 1970.

Joekes, A. M., Rose, G. A., and Sutor, J.: Multiple renal silica calculi. Br. Med. J., *1*:146, 1973.

Johansen, K., Gammelgard, P. A., and Jorgensen, F. S.: Treatment of cystinuria with alph-mercaptopropionylglycine. Scand. J. Urol. Nephrol., *14*:189, 1980.

Johansson, G., Backman, U., Danielson, B. G., Fellstrom, B., Ljunghall, S., and Wikstrom, B.: Biochemical and clinical effects of the prophylactic treatment of renal calcium stones with magnesium hydroxide. J. Urol., *124*:770, 1980.

Johansson, H., Thoren, L., Werner, I., et al.: Normocalcemic hyperparathyroidism, kidney stones, and idiopathic hypercalciuria. Surgery, *77*:691, 1975.

Joly, J. S.: Stone and Calculous Disease of the Urinary Organs. St. Louis, C. V. Mosby Co., 1931.

Jordan, W. R., Finlayson, B., and Luxenberg, M.: Kinetics of early time calcium oxalate nephrolithiasis. Invest. Urol., *15*:465, 1978.

Jorgensen, F. S.: Hypercalciuria and stone formation. N. Engl. J. Med., *292*:756, 1975.

Jorgensen, F. S., and Brunner, S.: The long-term effect of bendroflume-thiazide on renal calcium and magnesium excretion and stone formation in patients with recurring renal stones. Scand. J. Urol. Nephrol., *8*:128, 1974.

Jorgensen, F. S., and Transbol, I.: The effect of bendroflumethiazide on the renal handling of calcium, magnesium and phosphate in normocalcaemic renal stone formers and in hyperparathyroidism. Acta Med. Scand., *194*:327, 1973*a*.

Jorgensen, F. S., and Transbol, I.: The effect of bendroflumethiazide on the intestinal absorption of calcium in normocalcaemic renal stone formers and in hyperparathyroidism. Acta Med. Scand., *194*:323, 1973*b*.

Juuti, M., and Heinonen, O. P.: Incidence of urolithiasis and composition of household water in Southern Finland. Scand. J. Urol. Nephrol., *14*:181, 1980.

Kaminski, J. M., Katz, A. R., and Woodward, S. C.: Urinary bladder calculus formation on sutures in rabbits, cats and dogs. Surg. Gynecol. Obstet., *146*:353, 1978.

Kaplan, R. A., and Pak, C. Y.: Diagnosis and management of renal calculi. Tex. Med., *70*:88, 1974.

Karcz, J.: Urolithiasis as a complication of bone injuries in children. Pediatr. Pol., *45*:1239, 1973.

Karcz, J.: Staghorn urinary calculi in calices and kidney pelvis in children. Pol. Przegl. Chir., *46*:1459, 1974.

Kean, W. F.: Vitamin C and the stone. Lancet, *1*:364, 1974.

Keating, F. R., Jr.: Diagnosis of primary hyperparathyroidism. Clinical and laboratory aspects. JAMA, *178*:547, 1961.

Keutel, H. J.: Localization of uromucoid in human kidney and in sections of human kidney stones with the fluorescent antibody technique. J. Histochem. Cytochem., *13*:155, 1965.

Keutel, H. J., and King, J. S., Jr.: Further studies of matrix substance A. Invest. Urol., *2*:115, 1964.

Keyser, L. D., Schere, P. C., and Claffey, L. W.: Studies in the dissolution of urinary calculi; experimental and clinical study. J. Urol., *59*:826, 1948.

Kiesswetter, H., and Parkash, O.: The problem of stone formation in the upper urinary tract. A retrospective correlational study. Urol. Int., *27*:432, 1972.

King, J. S.: Currents in renal stone research. Clin. Chem., *17*:971, 1971.

King, J. S.: Etiologic factors involved in urolithiasis: A review of recent research. J. Urol., *97*:583, 1967.

King, J. S., and Wainer, J. S.: Glyoxylate metabolism in normal and stone forming humans and the effect of allopurinol therapy. Proc. Soc. Exper. Biol. Med., *128*:1162, 1968.

Kister, R., Terhorst, B., and Greiling, H.: Analysis of renal calculi by means of IR-spectroscopy. Z. Klin. Chem. Klin. Biochem., *12*:255, 1974.

Kleeman, C. R., Rockney, R. E., and Maxwell, M. H.: The effect of parathyroid extract (PTE) on the renal clearance of diffusible calculi. J. Clin. Invest., *37*:907, 1958.

Koff, S. A.: Mechanism of electrolyte imbalance following urointestinal anastomosis. Urology, *5*:109, 1975.

Kohman, E. F.: Oxalic acid in foods and its behavior and fate in the diets. J. Nutr., *18*:233, 1939.

Koide, T., Kinoshita, K., Takemoto, M., Yachiku, S., and Sonoda, T.: Conservative treatment of cystine calculi: Effect of oral alpha-mercaptopropionylglycine on cystine stone dissolution and on prevention of stone recurrence. J. Urol., *128*:513, 1982.

Kretschmer, H. L.: Stone in the ureter; clinical data based on 500 cases. Surg. Gynecol. Obstet., *74*:1065, 1942.

Kretschmer, H. L.: Xanthin calculi: A report of a case and review of the literature. J. Urol., *38*:183, 1937.

Kurkin, A. V.: Etiology and pathogenesis of endemic oxalate kidney stones in children. Arkh. Patol., *35*:44, 1973*a*.

Kurkin, A. V.: Nephrolithiasis and pyelonephritis in children. Pediatriia, *52*:13, 1973*b*.

Kutzmann, A. A.: Replacement lipomatosis of the kidney. Surg. Gynecol. Obstet., *52*:690, 1931.

Lackner, H., and Barton, L. J.: Cortical blood flow in ureteral obstruction. Invest. Urol., *8*:319, 1970.

Lafferty, F. W.: Primary hyperparathyroidism—changing clinical spectrum, prevalence of hypertension and discriminant analysis of laboratory tests. Arch. Intern. Med., *141*:1761, 1981.

Lagergren, C.: Biophysical investigations of urinary calculi. Acta Radiol. (Suppl), *129*:1, 1955.

Lalli, A. F.: Symposium on renal lithiasis. Roentgen aspects of renal calculous disease. Urol. Clin. North Am., *1*:213, 1974.

Landgrebe, A. R., Nyhan, W. L., and Coleman, M.: Urinary tract stones resulting from the excretion of oxypurinol. N. Engl. J. Med., *292*:626, 1975.

Laskowski, D. E.: Chemical microscopy of urinary calculi. Anal. Chem., *37*:1399, 1965.

Laubscher, H. H.: Giant vesical calculus—A case report. SA Med. J., *63*:209, 1983.

Lehtonen, T.: Effect of aminophylline on passage of ureteral concretions. Ann. Chir. Gynaecol. Fenn., *62*:90, 1973.

Lemann, J., Adams, N. D., and Gray, R. W.: Urinary calcium excretion in human beings. N. Engl. J. Med., *301*:535, 1979.

Lemann, J., Piering, W. F., and Lennon, E. J.: Possible role of carbohydrate-induced calciuria in calcium oxalate kidney stone formation. N. Engl. J. Med., *280*:232, 1969.

Lett, H.: On urinary calculus with special reference to stone in the bladder. Br. J. Urol., *8*:205, 1936.

Lewis, M., Thomas, W. C., Jr., and Tonuta, A.: Pyrophosphate and mineralizing potential of urine. Clin. Sci., *30*:389, 1966.

Liao, L. L., and Richardson, K. E.: The metabolism of oxalate precursors in isolated perfused rat livers. Arch. Biochem. Biophys., *153*:438, 1972.

Liberman, U. A., Sperling, O., Atsmon, A., Frank, M., Modan, M., and deVries, A.: Metabolic and calcium kinetic studies in idiopathic hypercalciuria. J. Clin. Invest., *47*:2580, 1968.

Libertino, J. A., Newman, H. R., Lytton, B., et al.: Staghorn calculi in solitary kidneys. J. Urol., *105*:753, 1971.

Lien, J., and Keane, P.: Urinary cAMP and calcium excretion in the fasting state and their response to oral calcium loading in patients with calcium urolithiasis. J. Urol., *129*:401, 1983.

Ljunghall, S., Backman, U., Danielson, B., Fellstrom, B., Johansson, G., and Wikstrom, B.: Calcium and magnesium metabolism during long-term treatment with thiazides. Scand. J. Urol. Nephrol., *15*:257, 1981.

Lonsdale, K.: Epitaxy as a growth factor in urinary calculi and gallstones. Nature, *217*:56, 1968*a*.

Lonsdale, K.: Human stones. Science, *159*:1199, 1968*b*.

Lonsdale, K., and Mason, P.: Uric acid, uric acid dihydrate, and urates in urinary calculi, ancient and modern. Science, *152*:1511, 1966.

Lonsdale, K., and Sutor, D. J.: Crystallographic studies of urinary and biliary calculi. Sov. Phys. Crystallogr., *16*:1060, 1972.

Lonsdale, K., Sutor, K. J., and Wooley, S.: Composition of urinary calculi by x-ray diffraction. Collected data from various localities. I. Norwich (England) and District, 1772-1961. Br. J. Urol., *40*:33, 1968*a*.

Lonsdale, K., Sutor, K. I., and Wooley, S.: Composition of urinary calculi by x-ray diffraction. Collected data from various localities. II-VI. Czechoslovakia. Br. J. Urol., *40*:402. 1968*b*.

Lotz, M., Potts, J. T., and Bartter, F. C.: Rapid, simple method for determining effectiveness of D-penicillamine therapy in cystinuria. Br. Med. J., *2*:521, 1965.

Loutfi, A.: Studies on bladder stone disease in Egyptian

children. VII. Suprapubic cystolithotomy in childhood without drainage. A new concept of treatment. J. Egypt. Med. Assoc., 57:146, 1974.

Loutfi, A., and Van Reen, R.: Studies of bladder stone disease in Egyptian children. J. Egypt Med. Assoc., 57:89, 1974.

Loutfi, A., Mansour, N., and Van Reen, R.: Studies on bladder stone disease in Egyptian children. III. Negative role of bilharziasis in pathogenesis. J. Egypt Med. Assoc., 57:109, 1974.

Loutfi, A., Van Reen, R., and Abdel-Hamid, G.: Studies on bladder stone disease in Egyptian children. II. Methodology and general aspects of the disease. J. Egypt Med. Assoc., 57:96, 1974a.

Loutfi, A., Van Reen, R., and Abdel-Hamid, G.: Studies on bladder stone disease in Egyptian children. V. Composition of bladder stones. J. Egypt Med. Assoc., 57:124, 1974b.

Loutfi, A., Van Reen, R., and Abdel-Hamid, G.: Studies on bladder stone disease in Egyptian children. VI. Crystalluria in the stone patients. J. Egypt Med. Assoc., 57:137, 1974c.

Loutfi, A., Waslien, C., and Van Reen, R.: Studies on bladder stone disease in Egyptian children. VI. Evaluation of vitamin A status. J. Egypt Med. Assoc., 57:116, 1974d.

Lyon, E. F., Borden, T. A., Ellis, J. E., et al.: Calcium oxalate lithiasis produced by pyridoxine deficiency and inhibition with high magnesium diets. Invest. Urol., 4:133, 1966.

Lyons, E. S., and Vermeulen, D. W.: Crystallization concepts and calculogenesis: Observations on artificial oxalate concretions. Invest. Urol., 3:309, 1965.

Malek, R. S., and Boyce, W. H.: Intranephronic calculosis: Its significance and relationships to matrix in nephrolithiasis. J. Urol., 109:551, 1973.

Malek, R. S., and Elder, J. S.: Xanthogranulomatous pyelonephritis: A critical analysis of 26 cases and of the literature. J. Urol., 119:589, 1978.

Malek, R. S., and Kelalis, P. P.: Pediatric nephrolithiasis. J. Urol., 113:545, 1975.

Mall, J. C., Collins, P. A., and Lyon, E. S.: Matrix calculi. Br. J. Radiol., 48:807, 1975.

Marquardt, H.: Incomplete renal tubular acidosis with recurrent nephrolithiasis and nephrocalcinosis. Urologe [A], 12:162, 1973.

Marshall, R. W., and Barry, H.: Urine saturation and the formation of calcium-containing renal calculi: The effects of various forms of therapy. In Cifuentes, L., Rapado, A., and Hodgkinson, A. (Eds.): Urinary Calculi. International Symposium on Renal Stone Research, p. 164. Basel, S. Karger, 1973.

Marshall, R. W., and Robertson, W. G.: Nomograms for the estimation of the saturation of urine with calcium oxalate, calcium phosphate, magnesium ammonium phosphate, uric acid, sodium acid urate, ammonium acid urate and cystine. Clin. Chim. Acta, 72:253, 1976.

Marshall, R. W., Cockran, M., Robertson, W. G., et al.: The relation between the concentration of calcium salts in the urine and renal stone composition in patients with calcium-containing renal stones. Clin. Sci., 43:433, 1972.

Marshall, V. F., and Green, J. L.: Aluminum gels with constant phosphorus intake for the control of renal phosphatic calculi. J. Urol., 67:611, 1952.

Marshall, V. F., Lavengood, R. W., Jr., and Kelly, D.: Complete longitudinal nephrolithotomy and the Shorr regimen in the management of staghorn calculi. Ann. Surg., 162:366, 1965.

Marshall, V. R., and Ryall, R. L.: Investigation of urinary calculi. Br. J. Hosp. Med., 9999:389, 1981.

Mates, J.: External factors in the genesis of urolithiasis. In Hodgkinson, A., and Nordin, B. E. C. (Eds.): Renal Stone Research Symposium, p. 59. London, J. & A. Churchill, Ltd., 1969.

Mathew, T.: Treatment of renal calculi. Drugs, 8:62, 1974.

May, P., and Schindler, E.: Methods and results of conservative treatment of uric acid stones. In Cifuentes, I., Rapado, A., and Hodgkinson, A. (Eds.): Urinary Calculi. International Symposium on Renal Stone Research, p. 111. Basel, S. Karger, 1973.

McGeown, M. G.: Heredity in renal stone disease. Clin. Sci., 19:465, 1960.

McGeown, M. G.: The urinary amino acids in relation to calculous disease. J. Urol., 78:318, 1957.

McLean, F. C., and Hastings, A. B.: Clinical estimation and significance of calcium ion concentration in the blood. Am. J. Med. Sci., 189:602, 1935.

Melick, R. A., and Henneman, P. H.: Clinical and laboratory studies of 207 consecutive patients in a kidney stone clinic. N. Engl. J. Med., 259:307, 1958.

Melnick, I., Landes, R. R., Hoffmann, A. A., et al.: Magnesium therapy for recurring calcium oxalate urinary calculi. J. Urol., 105:119, 1971.

Menon, M., and Krishnan, C. S.: Evaluation and medical management of patients with calcium stone disease. Urol. Clin. North Am., 10:595, 1983.

Menon, M., Mahle, C. J., Urinary citrate excretion in patients with renal calculi. J. Urol., 129:1158, 1983.

Meyer, A. S., Finlayson, B., and Dubois, L.: Direct observation of urinary stone ultrastructure. Br. J. Urol., 43:154, 1971.

Meyer, J. L., and Smith, L. H.: Growth of calcium oxalate crystals. I. A model for urinary stone growth. Invest. Urol., 13:31, 1975a.

Meyer, J. L., and Smith, L. H.: Growth of calcium oxalate crystals. II. Inhibition by natural urinary crystal growth inhibitors. Invest. Urol., 13:36, 1975b.

Middleton, A. W., Jr., and Pfister, R. C.: Stone-containing pyelocaliceal diverticulum: Embryogenic, anatomic, radiologic and clinical characteristics. J. Urol., 111:2, 1974.

Milkman, L. A.: Multiple spontaneous idiopathic symmetrical fractures. Am. J. Roentgenol., 32:622, 1934.

Miller, G. H., et al.: Calcium oxalate solubility in urine: Experimental urolithiasis, XIV. J. Urol., 79:607, 1958.

Miller, G. H., Jr.: Oral orthophosphate inhibition of induced urinary bladder calculi in the rat. Invest. Urol., 5:321, 1967.

Miller, J. D., Randolph, A. D., and Drach, G. W.: Observations upon calcium oxalate crystallization kinetics in simulated urine. J. Urol., 117:342, 1977.

Mitchell, J. P.: Lithiasis in children (Editorial). Eur. Urol., 7:121, 1981.

Mobley, J. E., and Hardison, W.: Nephrolithiasis following intestinal bypass for obesity. Urology, 3:639, 1974.

Modlin, M.: The aetiology of renal stone: A new concept arising from studies on a stone-free population. Ann. R. Coll. Surg. Engl., 40:155, 1967.

Modlin, M.: Renal stone: A study of 520 patients with special references to patterns of recurrence. S. Afr. Med. J., 312:824, 1956.

Mollard, P., and Chavrier, Y.: Surgical treatment of urinary lithiasis in children (74 cases). Lyon Chir., 67:338, 1971.

Montinari, M., Florio, G., Mangieri, C., et al.: Clinicostatistical data on urinary calculosis in childhood. Observations on 179 cases. Minerva Pediatr., 26:1590, 1974.

Moody, T. E., Vaugh, E. D., Jr., and Gillenwater, J. Y.: Relationship between renal blood flow and ureteral pressure during 18 hours of total unilateral ureteral occlusion. Invest. Urol., *13*:246, 1975.

Moore, C. A., and Bunce, G. E.: Reduction in frequency of renal calculous formation by oral magnesium administration. Invest. Urol., *2*:7, 1964.

Moore, S., and Gowland, G.: The immunological integrity of matrix substance A and its possible detection and quantitation in urine. Br. J. Urol., *47*:489, 1975.

Morrison, R. B.: Proceedings: Metabolic aspects of urinary calculi in Wellington. Br. J. Urol., *46*:177, 1974.

Mullin, E. M., Bonar, R. A., and Paulson, D. F.: Effect of transient hydro-nephrosis on subsequent compensatory renal growth. Invest. Urol., *13*:121, 1975.

Mullin, J. W.: Crystallization. 2nd ed., p. 150. Cleveland, Ohio, CRC Press, 1972.

Mulvaney, W. P.: The clinical use of Renacidin in urinary calcifications. J. Urol., *84*:206, 1960.

Mulvaney, W. P., and Henning, D. C.: Solvent treatment of urinary calculi: Refinements in technique. J. Urol., *88*:145, 1962.

Munster, A. M., and Hunter, J.: Urinary extravasation due to perforation of ureter by calculus. Arch. Surg., *97*:632, 1968.

Murad, F., and Pak, C. Y. C.: Urinary excretion of adenosine 3′,5′-monophosphate and guanosine 3′,5′ monophosphate. N. Engl. J. Med., *286*:1382, 1972.

Murphy, B. T., and Pyrah, L. N.: The composition, structure and mechanisms of the formation of urinary calculi. Br. J. Urol., *34*:129, 1962.

Murphy, K. J.: Prevention of recurring kidney stones. Br. J. Urol., *44*:730, 1972.

Nash, A. G., and Knight, M.: Ureterocele calculi. Br. J. Urol., *45*:404, 1973.

Naysan, P., Shulman, V., Pochaczevsky, R., et al.: Bladder stone in childhood. N.Y. State J. Med., *75*:1288, 1975.

Nemoy, N. J., and Stamey, T. A.: Surgical bacteriological and biochemical management of "infection stones." JAMA, *215*:1470, 1971.

Nicar, M. J., Skurla, C., Sakhaee, K., and Pak, C. Y. C.: Low urinary citrate excretion in nephrolithiasis. Urology, *21*:8, 1983:

Nichols, B. H., and Lower, W. E.: Roentgenographic studies of the urinary system. St. Louis, C. V. Mosby Co., 1933.

Noe, H. N., Stapleton, F. B., Jerkins, G., and Roy, S.: Clinical experience with pediatric urolithiasis. J. Urol., *129*:1166, 1983.

Nordin, B. A., Hodgkinson, A., Peacock, M., and Robertson, W. G.: Urinary tract calculi. *In* Hamburger, J., Crosnier, J., and Grunfeld, J. P. (Eds.): Nephrology. New York, John Wiley & Sons, 1979.

Nordin, B. E. C.: Pathogenesis and treatment of calcium stone disease. Br. J. Urol., *44*:729, 1972.

Nordin, B. E. C., and Hodgkinson, A.: Urolithiasis. Adv. Intern. Med., *13*:155, 1967.

Ohata, M., and Pak, C. Y.: Preliminary study of the treatment of nephrolithiasis (calcium stones) with diphosphonate. Metabolism, *23*:1176, 1974.

Okawa, T.: Proceedings: Primary hyperparathyroidism in urology. Calcif. Tissue Res., *15*:155, 1974.

O'Keefe, C. M., Cies, L., and Smith, L. H.: Inhibition of oxalate biosynthesis: In vivo studies in the rat. Biochem. Med., 7:299, 1973.

O'Leary, J. P., Thomas, E. C., Jr., and Woodward, E. R.: Urinary tract stone after small bowel bypass for morbid obesity. Am. J. Surg., *127*:142, 1974.

Ord, W. M., and Shattock, S. G.: On microscopic structure of urinary calculi of oxalate of lime. Trans. Pathol. Soc. London, *46*:91, 1895.

O'Regan, S., Homsy, Y., and Mongeau, J. G.: Urolithiasis in children. Can. J. Surg., *25*:566, 1982.

Oreopoulos, D. G., and Silverberg, S.: Calcium oxalate urinary tract stones in patients on maintenance dialysis. N. Engl. J. Med., *290*:1438, 1974.

Oreopoulos, D. G., Walker, D., Akriotis, D. J., et al.: Excretion of inhibitors of calcification in urine. Part I. Findings in control subjects and patients with renal stones. Can. Med. Assoc. J., *112*:827, 1975.

Ostergaard, A. H.: Analysis of a bladder stone in 1786. Acta Chir. Scand. (Suppl.), *433*:25, 1973.

Pak, C. Y.: Calcium Urolithiasis. New York, Plenum Press, 1978.

Pak, C. Y.: A cautious use of sodium cellulose phosphate in the management of calcium nephrolithiasis. Invest. Urol., *19*:187, 1981.

Pak, C. Y.: Hydrochlorothiazide therapy in nephrolithiasis. Effect on the urinary activity product and formation product of brushite. Clin. Pharmacol. Ther., *14*:209, 1973.

Pak, C. Y.: Physicochemical basis for formation of renal stone of calcium phosphate origin: Calculation of the degree of saturation of urine with respect to brushite. J. Clin. Invest., *48*:1914, 1969.

Pak, C. Y., and Chu, S.: A simple technique for the determination of urinary state of saturation with respect to brushite. Invest. Urol., *11*:211, 1973.

Pak, C. Y., Delea, C. S., and Bartter, F. C.: Successful treatment of recurrent nephrolithiasis (calcium stones) with cellulose phosphate. N. Engl. J. Med., *290*:175, 1974.

Pak, C. Y., Diller, E. C., Smith, G. W., II, et al.: Renal stones of calcium phosphate: Physicochemical basis for their formation. Proc. Soc. Exper. Biol. Med., *130*:753, 1969.

Pak, C. Y., East, D. A., Sanzenbacher, L. J., et al.: Gastrointestinal calcium absorption in nephrolithiasis. J. Clin. Endocrinol. Metab., *35*:261, 1972.

Pak, C. Y., Kaplan, R., Bone, H., et al.: A simple test for the diagnosis of absorptive, resorptive and renal hypercalciurias. N. Engl. J. Med., *292*:497, 1975.

Pak, C. Y., Kaplan, R., Bone, H., et al.: A simple test for the diagnosis of absorptive, in nephrolithiasis. J. Clin. Endocrinol. Metab., *35*:261, 1972.

Pak, C. Y., Ohata, M., Lawrence, E. C., et al.: The hypercalciurias: Causes, parathyroid functions and diagnostic criteria. J. Clin. Invest., *54*:387, 1974.

Pantanowitz, D., Pollen, J. J., Politzer, W. M., et al.: Urinary calculi. S. Afr. Med. J., *47*:128, 1973.

Parry, E. S., and Lister, I. S.: Sunlight and hypercalciuria. Lancet, *1*:1063, 1975.

Paterson, C. R.: Drugs for the treatment of hypercalcemia. Postgrad. Med. J., *50*:158, 1974.

Paulson, D. F.: Symposium on renal lithiasis. The challenge of calculi in children. Urol. Clin. North Am., *1*:365, 1974.

Paulson, D. F., Glen, J. F., Hughes, J., et al.: Pediatric urolithiasis. J. Urol., *108*:811, 1972.

Pavanello, L., Rizzoni, G., Dussini, N., Zacchello, G., and Passerini, G.: Cystinuria in children. Eur. Urol., *7*:139, 1981.

Pearlman, C. K.: Xanthine urinary calculus. J. Urol., *64*:799, 1950.

Peters, H. J., and Eckstein, W.: Possible pharmacological means of treating renal colic. Urol. Res., *3*:55, 1975.

Peters, J. P., and Van Slyke, D. D.: Cited in Gutman, A. B., and Yu, T. F.: Uric acid nephrolithiasis. Am. J. Med., *45*:756, 1968.

Peterson, H. O., and Holmes, G. W.: Roentgen analysis of 100 cases of ureteral calculi. Am. J. Roentgenol., *37*:479, 1937.

Peterson, L. J.: Urinary tract calculi associated with enteritis and intestinal bypass. Urology, *5*:172, 1975.

Pietrek, J., and Kokot, F.: Effect of cellulose phosphate on urinary excretion of calcium in patients with nephrolithiasis. Pol. Arch. Med. Wewn., *50*:29, 1973*a*.

Pietrek, J., and Kokot, F.: Treatment of patients with calcium-containing renal stones with cellulose phosphate. Br. J. Urol., *45*:136, 1973*b*.

Pinto, B., Crespi, G., Sole-Balcells, F., et al.: Patterns of oxalate metabolism in recurrent oxalate stone formers. Kidney Int., *5*:285, 1974.

Pirogov, A. B.: Diagnostic value of radioisotope methods of investigation of renal function in urolithiasis. Klin. Med. (Mosk.), *51*:80, 1973.

Poole-Wilson, P. A.: A new factor in urolithiasis: Long-term effects of severe respiratory poliomyelitis. Br. J. Urol., *45*:335, 1973.

Porter, P.: Colloidal properties of urates in relation to calculus formation. Res. Vet. Sci., *7*:128, 1966.

Powis, S. J., Black, J., Macdougall, J. A., et al.: Management of patients with urinary calculi. Br. Med. J., *1*:355, 1974.

Prien, E. L., Sr.: Symposium on renal lithiasis. The analysis of urinary calculi. Urol. Clin. North Am., *1*:229, 1974.

Prien, E. L., Sr.: The riddle of urinary stone disease. JAMA, *216*:503, 1971.

Prien, E. L., Sr.: Crystallographic analysis of urinary calculi: 23-year survey study. J. Urol., *89*:917, 1963.

Prien, E. L., and Frondel, C.: Studies in urolithiasis: The composition of urinary calculi. J. Urol., *57*:949, 1947.

Prien, E. L., Sr., and Gershoff, S. F.: Magnesium oxide–pyridoxine therapy for recurrent calcium oxalate calculi. J. Urol., *112*:509, 1974.

Prien, E. L., and Prien, E. L.: Composition and structure of urinary stone. Am. J. Med., *45*:654, 1968.

Priestley, J. T., and Osterberg, A. E.: The relationship between the chemical composition of renal calculi and associated bacteria. J. Urol., *36*:447, 1936.

Prince, C. L., and Scardino, P. L.: A statistical analysis of ureteral calculi. J. Urol., *83*:561, 1960.

Prince, C. L., Scardino, P. L., and Wolan, T. C.: The effect of temperature, humidity, and dehydration on the formation of renal calculi. J. Urol., *75*:209, 1956.

Puri, P., Guiney, E. J., and O'Donnel, B.: Urolithiasis in Irish children. Ir. Med. J., *68*:96, 1975.

Quencer, R. M., and Foster, S. C.: Perforated ureter secondary to a ureteral calculus: Report of a case. Radiology, *102*:561, 1972.

Raisz, L. G.: Leaving no (renal) stone unturned (Editorial). N. Engl. J. Med., *292*:528, 1975.

Rambar, A. C., and MacKenzie, R. G.: Urolithiasis in adolescents. Am. J. Dis. Child., *132*:1117, 1978.

Ramirez, C. T., Ruiz, J. A., Gomez, A. Z., Orgaz, R. E., and Samper, S. D.: Crystallographic study of prostatic calculi. J. Urol., *124*:840, 1980.

Rand, M. C.: General principles of chemical coagulation. Sewage Industrial Wastes, *31*:863, 1959.

Randall, A.: The origin and growth of renal calculi. Ann. Surg., *105*:1009, 1937.

Rapaport, A., Crasswell, P. O., Husdan, H., et al.: The renal excretion of hydrogen ion in uric acid stone formers. Metabolism, *16*:176, 1967.

Rattiazzi, L. C., Simmons, R. L., Markland, C., et al.: Calculi complicating renal transplantation into ileal conduits. Urology, *5*:29, 1975.

Ravich, R. A.: Relationship of colloids to the surface tension of urine. Science, *117*:561, 1953.

Reece, R. W., and Hackler, R. H.: Spontaneous rupture of the ureter. South. Med. J., *67*:739, 1974.

Rege, P. R., Levine, M. S., Oppenheimer, S., et al.: Renal calculi and biochemical abnormalities in children with myelomeningocele and ileoconduit diversion. Urology, *5*:12, 1975.

Reisner, G. S., Wilansky, D. L., and Schneiderman, C.: Uric acid lithiasis in the ilesotomy patient. Br. J. Urol., *45*:340, 1973.

Resnick, M., Pridgen, D. B., and Goodman, H. O.: Genetic pre-disposition to formation of calcium oxalate renal calculi. N. Engl. J. Med., *278*:1313, 1968.

Resnick, M. I., and Boyce, W. H.: Spherical calcium bodies in stone-forming urine. Invest. Urol., *15*:449, 1978.

Resnick, M. I., Oliver, J., and Drach, G. W.: Intranephronic calculosis in the Brazilian squirrel monkey. Invest. Urol., *15*:295, 1978.

Retief, P. J.: Proceedings: Urinary calculi in children. Br. J. Urol., *46*:118, 1974.

Revusova, V., Zvara, V., and Gratzlova, J.: Urinary zinc excretion in patients with urolithiasis. Urol. Int., *28*:72, 1973.

Reynolds, T. B., Lamman, G., and Tupikova, N.: Re-evaluation of phosphate excretion tests in the diagnosis of hyperparathyroidism. Arch. Intern. Med., *106*:48, 1960.

Riches, E.: The history of lithotomy and lithotrity. Ann. R. Coll. Surg. Engl., *43*:185, 1968.

Riddick, T. M.: Control of Colloid Stability Through Zeta Potential. Wynnewood, Pennsylvania, Livingston Publishing Co., 1968.

Rivera, J. V.: Urinary calculi in Puerto Rico. II. Seasonal incidence. Bull. Assoc. Med. Puerto Rico, *65*:28, 1973.

Robertson, W. G.: Measurement of ionized calcium in biological fluids. Clin. Chim. Acta, *24*:149, 1969.

Robertson, W. G., and Peacock, M.: Review of risk factors in calcium oxalate urolithiasis. World J. Urol., *1*:114, 1983.

Robertson, W. G., and Peacock, M.: Calcium oxalate crystalluria and inhibitors of crystallization in recurrent renal stone-formers. Clin. Sci., *43*:499, 1972.

Robertson, W. G., Hambleton, J., and Hodgkinson, A.: Peptide inhibitors of calcium phosphate precipitation in the urine of normal and stone-forming men. Clin. Chim. Acta, *25*:247, 1969.

Robertson, W. G., Heyburn, P. J., Peacock, M., Hanes, F. A., and Swaminathan, R.: The effect of high animal protein intake on the risk of calcium stone–formation in the urinary tract. Clin. Sci., *57*:285, 1979*a*.

Robertson, W. G., Peacock, M., and Heyburn, P. J.: Epidemiological risk-factors in calcium stone formation. Fortschr. Urol. Nephrol., *14*:105, 1979*b*.

Robertson, W. G., Peacock, M., Heyburn, P. J., Hanes, F. A., Rutherford, A., et al.: Should recurrent calcium oxalate stone–formers become vegetarians? Br. J. Urol., *51*:427, 1979*c*.

Robertson, W. G., Peacock, M., Heyburn, P. J., Speed, R., and Hanes, F.: The role of affluence in the genesis of calcium-containing stones. Fortschr. Urol. Nephrol., *14*:5, 1979*d*.

Robertson, W. G., Peacock, M., Marshall, R. W., et al.: Saturation-inhibition index as a measure of the risk of calcium oxalate stone formation in the urinary tract. N. Engl. J. Med., *294*:249, 1976.

Robertson, W. G., Peacock, M., Marshall, R. W., et al.:

The effect of ethane-1-hydroxy-1, 1-diphosphonate (EHDP) on calcium oxalate crystalluria in recurrent renal stone formers. Clin. Sci. Mol. Med., 47:13, 1974.

Robertson, W. G., Peacock, M., and Nordin, B. E. C.: Inhibitors of the growth and aggregation of calcium oxalate crystals in vitro. Clin. Chim. Acta, 43:31, 1973.

Robertson, W. G., Peacock, M., and Nordin, B. E. C.: Measurement of activity products in urine from stone-formers and normal subjects. In Finlayson, B., et al.: (Eds.): Urolithiasis: Physical Aspects, p. 79. Washington, D. C., National Academy of Sciences, 1972a.

Robertson, W. G., Peacock, M., and Nordin, B. E. C.: Crystalluria. In Finlayson, B., et al. (Eds.): Urolithiasis: Physical aspects, p. 243. Washington, D. C., National Academy of Sciences, 1972b.

Robertson, W. G., Peacock, M., and Nordin, B. E. C.: Activity products in stone-forming and non-stone-forming urine. Clin. Sci., 34:579, 1968.

Rokkones, T., and Skandsen, S.: Mineralogical and clinical investigation of stones from the urinary tract. Acta Med. Scand., 187:83, 1970.

Rollins, R., and Finlayson, B.: Mechanism of prevention of calcium oxalate encrustation by methylene blue and demonstration of the concentration dependence of its action. J. Urol., 110:459, 1973.

Rose, G. A., and Westbury, E. J.: The influence of calcium content of water, intake of vegetables and fruit and of other food factors upon the incidence of renal calculi. Urol. Res., 3:61, 1975.

Rose, J. G., Gillenwater, J. Y., and Wyker, A. T. L.: The recovery of function of chronically obstructed and infected ureters. Invest. Urol., 13:125, 1975.

Rose, M. B.: Renal stone formation. The inhibitory effect of urine on calcium oxalate precipitation. Invest. Urol., 12:428, 1975.

Rosenberg, J. C., Arnstein, A. R., Ing, T. S., et al.: Calculi complicating a renal transplant. Am. J. Surg., 129:326, 1975.

Roth, L. J., and Davidson, H. B.: Fibrous and fatty replacement of renal parenchyma. JAMA, 111:233, 1938.

Roth, R. A., and Finlayson, B.: Stones: Clinical Management of Urolithiasis. Baltimore, The Williams & Wilkins Co., 1983.

Roth, R., and Finlayson, B.: Observations on the radiopacity of stone substances with special reference to cystine. Invest. Urol., 11:186, 1973.

Rundles, R. W., Metz, E. N., and Silberman, H. R.: Allopurinol in the treatment of gout. Ann. Intern. Med., 64:229, 1966.

Russell, R. G. G., and Fleisch, G.: Pyrophosphate and stone formation. In Hodgkinson, A., and Nordin, B. E. C. (Eds.): Renal Stone Research Symposium, p. 165. London, J. & A. Churchill, Ltd., 1969.

Rutishauser, G.: Etiology of ureteral colic. Ther. Umsch., 28:790, 1971.

Sadre, M., Bastanfar, M., and Ziai, M.: Urinary calculi in Iran: Hospital experience over a 3 year period with special reference to bladder stones in children. Trans. S. Soc. Trop. Med. Hyg., 67:374, 1973.

Sandergard, E.: Prognosis of stone in the ureter. Acta Chir. Scand. (Suppl.), 219:30, 1956.

Sanjad, S., and Alterbarmakian, V.: Urinary tract lithiasis in children. J. Med. Liban., 26:31, 1973.

Sarig, S., Garti, M., Azoury, R., Wax, Y., and Perlberg, S.: A method for discrimination between calcium oxalate kidney stone formers and normals. J. Urol., 128:645, 1982.

Schmidt-Nielsen, K. S.: Desert Animals: Physiological Problems of Heat and Water. Oxford, Oxford University Press, 1964.

Schneider, H. J., and Hesse, A.: Modern methods in the analysis of urinary calculi. Z. Med. Labortech., 14:3, 1973.

Schneider, H. J., Berenyi, M., Hesse, A., et al.: Comparative urinary stone analyses. Quantitative chemical, x-ray diffraction, infrared spectroscopy and thermoanalytical procedures. Int. Urol. Nephrol., 5:9, 1973.

Scholl, A. J.: Stones in the kidney and ureter. In Cabot, B. (Ed.): Modern Urology, p. 598. Philadelphia, Lea & Febiger, 1936.

Scholten, H. G., Bakker, N. J., and Cornil, C.: Urolithiasis in childhood. J. Urol., 109:744, 1973.

Scholz, D., Schwille, P. O., Ulbrich, D., Bausch, W. M., and Sigel, A.: Composition of renal stones and their frequency in a stone clinic: Relationship to parameters of mineral metabolism in serum and urine. Urol. Res., 7:161, 1979.

Schrott, H. G., Jubiz, W., Frailey, J., et al.: Calcium infusion and phosphate deprivation tests in patients with primary hyperparathyroidism and with normocalcemia and nephrolithiasis. Metabolism, 21:205, 1972.

Schulze, U., Ritter, R., and Grunhagen, H.: Origin and composition of bladder calculi in childhood. Case report. Klin. Paediatr., 185:64, 1973.

Schweitzer, F. A. W.: Intra-pelvic pressure and renal function studies in experimental chronic partial ureteric obstruction. Br. J. Urol., 45:2, 1973.

Schwille, P. O., Baurle, H., and Baurle, U. G.: Study on urinary and serum enzymes in nephrolithiasis; LDH, LAP, MDH, and alpha-amylase. Urol. Int., 28:405, 1973.

Schwille, P. O., Jugelt, V., and Sigel, A.: Allopurinol-induced electrolyte and metabolism changes in urine of patients with kidney stones. Urologe, 11:185, 1972.

Schwille, P. O., Scholz, D., Hagemann, G., et al.: Metabolic and glucose load studies in uric acid, oxalic and hyperparathyroid stone formers. Isr. J. Med. Sci., 9:1116, 1973.

Schwille, P. O., Scholz, D., Schwille, K., Leutschaft, R., Goldberg, I., and Sigel, A.: Citrate in urine and serum and associated variables in subgroups of urolithiasis. Nephron, 31:194, 1982.

Scott, R.: Urinary tract stone disease. Classic studies. Urology, 6:667, 1975.

Seegmiller, J. E.: Metabolic basis of renal lithiasis from over-production of uric acid. In Cifuentes, L., Rapado, A., and Hodgkinson, A. (Eds.): Urinary Calculi. International Symposium on Renal Stone Research, p. 89. Basel, S. Karger, 1973.

Seifert, H.: Epitaxy of macromolecules on quartz surfaces. In Peiser, H. S. (Ed.): Crystal Growth. Proceedings of an International Conference on Crystal Growth, p. 543. New York, Pergamon Press, 1967.

Sengbusch, R. V., and Timmermann, A.: Die Bildung von Calcium-Oxalatmilrosteinen in menschlichen Harn und ihre Veranderung durch diätetische und medikamentose Massnahmen. Urol. Int., 5:218, 1957.

Sernia, O., Pezzano, A., and Bolgiani, M. P.: Urolithiasis in infancy. Case reports. Notes on etiopathogenesis, clinical aspects, diagnosis and therapy. Minerva Pediatr., 27:351, 1975.

Sharon, E., and Diamond, H. S.: Factitious uric acid urolithiasis as a feature of the munchausen syndrome. Mt. Sinai J. Med., N.Y., 41:698, 1974.

Sherwood, L. M.: Relative importance of parathyroid hormone and thyrocalcitonin in calcium homeostasis. N. Engl. J. Med., 278:663, 1968.

Sherwood, L. M., O'Riordan, J. L. H., Aurbach, G. D., et al.: Production of parathyroid hormone by nonparathyroid tumors. J. Clin. Endocrinol., 27:140, 1967.

Shorr, E., and Carter, A. C.: Aluminum gels in the management of renal phosphatic calculi. JAMA, 144:1549, 1950.

Shuster, J., Finlayson, B., Schaeffer, R., Sierakowski, R., Zoltek, J., and Dzegede, S.: Water hardness and urinary stone disease. J. Urol., 128:422, 1982.

Sierakowski, R., Finlayson, B., and Landes, R.: Stone incidence as related to water hardness in different geographical regions of the United States. Urol. Res., 7:157, 1978.

Silver, L., and Brendler, H.: Use of magnesium oxide in management of familial hyperoxaluria. J. Urol., 106:274, 1971.

Silver, T. M., Koff, S. A., and Thornbury, J.: An unusual pathway of urine extravasation associated with renal colic. Radiology, 109:537, 1973.

Simkiss, J.: Phosphates as crystal poisons of calcification. Biol. Rev., 39:487, 1964.

Simovic, N.: Familial predisposition to urolithiasis in infants. LiJec. Mjesn., 94:506, 1972.

Singer, A. M., Bennett, R. C., Carter, N. G., et al.: Blood and urinary changes in patients with ileostomies and ileorectal anastomoses. Br. Med. J., 3:141, 1973.

Singh, M., Chapman, R., Tresidder, G. C., et al.: The fate of the unoperated staghorn calculus. Br. J. Urol., 45:581, 1973.

Singh, P. P., Kothari, L. K., Sharma, D. C., et al.: Nutritional value of foods in relation to oxalic acid content. Am. J. Clin. Nutr., 25:1147, 1972.

Smith, D. R.: The management of cystinuria and cystine stone disease. J. Urol., 81:61, 1959.

Smith, J. M., and O'Flynn, J. D.: Vesical stone: The clinical features of 652 cases. Ir. Med. J., 68:85, 1975.

Smith, L. H.: Medical evaluation of urolithiasis. Etiologic aspects and diagnostic evaluation. Urol. Clin. North Am., 1:241, 1974a.

Smith, L. H.: Errors in membrane transport: cystinuria, renal glycosuria and renal tubular acidosis. In Principles of Internal Medicine. 7th ed., p. 600. New York, McGraw-Hill Book Co., 1974b.

Smith, L. H.: The diagnosis and treatment of metabolic stone disease. Med. Clin. North Am., 56:977, 1972.

Smith, L. H. (Ed.): Symposium on stones. Am. J. Med., 45:649, 1968.

Smith, L. H., and Hofman, A. F.: Acquired hyperoxaluria, urolithiasis, and intestinal disease: A new digestive disorder? Gastroenterology, 66:1257, 1974.

Smith, L. H., and McCall, J. T.: Chemical nature of peptide inhibition from urine. In Hodgkinson, A., and Nordin, B. E. C. (Eds.): Renal Stone Research Symposium, p. 153. London, J. & A. Churchill, Ltd., 1969.

Smith, L. H., Bauer, R. L., Craig, J. C., et al.: Inhibition of oxalate synthesis: In vitro studies using analogues of oxalate and glycolate. Biochem. Med., 6:317, 1972.

Smith, M. J. V.: Methylene blue in renal calculi. Urology, 6:676, 1975.

Smith, M. J. V.: The production and prophylaxis of calculi in Rana pipens. Invest. Urol., 10:69, 1972a.

Smith, M. J. V.: Basic considerations in calculous disease. Urol. Survey, 22:217, 1972b.

Smith, M. J. V.: Concretions and methylene blue. J. Urol., 107:164, 1972c.

Smith, M. J. V., and Boyce, W. H.: Allopurinol and urolithiasis. J. Urol., 102:750, 1969.

Smith, M. J. V., Hunt, L. D., King, J. S., et al.: Uricemia and urolithiasis. J. Urol., 101:637, 1969.

Solomons, C. C., Goodman, S. I., and Riley, C. M.: Calcium carbimide in the treatment of primary hyperoxaluria. N. Engl. J. Med., 276:207, 1967.

Sommerkamp, H., and Schwerk, W. B.: Incomplete tubular acidosis in recurrent urinary phosphate calculi. Urologe [A], 12:167, 1973.

Sotornik, I., Adamicka, V., Kocvara, S., et al.: Calcium excretion by each kidney separately in urolithiasis. Nephron, 9:318, 1972.

Sperling, O., DeVries, A., and Kadem, O.: Studies on the etiology of uric acid lithiasis. IV. Urinary nondialyzable substances in idiopathic uric acid lithiasis. J. Urol., 94:286, 1965.

Sperling, O., Persky-Brosh, S., Boer, P., et al.: Uric acid lithiasis associated with excessive purine production due to mutant phosphoribosylpyrophosphate synthetase. In Cifuentes, L., Rapado, A., and Hodgkinson, A. (Eds.): Urinary Calculi. International Symposium on Renal Stone Research, p. 96. Basel, S. Karger, 1973.

Stamey, T. A.: Urinary Infections. Baltimore, The Williams & Wilkins Co., 1972.

Stapleton, F. B., Noe, H. N., Roy, A., and Jerkins, G.: Hypercalciuria in children with urolithiasis. Am. J. Dis. Child., 136:675, 1982.

Starns, C. W., and Welsh, J. D.: Intestinal sucrose-isomaltase deficiency and renal calculi. N. Engl. J. Med., 282:1023, 1970.

Stecker, J. F., Jr., and Gillenwater, J. Y.: Experimental partial ureteral obstruction. I. Alteration in renal function. Invest. Urol., 8:377, 1971.

Steele, B. T., Lowe, P., Rance, C. P., Hardy, B. E., and Churchill, B. M.: Urinary tract calculi in children. Int. J. Pediatr. Nephrol., 4:47, 1983.

Stefan, H.: Nephro- and ureterolithiasis in congenital anomalies of the urinary tract in children. Rozhl. Hir., 52:500, 1973.

Stella, F. J., Massry, S. G., and Kleeman, C. R.: Medullary sponge kidney associated with parathyroid adenoma. A report of two cases. Nephron, 10:332, 1973.

Stewart, A. F., and Broadus, A. E.: The regulation of renal calcium excretion: An approach to hypercalciuria. Annu. Rev. Med., 32:457, 1981.

Stier, F. M., and Fried, F. A.: Effect of anoxia and ureteral obstruction on renal lysosomal stability. Invest. Urol., 11:225, 1973.

Strauss, A. L., Coe, F. L., Deutsch, L., and Parks, J. H.: Factors that predict relapse of calcium nephrolithiasis during treatment: A prospective study. Am. J. Med., 72:17, 1982.

Strauss, A. L., Coe, F. L., and Parks, J. H.: Formation of a single calcium stone of renal origin: clinical and laboratory characteristics of patients. Arch. Intern. Med., 142:504, 1982.

Streitz, J. M., Aufderheide, A. C., El Najjar, M., and Ortner, D.: A 1,500 year old bladder stone. J. Urol., 126:452, 1981.

Strott, C. A., and Nugent, C. A.: Laboratory tests in the diagnosis of hyperparathyroidism in hypercalcemic patients. Ann. Intern. Med., 68:188, 1968.

Stubbs, A. J., and Myers, R. T.: Experience with hyperparathyroidism. Surg. Gynecol. Obstet., 136:65, 1973.

Subramanyam, B. R., Megibow, A. J., Raghavendra, B. N., and Bosniak, M. A.: Diffuse xanthogranulomatous pyelonephritis: analysis by computed tomography and sonography. Urol. Radiol., 4:5, 1982.

Suby, H. I., and Albright, F.: Dissolution of phosphatic urinary calculi by the retrograde introduction of a citrate solution containing magnesium. N. Engl. J. Med., 228:81, 1943.

Suby, H. I., Suby, R. M., and Albright, F.: Properties of organic acid solutions which determine their irritability to the bladder mucosa and the effect of magnesium ions in overcoming this irritability. J. Urol., *48*:549, 1942.

Sutherland, J. W.: Recurrence following operations for upper tract stone. Br. J. Urol., *26*:22, 1954.

Sutor, D. J.: The nature of urinary stones. *In* Finlayson, B., et al. (Eds.): Urolithiasis: Physical Aspects, p. 43. Washington, D.C., National Academy of Sciences, 1972.

Sutor, D. J.: Growth studies of calcium oxalate in the presence of various ions and compounds. Br. J. Urol., *41*:171, 1969.

Sutor, D. J.: Difficulties in the identification of components of mixed urinary calculi using the ray method. Br. J. Urol., *40*:29, 1968.

Sutor, D. J., and O'Flynn, J. D.: Matrix formation in crystalline material *in vivo*. *In* Cifuentes, L., Rapado, A., and Hodgkinson, A. (Eds.): Urinary Calculi. International Symposium on Renal Stone Research, p. 280. Basel, S. Karger, 1973.

Sutor, D. J., and Scheidt, S.: Identification standards for human urinary calculus components using crystallographic methods. Br. J. Urol., *40*:22, 1968.

Sutor, D. J., and Wooley, S. E.: Some data on urinary stones which were passed. Br. J. Urol., *47*:131, 1975.

Sutor, D. J., and Wooley, S. E.: Composition of urinary calculi by x-ray diffraction. Collected data from various localities. XV-XVIII. Royal Navy; Bristol, England; and Dundee, Scotland. Br. J. Urol., *46*:229, 1974*a*.

Sutor, D. J., and Wooley, S. E.: The crystalline composition of prostatic calculi. Br. J. Urol., *46*:533, 1974*b*.

Sutor, D. J., and Wooley, S. E.: Composition of urinary calculi by x-ray diffraction. Collected data from various localities. IX-XI. (Glasgow, Scotland, United States of America, and Sudan.) Br. J. Urol., *43*:268, 1971.

Sutor, D. J., and Wooley, S. E.: Growth studies of calcium oxalate in the presence of various compounds and ions. Part II. Br. J. Urol., *42*:296, 1970*a*.

Sutor, D. J., and Wooley, S. E.: Composition of urinary calculi by x-ray diffraction. Collected data from various localities. VIII. Leeds, England. Br. J. Urol., *42*:302, 1970*b*.

Sutor, D. J., and Wooley, S. E.: Composition of urinary calculi by x-ray diffraction. Collected data from various localities. VII. The Sir Henry Thompson collection of bladder stones from the Royal College of Surgeons, London. Br. J. Urol., *41*:397, 1969.

Sutor, D. J., Wooley, S. E., and Illingworth, J. J.: Some aspects of the adult urinary stone problem in Great Britain and northern Ireland. Br. J. Urol., *46*:275, 1974*a*.

Sutor, D. J., Wooley, S. E., and Illingworth, J. J.: A geographical and historical survey of the composition of urinary stones. Br. J. Urol., *46*:393, 1974*b*.

Suvachittanont, O., et al.: The oxalic acid content of some vegetables in Thailand, its possible relationships with the bladder stone disease. J. Med. Assoc. Thailand, *56*:645, 1973.

Takasaki, E.: Urinary magnesium and oxalic acid excretion in patients with recurrent oxalate urolithiasis. Invest. Urol., *12*:251, 1975*a*.

Takasaki, E.: An observation on the composition and recurrence of urinary calculi. Urol. Int., *30*:228, 1975*b*.

Takasaki, E.: An observation on the analysis of urinary calculi by infrared spectroscopy. Calcif. Tissue Res., *7*:232, 1971.

Taneja, O. P., Mall, M. P., and Mittal, K. P.: Urologic aspects of endemic bladder stones in children. Aust. N. Z. J. Surg., *40*:130, 1970.

Taylor, J. S.: Early results in a detailed stone analysis. Br. J. Urol., *44*:730, 1972.

Tennant, C. E.: Ureteral stone of unusual size. JAMA, *82*:1122, 1924.

Teotia, M., and Teotia, S. P.: Inhibitor of calcium-oxalate crystal growth in primary bladder-stone disease. Lancet, *1*:599, 1972.

Teotia, S. P., Teotia, M., and Teotia, N. P.: Primary bladder stone disease in children—crystallization studies with special reference to urinary excretion of pyrophosphates. Indian J. Pediatr., *41*:293, 1974.

Thalut, K., Rizal, A., Brockis, J. G., Bowyer, R. C., Taylor, T. A., and Wisniewski, Z. S.: The endemic bladder stones of Indonesia—Epidemiology and clinical features. Br. J. Urol., *48*:617, 1976.

Thom, J. A., Morris, J. E., Bishop, A., and Blacklock, N. J.: The influence of refined carbohydrate on urinary calcium excretion. Br. J. Urol., *50*:459, 1978.

Thomas, J., Melon, J. M., Steg, A., et al.: Succinimide et lithiase oxalique premiers resultats biologiques. Ann. Urol., *5*:145, 1971.

Thomas, J., Thomas, E., Balau, L., et al.: Réalisation d'une lithiase oxalique expérimentale avec l'hydroxyproline. C.R. Soc. Biol. (Paris), *165*:264, 1971.

Thomas, W. C.: Effectiveness and mode of action of orthophosphates in patients with calcareous renal calculi. Trans. Clin. Climatol. Assoc., *83*:113, 1971.

Thomas, W. C., Jr.: Clinical concepts of renal calculous disease. J. Urol., *113*:423, 1975.

Thomas, W. C., Jr.: Symposium on renal lithiasis. Medical aspects of renal calculous disease. Treatment and prophylaxis. Urol. Clin. North Am., *1*:261, 1974.

Thomas, W. C., Jr.: Use of phosphates in patients with calcareous renal calculi. Kidney Int., *13*:390, 1978.

Thompson, J. C.: Urinary calculi at the Canton Hospital. Surg. Gynecol. Obstet., *32*:44, 1921.

Thompson, R. B., and Stamey, T. A.: Bacteriology of infected stones. Urology, *2*:267, 1973.

Thorwald, J.: The Century of the Surgeon, p. 24. New York, Pantheon, 1956.

Toor, M., et al.: The effect of fluid intake on the acidification of urine. Clin. Sci., *27*:259, 1964.

Transbol, I., and Frydendal, N.: Endocrine and metabolic aspects of urology. Aetiology of stone formation in 145 renal stone patients. Acta Chir. Scand. Suppl., *433*:137, 1973.

Troup, C. W., Lawnicki, C. C., Bourne, R. B., et al.: Renal calculus in children. J. Urol., *107*:306, 1972.

Twinern, F. P.: A study of recurrence following operation for nephrolithiasis. J. Urol., *37*:259, 1937.

Uhlmann, D. R.: Crystal growth from solution: Interface structure and interface kinetics. *In* Finlayson, B., et al. (Eds.): Urolithiasis: Physical Aspects, p. 169. Washington, D.C., National Academy of Sciences, 1972.

Uhlmann, D. R., and Chalmers, B.: The energetics of nucleation. Indust. Eng. Chem., *57*:19, 1965.

Valyasevi, A., and Dhanamitta, S.: Studies of bladder stone disease in Thailand. XVII. Effect of exogenous source of oxalate on crystalluria. Am. J. Clin. Nutr., *27*:877, 1974.

Valyasevi, A., Dhanamitta, S., and Van Reen, R.: Studies of bladder stone disease in Thailand. XVI. Effect of 4-hydroxy-1-proline and orthophosphate supplementations on urinary composition and crystalluria. Am. J. Clin. Nutr., *26*:1207, 1973.

Van Reen, R.: Geographical and nutritional aspects of endemic stones. *In* Brockis, J. G., and Finlayson, B. (Eds.): Urinary Lithiasis. Littleton, Mass. PSG Publishing Co., 1981.

Van Regemorter, G., and Hardy, J. C.: Extravasations at the level of the upper urinary tract. Acta Urol. Belg., 41:858, 1973.

Van't Reit, B., McKinney, W. M., Brandt, E. A., et al.: Dye effects on inhibition and dissolution of urinary calculi. Invest. Urol., 1:446, 1964.

Vaughan, E. D., Jr., Shenasky, J. H., II, and Gillenwater, J. Y.: Mechanism of acute hemodynamic response to ureteral occlusion. Invest. Urol., 9:109, 1971a.

Vaughan, E. D., Jr., Sorenson, E. J., and Gillenwater, J. Y.: Alterations in renal function immediately after release of acute total unilateral ureteral occlusion. Invest. Urol., 8:450, 1971b.

Vaughan, E. D., Jr., Sorenson, E. J., and Gillenwater, J. Y.: The renal hemodynamic response to chronic unilateral complete ureteral occlusion. Invest. Urol., 8:78, 1970.

Vermeulen, C. W., and Goetz, R.: Experimental urolithiasis. VII. Role of sex and genetic strain on determining chemical composition. J. Urol., 72:93, 1954.

Vermeulen, C. W., and Lyon, E. S.: Mechanism of genesis and growth of calculi. Am. J. Med., 45:684, 1968.

Vermeulen, C. W., Lyon, E. S., Ellis, J. E., et al.: The renal papilla and calculogenesis. J. Urol., 97:573, 1967.

Vermeulen, C. W., Lyon, E. S., and Fried, F. A.: On the nature of the stone-forming process. J. Urol., 94:176, 1965.

Vermeulen, C. W., Lyon, E. S., and Gill, W. B.: Artificial urinary concretions. Invest. Urol., 1:370, 1964.

Vermeulen, C. W., Ragins, H. D., Grove, W. J., et al.: Experimental urolithiasis. III. Prevention and dissolution of calculi by alteration of urinary pH. J. Urol., 66:1, 1951.

Vexler, L., Andrei, A., Cordunt, A. R., et al.: Parathyroid adenoma and renal lithiasis. Chirurgia (Bucur.), 23:9, 1974.

Viville, C., Halb, A., Sarrai, M., et al.: Urinary lithiasis in children. A propos of 40 cases. J. Urol. Nephrol. (Paris), 79:839, 1973.

Vogel, V. J.: American Indian Medicine. Norman, Oklahoma, University of Oklahoma Press, 1970.

Voogt, H. J., DeKamp, J. J., et al.: A xanthine calculus in a child with xanthinuria. Notes on a rare inborn error of metabolism. Ned. Tijdschr. Geneeskd., 117:976, 1973.

Wahlberg, J.: The renal response to ureteral obstruction. Scand. J. Urol. Nephrol. (Suppl.) 73: 1, 1983.

Wahlstrom, E. E.: Optical Crystallography. New York, John Wiley & Sons, 1943.

Walton, A. G.: The Formation and Properties of Precipitates. New York, Interscience Publisher, 1967.

Walton, A. G.: Nucleation of crystals from solution. Science, 148:601, 1965.

Wangensteen, O. H., et al.: Lithotomy and lithotomists: Progress in wound management from Franco to Lister. Surgery, 66:929, 1969.

Wart, F., Auvray, P., and Piront, A.: Extrarenal diffusion of contrast media during intravenous urography. Acta Urol. Belg., 41:564, 1973.

Watanabe, T.: Histochemical studies on mucosubstances in urinary stones. Tohoko J. Exp. Med., 107:345, 1972.

Waterhouse, C., and Heinig, R. E.: Parathormone function. N. Engl. J. Med., 294:545, 1976.

Watts, H. G.: Urinary tract stones in childhood. N.Z. Med. J., 80:533, 1974.

Watts, R. W.: Oxaluria. J. R. Coll. Physicians Lond., 7:161, 1973.

Watts, R. W.: Uric acid biosynthesis and its disorders. J. R. Coll. Physicians, 11:91, 1976.

Welshman, S. G., and McGeown, M. G.: Urinary citrate excretion in stone formers and normal controls. Br. J. Urol., 48:7, 1976.

Welshman, S. G., and McGeown, M. G.: The relationship of the urinary cations calcium, magnesium, sodium and potassium, in patients with renal calculi. Br. J. Urol., 47:237, 1975.

Werness, P. G., Bergert, J. H., and Smith, L. H.: Triamterene urolithiasis: solubility, pK, effect on crystal formation, and matrix binding of triamterene and its metabolites. J. Lab. Clin. Med., 99:254, 1982.

Wesson, M. B.: Renal calculi: Etiology and prophylaxis. J. Urol., 34:289, 1935.

Westbury, E. J.: Some observations on the quantitative analysis of over 1000 urinary calculi. Br. J. Urol., 46:215, 1974.

Wexler, B. C.: Histopathology of kidney stone formation in repeatedly bred rats. J. Urol., 90:527, 1963.

White, D. J., Jr., Christoffersen, J., Herman, T. S., Lanzalaco, A. C., and Nancollas, G. H.: Effects of urine pretreatment on calcium oxalate crystallization inhibition potentials. J. Urol., 129:175, 1983.

White, J. L.: Stones in the prostate and seminal vesicles. Texas J. Med., 23:581, 1928.

White, R. W., et al.: Minerals in the urine of stoneformers and their spouses. In Hodgkinson, A., and Nordin, B. E. C. (Eds.): Proceedings of the Renal Stone Research Symposium. London, J. & A. Churchill, Ltd., 1969.

Williams, F. E.: Long-term survey of 538 patients with upper urinary tract stone. Br. J. Urol., 35:416, 1963.

Williams, H. E.: Nephrolithiasis. N. Engl. J. Med., 290:33, 1974a.

Williams, H. E.: Calcium nephrolithiasis and cellulose phosphate. N. Engl. J. Med., 290:224, 1974b.

Williams, H. E., and Smith, L. H.: Disorders of oxalate metabolism. Am. J. Med., 45:715, 1968.

Williams, J. P., Mayo, M. E., and Harrison, N. W.: Massive bladder stone. Br. J. Urol., 49:51, 1977.

Wilson, D. M., Smith, L. H., Segura, J. M., et al.: Renal lithiasis. An optimistic outlook. Minn. Med., 57:368, 1974.

Witten, F. R., Morgan, J. W., Foster, J. G., and Glenn, J. F.: 2,8 hydroxyadenine urolithiasis: review of the literature and report of case in the United States. J. Urol., 130:938, 1983.

Wright, R. J., and Hodgkinson, A.: Oxalic acid, calcium and phosphorus in the renal papilla of normal and stone forming rats. Invest. Urol., 9:369, 1972.

Yanagawa, M., Ohkawa, H., and Tada, S.: The determination of urinary oxalate by gas chromatography. J. Urol., 129:1163, 1983.

Yendt, E. R.: Renal calculi. Can. Med. Assoc. J., 102:479, 1970.

Yendt, E. R., and Cohanim, M.: Ten years' experience with the use of thiazides in the prevention of kidney stones. Trans. Am. Clin. Climatol. Assoc., 85:65, 1973.

Yendt, E. R., Gagne, R. J., and Cohanim, M.: The effects of thiazides in idiopathic hypercalciuria. Am. J. Med. Sci., 251:449, 1966.

Young, J. D., Jr., and Martin, L. G.: Urinary calculi associated with incomplete renal tubular acidosis. J. Urol., 107:170, 1972.

Yu, F.: Urolithiasis in hyperuricemia and gout. J. Urol., 126:424, 1981.

Yu, T. F., and Gutman, A. B.: Relationship of renal production of ammonia to uric acid stone formation in primary gout. In Cifuentes, L., Rapado, A., and Hodgkinson, A. (Eds.): Urinary Calculi. International Symposium on Renal Stone Research, p. 101. Basel, S. Karger, 1973.

Zarembski, P. M., and Hodgkinson, A.: Some factors influencing the urinary excretion of oxalic acid in man. Clin. Chim. Acta, 25:1, 1969.

Zarembski, P. M., and Hodgkinson, A.: The oxalic acid content of English diets. Br. J. Nutr., 16:627, 1962.

Zhiugzhdaa, I. U., Radavichus, A. I., and Sinkevichusc, H. A.: Use of sequential mathematical analysis for establishing the threat of renal calculi disease in an endemic district. Urol. Nefrol. (Mosk.), 37:7, 1972.

Zinneman, H. H., and Jones, J. E.: Dietary methionine and its influence on cystine excretion in cystinuric patients. Metabolism, 15:915, 1966.

Zinsser, H. H., and Karp, F.: How to diminish endogenous oxalate excretion. I. Tyrosine administration. Invest. Urol., 10:249, 1973.

Zoller, N., and Griebsch, A.: Influence of various dietary purines on uric acid production. In Cifuentes, L., Rapado, A., and Hodgkinson, A. (Eds.): Urinary Calculi. International Symposium on Renal Stone Research, p. 84. Basel, S. Karger, 1973.

Selected Introductory Articles and Reviews

Boyce, W. H.: Organic matrix of human urinary concretions. Am. J. Med., 45:673, 1968.

Boyce, W. H.: Symposium on renal lithiasis. Urol. Clin. North Am., 1:179, 1974.

Busby, D. E.: Urinary calculus. Space Life Sci., 1:279, 1968.

Fleisch, H.: Some new concepts on the pathogenesis and the treatment of urolithiasis. Urol. Int., 19:372, 1965.

Gill, W. B.: Urolithiasis update: Biophysical and radiologic advances enhance antistone therapy. Am. J. Kidney Dis., 1:66, 1981.

Kaplan, R. A., and Pak, C. Y.: Diagnosis and management of renal calculi. Tex. Med., 70:88, 1974.

King, J. S.: Currents in renal stone research. Clin. Chem., 17:971, 1971.

King, J. S.: Etiologic factors involved in urolithiasis: A review of recent research. J. Urol., 97:583, 1967.

Malek, R. S.: Renal lithiasis: a practical approach. J. Urol., 118:893, 1977.

Nordin, B. E. C., and Hodgkinson, A.: Urolithiasis. Adv. Intern. Med., 13:155, 1967.

Pak, C. Y. C.: Medical management of nephrolithiasis. J. Urol., 128:1157, 1982.

Raisz, L. G.: Leaving no (renal) stone unturned (Editorial). N. Engl. J. Med., 292:529, 1975.

Robertson, W. G., Peacock, M., Marshall, R. W., et al.: Saturation-inhibition index as a measure of the risk of calcium oxalate stone formation in the urinary tract. N. Engl. J. Med., 294:249, 1976.

Scott, R.: Urinary tract stone disease. Classic studies. Urology, 6:667, 1975.

Smith, L. H.: Symposium on stones. Am. J. Med., 45:649, 1968.

Smith, M. J. V.: Basic considerations in calculous disease. Urol. Survey, 22:217, 1972.

Vermeulen, C. W., Ellis, J. E., and Hsu, T.: Experimental observations on the pathogenesis of urinary calculi. J. Urol., 95:681, 1966.

Williams, H. E.: Nephrolithiasis. N. Engl. J. Med., 290:33, 1974.

Yendt, E. R.: Renal calculi. Can. Med. Assoc. J., 102:479, 1970.

Research Seminars and Conferences, Proceedings

Hodgkinson, A., and Nordin, B. E. C.: Renal Stone Research Symposium (Leeds, 1968). London, J. & A. Churchill, Ltd., 1969.

Finlayson, B., Hench, L. L., and Smith, L. H.: Urolithiasis, Physical Aspects. Washington, D.C., National Academy of Sciences, 1972.

Cifuentes-DeLatte, L., Rapado, A., and Hodgkinson, A.: Urinary Calculi (Madrid, 1972). Basel, S. Karger, 1973.

Finlayson, B., and Thomas, W. C., Jr.: International Colloquium on Renal Lithiasis. Gainesville, University of Florida Press, 1976.

Brockis, J. G., and Finlayson, B.: Urinary calculus. In Finlayson, B., and Brockis, J. G. (Eds.): Urinary Lithiasis. Littleton, Mass. PSG Publishing Co., 1981.

Fleisch, H., Robertson, W. G., Smith, L. H., and Vahlensieck, W.: In Robertson, W. G., Fleisch, H., Smith, L. H., Vahlensieck, W. (Eds.) International symposium on urolithiasis research. New York, Plenum Press, 1976.

Smith, L. H., Robertson, W. G., and Finlayson, B.: Urolithiasis: Clinical and basic research. In Robertson, W. G., Smith, L. H., and Finlayson, B. (Eds.): Symposium. New York, Plenum Press, 1981.

Van Reen, R.: Idiopathic urinary bladder stone disease. In Van Reen, R. (Ed.): Symposium. Washington, D.C., DHEW, 1900.

APPENDIX A LOW PURINE DIET
(Carbohydrate—223, Protein—89, Fat—115: Cal. 2283)

BREAKFAST	
Fruit	1 serving
Cereal (no oatmeal)	1 serving
Eggs	2
Toast	1 slice
Butter or margarine	As desired
Beverage	Sanka, Kaffee Hag, or Postum
Milk	As desired
Cream	As desired
Sugar	As desired

LUNCHEON	
Soup	1 serving (see list)
Cheese	2 ounces
Vegetable (cooked)	1 serving
Vegetable (raw)	1 serving
Bread	1 slice
Butter or margarine	As desired
Dessert	1 serving (see list)
Milk	1 glassful

DINNER	
Allowed soup	If desired
Meat, fish, fowl	2 ounces (twice weekly)
Potato	1 serving
Vegetable (cooked or raw)	1 serving

DINNER *continued*	
Bread	1 slice
Butter or margarine	As desired
Dessert	1 serving (see list)
Milk	1 glassful

SPECIAL INSTRUCTIONS

1. Avoid liver, sweetbreads, brains, and kidney. A 2-ounce portion of any other meat, fish, or fowl may be served twice weekly.
2. Serve cheese and eggs as meat substitutes. Fish roe and caviar may be used as desired.
3. Use 1–2 pints of milk daily.
4. Omit all meat extracts, broth soups, and gravies.
5. Omit the following vegetables entirely from the diet:
   Dried beans, lentils, dried peas, spinach.
6. Avoid coffee, tea, chocolate, and cocoa.
7. Omit alcoholic beverages of all kinds.
8. Use fruits of all kinds—fresh, canned, and dried.
9. Allow cereals of all kinds except oatmeal.
10. Soups allowed are milk soups made with any vegetables except those forbidden.
11. Desserts allowed are fruit, puddings, cake, ice cream, gelatin desserts or pie.
12. Beverages allowed are milk or buttermilk, and any decaffeinated coffee or cereal coffee.

APPENDIX B   Low Methionine Diet

Foods Allowed

Soups	Soup made without meat stock or milk
Meat or meat substitute	Spaghetti or macaroni dish made without addition of meat, cheese, or milk. Peanut butter. *One serving per day:* Lamb, veal, beef, pork, crab, or bacon (3 strips)
Beverages	Soy milk, tea, coffee
Vegetables	Asparagus, artichoke, beans, beets, carrots, chicory, cucumber, eggplant, escarole, lettuce, onions, parsnips, potato, pumpkin, rhubarb, tomatoes, turnips
Fruits	Apples, apricots, bananas, berries, cherries, fruit cocktail, grapefruit, grapes, lemon juice, nectarines, oranges, peaches, pears, pineapple, plums, tangerines, watermelon, cantaloupe
Salads	Raw or cooked vegetable or fruit salad
Cereals	Marcaroni, spaghetti, noodles
Breads	Whole wheat, rye, white
Nuts	Peanuts
Desserts	Fresh or cooked fruit, ices, fruit pies
Concentrated sweets	Sugar, jams, jellies, syrup, honey, hard candies
Concentrated fats	Butter, oleomargarine, cream
Miscellaneous	Pepper, mustard, vinegar, garlic, oil, herbs and spices

Foods Not Allowed

Soups	Any soups made with meat broth
Meat or meat substitute	Fish and those meats not listed above
Vegetables	Those not listed above
Eggs	In any form
Cheese	All varieties
Nuts	All varieties, except peanuts
Beverages	Milk in any form
Fruits	Those not listed above

APPENDIX C LOW CALCIUM, LOW OXALATE DIET
(300 mg calcium)

Food Groups	Foods Allowed	Foods to Avoid
Beverage	Carbonated beverages, cereal beverages; limit tea and coffee to 3 cups daily of either	Malted beverages, milk, milk drinks, chocolate beverages
Breads and cereals	White and wheat bread, refined cereals, crackers, rye or variety breads, donuts, pastries, sweet rolls	Any cereal enriched with calcium, such as instant-type hot cereals; cereals containing bran, such as All-Bran or Granola; pancakes, waffles, and other "quick breads"; breads containing bran; 100% whole wheat bread
Desserts	Gelatin desserts made of allowed foods, fruit ices, sherbets. Cakes, cookies, or other products not made from milk	Desserts made with milk, such as custard, pudding, ice cream, ice milk; cream pies and cream-filled baked products
Fats	Butter or margarine, cream (up to ⅓ cup daily), salad oils, cooking fat, nondairy creamer, cream cheese (up to 2 oz per day)	Half-and-half, sour cream (can be included in ⅓ cup allowance)
Fruit	Canned, cooked, or fresh fruit except those excluded, dried fruit (up to ½ cup daily)	*Rhubarb, *cranberries, *plums, *gooseberries, and *raspberries
Meat and meat substitutes	Meat, fish, and fowl except those excluded. Not more than 2 eggs daily, including those used in cooking†	Sardines, shrimp, and oysters; cheese—yellow, natural, and processed; white cheese, including cottage cheese and Parmesan cheese; yoghurt
Potato or substitute	Potato, macaroni, noodles, spaghetti, refined rice	Whole grain rices
Soups	Broth, vegetable, or meat soup made from allowed foods	Bean or pea soup; cream or milk-based soups
Sweets and nuts	Candy without chocolate, almonds, or peanuts; honey, jam, jelly, syrups, and sugar; other nuts	*Chocolate, molasses, *cocoa, almonds, peanuts
Vegetables	Canned, cooked, or fresh vegetables or vegetable juice except those excluded	*Asparagus, dried beans and peas, broccoli, beet greens, swiss chard, collards, mustard greens, turnip greens, kale, *spinach
Miscellaneous	Salt, spices, and pepper (in moderation), vinegar	Cream sauce, milk gravy, peanut butter, ripe olives

*Foods high in oxalate.
†Robertson et al. (1979) believe that limited animal protein intake also benefits calcium stone formers.

APPENDIX D LOW PHOSPHATE DIET REGIMEN (SHORR REGIMEN)*

1. Daily dietary intake of phosphorus restricted to less than 300 mg/day; calcium restricted to less than 700 mg/day.
2. Patient takes 40 ml of basic aluminum carbonate gel four times daily.
3. Fluid intake of at least 3000 ml/day and more as needed to keep urinary output at 2000 ml/day.
4. Analysis of urinary phosphorus excretion, which should be less than 250 mg/day, is done at intervals.

*Modified from Marshall, V. F., Lavengood, R. W., Jr., and Kelly, D.: Ann. Surg., *162*:366, 1965.

GENITOURINARY TRAUMA

CHAPTER 26

Genitourinary Trauma

PAUL C. PETERS, M.D.,
ARTHUR I. SAGALOWSKY, M.D.

RENAL TRAUMA

Prompt recognition and accurate characterization of renal injuries are necessary to obtain maximal renal salvage and ensure general well-being of the patient. Delayed or missed diagnosis of renal injury may lead to excessive bleeding, urinary extravasation and intense tissue inflammation, and wound infection, all of which jeopardize renal function and recovery.

Anatomy

The kidneys are normally located high in the retroperitoneum and are protected posteriorly by the large psoas and quadratus lumborum muscles and anteriorly by the peritoneum and abdominal viscera. In addition, the kidneys are surrounded by cushioning perinephric fat inside Gerota's fascia and have a vertical mobility of one to three vertebral bodies. The lower rib cage (ribs 10 to 12) provides an outer barrier to the kidneys. Thus, in terms of surface anatomy and trauma one must consider the kidneys intrathoracic as well as retroperitoneal organs.

Etiology and Mechanisms of Injury

Traditionally, discussions of renal trauma diagnosis and management have dealt separately with blunt and penetrating injuries. The distinction by cause is important because of the differing renal and associated nonrenal injuries, and it will of necessity be maintained in this chapter. However, refinements in diagnostic modalities and surgical techniques allow increasing reliance on estimation of the extent of renal injury, as well as the cause, in deciding therapy. Thus, it is timely to present an overall approach to renal trauma.

Penetrating trauma accounted for 84 per cent of the 185 renal injuries that required surgery at Parkland Memorial Hospital, Dallas, between January 1, 1976 and August 8, 1980 (Table 26–1) (Sagalowsky et al., 1983). The great majority of penetrating renal injuries were due to gunshot wounds (79 per cent), and the remainder were due to stabbings. Every patient with renal trauma from a gunshot wound had accompanying intra-abdominal or intrathoracic injury (Table 26–2). Liver, small bowel, stomach, and colon injuries were the most common. Three combined renal and ureteral injuries occurred. During the same 56-month study period, 15 isolated ureteral injuries were treated (see further on). Renal injuries from gunshots had accompanying life-threatening aortic (4 per cent) or vena caval (7 per cent) trauma in 11 per cent of cases.

Stab wounds to the kidney also were associated with a high incidence of nonrenal injuries (77 per cent) in the same series (Table 26–3). Liver trauma was the most common injury associated with renal stab wounds. Trauma to the

TABLE 26–1. RENAL INJURIES REQUIRING SURGERY*

Etiology	No. Cases	Per Cent
Penetrating		
Gunshot	122	66
Stab	33	18
Blunt	30	16
Total	185	100

*Adapted from Sagalowsky, A. I., McConnell, J. D., an Peters, P. C.: J. Trauma, 23:128, 1983.

TABLE 26–2. ASSOCIATED NONRENAL INJURIES IN
GUNSHOT WOUNDS (122 CASES)*

Injured Organ	No. Cases	Per Cent
Liver	58	48
Small intestine/duodenum	47	38
Stomach	45	37
Colon	43	35
Spleen	28	23
Pancreas	25	20
Chest	12	10
Vena cava	9	7
Aorta	5	4
Ureter	3	2

*Adapted from Sagalowsky, A. I., McConnell, J. D.,
and Peters, P. C.: J. Trauma, *23*:128, 1983.

TABLE 26–3. ASSOCIATED NONRENAL INJURIES IN
STAB WOUNDS (33 CASES)*

Injured Organ	No. Cases	Per Cent
Liver	6	18
Colon	5	13
Spleen	5	13
Small intestine/duodenum	4	12
Vena cava	1	3
Ureter	1	3

*Adapted from Sagalowsky, A. I., McConnell, J. D.,
and Peters, P. C.: J. Trauma, *23*:128, 1983.

intestine or spleen was much less common in renal stabbings than in gunshot wounds. Ureteral or vena caval trauma was rare in stab wounds to the kidney, and associated aortic injury was not seen.

Carlton and associates reported similar findings in a series of 127 gunshot wounds and 54 stabbings with renal injuries treated at the Ben Taub Hospital in Houston during a 12-year period (Carlton, 1978). Renal injury was present in 8 and 6 per cent of abdominal gunshot wounds and stabbings, respectively. Associated nonrenal trauma was seen in 81 per cent of cases with penetrating renal injury (gunshot wounds,

90 per cent; stabbings, 56 per cent). The distribution of associated nonrenal injuries (in decreasing frequency, liver, colon, spleen, stomach, pancreas, small intestine) was essentially the same as that reported in the aforementioned Parkland experience. In an earlier Parkland Memorial Hospital series, 83 per cent of patients with penetrating renal trauma had nonrenal injuries (Peters and Bright, 1977).

The overt mechanism of renal injury from penetrating trauma is the obvious tissue disruption to parenchyma, collecting system, and vasculature (Fig. 26–1). In patients with gunshot wounds to the kidney, missile velocity and blast effect must be considered as well. High-velocity missiles (greater than 1100 feet per second) generally penetrate and exit from the body.

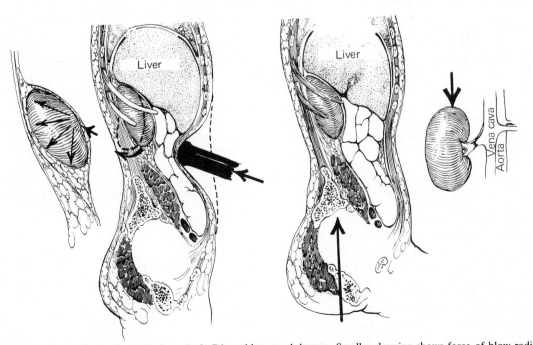

Figure 26–1. Mechanisms of renal injury. *Left*, Direct blow to abdomen. Smaller drawing shows force of blow radiating from the renal hilum. *Right*, Falling on buttocks from a height (contrecoup of kidney). Smaller drawing shows direction of force exerted upon the kidney from above. Tear of renal pedicle. (From McAninch, J. W.: *In* Smith, D. R. (Ed.): General Urology. Los Altos, Lange Medical Publications, 1981, p. 245. Used by permission.)

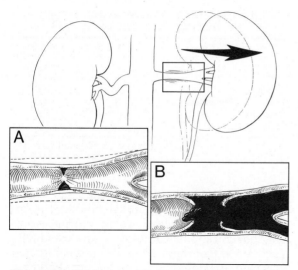

Figure 26–2. Mechanism of renal artery thrombosis in blunt traumatic injury. The kidney remains in motion in reference to the more stationary aorta. *A,* The media and adventitia, because of their elasticity, stretch readily. The intima, being less elastic, tears. *B,* The intimal flap initiates the clotting mechanism, and the thrombus is quickly propagated distally. (From Peters, P. C., and Bright, T. C., III: Urol. Clin. North Am., *4*:18, 1977.)

Such high-velocity trauma radiates a current of injury known as blast effect, which may cause delayed tissue necrosis, bleeding, and fistula formation in areas that appeared viable at the time of injury.

Blunt renal trauma usually is associated with sudden deceleration of the human body. Motor vehicle accidents of all types, falls from a height (Fig. 26–1), or blunt physical contact are the most common causes of this type of renal injury. Rib or upper lumbar vertebral transverse process fractures may lacerate or contuse renal parenchyma. Deceleration or crush injuries may thrust the kidneys internally against the rib cage or vertebrae or externally against the steering wheel or dashboard of a vehicle, resulting in contusion, laceration, or avulsion of renal parenchyma. A direct blow to the abdomen (Fig. 26–1) or flank during fighting or athletics is a common cause of blunt renal injury. Renal arterial intimal tear, with subsequent thrombosis, and disruption of the ureteropelvic junction are two unique renal injuries associated with deceleration (Fig. 26–2.) Children are prone to suffer the latter injury owing to the greater mobility of the longitudinal spinous ligaments, which permits hyperextension-flexion injuries in the young. In a Parkland Memorial Hospital series of 115 patients hospitalized with blunt renal trauma between 1965 and 1975, the specific etiology was: motor ve-

hicle accident, 86; fall, 15; fighting (fisticuffs), 7; football, 4; crush injury, 2; swing injury, 1 (Peters and Bright, 1977). Associated nonrenal injuries occurred in 44 per cent of cases and frequently were severe. In the more recent Parkland series, 100 per cent of the 30 cases of blunt renal trauma requiring surgery had associated nonrenal injuries (Table 26–4) (Sagalowksy et al., 1983). The higher incidence of splenic (57 per cent) and hepatic (40 per cent) injury and the lesser occurrence of bowel injury in association with blunt (as opposed to penetrating) renal trauma is noteworthy.

Pre-existing renal abnormality (hydronephrosis, tumor, vascular malformation, cystic disease) makes the kidney more susceptible to injury. One should always suspect predisposing factors when the renal injury is disproportionate to the trauma (Fig. 26–3).

Classification of Injury

Renal injuries may be classified as minor or major (Fig. 26–4). The most common nomenclature separates renal trauma into three classes: (1) minor parenchymal laceration or contusion (Fig. 26–4*A* to *C*); (2) major parenchymal laceration, usually through the corticomedullary junction and often involving the collecting system (Fig. 26–4*C*′ and *D*′); and (3) shattered kidney (Fig. 26–4*A*′) or renal pedicle injury (Fig. 26–4*B*′) (Peters and Bright, 1977). In general, 65 to 70 per cent of renal injuries are minor, 10 to 15 per cent are major parenchymal injuries, and the remaining 10 to 15 per cent are shattered kidneys or renal pedicle injuries. In the 115 patients reported in the Parkland series on blunt renal trauma requiring hospitalization, there were 54 Class 1 injuries (47 per cent), 36 Class 2 injuries (31 per cent), and 25 Class 3 injuries (22 per cent) (Peters and Bright, 1977). In the more recent Parkland series of 185 consecutive renal injuries that

TABLE 26–4. Associated Nonrenal Injuries in Blunt Trauma (30 Cases)*

Injured Organ	No. Cases	Per Cent
Spleen	17	57
Liver	12	40
Pancreas	4	13
Chest	4	13
Colon	2	7
Small intestine	1	3

*Adapted from Sagalowsky, A. I., McConnell, J. D., and Peters, P. C.: J. Trauma, *23*:128, 1983.

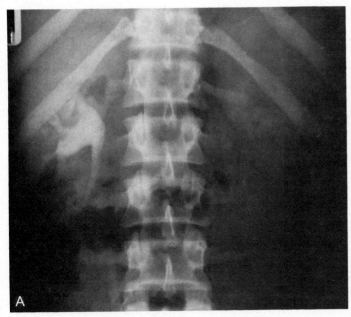

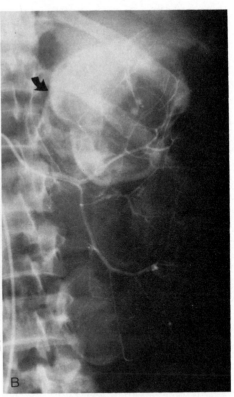

Figure 26–3. Patient with hematuria after minor left flank trauma in touch football game. *A,* Early pyelogram film shows poor visualization of left kidney and suggests mass effect or extravasation over upper pole. *B,* Arteriogram reveals changes of long-standing hydronephrosis from UPJ obstruction and extravasation (arrow).

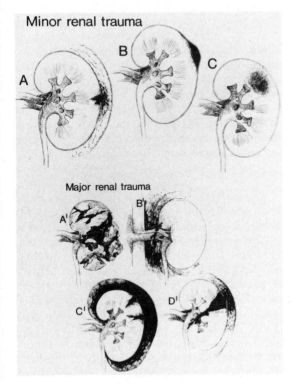

Figure 26–4. Minor renal injuries. *A,* Simple laceration. *B,* Subcapsular hematoma. *C,* Renal contusion. Major renal injuries: *A',* Renal rupture. *B',* Laceration of renal artery and vein. *C',* Perirenal hematoma. *D',* Laceration through collecting system. (From Peters, P. C., and Bright, T. C., III: Urol. Clin. North Am., *4:*19, 1977.)

required surgery, the incidence of renal pedicle trauma was 14 per cent—20, 12, and 15 per cent for blunt, gunshot, and stab injuries, respectively (Table 26–5) (Sagalowsky et al., 1983). Twenty of 26 renovascular injuries were due to penetrating trauma (77 per cent). From 1960 through 1979 a total of 94 patients with 96 renal pedicle injuries were treated at Parkland Memorial Hospital (Turner et al., 1983). The specific pedicle injury was to the renal artery, renal vein, or both in 18, 33, and 45 instances, respectively (19, 47, and 34 per cent, respectively). Sixty-four of these 94 patients (68 per cent) suffered penetrating trauma.

The greatest determinant of mortality in patients with renal trauma is the nature and extent of associated nonrenal injuries. The mortality rate was 10 per cent among 115 patients hospitalized at the Parkland Memorial Hospital for blunt renal trauma (Peters and Bright, 1977). Only 2 of 11 deaths were due primarily to renal injury–pedicle hemorrhage (Table 26–6). The mortality rate in patients requiring surgery for renal trauma in the most recent Parkland series was 5 per cent overall and 12 per cent in patients with renal pedicle injuries (Table 26–7). The mortality rate was 37 per cent in the 20-year retrospective Parkland review on renal pedicle trauma despite a high nephrectomy rate (44 per cent). Trauma resulting in renal pedicle injury has a high association with fatal nonrenal events.

TABLE 26–5. RENAL PEDICLE INJURIES IN RENAL TRAUMA REQUIRING SURGERY (185 CASES)*

Mechanism of Injury	No. Cases	Incidence (Per Cent)	Injury			Result	
			RENAL ARTERY	RENAL VEIN	BOTH	REPAIR	NEPHRECTOMY
Blunt	6	20					
			2				2
				3			3
					1		1
Gunshot	15	12					
			4			1	3
				5		1	4
					6	1	5
Stab	5	15					
				3		2	1
					2		2
Total	26	14					

*Adapted from Sagalowsky, A. I., McConnell, J. D., and Peters, P. C.: J. Trauma, 23:128, 1983.

Diagnosis

HISTORY

Trauma to the upper abdomen, back, flank, or lower rib cage may result in renal injury. A detailed history is essential in both blunt and penetrating trauma. In motor vehicle accidents, knowledge of vehicle speed and the victim's role as pedestrian, driver, or passenger helps the physician to estimate the degree of injury. A high index of suspicion of major renal injury is appropriate for all patients thrown from a vehicle or involved in a fall from a considerable height. The size or caliber of weapon is important in assessing penetrating injuries. Flank pain or history of hematuria after the injury requires evaluation regardless of the apparent location of trauma. Prior history of renal abnormality or hematuria makes renal trauma more likely after subsequent injury. Severe costovertebral pain may indicate renal ischemia from renal artery thrombosis.

PHYSICAL EXAMINATION

Flank or upper abdominal tenderness, contusion or palpable mass, and crepitance over the lower rib cage or lumbar vertebrae suggest renal injury and require evaluation. However, absence of these findings does not rule out major or even life-threatening renal trauma in a patient with a suggestive history.

URINALYSIS

Examination of the urine by the physician is part of the physical examination of the trauma patient and is the first diagnostic aid. Renal injury must be excluded in every patient with gross or microscopic hematuria following trauma. The degree of hematuria may bear no relationship to the severity of renal injury. Hematuria may be absent in 10 to 25 per cent of renal injuries. However, as seen in Table 26–8, the great majority of renal injuries without hematuria are Class 3 in type, and the severe nature of the trauma would alert the physician to possible renal injury in these cases.

RADIOGRAPHY

Occasionally patients with blunt or, more often, penetrating trauma are too unstable for preoperative studies. However, the following tests are desirable whenever possible. Chest and abdominal films are made. Rib or vertebral fractures were present in 32 and 7 per cent of our patients with blunt renal trauma, respectively (Fig. 26–5A) (Peters and Bright, 1977). Patterns of calcification over the kidney may suggest pre-existing pathology: mottled (neoplasm), solid (calculus), or curvilinear (aneurysm or cyst). Ground-glass density in the flank suggests urinary extravasation and/or hematoma or pre-existing mass, such as hydronephrosis or tumor. Absence of the psoas muscle shadow is a nonspecific but suggestive finding of renal injury.

TABLE 26–6. CAUSES OF DEATH IN BLUNT RENAL TRAUMA PATIENTS*

Head injury	3
Shock from blood loss	2
Multiple injuries, extreme	2
ATN from blood transfusion	1
Avulsion of the renal artery and vein	1
Avulsion of the renal vein only	1
Liver laceration	1

*From Peters, P. C., and Bright, T. C., III: Urol. Clin. North Am., 4:17, 1977.

TABLE 26–7. Mortality Rate with Renal Trauma

Series	Type of Renal Trauma	No. Cases	Mortality (Per Cent)
1960–1979 (Turner et al., 1983)	Pedicle injuries	94	37
1965–1979 (Peters and Bright, 1977)	Blunt trauma	115	10
1976–1980 (Sagalowsky et al., 1983)	Required renal surgery	185	5

TABLE 26–8. Absence of Hematuria in Renal Trauma*

Class of Injury	Cases Without Hematuria	
	Total Cases	Per Cent
1	3/52	5.8
2	1/36	2.8
3	9/14	64.3

*Adapted from Hai, M. A., Pontes, J. E., and Pierce, J. M., Jr.: J. Urol., *118*:7, 1977.

If urethral trauma has been excluded, a cystogram is performed by instilling 250 to 300 ml of 15 per cent iodinated contrast solution into the bladder per urethral catheter in all patients undergoing a urologic trauma evaluation (see lower tract injuries, later). The cystogram is evaluated for extraperitoneal or intraperitoneal extravasation or ureteral reflux.

Evaluation of the upper urinary tract proceeds with a high-dose infusion pyelogram or double-dose bolus pyelogram. Standard low-dose pyelography has a false negative rate of approximately 34 per cent in renal trauma (Carl-ton, 1978). We infuse 1 ml per pound body weight of 30 per cent iodinated contrast and obtain films at 1, 5, 15, and 30 minutes. The first film provides a nephrogram, and subsequent films help to identify calyceal and ureteral integrity or extravasation. Infusion pyelography identifies approximately 80 per cent of renal injuries (Peters and Bright, 1977; Carlton, 1978). The pyelogram has two equally important functions in the evaluation of renal trauma. First, the presence and function of a contralateral kidney are documented in unilateral injury. Second, the extent of injury to the affected renal unit(s) is classified, as depicted in Figure 26–4. Renal injury is suggested by (1) decreased excretion of contrast, (2) obliteration of psoas shadow or renal outline from extravasation of blood or urine, (3) scoliosis away from the injury as the result of ipsilateral psoas muscle spasm, and (4) extravasation of contrast (Fig. 26–6) (Carlton, 1978). A normal infusion pyelogram in a trauma patient with hematuria suggests minor renal contusion and rules out major renal injury (Fig. 26–7).

Incomplete or poor visualization of a por-

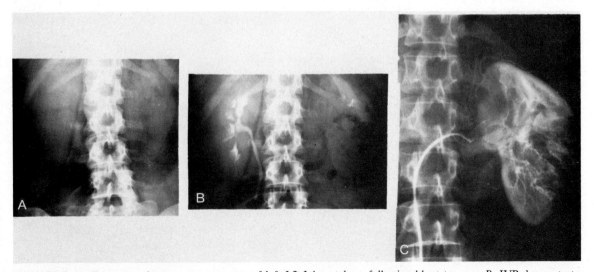

Figure 26–5. *A,* Fractures of transverse processes of left L2–L4 vertebrae following blunt trauma. *B,* IVP demonstrates poor excretion, loss of lower pole outline, and nonvisualization of lower calyces in left kidney. *C,* Arteriogram reveals major laceration through corticomedullary junction. (From Sagalowsky, A. I.: *In* Ehrlich, R. M. (Ed.): Modern Technics in Surgery. Mount Kisco, N.Y., Futura Publishing Co., 1984. Used by permission.)

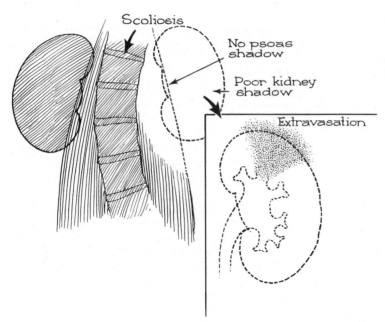

Scoliosis

No psoas shadow

Poor kidney shadow

Extravasation

Figure 26–6. Radiographic findings associated with renal parenchymal injury. (From Carlton, C. E., Jr.: *In* Harrison, J. H., et al. (Eds.): Campbell's Urology. Philadelphia, W. B. Saunders Co., 1978.)

tion of the kidney on infusion pyelography suggests major renal trauma, including deep laceration, avulsion, or vascular occlusion (Fig. 26–5B). Further delineation of the injury should be sought with selective angiography, whenever possible, if the pyelogram suggests a major injury. Arteriography in the patient shown in Figure 26–5B revealed a deep cortical laceration with preservation of the vasculature to all renal segments (Fig. 26–5C). Figure 26–8 reveals a major injury with laceration and avulsion of parenchyma. Arteriography may reveal complete parenchymal fracture with preserved vasculature to all of the kidney (Fig. 26–9). The identification of areas of renal devascularization is important because necrosis and abscess formation or hypertension are common sequelae (Fig. 26–10).

Figure 26–7. Normal infusion tomogram in patient with hematuria following an automobile accident. (From Carlton, C. E., Jr.: *In* Harrison, J. H., et al. (Eds.): Campbell's Urology. Philadelphia, W. B. Saunders Co., 1978.)

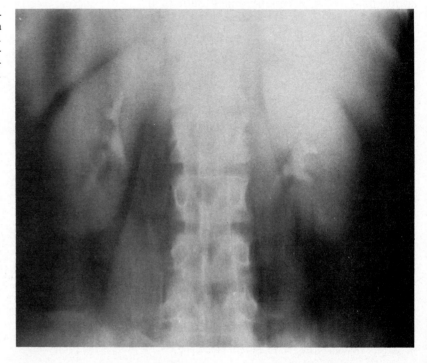

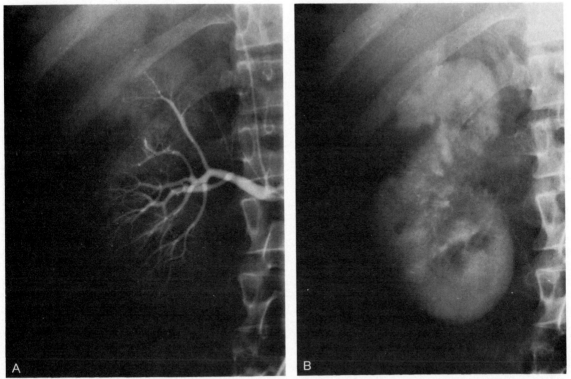

Figure 26–8. *A,* Arteriogram reveals major parenchymal laceration. *B,* Capillary phase of study clearly demonstrates avulsion injury and preservation of arterial supply to remaining parenchyma. (From Sagalowsky, A. I.: *In* Ehrlich, R. M. (Ed.): Modern Technics in Surgery. Mount Kisco, N.Y., Futura Publishing Co., 1984. Used by permission.)

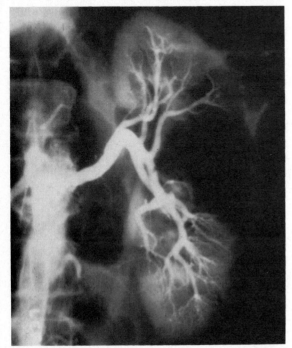

Figure 26–9. Major renal injury with complete parenchymal fracture and preservation of segmental blood supply.

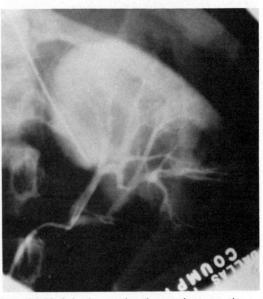

Figure 26–10. Selective renal angiogram demonstrating complete avulsion of the lower pole artery and associated parenchyma.

Nonvisualization of the kidney on pyelography requires immediate arteriography whenever possible. Although severe contusion and renal spasm may occasionally produce nonvisualization, renal artery intimal tear with thrombosis is the most common cause (Figs. 26–11 and 26–12). Pedicle injury was present in 7 of 14 instances of nonvisualization on pyelography in the Parkland series on blunt renal trauma (Table 26–9) (Peters and Bright, 1977). Arteriography is also useful to assess aortic or major visceral nonrenal trauma, especially hepatic and splenic injuries.

Computerized tomography (CT) is rightfully assuming an increasing role in the evaluation of abdominal and renal trauma. Some authors feel CT identifies urinary extravasation more often than does pyelography and more precisely defines the extent of injury (Table 26–10) (Federle et al., 1981; McAninch, 1983). However, pyelography rarely underestimates the extent or class of renal injury. Thus, it is debatable whether the additional precision offered by CT or one's basic philosophy of management is the real determinant of therapy. McAninch and associates believe that the diagnostic precision of CT allows nonoperative management of selected penetrating and blunt minor renal injuries confined to the flank (McAninch, 1983). The characteristics of specific renal injury

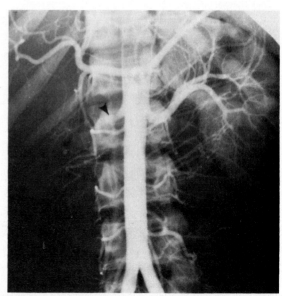

Figure 26–12. Total occlusion of right renal artery (arrow) following blunt renal trauma. (From Sagalowsky, A. I.: *In* Ehrlich, R. M. (Ed.): Modern Technics in Surgery. Mount Kisco, N.Y., Futura Publishing Co., 1984. Used by permission.)

on CT have been defined (Sandler and Toombs, 1981), and examples are presented. Intrarenal hematoma appears as a round, poorly marginated lesion, which has decreased attenuation in distinction to the contrast-induced enhancement of normal parenchyma (Figs. 26–13 and 26–14). Perinephric hematoma has a streaked or bubbly appearance from infiltration of blood into perinephric fat (Figs. 26–15, 26–16, and 26–17A). Renal lacerations with urine extravasation are well shown on films taken after the injection of intravenous contrast (Fig. 26–17B). Segmental devascularization or arterial spasm reveals a sharp margin on CT, unlike a contusion or intrarenal hematoma, and lacks subcapsular hematoma or enhancement after contrast administration. The availability, difficulty, and expense to the patient of CT are now in the same range as arteriography, and morbidity is low.

TABLE 26–9. Causes of Nonvisualizing Kidneys*

Renal artery thrombosis	3
Comminuted kidney	3
Renal vein avulsion with comminuted kidney	2
Renal contusion, severe	2
Polar rupture	2
Renal artery tear	1
Bivalve kidney	1
Avulsion of renal artery and vein	1

*From Peters , P. C., and Bright, T. C., III: Urol. Clin. North Am., *4*:17, 1977.

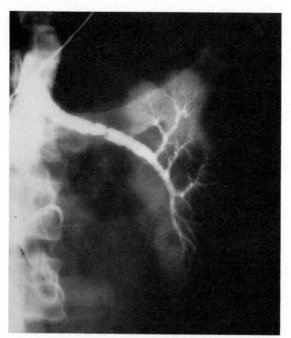

Figure 26–11. Irregular renal artery outline from traumatic intimal flap. This lesion is likely to progress to thrombosis if not repaired.

TABLE 26–10. RESULTS OF COMPUTED TOMOGRAPHY IN RENAL TRAUMA IN 24 PATIENTS WITH SUSPECTED MAJOR INJURY*

	Minor Laceration or Contusion	Major Laceration without Extravasation	Major Laceration with Extravasation	Total
Trauma				
Blunt	11	4	6	24
Penetrating		2	1	
IVP or Nephrotomography				
Poor visualization	11	6	6	24
Extravasation	0	(?)1	(?)2	
Computed Tomography				
Perirenal hematoma	11	6	7	
Intrarenal hematoma	2	6	6	24
Laceration	6	6	7	
Extravasation	0	0	7	
Operations	0	2	4	6

*From McAninch, J. W.: Monogr. Urol., *4*:43, 1983.

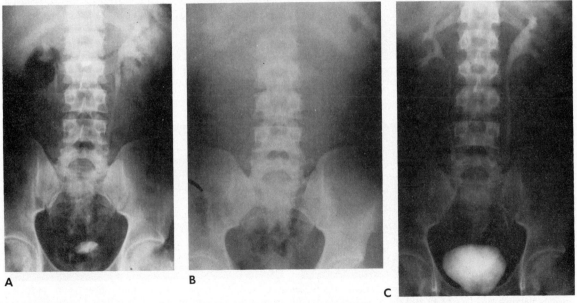

Figure 26–13. *A,* Initial infusion pyelogram following gunshot wound to left flank appears normal. Bullet is noted over L2 vertebral body. No renal injury was identified at the time of exploration. *B,* Abdominal plain film taken 5 days later, when patient developed fever and pain, shows generalized ground-glass appearance and paucity of bowel gas, suggesting urinary extravasation. *C,* Pyelogram taken the same day as *B* is still normal.

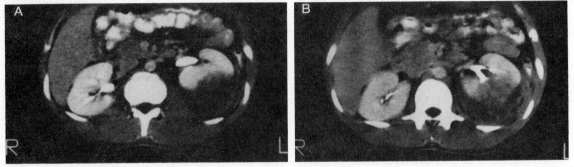

Figure 26–14. Abdominal CT of same patient as in Figure 26–13*C* reveals perirenal hematoma and urinoma *(A)* and intrarenal hematoma *(B).*

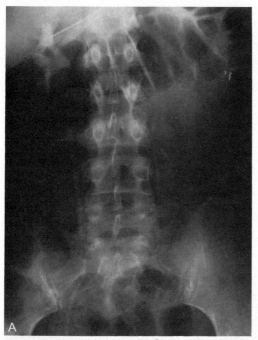
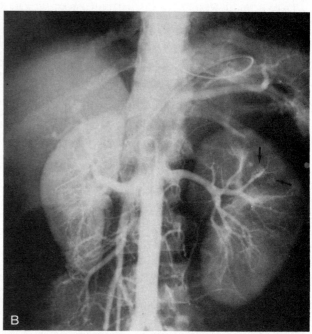

Figure 26–15. *A,* Pyelogram reveals poor visualization of left kidney in patient after automobile accident. *B,* Flush aortogram reveals left main renal artery and major segmental blood supply to be intact. A small amount of vascular extravasation (arrows) is demonstrated.

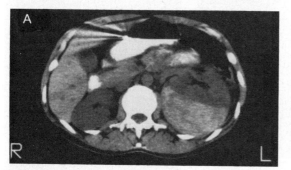

Figure 26–16. *A,* Abdominal CT of same patient as in Figure 26–15 reveals a large perirenal fluid collection. *B,* This view shows a parenchymal laceration and the characteristic bubbly appearance created by dissection of blood and urine in the perinephric fat.

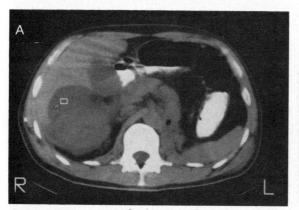
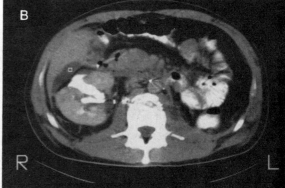

Figure 26–17. *A,* CT following trauma to the right flank shows perinephric collection. *B,* After the injection of intravenous iodinated contrast, deep parenchymal laceration extending into the collecting system is shown.

The ultimate use of CT vis-à-vis arteriography in the detection of renal and other abdominal trauma remains to be determined.

Retrograde pyelography is rarely useful in the diagnosis of renal parenchymal injury because sufficient information on function and parenchymal detail is not provided. In addition, the procedure is time-consuming and may introduce infection into the upper tracts. Retrograde pyelography may be indicated in the assessment of ureteral injuries (see further on).

Ultrasonography also is of limited value in the initial evaluation of renal trauma for the same reasons of imprecision and lack of functional correlation. Sonography is useful for identifying and following perinephric hematoma and urinoma; however, CT appears to be the preferred modality.

Radionuclide scans accurately depict renal blood flow (Fig. 26–18). However, parenchymal or collecting system defects are less precisely imaged with isotope scans than by the above-mentioned techniques. In addition, angiography would still be advised before repair of renovascular injuries. Thus, nuclear scans have only a limited role in the initial evaluation of renal trauma in patients with allergy to iodinated contrast materials.

Treatment

PHILOSOPHY

Surgical exploration of all penetrating renal injuries is recommended because of the high incidence of associated intra-abdominal injuries. As indicated earlier, some authors are observing on abdominal CT selected patients with penetrating trauma apparently confined to the flank. This approach is worth further careful study but should not yet be accepted as standard practice.

The management of blunt renal trauma depends upon the degree of injury. The great majority of patients have minor parenchymal injury and are best treated by observation. These patients are placed at bed rest until the urine grossly clears of blood, and vital signs, clinical examination, and hematocrit are serially monitored. Approximately 10 per cent of patients with blunt renal trauma have Class 3 injuries and uniformly require exploration to control hemorrhage and to have any chance of renal salvage. These injuries frequently require nephrectomy owing to extensive renal parenchymal trauma and other life-threatening nonrenal injuries that take precedence over renal vascular repairs.

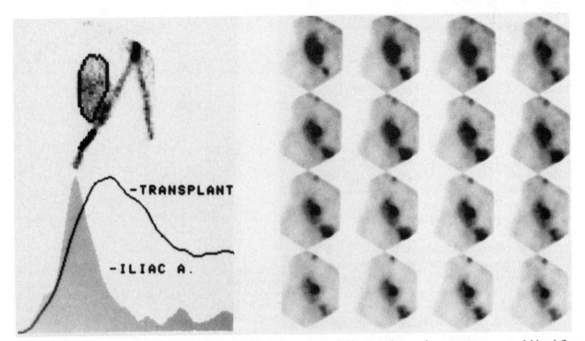

Figure 26–18. *Left,* Radionuclide image of renal allograft, aorta, and iliac arteries, and computer-generated blood flow curves of iliac artery and kidney. *Right,* Excretory phase of scan shows nephrogram, collecting system, and bladder.

Optimal management of the remaining 10 to 15 per cent of patients who have blunt major renal parenchymal injuries (Class 2) is controversial. Carlton has long proposed surgical repair of all major renal injuries, because 90 per cent of the delayed complications of nonoperative therapy (urinoma, abscess, delayed bleeding) occur in this group of patients (Carlton, 1978). In contrast, the reasons for nonoperative management of Class 2 blunt renal injuries are several. Nearly all small and many major urinary extravasations seal spontaneously. Careful monitoring of the patient's clinical status and use of sonography or CT allow early diagnosis of urinoma and percutaneous or open drainage and repair in those few patients who require specific treatment. Initial renal exploration at the time of injury also has the risk of sudden uncontrolled hemorrhage, requiring nephrectomy. Generalized practice of the surgical techniques to be described later allows early control of the renal pedicle before opening Gerota's fascia and greatly reduces the likelihood of such bleeding, making this argument against early exploration less compelling than it was in the past. In one series, the incidence of nephrectomy associated with renal exploration for trauma was reduced from 56 to 18 per cent after these surgical principles were applied (McAninch and Carroll, 1982). Major parenchymal lacerations heal spontaneously in the majority of cases, provided that the vasculature is intact. Devascularized renal segments should be debrided to prevent delayed abscess formation and bleeding. In Thompson's experience with nonoperative management of all blunt renal trauma except pedicle injuries in 43 patients, the incidence of delayed surgery and overall renal salvage was 4.7 and 96.5 per cent, respectively (Thompson, 1977).

Peters and Bright reported that 14.6 per cent of 41 patients hospitalized and observed for blunt renal trauma required delayed surgery, as follows: nephrectomy, two; heminephrectomy, two; repair of renal laceration, one; drainage of renal fossa, one (Peters and Bright, 1977). In the same series, the length of hospitalization was longer (10 to 21 days) in patients treated nonoperatively initially than in those requiring immediate surgery (7 to 12 days).

Frequently the urologist is first consulted during emergency exploratory laparotomy of a trauma patient in whom a large retroperitoneal hematoma is found. The urologist must decide on an approach to such potential renal injuries regardless of either the mechanism of injury or his treatment philosophy and with less diagnostic information than he would like. Our approach at Parkland Memorial Hospital is to explore and repair potential renal injuries if we are first consulted after the abdomen has already been opened by the General Surgery trauma team. Broad-spectrum antibiotics are given to all patients requiring surgery for renal trauma.

SURGICAL TECHNIQUES

A long vertical midline incision from xyphoid to pubis is chosen for speed in opening and closing the wound and to afford maximum exposure (Fig. 26–19). Rapid control of the renal pedicle before opening Gerota's fascia is the most important principle in surgery of renal trauma. The small intestine is mobilized out of the abdomen by incising the posterior parietal peritoneum from the cecum upward to the ligament of Treitz (Fig. 26–19). The inferior mesenteric vein may be ligated and transected where it joins the splenic vein to allow further cephalad retraction of the body of the pancreas and exposure of the left renal vein as it crosses over the aorta (Fig. 26–20). The left renal vein is mobilized by ligating and dividing adrenal, gonadal, and lumbar veins. The origin of both the right and the left renal arteries is found almost invariably posterior to the junction of the left

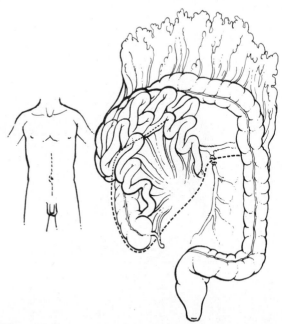

Figure 26–19. A long vertical midline incision allows rapid exposure in renal trauma cases. The entire small bowel and ascending colon may be rapidly mobilized by incising the posterior peritoneum, as shown. The inferior mesenteric vein may be ligated and divided to increase exposure to the renal vessels. (From Sagalowsky, A. I.: *In* Ehrlich, R. M. (Ed.): Modern Technics in Surgery. Mount Kisco, N.Y., Futura Publishing Co., 1984. Used by permission.)

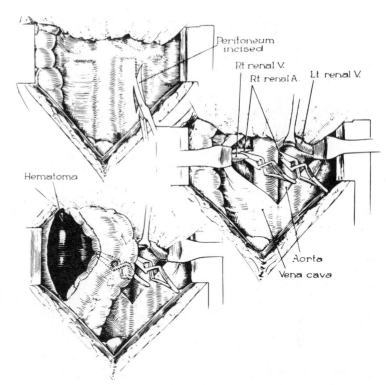

Figure 26–20. The posterior peritoneum is incised parallel to the inferior mesenteric vein. The left renal vein is mobilized and retracted cephalad to expose the origin of right and left renal arteries. The perirenal hematoma is entered only after the renal pedicle is controlled. (From Carlton, C. E., Jr.: *In* Harrison, J. H., et al. (Eds.): Campbell's Urology. Philadelphia, W. B. Saunders Co., 1978.)

renal vein and vena cava (Fig. 26–21). The course of the renal artery may be horizontal, cephalad, or caudad. Thus, the right renal artery may lie within a vertical span of several inches at the right lateral margin of the vena cava. The constant spatial relationship of the renal artery origin and the overlying left renal vein allows for rapid control of both renal arteries (Fig. 26–22). Multiple renal arteries occur in 25 per cent of patients, on right and left sides equally. The possibility of multiple renal arteries should be considered whenever the identified artery is smaller than anticipated. Multiple renal veins occur in 15 per cent of patients and are confined to the right side 80 per cent of the time.

Figure 26–21. Retroperitoneal node dissection demonstrates the nearly constant origin of right and left renal arteries dorsal to the left renal vein (retracted cephalad) as it crosses the aorta.

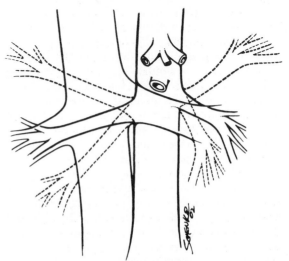

Figure 26–22. Variable course of renal arteries (particularly on the right side) is demonstrated. For rapid control, the renal artery is best located near the aorta.

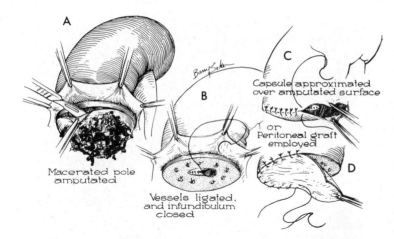

Figure 26–23. Surgical treatment of renal polar injury. *A,* Guillotine amputation of the injured parenchyma. *B,* Watertight closure of the collecting system and suture hemostasis. *C,* Reapproximation of renal capsule. *D,* Denuded surface covered with peritoneal patch graft. (From Carlton, C. E., Jr.: *In* Harrison, J. H., et al. (Eds.): Campbell's Urology. Philadelphia, W. B. Saunders Co., 1978.)

The renal artery on the affected side is carefully secured with a vascular clamp. Torque or crushing of the renal artery must be avoided. Following pedicle control, the colon is mobilized from the anterior surface of Gerota's fascia and the perirenal space is opened and the hematoma evacuated. The extent of renal injury is identified. If more than 30 minutes of renal artery occlusion is anticipated, renal cooling is advisable. Traumatized parenchyma is debrided sharply. Severe polar injuries are best treated by guillotine amputation to minimize delayed necrosis and fistula formation (Fig. 26–23). Openings into the collecting system are carefully closed with 4-0 and 5-0 chromic catgut (Fig. 26–23B). All injured intraparenchymal vessels are individually suture-ligated with 4-0 and 5-0 chromic catgut (Fig. 26–23B). When renal capsule is available, closure over the parenchymal injury is desirable (Fig. 26–23C). However, such closure is not mandatory if collecting system and vascular injuries have been properly repaired. Renal lacerations and avulsion injuries are treated in a similar manner. Devitalized tissue is debrided and collecting system and vascular injuries are repaired, as previously described. If hemostasis is adequate after these repairs, renal capsule may simply be closed. However, if further hemostasis is necessary, topical clotting agents such as Avitene or Oxycel may be applied and mattress sutures through parenchyma may be tied over bolsters. Saucerized defects in parenchyma may be covered with omental or peritoneal grafts (Figs. 26–23C and 26–24). Finally, the flank is drained with Penrose or closed suction drains in all surgical explorations of renal trauma.

Shattered kidneys require nephrectomy to prevent fatal hemorrhage. The extent of paren-chymal injury precludes reconstruction and renal salvage.

Renal vein lacerations may be repaired directly by venorrhaphy. Renal artery trauma may require a variety of repairs. Turner and coworkers (1983) reported the use of lateral arteriorrhaphy (5), or arterial resection and repair by primary reanastomosis (4), or bypass graft with saphenous vein (2), or autogenous artery (1) in 12 renal artery repairs attempted for 96 renal artery injuries occurring over a 20-year period (Turner et al., 1983).

INTERVENTIONAL RADIOLOGY

Percutaneous drainage affords effective initial treatment, and often definitive care, of both

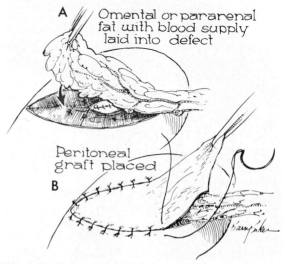

Figure 26–24. Placement of viable omentum or perirenal fat in large renal defect. (From Carlton, C. E., Jr.: *In* Harrison, J. H., et al. (Eds.): Campbell's Urology. Philadelphia, W. B. Saunders Co., 1978.)

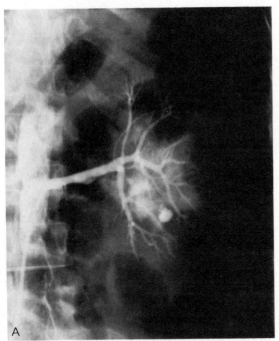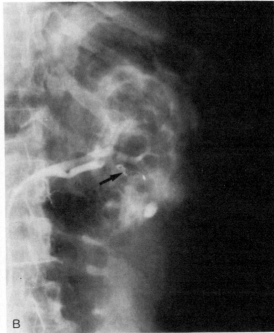

Figure 26–25. *A,* Renal arteriogram reveals bleeding false aneurysm from branch to left renal artery in patient 1 week after blunt trauma. *B,* Bleeding was arrested by selective embolization with Gianturco steel coil. (From Sagalowsky, A. I.: *In* Ehrlich, R. M. (Ed.): Modern Technics in Surgery. Mount Kisco, N.Y., Futura Publishing Co., 1984. Used by permission.)

urinoma and infected hematoma that occur after renal trauma. Delayed hemorrhage from segmental renal artery injury and false aneurysm formation (Fig. 26–25*A*) may be treated by specific embolization of the affected branch vessel with Gelfoam particles or a steel coil (Fig. 26–25*B*).

RESULTS

The specific renal operations performed for trauma at Parkland Memorial Hospital from 1976 to 1980 are shown in Table 26–11. The renal unit was salvaged in 85, 70, and 64 per cent of stab, gunshot, and blunt injuries, respectively. Management of renal pedicle trauma remains disappointing. Of the 12 renal artery repairs described by Turner, 4 were successful, 5 failed, and 3 cases lacked follow-up. The most recent results in 26 renal pedicle injuries managed at Parkland are shown in Table 26–5. One isolated renal artery injury, three isolated renal vein injuries, and one combined pedicle injury were repaired. In contrast to the experience at Parkland, others report that blunt trauma is the leading cause of renal pedicle injury (Maggio and Brosman, 1978; Cass, 1979). Renal pedicle trauma is associated with a high mortality rate (12 to 42 per cent), usually from associated nonrenal injuries.

COMPLICATIONS AND FOLLOW-UP

Abscess and urinoma may be heralded by pain and fever, and flank mass may be detected clinically or by sonography or CT. Dramatic

TABLE 26–11. RENAL OPERATIONS PERFORMED*

Operation	No. Cases	Per Cent
Gunshot		
Repair and drainage	58	47
Nephrectomy	34	28
Heminephrectomy	24	20
Aborted	4	3
Vascular repair	2	2
	122	100
Stab		
Repair and drainage	27	82
Nephrectomy	5	15
Heminephrectomy	1	3
	33	100
Blunt		
Repair and drainage	17	57
Nephrectomy	10	33
Heminephrectomy	1	3
Pyeloplasty	1	3
Aborted	1	3
	30	99

*Adapted from Sagalowsky, A. I., McConnell, J. D., and Peters, P. C.: J. Trauma, *23*:128, 1983.

transient fever and flank pain, without other signs of sepsis, may indicate renal infarction from renal artery thrombosis. Hypertension after renal parenchymal injury resolves over 2 to 6 weeks in most cases. However, persistent hypertension occurs in 1 to 5 per cent of renal trauma (Peters and Bright, 1977) and is caused by excess renin secretion due to renal artery stenosis or, less often, from a constricting perirenal hematoma (Page effect). An intravenous pyelogram and blood pressure determination are obtained 6 weeks and 1 year after renal injury. Patients suffering renovascular trauma may develop hypertension as late as 4 years after injury.

URETERAL INJURY

A simple classification allows one to organize the approach to the management of the patient with ureteral injury. In approaching the management of ureteral injury, the authors have found the following classification to be helpful: (1) site: upper, middle or lower third; (2) time of recognition: immediate or delayed; (3) nature of the injury: blunt trauma with laceration or avulsion, penetrating trauma (low-velocity or high-velocity missile); and (4) presence of concomitant injuries modifying treatment. Consideration of these four variables may result in different management for the same injury. For example, a midureteral injury might be managed by simple end-to-end anastomosis with an indwelling stent and nearby Penrose drain, or Hemovac if it were a solitary injury in a 30-year-old male patient, whereas the injury might require nephrectomy if associated with a colonic perforation and iliac artery injury in a 65-year-old patient.

Etiology

Ureteral injuries secondary to trauma are usually associated with a bullet wound, with 22-caliber and 38-caliber wounds being most common. In addition to urologic endoscopic manipulative injuries, such as avulsion during stone-basketing maneuvers, many abdominal operations are associated with urologic injury. Common among these are (1) abdominal hysterectomy; (2) cesarean section with or without inguinal hysterectomy; (3) colon resections, anterior and abdominoperineal; (4) surgery for large adnexal masses, including ovarian; (5) abdominal vascular procedures; and (6) herni-

TABLE 26–12. ETIOLOGY OF OPERATIVE URETERAL INJURIES, PARKLAND MEMORIAL HOSPITAL (10 YEARS)

Abdominal hysterectomy	8
Marshall-Marchetti vesical suspension	2
Colectomy	2
Exploratory laparotomy	3
Stone-basket manipulation	2
Ureterolithotomy and stone-basket manipulation	1
Vaginal hysterectomy	1
Wertheim hysterectomy	1
Iliofemoral thromboendarterectomy	1
Appendectomy	1
Colostomy closure	1
Transureteroureterostomy	1
Total	24

orrhaphy (Table 26–12). No surgery that involves operating on the trunk is exempt from causing ureteral injury; occasionally, ureteral injury occurs during laminectomy (neurosurgical or orthopedic). The incidence of ureteral injury following abdominal hysterectomy continues to be ten times the incidence following vaginal hysterectomy.

Diagnosis

The presence or absence of hematuria is of little help (Table 26–13). Ureteral injury due to penetrating missiles is usually suspected from the presence of extravasation on the excretory urogram. It must be suspected in all abdominal gunshot wounds. The excretory urogram is quite accurate as an aid to detection of ureteral injury. In a series of 49 patients reported by Carlton (1978), an abnormality was detected in 46 of 49 cases by excretory urography, and the site of extravasation could be localized in 25 of the 49 from the excretory urogram alone. Computerized axial tomography (CAT) is an accurate

TABLE 26–13. URETERAL INJURY: INCIDENCE OF HEMATURIA (29 PATIENTS)*

	Normal		Hematuria	
	No.	%	No.	%
External violence (10 patients)	1	10	9	90
Surgical trauma (19 patients)	17	89	2	11
Total	18	62	11	38

*From Carlton, C. E., Jr.: *In* Harrison, J. H., et al. (Eds.): Campbell's Urology. Philadelphia, W. B. Saunders Co., 1978.

means of diagnosing the extravasation preoperatively, although it is more commonly employed in the blunt trauma patients than in the penetrating missile ones. Penetrating injuries often are explored promptly because of associated injuries and shock, and there has not been time for preoperative CAT. At surgery, the use of 5 ml of indigo carmine intravenously will often disclose small areas of extravasation that may have been overlooked until the bluish discoloration appears in the tissues.

When ureteral injury is not suspected at the time of surgery when it occurs, or is not found at the time of exploration of the patient with multiple injuries, diagnosis may be delayed for a considerable time. Abdominal pain, tenderness, ileus, and fever are the most common signs and symptoms of unsuspected ureteral injury. Three to 5 per cent of patients have no symptoms at all, and months or years later a nonvisualizing kidney may be seen on excretory urography (Peters and Bright, 1976). In 7 to 10 per cent of patients, a hydronephrosis of varying size or the presence of a fluid collection (urinoma) may be the only clue to antecedent injury. Only about 10 per cent of patients show hematuria following surgical injury to the ureter.

Retrograde pyelography gives one the most precise preoperative study to localize the site and magnitude of extravasation. It determines whether the lesion is complete or partial. One may attempt passage of a ureteral stent or guidewire (Benson or Lunderquist) and subsequently a stent that will allow drainage and healing in partial or incomplete disruptions of the circumference of the ureter. Percutaneous puncture and antegrade insertion of guidewires, and subsequently stents over the guidewires, are an alternative to retrograde manipulation (Fig. 26–26).

Since percutaneous techniques may be performed under local anesthesia, the surgeon may prefer this approach in a patient who is gravely ill and no candidate for general anesthesia, especially if considerable hydronephrosis is present to facilitate the puncture of the collecting system. At times, a catheter can be passed down through the collecting system into the bladder when it is not possible to pass the ureteral catheter from below because of angulation of the ureter or edema of the intramural ureter. The degree of anatomic deformity and function, including functional recovery of the kidney by clearance techniques, can be assessed by urine collection via a nephrostomy tube introduced percutaneously over an indwelling catheter or guidewire.

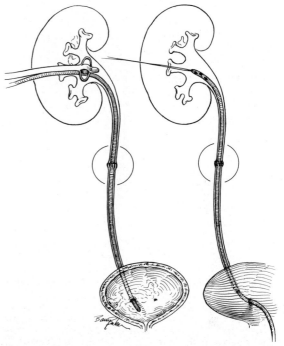

Figure 26–26. Preferred method of ureteral stenting. Ureteral stent alongside of and secured to nephrostomy. Indwelling ureteral stent secured to skin of the flank by nonabsorbable suture. (From Carlton, C. E., Jr.: *In* Harrison, J. H., et al. (Eds.): Campbell's Urology. Philadelphia, W. B. Saunders Co., 1978.)

Management

When ureteral injury is suspected, an excretory urogram is done. Delayed upright films after the intravenous injection of contrast material may show the level and magnitude of injury. An attempt should then be made to introduce a guidewire and retention ureteral catheter (double J catheter), which will serve as drain and stent. As noted earlier, retrograde or antegrade techniques may be used. CAT is of considerable value in the assessment of concomitant renal injury, showing extravasation not seen on the excretory urogram. Ureterography (antegrade or retrograde) more precisely localizes the area of ureteral injury. In patients in whom there is not complete disruption of ureteral continuity, passage of a double J ureteral and bladder stent with drainage down to the site of ureteral injury may be all that is necessary.

SURGICAL MANAGEMENT

At surgery, usually through a midline incision, the ureter should be divided (resected) superiorly and inferiorly to a point at which it bleeds freely or fluoresces with an ultraviolet

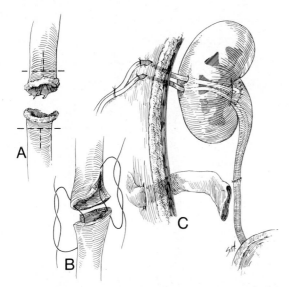

Figure 26–27. Ureteroureterostomy. *A,* The ureteral edges are debrided to viable bleeding tissue, and the ureter is longitudinally spatulated on opposite sides to prevent twisting. *B,* The apex of one spatulated side is sutured to the nonspatulated edge of the other ureteral end, with care taken to exclude the suture from the ureteral lumen. *C,* The anastomosis is completed with interrupted sutures. Urinary diversion is accomplished by nephrostomy drainage in connection with a Silastic ureteral stent placed through the anastomosis. (From Peters, P. C., and Bright, T. C., III: *In* Longmire, W. P., Jr. (Ed.): Advances in Surgery. Chicago, Year Book Medical Publishers, 1976.)

light after fluorescein dye is injected intravenously. This minimizes later fistulization because of failure to recognize areas of coagulation necrosis already present in the ureter. Ureteropelvic junction disruptions and major upper ureteral injuries (greater than 2-cm lacerations) are best treated by nephrostomy and stent after repair with fine-gut suture, as illustrated (Fig. 26–27). Drainage should always be provided down to the site of repair (Hoch et al., 1975). The authors prefer a Penrose drain with a urostomy bag placed over it at the skin level. Lower ureteral injuries usually require tunneled reimplantation into the bladder. If this cannot be done without tension on the anastomosis, using a psoas hitch of the urinary bladder when necessary, a full-thickness flap of bladder of suitable length should be turned cephalad and the ureter tunneled into it (Boari or Ockerblad flap) (Fig. 26–28). This is stented 7 to 10 days if there is considerable edema of the ureter or bladder flap. Again, the authors have tended to use indwelling double J stents and to avoid external stents, particularly in female patients. Female patients tolerate cystoscopic removal of stents without anesthesia better than do male patients.

When major ureteral loss is present, or when it is necessary to not have any ureteral leakage postoperatively (e.g., in the case of associated major vascular repair), one may ligate the ureter and perform nephrostomy either at the time or percutaneously within 24 hours, later doing a transureteroureterostomy if there is no contraindication (Hodges et al., 1963). Alternatively, one may choose substitution of a segment of tapered or nontapered ileum for the ureter. Stents used in the ureter in proximity to a repaired vascular injury should be very soft and flexible (Fig. 26–29) (Orkin, 1964). This is particularly necessary when major tissue loss is present and no omentum or retroperitoneal fat is available to interpose between injured tissues. Ordinary ureteral catheters are too rigid for this purpose, and erosion may occur with vascular leak. Although nephrectomy may be the procedure of choice when there is simultaneous injury to the colon, ureter, and iliac artery or aorta, it is seldom necessary in the 20- and 30-year-old trauma victims.

BLADDER INJURIES

Etiology and Classification

Owing to its location deep in the pelvis, the urinary bladder is an infrequently injured organ. The bladder is well protected by the surrounding bony structure of the pelvis laterally, by the urogenital diaphragm inferiorly, and by the rectum posteriorly. Its shape varies with the amount of urine contained within and the presence of intravesical obstruction or extrinsic pelvic disease. The type of injury that may occur depends on the volume of urine contained in the bladder at the time of insult.

Over a 10-year period at Parkland Memorial Hospital, 133 injuries to the urinary bladder were treated. Injuries to the bladder are secondary to penetrating or blunt trauma. The most common causes of penetrating injury are gunshot wounds, stab wounds, and iatrogenic injury secondary to attempted catheterization and urologic instrumentation (Table 26–14).

Bladder injuries secondary to blunt trauma may be classified as (1) contusion, (2) extraperitoneal rupture, or (3) intraperitoneal rupture. Bladder contusion secondary to blunt or penetrating trauma may be associated with gross hematuria but does not require surgical intervention. Extraperitoneal rupture of the urinary bladder occurs secondary to penetration of the bladder wall by a bone fragment when the pelvis

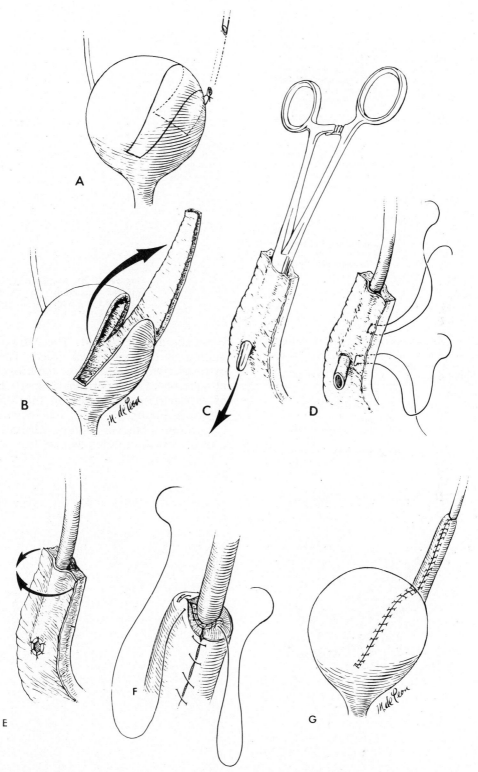

Figure 26–28. Technique of bladder flap ureteroplasty. *A* and *B*, Creation of broad-based bladder flap. *C,* Submucosal tunnel created for antireflux reimplantation of the ureter. *D,* Submucosal reimplantation of the ureter. Sutures in the posterior aspect of the flap rigidly fix the flap to the psoas muscle. *E,* Bladder flap rolled into tube. *F,* Ureter fixed to proximal flap. *G,* Completed bladder flap ureteroplasty. (From Carlton, C. E., Jr.: *In* Harrison, J. H., et al. (Eds.): Campbell's Urology. Philadelphia, W. B. Saunders Co., 1978.)

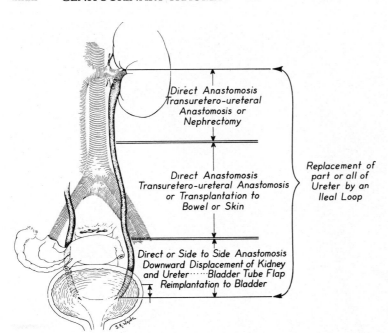

Figure 26–29. Management of ureteral injury, depending on location. (Reprinted and modified from Orkin, 1964.)

TABLE 26–14. Causes of 133 Urinary Bladder Injuries, Parkland Memorial Hospital

Penetrating Injury		Blunt Trauma	
Gunshot wound	58	Motor vehicle accident	53
Stab wound	6	Blow to abdomen	5
Iatrogenic	4	Fall	3
Spike	2	Spontaneous injury	1
Self-catheterization	1		

is fractured (Fig. 26–30). The extravasation is limited to the perivesical space. There is no extravasation of urine below the urogenital diaphragm or into the peritoneal cavity. Examples of extraperitoneal rupture of the bladder are shown in Figure 26–31. In our experience, extraperitoneal bladder rupture constitutes 44 per cent of vesical ruptures. Ninety-five per cent of

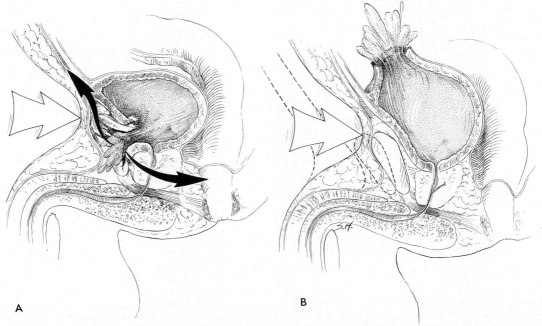

A   B

Figure 26–30. *A,* Mechanism of extraperitoneal urinary bladder rupture. The pubic rami are fractured, and the bladder is perforated by a bony fragment. *B,* Mechanism of intraperitoneal vesical rupture. A sharp blow is delivered to the lower abdomen of patient with distended urinary bladder. The distensive force is exerted equally on all surfaces of the bladder, and it ruptures as its weakest point, usually the dome.

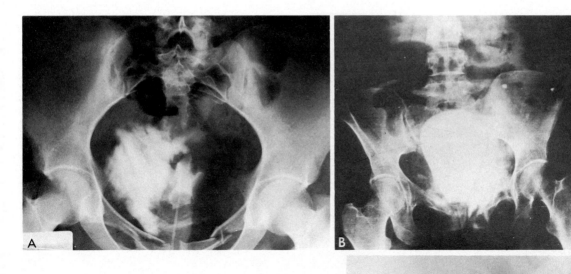

Figure 26–31. Cystographic appearance of extraperitoneal bladder rupture. *A,* Note the flame like wisps of extravasated contrast material with no filling of bladder lumen. *B,* Bladder filled with contrast material with perivesical extravasation. (From Shires, G. T. (Ed.): Care of the Trauma Patient. New York, McGraw Hill Book Co., 1966.) *C,* "Teardrop"–shaped bladder from compression by pelvic hematoma. Pyelogram taken after simultaneous intravenous injection of contrast agent. (From Longmire, W. P., Jr. (Ed.): Advances in Surgery, Vol. 10. Chicago, Year Book Medical Publishers, 1976.)

the extraperitoneal vesical ruptures due to blunt trauma in our series were associated with concomitant pelvic fractures. In contradistinction, 5 per cent (26 of 543) of patients with pelvic fractures displayed an extraperitoneal rupture of the urinary bladder.

Intraperitoneal rupture of the urinary bladder may have a different cause (Fig. 26–32). This injury usually occurs in a patient who sustains a blow to the lower abdomen while the bladder is distended with urine. The force of the blow is therefore directed equally toward all surfaces of the bladder, which will rupture at its weakest point, the dome. The bladder contents are evacuated into the peritoneal cavity, and free flow of urine into the peritoneal cavity continues, presenting as ascites if unrecognized.

Intraperitoneal vesical ruptures account for 48 per cent of bladder ruptures in our series. Eight per cent of patients suffered combined intra- and extraperitoneal rupture of the bladder. This occurs when there is a blow to the lower abdomen and concomitant pelvic fracture. Spontaneous rupture of the bladder may occur with acute or chronic urinary retention but is unusual in the absence of pre-existing bladder disease, such as neoplasm or inflammation.

Diagnosis

On initial presentation to the emergency room, the patient with bladder injury may complain of suprapubic pain or the absence of

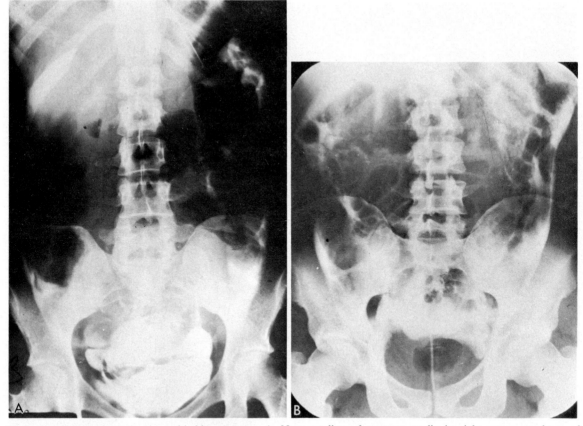

Figure 26–32. Intravesical urinary bladder rupture. *A,* Note pooling of contrast media in right upper quadrant of peritoneum. *B,* The contrast material outlines the peritoneal surface and the bowel interfaces.

micturition since injury, or he may give a history of a sharp, direct blow to the lower abdomen. Physical examination reveals suprapubic tenderness without any muscular rigidity or signs of peritoneal irritation unless associated visceral injuries are present. Bowel sounds are often normal. Only 3 per cent of patients present in shock from bladder injury alone; when shock is present, other causes of hypotension should be meticulously investigated (Reiser, 1963). The patient may not be able to void spontaneously because of pain or neurologic dysfunction or, in the case of intraperitoneal rupture, because there is urinary leakage into the peritoneal cavity so that the bladder is never distended enough for the act of micturition to occur. The presence of hematuria is a more reliable finding in the patient with bladder rupture than in other injuries of the genitourinary system. In our series, 94 per cent of patients with bladder rupture had hematuria.

After the patient has undergone initial assessment, the evaluation of the urinary tract proceeds as follows. A plain abdominal film is

made, and the presence of pelvic or other fractures is sought. Calcifications, foreign bodies, or missiles should be noted. Urethral trauma must be excluded by history, physical examination, and urethrography if indicated by history and blood at meatus. A soft retention catheter is then passed through the urethral meatus into the bladder. Next, 300 ml of 30 per cent iodine-containing, sterile, water-soluble contrast material is instilled through the catheter by gravity. Then an anteroposterior film is made, and the size and shape of the bladder are noted as well as any irregularity, trabeculation, or vesicoureteral reflux.

In the patient with a pelvic fracture, there is massive blood loss into the surrounding tissues, and the bladder will often be compressed into the "teardrop deformity" (Fig. 26–32). In patients with extraperitoneal rupture, flamelike wisps of urinary extravasation are noted on the film of the full bladder. Next, the bladder is allowed to drain, and an anteroposterior film is made. This postdrainage film may reveal subtle areas of urinary extravasation that were obscured when the bladder was filled with contrast material (Peters and Bright, 1976). After a satisfactory cystogram is made, evaluation of the upper urinary tract is performed by means of an intravenous infusion pyelogram. One ml per pound of body weight of a 30 per cent iodine-containing contrast material (Renografin) is infused over a 1-minute period. An abdominal film is made 1 minute after the completion of the injection for evaluation of the nephrographic appearance of the kidneys. Subsequent films are made at 5, 15, and 30 minutes after injection. The collecting systems will begin to fill at 5 minutes; however, 15 to 30 minutes are required for complete calyceal filling and subsequent ureteral filling with contrast material.

Treatment

The principles in the management of the patient with a ruptured bladder are (1) adequate urinary diversion from the area of the injury; (2) prompt, adequate drainage of the perivesical area or other areas of extravasation; and (3) closure of the defect in the vesical wall, if possible. In the patient with penetrating trauma, exploration should always be promptly performed, not only to evaluate and treat the bladder injury but also to assess the integrity of surrounding abdominal viscera and vasculature. The abdomen is usually opened with an appropriate midline incision and then explored. After any intra-abdominal injury is assessed, attention is directed to the bladder defect. In victims of penetrating trauma, after the bladder has been opened, the integrity of the ureteral orifices and lower ureter should be assessed. This may be done by injecting 5 ml of indigo carmine intravenously; after 3 to 8 minutes, its appearance should be noted at each ureteral orifice. If the vesical defect is in an inaccessible position that requires difficult external dissection and manipulation to expose, the defect in the bladder may be sutured intravesically with absorbable suture (chromic gut). If the penetrating missile has entered through the peritoneal surface of the bladder, the peritoneum is freed and the bladder defect closed in three layers. Running interlocking sutures are used. The mucosa is closed with 5-0 chromic catgut, the muscle with 3-0 chromic catgut, and the adventitial layer with 3-0 chromic catgut. In patients with bladder rupture, we prefer the use of a 28 or 30 French Malecot catheter as a suprapubic cystostomy tube. One-inch diameter Penrose drains are

placed on either side of the bladder neck in the space of Retzius and brought out through separate stab wounds.

Patients with intraperitoneal rupture of the bladder following blunt trauma are managed by exploratory laparotomy and bladder repair, as are those with extraperitoneal bladder rupture; however, prompt closure of the vesical defect is more important in the former group of patients.

Mulkey and Witherington (1974) have advocated nonoperative management of bladder rupture only for those patients who have a minimum of bleeding with no tendency to clot formation. These selected patients should have no evidence of sepsis, no protrusion of the bowel into the bladder, no other reason for abdominal surgery, and no urinary tract infection. The urethral catheter must be managed properly to make sure it is draining at all times.

In conservative (urethral catheter only) management of the patient with a small intraperitoneal rupture of the bladder, the surgeon need not be concerned with the small amount of urine that has leaked into the peritoneum, since fluid placed in the peritoneal cavity tends to approach the composition and osmolarity of the interstitial fluid (Evans and Brown, 1973). The electrolytes contained in this urine will diffuse across the peritoneal membrane into the interstitial fluid, and water will follow passively. The concentration of urea and creatinine in the peritoneum will increase as long as the leak continues, since these substances are not perfectly dialyzable across the peritoneum. If the urinary leak is decreased by catheter drainage or closure of the vesical defect, it can be anticipated that within 7 days the retained urea and creatinine will have equilibrated with the interstitial fluid. The composition of urea, creatinine, and electrolytes remains constant in the serum. The presence of sterile urine in the peritoneal cavity will not cause signs of peritonitis (Bourdeau et al., 1974). Bourdeau reported a patient with intraperitoneal urinary extravasation that was tolerated for 3 months without clinical or chemical abnormalities. Hayes and colleagues (1983) have shown that an extraperitoneal rupture of the bladder may be managed very well by urethral catheter drainage alone.

SURGICAL TECHNIQUES

Suprapubic Cystostomy (Fig. 26–33). Unless the abdomen has been previously opened for abdominal exploration, a small lower abdominal midline suprapubic incision should be made. The incision is extended sharply through the linea alba, and the rectus muscles are sep-

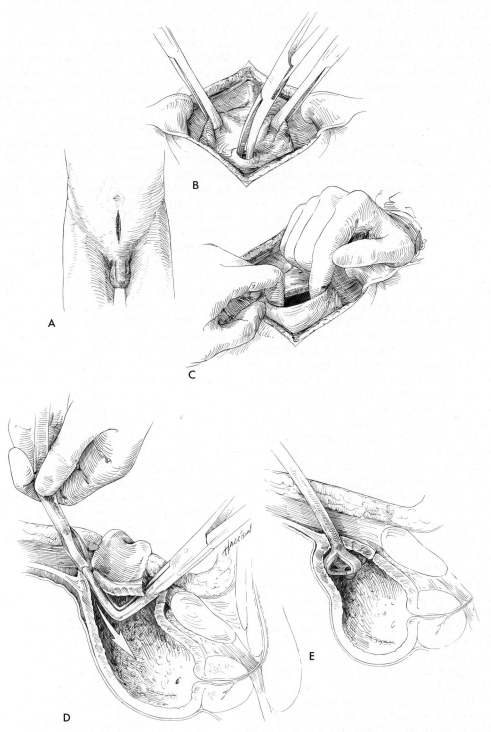

Figure 26–33. Technique of suprapubic cystostomy. *A,* A lower midline incision is made and the bladder exposed. *B,* Between two Allis forceps a tonsil forceps is inserted quickly through the bladder wall. Failure to insert with quick sustained motion results in dissection of bladder mucosa from muscle and complicates bladder entry. *C,* Opposing index fingers open bladder bluntly, thereby minimizing bleeding. *D,* A Malecot catheter is inserted obliquely through the bladder wall. Care is taken to dissect the peritoneum free of the bladder dome to avoid bowel injury. *E,* Cystostomy tube is placed in oblique tunnel to decrease chance of fistula formation.

arated to expose the perivesical space. The bladder is identified by the large interconnecting veins traversing its surface. An area over the anterior portion of the bladder is dissected free of its adventitial covering and grasped with two pairs of Allis forceps. A tonsil clamp is used to quickly puncture the bladder musculature and mucosa between the Allis forceps. If the bladder is not entered with a quick through-and-through insertion of the tonsil clamp, the bladder mucosa may be dissected from the bladder musculature and entry not be made into the bladder lumen.

After the initial opening in the bladder has been executed, opposing index fingers are inserted, and the bladder incision is bluntly extended. This minimizes bleeding. Inspection is then made of the interior of the bladder, the bladder neck, and the ureteral orifices, and the site of vesical rupture is sought. After the vesical rupture has been sutured, a right angle clamp is placed inside the bladder, extending out through the dome to draw the cystostomy tube into the bladder lumen. Care is taken to ensure that the dome of the bladder has been bluntly dissected away from the peritoneum at the point of exit of the right angle clamp. After the clamp has been brought through the bladder wall, the catheter is grasped and, keeping it taut, is brought into the lumen of the bladder so as to create as small a hole in the bladder as possible.

After the suprapubic tube has been separately placed, the original cystotomy incision is closed with running 2-0 chromic interlocking sutures through the mucosa and musculature, with a second layer of running 2-0 chromic sutures placed through the adventitia. One-inch Penrose drains are then placed in the space of Retzius on either side of the bladder neck, and the wound is closed by approximation of the rectus muscle bundles with interrupted 2-0 chromic sutures, followed by a rectus fascial closure of 0 Prolene or 0 chromic catgut interrupted sutures and closure of the skin and subcutaneous tissue. The suprapubic catheter should be brought out in an oblique fashion through the abdominal incision or separate stab wound, if desired, to allow for prompt closure of the cystostomy tract defect when the suprapubic tube is removed. Failure to bring this tube out through an oblique tunnel tends to increase the incidence of postoperative urinary fistula formation. These drains are removed on the fifth postoperative day, and the suprapubic tube is left in place for 7 to 10 days. A cystogram is made to check for extravasation of urine prior to its removal.

Complications

Prior to the advent of antimicrobial therapy and prompt surgical intervention, there was a high mortality rate associated with ruptured urinary bladder. Bacon (1943) reported a 44 per cent overall mortality rate. Nineteen of 21 patients managed conservatively in his series died. Culp (1942), reporting a series of bladder ruptures, the majority of which were secondary to endoscopic manipulation, showed a 64 per cent mortality and a 100 per cent mortality if the patients were treated with indwelling catheter alone. Most of his patients had pre-existing bladder disease. With the current treatment of vesical rupture by prompt surgical intervention and antibiotic coverage, the mortality rate is 9 per cent. This current high mortality rate is related not only to the bladder rupture itself but to the high incidence (50 per cent in our series) of associated visceral organ or vascular injuries (Guerriero, 1982). If intraperitoneal bladder rupture is unrecognized, continued extravasation of urine results in abdominal distention and nausea. These undrained collections of urine eventually become infected. Abscess formation follows.

URETHRAL INJURIES

Etiology and Anatomic Considerations

Rupture of the urethra is a rare injury. A 10-year experience from our institution is presented in Table 26–15. The anatomic relationships of the urethra are important because injuries to different areas assume varied clinical

TABLE 26–15. CAUSES OF URETHRAL TRAUMA, PARKLAND MEMORIAL HOSPITAL

Above Urogenital Diaphragm		Below Urogenital Diaphragm	
Motor vehicle accident	11	Iatrogenic manipulation	14
Foley catheter manipulation	1	Gunshot wound	10
Stab wound	1	Straddle injury or other direct perineal trauma	9
Total	13	Motor vehicle accident	3
		Self-manipulation	2
		Intercourse	2
		Bite (human)	1
		Total	41

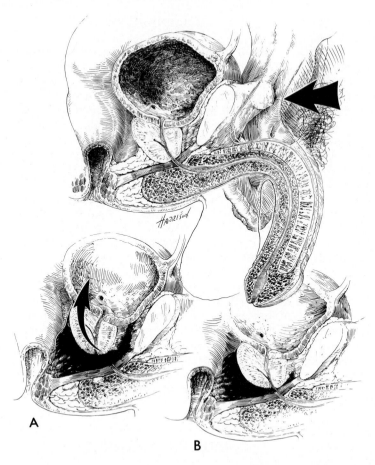

Figure 26–34. Rupture of urethra superior to urogenital diaphragm showing normal anatomy; arrow represents vector through which the force is applied.

A, Complete rupture of urethra with elevated prostate and large pelvic hematoma. *B*, Incomplete rupture of urethra with less distortion of normal anatomy. (From Longmire, W. P., Jr. (Ed.): Advances in Surgery, Vol. 10. Chicago, Year Book Medical Publishers, 1976.)

and prognostic significance. The urethra in the male is conveniently divided into four portions: (1) prostatic, (2) membranous, (3) bulbous, and (4) penile or pendulous. Etiologic agents that have been shown to cause urethral injuries are (1) blunt force, as in motor vehicle accidents or crush injuries; (2) penetrating missiles, such as gunshot wounds and stab wounds; (3) iatrogenic factors from urethral instrumentation; and (4) spontaneous urethral rupture associated with urethral stricture, with subsequent urinary extravasation and periurethral abscess formation.

In considering the classification of urethral injuries, it is convenient to group them into those occurring above the urogenital diaphragm and those occurring below the urogenital diaphragm. Urethral rupture superior to the urogenital diaphragm is most commonly a result of violent external force. The prostate is separated from its attachments to the urogenital diaphragm, and the puboprostatic ligaments are sheared off. The urethra is subsequently torn (Fig. 26–34). Over 90 per cent of these injuries are associated with a pelvic fracture. Tears of the urethra superior to the urogenital diaphragm

may be complete or incomplete. In the patient with complete disruption of the urethra above the urogenital diaphragm, the bladder and prostate ascend above the normal anatomic position, and the defect is filled with blood clots and urine. If the tear is incomplete and the puboprostatic ligaments are only partially severed, there may be a minimal degree of prostatic and bladder displacement. The distinction between a complete and an incomplete tear is important, and its significance in management will be discussed later. At the time of injury, the bladder neck frequently remains competent, and the degree of urinary extravasation may be minimal.

Urethral injuries inferior to the urogenital diaphragm usually result from a straddle-type injury or other direct blow to the perineum along the path of the urethra. This results in complete or partial severance of the urethra, and extravasation of blood and urine is usually confined to the fascial plane of the perineum (Fig. 26–35). If the superficial (Buck's) fascia remains intact, extravasation of blood and urine will be limited to the space between the tunica albuginea of the corpora spongiosa, essentially

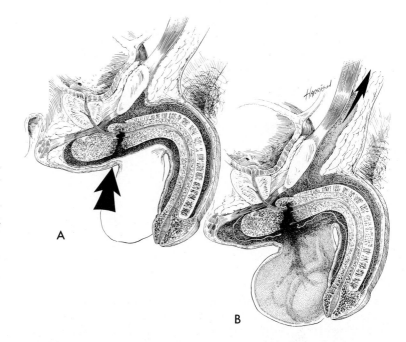

Figure 26–35. Rupture of urethra inferior to urogenital diaphragm. *A,* Rupture of urethra but not Buck's fascia, showing limitation of urine and blood extravasation. *B,* Rupture of urethra through Buck's fascia showing path of extravasation of blood and urine from Colles' fascial attachments at the perineal body into the scrotum and extending into the abdominal wall deep to Scarpa's fascia. (From Longmire, W. P., Jr. (Ed.): Advances in Surgery, Vol. 10. Chicago, Year Book Medical Publishers, 1976.)

a sleeve of the penis, and discoloration is confined to the penis (Fig. 26–36). If, in the process of injury, Buck's fascia is disrupted, subsequent extravasation of blood or urine is limited only by Colles' fascia with its attachment posteriorly at the triangular ligament, laterally to the fascia lata of the thigh, and superiorly and anteriorly to the attachments of the coracoclavicular fascia (Fig. 26–37). Colles' fascia is continuous with Scarpa's fascia. Therefore, if left untreated, urinary extravasation may extend over a wide area in the abdominal wall deep to Scarpa's fascia, but it does not extend into the thighs or buttocks.

Iatrogenic urethral injuries caused by misplaced catheters or overzealous manipulation of endoscopic instruments may occur anywhere along the urethra. Common sites for these injuries are the urethral meatus, the bulbous urethra, and the prostatomembranous urethra. If too large an instrument is forced through the urethra, ischemic necrosis at the meatal or bulbar region will ensue, with resultant inflammation, scarring, and stricture formation. Penetrating missiles may injure the urethra anywhere along its course, the location of injury being related to the path of the missile. The pendulous urethra is infrequently injured because of its mobility. Foreign bodies may be inserted into the urethra because of curiosity or for the purpose of erotic stimulation (Fig. 26–38). These may escape the patient's grasp and be retained, or they may damage the urethra, resulting in infection and scarring. Patients with urethral

stricture disease may rupture the urethra during voiding. This occurs because of extravasation of the urine under pressure through areas weakened by necrosis or inflammation. A localized area of urinary extravasation quickly becomes infected, and the resultant necrosis may allow spread of the infection through Buck's fascia and into the space limited by Colles' fascia. Massive spread of purulent material then occurs, limited only by Colles' fascial attachments.

Diagnosis

In the patient with a history of trauma to the perineum, a urethral injury should be sus-

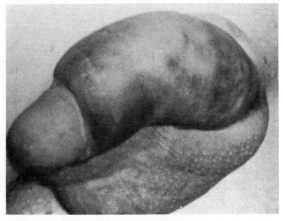

Figure 26–36. Traumatic rupture of the corpora cavernosa confined to Buck's fascia.

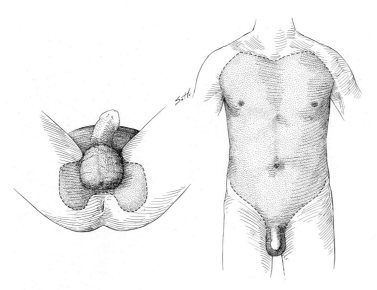

Figure 26–37. Areas of potential urine extravasation extending along Colles' fascial attachments.

pected. Careful questioning may reveal that the patient has noted a drop of blood at the meatus or has experienced difficulty in voiding. He may have noted swelling in the perineum during or after voiding, which represents the initial extravasation of urine. Physical examination may reveal swelling or discoloration of the genitalia, representing extravasation of blood or urine or both. A butterfly hematoma (Fig. 26–39) may be noted in the perineal region.

Rectal examination is mandatory in any patient with lower abdominal or perineal injury. The prostate may be elevated above its normal

position on rectal palpation in the patient with a urethral rupture superior to the urogenital diaphragm (Vermooten, 1946). A localized swelling in the area of the bulbous urethra should suggest urinary extravasation. A drop of blood at the urethral meatus may be seen; this is caused by contraction of the bulbocavernosus

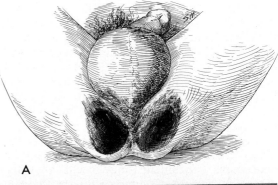

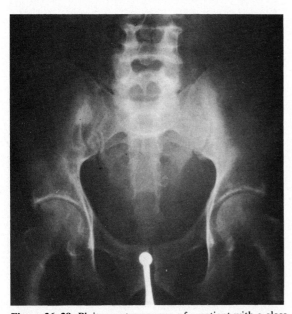

Figure 26–38. Plain roentgenogram of a patient with a glass cutter in urethra.

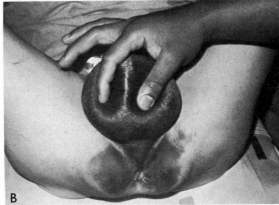

Figure 26–39. *A,* Diagram of a butterfly hematoma. *B,* Appearance of a patient with perineal butterfly hematoma.

muscle at the time of injury that delivers the blood to the meatus. Urinalysis will show hematuria if any urine is obtained. If, on the basis of history and physical examination, a urethral injury is suspected, an oblique retrograde urethrogram should be performed immediately (Fig. 26–40). An anteroposterior film of the pelvis is made, and any calcifications or pelvic fractures are noted. Next, with the patient in an oblique position, 25 to 30 ml of 29 per cent iodine-containing, water-soluble contrast material is introduced through a catheter-tip syringe placed in the urethral meatus. A film is taken during the injection to ensure that the urethra is full and is distended with contrast material. If a retention catheter has already been placed in the urethra and urine is draining, then injection of water-soluble contrast material alongside the catheter through a 16-gauge Angiocath will allow an adequate urethrogram to be obtained, and serious urethral injury may thus be demonstrated without removal of the catheter. If a catheter has been positioned properly, cystographic and pyelographic evaluation of the remainder of the urinary tract may be carried out after evaluation of the urethra, as described under bladder injuries.

Treatment

INITIAL MANAGEMENT

Treatment of urethral injuries above and below the urogenital diaphragm should be planned for both the initial management and the later reconstructive phase. The initial management of the urethra that has been ruptured superior to the urogenital diaphragm may be accomplished by one of three methods. First, a suprapubic cystotomy may be performed, with the urethra and bladder manipulated over interlocking sounds (Fig. 26–41) to allow the continuity of the urethra to be re-established, and an anastomosis then performed over an indwelling urethral catheter. A suprapubic tube is left in place. This procedure is carried out at the time of injury, and a Silastic retention catheter is used to minimize urethral inflammatory reaction. After the urethral catheter is in place, traction may be exerted upon it to approximate the prostatic apex with the urogenital diaphragm if an anastomosis could not be done. Turner-Warwick (1973) has modified this approach. After manipulation of the severed urethral edges and restoration of urethral continuity, he uses a proximally fenestrated urethral catheter

to provide more adequate drainage for urethral secretions than the conventional catheter affords. He also advocates the placement of perineal traction sutures through the bladder neck instead of balloon-catheter traction to approximate the prostatic urethra to the membranous urethra. He believes that the use of the fenestrated urethral catheter allows better drainage of urethral exudates than does the usual retention urethral catheter.

The second method of restoring urethral continuity is the dissection at the time of the injury of the severed urethral ends with primary urethral anastomosis, as advocated by Pierce (1972). A urethral catheter is left in place as a stent.

The third and most recent method for initial management of rupture of the urethra superior to the urogenital diaphragm is that advocated by Johanson (Morehouse and MacKinnon, 1969; Morehouse et al., 1972). It consists of the placement of a suprapubic cystostomy tube alone (Fig. 26–42) at the time of injury. No pelvic dissection, no perivesical drainage, and no urethral manipulation or urethral catheter placement are done. With this treatment, the pelvic hematoma is not disturbed by extensive dissection or manipulation, thereby simplifying the initial management of a serious injury. This method, by not disturbing the preformed pelvic hematoma, decreases the chance of further damage to the neurovascular structures of the pelvis. The chances of converting the rare incomplete tear to a complete one are minimized. Pelvic blood loss, which is already of large magnitude from fractures, will not be increased by disruption of a tamponaded hematoma.

Morehouse and MacKinnon and their associates (1969, 1972) have shown that after suprapubic cystostomy alone, the prostate will nearly always descend to its normal anatomic position as the body resolves the pelvic hematoma. If the urethral tear has been incomplete, the patient may require no further therapy. If the tear has been complete, then the invariable urethral stricture repair may be accomplished by a variety of methods. However, the urethral stricture that occurs following suprapubic cystostomy alone is usually accompanied by less inflammation, edema, and scar formation than if extensive perivesical dissection had been performed earlier. The urethral stricture may be repaired 3 to 6 months later. In addition, the placement of a suprapubic cystostomy tube alone, which is well within the capability of the occasional operator, decreases the chances of complications that follow the prolonged use of

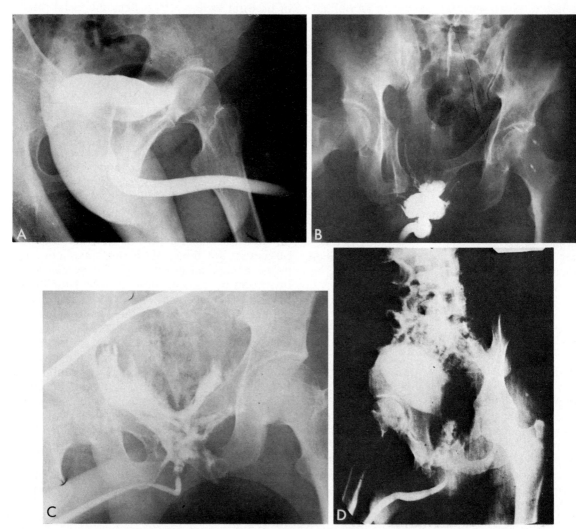

Figure 26–40. *A,* Normal retrograde urethrogram. Note that the contrast material has been injected *during* the exposure to ensure delineation of deep bulbar, membranous, and prostatic urethra. *B* to *D,* Rupture of urethra superior to urogenital diaphragm in male.

Illustration continued on the opposite page

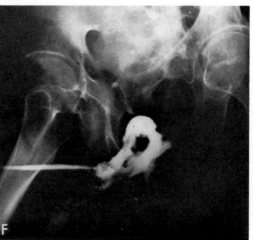

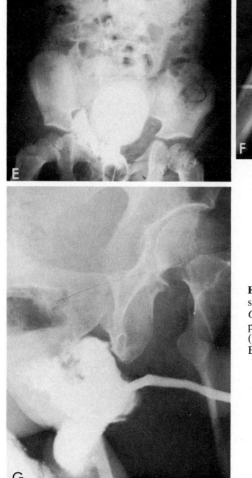

Figure 26–40 *Continued. E,* Rupture of urethra superior to urogenital diaphragm in female. *F* and *G,* Rupture of urethra inferior to urogenital diaphragm. (*F* reprinted from Longmire, W. P., Jr. (Ed.): Advances in Surgery, Vol. 10. Chicago, Year Book Medical Publishers, 1976.)

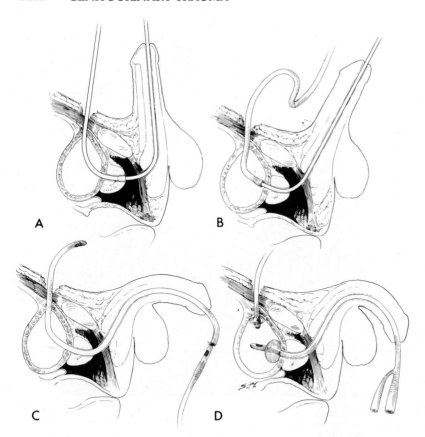

A

B

C

D

Figure 26–41. Method of urethral realignment with interlocking sounds.

urethral catheters, e.g., prostatitis, urethritis epididymitis. When realignment over a urethral catheter or primary anastomosis of the severed urethral ends is attempted at the time of injury, the incidence of stricture formation, inconti-

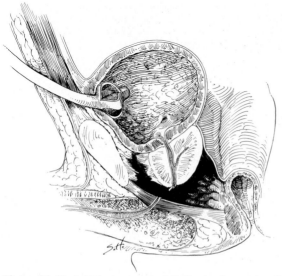

Figure 26–42. Initial placement of S–P tube for ruptured urethra. Note absence of pelvic dissection and perivesical drainage.

nence, and impotence is considerable (Table 26–16). If suprapubic cystostomy drainage is used initially and is followed by definitive urethral reconstruction, the incidence of these sequelae is reduced. Morehouse and MacKinnon and their coworkers have reported an incidence of zero in their initial series of 11 patients (1969, 1972). As Morehouse's experience has increased to more than 119 patients, stricture and incontinence rates are about 5 per cent, and the impotence rate is 8 per cent (Morehouse, 1984).

In the infant with urethral rupture above the urogenital diaphragm, cutaneous vesicostomy is a suitable alternative to the placement of a suprapubic catheter for urinary diversion. This technique is simple because the bladder of the infant is essentially an intraperitoneal organ and is easily approximated to the skin. This procedure offers the advantages of minimal pelvic dissection and prompt treatment of the suprapubic cystostomy but avoids the problems of bladder irritability and infection that occur in infants with suprapubic catheters. It also avoids the problems associated with long-term indwelling urethral catheter placement in the small male urethra.

The technique of cutaneous vesicostomy (Fig. 26–43) begins with a short (5 cm) trans-

TABLE 26–16. REPAIR OF URETHRAL RUPTURE

Author	Method*	Incidence of Stricture	Incidence of Impotence	Incidence of Incontinence
Peters (1983)	1	4/6 (66%)	3/6 (50%)	2/6 (33%)
Peter and Allen (1984, unpublished data)	4	2/29 (6%)	3/29 (10%)	0/29
Meyers and DeWeerd (1972)	2	2/22 (18%)	—	—
Morehouse (1970)	2	27/27 (100%)	15/27 (55%)	18/27 (65%)
Morehouse (unpublished data)	4	112/119 (7%)	92/109 (8%)	113/119 (5%)
Pierce (1972)	3	2/4 (50%)	—	—
Waterhouse (1980)	4	4/54 (7%)	0/54	2/54 (2%)
Witherington (1984, unpublished data)	3	0/8	0	0

*1 = Realignment over urethral catheter
2 = Realignment over urethral catheter plus traction
3 = Primary reanastomosis
4 = Suprapubic tube alone plus delayed repair

verse incision below the umbilicus (4 to 5 cm). After the perivesical space is entered, the bladder is grasped with two pairs of Allis forceps, and a tonsil hemostat is quickly inserted between the Allis forceps and into the bladder lumen. Failure to insert the tonsil quickly into the lumen will cause the bladder mucosa to dissect from the muscular layers, complicating entry into the bladder. After the bladder has been opened, the bladder mucosa is anastomosed to the skin with 4-0 interrupted chromic sutures, creating a 1-cm stoma approximately 2 to 3 cm below the umbilicus. An exemplary case is presented in Figure 26–44.

Michie (1972) has suggested the placement of traction sutures between the rectus fascia and the vesical wall to give added stability to the vesicostomy. Other points stressed by Michie are (1) the hole must be the proper size to allow complete bladder drainage but should not be too large, or herniation of the posterior bladder wall will occur; (2) skin sutures should be placed a few millimeters from the skin edge to prevent calcific granules from forming; (3) the perivesi-

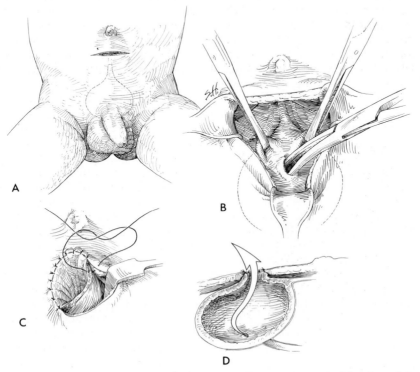

Figure 26–43. Operative technique of cutaneous vesicostomy. *A,* Short transverse incision 2 cm below umbilicus. *B,* Bladder grasped with Allis forceps and entered. *C,* Vesicocutaneous anastomosis. *D,* Path of urine exit.

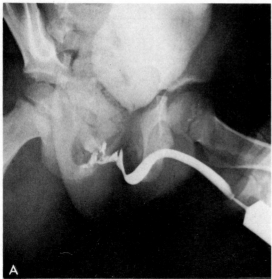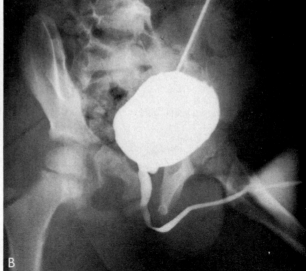

Figure 26–44. *A,* Retrograde urethrogram in a child with urethral rupture above the urogenital diaphragm. *B,* Voiding cystourethrogram: 1-month postoperative appearance of urethra after treatment with a cutaneous vesicostomy alone. No urethral reconstruction was necessary. (Courtesy of Dr. Dymis Lawrence, Compton, California.)

cal dissection should be minimized; (4) antibiotics are administered 2 hours prior to and for 14 days after surgery; (5) traction sutures should be placed at 3, 6, 9, and 12 o'clock positions about the stoma, or necrosis of the bladder wall may occur.

After the diagnosis of rupture of the urethra inferior to the urogenital diaphragm has been made by urethrography, several modes of treatment are available. If the injury is a small laceration, as produced by a foreign body or cystoscopic instrument, a urethral catheter may be placed as a stent for urinary diversion, and the surrounding urethra will heal without incident. The catheter should be left in place for 3 to 5 days. If the urethral disruption appears to be more extensive but a urethral catheter is already in place and is draining well, no further treatment may be necessary. However, close observation of this type of patient should be maintained so that any urinary extravasation with subsequent abscess formation will be recognized promptly. If there is any doubt about the position of the urethral catheter in the treatment of a urethral injury, a suprapubic cystostomy should be performed. If a complete urethral disruption is found, the placement of a suprapubic catheter is recommended. This is accompanied by primary end-to-end anastomosis of the severed urethral segments (Fig. 26–45).

In order to reduce infection, foreign bodies inserted vicariously into the urethra should be removed promptly after diagnosis. Foreign bodies that have reached the posterior urethra can be more easily removed by pushing them into the bladder and removing them in the direction of least transverse diameter with grasping endoscopic forceps or Strong-Alcock forceps. If the foreign body is a slender metallic object, such as a pin, cystoscopic manipulation with grasping forceps may allow easy removal. Figure 26–37 illustrates a case in which a glass cutter was inserted into the urethra. The distal tip of the foreign body could be palpated in the perineum, and rather than cystoscopic manipulation or suprapubic cystostomy, a perineal urethrostomy was performed, allowing easy removal of the foreign body.

Initial management of the patient with a spontaneous rupture of the urethra consists of prompt drainage of the urinary extravasation. These lesions are frequently associated with urethral stricture formation and bacteriuria. A small amount of extravasated urine or blood with subsequent infection may serve as a nidus for abscess formation that is resistant to antibiotic therapy alone. Surgical drainage and adequate débridement are mandatory. If the patient presents late with a spontaneously ruptured urethra and massive periurethral phlegmon, the preferred treatment is bivalving of the scrotum and excision of the necrotic urethra with the creation of a proximal and distal urethrostomy, if possible. Unrecognized urethral injury below the urogenital diaphragm will result in urinary

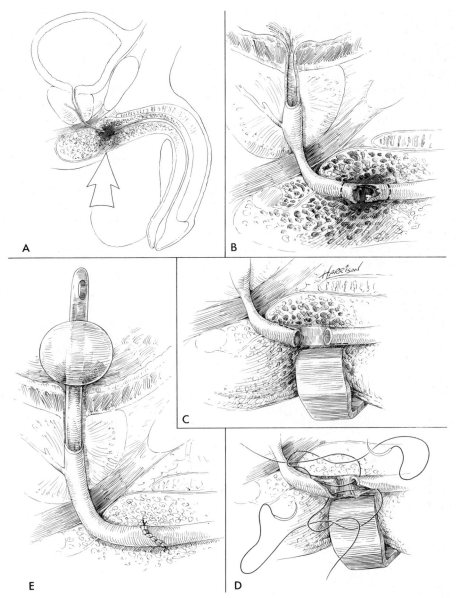

Figure 26–45. Technique of primary urethral repair with end-to-end anastomosis of rupture below urogenital diaphragm. *A,* Appearance of injury. *B,* Urethral ends excised transversely to viable bleeding tissue. *C,* Urethral ends spatulated 1 to 2 cm. *D* and *E,* Interrupted suture line with Silastic catheter in place.

extravasation with infection and necrotizing abscess formation early and stricture formation later and will require staged reconstructive procedures.

URETHRAL RECONSTRUCTION

After the initial management of an acutely severed urethra, the most common subsequent complication is urethral stricture. Stricture formation following rupture of the urethra superior to the urogenital diaphragm has been estimated in various series to occur in from 25 per cent to 100 per cent of cases (Table 26–16). The incidence of stricture following injury to the urethra below the urogenital diaphragm secondary to the typical straddle injury is 44 per cent in our series. Therefore, the reconstruction of the urethral stricture is of vital importance in the overall management of the patient who has experienced urethral trauma. Initial management of the traumatized urethra is followed by a variable period before the clinical manifestation of the stricture. If the initial injury has been managed by suprapubic cystostomy alone, an interval of

3 months following the injury is usually adequate for the resolution of pelvic hematoma and tissue damage. Urethral reconstruction should be delayed for at least this long to (1) allow a precise assessment of the degree and extent of urethral stricture formation; and (2) allow the tissue edema to subside, the blood supply to be restored, and tensile strength of the tissues to recover sufficiently to permit the sutures used in reconstruction to hold. After the diagnosis of stricture formation has been made by urethral calibration or retrograde urethrography, some patients may be managed successfully with periodic urethral dilation with steel sounds. However, a large number of these strictures are resistant to dilation, and definitive urethral reconstruction must be undertaken. Strictures that are initially filiform in caliber should be repaired.

Once the decision has been made to reconstruct the damaged urethra, a number of techniques are available to the well-trained urologist. The classic Johanson urethroplasty (Johanson, 1953), which has been modified in recent years by Turner-Warwick (1983), Leadbetter (1960), Blandy and associates (1968), and others, is still, when properly performed, the procedure against which all other urethral reconstructions must be measured. This urethral

reconstruction consists of two separate operations with a 3- to 6-month interval between the first and second stages.

During the first stage (Fig. 26–46), an incision is made on the ventral surface of the penis overlying the area of stricture. In the patient with a stricture of the penile urethra or distal bulbous urethra, the incision is carried in a longitudinal fashion through the urethral mucosa, and the urethra is opened through the length of the stricture to include 0.5 to 1 cm of normal urethral mucosa on each side of the strictured area. Next, the edges of the penile skin incision are approximated to the edges of the urethral mucosa throughout the length of the incision. After a period of at least 3 months, these indurated, scarred areas of urethral mucosa will become soft and pliable and are easily manipulated surgically. When they are "as soft as a baby's bottom," they are ready for repair.

In the patient with a deep bulbar or membranous urethral stricture, a scrotal inlay is constructed as a first stage. To perform this procedure, a segment of the strictured urethra is first exposed through a perineal incision (Fig. 26–47). Through a second incision oriented perpendicular to the first, an area of soft, pliable scrotal tissue is incised, and the edges of the scrotal inlay are sutured circumferentially to the

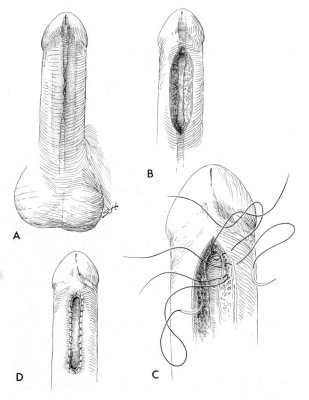

Figure 26–46. Johanson urethroplasty. First stage, applicable to distal urethral strictures. (From Longmire, W. P., Jr. (Ed.): Advances in Surgery. Chicago, Year Book Medical Publishers, 1976.)

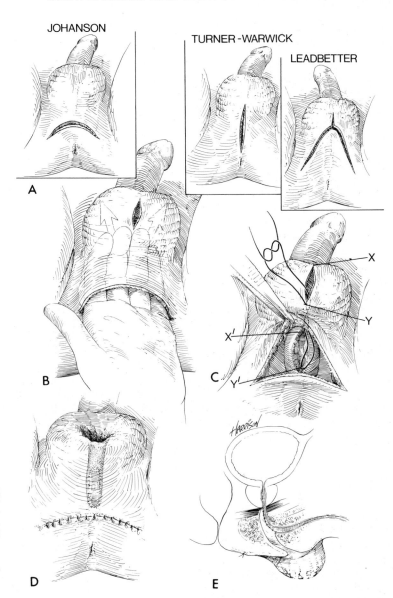

Figure 26–47. Johanson urethroplasty. *A,* Skin incision (insets show alternative incisions). *B,* Mobilization of scrotal flap and counterincision. *C,* Edge of scrotal skin approximated to urethral mucosa (*X′* to *X* and *Y′* to *Y*). *D,* Finished inlay. *E,* Cross-sectioned view. (From Longmire, W. P., Jr. (Ed.): Advances in Surgery, Vol. 10. Chicago, Year Book Medical Publishers, 1976.)

edges of the urethral mucosa after the operator is certain that he has cut proximally and distally into healthy urethral tissue. As with distal urethral strictures, an interval of 3 to 6 months is desirable between the first and second stages, as this allows adequate healing and resolution of inflammatory processes to make the tissues of the urethra more pliable; restoration of blood supply and tensile strength are also optimal.

The second stage of the reconstruction is then performed (Fig. 26–48). Care must be taken at this time to note that the proximal and distal urethral openings of the first-stage procedure are adequate by calibration with steel sounds. The operative site should be free of residual infection, inflammation, scarring, and

tendency to stenosis, both proximally and distally. If there is some evidence of recurrent stricture formation or inflammation, the first-stage urethroplasty should be revised, and an area of healthy urethra should be included to protect against subsequent scar formation. In the second-stage urethroplasty, an incision is made, and the proximal and distal urethral apertures and a strip of intervening epithelium are incised. Browne (1949) and Johanson (1953) have shown in reconstruction of the hypospadiac urethra that a buried strip of epithelium will form a tube, the circumference of which is at least 30 per cent greater than the diameter of the buried strip. The width of this buried strip should be two-thirds the size of the desired

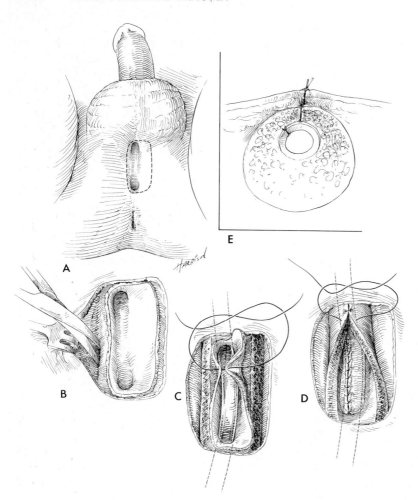

Figure 26–48. Second stage for closure of defect. *A*, Eccentric skin incision around proximal and distal urethral openings. *B*, Mobilization of urethra. *C*, Closure of urethral lumen over Silastic catheter. *D*, Approximation of bulbocavernous muscles. *E*, Cross section, showing offset suture lines.

urethral diameter. However, operative tubularization of this epithelial strip provides a more satisfactory result.

An eccentric circumferential incision (Fig. 26–48) should be made around the ostium of the first stage so that the suture line of the epithelial tube that is subsequently constructed will not be directly in the midline. The incision should be generous enough to allow the cut edges to be sutured together without tension. In addition, there should not be a tendency to sacculation at this point, or a diverticulum of the urethra will develop as a result. To avoid this, the diameter needed should be measured with a vernier caliper or malleable ruler and marked with a blue tissue-marking pencil before the incision is made.

After the strip of epithelium has been tubularized with 4-0 Dexon suture, constructing a new urethra, the edges of the corpora spongiosa should be approximated over the newly formed urethral tube with 4-0 absorbable catgut suture.

Another layer of support is provided by approximation of the bulbocavernosa muscles with 4-0 chromic gut sutures. The subcutaneous tissue is closed with fine chromic suture and the skin with 4-0 or 5-0 chromic sutures. We prefer to leave an indwelling urethral catheter of appropriate size in place for urinary diversion. It should be at least 2-French smaller than the caliber of the reconstructed urethra. As an alternative, a suprapubic tube may be used for urinary diversion if it is not already in place. A small cystotomy incision may be made over a perforated sound, or the curved Lowsley prostatic tractor may be introduced through the urethra and a catheter pulled into the bladder for use as a suprapubic tube.

Allen (1975) and Pierce (1962) have advocated the use of the transpubic approach for reconstruction of strictures of the membranous urethra (Fig. 26–49). In this procedure, a low midline incision is made, and the lower end partially encompasses the base of the penis and

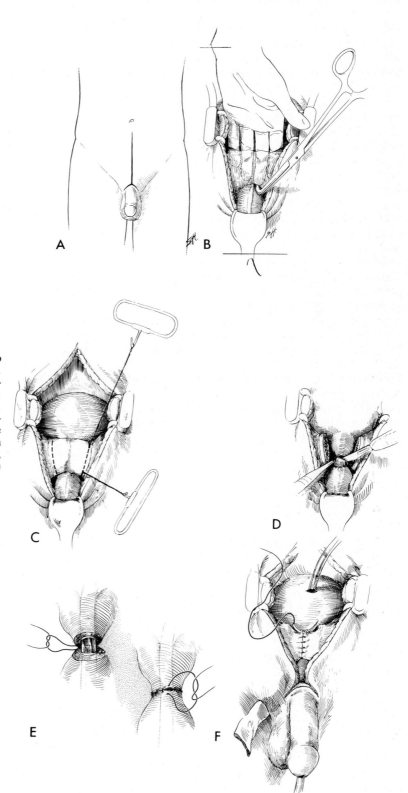

Figure 26–49. Transpubic approach to membranous urethral strictures. *A*, Incision from umbilicus to and partially surrounding base of penis. *B*, Development of retropubic space. *C*, Pubectomy with Gigli's saw. *D*, Excision of area of stricture. *E*, Closure of urethra. *F*, Closure of periosteum and placement of drain. (From Allen, T. D., et al.: J. Urol., *111*:830, 1974.)

suspensory ligament. After the perivesical space is entered, the pubic symphysis is exposed. The fingers are passed through the retropubic space after the suspensory ligaments of the penis are incised, and a right angle clamp is pushed through the urogenital diaphragm beneath the pubic arch, avoiding the dorsal vein of the penis and the retropubic venous plexus. After an avascular plane is demonstrated, it is enlarged. With the pubis isolated, the periosteum is stripped off the pubic bone about ¾-inch to each side of the midline. With the Gigli saw, a segment of the bone is removed. After a pubic bone segment of about 1½ inches in diameter is removed, excellent exposure of the prostatic and membranous urethra is obtained. The area of stricture may then be excised and the margins and the edges of the urethra mobilized and reanastomosed without tension over a urethral catheter. After urethral reanastomosis, a suprapubic tube is left in place and a Penrose drain is brought out laterally through the scrotum posterior to the spermatic cord. The edges of the periosteum, which has been stripped from the pubis, are reapproximated. Regeneration of the excised pubic bone segment will occur if periosteum can be reapproximated. The wound is then closed. An advantage of this reconstruction is the preservation of the urethral sphincter, which may be identified and avoided, thus decreasing the chances of urinary incontinence following urethral reconstruction.

Waterhouse and coworkers (1973, 1980) have proposed a method for urethral reconstruction (Fig. 26–50) following traumatic stricture formation, which consists of a transpubic exposure of the membranous urethra and transposition of the transected bulbous urethra to an anterior position on the prostate. The transected anterior urethra is mobilized to some extent to allow it to pass anterior to the area of stricture; under direct vision it is reanastomosed to the prostatic urethra. The distal urethra is approached perineally through a vertical incision. After it is mobilized to the level of the triangular ligament, it is transected. Anterior urethral mobilization is continued to the glans penis. The septum between the diverging corpora cavernosa is incised, and the mobilized anterior urethra is then passed through this incision. The prostatic urethra is then identified, and the urethral ends are spatulated and anastomosed to the distal transected urethra. A Silastic indwelling urethral catheter is left in place. Waterhouse has reported that eight of eight patients were continent after this procedure. Stricture formation resulted in one of eight patients, and two of six were impotent. However, if a TUR is required subsequently, incontinence may result.

An entirely acceptable procedure that we have recently used for reconstruction of a membranous urethral stricture is a modification of the patch graft urethroplasty, in which a free

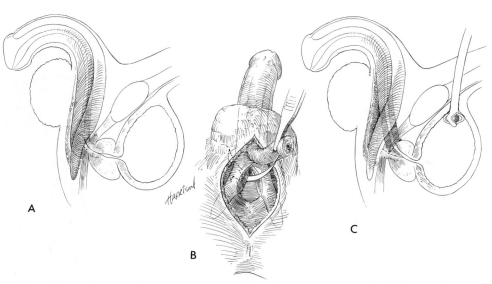

Figure 26–50. Waterhouse's method of transpubic urethral stricture repair. *A*, Preoperative view of stricture. *B*, Urethra transected and placed through divided and mobilized corpora cavernosa. *C*, Healthy urethra sutured to neoprostatic urethra.

dermal graft is tubularized to substitute for an obliterated urethra (Fig. 26–51). Ten ml of methylene blue per urethra is injected. This methylene blue will stain the area of scarred urethral tissue and will make its extent more easily identifiable. It also makes it possible to identify a urethra that may be narrowed to a diameter of 1 mm or less. A longitudinal incision is then made over the length of the stricture, and the healthy urethra is identified and incised a length of 1 cm beyond the proximal and distal extent of the stricture.

After the extent of the stricture has been determined and the urethra has been opened, a free full-thickness graft is taken from the dorsal penile skin, prepuce, or other area of soft, relatively thin-skinned, non-hair-bearing area, e.g., the inner arm. The most appropriate size and shape of the skin for urethral repair are best measured by using a piece of tinfoil, as from a suture package, and cutting it to the size and shape of the urethral defect. The area may

then be marked on the donor site around this template with a blue tissue-marking pencil. By sharp dissection, a full-thickness graft of skin is obtained. This piece of skin is then stretched on a plastic board, e.g., a Dermacarrier, and pinned down with several 25-gauge needles. This prevents rolling of the graft while it is being defatted. Meticulous attention should be given to defatting the entire graft, as its survival depends on the osmotic forces surrounding it to supply nutrition, and fat acts as a barrier to the overlying epithelium.

After the free graft has been obtained, it is sutured to the edges of the urethral mucosa, with the epithelial surface corresponding to the urethral lumen and the dermal surface outside. This anastomosis is best made by the placement of an apical stitch, followed by sutures of interrupted 4-0 Dexon (or Vicryl) along the edges. If four-quadrant stay sutures are placed, it is more difficult to trim the graft properly to fit the recipient site exactly as closure proceeds. It

Figure 26–51. Patch graft urethroplasty. *A,* Midline perineal incision extended down into urethral lumen. *B* and *C,* Placement of dermal graft with epidermal surface toward the lumen. Edges of graft sutured to urethral edges. The fat of the dermal graft has been meticulously removed. *D,* Corpora spongiosa closed over graft as separate layer. (From Kibbey, R. G., et al.: J. Urol., *115*:155, 1976; and Devine, P. C., et al.: J. Urol., *121*:282, 1979.)

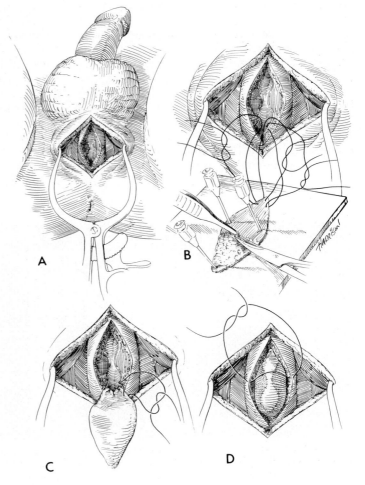

is preferable to start at one end and work toward the other to allow for appropriate trimming. After the urethral edges are sutured to the dermal graft over an appropriately sized Silastic urethral catheter (2-French less than the urethral caliber), the corpora spongiosa are closed over the free graft for support, as are the layers of the bulbocavernosus muscle. The subcutaneous tissues are closed with absorbable suture and the skin with fine nonabsorbable suture. The Silastic urethral catheter is left indwelling for 14 days, at which time a voiding urethrogram is obtained to determine whether there is any extravasation. If extravasation is demonstrated, a Silastic catheter is reinserted for an additional week.

Complications of urethral reconstruction include wound infection and hematoma formation initially, recurrent stricture formation, urethrocutaneous fistula, urethral diverticulum, periurethral abscesses, and epididymitis. Therefore, meticulous attention to hemostasis and exactness of surgical technique is essential in reconstruction of urethral strictures to prevent further complications of the operative procedure.

Urethral avulsion is an infrequent injury. In extreme cases, an entire segment of the urethra may telescope from the meatus. A recent case has been cited by Witherington and McKinney (1983) (Fig. 26–52). The Badenoch type repair may also be used to correct this (Fig. 26–53). As Judd and Donohue (1970) have stressed, one must be careful in distal immobilization of too much urethra, or telescoping of the penis back into the scrotal recesses will occur (Fig. 26–54).

INJURIES TO THE EXTERNAL GENITALIA

Penile Trauma

Injury of the penis is unusual owing to its mobility and well-guarded position. Penile anatomy has been previously described in this text, but a review will be presented here since injuries of different components of the penis vary in clinical significance.

The main structures that form the penis are the two corpora cavernosa and the corpus spongiosum with the enclosed urethra. The corpora cavernosa are thick bodies of vascular erectile tissue surrounded by a sturdy tunica albuginea. The three erectile bodies are surrounded by a distinct fascial layer (Buck's fascia), which is attached distally at the corona and proximally at the triangular ligament. Superficial to Buck's fascia lies Colles' fascia, which attaches posteriorly at the triangular ligament and laterally with the fascia lata at the inguinal ligament; it continues anteriorly as Scarpa's fascia to the level of the coracoclavicular fascia (Figs. 26–55 and 26–56). Trauma involving the penis may affect one or all of its structural components. The causes of penile trauma are most often penetrating missiles, either bullet wounds or stab wounds, or avulsing power takeoff injuries that occur when the clothing of the patient is caught in large machines, such as those used in farming or industry (Fig. 26–57). Strangulation (Fig. 26–58) of the penis with resultant ischemia and distal necrosis may be caused by condom catheters, strings wrapped about the penis, or various constricting metal bands, such as finger

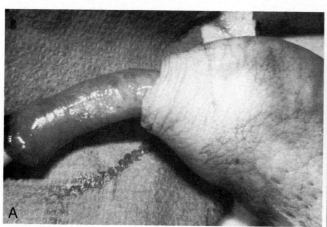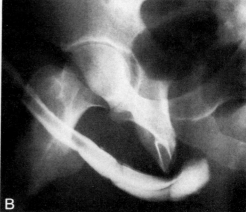

Figure 26–52. *A,* Tubular portion of tissue protruding from meatus with indwelling catheter. *B,* Pericatheter retrograde urethrogram reveals contrast medium confined to limited area without much extravasation. Buck's fascia is believed to be intact. (From Witherington, R., and McKinney, J. E.: J. Urol., *130*:564, 1983.)

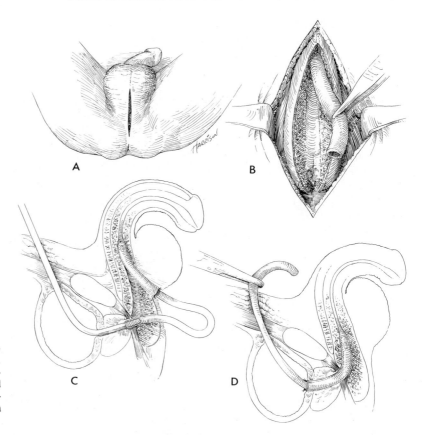

Figure 26–53. Badenoch urethroplasty. *A*, Midline perineal incision. *B*, Distal urethra mobilized. *C*, Distal urethra sutured to catheter and telescoped through prostatic urethra. *D*, Urethra sutured to mucosa at bladder neck.

rings or workmen's tools. Blunt injury to the erect penis, such as may occur during intercourse, may result in corporal or urethral rupture (See Fig. 26–36).

DIAGNOSIS

Although a history of the nature of the incident responsible for the injury is important, the physical examination of the penis will usually reveal the type and extent of the injury. The entrance of a penetrating missile will be obvious. The extent of extravasation of blood and urine in blunt penile trauma is determined by the integrity of Buck's fascia. If this layer remains intact, the bleeding from a ruptured corpus cavernosum or urethra (see Fig. 26–36) will be limited to Buck's fascia. If, however, Buck's fascia has been violated, the extravasation will extend to Colles' fascial attachments (Fig. 26–55).

TREATMENT

The portion of the penis that is injured determines the type of repair that is required. In patients who have sustained circumferential avulsion of the penile skin, all skin proximal to the injury should be saved (Peters and Bright,

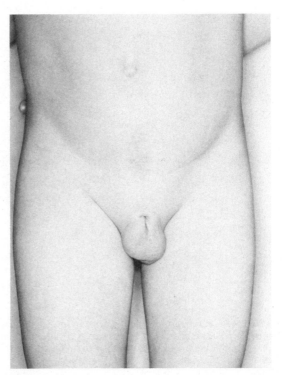

Figure 26–54. Recession of the penis back into the scrotal folds following too much mobilization of distal urethra for a Badenoch type repair.

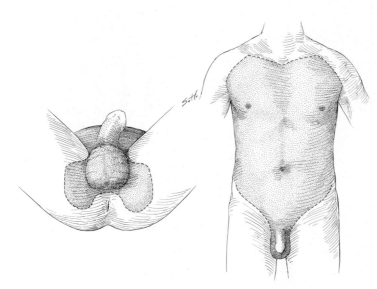

Figure 26–55. Areas of potential urine extravasation that extend along Colles' fascial attachments.

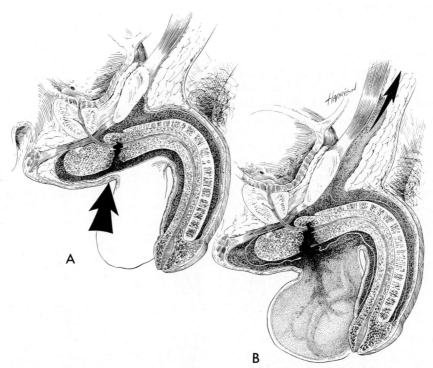

Figure 26–56. Rupture of urethra inferior to urogenital diaphragm. *A,* Rupture of urethra but not Buck's fascia, showing limitation of urine and blood extravasation. *B,* Rupture of urethra through Buck's fascia, showing path of extravasation of blood and urine from Colles' fascial attachments at the perineal body into the scrotum and extending onto the abdominal wall deep to Scarpa's fascia. (From Longmire, W. P., Jr. (Ed.): Advances in Surgery, Vol. 10. Chicago, Year Book Medical Publishers, 1976.)

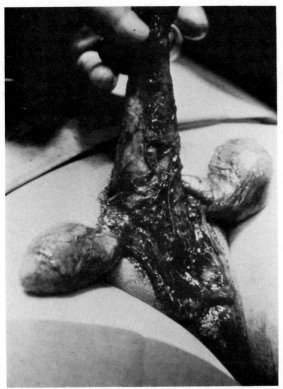

Figure 26–57. Power takeoff injury to genitalia.

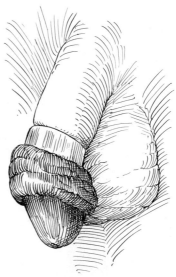

Figure 26–58. Strangulation of distal penis due to constricting band.

1976). The skin distal to the injury (Fig. 26–59) should be removed, and a split-thickness skin graft, 0.015-inch thick, should be used to cover the defect from its proximal origin to the coronal sulcus. If the distal skin is not removed, the interposed split-thickness skin graft will cause obstruction of the normal lymphatic drainage of this distal skin, and lymphedema will result.

Penetrating penile injury that involves layers deep to the skin and Colles' fascia should be surgically explored. A convenient method of complete penile exploration consists of a circumcising incision at the coronal sulcus, allowing the skin of the penis to be telescoped back to its base with a minimum of dissection and blood loss. This incision also allows full exposure of all components of the penis, thereby simplifying the proper débridement and repair of the injury. If the corpora cavernosa have been violated either by a penetrating missile or by blunt trauma, they should be immediately explored and sutured with interrupted 3-0 buried permanent sutures, such as Prolene, for prompt hemostasis and return of function. After completion of the repair, the penile skin may be returned to its normal position, and the circumcising incision may be closed with 4-0 interrupted chromic sutures. In these wounds, adequate drainage should be provided by means of a Penrose drain to allow decompression of the anticipated hematoma.

In the patient with strangulation of a portion of the penis, the offending material should be removed immediately. This is usually easy when strangulation is secondary to a condom catheter or a piece of thread. However, the removal of circular metal objects may be more difficult, particularly if edema has developed in the distal penis. These patients should be taken to the operating room and placed under general anesthesia; the object (e.g., a wrench) may then be removed with appropriate metal-cutting devices. Even though the distal penis appears necrotic, the injury should be treated conservatively, as satisfactory results can be anticipated in most cases. Occasionally, compressing the glans for a prolonged period, or wrapping it with string from distal to proximal, or using agents to decrease glandular edema, i.e., diuretics or hyaluronidase subcutaneously, may resolve enough edema to allow the constricting agent to slip over the glans with instant relief of the obstruction. If the patient has incarcerated his prepuce in a zipper, a circumcision may be performed to remove it.

Amputation of the penis may be attempted by mentally ill patients. Even when the complete shaft has been amputated, repair may be attempted. If proximal and distal arterial patency

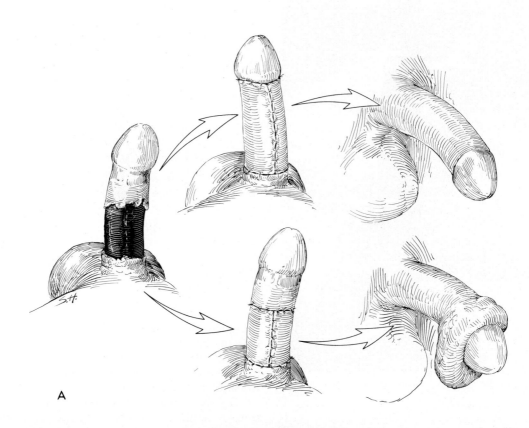

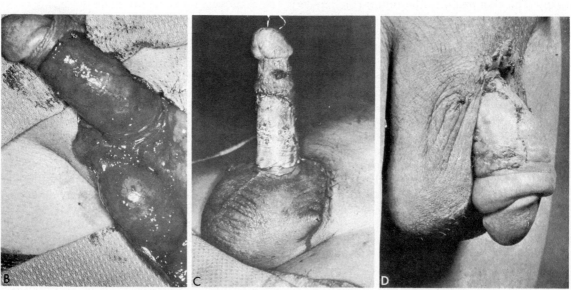

Figure 26–59. *A,* Correct *(above)* and incorrect *(below)* management of partial avulsion of penile skin. If distal remnant of penile skin is left in place, lymphedema of distal segment will occur secondary to obstruction of lymphatic drainage. (From Smith, R. B., and Skinner, D. G. (Eds.): Complications of Urologic Surgery. Philadelphia, W. B. Saunders Co., 1976.) *B–D,* Operative and postoperative appearance of *incorrect* management of avulsion of penile skin. Note distal penile edema caused by lymphatic obstruction.

can be established, arterial repair may be attempted if magnification techniques are available. It is difficult to maintain patency of vessels that are 2 mm or less in diameter. A 6-0 or 7-0 Prolene interrupted everting simple suture is recommended for vascular repair. Continuity of one deep or superficial vein should be established, if at all possible. Frequently, all that is possible is reanastomosis of the tunica albuginea of the corpora cavernosa and the penile skin and urethra. Proximal cystostomy is recommended. If distal gangrene supervenes, amputation and repair should be performed.

Steps in penile amputation (Fig. 26–60) recommended to minimize complications are (1) incision of the penile skin so that the dorsal flap overlaps the ventral flap by 0.5 to 1 cm more than the diameter of the corpus cavernosus; (2) amputation of the corpora cavernosa after proximal tourniquet control at the base of the penis and closure of the tunica albuginea with substantial absorbable sutures, i.e., 2-0 chromic; (3) amputation of the urethra 1.5 cm distal to the point of amputation of the corpora cavernosa; and (4) excision of a 1-cm ellipse of distal penile skin on the ventral inferior aspect and subsequent mucocutaneous anastomosis with 4-0 chromic gut, interposing a 1-cm ovoid flap of penile skin. After the amputation site has healed, staged genital reconstruction may begin.

The reconstruction of the amputated genitalia (Fig. 26–61) begins with the formation of a tube pedicle graft in the left lower quadrant of abdominal skin. After this tube has been formed, its caudal end is separated from the abdominal wall. To provide an erectile body, Small-Carrion Silastic prostheses are placed in the remnants of the corpora cavernosa and burrowed into the pedicle flap. After the prostheses are in place, the caudal end of the tube graft is sutured to the distal end of the penis. After all wounds have healed, the cephalic end of the tube graft is severed from the abdominal wall. Urethral reconstruction may be performed later, if desired. Recently, cooperative techniques in conjunction with plastic surgeons using musculoskeletal flaps have greatly enhanced techniques of penile reconstruction (see Chapter 81). An elliptical musculoskeletal flap from the shoulder area posteriorly is especially applicable to penile reconstruction.

Stenosis of the urethral meatus often follows partial amputation of the penis. Again, this is related to a deficient blood supply to the mucosa leading to retraction during healing. Unsatisfactory results may be minimized by transecting the urethra at least 1 cm distal to the point of transection of the corpora cavernosa. A spatulated mucocutaneous anastomosis may be used, with a flap of skin interposed at some point in the circumference. When meatal stenosis has occurred, it is best corrected by a formal meatoplasty using a rotational flap technique, such as a Z-plasty.

INJURIES TO THE SCROTUM AND TESTIS

The fascial layers of the abdominal wall descend into the scrotum and are continuous with the layers of the scrotum, as shown in Figure 26–62. A thorough knowledge of these fascial planes is mandatory for the management of injuries to the testis and scrotal contents. Because of its mobility and position, the scrotum is infrequently injured. Injuries may be caused

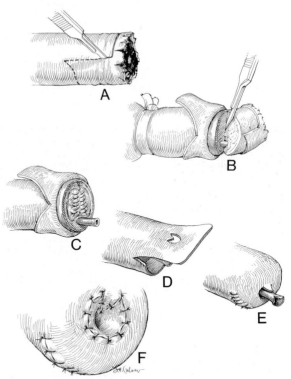

Figure 26–60. Partial amputation traumatized. *A,* Appearance of injury. *B,* Amputation of involved area so that urethra is 1 cm longer than corporal bodies. *C,* Urethra projecting 1 cm beyond cut edge of corpora. *D,* Buttonhole on skin for new meatus. *E,* Closure of ventral sin. *F,* Anastomosis of mucous membrane to skin to include wedge of skin in circumference. (*C* to *F,* From Smith, R. B., and Skinner, D. G. (Eds.): Complications of Urologic Surgery. Philadelphia, W. B. Saunders Co., 1976.)

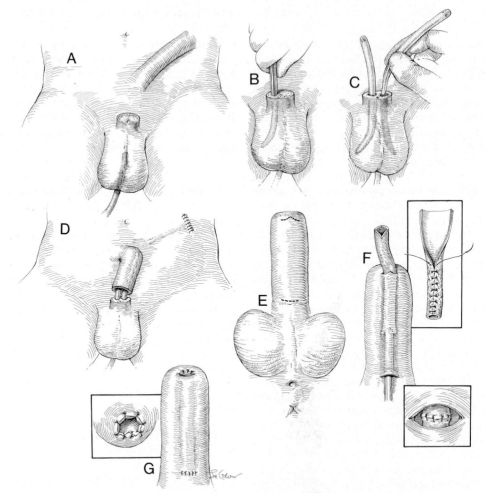

Figure 26–61. Reconstruction of complete amputation. *A,* Development of skin tube. *B* to *D,* Insertion of Small-Carrion prosthesis into dilated pedicle tube. *E* to *G,* Formation of distal urethra with full-thickness donor graft from inner arm or abdomen. (From Smith, R. B., and Skinner, D. G. (Eds.): Complications of Urologic Surgery. Philadelphia, W. B. Saunders Co., 1976.)

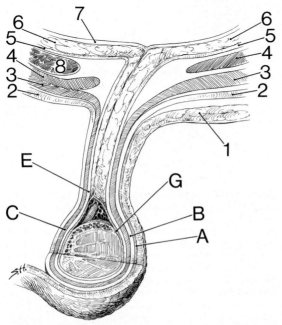

Figure 26–62. Layers of abdominal wall and corresponding layers in scrotum. (1) Skin and subcutaneous tissue; (2) external oblique muscle and aponeurosis; (3) internal oblique muscle; (4) transversus abdominis muscle; (5) transversalis fascia; (6) extraperitoneal connective tissue; (7) peritoneum; (8) rectus abdominis muscle.

(A) Skin and tunica dartos; (B) external spermatic fascia; (C) cremaster muscle; (E) internal spermatic fascia; (G) tunica vaginalis testis.

by penetrating missiles, e.g., gunshot wounds and stab wounds, or by blunt trauma. If the scrotal skin has been lacerated, treatment consists of primary débridement and closure of the wound. If the dartos layer has been violated, it should be closed separately to decrease the risk of hematoma formation. Penetrating scrotal wounds that extend deeper than the dartos layer should be explored in the operating room. If the tunica albuginea of the testicle has been violated, seminiferous tubules will be extruding from the wound. The necrotic and devitalized tubules should be sharply debrided (Fig. 26–63) and the tunica albuginea closed primarily with absorbable sutures. If the tunica vaginalis has been entered, a small Penrose drain should be

placed within the cavity and brought out through a dependent portion of the scrotum. If, on scrotal examination, the testis seems to be intact but the structures of the spermatic cord have been damaged, exploration should be carried out with appropriate ligation of vessels to decrease the chances of massive scrotal hematoma formation.

Blunt trauma to the scrotum requires individualized treatment. In the blunt trauma patient, the differential diagnosis of testicular torsion and epididymitis must be considered (Table 26–17). These patients often attribute the swelling and pain to an episode of minor trauma. The alert clinician can often make a clear differential diagnosis by means of urinalysis and

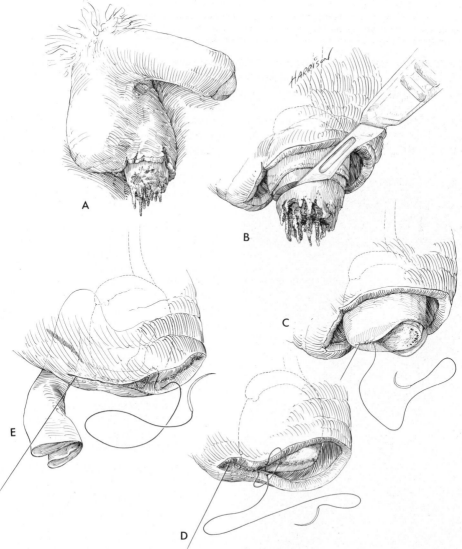

Figure 26–63. Technique of closure of traumatic scrotal and testicular defect. *A,* Appearance of injury. *B,* Sharp débridement of seminiferous tubules. *C,* Closure of tunica albuginea. *D,* Closure of dartos layer—important in prevention of scrotal hematoma. *E,* Skin closure, with drain in tunica vaginalis.

TABLE 26–17. DIFFERENTIAL DIAGNOSIS OF TESTICULAR TRAUMA, TORSION, TUMOR, AND EPIDIDYMITIS

	Torsion	Trauma	Tumor	Epididymitis
Urine	Normal	Normal	Normal	Pyuria Bacteriuria

Palpation	1. Pain
	2. Indefinable
	   structures
	3. Horizontal lie
		1. Pain and
		   swelling
		2. Related to
		   nature of
		   injury
			1. Painless unless
			   hemorrhage
			2. Diffuse or local
			   testicular
			   swelling
				1. Discrete epididymis
				2. Soft testis (early)

Onset	1. Sudden
	2. Previous
	   episodes
	3. During sleep or
	   vehicle ride
		Sudden	Gradual unless
			hemorrhagic
				1. Gradual
				2. Groin pain
				3. Previous funiculitis

Scan (Stage et al., 1981)	Decreased activity	Depends on injury	Normal	Increased activity
Small parts sonography	↑ Size	Rupture seen	Complex pattern	Enlarged epididymis
Doppler (Thompson et al., 1975)	Flow	Depends on injury	Normal	Normal

rectal palpation. One finds infection in the urine in the patient with epididymitis secondary to prostatitis and a microscopically normal urine in the patient with testicular torsion. In our series, 2 of 33 patients with torsion had microscopic pyuria. Unless only minimal swelling and tenderness are present, prompt exploration is recommended. Preoperative small parts sonography is helpful in diagnosis. A ruptured testis may result from blunt trauma, and any chance for salvage of the testes will be lost with conservative treatment. Prompt exploration in cases of blunt scrotal trauma decreases not only the chances of testicular loss but also the morbidity to the patient. Conservative management with elevation of the scrotum and application of ice bags has resulted in a high percentage of testicular loss.

If there has been significant avulsion of scrotal skin but the testes are still viable, the testis should be implanted into a subcutaneous pouch in the thigh (Fig. 26–64). The temperature in a superficial pouch in the thigh is 89° F as compared with 98° F in the abdominal or inguinal subcutaneous pouch, as shown by Culp and Huffman (1956) (Table 26–18). A recent

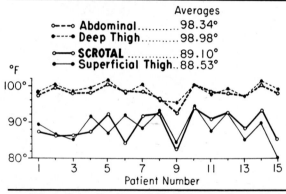

Figure 26–64. Appearance of patient with testis implanted into subcutaneous thigh pouch.

TABLE 26–18. ABDOMINAL, DEEP THIGH, SCROTAL, AND SUPERFICIAL THIGH TEMPERATURE*

	Averages
○– – –○ Abdominal	98.34°
●– – –● Deep Thigh	98.98°
○——○ SCROTAL	89.10°
●——● Superficial Thigh	88.53°

*From Culp, D. A., and Huffman, W. C.: J. Urol., 76:436, 1956.

ingenious method of using perineal skin flaps for immediate coverage of the testis in massive scrotal loss has been devised by McDougal (1983) (Fig. 26–65).

THERMAL, CHEMICAL, AND ELECTRICAL INJURY TO THE GENITALIA

Owing to the recent advances in burn wound therapy and the subsequent survival of more patients who have suffered serious burns, the urologist is called upon more frequently to treat and reconstruct the injured genitalia.

Burns of the genitalia consist of three types: (1) those caused by thermal injury, (2) those secondary to chemical injury, and (3) those secondary to electrical forces. Thermal injury produces the typical burn wound that involves the skin and subcutaneous tissue with a deeper area of necrosis.

The injury caused by an electrical burn is quite different. The nature of an electrical burn stems from the creation of a path for electrical current that produces tissue damage at entrance and exit sites with a variable amount of intervening tissue destruction. This intervening tissue damage is related to the characteristics of the current and the resistance of the particular tissue through which the current courses. When the body becomes the conduit for electrical current to the ground, the injuries that are produced result from conversion of electrical energy to heat energy (Baxter, 1970). The genitalia are potential exit sites of electrical burns. In addition to the damage to the skin and subcutaneous tissues, injury may involve the bulbocavernosus muscles or the corporal bodies, and variable degrees of ischemia, necrosis, and thrombosis may occur. Therefore, an apparently minor entrance or exit wound may overlie extensive and deep necrotic soft tissue injury.

When seen initially, the patient with a serious burn should have a urethral catheter inserted to monitor urine output and to prevent urinary retention when the genitalia are involved. If the genitalia are charred or otherwise badly damaged, the placement of a suprapubic catheter is indicated; care should be taken to place it through an uninvolved area of the abdominal wall, if possible.

Initial treatment of the burn wound consists of débridement of devitalized tissue followed by topical therapy with silver sulfadiazine or Sulfamylon. One should not cover more than 20 per cent of the body surface with Sulfamylon at one time in order to avert a tendency to severe metabolic acidosis. Serious thermal injuries, and especially electrical injuries, may require repeated débridement, since the areas surrounding the necrotic burn wounds are involved by variable amounts of ischemia, which may progress to further necrosis.

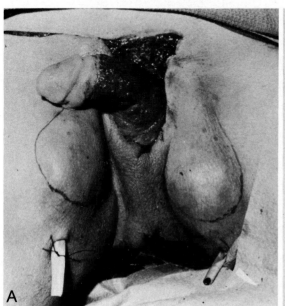 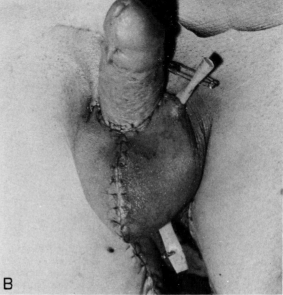

Figure 26–65. *A,* Penis and perineum are covered with split-thickness skin. Scrotal reconstruction is begun 4 to 6 weeks after thigh implantation of testes. All wounds should be healed before this stage is undertaken. Proposed flaps are outlined. *B,* Closure of thigh defects and drainage of reconstructed scrotum complete procedure. (From McDougal, W. S.: J. Urol., *129*:757, 1983.)

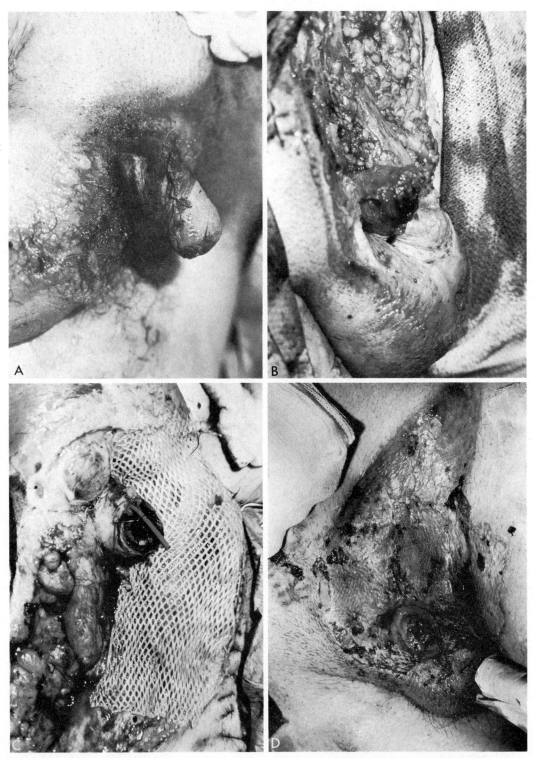

Figure 26–66. Appearance of massive electrical burn to penis. *A,* Initial postburn appearance. The penis was the exit site for the electric current. *B,* Five days post injury. *Note:* Extensive debridement has been necessary because of delayed necrosis. *C,* Later appearance, with split-thickness mesh graft covering part of defect. The catheter in the middle of the picture is in the urethral lumen. *D,* Late appearance after grafting is complete. Remaining penile stump is visible in the center of the figure. Tape at right lower edge of picture is unrelated to discussion.

If the injury is a first- or second-degree burn, it will heal primarily with adequate wound care and prevention of burn wound sepsis. A split-thickness burn may be converted to a full-thickness defect if local infection is not controlled. If the burn is full-thickness, sequential homograft or heterograft application after adequate débridement and wound care is needed; this should be followed by split-thickness autografting (0.015-inch) to cover the defect (Fig. 26–66). The heterograft or homograft that shows a 100 per cent "take" is evidence that the burn wound is sterile. A full-thickness pedicle flap to cover a burned area may be rotated with confidence if the heterograft or homograft over the area demonstrates a 100 per cent "take."

If the patient has suffered extensive necrosis of the genitalia, the penis may have to be amputated to effect proper débridement. In this event, the pubic and perineal wounds should be allowed to heal with or without skin grafts, and the reconstruction of the genitalia is performed after the area is completely healed.

If the phallus is completely destroyed, reconstruction of a structure adequate for intercourse is performed in several stages, as described earlier in this chapter.

References

Allen, T. D.: The transpubic approach for strictures of membranous urethra. J. Urol., *114*:63, 1975.

Bacon, S. K.: Rupture of the urinary bladder: clinical analysis of 147 cases in the past 10 years. J. Urol., *49*:432, 1943.

Baxter, C. R.: Present concepts in the management of major electrical injury. Surg. Clin. North Am., *50*:1401, 1970.

Blandy, J. P., Singh, M., and Tressider, G. C.: Urethroplasty by scrotal flap for long urethral strictures. Br. J. Urol., *40*:261, 1968.

Bourdeau, G. V., Jindal, S. L., Gillies, R. R., and Berry, J. V.: Urinary ascites secondary to ureteroperitoneal fistula. Urology, *6*:209, 1974.

Browne, D.: An operation for hypospadias. Proc. R. Soc. Med., *42*:466, 1949.

Carlton, C. E., Jr.: Injuries of the kidney and ureter. *In* Harrison, J. H., et al. (Eds.): Campbell's Urology, Vol. 1., 4th ed. Philadelphia, W. B. Saunders Co., 1978.

Cass, A. S., Susset, J., Khan, A., et al.: Renal pedicle injury in the multiple injured patient. J. Urol., *122*:728, 1979.

Cass, A. S., Susset, J., Khan, A., et al.: The role of computed tomography in renal trauma. Radiology, *141*:455, 1981.

Culp, D. A., and Huffman, W. C.: Treatment determination in the thigh with regard to burying the traumatically exposed testes. J. Urol., *76*:436, 1956.

Culp, O. S.: Treatment of ruptured bladder and urethra: analysis of 86 cases of urinary extravasation. J. Urol., *48*:266, 1942.

Devine, P. C., Wendelken, J. R., and Devine, C. J., Jr.: Free full thickness skin graft urethroplasty: current technique. J. Urol., *121*:282, 1979.

Evans, R. J., and Brown, H. E.: Ascites in newborn infants. Urology, *1*:386, 1973.

Federle, M. P., Kaiser, J. A., McAninch, J. W., et al.: The role of computed tomography in renal trauma. Radiology, *141*:455, 1981.

Guerriero, W. J.: Trauma to the kidneys, ureters, bladder and urethra. Surg. Clin. North Am., *62*:1047, 1982.

Hai, M. A., Pontes, J. E., and Pierce, J. M., Jr.: Surgical management of major renal trauma. J. Urol., *118*:7, 1977.

Hayes, E. E., Sandler, C. M., and Corriere, J. N., Jr.: Management of the ruptured bladder secondary to blunt abdominal trauma. J. Urol., *129*:946, 1983.

Hoch, W. H., Kursh, L., and Persky, L.: Early aggressive management of intraoperative ureteral injuries. J. Urol., *144*:530, 1975.

Hodges, C. V., Moore, R. J., Lehman, T. H., and Benham, A. M.: Clinical experience with transureteroureterostomy. J. Urol., *90*:552, 1963.

Johanson, B.: Reconstruction of the male urethra in stricture. Acta Chir. Scand. (Suppl.) *176*:1, 1953.

Judd, R., and Donohue, J. P.: Micropenis following Badenoch pullthrough procedure. J. Urol., *103*:104, 1970.

Leadbetter, G. W.: A simplified urethroplasty for strictures of the bulbous urethra. J. Urol., *83*:54, 1960.

Maggio, A. J., Jr., and Brosman, S.: Renal artery trauma. Urology, *11*:125, 1978.

McAninch, J. W.: The injured kidney. *In* Stamey, T. A. (Ed.): Monographs in Urology. Princeton, N.J., Custom Publishing Services, 1983.

McAninch, J. W., and Carroll, P. R.: Renal trauma: kidney preservation through improved vascular control—a refined approach. J. Trauma, *22*:285, 1982.

McDougal, W.S.: Scrotal reconstruction using thigh pedicle flaps. J. Urol., *129*:757, 1983.

Michie, A. J.: Technique of tubeless cystostomy. Annual report of the Harrison Department of Surgical Research and the Department of Surgery of the University of Pennsylvania, Philadelphia, 1972, p. 164.

Morehouse, D. D.: Personal communication, 1984.

Morehouse, D. D., and MacKinnon, K. J.: Urologic injuries associated with pelvic fractures. J. Trauma, *9*:479, 1969.

Morehouse, D. D., Belitsky, P., and MacKinnon, K. J.: Rupture of posterior urethra. J. Urol., *107*:255, 1972.

Mulkey, A. P., and Witherington, R.: Conservative management of vesical rupture. Urology, *4*:426, 1974.

Orkin, L. A.: Trauma to the ureter: Pathogenesis and Management. Philadelphia, F. A. Davis Co., 1964.

Peters, P. C., and Bright, T. C., III: Management of trauma to the urinary tract. *In* Longmire, W. P., Jr. (Ed.): Advances in Surgery, Vol. 10, Chicago, Year Book Medical Publishers, 1976.

Peters, P. C., and Bright, T. C., III: Blunt renal injuries. Urol. Clin. North Am., *4*:17, 1977.

Pierce, J. M.: Exposure of membranous and posterior urethra by total pubectomy. J. Urol., *88*:256, 1962.

Pierce, J. M.: Management of dismemberment of the prostatic membranous urethra and ensuing stricture disease. J. Urol., *107*:259, 1972.

Reiser, C., and Nichols, E.: Rupture of the bladder: unusual features. J. Urol., *90*:53, 1963.

Sagalowsky, A. I., McConnell, J. D., and Peters, P. C.: Renal trauma requiring surgery. J. Trauma, *23*:128, 1983.

Sandler, C. M., and Toombs, B. D.: Computed tomographic evaluation of blunt renal injuries. Radiology, *141*:461, 1981.

Stage, K. H., Schoenvogel, R., and Lewis, S.: Testicular scanning: clinical experience with 72 patients. J. Urol., *125*:334, 1981.

Thompson, I. M.: Expectant management of blunt renal trauma. Urol. Clin. North Am., *4*:29, 1977.

Turner, W. J., Jr., Snyder, W. H., III, and Fry, W. J.: Mortality and renal salvage after renovascular trauma. Am. J. Surg., *146*:848, 1983.

Turner-Warwick, R.: Observations on the treatment of traumatic urethral injuries and the value of the fenestrated urethral catheter. Br. J. Surg., *60*:775, 1973.

Turner-Warwick, R.: Urethral stricture surgery. *In* Glenn, J. F. (Ed.): Urologic Surgery, 3rd ed. Philadelphia, J. B. Lippincott Co., 1983.

Vermooten, V.: Rupture of the urethra: a new diagnostic sign. J. Urol., *56*:228, 1946.

Waterhouse, K., et al.: The transpubic approach to the lower urinary tract. J. Urol., *109*:486, 1973.

Waterhouse, K., Laungani, G., and Patil, U.: The surgical repair of membranous urethral strictures: experience with 105 consecutive cases. J. Urol., *123*:500, 1980.

Witherington, R., and McKinney, J. E.: An unusual case of anterior urethral injury. J. Urol., *130*:564, 1983.

INDEX

Gonadotropin-releasing hormone (GnRH), 186, 188–189, 242
  for cryptorchidism, 1957
Gonadotropin-releasing hormone (GnRH) agonists, for prostate cancer, 1507
  antagonists, for prostate cancer, 1507–1508
Gonadotropins, 186, 187, 188
  deficiency of, in male infertility, 677
    idiopathic, 680t, 681–683
    postpubertal, 659
  diurnal rhythm of, 187
  feedback control of, *191*, 191–192
  influence of amines on secretion of, 188
  production of, 248–249
  prolactin and, relationship between, 190–191
  role of, in spermatogenesis, 215
  secretion and measurement of, 189–190, 189t, *190*
Gonads, embryonic, cell types in, 1805–1806
Gonococcal prostatitis, 883
Gonococcal urethritis. See *Urethritis, gonococcal*
Goodwin's transcolonic technique, of ureterosigmoidostomy, 2603, *2603*
Gracilis sartorius, used in scrotal repair, 2957, *2958*
Grafts. See also specific types
  rejection of, immunologic considerations in, 2550–2553
  renal, implantation of, 2543–2549
  skin, for treatment of urethral strictures, 2876, 2878–2879, *2879*
    failure of, 2878
  tube, 2880–2882, *2880–2883*, 2884–2886, *2885*
Gram-negative bacteremia, 769–772
Granuloma, nonspecific, of external genitalia, *960*, 962
  pyogenic, of external genitalia, 967
  schistosome, 987–988, *988–989*
Granuloma inguinale, *947*, 953–955
Granulomatous bowel disease, and ureteral obstruction, 592–594, *593*
Granulomatous caruncle, 1441
Granulomatous disease, partial nephrectomy for, 2455
Granulomatous prostatitis, 883–884
  nonspecific, 884
Grayhack procedure, for priapism, 2895–2896, *2896*
Groin, hanging, onchocercal infection and, 1015–1016
Growth, of benign prostatic hyperplasia, 1250
  of germinal testicular tumors, 1543
  of prostate gland, factors controlling, 241–253
  of urinary crystals, 1107
    and passage size, *1108*, 1109–1110
  renal, compensatory, in hydronephrosis, 545–547, *546*
  renotrophic factor and, 546
Growth theory, of testicular descent, 1949
Gruntzig balloon catheter, renal artery dilation using, 2565, *2565*
Gubernaculum, *1809*, 1810
Guidewire sliding-catheter dilation, *511*, 520–522, *523*
Gunshot wounds, nonrenal injury due to, 1192, 1193t
  renal injury due to, 1192, 1192t
Gynecomastia, 3017, *3018*
  estrogen therapy and, 1504

Gynecomastia (*Continued*)
  in Klinefelter syndrome, 1820
  Leydig cell tumors associated with, 2286
  with germinal testicular tumors, 1544

Haemophilus ducreyi, infection caused by, 949–950
  sexually transmitted disease caused by, 901t
Hamartoma, metanephric, 2253
  renal, 1300–1301, *1300–1304*
Hamilton Russell operation, for urethral strictures, 2869, *2870*
Headache, vasodilating, of pheochromocytoma, 3032
Healing and regeneration, of ureter, 2582–2584
Heart, abnormalities of, in prune-belly syndrome, 2164
  damage to, doxorubicin for Wilms' tumor and, 2263
  perioperative care of. See *Perioperative care, in cardiac patient*
Heart disease, valvular, perioperative care of, 2364–2365
Heart failure, congestive, perioperative care of, 2362–2363
Heitz-Boyer and Hovelacque procedure, for bladder exstrophy, 1889
Helical artery, 701
Hellstrom procedure, for ureteropelvic junction repair, 2527, *2527*
Hemangioma, of external genitalia, 967, *968*
  urethral, excision of, *2857*, 2857–2858
Hemangiopericytoma, renal, 1334
Hematocele, testicular, 2960
Hematologic considerations, in urologic surgery, 2382–2384
Hematologic study, of neuroblastoma, 2270–2271
Hematologic toxicity, due to chemotherapy for Wilms' tumor, 2262
Hematoma, as complication of circumcision, 2891
  butterfly, perineal, in urethral injury, 1220, *1220*
  causing failure of skin graft, 2878
  of rectus abdominis muscle, ureteral obstruction and, 602–603
  retroperitoneal, primary, 602
  traumatic, of external genitalia, *968*, 969
  ultrasound studies of, 391–392, *392*
Hematoporphyrin derivative (HPD), for bladder cancer, 1386
Hematospermia, history of, 278
  in genitourinary tuberculosis, 1049
Hematuria, 2342–2349
  absence of, in renal trauma, 1196, 1197t
  as neonatal emergency, 2221–2223, 2222t, 2223t
  calculi causing, surgery for, 2480
  definition of, 284, 2342
  detection and quantification of, 2342
  essential, unilateral, partial nephrectomy for, 2457–2459, *2459–2460*
  glomerular, 2343, 2343t, 2345
    assessment of, 2344t
  history of, 278
  idiopathic, benign, 2345
  in adult polycystic disease, 1773